# A
# DRUG
# HANDBOOK

## Second Edition

American Society of
Health-System Pharmacists
Bethesda, Maryland

LIPPINCOTT WILLIAMS & WILKINS
A **Wolters Kluwer** Company

Philadelphia • Baltimore • New York • London
Buenos Aires • Hong Kong • Sydney • Tokyo

## Staff

**Publisher**
Judith A. Schilling McCann, RN, MSN

**Editorial Director**
William J. Kelly

**Clinical Director**
Marguerite S. Ambrose, RN, MSN

**Art Director**
Elaine Kasmer

**Clinical Manager**
Eileen Cassin Gallen, RN, BSN

**Drug Information Editor**
Melissa M. Devlin, PharmD

**Senior Associate Editor**
Anne Stuart Dawson

**Editors**
Lynne Christensen, Karen Comerford,
Catherine Harold, Patricia Nale

**Clinical Editors**
Nancy LaPlante, RN, BSN; Pamela S. Messer,
RN, MSN; Lisa Morris Bonsall, RN, MSN,
CRNP

**Copy Editors**
Leslie Dworkin, Caryl Knutsen, Dolores
Connors Matthews, Beth Pitcher, Louise
Quinn, Jenifer F. Walker

**Designers**
Arlene Putterman (senior art director), Donald
G. Knauss

**Electronic Production Services**
Diane Paluba (manager), Joy Rossi Biletz
(technician)

**Manufacturing**
Patricia K. Dorshaw (manager), Beth Janae
Orr (book production manager)

**Editorial Assistants**
Danielle J. Barsky, Carol A. Caputo, Arlene P.
Claffee

**Indexer**
Barbara Hodgson

Visit eDrugInfo.com and AHFSDrugInformation.com

AHFSDH—D  N  O  S  A  J
03  02    10  9  8  7  6  5  4  3  2  1
ISBN 1-58255-202-9

**Library of Congress Cataloging-in Publication Data**

AHFS drug handbook.— 2nd ed.
   p. ; cm.
  Rev. ed. of: Pharmacist's drug handbook. c2001.
  Includes index.
  1. Pharmacy—Handbooks, manuals, etc. 2.
Drugs—Handbooks, manuals, etc.
I. Title: Drug handbook. II. American Society of
Health-System Pharmacists. III. Pharmacist's drug
handbook.
  [DNLM: 1. Pharmaceutical Preparations—Handbooks. QV 735 A285 2003]
RS156 .P48 2003
615'.1—dc21          2002005394
ISBN 1-58255-202-9 (pbk. : alk. paper)

# Contents

# American Society of Health-System Pharmacists Consultants and Contributors

**Gerald K. McEvoy, PharmD**
Editor

**Jane L. Miller, PharmD**
Associate Editor

**Olin H. Welsh, PharmD**
Associate Editor
Editorial Development

**Elaine K. Snow, BS**
Associate Editor

**Kathy Litvak, MS**
Assistant Editor

**Donald R. Dewey, BS**
Senior Drug Information Analyst

**Phillip A. Fong, PharmD**
Senior Drug Information Analyst

**Anne O'Rourke, BS**
Senior Drug Information Analyst

**Laura A. Bollinger, MS**
Drug Information Analyst

**Janie Kim, PharmD**
Drug Information Analyst

**Tran Le, PharmD**
Drug Information Analyst

**Gerald Scott Melton, DVM**
Drug Information Analyst

**Barbara F. Young, PharmD, MHA**
Drug Information Analyst

**Jeffery Shick, BS**
Director
Database Services

**Edward D. Millikan, PharmD**
Clinical Informaticist
Database Services

**P.M. Douglas, RN, BSc**
Associate Editor
Database Services

**M.E. Ford, MD, MPH**
Contributing Editor

**Linda Kester, MS**
Contributing Editor

**Linda Bedford Arcuri, PharmD**
Contributor

**Laura Brady Sullivan, PharmD**
Contributor

**Susan Braun, PharmD**
Contributor

**Marjorie Kay Frederickson, BS**
Contributor

**Julia A. Leszko, BS**
Contributor

**Amy L. Schroeder, BS**
Contributor

# Lippincott Williams & Wilkins Consultants

**Steven R. Abel, RPh, PharmD**
Professor and Head
Department of Pharmacy Practice
Purdue University
West Lafayette, Ind.

**Tricia M. Berry, PharmD, BCPS**
Assistant Professor of Pharmacy
  Practice
St. Louis College of Pharmacy
St. Louis, Mo.

**James Caldwell, PharmD**
Clinical Pharmacy Professor
Anne Arundel Medical Center
Annapolis, Md.

**Lawrence Carey, PharmD**
Clinical Pharmacist Supervisor
Jefferson Home Infusion Service
Philadelphia

**Jennifer L. Defilippi, PharmD**
Clinical Pharmacy Specialist, Psychiatry
Central Texas Veteran's Health Care
  System
Waco, Tex.

**Tatyana Gurvich, PharmD**
Clinical Pharmacologist
Glendale Adventist Family Practice
Residency Program
Glendale, Calif.

**AnnThu Hoang, PharmD**
Medical Director
IntraMed Educational Group
New York

**Maureen Ketz, PharmD**
Independent Consultant
North Royalton, Ohio

**Michelle Kosich, PharmD**
Clinical Pharmacist
Mercy Community Hospital
Havertown, Pa.

**Kristy H. Lucas, PharmD**
Clinical Assistant Professor
West Virginia University
Charleston, W.Va.

**Randall A. Lynch, RPh, PharmD**
Assistant Director, Pharmacy Services
Presbyterian Medical Center
University of Pennsylvania
  Health System
Philadelphia

**Marie Maloney, PharmD**
Clinical Pharmacist
University Medical Center
Tucson, Ariz.

**George Melko, RPh, PharmD**
Independent Consultant
West Chester, Pa.

**Christine K. O'Neil, PharmD, BCPS**
Associate Professor
Duquesne University
Pittsburgh

**David Pipher, PharmD**
Director of Pharmacy
Forbes Regional Hospital
Monroeville, Pa.

**Christine Price, PharmD**
Clinical Coordinator
Morton Plant Mease Health Care
Dunedin, Fla.

**Gary Smith, RPh, PharmD**
Manager, Clinical Pharmacy Services
Fairview Physician Associates
Edina, Minn.

**Joseph F. Steiner, RPh, PharmD**
Dean and Professor of Pharmacy
  Practice
College of Pharmacy
Idaho State University
Pocactello, Idaho

**Barbara S. Wiggins, RPh, PharmD**
Clinical Pharmacist, Cardiology
Clinical Instructor
University of Washington Medical
  Center
Seattle

# Foreword

Pharmacists must have valid, up-to-date drug information in an easily accessible format to provide excellent pharmaceutical care. With the current challenges to providing pharmaceutical care, collaborative practice agreements, and disease state management, pharmacists have increasing responsibility for managing drug therapies. With these responsibilities, it is of the utmost importance to have access to a drug data source that can be trusted to provide thorough and unbiased information. Created as a carry-along version of the well-established and highly regarded *AHFS Drug Information,* the *AHFS Drug Handbook* is that source.

The *AHFS Drug Handbook,* Second Edition provides a unique and valuable reference for pharmacists and other health care professionals by effectively combining drug information with therapeutic monitoring guidelines in a portable, clear format. This concise and informative handbook is a joint publishing effort by Lippincott Williams & Wilkins and the American Society of Health-System Pharmacists, who publish the well-established and continually updated reference source *AHFS Drug Information.* And while that book is an outstanding authoritative desktop reference, *AHFS Drug Handbook* provides many of its benefits in a compact, convenient size. This handbook gives you comprehensive drug profiles—more than 900 generic and 2,000 brand-name drugs—as well as valuable information on 39 pharmacologic classes. This edition has several new features, including 64 more pages of drug information, I.V. administration guidelines and compatibilities, more unlabeled uses, more drug-herb interactions, and more alerts for soundalike drug names and other potential dangers.

The book also features informative appendices that every pharmacist should have but that aren't found in such a readily accessible format in other books. All of the appendices are useful in addressing common health care issues, and all have been updated to provide the latest information in an easy-to-read format. The appendices on subcutaneous, intramuscular, and intravenous injection techniques; cytochrome P-450 enzymes and common drug interactions; and herbal medicines are particularly beneficial supplements to the book. The appendix on therapeutic drug monitoring guidelines provides a useful, drug-focused structure for monitoring individual drugs. And there are also guidelines for using selected antimicrobials, now with a revised layout based on morphologic organization and a list of selected narcotic analgesic combination products. A new appendix features dosage equivalents for opioids. And by visiting eDrugInfo.com or AHFSDrugInformation.com, you can easily access changes and updates to the drug information.

Pharmacists need a comprehensive resource that gives them all the up-to-date information they need in an easy-to-use format. The *AHFS Drug Handbook* is a valuable tool for any pharmacist looking to ensure positive therapeutic outcomes while providing the highest quality of pharmaceutical care.

**Joseph T. DiPiro, PharmD**
Panoz Professor of Pharmacy
University of Georgia
College of Pharmacy
Clinical Professor of Surgery
Medical College of Georgia
Augusta, Georgia

# How to use this book

The *AHFS Drug Handbook* provides up-to-date information on virtually every drug in current clinical use. It covers aspects of drug information from fundamental pharmacology to specific management of toxicity and overdose. It also includes several indispensable features—individual entries that describe major pharmacologic classes; interactions categorized as drug-drug, drug-herb, drug-food, and drug-lifestyle; special guidance for drug therapy in pregnant, breast-feeding, pediatric, and geriatric patients; and therapeutic management guidelines. If you need more detailed information on a particular drug, consult *AHFS Drug Information.*

## Pharmacologic class entries

Listed alphabetically as a separate section, 39 entries describe the clinical indications and actions, pharmacology, adverse effects, and special implications of drugs in major pharmacologic groups. This allows the reader to compare the effects and uses of drugs within each class. Pharmacologic class entries list special considerations common to all generic members of the class, including geriatric, pediatric, and breast-feeding considerations. If specific considerations are unknown, these headings are omitted.

Representative combinations appear at the end of each class entry. These lists show combinations of generic drugs in the class with other generics of the same or another class, followed by trade names of products that contain each combination of generics.

## Generic drug entries

The individual drug entries provide detailed information on virtually all drugs in current clinical use, arranged alphabetically by generic name for easy access. A guide word at the top of each page identifies the generic drug presented on that page. Each generic entry is complete where it falls alphabetically and doesn't require cross-referencing to other sections of the book.

In each drug entry, the generic name, with alternative generic names following in parentheses, precedes an alphabetically arranged list of current trade names (an asterisk * signals products available only in Canada). Several narcotic analgesic combination products—such as Percocet (acetaminophen and oxycodone hydrochloride)—are listed in an appendix.

The **pharmacologic and therapeutic classifications** identify the pharmacologic or chemical category of the drug and its major clinical uses. Listing both classifications helps the reader grasp the multiple, varying, and sometimes overlapping uses of drugs within a single pharmacologic class and among different classes.

The **pregnancy risk category** identifies the potential risk to the fetus. Drugs in category A usually are considered safe to use in pregnancy; drugs in category X usually are contraindicated.

*Pregnancy risk category A:* Adequate studies in pregnant women have failed to show a risk to the fetus in the first trimester of pregnancy—and there's no evidence of risk in later trimesters.

*Pregnancy risk category B:* Animal studies haven't shown an adverse effect on the fetus, but there are no adequate clinical studies in pregnant women.

*Pregnancy risk category C:* Animal studies have shown an adverse effect on the fetus, but there are no adequate studies in humans. The drug may be useful in pregnant women despite its potential risks.

*Pregnancy risk category D:* There is evidence of risk to the human fetus, but the potential benefits of use in pregnant women may be acceptable despite potential risks.

*Pregnancy risk category X:* Studies in animals or humans show fetal abnormalities, or adverse reaction reports indicate evidence of fetal risk. The risks involved clearly outweigh potential benefits.

*Pregnancy risk category NR:* Not rated.

If appropriate, the next line identifies any drug that the Drug Enforcement Agency (DEA) lists as a controlled substance and specifies the schedule of control as II, III, IV, or V.

■ **Available forms** lists the preparations available for each drug, such as tablets, capsules, solution, or injection, specifying available dosage forms and strengths. Its prescription or nonprescription status is also indicated.

■ **Indications and dosages** presents all clinically accepted indications for use with general dosage recommendations for adults and children; dosage adjustments for specific patient groups, such as the elderly or patients with renal or hepatic impairment, are included, when appropriate, using the **≡Dosage adjustment** logo. (Note that additional information may be found in the *Clinical considerations* section.) A preceding open diamond ◇ signals a clinically accepted but unlabeled use. Dosage instructions reflect current clinical trends in therapeutics and shouldn't be considered as absolute and universal recommendations. For individual application, dosage must be considered according to the patient's condition.

■ **I.V. administration**, when applicable, includes guidelines for safely mixing and administering I.V. drugs.

■ **Mechanism of action** explains the mechanism and effects of the physiologic action of the drug.

■ **Pharmacokinetics** describes absorption, distribution, metabolism, and excretion of the drug; it specifies peak levels and half-life, as appropriate. A table outlining the route, onset, peak, and duration of action is also included.

■ **Contraindications and precautions** lists conditions associated with special risks in patients who receive the drug.

■ **Interactions** specifies the clinically significant additive, synergistic, or antagonistic effects that result from interactions, which are broken down into four categories: drug-drug, drug-herb, drug-food, and drug-lifestyle. The interacting agent is italicized.

■ **Adverse reactions** lists the undesirable effects that may follow use of the drug; these effects are arranged by body systems (CNS, CV, EENT, GI, GU, Hematologic, Hepatic, Metabolic, Musculoskeletal, Respiratory, Skin, and Other). Local effects occur at the site of drug administration (by application, infusion, or injection); adverse reactions not specific to a single body system (for example, the effects of hypersensitivity) are listed under Other. The most common adverse reactions (those experienced by at least 10% of all people taking the drug in clinical trials) are in *italic* type; less common reactions are in roman type; life-threatening reactions are in ***bold italic*** type; and reactions that are both common and life-threatening are in **BOLD CAPITAL** letters.

■ **Overdose and treatment** summarizes the signs and symptoms of a drug overdose and recommends specific treatment, as appropriate. Usually, this segment recommends emesis or gastric lavage, followed by activated charcoal to reduce the amount of drug absorbed and possibly a cathartic to eliminate the toxin. This section specifies antidotes, drug therapy, and other special care, if known. It also specifies the effects of hemodialysis or peritoneal dialysis for dialyzable drugs.

■ **Clinical considerations** offers recommendations specific to the drug for preparation and administration and for care and teaching of the patient during therapy. This section includes pointers for preventing and treating adverse reactions and for promoting patient comfort. Recommendations common to all members of the pharmacologic class of the drug are listed only in the relevant pharmacologic class entry. This section also uses an **H ALERT** logo to point out drugs that are likely to cause medication errors, such as those with soundalike drug names. If applicable, the last bullet in this section lists any significant interference with a diagnostic test or its result by direct effects on the test itself or by systemic drug effects that lead to misleading test results.

■ **Therapeutic monitoring** provides recommendations for monitoring the effects of drug therapy.

■ **Special populations** offers recommendations for drug therapy in pregnant, breast-feeding, pediatric, and geriatric patients.

■ **Patient counseling** provides patient-teaching guidelines to use during drug therapy.

## Appendices

The appendices include a review of subcutaneous, intramuscular, and intravenous injection techniques; therapeutic drug monitoring guidelines; guidelines for use of selected antimicrobials; a summary of selected narcotic analgesic combination products; a table of cytochrome P-450 enzymes and common drug interactions; dosage equivalents for opioids; and a guide to herbal medicines.

## Index

The index lists both generic and trade names, diseases, and pharmacologic classes.

# Guide to abbreviations

| | | | |
|---|---|---|---|
| ACE | angiotensin-converting enzyme | I.D. | intradermal |
| AIDS | acquired immunodeficiency syndrome | I.M. | intramuscular |
| | | INR | international normalized ratio |
| ALT | alanine aminotransferase | IU | international unit |
| aPTT | activated partial thromboplastin time | I.V. | intravenous |
| | | kg | kilogram |
| AST | aspartate aminotransferase | L | liter |
| ATP | adenosine triphosphate | LDH | lactate dehydrogenase |
| AUC | area under the curve | $m^2$ | square meter |
| AV | atrioventricular | $mm^3$ | cubic millimeter |
| b.i.d. | twice a day | MAO | monoamine oxidase |
| BPH | benign prostatic hypertrophy | mcg | microgram |
| BUN | blood urea nitrogen | mEq | milliequivalent |
| cAMP | cyclic 3', 5' adenosine monophosphate | mg | milligram |
| | | MI | myocardial infarction |
| CBC | complete blood count | ml | milliliter |
| CK | creatine kinase | ng | nanogram (millimicrogram) |
| CMV | cytomegalovirus | NSAID | nonsteroidal anti-inflammatory drug |
| CNS | central nervous system | | |
| COPD | chronic obstructive pulmonary disease | OTC | over-the-counter |
| CPR | cardiopulmonary resuscitation | P.O. | by mouth |
| CSF | cerebrospinal fluid | P.R. | per rectum |
| CV | cardiovascular | p.r.n. | as needed |
| CVA | cerebrovascular accident | PT | prothrombin time |
| CVP | central venous pressure | PTT | partial thromboplastin time |
| $D_5W$ | dextrose 5% in water | PVC | premature ventricular contraction |
| DIC | disseminated intravascular coagulation | | |
| | | q | every |
| DNA | deoxyribonucleic acid | q.i.d. | four times a day |
| ECG | electrocardiogram | RBC | red blood cell |
| EEG | electroencephalogram | RDA | recommended daily allowance |
| EENT | eye, ear, nose, and throat | RNA | ribonucleic acid |
| FDA | Food and Drug Administration | SA | sinoatrial |
| g | gram | S.C. | subcutaneous |
| G | gauge | SIADH | syndrome of inappropriate antidiuretic hormone |
| GGT | gamma glutamyltransferase | | |
| G6PD | glucose-6-phosphate dehydrogenase | S.L. | sublingual, sublingually |
| | | SSRI | selective serotonin reuptake inhibitor |
| GI | gastrointestinal | | |
| GU | genitourinary | $T_3$ | triiodothyronine |
| HF | heart failure | $T_4$ | thyroxine |
| HIV | human immunodeficiency virus | t.i.d. | three times a day |
| h.s. | at bedtime | WBC | white blood cell |

# Pharmacologic classes

## adrenergics, direct and indirect acting

albuterol sulfate, arbutamine hydrochloride, bitolterol mesylate, brimonidine tartrate, dobutamine hydrochloride, dopamine hydrochloride, ephedrine, ephedrine hydrochloride, ephedrine sulfate, epinephrine, epinephrine bitartrate, epinephrine hydrochloride, epinephryl borate, isoetharine hydrochloride, isoetharine mesylate, isoproterenol, isoproterenol hydrochloride, isoproterenol sulfate, metaproterenol sulfate, metaraminol bitartrate, naphazoline hydrochloride, norepinephrine bitartrate, phenylephrine hydrochloride, pirbuterol acetate, pseudoephedrine hydrochloride, pseudoephedrine sulfate, ritodrine hydrochloride, salmeterol xinafoate, terbutaline sulfate, tetrahydrozoline hydrochloride, xylometazoline hydrochloride

Beta-receptor activation is associated with activation of adenylate cyclase and accumulation of cAMP. Beta$_1$ receptors are excitatory and are located in cardiac tissues. Beta$_2$ receptors are inhibitory and are located primarily on smooth muscle and glands.

The cellular consequences of alpha-receptor activation are less understood. Alpha$_1$ receptors are excitatory and are located on smooth muscle and glands. Alpha$_2$ receptors are prejunctional regulatory receptors in the CNS and postjunctional receptors in many peripheral tissues.

Adrenergic drugs may mimic the naturally occurring catecholamines norepinephrine, epinephrine, and dopamine or may function by stimulating the release of norepinephrine.

## Clinical indications and actions

Most adrenergic drugs act on two or more receptor sites; the net effect is the sum of alpha and beta activity. Dopaminergic and serotonergic activity may occur, possibly stimulating receptors in the CNS to release histamine.

Temporary appetite suppression is another effect, often resulting in a rebound weight gain after tolerance to the anorexic effect develops or after the drug is withdrawn. Other uses include support of blood pressure, suppression of urinary incontinence and enuresis, and relief from dysmenorrhea pain.

### Hypotension

Alpha agonists, such as norepinephrine, metaraminol, phenylephrine, and pseudoephedrine, cause arteriolar and venous constriction, resulting in increased blood pressure. This action helps support blood pressure in hypotension and helps manage serious allergic conditions. Topical formulations are used to induce local vasoconstriction (decongestion), arrest superficial hemorrhage (styptic), stimulate radial smooth muscle of the iris (mydriasis), and, with local anesthetics, localize anesthesia and prolong duration of action. Ophthalmic preparations reduce aqueous humor production and increase uveoscleral outflow.

### Cardiac stimulation

Beta$_1$ agonists, such as dobutamine, act primarily in the heart, producing a positive inotropic effect. Because they increase heart rate, enhance AV conduction, and increase the strength of the heartbeat, beta$_1$ agonists may be used to restore heartbeat in cardiac arrest or to treat acute heart failure and cardiogenic or other types of shock. Beta$_1$ agonists may also be used for heart block in syncopal seizures, but they aren't the treatment of choice. Their use in shock is somewhat controversial because beta$_1$ agonists induce lipolysis (the increase of free fatty acids in plasma), which promotes a metabolic acidosis, and because they favor arrhythmias, which pose a special threat in cardiogenic shock.

### Bronchodilation

Beta$_2$ agonists, such as albuterol, bitolterol, isoetharine, metaproterenol, salmeterol, pirbuterol, and terbutaline, act primarily on smooth muscle of the bronchial tree, vasculature, intestines, and uterus. They also induce hepatic and muscle glycogenolysis, which results in hyperglycemia (sometimes useful in insulin overdose) and hyperlactic acidemia.

Some are used as bronchodilators, some as vasodilators. They're also used to relax the uterus, to delay delivery in premature labor, and for dysmenorrhea. Some degree of cardiostimulation may occur, because all beta$_2$ agonists have some degree of beta$_1$ activity.

### Renal vasodilation

Dopamine is the only commercially available sympathomimetic with significant dopaminergic activity, although some other sympathomimetics appear to act on dopamine receptors in the CNS. Dopamine receptors are prominent in the periphery (splanchnic and renal vasculature), where they mediate vasodilation, which is useful in inducing diuresis in patients with acute renal failure, heart failure, and shock.

## Pharmacology

Most actions of adrenergic drugs involve the following: peripheral excitatory actions on glands and vascular smooth muscle; cardiac and CNS excitatory actions; peripheral inhibitory actions on smooth muscle of the bronchial tree and blood vessels supplying skeletal muscles and the gut; and metabolic and endocrine effects. Because different tissues respond in varying degrees to adrenergic agonists, differences in the actions of catecholamines are attributed to the presence of different receptor types (alpha and beta) within the tissues.

## Overview of adverse reactions

Geriatric patients, infants, and patients with thyrotoxicosis or CV disease are more sensitive to the effects of these drugs.

Alpha agonists commonly produce CV reactions. An excessive increase in blood pressure is a major adverse reaction of systemically administered alpha agonists. Exaggerated pressor response may occur in hypertensive or geriatric patients, which may evoke vagal reflex responses and cause bradycardia and AV block. Alpha agonists also interfere with lactation and may cause nausea, vomiting, sweating, piloerection, rebound congestion or miosis, difficult urination, and headache. Ophthalmic use may cause mydriasis, photophobia, burning, stinging, and blurring.

Beta agonists most frequently cause tachycardia, palpitations, and other arrhythmias. Their other effects include premature atrial and ventricular contractions, tachyarrhythmias, and myocardial necrosis. Reflex tachycardia and palpitations occur with beta$_2$ agonists because of decreased blood pressure.

Metabolic reactions to beta agonists include hyperglycemia, increased metabolic rate, hyperlactic acidosis, and local and systemic acidosis (decreased bronchodilator response).

Respiratory reactions include increased perfusion of nonfunctioning portions of lungs (COPD); mucous plugs may develop as a result of increased mucus secretion. Other reactions include tremors, vertigo, insomnia, sweating, headache, nausea, vomiting, and anxiety.

Centrally acting adrenergics have similar effects, as well as dry mouth, flushing, diarrhea, impotence, hyperthermia (excessive doses), agitation, anorexia, dizziness, dyskinesia, and changes in libido. Chronic use of adrenergics in children may cause endocrine disturbances that arrest growth; however, growth usually rebounds after withdrawal of drug.

## Clinical considerations
### Parenteral preparations

■ If used as a pressor drug, advise clinician to correct fluid volume depletion before giving drug. Adrenergics aren't a substitute for blood, plasma, fluid, or electrolytes.
■ Advise clinician to carefully monitor blood pressure, pulse, and respiratory and urinary output during therapy.

■ Tachyphylaxis or tolerance may develop after prolonged or excessive use.

### Inhalation therapy

■ The preservative sodium bisulfite is present in many adrenergic formulations. Patients with an allergy to sulfites should avoid drugs that contain this preservative.
■ Advise clinician to give drug when patient arises in morning and before meals, to improve ventilation and reduce fatigue.
■ For unknown reasons, paradoxical airway resistance, manifested by sudden increase in dyspnea, may result from repeated, excessive use of isoetharine. If this occurs, patient should stop taking drug and use alternative therapy, such as epinephrine.
■ Adrenergic inhalation may be alternated with other drug administration (steroids, other adrenergics) if needed, but shouldn't be given simultaneously because of the danger of excessive tachycardia.
■ Don't use discolored or precipitated solutions.
■ Protect solutions from light, freezing, and heat. Store at controlled room temperature.
■ Systemic absorption, although infrequent, can follow applications to nasal and conjunctival membranes. Advise patient to stop drug if symptoms of systemic absorption occur.
■ Prolonged or too-frequent use may cause tolerance to bronchodilation and cardiac stimulant effect. Rebound bronchospasm may follow end of drug effect.
■ Advise patient not to use drug for longer than 48 to 72 hours without consulting a prescriber.

### Special populations

**Pregnant patients.** Pregnancy risk categories range from B to D in this group. Refer to specific package insert for manufacturer recommendations.
**Breast-feeding patients.** The use of adrenergics during breast-feeding usually isn't recommended.
**Pediatric patients.** Lower doses of adrenergics are recommended.
**Geriatric patients.** May be more sensitive to therapeutic and adverse effects of some adrenergics and may require lower doses.

## Patient counseling
### Inhalation therapy

■ Instruct patient in correct use of nebulizer and warn patient to use lowest effective dose.
■ Explain that overuse of adrenergic bronchodilators may cause tachycardia, headache, nausea and dizziness, loss of effectiveness, possible paradoxical reaction, and cardiac arrest.
■ Tell patient to contact prescriber if bronchodilator causes dizziness, chest pain, or lack of therapeutic response to usual dose.
■ Advise patient to avoid other adrenergics unless they're prescribed.

- Inform patient that saliva and sputum may appear pink after inhalation treatment.
- Instruct patient to begin treatment with first symptoms of bronchospasm.
- Caution patient to keep spray away from eyes.
- Tell patient not to discard drug applicator. Refill units are available.

**Nasal therapy**
- Instruct patient to blow nose gently, with both nostrils open, to clear nasal passages before administration of drug.
- Instruct patient on proper method of instillation, as follows:
— Drops: Tilt head back while sitting or standing up, or lie on bed with head over side. Stay in position a few minutes to permit drug to spread through nose.
— Spray: With head upright, squeeze bottle quickly and firmly to produce 1 or 2 sprays into each nostril; wait 3 to 5 minutes, blow nose, and repeat dose.
— Jelly: Place in each nostril and sniff the jelly as far back into the nose as possible.
- Tell patient not to use nasal decongestant for longer than 3 to 5 days.

**Ophthalmic therapy**
- Tell patient to apply pressure to lacrimal sac during instillation of drops and for 1 to 2 minutes afterward to avoid excessive systemic absorption.
- Inform patient that after instillation of ophthalmic preparation, pupils of eyes will be very large and eyes may be more sensitive to light than usual. Advise patient to wear dark glasses until pupils return to normal.
- Warn patient to use drug only as directed.
- Instruct patient to contact his prescriber if no relief occurs or condition worsens.
- Tell patient to store drug away from heat and light and out of reach of children.

## Representative combinations

*Ephedrine sulfate* with guaifenesin and theophylline: Bronkolixir; with guaifenesin, theophylline, and phenobarbital: Bronkotabs; with belladonna extract, boric acid, zinc oxide, beeswax, and cocoa butter: Wyanoids Relief Factor.

*Epinephrine* with benzalkonium chloride: Glaucon; with pilocarpine: E-Pilo.

*Isoproterenol hydrochloride* with phenylephrine bitartrate: Duo-Medihaler.

*Naphazoline* with antazoline phosphate, boric acid, phenylmercuric acetate, and carbonate anhydrous: Vasocon-A Solution; with pheniramine maleate: Naphcon-A; with phenylephrine hydrochloride, pyrilamine maleate, and phenylpropanolamine hydrochloride: 4-Way Long Lasting Spray; with polyvinyl alcohol: Albalon.

*Pseudoephedrine* with chlorpheniramine maleate: Chlor-Trimeton; with codeine phosphate and guaifenesin: Alamine Expectorant,

Deproist Expectorant with Codeine, Guiatussin DAC, Isoclor Expectorant, Novahistine Expectorant, Robitussin-DAC; with dextromethorphan and acetaminophen: Contac Severe Cold and Flu Nighttime; with dextromethorphan, acetaminophen, and guaifenesin: Vicks 44M Cough, Cold, and Flu Relief; with dexbrompheniramine: Disophrol, Drixoral; with dexchlorpheniramine: Polaramine; with guaifenesin: Robitussin-PE, Zephrex; with hydrocordone bitartrate: De-Tuss, Detussin Liquid, Entuss-D, Tussend; with triprolidine: Actagen, Actamin, Actifed, Allerfrim Tablets, Aprodine, Cenafed Plus, Triposed.

See also *antihistamines, barbiturates,* and *xanthine derivatives.*

---

# adrenocorticoids (nasal and oral inhalation)

*Nasal:* **beclomethasone dipropionate, budesonide, flunisolide, fluticasone propionate, triamcinolone acetonide**

*Oral:* **beclomethasone dipropionate, budesonide, flunisolide, fluticasone propionate, triamcinolone acetonide**

Topical administration through oral aerosol and nasal spray delivers adrenocorticoids to sites of inflammation in the nasal passages or the tracheobronchial tree. Because smaller doses are given, less drug is absorbed systemically, with fewer systemic adverse effects.

## Clinical indications and actions
*Nasal inflammation*
Nasal solutions are used to relieve symptoms of seasonal or perennial rhinitis when antihistamines and decongestants are ineffective, to treat inflammatory conditions of the nasal passages, and to prevent recurrence after surgical removal of nasal polyps. (See *Nasal adrenocorticoids for inflammation from allergic rhinitis,* page 4.)

*Chronic bronchial asthma*
Aerosols are used to treat chronic bronchial asthma not controlled by bronchodilators and other nonsteroidal drugs. (See *Oral inhalation adrenocorticoids for chronic bronchial asthma,* page 5.)

## Pharmacology
Inhaled glucocorticoid is absorbed through the nasal mucosa or through the trachea, bronchi, and alveoli. The anti-inflammatory effects of glucocorticoids depend on the direct local action of the steroid. Glucocorticoids stimulate transcription of messenger RNA in individual cell nuclei to synthesize enzymes that decrease inflammation. These enzymes stimulate bio-

---

* Canada only    ◇ Unlabeled clinical use

**NASAL ADRENOCORTICOIDS FOR
INFLAMMATION FROM ALLERGIC RHINITIS**

| Drug | Pediatric daily dose* | Adult daily dose* |
|---|---|---|
| beclomethasone dipropionate | **Nasal aerosol:**<br>Under age 6: not recommended<br>Ages 6-12: 84 mcg b.i.d. to q.i.d.<br>Maximum dose: 168-336 mcg/day<br>**Nasal solution:**<br>Under age 6: not recommended<br>Ages 6-12: 84 mcg t.i.d.<br>Maximum dose: 252 mcg/day | **Nasal aerosol:**<br>84 mcg b.i.d. to q.i.d.<br>Maximum dose: 168-336 mcg/day<br>**Nasal solution:**<br>84-168 mcg b.i.d.<br>Maximum dose: 336 mcg/day |
| budesonide | **Nasal powder:**<br>Under age 6: not recommended<br>Ages 6-12: 200-400 mcg/day<br>Maximum dose: 400 mcg/day<br>**Nasal solution:**<br>Under age 6: not recommended<br>Ages 6-12: 64-256 mcg/day<br>Maximum dose: 256 mcg/day | **Nasal powder:**<br>200-400 mcg/day<br>Maximum dose: 800 mcg/day<br>**Nasal solution:**<br>64-256 mcg/day<br>Maximum dose: 256 mcg/day |
| flunisolide | **Nasal solution:**<br>Under age 6: not recommended<br>Ages 6-14: 50-100 mcg b.i.d.<br>Maximum dose: 200 mcg/day | **Nasal solution:**<br>50-100 mcg b.i.d. to t.i.d.<br>Maximum dose: 400 mcg/day |
| fluticasone propionate | **Nasal solution:**<br>Under age 4: not recommended<br>Ages 4-12: 100-200 mcg once daily<br>Maximum dose: 200 mcg/day | **Nasal solution:**<br>100-200 mcg once daily<br>Maximum dose: 200 mcg daily |
| triamcinolone acetonide | **Nasal aerosol:**<br>Under age 5: not recommended<br>Ages 6-12: 110-220 mcg once daily<br>Maximum dose: 220 mcg/day<br>**Nasal solution:**<br>Under age 6: not recommended<br>Ages 6-12: 110-220 mcg/day<br>Maximum dose: 220 mcg/day | **Nasal aerosol:**<br>110-220 mcg once daily<br>Maximum dose: 440 mcg/day<br>**Nasal solution:**<br>110-220 mcg/day<br>Maximum dose: 220 mcg/day |

* Total doses to both nostrils.

chemical pathways that decrease the inflammatory response by stabilizing leukocyte lysosomal membranes, which prevents the release of destructive acid hydrolases from leukocytes; inhibiting macrophage accumulation in inflamed areas; reducing leukocyte adhesion to the capillary endothelium; reducing capillary wall permeability and edema formation; decreasing complement components; antagonizing histamine activity and release of kinin from substrates; reducing fibroblast proliferation, collagen deposition, and scar tissue formation; and other unknown mechanisms.

## Overview of adverse reactions

*Nasal:* Local sensations of nasal burning and irritation occur in about 10% of patients; sneezing attacks occur immediately after nasal application in about 10% of patients; transient mild nosebleeds occur in 10% to 15% of patients. It's unknown if these are effects of the nasal solution or of the dryness it induces in the nasal passages. Localized candidal infections of the nose or pharynx rarely occur.
*Oral:* Localized infections with *Candida albicans* or *Aspergillus niger* occur commonly in the mouth and pharynx and occasionally in the larynx.
*Systemic:* Systemic absorption may occur, potentially leading to hypothalamic-pituitary-adrenal (HPA) axis suppression. This is more likely to occur with large doses or with combined nasal and oral corticosteroid therapy.
*Other:* Hypersensitivity reactions are possible. Some patients may be intolerant of the fluorocarbon propellants in the preparations.

## Clinical considerations

■ Full therapeutic benefit requires regular use and is usually evident within a few days, although a few patients may require up to 3 weeks of therapy for maximum benefit. Therapy should be stopped in the absence of significant symptomatic improvement within recommended time frame (varies with drug used).

### ORAL INHALATION ADRENOCORTICOIDS FOR CHRONIC BRONCHIAL ASTHMA

| Drug | Pediatric daily dose | Adult daily dose |
|---|---|---|
| beclomethasone dipropionate | **Inhalation aerosol:** <br> Under age 6: not recommended <br> Ages 6-12: 42-84 mcg t.i.d. to q.i.d. or 168 mcg b.i.d. <br> Maximum dose: 420 mcg/day | **Inhalation aerosol:** <br> 84 mcg t.i.d. to q.i.d. or 168 mcg b.i.d. <br> Maximum dose: 840 mcg/day |
| budesonide | **Inhalation powder:** <br> Under age 6: not recommended <br> Ages 6-12: 200-400 mcg b.i.d. <br> Maximum dose: 800 mcg/day | **Inhalation powder:** <br> 200-400 mcg b.i.d. <br> Maximum dose: 1,600 mcg/day |
| flunisolide | **Inhalation aerosol:** <br> Under age 6: not recommended <br> Over age 6: 500 mcg b.i.d. <br> Maximum dose: 1 mg/day | **Inhalation aerosol:** <br> 500 mcg b.i.d. <br> Maximum dose: 2 mg/day |
| fluticasone propionate | **Inhalation aerosol:** <br> Under age 12: not recommended <br> **Inhalation powder:** <br> Under age 4: not recommended <br> Ages 4-11: 50 mcg b.i.d. <br> Maximum dose: 200 mcg/day | **Inhalation aerosol:** <br> 88-440 mcg b.i.d. <br> Maximum dose: 1,760 mcg/day <br> **Inhalation powder:** <br> 100-500 mcg b.i.d. <br> Maximum dose: 2 mg/day |
| triamcinolone acetonide | **Inhalation aerosol:** <br> Under age 6: not recommended <br> Ages 6-12: 100-200 mcg t.i.d. or q.i.d., or 200-400 mcg b.i.d. <br> Maximum dose: 1,200 mcg/day | **Inhalation aerosol:** <br> 200 mcg t.i.d. or q.i.d., or 400 mcg b.i.d. <br> Maximum dose: 1,600 mcg/day |

■ A patient who uses nasal or oral inhalation therapy may be allowed to discontinue systemic corticosteroid therapy.

■ After the desired clinical effect is obtained, the maintenance dosage should be reduced to the smallest amount needed to control symptoms.

■ Drug should be discontinued if the patient develops signs of systemic absorption (such as Cushing's syndrome, hyperglycemia, or glucosuria), mucosal irritation or ulceration, hypersensitivity, or infection. If antifungals or antibiotics are being used with corticosteroids and the infection doesn't respond immediately, corticosteroids should be discontinued until the infection is controlled.

#### Special populations

**Pregnant patients.** Corticosteroids shouldn't be used, especially in large doses or for long periods of time. They should only be used when the potential benefits outweigh the potential risks.

**Breast-feeding patients.** Should be used with caution. Corticosteroids may cause growth suppression in infants if drug appears in breast milk.

**Pediatric patients.** Nasal or oral inhalant corticosteroid therapy may be successfully substituted for systemic corticosteroid therapy. However, the risk of HPA axis suppression and Cushing's syndrome still exists.

**Geriatric patients.** Many geriatric patients have conditions that could be aggravated by the excessive use of corticosteroid inhalant therapy. Geriatric patients have a reduced ability to metabolize and eliminate drugs; advise clinician to monitor patient closely for adverse effects.

### Patient counseling

**Nasal therapy**

■ Instruct patient to use only as directed. Inform him that full therapeutic effect isn't immediate but requires regular use of inhaler.

■ Encourage patient with blocked nasal passages to use an oral decongestant 30 minutes before intranasal corticosteroid administration to ensure adequate penetration. Advise patient to clear nasal passages of secretions before using the inhaler.

■ Instruct patient to clean inhaler according to manufacturer's instructions.

**Oral therapy**

■ Instruct patient to use only as directed.

■ Advise patient receiving bronchodilators by inhalation to use the bronchodilator before the corticosteroid to enhance penetration of the corticosteroid into the bronchial tree. He should wait several minutes to allow the bronchodilator to relax the smooth muscle.

■ Instruct patient to hold his breath for a few seconds to enhance placement and action of the drug and to wait 1 minute before taking subsequent puffs of drug.

■ Tell patient to rinse mouth with water after using the inhaler to decrease the chance of oral fungal infections. Tell him to check nasal and oral mucous membranes frequently for signs of fungal infection.

■ Instruct patient to clean inhaler properly.

■ Warn asthmatic patient not to increase use of corticosteroid inhaler during a severe asthma attack, but to call prescriber for adjustment of therapy and possibly the addition of a systemic steroid.

■ Inform patient that drug is for preventive therapy, not to abort an acute attack.

**Nasal or oral therapy**

■ Tell patient to report decreased response. Dosage adjustment or discontinuation of drug may be needed.

■ Instruct patient to observe for adverse effects and, if fever or local irritation develops, to discontinue use and report the effect promptly.

## Representative combinations
None.

---

## adrenocorticoids (systemic)

*Glucocorticoids:* **betamethasone, betamethasone sodium phosphate, betamethasone sodium phosphate and betamethasone acetate, cortisone acetate, dexamethasone, dexamethasone acetate, dexamethasone sodium phosphate, hydrocortisone, hydrocortisone acetate, hydrocortisone cypionate, hydrocortisone sodium phosphate, hydrocortisone sodium succinate, methylprednisolone, methylprednisolone acetate, methylprednisolone sodium succinate, prednisolone, prednisolone acetate, prednisolone sodium phosphate, prednisolone tebutate, prednisone, triamcinolone, triamcinolone acetonide, triamcinolone diacetate, triamcinolone hexacetonide**

*Mineralocorticoid:* **fludrocortisone acetate**

---

Adrenocorticoids, also called adrenocortical hormones, are classified according to their activity into two groups: mineralocorticoids and glucocorticoids. Mineralocorticoids regulate electrolyte homeostasis. Glucocorticoids regulate inflammation, the body's immune responses to diverse stimuli, and carbohydrate, lipid, and protein metabolism. Many cortico-steroids exert both kinds of activity. (See *Comparing systemic glucocorticoids.*)

## Clinical indications and actions
### Asthma
Systemic glucocorticoids are used to treat status asthmaticus and acute asthma episodes. Therapy is combined with sympathomimetics and aminophylline.

### Sarcoidosis
Therapy is aimed at the management of ocular, CNS, glandular, myocardial, or severe pulmonary involvement. Systemic glucocorticoids may also be used for hypercalcemia or severe skin lesions.

### Advanced pulmonary or extrapulmonary tuberculosis
Systemic glucocorticoids have been used to help decrease inflammation caused by *Mycobacterium tuberculosis.*

### Pericarditis
Unlabeled uses for systemic glucocorticoids include treatment of pain, fever, and inflammation of pericarditis.

### Inflammation
A major pharmacologic use of glucocorticoids is treatment of inflammation. The anti-inflammatory effects depend on the direct local action of the steroids. Glucocorticoids decrease the inflammatory response by stabilizing leukocyte lysosomal membranes, which prevents the release of destructive acid hydrolases from leukocytes; inhibiting macrophage accumulation in inflamed areas; reducing leukocyte adhesion to the capillary endothelium; reducing capillary wall permeability and edema formation; decreasing complement components; antagonizing histamine activity and release of kinin from substrates; reducing fibroblast proliferation, collagen deposition, and subsequent scar tissue formation; and other unknown mechanisms.

### Immunosuppression
The full mechanisms of immunosuppressive actions are unknown. Glucocorticoids reduce activity and volume of the lymphatic system, producing lymphocytopenia, decreasing immunoglobulin and complement concentrations, decreasing passage of immune complexes through basement membranes, and possibly depressing reactivity of tissue to antigen-antibody interaction.

### Adrenal insufficiency
Combined mineralocorticoid and glucocorticoid therapy is used in treating adrenal insufficiency and in salt-losing forms of congenital adrenogenital syndrome.

### Rheumatic and collagen diseases; other severe diseases
Glucocorticoids are used to treat rheumatic and collagen diseases, such as arthritis, polyarteritis nodosa, and systemic lupus erythematosus; thyroiditis; severe dermatologic diseases, such as pemphigus, exfoliative dermatitis, lichen

## COMPARING SYSTEMIC GLUCOCORTICOIDS

| Drug | Approximate equivalent dose (mg) | Relative glucocorticoid (anti-inflammatory) potency | Relative mineralocorticoid potency | Plasma half-life (hr) | Biological half-life (hr) |
|------|------|------|------|------|------|
| betamethasone, oral | 0.6-0.75 | 20-30 | 0 | > 5 | 36-54 |
| betamethasone acetate | 0.6-0.75 | 20-30 | 0 | > 5 | 36-54 |
| betamethasone sodium phosphate | 0.6-0.75 | 20-30 | 0 | > 5 | 36-54 |
| cortisone acetate | 25 | 0.8 | 2 | ½ | 8-12 |
| dexamethasone, oral | 0.5-0.75 | 20-30 | 0 | 2-3½ | 36-54 |
| dexamethasone acetate | 0.5-0.75 | 20-30 | 0 | 2-3½ | 36-54 |
| dexamethasone sodium phosphate | 0.5-0.75 | 20-30 | 0 | 2-3½ | 36-54 |
| hydrocortisone, oral | 20 | 1 | 2 | 1½-2 | 8-12 |
| hydrocortisone acetate | 20 | 1 | 2 | 1½-2 | 8-12 |
| hydrocortisone cypionate | 20 | 1 | 2 | 1½-2 | 8-12 |
| hydrocortisone sodium phosphate | 20 | 1 | 2 | 1½-2 | 8-12 |
| hydrocortisone sodium succinate | 20 | 1 | 2 | 1½-2 | 8-12 |
| methylprednisolone, oral | 4 | 5 | 0 | 1-3 | 18-6 |
| methylprednisolone acetate | 4 | 5 | 0 | 1-3 | 18-36 |
| methylprednisolone sodium succinate | 4 | 5 | 0 | 1-3 | 18-36 |
| prednisolone, oral | 5 | 4 | 1 | 2¼-3½ | 18-36 |
| prednisolone acetate | 5 | 4 | 1 | 2¼-3½ | 18-36 |
| prednisolone sodium phosphate | 5 | 4 | 1 | 2¼-3½ | 18-36 |
| prednisolone tebutate | 5 | 4 | 1 | 2¼-3½ | 18-36 |
| prednisone | 5 | 4 | 1 | 1 | 18-36 |
| triamcinolone, oral | 4 | 5 | 0 | > 3⅓ | 18-36 |
| triamcinolone acetonide | 4 | 5 | 0 | > 3⅓ | 18-36 |
| triamcinolone diacetate | 4 | 5 | 0 | > 3⅓ | 18-36 |
| triamcinolone hexacetonide | 4 | 5 | 0 | > 3⅓ | 18-36 |

planus, and psoriasis; allergic reactions; ocular disorders, such as inflammations; respiratory diseases, such as asthma, sarcoidosis, and lipid pneumonitis; hematologic diseases, such as autoimmune hemolytic anemia and idiopathic thrombocytopenia; neoplastic diseases, such as leukemias and lymphomas; and GI diseases, such as ulcerative colitis, regional enteritis, and celiac disease. Other indications include myasthenia gravis, organ transplant, nephrotic syndrome, and septic shock.

*Antenatal use in preterm labor*
Dexamethasone and betamethasone have been used as short-course I.M. therapy in women with preterm labor to hasten fetal maturation of lungs and cerebral blood vessels.

*Hypercalcemia*
Glucocorticoids are used to treat hypercalcemia secondary to sarcoidosis, vitamin D intoxication, multiple myeloma, and breast cancer in postmenopausal women.

*Cerebral edema*
High-dose parenteral glucocorticoid administration may decrease cerebral edema in brain tumors and during neurosurgery.

*Acute spinal cord injury*
Large I.V. doses of glucocorticoids, when given shortly after injury, may improve motor and sensory function in patients with acute spinal cord injury.

## Pharmacology

Corticosteroids dramatically affect almost all body systems. They control the rate of protein synthesis, reacting with receptor proteins in the cytoplasm of sensitive cells to form a steroid-receptor complex. Steroid receptors have been identified in many tissues. The steroid-receptor complex migrates into the nucleus of the cell, where it binds to chromatin. Information carried by the steroid of the receptor protein directs the genetic apparatus to transcribe RNA, resulting in the synthesis of specific proteins that serve as enzymes in various biochemical pathways. Because the maximum pharmacologic activity lags behind peak blood levels, the effects of corticosteroids may result from modification of enzyme activity rather than from direct action by the drugs.

Glucocorticoids stimulate transcription of messenger RNA in individual cell nuclei to synthesize enzymes that decrease inflammation. These enzymes stimulate biochemical pathways that decrease the inflammatory response by stabilizing leukocyte lysosomal membranes, which prevents the release of destructive acid hydrolases from leukocytes; inhibiting macrophage accumulation in inflamed areas; reducing leukocyte adhesion to the capillary endothelium; reducing capillary wall permeability and edema formation; decreasing complement components; antagonizing histamine activity and release of kinin from substrates; reducing fibroblast proliferation, collagen deposition, and scar tissue formation; and other unknown mechanisms.

Mineralocorticoids act renally at the distal tubules to enhance the reabsorption of sodium ions, and thus water, from the tubular fluid into the plasma, and enhance the urinary excretion of both potassium and hydrogen ions. The primary features of excess mineralocorticoid activity are positive sodium balance and expansion of the extracellular fluid volume, normal or slight increase in the plasma sodium level, hypokalemia, and alkalosis. In contrast, mineralocorticoid deficiency produces sodium loss, hyponatremia, hyperkalemia, contraction of the extracellular fluid volume, and cellular dehydration.

## Overview of adverse reactions

Suppression of the hypothalamic-pituitary-adrenal (HPA) axis is the major effect of systemic therapy with corticosteroids. When given in high doses or for prolonged therapy, glucocorticoids suppress release of corticotropin from the pituitary gland; subsequently, the adrenal cortex stops secreting endogenous corticosteroids. The degree and duration of HPA-axis suppression produced by the drugs are highly variable among patients and depend on the dose, frequency and time of administration, and duration of therapy.

Patients with a suppressed HPA axis from exogenous glucocorticoid administration who abruptly stop therapy may experience severe withdrawal symptoms, such as fever, myalgia, arthralgia, malaise, anorexia, nausea, desquamation of skin, orthostatic hypotension, dizziness, fainting, dyspnea, and hypoglycemia. Therefore, corticosteroid therapy should always be withdrawn gradually.

Adrenal suppression may persist for as long as 12 months in patients who have received large doses for prolonged periods. Until complete recovery occurs, patients under stress may show signs and symptoms of adrenal insufficiency and may need glucocorticoid and mineralocorticoid replacement therapy.

Cushingoid symptoms, the effects of excessive glucocorticoid therapy, may develop in patients receiving large doses of glucocorticoids over several weeks or longer. These include moon face, central obesity, striae, hirsutism, acne, ecchymoses, hypertension, osteoporosis, muscle atrophy, sexual dysfunction, diabetes, cataracts, hyperlipidemia, peptic ulcer, increased susceptibility to infection, and fluid and electrolyte imbalances.

Other adverse reactions to normal or high doses of corticosteroids may include CNS effects (euphoria, insomnia, psychotic behavior, pseudotumor cerebri, mental changes, nervousness, restlessness); CV effects (heart failure, hypertension, edema); GI effects (peptic ulcer, irritation, increased appetite); metabolic effects (hypokalemia, sodium retention, fluid retention, weight gain, hyperglycemia, osteoporosis); musculoskeletal effects (acute tendon rupture, muscle wasting and pain, myopathy); skin effects (delayed wound healing, acne, skin eruptions, muscle atrophy, striae, Kaposi's sarcoma); and immunosuppression (increased susceptibility to infection, activation of latent infection, exacerbation of intercurrent infections).

## Clinical considerations

■ The patient may experience sudden weight gain, edema, change in blood pressure, or change in electrolyte status.
■ During times of physiologic stress, such as trauma, surgery, and infection, the patient may require additional steroids and may experience signs of steroid withdrawal; patients who were previously steroid-dependent may need systemic corticosteroids to prevent adrenal insufficiency.

■ Drug needs to be reduced gradually in long-term therapy. Rapid reduction may cause withdrawal symptoms.

■ Caregivers should be aware of patient's psychological history and watch for behavioral changes.

■ Patient should be observed for infection or delayed wound healing.

### Special populations
**Pregnant patients.** Glucocorticoids may cause fetal abnormalities; avoid use if possible.

**Breast-feeding patients.** Women taking pharmacologic doses of corticosteroids shouldn't breast-feed.

**Pediatric patients.** Long-term administration of pharmacologic doses of glucocorticoids may retard bone growth. Signs and symptoms of adrenal suppression include retardation of linear growth, delayed weight gain, low plasma cortisol levels, and lack of response to corticotropin stimulation. Alternate-day therapy is recommended to minimize growth suppression. Benefits of therapy should strongly outweigh side effects.

**Geriatric patients.** Many geriatric patients have conditions that could easily be aggravated by corticosteroid therapy. Geriatric patients have a reduced ability to metabolize and eliminate drugs; advise clinician to monitor patient closely.

### Patient counseling
■ Explain the need to take the adrenocorticoid as prescribed. Give patient instructions on what to do if a dose is inadvertently missed.

■ Warn patient not to stop drug abruptly.

■ Inform patient of therapeutic and adverse effects of drug and tell him to report complications immediately.

■ Tell patient to carry a medical identification card noting the need for more adrenocorticoids during stress.

### Representative combinations
*Betamethasone sodium phosphate* with betamethasone acetate: Celestone Soluspan.

*Dexamethasone sodium phosphate* with lidocaine hydrochloride: Decadron with Xylocaine.

---

# adrenocorticoids (topical)

**alclometasone dipropionate, amcinonide, betamethasone benzoate, betamethasone dipropionate, betamethasone valerate, clobetasol propionate, clocortolone pivalate, desonide, desoximetasone, dexamethasone, dexamethasone sodium phosphate, diflorasone diacetate, fluocinolone acetonide, fluocinonide,**

**flurandrenolide, fluticasone propionate, halcinonide, halobetasol propionate, hydrocortisone, hydrocortisone acetate, hydrocortisone butyrate, hydrocortisone valerate, methylprednisolone acetate, triamcinolone acetonide**

Numerous analogues of topical hydrocortisone provide a wide range of potencies in creams, ointments, lotions, and gels.

### Clinical indications and actions
*Inflammatory disorders of skin and mucous membranes*

Topical adrenocorticoids relieve inflammatory and pruritic skin disorders, including localized neurodermatitis, psoriasis, atopic or seborrheic dermatitis, the inflammatory phase of xerosis, anogenital pruritus, discoid lupus erythematosus, lichen planus, granuloma annulare, and lupus erythematosus.

These drugs may also relieve irritant or allergic contact dermatitis; however, relief of acute dermatosis may require systemic adrenocorticoids.

Rectal disorders responsive to this class of drugs include ulcerative colitis, cryptitis, inflamed hemorrhoids, postirradiation or factitial proctitis, and pruritus ani.

Oral lesions, such as nonherpetic oral inflammatory and ulcerative lesions and routine gingivitis, may respond to treatment with topical adrenocorticoids.

OTC forms of topical corticosteroids are indicated for minor skin irritation, such as itching; rash caused by eczema, dermatitis, insect bites, poison ivy, poison oak, or poison sumac; or dermatitis caused by exposure to soaps, detergents, cosmetics, and jewelry.

### Pharmacology
The anti-inflammatory effects of topical glucocorticoids depend on the direct local action of the steroid. Although the exact mechanism of action is unclear, many researchers believe that glucocorticoids stimulate transcription of messenger RNA in individual cell nuclei to synthesize enzymes that decrease inflammation. These enzymes stimulate biochemical pathways that decrease the inflammatory response by stabilizing leukocyte lysosomal membranes, which prevents the release of destructive acid hydrolases from leukocytes; inhibiting macrophage accumulation in inflamed areas; reducing leukocyte adhesion to the capillary endothelium; reducing capillary wall permeability and edema formation; decreasing complement components; antagonizing histamine activity and release of kinin from substrates; reducing fibroblast proliferation, collagen deposition, and subsequent scar tissue formation; and other unknown mechanisms.

## POTENCIES OF TOPICAL CORTICOSTEROIDS

Topical corticosteroid preparations can be grouped according to relative anti-inflammatory activity. The following list arranges groups of topical corticosteroids in decreasing order of potency (based mainly on vasoconstrictor assay or clinical effectiveness in psoriasis). Preparations within each group are approximately equivalent.

| Group | Drug | Concentration (%) |
|-------|------|-------------------|
| I | betamethasone dipropionate (Diprolene) | 0.05 |
| | betamethasone dipropionate (Diprolene AF) | 0.05 |
| | clobetasol propionate (Temovate) | 0.05 |
| | diflorasone diacetate (Psorcon) | 0.05 |
| II | amcinonide (Cyclocort) | 0.1 |
| | betamethasone dipropionate ointment (Diprosone) | 0.05 |
| | desoximetasone (Topicort) | 0.05, 0.25 |
| | diflorasone diacetate (Florone, Maxiflor) | 0.05 |
| | fluocinonide (Lidex) | 0.05 |
| | fluocinonide gel | 0.05 |
| | halcinonide (Halog) | 0.1 |
| III | betamethasone benzoate gel | 0.025 |
| | betamethasone dipropionate cream (Diprosone) | 0.05 |
| | betamethasone valerate ointment (Valisone) | 0.1 |
| | diflorasone diacetate cream (Florone, Maxiflor) | 0.05 |
| | triamcinolone acetonide cream (Aristocort) | 0.5 |
| IV | desoximetasone (Topicort LP) | 0.05 |
| | fluocinolone acetonide (Synalar-HP) | 0.2 |
| | fluocinolone acetonide ointment (Synalar) | 0.025 |
| | flurandrenolide (Cordran) | 0.05 |
| | fluticasone propionate (Cutivate) | 0.005, 0.05 |
| | triamcinolone acetonide ointment (Aristocort, Kenalog) | 0.1 |
| V | betamethasone benzoate cream | 0.025 |
| | betamethasone dipropionate lotion (Diprosone) | 0.05 |
| | betamethasone valerate cream or lotion (Valisone) | 0.1 |
| | fluocinolone acetonide cream (Synalar) | 0.025 |
| | flurandrenolide (Cordran) | 0.05 |
| | hydrocortisone butyrate (Locoid) | 0.1 |
| | hydrocortisone valerate (Westcort) | 0.2 |
| | triamcinolone acetonide cream or lotion (Kenalog) | 0.1 |
| VI | alclometasone dipropionate (Aclovate) | 0.05 |
| | desonide (Tridesilon) | 0.05 |
| | fluocinolone acetonide solution (Synalar) | 0.01 |

Topical corticosteroids are minimally absorbed systemically and cause fewer adverse effects than systemic corticosteroids. Fluorinated derivatives are absorbed to a greater extent than are other topical steroids. The degree of absorption depends on the site of application, the amount applied, the relative potency, the presence of an occlusive dressing (may increase penetration by 10%), skin condition, and the vehicle carrying the drug. Topical corticosteroids are used to relieve pruritus, inflammation, and other signs of corticosteroid-responsive dermatoses.

Ointments are preferred for dry, scaly areas; solutions, gels, aerosols, and lotions are used for hairy areas. Creams can be used for most areas except those in which dampness may cause maceration. Gels and lotions can be used for moist lesions. However, gels may contain alcohol, which can dry and irritate skin. The topical preparations are classified by potency into six groups: group I is the most potent and group VI the least potent. (See *Potencies of topical corticosteroids*.)

## Overview of adverse reactions

Local effects include burning, itching, irritation, dryness, folliculitis, striae, miliaria, acne, perioral dermatitis, hypopigmentation, hypertrichosis, allergic contact dermatitis, secondary infection, and atrophy.

Systemic absorption may occur, leading to hypothalamic-pituitary-adrenal (HPA) axis suppression.

The risk of adverse reactions increases with the use of occlusive dressings or more potent steroids, in patients with liver disease, and in children (because of their greater ratio of skin surface to body weight).

Prolonged application around the eyes may lead to cataracts or glaucoma.

## Clinical considerations
- Recommend washing hands before and after applying the drug.
- Recommend gently cleaning the area of application. Washing or soaking the area before application may increase drug penetration.
- Recommend applying sparingly in a light film and rubbing in lightly. Recommend avoiding contact with eyes, unless using an ophthalmic product.
- Prolonged application of drug in areas near the eyes, genitals, rectum, face, and skin folds should be avoided. High-potency topical corticosteroids are more likely to cause striae and atrophy in these areas because of their higher rates of absorption.
- Advise clinician to monitor response. Advise clinician to observe area of inflammation.
- Occlusive dressings shouldn't be applied over topical steroids.
- Drug should be stopped if signs of systemic absorption develop.

### Special populations
**Pregnant patients.** Safe use of topical steroids during pregnancy hasn't been established. It's unknown if topical steroids affect fertility.
**Breast-feeding patients.** Use topical corticosteroids with caution.
**Pediatric patients.** Limit topical corticosteroid therapy to the minimum amount needed for therapeutic efficacy. Advise parents not to use tight-fitting diapers or plastic pants on a child whose diaper area is being treated, because such garments may act as occlusive dressings. Pediatric patients may be more susceptible than adults to topical corticosteroid-induced, HPA-axis suppression and Cushing's syndrome because of a greater skin surface area-to-body weight ratio.
**Geriatric patients.** Loss of collagen may lead to friable and transparent skin with increased epidermal permeability to water and certain chemicals. Topically applied drugs such as steroid creams may have a greater effect locally than in younger patients. Geriatric patients also have a reduced ability to metabolize and eliminate drugs and may have higher plasma drug levels and more adverse reactions. Patient should be monitored closely.

### Patient counseling
- Instruct patient on use of drug.
- Advise patient to discontinue drug and report local or systemic adverse reactions, worsening condition, or persistent symptoms.
- Warn patient not to use OTC topical products other than those specifically recommended.
- Tell patient to apply a missed dose as soon as it's remembered and to continue with the regular schedule of application. However, if it's almost time for the next application, tell patient to wait and continue regular schedule. He shouldn't apply a double dose.

## Representative combinations
*Betamethasone dipropionate* with clotrimazole: Lotrisone.

*Dexamethasone* with neomycin sulfate: NeoDecadron Cream; with neomycin sulfate and polymyxin B sulfate: Dexacidin Ointment.

*Fluocinolone acetonide* with neomycin: Neo-Synalar.

*Flurandrenolide* with neomycin: Cordran.

*Hydrocortisone with iodoquinol:* Vytone Cream; with iodochlorhydroxyquin: Vioform-Hydrocortisone Cream, AP, Corque Cream, Hysone; with neomycin: Hydrocortisone-Neomycin, Neo-Cortef; with pramoxine: Pramosone, Zone-A Forte; with neomycin and polymyxin B: Cortisporin Cream; with neomycin, bacitracin, and polymyxin B sulfate: Cortisporin Ointment; with neomycin sulfate and polymyxin B sulfate: Cortisporin; with dibucaine: Corticaine; with pyrilamine maleate and chlorpheniramine maleate: HC Derma-Pax; with benzoyl peroxide and mineral oil: Vanoxide-HC; with lidocaine and glycerin: Lida-Mantle-HC; with sulfur and salicylic acid: Therac Lotion.

*Methylprednisolone* with neomycin: Neo-Medrol Acetate.

*Triamcinolone acetonide* with nystatin: Mykacet, Myco II, Myco-Biotic II, Mycogen II, Mycolog-II, Myco-Triacet II, Mytrex, Nystatin-Triamcinolone Acetonide, N.G.T.; with neomycin, gramicidin, and nystatin: Myco-Triacet II, Tri-Statin II.

# alpha adrenergic blockers

**dihydroergotamine mesylate, doxazosin mesylate, ergotamine tartrate, phentolamine mesylate, prazosin hydrochloride, tamsulosin hydrochloride, terazosin hydrochloride, tolazoline hydrochloride**

Drugs that block the effects of peripheral neurohormonal transmitters (such as norepinephrine, epinephrine, and related sympathomimetic amines) on adrenergic receptors in various effector systems are designated as adrenergic blockers. Like adrenoreceptors, blockers are classified into two subtypes—alpha and beta. Essentially, alpha adrenergic blockers are those drugs that antagonize mydriasis, vasoconstriction, nonvascular smooth-muscle excitation, and other adrenergic responses caused by alpha receptor stimulation.

## Clinical indications and actions
### Peripheral vascular disorders
Alpha adrenergic blockers are indicated for treating peripheral vascular disorders, including Raynaud's disease, acrocyanosis, frostbite,

acute atrial occlusion, phlebitis, and diabetic gangrene. Dihydroergotamine and ergotamine have been used to treat vascular headaches. Prazosin has been used to treat Raynaud's disease. Phentolamine is indicated to treat dermal necrosis caused by extravasation of norepinephrine, dopamine, or phenylephrine (alpha agonists).

*Hypertension*

Tolazoline is indicated to treat persistent pulmonary hypertension in neonates. Prazosin, carvedilol, doxazosin, and terazosin are used to manage essential hypertension. Phentolamine is used to control hypertension and is a useful adjunct in the surgical treatment of pheochromocytoma.

*BPH*

Terazosin, tamsulosin, and doxazosin are used to control mild to moderate urinary obstructive symptoms in men with BPH.

## Pharmacology

*Nonselective alpha adrenergic blockers*

Ergotamine, phentolamine, and tolazoline antagonize both alpha$_1$ adrenergic and alpha$_2$ adrenergic receptors. Generally, alpha blockade results in tachycardia, palpitations, and increased secretion of renin caused by the abnormally large amounts of norepinephrine (transmitter "overflow") released from adrenergic nerve endings as a result of the concurrent blockade of alpha$_1$ adrenergic and alpha$_2$ adrenergic receptors. The effects of norepinephrine are clinically counterproductive to the major uses of nonselective alpha adrenergic blockers, which include treating peripheral vascular disorders such as Raynaud's disease, acrocyanosis, frostbite, acute atrial occlusion, phlebitis, phlebothrombosis, diabetic gangrene, shock, and pheochromocytoma.

*Selective alpha adrenergic blockers*

Alpha$_1$ adrenergic blockers have readily observable effects and are currently the only alpha-adrenergic drugs with known clinical uses. They decrease vascular resistance and increase venous capacitance, lowering blood pressure and causing pink, warm skin; nasal and scleroconjunctival congestion; ptosis; orthostatic and exercise hypotension; mild to moderate miosis; and interference with ejaculation. They also relax nonvascular smooth muscle, notably in the prostate capsule, reducing urinary symptoms in men with BPH. Because alpha$_1$ adrenergic blockers don't block alpha$_2$ adrenergic receptors, they don't cause transmitter overflow. In theory, alpha$_1$ adrenergic blockers should be useful in the same conditions as nonselective alpha adrenergic blockers; however, doxazosin, prazosin, and terazosin are approved to treat hypertension. Terazosin and doxazosin are approved to treat prostatic outflow obstruction secondary to BPH.

Alpha$_2$ adrenergic blockers, such as yohimbine, produce more subtle physiologic effects and currently have no therapeutic applications.

## Overview of adverse reactions

Nonselective alpha adrenergic blockers typically cause orthostatic hypotension, tachycardia, palpitations, fluid retention (from excess renin secretion), nasal and ocular congestion, and aggravation of the signs and symptoms of respiratory infection. Use of these drugs is contraindicated in patients with renal insufficiency and severe cerebral and coronary atherosclerosis.

Selective alpha adrenergic blockers may cause severe orthostatic hypotension and syncope, especially with the first dose. The most common adverse effects of alpha-adrenergic blockers are dizziness, headache, and malaise.

## Clinical considerations

■ Vital signs, especially blood pressure, should be monitored.

■ Dose should be given at bedtime to reduce potential of dizziness or light-headedness.

■ To avoid first-dose syncope, advise clinician to begin with a small dose.

### Special populations

**Pregnant patients.** Avoid use in pregnant women.

**Breast-feeding patients.** Women taking these drugs shouldn't breast-feed.

**Pediatric patients.** Safety and efficacy of many of these drugs haven't been established for use in children. Refer to specific drug monograph for more information.

**Geriatric patients.** Hypotensive effects may be more pronounced.

## Patient counseling

■ Warn patient about orthostatic hypotension. Tell him to avoid suddenly moving to an upright position.

■ Tell patient to promptly report dizziness or irregular heartbeat.

■ Advise patient to take dose at bedtime to reduce potential for dizziness or light-headedness.

■ Warn patient to avoid driving and other hazardous tasks that require mental alertness until effects of drug are established.

■ Reassure patient that adverse effects, including dizziness, should lessen after several doses.

■ Tell patient that alcohol use, excessive exercise, prolonged standing, and exposure to heat will intensify adverse effects.

■ Advise patient of the reason for taking the drug.

## Representative combinations

None.

# aminoglycosides

**amikacin sulfate, gentamicin sulfate, kanamycin sulfate, neomycin sulfate, paromycin, streptomycin sulfate, tobramycin sulfate**

The basic structure of aminoglycosides is an aminocyclitol nucleus joined with one to two amino sugars by glycosidic linkage.

Aminoglycosides share certain pharmacokinetic properties, such as renal excretion, poor oral absorption, poor CNS penetration, and serious adverse reactions and toxicity; their clinical use may require close monitoring of serum levels.

## Clinical indications and actions

*Infection caused by susceptible organisms*
Aminoglycosides are used as sole therapy for:
■ infections caused by susceptible aerobic gram-negative bacilli, including septicemia; postoperative, pulmonary, intra-abdominal, and serious, recurrent urinary tract infections; and infections of skin, soft tissue, bones, and joints
■ infections from aerobic gram-negative bacillary meningitis (not susceptible to other antibiotics); because of poor CNS penetration, drugs are given intrathecally or intraventricularly (in ventriculitis)
■ kanamycin or paromycin (used orally) and neomycin (used orally or as a retention enema) as adjunct therapy to inhibit ammonia-forming bacteria in the GI tract of patients with hepatic encephalopathy
■ gentamicin encapsulated in liposomes is being evaluated for the treatment of disseminated *Mycobacterium avium* complex infections.

Aminoglycosides are combined with other antibacterials in many other types of infection, including:
■ serious staphylococcal infections (with an antistaphylococcal penicillin)
■ serious *Pseudomonas aeruginosa* infections (with such drugs as an antipseudomonal penicillin or cephalosporin)
■ enterococcal infections, including endocarditis (with such drugs as penicillin G, ampicillin, or vancomycin)
■ as initial empiric therapy in febrile, leukopenic compromised host (with an antipseudomonal penicillin or cephalosporin)
■ serious *Klebsiella* infections (with a cephalosporin)
■ nosocomial pneumonia (with a cephalosporin)
■ anaerobic infections involving *Bacteroides fragilis* (with drugs such as clindamycin, metronidazole, cefoxitin, doxycycline, chloramphenicol, or ticarcillin)

■ tuberculosis (use of parenteral amikacin, kanamycin or streptomycin with other antitubercular drugs)
■ treatment of pelvic inflammatory disease (PID) (gentamicin with clindamycin).

## Pharmacology
Aminoglycosides are bactericidal. Although the exact mechanism of action isn't fully known, the drugs appear to bind directly and irreversibly to 30S ribosomal subunits, inhibiting bacterial protein synthesis. Bacterial resistance to aminoglycosides may be from decreased bacterial cell wall permeability, low affinity of the drug for ribosomal binding sites, or enzymatic degradation by microbial enzymes.

Aminoglycosides are active against many aerobic gram-negative organisms and some aerobic gram-positive organisms. They don't kill fungi, viruses, or anaerobic bacteria.

Gram-negative organisms susceptible to aminoglycosides include *Acinetobacter, Citrobacter, Enterobacter, Escherichia coli, Klebsiella,* indole-positive and indole-negative *Proteus, Providencia, Pseudomonas aeruginosa, Salmonella, Serratia,* and *Shigella.* Streptomycin is active against *Brucella, Calymmatobacterium granulomatis, Francisella tularensis, Haemophilus influenzae, Haemophilus ducreyi, Pasteurella multocida,* and *Yersinia pestis.*

Susceptible aerobic gram-positive organisms include *Staphylococcus aureus* and *S. epidermidis.* Streptomycin is active against *Nocardia, Erysipelothrix, Enterococcus faecalis,* and some mycobacteria, including *Mycobacterium tuberculosis, M. marinum,* and certain strains of *Mycobacterium kansasii* and *M. leprae.*

Paromycin is active against protozoa, especially *Entamoeba histolytica,* and is somewhat effective against *Taenia saginata, Hymenolepsis nana, Diphyllobothrium latum,* and *Taenia solium.* Neomycin and paromycin have some activity against *Acanthamoeba.*

Aminoglycosides aren't systemically absorbed after oral administration in patients with intact GI mucosa and are usually used parenterally for systemic infections. Intraventricular or intrathecal administration is needed for CNS infections. Kanamycin and neomycin are given orally for bowel sterilization.

Aminoglycosides are distributed widely throughout the body after parenteral administration; CSF levels are minimal even in patients with inflamed meninges. Over time, aminoglycosides accumulate in body tissue, especially the kidney and inner ear, causing drug saturation. The drug is released slowly from these tissues. Most aminoglycosides are minimally protein bound and aren't metabolized. They don't penetrate abscesses well.

## AMINOGLYCOSIDES: RENAL FUNCTION AND HALF-LIFE

As the table shows, aminoglycosides, which are excreted by the kidneys, have significantly prolonged half-lives in patients with end-stage renal disease. Knowing this can help you assess the patient's potential for drug accumulation and toxicity. Nephrotoxicity, a major hazard of therapy with aminoglycosides, is linked to serum levels that exceed the therapeutic levels listed below. Therefore, monitoring peak and trough levels is essential for safe use of these drugs.

| Drug and route | Half-life (hr) | | Therapeutic levels (mcg/ml) | |
| | Normal renal function | End-stage renal disease | Peak | Trough |
|---|---|---|---|---|
| amikacin I.M., I.V. | 2-3 | 24-60 | 16-32 | < 10 |
| gentamicin I.M., I.V., topical | 2 | 24-60 | 4-8 | < 2 |
| kanamycin I.M., I.V., topical | 2-3 | 24-60 | 15-40 | < 10 |
| neomycin oral, topical | 2-3 | 12-24 | Not applicable | Not applicable |
| netilmicin I.M., I.V. | 2-2½ | < 10 | 6-10 | < 2 |
| streptomycin I.M., I.V. | 2½ | 100 | 20-30 | Not applicable |
| tobramycin I.M., I.V., topical | 2-2½ | 24-60 | 4-8 | < 2 |

Aminoglycosides are excreted primarily in urine, chiefly by glomerular filtration. Neomycin is chiefly excreted unchanged in feces when taken orally. Elimination half-life ranges between 2 and 4 hours and is prolonged in patients with decreased renal function. (See *Aminoglycosides: Renal function and half-life.*)

### Overview of adverse reactions

*Systemic:* Ototoxicity and nephrotoxicity are the most serious complications of aminoglycoside therapy. Ototoxicity involves both vestibular and auditory functions and is usually related to persistently high serum drug levels. Damage is reversible only if detected early and if drug is discontinued promptly.

Any aminoglycoside may cause usually reversible nephrotoxicity. The damage results in tubular necrosis. Mild proteinuria and casts are early signs of declining renal function, followed several days later by elevated serum creatinine levels. Nephrotoxicity usually begins on day 4 to 7 of therapy and appears to be dose-related.

Neuromuscular blockade results in skeletal weakness and respiratory distress similar to that seen with the use of neuromuscular blockers, such as tubocurarine and succinylcholine.

Oral aminoglycoside therapy often causes nausea, vomiting, and diarrhea. Less common adverse reactions include hypersensitivity reactions (ranging from mild rashes, fever, and eosinophilia to fatal anaphylaxis) and hematologic reactions (hemolytic anemia, transient neutropenia, leukopenia, and thrombocytopenia). Transient elevations of liver function values also occur.

*Local:* Parenterally administered forms of aminoglycosides may cause vein irritation, phlebitis, and sterile abscess.

### Clinical considerations

■ Don't give an aminoglycoside to a patient with hypersensitive reactions to any aminoglycoside.
■ Culture and sensitivity tests should be performed before first dose.
■ Vital signs, electrolyte levels, and renal function test results should be monitored before and during therapy; be sure patient is well hydrated to minimize chemical irritation of renal tubules; advise clinician to watch for signs of declining renal function.
■ Advise clinician to keep peak serum levels and trough serum levels at recommended concentrations, especially in patients with decreased renal function. Blood is drawn for peak level 1 hour after I.M. injection (30 minutes to 1 hour after I.V. infusion); for trough level, sample is drawn just before the next dose. Time and date all blood samples. Don't use he-

parinized tube to collect blood samples; it interferes with results.
- Recommend that patient's hearing be evaluated before and during therapy; advise clinician to monitor for complaints of tinnitus, vertigo, or hearing loss.
- Avoid use of aminoglycosides with other ototoxic or nephrotoxic drugs.
- Usual duration of therapy is 7 to 10 days; if no response occurs in 3 to 5 days, advise clinician to discontinue drug and repeat cultures for reevaluation of therapy.
- Recommend that patients on long-term therapy be closely monitored—especially geriatric and debilitated patients and others receiving immunosuppressant or radiation therapy—for possible bacterial or fungal superinfection; patient should be monitored for fever.
- Don't add or mix other drugs with I.V. infusions, particularly penicillins, which inactivate aminoglycosides; the two groups are chemically and physically incompatible. If other drugs must be given I.V., temporarily stop infusion of primary drug.
- Oral aminoglycosides may be absorbed systemically in patients with ulcerative GI lesions; significant absorption may endanger patients with decreased renal function.

**Oral and parenteral administration**
- Rapid I.V. administration may cause neuromuscular blockade. Infuse I.V. drug continuously or intermittently over 30 to 60 minutes for adults, 1 to 2 hours for infants; dilution volume for children is determined individually.
- Solutions should always be clear, colorless to pale yellow (in most cases, darkening indicates deterioration), and free of particles; don't give solutions containing precipitates or other foreign matter.
- Amikacin, gentamicin (without preservatives), kanamycin, and tobramycin have been given intrathecally or intraventricularly. Some clinicians prefer intraventricular administration to ensure adequate CSF levels in the treatment of ventriculitis.

*Special populations*
**Pregnant patients.** Pregnancy risk category is D; drugs cross the placenta, creating the potential for fetal toxicity and congenital deafness.
**Breast-feeding patients.** Small amounts of drugs appear in breast milk; advise patient to use an alternative feeding method during therapy.
**Pediatric patients.** Half-life of aminoglycosides is prolonged in neonates and premature infants because of immaturity of their renal systems; dosage alterations may be needed.
**Geriatric patients.** Geriatric patients often have decreased renal function and are at greater risk for nephrotoxicity; they often require lower drug dose and longer dosing intervals.

They're also susceptible to ototoxicity and superinfection.

## Patient counseling
- Tell patient signs and symptoms of hypersensitivity and other adverse reactions to aminoglycosides.
- Teach signs and symptoms of bacterial or fungal superinfection to geriatric patients, debilitated patients, and patients with low resistance from immunosuppressants or irradiation; emphasize the need to report these conditions promptly.

## Representative combinations
*Neomycin* with polymyxin B sulfates and bacitracin: Neosporin, Mycitracin, Foille Plus; with polymyxin B sulfates and gramicidin: Neosporin; with polymyxin B sulfates and hydrocortisone: Cortisporin, Drotic, Octicair, Otocort; with dexamethasone sodium phosphate: Neo-Decadron; with flurandrenolide: Cordran SP.

(See also *adrenocorticoids [topical]*, pages 9 to 11.)

---

# androgens

**danazol, fluoxymesterone, methyltestosterone, testosterone, testosterone cypionate, testosterone enanthate, testosterone propionate, testosterone transdermal system**

---

Testosterone is the endogenous androgen, or male sex hormone. The testosterone esters (cypionate, enanthate, propionate), methyltestosterone, and fluoxymesterone are synthetic derivatives with greater potency or longer duration of action than testosterone.

## Clinical indications and actions
*Androgen deficiency*
Androgens (testosterone, all testosterone esters, methyltestosterone, fluoxymesterone) are indicated to treat androgen deficiency from testicular failure or castration, or gonadotropin or luteinizing hormone-releasing hormone deficiency of pituitary origin. Methyltestosterone and testosterone cypionate are also indicated to treat male climacteric symptoms and impotence when these are caused by androgen deficiency.
*Delayed male puberty*
All androgens may be used to stimulate the onset of puberty when it's significantly delayed and psychological support proves insufficient.
*Breast cancer*
Testosterone, all testosterone esters, and fluoxymesterone are indicated for palliative treatment of metastatic breast cancer in women dur-

ing the first 5 postmenopausal years. Androgens also may be used in premenopausal women with metastatic disease if the tumor is hormone-responsive.

*Postpartum breast engorgement*
Fluoxymesterone, testosterone, methyltestosterone, and testosterone propionate are indicated to treat painful postpartum breast engorgement in non–breast-feeding women.

*Hereditary angioedema*
Danazol is indicated in the prophylaxis of angioedema attacks.

*Endometriosis*
Danazol is indicated for palliative treatment of endometriosis. Danazol relieves pain and helps resolve endometrial lesions in 30% to 80% of patients who receive it. Endometriosis usually recurs 8 to 12 months after danazol is discontinued.

*Fibrocystic breast disease*
Danazol is indicated for palliative treatment of fibrocystic breast disease that's unresponsive to simple therapy. It usually relieves pain before it reduces nodularity. Fibrocystic breast disease recurs in about half of patients who have undergone successful treatment with danazol, usually 1 year after discontinuing the drug.

Danazol has been used for palliative treatment of virginal breast hypertrophy, for gynecomastia, and for excessive menstrual blood loss; for contraception in men (with testosterone) and women; for treatment of alpha$_1$-antitrypsin deficiency, systemic lupus erythematosus, gynecomastia in men, and Melkersson-Rosenthal syndrome; and for management of patients with hemophilia A (factor VIII deficiency, classic hemophilia), hemophilia B (factor IX deficiency, Christmas disease), and idiopathic thrombocytopenic purpura (ITP).

## Pharmacology

Testosterone promotes maturation of the male sexual organs and the development of secondary sexual characteristics (facial and body hair and vocal cord thickening). Testosterone also causes the growth spurt of adolescence and terminates growth of the long bones by closing the epiphyses (growth plates at the ends of bones). Testosterone promotes retention of calcium, nitrogen, phosphorus, sodium, and potassium and enhances anabolism (tissue building). Through negative feedback on the pituitary, exogenously administered testosterone (and other androgenic drugs) decreases endogenous testosterone production and to some degree inhibits spermatogenesis in men. Androgens repeatedly stimulate production of erythrocytes by enhancing the production of erythropoietic stimulating factor.

## Overview of adverse reactions

The most common adverse effects caused by androgen therapy are extensions of the hormonal action. In men, frequent and prolonged erections, bladder irritability (causing frequent urination), and gynecomastia (swelling or tenderness of breast tissue) may occur. In women, clitoral enlargement, deepening of the voice, growth of facial or body hair, unusual hair loss, and irregular or absent menses may occur. Virilization, including hirsutism, deepening of voice, or clitoral enlargement may be irreversible even with prompt discontinuation of the drug. Oily skin or acne occurs commonly in both sexes.

Metabolic adverse effects include retention of fluid and electrolytes (occasionally resulting in edema), increased serum calcium levels (hypercalcemia may occur, especially in women receiving the drug for breast cancer metastatic to bone), decreased glucose levels, and increased serum cholesterol levels.

Long-term administration of androgens may cause loss of libido and suppression of spermatogenesis in men. Although rare, serious hepatic dysfunction, including hepatic necrosis and hepatocellular carcinoma, has been reported in prolonged androgen administration.

## Clinical considerations

■ Don't give androgens to men with breast or prostatic cancer or with symptomatic prostatic hypertrophy; to patients with severe cardiac, renal, or hepatic disease; or to patients with undiagnosed abnormal genital bleeding.

■ Hypercalcemia symptoms may be difficult to distinguish from symptoms of the condition being treated unless anticipated and thought of as a cluster. Hypercalcemia is most likely to occur in women with breast cancer, particularly when metastatic to bone.

■ Priapism indicates that dose is excessive.

■ Yellowing of skin or sclera of the eyes may indicate hepatic dysfunction from androgens.

### *Special populations*

**Pregnant patients.** Don't give androgens during pregnancy because they may cause masculinization of a female fetus or other fetal harm.

**Breast-feeding patients.** The degree that androgen appears in breast milk is unknown. Because androgens may induce premature sexual development in boys or virilization in girls, women receiving androgens shouldn't breast-feed.

**Pediatric patients.** Advise clinician to observe children receiving androgens carefully for excessive virilization and precocious puberty. Androgen therapy may cause premature epiphyseal closure and short stature. Regular X-ray examinations of hand bones may be used to monitor skeletal maturation during therapy.

**Geriatric patients.** Elderly men receiving androgens may be at increased risk for prostatic hypertrophy and prostatic carcinoma. Androgens may aggravate prostatic hypertrophy with obstruction and are contraindicated in these cases.

## Patient counseling

- Warn patient against using androgens to improve athletic performance. Androgens are classified as Schedule III controlled substances and their distribution is regulated by the Drug Enforcement Agency.
- Advise patient to report GI upset.
- Tell patient that virilization, including hirsutism, deepening of voice, or clitoral enlargement, may not be reversible.
- Explain that drug may cause menstrual cycle irregularities in premenopausal women and withdrawal bleeding in postmenopausal women.

## Representative combinations

*Fluoxymesterone* with ethinyl estradiol: Halodrin.

*Testosterone cypionate* with estradiol cypionate: De-Comberol, depAndrogyn, Depo-Testadiol, Depotestogen, Duo-Cyp, Duratestin, Menoject-L.A., Test-Estro Cypionate.

*Testosterone enanthate* with estradiol valerate: Andrest 90-4, Andro-Estro 90-4, Androgyn L.A., Duo-Gen L.A., Duogex L.A.*, Neo-Pause*, Teev, Valertest No. 1

# angiotensin-converting enzyme (ACE) inhibitors

**benazepril hydrochloride, captopril, enalapril maleate, fosinopril sodium, lisinopril, moexipril hydrochloride, perindopril erbumine, quinapril hydrochloride, ramipril, trandolapril**

ACE inhibitors are used to manage hypertension, and most are used to treat heart failure. Captopril is indicated for the prevention of diabetic nephropathy, and captopril and lisinopril are useful in improving survival rate in patients after an MI.

## Clinical indications and actions
### Hypertension, heart failure

ACE inhibitors are used to treat hypertension. Their antihypertensive effects are secondary to decreased peripheral resistance and decreased sodium and water retention.

ACE inhibitors are also used to manage heart failure because they decrease systemic vascular resistance (afterload) and pulmonary capillary wedge pressure (preload). After MI, ACE inhibitors are used to decrease mortality rate and to prevent diabetic nephropathy. (See *Comparing doses of angiotensin-converting enzyme inhibitors,* page 18.)

## Pharmacology

ACE inhibitors prevent the conversion of angiotensin I to angiotensin II, a potent vasoconstrictor. Inhibition of angiotensin II decreases vasoconstriction, reducing peripheral arterial resistance, and decreases adrenocortical secretion of aldosterone. This results in decreased sodium and water retention and extracellular fluid volume.

## Overview of adverse reactions

The most common adverse effects of therapeutic doses of ACE inhibitors are headache, fatigue, hypotension, tachycardia, dysgeusia, proteinuria, hyperkalemia, rash, cough, and angioedema of the face and limbs. Severe hypotension may occur at toxic drug levels. ACE inhibitors should be used cautiously in patients with impaired renal function or serious autoimmune disease and in patients taking other drugs known to depress WBC count or immune response.

## Clinical considerations

- Diuretic therapy should be discontinued 2 to 3 days before starting ACE inhibitor therapy to reduce risk of hypotension; if drug doesn't adequately control blood pressure, reinstate diuretics. If diuretics can't be stopped, begin ACE inhibitor at lowest dose.
- Advise clinician to periodically monitor WBC counts.
- Lower doses are needed in patients with impaired renal function.
- Advise patients to use potassium supplements with caution because ACE inhibitors may cause potassium retention.

### Special populations

**Pregnant patients.** Discontinue ACE inhibitors if pregnancy is detected. Drug may harm or cause fetal death during the second or third trimesters.

**Breast-feeding patients.** Captopril and enalapril appear in breast milk. An alternative feeding method is recommended during therapy.

**Pediatric patients.** Safety and efficacy of ACE inhibitors in children haven't been established. Use only if potential benefit outweighs risk.

**Geriatric patients.** Geriatric patients may need lower doses because of impaired drug clearance. These patients may be more sensitive to hypotensive effects.

## Patient counseling

- Tell patient that the drugs may cause a dry, persistent, tickling cough, which is reversible when therapy is discontinued.
- Tell patient to report feelings of lightheadedness, especially in the first few days, so dosage can be adjusted; signs of infection, such as sore throat and fever, because drugs may decrease WBC count; facial swelling or difficulty breathing because drugs may cause an-

---

* Canada only    ◇ Unlabeled clinical use

## COMPARING DOSES OF ANGIOTENSIN-CONVERTING ENZYME INHIBITORS

| Drug | Target adult daily dose | Dosage adjustments |
|------|------------------------|--------------------|
| benazepril | 10-40 mg in single or divided doses | Creatinine clearance < 30 ml/min or on concurrent diuretic: initially, 5 mg per day |
| captopril | 25-150 mg in single or divided doses | Renal impairment, hyponatremia or hypovolemia: 6.25-12.5 mg b.i.d. or t.i.d. |
| enalapril | P.O.: 10-40 mg in single or divided doses I.V.: 1.25 mg (≥ 5 minutes) q 6 hours | Creatinine clearance ≤ 30 ml/min or on concurrent diuretic: initially, 2.5 mg per day |
| fosinopril | 20-40 mg in single or divided doses | Use cautiously if on concurrent diuretic: initially, 10 mg per day |
| lisinopril | 20-40 mg in a single dose | Creatinine clearance ≤ 10-30 ml/min or concurrent diuretic: initially, 5 mg per day Creatinine clearance < 10 ml/min: initially, 2.5 mg per day |
| moexipril | 7.5-30 mg in single or divided doses | Creatinine clearance < 40 ml/min: initially, 3.75 mg per day |
| perindopril | 4-8 mg in single or divided doses | Creatinine clearance of 30-60 ml/min: initially, 2 mg per day |
| quinapril | 20-80 mg in single or divided doses | Creatinine clearance of 30-60 ml/min or on concurrent diuretic: initially, 5 mg per day Creatinine clearance of 10-30 ml/min: initially, 2.5 mg per day |
| ramipril | 2.5-20 mg in single or divided doses | Creatinine clearance < 40 ml/min or serum creatinine > 2.5 mg/dl: initially, 1.25 mg per day |
| trandolapril | 1-4 mg in a single dose | Creatinine clearance < 30 ml/min, on concurrent diuretic, hepatic cirrhosis: initially, 0.5 mg per day |

gioedema; and loss of taste, which may necessitate discontinuation of drug.
▪ Advise patient to avoid sudden position changes to minimize orthostatic hypotension.
▪ Warn patient to seek medical approval before taking OTC cold preparations.
▪ Tell patient to call prescriber if troublesome cough develops.
▪ Instruct patient to promptly report pregnancy.
▪ Tell patient not to take potassium-containing salt substitutes without medical approval.

### Representative combinations
*Captopril* with hydrochlorothiazide: Capozide.
*Benazepril hydrochloride* with amlodipine: Lotrel; with hydrochlorothiazide: Lotensin HCT.
*Enalapril* with hydrochlorothiazide: Vaseretic.
*Lisinopril* with hydrochlorothiazide: Prinzide, Zestoretic.

# angiotensin II receptor antagonists

**candesartan cilexetil, irbesartan, losartan potassium, telmisartan, valsartan**

Angiotensin II receptor antagonists (AIIRAs) are a class of antihypertensive drugs that exert their therapeutic effects by selectively blocking the binding of angiotensin II to the angiotensin II type 1 ($AT_1$) receptor. They're indicated both as monotherapy and combined with other antihypertensives. Compared with ACE inhibitors, AIIRAs cause fewer side effects, such as cough and angioedema.

## Clinical indications and actions
### Hypertension
All AIIRAs are indicated for hypertension, either as monotherapy or with other drugs. AIIRAs act by selectively blocking the binding of angiotensin II to the $AT_1$ receptor, causing vasodilation.

## COMPARING ANGIOTENSIN II RECEPTOR ANTAGONISTS

| Drug | Oral bio-availability (%) | Effect of food | Prodrug | Metabolized by cytochrome P-450 isoenzymes | Protein binding (%) | Half-life (hr) |
|------|------|------|------|------|------|------|
| candesartan | 15 | No effect | Yes | Unknown | >99 | 9 |
| irbesartan | 60-80 | No effect | No | Yes CYP2C9 | 90 | 11-15 |
| losartan | 33 | ↓AUC ~10% | Yes | Yes CYP2C9 and CYP3A4 | ~ 99 | 2 (6-9 for active metabolite) |
| telmisartan | 42-58 | ↓AUC 6%-20% | No | No | >99.5 | 24 |
| valsartan | 25 | ↓AUC ~ 40% | No | Unknown | 95 | 6 |

### Heart failure

Heart failure is related to elevated levels of angiotensin II and aldosterone. ACE inhibitors have been shown to decrease mortality rates in patients with heart failure and to improve quality of life because they inhibit the renin-angiotensin-aldosterone-system (RAAS). Studies are being conducted to determine if AIIRAs will have similar effects as ACE inhibitors on mortality rates in patients with heart failure. Until more information is available, reserve IIRAs for patients unable to tolerate ACE inhibitors.

### Pharmacology

Angiotensin II is a potent vasoconstrictor that's formed from angiotensin I by the enzyme ACE. Angiotensin II causes vasoconstriction, increased aldosterone secretion, cardiac stimulation, and reabsorption of sodium by the kidney. AIIRAs selectively block the binding of angiotensin II to the $AT_1$ receptor. $AT_1$ receptors are found in many tissues throughout the body, including vascular smooth muscle and the adrenal gland. Blockade of $AT_1$ receptors by the AIIRAs results in vasodilation, decreased aldosterone secretion, a 2- to 3-fold increase in plasma renin activity, and an increase in angiotensin II. The increase in renin and angiotensin II results from removal of the negative feedback of angiotensin II and isn't enough to overcome the antihypertensive effects of AIIRAs. Another type of receptor is called the $AT_2$ receptor. The role of the $AT_2$ receptor isn't known, but it doesn't appear to be involved in CV homeostasis. AIIRAs are 1,000- to 20,000-fold more selective for the $AT_1$ than the $AT_2$ receptor. (See Comparing angiotensin II receptor antagonists.)

### Overview of adverse reactions

AIIRAs are well tolerated, with side effects similar to those of placebos. Adverse effects include dizziness, insomnia, headache, fatigue, anxiety, nervousness, diarrhea, dyspepsia, heartburn, nausea, vomiting, arthralgia, back or leg pain, muscle cramps, myalgia, upper respiratory infection, cough, nasal congestion, sinusitis, pharyngitis, rhinitis, influenza, bronchitis, viral infection, edema, chest pain, rash, tachycardia, urinary tract infection, peripheral edema, and albuminuria.

Symptomatic hypotension may occur in patients who are volume- or salt-depleted (such as those taking diuretics). AIIRAs can cause deterioration in renal function, including oliguria, acute renal failure, and progressive azotemia. Decreased hemoglobin and hematocrit, increased serum potassium levels, and occasional increases in liver function test results have occurred in patients receiving valsartan.

### Clinical considerations

- Use extreme caution when giving AIIRAs with potassium supplements or potassium-sparing diuretics.
- Use caution in volume-depleted patients (such as those taking diuretics); advise clinician to correct volume depletion before administration and use a lower starting dose.
- Use caution in patients with hepatic dysfunction; losartan requires dosing adjustment.
- Use with caution in patients whose renal function may be dependent on the RAAS; a worsening of renal function may occur (such as heart failure or renal artery stenosis).
- Telmisartan increases peak digoxin level by 49% and trough by 20%. Advise clinician to monitor digoxin level more frequently.

### Special populations

**Pregnant patients.** AIIRAs are pregnancy risk category C in the first trimester and category D in the second and third trimesters. Drugs that act on the RAAS have been linked to fetal and neonatal injury, and death when intrauterine exposure occurred during the second and third trimesters of pregnancy. Patients taking AI-

IRAs who become pregnant should have the drug discontinued by their prescriber unless use is considered life-saving.

**Breast-feeding patients.** It isn't known if AIIRAs appear in breast milk; because of potential risk to the nursing infant, a decision should be made regarding drug discontinuation.

**Pediatric patients.** The safety and efficacy of AIIRAs haven't been established in patients under age 18.

**Geriatric patients.** No dosing adjustments are required.

## Patient counseling

- Inform women about the risks associated with exposure to AIIRAs during the second and third trimesters of pregnancy; adverse effects on the fetus don't appear to occur when intrauterine exposure is limited to the first trimester.
- Tell patient to report pregnancy to her prescriber as soon as possible.
- Advise patient to continue taking drugs unless a prescriber instructs her to stop.
- Instruct patient to take missed doses as soon as they're remembered unless it's almost time for the next dose.
- Tell patient to call prescriber if signs of allergy or dizziness develop.

## Representative combinations

*Hydrochlorothiazide and losartan:* Hyzaar.

*Hydrochlorothiazide and irbesartan:* Avapro HCT.

*Hydrochlorothiazide and valsartan:* Diovan HCT.

---

# anticholinergics

*Belladonna alkaloids:* **atropine sulfate, hyoscyamine sulfate, scopolamine hydrobromide**

*Synthetic quaternary anticholinergics:* **clidinium bromide, glycopyrrolate, ipratropium bromide, mepenzolate bromide, methoscopalamine bromide, propantheline bromide**

*Tertiary synthetic and semisynthetic (antispasmodic) derivatives:* **dicyclomine hydrochloride, homatropine, oxybutynin chloride, tolterodine tartrate**

*Antiparkinsonian agents:* **benztropine mesylate, biperidenhydrochloride, biperiden lactate, trihexyphenidyl hydrochloride**

Anticholinergics are used to treat various spastic conditions, including acute dystonic reactions, muscle rigidity, parkinsonism, and extrapyramidal disorders. They're also used to reverse neuromuscular blockade, prevent nausea and vomiting from motion sickness, as adjunctive treatment for peptic ulcer disease and other GI disorders, and preoperatively to decrease secretions and block cardiac reflexes. Belladonna alkaloids are naturally occurring anticholinergics that have been used for centuries. Many semisynthetic alkaloids and synthetic anticholinergic compounds are available; however, most offer few advantages over naturally occurring alkaloids. (See *Comparing systemic anticholinergics.*)

## Clinical indications and actions
### Hypersecretory conditions

Many anticholinergics, such as atropine, belladonna leaf, glycopyrrolate, hyoscyamine, levorotatory alkaloids of belladonna, and mepenzolate, are used therapeutically for their antisecretory properties. These properties derive from competitive blockade of cholinergic receptor sites, causing decreased gastric acid secretion, salivation, bronchial secretions, and sweating.

### GI tract disorders

Some anticholinergics, such as atropine, belladonna leaf, glycopyrrolate, hyoscyamine, levorotatory alkaloids of belladonna, mepenzolate, and propantheline, as well as the antispasmodics such as dicyclomine, are used to treat spasms and other GI tract disorders. These drugs competitively block the actions of acetylcholine at cholinergic receptor sites. Antispasmodics presumably act by a nonspecific, direct spasmolytic action on smooth muscle. These drugs are useful in treating pylorospasm, ileitis, and irritable bowel syndrome. Transdermal scopolamine is used to prevent nausea and vomiting caused by anesthesia and surgery. Atropine may be useful in treating nausea and vomiting caused by morphine used in treatment of an MI.

### Sinus bradycardia

Atropine is used to treat sinus bradycardia caused by drugs, poisons, or sinus node dysfunction. It blocks normal vagal inhibition of the SA node and causes an increase in heart rate. Atropine may be used for the treatment of sustained bradycardia and hypotension caused by nitroglycerin used in treatment of an MI.

### Dystonia and parkinsonism

Biperiden, benztropine, and trihexyphenidyl hydrochloride are used to treat acute dystonic reactions and drug-induced extrapyramidal adverse effects. They act centrally by blocking cholinergic receptor sites, balancing cholinergic activity with dopamine.

## COMPARING SYSTEMIC ANTICHOLINERGICS

| Drug | Plasma half-life (hr) | Onset of action | Duration of action |
|---|---|---|---|
| atropine, oral | 2½ | Inhibition of saliva occurs in 30-60 min | 4-6 hr |
| atropine, parenteral | 2½ | Peak increase in heart rate occurs after 2-4 min | Brief |
| benztropine | Unknown | P.O.: 1-2 hr I.V., I.M.: 15 min | 24 hr |
| clidinium | Biphasic with initial half-life of 2½ and terminal half-life of 20 | 1 hr | 3 hr |
| dicyclomine | 9-10 | Unknown | Unknown |
| glycopyrrolate | ½-4½ I.V. 15-30 min I.M. | 1 min I.V. | 2-7 hr |
| homatropine | Unknown | 40-60 min | 1-3 days |
| hyoscyamine, oral | 3½ | 20-30 min | 4-6 hr |
| hyoscyamine, parenteral | 3½ | 2-3 min | 4-6 hr |
| mepenzolate | Unknown | Unknown | Unknown |
| methoscopolamine | Unknown | 1 hr | 6-8 hr |
| oxybutynin | Unknown | 30-60 min | 6-10 hr |
| propantheline | 1½ | 1½ hr | 6 hr |
| scopolamine, oral | 1 hr | 4-6 hr | |
| scopolamine, parenteral | 30 min | 4 hr | |
| tolterodine | Unknown | 1 hr | 5 hr |
| trihexyphenidyl | Unknown | Within 1 hr | 6-12 hr |

### Perioperative use

Atropine, glycopyrrolate, and hyoscyamine are used postoperatively with anticholinesterase agents to reverse nondepolarizing neuromuscular blockade. These drugs block muscarinic effects of anticholinesterase agents by competitively blocking muscarinic receptor sites.

Atropine, glycopyrrolate, and scopolamine are used preoperatively to decrease secretions and block cardiac vagal reflexes. They diminish secretions by competitively inhibiting muscarinic receptor sites; they block cardiac vagal reflexes by preventing normal vagal inhibition of the SA node.

### Bronchospasm

Atropine and ipratropium are potent bronchodilators and are used to treat antigen-, methacholine-, histamine-, or exercise-induced bronchospasm (oral inhalation and I.M. atropine); oral inhalation of atropine or ipratropium is effective in the treatment of chronic bronchitis and asthma; oral inhalation of atropine sulfate has been used for the short-term treatment and prevention of bronchospasm caused by chronic bronchial asthma, bronchitis, and chronic obstructive pulmonary disease.

### Genitourinary tract disorders

Atropine, oxybutynin, tolterodine, and propantheline have been used to treat reflex neurogenic bladder.

### Poisoning

Atropine is used to reverse the cholinergic effects of toxic exposure to organophosphate, carbamate anticholinesterase pesticides, and ingestion of cholinomimetic plants and fungi.

### Motion sickness

Scopolamine is effective in preventing nausea and vomiting from motion sickness. Its exact mechanism of action is unknown, but it's thought to affect neural pathways originating in the labyrinth of the ear.

## Pharmacology

Anticholinergics competitively antagonize the actions of acetylcholine and other cholinergics at muscarinic and nicotinic receptors within the parasympathetic nervous system and smooth muscles that lack cholinergic innervation. Lack of specificity for site of action increases the hazard of adverse effects in association with therapeutic effects.

Antispasmodics are structurally similar to anticholinergics; however, their anticholinergic activity usually occurs only at high doses. Their mechanism of action is unknown, but they're believed to directly relax smooth muscle.

## Overview of adverse reactions

Dry mouth, decreased sweating or anhidrosis, headache, mydriasis, blurred vision, cycloplegia, xerophthalmia, dry skin, urinary hesitancy and retention, constipation, palpitations, and tachycardia most commonly occur with therapeutic doses of anticholinergics and usually disappear once the drug is discontinued. Signs of drug toxicity include CNS signs resembling psychosis (disorientation, confusion, hallucinations, delusions, anxiety, agitation, and restlessness) and peripheral effects such as dilated, nonreactive pupils; blurred vision; hot, dry, flushed skin; dry mucous membranes; dysphagia; stupor; seizures; decreased or absent bowel sounds; urine retention; hyperthermia; tachycardia; hypertension; and increased respiration.

## Clinical considerations

■ Patient's vital signs, urine output, visual changes, and signs of impending toxicity should be monitored.
■ Constipation may be relieved by stool softeners or bulk laxatives.

### Special populations

**Pregnant patients.** The safety of anticholinergic therapy during pregnancy hasn't been determined. Use by pregnant women is indicated only when the benefits of drug outweigh potential risks to the fetus.
**Breast-feeding patients.** Some anticholinergics may appear in breast milk, possibly resulting in infant toxicity; breast-feeding women should avoid these drugs. Anticholinergics may decrease milk production.
**Pediatric patients.** Safety and efficacy haven't been established.
**Geriatric patients.** Give cautiously. Lower doses are usually indicated. Patients over age 40 may be more sensitive to the effects of these drugs.

## Patient counseling

■ Teach patient how and when to take drug.
■ Warn patient to avoid driving and other hazardous tasks if he experiences dizziness, drowsiness, or blurred vision.
■ Advise patient to avoid alcoholic beverages, because they may cause additive CNS effects.
■ Advise patient to consume plenty of fluids and dietary fiber to help avoid constipation.
■ Tell patient to promptly report dry mouth, blurred vision, rash, eye pain, or significant changes in urine volume, or pain or difficulty during urination.
■ Warn patient that drug may cause increased sensitivity or intolerance to high temperatures, resulting in dizziness.
■ Instruct patient to report confusion and rapid or pounding heartbeat.
■ Advise women to report pregnancy or intent to conceive.
■ Warn patient to avoid OTC drugs such as Benadryl or Nytol, which also have anticholinergic activity.

## Representative combinations

*Atropine* with meperidine: Atropine/Demerol injection; with scopolamine hydrobromide (hyoscine hydrobromide), hyoscyamine sulfate, and phenobarbital: Antispasmodic Elixir, Donnatal No. 2, Phenobarbital with Belladonna Alkaloids Elixir, Bellalphen, Donnatal, Haponal, Kinesed, Spasmolin; with scopolamine hydrobromide (hyoscine hydrobromide), hyoscyamine sulfate, kaolin, pectin, sodium benzoate, alcohol, and powdered opium: Donnagel-PG; with phenazopyridine, hyoscyamine, and scopolamine: Urogesic; with hyoscyamine, methenamine, phenyl salicylate, methylene blue, and benzoic acid: Urised; with scopolamine hydrobromide, hyoscyamine hydrobromide, and phenobarbital: Barbidonna No. 2 Tablets, Barbidonna Tablets, Belladonna Alkaloids with Phenobarbital Tablets, Barophen, Donnamor, Donnapine, Donnatal Extentabs, Hyosophen Tablets, Malatal Tablets, Spasmophen, Spasquid, Susano.

*Belladonna alkaloids* with ergotamine tartrate, caffeine, and phenacetin: Wigraine; with phenobarbital: Chardonna-2, Butibel Elixir; with powdered opium: B&O Supprettes No. 15A, B&O Supprettes No. 16A.

*Belladonna* extract with butabarbital: Butibel.

*Hyoscyamine sulfate* with phenobarbital: Levsin with Phenobarbital Tablets, Levsin-PB, Bellacane Tablets.

---

# antihistamines

**azelastine hydrochloride, brompheniramine maleate, cetirizine hydrochloride, chlorpheniramine maleate, clemastine fumarate, cyclizine hydrochloride, cyclizine lactate, cyproheptadine hydrochloride, dimenhydrinate, diphenhydramine hydrochloride, fexofenadine hydrochloride, loratadine, meclizine hydrochloride, promethazine hydrochloride, tripelennamine hydrochloride, triprolidine hydrochloride**

Antihistamines—synthetically produced $H_1$-receptor antagonists—have many applications related specifically to their chemical structure. Their widespread use testifies to their versatility and relative safety. Some antihistamines are used primarily to treat rhinitis or pruritus, whereas others are used more for their antiemetic and antivertigo effects; still others are used as sedative-hypnotics, local anesthetics, and antitussives.

## Clinical indications and actions

### Allergy
Most antihistamines (azelastine, brompheniramine, chlorpheniramine, clemastine, cyproheptadine, diphenhydramine, promethazine, and triprolidine) are used to treat allergic symptoms, such as rhinitis and urticaria. By preventing access of histamine to $H_1$-receptor sites, they suppress histamine-induced allergic symptoms.

### Pruritus
Cyproheptadine and hydroxyzine are used systemically. It is believed that these drugs counteract histamine-induced pruritus by a combination of peripheral effects on nerve endings and local anesthetic and sedative activity.

Tripelennamine and diphenhydramine are used topically to relieve itching from minor skin irritation. Structurally related to local anesthetics, these compounds prevent initiation and transmission of nerve impulses.

### Vertigo, nausea, and vomiting
Cyclizine, dimenhydrinate, and meclizine are used only as antiemetic and antivertigo drugs. Their antihistaminic activity is unknown. Diphenhydramine and promethazine are used as antiallergic and antivertigo drugs and as antiemetics and antinauseants. Although the mechanisms aren't fully understood, antiemetic and antivertigo effects probably result from central antimuscarinic activity.

### Sedation
Diphenhydramine and promethazine are used for their sedative action; the mechanism of antihistamine-induced CNS depression is unknown.

### Suppression of cough
Diphenhydramine syrup is used as an antitussive. The cough reflex is suppressed by a direct effect on the medullary cough center.

### Dyskinesia
The central antimuscarinic action of diphenhydramine reduces drug-induced dyskinesias and parkinsonism by inhibiting acetylcholine (anticholinergic effect).

## Pharmacology
Antihistamines are structurally related chemicals that compete with histamine for $H_1$-receptor sites on the smooth muscle of the bronchi, GI tract, uterus, and large blood vessels, binding to the cellular receptors and pre

venting access and subsequent activity of histamine. They don't directly alter histamine or prevent its release. Also, antihistamines antagonize the action of histamine that causes increased capillary permeability and resultant edema and suppress flare and pruritus caused by the endogenous release of histamine.

## Overview of adverse reactions
At therapeutic dosage levels, all antihistamines except astemizole and loratadine are likely to cause drowsiness and impaired motor function during initial therapy. Also, their anticholinergic action usually causes dry mouth and throat, blurred vision, and constipation. Antihistamines that are also phenothiazines, such as promethazine, may cause other adverse effects, including cholestatic jaundice (thought to be a hypersensitivity reaction), and may predispose patients to photosensitivity; patients taking such drugs should avoid prolonged exposure to sunlight. Adverse GI effects of hepatic failure and hepatic function abnormality have been reported.

Toxic doses elicit a combination of CNS depression and excitation as well as atropine-like symptoms, including sedation, reduced mental alertness, apnea, CV collapse, hallucinations, tremors, seizures, dry mouth, flushed skin, and fixed, dilated pupils. Toxic effects reverse when drug is discontinued. Used appropriately, in correct doses, antihistamines are safe for prolonged use.

## Clinical considerations
■ Do not use antihistamines during an acute asthma attack because they may not alleviate the symptoms, and antimuscarinic effects can cause thickening of secretions.
■ Use antihistamines with caution in geriatric patients and in those with increased intraocular pressure, hyperthyroidism, CV or renal disease, diabetes, hypertension, bronchial asthma, urine retention, prostatic hypertrophy, bladder neck obstruction, or stenosing peptic ulcers.
■ Blood counts should be monitored during long-term therapy; advise clinician to watch for signs of blood dyscrasias.
■ Antihistamines should be given with food to reduce GI distress; recommend sugarless gum, sour hard candy, or ice chips to relieve dry mouth; recommend increasing fluid intake (if allowed) or humidifying air to decrease adverse effect of thickened secretions.
■ If tolerance develops to one antihistamine, another may be substituted.
■ Some antihistamines may mask ototoxicity from high doses of aspirin and other salicylates.

### Special populations

**Pregnant patients.** Safe use of antihistamines during pregnancy hasn't been established. Some manufacturers recommend that drugs not be used during the third trimester of pregnancy because of the risk of severe reactions, such as seizures, in neonates and premature infants.

**Breast-feeding patients.** Antihistamines shouldn't be used during breast-feeding.

**Pediatric patients.** Children, especially those under age 6, may experience paradoxical hyperexcitability with restlessness, insomnia, nervousness, euphoria, tremors, and seizures.

**Geriatric patients.** Geriatric patients are usually more sensitive to adverse effects of antihistamines and are especially likely to experience a greater degree of dizziness, sedation, hypotension, and urine retention.

### Patient counseling

▪ Advise patient to take drug with meals or snacks to prevent gastric upset and to use any of the following measures to relieve dry mouth: warm water rinses, artificial saliva, ice chips, or sugarless gum or candy. The patient should avoid overusing mouthwash, which may add to dryness (alcohol content) and destroy normal flora.

▪ Warn patient to avoid hazardous activities, such as driving a car or operating machinery, until extent of CNS effects are known and to seek medical approval before using alcoholic beverages, tranquilizers, sedatives, pain relievers, or sleeping aids.

▪ Warn patient to stop taking antihistamines 4 days before diagnostic skin tests to preserve accuracy of tests.

### Representative combinations

*Carbinoxamine maleate* with pseudoephedrine and dextromethorphan: Carbodec DM, Pseudo-Car DM, Rondec-DM, Tussafed; with pseudoephedrine hydrochloride: Rondec, Rondec-TR; with pseudoephedrine and guaifenesin: Brexin L.A.

*Chlorpheniramine* with phenylephrine and phenylpropanolamine: Naldecon; with dextromethorphan: Vicks Formula 44 Cough Mixture; with codeine and guaifenesin: Tussar SF; with acetaminophen: Coricidin Tablets; with pseudoephedrine and dextromethorphan: Rhinosyn-DM; with pseudoephedrine, dextromethorphan, and acetaminophen: Co-Apap; with phenylpropanolamine: Contac 12-hour, Ornade, Resaid S.R., Triaminic-12, Dura-Vent; with pseudoephedrine hydrochloride: Cophene No. 2, Rescon Capsules, Chlordrine S.R., Chlorphendrine SR, Colfed-A, Duralex, Klerist-D, Kronofed-A, N-D Clear, Pseudo-Clor, Rescon-ED, Time-Hist, Chlorpheniramine Maleate/Pseudoephedrine HCl.

*Diphenhydramine* with pseudoephedrine: Benadryl Decongestant, Benylin DM; with acetaminophen: Tylenol Severe Allergy.

*Promethazine* with codeine: Phenergan with codeine; with dextromethorphan: Phenergan with Dextromethorphan; with phenylephrine: Phenergan VC; with phenylephrine and codeine: Phenergan VC with codeine.

*Pyrilamine maleate* with codeine: Tricodene Cough and Cold; with phenylephrine and codeine: Codimal; with phenylephrine and dextromethorphan: Codimal DM; with phenylephrine, dextromethorphan, and acetaminophen: Robitussin Night Relief; with phenylephrine and hydrocodone: Codimal; with phenylpropanolamine, chlorpheniramine maleate, and dextromethorphan: Tricodene Forte, Tricodene NN, Triminol Cough.

*Triprolidine* with pseudoephedrine and codeine: Actifed with Codeine, CoActifed*, Pseudodine C Cough; with pseudoephedrine: Actagen, Actifed, Allerfrin, Novafed, Triacin-C, Triafed with Codeine, Trifed-C, Trifed-C Cough, Triofed, Triposed.

# barbiturates

**amobarbital, amobarbital sodium, aprobarbital, butabarbital sodium, mephobarbital, metharbital, phenobarbital, pentobarbital sodium, phenobarbital sodium, primidone, secobarbital sodium**

Although barbiturates have been used extensively as sedative-hypnotics and antianxiety drugs, benzodiazepines are the current drugs of choice for sedative-hypnotic effects. Phenobarbital, mephobarbital, and metharbital remain effective for anticonvulsant therapy. A few short-acting barbiturates are used as general anesthetics.

## Clinical indications and actions

### Seizure disorders

Phenobarbital is used in the prophylactic treatment and acute management of seizure disorders. It's used mainly in tonic-clonic (grand mal) and partial seizures. At anesthetic doses, all barbiturates have anticonvulsant activity. Phenobarbital is an effective parenteral drug for status epilepticus (with airway support). Mephobarbital and metharbital may also be used.

Barbiturates suppress the spread of seizure activity produced by epileptogenic foci in the cortex, thalamus, and limbic systems by enhancing the effects of gamma-aminobutyric acid (GABA).

### Sedation, hypnosis

Most currently available barbiturates are used as sedative-hypnotics for short-term (up to 2 weeks) treatment of insomnia because of their nonspecific CNS effects.

Barbiturates aren't used routinely as sedatives. Barbiturate-induced sleep differs from physiologic sleep in that rapid-eye-movement sleep cycles are reduced.

### Preanesthesia sedation
Barbiturates are also used as preanesthetic sedatives and for relief of anxiety.

### Psychiatric use
Barbiturates (especially amobarbital) have been used parenterally in narcoanalysis and narcotherapy and in identifying schizophrenia.

## Pharmacology
Barbiturates are structurally related compounds that act throughout the CNS, particularly in the mesencephalic reticular activating system, which controls the CNS arousal mechanism. Barbiturates induce an imbalance in central inhibitory and facilitatory mechanisms, which, in turn, influence the cerebral cortex and the reticular formation. Barbiturates decrease both presynaptic and postsynaptic membrane excitability.

The exact mechanisms of action of barbiturates at these sites aren't known, nor is it clear which cellular and synaptic actions result in sedative-hypnotic effects. Barbiturates can produce all levels of CNS depression, from mild sedation to coma to death. Barbiturates exert their effects by facilitating the actions of GABA. Barbiturates also exert a central effect, which depresses respiration and GI motility. Barbiturates have no analgesic action and may increase the reaction to painful stimuli at subanesthetic doses. The principal anticonvulsant mechanism of action is reduction of nerve transmission and decreased excitability of the nerve cell. Barbiturates also raise the seizure threshold.

## Overview of adverse reactions
Drowsiness, lethargy, vertigo, headache, and CNS depression are common with barbiturates. After hypnotic doses, a hangover effect, subtle distortion of mood, and impairment of judgment or motor skills may continue for many hours. After a decrease in dose or discontinuation of barbiturates used for hypnosis, rebound insomnia or increased dreaming or nightmares may occur. Barbiturates cause hyperalgesia in subhypnotic doses. Hypersensitivity reactions (rash, fever, serum sickness) aren't common and are more likely to occur in patients with a history of asthma or allergies to other drugs; reactions include urticaria, rash, angioedema, and Stevens-Johnson syndrome. Barbiturates can cause paradoxical excitement at low doses, confusion in geriatric patients, and hyperactivity in children. High fever, severe headache, stomatitis, conjunctivitis, or rhinitis may precede skin eruptions. Because of the potential for fatal consequences, discontinue barbiturates if dermatologic reactions occur.

Withdrawal symptoms may occur after as little as 2 weeks of uninterrupted therapy. Symptoms of abstinence usually occur within 8 to 12 hours after the last dose, but may be delayed up to 5 days. They include weakness, anxiety, nausea, vomiting, insomnia, hallucinations, and possibly seizures.

## Clinical considerations
■ Doses of barbiturates must be individualized.

■ Don't use barbiturates in patients with porphyria, liver impairment, severe respiratory disease, or previous addiction to barbiturates or in nephritic patients.

■ Use barbiturates cautiously, if at all, in patients who are mentally depressed or have suicidal tendencies or history of drug abuse.

■ Avoid giving barbiturates to patients with status asthmaticus.

■ Parenteral solutions are highly alkaline and contain organic solvents (propylene glycol); infuse at 100 mg/min or less; avoid extravasation, which may cause local tissue damage and tissue necrosis; inject I.V. or deep I.M. only. Don't exceed 5 ml per I.M. injection site to avoid tissue damage.

■ Rapid I.V. administration of barbiturates may cause respiratory depression, apnea, laryngospasm, or hypotension. Resuscitative measures should be available. I.V. site should be assessed for signs of infiltration or phlebitis.

■ Drug may be given P.R. if oral or parenteral route is inappropriate; it shouldn't be given intra-arterially or S.C.

■ Advise clinician to assess level of consciousness before and frequently during therapy to evaluate effectiveness of drug. Advise clinician to monitor neurologic status for possible alterations or deteriorations and monitor seizure character, frequency, and duration for changes.

■ Vital signs must be checked frequently, especially during I.V. administration.

■ Patient's sleeping patterns should be assessed before and during therapy to ensure effectiveness of drug.

■ Recommend safety measures—side rails, assistance when out of bed, call light within reach—to prevent falls and injury.

■ Airway support should be considered during I.V. administration.

■ Anticipate possible rebound confusion and excitatory reactions in patient.

■ Patient should be monitored for complaints of constipation. Recommend diet high in fiber, if indicated.

■ Advise clinician to carefully monitor PT and INR in patients taking anticoagulants; dose of anticoagulant may require adjustment to counteract possible interaction.

■ Abrupt discontinuation may cause withdrawal symptoms; discontinue slowly.

■ Death is common with an overdose of 2 to 10 g; it may occur at much smaller doses if alcohol is also ingested.

■ Explain that a morning hangover is common after therapeutic use of barbiturates.

### Special populations

**Pregnant patients.** Barbiturates may cause fetal harm. Postpartum hemorrhage and hemorrhagic disease of the newborn have occurred. The latter can be reversed with vitamin K therapy. If a woman is taking these drugs in the last trimester of pregnancy, neonates may exhibit withdrawal symptoms.

**Breast-feeding patients.** Barbiturates appear in breast milk and may result in infant CNS depression. Use with caution.

**Pediatric patients.** Premature infants are more susceptible to the depressant effects of barbiturates because of immature hepatic metabolism. Children receiving barbiturates may experience hyperactivity, excitement, or hyperalgia.

**Geriatric patients.** Geriatric patients and patients receiving subhypnotic doses may experience hyperactivity, excitement, confusion, depression, or hyperalgesia. Use with caution.

### Patient counseling

■ Warn patient to avoid use of other drugs with CNS depressant effects, such as antihistamines, analgesics, and alcohol, because they have additive effects and result in increased drowsiness. Instruct patient to seek prescriber approval before taking OTC cold or allergy preparations.

■ Caution patient not to change dose or frequency without medical approval; abrupt discontinuation of drug may trigger rebound insomnia, with increased dreaming, nightmares, or seizures.

■ Warn patient against driving and other hazardous tasks that require alertness while taking barbiturates. Instruct him in safety measures to prevent injury.

■ Be sure women understand that barbiturates are capable of causing physical or psychological dependence (addiction), and that these effects may be transmitted to a fetus; withdrawal symptoms can occur in neonates whose mothers took barbiturates in the third trimester.

■ Instruct patient to report skin eruption or other marked adverse effect.

### Representative combinations

*Amobarbital* with secobarbital: Tuinal 100 mg Pulvules, Tuinal 200 mg Pulvules.

*Butabarbital* with acetaminophen: Sedapap; with belladonna: Butibel.

*Phenobarbital* with CNS stimulants: Bronkolixir, Bronkotabs, Quadrinal; with ergotamine tartrate: Bellergal-S; with phenytoin: Dilantin Kapseals; with aminophylline and ephedrine hydrochloride: Mudrane; with belladonna: Chardonna-2, Butibel, Butibel Elixir;

with atropine: Antrocol; with hyoscyamine: Levsin-PB, Levsin and Phenobarbital, Bellacane; with acetylsalicylic acid and codeine phosphate: Phenaphen with Codeine No. 3, Phenaphen with Codeine No. 4; with atropine, hyoscyamine, and scopolamine hydrobromide: Donnatal, Donnatol No. 2, Donnamor, Donnapine, Donnatal Extentabs, Barbidonna, Barophen, Hyosophen, Kinesed, Spasmophen, Spasquid, Susano, Barbidonna No. 2, Belladonna Alkaloids with Phenobarbital Tablets, Malatal, Antispasmodic Elixir, Hyoscyamine Compound, Phenobarbital with Belladonna Alkaloids Elixir.

*Pentobarbital sodium* with ephedrine: Ephedrine and Nembutal Sodium; with ergotamine tartrate and caffeine: Cafergot-PB.

(See also *anticholinergics [belladonna alkaloids]*, page 20.)

# benzodiazepines

**alprazolam, chlordiazepoxide hydrochloride, clonazepam, clorazepate dipotassium, diazepam, estazolam, flurazepam hydrochloride, lorazepam, midazolam hydrochloride, oxazepam, quazepam, temazepam, triazolam**

Benzodiazepines—synthetically produced sedative-hypnotics—are the treatment of choice for anxiety, convulsive disorders, and sedation. These drugs are preferred over barbiturates because therapeutic doses produce less drowsiness, respiratory depression, and impairment of motor function, and toxic doses are less likely to be fatal.

### Clinical indications and actions

#### Seizure disorders

Four of the benzodiazepines (diazepam, clonazepam, clorazepate, and parenteral lorazepam) are used as anticonvulsants. Their anticonvulsant properties are derived from an ability to suppress the spread of seizure activity produced by epileptogenic foci in the cortex, thalamus, and limbic systems by enhancing presynaptic inhibition. Clonazepam is useful in the adjunctive treatment of petit mal variant (Lennox-Gastaut syndrome), myoclonic, or akinetic seizures. Benzodiazepines are also useful adjuncts for the prophylactic management of partial seizures with elementary symptoms (jacksonian seizures), psychomotor seizures, and petit mal seizures. Parenteral diazepam is indicated to treat status epilepticus.

#### Anxiety, tension, and insomnia

Most benzodiazepines (alprazolam, chlordiazepoxide, clorazepate, diazepam, estazolam, flurazepam, lorazepam, oxazepam, quazepam, temazepam, and triazolam) are useful as antianxiety drugs or sedative-hypnotic drugs. They have a similar mechanism of action; they're believed to facilitate the effects of gamma-aminobutyric acid (GABA) in the ascending reticular activating system, increasing inhibition and blocking both cortical and limbic arousal.

They're used to treat anxiety and tension that occur alone or as an adverse effect of a primary disorder. They aren't recommended for tension associated with everyday stress. The choice of a specific benzodiazepine depends on individual metabolic characteristics of the drug. For instance, in patients with depressed renal or hepatic function, alprazolam, lorazepam, or oxazepam may be selected because they have a relatively short duration of action and have no active metabolites.

The sedative-hypnotic properties of chlordiazepoxide, clorazepate, diazepam, lorazepam, and oxazepam make these the drugs of choice as preoperative drug and as an adjunct in the rehabilitation of alcoholics.

### Surgical adjuncts for conscious sedation or amnesia

Diazepam, midazolam, and lorazepam have amnesic effects. The mechanism of such action isn't known. Parenteral administration before such procedures as endoscopy or elective cardioversion causes impairment of recent memory and interferes with the establishment of memory trace, producing anterograde amnesia.

### Skeletal muscle spasm, tremor

Because oral forms of diazepam and chlordiazepoxide have skeletal muscle relaxant properties, they're often used to treat neurologic conditions involving muscle spasms and tetanus. The mechanism of such action is unknown, but they're believed to inhibit spinal polysynaptic and monosynaptic afferent pathways.

### Delirium

Benzodiazepines may be beneficial alone or with antipsychotic drugs to treat delirium. However, caution should be used because benzodiazepines can also exacerbate delirium.

### ◇ Schizophrenia

Benzodiazepines have been used as an adjunct to antipsychotic drugs in the management of schizophrenia.

### ◇ Cancer chemotherapy-induced nausea and vomiting

Benzodiazepines have been used as an adjunct to control nausea and vomiting caused by emetogenic cancer chemotherapy.

### ◇ Neonatal opiate withdrawal

Parenteral diazepam has been used to relieve agitation caused by neonatal opiate withdrawal.

### ◇ Drug-induced CV emergencies

Benzodiazepines are used as adjuncts in the treatment of certain drug-induced CV emergencies, such as hemodynamically significant

tachycardia, acute coronary syndrome, and hypertensive emergency.

## Pharmacology

Benzodiazepines are a group of structurally related chemicals that selectively act on polysynaptic neuronal pathways throughout the CNS. Their precise sites and mechanisms of action aren't completely known. However, the benzodiazepines enhance or facilitate the action of GABA, an inhibitory neurotransmitter in the CNS. The drugs appear to act at the limbic, thalamic, and hypothalamic levels of the CNS. These drugs produce anxiolytic, sedative, hypnotic, skeletal muscle relaxant, and anticonvulsant effects. All of the benzodiazepines have CNS-depressant activities; however, individual derivatives act more selectively at specific sites, allowing them to be subclassified into five categories based on their predominant clinical use.

## Overview of adverse reactions

Therapeutic dosage of the benzodiazepines usually causes drowsiness and impaired motor function, which should be monitored early in treatment. It may be persistent. GI discomfort, such as constipation, diarrhea, vomiting, and changes in appetite, with urinary alterations, have also been reported. Visual disturbances and CV irregularities are also common. Continuing problems with short-term memory, confusion, severe depression, shakiness, vertigo, slurred speech, staggering, bradycardia, shortness of breath or difficulty breathing, and severe weakness usually indicate a toxic dose level. Prolonged or frequent use of benzodiazepines can cause physical dependency and withdrawal syndrome when drug use is discontinued.

## Clinical considerations

■ Benzodiazepines shouldn't be used in patients with chronic pulmonary insufficiency, sleep apnea, depressive neuroses or psychotic reactions without predominant anxiety, or acute alcohol intoxication.

■ Advise clinician to assess level of consciousness and neurologic status before and frequently during therapy for changes. Patient should be monitored for paradoxical reactions, especially early in therapy.

■ Advise clinician to observe sleep patterns and quality, and for changes in seizure character, frequency, or duration.

■ Advise clinician to assess vital signs frequently during therapy. Significant changes in blood pressure and heart rate may indicate impending toxicity.

■ Advise clinician to give dose with milk or immediately after meals to prevent GI upset. An antacid may be given, if needed, at least 1 hour before or after dose to prevent interaction and ensure maximum drug absorption and effectiveness.

■ Advise clinician to periodically monitor renal and hepatic function to ensure adequate drug removal and prevent cumulative effects.

■ Recommend that safety measures be instituted—raised side rails and ambulatory assistance—to prevent injury. Anticipate possible rebound excitement reactions.

■ After prolonged use, abrupt discontinuation may cause withdrawal symptoms; recommend stopping gradually.

### Special populations

**Pregnant patients.** Benzodiazepines may cause fetal harm if given during pregnancy. There's an increased risk of congenital malformation if given during the first trimester. Use of benzodiazepines during labor may cause neonatal flaccidity. Use should be determined if benefits outweigh risks.

**Breast-feeding patients.** The breast-fed infant of a mother who uses a benzodiazepine drug may show sedation, feeding difficulties, and weight loss. Safe use hasn't been established.

**Pediatric patients.** Because children, particularly very young ones, are sensitive to the CNS-depressant effects of benzodiazepines, use caution. A neonate whose mother took a benzodiazepine during pregnancy may exhibit withdrawal symptoms.

**Geriatric patients.** Geriatric patients receiving benzodiazepines require lower doses because they're sensitive to CNS effects; use with caution.

Parenteral administration of these drugs is more likely to cause apnea, hypotension, bradycardia, and cardiac arrest.

Geriatric patients may show prolonged elimination of benzodiazepines, except possibly of oxazepam, lorazepam, temazepam, and triazolam.

### Patient counseling

■ Warn patient to avoid alcohol or other CNS depressants, such as antihistamines, analgesics, MAO inhibitors, antidepressants, and barbiturates, to prevent additive depressant effects.

■ Caution patient to take drug as prescribed and not to give drug to others. Tell him not to change the dose or frequency and to call before taking OTC cold or allergy preparations that may potentiate CNS depressant effects.

■ Warn patient to avoid activities requiring alertness and good psychomotor coordination until the CNS response to the drug is determined. Instruct him in safety measures to prevent injury.

■ Tell patient to avoid using antacids, which may delay drug absorption, unless prescribed.

■ Be sure patient understands that benzodiazepines are capable of causing physical and psychological dependence with prolonged use.

■ Warn patient not to stop taking the drug abruptly to prevent withdrawal symptoms after prolonged therapy.

■ Tell patient that smoking decreases the effectiveness of the drug. Encourage patient to stop smoking during therapy.

■ Tell patient to report adverse effects. These are often dose-related and can be relieved by dosage adjustments.

■ Advise a woman of child-bearing age who is taking drug to inform prescriber if she suspects pregnancy or intends to become pregnant during therapy.

### Representative combinations

*Chlordiazepoxide* with amitriptyline hydrochloride: Limbitrol DS; with clidinium bromide: Librax; with esterified estrogens: Menrium.

# beta blockers

*beta₁ blockers:* **acebutolol, atenolol, betaxolol hydrochloride, bisoprolol, esmolol, metoprolol tartrate**

*beta₁ and beta₂ blockers:* **carteolol hydrochloride, carvedilol, labetalol, levobunolol hydrochloride, metipranolol hydrochloride, nadolol, penbutolol sulfate, pindolol, propranolol, sotalol, timolol maleate**

Beta blockers are widely used to treat hypertension, angina pectoris, and arrhythmias. These drugs are well tolerated by most patients.

### Clinical indications and actions

#### Hypertension

Most beta blockers are used to treat hypertension. Although the exact mechanism of their antihypertensive effect is unknown, the action is thought to result from decreased cardiac output, decreased sympathetic outflow from the CNS, and suppression of renin release.

#### Angina

Propranolol, atenolol, nadolol, and metoprolol are used to treat angina pectoris; they decrease myocardial oxygen requirements through the blockade of catecholamine-induced increases in heart rate, blood pressure, and the extent of myocardial contraction.

#### Arrhythmias

Propranolol, acebutolol, sotalol, and esmolol are used to treat arrhythmias; they prolong the refractory period of the AV node and slow AV conduction.

#### Glaucoma

Betaxolol, levobunolol, metipranolol, and timolol reduce intraocular pressure by an unknown mechanism, but the drug effect is at least par-

## COMPARING ORAL CALCIUM CHANNEL BLOCKERS

| Drug | Onset of action | Peak serum level | Half-life | Therapeutic serum level |
|------|------|------|------|------|
| bepridil | 1 hr | 2-3 hr | 24 hr | 1-2 ng/ml |
| diltiazem | 15 min | 30 min | 3-4 hr | 50-200 ng/ml |
| felodipine | 2-5 hr | 2.5-5 hr | 11-16 hr | unknown |
| nicardipine | 20 min | 1 hr | 8.6 hr | 28-50 ng/ml |
| nifedipine | 5-30 min | 30 min-2 hr | 2-5 hr | 25-100 ng/ml |
| nimodipine | unknown | < 1 hr | 1-2 hr | unknown |
| nisoldipine | unknown | 6-12 hr | 7-12 hr | unknown |
| verapamil | 30 min | 1-2.2 hr | 6-12 hr | 80-300 ng/ml |

administration. Prolonged oral verapamil therapy may cause constipation.

Adverse effects of nifedipine include hypotension, reflex tachycardia, peripheral edema, flushing, light-headedness, and headache.

Diltiazem most commonly causes anorexia, nausea, various degrees of heart block, bradycardia, heart failure, and peripheral edema.

### Clinical considerations

- Advise clinician to monitor cardiac rate and rhythm and blood pressure carefully when starting or changing therapy.
- Use of calcium supplements may decrease the effectiveness of calcium channel blockers.
- Use cautiously in patients with impaired left ventricular function.

#### Special populations

**Pregnant patients.** Pregnancy risk category is C. Avoid use in pregnant women.

**Breast-feeding patients.** Calcium channel blockers (verapamil and diltiazem) may appear in breast milk. To avoid possible adverse effects in infants, discontinue breast-feeding during therapy with these drugs.

**Pediatric patients.** Adverse hemodynamic effects of parenteral verapamil have been observed in neonates and infants. Safety and effectiveness of diltiazem and nifedipine haven't been established.

**Geriatric patients.** Use with caution because the half-life of calcium channel blockers may be increased as a result of decreased clearance.

### Patient counseling

- Tell patient not to abruptly discontinue drug; gradual dose reduction may be needed.
- Instruct patient to report irregular heartbeat, shortness of breath, swelling of hands and feet, pronounced dizziness, constipation, nausea, or hypotension.
- Warn patient not to double the dose.

### Representative combinations

Amlodipine and benazepril hydrochloride: Lotrel.

## cephalosporins

**First-generation cephalosporins:**
cefadroxil, cefazolin sodium, cephalexin monohydrate, cephalothin sodium, cephradine

**Second-generation cephalosporins:**
cefaclor, cefamandole nafate, cefmetazole sodium, cefonicid sodium, cefotetan disodium, cefoxitin sodium, cefprozil, ceftibuten, cefuroxime axetil, cefuroxime sodium

**Third-generation cephalosporins:**
cefdinir, cefixime, cefoperazone sodium, cefotaxime sodium, cefpodoxime proxetil, ceftazidime, ceftizoxime sodium, ceftriaxone sodium

**Fourth-generation cephalosporin:**
cefepime hydrochloride

Cephalosporins are beta-lactam antibiotics isolated from the fungus *Cephalosporium acremonium*. Their mechanism of action is similar to that of penicillins, but their antibacterial spectra differ.

### Clinical indications and actions

*Infection caused by susceptible organisms*

*Parenteral cephalosporins:* Cephalosporins are used to treat serious infections of the lungs, skin, soft tissue, bones, joints, urinary tract, blood (septicemia), abdomen, and ◇ heart (endocarditis).

Third-generation cephalosporins (except moxalactam and cefoperazone) and the second-generation drug cefuroxime are used to treat CNS infections caused by susceptible strains of *Neisseria meningitidis, Haemophilus influenzae,* and *Streptococcus pneumoniae;* meningitis caused by *Escherichia coli* or *Klebsiella* can be treated with ceftriaxone, cefotaxime, or ceftizoxime.

First-generation and some second-generation cephalosporins also can be given prophylactically to reduce postoperative infection after surgical procedures classified as contaminated or potentially contaminated; third-generation drugs aren't usually indicated.

Penicillinase-producing *N. gonorrhoeae* can be treated with cefoxitin, cefotaxime, ceftriaxone, ceftizoxime, or cefuroxime.

*Oral cephalosporins:* Cephalosporins can be used to treat otitis media and infections of the respiratory tract, urinary tract, and skin and soft tissue.

◇ Ceftriaxone, cefotaxime, or cefuroxime axetil has been used in the treatment of Lyme disease.

Cefepime, ceftazidime, and ceftriaxone have been used parenterally for empiric anti-infective therapy of probable bacterial infections in febrile neutropenic patients.

## Pharmacology

Cephalosporins are chemically and pharmacologically similar to penicillin; their structure contains a beta-lactam ring, a dihydrothiazine ring, and side chains, and they act by inhibiting bacterial cell wall synthesis, causing rapid cell lysis. (See *Comparing cephalosporins.*)

The sites of action for cephalosporins are enzymes known as penicillin-binding proteins (PBP). The affinity of certain cephalosporins for PBP in various microorganisms helps explain the differing spectra of activity in this class of antibiotics.

Bacterial resistance to beta-lactam antibiotics is conferred most significantly by production of beta-lactamase enzymes (by both gram-negative and gram-positive bacteria) that destroy the beta-lactam ring and thus inactivate cephalosporins; decreased cell wall permeability and alteration in binding affinity to PBP also contribute to bacterial resistance.

Cephalosporins are bactericidal; they act against many gram-positive and gram-negative bacteria, and some anaerobic bacteria. They don't kill fungi or viruses.

First-generation cephalosporins act against many gram-positive cocci, including penicillinase-producing *S. aureus* and *S. epidermidis; S. pneumoniae, S. agalactiae* (group B streptococci), and *S. pyogenes* (group A beta-hemolytic streptococci); susceptible gram-negative organisms include *Klebsiella pneumoniae, E. coli, Proteus mirabilis,* and *Shigella.*

Second-generation cephalosporins are effective against all organisms attacked by first-generation drugs and have additional activity against *Moraxella catarrhalis, H. influenzae, Enterobacter, Citrobacter, Providencia, Acinetobacter, Serratia,* and *Neisseria; Bacteroides fragilis* is susceptible to cefotetan and cefoxitin.

Third-generation cephalosporins are less active than first- and second-generation drugs against gram-positive bacteria, but are more active against gram-negative organisms, including those resistant to first- and second-generation drugs; they have the greatest stability against beta-lactamases produced by gram-negative bacteria. Susceptible gram-negative organisms *include E. coli, Klebsiella, Enterobacter, Providencia, Acinetobacter, Serratia, Proteus, Morganella,* and *Neisseria;* some third-generation drugs are active against *B. fragilis* and *Pseudomonas.*

The fourth-generation cephalosporin cefepime is active against a wide range of gram-positive and gram-negative bacteria. Susceptible gram-negative organisms include *Enterobacter* spp., *E. coli, K. pneumoniae, P. mirabilis,* and *Pseudomonas aeruginosa;* susceptible gram-positive organisms include *S. aureus* (methicillin-susceptible strains only), *S. pneumoniae,* and *S. pyogenes* (Lancefield's group A streptococci).

Oral absorption of cephalosporins varies widely; many must be given parenterally. Most are distributed widely into the body, the actual amount varying with individual drugs. CSF penetration by first- and second-generation drugs is minimal; third-generation drugs achieve much greater penetration, and although the fourth-generation drug cefepime is known to cross the blood-brain barrier, it isn't known to what degree. Cephalosporins cross the placenta. Degree of metabolism varies with individual drugs; some aren't metabolized at all, whereas others are extensively metabolized.

Cephalosporins are excreted primarily in urine, chiefly by renal tubular effects; elimination half-life ranges from 30 minutes to 10 hours in patients with normal renal function. Some of the drug appears in breast milk. Most cephalosporins can be removed by hemodialysis or peritoneal dialysis. Patients on dialysis may require dosage adjustment.

## Overview of adverse reactions

Hypersensitivity reactions range from mild rash, fever, and eosinophilia to fatal anaphylaxis, and are more common in patients with penicillin allergy. Hematologic reactions include positive direct and indirect antiglobulin (Coombs' test), thrombocytopenia or thrombocythemia, transient neutropenia, and reversible leukopenia. Adverse renal effects, nausea, vomiting, diarrhea, abdominal pain, glossitis, dyspepsia, tenesmus, and minimal elevation of liver function test results have occurred. Hemolytic anemia with extravascular

## COMPARING CEPHALOSPORINS

| Drug and route | Elimination half-life (hr) Normal renal function | End-stage renal disease | Sodium (mEq/g) | CSF Penetration |
|---|---|---|---|---|
| cefaclor oral | 0.5-1 | 3-5.5 | Unknown | No |
| cefadroxil oral | 1-2 | 20-25 | Unknown | No |
| cefamandole I.M., I.V. | 0.5-2 | 12-18 | 3.3 | No |
| cefazolin I.M., I.V. | 1.2-2.2 | 3-7 | 2.0-2.1 | No |
| cefdinir P.O. | 1.5 | 16 | Unknown | Unknown |
| cefepime I.M., I.V. | 2 | 17-21 | Unknown | Yes |
| cefixime oral | 3-4 | 11.5 | Unknown | Unknown |
| cefmetazole I.V. | 1.2 | Unknown | 2 | Unknown |
| cefonicid I.M., I.V. | 3.5-5.8 | 11 | 3.7 | No |
| cefoperazone I.M., I.V. | 1.5-2.5 | 1.3-2.9 | 1.5 | Sometimes |
| cefotaxime I.M., I.V. | 1-1.5 | 3-11 | 2.2 | Yes |
| cefotetan I.M., I.V. | 2.8-4.6 | 13-35 | 3.5 | No |
| cefoxitin I.M., I.V. | 0.5-1 | 6.5-21.5 | 2.3 | No |
| cefpodoxime oral | 2-3 | 9.8 | Unknown | Unknown |
| cefprozil oral | 1-1.5 | 5.2-5.9 | Unknown | Unknown |
| ceftazidime I.M., I.V. | 1.5-2 | 35 | 2.3 | Yes |
| ceftibuten oral | 2.4 | 13.4-22.3 | Unknown | Unknown |
| ceftizoxime I.M., I.V. | 1.5-2 | 30 | 2.6 | Yes |
| ceftriaxone I.M., I.V. | 5.5-11 | 15.7 | 3.6 | Yes |
| cefuroxime I.M., I.V. | 1-2 | 15-22 | 2.4 | Yes |
| cephalexin oral | 0.5-1 | 19-22 | Unknown | No |
| cephalothin I.M., I.V. | 0.5-1 | 19 | 2.8 | No |
| cephapirin I.M., I.V. | 0.5-1 | 1.0-1.5 | 2.4 | No |
| cephradine oral, I.M., I.V. | 0.5-2 | 8-15 | 6 | No |

hemoysis and some fatalities have occurred in patients receiving cefotaxime, ceftizoxime, ceftriaxone, and cerotetan.

Local venous pain and irritation are common after I.M. injection; such reactions occur more often with higher doses and long-term therapy.

Disulfiram-type reactions occur when cefamandole, cefoperazone, moxalactam, cefonicid, or cefotetan is given within 48 to 72 hours of alcohol ingestion.

Bacterial and fungal superinfection results from suppression of normal flora.

Cross-sensitivity may occur in up to 15% of patients hypersensitive to penicillin.

## Clinical considerations

■ Review patient's history of allergies.
■ Advise clinician to monitor patient continuously for possible hypersensitivity reactions or other untoward effects.
■ Advise clinician to monitor renal function test results; doses of certain cephalosporins must be lowered in patients with severe renal impairment. In decreased renal function, advise clinician to monitor BUN levels, serum creatinine levels, and urine output for significant changes.
■ Advise clinician to monitor PT and platelet counts and assess patient for signs of hypoprothrombinemia, which may occur, with or without bleeding, during therapy with cefamandole, cefepime, cefoperazone, cefonicid, or cefotetan, usually in geriatric, debilitated, or malnourished patients.
■ Advise clinician to monitor patients on long-term therapy for possible bacterial and fungal superinfection, especially geriatric and debilitated patients and others receiving immunosuppressants or radiation therapy.
■ Advise clinician to monitor susceptible patients receiving sodium salts of cephalosporins for possible fluid retention; consult individual drug entry for sodium content.
■ Cephalosporins cause false-positive results in urine glucose tests using cupric sulfate solutions (Benedict's reagent or Clinitest); glucose oxidase tests aren't affected. Consult individual drug entries for other possible test interactions.

### Administration

■ Advise clinician to give cephalosporins at least 1 hour before giving bacteriostatic antibiotics (tetracyclines, erythromycins, and chloramphenicol); these drugs inhibit bacterial cell growth, decreasing cephalosporin uptake by bacterial cell walls.
■ Advise clinician to give oral cephalosporin at least 1 hour before or 2 hours after meals for maximum absorption.
■ Refrigerate oral suspensions; shake well before administering to assure correct dose.
■ Advise clinician to administer I.M. dose deep into large muscle mass (gluteal or midlateral thigh) and rotate injection sites.

■ Don't add or mix other drugs with I.V. infusions, particularly aminoglycosides, which are inactivated if mixed with cephalosporins; if other drugs must be given I.V., temporarily stop infusion of primary drug.
■ Adequate dilution of I.V. infusion and rotation of the site every 48 hours help minimize local vein irritation; use of small-gauge needle in larger available vein may be helpful.

### Special populations

**Pregnant patients.** Safety in pregnancy hasn't been established. Use only when clearly needed.
**Breast-feeding patients.** Cephalosporins appear in breast milk; use with caution in breast-feeding women.
**Pediatric patients.** Serum half-life is prolonged in neonates and in infants up to age 1 year.
**Geriatric patients.** Use with caution; geriatric patients are susceptible to superinfection and to coagulopathies. Geriatric patients commonly have renal impairment and may require lower doses of cephalosporins.

## Patient counseling

■ Explain the disease process and reason for therapy.
■ Teach patient signs and symptoms of hypersensitivity and other adverse reactions, and emphasize need to report any unusual effects.
■ Teach patient signs and symptoms of bacterial and fungal superinfection to geriatric and debilitated patients and others with low resistance from immunosuppressants or irradiation; emphasize need to report them promptly.
■ Warn patient not to ingest alcohol in any form within 72 hours of treatment with cefamandole, cefoperazone, moxalactam, cefonicid, or cefotetan.
■ Suggest patient add yogurt or buttermilk to diet to prevent intestinal superinfection from suppression of normal intestinal flora.
■ Advise diabetic patients to monitor urine glucose level with Diastix, Chemstrip uG, or glucose enzymatic test strip and not to use Clinitest.
■ Tell patient to take oral drug with food if GI irritation occurs.
■ Be sure patient understands how and when to take drug; urge patient to complete entire prescribed regimen, to comply with instructions for around-the-clock dosing, and to keep follow-up appointments.
■ Counsel patient to check expiration date of drug, how to store drug, and to discard unused drug.

## Representative combinations
None.

## COMPARING LOOP DIURETICS

| Drug and route | Usual dosage | Onset (min) | Peak (hr) | Duration (hr) |
|---|---|---|---|---|
| **bumetanide** | | | | |
| I.V. | 0.5-1 mg ≤ t.i.d | ≤ 5 | ¼-¾ | 4-6 |
| P.O. | 0.5-2 mg/day | 30-60 | 1-2 | ½-1 |
| **ethacrynic acid** | | | | |
| I.V. | 50 mg/day | ≤ 5 | ¼-½ | 2 |
| P.O. | 50-100 mg/day | ≤ 30 | 2 | 6-8 |
| **furosemide** | | | | |
| I.V. | 20-40 mg q 2 hr, p.r.n. | ≤ 5 | ⅓-1 | 2 |
| P.O. | 20-80 mg ≤ b.i.d. | 30-60 | 1-2 | 6-8 |
| **torsemide** | | | | |
| I.V. | 5-20 mg/day | ≤ 10 | ≤ 1 | 6-8 |
| P.O. | 5-20 mg/day | ≤ 60 | 1-2 | 6-8 |

# diuretics, loop

**bumetanide, ethacrynate sodium, ethacrynic acid, furosemide, torsemide**

Loop diuretics are sometimes referred to as high-ceiling diuretics because they produce a peak diuresis greater than that produced by other drugs. Loop diuretics are particularly useful in edema caused by heart failure, hepatic cirrhosis, and renal disease. Ethacrynic acid was synthesized during the search for compounds that might interact with renal sulfhydryl groups like mercurial diuretics. However, ethacrynic acid causes ototoxicity and a higher risk of GI reactions and is therefore used less frequently. Structurally similar to furosemide, bumetanide is about 40 times more potent. Torsemide is the newest loop diuretic. (See *Comparing loop diuretics.*)

## Clinical indications and actions
### Edema
Loop diuretics effectively relieve edema caused by heart failure. They may be useful in patients who are refractory to other diuretics. Because furosemide and bumetanide may increase glomerular filtration rate, they're useful in patients with renal impairment. I.V. loop diuretics are used adjunctively in acute pulmonary edema to decrease peripheral vascular resistance. Loop diuretics also are used to treat edema associated with hepatic cirrhosis and nephrotic syndrome.
### Hypertension
Loop diuretics are used in patients with mild to moderate hypertension, although thiazides are the initial diuretics of choice in most pa-

tients. Loop diuretics are preferred in patients with heart failure or renal impairment; used I.V., they're a helpful adjunct in managing hypertensive crises.
◇ Loop diuretics have been used to increase excretion of calcium in patients with hypercalcemia.

Loop diuretics have been used to enhance the elimination of drugs and toxic substances after intoxication.

## Pharmacology
Loop diuretics inhibit sodium and chloride reabsorption in the ascending loop of Henle, thus increasing renal excretion of sodium, chloride, and water; like thiazide diuretics, loop diuretics increase excretion of potassium. Loop diuretics produce greater maximum diuresis and electrolyte loss than thiazide diuretics.

## Overview of adverse reactions
The most common adverse effects caused by therapeutic doses of loop diuretics are metabolic and electrolyte disturbances (particularly potassium depletion), hypochloremic alkalosis, hyperglycemia, hyperuricemia, and hypomagnesemia. Rapid parenteral administration of loop diuretics may cause hearing loss (including deafness) and tinnitus. High doses may produce profound diuresis, leading to hypovolemia and CV collapse.

## Clinical considerations
■ Recommend safety measures for all ambulatory patients until response to the diuretic is known.
■ Patients taking cardiac glycosides are at increased risk of digitalis toxicity from potassium depletion.
■ Patients with hepatic disease are especially susceptible to diuretic-induced electrolyte im-

---

balance; in extreme cases, stupor, coma, and death can result.

■ Consider possible dosage adjustment in the following circumstances: reduced doses for patients with hepatic dysfunction; increased doses in patients with renal impairment, oliguria, or decreased diuresis (inadequate urine output may result in circulatory overload, causing water intoxication, pulmonary edema, and heart failure); increased doses of insulin or oral hypoglycemics in diabetic patients; and reduced doses of other antihypertensives.

■ Advise clinician to monitor blood pressure and pulse rate (especially during rapid diuresis), establish baseline values before therapy, and watch for significant changes.

■ Advise clinician to establish baseline and periodically reviewing CBC, including WBC count; serum electrolytes; carbon dioxide; magnesium; BUN and creatinine levels; and results of liver function tests.

■ Advise clinician to give diuretics in the morning so major diuresis occurs before bedtime. To prevent nocturia, diuretics shouldn't be prescribed for use after 6 p.m.

■ Advise clinician to monitor patient for signs of excessive diuresis: hypotension, tachycardia, poor skin turgor, and excessive thirst.

■ Advise clinician to monitor patient for edema and ascites.

### Special populations
**Pregnant patients.** There are no adequately controlled studies for use of loop diuretics in pregnant women. Avoid use if possible.
**Breast-feeding patients.** Don't use loop diuretics in breast-feeding women.
**Pediatric patients.** Use loop diuretics with caution in neonates; don't use ethacrynic acid and ethacrynate sodium in infants. The usual pediatric dose can be used, but extend dose intervals.
**Geriatric patients.** Geriatric and debilitated patients require close observation because they're more susceptible to drug-induced diuresis. Excessive diuresis can quickly lead to dehydration, hypovolemia, hypokalemia, and hyponatremia and may cause circulatory collapse. Reduced doses may be indicated.

### Patient counseling
■ Explain to patient the reason for therapy and diuretic effect of these drugs (increased volume and frequency of urination).

■ Teach patient signs of adverse effects, especially hypokalemia (weakness, fatigue, muscle cramps, paresthesias, confusion, nausea, vomiting, diarrhea, headache, dizziness, or palpitations), and importance of reporting such symptoms promptly.

■ Advise patient to eat potassium-rich foods.

■ Tell patient to report increased edema or weight or excess diuresis (more than 2-lb [0.9-kg] weight loss per day).

■ With initial doses, caution patient to change position slowly, especially when rising to upright position, to prevent dizziness from orthostatic hypotension.

■ Instruct patient to call prescriber immediately if he experiences chest, back, or leg pain; shortness of breath; or dyspnea.

■ Inform patient that photosensitivity may occur in some patients. Caution patient to take protective measures against exposure to ultraviolet light or sunlight, such as using sunblock and wearing protective clothing.

## Representative combinations
None.

# diuretics, potassium-sparing

**amiloride hydrochloride, spironolactone, triamterene**

Potassium-sparing diuretics are less potent than many others; in particular, amiloride and triamterene have little clinical effect when used alone. However, they protect against potassium loss and are used with more potent diuretics. Spironolactone, an aldosterone antagonist, is particularly useful in patients with edema and hypertension associated with hyperaldosteronism.

## Clinical indications and actions
*Edema*
All potassium-sparing diuretics are used to manage edema caused by hepatic cirrhosis, nephrotic syndrome, and heart failure.
*Hypertension*
Amiloride and spironolactone are used to treat mild and moderate hypertension; the exact mechanism is unknown. Spironolactone may block the effect of aldosterone on arteriolar smooth muscle.
*Diagnosis of primary hyperaldosteronism*
Because spironolactone inhibits aldosterone, correction of hypokalemia and hypertension is presumptive evidence of primary hyperaldosteronism.
*Other uses*
Amiloride has been used to correct metabolic alkalosis caused by thiazide and other kaliuretic diuretics, and with hydrochlorothiazide in patients with recurrent calcium nephrolithiasis. It has also been used to manage lithium-induced polyuria secondary to lithium-induced nephrogenic diabetes insipidus.

Spironolactone has been used to aid in the treatment of hypokalemia and for prophylaxis of hypokalemia in patients taking cardiac glycosides. It has also been used in the treatment of precocious puberty, female hirsutism, and as an adjunct to treatment in myasthenia gravis and familial periodic paralysis.

## Pharmacology
Amiloride and triamterene act directly on the distal renal tubules, inhibiting sodium reabsorption and potassium excretion, thereby reducing potassium loss. Spironolactone competitively inhibits aldosterone at the distal renal tubules, also promoting sodium excretion and potassium retention.

## Overview of adverse reactions
Hyperkalemia is the most important adverse reaction; it may occur with all drugs in this class and could lead to arrhythmias. Other adverse reactions include nausea, vomiting, headache, weakness, fatigue, bowel disturbances, cough, and dyspnea.

Potassium-sparing diuretics are contraindicated in patients with serum potassium levels above 5.5 mEq/L, in those receiving other potassium-sparing diuretics or potassium supplements, and in patients with anuria, acute or chronic renal insufficiency, diabetic nephropathy, or those hypersensitive to the drug. They should be used cautiously in patients with severe hepatic insufficiency because electrolyte imbalance may precipitate hepatic encephalopathy, and in patients with diabetes, who are at increased risk of hyperkalemia.

## Clinical considerations
■ Give diuretics in the morning to ensure that major diuresis occurs before bedtime. To prevent nocturia, don't prescribe diuretics for use after 6 p.m.
■ Recommend establishing safety measures for ambulatory patients until response is known; diuretics may cause orthostatic hypotension, weakness, ataxia, and confusion.
■ Consider possible dosage adjustments in the following circumstances: reduced doses for patients with hepatic dysfunction and for those taking other antihypertensives; increased doses in patients with renal impairment; and changes in insulin requirements in diabetic patients.
■ Advise clinician to monitor patient for hyperkalemia and arrhythmias, measure serum potassium and other electrolyte levels frequently, and check for significant changes. Advise clinician to monitor the following at baseline and periodic intervals: CBC including WBC count, carbon dioxide, BUN, and creatinine levels and, especially, liver function test results.
■ Advise clinician to monitor vital signs, intake and output, weight, and blood pressure daily; also recommend checking patient for edema, oliguria, or lack of diuresis, which may indicate drug tolerance.
■ Advise clinician to monitor patient with hepatic disease in whom mild drug-induced acidosis may be hazardous; also recommend watching for mental confusion, lethargy, or stupor. Patients with hepatic disease are especially susceptible to diuretic-induced electrolyte imbalance; in extreme cases, coma and death can result.
■ Advise clinician to monitor patient for other signs of toxicity.

### Special populations
**Pregnant patients.** There are no adequately controlled studies for use in pregnant women.
**Breast-feeding patients.** Safety hasn't been established; drug may appear in breast milk.
**Pediatric patients.** If indicated, use drugs with caution; children are more susceptible to hyperkalemia.
**Geriatric patients.** Geriatric and debilitated patients require close observation because they're more susceptible to drug-induced diuresis and hyperkalemia. Reduced doses may be indicated.

## Patient counseling
■ Explain to patient the signs and symptoms of possible adverse effects and the importance of reporting unusual effects.
■ Tell patient to report increased edema or weight loss (more than 2-lb [0.9-kg ] per day) or excess diuresis and to record weight each morning after voiding and before dressing and breakfast, using the same scale.
■ Teach patient how to minimize dizziness from orthostatic hypotension by avoiding sudden postural changes.
■ Advise patient to avoid potassium-rich food and potassium-containing salt substitutes or supplements, which increase the hazard of hyperkalemia.
■ Tell patient to take drug at same time each morning to avoid interrupted sleep from nighttime diuresis.
■ Advise patient to take drug with or after meals to minimize GI distress.
■ Caution patient to avoid hazardous activities, such as driving or operating machinery, until response to drug is known.
■ Tell patient to seek medical approval before taking OTC drugs; many contain sodium and potassium and can cause electrolyte imbalance.

## Representative combinations
*Amiloride* with hydrochlorothiazide: Moduretic.

*Spironolactone* with hydrochlorothiazide: Aldactazide.

*Triamterene* with hydrochlorothiazide: Dyazide, Maxzide.

## COMPARING THIAZIDE DIURETICS

| Drug | Equivalent dose (mg) | Onset (hr) | Peak (hr) | Duration (hr) |
|------|------|------|------|------|
| bendroflumethiazide | 5 | ≤ 2 | 4 | 6-12 |
| chlorothiazide | 500 | ≤ 2 | 4 | 6-12 |
| hydrochlorothiazide | 50 | ≤ 2 | 4-6 | 6-12 |
| methyclothiazide | 5 | ≤ 2 | 4-6 | 24 |

# diuretics, thiazide

bendroflumethiazide,
chlorothiazide, chlorothiazide
sodium, hydrochlorothiazide,
hydroflumethiazide,
methyclothiazide, polythiazide,
trichlormethiazide

# diuretics, thiazide-like

chlorthalidone, indapamide,
metolazone

Thiazide diuretics were the first potent and safe diuretics.

## Clinical indications and actions
### Edema
Thiazide diuretics are used to treat edema caused by congestive heart failure and nephrotic syndrome and, with spironolactone, to treat edema and ascites secondary to hepatic cirrhosis. Thiazides may also be used to control edema during pregnancy except if caused by renal disease. This treatment isn't indicated for mild edema.

Efficacy and toxicity profiles of thiazide and thiazide-like diuretics are equivalent at comparable doses; the single exception is metolazone, which may be more effective in patients with impaired renal function. Usually, thiazide diuretics are less effective than loop diuretics in patients with renal insufficiency.
### Hypertension
Thiazide diuretics are commonly used for initial management of all degrees of hypertension. Used alone, they reduce mean blood pressure by only 10 to 15 mm Hg. For mild hypertension, thiazide diuresis alone will usually reduce blood pressure to desired levels. However, in moderate to severe hypertension that doesn't respond to thiazides alone, therapy with another antihypertensive is needed.
### ◇ Diabetes insipidus
In diabetes insipidus, thiazides cause a paradoxical decrease in urine volume; urine becomes more concentrated, possibly because of sodium depletion and decreased plasma volume. Thiazides are particularly effective in nephrogenic diabetes insipidus.
### Other uses
Also used as prophylaxis of renal calculi formation caused by hypercalciuria and in the treatment of electrolyte disturbances caused by renal tubular necrosis.

## Pharmacology
Thiazide diuretics interfere with sodium transport across tubules of the cortical diluting segment of the nephron, thereby increasing renal excretion of sodium, chloride, water, potassium, and calcium. Bicarbonate, magnesium, phosphate, bromide, and iodide excretion are also increased. These drugs may also decrease excretion of ammonia, causing increased serum ammonia levels. Long-term thiazide therapy can cause mild metabolic alkalosis associated with hypokalemia and hypochloremia.

The exact mechanism of thiazides' antihypertensive effect is unknown; it's thought to be partially caused by direct arteriolar dilatation. Thiazides initially decrease extracellular fluid volume, plasma volume, and cardiac output; extracellular fluid volume and plasma volume revert to near baseline levels in several weeks but remain slightly below normal. Cardiac output returns to normal or slightly above. Total body sodium level remains slightly below pretreatment levels. Peripheral vascular resistance is initially elevated but falls below pretreatment levels with long-term diuretic therapy. (See Comparing thiazide diuretics.)

In patients with diabetes insipidus, thiazides cause a paradoxical decrease in urine volume and increase in renal level of urine, possibly because of sodium depletion and decreased plasma volume, which leads to an increase in renal water and sodium reabsorption. In addition, thiazides can cause hyperglycemia, exacerbation of diabetes mellitus, or precipitation of diabetes mellitus.

## Overview of adverse reactions
Therapeutic doses of thiazide diuretics cause electrolyte and metabolic disturbances, most commonly potassium depletion; patients may require dietary supplementation.

Other abnormalities include hypochloremic alkalosis, hypomagnesemia, hyponatremia, hypercalcemia, hyperuricemia, elevated cholesterol levels, and hyperglycemia. Overdose of thiazides may produce lethargy that can progress to coma within a few hours. Also, type 2 diabetes mellitus has been precipitated in prediabetic patients.

## Clinical considerations

- Thiazides and thiazide-like diuretics (except metolazone) are ineffective in patients with a glomerular filtration rate below 25 ml per minute.
- Because thiazides may cause adverse lipid effects, consider an alternative drug in patients with significant hyperlipidemia.
- Advise clinician to monitor intake and output, weight, and electrolyte levels regularly.
- Advise clinician to monitor potassium levels and consult a dietitian to provide high-potassium diet. Foods rich in potassium include citrus fruits, tomatoes, bananas, dates, and apricots. Watch for signs of hypokalemia, such as muscle weakness or cramps. Patients also taking a cardiac glycoside have an increased risk of digitalis toxicity from the potassium-depleting effect of these diuretics.
- Thiazides may be used with potassium-sparing diuretics or potassium supplements to prevent potassium loss.
- Advise clinician to monitor glucose levels in diabetic patients. Thiazides may cause hyperglycemia and a need to adjust insulin or oral hypoglycemic doses.
- Advise clinician to monitor serum creatinine and BUN levels regularly. Drug isn't as effective if these levels are more than twice normal.
- Advise clinician to monitor uric acid levels, especially in patients with history of gout; these drugs may cause an increase in uric acid levels.
- Antihypertensive effects persist for about 1 week after discontinuation of drug.

### Special populations

**Pregnant patients.** Thiazides cross the placenta and appear in cord blood. Risks and benefits must be evaluated. There are some reports of teratogenic effects, but they're inconclusive. Some clinicians advise patients to avoid use in the first trimester. Routine use isn't recommended with mild edema.

**Breast-feeding patients.** Thiazides appear in breast milk; safety and effectiveness in breast-feeding women haven't been established.

**Pediatric patients.** Safety and effectiveness in children haven't been established for all thiazide diuretics. Indapamide and metolazone aren't recommended for use in children.

**Geriatric patients.** Geriatric and debilitated patients require close observation and may require reduced doses. They're more sensitive to excess diuresis because of age-related changes in CV and renal function. In geriatric patients, excess diuresis can quickly lead to dehydration, hypovolemia, hyponatremia, hypomagnesemia, and hypokalemia.

## Patient counseling

- Explain reason for therapy and diuretic effects of these drugs (increased volume and frequency of urination).
- Instruct patient to report joint swelling, pain, or redness; these signs may indicate hyperuricemia.
- Warn patient to call prescriber immediately if signs of electrolyte imbalance occur; these include weakness, fatigue, muscle cramps, paresthesia, confusion, nausea, vomiting, diarrhea, headache, dizziness, and palpitations.
- Tell patient to report increased edema, excess diuresis, or weight loss (more than a 2-lb [0.9-kg] per day); advise him to record weight each morning after voiding and before dressing and breakfast, using the same scale.
- Advise patient to take drug in the morning to prevent nocturia.
- Instruct patient to take drug with food to minimize gastric irritation; to eat potassium-rich foods; and not to add salt to foods. Recommend use of salt substitutes.
- Counsel patient to avoid smoking because nicotine increases blood pressure.
- Tell patient to seek medical approval before taking OTC drugs.
- Advise patient to use sunblock.

**With initial doses**
- Caution patient to change position slowly, especially when rising to upright position, to prevent dizziness from orthostatic hypotension.
- Instruct patient to call prescriber immediately if he experiences chest, back, or leg pain; shortness of breath; or dyspnea.
- Tell patient to take drug only as prescribed and at the same time each day, to prevent nighttime diuresis and interrupted sleep.

## Representative combinations

*Chlorthalidone* with atenolol: Tenoretic, Atenolol/Chlorthalidone Tablets; with reserpine: Regroton.

*Hydrochlorothiazide* with bisoprolol: Ziac Tablets; with deserpidine: Oreticyl; with guanethidine monosulfate: Esimil; with hydralazine: Apresazide, Hydrochlorothiazide/Hydralazine Caps; with hydralazine hydrochloride and reserpine: Hydrap-ES Tablets, Marpres Tablets, Tri-Hydroserpine Tablets; with methyldopa: Aldoril, Methyldopa and Hydrochlorothiazide Tablets; with propranolol: Inderide, Propranolol/Hydrochlorothiazide Tablets; with reserpine: Hydrochlorothiazide/Reserpine Tablets, Hydropine, Hydropres, Hydro-Serp, Hydroserpine, Hydrotensin, Mallopres; with hydralazine and reserpine: Ser-Ap-Es, Unipres; with spironolactone: Aldactazide; with timolol maleate: Timolide; with triamterene: Dyazide, Maxzide; with amiloride hydrochloride: Moduretic.

*Hydroflumethiazide* with reserpine: Salutensin Tablets.

# estrogens

**dienestrol, diethylstilbestrol, diethylstilbestrol diphosphate, esterified estrogens, estradiol, estradiol cypionate, estradiol valerate, estrogen and progestin, estrogenic substances (conjugated), estropipate, ethinyl estradiol**

Numerous synthetic modifications of naturally occurring estrogen molecules and completely synthetic estrogenic compounds have been developed.

Estrogens have several uses: in treating the symptoms of menopause, atrophic vaginitis, breast cancer, and other diseases; in the prophylaxis of osteoporosis; and as contraceptives when used with progestins.

## Clinical indications and actions
*Moderate to severe vasomotor symptoms of menopause*
Endogenous estrogen levels are markedly reduced after menopause. This commonly results in vasomotor symptoms, such as hot flashes and dizziness. Diethylstilbestrol, estradiol cypionate, and ethinyl estradiol serve to mimic the action of endogenous estrogens in preventing these symptoms.
*Atrophic vaginitis; kraurosis vulvae*
Diethylstilbestrol stimulates development, cornification, and secretory activity in vaginal tissues.
*Carcinoma of the breast*
Conjugated estrogens, diethylstilbestrol, esterified estrogens, estradiol, and ethinyl estradiol inhibit the growth of hormone-sensitive cancers in certain carefully selected men and postmenopausal women.
*Carcinoma of the prostate*
Conjugated estrogens, diethylstilbestrol, esterified estrogens, estradiol, estradiol valerate, and ethinyl estradiol inhibit growth of hormone-sensitive cancer tissue in men with advanced disease.
*CV risk prevention*
Although somewhat controversial, estrogen and estrogen/progestin has shown to reduce the risk of ischemic heart disease by 50%. Therapy initiation should be highly individualized.
*Prophylaxis of postmenopausal osteoporosis*
Conjugated estrogens replace or augment activity of endogenous estrogen in causing calcium and phosphate retention and preventing bone decalcification.

*Contraception*
Estrogens are also used with progestins for ovulation control to prevent conception.

## Pharmacology
Estrogens are hormones secreted by ovarian follicles and also by the adrenals, corpeus luteum, placenta, and testes. Conjugated estrogens and estrogenic substances are normally obtained from the urine of pregnant mares. Other estrogens are manufactured synthetically. Of the six naturally occurring estrogens, three (estradiol, estrone, and estriol) are present in significant quantities.

Estrogens promote the development and maintenance of the female reproductive system and secondary sexual characteristics. Estrogens inhibit the release of pituitary gonadotropins and also have various metabolic effects, including retention of fluid and electrolytes, retention and deposition in bone of calcium and phosphorus, and mild anabolic activity. They also increase high-density lipoproteins and decrease low-density lipoproteins.

Estrogens and estrogenic substances given as drugs have effects related to endogenous estrogen's mechanism of action. They can mimic the action of endogenous estrogen when used as replacement therapy or produce such useful effects as inhibiting ovulation or inhibiting growth of certain hormone-sensitive cancers.

Use of estrogens isn't without risk. Long-term use is associated with an increased risk of endometrial cancer, gallbladder disease, and thromboembolic disease. Elevations in blood pressure often occur as well.

## Overview of adverse reactions
Acute reactions include changes in menstrual bleeding patterns (spotting, prolongation or absence of bleeding), abdominal cramps, swollen feet or ankles, bloated sensation (fluid and electrolyte retention), breast swelling and tenderness, weight gain, nausea, loss of appetite, headache, photosensitivity, and loss of libido.

With chronic administration, adverse reactions include increased blood pressure (sometimes into the hypertensive range), thromboembolic disease, cholestatic jaundice, benign hepatomas, and endometrial carcinoma (rare). Risk of thromboembolic disease increases markedly with cigarette smoking, especially in women over age 35. Increased risk of thromboembolic events is also seen in postmenopausal women, women undergoing surgery, and those with fractures or who are immobilized.

## Clinical considerations
■ Some clinicians advise women to discontinue estrogen replacement therapy during immobilization from fracture, CVA, or severe illness; estrogen replacement therapy can be restarted when normal activity is resumed.

■ Don't use estrogens in patients with thrombophlebitis or thromboembolic disorders; cancer of the breast, reproductive organs, or genitals; or undiagnosed abnormal genital bleeding.

■ Use with caution in patients with hypertension, asthma, mental depression, bone disease, blood dyscrasias, gallbladder disease, migraine, seizures, diabetes mellitus, amenorrhea, heart failure, hepatic or renal dysfunction, or a family history of breast or genital tract cancer. Development or worsening of these conditions may require discontinuation of the drug.

■ Give patient package insert describing estrogen adverse reactions, and also provide verbal explanation.

■ Recommend monitoring patients with diabetes mellitus for loss of diabetes control.

■ If patient is receiving a warfarin-type anticoagulant, advise clinician to monitor PT and INR for anticoagulant dosage adjustment.

■ Estrogen therapy is usually given cyclically. The drugs are usually given once daily for 3 weeks, followed by 1 week without the drugs; this regimen is repeated p.r.n.

### Special populations

**Pregnant patients.** Estrogens are contraindicated for use in pregnancy.

**Breast-feeding patients.** Estrogens are contraindicated in breast-feeding women.

**Pediatric patients.** Because of the effects of estrogen on epiphyseal closure, use estrogens with caution in adolescents whose bone growth isn't complete. Estrogens aren't used in children.

**Geriatric patients.** Postmenopausal women with long-term estrogen use have an increased risk of endometrial cancer if they have a uterus. This risk can be reduced by adding a progestin to the regimen.

### Patient counseling

■ Warn patient to report adverse reactions immediately.

■ Tell men on long-term therapy about possible gynecomastia and impotence.

■ Explain to patient on cyclic therapy for postmenopausal symptoms that, although withdrawal bleeding may occur in week off drug, fertility hasn't been restored; ovulation doesn't occur.

■ Diabetic patients should report symptoms of hyperglycemia or glycosuria.

■ Tell women who are planning to breast-feed not to take estrogens.

### Representative combinations

*Estradiol cypionate* with testosterone cypionate and chlorobutanol: Depo-testadiol, Duo-cyp, Menoject, testosterone cypionate and estradiol cypionate, depAndrogyn, Depotestogen, Duratestrin, T-E Cypionates, Test-Estro Cypionate.

*Estradiol valerate* with testosterone enanthate: Deladumone, Delatestadiol, Teev, Testos-terone Enanthate and Estradiol Valerate Injection, Valertest.

*Estrogen* with methyltestosterone: Estratest, Estratest H.S.

*Estrogenic substances (conjugated)* with meprobamate: Milprem, PMB; with methyltestosterone: Premarin with methyltestosterone; with medroxyprogesterone: Premphase, Prempro.

*Esterified estrogens* with chlordiazepoxide: Menrium.

*Ethinyl estradiol* with norethindrone: Brevicon, Genora 1/35, Jenest, Loestrin Fe 1.5/30, ModiCon, Nelova1/35E, Ortho-Novum 1/35, Ortho-Novum 7/7/7, Ortho-Novum 10/11; with norgestimate: Cyclen; with ethynodiol diacetate: Demulen 1/35, Demulen 1/50; with desogestrel: Desogen, Marvelon; with norgestrel: Lo/Ovral, Ovral; with levonorgestrel: Levlen, Min-Ovral, Nordette, Tri-Levlen, Triphasil, Triquilar.

*Ethynodiol diacetate* with ethinyl estradiol: Demulen 1/35, Demulen 1/50.

# fluoroquinolones

**ciprofloxacin, enoxacin,
gatifloxacine, levofloxacin,
lomefloxacin hydrochloride,
moxifloxacin, norfloxacin, ofloxacin,
sparfloxacin, trovafloxacin
mesylate/alatrofloxacin mesylate**

Fluoroquinolones are broad-spectrum, systemic antibacterial drugs active against a wide range of aerobic gram-positive and gram-negative organisms. Gram-positive aerobic bacteria include S*taphylococcus aureus, S. epidermis, S. saprophyticus, S. hemolyticus,* penicillinase- and non–penicillinase-producing staphylococci as well as some methicillin-resistant strains, *Streptococcus pneumoniae,* group A (beta) hemolytic streptococci *(S. pyogenes),* group B streptococci *(S. agalactiae),* viridans streptococci, groups C, F, and G streptococci and nonenterococcal group D streptococci, and *Enterococcus faecalis.* These drugs are active against gram-positive aerobic bacilli including *Corynebacterium, Listeria monocytogenes,* and *Nocardia asteroides.*

Fluoroquinolones are effective against gram-negative aerobic bacteria including, but not limited to, *Neisseria meningitidis* and most strains of penicillinase- and non–penicillinase-producing *Neisseria gonorrhoeae, Haemophilus influenzae, Haemophilus parainfluenzae, Haemophilus ducreyi, Moraxella catarrhalis,* and most clinically important Enterobacteriaceae, *P. aeruginosa, Vibrio cholerae,* and *Vibrio parahaemolyticus.* Certain fluoroquinolones are active against *Chlamydia trachomatis, Mycoplasma hominis, Mycoplasma pneumoniae,*

## COMPARING FLUOROQUINOLONES

| Drug | Oral bioavailability (%) | Plasma protein–binding (%) | Half-life (hr) |
|------|--------------------------|----------------------------|----------------|
| ciprofloxacin | 70-80 | 20-40 | Normal renal function: 4-6<br>Severe renal failure: 6-8 |
| enoxacin | 90 | 40 | Normal renal function: 3-6<br>Severe renal failure: 9-10 |
| levofloxacin | 100 (without regard to food) | 50 | Normal renal function: 6 |
| lomefloxacin | 78-86 (may take with or without food) | 10 | Normal renal function: not stated<br>Severe renal failure: 21-45 |
| norfloxacin | Not stated | 10-15 | Normal renal function: 3-4<br>Severe renal failure: 9-10 |
| ofloxacin | Not stated | 20-25 | Normal renal function: 4½-7<br>Severe renal failure: 15-16 |
| sparfloxacin | 92 | 45 | Normal renal function: 16-30 |
| trovafloxacin/alatrofloxacin | 88 (without regard to food) | 76 | Normal renal function: 9-11¼ |

*Legionella pneumophila*, and *Mycobacterium avium-intracellulare.*

### Clinical indications and actions

Fluoroquinolones are indicated for the treatment of the following infections when caused by susceptible organisms: bone and joint infections, bacterial bronchitis, endocervical and urethral chlamydial infections, bacterial gastroenteritis, endocervical and urethral gonorrhea, intra-abdominal infections, empiric therapy for febrile neutropenia, pelvic inflammatory disease, bacterial pneumonia, bacterial prostatitis, acute sinusitis, skin and soft-tissue infections, typhoid fever, bacterial urinary tract infections, chancroid, meningococcal carriers, and bacterial septicemia. Fluoroquinolones may be used for the prevention of bacterial urinary tract infections.

### Pharmacology

Fluoroquinolones produce a bactericidal effect by inhibiting intracellular DNA topoisomerase II (DNA gyrase) or topoisomerase IV. These enzymes are essential catalysts in the duplication, transcription, and repair of bacterial DNA. (See *Comparing fluoroquinolones.*)

### Overview of adverse reactions

The following side effects are observed rarely with fluoroquinolones, but require medical attention: CNS stimulation (acute psychosis, agitation, hallucinations, tremors), hepatotoxicity, hypersensitivity reactions, interstitial nephritis, phlebitis, pseudomembranous colitis, and tendinitis or tendon rupture. The following side effects don't require medical attention unless they persist or become intolerable: CNS adverse effects (dizziness, headache, nervousness, drowsiness, insomnia); GI reactions; and photosensitivity.

### Clinical considerations

■ Consider the risk-benefit ratio of therapy with fluoroquinolones on an individual basis when any of the following conditions is present: seizure disorders, cerebral ischemia, severe hepatic dysfunction, or renal insufficiency.
■ Renal and liver function test results should be monitored in patients with impaired renal or hepatic function.
■ Achilles and other tendon ruptures may occur. Discontinue drug if patient experiences pain, inflammation, or rupture of a tendon.

### Special populations

**Pregnant patients.** Pregnancy risk category is C. Adequate, well-controlled trials haven't been completed, but these drugs cross the placenta and may cause arthropathies.
**Breast-feeding patients.** It's unknown if fluoroquinolones appear in breast milk. Therefore, their use in nursing mothers isn't recommended because these drugs may cause arthropathies in newborns and infants.
**Pediatric patients.** Fluoroquinolones aren't recommended because they can cause joint problems.
**Geriatric patients.** Because renal function deteriorates over time, geriatric patients may require a reduction in their daily dose.

| Peak concentration (hr) | Elimination | Dosage adjustment | Dialyzability |
|---|---|---|---|
| 1-2 | 40-70% of drug is cleared unchanged by the kidneys in 24 hr | Renal failure | < 10% removed by hemodialysis |
| 1-3 | 40-60% of drug is cleared unchanged by the kidneys in 48 hr | Renal failure | < 5% removed by hemodialysis |
| 1 | Almost entirely eliminated unchanged in the urine | Renal failure | Not defined |
| 1½ | 60-80% of drug is cleared unchanged by the kidneys in 48 hr | Renal failure | < 3% removed by hemodialysis |
| 1-2 | 26% of drug is cleared unchanged by the kidneys in 24 hr | Renal failure | < 10% removed by hemodialysis |
| 1-2 | 70-90% of drug is cleared unchanged by the kidneys in 36 hr | Renal failure | < 10-30% removed by hemodialysis |
| 3-6 | 10% is excreted unchanged in the urine | Renal failure | Not defined |
| 1-2 | 50% of oral dose (43% in feces and 6% in urine) excreted as unchanged drug | Cirrhosis | Not efficiently removed by dialysis |

## Patient counseling

■ Instruct patient to take this drug as prescribed and to finish the full course of therapy.

■ Tell patient to take the drug with an 8-ounce glass of water.

■ Enoxacin and norfloxacin should be taken on an empty stomach.

■ Instruct patient that if a dose is missed, the next dose should be taken as soon as possible; dose shouldn't be doubled.

■ Advise patient to avoid concurrent use of antacids or sucralfate and orally administered fluoroquinolones.

■ Advise patient not to take other drugs concurrently without first checking with a pharmacist or prescriber.

## Representative combinations

None.

# histamine$_2$ (H$_2$)-receptor antagonists

## cimetidine, famotidine, nizatidine, ranitidine, ranitidine bismuth citrate

H$_2$-receptor antagonists have revolutionized the treatment of peptic ulcer disease. These drugs structurally resemble histamine and competitively inhibit the action of histamine on gastric H$_2$ receptors. Cimetidine is the prototype of this class. (See *Adult dosages of histamine$_2$-receptor antagonists,* page 44.)

## Clinical indications and actions

### Duodenal ulcer

Cimetidine, famotidine, nizatidine, and ranitidine are used to treat acute duodenal ulcer and to prevent ulcer recurrence. Ranitidine bismuth citrate is used with clarithromycin to treat active duodenal ulcer associated with *Helicobacter pylori* infection.

### Gastric ulcer

Cimetidine famotidine, nizatidine, and ranitidine are indicated for acute gastric ulcer. However, the benefits of long-term therapy (over 8 weeks) with these drugs remain unproven.

### Hypersecretory states

Cimetidine, famotidine, nizatidine, and ranitidine are used to treat hypersecretory states such as Zollinger-Ellison syndrome. Because patients with these conditions require much higher doses than patients with peptic ulcer disease, they may experience more pronounced adverse effects.

### Reflux esophagitis

Cimetidine, famotidine, nizatidine, and ranitidine are used to provide short-term relief from gastroesophageal reflux in patients who don't respond to conventional therapy (lifestyle changes, antacids, diet modification). They act by raising the stomach pH. Some clinicians prefer to combine the H$_2$-receptor antagonist with metoclopramide, but further study is needed to confirm effectiveness of the combination.

### ◊ Stress ulcer prophylaxis

Cimetidine, famotidine, nizatidine, and ranitidine are used to prevent stress ulcers in critically ill patients, particularly those in intensive care units. However, this indication remains unlabeled (FDA-unapproved); some prescribers

## ADULT DOSAGES OF HISTAMINE$_2$-RECEPTOR ANTAGONISTS

| Indication | cimetidine | famotidine | nizatidine | ranitidine |
|---|---|---|---|---|
| Duodenal ulcer | P.O. 800 mg h.s. or 300 mg q.i.d. with meals and h.s. or 400 mg b.i.d. | P.O. 40 mg h.s. or 20 mg b.i.d. | P.O. 300 mg h.s. or 150 mg b.i.d. | P.O. 150 mg b.i.d. or 300 mg once per day after evening meal or h.s. |
| Duodenal ulcer maintenance | P.O. 400 mg h.s. | P.O. 20 mg h.s. | P.O. 150 mg h.s. | P.O. 150 mg h.s. |
| Gastric ulcer | P.O. 800 mg h.s. or 300 mg q.i.d. with meals and h.s. | P.O. 4 0 mg h.s. | P.O. 300 mg h.s. or 150 mg b.i.d. | P.O. 150 mg b.i.d. |
| Gastric ulcer maintenance | NA | NA | NA | P.O. 150 mg h.s. |
| Gastroesophageal reflux disease | P.O. 400 mg q.i.d. or 800 mg b.i.d. | P.O. 20 mg b.i.d. | P.O. 150 mg b.i.d. | P.O. 150 mg b.i.d. |
| Erosive esophagitis | P.O. 400 mg q.i.d. or 800 mg b.i.d. | P.O. 20-40 mg b.i.d. | P.O. 150 mg b.i.d. | P.O. 150 mg q.i.d. |
| Erosive esophagitis healing maintenance | NA | NA | NA | P.O. 150 mg b.i.d. |
| Pathological hypersecretory conditions | P.O. 300 mg q.i.d. with meals and h.s. | P.O. 20 mg q 6 hrs | NA | P.O. 150 mg b.i.d. |
| Prevention of upper GI bleeding | I.V.: 50 mg/hr continuous infusion | NA | NA | NA |
| Heartburn, acid indigestion, sour stomach | P.O. 200 mg, p.r.n., up to 200 mg b.i.d. | P.O. 10 mg, p.r.n., up to 10 mg b.i.d. | P.O. 75 mg, p.r.n., up to 75 mg b.i.d. | P.O. 75 mg, p.r.n., up to 75 mg b.i.d. |
| Product information | Tablet: 100 mg (OTC), 200 mg, 300 mg, 400 mg, 800 mg Liquid: 300 mg/5 ml Injection: 300 mg/ 2 ml Injection, premixed: 300 mg/50 ml normal saline, 300 mg/2 ml | Tablet: 10 mg (OTC), 20 mg, 40 mg Oral suspension: 40 mg/5 ml Injection: 10 mg/ml Injection, premixed: 20 mg/50 ml in normal saline | Capsule: 75 mg (OTC), 150 mg, 300 mg | Tablet: 75 mg (OTC), 150 mg, 300 mg Effervescent tablet: 150 mg Effervescent granule: 150 mg Capsule: 150 mg, 300 mg Syrup: 15 mg/ml Injection: 0.5 mg/ ml, 25 mg/ml |

NA: Not FDA-approved.

prefer intensive antacid therapy for such patients.

◇ *Other uses*

H$_2$-receptor antagonists have been used for a number of other unlabeled indications, including short-bowel syndrome, prophylaxis for allergic reactions to I.V. contrast medium, and eradication of *H. pylori* in treatment of peptic ulcers. Ranitidine bismuth citrate with clarithromycin is used to treat *H. pylori* infection.

Other uses include relief of occasional heartburn, acid indigestion, or sour stomach.

## Pharmacology

All H$_2$-receptor antagonists inhibit the action of histamine at H$_2$ receptors in gastric parietal cells, reducing gastric acid output and level regardless of the stimulatory agent (histamine, food, insulin, caffeine, betazole, pentagastrin) or basal conditions.

## Overview of adverse reactions

H$_2$-receptor antagonists rarely cause adverse reactions. However, mild transient diarrhea, neutropenia, dizziness, fatigue, arrhythmias, and gynecomastia have been reported.

## HISTAMINE$_2$-RECEPTOR ANTAGONISTS: DOSAGE ADJUSTMENTS FOR RENAL IMPAIRMENT

| Drug | Estimated creatinine clearance (ml/min) | Recommended dosage adjustment |
|------|------------------------------------------|-------------------------------|
| cimetidine | 20-40 | q 8 hr or 75% of normal dose |
| famotidine | < 10 | q 24 hr or 50% of normal dose |
| nizatidine | 20-50 | 150 mg/day (active treatment) or 150 mg q other day (maintenance) |
| ranitidine | < 50 | 150 mg q 24 hr; increase to every 12 hr as tolerated |

Cimetidine may inhibit hepatic enzymes, thereby impairing the metabolism of certain drugs. Ranitidine may also produce this effect, but to a lesser extent. Famotidine and nizatidine haven't been shown to inhibit hepatic enzymes or drug clearance.

### Clinical considerations
■ Give a single daily dose h.s., twice-daily doses morning and evening, and multiple doses with meals and h.s. Most prescribers prefer the once-daily dose h.s. regimen for improved compliance.
■ Advise clinician that when administering drugs I.V., not to exceed recommended infusion rates because this may increase the risk of adverse CV effects. Continuous I.V. infusion may yield better suppression of acid secretion.
■ Advise clinician that because antacids may decrease drug absorption, they should be given at least 1 hour apart from H$_2$-receptor antagonists.
■ Patients with renal disease may require a modified schedule. (See *Histamine$_2$-receptor antagonists: Dosage adjustments for renal impairment.*)
■ Avoid discontinuing these drugs abruptly.
■ Many investigational uses for these drugs (particularly cimetidine) are being evaluated. Ranitidine bismuth citrate shouldn't be prescribed alone for the treatment of active duodenal ulcers.
■ Symptomatic response to therapy doesn't rule out gastric malignancy.

### Special populations
**Pregnant patients.** There are no adequate controlled studies in pregnant women. Cimetidine may potentially result in reversible decreased sperm levels in men.
**Breast-feeding patients.** H$_2$-receptor antagonists may appear in breast milk. Ratio of risk to benefit must be considered.
**Pediatric patients.** Safety and efficacy in children are unknown.
**Geriatric patients.** Use caution when giving these drugs to geriatric patients because of the increased risk of adverse reactions, particularly those affecting the CNS. Dosage adjustment

is required in patients with impaired renal function.

### Patient counseling
Instruct patient to avoid smoking during drug therapy because smoking stimulates gastric acid secretion and worsens the disease.

### Representative combinations
None.

# HMG-CoA reductase inhibitors

**atorvastatin calcium, fluvastatin sodium, lovastatin, pravastatin sodium, simvastatin**

HMG-CoA reductase inhibitors, also known as statins, are a highly effective class of drugs that have become first-line pharmacologic therapy for the management of hypercholesterolemia, and primary and secondary coronary heart disease.

### Clinical indications and actions
*CV events*
All statins are indicated for the treatment of primary hypercholesterolemia and mixed dyslipidemia. Atorvastatin, pravastatin, and simvastatin are indicated for hypertriglyceridemia and primary dysbetalipoproteinemia. Atorvastatin and simvastatin are indicated for homozygous familial hyperlipidemia. Lovastatin and pravastatin are indicated for the primary prevention of coronary events. All statins except atorvastatin and cerivastatin are indicated for the secondary prevention of CV events.
*Other uses*
◊ *Lovastatin:* diabetic dyslipidemia, nephrotic hyperlipidemia, neck artery disease, familial beta dysbetalipoproteinemia, and familial combined hyperlipidemia.
◊ *Pravastatin:* heterozygous familial hypercholesterolemia, diabetic dyslipidemia in non–insulin-dependent diabetes, hypercholesterolemia secondary to the nephrotic syn-

## COMPARING HMG-CoA REDUCTASE INHIBITORS

| Drug | Usual dose | Absolute bioavailability | Metabolism enzymes | Active metabolite | Excretion (%) |
|------|-----------|-------------------------|-------------------|-------------------|---------------|
| atorvastatin | 10-80 mg/day | 14 | CYP3A4 | Yes | < 2 (urine) |
| fluvastatin | 20-80 mg/day h.s. | 24 | CYP2C9, 2C8, 3A4 | Yes | < 6 (urine) ~90 (feces) |
| lovastatin | 20-80 mg/day with evening meal | < 5 | CYP3A4 | No | 10 (urine) 83 (feces) |
| pravastatin | 10-40 mg/day | 17 | Not reported | No | ~ 20 (urine) 70 (feces) |
| simvastatin | 5-80 mg/day in evening | < 5 | CYP3A4 | No | 13 (urine) 60 (feces) |

drome, and homozygous hypercholesterolemia in patients with reduced low-density lipoprotein (LDL) receptor activity.
◇ *Simvastatin:* heterozygous familial hypercholesterolemia, familial combined hyperlipidemia, diabetic dyslipidemia in type II diabetes, hyperlipidemia secondary to the nephrotic syndrome, and homozygous familial hypercholesterolemia in patients with defective LDL receptors.

## Pharmacology

Statins lower cholesterol by competitively inhibiting the enzyme HMG-CoA reductase. This enzyme catalyzes the conversion of HMG-CoA to mevalonate, which is an early rate-limiting step in cholesterol biosynthesis. Statins decrease LDL cholesterol (LDL-C), total cholesterol (total-C), apoprotein B (apo-B), very low-density lipoprotein (VLDL) cholesterol, and plasma triglycerides, and increase high-density lipoprotein cholesterol (HDL-C). Coronary artery disease may be caused by increased levels of total cholesterol, apo-B, and LDL-C, as well as by decreased levels of HDL-C. In addition, CV morbidity and mortality rates vary directly with the level of total-C and LDL-C, and inversely with the level of HDL-C. The mechanism by which statins lower LDL-C may be related to both a reduction of VLDL cholesterol and an induction of the LDL receptor, which results in reduced synthesis or increased breakdown of LDL-C.

Statins are highly effective at lowering total-C and LDL-C in patients with heterozygous familial and nonfamilial forms of hypercholesterolemia. Initial cholesterol-lowering effects are seen within 1 to 2 weeks, with maximum lowering effects seen within 4 to 6 weeks. Because cholesterol synthesis occurs mainly at night, single daily doses of all the drugs except atorvastatin and pravastatin should be given in the evening or h.s. Lovastatin should be taken with the evening meal because food increases its absorption. (See *Comparing HMG-CoA reductase inhibitors.*)

## Overview of adverse reactions

Statins are well-tolerated and have very few side effects. Adverse reactions include photosensitivity; hepatotoxicity defined as an increase in transaminase levels to greater than 3 times normal; mild, nonspecific GI complaints; transient and mild increase in creatine phosphokinase (CPK) levels; myopathy characterized by myalgia; and muscle weakness associated with CPK values greater than 10 times the upper limit of normal. Lovastatin and simvastatin may cause insomnia.

A rare hypersensitivity syndrome has been reported. It's characterized by at least one of the following features: anaphylaxis, angioedema, lupus erythematosus-like syndrome, polymyalgia rheumatica, vasculitis, purpura, thrombocytopenia, leukopenia, hemolytic anemia, positive antinuclear antibodies, increased erythrocyte sedimentation rate, eosinophilia, arthritis, asthenia, photosensitivity, fever, chills, flushing, malaise, dyspnea, toxic epidermal necrolysis, erythema multiforme, and dermatomyositis.

## Clinical considerations

■ Statins are contraindicated in pregnancy and lactation, as well as in patients with active liver disease or unexplained persistent elevations of liver function test (LFT) results.
■ Consider myopathy in any patient with diffuse myalgias, muscle tenderness, weakness, or CPK increases greater than 10 times the upper limit of normal. Discontinue drug if markedly elevated CPK levels occur or if myopathy is suspected. Don't exceed 20 mg/day of lovastatin or 10 mg/day of simvastatin in patients taking cyclosporine or itraconazole.
■ Suggest withholding or discontinuing statins in patients with risk factors for renal failure secondary to rhabdomyolysis, including severe acute infection, sepsis, hypotension, major surgery, trauma, uncontrolled seizures, and severe metabolic, endocrine, or electrolyte disorders.

- Use statins with caution in patients who consume large quantities of alcohol.
- Advise clinician to monitor liver function test results before the initiation of statins and at 6 and 12 weeks after the start or change of treatment, and periodically (such as semiannually) thereafter. Drug should be stopped if AST increases more than 3 times upper limits of normal.
- Advise clinician to closely monitor patients taking pravastatin with renal insufficiency.
- The absorption of lovastatin is increased when taken with food, and it should be taken with the evening meal. All other statins, except atorvastatin and pravastatin, may be taken without regard to meals, but should be taken in the evening or at bedtime, because most cholesterol synthesis occurs at night.
- The risk of myopathy is increased when statins are taken with cyclosporine, erythromycin, gemfibrozil, fibric acid derivatives, azole antifungals, certain macrolides or lipid-lowering doses of niacin.
- Because of increased risk of myopathy, avoid concurrent use of statins with fibrates.

### Special populations
**Pregnant patients.** Statin drugs are pregnancy category X and are contraindicated during pregnancy. Cholesterol is essential for fetal development and drugs that inhibit cholesterol synthesis may have adverse effects on the developing fetus. If patients become pregnant while taking a statin, discontinue the drug immediately.
**Breast-feeding patients.** Some statins appear in breast milk. Because of the potential adverse effects, women shouldn't take statins while breast-feeding.
**Pediatric patients.** Safety and efficacy in patients under age 18 haven't been established; use isn't recommended.
**Geriatric patients.** Plasma levels don't vary with age for cerivastatin, fluvastatin, and atorvastatin. In patients over age 70, the area under the curve is increased with lovastatin and simvastatin. For pravastatin, patients over age 65 show a greater effect on LDL-C, total-C, and LDL:HDL ratio compared to patients under age 65.

### Patient counseling
- Tell patient that statin drugs may cause photosensitivity and to avoid prolonged exposure to sun and other sources of ultraviolet light. Advise patient to wear protective clothing and use sunblock.
- Instruct a woman of child-bearing age on the potential hazards of statin drugs in pregnancy. Tell her to discontinue drug immediately if she becomes pregnant and to notify her prescriber.
- Instruct patient to promptly notify prescriber if he experiences any unexplained muscle pain,

tenderness, or weakness, especially if accompanied by malaise or fever.
- Instruct patient on the importance of adhering to dietary recommendations.
- Tell patient to take lovastatin with the evening meal; fluvastatin and simvastatin may be taken without regard to meals but should be taken in the evening or h.s. for best results; atorvastatin or pravastatin may be taken without regard to meals and at any time of the day.

### Representative combinations
None.

---

# nitrates

### amyl nitrite, isosorbide dinitrate, isosorbide mononitrate, nitroglycerin, pentaerythritol tetranitrate

---

Nitrates have been recognized as effective vasodilators for longer than 100 years. The best-known drug of this group, nitroglycerin, remains the therapeutic mainstay for classic and variant angina. With the availability of a commercial I.V. nitroglycerin form, use of the drug in reducing afterload and preload in various cardiac disorders has generated renewed enthusiasm. Various other dosage forms of nitroglycerin and of other nitrates also are available, thereby improving and extending their clinical usefulness.

### Clinical indications and actions
*Angina pectoris*
By relaxing vascular smooth muscle in both the venous and arterial beds, nitrates cause a net decrease in myocardial oxygen consumption; by dilating coronary vessels, they lead to redistribution of blood flow to ischemic tissue. Although systemic and coronary vascular effects may vary slightly, depending on which nitrate is used, both smooth muscle relaxation and vasodilation probably account for the value of nitrates in treating angina. Because individual nitrates have similar pharmacologic and therapeutic properties, the best nitrate to use in a specific situation depends mainly on the onset of action and duration of effect required.

S.L. nitroglycerin is considered the drug of choice to treat acute angina pectoris because of its rapid onset of action, relatively low cost, and well-established effectiveness. Lingual or buccal nitroglycerin and other rapidly acting nitrates, such as amyl nitrite and S.L. or chewable isosorbide dinitrate, also may be useful for this indication. Amyl nitrite is rarely used because it's expensive, inconvenient, and carries a high risk of adverse effects. S.L., lingual, or buccal nitroglycerin, or S.L. or chewable isosorbide dinitrate or mononitrate is typically effective in circumstances likely to provoke an angina attack.

Beta blockers are usually considered the drug of choice in the prophylactic management of angina pectoris. Nitrates with a relatively long duration of effect include oral preparations of isosorbide mononitrate and isosorbide dinitrate, and oral or topical nitroglycerin. Combination treatment of beta blockers and nitrates appears to be the therapy of choice.

The effectiveness of oral nitrates is debatable, although isosorbide dinitrate, isosorbide mononitrate, and nitroglycerin generally are considered effective. However, the effectiveness of topical nitroglycerin preparations hasn't been fully determined. Some experts believe oral nitrates are ineffective or less effective than rapidly acting I.V. nitrates in reducing frequency of angina and increasing exercise tolerance. Also, prolonged use of oral nitrates may cause cross-tolerance to S.L. nitrates.

I.V. nitroglycerin may be used to treat unstable angina pectoris, Prinzmetal's angina, and angina pectoris in patients who haven't responded to recommended doses of nitrates or a beta blocker.

Sedatives may be useful in the adjunctive management of angina pectoris caused by psychogenic factors. However, if combination therapy is required, each drug should be adjusted individually; fixed combinations of oral nitrates and sedatives should be avoided.

*Acute MI*

The hemodynamic effects of I.V., S.L., or topical nitroglycerin may prove beneficial in treating left ventricular failure and pulmonary congestion associated with acute MI. However, the effects of the drug on morbidity and mortality in patients with these conditions is controversial.

I.V., S.L., and topical nitroglycerin and isosorbide dinitrate are effective adjunctive agents in managing acute and chronic heart failure. S.L. administration can quickly reverse the signs and symptoms of pulmonary congestion in acute pulmonary edema; however, the I.V. form may control hemodynamic status more accurately.

*Other uses*

I.V. nitroglycerin is used to control perioperative hypertension, hypertensive emergencies, HF, and pulmonary edema caused by MI.

◊ I.V. nitroglycerin has been used to treat severe hypertension and hypertensive crises; other forms have been used to treat refractory HF. Nitroglycerin also has been used for relief of pain, dysphagia, and spasm in patients with diffuse esophageal spasm without gastroesophageal reflux.

Nitroglycerin treatment has also been instituted for cocaine overdose to reverse coronary vasoconstriction.

## Pharmacology

The major pharmacologic property of nitrates is vascular smooth muscle relaxation, resulting in generalized vasodilation. Venous effects predominate; however, nitroglycerin produces dose-dependent dilatation of both arterial and venous beds. Nitrates are metabolized to a free radical nitric oxide, thought to be an endothelium-derived relaxing factor (EDRF), which is usually impaired in patients with coronary artery disease. Decreased peripheral venous resistance results in venous pooling of blood and decreased venous return to the heart (preload); decreased arteriolar resistance reduces systemic vascular resistance and arterial pressure (afterload). These vascular effects lead to reduction of myocardial oxygen consumption, promoting a more favorable oxygen supply-demand ratio. Although nitrates reflexively increase heart rate and myocardial contractility, reduced ventricular wall tension results in a net decrease in myocardial oxygen consumption. In the coronary circulation, nitrates redistribute circulating blood flow along collateral channels and preferentially increase subendocardial blood flow, improving perfusion to the ischemic myocardium.

Nitrates relax all smooth muscle—not just vascular smooth muscle—regardless of autonomic innervation, including bronchial, biliary, GI, ureteral, and uterine smooth muscle. Nitrates may also have antiplatelet and antithrombic effects.

## Overview of adverse reactions

Headache is most common early in therapy; it may be severe, but usually diminishes rapidly. Orthostatic hypotension, dizziness, weakness, and transient flushing may occur. In patients sensitive to hypotensive effects, nausea, vomiting, weakness, restlessness, pallor, cold sweats, tachycardia, syncope, or CV collapse may occur. Dose reduction may control GI upset; discontinue therapy if blurred vision, dry mouth, or rash develops. Tolerance and dependence can occur with repeated, prolonged use.

Tolerance to both the vascular and antianginal effects of the drugs can develop, and cross-tolerance between the nitrates and nitrites has been demonstrated. Tolerance is associated with a high or sustained plasma drug level and occurs with oral, I.V., and topical therapy. It rarely occurs with intermittent S.L. use. However, patients taking oral isosorbide dinitrate or topical nitroglycerin haven't exhibited cross-tolerance to S.L. nitroglycerin.

Localized effects of tingling or burning may occur with S.L. administration.

To prevent tolerance, the lowest effective dose and an intermittent dosing schedule should be used. A nitrate-free interval of 10 to 12 hours daily may also be helpful.

- Advise patient on chronic NSAID therapy to arrange for monitoring of laboratory parameters, especially BUN, serum creatinine, liver function test results, and CBC.
- Warn patient with current rectal bleeding or history of rectal bleeding to avoid using rectal NSAID suppositories. They may cause irritation and bleeding because they must be retained in the rectum for at least 1 hour.
- Warn patient that use of alcoholic beverages while on NSAID therapy may increase GI irritation and, possibly, GI bleeding.

### Representative combinations
*Diclofenac sodium* and misoprostil: Arthrotec.

# nucleoside reverse transcriptase inhibitors

**abacavir sulfate, didanosine, lamivudine, stavudine, zalcitidine, zidovudine**

These antiviral drugs act specifically against HIV through inhibition of HIV DNA polymerase (reverse transcriptase).

### Clinical indications and actions
*HIV infection and AIDS*
Nucleoside reverse transcriptase inhibitors (NRTIs) are indicated for the treatment of HIV infection and AIDS. Note that two drug regimens containing only nucleoside reverse transcriptase inhibitors are now considered suboptimal. Combination therapy, including protease inhibitors or nonnucleoside reverse transcriptase inhibitors, is recommended. These drugs may also be used for the prevention of maternal-fetal HIV transmission and in the prevention of HIV infection after occupational exposure (such as needlesticks or other parenteral exposures).

### Pharmacology
Nucleoside reverse transcriptase inhibitors suppress HIV replication by inhibition of HIV DNA polymerase. Competitive inhibition of nucleoside reverse transcriptase inhibits DNA viral replication by chain termination, competitive inhibition of reverse transcriptase, or both. (See *Comparing nucleoside reverse transcriptase inhibitors,* pages 52 and 53.)

### Overview of adverse reactions
Because of the complexity of HIV infection, it's often difficult to distinguish between disease-related symptoms and adverse drug reactions. The most frequently reported side effects of nucleoside reverse transcriptase inhibitors include anemia, leukopenia, and neutropenia. Less frequent side effects include thrombocytopenia. Rare side effects include hepatotoxicity, myopathy, and neurotoxicity. There have also been reports of lactic acidosis and hepatomegaly, including fatalities. The occurrence of any of the aforementioned side effects requires prompt medical attention. The following side effects don't require medical attention unless they persist or are bothersome: headache, severe insomnia, myalgias, nausea, or hyperpigmentation of nails.

### Clinical considerations
- Consider the risk-benefit ratio of therapy with nucleoside reverse transcriptase inhibitors on an individual basis when any of the following conditions are present: alcoholism, cardiac disease, hypertriglyceridemia, pancreatitis, bone marrow suppression, fluid overload, folic acid or vitamin $B_{12}$ deficiency, liver dysfunction, peripheral neuropathy, or renal or hepatic dysfunction. These conditions may predispose the patient to adverse drug reactions during treatment.
- The bone marrow suppressant action of the nucleoside reverse transcriptase inhibitors may cause increased susceptibility to certain microbial infections; this effect may be accentuated by other drugs that also cause bone marrow suppression.

#### Special populations
**Pregnant patients.** Pregnancy risk category is C (didanosine is category B). Adequate, well-controlled trials haven't been completed, but the risk of HIV transmission to the fetus is decreased with the use of nucleoside reverse transcriptase inhibitors during pregnancy. Teratogenicity or ill effects haven't been seen in neonates. This drug crosses the placenta and decreases the perinatal transmission of HIV. Prescribers are encouraged to contact the Antiretroviral Pregnancy Registry at 1-800-258-4263 to report pregnant women on therapy.
**Breast-feeding patients.** The rate and extent of excretion of nucleoside reverse transcriptase inhibitors into breast milk is unknown. Therefore, their use in breast-feeding women isn't recommended. However, the risks and benefits to both the woman and infant must be considered in each case.
**Pediatric patients.** Nucleoside reverse transcriptase inhibitors may be used in children age 3 months or older. The half-life of these drugs may be prolonged in neonates, but otherwise the pharmacokinetic and safety profile of the drug is similar in children and adults.
**Geriatric patients.** Safety and efficacy of nucleoside reverse transcriptase inhibitors in geriatric patients are unknown. Anecdotal evidence suggests that geriatric patients respond well to this therapy, but that they may experience a more prolonged half-life of elimination.

## COMPARING NUCLEOSIDE REVERSE TRANSCRIPTASE INHIBITORS

| Drug | Dosage | Dosage adjustment |
|------|--------|-------------------|
| abacavir sulfate | Adults: 300 mg b.i.d.<br>Children: 8 mg/kg b.i.d. up to a maximum of 300 mg b.i.d. | Not known |
| didanosine | Adults > 132 lb (60 kg): 200 mg (tablets) q 12 hr, or 250 mg (buffered powder) q 12 hr<br>Adults < 132 lb (60 kg): 125 mg (tablets) q 12 hr, or 167 mg (buffered powder) q 12 hr<br>Children: 31 to 125 mg q 8-12 hr based on body surface area | No adjustment for renal or hepatic failure. |
| lamivudine | Adults > 110 lb (50 kg): 150 mg b.i.d.<br>Adults < 110 lb (50 kg): 2 mg/kg b.i.d.<br>Children: 4 mg/kg b.i.d. to maximum of 150 mg q 12 hr | Patients 16 or older with renal impairment require dosage adjustment. |
| stavudine | Adults < 132 lb (60 kg): 30 mg q 12 hr<br>Adults ≥ 132 lb (60 kg): 40 mg q 12 hr<br>Children 66-132 lb (30-60 kg): 30 mg q 12 hr<br>Children < 66 lb (30 kg): 1 mg/kg q 12 hr | Patients with CrCl < 50 ml/min may require dosage adjustment. |
| zalcitidine | Adults ≥ 66 lb (30 kg): 0.75 mg q 8 hr | Patients with CrCl < 50 ml/min may require dosage adjustment. |
| zidovudine | Adults: 600 mg/day in divided doses<br>Children: 3 months to 12 years: 180 mg/m$^2$ q 6 hr (720 mg/m$^2$/day), not to exceed 200 mg q 6 hr | Anemia, neutropenia, renal disease patients may require adjustment. |

## Patient counseling

■ Tell the patient to take the drug as prescribed, that it's important not to take more or less drug than instructed, and to finish the full course of therapy.

■ Instruct patient not to miss a dose but, if a dose is missed, to take the next dose as soon as possible; the dose shouldn't be doubled.

■ Advise patient to adhere to scheduled prescriber's appointments because important blood tests are needed to evaluate the response to this drug.

■ Tell patient not to take other drugs concurrently without first checking with the pharmacist or prescriber.

■ Instruct patient to floss and brush teeth carefully to prevent unneeded bleeding from the gums.

■ Tell patient to avoid sexual intercourse or to use a condom to decrease the risk of HIV transmission.

## Representative combinations

*Lamivudine and zidovudine* combination (Combivir).

# opioids

**alfentanil hydrochloride, codeine phosphate, codeine sulfate, difenoxin hydrochloride, diphenoxylate hydrochloride, fentanyl citrate, hydromorphone hydrochloride, levomethadyl acetate hydrochloride, meperidine hydrochloride, methadone hydrochloride, morphine sulfate, oxycodone hydrochloride, oxymorphone hydrochloride, propoxyphene hydrochloride, propoxyphene napsylate, remifentanil hydrochloride, sufentanil citrate**

Opioids, previously called narcotic agonists, are usually understood to include natural and semisynthetic alkaloid derivatives from opium and their synthetic surrogates, whose actions mimic those of morphine. Most of these drugs are classified as Schedule II by the Drug Enforcement Agency because they have a high potential for addiction and abuse. In the past, opioids were used indiscriminately for analgesia and sedation and to control diarrhea and cough. (See *Comparing opioids,* page 54.)

| Oral bioavailability | Plasma protein–binding (%) | Half-life (hr) | Elimination | Dialyzability |
|---|---|---|---|---|
| 83%; may be taken with or without food | About 50 | 1½ | Renal clearance accounts for 82.2%; fecal elimination is 16% | Not known |
| Acid labile, variable absorption, take on an empty stomach | < 5 | Adults: ¾-2¾ Children: ½-1¼ Severe renal failure: 4½ | Renal clearance by glomerular filtration and active tubular secretion accounts for 50% of total body clearance | 20% loss following a 4-hr dialysis |
| 60%-88%; food reduces the rate but not the extent of absorption | 36 | Adults: 2-11 Children: 1¾-2 CrCl 10-40 ml/min: 13½ CrCl < 10 ml/min: 19½ | Renal clearance by glomerular filtration and active tubular secretion accounts for 68%-71% of total body clearance | Not known |
| 78%-86%; may take with or without food | Negligible | Adults: 1-1½ Children: 1-1¼ CrCl < 25 ml/min: 4¾ | Renal clearance by glomerular filtration and active tubular secretion; 40% is excreted unchanged in 6-24 hr | Not known |
| 80% in adults; 54% in children. Food decreases bioavailability by 14% | < 4 | Adults: 1-3 Children: ¾ CrCl < 55 ml/min: 8½ | 70% excreted unchanged in urine | Not known |
| 65%; unknown effect of food on bioavailability | 34-38 | Adults: 1 CrCl < 20 ml/min: 1½ | 90% excreted in urine | Negligible effect |

## Clinical indications and actions

The opioids produce varying degrees of analgesia and have antitussive, antidiarrheal, and sedative effects. Clinical response is dose-related and varies with each patient.

### Analgesia

Opioids may be used in the symptomatic management of moderate to severe pain associated with acute and some chronic disorders, including renal or biliary colic, MI, acute trauma, postoperative pain, or terminal cancer. They also may be used to provide analgesia during diagnostic and orthopedic procedures and during labor. Drug selection, route of administration, and dose depend on a variety of factors. For example, in mild pain, oral therapy with codeine or oxycodone usually suffices. In acute pain of known short duration, such as that caused by diagnostic procedures or orthopedic manipulation, a short-acting drug such as meperidine or fentanyl is effective. These drugs are often given to alleviate postoperative pain, but because they influence CNS function, special care should be taken to monitor the course of recovery and to detect early signs of complications. Opioids are commonly used to manage severe, chronic pain from terminal cancer; this treatment requires careful evaluation and titration of drug, dose, and route of administration.

### Pulmonary edema

Morphine, meperidine, oxymorphone, hydromorphone, and other similar drugs have been used to relieve anxiety in patients with dyspnea from acute pulmonary edema and acute left ventricular failure. These drugs shouldn't be used to treat pulmonary edema from a chemical respiratory stimulant. Opioids decrease peripheral resistance, causing pooling of blood in the limbs and decreased venous return, cardiac workload, and pulmonary venous pressure; blood is shifted from the central to the peripheral circulation.

### Preoperative sedation

Routine use of opioids for preoperative sedation in patients without pain isn't recommended because it may cause complications during and after surgery. To allay preoperative anxiety, a barbiturate or benzodiazepine is equally effective, with a lower risk of postoperative vomiting.

### Anesthesia

Certain opioids, including alfentanil, fentanyl, remifentanil, and sufentanil, may be used for induction of anesthesia, as an adjunct in the maintenance of general and regional anesthesia, or as the primary anesthetic drug in surgery.

## COMPARING OPIOIDS

| Drug | Route | Onset (min) | Peak | Duration (hr) |
|------|-------|-------------|------|---------------|
| alfentanil | I.V. | Immediate | Not available | Not available |
| codeine | I.M., P.O., S.C. | 15-30 | 30-60 min | 4-6 |
| fentanyl | I.M., I.V. | 7-8 | Not available | 1-2 |
| hydrocodone | P.O. | 30 | 60 min | 4-6 |
| hydromorphone | I.M., I.V., S.C. | 15 | 30 min | 4-5 |
|  | P.O., rectal | 30 | 60 min | 4-5 |
| meperidine | I.M. | 10-15 | 30-50 min | 2-4 |
|  | P.O. | 15-30 | 60 min | 2-4 |
|  | S.C. | 10-15 | 40-60 min | 2-4 |
| methadone | I.M., P.O., S.C. | 30-60 | 30-60 min | 4-6 † |
| morphine | I.M. | ≤ 20 | 30-60 min | 3-7 |
|  | P.O., rectal | ≤ 20 | ≤ 60 min | 3-7 |
|  | S.C. | ≤ 20 | 50-90 min | 3-7 |
| oxycodone | P.O. | 15-30 | 30-60 min | 4-6 |
| oxymorphone | I.M., S.C. | 10-15 | 30-60 min | 3-6 |
|  | I.V. | 5-10 | 30-60 min | 3-6 |
|  | rectal | 15-30 | 30-60 min | 3-6 |
| propoxyphene | P.O. | 20-60 | 2-2½ hr | 4-6 |
| remifentanil | I.V. | Immediate | Not available | Not available |
| sufentanil | I.V. | 1.3-3 | Not available | Not available |

† Because of cumulative effects, duration of action increases with repeated doses.

### Cough suppression

Some opioids, most commonly codeine and its derivative, hydrocodone, are used as antitussives to relieve dry, nonproductive cough.

### Diarrhea

Diphenoxylate and other opioids are used as antidiarrheal drugs. All opioids cause constipation to some degree; however, only a few are indicated for this use. Usually, opiate antidiarrheals are empirically combined with antacids, absorbing agents, and belladonna alkaloids in commercial preparations.

## Pharmacology

Opioids act as agonists at specific opiate receptor binding sites in the CNS and other tissues; these are the same receptors occupied by endogenous opioid peptides (enkephalins and endorphins) to alter CNS response to painful stimuli. Opiate agonists don't alter the cause of pain, but instead the patient's perception of the pain; they relieve pain without affecting other sensory functions. Opiate receptors are present in highest levels in the limbic system, thalamus, striatum, hypothalamus, midbrain, and spinal cord.

Opioids produce respiratory depression by a direct effect on the respiratory centers in the brain stem, resulting in decreased sensitivity and responsiveness to increases in carbon dioxide tension. The antitussive effects of these drugs are mediated by a direct suppression of the cough reflex center. They cause nausea, probably by stimulation of the chemoreceptor trigger zone in the medulla oblongata; through orthostatic hypotension, which causes dizziness; and possibly by increasing vestibular sensitivity.

Opioids also cause drowsiness, sedation, euphoria, dysphoria, mental clouding, and EEG changes; higher than usual analgesic doses cause anesthesia. Most opioids cause miosis, although meperidine and its derivatives may also cause mydriasis or no pupillary change.

Because opioids decrease gastric, biliary, and pancreatic secretions and delay digestion, constipation is a common adverse reaction. At the same time, these drugs increase tone in the biliary tract and may cause biliary spasms. Some patients may have no biliary effects, whereas others may have biliary spasms that increase plasma amylase and lipase levels up to 15 times normal values.

Opioids increase smooth muscle tone in the urinary tract and induce spasms, causing urinary urgency. These drugs have little CV effect in a supine patient, but may cause orthostatic hypotension when the patient assumes upright posture. These drugs are also associated with manifestations of histamine release or peripheral vasodilation, including pruritus, flushing, red eyes, and sweating. These effects are often mistakenly attributed to allergy and should be evaluated carefully.

Opiates can be divided chemically into three groups: phenanthrenes (codeine, hydrocodone, hydromorphone, morphine, oxycodone, and oxymorphone); diphenylheptanes (levomethadyl, methadone, and propoxyphene); and phenylpiperidines (alfentanil, diphenoxylate, fentanyl, meperidine, and remifentanil, sufentanil). If a patient is hypersensitive to an opioid, agonist-antagonist, or antagonist of a given chemical group, use extreme caution in considering the use of another drug from the same chemical group; however, a drug from the other groups might be well tolerated.

Some opioids are well absorbed after oral or rectal administration; others must be given parenterally. I.V. dosing is the most rapidly effective and reliable; absorption after I.M. or S.C. dosing may be erratic. Opioids vary in onset and duration of action; they are removed rapidly from the bloodstream and distributed, in decreasing order of concentration, into skeletal muscle, kidneys, liver, intestinal tract, lungs, spleen, and brain; they readily cross the placenta.

Opioids are metabolized mainly in the microsomes in the endoplasmic reticulum of the liver (first-pass effect) and also in the CNS, kidneys, lungs, and placenta. They undergo conjugation with glucuronic acid, hydrolysis, oxidation, or N-dealkylation. They are excreted primarily in the urine; small amounts are excreted in the feces.

## Overview of adverse reactions

Respiratory depression and, to a lesser extent, circulatory depression (including orthostatic hypotension) are the major hazards of treatment with opioids. Rapid I.V. administration increases the risk and severity of these serious adverse effects. Respiratory arrest, shock, and cardiac arrest have occurred. It's likely that equianalgesic doses of individual opiates produce a comparable degree of respiratory depression, but its duration may vary. Other adverse CNS effects include dizziness, visual disturbances, mental clouding or depression, sedation, coma, euphoria, dysphoria, weakness, faintness, agitation, restlessness, nervousness, seizures, and, rarely, delirium and insomnia. Adverse effects seem to be more prevalent in ambulatory patients and those without severe pain. Adverse GI effects include nausea, vomiting, and constipation, as well as increased biliary tract pressure that may result in biliary spasm or colic. Tolerance, psychological dependence, and physical dependence (addiction) may follow prolonged, high-dose therapy (more than 100 mg of morphine daily for longer than 1 month).

Use opiate agonists with extreme caution during pregnancy and labor, because they readily cross the placenta. Premature infants appear especially sensitive to their respiratory and CNS depressant effects when used during delivery.

Opiate agonists have a high potential for addiction and should always be given with caution in patients susceptible to physical or psychological dependence. The agonist-antagonists have a lower potential for addiction and abuse, but the liability still exists.

## Clinical considerations

- Advise clinician to administer with extreme caution to patients with head injury, increased intracranial pressure, seizures, asthma, COPD, alcoholism, prostatic hypertrophy, severe hepatic or renal disease, acute abdominal conditions, arrhythmias, hypovolemia, or psychiatric disorders, and to geriatric or debilitated patients. Reduced doses may be needed.
- Resuscitative equipment and a narcotic antagonist (naloxone) should be available. Prescribers should be prepared to provide support of ventilation and gastric lavage.
- Parenteral administration of opiates provides better analgesia than oral administration. Give I.V. administration by slow injection, preferably in diluted solution. Rapid I.V. injection increases the risk of adverse effects.
- Advise clinician to give parenteral injections by I.M. or S.C. route cautiously to patients who are chilled, hypovolemic, or in shock, because decreased perfusion may lead to accumulation of the drug and toxic effects. I.M. or S.C. injection sites should be rotated to avoid induration.
- A regular dosing schedule (rather than "as needed for pain") is preferred to alleviate the symptoms and anxiety that accompany pain.
- Duration of respiratory depression may be longer than the analgesic effect. Advise clinician to monitor patient closely with repeated dosing.
- With chronic administration, advise clinician that the patient's respiratory status be evaluated before each dose. Because severe respiratory depression may occur (especially with accumulation from chronic dosing), watch for respiratory rate below the patient's baseline level. Evaluate the patient for restlessness, which may be a sign of compensatory response for hypoxia.
- Opiates or agonist-antagonists may cause orthostatic hypotension in ambulatory patients. The patient should sit or lie down to relieve dizziness or fainting.
- Because opiates depress respiration when used postoperatively, encourage patient turning, coughing, and deep breathing to avoid atelectasis.

■ Advise clinician that if gastric irritation occurs, give oral products with food; food delays absorption and onset of analgesia.

■ Opiates may obscure the signs and symptoms of an acute abdominal condition or worsen gallbladder pain.

■ The antitussive activity of opiates is used to control persistent, exhausting cough or dry, nonproductive cough.

■ The first sign of tolerance to the therapeutic effect of opioid agonists or agonist-antagonists is usually a shortened duration of effect.

■ Preservative-free morphine (Astramorph, Duramorph) is available for epidural or intrathecal use.

### Special populations

**Pregnant patients.** Meperidine and oxymorphone hydrochloride are classified as pregnancy risk category B, but D if used for a prolonged time or for high doses used at term. Most opioids are listed as pregnancy risk category C. Administration of an opiate to a woman shortly before delivery may cause respiratory depression in the neonate. Monitor closely and be prepared to resuscitate. In animal studies, some opiate antagonists have been shown to be teratogenic.

**Breast-feeding patients.** Codeine, meperidine, methadone, morphine, and propoxyphene appear in breast milk and should be used with caution in breast-feeding women. Methadone has been shown to cause physical dependence in breast-feeding infants of women maintained on methadone.

**Pediatric patients.** Safety and efficacy in children haven't been established. Use care when giving to children.

**Geriatric patients.** Lower doses are usually indicated for geriatric patients, who may be more sensitive to the therapeutic and adverse effects of drug.

### Patient counseling

■ Instruct patient to use drug with caution and to avoid hazardous activities that require full alertness and coordination.

■ Tell patient to avoid drinking alcohol when taking opioid agonists, because alcohol causes additive CNS depression.

■ Explain that constipation may result from taking an opiate. Suggest measures to increase dietary fiber content, or recommend a stool softener.

■ If patient's condition allows, instruct patient to breathe deeply, cough, and change position every 2 hours to avoid respiratory complications.

■ Encourage patient to void at least every 4 hours to avoid urine retention.

■ Tell the patient to take drug as prescribed and to call prescriber if significant adverse effects occur.

■ Tell patient not to increase dose if he isn't experiencing the desired effect, but to call for prescribed dosage adjustment.

■ Instruct the patient not to double the dose. Tell him to take a missed dose as soon as he remembers unless it's almost time for the next dose. If this is the case, he should skip the missed dose and go back to the regular dosing schedule.

■ Tell patient to call immediately for emergency help if he thinks he or someone else has taken an overdose.

■ Explain signs of overdose to patient and his family.

### Representative combinations

*Codeine* with acetaminophen: Phenaphen with codeine, Tylenol with codeine, Capital with codeine, Aceta with codeine, Acetaminophen with Codeine Oral Solution, Acetaminophen with Codeine Tablets, Margesic No. 3, Tylenol with Codeine No. 4, Phenaphen with Codeine No. 4; with caffeine: Fioricet with codeine; with calcium iodide and alcohol: Calcidrine.

*Codeine phosphate* with guaifenesin: Cheracol, Guiatuss AC, Guiatussin with Codeine Liquid, Mytussin AC, Robitussin A-C, Tolu-Sed Cough; with iodinated glycerol: Tussi-Organidin NR; with triprolidine hydrochloride and pseudoephedrine hydrochloride: Actifed with Codeine.

*Codeine* with aspirin: Empirin with codeine, Aspirin with Codeine No. 3, Aspirin with Codeine No. 4.

*Codeine and aspirin* with caffeine and butalbital: Fiorinal with Codeine; with carisoprodol: Soma Compound with Codeine.

*Dihydrocodeine* with acetaminophen and caffeine: Synalgos-DC.

*Fentanyl* with droperidol: Innovar, Fentanyl Citrate and Droperidol.

*Hydrocodone bitartrate* with acetaminophen: Anexsia 5/500 Tablets, Anexsia 7.5/650 Tablets, Anexsia 10/660 Tablets, Bancap HC, Dolacet, Duocet, Hydrocet, Lorcet-HD, Lorcet Plus, Zydone, Lortab, Lortab Elixir, Co-Gesic, Damason-P, Hydrogesic, Hy-Phen, Vicodin, Vicodin ES, Hydrocodone Bitartrate and Acetaminophen Tablets; with aspirin: Lortab ASA, Panasal 5/500; with aspirin and caffeine: Damason-P; with aspirin, acetaminophen, and caffeine: Hyco-Pap; with guaifenesin: Hycotuss Expectorant Syrup (with alcohol); with guaifenesin and pseudoephedrine hydrochloride: Detussin Expectorant, Entuss-D; with guaifenesin and phenindamine tartrate: P-V-Tussin tablets; with guaifenesin and phenylephrine: Donatussin DC; with potassium guaiacosulfonate: Codiclear DH, Entuss-D Liquid; with pseudoephedrine hydrochloride: Detussin Liquid; with homatropine methylbromide: Hycodan; with phenylephrine hydrochloride and pyrilamine maleate: Codimal DH; with phenylpropanolamine hydrochloride: Hycomine; with phenylephrine hydrochloride, pyrilamine maleate, chlorpheniramine maleate salicylamide, citric acid, and caffeine: Citra Forte; with pheniramine maleate, pyrilamine maleate, potassium citrate, and ascorbic acid: Citra forte; with phenylephrine hydrochloride, phenylpropanolamine hydrochloride, pheniramine maleate, pyrilamine maleate, and alcohol: Ru-Tuss with hydrocodone; with guaifenesin and alcohol: S-T forte; with phenyltoloxamine: Tussionex.

*Hydromorphone* with guaifenesin: Dilaudid Cough.

*Meperidine* with promethazine: Mepergan, Mepergan Fortis; with atropine sulfate: Atropine and Demerol Injection.

*Oxycodone hydrochloride* with acetaminophen: Tylox, Roxicet, Roxicet 5/500 Caplets, Roxicet Oral Solution, Oxycodone with Acetaminophen Capsules, Roxilox Capsules, Oxycocet*, Percocet, Percocet-Demi; with aspirin: Oxycodone with Aspirin Tablets, Roxiprin Tablets; with oxycodone terephthalate and aspirin: Percodan, Percodan-Demi.

*Propoxyphene* with acetaminophen: Lorcet, Wygesic, Darvocet-N, Propacet 100, Propoxyphene Napsylate and Acetaminophen, E-Lor Tablets, Genagesic.

*Propoxyphene napsylate* with acetaminophen: Darvocet-N 50, Darvocet-N 100, Propocet 100; with aspirin: Propoxyphene HCl Compound Capsules; with aspirin and caffeine: Darvon Compound, Propoxyphene Compound, PC-CAP.

# opioid (narcotic) agonist-antagonists

**buprenorphine hydrochloride, butorphanol tartate, nalbuphine hydrochloride, pentazocine hydrochloride**

The term "opioid (or narcotic) agonist-antagonist" is somewhat imprecise. This class of drugs has varying degrees of agonist and antagonist activity. These drugs are potent analgesics, with somewhat less addiction potential than the pure narcotic agonists.

## Clinical indications and actions
### Pain
Opioid agonist-antagonists are primarily used as analgesics, particularly in patients at high risk for drug dependence or abuse. Some are used as preoperative or preanesthetic drugs, to supplement balanced anesthesia, or to relieve prepartum pain.

### Other uses
◇ Buprenorphine has been used to reverse fentanyl-induced anesthesia. Buprenorphine and naloxone have been used to reduce opiate consumption in patients who are physically dependent on opiates.

## Pharmacology
The detailed pharmacology of these drugs is poorly understood. Each drug is believed to act on different opiate receptors in the CNS to a greater or lesser degree, thus yielding slightly different effects. Like the opioid agonists, these drugs can be divided into related chemical groups. Buprenorphine, butorphanol, and nalbuphine are phenanthrenes, like morphine, whereas pentazocine falls into a unique class, the benzmorphans.

## Overview of adverse reactions
Major hazards of agonist-antagonists are respiratory depression, apnea, shock, and cardiopulmonary arrest, possibly causing death. All opioid agonist-antagonists can cause respiratory depression, but the severity of such depression each drug can cause has a "ceiling"; for example, each drug depresses respiration to a certain point, but increased doses don't depress it further. All opioid agonist-antagonists have been reported to cause withdrawal symptoms after abrupt discontinuation of long-term use; they appear to have some addiction potential, but less than that of the pure opioid agonists.

CNS effects are the most common adverse reactions and may include drowsiness, sedation, light-headedness, dizziness, hallucinations, disorientation, agitation, euphoria, dysphoria, insomnia, confusion, headache, tremor, miosis, seizures, and psychological dependence. CV reactions may include tachycardia, bradycardia, palpitations, chest wall rigidity, hypertension, hypotension, syncope, and edema. GI reactions may include nausea, vomiting, and constipation (most common), dry mouth, anorexia, and biliary spasms (colic). Other effects include urine retention or hesitancy, decreased libido, flushing, rash, pruritus, and pain at the injection site.

Opioid agonist-antagonists have abuse potential because they can produce morphine-like dependence. Psychological and physiologic dependence with drug tolerance can develop with long-term, repeated administration. Patients with dependence or tolerance to narcotic agonist-antagonists usually present with an acute abstinence syndrome or withdrawal signs and symptoms, of which the severity is related to the degree of dependence, abruptness of withdrawal, and the drug used.

Common signs and symptoms of withdrawal are yawning, lacrimation, and sweating (early); mydriasis, piloerection, flushing of face, tachycardia, tremor, irritability, and anorexia (intermediate); and muscle spasms, fever, nausea, vomiting, and diarrhea (late).

## Clinical considerations

- Opioid agonist-antagonists are contraindicated in patients hypersensitive to any drug of the same chemical group.
- Use these drugs with extreme caution in patients with supraventricular arrhythmias. Avoid or give drug with extreme caution in patients with head injury or increased intracranial pressure, because neurologic parameters are obscured, and during pregnancy and labor, because drug crosses the placenta readily (premature infants are especially sensitive to respiratory and CNS depressant effects of opioid agonist-antagonists).
- Use opioid agonist-antagonists cautiously in patients with renal or hepatic dysfunction, because drug accumulation or prolonged duration of action may occur; in patients with pulmonary disease (asthma, COPD) because drug depresses respiration and suppresses cough reflex; in patients undergoing biliary tract surgery because drug may cause biliary spasm; in patients with convulsive disorders because drug may precipitate seizures; in geriatric and debilitated patients, who are more sensitive to both therapeutic and adverse drug effects; and in patients susceptible to physical or psychological addiction because of the high risk of addiction to this drug.
- Opioid agonist-antagonists have a lower potential for abuse than do opioid agonists, but the risk still exists.
- Before administration, all parenteral products should be visually inspected for particles and discoloration and the strength of the solution noted.
- Parenteral administration of opioid agonist-antagonists provides better analgesia than does oral dosing. Give I.V. dosing by very slow injections, preferably in diluted solution. Rapid I.V. injection increases the risk of adverse effects.
- Give I.M. or S.C. injections cautiously to patients who are chilled, hypovolemic, or in shock, because decreased perfusion may lead to accumulation.
- Opioid agonist-antagonists, as well as opioid antagonists, can reverse the desired effects of opioids; thus, members of different pharmacologic groups (such as meperidine and buprenorphine) shouldn't be prescribed at the same time.
- Advise clinician that resuscitative equipment should be on hand and an opioid antagonist (naloxone) available. Prescribers should be prepared to provide ventilation and gastric lavage.
- Patient tolerance may develop to the opiate agonist activity but doesn't develop to opiate antagonist activity.
- A regular dosing schedule (rather than an "as needed for pain" regimen) is preferable to alleviate the symptoms and anxiety that accompany pain.

- The duration of respiratory depression may be longer than the analgesic effect. Advise clinician to monitor patient closely with repeated dosing.
- During chronic administration, the patient's respiratory status should be regularly evaluated. Because severe respiratory depression may occur (especially with accumulation on chronic dosing), watch for a respiratory rate that's less than the patient's baseline respiratory rate. Patient should also be evaluated for restlessness, which may be a compensatory response to hypoxia.
- Opioid agonist-antagonists may cause orthostatic hypotension in ambulatory patients. Advise patient to sit or lie down to relieve dizziness or fainting.
- Because opioid agonist-antagonists can depress respiration when used postoperatively, strongly encourage patient turning, coughing, and deep breathing to avoid atelectasis. Monitor respiratory status.
- Oral opioid agonist-antagonists may be taken with food to prevent gastric irritation. Food delays absorption and the onset of analgesia.
- Opioid agonist-antagonists may obscure the signs and symptoms of an acute abdominal condition or worsen gallbladder pain.
- The first sign of tolerance to the therapeutic effect of opioid agonist-antagonists is usually a reduced duration of effect.

### Special populations

**Pregnant patients.** Most drugs in this class are pregnancy risk category C. Administering an opiate agonist-antagonist to a woman shortly before delivery may cause respiratory depression in the neonate. The infant must be closely monitored and staff should be prepared to resuscitate.
**Breast-feeding patients.** These drugs aren't recommended for use in breast-feeding women.
**Pediatric patients.** Neonates may be more susceptible to the respiratory depressant effects of opiate agonist-antagonists.
**Geriatric patients.** Lower doses are usually indicated for geriatric patients, who may be more sensitive to the therapeutic and adverse effects of these drugs.

## Patient counseling

- Advise ambulatory patients to be cautious when performing tasks that require alertness, such as driving, if they're taking an opioid agonist-antagonist.
- Warn patient not to stop taking an opioid agonist-antagonist abruptly if he's been taking it for a prolonged period or at a high dose.
- Tell patient not to increase dose if it isn't producing the desired effect, but to call for prescribed dosage adjustment.
- Advise patient to avoid drinking alcohol when taking opioid agonist-antagonists because additive CNS depression will occur.

- Tell patient that constipation may result. Suggest measures to increase dietary fiber content or recommend a stool softener.
- Instruct patient not to double the dose. Tell him to take a missed dose as soon as he remembers unless it's almost time for the next dose. If this is the case, tell him to skip the missed dose and go back to regular dosing schedule.
- Tell patient to call for emergency help if he thinks he or someone else has taken an overdose.
- Explain signs of overdose to patient and to his family.
- Instruct patient to breathe deeply, cough, and change position every 2 hours to avoid respiratory complications.
- Encourage patient to void at least every 4 hours to avoid urine retention.
- Tell patient to take the drug as prescribed and to promptly report any significant adverse effects.
- Inform a woman taking an opioid agonist-antagonist to call prescriber promptly if she is planning or suspects pregnancy; warn that her fetus may become addicted to drug.

### Representative combinations
*Pentazocine* with acetaminophen: Talacen; with aspirin: Talwin Compound; with naloxone: Talwin Nx.
*Buprenorphine* and naloxone.

# penicillins

**Natural penicillins:** penicillin G benzathine, penicillin G potassium, penicillin G procaine, penicillin G sodium, penicillin V potassium

**Aminopenicillins:** amoxicillin trihydrate with clavulanate potassium, ampicillin, ampicillin sodium with sulbactam sodium, ampicillin trihydrate

**Penicillinase-resistant penicillins:** cloxacillin sodium, dicloxacillin sodium, nafcillin sodium, oxacillin sodium

**Extended spectrum penicillins:** carbenicillin indanyl sodium, mezlocillin sodium, piperacillin sodium, piperacillin sodium with tazobactam sodium, ticarcillin disodium, ticarcillin with clavulanate potassium

Penicillin is naturally derived from the mold *Penicillium chrysogenum.* New synthetic derivatives are created by chemical reactions that modify their structure, resulting in increased GI absorption, resistance to destruction by beta-lactamase (penicillinase), and a broader spectrum of susceptible organisms. Penicillins are very effective antibiotics with low toxicity.

## Clinical indications and actions
*Infection caused by susceptible organisms*
*Natural penicillins.* Penicillin G is the prototype of this group; derivatives such as penicillin V are more acid stable and thus better absorbed by the oral route. All natural penicillins are vulnerable to inactivation by beta-lactamase–producing bacteria. Natural penicillins act primarily against gram-positive organisms.

Clinical indications for natural penicillins include streptococcal pneumonia, enterococcal and nonenterococcal group D endocarditis, diphtheria, anthrax, meningitis, tetanus, botulism, actinomycosis, syphilis, relapsing fever, Lyme disease, rat-bite fever, and Whipple's disease. Natural penicillins are used prophylactically against pneumococcal infections, rheumatic fever, bacterial endocarditis, and neonatal group B streptococcal disease.

Susceptible aerobic gram-positive cocci include non–penicillinase-producing *Staphylococcus aureus, Staphylococcus epidermis;* nonenterococcal group D streptococci, groups A, B, C, D, G, H, K, L, and M streptococci, *Streptococcus viridans;* and enterococcus (usually with an aminoglycoside). Susceptible aerobic gram-negative cocci include *Neisseria meningitidis* and non–penicillinase-producing *N. gonorrhoeae.*

Susceptible aerobic gram-positive bacilli include *Corynebacterium* (both diphtheria and opportunistic species), *Listeria,* and *Bacillus anthracis.* Susceptible anaerobes include *Peptococcus, Peptostreptococcus, Actinomyces, Clostridium, Fusobacterium, Veillonella,* and non–beta-lactamase-producing strains of *Streptococcus pneumoniae.* The drugs are also active against some gram-negative aerobic bacilli including some strains of *Haemophilus influenzae, Pasturella multocida, Streptobacillus moniliformis,* and *Spirillum minus.*

Susceptible spirochetes include *Treponema pallidum, Treponema pertenue, Leptospira,* and *Borrelia recurrentis* and possibly *Borrelia burgdorferi.*

*Aminopenicillins* (amoxicillin and ampicillin) offer a broader spectrum of activity including many gram-negative organisms. Like natural penicillins, aminopenicillins are vulnerable to inactivation by penicillinase. They are primarily used to treat septicemia, gynecologic infections, and infections of the urinary, respiratory, and GI tracts, and skin, soft tissue, bones, and joints. Their activity spectrum includes *Escherichia coli, Proteus mirabilis, Shigella, Salmonella, S. pneumoniae, N. gonorrhoeae, H. influenzae, S. aureus,*

*S. epidermidis* (non–penicillinase-producing *Staphylococcus*), and *Listeria monocytogenes*.

*Penicillinase-resistant penicillins* (cloxacillin, dicloxacillin, oxacillin, and nafcillin) are semisynthetic penicillins designed to remain stable against hydrolysis by most staphylococcal penicillinases and thus are the drugs of choice against susceptible penicillinase-producing staphylococci. They also retain activity against most organisms susceptible to natural penicillins. Clinical indications are much the same as for aminopenicillins.

*Extended-spectrum penicillins* (carbenicillin, mezlocillin, piperacillin, and ticarcillin), as their name implies, offer a wider range of bactericidal action than the other three classes, are used in hard-to-treat gram-negative infections, and are usually given with aminoglycosides. They are used most often against susceptible strains of *Enterobacter, Klebsiella, Citrobacter, Serratia, Bacteroides fragilis, and Pseudomonas aeruginosa;* their gram-negative spectrum also includes *Proteus vulgaris, Proteus mirabilis, Providencia rettgeri, Salmonella, Shigella,* and *Morganella morganii.* These penicillins are also vulnerable to destruction by beta-lactamase or penicillinases.

## Pharmacology

The basic structure of penicillin is a thiazolidine ring connected to a beta-lactam ring that contains a side chain. This nucleus is the main structural requirement for antibacterial activity; modifications of the side chain alter the antibacterial and pharmacologic effects of penicillin.

Penicillins are generally bactericidal. They inhibit synthesis of the bacterial cell wall, causing rapid cell lysis, and are most effective against fast-growing susceptible bacteria.

The sites of action for penicillins are enzymes known as penicillin-binding proteins (PBPs). The affinity of certain penicillins for PBPs in various microorganisms helps explain differing spectra of activity in this class of antibiotics.

Bacterial resistance to beta-lactam antibiotics is conferred most significantly by bacterial production of beta-lactamase enzymes, which destroy the beta-lactam ring and thus inactivate penicillin; decreased cell wall permeability and alteration in binding affinity to PBP also contribute to such resistance.

Oral absorption of penicillin varies widely; penicillin G is the most acid labile. Side-chain modifications in penicillin V, ampicillin, amoxicillin, and other orally administered penicillins are more stable in gastric acid and permit better absorption from the GI tract. (See *Comparing penicillins.*)

Penicillins are distributed widely throughout the body; CSF penetration is minimal but is enhanced in patients with inflamed meninges. Most penicillins are only partially metabolized.

With the exception of nafcillin, penicillins are excreted primarily in urine, chiefly through renal tubular effects; nafcillin undergoes enterohepatic circulation and is excreted chiefly through the biliary tract.

## Overview of adverse reactions

*Systemic:* Hypersensitivity reactions range from mild rash, fever, and eosinophilia to fatal anaphylaxis. Hematologic reactions include hemolytic anemia, transient neutropenia, leukopenia, and thrombocytopenia.

Certain adverse reactions are more common with specific classes of penicillin: bleeding episodes are usually seen at high-dose levels of extended-spectrum penicillins; acute interstitial nephritis is reported most often with methicillin; GI adverse effects are most common with but not limited to ampicillin. High doses, especially of penicillin G, irritate the CNS in patients with renal disease, causing confusion, twitching, lethargy, dysphagia, seizures, and coma. Hepatotoxicity is most common with penicillinase-resistant penicillins; hyperkalemia and hypernatremia are most common with extended-spectrum penicillins.

Jarisch-Herxheimer reaction can occur when penicillin G is used in secondary syphilis; signs and symptoms are chills, fever, headache, myalgia, tachycardia, malaise, sweating, hypotension, and sore throat, attributed to release of endotoxin following spirochete death.

*Local:* Local irritation from parenteral therapy may be severe enough to require discontinuation of the drug or administration by subclavian catheter if drug therapy is to continue.

## Clinical considerations

■ Assess patient's history of allergies.

■ Keep in mind that a negative history for penicillin hypersensitivity doesn't preclude future allergic reactions; advise clinician to monitor patient continuously for possible allergic reactions or other untoward effects.

■ Reduced dosage is needed in patients with renal impairment based on creatinine clearance and manufacturer's guidelines.

■ Advise clinician to assess level of consciousness, neurologic status, and renal function when high doses are used, because excessive blood levels can cause CNS toxicity.

■ Advise clinician to monitor vital signs, electrolytes, and renal function test results; monitor body weight for fluid retention with extended-spectrum penicillins for possible hypokalemia or hypernatremia.

■ Coagulation abnormalities, even frank bleeding, can follow high doses, especially of extended-spectrum penicillins. Advise clinician to monitor PT and platelet counts and assess patient for signs of occult or frank bleeding.

■ Advise clinician to monitor patients on long-term therapy for possible superinfection, es-

## COMPARING PENICILLINS

| Drug | Route | Adult dose | Frequency | Penicillinase-resistant |
|------|-------|-----------|-----------|-------------------------|
| amoxicillin | P.O. | 250-500 mg<br>3 g with 1 g probenecid for gonorrhea | q 8 hr<br>single dose | No |
| amoxicillin/ clavulanate potassium | P.O. | 250 mg<br>500 mg | q 8 hr<br>q 12 hr | Yes |
| ampicillin | I.M., I.V.<br><br>P.O. | 2-14 g daily<br><br>250-500 mg<br>2.5 g with 1 g probenecid (for gonorrhea) | divided doses given q 4-6 hr<br>q 6 hr<br>single dose | No |
| ampicillin sodium/ sulbactam sodium | I.M., I.V. | 1.5-3 g | q 6-8 hr | Yes |
| carbenicillin | P.O. | 382-764 mg | q 6 hr | No |
| cloxacillin | P.O. | 250 mg-1 g | q 6 hr | Yes |
| dicloxacillin | P.O. | 125-500 mg | q 6 hr | Yes |
| mezlocillin | I.M., I.V. | 3-4 g | q 4-6 hr | No |
| nafcillin | I.M., I.V.<br>P.O. | 250 mg-2 g<br>500 mg-1 g | q 4-6 hr<br>q 6 hr | Yes |
| oxacillin | I.M., I.V.<br>P.O. | 250 mg-2 g<br>500 mg-1 g | q 4-6 hr<br>q 6 hr | Yes |
| penicillin G benzathine | I.M. | 1.2-2.4 million units | single dose | No |
| penicillin G potassium | I.M., I.V. | 200,000-4 million units | q 4 hr | No |
| penicillin G procaine | I.M. | 600,000-1.2 million units<br>4.8 million units with 1 g probenecid (for syphilis) | q 1-3 days<br><br>single dose for primary, secondary, and early latent syphilis; weekly for 3 weeks for late latent syphilis | No |
| penicillin G sodium | I.M., I.V. | 200,000-4 million units | q 4 hr | No |
| penicillin V potassium | P.O. | 250-500 mg | q 6-8 hr | No |
| piperacillin | I.M., I.V. | 100-300 mg/kg daily | divided dose given q 4-6 hr | No |
| piperacillin sodium/ tazobactam sodium | I.V. | 3.375 g | q 6 hr | Yes |
| ticarcillin | I.M., I.V. | 150-300 mg/kg daily | divided doses given q 3-6 hr | No |
| ticarcillin/ clavulanate potassium | I.V. | 3.1 g | q 4-6 hr | Yes |

pecially geriatric and debilitated patients and others receiving immunosuppressants or radiation therapy; monitor closely, especially for fever.

**Oral and parenteral administration**

■ Advise clinician to give penicillins at least 1 hour before giving bacteriostatic antibiotics (tetracyclines, erythromycins, and chloramphenicol); these drugs inhibit bacterial cell growth, decreasing rate of penicillin uptake by bacterial cell walls.

■ Refrigerate oral suspensions; shake well before administering to ensure correct dose.

■ Advise clinician to give oral penicillin at least 1 hour before or 2 hours after meals to enhance gastric absorption; food may decrease absorption.

■ Advise clinician to give I.M. dose deep into large muscle mass (gluteal or midlateral thigh); rotate injection sites to minimize tissue injury; don't inject more than 2 g of drug per injection site. Ice should be applied to injection site for pain.

■ Don't add or mix other drugs with I.V. infusions, particularly aminoglycosides, which are inactivated if mixed with penicillins; they're chemically and physically incompatible. If other drugs must be given I.V., temporarily stop infusion of primary drug.

■ Infuse I.V. drug continuously or intermittently (over 30 minutes) and assess I.V. site frequently to prevent infiltration or phlebitis; rotate infusion site every 48 hours; intermittent I.V. infusion may be diluted in 50 to 100 ml sterile water, normal saline solution, $D_5W$, $D_5W$ and 0.45% saline, or lactated Ringer's solution.

## *Special populations*

**Pregnant patients.** Safe use of penicillins in pregnancy hasn't been definitely established. However, penicillin G has been used for the treatment of syphilis without adverse effects, and amoxicillin and ampicillin have been used for the treatment of urinary tract infections without adverse effects.

**Breast-feeding patients.** Consult individual drug recommendations.

**Pediatric patients.** Specific dosage recommendations have been established for most penicillins.

**Geriatric patients.** Use with caution; geriatric patients are susceptible to superinfection. Many geriatric patients have renal impairment, which decreases excretion of penicillins; lower the dose in geriatric patients with diminished creatinine clearance.

## **Patient counseling**

■ Explain to patient disease process and reason for therapy.

■ Teach patient signs and symptoms of hypersensitivity and other adverse reactions; emphasize need to report unusual reactions.

■ Teach patient signs and symptoms of bacterial and fungal superinfection to patients, especially geriatric and debilitated patients and others with low resistance from immunosuppressants or irradiation; emphasize need to report signs of infection.

■ Be sure patient understands how and when to take drugs; urge him to complete entire prescribed regimen, to comply with instructions for around-the-clock dosing, and to keep follow-up appointments.

■ Counsel patient to check expiration date of drug and to discard unused drug and not give it to family members or friends.

## **Representative combinations**

*Amoxicillin* with clavulanate potassium: Augmentin.

*Ampicillin* with probenecid: Polycillin-PRB, Probampacin.

*Ampicillin sodium* with sulbactam sodium: Unasyn.

*Ampicillin trihydrate* with probenecid: Polycillin-PRB, Principen with Probenecid, Probampacin.

*Penicillin G benzathine* with penicillin G procaine: Bicillin C-R, Bicillin C-R 900/300.

*Piperacillin sodium* with tazobactam sodium: Zosyn.

*Ticarcillin disodium* with clavulanate potassium: Timentin.

# phenothiazines

*Aliphatic derivatives:*
**chlorpromazine hydrochloride,
promethazine hydrochloride,
trimeprazine, triflupromazine**

*Piperazine derivatives:* **fluphenazine
hydrochloride, perphenazine,
prochlorperazine, trifluoperazine
hydrochloride**

*Piperidine derivatives:* **mesoridazine
besylate, thioridazine**

*Thioxanthene:* **thiothixene**

Phenothiazines were originally found to have sedative, antihistaminic, and narcotic-potentiating effects. Chlorpromazine has many effects, among them strong antipsychotic activity.

## Clinical indications and actions
### *Psychoses*

Phenothiazines (except promethazine) and thiothixene are indicated to treat agitated psychotic states. They're especially effective in controlling hallucinations in schizophrenic patients, the manic phase of manic-depressive illness, and excessive motor and autonomic activity.

**Nausea and vomiting**

Chlorpromazine, perphenazine, promethazine, and prochlorperazine are effective in controlling severe nausea and vomiting induced by CNS disturbances. They don't prevent motion sickness or vertigo.

**◇ Anxiety**

Chlorpromazine, mesoridazine, promethazine, prochlorperazine, and trifluoperazine also may be used for short-term treatment of moderate anxiety in selected nonpsychotic patients, for example, to control anxiety before surgery.

**Severe behavior problems**

Chlorpromazine and thioridazine are indicated to control combativeness and hyperexcitability in children with severe behavior problems. They're also used in hyperactive children for short-term treatment of excessive motor activity with labile moods, impulsive behavior, aggressiveness, attention deficit, and poor tolerance of frustration. Mesoridazine is used to manage hypersensitivity and to promote cooperative behavior in patients with mental deficiency and chronic brain syndrome.

**Tetanus**

Chlorpromazine is an effective adjunct in treating tetanus.

**Porphyria**

Because of its effects on the autonomic nervous system, chlorpromazine is effective in controlling abdominal pain in patients with acute intermittent porphyria.

**Delirium**

Phenothiazines have been used in the treatment of delirium. Antipsychotics remain first-line therapy.

**Intractable hiccups**

Chlorpromazine has been used to treat patients with intractable hiccups. The mechanism is unknown.

**Neurogenic pain**

Fluphenazine is a useful adjunct to manage selected chronic pain states.

**Allergies and pruritus**

Because of their potent antihistaminic effects, many of these drugs (including promethazine and trimeprazine) are used to relieve itching or symptomatic rhinitis.

## Pharmacology

Phenothiazines are classified in terms of chemical structure: the aliphatic drug (chlorpromazine) has a greater sedative, hypotensive, and allergic activity. Piperazines (perphenazine, prochlorperazine, fluphenazine, and trifluoperazine) are more likely to produce extrapyramidal symptoms. Piperidines (thioridazine and mesoridazine) have intermediate effects. Thioxanthenes are chemically similar to phenothiazines and are pharmacologically similar to piperazine phenothiazines. Promethazine is a derivative that has antihistamine qualities.

All antipsychotics have fundamentally similar mechanisms of action. They're believed to function as dopamine antagonists, blocking postsynaptic dopamine receptors in various parts of the CNS. Their antiemetic effects result from blockage of the chemoreceptor trigger zone. They also produce varying degrees of anticholinergic and alpha-adrenergic receptor blocking actions. The drugs are structurally similar to tricyclic antidepressants (TCAs) and share many adverse reactions.

All antipsychotics have equal clinical efficacy when given in equivalent doses. The choice of specific therapy is determined primarily by the individual patient's response and adverse reaction profile. A patient who doesn't respond to one drug may respond to another.

Onset of full therapeutic effects requires 6 weeks to 6 months; therefore, dosage adjustment is recommended at no less than weekly intervals.

## Overview of adverse reactions

Phenothiazines may produce extrapyramidal symptoms (dystonic movements, torticollis, oculogyric crises, parkinsonian symptoms) from akathisia during early treatment, to tardive dyskinesia after long-term use.

In rare cases, a neuroleptic malignant syndrome resembling severe parkinsonism may occur; it consists of rapid onset of hyperthermia, muscular hyperreflexia, marked extrapyramidal and autonomic dysfunction, arrhythmias, and sweating.

Other adverse reactions are similar to those seen with TCAs, including sedative and anticholinergic effects, orthostatic hypotension, reflex tachycardia, fainting, dizziness, arrhythmias, anorexia, nausea, vomiting, abdominal pain, local gastric irritation, seizures, endocrine effects, hematologic disorders, ocular changes, skin eruptions, and photosensitivity. Allergic manifestations are usually marked by elevation of liver enzyme levels progressing to obstructive jaundice.

Piperidine derivatives have the most pronounced CV effects; piperazine derivatives have the least. Parenteral administration is often associated with CV effects because of more rapid absorption. Seizures are common with aliphatic derivatives.

There is the potential for dose-related, serious cardiac effects and arrhythmias, such as prolonged QT interval and atypical ventricular tachycardia. Cautiously evaluate patients with a history of these conditions and patients prone to them.

Concomitant use with CNS depressants (additive effects) or lithium (potential for acute encephalopathic syndrome) requires close evaluation and monitoring of patient for adverse effects.

---

## Clinical considerations

■ Phenothiazines are contraindicated in patients hypersensitive to phenothiazines and related compounds.

■ Use with caution in patients with cardiac disease (arrhythmias, heart failure, angina pectoris, valvular disease, or heart block).

■ Use cautiously in patients with encephalitis, Reye's syndrome, head injury, epilepsy, or other seizure disorders.

■ Use phenothiazines cautiously in patients with glaucoma, prostatic hypertrophy, paralytic ileus, urine retention, hepatic or renal dysfunction, Parkinson's disease, pheochromocytoma, and hypocalcemia.

■ Advise clinician that vital signs should be checked regularly for decreased blood pressure (especially before and after parenteral therapy) or tachycardia; advise clinician to observe patient carefully for other adverse reactions.

■ Advise clinician to monitor intake and output for urine retention or constipation, which may require dosage reduction.

■ Advise clinician to monitor bilirubin levels weekly for first 4 weeks and monitor CBC, ECG (for quinidine-like effects), liver and renal function test results, electrolyte levels (especially potassium), and eye examination results at baseline and periodically thereafter, especially in patients on long-term therapy.

■ Advise clinician to observe patient for mood changes to monitor progress; benefits may not be apparent for several weeks.

■ Advise clinician to monitor patient for involuntary movements. Patient receiving prolonged treatment should be checked at least once every 6 months.

■ Advise clinician that drug shouldn't be withdrawn abruptly; although physical dependence doesn't occur with antipsychotic drugs, rebound exacerbation of psychotic symptoms may occur, and many drug effects persist.

■ Carefully follow manufacturer's instructions regarding drug color for reconstitution, dilution, administration, and storage of drugs; slightly discolored liquids may or may not be usable.

### Special populations

**Pregnant patients.** Safety of phenothiazine use during pregnancy isn't known.

**Breast-feeding patients.** If possible, patient shouldn't breast-feed while taking antipsychotics; most phenothiazines appear in breast milk and have a direct effect on prolactin levels. Benefit to mother must outweigh hazard to infant.

**Pediatric patients.** Unless otherwise specified, antipsychotics aren't recommended for children under age 12; be careful when using phenothiazines for nausea and vomiting because acutely ill children (suffering from chickenpox, measles, CNS infections, dehydration) are at greatly increased risk of dystonic reactions.

**Geriatric patients.** Lower doses are indicated in geriatric patients, who are more sensitive to therapeutic and adverse effects, especially cardiac toxicity, tardive dyskinesia, and other extrapyramidal effects. Adjust dosage to patient response.

## Patient counseling

■ Explain to patient reasons for and anticipated risks and benefits of therapy, and that full therapeutic effect may not occur for several weeks.

■ Teach patient signs and symptoms of adverse reactions and importance of reporting unusual effects, especially involuntary movements.

■ Tell patient to avoid beverages and drugs containing alcohol, and not to take other drugs (especially CNS depressants), including OTC products, without medical approval.

■ Instruct diabetic patient to monitor blood glucose level because drug may alter insulin needs.

■ Teach patient how and when to take drug, not to increase dose without medical approval, and never to discontinue drug abruptly; suggest taking full dose h.s. if daytime sedation is troublesome.

■ Advise patient to lie down for 30 minutes after first dose (1 hour if I.M.) and to rise slowly from sitting or supine position to prevent orthostatic hypotension.

■ Warn patient to avoid tasks requiring mental alertness and psychomotor coordination such as driving until full effects of drug are established; emphasize that sedative effects will lessen after several weeks.

■ Advise patient to take drug with milk or food to minimize GI distress because drugs are locally irritating. Warn that oral concentrates and solutions will irritate skin, and tell patient not to crush or open sustained-release products, but to swallow them whole.

■ Warn patient that photosensitivity reactions, such as burns and abnormal hyperpigmentation, may occur.

■ Tell patient to avoid exposure to extremes of heat or cold, because of risk of hypothermia or hyperthermia induced by alteration in thermoregulatory function.

■ Explain to patient that phenothiazines may cause pink to brown urine.

## Representative combinations

None.

# progestins

**hydroxyprogesterone caproate,
medroxyprogesterone acetate,
megestrol acetate, norethindrone,
norethindrone acetate, norgestrel,
progesterone**

Progesterone is the endogenous progestin secreted by the corpus luteum within the female ovary. Several synthetic progesterone derivatives with greater potency or duration of action have been synthesized. Some of these derivatives also possess weak androgenic or estrogenic activity. Progestins are used to treat dysfunctional uterine bleeding and certain cancers. They're also used as contraceptives, either alone or with estrogens.

## Clinical indications and actions
### Hormonal imbalance, female
Hydroxyprogesterone, medroxyprogesterone, norethindrone, and progesterone are indicated to treat amenorrhea and dysfunctional uterine bleeding caused by hormonal imbalance. Hydroxyprogesterone is also indicated to produce desquamation and a secretory endometrium.
### Endometriosis
Norethindrone and norethindrone acetate are used to treat endometriosis.
### Carcinoma
Hydroxyprogesterone, medroxyprogesterone, and megestrol are used in the adjunctive and palliative treatment of certain types of metastatic tumors. They're not considered primary therapy. See individual drugs for specific indications.
### Contraception
Norethindrone, medroxyprogesterone acetate, and norgestrel are approved for use with estrogens or alone as oral contraceptives.

Progestins are no longer indicated to detect pregnancy (because of teratogenicity) or to treat threatened or habitual abortion, for which they're not effective.

## Pharmacology
Progesterone is formed from steroid precursors in the ovary, testis, adrenal cortex, and placenta. Luteinizing hormone stimulates the synthesis and secretion of progesterone from the corpus luteum. Progesterone causes secretory changes in the endometrium, changes in the vaginal epithelium, increases in body temperature, relaxation of uterine smooth muscle, stimulation of growth of breast alveolar tissue, inhibition of gonadotropin release from the pituitary, and withdrawal bleeding (in the presence of estrogens). Synthetic progesterone derivatives have these properties as well.

## Overview of adverse reactions
The most common adverse effect is a change in menstrual bleeding pattern, ranging from spotting or breakthrough bleeding to complete amenorrhea. Other reactions include breast tenderness and secretion, weight changes, increases in body temperature, edema, nausea, acne, somnolence, insomnia, hirsutism, hair loss, depression, cholestatic jaundice, and allergic reactions (rare). Some patients taking parenteral progestins have also suffered localized reactions at the injection site.

## Clinical considerations
- Progestins are contraindicated during pregnancy and in patients with thromboembolic disorders, breast cancer, undiagnosed abnormal vaginal bleeding, or severe hepatic disease.
- Progestins should be used cautiously in patients with diabetes mellitus, cardiac or renal disease, seizure disorder, migraine, or mental depression.
- Recommend giving oil injections deep I.M. in gluteal muscles. I.M. injections may be painful; observe injection site for sterile abscess formation.
- Glucose tolerance may be altered in diabetic patients. Advise clinician to monitor patient closely because antidiabetic may need to be adjusted.
- When used as an oral contraceptive, progestins are given daily without interruption, regardless of menstrual cycle.
- Use of progestins may lead to gingival bleeding and hyperplasia.
- A patient who is exposed to progestins during the first 4 months of pregnancy or who becomes pregnant while receiving the drug should be informed of the potential risks to the fetus.
- Because oral contraceptive combinations contain progestins, consider the precautions associated with oral contraceptives in patients receiving progestins.

### Special populations
**Pregnant patients.** Progestins are listed as pregnancy category X. Potential adverse effects include masculinization of the female fetus, hypospadias in males, and potential CV and limb defects.
**Breast-feeding patients.** Don't use progestins in breast-feeding women, except for Depo-Provera, which may be used in breast-feeding women after 6 weeks.

## Patient counseling
- Tell patient that GI distress may subside with use, after a few cycles.
- Instruct patient receiving progestins to have a full physical examination, including a gynecologic examination and a Papanicolaou test, every 6 to 12 months.
- Advise patient to discontinue therapy and call prescriber immediately if migraine or vi-

## COMPARING PROTEASE INHIBITORS

| Drug | Dosage | Dosage adjustment | Oral bioavailability |
|------|--------|-------------------|---------------------|
| imprenavir | Adults: 1,200 mg b.i.d.<br>Children: 20-22.5 mg/kg b.i.d. | Reduce dose with impaired hepatic function. | May be taken without food, but shouldn't be taken with a high-fat meal, which reduces absorption. Absolute bioavailability hasn't been established. |
| indinavir | Adults: 800 mg q 8 hr<br>Adults with cirrhosis: 600 mg q 8 hr | Reduce dose in cirrhosis | Meals rich in fats, proteins, or calories reduce bioavailability by 77%. |
| nelfinavir | Adults: 750 mg t.i.d. with food<br>Children: 20-30 mg/kg t.i.d. with food | None | Food produces 2- to 3-fold increase in bioavailability. |
| ritonavir | Adults: 600 mg b.i.d. with food<br>Children > 2: 250 mg/m$^2$-400 mg/m$^2$ b.i.d. with food | None | Food produces 15% increase in bioavailability. |
| saquinavir | Fortovase: 1,200 mg t.i.d. with food or within 2 hr of a meal<br>Invirase: 600 mg t.i.d. with food or within 2 hr of a meal | None | High fat meals produce a 4% increase in bioavailability of Invirase. Soft gelatin capsule formulation (Fortovase) has a 33% increase in bioavailability. |

sual disturbances occur, or if sudden severe headache or vomiting develops.

■ Teach patient how to perform breast self-examination.

■ Tell patient to call promptly if period is missed or unusual bleeding occurs and to call and discontinue drug immediately if pregnancy is suspected.

■ Advise patient who misses a dose to take the missed dose as soon as possible or omit it.

■ Advise patient who misses consecutive doses when used as a contraceptive to discontinue the drug and use an alternative contraception method until period begins or pregnancy is ruled out.

■ Inform patient that drug may cause possible dental problems (tenderness, swelling, or bleeding of gums). Advise patient to brush and floss teeth, massage gums, and have dentist clean teeth regularly. She should refer to dentist with questions about care of teeth or gums or if tenderness, swelling, or bleeding of gums is noticed.

■ Advise patient to use extra care to avoid pregnancy when starting use of drug as an oral contraceptive and for at least 3 months after discontinuing it.

■ Advise patient to keep an extra 1-month supply available.

■ Tell patient to keep tablets in original container.

■ Emphasize to patient the importance of not giving drug to anyone else.

### Representative combinations

*Hydroxyprogesterone caproate* with estradiol valerate: Hylutin.

*Norethindrone acetate* with ethinyl estradiol: Brevicon, Loestrin 1.5/30, Loestrin Fe 1.5/30, Loestrin 21 1/20, Loestrin Fe 1/20, Modicon, Norinyl 1 + 35, Ortho 1/35*, Ortho 7/7/7*, Ortho 10/11*, Ortho-Novum 7/7/7, Ovcon-35, Ovcon-50, Tri-Norinyl; with mestranol: Norinyl 1/50, Ortho-Novum 0.5/35*, Ortho-Novum 1/50, Ortho-Novum 1/35.

*Norgestrel* with ethinyl estradiol: Lo/Ovral, Ovral.

# protease inhibitors

## amprenavir, indinavir sulfate, nelfinavir mesylate, ritonavir, saquinavir, saquinavir mesylate

These antiviral drugs act specifically against HIV through inhibition of HIV protease.

## Clinical indications and actions
### HIV infection and AIDS

Protease inhibitors are used as monotherapy or with nucleoside analogues for the treatment of HIV infection and AIDS.

◇ Protease inhibitors may be used in conjunction with zidovudine and lamivudine for postexposure prophylaxis of HIV infection.

## Pharmacology

Protease inhibitors bind to the protease active site and inhibit the activity of HIV protease. This enzyme is required for the proteolysis of viral polyprotein precursors into individual functional proteins found in infectious HIV. The net effect is formation of noninfectious,

| Plasma protein–binding (%) | Half-life (hr) | Peak concentration (hr) | Elimination |
|---|---|---|---|
| 90 | Adults: 7-10½ | 1-2 | 14% renal, 75% fecal elimination |
| 60 | Adults: 1¾ | Fasting: ¾ | 83% hepatic; 19% renal |
| >98 | Adults: 3½-5 | Fed: 2-4 | 87% fecal elimination; 78% as metabolites; 1%-2% recovered unchanged in urine |
| 98-99 | Adults: 3-5 | Fasted: 2<br>Fed: 4 | 88% fecal elimination; 34% as unchanged drug; 11% excreted in urine; 4% as unchanged drug |
| 98 | Not defined | Not defined | 88% fecal elimination as unchanged drug and metabolites; 1% recovered unchanged in urine |

immature viral particles. Note that two drug regimens containing only nucleoside reverse transcriptase inhibitors are now considered suboptimal. Combination therapy including protease inhibitors or nonnucleoside reverse transcriptase inhibitors are recommended. (See *Comparing protease inhibitors.*)

## Overview of adverse reactions

The most frequently reported side effects of protease inhibitors, for which immediate medical attention should be sought, include kidney stones, diabetes or hyperglycemia, ketoacidosis, or paresthesias. Frequently reported side effects that don't require medical attention unless they persist or are bothersome include generalized weakness, GI disturbances, headache, insomnia, and taste perversion. Less frequent side effects include dizziness and somnolence.

## Clinical considerations

■ Consider the risk-benefit ratio of therapy with protease inhibitors on an individual basis when the patient has hemophilia or liver dysfunction.

■ Indinavir may cause nephrolithiasis. Advise patient to increase fluid intake.

The potential benefits will be better achieved with patient compliance to drug therapy.

### Special populations

**Pregnant patients.** Pregnancy risk categories are B and C. Adequate, well-controlled trials haven't been completed because the drug can produce hyperbilirubinemia; exercise caution in pregnant women to prevent ill effects in neonates. Prescribers are encouraged to con-

tact the registry at 1-800-258-4263 to report pregnant women on therapy.

**Breast-feeding patients.** The rate and extent of excretion of protease inhibitors into breast milk is unknown. Therefore, their use in breast-feeding women isn't recommended. However, the risks and benefits to both the woman and infant must be considered in each case.

**Pediatric patients.** Refer to specific drug monographs for dosing information.

**Geriatric patients.** Safety and efficacy haven't been evaluated systemically.

## Patient counseling

■ Instruct patient to take drug as prescribed and to finish the full course of therapy.

■ Tell patient to take the next dose as soon as possible after a missed dose, but not to double the dose.

■ Tell patient that drug should be taken with plenty of water, 1 or 2 hours before meals, and he should drink about 48 ounces of water daily.

■ Instruct patient not to take other drugs concurrently without first checking with the pharmacist or prescriber.

## Representative combinations

None.

## COMPARING SELECTIVE SEROTONIN REUPTAKE INHIBITORS

| Drug | Adult dosage | Dosage adjustment | Oral bioavailability |
|------|-------------|-------------------|---------------------|
| citalopram | 20-40 mg/day | Lower dosing recommended in the elderly | No food effect |
| fluoxetine | 20-60 mg/day in single or divided doses | No adjustment for renal or hepatic failure | Well absorbed; no food effect |
| fluvoxamine | 50-300 mg/day at h.s. Total daily dose of >100 mg/day should be given in two divided doses | Reduction of initial dosage and modification of subsequent doses in renal and hepatic impairment | No food effect |
| paroxetine | 20-60 mg/day in single or divided doses | Maximum dose of 40 mg/day in severe renal or hepatic failure | 50%-100%, no food effect |
| sertraline | 25-50 mg once daily | Reduce dose or increase interval in severe hepatic failure | Food increase rate and extent of absorption |

# selective serotonin reuptake inhibitors (SSRIs)

**citalopram hydrobromide, fluoxetine, fluvoxamine maleate, paroxetine, sertraline hydrochloride**

These drugs are antidepressant, antiobsessional, antipanic drugs that selectively inhibit the reuptake of serotonin with little or no effects on other neurotransmitters such as norepinephrine or dopamine. (See *Comparing selective serotonin reuptake inhibitors.*)

## Clinical indications and actions
*Major depression, obsessive-compulsive disorder (OCD), bulimia nervosa, premenstrual dysphoric disorders, and panic disorders.*
SSRIs are used to treat these disorders; sertraline is also the first drug approved for the treatment of posttraumatic stress disorder (PTSD).
*Other disorders*
◇ Fluoxetine has been used for the treatment of bipolar disorder, symptomatic management of cataplexy, and management of alcohol dependence.
◇ Paroxetine and sertraline have been used for the treatment of premature ejaculation and chronic headache; paroxetine for the symptoms of diabetic neuropathy.

## Pharmacology
The antidepressant, antiobsessional, antipanic actions of fluoxetine, fluvoxamine maleate, sertraline, and paroxetine are thought to be related to the potent and selective inhibition of serotonin uptake, but not related to norepinephrine or dopamine uptake, in the central nervous system. These drugs lack affinity for alpha-adrenergic receptors and muscarinic receptors.

## Overview of adverse reactions
Frequent side effects include headache, tremor, dizziness, sleep disturbances, GI disturbances, and sexual dysfunction. Less frequent side effects include bleeding (red spots on skin, nose bleeds), akathesia (restlessness), breast tenderness or enlargement, extrapyramidal effects, dystonia, fever, hyponatremia, mania or hypomania, palpitations, serotonin syndrome, weight gain or loss, skin rash, hives, or itching.

## Clinical considerations
■ Hyponatremia is usually caused by inappropriate secretion of antidiuretic hormone. This problem is most often seen in geriatric patients and those treated with diuretics.
■ Diarrhea, fever, palpitations, mood swings or behavioral changes, restlessness, shaking, and shivering characterize serotonin syndrome. Hypertension and seizures may accompany the serotonin syndrome. This syndrome is most commonly seen within days following dosage increases or concurrent administration of a serotonergic drug.

### Special populations
**Pregnant patients.** Pregnancy risk category is C. Data haven't shown evidence of teratogenicity or ill effects in neonates of women given SSRIs during the first trimester of pregnancy or throughout gestation. The effects of SSRIs on labor and delivery aren't known.
**Breast-feeding patients.** SSRIs appear in breast milk and may cause diarrhea and sleep

| Plasma protein–binding (%) | Half-life (hr) | Onset of action (wk) | Peak concentration (hr) | Elimination |
|---|---|---|---|---|
| 80 | 35 | 1-4 | 4 (after a single dose) | 35% excreted in urine; 65% in feces |
| 94½ | 2-3 days for fluoxetine and 7-9 days for nor-fluoxetine | 1-3, may be 5 for OCD | 6-8 (after a single dose) | 80% excreted in urine; 15% in feces |
| 80 | 13½-15½ | 4-5 | 3-8 | 94% renal excretion |
| 95 | Average of 21-24 | 1-3 | 2-8 | 64% excreted in urine; 36% in feces |
| 98 | Sertraline: 24-26 N-desmethyl-sertraline: 62-104 | 2-4 | 4½-8½ | 45% renal; 45% in feces |

disturbance in neonates. Use of SSRIs in breast-feeding women isn't recommended. However, the risks and benefits to both the woman and infant must be considered in each case.
**Pediatric patients.** There's insufficient information to establish the safety and efficacy of SSRIs in children, but there's evidence of beneficial response following SSRI treatment for depression or OCD in children. Pediatric patients appear to be more susceptible than adults to the behavioral adverse reactions of SSRIs (mania, social inhibition, irritability, restlessness, and insomnia).
**Geriatric patients.** The use of SSRIs is safe and effective in geriatric patients. Geriatric patients are more sensitive to the insomniac effects of SSRIs. Sertraline plasma level may be decreased in these patients.

### Patient counseling

■ Tell patient that drug may take 4 to 5 weeks to produce its fully intended benefit. Drug should be taken as prescribed. If a dose is missed, dose shouldn't be doubled.
■ Instruct patient to stop taking drug and contact a prescriber or pharmacist as soon as possible if a rash or hives develops.
■ Advise patient to avoid alcohol and the use of serotonergic drugs or substances.
■ Tell patient to use caution when driving or doing jobs requiring alertness because this drug may cause drowsiness or impairment of judgment or motor skills.

### Representative combinations

None.

## sulfonamides

**co-trimoxazole (trimethoprim-sulfamethoxazole), sulfadiazine, sulfamethoxazole, sulfasalazine, sulfisoxazole**

Sulfonamides were the first effective drugs used to treat systemic bacterial infections. Many derivatives have been synthesized, and many therapeutic milestones have been reached, including improved solubility of sulfonamides in urine (which reduces renal toxicity) and discovery of the advantages of combinations such as triple sulfa and, especially, of combined trimethoprim and sulfamethoxazole (co-trimoxazole). Development of other major antibiotics has reduced the clinical impact of sulfonamides. However, introduction of the combination drug co-trimoxazole has increased their usefulness in certain infections.

### Clinical indications and actions
*Bacterial infections*
When first introduced, sulfonamides were active against many gram-positive and gram-negative organisms; over time, many bacteria have become resistant. Currently, sulfonamides are active against some strains of staphylococci, streptococci, *Nocardia asteroides, Nocardia brasiliensis, Clostridium tetani, Clostridium perfringens, Bacillus anthracis, Escherichia coli, Neisseria gonorrhoeae,* and *Neisseria meningitidis.* Resistance to sulfonamides is common if therapy continues beyond 2 weeks; resistance to one sulfonamide usually means cross-resistance to others.

Sulfonamides are used to treat urinary tract infections caused by *E. coli, Proteus mirabilis,*

*Proteus vulgaris, Klebsiella, Enterobacter,* and *Staphylococcus aureus,* and genital lesions caused by *Haemophilus ducreyi* (chancroid). They're the drugs of choice in nocardiosis, usually with surgical drainage or combined with other antibiotics, including ampicillin, erythromycin, cycloserine, or minocycline. Sulfonamides also are used to treat otitis media. Sulfadiazine is used to eradicate meningococci from the nasopharynx of asymptomatic carriers of *N. meningitidis.*

Co-trimoxazole is used to treat infections of the urinary tract, respiratory tract, and ear; to treat chronic bacterial prostatitis; and to prevent recurrent urinary tract infection in women and "traveler's diarrhea."

Co-trimoxazole is also used to treat *Pneumocystis carinii* pneumonia.

***Parasitic infections***
Sulfonamides combined with pyrimethamine are used to treat toxoplasmosis; certain sulfonamides are combined with quinine and pyrimethamine to treat chloroquine-resistant *Plasmodium falciparum* malaria.

***Inflammation***
Sulfasalazine, used to treat inflammatory bowel disease, is cleaved to sulfapyridine and 5-aminosalicylic acid in the intestine.

***Plague***
Co-trimazole is recommended by the Centers for Disease Control and Prevention for anti-infective prophylaxis in adults 18 and over and children 2 months or over who are at high risk for exposure to pneumonic plague.

## Pharmacology

Sulfonamides are bacteriostatic. Their mechanism of action correlates directly with the structural similarities they share with para-aminobenzoic acid. They inhibit biosynthesis of folic acid, which is needed for cell growth. Susceptible bacteria are those that synthesize folic acid.

Sulfonamides are well absorbed from the GI tract after oral administration, except for sulfasalazine, which is absorbed minimally by the oral route. Sulfonamides are distributed widely into tissues and fluids, including pleural, peritoneal, synovial, and ocular fluids; some, including sulfisoxazole, penetrate CSF. Sulfonamides readily cross the placenta and appear in low levels in breast milk. Sulfonamides are metabolized by the liver and the parent drug and metabolites are excreted in urine by glomerular filtration. Hemodialysis removes both sulfamethoxazole and sulfisoxazole, but peritoneal dialysis removes only sulfisoxazole.

## Overview of adverse reactions

Sulfonamides cause adverse reactions affecting many organs and systems. Many are considered to be caused by hypersensitivity, including the following: rash, fever, pruritus, erythema multiforme, erythema nodosum, Stevens-Johnson syndrome, Lyell's syndrome, exfoliative dermatitis, photosensitivity, joint pain, conjunctivitis, leukopenia, and bronchospasm. Hematologic reactions include granulocytopenia, thrombocytopenia, agranulocytosis, hypoprothrombinemia, and, in G6PD deficiency, hemolytic anemia. Renal effects usually result from crystalluria (precipitation of the sulfonamide in the renal system). GI reactions include anorexia, stomatitis, pancreatitis, diarrhea, and folic acid malabsorption. Oral therapy commonly causes nausea and vomiting. Hepatotoxicity and CNS reactions (dizziness, confusion, headache, ataxia, drowsiness, and insomnia) are rare.

## Clinical considerations

■ Assess patient's history of allergies; don't give a sulfonamide to patient hypersensitive to it or to other drugs containing sulfur.

■ Sulfonamides are also contraindicated in patients with severe renal or hepatic dysfunction or porphyria, during pregnancy at term, and during breast-feeding. Sulfonamides may cause kernicterus in infants because they displace bilirubin at the binding site, cross the placenta, and appear in breast milk. Don't use in infants under age 2 months (except in the treatment of congenital toxoplasmosis as adjunctive therapy with pyrimethamine).

■ Advise clinician to administer sulfonamides with caution in patients with the following conditions: mild to moderate renal or hepatic impairment; urinary obstruction, because of the risk of drug accumulation; severe allergies; asthma; blood dyscrasia; or G6PD deficiency.

■ Advise clinician to continuously monitor patient for possible hypersensitivity reactions or other untoward effects; patients with AIDS have a much higher risk of adverse reactions.

■ Advise clinician to obtain cultures and sensitivity test results before giving first dose, but therapy may begin before laboratory tests are complete; test results should be checked periodically to assess drug efficacy. Advise clinician to monitor urine cultures, CBCs, and urinalysis before and during therapy.

■ Advise clinician to monitor patients on prolonged therapy for superinfection, especially geriatric and debilitated patients and others receiving immunosuppressants or radiation therapy.

■ Sulfonamides may interact with other drugs (oral anticoagulants, cyclosporine, digoxin, folic acid, hydantoins, methotrexate, and sulfonylureas) and may alter test results; consult individual drug entries for possible test interactions.

**Administration**
■ Advise clinician to give oral dose with full 8-ounce (240-ml) glass of water and force fluids to 12 to 16 glasses per day, depending on the drug; patient's urine output should be at least 1,500 ml/day.

- Follow manufacturer's directions for reconstitution, dilution, and storage of drugs; check expiration dates.
- Advise clinician to give oral sulfonamide at least 1 hour before or 2 hours after meals for maximum absorption.
- Shake oral suspensions well before administering to ensure correct dose.

### Special populations

**Pregnant patients.** Safe use during pregnancy hasn't been established. There is potential for cleft palate, other bony abnormalities, and kernicterus in the infant.

**Breast-feeding patients.** Because sulfonamides appear in breast milk, a decision should be made to discontinue either breast-feeding or the drug, taking into account the importance of the drug to the woman. Premature infants, infants with hyperbilirubinemia, and those with G6PD deficiency are at risk for kernicterus.

**Pediatric patients.** Sulfonamides are contraindicated in infants under age 2 months, unless there's no therapeutic alternative.

Give sulfonamides with caution to children with fragile X chromosome and mental retardation because they're vulnerable to psychomotor depression from folate depletion.

**Geriatric patients.** Use with caution; geriatric patients are susceptible to bacterial and fungal superinfection, are at greater risk of folate deficiency anemia after sulfonamide therapy, and commonly are at greater risk of renal and hematologic effects because of diminished renal function.

### Patient counseling

- Teach patient the signs and symptoms of hypersensitivity and other adverse reactions, and emphasize the need to report these; specifically, urge patient to report bloody urine, difficulty breathing, rash, fever, chills, or severe fatigue.
- Teach the signs and symptoms of bacterial and fungal superinfection to geriatric and debilitated patients and others with low resistance from immunosuppressants or irradiation; emphasize the need to report them.
- Advise diabetic patient that sulfonamides may increase effects of oral hypoglycemic and not to monitor urine glucose levels with Clinitest; sulfonamides alter results of tests using cupric sulfate.
- Advise patient to avoid exposure to direct sunlight because of risk of photosensitivity reaction.
- Tell patient to take oral drug with a full glass of water and to drink at least twelve to sixteen 8-ounce (240-ml) glasses of water daily depending on the drug; explain that tablet may be crushed and swallowed with water to ensure maximal absorption.
- Be sure patient understands how and when to take drugs; urge him to complete entire prescribed regimen, to comply with instructions for around-the-clock dosing, and to keep follow-up appointments.
- Teach patient to check expiration date of drug and how to store drug, and to discard unused drug.
- For sulfasalazine, inform patient to take with food if GI irritation occurs and tell him that it may cause an orange-yellow discoloration of the urine or skin and may permanently stain soft contact lenses yellow.
- Photosensitization may occur; therefore, caution patient to take protective measures (such as wearing sunblock and protective clothing) against exposure to ultraviolet light or sunlight until tolerance is determined.

### Representative combinations

*Sulfadiazine* with sulfamerazine and sulfamethazine: Triple Sulfa.

*Sulfamethizole* with oxytetracycline hydrochloride and phenazopyridine: Urobiotic-250; with sulfathiazole, sulfacetamide, sulfabenzamide, and urea: Triple Sulfa, V.V.S., Trysul, Gyne-Sulf, Sultrin.

*Sulfamethoxazole* with phenazopyridine hydrochloride: Azo Gantanol, Azo-Sulfamethoxazole; with trimethoprim: Bactrim, Cotrim, Co-Trimoxazole, Septra, SMZ-TMP.

*Sulfisoxazole* with erythromycin ethylsuccinate: Pediazole; with phenazopyridine hydrochloride: Azo Gantrisin.

*Sulfadoxine* with pyrimethamine: Fansidar.

---

# sulfonylureas

### acetohexamide, chlorpropamide, glimepiride, glipizide, glyburide, tolazamide, tolbutamide

---

Sulfonylureas, which have hypoglycemic effects, are useful only in patients with mild to moderately severe, stable, non–insulin-dependent diabetes mellitus (NIDDM). These drugs can be used only in patients with functioning beta cells of the pancreas.

### Clinical indications and actions

*Diabetes mellitus, non–insulin-dependent*
Sulfonylureas are used to manage mild to moderately severe, stable, nonketotic NIDDM that can't be controlled by diet alone. Sulfonylureas stimulate insulin release from the pancreas. After long-term therapy, extrapancreatic hypoglycemic effects include reduced hepatic glucose production, an increased number of insulin receptors, and changes in insulin binding.

◊ *Neurogenic diabetes insipidus*
Although an unlabeled indication, chlorpropamide has been used in selected patients to treat neurogenic diabetes insipidus. The drug

## COMPARING SULFONYLUREAS

Typically, sulfonylureas have similar actions and produce similar effects. They differ mainly in duration of action and dosage.

| Drug | Usual daily dosage | Onset (hr) | Peak (hr) | Duration (hr) |
|------|--------------------|-----------|-----------|----------------|
| **First generation** | | | | |
| acetohexamide | 500 mg once daily or b.i.d. | 1 | 2 | 12-24 |
| chlorpropamide | 250 mg once daily | 1 | 3-6 | 24-60 |
| tolazamide | 250 mg once daily or b.i.d. | 4-6 | 6-10 | 12-24 |
| tolbutamide | 1,000 mg b.i.d. or t.i.d. | ½-1 | 4-8 | 6-12 |
| **Second generation** | | | | |
| glimepiride | 1-4 mg once daily | 1 | 2-3 | 24 |
| glipizide | 5 mg once daily | 1-3 | 2-3 | 10-24 |
| glyburide | 5 mg once daily | 2 | 3-4 | 12-24 |

appears to potentiate the effect of minimal levels of antidiuretic hormone.

## Pharmacology

Sulfonylurea antidiabetics are sulfonamide derivatives that exert no antibacterial activity.

Sulfonylureas lower blood glucose levels by stimulating insulin release from the pancreas. These drugs work only in the presence of functioning beta cells in the islet tissue of the pancreas. After prolonged administration, they produce hypoglycemia through significant extrapancreatic effects, including reduction of hepatic glucose production and enhanced peripheral sensitivity to insulin. The latter may result from an increase in the number of insulin receptors or from changes in events after insulin binding. (See *Comparing sulfonylureas*.)

Sulfonylureas are divided into first-generation drugs (chlorpropamide) and second-generation drugs (glyburide, glipizide, and glimepiride). Although their mechanisms of action are similar, the second-generation drugs carry a more lipophilic side chain, are more potent, and cause fewer adverse reactions. Their most important differences are their durations of action.

## Overview of adverse reactions

Dose-related adverse effects, which usually aren't serious and respond to decreased doses, include headache, nausea, vomiting, anorexia, heartburn, weakness, and paresthesia. Hypoglycemia may follow excessive doses, increased exercise, decreased food intake, or consumption of alcohol. Signs and symptoms of overdose include anxiety, chills, cold sweats, confusion, cool pale skin, difficulty concentrating, drowsiness, excessive hunger, headache, nausea, nervousness, rapid heartbeat, shakiness, unsteady gait, weakness, and unusual fatigue.

## Clinical considerations

- Advise clinician to administer sulfonylureas 30 minutes before morning meal for once-daily dosing, or 30 minutes before morning and evening meals for twice-daily dosing.
- Contraindicated in patients with juvenile-onset, brittle, or severe diabetes; diabetes mellitus adequately controlled by diet; and maturity-onset diabetes complicated by ketosis, acidosis, diabetic coma, Raynaud's gangrene, renal or hepatic impairment, or thyroid or other endocrine dysfunction.
- Use cautiously in patients hypersensitive to sulfonamide.
- For patients transferring from insulin therapy to a sulfonylurea drug, advise clinician to monitor for urine glucose and ketones at least three times daily, before meals; emphasize the need for testing a double-voided specimen. Patients may require hospitalization during such changes in therapy.
- Patients transferring from another sulfonylurea (except chlorpropamide) usually need no transition period.
- NIDDM patients may require insulin therapy during periods of increased stress, such as infection, fever, surgery, or trauma. Advise clinician to monitor patients closely for hyperglycemia in these situations.

should be checked periodically to assess drug efficacy.

- Advise clinician to monitor vital signs, electrolytes, and renal function test results before and during therapy.
- Check expiration dates. Outdated tetracyclines may cause nephrotoxicity.
- Advise clinician to monitor patient for bacterial and fungal superinfection, especially in geriatric, debilitated, and other patients receiving immunosuppressants or radiation therapy; watch especially for oral candidiasis. If symptoms occur, drug should be stopped.
- Tetracyclines may interfere with certain laboratory tests; consult individual drug entry.

**Administration**

- Oral drugs should be given 1 hour before or 2 hours after meals for maximum absorption; don't give with food, milk or other dairy products, sodium bicarbonate, iron compounds, or antacids, which may impair absorption.
- Advise clinician to give water with and after oral drug to facilitate passage to stomach because incomplete swallowing can cause severe esophageal irritation; don't give within 1 hour of bedtime, to prevent esophageal reflux.
- Follow manufacturer's directions for reconstitution and storage; keep product refrigerated and out of light.
- Avoid I.V. use of drug in patients with decreased renal function.
- I.V. use of tetracyclines in pregnancy or in patients with renal impairment, especially when dose exceeds 2 g/day, can cause hepatic failure.
- Advise clinician to monitor I.V. injection sites and rotate routinely to reduce local irritation. I.V. use may cause severe phlebitis.

### Special populations

**Pregnant patients.** Tetracyclines may cause fetal toxicity in pregnant women.
**Breast-feeding patients.** Breast-feeding women shouldn't use tetracyclines.
**Pediatric patients.** Tetracyclines shouldn't be used in children under age 8 unless there's no alternative. They may cause permanent discoloration of teeth, enamel hypoplasia, and a reversible decrease in bone calcification.
**Geriatric patients.** Some geriatric patients have decreased esophageal motility; use tetracyclines cautiously and monitor for local irritation from slowly passing oral dosage forms. Geriatric patients are more susceptible to superinfection.

### Patient counseling

- Explain to patient the disease process and reason for therapy.
- Teach patient signs and symptoms of adverse reactions, and emphasize need to report these promptly; urge patient to report unusual effects.

- Teach signs and symptoms of bacterial and fungal superinfection to geriatric and debilitated patients and others with low resistance from immunosuppressants or irradiation.
- Advise patient using oral contraceptives to use a backup method of contraception during drug therapy.
- Advise patient to avoid direct sunlight and to use a sunblock to prevent photosensitivity reactions.
- Tell patient to take oral tetracyclines with a full 8-ounce (240-ml) glass of water (to facilitate passage to the stomach) 1 hour before or 2 hours after meals for maximum absorption, and not less than 1 hour before bedtime (to prevent irritation from esophageal reflux).
- Emphasize that taking drug with food, milk or other dairy products, sodium bicarbonate, or iron compounds may interfere with absorption. Tell patient to take antacids 3 hours after tetracycline.
- Stress importance of completing prescribed regimen exactly as ordered and keeping follow-up appointments.
- Tell patient that doxycycline and monocycline may be taken with food.
- Instruct patient to check expiration date before use.

### Representative combinations

*Oxytetracycline* with polymyxin B sulfate: Terramycin with polymyxin B, Terramycin topical ointment.

*Oxytetracycline* hydrochloride with phenazopyridine hydrochloride and sulfamethizole: Urobiotic-250.

*Tetracycline hydrochloride* with citric acid: Achromycin V.

# thrombolytic enzymes

**alteplase, anistreplase, reteplase (recombinant), streptokinase, urokinase**

When a thrombus obstructs a blood vessel, permanent damage to the ischemic area may occur before the body can dissolve the clot. Thrombolytics were developed in the hope that speeding lysis of the clot would prevent permanent ischemic damage. The effects of this compound on various kinds of clots have been studied. It isn't clear if such drugs significantly reduce thrombosis-induced ischemic damage in all situations for which the drugs are currently used. (See *Comparing thrombolytic enzymes,* page 76.)

### Clinical indications and actions
*Thrombosis, thromboembolism*
Alteplase, streptokinase, and urokinase are used to treat acute pulmonary thromboembolism;

## COMPARING THROMBOLYTIC ENZYMES

Thrombolytic enzymes dissolve clots by accelerating the formation of plasmin by activated plasminogen. Plasminogen activators, found in most tissues and body fluids, help plasminogen (an inactive enzyme) convert to plasmin (an active enzyme), which dissolves the clot.

Doses of five enzymes listed below may vary according to the patient's condition.

| Drug | Action | Initial dose | Maintenance therapy |
|------|--------|--------------|---------------------|
| alteplase | Directly converts plasminogen to plasmin | I.V. bolus: 6 to 10 mg over 1-2 min | I.V. infusion: 60 mg/hr in the 1st hr; then 20 mg/hr for the next 2 hr for a total of 100 mg |
| anistreplase | Directly converts plasminogen to plasmin | I.V. push: 30 units over 2-5 min | Not necessary |
| reteplase | Enhances the cleavage of plasminogen to generate plasmin | Double I.V. bolus injection of 10 + 10 units | Not necessary |
| streptokinase | Indirectly activates plasminogen, which converts to plasmin | Intracoronary bolus: 15,000-20,000 IU<br><br>I.V. bolus: none needed | Intracoronary infusion: 2,000-4,000 IU/min over 1 hr; total dose 140,000 IU<br><br>I.V. infusion: 1,500,000 units over 1 hr |
| urokinase | Directly converts plasminogen to plasmin | Intracoronary bolus: none needed | Intracoronary infusion: 2,000 units/lb/hr (4,400 units/kg/hr); rate of 15 ml of solution/hr for total of 12 hr (total volume shouldn't exceed 200 ml) |

streptokinase and urokinase are used to treat deep vein thrombosis, acute arterial thromboembolism, or acute coronary arterial thrombosis and to clear arteriovenous cannula occlusion and venous catheter obstruction. Anistreplase, alteplase, reteplase, streptokinase, and urokinase are indicated in acute MI. These drugs are given to lyse coronary artery thrombi, which may result in improved ventricular function and decreased risk of heart failure. Alteplase is used in the management of acute ischemic CVA.

## Pharmacology

Streptokinase is a protein-like substance produced by group C beta-hemolytic streptococci; urokinase is an enzyme isolated from human kidney tissue cultures. Alteplase is a tissue-type plasminogen activator synthesized by recombinant DNA technology. Anistreplase is anisoylated streptokinase-plasminogen activated complex; it's a fibrinolytic enzyme (plasminogen) plus activator complex (streptokinase) with the activator temporarily blocked by an anisoyl group. Reteplase is a recombinant-plasminogen activator. Thrombolytics act to lyse clots chiefly by converting plasminogen to plasmin; in contrast, anticoagulants act by preventing thrombi from developing. Thrombolytics are more likely to produce clinical bleeding than are oral anticoagulants.

## Overview of adverse reactions

Adverse reactions to these drugs are essentially an extension of their actions; hemorrhage is the most common adverse effect. These drugs cause bleeding twice as often as does heparin. Streptokinase is more likely to cause an allergic reaction than urokinase. Information regarding hypersensitivity to alteplase is limited.

## Clinical considerations

■ Thrombolytic therapy requires medical supervision with continuous clinical and laboratory monitoring.

■ Thrombolytics act only on fibrin clots, not those formed by a precipitated drug.

■ Advise clinician to precisely follow instructions for reconstitution and passing solution through a filter 0.45 micron or smaller to remove filaments in the solution; don't use with dextran because it can interfere with coagulation as well as blood typing and crossmatching.

■ Advise clinician to obtain pretherapy baseline determinations of thrombin time, activated partial thromboplastin time, PT, INR, hematocrit, and platelet count for subsequent blood monitoring. During systemic thrombolytic therapy, as in pulmonary embolism or venous thrombosis, PT, INR, or thrombin time after 4 hours of therapy should be about twice the pretreatment value.

■ Advise clinician to give drugs by infusion pump to ensure accuracy; I.M. injections are contraindicated during therapy because of increased risk of bleeding at the injection site.

■ Advise clinician to check vital signs frequently, monitor patient for blood pressure alterations in excess of 25 mm Hg and any change in cardiac rhythm; check pulses, color, and sensitivity of limbs every hour; monitor patient for excessive bleeding every 15 minutes for first hour, every 30 minutes for second through eighth hours; then at least once every 8 hours. Advise clinician to stop therapy if bleeding is evident; pretreatment with heparin or drugs affecting platelets increases risk.

■ Advise clinician to monitor patient for hypersensitivity as well as hemorrhage; advise clinician to keep available typed and cross-matched packed RBCs and whole blood, aminocaproic acid to treat bleeding, and corticosteroids to treat allergic reactions.

■ Advise patient to keep involved extremity in straight alignment to prevent bleeding from infusion site. Establish precautions to prevent injury and avoid unneeded handling of patient because bruising is likely.

■ At end of infusion, flush remaining dose from pump tubing with I.V. D$_5$W or normal saline solution.

■ Continuous heparin infusion usually is started with the prescribed thrombolytic.

■ Before using thrombolytic to clear an occluded catheter, recommend trying to gently aspirate or flush with heparinized saline solution. Avoid forcible flushing or vigorous suction, which could rupture the catheter or expel the clot into the circulation.

■ When treating MI or CVA, the sooner the treatment is given, the greater the benefit.

### Special populations
**Pregnant patients.** Thrombolytics should be used in pregnancy only if clearly indicated.
**Breast-feeding patients.** Safety in breast-feeding women isn't known.
**Pediatric patients.** Safety in children isn't known.
**Geriatric patients.** Patients age 75 or over are at greater risk of cerebral hemorrhage because they're more apt to have preexisting cerebrovascular disease.

### Patient counseling
■ Explain to patient the reason for treatment and procedure, and necessity for bed rest.
■ Ask patient to be alert for signs of bleeding.
■ When using these drugs to clear catheter, tell patient to exhale and hold breath at any time catheter isn't connected, to prevent air from entering the open catheter.

### Representative combinations
None.

# tricyclic antidepressants (TCAs)

**amitriptyline hydrochloride, amoxapine, clomipramine hydrochloride, desipramine hydrochloride, doxepin hydrochloride, imipramine hydrochloride, imipramine pamoate, nortriptyline hydrochloride, protriptyline, trimipramine maleate**

Clinical trials with the TCA class prototype, imipramine, found no antipsychotic activity, but showed marked mood-elevating effects.

## Clinical indications and actions
### Depression
TCAs are used to treat major depression and dysthymic disorder. Depressed patients who are also anxious are helped most by the more sedative drugs: doxepin, imipramine, and trimipramine. Protriptyline has a stimulant effect that evokes a favorable response in withdrawn depressed patients; only maprotiline has FDA approval for use in depression mixed with anxiety.
### Obsessive-compulsive disorder (OCD)
Clomipramine is used in the treatment of OCD.
### Enuresis
Imipramine is used for enuresis in children over age 6.
### Severe, chronic pain
TCAs, especially amitriptyline, desipramine, doxepin, imipramine, and nortriptyline, are useful in the management of severe chronic pain.
### Other psychiatric disorders
◊ TCAs have been used to treat phobic disorders with panic attacks, eating disorders (bulimia nervosa), and in the short-term treatment of duodenal or gastric ulcer.

TCAs have also been used for the management of nicotine dependence.

## Pharmacology
Although the precise mechanism of their CNS effects isn't established, TCAs may exert their effects by inhibiting reuptake of the neurotransmitters norepinephrine and serotonin in CNS nerve terminals (presynaptic neurons), increasing levels and enhancing activity of neurotransmitters in the synaptic cleft. TCAs also have antihistaminic, sedative, anticholinergic, vasodilatory, and quinidine-like effects; the drugs are structurally similar to phenothiazines and share similar adverse reactions.

Individual TCAs differ somewhat in their degree of CNS inhibitory effect. The tertiary amines (amitriptyline, doxepin, imipramine, and trimipramine) exert greater sedative effects; tertiary amines and protriptyline have more profound effects on cardiac conduction, whereas desipramine has the least anticholinergic activity. All of the currently available TCAs have equal clinical efficacy when given in equivalent therapeutic doses; choice of specific therapy is determined primarily by pharmacokinetic properties and the patient's adverse reaction profile. Patients may respond to some TCAs and not others; if patient doesn't respond to one drug, another should be tried.

## Overview of adverse reactions

Adverse reactions to TCAs are similar to those seen with phenothiazine antipsychotics, including varying degrees of sedation, anticholinergic effects, and orthostatic hypotension. The tertiary amines have the strongest sedative effects; tolerance to these effects usually develops in a few weeks. Protriptyline has the least sedative effect (and may be stimulatory), but shares with the tertiary amines the most pronounced effects on blood pressure and cardiac tissue. Maprotiline and amoxapine are most likely to cause seizures, especially in overdose situations. Desipramine has a greater margin of safety in patients with prostatic hypertrophy, paralytic ileus, glaucoma, and urine retention because of its relatively low level of anticholinergic activity.

## Clinical considerations

■ TCAs impair ability to perform tasks requiring mental alertness, such as driving a car.
■ Advise clinician to check vital signs regularly for decreased blood pressure or tachycardia; observe patient carefully for adverse reactions and report changes. ECG should be obtained in patients over age 40 before starting therapy.
■ Advise clinician to have the patient take the first dose in the office to allow close observation for adverse reactions.
■ Suggest checking for anticholinergic adverse reactions, which may require dose reduction.
■ Caregiver should be sure patient swallows each dose of drug when given; as depressed patients begin to improve, they may hoard pills for suicide attempt.
■ Advise clinician to observe patients for mood changes to monitor progress; benefits may not occur for several (3 to 6) weeks.
■ Full dose of drug shouldn't be withdrawn abruptly; dose should be gradually reduced over a period of weeks to avoid rebound effect or other adverse reactions.
■ Carefully follow manufacturer's instructions for reconstitution, dilution, and storage of drugs.
■ Investigational uses include treating peptic ulcer, migraine prophylaxis, and allergy. Potential toxicity has, to date, outweighed most advantages.
■ Because suicidal overdose with TCAs is usually fatal, only small amounts should be prescribed. If possible, entrust a reliable family member with the drug and warn him to store drug safely away from children.

### Special populations

**Pregnant patients.** Safe use of TCAs in pregnancy hasn't been established. Fetal malformations, urinary retention, CNS effects (lethargy), developmental delay, and withdrawal symptoms have occurred in neonates born to women taking TCAs during pregnancy.
**Breast-feeding patients.** Safety in breast-feeding women hasn't been established.
**Pediatric patients.** TCAs aren't advised for children under age 12.
**Geriatric patients.** Use lower doses because these patients are more sensitive to both therapeutic and adverse effects of TCAs.

### Patient counseling

■ Explain to patient the reason for therapy and anticipated risks and benefits; also explain that full therapeutic effect may not occur for several weeks.
■ Teach patient the signs and symptoms of adverse reactions and the importance of reporting them.
■ Tell patient to avoid beverages and drugs containing alcohol and not to take other drugs (including OTC products) without medical approval.
■ Teach patient how and when to take drug, not to increase dose without medical approval, and never to discontinue drug abruptly.
■ Tell patient to lie down for 30 minutes after first dose and to rise slowly to avoid orthostatic hypotension.
■ Recommend taking drug with milk or food to minimize GI distress; suggest taking full dose at bedtime if daytime sedation is troublesome.
■ Urge diabetic patients to monitor blood glucose level because drug may alter insulin needs.
■ Advise patient to avoid tasks that require mental alertness until full effect of drug is determined.
■ Warn patient that excessive exposure to sunlight, heat lamps, or tanning beds may cause burns and abnormal hyperpigmentation.
■ Recommend sugarless gum or hard candy, artificial saliva, or ice chips to relieve dry mouth.
■ Advise patient that unpleasant adverse effects (except dry mouth) generally diminish over time.

### Representative combinations

*Amitriptyline hydrochloride* with perphenazine: Etrafon, Triavil; with chlordiazepoxide: Limbitrol.

# vitamins

**Fat-soluble:** vitamin A (retinol), vitamin A acid (retinoic acid), vitamin D, vitamin D$_2$ (ergocalciferol), vitamin D$_3$ (calcipotriene), vitamin E, vitamin K (phytonadione)

**Water-soluble:** vitamin B$_1$ (thiamine), vitamin B$_2$ (riboflavin), vitamin B$_3$ (niacin), vitamin B$_6$ (pyridoxine), vitamin B$_9$ (folic acid, folacin), vitamin B$_{12}$ (cyanocobalamin), vitamin C (ascorbic acid)

---

Vitamins are chemically unrelated organic compounds that are required for normal growth and maintenance of metabolic functions. Because the body is unable to synthesize many vitamins, it must obtain them from exogenous sources. Vitamins don't furnish energy and aren't essential building blocks for the body; however, they're essential for the transformation of energy and for the regulation of metabolic processes.

Vitamins are classified as fat-soluble or water-soluble, and the Food and Nutrition Board of the National Research Council determines the RDAs for each. These RDAs represent amounts that will provide adequate nutrition in most healthy persons; they're not minimum requirements. Note that a diet that includes ample intake of the major food groups provides sufficient amounts of vitamins. If needed, vitamins should be used as an adjunct to a regular diet and not as a food substitute.

Controversy has existed for years over use of vitamins. Some argue that vitamin supplementation is unnecessary; some recommend moderate supplementation; still others advocate the use of megavitamins.

## Clinical indications and actions
*Vitamin deficiency or malabsorption; conditions of metabolic stress*
Vitamin supplementation is required when deficiencies exist, in malabsorption syndrome, in hypermetabolic disease states, during pregnancy and lactation, and in the elderly, alcoholics, or dieters. Multiple vitamins may be indicated for patients taking oral contraceptives, estrogens, prolonged antibiotic therapy, isoniazid, or for patients receiving prolonged total parenteral nutrition.

Persons with increased metabolic requirements, such as infants and those suffering severe injury, trauma, major surgery, or severe infection also require supplementation. Prolonged diarrhea, severe GI disorders, malignancy, surgical removal of sections of GI tract, obstructive jaundice, cystic fibrosis, and other conditions leading to reduced or poor absorption are indications for multiple vitamin therapy. Refer to individual vitamins for specific indications.

## Pharmacology
Vitamins are available as single drugs or with several other vitamins with or without minerals, trace elements, iron, fluoride, or other nutritional supplements. Often, diets deficient in one vitamin are also deficient in other vitamins of similar dietary source. Malabsorption syndromes also affect the usage of several vitamins as do certain disease states that increase metabolic rates. Therefore, multiple vitamin therapy may be useful in these situations.

Fat-soluble vitamins are absorbed with dietary fats and stored in the body in moderate amounts; they aren't normally excreted in urine. Chronic ingestion leads to excessive build-up of these vitamins and toxicity.

Water-soluble vitamins aren't stored in the body in any appreciable amounts and are excreted in urine. These vitamins seldom cause toxicity in patients with normal renal function.

Both types of vitamins are needed for the maintenance of normal structure and metabolic functions of the body. (See *Recommended daily allowances for adults ages 23 to 50.*)

## Overview of adverse reactions
Common adverse reactions seen with both fat-soluble and water-soluble vitamins include nausea, vomiting, diarrhea, tiredness, weakness, headache, loss of appetite, rash, and itching.

## Clinical considerations
■ Monitoring may be required. See specific vitamin entries for details.
■ Vitamins containing iron may cause constipation and black, tarry stools.
■ Excessive fluoride supplements can cause hypocalcemia and tetany.
■ Recommend giving with food or after meals to reduce GI distress associated with vitamin therapy.

## Special populations
**Pregnant patients.** Vitamin supplementation in pregnancy should be regulated by a prescriber.
**Breast-feeding patients.** RDAs may be increased in breast-feeding women.
**Pediatric patients.** RDAs vary with age. Excessive amounts of vitamins, particularly in neonates, may be toxic.

## Patient counseling
■ Stress to patient the importance of adequate dietary intake. Vitamins aren't food substitutes.
■ Tell patient to take vitamins only as directed, not to exceed RDA, and to take with food,

---

## RECOMMENDED DAILY ALLOWANCES FOR ADULTS AGES 23 TO 50

| Vitamin | Men | Women | Pregnant women† | Lactating women† |
|---|---|---|---|---|
| A | 1,000 mcg | 800 mcg | 800 mcg | 1,300 mcg |
| $B_1$ | 1.5 mg | 1.1 mg | 1.5 mg | 1.6 mg |
| $B_2$ | 1.7 mg | 1.3 mg | 1.6 mg | 1.8 mg |
| $B_6$ | 2 mg | 1.6 mg | 2.2 mg | 2.1 mg |
| $B_{12}$ | 2 mcg | 2 mcg | 2.2 mcg | 2.6 mcg |
| C | 60 mg | 60 mg | 70 mg | 95 mg |
| D | 200 IU | 200 IU | 400 IU | 400 IU |
| E | 15 IU | 12 IU | 15 IU | 18 IU |
| K | 80 mcg | 65 mcg | 65 mcg | 65 mcg |
| folic acid | 200 mcg | 180 mcg | 400 mcg | 280 mcg |
| niacin | 19 mg | 15 mg | 17 mg | 20 mg |

† First 6 months.

milk, or after meals to reduce chance of stomach upset.
■ Store vitamins away from heat and light and out of the reach of small children.
■ Warn patient that vitamins with iron may cause constipation and black, tarry stools.
■ Tell patient to read all label directions. Warn him not to take large doses unless prescribed.
■ Inform patient that liquid vitamins may be mixed with food or juice.
■ Advise patient not to refer to vitamins or other drugs as candy and to avoid taking them indiscriminately.

### Representative combinations
The following list includes selected combinations that are available only by prescription.

*B vitamins* (oral) niacin ($B_3$), pantothenic acid ($B_5$), pyridoxine ($B_6$), and cyanocobalamin ($B_{12}$), with folic acid ($B_9$), iron, manganese, zinc, and 13% alcohol: Megaton Elixir; with thiamine ($B_1$), riboflavin ($B_2$), ferric pyrophosphate, and 15% alcohol: Senilezol Liquid; with thiamine ($B_1$), riboflavin ($B_2$), ascorbic acid, and folic acid: Berocca, B-Plex, Strovite, B-C with folic acid; with thiamine ($B_1$), riboflavin ($B_2$), ascorbic acid, folic acid, and biotin: Nephrocaps.

*B vitamins* (parenteral) with riboflavin ($B_2$), niacin ($B_3$), pantothenic acid ($B_5$), pyridoxine ($B_6$), and ascorbic acid: Becomject-100.

*Multivitamins* (oral) vitamins E, thiamine ($B_1$), riboflavin ($B_2$), niacin ($B_3$), pantothenic acid ($B_5$), pyridoxine ($B_6$), cyanocobalamin ($B_{12}$), ascorbic acid, and folic acid: Cefol Filmtabs; with vitamins A, D, E, thiamine ($B_1$), riboflavin ($B_2$), niacin ($B_3$), pantothenic acid ($B_5$), pyridoxine ($B_6$), cyanocobalamin ($B_{12}$), ascorbic acid, iron, and folic acid: Unicomplex-

T&M Tablets, Cerovite Jr., Quintabs-M, Centrum Jr. with Iron, Monocaps, Unicap Sr., Hi-Po-Vites.

*Multivitamins* (parenteral) vitamins A, D, E, thiamine ($B_1$), riboflavin ($B_2$), niacin ($B_3$), pantothenic acid ($B_5$), pyridoxine ($B_6$), anocobalamin ($B_{12}$), ascorbic acid, biotin, and folic acid: Berocca Parenteral Nutrition, M.V.I.-12.

*Multivitamins* with fluoride (oral) vitamins A, D, thiamine ($B_1$), riboflavin ($B_2$), niacin ($B_3$), pantothenic acid ($B_5$), pyridoxine ($B_6$), cyanocobalamin ($B_{12}$), ascorbic acid, folic acid, and fluoride: Polyvitamin Fluoride, Mulvidren-F Softab Tablets, Polytabs-F; vitamins A, D, E, thiamine ($B_1$), riboflavin ($B_2$), niacin ($B_3$), pyridoxine ($B_6$), cyanocobalamin ($B_{12}$), ascorbic acid, folic acid, and fluoride: Poly-Vi-Flor, Florvite, Vi-Daylin/F.

# abacavir sulfate
Ziagen

*Pharmacologic classification:* nucleoside analogue reverse transcriptase inhibitor (NRTI)
*Therapeutic classification:* antiviral
*Pregnancy risk category C*

## Available forms
Available by prescription only
*Tablets:* 300 mg
*Oral solution:* 20 mg/ml

## Indications and dosages
*HIV-1 infection*
*Adults:* 300 mg P.O. b.i.d. with other antiretrovirals.
*Children ages 3 months to 16 years:* 8 mg/kg P.O. b.i.d. (up to maximum of 300 mg P.O. b.i.d.) with other antiretrovirals.

## Mechanism of action
*Antiviral action:* Converted intracellularly to an active metabolite, carbovir triphosphate, which inhibits the activity of HIV-1 reverse transcriptase by competing with the natural substrate deoxyguanosine-5′-triphosphate (dGTP) and by incorporation into viral DNA.

## Pharmacokinetics
*Absorption:* Rapidly and extensively absorbed after oral administration; the mean absolute bioavailability of the tablet is 83%.
*Distribution:* Distributed in the extravascular space. About 50% of drug binds to plasma proteins.
*Metabolism:* Primarily metabolized by alcohol dehydrogenase and glucuronyl transferase to form two metabolites that lack antiviral activity.
*Excretion:* Primarily excreted in urine; about 16% of dose is excreted in feces. Elimination half-life in single-dose studies was 1 to 2 hours.

| Route | Onset | Peak | Duration |
|-------|-------|------|----------|
| P.O. | Unknown | Unknown | Unknown |

## Contraindications and precautions
Contraindicated in patients hypersensitive to the drug or its components. Use cautiously in patients with known risk factors for liver disease.

## Interactions
None known.

## Adverse reactions
**CNS:** insomnia and sleep disorders, headache.
**GI:** *nausea, vomiting,* diarrhea, anorexia.
**Skin:** rash.
**Other:** *hypersensitivity reaction,* fever.

## Overdose and treatment
There's no known antidote, and it isn't known if the drug is removed by peritoneal dialysis or hemodialysis.

## Clinical considerations
■ Abacavir should always be used with other antiretrovirals and shouldn't be added as a single drug when antiretroviral regimens are changed as a result of loss of virologic response.
■ Because the drug is absorbed equally well from both dosage forms, solution and tablets can be used interchangeably.
**⚕ ALERT** Drug has caused fatal hypersensitivity reactions. If signs or symptoms of hypersensitivity (fever, skin rash, fatigue, GI symptoms such as nausea, vomiting, diarrhea, or abdominal pain) develop, drug should be stopped as soon as a reaction is suspected, and patient should seek immediate medical attention.
■ Drug should be stopped if hypersensitivity cannot be ruled out.
**⚕ ALERT** Drug shouldn't be started following a hypersensitivity reaction because more severe symptoms will recur within hours and may include life-threatening hypotension and death. Symptoms usually appear within the first 6 weeks of treatment, but may occur at any time.
■ Drug may be reintroduced only in patients without prior hypersensitivity.
■ To facilitate reporting of hypersensitivity reactions and collection of information on each case, an abacavir hypersensitivity registry has been established at 1-800-270-0425.

### *Therapeutic monitoring*
■ Lactic acidosis and severe (even fatal) hepatomegaly with steatosis have been reported with use of nucleoside analogues alone or in combination, including abacavir and other antiretrovirals. Advise clinician to stop treatment if a patient develops clinical or laboratory findings suggestive of lactic acidosis or pronounced

hepatotoxicity (which may include hepatomegaly and steatosis even in the absence of marked transaminase elevations).

■ Advise clinician to monitor patient for hypersensitivity reactions.

### Special populations

**Pregnant patients.** There are no adequate controlled studies in pregnant women. Report maternal-fetal outcomes of pregnant women exposed to drug to the Antiretroviral Pregnancy Registry at 1-800-258-4263.

**Breast-feeding patients.** Because of the potential for HIV transmission through breastfeeding and because of the possible adverse effects of abacavir, women receiving this drug shouldn't breast-feed.

**Pediatric patients.** Safety and efficacy haven't been established in children age 3 months to 13 years.

**Geriatric patients.** Dose selection for a geriatric patient should be cautious, taking into account greater frequency of decreased hepatic, renal, or cardiac function, and of concomitant disease or other drug therapy in this age group.

### Patient counseling

■ Advise patient of the risk of a life-threatening hypersensitivity reaction with this drug.

■ Advise patient (in whom treatment has been stopped for reasons other than hypersensitivity) that severe or fatal hypersensitivity reactions can occur following the reintroduction of treatment.

■ Tell patient to immediately contact the prescriber if signs or symptoms of hypersensitivity (fever; skin rash; severe tiredness; GI symptoms such as nausea, vomiting, diarrhea or stomach pain; achiness; or generally ill feeling) develop.

■ Instruct patient to always carry a medical alert card summarizing the symptoms of the hypersensitivity reaction.

■ Explain that this drug isn't a cure for HIV infection nor does it reduce the risk of transmission of HIV to others through sexual contact or blood contamination. Advise patient to remain under a prescriber's care throughout drug therapy and to use safe sex practices.

■ Inform patient that long-term effects of this drug are unknown.

■ Advise patient to take drug exactly as prescribed.

■ Urge patient to read the drug guide that comes with each new prescription and refill.

■ Tell patient that the drug may be taken without regard to meals.

# acarbose

Precose

*Pharmacologic classification:* alpha-glucosidase inhibitor
*Therapeutic classification:* antidiabetic
*Pregnancy risk category B*

## Available forms

Available by prescription only
*Tablets:* 25 mg, 50 mg, 100 mg

## Indications and dosages

*Dietary adjunct to lower blood glucose levels in patients with type 2 (non–insulin-dependent) diabetes mellitus whose hyperglycemia can't be managed by diet alone or by diet and a sulfonylurea*
*Adults:* Initially, 25 mg P.O. t.i.d. with the first bite of each main meal. Subsequent dosage adjustment made at 4- to 8-week intervals based on 1-hour postprandial glucose levels and tolerance. Maintenance dosage is 50 to 100 mg P.O. t.i.d. depending on patient's weight. Maximum dose for patients weighing 60 kg (132 lb) or less is 50 mg P.O. t.i.d.; for patients weighing over 60 kg, maximum dose is 100 mg P.O. t.i.d.

*Adjunct to insulin or metformin therapy in patients with type 2 (non–insulin-dependent) diabetes mellitus whose hyperglycemia can't be managed by diet, exercise, and insulin or metformin alone*
*Adults:* Initially, 25 mg P.O. t.i.d. with first bite of each main meal. Adjust dosage at 4- to 8-week intervals based on 1-hour postprandial glucose levels and tolerance to determine minimum effective dosage of each drug. Maintenance dosage is 50 to 100 mg P.O. t.i.d. based on patient's weight. Maximum dose for patients weighing 60 kg (132 lb) or less is 50 mg P.O. t.i.d.; for patients weighing over 60 kg, maximum dose is 100 mg P.O. t.i.d.

## Mechanism of action

*Antidiabetic action:* The ability of acarbose to lower blood glucose levels results from a competitive, reversible inhibition of pancreatic alpha-amylase and membrane-bound intestinal alpha-glucoside hydrolase enzymes. In diabetic patients, this enzyme inhibition results in delayed glucose absorption and a lowering of postprandial hyperglycemia. The drug doesn't enhance insulin secretion.

## Pharmacokinetics

*Absorption:* Minimally absorbed.
*Distribution:* Acts locally within the GI tract.
*Metabolism:* Metabolized exclusively within the GI tract, principally by intestinal bacteria with some metabolized action caused by digestive enzymes.

*Excretion:* Within 96 hours, 51% of dose is excreted in feces as unabsorbed drug. The fraction of drug absorbed is almost completely excreted by the kidneys. Plasma elimination half-life of acarbose is about 2 hours. Drug accumulation doesn't occur with t.i.d. oral dosing.

| Route | Onset | Peak | Duration |
|-------|-------|------|----------|
| P.O. | Unknown | 1 hr | 2-4 hr |

## Contraindications and precautions

Contraindicated in patients hypersensitive to drug, diabetic ketoacidosis, cirrhosis, inflammatory bowel disease, colonic ulceration, or partial intestinal obstruction and in those predisposed to intestinal obstruction. Also contraindicated in patients with chronic intestinal diseases associated with marked disorders of digestion or absorption and in those with conditions that may deteriorate because of increased gas formation in the intestine. Avoid using drug in patients with serum creatinine levels exceeding 2 mg/dl and in breast-feeding or pregnant women.

Use cautiously in patients with mild to moderate renal impairment.

## Interactions

**Drug-drug.** *Calcium channel blockers, corticosteroids, estrogens, isoniazid, nicotinic acid, oral contraceptives, phenothiazines, phenytoin, sympathomimetics, thiazides, other diuretics, and thyroid hormones:* May cause hyperglycemia or hypoglycemia when withdrawn. Advise clinician to monitor patient's blood glucose levels.

*Digestive enzyme preparations containing carbohydrate-splitting enzymes (amylase, pancreatin), intestinal adsorbents (activated charcoal):* May reduce the effect of acarbose. Don't give together.

*Sulfonylureas or insulin:* When used with acarbose, the hypoglycemic potential of these drugs may be increased. Advise clinician to monitor patient's blood glucose level closely.

**Drug-herb.** *Aloe, bilberry leaf, bitter melon, burdock, dandelion, fenugreek, garlic,* and *ginseng:* Concomitant use may improve blood glucose control, requiring a reduction of antidiabetics. Advise patient to discuss the use of herbal medicines with prescriber before use.

## Adverse reactions

**GI:** *abdominal pain, diarrhea, flatulence.*
**Hepatic:** elevated serum transaminase levels.

## Overdose and treatment

Unlike sulfonylureas or insulin, acarbose overdose doesn't result in hypoglycemia. An overdose may result in transient increases in flatulence, diarrhea, and abdominal discomfort, which quickly subside.

## Clinical considerations

■ Recommend maintaining exercise and diet control with acarbose therapy.
■ Acarbose isn't effective as sole therapy in patients with diabetes mellitus complicated by acidosis, ketosis, or coma; management of these conditions requires insulin.
■ Because of its mechanism of action, acarbose shouldn't cause hypoglycemia when administered alone in the fasted or postprandial state.

### Therapeutic monitoring

■ Acarbose alone doesn't cause hypoglycemia. However, when given with a sulfonylurea or insulin, it may increase the hypoglycemic potential of the sulfonylurea. Advise clinician to closely monitor patient receiving both drugs. If hypoglycemia occurs, it should be treated with oral glucose (dextrose), whose absorption isn't inhibited by acarbose, rather than sucrose (cane sugar). Severe hypoglycemia may require I.V. glucose infusion or glucagon administration. Dosage adjustment in acarbose and sulfonylurea may be required to prevent further episodes of hypoglycemia.
■ During stress, such as infection, fever, surgery, or trauma, patient may require insulin therapy. Advise clinician to monitor patient closely for hyperglycemia in these situations.
■ Advise clinician to monitor patient's 1-hour postprandial plasma glucose levels to determine therapeutic effectiveness of acarbose and to identify appropriate dose. Thereafter, measure glycosylated hemoglobin every 3 months. Treatment goals include decreasing both postprandial plasma glucose and glycosylated hemoglobin levels to normal or near normal by using the lowest effective dose of acarbose either as monotherapy or with sulfonylureas.
■ Advise clinician to monitor serum transaminase levels every 3 months during first year of therapy and then periodically thereafter in patients receiving doses exceeding 50 mg t.i.d. Abnormalities may require dosage adjustment or withdrawal of drug.

### Special populations

**Breast-feeding patients.** It isn't known if drug appears in breast milk. Acarbose shouldn't be given to breast-feeding women.
**Pediatric patients.** Safety and efficacy in pediatric patients under age 18 haven't been established.

## Patient counseling

■ Tell patient to take drug with the first bite of each of three main meals daily.
■ Make sure patient understands that therapy relieves symptoms but doesn't cure disease.
■ Stress the importance of adhering to specific diet, reducing weight, exercising, and following personal hygiene programs. Explain how and when to perform self-monitoring of

blood glucose level and teach recognition of and intervention for hyperglycemia.

■ Teach patient to recognize and intervene for hypoglycemia if a sulfonylurea drug is also taken. Tell patient to treat symptoms of low blood glucose with a form of dextrose instead of products containing table sugar.

■ Advise patient to carry medical identification regarding diabetic status.

# acebutolol
Sectral

*Pharmacologic classification*: beta blocker
*Therapeutic classification*: antihypertensive, antiarrhythmic
*Pregnancy risk category B*

## Available forms
Available by prescription only
*Capsules*: 200 mg, 400 mg

## Indications and dosages
**Hypertension**
*Adults*: 400 mg P.O. either as a single daily dose or 200 mg b.i.d. Patients may receive as much as 1,200 mg divided b.i.d.
**Ventricular arrhythmias**
*Adults*: 200 mg P.O. b.i.d. Increase dosage to provide an adequate clinical response. Usual daily dose is 600 to 1,200 mg.
◊ *Angina*
*Adults*: Initially, 200 mg b.i.d. Increase up to 800 mg daily until angina is controlled. Patients with severe angina may require higher doses.
≡ *Dosage adjustment.* Reduce dosage in geriatric patients and in those with impaired renal function. If creatinine clearance is 25 to 49 ml/minute, decrease dose by 50%. If creatinine clearance is less than 25 ml/minute, decrease dose by 75%. Avoid doses over 800 mg/day in geriatric patients.

## Mechanism of action
*Antihypertensive action:* Exact mechanism of antihypertensive beta$_1$ blocker effect is unknown. Drug has cardioselective beta blocking properties and mild intrinsic sympathomimetic activity.
*Antiarrhythmic action:* Drug decreases heart rate and prevents exercise-induced increases in heart rate; it also decreases myocardial contractility, cardiac output, and SA and AV nodal conduction velocity.

## Pharmacokinetics
*Absorption:* Well absorbed after oral administration.
*Distribution:* About 26% protein-bound; minimal quantities are detected in CSF.

*Metabolism:* Undergoes extensive first-pass metabolism in the liver; peak levels of its major active metabolite, diacetolol, occur at about 3½ hours.
*Excretion:* From 30% to 40% of a given dose is excreted in urine; remainder occurs in feces and bile. Half-life of acebutolol is 3 to 4 hours; half-life of diacetolol is 8 to 13 hours.

| Route | Onset | Peak | Duration |
|-------|-------|------|----------|
| P.O. | 1½ hr | 2½ hr | 24 hr |

## Contraindications and precautions
Contraindicated in patients with persistent severe bradycardia, second- and third-degree heart block, overt cardiac failure, and cardiogenic shock. Use cautiously in patients at risk for heart failure and in patients with bronchospastic disease, diabetes, hyperthyroidism, and peripheral vascular disease, and in patients with impaired hepatic function.

## Interactions
**Drug-drug.** *Other antihypertensives:* Acebutolol may potentiate hypotensive effects. Advise clinician to monitor blood pressure.
*Insulin or oral antidiabetics:* Dosage requirements in stable diabetic patients may be altered. Advise clinician to monitor blood glucose levels.
*Indomethacin, NSAIDs, and alpha-adrenergic stimulants such as those in OTC cold remedies:* Hypotensive effects of acebutolol may be antagonized by these drugs. Use together cautiously.

## Adverse reactions
**CNS:** depression, dizziness, fatigue, headache, hyperesthesia, hypoesthesia, insomnia.
**CV:** *bradycardia,* chest pain, edema, *heart failure,* hypotension.
**GI:** abdominal pain, constipation, diarrhea, dyspepsia, flatulence, nausea, vomiting.
**Metabolic:** *hypoglycemia, increased risk for developing type 2 diabetes mellitus.*
**Musculoskeletal:** arthralgia, myalgia.
**Respiratory:** *bronchospasm,* cough, dyspnea.
**Skin:** rash.
**Other:** impotence.

## Overdose and treatment
Signs of overdose include severe hypotension, bradycardia, heart failure, and bronchospasm.

After acute ingestion, advise clinician to empty stomach by emesis or gastric lavage and follow with activated charcoal to reduce absorption. Symptomatic and supportive treatment should be provided.

## Clinical considerations
■ Store capsules in well-closed containers, protected from light at controlled room temperature.

---

*Reactions may be* common, uncommon, *life-threatening,* or COMMON AND LIFE-THREATENING.

- Dose should be adjusted every 1 to 2 months if blood pressure control is inadequate.
- Drug shouldn't be stopped abruptly because it may exacerbate angina symptoms or precipitate MI in patients with coronary artery disease. Advise clinician to discontinue drug gradually over 2 weeks.
- Beta blockers may mask the symptoms of hypoglycemia.
- Acebutolol may cause positive antinuclear antibody titers.

### Therapeutic monitoring
Advise clinician to carefully monitor blood pressure during dosage adjustment.

### Special populations
**Pregnant patients.** There are no adequate and controlled studies in pregnant women. Infants born to women receiving acebutolol during pregnancy had low birth weights and decreased systolic blood pressures and heart rates during the first 72 hours after delivery.
**Breast-feeding patients.** Both acebutolol and its metabolite, diacetolol, appear in breast milk; breast-feeding isn't recommended.
**Pediatric patients.** Safety and efficacy in children under age 12 haven't been established.
**Geriatric patients.** Avoid doses over 800 mg.

### Patient counseling
Advise patient to promptly report wheezing.

---

# acetaminophen
Acephen, Aceta, Anacin Aspirin Free, Feverall, Genapap, Panadol, PediApap, Suppap, Tylenol

*Pharmacologic classification:* para-aminophenol derivative
*Therapeutic classification:* nonnarcotic analgesic, antipyretic
*Pregnancy risk category B*

### Available forms
Available without a prescription
*Tablets:* 325 mg, 500 mg, 650 mg
*Tablets (chewable):* 80 mg, 160 mg
*Tablets (extended-release):* 650 mg
*Capsules:* 500 mg
*Suppositories:* 80 mg, 120 mg, 125 mg, 325 mg, 650 mg
*Solution:* 48 mg/ml, 80 mg/ml*, 100 mg/ml, 80 mg/5 ml, 120 mg/5 ml, 160 mg/5 ml, 167 mg/5 ml, 500 mg/15 ml
*Suspension:* 80 mg/ml*, 100 mg/ml, 80 mg/5 ml*, 160 mg/5 ml
*Caplets:* 160 mg, 325 mg, 500 mg
*Syrup:* 16 mg/ml
*Sprinkle capsules:* 80 mg, 160 mg

## Indications and dosages
*Mild pain, fever*
*Adults and children over age 12:* 325 to 650 mg P.O. or P.R. q 4 to 6 hours p.r.n. Maximum dose shouldn't exceed 4 g daily. Maximum dose for long-term therapy is 2.6 g daily; alternatively, two 650-mg extended-release tablets every 8 hours p.r.n., not to exceed 4 g per day.
*Children ages 11 to 12:* 480 mg/dose P.O. or P.R. q 4 to 6 hours, p.r.n.
*Children ages 9 to 10:* 400 mg/dose P.O. or P.R. q 4 to 6 hours, p.r.n.
*Children ages 6 to 8:* 320 mg/dose P.O. or P.R. q 4 to 6 hours, p.r.n.
*Children ages 4 to 5:* 240 mg/dose P.O. or P.R. q 4 to 6 hours, p.r.n.
*Children ages 2 to 3:* 160 mg/dose P.O. or P.R. q 4 to 6 hours, p.r.n.
*Children ages 12 to 23 months:* 120 mg/dose P.O. or P.R. q 4 to 6 hours, p.r.n.
*Children ages 4 to 11 months:* 80 mg/dose P.O. or P.R. q 4 to 6 hours, p.r.n.
*Children ages 3 months or younger:* 40 mg/dose P.O. or P.R. q 4 to 6 hours, p.r.n.
*Osteoarthritis*
*Adults:* Up to 1 g P.O. q.i.d.; doses of 3 to 4 g per day common in these patients.

## Mechanism of action
Mechanism and site of action may be related to inhibition of prostaglandin synthesis in CNS.
*Analgesic action:* Analgesic effect may be related to an elevation of the pain threshold.
*Antipyretic action:* Drug may exert antipyretic effect by direct action on hypothalamic heat-regulating center to block effects of endogenous pyrogen. This results in increased heat dissipation through sweating and vasodilation.

## Pharmacokinetics
*Absorption:* Absorbed rapidly and completely via the GI tract.
*Distribution:* 25% protein-bound. Plasma levels don't correlate well with analgesic effect, but do correlate with toxicity.
*Metabolism:* About 90% to 95% is metabolized in the liver.
*Excretion:* Excreted in urine. Average elimination half-life ranges from 1 to 4 hours. In acute overdose, prolongation of elimination half-life is correlated with toxic effects. Half-life over 4 hours is linked to hepatic necrosis; over 12 hours is linked to coma.

| Route | Onset | Peak | Duration |
|---|---|---|---|
| P.O., P.R. | Unknown | 1-3 hr | 3-4 hr |

## Contraindications and precautions
No known contraindications. Should be used cautiously in patients with history of chronic alcohol abuse because hepatotoxicity has occurred after therapeutic doses. Should also be used cautiously in patients with hepatic or CV

disease, renal function impairment, or viral infection.

## Interactions

**Drug-drug.** *Antacids:* Delay and decrease the absorption of acetaminophen. Separate administration times.

*Anticoagulants and thrombolytic drugs:* May potentiate effects of these drugs, but this appears to be clinically insignificant.

*Anticonvulsants and isoniazid:* Increased risk of hepatotoxicity. Use together cautiously.

*Phenothiazines:* If used with acetaminophen in large doses, hypothermia may result. Use together cautiously.

**Drug-herb.** *Watercress:* May inhibit oxidative metabolism of acetaminophen. Discourage use together.

**Drug-food.** *Foods:* Delay and decrease absorption of acetaminophen. Advise patient to take drug on an empty stomach.

*Caffeine:* May enhance therapeutic effect of acetaminophen. Inform patient of this effect.

**Drug-lifestyle.** *Alcohol use:* Increases the risk of liver toxicity. Advise patient to avoid alcohol.

## Adverse reactions

**Hematologic:** hemolytic anemia, *neutropenia, leukopenia, pancytopenia, thrombocytopenia*.

**Hepatic:** jaundice, *liver damage* (with toxic doses).

**Metabolic:** hypoglycemia.

**Skin:** rash, urticaria.

## Overdose and treatment

In all cases of suspected acetaminophen overdose, a regional poison center or the Rocky Mountain Poison and Drug Center (1-800-332-3073) may be called for assistance. In acute overdose, plasma levels of 300 mcg/ml 4 hours postinjection or 50 mcg/ml 12 hours postinjection indicate hepatotoxicity. Signs and symptoms of overdose include cyanosis, anemia, jaundice, skin eruptions, fever, emesis, CNS stimulation, delirium, methemoglobinemia progressing to depression, coma, vascular collapse, seizures, and death. Acetaminophen poisoning develops in stages:

*Stage 1* (12 to 24 hours after ingestion): nausea, vomiting, diaphoresis, anorexia

*Stage 2* (24 to 48 hours after ingestion): clinically improved but elevated liver function tests

*Stage 3* (72 to 96 hours after ingestion): peak hepatotoxicity

*Stage 4* (7 to 8 days after ingestion): recovery.

To treat toxic overdose of acetaminophen, advise clinician to empty stomach immediately by inducing emesis with ipecac syrup if patient is conscious or by gastric lavage. Advise clinician to give activated charcoal by way of nasogastric tube. Oral acetylcysteine (Mucomyst) is a specific antidote for acetaminophen

poisoning and is most effective if started within 10 to 12 hours after ingestion, but it can help if started within 24 hours after ingestion. Recommend giving a Mucomyst loading dose of 140 mg/kg P.O., followed by maintenance dosages of 70 mg/kg P.O. every 4 hours for an additional 17 doses. Doses vomited within 1 hour of administration must be repeated. Advise clinician to remove charcoal before giving acetylcysteine because it may interfere with absorption of this antidote.

Acetylcysteine minimizes hepatic injury by supplying sulfydryl groups that bind with acetaminophen metabolites. Hemodialysis may be helpful to remove acetaminophen from the body. Advise clinician to monitor laboratory parameters and vital signs closely. Symptomatic and supportive measures (respiratory support, correction of fluid and electrolyte imbalances) should be provided. Plasma acetaminophen levels should be determined at least 4 hours after overdose. If plasma acetaminophen levels indicate hepatotoxicity, advise clinician to perform liver function tests every 24 hours for at least 96 hours.

## Clinical considerations

■ Acetaminophen has no significant anti-inflammatory effect. Even so, studies have shown substantial benefit in patients with osteoarthritis of the knee. Therapeutic benefits may stem from the analgesic effects of the drug.

■ Many OTC products contain acetaminophen. Be aware of this when dispensing this drug.

**H ALERT** Be aware of patient's total daily intake of acetaminophen, especially if he is also prescribed other drugs containing this component, such as Percocet. Toxicity can occur.

■ Patients unable to tolerate aspirin may be able to tolerate acetaminophen.

■ When buffered acetaminophen effervescent granules are prescribed, consider sodium content for sodium-restricted patients.

■ Advise patients with phenylketonuria that many preparations contain aspartame.

■ Many acetaminophen preparations contain sulfites.

■ The extended-release tablet shouldn't be crushed, chewed, or dissolved in liquid.

■ Store rectal acetaminophen suppositories in refrigerator.

■ Acetaminophen may cause a false-positive test result for urinary 5-hydroxyindoleacetic acid.

### *Therapeutic monitoring*

■ Address patient's level of pain and response before and after drug administration.

■ Advise clinician to monitor vital signs, especially temperature, to evaluate effectiveness of drug.

■ Advise clinician to monitor PT and INR values in patients receiving oral anticoagulants and sustained acetaminophen therapy.

## Special populations
**Breast-feeding patients.** Drug appears in breast milk in low levels. No adverse effects have been reported.
**Pediatric patients.** Children shouldn't take more than five doses per day or take drug for longer than 5 days unless prescribed. Instruct caregivers on weight-based acetaminophen dosing, to use the provided calibrated measuring device with the preparation, and not to give more than the recommended dose.
**Geriatric patients.** Geriatric patients are more sensitive to drug. Use with caution.

## Patient counseling
■ Instruct patient in proper administration of prescribed form of drug.
■ Advise patient on chronic high-dose drug therapy to arrange for monitoring of laboratory parameters, especially BUN, serum creatinine, liver function tests, and CBC.
■ Warn patient with current or past rectal bleeding to avoid using rectal acetaminophen suppositories. If they're used, they must be retained in the rectum for at least 1 hour.
■ Warn patient that high doses or unsupervised chronic use of acetaminophen can cause liver damage. Use of alcoholic beverages increases the risk of liver toxicity.
■ Tell patient to avoid use with temperature of more than 103° F (39° C), a fever persisting longer than 3 days, or a recurrent fever.
■ Caution patient and parent not to use other OTC preparations that contain acetaminophen, because toxicity may occur.
■ Tell patient not to take NSAIDs with acetaminophen on a regular basis.
■ Warn patient to avoid taking tetracycline antibiotics within 1 hour after taking buffered acetaminophen effervescent granules.
■ Tell patient not to use drug for arthritic or rheumatic conditions without medical approval. Drug may relieve pain but not other symptoms.
■ Advise adult patient not to take drug for longer than 10 days without medical approval.
■ Tell patient on high-dose or long-term therapy that regular follow-up visits are essential.

---

# acetazolamide
# acetazolamide sodium
Diamox, Diamox Sequels

*Pharmacologic classification:* carbonic anhydrase inhibitor
*Therapeutic classification:* antiglaucoma drug, anticonvulsant, diuretic, altitude sickness agent
*Pregnancy risk category C*

## Available forms
Available by prescription only
*Tablets:* 125 mg, 250 mg
*Capsules (extended-release):* 500 mg
*Injection:* 500 mg

## Indications and dosages
*Secondary glaucoma and preoperative management of acute angle-closure glaucoma*
*Adults:* 250 mg P.O. q 4 hours, or 250 mg P.O. b.i.d. for short-term therapy. In acute cases, 500 mg P.O. followed by 125 to 250 mg P.O. q 4 hours. To rapidly lower intraocular pressure, 500 mg I.V., which may be repeated in 2 to 4 hours, if needed, followed by 125 to 250 mg P.O. q 4 hours.
*Children:* 5 to 10 mg/kg I.V. q 6 hours.
*Edema in heart failure*
*Adults:* 250 to 375 mg P.O. daily in morning.
*Children:* 5 mg/kg or 150 mg/m$^2$ P.O. or I.V. daily in morning.
*Drug-induced edema*
*Adults:* 250 to 375 mg (5 mg/kg) P.O. as single daily dose for 1 to 2 days alternating with 1 drug-free day.
*Chronic open-angle glaucoma*
*Adults:* 250 mg to 1 g P.O. daily in divided doses, or 500 mg (extended-release) P.O. once daily or b.i.d. Doses over 1 g daily don't produce an increased effect.
*Children:* 8 to 30 mg/kg P.O. or 300 to 900 mg/m$^2$ daily in three divided doses.
*Prevention or amelioration of acute mountain sickness*
*Adults:* 250 mg to 1 g P.O. daily in divided doses (such as 250 mg q 8 to 12 hours) or 500 mg (extended-release) P.O. q 12 to 24 hours, taken preferably 48 hours before ascent and continued for at least 48 hours after arrival at high altitude.
*Myoclonic seizures, refractory generalized tonic-clonic (grand mal) or absence (petit mal) seizures, mixed seizures*
*Adults and children:* 8 to 30 mg/kg P.O. daily, divided into one to four doses. The optimum dose range is 375 mg to 1 g P.O. daily. When given with other anticonvulsants, the initial dose is 250 mg daily.
*Periodic paralysis*
*Adults:* 250 mg P.O. b.i.d. or t.i.d. Maximum dose, 1.5 g daily.

## I.V. administration
■ Reconstitute powder by adding at least 5 ml sterile water for injection.
■ Direct I.V. administration is preferred if drug must be given parenterally.

## Incompatibilities
Incompatible with multivitamins.

## Mechanism of action
*Antiglaucoma action:* In open-angle glaucoma and perioperatively for acute angle-closure glaucoma, acetazolamide and acetazolamide

sodium decrease the formation of aqueous humor, lowering intraocular pressure.

*Anticonvulsant action:* Inhibition of carbonic anhydrase in the CNS appears to slow down abnormal paroxysmal discharge from the neurons.

*Diuretic action:* Acetazolamide and acetazolamide sodium act by noncompetitive reversible inhibition of the enzyme carbonic anhydrase, which is responsible for formation of hydrogen and bicarbonate ions from carbon dioxide and water. This inhibition results in decreased hydrogen level in the renal tubules, promoting excretion of bicarbonate, sodium, potassium, and water; systemic acidosis may occur because carbon dioxide isn't eliminated as rapidly.

*Altitude sickness drug:* Acetazolamide shortens the period of high-altitude acclimatization; by inhibiting conversion of carbon dioxide to bicarbonate, it may increase carbon dioxide tension in tissues and decrease it in the lungs. The resultant metabolic acidosis may also increase oxygenation during hypoxia.

## Pharmacokinetics

*Absorption:* Well absorbed from the GI tract after oral administration.

*Distribution:* Distributed throughout body tissues.

*Metabolism:* None.

*Excretion:* Excreted primarily in urine via tubular secretion and passive reabsorption.

| Route | Onset | Peak | Duration |
|---|---|---|---|
| P.O. | 1-1½ hr | 2-4 hr | 8-12 hr |
| P.O. (extended) | 2 hr | 3-6 hr | 18-24 hr |
| I.V. | 2 min | 15 min | 1-5 hr |

## Contraindications and precautions

Contraindicated in patients hypersensitive to drug; in long-term therapy for chronic noncongestive angle-closure glaucoma; and in those with hyponatremia or hypokalemia, renal or hepatic disease or dysfunction, adrenal gland failure, and hyperchloremic acidosis. Use cautiously in patients with respiratory acidosis, emphysema, diabetes, or COPD and in those receiving other diuretics.

## Interactions

**Drug-drug.** *Amphetamines, flecainide, procainamide, and quinidine:* Acetazolamide alkalinizes urine and thus may decrease excretion of these drugs. Advise clinician to monitor patient closely.

*Lithium, phenobarbital, and salicylates:* Increased excretion of these drugs causes low plasma levels, possibly necessitating dosage adjustments.

**Drug-lifestyle.** *Sun exposure:* May cause phototoxicity. Advise patient to take precautions, such as wearing protective clothing, using sunblock, and limiting exposure to sunlight.

## Adverse reactions

**CNS:** confusion, drowsiness, paresthesia.
**EENT:** hearing dysfunction, transient myopia, tinnitus.
**GI:** anorexia, altered taste, diarrhea, nausea, vomiting.
**GU:** hematuria, polyuria.
**Hematologic:** *aplastic anemia,* hemolytic anemia, *leukopenia.*
**Metabolic:** asymptomatic hyperuricemia, hyperchloremic acidosis, hypokalemia, decreased thyroid iodine uptake.
**Skin:** rash.

## Overdose and treatment

Specific recommendations are unavailable. Treatment is supportive and symptomatic. Acetazolamide increases bicarbonate excretion and may cause hypokalemia and hyperchloremic acidosis. Advise clinician to induce emesis or perform gastric lavage. Catharsis shouldn't be induced because this may exacerbate electrolyte disturbances. Advise clinician to monitor fluid and electrolyte levels.

## Clinical considerations

■ Suspensions containing 250 mg/5 ml of syrup are the most palatable. These remain stable for about 1 week.
■ Tablets don't dissolve in fruit juice.
■ Because it alkalinizes urine, acetazolamide may cause false-positive proteinuria in Albustix or Albutest.

### Therapeutic monitoring

■ Advise clinician to monitor electrolyte and glucose levels.
■ Advise clinician to monitor patient for hepatic coma or precoma in patients with hepatic cirrhosis, hypokalemia, or elevations in blood ammonia levels caused by drug therapy.

### Special populations

**Pregnant patients.** Acetazolamide may cause fetal toxicity when administered to pregnant women.

**Breast-feeding patients.** Safety of drug in breast-feeding women hasn't been established.

**Geriatric patients.** Advise clinician to observe geriatric and debilitated patients closely because they're more susceptible to drug-induced diuresis. Excessive diuresis promotes rapid dehydration, leading to hypovolemia, hypokalemia, and hyponatremia and may cause circulatory collapse. Reduced dosages may be indicated.

## Patient counseling

Warn patient to use caution while driving or performing tasks that require alertness, coor-

---

dination, or physical dexterity because drug may cause drowsiness.

# acetylcysteine
Mucomyst, Mucosil, Parvolex*

*Pharmacologic classification:* amino acid (L-cysteine) derivative
*Therapeutic classification:* mucolytic, antidote for acetaminophen overdose
*Pregnancy risk category B*

## Available forms
Available by prescription only
*Solution:* 10%, 20%
*Injection*:* 200 mg/ml

## Indications and dosages
*Acute and chronic bronchopulmonary disease, tracheostomy care, pulmonary complications of surgery, diagnostic bronchial studies*
Give by nebulization, direct application, or intratracheal instillation.
*Adults and children:* 1 to 2 ml of 10% or 20% solution by direct instillation into trachea as often as hourly; or 3 to 5 ml of 20% solution or 6 to 10 ml of 10% solution administered by nebulizer q 2 to 3 hours. For instillation via percutaneous intratracheal catheter, give 1 to 2 ml of 20% solution or 2 to 4 ml of 10% solution q 1 to 4 hours; via tracheal catheter to treat a specific bronchopulmonary tree segment, give 2 to 5 ml of 20% solution. For diagnostic bronchial studies (administered before procedure), give 1 to 2 ml of 20% solution or 2 to 4 ml of 10% solution for two or three doses.
*Acetaminophen toxicity*
*Adults and children:* Initially, 140 mg/kg P.O., followed by 70 mg/kg q 4 hours for 17 doses (a total of 1,330 mg/kg) or until acetaminophen assay reveals nontoxic level.
*Alternatively, drug may be administered I.V. in three doses: Loading dose 150 mg/kg I.V., followed by 50 mg/kg I.V., and final dose of 100 mg/kg I.V.
◊ *Prevention of acute renal failure associated with radiographic contrast media*
*Adults:* 600 mg P.O. b.i.d., given the day before and on the day of contrast media administration for total of four doses. For hydration: acetylcysteine has been given with 0.45% NaCl injection, given by IV infusion at 1 mL/kg per hour for 12 hours before and 12 hours after administration of contrast media.

## I.V. administration
- Drug is given in 3 doses.
- Mix the loading dose in 200 ml D₅W and infuse over 15 minutes.
- Follow with second dose mixed in 500 ml D₅W and infuse over 4 hours.

- Final dose mixed in 1,000 ml D₅W and infused over 16 hours.
- Volume and rate of infusion for use in children will need to reflect the child's weight and fluid restrictions.

## Incompatibilities
None reported.

## Mechanism of action
*Mucolytic action:* Drug produces its mucolytic effect by splitting the disulfide bonds of mucoprotein, the substance responsible for increased viscosity of mucus secretions in the lungs; thus, pulmonary secretions become less viscous and more liquid.
*Acetaminophen antidote:* Mechanism by which acetylcysteine reduces acetaminophen toxicity isn't fully understood; it's thought that acetylcysteine restores hepatic stores of glutathione or inactivates the toxic metabolite of acetaminophen via a chemical interaction, thereby preventing hepatic damage.

## Pharmacokinetics
*Absorption:* Most inhaled acetylcysteine acts directly on mucus in the lungs; the remainder is absorbed by pulmonary epithelium. After oral administration, drug is absorbed from the GI tract.
*Distribution:* Unknown.
*Metabolism:* Metabolized in the liver.
*Excretion:* Unknown.

| Route | Onset | Peak | Duration |
|---|---|---|---|
| P.O., I.V., inhalation | Unknown | Unknown | Unknown |

## Contraindications and precautions
Contraindicated in patients hypersensitive to drug. Use cautiously in geriatric or debilitated patients with severe respiratory insufficiency.

## Interactions
**Drug-drug.** *Activated charcoal:* Absorbs orally administered acetylcysteine, preventing its absorption. Charcoal should be removed before acetylcysteine administration.
*Amphotericin B, ampicillin, chlortetracycline, chymotrypsin, erythromycin lactobionate, hydrogen peroxide, iodized oil, oxytetracycline, tetracycline, and trypsin:* Incompatible with these drugs. Drugs should be given separately.

## Adverse reactions
**CV:** chest tightness, hypotension, hypertension, tachycardia.
**EENT:** *rhinorrhea.*
**GI:** nausea, stomatitis, vomiting.
**Respiratory:** *bronchospasm.*
**Other:** clamminess, fever.

## Overdose and treatment
No information available.

## Clinical considerations

■ Acetylcysteine solutions release hydrogen sulfide and discolor on contact with rubber and some metals (especially iron, nickel, and copper); drug tarnishes silver (this doesn't affect drug potency).

■ Solution may turn light purple; this doesn't affect safety or efficacy of the drug. Use plastic or stainless steel or other inert metal when administering drug by nebulization. Don't use hand-held bulb nebulizers; output is too small and particle size too large.

■ After opening, store in refrigerator or use within 96 hours.

■ When used orally for acetaminophen overdose, recommend diluting with cola, fruit juice, or water to a 5% concentration and give within 1 hour.

■ Don't place directly in the chamber of a heated (hot pot) nebulizer.

■ Optimal results occur when acetylcysteine is administered within 16 hours of acetaminophen ingestion, but preferably 8 hours; however, drug may be administered up to 24 hours after acetaminophen ingestion. A regional poison center or the Rocky Mountain Poison and Drug Center may be contacted at 1-800-332-3073 for assistance for use of acetylcysteine as an antidote.

### Therapeutic monitoring

■ Advise clinician to monitor cough type and frequency; for maximum effect, instruct patient to clear airway by coughing before aerosol administration. Many clinicians pretreat with bronchodilators before administration of acetylcysteine. Suction equipment should be available; if patient has insufficient cough to clear increased secretions, suction will be needed to maintain open airway.

■ If encephalopathy develops as a result of hepatic failure, acetylcysteine therapy should be stopped to prevent further accumulation of nitrogenous substances.

■ Advise clinician to obtain a 4-hour postingestion acetaminophen level (for peak level); the results are used with a nomogram to estimate the potential for hepatotoxicity. This guides the administration of acetylcysteine.

### Special populations

**Pregnant patients.** There are no adequate studies in pregnant women. Use only if clearly indicated.

**Breast-feeding patients.** It's unknown if drug appears in breast milk.

**Pediatric patients.** Drug may be given by tent or croupette. Use a sufficient volume (up to 300 ml) of a 10% or 20% solution to maintain a heavy mist in the tent for the time prescribed. Administration may be continuous or intermittent.

**Geriatric patients.** Geriatric patients may have inadequate cough and be unable to clear airway completely of mucus. Advise clinician to keep suction equipment available and monitor patient closely.

## Patient counseling

Warn patient of unpleasant odor (rotten egg odor of hydrogen sulfide), and explain that increased amounts of liquefied bronchial secretion plus unpleasant odor may cause nausea and vomiting; have patient rinse mouth with water after nebulizer treatment.

# activated charcoal

Actidose-Aqua, Charco Aid, Charco Caps, Insta-Char Pediatric

*Pharmacologic classification:* adsorbent
*Therapeutic classification:* antidote, antidiarrheal, antiflatulent
*Pregnancy risk category NR*

## Available forms

Available without a prescription
*Tablets:* 325 mg, 650 mg
*Tablets with 40 mg simethicone (delayed-release):* 200 mg
*Tablets (delayed-release) with 80 mg simethicone:* 250 mg
*Capsules:* 260 mg
*Powder:* 30 g, 50 g
*Suspension:* 0.625 g/5 ml, 0.7 g/5 ml (50 g), 1 g/5 ml, 1.25 g/5 ml
*Hemoperfusion system:* 300 g

## Indications and dosages

### Flatulence or dyspepsia

*Adults:* 600 mg to 5 g P.O. as a single dose, or 975 mg to 3.9 g t.i.d. after meals.

### Poisoning

*Adults and children:* Five to ten times the estimated weight of drug or chemical ingested. Dose is 30 to 100 g in 250 ml water to make a slurry.

Give orally, preferably within 30 minutes of ingestion. Larger doses are needed if food is in the stomach. Drug is used adjunctively in treating poisoning or overdose with acetaminophen, amphetamines, antimony, aspirin, atropine, arsenic, barbiturates, camphor, cocaine, cardiac glycosides, glutethimide, ipecac, malathion, morphine, opium, oxalic acid, parathion, phenol, phenothiazines, phenytoin, poisonous mushrooms, potassium permanganate, propoxyphene, quinine, strychnine, sulfonamides, or tricyclic antidepressants.

Activated charcoal may be given 20 to 60 g q 4 to 12 hours (gastric dialysis) to enhance removal of some drugs from the bloodstream. Advise clinician to monitor serum drug level.

◇ *To relieve GI disturbances (halitosis, anorexia, nausea, vomiting) in uremic patients*
*Adults:* 20 to 50 g P.O. daily.

## Mechanism of action
*Antidote action:* Drug adsorbs ingested toxins, inhibiting GI absorption.
*Antidiarrheal action:* Activated charcoal adsorbs toxic and nontoxic irritants that cause diarrhea or GI discomfort.
*Antiflatulent action:* Activated charcoal adsorbs intestinal gas to relieve discomfort.

## Pharmacokinetics
*Absorption:* Not absorbed from the GI tract.
*Distribution:* None.
*Metabolism:* None.
*Excretion:* Excreted in feces.

| Route | Onset | Peak | Duration |
|-------|-------|------|----------|
| P.O. | Immediate | Unknown | Unknown |

## Contraindications and precautions
No known contraindications.

## Interactions
**Drug-drug.** *Orally administered acetylcysteine, syrup of ipecac:* Activated charcoal inactivates these drugs and many other orally administered drugs. Charcoal should be removed by gastric lavage before acetylcysteine is administered.
**Drug-food.** *Milk products:* Decrease the effectiveness of activated charcoal. Don't dilute drug with dairy products.

## Adverse reactions
**GI:** *black stools,* constipation, nausea, intestinal obstruction.

## Overdose and treatment
No information available.

## Clinical considerations
**◪ ALERT** Don't use activated charcoal if poisoning involves corrosive agents, cyanide, iron, mineral acids, or organic solvents.
■ Don't give activated charcoal P.O. to a semiconscious or unconscious patient; instead, the drug should be given through a nasogastric tube.
■ Because activated charcoal adsorbs and inactivates syrup of ipecac, it should be given only after emesis is complete.
■ Dose may need to be repeated if patient vomits shortly after administration.
■ Activated charcoal is most effective when used within 30 minutes of toxin ingestion; a cathartic is commonly administered with or after activated charcoal to speed removal of the toxin and charcoal complex.
■ Powder form is most effective. Mix with tap water to form consistency of thick syrup. A small amount of fruit juice or flavoring may be added to make mixture more palatable.
■ If administering drug for indications other than poisoning, be sure to give other drugs 1 hour before or 2 hours after activated charcoal.
■ Activated charcoal may be used orally to decrease colostomy odor.

### Therapeutic monitoring
■ Advise clinician to monitor patient's nutritional status; prolonged use (over 72 hours) may impair patient's nutritional status.
■ Advise clinician to monitor serum electrolyte levels if it's a repeated dosing of charcoal with sorbitol or in children who may be more sensitive to sorbitol.

### Special populations
**Pediatric patients.** Don't use charcoal with sorbitol in children under 1 year old.

## Patient counseling
■ Tell patient to call poison information center or hospital emergency department before taking activated charcoal as an antidote.
■ If patient is using activated charcoal as an antidiarrheal or antiflatulent, instruct him to take drugs 1 hour before or 2 hours after activated charcoal. For antidiarrheal use, advise patient to report diarrhea that persists after 2 days of therapy; fever; or flatulence that persists after 7 days.
■ Warn patient that activated charcoal turns stools black.
■ Advise patient not to mix drug with milk products, which may lessen its effectiveness.

---

# acyclovir (acycloguanosine)
# acyclovir sodium
Zovirax

*Pharmacologic classification:* synthetic purine nucleoside
*Therapeutic classification:* antiviral
*Pregnancy risk category C*

## Available forms
Available by prescription only
*Tablets:* 400 mg, 800 mg
*Capsules:* 200 mg
*Oral suspension:* 200 mg/5 ml
*Injection:* 500 mg/vial, 1 g/vial
*Ointment:* 5%
*Injection concentrate for I.V. infusion:* 25 mg/ml, 50 mg/ml
*Redi-infusion:* 5 mg/ml

## Indications and dosages
*Initial and recurrent mucocutaneous herpes simplex virus (HSV type 1 and HSV type 2) or severe initial genital herpes or*

*herpes simplex in immunocompromised patient*
*Adults and children over age 12:* 5 mg/kg, given at a constant rate over 1 hour by I.V. infusion q 8 hours for 7 days (5 days for genital herpes).
*Children under age 12:* 10 mg/kg infused at a constant rate over 1 hour by I.V. infusion q 8 hours for 7 days (5 days for genital herpes).
◇ *Mucocutaneous HSV type 1 and HSV type 2 in immunocompromised patient*
*Adults:* 400 mg P.O. q 4 hours while awake (5 times daily).
*Children:* 1 g P.O. daily divided into three to five doses for 7 to 14 days; dose shouldn't exceed 80 mg/kg daily.
◇ *Disseminated herpes zoster*
*Adults:* 5 to 10 mg/kg I.V. q 8 hours for 7 to 10 days. Infuse over at least 1 hour.
*Initial genital herpes*
*Adults:* 200 mg P.O. q 4 hours while awake (a total of five capsules daily). Treatment should continue for 10 days. Alternatively, 400 mg P.O. t.i.d. for 7 to 10 days.
◇ *Genital herpes in the immunocompromised patient*
*Adults:* 400 mg P.O. 3 to 5 times daily.
◇ *Rectal herpes infection*
*Adults:* 400 mg P.O. 5 times daily for 10 days or until resolution; alternatively, 800 mg P.O. q 8 hours for 7 to 10 days for initial infections.
*Acute herpes zoster infections*
*Adults:* 800 mg P.O. five times daily for 7 to 10 days. Initiate therapy within 48 hours of rash onset.
*Intermittent therapy for recurrent genital herpes*
*Adults:* 200 mg P.O. q 4 hours while awake (a total of five capsules daily). Continue treatment for 5 days. Begin therapy at first sign of recurrence.
*Chronic suppressive therapy for recurrent genital herpes*
*Adults:* 400 mg P.O. b.i.d. for up to 1 year, followed by reevaluation.
*Genital herpes; non–life-threatening herpes simplex infection in immunocompromised patients*
*Adults and children:* Apply sufficient quantity of ointment to adequately cover all lesions q 3 hours, six times daily for 7 days.
*Neonatal herpes simplex virus infection*
*Neonates and infants up to 3 months:* 10 mg/kg I.V. every 8 hours for 10 days.
*Preterm neonates:* 10 mg/kg I.V. q 12 hours.
*Primary or recurrent HSV infections in patients with HIV*
*Adults:* 200 to 800 mg P.O. 5 times daily.
◇ *Chronic suppressive or maintenance prophylaxis therapy for recurrent HSV infections in patients with HIV*
*Adults and adolescents:* 200 mg P.O. t.i.d. or 400 mg P.O. b.i.d.

*Infants and children:* 600 to 1,000 mg P.O. daily in three to five divided doses; alternatively, 80 mg/kg in three to four divided doses.
*Acute varicella (chickenpox) infections*
*Adults and children age 2 and older weighing over 40 kg (88 lb):* 800 mg P.O. q.i.d. for 5 days.
*Children age 2 or over weighing under 40 kg:* 20 mg/kg P.O. q.i.d. for 5 days.
◇ *Acute herpes zoster ophthalmicus*
*Adults:* 600 mg P.O. q 4 hours 5 times daily for 10 days; preferably within 72 hours of rash onset, but no longer than 7 days.
*Varicella in the immunocompromised patient*
*Adults and children over age 12:* 10 mg/kg I.V. over 1 hour q 8 hours for 7 days.
*Children under age 12:* 20 mg/kg I.V. over 1 hour q 8 hours for 7 days.
*Herpes simplex encephalitis*
*Adults and children over age 12:* 10 mg/kg I.V. over 1 hour q 8 hours for 10 days.
*Children age 3 months to 12 years:* 20 mg/kg q 8 hours I.V. over at least 1 hour for 10 days.
≣ *Dosage adjustment.* In patients with renal failure, adjust normal oral dose (200 to 400 mg) to 200 mg q 12 hours if creatinine clearance drops below 10 ml/minute. For normal doses exceeding 400 mg, refer to package insert.

In patients with renal failure, give 100% of the I.V. dose q 8 hours if creatinine clearance exceeds 50 ml/minute; 100% of the dose q 12 hours if it ranges between 25 and 50 ml/minute; 100% of the dose q 24 hours if it ranges between 10 and 25 ml/minute; and 50% of the dose q 24 hours if it falls below 10 ml/minute.

## I.V. administration
■ Reconstitute drug by adding 10 to 20 ml of sterile water for injection to a 500-mg or 1-g acyclovir vial, respectively, to provide a solution of 50 mg/ml.
■ Don't use bacteriostatic water for injection.
■ Use reconstituted solution within 12 hours. Further dilute in 50 to 125 ml of a compatible I.V. solution to a level of no more than 7 mg/ml.
■ Infuse I.V. dose over at least 1 hour to prevent renal tubular damage.

### Incompatibilities
May form a precipitate when combined with parabens. Also incompatible with biological or colloidal solutions and idarubicin hydrochloride.

## Mechanism of action
*Antiviral action:* Acyclovir is converted by the viral cell into its active form (triphosphate) and inhibits viral DNA polymerase.

In vitro, acyclovir is active against HSV type 1, HSV type 2, varicella-zoster virus, Epstein-Barr virus, and cytomegalovirus. In vivo, acyclovir may reduce the duration of acute infection and speed lesion healing in initial genital herpes episodes. Patients with frequent herpes recurrences (more than six episodes a year) may receive oral acyclovir prophylactically to prevent recurrences or reduce their frequency.

## Pharmacokinetics

*Absorption:* With oral administration, absorbed slowly and incompletely (15% to 30%). Absorption isn't affected by food. With topical administration, absorption is minimal.

*Distribution:* Distributed widely to organ tissues and body fluids. CSF levels equal about 50% of serum levels. About 9% to 33% plasma protein–bound.

*Metabolism:* Metabolized inside the viral cell to its active form. About 10% of dose is metabolized extracellularly.

*Excretion:* Up to 92% of systemically absorbed acyclovir is excreted as unchanged drug by the kidneys by glomerular filtration and tubular secretion. In patients with normal renal function, half-life is 2 to 3½ hours. Renal failure may extend half-life to 19 hours.

| Route | Onset | Peak | Duration |
|---|---|---|---|
| P.O. | Unknown | 2-5 hr | Unknown |
| I.V. | Immediate | Immediate | Unknown |
| Topical | Unknown | Unknown | Unknown |

## Contraindications and precautions

Contraindicated in patients hypersensitive to drug. Use cautiously in patients with underlying neurologic problems, renal disease, or dehydration and in those receiving nephrotoxic drugs.

## Interactions

**Drug-drug.** *Methotrexate:* Possible reaction in patients who have had a previous neurologic reaction to intrathecal methotrexate administration. Use I.V. acyclovir with caution in these patients.

*Probenecid:* May result in reduced renal tubular secretion of acyclovir, leading to increased drug half-life, reduced elimination rate, and decreased urine excretion. This reduced clearance causes more sustained serum drug levels. Avoid use together.

*Zidovudine:* May result in increased levels of acyclovir, causing toxicity. Advise clinician to monitor acyclovir levels closely.

## Adverse reactions

**CNS:** *encephalopathic changes (lethargy, obtundation, tremor, confusion, hallucinations, agitation,* **seizures,** *coma),* headache, malaise.
**GI:** diarrhea, *nausea, vomiting.*
**GU:** hematuria, *transient elevations of serum creatinine and BUN levels.*

**Hematologic:** *bone marrow hypoplasia,* **leukopenia,** megaloblastic hematopoiesis, thrombocytosis, **thrombocytopenia.**
**Skin:** itching, rash, transient burning and stinging, pruritus, urticaria, vulvitis.
**Other:** *inflammation, phlebitis* (at injection site).

## Overdose and treatment

Overdose has followed I.V. bolus administration in patients with unmonitored fluid status or in patients receiving inappropriately high parenteral dosages. Acute toxicity hasn't been reported after high oral dosage. Hemodialysis decreases drug plasma level by 60%.

Clinical effects of overdose include signs of nephrotoxicity, including elevated serum creatinine and BUN levels, progressing to renal failure.

## Clinical considerations

■ Drug shouldn't be administered S.C., I.M., by I.V. bolus, or ophthalmically.
■ Solubility of acyclovir in urine is low. Ensure that patient taking the systemic form of drug is well hydrated to prevent nephrotoxicity.
■ Don't apply topical preparation to vagina or cervix.

### Therapeutic monitoring

■ Advise clinician to monitor serum creatinine level. If level doesn't return to normal within a few days after therapy begins, advise clinician to increase hydration, adjust dose, or discontinue drug.
■ Advise clinician to monitor patient for encephalopathic signs; they're more likely in patients who have experienced neurologic reactions to cytotoxic drugs.

### Special populations

**Pregnant patients.** Use only if benefits outweigh the risks.
**Pediatric patients.** Safety and effectiveness of oral and topical acyclovir in children haven't been established. I.V. acyclovir has been used in only a few children. To reconstitute acyclovir for children, don't use bacteriostatic water for injection that contains benzyl alcohol.
**Geriatric patients.** Give drug cautiously to geriatric patients because they may suffer from renal dysfunction or dehydration.

## Patient counseling

■ Warn patient that although drug helps manage the disease, it doesn't cure it or prevent its spread to others.
■ Tell patient to begin taking drug when early infection symptoms, such as tingling, itching, or pain, occur.
■ Instruct patient taking ointment to use a finger cot or rubber glove and to apply about a ½″ ribbon of ointment for every 4 square inch-

es of area to be covered. Ointment should thoroughly cover each lesion. Warn patient to avoid getting ointment in the eye.

■ Instruct patient to avoid sexual intercourse during active genital infection.

# adenosine
Adenocard

*Pharmacologic classification:* nucleoside
*Therapeutic classification:* antiarrhythmic
*Pregnancy risk category C*

## Available forms
Available by prescription only
*Injection:* 3 mg/ml in 2-ml and 5-ml vials

## Indications and dosages
***Conversion of paroxysmal supraventricular tachycardia (PSVT) to sinus rhythm***
*Adults:* 6 mg I.V. by rapid bolus injection (over 1 to 2 seconds). If PSVT isn't eliminated in 1 to 2 minutes, give 12 mg by rapid I.V. push. Repeat 12-mg dose if needed. Single doses over 12 mg aren't recommended.

## I.V. administration
■ Rapid I.V. injection is needed for drug action.
■ Give directly into a vein if possible; if an I.V. line is used, use the most proximal port and follow with a rapid normal saline flush to ensure that drug reaches the systemic circulation rapidly.

### *Incompatibilities*
Don't mix with other drugs.

## Mechanism of action
*Antiarrhythmic action:* Adenosine is a naturally occurring nucleoside. In the heart, it acts on the AV node to slow conduction and inhibit reentry pathways. Adenosine is also useful for the treatment of PSVT caused by accessory bypass tracts (Wolff-Parkinson-White syndrome).

## Pharmacokinetics
*Absorption:* Administered by rapid I.V. injection.
*Distribution:* Rapidly taken up by erythrocytes and vascular endothelial cells.
*Metabolism:* Metabolized within tissues to inosine and adenosine monophosphate.
*Excretion:* Unknown; circulating plasma half-life is less than 10 seconds.

| Route | Onset | Peak | Duration |
|-------|-------|------|----------|
| I.V. | Immediate | Immediate | Unknown |

## Contraindications and precautions
Contraindicated in patients hypersensitive to drug and in those with second- or third-degree heart block or sick sinus syndrome, unless an artificial pacemaker is present, because adenosine decreases conduction through the AV node and may produce first-, second-, or third-degree heart block. These effects are usually transient; however, patients in whom significant heart block develops after a dose of adenosine shouldn't receive additional doses.

Don't use in atrial fibrillation or atrial flutter. Use cautiously in patients with asthma because bronchoconstriction may occur.

## Interactions
**Drug-drug.** *Carbamazepine:* Higher degrees of heart block occur in patients receiving concurrent therapy. Avoid use together.
*Dipyridamole:* May potentiate the effects of the drug; smaller doses may be needed.
*Methylxanthines:* Antagonize effects of adenosine. Therefore, patients receiving theophylline may require higher doses or may not respond to adenosine therapy.
**Drug-herb.** *Guarana:* May decrease response of adenosine. Advise clinician to monitor patient closely.
**Drug-food.** *Caffeine:* May antagonize the effects of adenosine. Patient may require higher doses or may not respond to adenosine therapy.

## Adverse reactions
**CNS:** apprehension, back pain, blurred vision, burning sensation, dizziness, heaviness in arms, light-headedness, neck pain, numbness, tingling in arms.
**CV:** chest pain, *facial flushing,* headache, hypotension, palpitations.
**GI:** metallic taste, nausea.
**Respiratory:** *chest pressure, dyspnea, shortness of breath,* hyperventilation.
**Skin:** diaphoresis.
**Other:** *throat tightness, groin pressure.*

## Overdose and treatment
Because the half-life of adenosine is less than 10 seconds, the adverse effects of overdose usually dissipate rapidly and are self-limiting. Lingering adverse effects should be treated symptomatically.

## Clinical considerations
■ Recommend using caution in using Adenocard in patients with previous history of ventricular fibrillation or those taking digoxin and verapamil.
■ Check solution for crystals, which may occur if solution is cold. If crystals are visible, gently warm solution to controlled room temperature. Don't use solutions that aren't clear.
■ Discard unused drug because it contains no preservatives.

**H ALERT** Don't confuse adenosine phosphate with adenosine (Adenocard).

### Therapeutic monitoring
■ Advise clinician to monitor ECG rhythm during administration; drug may cause short-lasting first-, second-, or third-degree heart block or asystole.

### Patient counseling
Warn patient of adverse reactions.

# albumin, human (normal serum albumin, human)
Albuminar-5, Albuminar-25, Albutein 5%, Albutein 25%, Buminate 5%, Buminate 25%, Plasbumin-5, Plasbumin-25

*Pharmacologic classification:* blood derivative
*Therapeutic classification:* plasma protein
*Pregnancy risk category C*

### Available forms
*Injection:* 5% (50 mg/ml) in 50-ml, 250-ml, 500-ml, 1,000-ml vials; 25% (250 mg/ml) in 20-ml, 50-ml, 100-ml vials

### Indications and dosages
*Shock*
*Adults:* Initially, 500 ml (5% solution) by I.V. infusion, may repeat after 30 minutes. Dosage varies with patient's condition and response. Don't exceed 250 g in 48 hours.
*Children:* 10 to 20 ml/kg (5% solution) by I.V. infusion, at a rate up to 5 to 10 ml/minute.
*Hypoproteinemia*
*Adults:* 1,000 to 1,500 ml 5% solution by I.V. infusion daily, maximum rate 5 to 10 ml/minute; or 200 to 300 ml of 25% solution by I.V. infusion daily, maximum rate 3 ml/minute. Dosage varies with patient's condition and response.
*Burns*
*Adults and children:* Dosage varies based on extent of burn and patient's condition. Usually maintain plasma albumin level at 2 to 3 g/dl.
*Hyperbilirubinemia*
*Infants:* 1 g/kg albumin (4 ml/kg of 25% solution) by I.V. infusion 1 to 2 hours before transfusion.
◇ *High-risk neonates with low serum protein level:* 1.4 to 1.8 ml/kg by I.V. infusion of 25% solution.

### I.V. administration
■ Dilute if necessary with normal saline solution or D₅W. Use 5-micron or larger filter; don't give through 0.22-micron I.V. filter.

■ Avoid rapid I.V. infusion; rate is individualized based on patient's age, condition, and diagnosis. In patients with hypovolemic shock, infuse 5% solution at a rate not exceeding 2 to 4 ml/minute, and 25% solution (diluted or undiluted) at a rate not exceeding 1 ml/minute; in patients with normal blood volume, infuse 5% solution at a rate not exceeding 5 to 10 ml/minute, and 25% solution (diluted or undiluted) at a rate not exceeding 2 to 3 ml/minute. Don't give more than 250 g in 48 hours.
■ Solution should be a clear amber color; don't use if cloudy or contains sediment. Store at controlled room temperature; freezing may break bottle.
■ Use opened solution promptly, discarding unused portion after 4 hours; solution contains no preservatives and becomes unstable.

### Incompatibilities
Incompatible with verapamil hydrochloride.

### Mechanism of action
*Plasma volume-expanding action:* Albumin 5% supplies colloid to the blood and expands plasma volume. Albumin 25% provides intravascular oncotic pressure at 5:1, causing fluid to shift from interstitial space to circulation and slightly increasing plasma protein level.

### Pharmacokinetics
*Absorption:* Administered I.V.
*Distribution:* Accounts for about 50% of plasma proteins; distributed into the intravascular space and extravascular sites, including skin, muscle, and lungs. In patients with reduced circulating blood volume, hemodilution secondary to albumin administration persists for many hours; in patients with normal blood volume, excess fluid and protein are lost.
*Metabolism:* Although synthesized in the liver, liver isn't involved in clearance of albumin from plasma in healthy individuals.
*Excretion:* Little is known about excretion in healthy individuals. Administration of albumin decreases hepatic albumin synthesis and increases albumin clearance if plasma oncotic pressure is high. In certain pathologic states, the liver, kidneys, or intestines may provide elimination mechanisms for albumin.

| Route | Onset | Peak | Duration |
|-------|-------|------|----------|
| I.V. | < 15 min | < 15 min | Several hr |

### Contraindications and precautions
Contraindicated in patients hypersensitive to drug. Use with extreme caution in patients with hypertension, cardiac disease, severe pulmonary infection, severe chronic anemia, or hypoalbuminemia with peripheral edema.

---

## Interactions
**Drug-drug.** *ACE inhibitors:* Atypical reactions when used with plasma exchange of large volumes of albumin. Advise clinician to withhold ACE inhibitors for 24 hours before plasma exchange.

## Adverse reactions
**CNS:** headache.
**CV:** hypotension, tachycardia, *vascular overload after rapid infusion.*
**GI:** increased salivation, nausea, vomiting.
**Metabolic:** increased serum alkaline phosphatase level, slightly increased plasma albumin level.
**Respiratory:** altered respiration, dyspnea, *pulmonary edema.*
**Skin:** urticaria, rash.
**Other:** chills, fever, back pain.

## Overdose and treatment
Symptoms of overdose include signs of circulatory overload, such as increased venous pressure and distended neck veins, or pulmonary edema; slow flow to a keep-vein-open rate and reevaluate therapy.

## Clinical considerations
■ One volume of 25% albumin produces the same hemodilution and relative anemia as five volumes of 5% albumin; reference to "1 unit" albumin usually indicates 50 ml of the 25% concentration containing 12.5 g of albumin.
■ Patient should be properly hydrated before infusion starts; product may be administered without regard to blood typing and cross-matching.
■ Each liter contains 130 to 160 mEq of sodium before dilution with any additional I.V. fluids; a 50-ml bottle of solution contains 7 to 8 mEq sodium. This preparation was once known as "salt-poor albumin."

### Therapeutic monitoring
■ Vital signs must be monitored carefully and the patient observed for adverse reactions.
■ Advise clinician to monitor intake and output, hematocrit, serum protein, hemoglobin, and electrolyte levels to help determine continuing dosage.
■ The goal is to maintain plasma albumin levels at 2 to 3 g/dl or an oncotic pressure of 20 (total serum protein level of 5.2 g/dl).

### Special populations
**Pediatric patients.** Premature infants with low serum protein levels may receive 1.4 to 1.8 ml/kg of a 25% albumin solution/kg by I.V. infusion (350 to 450 mg albumin).

## Patient counseling
■ Explain use and administration to patient and family.

■ Tell patient to report adverse effects promptly.

# albuterol sulfate
Airet, Proventil, Proventil HFA, Proventil Repetabs, Proventil Syrup, Ventolin, Ventolin HFA, Ventolin Syrup, Volmax

*Pharmacologic classification:* adrenergic
*Therapeutic classification:* bronchodilator
*Pregnancy risk category C*

## Available forms
Available by prescription only
*Tablets:* 2 mg, 4 mg
*Tablets (sustained-release):* 4 mg, 8 mg
*Syrup:* 2 mg/5 ml
*Aerosol inhaler:* 90 mcg/metered spray
*Solution for nebulization:* 0.083%, 0.5%
*Capsules for inhalation:* 200 mcg microfine

## Indications and dosages
**Bronchospasm in patients with reversible obstructive airway disease**
*Adults and children age 12 and older:* Tablets: give 2 to 4 mg (immediate-release) P.O. t.i.d. or q.i.d.; maximum dose, 8 mg q.i.d. Alternatively, use sustained-release tablets. Usual starting dose is 4 mg q 12 hours. Increase to 8 mg q 12 hours if patient fails to respond. Cautiously increase stepwise as needed and tolerated to 16 mg q 12 hours.
*Children ages 6 to 14:* Oral solution: 2 mg P.O. t.i.d. to q.i.d.; may increase to 24 mg/day in divided doses.
*Adults and children age 4 and older:* Aerosol inhalation: One to two inhalations q 4 to 6 hours. More frequent administration or a greater number of inhalations isn't usually recommended. However, because deposition of inhaled drugs is variable, higher doses are occasionally used, especially in patients with acute bronchospasm.
*Adults:* Solution for inhalation: 2.5 mg t.i.d. or q.i.d. by nebulizer.
*Children ages 2 to 12:* 0.1 mg/kg to 0.15 mg/kg to maximum of 2.5 mg t.i.d. to q.i.d.
*Adults and children age 4 and older:* Capsules for inhalation: 200 mcg inhaled q 4 to 6 hours using a Rotahaler inhalation device.
*Children ages 6 to 11:* Give 2 mg P.O. t.i.d. or q.i.d. or 4 mg extended-release preparation q 12 hours.
*Children ages 2 to 5:* Give 0.1 mg/kg P.O. t.i.d., not to exceed 2 mg t.i.d.
≡**Dosage adjustment.** In adults over age 65, give 2 mg P.O. t.i.d. or q.i.d.
**To prevent exercise-induced bronchospasm**
*Adults and children age 4 and older:* Two inhalations 15 minutes before exercise.

## Mechanism of action

*Bronchodilator action:* Selectively stimulates beta receptors of the lungs, uterus, and vascular smooth muscle. Bronchodilation results from relaxation of bronchial smooth muscles, which relieves bronchospasm and reduces airway resistance.

## Pharmacokinetics

*Absorption:* After oral inhalation, appears to be absorbed gradually, over several hours, from the respiratory tract; however, dose is mostly swallowed and absorbed through the GI tract.
*Distribution:* Doesn't cross the blood-brain barrier.
*Metabolism:* Extensively metabolized in the liver to inactive compounds.
*Excretion:* Rapidly excreted in urine and feces. After oral inhalation, 70% of dose is excreted in urine unchanged and as metabolites within 24 hours; 10% in feces. Elimination half-life is about 4 hours. After oral administration, 75% of dose is excreted in urine within 72 hours as metabolites; 4% in feces.

| Route | Onset | Peak | Duration |
|-------|-------|------|----------|
| P.O. | 15-30 min | 2-3 hr | 6-12 hr |
| I.V. | Variable | Unknown | 4-6 hr |
| Inhalation | 5-15 min | ½-2 hr | 2-6 hr |

## Contraindications and precautions

Contraindicated in patients hypersensitive to drug or any component of its formulation. Use cautiously in patients with CV disorders, including coronary insufficiency and hypertension; in patients with hyperthyroidism or diabetes mellitus; and in those who are unusually responsive to adrenergics.

## Interactions

**Drug-drug.** *Epinephrine and other orally inhaled sympathomimetic amines:* May increase sympathomimetic effects and risk of toxicity. Avoid use together.
*MAO inhibitors and tricyclic antidepressants:* Serious CV effects may follow use. Avoid use together.
*Propranolol and other beta blockers:* May antagonize the effects of albuterol. Use caution when used together.

## Adverse reactions

**CNS:** *tremor, nervousness,* dizziness, insomnia, *headache, hyperactivity,* weakness, CNS stimulation, malaise, hypesthesia, migraine, hypertonia.
**CV:** *tachycardia, palpitations,* hypertension.
**EENT:** dry and irritated nose and throat (with inhaled form), nasal congestion, epistaxis, hoarseness.
**GI:** heartburn, increased appetite, taste perversion, *nausea, vomiting,* anorexia.
**Metabolic:** hypokalemia (with high doses).

**Musculoskeletal:** muscle cramps.
**Respiratory:** *bronchospasm,* cough, wheezing, dyspnea, bronchitis, increased sputum.
**Other:** hypersensitivity reactions.

## Overdose and treatment

Signs and symptoms of overdose include exaggeration of common adverse reactions, particularly angina, hypertension, hypokalemia, and seizures. Cardiac arrest may occur.

To treat, advise clinician to use selective beta blockers (such as metoprolol) with extreme caution; they may induce asthmatic attack. Dialysis isn't appropriate. Advise clinician to monitor vital signs and electrolyte levels closely.

## Clinical considerations

- Orally inhaled albuterol has been used investigationally to prevent or alleviate episodes of muscle paralysis in the treatment of some patients with hyperkalemic familial periodic paralysis.
- Albuterol may decrease the sensitivity of spirometry used for the diagnosis of asthma.

### Therapeutic monitoring

- Small, transient increases in blood glucose levels may occur after oral inhalation.
- Serum potassium levels may decrease after inhalation therapy administration, but potassium supplementation is usually unnecessary.
- Effectiveness of treatment is measured by periodic monitoring of patient's pulmonary function. Advise clinician to monitor patient for worsening symptoms or loss of control.

### Special populations

**Pregnant patients.** The potential exists for cleft palate and limb defects; however, there's no consistent pattern of congenital abnormalities.
**Breast-feeding patients.** Because it's unknown if albuterol appears in breast milk, alternative feeding methods are recommended.
**Pediatric patients.** Safety and efficacy of extended-release tablets or immediate-release tablets in children under age 6 haven't been established.
**Geriatric patients.** Lower doses may be required because geriatric patients are more sensitive to sympathomimetic amines.

## Patient counseling

- Instruct patient in proper use of inhaler. Tell him to read directions before use, that dryness of mouth and throat may occur, and that rinsing with water after each dose may help.
*Administration by metered-dose nebulizers:* Instruct patient to shake canister thoroughly to activate; place mouthpiece well into mouth, aimed at back of throat. Close lips and teeth around mouthpiece. Exhale through nose as completely as possible, then inhale through

mouth slowly and deeply while actuating the nebulizer to release dose. Hold breath 10 seconds (count "1-100, 2-100, 3-100," until "10-100" is reached). Remove mouthpiece, and exhale slowly.

*Administration by metered powder inhaler:* Caution patient not to take forced deep breath, but to breathe with normal force and depth. Advise clinician to observe patient closely for exaggerated systemic drug action.

*Administration by oxygen aerosolization:* Give over 15- to 20-minute period, with oxygen flow rate adjusted to 4 L/minute. Advise clinician to turn on oxygen supply before patient places nebulizer in mouth. Lips don't have to be closed tightly around nebulizer opening. Placement of Y tube in rubber tubing permits patient to control administration. Advise patient to rinse mouth immediately after inhalation therapy to help prevent dryness and throat irritation. Rinse mouthpiece thoroughly with warm running water at least once daily to prevent clogging (it isn't dishwasher-safe). After cleaning, wait until mouthpiece is completely dry before storing. Don't place near artificial heat, such as a dishwasher or oven. Replace reservoir bag every 2 to 3 weeks or p.r.n.; replace mouthpiece every 6 to 9 months or p.r.n. Replacement of bags or mouthpieces may require a prescription.

■ Advise patient that repeated use may result in paradoxical bronchospasm. In such a case, patient should discontinue drug and contact his prescriber immediately.

■ Tell patient to contact his prescriber if troubled breathing persists 1 hour after using drug, if symptoms return within 4 hours, if condition worsens, or if new (refill) canister is needed within 2 weeks.

■ Advise patient to wait 15 minutes after using inhaled albuterol before using adrenocorticoids (beclomethasone, dexamethasone, flunisolide, or triamcinolone).

■ Warn patient to use only as directed and not to use more than prescribed amount or more often than prescribed.

# aldesleukin (interleukin-2, IL-2)
Proleukin

*Pharmacologic classification:* lymphokine
*Therapeutic classification:* immunoregulatory drug
*Pregnancy risk category C*

## Available forms
Available by prescription only
*Injection:* 22 million IU/vial

## Indications and dosages
*Metastatic renal cell carcinoma, metastatic melanoma*
*Adults:* 600,000 IU/kg (0.037 mg/kg) I.V. q 8 hours for 5 days (a total of 14 doses). After a 9-day rest, repeat sequence for another 14 doses. Repeat courses may be administered after a rest period of at least 7 weeks from hospital discharge.
◊ *Adults:* Continuous I.V. infusion of 18 million IU/m² for two 5-day cycles with a 5- to 8-day rest between cycles.
◊ *Adults:* 18 million IU S.C. daily for 5 days, followed by 2-day rest period.

## I.V. administration
■ Reconstitute and dilute carefully to avoid altering the pharmacologic properties of drug; follow manufacturer's recommendations. Don't mix with other drugs.
■ Reconstitute vial containing 22 million IU (1.3 mg) with 1.2 ml sterile water for injection. Don't use bacteriostatic water or normal saline injection because these diluents cause increased aggregation of drug. Direct the stream at the sides of the vial and gently swirl to reconstitute. Don't shake.
■ Reconstituted solution will have a level of 18 million IU (1.1 mg)/ml. Reconstituted drug should be particle-free and colorless to slightly yellow.
■ Add the correct dose of reconstituted drug to 50 ml D₅W and infuse over 15 minutes. Don't use an in-line filter. Plastic infusion bags are preferred because they provide consistent drug delivery.
■ Vials are for single-use only and contain no preservatives. Discard unused drug.
■ Powder for injection or reconstituted solutions must be stored in the refrigerator. After reconstitution and dilution, drug must be administered within 48 hours. Be sure that solutions are returned to controlled room temperature before administering drug to patient.

## Incompatibilities
Incompatible with albumin, bacteriostatic water for injection, and normal saline solution. Avoid mixing with other drugs.

## Mechanism of action
*Immunoregulatory action:* Aldesleukin is a lymphokine, a highly purified immunoregulatory protein synthesized using genetically engineered *Escherichia coli*. The drug produced is similar to human IL-2: it enhances lymphocyte mitogenesis, stimulates long-term growth of IL-2–dependent cell lines, enhances lymphocyte cytotoxicity, induces both lymphokine-activated and natural killer cell activity, and induces the production of interferon gamma.

## Pharmacokinetics
*Absorption:* Administered I.V.

*Distribution:* Peak serum levels are proportional to dose. About 30% is rapidly distributed in plasma; the balance is rapidly distributed to the liver, kidneys, and lungs. Initial studies indicate that the distribution half-life is 13 minutes after a 5-minute I.V. infusion.
*Metabolism:* Metabolized by the kidneys to amino acids within the cells lining the proximal convoluted tubules.
*Excretion:* Excreted through the kidneys by peritubular extraction and glomerular filtration. Peritubular extraction ensures drug clearance as renal function diminishes and serum creatinine increases. Elimination half-life is 85 minutes.

| Route | Onset | Peak | Duration |
|-------|-------|------|----------|
| I.V. | 4 wk | Unknown | < 12 mo |

## Contraindications and precautions

Contraindicated in patients hypersensitive to drug or any component of the formulation and in those with abnormal cardiac (thallium) stress test or pulmonary function tests or organ allografts. Retreatment is contraindicated in patients who experience the following adverse effects: pericardial tamponade; respiratory dysfunction requiring intubation; disturbances in cardiac rhythm that were uncontrolled or unresponsive to intervention; sustained ventricular tachycardia (five beats or more); chest pain accompanied by ECG changes, indicating MI or angina pectoris; renal dysfunction requiring dialysis for 72 hours or longer; coma or toxic psychosis lasting 48 hours or longer; seizures that are repetitive or difficult to control; ischemia or perforation of the bowel; GI bleeding requiring surgery.

Use with extreme caution in patients with cardiac or pulmonary disease or seizure disorders.

## Interactions

**Drug-drug.** *Antihypertensives:* May increase risk of hypotension. Use together cautiously.
*Corticosteroids:* May decrease antitumor effectiveness of aldesleukin. Advise clinician to monitor drug effect.
*Cardiotoxic, hepatotoxic, myelotoxic, or nephrotoxic drugs:* May enhance the toxicity of these drugs. Use together cautiously.
*Psychotropic agents:* Altered CNS function. Use together cautiously.

## Adverse reactions

**CNS:** *malaise, headache, mental status changes, dizziness,* **CVA,** *sensory dysfunction, special senses disorders, syncope, motor dysfunction,* **coma,** fatigue, *seizures.*
**CV:** *hypotension, sinus tachycardia,* **arrhythmias, bradycardia,** *PVCs, premature atrial contractions,* chest pain, **MI, heart failure, cardiac arrest,** myocarditis, endocarditis, peri-

cardial effusion, thrombosis, **capillary leak syndrome (CLS).**
**EENT:** conjunctivitis.
**GI:** *nausea, vomiting, diarrhea,* abdominal pain, *stomatitis, anorexia, bleeding, dyspepsia, constipation,* **bowel perforation, infarction.**
**GU:** *elevated BUN and serum creatinine levels, oliguria, anuria, proteinuria, hematuria, dysuria,* urine retention, urinary frequency, urinary tract infection (UTI).
**Hematologic:** *anemia,* THROMBOCYTOPENIA, LEUKOPENIA, *coagulation disorders,* leukocytosis, eosinophilia.
**Hepatic:** *jaundice,* ascites, hepatomegaly, *elevated bilirubin, serum transaminase, and alkaline phosphatase levels.*
**Metabolic:** weight gain or loss, *hypomagnesemia, acidosis, hypocalcemia, hypophosphatemia, hypokalemia, hyperuricemia, hypoalbuminemia,* hypoproteinemia, hyponatremia, hyperkalemia.
**Musculoskeletal:** arthralgia, myalgia, back pain.
**Respiratory:** pulmonary congestion, dyspnea, **pulmonary edema, respiratory failure, pleural effusion, apnea,** pneumothorax, tachypnea.
**Skin:** pruritus, erythema, rash, dryness, exfoliative dermatitis, purpura, alopecia, petechiae.
**Other:** fever, chills, weakness, edema, infections of catheter tip or injection site, phlebitis, SEPSIS, *gangrene.*

## Overdose and treatment

Administration of high doses produces rapid onset of expected adverse reactions, including cardiac, renal, and hepatic toxicity.

Drug toxicity is dose-related. Treatment is supportive. Because of short serum half-life of drug, discontinuation may ameliorate many of the adverse effects. Dexamethasone may decrease the toxicity of drug but may also impair effectiveness.

## Clinical considerations

- Patients should be neurologically stable with a negative computed tomography scan for CNS metastases. Drug may exacerbate symptoms in patients with unrecognized or undiagnosed CNS metastases.
- Renal and hepatic impairment occur during treatment. Avoid administering other hepatotoxic or nephrotoxic drugs because toxicity may be additive. Clinician should be prepared to adjust dosage of other drugs to compensate for this impairment. Dosage modification because of toxicity is usually accomplished by holding a dose or interrupting therapy rather than by reducing the dose to be administered.
- Severe anemia or thrombocytopenia may occur. Packed RBCs or platelets may be needed.
- Advise clinician to treat previous infections before therapy starts.

---

* Canada only ◇ Unlabeled clinical use

■ Advise clinician to treat CLS with careful monitoring of fluid status, pulse, mental status, urine output, and organ perfusion. Central venous pressure monitoring is needed.

■ Because fluid management or administration of pressor agents may be essential to treat CLS, use cautiously in patients who require large volumes of fluid (such as patients with hypercalcemia).

■ Preliminary studies indicate that a high percentage of patients (over 75%) develop non-neutralizing antibodies to aldesleukin when treated with the every-8-hour dosing regimen. Neutralizing antibodies develop in less than 1%. The clinical significance of this finding isn't yet known.

■ Aldesleukin has been investigated for various cancers, including Kaposi's sarcoma, metastatic melanoma, colorectal cancer, and malignant lymphoma.

### Therapeutic monitoring

■ Advise clinician to perform standard hematologic tests, including CBC, differential, and platelet counts; serum electrolytes; and renal and hepatic function tests before therapy. Also advise clinician to obtain chest X-ray. This should be repeated daily during drug administration.

■ Advise clinician to monitor CNS effects of drug and discontinuing drug if moderate to severe lethargy or somnolence develops because continued administration can result in coma.

■ Advise clinician to take vital signs, including patient's temperature, every 4 hours and weigh patient daily.

### Special populations

**Pregnant patients.** It's unknown if drug causes fetal harm. Don't use in pregnancy if possible.

**Breast-feeding patients.** It's unknown if drug appears in breast milk. Consider risk and benefit and decide whether to discontinue drug or breast-feeding because of risk of serious adverse effects to the infant.

**Pediatric patients.** Safety and efficacy haven't been established in children under age 18.

### Patient counseling

■ Make sure patient understands the serious toxicity of drug. Adverse effects are expected with normal doses, and serious toxicity may occur despite close clinical monitoring.

# alemtuzumab
Campath

*Pharmacologic classification:* monoclonal antibody
*Therapeutic classification:* antineoplastic
*Pregnancy risk category C*

## Available forms
*Ampules:* 10 mg/ml, 3-ml ampules

## Indications and dosages
**B-cell chronic lymphocytic leukemia in patients treated with alkylating drugs, in whom fludarabine therapy has failed**
*Adults:* Initially, 3 mg I.V. infusion over 2 hours daily; if tolerated (infusion-related toxicities are grade 2 or less), increase dose to 10 mg daily and continue, as tolerated; then increase to 30 mg daily. As maintenance, give 30 mg I.V. three times weekly on nonconsecutive days (such as Monday, Wednesday, Friday) for up to 12 weeks. Don't give single doses greater than 30 mg or weekly doses greater than 90 mg.

≡ *Dosage adjustment.* For patients with hematologic toxicity, see the table below.

| Hematologic toxicity | Dose modification and reinitiation |
|---|---|
| First occurrence of absolute neutrophil count (ANC) ≤ 250/mm³ or platelets ≤ 25,000/mm³ | Withhold therapy; resume at same dose when ANC ≥ 500/mm³ or platelets ≥ 50,000/mm³. If delay between doses is ≥ 7 days, start therapy at 3 mg; escalate to 10 mg then 30 mg as tolerated. |
| Second occurrence of ANC ≤ 250/mm³ or platelets ≤ 25,000/mm³ | Withhold therapy; when ANC ≥ 500/mm³ or platelets ≥ 50,000/mm³, resume at 10 mg. If delay between doses is ≥ 7 days, start therapy at 3 mg; escalate to 10 mg only. |
| Third occurrence of ANC ≤ 250/mm³ or platelets ≤ 25,000/mm³ | Discontinue therapy. |
| For a decrease of ANC or platelet count ≤ 50% of the baseline value in patients starting therapy with ANC ≤ 500/mm³ or platelet count ≤ 25,000/mm³ | Withhold therapy; when ANC or platelet count returns to baseline, resume therapy. If delay between dosing is ≥ 7 days, start therapy at 3 mg and escalate to 10 mg, then 30 mg as tolerated. |

## I.V. administration
- Don't give as I.V. push or bolus. Infuse over 2 hours.
- Advise premedicating with diphenhydramine 50 mg and acetaminophen 650 mg 30 minutes before infusion; advise clinician to give hydrocortisone 200 mg to decrease severe infusion-related events. Advise clinician to give anti-infective prophylaxis while patient is on therapy. TMP-sulfa DS b.i.d. three times a week and famciclovir (or equivalent) 250 mg b.i.d. have been used at start of alemtuzumab therapy. Continue for 2 months, or until CD4+ count is 200 cells/mm$^3$ or more, whichever occurs later.
- Don't shake ampule before use; filter with a sterile, low–protein binding, 5-micron filter before dilution. Add to 100 ml normal saline or D$_5$W solution. Gently invert bag to mix solution. Use within 8 hours of preparation.

### Incompatibilities
None reported.

### Mechanism of action
*Antineoplastic action:* The action is thought to be antibody-dependent lysis of leukemic cells following cell-surface binding.

### Pharmacokinetics
*Absorption:* Administered I.V.
*Distribution:* Binds to various tissues.
*Metabolism:* Unknown.
*Excretion:* Average half-life is about 12 days.

| Route | Onset | Peak | Duration |
|---|---|---|---|
| I.V. | Unknown | Unknown | Unknown |

### Contraindications and precautions
Contraindicated in patients with active systemic infections, underlying immunodeficiency (such as HIV), or type I hypersensitivity or anaphylactic reactions to alemtuzumab or its components.

### Interactions
None reported.

### Adverse reactions
**CNS:** *insomnia,* depression, somnolence, *asthenia, headache, dysthenias, dizziness, fatigue,* malaise, tremor.
**CV:** *edema, peripheral edema, hypotension, hypertension, tachycardia, supraventricular tachycardia.*
**EENT:** epistaxis, rhinitis, *pharyngitis.*
**GI:** *anorexia, nausea, vomiting, diarrhea, stomatitis, ulcerative stomatitis, mucositis, abdominal pain, dyspepsia,* constipation.
**Hematologic:** NEUTROPENIA, *anemia,* **pancytopenia,** THROMBOCYTOPENIA, purpura.
**Musculoskeletal:** *pain, skeletal pain, back pain, myalgias.*
**Respiratory:** *dyspnea, cough, bronchitis, pneumonitis,* **bronchospasm.**

**Skin:** *rash, urticaria, pruritus, increased sweating.*
**Other:** INFECTION, SEPSIS, *herpes simplex, rigors, fever,* temperature change sensation, candidiasis.

### Overdose and treatment
Even in normal dosages, patients may experience signs and symptoms of hematologic toxicity, including myelosuppression, bone marrow dysplasia, and thrombocytopenia. Initial doses of greater than 3 mg are not well tolerated. Extremely high doses can cause acute bronchospasm, cough, and shortness of breath, then anuria and death.

Advise clinician to stop drug; treatment should be supportive.

### Clinical considerations
- Drug may interfere with diagnostic serum tests that use antibodies.
- Drug should be started at low dose and increased as tolerated.
- Blood should be irradiated if transfusions are needed to protect against graft versus host disease. Advise clinician to monitor hematologic studies carefully.
- Don't exceed recommended doses.
- Don't give drug if patient has systemic infection at scheduled dose time.
- Don't immunize with live viral vaccines.
- If therapy is interrupted for ≥ 7 days, advise clinician to restart with gradual dose escalation.

### Therapeutic monitoring
- Advise clinician to monitor blood pressure and hypotensive symptoms during administration.
- Advise clinician to obtain CBC and platelet counts weekly during therapy and more frequently if anemia, neutropenia, or thrombocytopenia worsens.
- Advise clinician to obtain CD4+ counts after treatment until CD4+ count is ≥ 200 cells/mm$^3$.

### Special populations
**Breast-feeding patients.** It's unknown if drug appears in breast milk. Advise patient to stop breast-feeding during treatment and for at least 3 months after taking last dose of drug.
**Pediatric patients.** Safety and efficacy in children are unknown.
**Geriatric patients.** No substantial differences among age groups have been observed.

### Patient counseling
- Tell patient to report immediately any infusion reactions, such as rigors, chills, fever, nausea, or vomiting.
- Advise patient that blood tests will be performed during therapy to monitor for adverse effects.

■ Advise patient to report immediately any signs or symptoms of infection.

---

# alendronate sodium
Fosamax

*Pharmacologic classification:* osteoclast-mediated bone resorption inhibitor
*Therapeutic classification:* antiosteoporotic
*Pregnancy risk category C*

---

## Available forms
Available by prescription only
*Tablets:* 5 mg, 10 mg, 35 mg, 40 mg, 70 mg

## Indications and dosages
*Osteoporosis in postmenopausal women*
*Adults:* 10 mg P.O. daily or 70 mg P.O. once weekly taken with water at least 30 minutes before first food, beverage, or drug of the day.
*Prevention of osteoporosis in post-menopausal women*
*Adults:* 5 mg P.O. daily or 35 mg P.O. weekly taken with water at least 30 minutes before first food, beverage, or drug of the day.
*Conjunction with calcium and vitamin D supplementation in the treatment of corti-costeroid-induced osteoporosis*
*Adults:* 5 mg P.O. daily. In postmenopausal women not receiving estrogen replacement therapy, dose is 10 mg P.O. daily.
*Paget's disease of bone*
*Adults:* 40 mg P.O. daily for 6 months taken with water at least 30 minutes before first food, beverage, or drug of the day.
*Treatment to increase bone mass in men with osteoporosis*
*Adults:* 10 mg P.O. daily; alternatively, 70 mg P.O. once weekly.

## Mechanism of action
*Antiosteoporotic action:* At the cellular level, alendronate suppresses osteoclast activity on newly formed resorption surfaces, which reduces bone turnover. Bone formation exceeds bone resorption at bone remodeling sites and thus leads to progressive gains in bone mass.

## Pharmacokinetics
*Absorption:* Absorbed from the GI tract. Food or beverages can decrease bioavailability significantly.
*Distribution:* Distribution is to soft tissues but is then rapidly redistributed to bone or excreted in urine. Protein binding is about 78%.
*Metabolism:* Doesn't appear to be metabolized.
*Excretion:* Excreted in urine.

| Route | Onset | Peak | Duration |
|-------|-------|------|----------|
| P.O. | Unknown | Unknown | Unknown |

## Contraindications and precautions
Contraindicated in patients hypersensitive to any component of drug, hypocalcemia, or severe renal insufficiency (creatinine clearance below 35 ml/minute).
Use cautiously in patients with active upper GI problems, such as dysphagia, symptomatic esophageal diseases, gastritis, duodenitis, or ulcers, and in patients with mild to moderate renal insufficiency (creatinine clearance between 35 and 60 ml/minute).

## Interactions
**Drug-drug.** *Antacids and calcium supplements:* Interfere with absorption of alendronate. Instruct patient to wait at least 30 minutes after taking alendronate before consuming other drugs.
*Aspirin and NSAIDs:* Increase risk of upper GI adverse reactions with alendronate doses above 10 mg daily. Advise clinician to monitor patient closely.
*Hormone replacement therapy:* Not recommended when used in treatment of osteoporosis with alendronate because of lack of clinical evidence regarding effectiveness.

## Adverse reactions
**CNS:** headache.
**GI:** taste perversion, abdominal pain, nausea, dyspepsia, constipation, diarrhea, flatulence, acid regurgitation, esophageal ulcer, vomiting, dysphagia, abdominal distention, gastritis.
**Musculoskeletal:** musculoskeletal pain.

## Overdose and treatment
Hypocalcemia, hypophosphatemia, and upper GI adverse effects, such as upset stomach, heartburn, esophagitis, gastritis, or ulcer, may result from oral overdose. Specific information isn't available, but consider administration of milk or antacids (to bind alendronate). Dialysis isn't beneficial.

## Clinical considerations
■ Hypocalcemia must be corrected before drug therapy starts. Other disturbances of mineral metabolism (such as vitamin D deficiency) should also be corrected before therapy starts.
■ When drug is used to treat osteoporosis in postmenopausal women, disease is confirmed by low bone mass findings on diagnostic studies or history of an osteoporotic fracture.
■ Drug is indicated for patients with Paget's disease who have alkaline phosphatase levels at least twice the upper limit for normal, in those who are symptomatic, or in those at risk for future complications from the disease.
**◄ ALERT** Advise patient to take with a full glass of water and sit upright for 30 minutes to avoid esophageal ulcer formation.

---

pertension; and hemiplegic or basilar migraine. Don't give within 24 hours after treatment with other serotonin agonists or ergotamine drugs.

Use cautiously in patients with renal or hepatic impairment and in those with cataracts because of the potential for corneal opacities. Use cautiously also in patients with risk factors for coronary artery disease (CAD), such as obesity, diabetes, and family history of CAD.

### Interactions

**Drug-drug.** *CYP2D6 inhibitors, MAO inhibitors:* May increase levels of almotriptan. Although no adverse clinical effects have been reported, advise clinician to monitor patient for potential adverse reaction. Reduced dosage may be needed.

*CYP3A4 inhibitors such as ketoconazole:* May increase levels of almotriptan. Advise clinician to monitor patient for potential adverse reaction. Reduced dosage may be needed.

*Ergot-containing drugs:* May cause additive effects. Avoid using together.

*Serotonin $_{1B/1D}$ agonists:* May cause additive effects. Avoid using together.

*SSRIs:* May cause additive serotonin effects, resulting in weakness, hyperreflexia, or incoordination. Advise clinician to monitor patient closely if given together.

### Adverse reactions

**CNS:** paresthesia, headache, dizziness, somnolence.
**GI:** nausea, dry mouth.

### Overdose and treatment

No adverse effects have been reported in patients ingesting up to 200 mg. Based on the drug's pharmacodynamics, an overdose could cause hypertension and other CV symptoms.

Gastric lavage and activated charcoal may help treat overdose. It's unclear if dialysis is effective. Supportive measures include clinical and ECG monitoring for at least 20 hours, even if symptoms don't occur.

### Clinical considerations

■ Dosage should be reduced in patients with poor renal or hepatic function.
■ Dose should be repeated after 2 hours if needed.
■ Don't give more than 2 doses within 24 hours.
■ Drug shouldn't be prescribed with other serotonin agonist drugs or with ergotamine derivatives.
■ Drug shouldn't be prescribed for patient with ischemic heart disease or hemiplegic or basilar migraine.
■ Drug can be taken with or without food.

### Therapeutic monitoring

■ Caution should be used when prescribing drug to patient who is taking an MAO inhibitor or a CYP-450 3A4 or 2D6 inhibitor.

■ Advise clinician to monitor ECG in patients with risk factors for CAD or with symptoms similar to those of CAD, such as chest or throat tightness, pain, and heaviness.

### Special poulations

**Breast-feeding patients.** It's unknown if drug appears in breast milk. Use cautiously in breast-feeding women.
**Pediatric patients.** Drug hasn't been studied in children.
**Geriatric patients.** No adjustments are needed unless patient has renal or hepatic impairment.

### Patient counseling

■ Advise patient to take drug only when he is having a migraine and that drug isn't taken on a regular schedule.
■ Tell patient that drug can be taken with or without food.
■ Teach patient to avoid possible migraine triggers, such as cheese, chocolate, citrus fruits, caffeine, and alcohol.
■ Advise patient to repeat dose only once within 24 hours.
■ Inform patient that repeat dose should be taken no sooner than 2 hours after initial dose.
■ Warn patient that other commonly prescribed migraine drugs can interact with almotriptan.
■ Tell patient to report a history of heart disease or uncontrolled high blood pressure to prescriber and advise him not to take drug.
■ Advise patient to report chest or throat tightness, pain, or heaviness.

# alprazolam

Alprazolam Intensol, Apo-Alpraz*, Novo-Alprazol*, Xanax

*Pharmacologic classification:* benzodiazepine
*Therapeutic classification:* anxiolytic
*Pregnancy risk category D*
*Controlled substance schedule IV*

### Available forms

Available by prescription only
*Tablets:* 0.25 mg, 0.5 mg, 1 mg, 2 mg
*Oral solution:* 0.1 mg/1 ml, 1 mg/1 ml

### Indications and dosages

*Anxiety*
*Adults:* Usual starting dose is 0.25 to 0.5 mg P.O. t.i.d. Increase dose p.r.n. q 3 to 4 days. Maximum total daily dose, 4 mg in divided doses.

≡*Dosage adjustment.* In geriatric or debilitated patients or those with hepatic impairment, initial dose is 0.25 mg P.O. b.i.d. or t.i.d.
*Panic disorder*
*Adults:* Initially, 0.5 mg P.O. t.i.d. Increase as needed and tolerated at intervals of 3 to 4 days

in increments of 1 mg daily. Most patients require more than 4 mg daily; however, doses from 1 to 10 mg daily have been reported.

## Mechanism of action
*Anxiolytic action:* Alprazolam depresses the CNS at the limbic and subcortical levels of the brain. It produces an antianxiety effect by enhancing the effect of the neurotransmitter gamma-aminobutyric acid on its receptor in the ascending reticular activating system, which increases inhibition and blocks both cortical and limbic arousal.

## Pharmacokinetics
*Absorption:* Well absorbed when administered orally.
*Distribution:* Distributed widely throughout the body. About 80% to 90% of an administered dose is plasma protein–bound.
*Metabolism:* Metabolized in the liver equally to alpha-hydroxyalprazolam and inactive metabolites.
*Excretion:* Excreted in urine. Half-life of alprazolam is 12 to 15 hours.

| Route | Onset | Peak | Duration |
|---|---|---|---|
| P.O. | 15-30 min | 1-2 hr | Unknown |

## Contraindications and precautions
Contraindicated in patients hypersensitive to drug or other benzodiazepines or acute angle-closure glaucoma. Use cautiously in patients with hepatic, renal, or pulmonary disease.

## Interactions
**Drug-drug.** *Cimetidine and possibly disulfiram:* Diminished hepatic metabolism of alprazolam, increasing its plasma level. Advise clinician to monitor patient carefully.
*Digoxin:* Plasma levels of digoxin may increase. Advise clinician to monitor serum digoxin levels.
*Haloperidol:* Benzodiazepines may decrease serum levels of haloperidol.
*Phenothiazines, narcotics, barbiturates, general anesthetics, antihistamines, MAO inhibitors, and antidepressants:* Alprazolam potentiates the CNS depressant effects of these drugs. Avoid use together.
*Rifampin:* The effects of alprazolam may decrease with use of rifampin. Advise clinician to monitor patient for clinical effect.
*Theophylline:* May increase the sedative effects of alprazolam. Use together cautiously.
**Drug-herb.** *Kava:* May induce coma if taken with alprazolam. Discourage use together.
**Drug-lifestyle.** *Heavy smoking:* Accelerates alprazolam metabolism, thus lowering clinical effectiveness. Discourage smoking.
*Alcohol use:* Alprazolam potentiates the CNS depressant effects of alcohol. Advise patient to avoid alcohol.

## Adverse reactions
**CNS:** *drowsiness, light-headedness,* minor changes in EEG patterns, headache, confusion, tremor, dizziness, syncope, *depression,* insomnia, nervousness.
**CV:** hypotension, tachycardia.
**EENT:** blurred vision, nasal congestion.
**GI:** *dry mouth,* nausea, vomiting, *diarrhea, constipation.*
**Hepatic:** elevated liver function test results.
**Metabolic:** weight gain or loss.
**Musculoskeletal:** muscle rigidity.
**Skin:** dermatitis.

## Overdose and treatment
Signs and symptoms of overdose include somnolence, confusion, coma, hypoactive reflexes, dyspnea, labored breathing, hypotension, bradycardia, slurred speech, unsteady gait, and impaired coordination.

Advise clinician to support blood pressure and respiration until drug effects subside; advise clinician to monitor vital signs. Flumazenil, a specific benzodiazepine antagonist, may be useful. Mechanical ventilatory assistance via endotracheal tube may be required to maintain a patent airway and support adequate oxygenation. As needed, recommend using I.V. fluids and vasopressors, such as dopamine and phenylephrine, to treat hypotension. If the patient is conscious, emesis should be induced. Advise clinician to use gastric lavage if ingestion was recent, but only if an endotracheal tube is in place to prevent aspiration. After emesis or lavage, advise clinician to give activated charcoal with a cathartic as a single dose. Dialysis is of limited value. Don't use barbiturates if excitation occurs because of possible exacerbation of excitation or CNS depression.

## Clinical considerations
■ Lower doses are effective in geriatric patients and patients with renal or hepatic dysfunction.
■ Anxiety with depression is also responsive to alprazolam but may require more frequent dosing.
■ Store drug in a cool, dry place away from direct light.

### Therapeutic monitoring
■ Advise clinician to monitor patients receiving prolonged therapy with high doses because they should be weaned from the drug gradually to prevent withdrawal symptoms. A 2- to 3-month withdrawal may be needed at a decreasing rate of no more than 0.5 mg q 3 days.

### Special populations
**Breast-feeding patients.** The breast-fed infant of a woman taking alprazolam may become sedated, have feeding difficulties, or lose weight. Avoid use in breast-feeding women.

---

**Pediatric patients.** Advise clinician to closely observe neonate for withdrawal symptoms if mother took alprazolam during pregnancy. Use of alprazolam during labor may cause neonatal flaccidity. Safety hasn't been established in children or adolescents under age 18. **Geriatric patients.** Lower doses are usually effective in geriatric patients because of decreased elimination. When therapy starts or changes, geriatric patients who receive drug require supervision with ambulation and activities of daily living.

## Patient counseling

- Be sure patient understands potential for physical and psychological dependence with chronic use of alprazolam.
- Instruct patient not to alter drug regimen.
- Warn patient that sudden changes in position may cause dizziness. Advise him to dangle legs for a few minutes before getting out of bed to prevent falls and injury.

# alprostadil

Prostin VR Pediatric

*Pharmacologic classification:* prostaglandin
*Therapeutic classification:* corrective drug for patent ductus arteriosus
*Pregnancy risk category NR*

## Available forms

Available by prescription only
*Injection:* 500 mcg/ml

## Indications and dosages

*Temporary maintenance of patency of ductus arteriosus until surgery can be performed*
*Infants:* Initial I.V. infusion of 0.05 to 0.1 mcg/kg/minute via infusion pump. After satisfactory response is achieved, reduce infusion rate to the lowest dose that will maintain response. Maintenance dosages vary. Infusion rate should be the lowest possible dose and is usually achieved by progressively halving the initial dose. Rates as low as 0.002 to 0.005 mcg/kg/minute have been effective.

## I.V. administration

- Adding a 500-mcg solution to 50 ml of $D_5W$ or normal saline solution provides a level of 10 mcg/ml. At this level, a 0.01-ml/kg/minute infusion rate delivers 0.1 mcg/kg/minute of alprostadil.
- During dilution, take care to avoid direct contact of the concentrate with the wall of the plastic volumetric infusion chamber; if a hazy solution develops, discard the chamber and solution.

**⚠ ALERT** Dilute drug before administration. Discard prepared solution after 24 hours.

## Incompatibilities
None reported.

## Mechanism of action
*Ductus arteriosus patency adjunct action:* Alprostadil, also known as prostaglandin $E_1$ or $PGE_1$ is a prostaglandin that relaxes or dilates the rings of smooth muscle of the ductus arteriosus and maintains patency in neonates when infused before natural closure.

## Pharmacokinetics
*Absorption:* Administered I.V.
*Distribution:* Distributed rapidly throughout the body.
*Metabolism:* 68% of dose is metabolized in one pass through the lung, primarily by oxidation; 100% is metabolized within 24 hours.
*Excretion:* Excreted in urine within 24 hours.

| Route | Onset | Peak | Duration |
|-------|-------|------|----------|
| I.V. | 20 min | 1-2 hr | Length of infusion |

## Contraindications and precautions
Contraindicated in neonates with respiratory distress syndrome.
Use cautiously in neonates with bleeding disorders.

## Interactions
None reported.

## Adverse reactions
CNS: *seizures.*
CV: **bradycardia,** hypotension, tachycardia, **cardiac arrest,** edema.
GI: diarrhea.
Hematologic: *DIC.*
Metabolic: *hypokalemia.*
Respiratory: APNEA.
Other: *flushing, fever, sepsis.*

## Overdose and treatment
Signs and symptoms are similar to the adverse reactions and include apnea, bradycardia, pyrexia, hypotension, and flushing. Apnea most commonly occurs in neonates weighing under 2 kg (4.4 lb) at birth and usually develops during the first hour of drug therapy.

Treatment of apnea or bradycardia requires discontinuance of the infusion and appropriate supportive therapy, including mechanical ventilation, p.r.n. Pyrexia or hypotension may be treated by reducing the infusion rate. Flushing should be corrected by repositioning the intra-arterial catheter.

## Clinical considerations
- In infants with restricted pulmonary blood flow, advise clinician to measure effectiveness of drug by monitoring blood oxygenation. In infants with restricted systemic blood flow, advise clinician to measure effectiveness of drug

by monitoring systemic blood pressure and blood pH.
- Apnea and bradycardia may reflect drug overdose. Advise clinician that the infusion be stopped immediately if they occur.
- Peripheral arterial vasodilation (flushing) may respond to repositioning of the catheter.
- Drug should be administered only by personnel trained in pediatric intensive care.
- Store ampules in refrigerator.

### Therapeutic monitoring
- Advise clinician to assess all vital functions closely and frequently to prevent adverse effects.
- Advise clinician to monitor arterial pressure by umbilical artery catheter, auscultation, or Doppler transducer. The rate of infusion should be slowed if arterial pressure decreases significantly.
- Advise clinician to closely monitor respiratory status during treatment and have ventilatory assistance immediately available.

### Patient counseling
- Inform parents of need for drug and its use.
- Encourage parents to ask questions and express concerns.

---

# alprostadil
Caverject, Edex, Muse

*Pharmacologic classification:* prostaglandin
*Therapeutic classification:* corrective drug for impotence
*Pregnancy risk category NR*

### Available forms
Available by prescription only
*Sterile powder for intracavernosal injection for intracavernosal use:* 6.15-mcg, 6.225-mcg, 10.75-mcg, 11.9-mcg, 12.45-mcg, 21.5-mcg, 23.2-mcg, 24.9-mcg, 43-mcg, 49.8-mcg vials
*Injection (frozen) intracavitary:* 10.2 mcg/ml, 20.2 mcg/ml, 40.4 mcg/ml
*Urethral suppository pellet:* 125 mcg, 250 mcg, 500 mcg, 1,000 mcg

### Indications and dosages
*Erectile dysfunction of vasculogenic, psychogenic, or mixed etiology*
*Adults:* Dosages are highly individualized. For injection: Initial dose is 2.5 mcg intracavernously. If partial response occurs, increase second dose by 2.5 to 5 mcg, and then increase dose further in increments of 5 to 10 mcg until patient achieves an erection (suitable for intercourse but not lasting over 1 hour). If initial dose isn't effective, increase second dose to 7.5 mcg within 1 hour; then increase dose further in 5- to 10-mcg increments until patient achieves an erection. Patient must remain in

prescriber's office until complete detumescence occurs. If patient responds, don't repeat procedure for 24 hours. For pellet, start initially with lower doses (125 or 250 mcg). Increases or decreases should be made on separate occasions in a stepwise manner until patient achieves an erection that's sufficient for sexual intercourse.
*Erectile dysfunction of pure neurologic etiology (spinal cord injury)*
*Adults:* Dosages are highly individualized. Initial dose is 1.25 mcg intracavernously. If partial response occurs, give second dose of 1.25 mcg and then a third dose of 2.5 mcg; increase dose further in 5-mcg increments until patient achieves an erection (suitable for intercourse but not lasting over 1 hour). If initial dose isn't effective, increase second dose to 2.5 mcg within 1 hour; then increase further in 5-mcg increments until patient achieves an erection. Patient must remain in prescriber's office until complete detumescence occurs. No more than two doses administered 1 hour apart should be given in 1 day. If patient responds, don't repeat procedure for 24 hours.

### Mechanism of action
*Corrective action in impotence:* A prostaglandin derivative that induces erection by relaxation of trabecular smooth muscle and by dilation of cavernosal arteries. This leads to expansion of lacunar spaces and entrapment of blood by compressing the venules against the tunica albuginea, a process referred to as the corporal veno-occlusive mechanism.

### Pharmacokinetics
*Absorption:* Absolute bioavailability hasn't been determined.
*Distribution:* Plasma protein–bound primarily to albumin (81%).
*Metabolism:* Rapidly converted to compounds that are further metabolized before excretion.
*Excretion:* Excreted primarily in urine, the remainder in feces.

| Route | Onset | Peak | Duration |
|---|---|---|---|
| Intra-cavernous | Unknown | 2-5 min | 2 hr |
| P.R. | 10 min | 16 min | 1-2 hr |

### Contraindications and precautions
Contraindicated in patients hypersensitive to drug, conditions associated with disposition to priapism (sickle cell anemia or trait, multiple myeloma, or leukemia), or penile deformation (angulation, cavernosal fibrosis, or Peyronie's disease). Don't give to men with penile implants or when sexual activity is contraindicated. Also avoid use in women, children, and neonates. Muse shouldn't be used for sexual intercourse with a pregnant woman unless the couple uses a condom barrier.

## Interactions
**Drug-drug.** *Anticoagulants:* Increased risk of bleeding from intracavernosal injection site. Advise clinician to monitor patient closely.
*Cyclosporine:* Decreased cyclosporine level. Use together cautiously.
*Vasoactive drugs:* Safety and efficacy of use with other drugs haven't been studied and, therefore, combined use isn't recommended.

## Adverse reactions
**CNS:** headache, dizziness, fainting.
**CV:** hypertension, hypotension, swelling of leg veins.
**GU:** *penile pain,* prolonged erection, penile fibrosis, penis disorder, penile rash, penile edema, prostatic disorder, testicular and perineal aching, burning of urethra, minor urethral burning.
**Musculoskeletal:** back pain.
**Respiratory:** upper respiratory infection, flu syndrome, sinusitis, nasal congestion, cough.
**Other:** injection site hematoma, injection site ecchymosis, localized trauma, localized pain.

## Overdose and treatment
If intracavernous overdose of drug occurs, patient should be under medical supervision until systemic effects have resolved or penile detumescence has occurred. Symptomatic treatment of systemic symptoms is appropriate.

## Clinical considerations
■ Patient must have underlying treatable medical causes of erectile dysfunction diagnosed and treated before therapy starts.
■ Regular follow up of patient with careful examination of the penis is strongly recommended to detect signs of penile fibrosis. Drug should be stopped in patients who develop penile angulation, cavernosal fibrosis, or Peyronie's disease.
■ Female partners of users of Muse may experience vaginal itching and burning.
■ Intercavernosal alprostadil has been used as an adjunct to different diagnoses of erectile dysfunction and in evaluating hemodynamic status of erectile tissue.

### *Therapeutic monitoring*
■ Advise clinician to monitor patient for hypotension and adjust drug to the lowest effective dose.
■ Advise clinician to monitor patient for adverse effects and discontinue immediately if penile angulation, cavernosal fibrosis, or Peyronie's disease develops.

### *Special populations*
Drug isn't indicated for use in women, neonates, or children.

## Patient counseling
■ To ensure safe and effective use, thoroughly instruct patient how to prepare and give alprostadil before beginning intracavernosal treatment at home. Stress importance of following instructions carefully.
■ Tell patient to discard vials with precipitates or discoloration. Reconstituted vial is designed for one use only and should be discarded after withdrawal of proper volume of the solution.
■ Instruct patient not to shake the contents of reconstituted vial.
■ Stress importance of not reusing or sharing needles or syringes as well as not sharing drug.
■ Ensure that patient has the manufacturer's instructions for administration included in each package of alprostadil.
■ Tell patient that desirable dose will be established in the prescriber's office. Patient shouldn't change the dose without medical approval.
■ Inform patient that he can expect an erection to occur within 5 to 20 minutes after drug administration and that standard treatment goal is to produce an erection not lasting over 1 hour.
■ Warn patient that an erection lasting over 6 hours has been known to occur after alprostadil injection. If this occurs, instruct patient to seek medical attention immediately.
■ Tell patient that Caverject and Edex shouldn't be used more than three times weekly, with at least 24 hours between each use. The maximum frequency of use of Muse is two administrations per 24-hour period.
■ Review possible adverse reactions with patient. Tell patient to immediately report priapism, penile pain that wasn't present before or that's increased in intensity, and the occurrence of nodules or hard tissue in the penis.
■ Instruct patient to inspect penis daily for signs or symptoms of redness, swelling, tenderness, or curvature of the erect penis, which might suggest an infection. The patient should contact his prescriber if he suspects infection.
■ Remind patient that regular follow-up visits are needed to evaluate effectiveness and safety of therapy.
■ Inform patient that drug doesn't offer protection from transmission of sexually transmitted diseases and that protective measures continue to be necessary.
■ Warn patient that a small amount of bleeding can occur at the injection site. This can increase the risk of transmitting blood-borne diseases, if present, to his sexual partner.
■ Caution patient using Muse to use a condom when having sexual intercourse with a pregnant partner; this will also prevent potential vaginal burning and itching in female partner.

# alteplase (recombinant alteplase, tissue plasminogen activator)

Activase, Cathflo Activase

*Pharmacologic classification:* enzyme
*Therapeutic classification:* thrombolytic enzyme
*Pregnancy risk category C*

## Available forms

Available by prescription only
*Injection:* 50-mg (29 million IU), 100-mg (58 million IU) vials
*Intracatheter instillation:* 2 mg/vial (lyophilized powder)

## Indications and dosages

*Lysis of thrombi obstructing coronary arteries in management of acute MI*
**Three-hour infusion**
*Adults weighing over 65 kg (143 lb):* 60 mg in first hour, with 6 to 10 mg I.V. bolus over first 1 to 2 minutes; then 20 mg/hour for an additional 2 hours. Total dose, 100 mg.
*Adults weighing 65 kg or less:* 1.25 mg/kg given over 3 hours as described above.
**Accelerated infusion**
*Adults weighing over 67 kg (148 lb):* 15 mg I.V. push, 50 mg over 30 minutes, then 35 mg over 60 minutes.
*Adults weighing 67 kg or less:* 15 mg I.V. push, 0.75 mg/kg over 30 minutes (not to exceed 50 mg), then 0.5 mg/kg over 60 minutes (not to exceed 35 mg).
◇ *Prevention of reocclusion after thrombolysis for acute MI*
*Adults:* 3.3 mcg/kg/min by I.V. infusion for 4 hours with heparin therapy immediately after initial thrombolytic infusion.
*Pulmonary embolism*
*Adults:* 100 mg by I.V. infusion over 2 hours. Begin heparin therapy at the end of infusion.
◇ *Adults:* 30 to 50 mg infused via the intrapulmonary artery over 1½ or 2 hours, respectively, in conjunction with heparin therapy.
◇ *Lysis of arterial occlusion in a peripheral vessel or bypass graft*
*Adults:* 0.5 to 0.1 mg/kg/hour infused via the intrapulmonary artery for 1 to 8 hours.
*Acute ischemic stroke*
*Adults:* 0.9 mg/kg (maximum dose, 90 mg). Give 10% of dose as an I.V. bolus over 1 minute; remaining 90% over 1 hour.
*Restoration of function to central venous access devices as assessed by the ability to withdraw blood (Cathflo Activase only)*
*Adults and children over age 2:* If > 30 kg, instill 2 mg in 2 ml sterile water into catheter. If > 10 kg and ≤ 30 kg, instill 110% of the internal lumen volume of the catheter. Don't exceed 2 mg. Aspirate after 30 minutes. If func-

tion was restored, aspirate 4 to 5 ml of blood and irrigate with normal saline solution. If function not restored after 120 minutes, instill a second dose.

## I.V. administration

■ Prepare solution using supplied sterile water for injection. Don't use bacteriostatic water for injection.
■ Don't mix other drugs with alteplase. Use 18G needle for preparing solution—aim water stream at lyophilized cake. Expect a slight foaming to occur. Don't use if vacuum isn't present.
■ Drug may be further diluted with normal saline solution injection or $D_5W$ to yield a level of 0.5 mg/ml. Reconstituted or diluted solutions are stable for up to 8 hours at controlled room temperature.
■ The accelerated infusion method is preferred over the 3-hour infusion because greater patency of the infarct-related artery has been reported.

## Incompatibilities

None reported, but don't mix with other drugs.

## Mechanism of action

*Thrombolytic action:* Alteplase is an enzyme that catalyzes the conversion of tissue plasminogen to plasmin in the presence of fibrin. This fibrin specificity produces local fibrinolysis in the area of recent clot formation, with limited systemic proteolysis. In patients with acute MI, this allows for reperfusion of ischemic cardiac muscle and improved left ventricular function with a decreased risk of heart failure after an MI.

## Pharmacokinetics

*Absorption:* Administered I.V.
*Distribution:* Rapidly cleared from the plasma by the liver; 80% of dose is cleared within 10 minutes after infusion is discontinued.
*Metabolism:* Primarily hepatic.
*Excretion:* Over 85% of drug is excreted in urine; 5% in feces. Plasma half-life is under 10 minutes.

| Route | Onset | Peak | Duration |
|-------|-------|------|----------|
| I.V. | Immediate | 45 min | 4 hr |

## Contraindications and precautions

Contraindicated in patients with history or evidence of intracranial hemorrhage, suspected subarachnoid hemorrhage, seizure at the onset of stroke, active internal bleeding, intracranial neoplasm, arteriovenous malformation, aneurysm, and severe uncontrolled hypertension (more than 185 mm Hg systolic or 110 mm Hg diastolic). Also contraindicated in patients with a history of CVA, recent (within 2 months) intraspinal or intracranial trauma or surgery, or known bleeding diathesis (see package insert).

Use cautiously in patients with recent (within 10 days) major surgery; in pregnancy and first 10 days postpartum; organ biopsy; trauma (including cardiopulmonary resuscitation); GI or GU bleeding; cerebrovascular disease; hypertension; likelihood of left-sided heart thrombus; hemostatic defects, including those secondary to severe hepatic or renal disease; hepatic dysfunction; occluded AV cannula; severe neurologic deficit (National Institutes of Health Stroke Scale over 22); signs of major early infarct on a computed tomographic (CT) scan; mitral stenosis; atrial fibrillation; acute pericarditis or subacute bacterial endocarditis; septic thrombophlebitis; diabetic hemorrhagic retinopathy or other hemorrhagic ophthalmic conditions; in those receiving anticoagulants; and in patients age 75 and older.

## Interactions

**Drug-drug.** *Drugs that antagonize platelet function (abciximab, aspirin, dipyridamole):* May increase risk of bleeding if given before, during, or after alteplase therapy. Use together cautiously.

## Adverse reactions

**CNS:** *cerebral hemorrhage,* fever.
**CV:** hypotension, *arrhythmias,* edema, *AV block, cardiac arrest, new ischemic stroke, thromboembolism, recurrent thromboembolic events.*
**GI:** nausea, vomiting.
**Hematologic:** *severe, spontaneous bleeding (cerebral, retroperitoneal, GU, GI).*
**Other:** bleeding at puncture sites, hypersensitivity reactions, *anaphylaxis.*

## Overdose and treatment

No information is available regarding accidental ingestion.

Excessive I.V. dosage can lead to bleeding problems. Doses of 150 mg have caused an increased risk of intracranial bleeding. Infusion should be stopped immediately if signs or symptoms of bleeding are observed.

## Clinical considerations

- Reconstitute Cathflo Activase with 2.2 ml sterile water and dissolve completely into a colorless to pale yellow solution that yields a concentration of 1 mg/ml. Solutions are stable for up to 8 hours at controlled room temperature.
- Assess the cause of catheter dysfunction before using Cathflo Activase. Some conditions that occluded the catheter include catheter malposition, mechanical failure, constriction by a suture, and lipid deposits or drug precipitates within the catheter lumen. Do not attempt to suction because of the risk of damage to the vascular wall or collapse of soft-walled catheters.

- Do not use excessive pressure while instilling Cathflo Activase into the catheter, which could cause catheter rupture or expulsion of the clot into the circulation.
- Expect to begin alteplase infusions as soon as possible after onset of MI symptoms, such as angina pain or equivalent greater than 30 minutes' duration; angina that's unresponsive to nitroglycerin; or ECG evidence of MI.
- Advise clinician to give drug within 3 to 6 hours after onset of stroke symptoms after exclusion of intracranial hemorrhage by CT scan or other diagnostic imaging methods capable of detecting presence of hemorrhage. Treatment should be performed only in facilities that can provide appropriate evaluation and management of intracranial hemorrhage. Therapy that is started within 7 to 12 hours may be beneficial in reducing mortality.
- Heparin is usually administered during or after alteplase as part of the treatment regimen for acute MI or pulmonary embolism. The use of anticoagulant or antiplatelet therapy for 24 hours is contraindicated when alteplase is used for acute ischemic stroke.
- Drug therapy for acute ischemic stroke should be stopped in patients who haven't recently used oral anticoagulants or heparin if pretreatment PT exceeds 15 seconds or if an elevated aPTT is identified.
- Staff should avoid I.M. injections, venipuncture, and arterial puncture during therapy. Use pressure dressings or ice packs on recent puncture sites to prevent bleeding. If arterial puncture is needed, select a site on the arm and apply pressure for 30 minutes afterward.
- Altered results may be expected in coagulation and fibrinolytic tests. The use of aprotinin (150 to 200 U/ml) in the blood sample may attenuate this interference.

### Therapeutic monitoring

- Advise clinician to monitor patient for bleeding or hemorrhage.
- Advise clinician to monitor ECG for transient arrhythmias (sinus bradycardia, ventricular tachycardia, accelerated idioventricular rhythm, ventricular premature depolarizations) associated with reperfusion after coronary thrombolysis. Antiarrhythmics should be available.

### Special populations

**Pediatric patients.** Safety and efficacy for use in children haven't been established, but the drug has been used investigationally in children with some success.
**Geriatric patients.** Use cautiously in patients over age 75 because of the potential of CV side effects.

## Patient counseling

- Teach patient signs and symptoms of internal bleeding and tell him to report these immediately.

- Advise patient about proper dental care to avoid excessive gum trauma resulting from vigorous brushing; drug increases chances of bleeding.

# aluminum carbonate
Basaljel

*Pharmacologic classification:* inorganic aluminum salt
*Therapeutic classification:* antacid, hypophosphatemic agent
*Pregnancy risk category NR*

## Available forms
Available without a prescription
*Tablets or capsules:* aluminum hydroxide equivalent 500 mg
*Suspension:* aluminum hydroxide equivalent 400 mg/5 ml

## Indications and dosages
*Antacid*
Adults: 10 ml suspension P.O. q 2 hours p.r.n. or 1 to 2 tablets or capsules q 2 hours p.r.n.
*Hyperphosphatemia and prevention of urinary phosphate stones formation (with low-phosphate diet)*
Adults: 1 g P.O. t.i.d. or q.i.d.; adjust to lowest possible dose after therapy starts, monitoring diet and serum levels.

## Mechanism of action
*Antacid action:* Exerts its antacid effect by neutralizing gastric acid; this increases pH, thereby decreasing pepsin activity.
*Hypophosphatemic action:* Aluminum carbonate reduces serum phosphate levels by complexing with phosphate in the gut. This results in formation of insoluble, nonabsorbable aluminum phosphate, which is then excreted in feces. Calcium absorption increases secondary to reduced phosphate absorption.

## Pharmacokinetics
*Absorption:* Largely unabsorbed; small amounts may be absorbed systemically.
*Distribution:* None.
*Metabolism:* None.
*Excretion:* Excreted in feces; some may appear in breast milk.

| Route | Onset | Peak | Duration |
|-------|-------|------|----------|
| P.O. | 20 min | Unknown | 20-180 min |

## Contraindications and precautions
No known contraindications. Use cautiously in patients with chronic renal disease.

## Interactions
**Drug-drug.** *Antimuscarinics, chenodiol, chlordiazepoxide, coumarin anticoagulants, diazepam, digoxin, indomethacin, iron salts, iso-niazid, phenothiazines (especially chlorpromazine), quinolones, sodium or potassium phosphate, tetracycline, and vitamin A:* Aluminum carbonate may decrease absorption of many drugs, thereby lessening their effectiveness. Separate administration by at least 2 hours.
*Enterically coated drugs:* Premature drug release. Separate administration times by 1 hour.

## Adverse reactions
**CNS:** encephalopathy.
**GI:** *constipation, **intestinal obstruction,** in*creased serum gastrin levels.
**Metabolic:** hypophosphatemia.
**Musculoskeletal:** osteomalacia.

## Overdose and treatment
No information available. Patients with impaired renal function are at a higher risk of aluminum toxicity to brain, bone, and parathyroid glands.

## Clinical considerations
- When administering suspension, recommend shaking well and giving with small amounts of water or fruit juice.
- After administration through a nasogastric tube, recommend flushing tube with water to prevent obstruction.
- When administering drug as an antiurolithic, encourage increased fluid intake to enhance drug effectiveness.
- Constipation may be managed with stool softeners or bulk laxatives, or advise clinician to give alternately with magnesium-containing antacids (unless patient has renal disease).
- Long-term aluminum carbonate use can lead to calcium resorption and subsequent bone demineralization.
- Aluminum carbonate may interfere with imaging techniques using sodium pertechnetate Tc99m and thus impair evaluation of Meckel's diverticulum. It may also interfere with reticuloendothelial imaging of liver, spleen, or bone marrow using technetium Tc99m sulfur colloid. It may antagonize the effect of pentagastrin during gastric acid secretion tests.

## Therapeutic monitoring
Advise clinician to monitor serum calcium and phosphate levels periodically; reduced serum phosphate levels may lead to increased serum calcium levels.

## Special populations
**Pediatric patients.** Use cautiously in children under age 6. Safety and efficacy haven't been established in children, but drug has been used in a few cases.
**Geriatric patients.** Because geriatric patients commonly have decreased GI motility, they may become constipated from this drug.

## Patient counseling
- Advise patient to take drug only as directed and not to take more than 24 capsules or tablets or 120 ml of regular suspension in a 24-hour period. Instruct patient to shake suspension well.
- As needed, advise patient to restrict sodium intake, to drink plenty of fluids, and to follow a low-phosphate diet.
- Advise patient not to switch antacids without medical approval.

# aluminum hydroxide
ALterna GEL, Alu-Cap, Alu-Tab, Amphojel, Dialume, Nephrox

*Pharmacologic classification:* aluminum salt
*Therapeutic classification:* antacid, hypophosphatemic agent
*Pregnancy risk category C*

## Available forms
Available without a prescription
*Tablets:* 300 mg, 500 mg, 600 mg
*Capsules:* 475 mg, 500 mg
*Liquid:* 600 mg/5 ml
*Suspension:* 320 mg/5 ml, 450 mg/5 ml, 675 mg/5 ml

## Indications and dosages
*Antacid; hyperphosphatemia*
*Adults:* 500 to 1,500 mg P.O. (tablet or capsule) 1 hour after meals and h.s.; or 5 to 30 ml of suspension p.r.n. 1 hour after meals and h.s.

## Mechanism of action
*Antacid action:* Aluminum hydroxide neutralizes gastric acid, reducing the direct acid irritant effect. This increases pH, which decreases pepsin activity.
*Hypophosphatemic action:* Aluminum hydroxide reduces serum phosphate levels by complexing with phosphate in the gut, resulting in insoluble, nonabsorbable aluminum phosphate, which is then excreted in feces. Calcium absorption increases as a result of decreased phosphate absorption.

## Pharmacokinetics
*Absorption:* Absorbed minimally; small amounts may be absorbed systemically.
*Distribution:* None.
*Metabolism:* None.
*Excretion:* Excreted in feces; some may appear in breast milk.

| Route | Onset | Peak | Duration |
|-------|-------|------|----------|
| P.O. | Variable | Unknown | 20-180 min |

## Contraindications and precautions
No known contraindications. Use cautiously in patients with renal disease.

## Interactions
**Drug-drug.** *Antimuscarinics, chenodiol, chlordiazepoxide, coumarin anticoagulants, diazepam, digoxin, iron salts, isoniazid, phenothiazines (especially chlorpromazine), quinolones, sodium or potassium phosphate, tetracycline, and vitamin A:* Aluminum hydroxide may decrease absorption of many drugs, thereby decreasing their effectiveness; separate administration by at least 2 hours.
*Enterically coated drugs:* Aluminum hydroxide causes premature release of these drugs. Separate doses by 1 hour.

## Adverse reactions
**CNS:** encephalopathy.
**GI:** *constipation, intestinal obstruction,* elevated serum gastrin levels.
**Metabolic:** hypophosphatemia.
**Musculoskeletal:** osteomalacia.

## Overdose and treatment
No information available. Patients with impaired renal function are at a higher risk of aluminum toxicity to brain, bone, and parathyroid glands.

## Clinical considerations
- Shake suspension well (especially extra-strength suspension) and give with small amounts of water or fruit juice.
- After administering through nasogastric tube, recommend flushing tube with water to prevent obstruction.
- When drug is used as an antiurolithic, encourage increased fluid intake to enhance drug effectiveness.
- Constipation may be managed with stool softeners or bulk laxatives. Suggest alternating aluminum hydroxide with magnesium-containing antacids (unless patient has renal disease).
- Drug therapy may interfere with imaging techniques using sodium pertechnetate Tc99m and thus impair evaluation of Meckel's diverticulum. It may also interfere with reticuloendothelial imaging of liver, spleen, and bone marrow using technetium Tc99m sulfur colloid. It may antagonize the effect of pentagastrin during gastric acid secretion tests.

### Therapeutic monitoring
- Recommend periodically monitoring serum calcium and phosphate levels; decreased serum phosphate levels may lead to increased serum calcium levels.
- Advise clinician to observe patient for hypophosphatemia signs and symptoms (anorexia, muscle weakness, and malaise).

### Special populations
**Breast-feeding patients.** Although drug may appear in breast milk, no problems have been caused by its use in breast-feeding women.

**Pediatric patients.** Use with caution in children under age 6.

**Geriatric patients.** Because geriatric patients commonly have decreased GI motility, they may become constipated from this drug.

## Patient counseling

■ Caution patient to take drug only as directed; to shake suspension well or chew tablets thoroughly; and to follow with sips of water or juice.

■ Instruct patient to restrict sodium intake, drink plenty of fluids, or follow a low-phosphate diet.

■ Advise patient not to switch to another antacid without medical approval.

---

# amantadine hydrochloride
Symmetrel

*Pharmacologic classification:* synthetic cyclic primary amine
*Therapeutic classification:* antiviral, antiparkinsonian
*Pregnancy risk category C*

## Available forms
Available by prescription only
*Capsules:* 100 mg
*Syrup:* 50 mg/5 ml
*Tablets:* 100 mg

## Indications and dosages
**Prophylaxis or symptomatic treatment of influenza type A virus, respiratory tract illnesses in geriatric or debilitated patients**
*Adults up to age 64 and children age 10 and older weighing over 40 kg (88 lb):* 200 mg P.O. daily in a single dose or divided b.i.d.
*Children ages 1 to 9:* 4.4 to 8.8 mg/kg P.O. daily up to a maximum of 150 mg/day. To reduce toxicity, it is recommended for children of any age who weigh < 40 kg to receive 5 mg/kg/day given in one or two divided doses (up to a maximum of 150 mg/day is recommended).
*Adults over age 64:* 100 mg P.O. once daily. Continue treatment for 24 to 48 hours after symptoms disappear. Prophylaxis should start as soon as possible after initial exposure and continue for at least 10 days after exposure. Prophylactic treatment may be continued up to 90 days for repeated or suspected exposures if influenza virus vaccine is unavailable. If used with influenza virus vaccine, continue dose for 2 to 4 weeks until protection from vaccine develops.
**Drug-induced extrapyramidal reactions**
*Adults:* 100 to 300 mg/day P.O. in divided doses.
**Idiopathic parkinsonism, parkinsonian syndrome**
*Adults:* 100 mg P.O. b.i.d.; in patients who are seriously ill or receiving other antiparkinsonians, 100 mg/day for at least 1 week, then

100 mg b.i.d., p.r.n. Patient may benefit from as much as 400 mg/day, but doses over 200 mg must be closely supervised.
≡*Dosage adjustment.* In patients with renal dysfunction, base maintenance dosage on creatinine clearance value, as follows:
For syrup, give 200 mg P.O. on the first day; for capsules, give 200 mg P.O the first day, and then 100 mg daily if creatinine clearance is between 30 and 50 ml/minute; 200 mg on the first day and 100 mg q alternating day if it ranges between 15 to 29 ml/minute; and 200 mg q 7 days if it's below 15 ml/minute.
Patients on chronic hemodialysis should receive 200 mg P.O. q 7 days.

## Mechanism of action
*Antiviral action:* Amantadine interferes with viral uncoating of the RNA in lysosomes. In vitro, amantadine is active only against influenza type A virus. (However, spontaneous resistance commonly occurs.) In vivo, amantadine may protect against influenza type A virus in 70% to 90% of patients; when administered within 24 to 48 hours of onset of illness, it reduces duration of fever and other systemic symptoms.
*Antiparkinsonian action:* Amantadine is thought to cause the release of dopamine in the substantia nigra.

## Pharmacokinetics
*Absorption:* Well absorbed from the GI tract with oral administration. Usual serum level is 0.2 to 0.9 mcg/ml. (Neurotoxicity may occur at levels exceeding 1.5 mcg/ml.)
*Distribution:* Distributed widely throughout body; crosses the blood-brain barrier.
*Metabolism:* About 10% of dose is metabolized.
*Excretion:* About 90% of dose is excreted unchanged in urine, primarily by tubular secretion. Portion of drug may appear in breast milk. Excretion rate depends on urine pH (acidic pH enhances excretion). Elimination half-life in patients with normal renal function is about 24 hours; in those with renal dysfunction, it may be prolonged to 10 days.

| Route | Onset | Peak | Duration |
|-------|-------|------|----------|
| P.O. | Unknown | 1-4 hr | Unknown |

## Contraindications and precautions
Contraindicated in patients hypersensitive to drug. Don't use in patients with untreated angle-closure glaucoma.

Use cautiously in patients with seizure disorders, heart failure, peripheral edema, hepatic disease, mental illness, eczematoid rash, renal impairment, orthostatic hypotension, and CV disease, and in the elderly.

## Interactions
**Drug-drug.** *Benztropine and trihexyphenidyl (when these drugs are given in high doses):* When used together, amantadine may potentiate anticholinergic adverse effects, possibly causing confusion and hallucinations.
*CNS stimulants:* May cause additive stimulation. Avoid use together.
*Co-trimoxazole:* Decreased renal clearance of amantadine with the potential for toxic delirium. Avoid use together.
*Hydrochlorothiazide and triamterene:* A combination of these drugs may decrease urinary amantadine excretion, resulting in increased serum amantadine levels and possible toxicity. Avoid use together.
**Drug-herb.** *Jimsonweed:* May adversely affect CV system function. Discourage use together.
**Drug-lifestyle.** *Alcohol use:* May result in lightheadedness, confusion, fainting, and hypotension. Advise patient to avoid alcohol.

## Adverse reactions
**CNS:** depression, fatigue, confusion, *dizziness,* hallucinations, anxiety, *irritability,* ataxia, *insomnia,* headache, *light-headedness.*
**CV:** peripheral edema, orthostatic hypotension, *heart failure.*
**GI:** anorexia, *nausea,* constipation, vomiting, dry mouth.
**Skin:** livedo reticularis (with prolonged use).

## Overdose and treatment
Clinical effects of overdose include nausea, vomiting, anorexia, hyperexcitability, tremors, slurred speech, blurred vision, lethargy, anticholinergic symptoms, seizures, and possible ventricular arrhythmias, including torsades de pointes and ventricular fibrillation. CNS effects result from increased levels of dopamine in the brain.

Treatment includes immediate gastric lavage or emesis induction along with supportive measures, forced fluids, and, if needed, I.V. administration of fluids. Urine acidification may be used to increase drug excretion. Physostigmine may be given (1 to 2 mg by slow I.V. infusion at 1- to 2-hour intervals) to counteract CNS toxicity. Seizures or arrhythmias may be treated with conventional therapy. Advise clinician to monitor patient closely.

## Clinical considerations
■ To prevent orthostatic hypotension, advise patient to move slowly when changing position (especially when rising to standing position).
■ If patient experiences insomnia, dose should be given several hours before bedtime.
■ Prophylactic drug use is recommended for selected high-risk patients who can't receive influenza virus vaccine. Manufacturer recommends prophylactic therapy lasting up to 90 days with possible repeated or unknown exposure.

### Therapeutic monitoring
Advise clinician to monitor patient's blood pressure if dizziness or lightheadedness occurs.

### Special populations
**Pregnant patients.** There are no adequate controlled studies in pregnant women. Use drug only when benefits outweigh the risks.
**Breast-feeding patients.** Drug appears in breast milk. Avoid breast-feeding during therapy with amantadine.
**Pediatric patients.** Safety and effectiveness of drug in children under age 1 haven't been established.
**Geriatric patients.** Geriatric patients are more susceptible to adverse neurologic effects; dividing daily dosage into two doses may reduce risk.

## Patient counseling
■ Warn patient that drug may impair mental alertness.
■ Advise patient to take drug after meals to ensure best absorption.
■ Caution patient to avoid abrupt position changes because these may cause lightheadedness or dizziness.
■ If drug is being taken to treat parkinsonism, warn patient not to discontinue it abruptly because that might precipitate a parkinsonian crisis.
■ Warn patient to avoid alcohol while taking drug.
■ Instruct patient to report adverse effects promptly, especially dizziness, depression, anxiety, nausea, and urine retention.

---

# amikacin sulfate
Amikin

*Pharmacologic classification:* aminoglycoside
*Therapeutic classification:* antibiotic
*Pregnancy risk category D*

## Available forms
Available by prescription only
*Injection:* 50 mg/ml, 250 mg/ml
*Injection for I.V. infusion:* 5 mg/ml

## Indications and dosages
*Serious infections caused by susceptible organisms*
*Adults and children with normal renal function:* 15 mg/kg/day divided q 8 to 12 hours I.M. or I.V. Don't exceed 1.5 g/day or 15 mg/kg.
◇ *Adults:* 4 to 20 mg given intrathecally or intraventricularly as a single dose in conjunction with I.M. or I.V. administration.

*Neonates with normal renal function:* Initially, 10 mg/kg I.M. or I.V., then 7.5 mg/kg q 12 hours.

**Uncomplicated urinary tract infections**
*Adults:* 250 mg I.M. or I.V. b.i.d.
◇ *Clinical tuberculosis*
*Adults, children, and older infants:* 15 mg/kg I.M. daily, 5 times weekly as an adjunct to other antitubercular drugs.
≡ *Dosage adjustment.* In renal impairment, initially, 7.5 mg/kg. Subsequent doses and frequency determined by blood amikacin levels and renal function test results. One method is to give additional 7.5-mg/kg doses and alter dosing interval based on steady-state serum creatinine. 7.5-mg/kg doses can be given at intervals (in hours) calculated by multiplying the patient's steady-state serum creatinine (in mg/dL) by 9.

Keep peak serum levels between 15 and 35 mcg/ml; trough serum levels shouldn't exceed 5 to 10 mcg/ml.

## I.V. administration
■ Prepare I.V. infusion by adding 500 mg of amikacin to 100 to 200 ml of $D_5W$ or normal saline solution.
■ Alternatively, prepare ADD-Vantage vials per manufacturer instructions. Infuse over 30 to 60 minutes. For infants, dilute enough to allow an infusion period of 1 to 2 hours.

### Incompatibilities
Incompatible with amphotericin B, bacitracin, cephalothin, cephapirin, cisplatin, heparin sodium, phenytoin, thiopental, vancomycin, and vitamin B complex with C. Manufacturer recommends that amikacin not be mixed with other drugs.

## Mechanism of action
*Antibiotic action:* Amikacin is bactericidal; it binds directly to the 30S ribosomal subunit, inhibiting bacterial protein synthesis. Its spectrum of activity includes many aerobic gram-negative organisms (including most strains of *Pseudomonas aeruginosa*) and some aerobic gram-positive organisms. Amikacin may act against some organisms resistant to other aminoglycosides, such as *Proteus, Pseudomonas,* and *Serratia;* some strains of these may be resistant to amikacin. Drug is ineffective against anaerobes.

## Pharmacokinetics
*Absorption:* Poorly absorbed after oral administration and is given parenterally.
*Distribution:* Distributed widely after parenteral administration; intraocular penetration is poor. Factors that increase volume of distribution (burns, peritonitis) may increase dosage requirements. CSF penetration is low, even in patients with inflamed meninges. Intraventricular administration produces high levels

throughout the CNS. Protein binding is minimal. Amikacin crosses the placenta.
*Metabolism:* Not metabolized.
*Excretion:* Excreted primarily in urine by glomerular filtration; small amounts may be excreted in bile and breast milk. Elimination half-life in adults is 2 to 3 hours. In patients with severe renal damage, half-life may extend to 30 to 86 hours. Over time, amikacin accumulates in inner ear and kidneys; urine levels approach 800 mcg/ml 6 hours after a 500-mg I.M. dose.

| Route | Onset | Peak | Duration |
|-------|-------|------|----------|
| I.V. | Immediate | Immediate | 8-12 hr |
| I.M. | Unknown | 1 hr | 8-12 hr |

## Contraindications and precautions
Contraindicated in patients hypersensitive to drug or other aminoglycosides.

Use cautiously in patients with impaired renal function or neuromuscular disorders, in neonates and infants, and in the elderly.

## Interactions
**Drug-drug.** *Amphotericin B, capreomycin, cisplatin, cephalosporins, loop diuretics, methoxyflurane, polymyxin B, vancomycin, and other aminoglycosides:* Concurrent use may increase the hazard of nephrotoxicity, ototoxicity, and neurotoxicity. Use together cautiously.
*Dimenhydrinate, other antiemetics, and antivertigo drugs:* May mask amikacin-induced ototoxicity. Advise clinician to monitor patient closely.
*Bumetanide, ethacrynic acid, furosemide, mannitol, or urea:* Increased hazard of ototoxicity. Use together cautiously.
*General anesthetics or neuromuscular blockers such as succinylcholine and tubocurarine:* Amikacin may potentiate neuromuscular blockade. Advise clinician to monitor patient closely.
*Penicillins:* Results in a synergistic bactericidal effect against *Pseudomonas aeruginosa, Escherichia coli, Klebsiella, Citrobacter, Enterobacter, Serratia,* and *Proteus mirabilis.* However, the drugs are physically and chemically incompatible and are inactivated when mixed or given together. Avoid use together.

## Adverse reactions
**CNS:** *neuromuscular blockade.*
**EENT:** *ototoxicity.*
**GU:** *nephrotoxicity, azotemia.*
**Musculoskeletal:** arthralgia, acute muscular paralysis.

## Overdose and treatment
Clinical signs of overdose include ototoxicity, nephrotoxicity, and neuromuscular toxicity. Drug can be removed by hemodialysis or peritoneal dialysis.

---

Reactions may be *common,* uncommon, *life-threatening,* or COMMON AND LIFE-THREATENING.

Treatment with calcium salts or anticholinesterases reverses neuromuscular blockade.

## Clinical considerations

■ Because drug is dialyzable, patients undergoing hemodialysis need dosage adjustments.
■ Recommendations for care and teaching of patients during therapy and use in geriatric patients and breast-feeding women are the same as for all aminoglycosides.
**H ALERT** Amikacin may be mistaken as Amicar.

### Therapeutic monitoring

Advise clinician to monitor peak and trough levels. Peak serum levels should be no more than 35 mcg/ml and trough serum levels no more than 10 mcg/ml.

### Special populations

**Pediatric patients.** Because potential for ototoxicity is unknown, use amikacin in infants only when other drugs are ineffective or contraindicated. Advise clinician to monitor patient closely during therapy.

## Patient counseling

■ Instruct patient to report adverse reactions promptly.
■ Encourage adequate fluid intake.

---

# amiloride hydrochloride
Midamor

*Pharmacologic classification:* potassium-sparing diuretic
*Therapeutic classification:* diuretic, antihypertensive
*Pregnancy risk category B*

## Available forms

Available by prescription only
*Tablets:* 5 mg

## Indications and dosages

**Hypertension; edema caused by heart failure, usually in patients who are also taking thiazide or other potassium-wasting diuretics**
*Adults:* Usually 5 mg P.O. daily. Dose may be increased to 10 mg daily, if needed. Don't exceed 20 mg daily.
◇ **Lithium-induced polyuria**
*Adults:* 5 to 10 mg P.O. b.i.d.

## Mechanism of action

*Diuretic action:* Amiloride acts directly on the distal renal tubule to inhibit sodium reabsorption and potassium excretion, reducing potassium loss.

*Antihypertensive action:* Amiloride is commonly used with more effective diuretics to manage edema caused by heart failure, hepat-

ic cirrhosis, and hyperaldosteronism. Mechanism of amiloride's hypotensive effect is unknown.

## Pharmacokinetics

*Absorption:* About 50% is absorbed from GI tract. Food decreases absorption to 30%.
*Distribution:* Wide extravascular distribution.
*Metabolism:* Insignificant.
*Excretion:* Most is excreted in urine; half-life is 6 to 9 hours in patients with normal renal function.

| Route | Onset | Peak | Duration |
|-------|-------|------|----------|
| P.O. | 2 hr | 6-10 hr | 24 hr |

## Contraindications and precautions

Contraindicated in patients with elevated serum potassium level (over 5.5 mEq/L). Don't give to patients receiving other potassium-sparing diuretics, such as spironolactone and triamterene. Also contraindicated in patients with anuria, acute or chronic renal insufficiency, diabetic nephropathy, and hypersensitivity to drug.

Use with extreme caution in patients with diabetes mellitus.

## Interactions

**Drug-drug.** *Angiotensin-converting enzyme inhibitors, potassium-containing drugs (parenteral penicillin G) or potassium-sparing diuretics:* Amiloride increases the risk of hyperkalemia when administered with other drugs. Use together cautiously.
*Antihypertensives:* Amiloride may potentiate hypotensive effects. This may be used to therapeutic advantage.
*Digoxin:* Renal clearance of digoxin may be decreased, along with the inotropic effect. Use together cautiously.
*Lithium:* Amiloride may reduce renal clearance of lithium and increase lithium blood levels. Use together cautiously.
*NSAIDs, such as ibuprofen or indomethacin:* May alter renal function and thus affect potassium excretion. Use together cautiously.
**Drug-herb.** *Licorice:* Increased risk of hypokalemia. Discourage use together.
**Drug-food.** *Potassium-containing salt substitutes:* Increased risk of hyperkalemia. Avoid use together.

## Adverse reactions

**CNS:** *headache,* weakness, dizziness, fatigue, encephalopathy.
**CV:** orthostatic hypotension.
**GI:** *nausea, anorexia, diarrhea, vomiting,* abdominal pain, constipation, appetite changes.
**GU:** impotence, abnormal renal function tests.
**Hematologic:** *aplastic anemia, neutropenia.*
**Hepatic:** abnormal liver function test results.
**Metabolic:** hyperkalemia.

---

* Canada only    ◇ Unlabeled clinical use

**Musculoskeletal:** muscle cramps.
**Respiratory:** dyspnea.

## Overdose and treatment
Signs and symptoms of overdose are consistent with dehydration and electrolyte disturbance.

Treatment is supportive and symptomatic. In acute ingestion, recommend emptying stomach by emesis or lavage. In severe hyperkalemia (6.5 mEq/L or more), advise clinician to reduce serum potassium levels with I.V. sodium bicarbonate or glucose with insulin. A cation exchange resin, sodium polystyrene sulfonate (Kayexalate), given orally or as a retention enema, may also reduce serum potassium levels.

## Clinical considerations
■ Recommendations for use of amiloride and for care and teaching of the patient during therapy are the same as those for all potassium-sparing diuretics.
■ Amiloride therapy causes severe hyperkalemia in diabetic patients following I.V. glucose tolerance testing; drug should be stopped at least 3 days before testing.

### Therapeutic monitoring
Advise clinician to monitor patient for signs of hyperkalemia, including paresthesia, muscular weakness, fatigue, flaccid paralysis of the extremities, bradycardia, shock, and ECG abnormalities.

### Special populations
**Pregnant patients.** There are no adequate studies involving pregnant women.
**Breast-feeding patients.** Amiloride appears in breast milk in animals; no human data are available.
**Pediatric patients.** Safety and efficacy in children haven't been established, but a dose of 0.625 mg/kg/day has been used in children weighing 6 to 20 kg.
**Geriatric patients.** Geriatric and debilitated patients require close observation because they're more susceptible to drug-induced diuresis and hyperkalemia. Reduced dosages may be indicated.

## Patient counseling
■ Tell patient to take tablets or single-dose packets with food because it may cause stomach upset. Multidose suspension should be taken on an empty stomach.
■ Advise patient to avoid consumption of large quantities of foods that are high in potassium.
■ Tell patient to notify prescriber if symptoms of dehydration occur.

# aminocaproic acid
Amicar

*Pharmacologic classification:* carboxylic acid derivative
*Therapeutic classification:* fibrinolysis inhibitor
*Pregnancy risk category C*

## Available forms
Available by prescription only
*Tablets:* 500 mg
*Syrup:* 1.25 g/5 ml
*Injection:* 250 mg/ ml (20 ml vial)

## Indications and dosages
*Excessive acute bleeding from hyperfibrinolysis*
*Adults:* 4 to 5 g I.V. or P.O. over first hour, followed with constant infusion of 1 g/hour for about 8 hours or until bleeding is controlled. Maximum dose, 30 g/24 hours.
◊ *Children:* 100 mg/kg I.V., or 3 g/m$^2$ I.V. first hour, followed by constant infusion of 33.3 mg/kg/hour or 1 g/m$^2$/hour. Maximum dose, 18 g/m$^2$ for 24 hours.
*Chronic bleeding tendency*
*Adults:* 5 to 30 g/day P.O. in divided doses at 3- to 6-hour intervals.
◊ *Antidote for excessive thrombolysis from administration of streptokinase or urokinase*
*Adults:* 4 to 5 g I.V. in first hour, followed by continuous infusion of 1 g/hour. Continue treatment for 8 hours or until hemorrhage is controlled.
◊ *Secondary ocular hemorrhage in non-perforating traumatic hyphema*
*Adults:* 100 mg/kg P.O. q 4 hours for 5 days; maximum, 5 g/dose and 30 g/day.
◊ *Hereditary hemorrhagic telangiectasia*
*Adults:* 1 to 1.5 g P.O. b.i.d. for 1 to 2 months followed by 1 to 2 g daily.

## I.V. administration
**⚠ ALERT** Bulk doses and bulk packages must be further diluted.
■ To prepare an I.V. infusion, use normal saline injection, D$_5$W injection, or lactated Ringer's injection for dilution. Dilute doses up to 5 g with 250 ml of solution, doses of 5 g or greater with at least 500 ml.
**⚠ ALERT** Avoid rapid I.V. infusion to minimize risk of CV adverse reactions, such as hypotension, bradycardia, and arrhythmias; use infusion pump to ensure constancy of infusion.

### Incompatibilities
Incompatible with fructose solution.

## Mechanism of action
*Hemostatic action:* Aminocaproic acid inhibits plasminogen activators; to a lesser degree, it

blocks antiplasmin activity by inhibiting fibrinolysis.

## Pharmacokinetics
*Absorption:* Rapidly and completely absorbed from GI tract.
*Distribution:* Readily permeates human blood cells and other body cells; not protein-bound.
*Metabolism:* Insignificant.
*Excretion:* 40% to 60% of a single oral dose is excreted unchanged in urine in 12 hours.

| Route | Onset | Peak | Duration |
|-------|-------|------|----------|
| P.O. | 1 hr | 2 hr | Unknown |
| I.V. | 1 hr | Unknown | 3 hr |

## Contraindications and precautions
Contraindicated in patients with active intravascular clotting or presence of DIC unless heparin is used concomitantly. Injectable form is contraindicated in neonates.

Use cautiously in patients with cardiac, renal, or hepatic disease.

## Interactions
**Drug-drug.** *Estrogens and oral contraceptives containing estrogen:* Increases risk of hypercoagulability. Use with caution.

## Adverse reactions
**CNS:** dizziness, malaise, headache, delirium, *seizures,* hallucinations, weakness.
**CV:** hypotension, *bradycardia, arrhythmias* (with rapid I.V. infusion), generalized thrombosis.
**EENT:** tinnitus, nasal congestion, conjunctival suffusion.
**GI:** nausea, cramps, diarrhea.
**GU:** *acute renal failure.*
**Hepatic:** increased AST, ALT.
**Metabolic:** *hyperkalemia.*
**Musculoskeletal:** myopathy.
**Skin:** rash.

## Overdose and treatment
Signs and symptoms of overdose include nausea, diarrhea, delirium, thrombotic episodes, and cardiac and hepatic necrosis. Drug should be stopped immediately.

## Clinical considerations
■ Aminocaproic acid has been used investigationally to treat missed abortion, allergic reaction, dermatitides, prophylaxis for blood transfusion reaction, connective tissue disease, and rheumatoid arthritis.

### Therapeutic monitoring
■ Advise clinician to monitor coagulation studies, heart rhythm, and blood pressure. Chronic use of drug requires routine creatine kinase determinations.
■ Be alert for signs of phlebitis. If skeletal myopathy occurs, consider cardiomyopathy.

■ Be alert for signs of overdose.

### Special populations
**Pediatric patients.** Safety and efficacy in children haven't been established.

## Patient counseling
■ Advise patient to change positions slowly to minimize dizziness.
■ Tell patient that routine CK determinations will be needed with long-term use.
■ Teach patient signs and symptoms of thrombophlebitis, and advise him to report them promptly.

# aminophylline
Phyllocontin, Truphylline

*Pharmacologic classification:* xanthine derivative
*Therapeutic classification:* bronchodilator
*Pregnancy risk category C*

## Available forms
Available by prescription only
*Tablets:* 100 mg, 200 mg
*Tablets (controlled-release):* 225 mg
*Liquid:* 105 mg/5 ml
*Injection:* 250-mg, 500-mg vials and ampules
*Rectal suppositories:* 250 mg, 500 mg

## Indications and dosages
*Symptomatic relief of acute bronchospasm*
*Patients not currently receiving theophylline who require rapid relief of symptoms:* Loading dose is 6 mg/kg (equivalent to 4.7 mg/kg anhydrous theophylline) I.V. slowly (25 mg/minute or less), then maintenance infusion.
**Maintenance infusions**
*Adults (nonsmokers):* 0.7 mg/kg/hour I.V. for 12 hours, then 0.5 mg/kg/hour I.V.; or 3 mg/kg P.O. q 6 hours for two doses, then 3 mg/kg P.O. q 8 hours.
*Otherwise healthy adult smokers:* 1 mg/kg/hour I.V. for 12 hours, then 0.8 mg/kg/hour I.V.; or 3 mg/kg P.O. q 4 hours for three doses, then 3 mg/kg P.O. q 6 hours.
*Older patients; adults with cor pulmonale:* 0.6 mg/kg/hour I.V. for 12 hours, then 0.3 mg/kg/hour I.V.; or 2 mg/kg P.O. q 6 hours for two doses, then 2 mg/kg P.O. q 8 hours.
*Adults with heart failure or liver disease:* 0.5 mg/kg/hour I.V. for 12 hours, then 0.1 to 0.2 mg/kg/hour I.V.; or 2 mg/kg P.O. q 8 hours for two doses, then 1 to 2 mg/kg P.O. q 12 hours.
*Children ages 9 to 16 years:* 1 mg/kg/hour I.V. for 12 hours, then 0.8 mg/kg/hour I.V.; or 3 mg/kg P.O. q 4 hours for three doses, then 3 mg/kg P.O. q 6 hours.
*Children ages 6 months to 9 years:* 1.2 mg/kg/hour I.V. for 12 hours, then 1 mg/kg/hour I.V.;

or 4 mg/kg P.O. q 4 hours for three doses, then 4 mg/kg P.O. q 6 hours.

*Patients currently receiving theophylline:* Aminophylline loading infusions of 0.63 mg/kg (0.5 mg/kg anhydrous theophylline) will increase plasma levels of theophylline by 1 mcg/ml, after serum levels have been evaluated. Some clinicians recommend a loading dose of 3.1 mg/kg I.V. (2.5 mg/kg anhydrous theophylline) if no obvious signs of theophylline toxicity are present, then maintenance infusion.

*Chronic bronchial asthma*

*Adults and children:* 16 mg/kg or 400 mg (whichever is less) P.O. daily in three or four divided doses q 6 to 8 hours if using rapidly absorbed dosage forms. Dosage may be increased, if tolerated, in increments of 25% q 2 to 3 days. Alternatively, if using extended-release preparations, 12 mg/kg or 400 mg (whichever is less) P.O. daily in two or three divided doses q 8 to 12 hours. Dosage may be increased, if tolerated, by 2 to 3 mg/kg daily q 3 days.

Regardless of dosage form, the following are recommended maximum doses. For adults and children age 16 and older, 13 mg/kg daily or 900 mg/day (whichever is less); children ages 12 to 16, 18 mg/kg daily; children ages 9 to 12, 20 mg/kg daily; and children ages 1 to 9, 24 mg/kg daily.

When recommended maximum dose is reached, dosage adjustment is based on peak serum theophylline levels. Advise clinician to monitor serum levels to ensure that theophylline levels range from 10 to 20 mcg/ml.

Note: Rectal dose is the same as that recommended for oral dose.

◊ *Periodic apnea associated with Cheyne-Stokes respirations, promote diuresis, paroxysmal nocturnal dyspnea*

*Adults:* 200 to 400 mg I.V. bolus.

◊ *Reduction of severe bronchospasm in infants with cystic fibrosis*

*Infants:* 10 to 12 mg/kg I.V. daily.

## I.V. administration

■ I.V. drug administration includes I.V. push at a very slow rate or an infusion with 100 to 200 ml of $D_5W$ or normal saline.

## Incompatibilities

Incompatible with amikacin, amiodarone, ascorbic acid, bleomycin, cephapirin, chlorpromazine, ciprofloxacin, clindamycin phosphate, codeine phosphate, corticotropin, dimenhydrinate, dobutamine, doxapram, doxorubicin, epinephrine hydrochloride, fat emulsion 10%, fructose 10% in normal saline injection, invert sugar 10% in water, levorphanol, meperidine, methadone, methylprednisolone sodium succinate, morphine, nafcillin, norepinephrine, ondansetron, papaverine, penicillin G potassium, pentazocine lactate, phenobarbital sodium, phenytoin sodium, procaine, prochlorperazine edisylate, promazine, promethazine hydrochloride, regular insulin, vancomycin, verapamil hydrochloride, and vitamin B complex with C.

## Mechanism of action

*Bronchodilating action:* Aminophylline acts at the cellular level after it's converted to theophylline. (Aminophylline [theophylline ethylenediamine] is 79% theophylline). Theophylline acts by either inhibiting phosphodiesterase or blocking adenosine receptors in the bronchi, thereby relaxing smooth muscle. Drug also stimulates the respiratory center in the medulla and prevents diaphragmatic fatigue.

## Pharmacokinetics

*Absorption:* Most dosage forms are absorbed well; absorption of the suppository, however, is unreliable and slow. Rate and onset of action also depend on the dosage form selected. Food may alter the rate, but not the extent, of absorption, of oral doses.

*Distribution:* Distributed in all tissues and extracellular fluids except fatty tissue.

*Metabolism:* Converted to theophylline, then metabolized to inactive compounds.

*Excretion:* Excreted in urine as theophylline (10%).

| Route | Onset | Peak | Duration |
|-------|-------|------|----------|
| P.O. | 15-60 min | 1-7 hr | Variable |
| I.V. | 15 min | Immediate | Variable |
| P.R. | Unknown | Unknown | Unknown |

## Contraindications and precautions

Contraindicated in patients hypersensitive to xanthine compounds (caffeine, theobromine) and ethylenediamine and in patients with active peptic ulcer disease and seizure disorders (unless adequate anticonvulsant therapy is given). Rectal suppositories are also contraindicated in patients who have an irritation or infection of the rectum or lower colon.

Use cautiously in neonates and infants under age 1, young children, the elderly, and patients with heart failure, CV disorders, COPD, cor pulmonale, renal or hepatic disease, hyperthyroidism, diabetes mellitus, peptic ulcer, severe hypoxemia, or hypertension.

## Interactions

**Drug-drug.** *Alkali-sensitive drugs:* Reduced activity of aminophylline. Don't add these drugs to I.V. fluids containing aminophylline.

*Allopurinol (high dose), cimetidine, erythromycin, propranolol, quinolones, or troleandomycin:* May increase serum level of aminophylline by decreasing hepatic clearance. Use together cautiously.

Overdose with amoxapine produces a much higher risk of CNS toxicity than do other antidepressants. Acute deterioration of renal function (evidenced by myoglobin in urine) occurs in 5% of overdosed patients; this is most likely to occur in patients with repeated seizures after the overdose. Seizures may progress to status epilepticus within 12 hours.

Severity of overdose is best indicated by widening of the QRS complex, which generally represents a serum level in excess of 1,000 ng/ml; serum levels aren't usually helpful. Metabolic acidosis may follow hypotension, hypoventilation, and seizures.

Treatment is symptomatic and supportive, including maintaining airway, stable body temperature, and fluid and electrolyte balance; advise clinician to monitor renal status because of the risk of renal failure. Advise clinician to induce emesis with ipecac if patient is conscious and following with gastric lavage and activated charcoal to prevent further absorption. Dialysis is of little use. Seizures should be treated with parenteral diazepam or phenytoin (the value of physostigmine is less certain); arrhythmias, with parenteral phenytoin or lidocaine; and acidosis, with sodium bicarbonate. Barbiturates shouldn't be given; these may enhance CNS and respiratory depressant effects.

## Clinical considerations

**⚠ ALERT** Be aware of sound-alikes: amoxicillin and amoxapine.
■ Amoxapine causes a high risk of seizures.
■ Antidepressants may cause manic episodes during the depressed phase in patients with bipolar disorder.
■ The full dose may be given h.s. to help reduce daytime sedation.
■ The full dose shouldn't be withdrawn abruptly. After abrupt withdrawal of long-term therapy, patient may experience nausea, headache, and malaise. This doesn't indicate addiction.
■ Tolerance to sedative effects usually develops over the first few weeks of therapy.
■ Drug should be stopped at least 48 hours before surgical procedures.
■ Sugarless chewing gum, hard candy, or ice may alleviate dry mouth.

### Therapeutic monitoring
■ Advise clinician to monitor patient for tardive dyskinesia and other extrapyramidal effects that may occur because of the dopamine-blocking activity of amoxapine.
■ Advise clinician to monitor patient for gynecomastia in men because amoxapine may increase cellular division in breast tissue.

### Special populations
**Pregnant patients.** Safe use of tricyclic antidepressants in pregnancy hasn't been established. Fetal malformations, urinary retention, CNS effects (lethargy), developmental delay, and withdrawal symptoms have occurred in neonates born to mothers taking tricyclic antidepressants during pregnancy.
**Breast-feeding patients.** Amoxapine appears in breast milk in levels of 20% of maternal serum as parent drug and 30% as metabolites. The potential benefits to the woman should outweigh the possible adverse reactions in the infant.
**Pediatric patients.** Drug isn't recommended for patients under age 16.
**Geriatric patients.** Lower doses are indicated because older patients are more sensitive to the therapeutic and adverse effects of drug. Geriatric patients are much more susceptible to tardive dyskinesia and extrapyramidal symptoms.

## Patient counseling

■ Explain that full effects of drug may not become apparent for at least 2 weeks or more after therapy begins, perhaps not for 4 to 6 weeks.
■ Tell patient to take drug exactly as prescribed; however, full dose may be taken at bedtime to alleviate daytime sedation. Patient shouldn't double the dose for missed ones.
■ Warn patient that hazardous activities that require alertness should be avoided until the full effects of the drug are known because drug may cause drowsiness or dizziness.
■ Tell patient not to drink alcoholic beverages while taking drug.
■ Suggest that patient take drug with food or milk if it causes stomach upset; dry mouth can be relieved with sugarless gum or hard candy.
■ After initial doses, tell patient to lie down for about 30 minutes and rise slowly to prevent dizziness.
■ Warn patient not to discontinue drug suddenly.
■ Encourage patient to report unusual or troublesome reactions immediately, especially confusion, movement disorders, rapid heartbeat, dizziness, fainting, or difficulty urinating.
■ Inform patient that exposure to sunlight, sunlamps, or tanning beds may cause burning of the skin or abnormal pigmentary changes.

# amoxicillin/clavulanate potassium
Augmentin, Augmentin ES-600, Clavulin*

*Pharmacologic classification:* aminopenicillin and beta-lactamase inhibitor
*Therapeutic classification:* antibiotic
*Pregnancy risk category B*

## Available forms
Available by prescription only
*Tablets (chewable):* 125 mg amoxicillin trihydrate, 31.25 mg clavulanic acid; 200 mg amoxicillin trihydrate, 28.5 mg clavulanic acid;

250 mg amoxicillin trihydrate, 62.5 mg clavulanic acid; 400 mg amoxicillin trihydrate, 57 mg clavulanic acid

*Tablets:* 250 mg amoxicillin trihydrate, 125 mg clavulanic acid; 500 mg amoxicillin trihydrate, 125 mg clavulanic acid; 875 mg amoxicillin trihydrate, 125 mg clavulanic acid

*Oral suspension:* 125 mg amoxicillin trihydrate and 31.25 mg clavulanic acid/5 ml (after reconstitution); 200 mg amoxicillin trihydrate and 28.5 mg clavulanic acid/5 ml (after reconstitution); 250 mg amoxicillin trihydrate and 62.5 mg clavulanic acid/5 ml (after reconstitution); 400 mg amoxicillin trihydrate and 57 mg clavulanic acid/5 ml (after reconstitution); 600 mg amoxicillin trihydrate and 42.9 mg clavulanic acid/5 ml (after reconstitution)

## Indications and dosages
*Lower respiratory tract infections, otitis media, sinusitis, skin and skin structure infections, and urinary tract infections caused by susceptible organisms*
*Adults and children weighing over 40 kg (88 lb):* 250 mg (based on amoxicillin component) P.O. q 8 hours or one 500-mg tablet q 12 hours. For more severe infections, 500 mg q 8 hours or 875 mg q 12 hours.
*Children weighing under 40 kg:* 25 to 45 mg/kg/day P.O. (based on amoxicillin component) given in divided doses q 8 to 12 hours. For acute otitis media, the usual dosage range is 40 to 45 mg/kg/daily in 2 or 3 divided doses for 10 days.
*Neonates and infants under 12 weeks:* 30 mg/kg daily in divided doses q 12 hours.
*Recurrent or persistent acute otitis media with antibiotic exposure within the last 3 months, in patients ≤ 2 years or in daycare facilities, caused by* **Streptococcus pneumoniae, Haemophilus influenzae,** *or* **Moraxella catarrhalis.**
*Infants and children ages 3 months to 12 years:* 90 mg/kg/day Augmentin ES-600 (based on amoxicillin component) P.O. q 12 hours for 10 days. Experience with this drug in patients > 40 kg is unavailable.
≡ *Dosage adjustment.* In patients with creatinine clearance of 15 to 30 ml/min, usual dose q 12 to 18 hours; 5 to 15 ml/min, usual dose q 20 to 36 hours; less than 5 ml/min, usual dose every 48 hours. Some clinicians recommend not using if creatinine clearance is less than 30 ml/min.
In hemodialysis patients, give 500 mg P.O. midway through treatment and then 500 mg P.O. at the end of treatment.

## Mechanism of action
*Antibiotic action:* Amoxicillin is bactericidal; it adheres to bacterial penicillin-binding proteins, inhibiting bacterial cell wall synthesis.

Clavulanate has only weak antibacterial activity and doesn't affect mechanism of action of amoxicillin. However, clavulanic acid has a beta-lactam ring and is structurally similar to penicillin and cephalosporins; it binds irreversibly with certain beta-lactamases and prevents them from inactivating amoxicillin, enhancing its bactericidal activity.

This combination acts against penicillinase- and non–penicillinase-producing gram-positive bacteria, *Neisseria gonorrhoeae, Neisseria meningitidis, Haemophilus influenzae, Moraxella catarrhalis, Escherichia coli, Proteus mirabilis, Citrobacter diversus, Klebsiella pneumoniae, Proteus vulgaris, Salmonella,* and *Shigella, Clostridium, Peptococcus,* and *Peptostreptococcus.*

## Pharmacokinetics
*Absorption:* Well absorbed after oral administration.
*Distribution:* Distributes into pleural fluid, lungs, and peritoneal fluid; high urine levels are attained. Amoxicillin also distributes into synovial fluid, liver, prostate, muscle, and gallbladder; and penetrates into middle ear effusions, maxillary sinus secretions, tonsils, sputum, and bronchial secretions. Amoxicillin and clavulanate cross the placenta and low levels appear in breast milk. Amoxicillin and clavulanate potassium have minimal protein-binding of 17% to 20% and 22% to 30%, respectively.
*Metabolism:* Amoxicillin is metabolized only partially. The metabolic fate of clavulanate potassium isn't completely identified, but it appears to undergo extensive metabolism.
*Excretion:* Amoxicillin is excreted principally in urine by renal tubular secretion and glomerular filtration; drug also appears in breast milk.

Clavulanate potassium is excreted by glomerular filtration. Elimination half-life of amoxicillin in adults is 1 to 1½ hours; it's prolonged to 7½ hours in patients with severe renal impairment. Half-life of clavulanate in adults is about 1 to 1½ hours, prolonged to 4½ hours in patients with severe renal impairment.

Both drugs are removed readily by hemodialysis and minimally removed by peritoneal dialysis.

| Route | Onset | Peak | Duration |
|-------|-------|------|----------|
| P.O. | Unknown | 1-2½ hr | 6-8 hr |

## Contraindications and precautions
Contraindicated in patients hypersensitive to drug or other penicillins and in those with a previous history of amoxicillin-associated cholestatic jaundice or hepatic dysfunction. An oral penicillin shouldn't be used in patients with severe pneumonia, empyema, bacteremia, pericarditis, meningitis, and purulent or septic arthritis. Use with caution in patients with mononucleosis.

## Interactions

**Drug-drug.** *Allopurinol:* Appears to increase risk of rash from both drugs. Avoid use together.
*Methotrexate:* Large doses of penicillins may interfere with renal tubular secretion of methotrexate, delaying elimination and prolonging elevated serum levels of methotrexate. Advise clinician to monitor patient for adverse effects.
*Oral contraceptives:* Effectiveness of oral contraceptives may be reduced. Recommend using alternative barrier method.
*Probenecid:* Blocks tubular secretion of amoxicillin, raising its serum levels; it has no effect on clavulanate. Avoid use together.

## Adverse reactions

**CNS:** agitation, anxiety, insomnia, confusion, behavioral changes, dizziness.
**GI:** *nausea,* vomiting, *diarrhea,* indigestion, gastritis, stomatitis, glossitis, black "hairy" tongue, enterocolitis, pseudomembranous colitis.
**GU:** vaginitis.
**Hematologic:** anemia, ***thrombocytopenia,*** thrombocytopenic purpura, eosinophilia, ***leukopenia, agranulocytosis.***
**Other:** hypersensitivity reactions (erythematous maculopapular rash, urticaria, ***anaphylaxis***), overgrowth of nonsusceptible organisms.

## Overdose and treatment

Clinical signs of overdose include neuromuscular sensitivity or seizures.

After recent ingestion (4 hours or less), advise clinician to empty the stomach by induced emesis or gastric lavage and follow with activated charcoal to reduce absorption. Amoxicillin/clavulanate potassium can be removed by hemodialysis.

## Clinical considerations

■ Amoxicillin/clavulanate potassium has been used to treat infections caused by *Eikenella corrodens* or *Pasteurella multocida* and infections caused by anaerobic and mixed aerobic-anaerobic bacterial infections.
**ℍ ALERT** Both 250-mg and 500-mg film-coated tablets contain the same amount of clavulanic acid (125 mg). Therefore, two 250-mg tablets aren't equivalent to one 500-mg tablet. Also, don't interchange the oral suspensions because of the clavulanic acid content.
■ Oral dosage is maximally absorbed from an empty stomach, but food doesn't cause significant impairment of absorption.
■ For reconstitution, add specified water in two parts and agitate well after each addition.
■ Suspension is stable for 10 days in refrigerator after reconstitution.
■ Commercial products containing aspartame shouldn't be used in pediatric patients with phenylketonuria.

■ Because amoxicillin/clavulanate potassium is dialyzable, patients undergoing hemodialysis may need dosage adjustments.
■ Amoxicillin/potassium clavulanate alters results of urine glucose tests that use cupric sulfate (Benedict's reagent or Clinitest). Urine glucose determinations should be made with glucose oxidase methods (Chemstrip uG or Diastix or glucose enzymatic test strip). Positive Coombs' tests have been reported with other clavulanate combinations. Amoxicillin/potassium clavulanate may produce a positive direct antiglobulin test (DAT).

### Therapeutic monitoring

■ Advise clinician to monitor renal, hepatic, and hematologic function periodically.
■ Recommend testing for *Clostridium difficile* in patients with diarrhea.

### Special populations

**Pregnant patients.** There are no adequate and controlled studies of use of this drug in pregnant women. Only use in pregnant women if clearly needed.
**Breast-feeding patients.** Both amoxicillin and potassium clavulanate appear in breast milk; use with caution in breast-feeding women.
**Geriatric patients.** In geriatric patients, diminished renal tubular secretion may prolong half-life of amoxicillin.

## Patient counseling

■ Tell patient to chew chewable tablets thoroughly or crush before swallowing and wash down with liquid to ensure adequate absorption of drug; capsule may be emptied and contents swallowed with water.
■ Instruct patient to report diarrhea promptly.
■ Inform patient to complete full course of drug.

# amoxicillin trihydrate

Amoxil, Polymox, Trimox

*Pharmacologic classification:* aminopenicillin
*Therapeutic classification:* antibiotic
*Pregnancy risk category B*

## Available forms

Available by prescription only
*Tablets (chewable):* 125 mg, 200 mg, 250 mg, 400 mg
*Tablets (film-coated):* 500 mg, 875 mg
*Capsules:* 250 mg, 500 mg
*Suspension:* 125 mg/5 ml, 250 mg/5 ml
*Pediatric drops:* 50 mg/ml (after reconstitution)

## Indications and dosages

*Systemic infections, acute and chronic urinary or respiratory tract infections caused*

*by susceptible organisms, uncomplicated
urinary tract infections caused by susceptible organisms*
*Adults:* 250 mg P.O. q 8 hours or 500 mg q 12
hours. In adults who have severe infections or
those caused by susceptible organisms, 500 mg
q 8 hours or 875 mg q 12 hours may be needed.
*Children age 3 months and older:* 20 to
45 mg/kg based on amoxicillin component and
severity of infection P.O. daily in divided doses
q 8 to 12 hours.
*Neonates and infants up to 12 weeks:* 30 mg/kg
P.O. daily in divided doses q 12 hours.
**Pediatric drops**
*Children weighing under 6 kg (13 lb):* 0.75 ml
q 8 hours.
*Children weighing 6 to 7 kg (13 to 15 lb):* 1 ml
q 8 hours.
*Children weighing 7 to 8 kg (16 to 18 lb):* 1.25
ml q 8 hours.
*Children with lower respiratory tract infection
weighing under 6 kg:* 1.25 ml q 8 hours.
*Children with lower respiratory tract infection
weighing 6 to 7 kg:* 1.75 ml q 8 hours.
*Children with lower respiratory tract infection
weighing 7 to 8 kg:* 2.25 ml q 8 hours.
*Uncomplicated gonorrhea*
*Adults and children weighing over 40 kg:* 3 g
P.O. as a single dose.
*Children over age 2 or under 40 kg:* 50 mg/kg
given with 25 mg/kg probenecid as a single
dose.
*Chlamydial and mycoplasmal infections
during pregnancy*
*Adults:* 500 mg P.O. t.i.d. for 7 to 10 days.
◇ *Lyme disease*
*Adults:* 250 to 500 mg P.O. t.i.d. to q.i.d. for
10 to 30 days.
*Children:* 25 to 50 mg/kg daily (maximum 1
to 2 g daily) P.O. in three divided doses for 10
to 30 days.
*Post-exposure prophylaxis to penicillin-
susceptible anthrax*
*Adults and children over age 9:* 500 mg P.O.
t.i.d. for 60 days.
*Children under age 9:* 80 mg/kg daily P.O.
in three divided doses for 60 days.
◇ *Acute uncomplicated urinary tract infection in nonpregnant women*
*Adults:* 3 g P.O. as one single dose.
≡ *Dosage adjustment.* In renal failure, patients
who require repeated doses may need adjustment of dosing interval. If creatinine clearance
is 10 to 30 ml/minute, increase interval to q 12
hours; if creatinine clearance is less than 10
ml/minute, give q 24 hours. Supplemental doses may be needed after hemodialysis.
*Oral prophylaxis of bacterial endocarditis*
Consult current American Heart Association
recommendations before administering drug.
*Adults:* 2 g P.O. 1 hour before procedure.
*Children:* 50 mg/kg P.O. 1 hour before procedure.

## Mechanism of action
*Antibacterial action:* Amoxicillin is bactericidal; it adheres to bacterial penicillin-binding
proteins, inhibiting bacterial cell wall synthesis.

Spectrum of action of amoxicillin includes
non–penicillinase-producing gram-positive
bacteria, *Streptococcus* group B, *Neisseria gonorrhoeae, Proteus mirabilis, Salmonella,* and
*Haemophilus influenzae.* It's also effective
against non–penicillinase-producing *Staphylococcus aureus, Streptococcus pyogenes, Streptococcus bovis, Streptococcus pneumoniae,
Streptococcus viridans, N. meningitidis, Escherichia coli, Salmonella typhi, Bordetella pertussis, Peptococcus,* and *Peptostreptococcus.*

## Pharmacokinetics
*Absorption:* About 80% absorbed after oral
administration.
*Distribution:* Widely distributed. Amoxicillin
readily crosses the placenta; about 17% to 20%
is protein-bound.
*Metabolism:* Metabolized only partially.
*Excretion:* Excreted principally in urine by renal tubular secretion and glomerular filtration;
appears in breast milk. Elimination half-life in
adults is about 1 to 1¼ hours; severe renal impairment increases half-life to 7¼ hours.

| Route | Onset | Peak | Duration |
|-------|-------|------|----------|
| P.O. | Unknown | 1-2 hr | 6-8 hr |

## Contraindications and precautions
Contraindicated in patients hypersensitive to
drug or other penicillins. Use with caution in
patients with mononucleosis.

## Interactions
**Drug-drug.** *Allopurinol:* Increased risk of rash
from both drugs. Advise clinician to monitor
patient.
*Clavulanate potassium:* Enhances effect of
amoxicillin against certain beta-lactamase–
producing bacteria. Advise patient of therapeutic benefits.
*Methotrexate:* Large doses of penicillins may
interfere with renal tubular secretion of methotrexate, delaying elimination and prolonging
elevated serum levels of methotrexate. Advise
clinician to monitor patient for toxicity.
*Oral contraceptives:* Effectiveness of oral contraceptives may be decreased. Recommend using alternative barrier method.
*Probenecid:* Blocks renal tubular secretion of
amoxicillin, raising its serum levels. Probenecid
may be used for this purpose.

## Adverse reactions
**CNS:** lethargy, hallucinations, *seizures,* anxiety, confusion, agitation, depression, dizziness,
fatigue.
**GI:** *nausea,* vomiting, *diarrhea,* glossitis, stomatitis, gastritis, abdominal pain, enterocolitis,

---

Reactions may be *common,* uncommon, *life-threatening,* or COMMON AND LIFE-THREATENING.

■ Tell patient to expect frequent laboratory testing to monitor kidney and liver function.

# amphotericin B liposomal

AmBisome

*Pharmacologic classification:* polyene antibiotic
*Therapeutic classification:* antifungal
*Pregnancy risk category B*

## Available forms

Available by prescription only
*Injection:* 50-mg vial

## Indications and dosages

**Cryptococcal meningitis in HIV-infected patients**
*Adults and children:* 6 mg/kg/day over 2 hours.
**Empirical therapy for presumed fungal infection in febrile, neutropenic patients**
*Adults and children:* 3 mg/kg I.V. infusion daily.
**Systemic fungal infections from Aspergillus sp., Candida *sp.,* or Cryptococcus *sp.* refractory to amphotericin B deoxycholate or in patients for whom renal impairment or unacceptable toxicity precludes use of amphotericin B deoxycholate**
*Adults and children:* 3 to 5 mg/kg I.V. infusion daily.
**Visceral leishmaniasis in immunocompetent patients**
*Adults and children:* 3 mg/kg I.V. infusion daily on days 1 to 5, 14, and 21. A repeat course of therapy may be beneficial if initial treatment fails to achieve parasitic clearance.
**Visceral leishmaniasis in immunocompromised patients**
*Adults and children:* 4 mg/kg I.V. infusion daily on days 1 to 5, 10, 17, 24, 31, and 38. Expert advice regarding further treatment is recommended if initial therapy fails or patient experiences relapse.

## I.V. administration

■ Reconstitute each 50-mg vial of amphotericin B liposomal with 12 ml of sterile water for injection to yield a solution of 4 mg amphotericin B/ml.
**ℍ ALERT** Don't reconstitute with bacteriostatic water for injection and don't allow bacteriostatic drug in solution. Don't reconstitute with saline or add saline to reconstituted concentration or mix with other drugs.
■ After reconstitution, shake vial vigorously for 30 seconds or until particulate matter is dispersed.
■ Withdraw calculated amount of reconstituted solution into a sterile syringe and inject through a 5-micron filter into the appropriate amount of $D_5W$ to further dilute to a final level of 1 to 2 mg/ml. Lower levels (0.2 to 0.5 mg/ml)

may be appropriate for pediatric patients to provide sufficient volume of infusion.
■ An existing I.V. line must be flushed with $D_5W$ before infusion of drug. If this isn't feasible, give drug through a separate line.
■ Use a controlled infusion device and an in-line filter with a mean pore diameter larger than 1 micron. Initially, infuse drug over at least 2 hours. Infusion time may be reduced to 1 hour if treatment is well tolerated. If patient experiences discomfort during infusion, duration of infusion may be increased.

### Incompatibilities

Don't reconstitute with saline, add saline to the reconstituted concentration, or mix with other drugs.

## Mechanism of action

*Antifungal activity:* Amphotericin B, the active component of AmBisome, binds to the sterol component of a fungal cell membrane leading to alterations in cell permeability and cell death.

## Pharmacokinetics

*Absorption:* Administered I.V.
*Distribution:* Unknown.
*Metabolism:* Unknown.
*Excretion:* The initial half-life is 7 to 10 hours with 24 hour dosing; terminal elimination half-life is 100 to 153 hours.

| Route | Onset | Peak | Duration |
|-------|-------|------|----------|
| I.V. | Unknown | Unknown | Unknown |

## Contraindications and precautions

Contraindicated in patients hypersensitive to drug or its components.

Use cautiously in patients with impaired renal function, in geriatric patients, and in pregnant women.

## Interactions

**Drug-drug.** *Antineoplastics:* May enhance potential for renal toxicity, bronchospasm, and hypotension. Recommend using cautiously.
*Cardiac glycosides:* Increased risk of digitalis toxicity from amphotericin B–induced hypokalemia. Advise clinician to monitor serum potassium level closely.
*Clotrimazole, fluconazole, ketoconazole, miconazole:* May induce fungal resistance to amphotericin B. Use together cautiously.
*Corticosteroids, corticotropin:* May potentiate potassium depletion, which could result in cardiac dysfunction. Advise clinician to monitor serum electrolyte level and cardiac function.
*Flucytosine:* May increase flucytosine toxicity by increasing cellular reuptake or impairing renal excretion of flucytosine. Use together cautiously.
*Other nephrotoxic drugs, such as antibiotics, antineoplastics:* May cause additive nephro-

toxicity. Give cautiously. Advise clinician to monitor renal function closely.

*Skeletal muscle relaxants:* Enhanced effects of skeletal muscle relaxants resulting from amphotericin B–induced hypokalemia. Advise clinician to monitor serum potassium levels.

## Adverse reactions

**CNS:** *anxiety, confusion, headache, insomnia, asthenia.*

**CV:** *chest pain, hypotension, tachycardia,* hypertension, *edema.*

**EENT:** *epistaxis, rhinitis.*

**GI:** *nausea, vomiting, abdominal pain, diarrhea,* **GI hemorrhage.**

**GU:** *hematuria, elevated creatinine and BUN levels.*

**Hepatic:** *elevated ALT and AST levels, increased alkaline phosphatase level, bilirubinemia.*

**Metabolic:** *hyperglycemia,* hypernatremia, *hypocalcemia, hypokalemia, hypomagnesemia.*

**Musculoskeletal:** *back pain.*

**Respiratory:** *increased cough, dyspnea,* hypoxia, *pleural effusion, lung disorder,* hyperventilation.

**Skin:** *pruritus, rash, sweating.*

**Other:** *chills, infection, flushing,* **anaphylaxis,** *pain,* **sepsis,** *fever, blood product infusion reaction.*

## Overdose and treatment

Repeated daily doses of up to 7.5 mg/kg have been given without toxicity. If overdose occurs, advise clinician to stop drug immediately. Symptomatic supportive measures should be instituted. Particular attention should be paid to monitor renal function. The drug isn't hemodialyzable.

## Clinical considerations

■ Patients also receiving chemotherapy or bone marrow transplantation are at greater risk for additional adverse reactions, including seizures, arrhythmias, and thrombocytopenia.

■ Leukocyte transfusions shouldn't be given with drug because acute pulmonary toxicity has been reported with concurrent administration.

■ To lessen risk or severity of adverse reactions, premedication with antipyretics, antihistamines, antiemetics, or corticosteroids can be ordered.

**⊌ ALERT** The different amphotericin B preparations aren't interchangeable, and dosages will vary.

■ Patients given amphotericin B liposomal had a lower risk of chills, elevated BUN, hypokalemia, hypertension, and vomiting than patients treated with conventional amphotericin B.

■ Advise clinician to observe patient closely for adverse reactions during infusion. If anaphylaxis occurs, advise clinician to stop infusion immediately, provide supportive therapy, and notify prescriber.

■ Unopened drug is stored under refrigeration at 36° to 46° F (2° to 8° C). Once reconstituted, vial of reconstituted concentrate may be stored for up to 24 hours at 36° to 46° F. Don't freeze.

■ HIV-infected patients may experience elevated creatinine levels.

### Therapeutic monitoring

■ Advise clinician to monitor BUN and serum creatinine and electrolyte levels (particularly magnesium and potassium), liver function, and CBC. Therapy may take several weeks to months.

■ Patient requires close observation for signs of hypokalemia (ECG changes, muscle weakness, cramping, drowsiness).

### Special populations

**Breast-feeding patients.** It's unknown if drug appears in milk, but because of the potential for serious adverse reactions in breast-fed infants, a decision should be made whether to discontinue nursing or to discontinue the drug.

**Pediatric patients.** Safety and efficacy in pediatric patients under age 1 month haven't been established.

**Geriatric patients.** No dosage alteration is needed. Recommend carefully monitoring geriatric patients.

## Patient counseling

■ Teach patient signs and symptoms of hypersensitivity, and stress importance of reporting them immediately.

■ Warn patient that acute infusion reaction may occur 1 to 3 hours after I.V. infusion begins.

■ Warn patient that therapy may take several months; teach personal hygiene and other measures to prevent spread and recurrence of lesions.

■ Instruct patient to report any adverse reactions that occur while receiving drug.

■ Instruct patient to watch for and report signs of hypokalemia (muscle weakness, cramping, drowsiness).

■ Advise patient that frequent laboratory testing will be needed.

---

## ampicillin
Apo-Ampi*, Novo-Ampicillin*, Omnipen, Penbritin*

## ampicillin sodium
Ampicin*, Omnipen-N, Penbritin*

## ampicillin trihydrate
Omnipen, Principen, Totacillin

---

*Pharmacologic classification:*
aminopenicillin
*Therapeutic classification:* antibiotic
*Pregnancy risk category B*

## Available forms
Available by prescription only
*Capsules:* 250 mg, 500 mg
*Suspension:* 125 mg/5 ml, 250 mg/5 ml, 500 mg/5 ml (after reconstitution)
*Parenteral:* 125 mg, 250 mg, 500 mg, 1 g, 2 g
*Infusion:* 500 mg, 1 g, 2 g

## Indications and dosages
*Systemic infections, acute and chronic urinary tract infections caused by susceptible organisms*
*Adults:* 250 to 500 mg P.O. q 6 hours.
*Children under 40 kg (88 lb):* 25 to 100 mg/kg P.O. daily, divided into doses given q 6 hours; or 100 to 200 mg/kg I.V. daily for 3 days and then I.M., divided into doses given q 6 to 8 hours.
*Meningitis*
*Adults:* 8 to 14 g I.V. or 150 to 200 mg/kg/day divided q 3 to 4 hours for 3 days; then may give I.M. if desired.
*Children ages 2 months to 12 years:* 200 to 400 mg/kg I.V. daily in divided doses q 4 to 6 hours. May be given along with chloramphenicol, pending culture results.
*Neonates under 1 week old:* 50 to 75 mg/kg I.V. q 12 hours (weight under 2 kg) or q 8 hours (weight over 2 kg).
*Neonates over 1 week old:* 50 mg/kg I.V. q 8 hours (weight under 2 kg) or q 6 hours (weight over 2 kg).
*Neonatal group B streptococcal meningitis*
*Neonates ages 7 days or younger:* 200 mg/kg/daily I.V. given in three divided doses.
*Neonates ages 7 days or older:* 300 mg/kg/daily I.V. given in 4 to 6 divided doses.
*Uncomplicated gonorrhea*
*Adults:* 3.5 g P.O. with 1 g probenecid given as a single dose.
≡*Dosage adjustment.* Increase dosing interval to q 12 hours in patients with severe renal impairment (creatinine clearance 10 ml/minute or less).
*Prophylaxis for bacterial endocarditis before dental or minor respiratory procedures*
*Adults:* 2 g (I.V. or I.M.) 30 minutes before procedure.
*Children:* 50 mg/kg I.V. or I.M. 30 minutes before procedure.
*Treatment of enterococcal endocarditis*
*Adults:* 12 g daily by continuous I.V. infusion or in six equally divided doses in conjunction with gentamicin for 4 to 6 weeks.

◇ *Prophylaxis of neonatal group B streptococcus infections*
*Adult:* 2 g I.V. given to the mother 4 hours before delivery, then 1 to 2 g I.V. q 4 to 6 hours until delivery.

## I.V. administration
■ For I.V. injection, reconstitute with bacteriostatic water for injection. Use 5 ml for the 125-mg, 250-mg, or 500-mg vials; 7.4 ml for the 1-g vials; or 14.8 ml for the 2-g vials.
■ Give direct I.V. injections over 10 to 15 minutes to avoid the possibility of seizures. Don't exceed 100 mg/minute.
■ Or, dilute in 50 to 100 ml of normal saline solution for injection and give by intermittent infusion over 15 to 30 minutes.
■ Use initial dilution within 1 hour. Follow manufacturer's directions for stability data when ampicillin is further diluted for I.V. infusion.
■ Give I.V. intermittently to prevent vein irritation. Change site every 48 hours.

## Incompatibilities
Don't mix with solutions containing dextrose or fructose; these substances promote rapid breakdown of ampicillin. Incompatible with amikacin, amino acid solutions, chlorpromazine, dextran solutions, dopamine, erythromycin lactobionate, 10% fat emulsions, fructose, gentamicin, heparin sodium, hetastarch, hydrocortisone sodium succinate, hydromorphone, kanamycin, lidocaine, lincomycin, polymyxin B, prochlorperazine edisylate, sodium bicarbonate, streptomycin, and tobramycin.

## Mechanism of action
*Antibiotic action:* Ampicillin is bactericidal; it adheres to bacterial penicillin-binding proteins, inhibiting bacterial cell wall synthesis.

Spectrum of action includes non–penicillinase-producing gram-positive bacteria. It's also effective against many gram-negative organisms, including *Neisseria gonorrhoeae, Neisseria meningitidis, Haemophilus influenzae, Escherichia coli, Proteus mirabilis, Salmonella,* and *Shigella.* Ampicillin should be used in gram-negative systemic infections only when organism sensitivity is known.

## Pharmacokinetics
*Absorption:* About 42% of ampicillin is absorbed after an oral dose.
*Distribution:* Distributes into pleural, peritoneal and synovial fluids, lungs, prostate, liver, and gallbladder; it also penetrates middle ear effusions, maxillary sinus and bronchial secretions, tonsils, and sputum. Readily crosses the placenta; minimally protein-bound (15% to 25%).
*Metabolism:* Only partially metabolized.
*Excretion:* Excreted in urine by renal tubular secretion and glomerular filtration. It also ap-

---

pears in breast milk. Elimination half-life is about 1 to 1½ hours; in patients with extensive renal impairment, half-life is extended to 10 to 24 hours.

| Route | Onset | Peak | Duration |
|-------|-------|------|----------|
| P.O. | Unknown | 2 hr | 6-8 hr |
| I.V. | Immediate | Immediate | Unknown |
| I.M. | Unknown | 1 hr | Unknown |

## Contraindications and precautions

Contraindicated in patients hypersensitive to drug or other penicillins. Use with caution in patients with mononucleosis.

## Interactions

**Drug-drug.** *Allopurinol:* Appears to increase risk of rash from both drugs. Advise clinician to monitor patient closely.

*Aminoglycoside antibiotic:* A synergistic bactericidal effect against some strains of enterococci and group B streptococci. However, the drugs are physically and chemically incompatible and are inactivated if mixed or given together. Don't mix together.

*Clavulanate:* Results in increased bactericidal effects because clavulanic acid is a beta-lactamase inhibitor. Use drugs together for clinical effect.

*Methotrexate:* Large doses of penicillins may interfere with renal tubular secretion of methotrexate, delaying elimination and elevating serum levels of methotrexate. Advise clinician to monitor patient for methotrexate toxicity.

*Oral contraceptives:* Effects of oral contraceptives may be decreased. Recommend using alternative barrier method.

*Probenecid:* Inhibits renal tubular secretion of ampicillin, raising its serum levels. Avoid use together.

## Adverse reactions

**CNS:** lethargy, hallucinations, *seizures,* anxiety, confusion, agitation, depression, dizziness, fatigue.

**GI:** *nausea,* vomiting, *diarrhea,* glossitis, stomatitis, gastritis, abdominal pain, enterocolitis, pseudomembranous colitis, black "hairy" tongue.

**GU:** interstitial nephritis, nephropathy, vaginitis.

**Hematologic:** anemia, *thrombocytopenia, thrombocytopenic purpura,* eosinophilia, *leukopenia, hemolytic anemia, agranulocytosis.*

**Other:** hypersensitivity reactions (erythematous maculopapular rash, urticaria, *anaphylaxis*), overgrowth of nonsusceptible organisms, pain at injection site, vein irritation, thrombophlebitis.

## Overdose and treatment

Clinical signs of overdose include neuromuscular sensitivity or seizures. After recent ingestion (within 4 hours), advise emptying the stomach by inducing emesis or gastric lavage, followed by activated charcoal to reduce absorption. Drug can be removed by hemodialysis.

## Clinical considerations

- Consider the recommendations relevant to all penicillins.
- Obtain patient's allergy history before dispensing drug.
- Ampicillin alters results of urine glucose tests that use cupric sulfate (Benedict's reagent or Clinitest). Urine glucose determinations should be done with glucose oxidase methods (Chemstrip uG, Diastix, or glucose enzymatic test strip).

### Therapeutic monitoring

Advise clinician to monitor renal, hepatic, hematologic systems during prolonged therapy.

### Special populations

**Pregnant patients.** Safe use during pregnancy hasn't been established, but drug has been used to treat urinary tract infections in pregnant women without affecting the fetus.

**Breast-feeding patients.** Use cautiously. Ampicillin appears in breast milk; safety in breast-feeding women hasn't been established.

**Geriatric patients.** Because of diminished renal tubular secretion in geriatric patients, half-life of drug may be prolonged.

## Patient counseling

- Advise patient to report diarrhea promptly.
- Instruct patient to complete all of the prescribed drug.

# ampicillin sodium/ sulbactam sodium

Unasyn

*Pharmacologic classification:* aminopenicillin/beta-lactamase inhibitor combination
*Therapeutic classification:* antibiotic
*Pregnancy risk category B*

## Available forms

Available by prescription only
*Injection:* vials and piggyback vials containing 1.5 g (1 g ampicillin sodium with 500 mg sulbactam sodium) and 3 g (2 g ampicillin sodium with 1 g sulbactam sodium)

---

## Indications and dosages

### Pelvic inflammatory disease

*Adults and children*: 3 g (2 g ampicillin and 1 g sulbactam) I.V. or I.M. q 6 hours given with doxycycline 100 mg P.O. q 12 hours. Continue parenteral therapy for 24 hours after clinical improvement. Continue therapy with oral doxycycline 100 mg P.O. b.i.d. to complete 14-day cycle.

### Skin and skin-structure infections, intra-abdominal and gynecologic infections caused by susceptible gram-positive bacteria, gram-negative bacteria, and beta-lactamase–producing strains of Staphylococcus aureus, Escherichia coli, Klebsiella (including K. pneumoniae), Proteus mirabilis, Bacteroides (including B. fragilis), Enterobacter, Neisseria meningitidis, Neisseria gonorrhoeae, Moraxella catarrhalis, and Acinetobacter calcoaceticus

*Adults*: 1.5 to 3 g I.M. or I.V. q 6 hours. Don't exceed 4 g/day sulbactam sodium.

### Skin and skin-structure infections caused by susceptible organisms

*Children weighing under 40 kg (88 lb):* Same as adult dose.

*Children 1 year and older weighing under 40 kg:* 300 mg/kg I.V. daily in divided doses q 6 hours not to exceed 14 days of therapy.

≡ *Dosage adjustment.* For patients with renal impairment, give the usually recommended doses, but less frequently. Patients with creatinine clearances ≥ 30 ml/min receive 1.5 to 3 g of the drug q 6 to 8 hours; patients with creatinine clearances of 15 to 29 ml/min receive 1.5 to 3 g q 12 hours; patients with creatinine clearances of 5 to 14 ml/min receive 1.5 to 3 g q 24 hours. Patients undergoing hemodialysis should receive 1.5 g to 3 g once q 24 hours—preferably immediately following dialysis.

## I.V. administration

- For I.V. use, reconstitute powder in piggyback units to desired levels with sterile water for injection, normal saline injection, $D_5W$, lactated Ringer's injection, 1/6 M sodium lactate injection, 5% dextrose in 0.45% saline, or 10% invert sugar.

**H** *ALERT* Give I.V. administration by slow injection over at least 10 to 15 minutes or infused in greater dilutions with 50 to 100 ml of a compatible diluent over 15 to 30 minutes to avoid risk for seizures.

- Store powder at 86° F (30° C) or colder.

### Incompatibilities

Incompatible with amikacin, amino acid solutions, chlorpromazine, dextran solutions, dopamine, erythromycin, lactobionate, 10% fat emulsions, fructose, gentamicin, heparin sodium, hetastarch, hydrocortisone sodium succinate, kanamycin, lidocaine, lincomycin, netilmicin, polymyxin B, prochlorperazine edisylate, sodium bicarbonate, streptomycin, or tobramycin.

## Mechanism of action

*Antibiotic action:* Ampicillin is bactericidal; it adheres to bacterial penicillin-binding proteins, inhibiting bacterial cell wall synthesis. Sulbactam inhibits beta-lactamase, an enzyme produced by ampicillin-resistant bacteria that degrades ampicillin.

## Pharmacokinetics

*Absorption:* Well absorbed after I.M. administration.

*Distribution:* Both are distributed into pleural, peritoneal and synovial fluids, lungs, prostate, liver, and gallbladder; they also penetrate middle ear effusions, maxillary sinus and bronchial secretions, tonsils, and sputum. Ampicillin readily crosses the placenta; it's minimally protein-bound at 15% to 25%; sulbactam is about 38% bound.

*Metabolism:* Both are metabolized only partially; only 15% to 25% of both is metabolized.

*Excretion:* Both are excreted in the urine by renal tubular secretion and glomerular filtration. It also appears in breast milk. Elimination half-life is 1 to 1¼ hours; in patients with extensive renal impairment, half-life can be as long as 10 to 24 hours.

| Route | Onset | Peak | Duration |
|-------|-------|------|----------|
| I.V. | 15 min | Immediate | Unknown |
| I.M. | Unknown | Unknown | Unknown |

## Contraindications and precautions

Contraindicated in patients hypersensitive to drug or other penicillins.

Use cautiously in patients with maculopapular rash.

## Interactions

**Drug-drug.** *Allopurinol:* May lead to an increased risk of rash. Advise clinician to monitor patient closely.

*Aminoglycosides:* The ampicillin component may cause in vitro inactivation of aminoglycosides if these antibiotics are mixed in the same infusion container. Don't mix together.

*Anticoagulants:* Large doses of I.V. penicillins can increase bleeding risks of anticoagulants because of a prolongation of bleeding times. Advise clinician to monitor PT and INR.

*Probenecid:* Decreases excretion of both ampicillin and sulbactam. Advise clinician to monitor patient for toxicity.

## Adverse reactions

**CV:** vein irritation, thrombophlebitis.

**GI:** *nausea*, vomiting, *diarrhea*, glossitis, stomatitis, gastritis, black "hairy" tongue, enterocolitis, pseudomembranous colitis.

---

* Canada only    ◇ Unlabeled clinical use

**Hematologic:** anemia, *thrombocytopenia*, thrombocytopenic purpura, eosinophilia, *leukopenia, agranulocytosis.*
**Other:** hypersensitivity reactions (erythematous maculopapular rash, urticaria, *anaphylaxis*), *overgrowth of nonsusceptible organisms,* pain at injection site.

## Overdose and treatment
Neurologic adverse reactions, including seizures, are likely. Treatment is supportive. Ampicillin and sulbactam are likely to be removed by hemodialysis.

## Clinical considerations
■ For I.M. injection, reconstitute with sterile water for injection, or 0.5% or 2% lidocaine hydrochloride injection. To obtain 375 mg/ml solutions (250 mg ampicillin/125 mg sulbactam/ml), add contents of the 1.5-g vial to 3.2 ml of diluent to produce 4 ml withdrawal volume; add 3-g vial to 6.4 ml of diluent to produce 8 ml withdrawal volume.
■ Reconstituted solutions are stable for varying periods (from 2 to 72 hours) depending on diluent used. Refer to package insert for specific information. For patients on sodium restriction, note that a 1.5-g dose of ampicillin sodium/sulbactam sodium yields 5 mEq of sodium.
■ Ampicillin alters results of urine glucose tests that use cupric sulfate (Benedict's reagent or Clinitest). Make urine glucose determinations with glucose oxidase methods (Chemstrip uG, Diastix, or glucose enzymatic test strip).
■ In pregnant women, transient decreases in serum estradiol, conjugated estrone, conjugated estriol, and estriol glucuronide may occur.

### Therapeutic monitoring
■ Recommend testing for *Clostridium difficile* in patients with persistent diarrhea.
■ Advise clinician to monitor patient for overgrowth of nonsusceptible organisms.

### Special populations
**Pregnant patients.** Safety in pregnant women hasn't been established.
**Breast-feeding patients.** Appears in breast milk; safety in breast-feeding women hasn't been established. Alternative feeding method is recommended during therapy.
**Pediatric patients.** Safety in children under age 1 hasn't been established. Safety and efficacy for use in children for treatment of skin and skin structure infections has been established. Not for use for other infections or for I.M. use.
**Geriatric patients.** Because of diminished renal tubular secretion in geriatric patients, half-life of drug may be prolonged.

## Patient counseling
■ Tell patient to report a rash, fever, chills. A rash is the most frequent allergic reaction.
■ Advise patient to report discomfort at insertion site.
■ Warn patient that I.M. injection may cause pain at the injection site.

# amprenavir
Agenerase

*Pharmacologic classification:* protease inhibitor
*Therapeutic classification:* antiretroviral
*Pregnancy risk category C*

## Available forms
Available by prescription only
*Capsules:* 50 mg, 150 mg
*Oral solution:* 15 mg/ml

## Indications and dosages
*Treatment of HIV-1 infection with other antiretroviral drugs*
*Adults and children ages 13 to 16 weighing 50 kg (110 lb) or more:* 1,200 mg P.O. (eight 150-mg capsules) or 1,400 mg as oral solution P.O. b.i.d. with other antiretroviral drugs.
*Children ages 4 to 12 or 13 to 16 weighing under 50 kg: Capsules:* 20 mg/kg P.O. b.i.d. or 15 mg/kg P.O. t.i.d. (to a maximum daily dose of 2,400 mg) with other antiretroviral drugs.
*Oral solution:* 22.5 mg/kg P.O. (1.5 ml/kg) b.i.d. or 17 mg/kg P.O. (1.1 ml/kg) t.i.d. (to a maximum daily dose of 2,800 mg) with other antiretroviral drugs.
≣ *Dosage adjustment.* Patients with moderate or severe hepatic impairment should receive reduced dosage. Note: Oral solution is contraindicated in patients with hepatic or renal failure.
*Patients with Child-Pugh score of 5 to 8:* 450 mg (capsules) P.O. b.i.d; or, oral solution 513 mg (34 ml) b.i.d.
*Patients with Child-Pugh score of 9 to 12:* 300 mg (capsules) P.O. b.i.d.; or, oral solution 342 mg (23 ml) b.i.d.

## Mechanism of action
*Antiretroviral action:* Amprenavir binds to the active site of HIV-1 protease and thereby prevents the processing of viral *gag* and *gag-pol* polyprotein precursors, resulting in the formation of immature noninfectious viral particles.

## Pharmacokinetics
*Absorption:* Rapidly absorbed.
*Distribution:* About 90% plasma protein–bound.
*Metabolism:* Metabolized in the liver by the cytochrome P-450 CYP3A4 enzyme system.

---

*Excretion:* Excretion of unchanged amprenavir in urine and feces is minimal. The plasma elimination half-life ranges from 7.1 to 10.6 hours.

| Route | Onset | Peak | Duration |
|-------|-------|------|----------|
| P.O. | Unknown | 1-2 hr | Unknown |

## Contraindications and precautions

Contraindicated in patients hypersensitive to drug or any of its components. Also contraindicated in infants, children under 4 years of age, pregnant women, patients with liver or kidney failure, and patients being treated with disulfuram or Flagyl.

Use cautiously in patients with a known sulfonamide allergy, those with hepatic impairment, and those with hemophilia A and B.

## Interactions

**Drug-drug.** *Antacids:* Recommend separating administration of antacids and drug by at least 1 hour to avoid possible interference with absorption.

*Antiarrhythmics, such as amiodarone, lidocaine (systemic), quinidine; anticoagulants such as warfarin; and tricyclic antidepressants:* When used together, amprenavir serum levels may be affected. Advise clinician to monitor closely.

*Bepridil, dihydroergotamine, midazolam, rifampin, and triazolam:* Serious and life-threatening interactions may occur. Avoid use together.

*Efavirenz, saquinavir:* Decreased AUC of amprenavir. Advise clinician to monitor patient closely. Efavirenz dosage may need adjustment.

*HMG-CoA reductase inhibitors:* Increased levels of these drugs; therefore, increased risk of myopathy, including rhabdomyolysis. Avoid use together.

*Indinavir, nelfinavir, ritonavir:* Increased plasma levels of amprenavir. Advise clinician to monitor patient closely.

*Ketoconazole:* Increases plasma levels of both drugs. Advise clinician to monitor patient closely.

*Macrolides:* Increased amprenavir plasma levels. Dosage adjustment may be required.

*Oral contraceptives:* Potential for metabolic interactions. Use alternative or additional methods of birth control.

*Psychotherapeutic drugs:* May cause increased CNS effects. Advise clinician to monitor patient closely.

*Rifabutin:* Decreased amprenavir levels and a substantial increase in rifabutin levels. Recommend reducing dosage.

*Sildenafil:* Substantially increased sildenafil levels, which may cause an increase in effects from sildenafil, including hypotension, visual changes, and priapism. Patient shouldn't exceed 25 mg of sildenafil in a 48-hour period.

*Vitamin E:* Amprenavir contains high doses of vitamin E; concomitant use would further elevate vitamin E levels in these patients. Advise patient not to take supplemental vitamin E while on amprenavir therapy.

**Drug-herb.** *St. John's wort:* Use together may lower amprenavir level, which could result in loss of drug's therapeutic response. Warn patient not to use these together.

**Drug-food.** *High-fat meals:* Reduce drug absorption. Advise patient not to take drug with a high-fat meal.

*Grapefruit juice:* Recommend taking with liquid other than grapefruit juice. May change the pharmacokinetics of the drug. Advise patient not to take with grapefruit juice.

**Drug-lifestyle.** *Alcohol intake:* Use together may increase the risk of adverse effects because of the propylene glycol content. Advise patient to avoid alcohol.

## Adverse reactions

**CNS:** *paresthesia,* depressive or mood disorders, headache.

**GI:** *nausea, vomiting, diarrhea or loose stools,* taste disorders.

**Metabolic:** *hyperglycemia, hypertriglyceridemia,* hypercholesterolemia.

**Skin:** *rash, Stevens-Johnson syndrome.*

## Overdose and treatment

No known antidote. It isn't known if amprenavir can be removed by peritoneal lavage or hemodialysis. If overdose occurs, advise clinician to monitor patient for evidence of toxicity and give supportive treatment, p.r.n.

## Clinical considerations

■ Drug is a sulfonamide. Patients with a known sulfonamide allergy should be treated with caution.

**◪ ALERT** Capsules and oral solution aren't interchangeable on milligram-per-milligram basis.

**◪ ALERT** The oral solution contains large amounts of propylene glycol. Propylene glycol adverse effects include hyperosmolality, lactic acidosis, respiratory depression, and seizures.

■ Store capsules and oral solution at controlled room temperature.

### Therapeutic monitoring

■ Advise clinician to monitor patient for adverse reactions. Drug may cause redistribution or accumulation of body fat, including central obesity, dorsocervical fat enlargement (buffalo hump), peripheral wasting, breast enlargement, or cushingoid appearance. Severe and life-threatening reactions, including Stevens-Johnson syndrome, have occurred.

■ Advise clinician to perform CBC weekly and as clinically indicated to monitor for neutropenia in patients also receiving rifabutin.

---

## Special populations

**Pregnant patients.** To monitor maternal-fetal outcomes of pregnant women exposed to drug, an Antiretroviral Pregnancy Registry has been established. Prescribers may call 1-800-258-4263 to register patients who have been exposed to drug during pregnancy.

**Breast-feeding patients.** It isn't known if drug appears in breast milk, so instruct breast-feeding women not to breast-feed if they're receiving drug. In addition, it's recommended that HIV-infected women not breast-feed their infants to avoid risking postnatal transmission of HIV.

**Pediatric patients.** An adverse event profile similar to that in adults is seen in pediatric patients. Safety, efficacy, and pharmacokinetics of drug haven't been evaluated in children under age 4.

**Geriatric patients.** Dosing in the elderly should be cautious, reflecting the greater frequency of decreased hepatic, renal, or cardiac function, and of concomitant disease or other drug therapy.

## Patient counseling

- Inform patient that drug isn't a cure for HIV infection and opportunistic infections and other complications from HIV may continue to develop. The drug doesn't reduce the risk of transmitting HIV to others through sexual contact.
- Tell patient he may take drug without regard to meals but to avoid taking with high-fat meals because absorption may be decreased.
- Advise patient to take drug each day as prescribed. It must always be taken with other antiretroviral drugs. Dose must not be altered or discontinued without consulting a prescriber.
- Tell patient if a dose is missed to take the dose as soon as possible and then return to the normal schedule. However, if a dose is skipped, don't double the next dose.
- Instruct patients taking hormonal contraceptives to use alternate contraceptive measures during drug therapy.

# anastrozole

Arimidex

*Pharmacologic classification:* nonsteroidal aromatase inhibitor
*Therapeutic classification:* antineoplastic
*Pregnancy risk category D*

## Available forms

Available by prescription only
*Tablets:* 1 mg

## Indications and dosages

*Treatment of advanced breast cancer in postmenopausal women with disease progression after tamoxifen therapy*
*Adults:* 1 mg P.O. daily.
*First-line therapy for hormone receptor–positive or hormone receptor–unknown locally advanced or metastatic breast cancer in postmenopausal women*
*Adults:* 1 mg P.O. daily. Therapy continues until tumor progression is evident.

## Mechanism of action

*Antineoplastic action:* A potent and selective nonsteroidal aromatase inhibitor, anastrozole significantly lowers serum estradiol levels. Estradiol is the principal estrogen circulating in postmenopausal women that has the ability to stimulate breast cancer cell growth.

## Pharmacokinetics

*Absorption:* Absorbed from the GI tract; food affects the extent of absorption.
*Distribution:* 40% plasma protein–bound in the therapeutic range.
*Metabolism:* Metabolized in the liver.
*Excretion:* About 11% of anastrozole is excreted in urine as parent drug and about 60% is excreted in urine as metabolites. Half-life is about 50 hours.

| Route | Onset | Peak | Duration |
|-------|-------|------|----------|
| P.O. | < 24 hr | Unknown | < 6 days |

## Contraindications and precautions

Contraindicated in pregnant women.

## Interactions

None reported.

## Adverse reactions

**CNS:** *asthenia, headache,* dizziness, depression, paresthesia.
**CV:** chest pain, edema, thromboembolic disease.
**EENT:** pharyngitis.
**GI:** increased appetite, dry mouth, *nausea,* vomiting, diarrhea, constipation, abdominal pain, anorexia.
**GU:** vaginal hemorrhage, vaginal dryness.
**Metabolic:** weight gain.
**Musculoskeletal:** *back pain,* bone pain, pelvic pain.
**Respiratory:** dyspnea, increased cough.
**Skin:** *hot flashes,* rash, sweating.
**Other:** *pain,* peripheral edema.

## Overdose and treatment

A single dose of anastrozole that results in life-threatening symptoms hasn't been established. Single oral doses that exceeded 100 mg/kg caused severe irritation of the stomach (necrosis, gastritis, ulceration, and hemorrhage) in animals.

---

Reactions may be *common,* uncommon, *life-threatening,* or COMMON AND LIFE-THREATENING.

There is no specific antidote to overdose; treatment must be symptomatic. Vomiting may be induced if the patient is alert. Dialysis may be helpful. General supportive care, including frequent monitoring of vital signs and close observation of the patient, is indicated.

## Clinical considerations
- Pregnancy must be excluded before treatment starts with anastrozole.
- Give drug under supervision of qualified staff experienced in the use of anticancer drugs.
- Patients treated with drug don't require glucocorticoid or mineralocorticoid therapy.

### Therapeutic monitoring
For patients with mild to moderate hepatic impairment, advise clinician to monitor for side effects.

### Special populations
**Breast-feeding patients.** It isn't known if anastrozole appears in breast milk. Drug shouldn't be given to breast-feeding women.
**Pediatric patients.** Safety and efficacy in pediatric patients haven't been established.

## Patient counseling
- Instruct patient to report adverse reactions.
- Stress importance of follow-up care.

# argatroban
Acova

*Pharmacologic classification:* direct thrombin inhibitor
*Therapeutic classification:* anticoagulant
*Pregnancy risk category B*

## Available forms
Available by prescription only
*Injection:* 100 mg/ml

## Indications and dosages
***Prophylaxis or treatment of thrombosis in patients with heparin-induced thrombocytopenia***
*Adults:* 2 mcg/kg/minute, given as a continuous I.V. infusion; adjust dosage until the steady state aPTT is 1.5 to 3 times the initial baseline value, not to exceed 100 seconds; maximum dose 10 mcg/kg/minute.
≡ *Dosage adjustment.* For patients with moderate hepatic impairment, the initial dose should be reduced to 0.5 mcg/kg/min, given as a continuous infusion. The PTT should be monitored closely and the dosage should be adjusted as clinically indicated.

## I.V. administration
- Dilute in normal saline solution, $D_5W$, or lactated Ringer's injection to a final level of 1 mg/ml.
- Each 2.5-ml vial should be diluted 100-fold by mixing it with 250 ml of diluent.
- Mix the constituted solution by repeated inversion of the diluent bag for 1 minute.
- Prepared solutions are stable for up to 24 hours at 25° C (77° F).

### Incompatibilities
None reported.

## Mechanism of action
*Antithrombin action:* Reversibly binds to the thrombin active site and inhibits thrombin-catalyzed or induced reactions, including fibrin formation, activation of coagulation factors V, VIII, and XIII, and protein C and platelet aggregation. Argatroban is capable of inhibiting the action of both free and clot-associated thrombin.

## Pharmacokinetics
*Absorption:* Administered I.V.
*Distribution:* Argatroban distributes mainly in the extracellular fluid. Argatroban is 54% bound to human proteins, of which 34% is bound to α-acid glycoprotein and 20% to albumin.
*Metabolism:* Argatroban is primarily metabolized in the liver by hydroxylation. The formation of four metabolites is catalyzed in the liver by the cytochrome P450 enzymes CYP3A4/5. The primary metabolite (M1) is 20% weaker than that of the parent drug. The other metabolites are detected in low levels in the urine. The terminal elimination half-life ranges from 39 to 51 minutes.
*Excretion:* Primary excretion of argatroban is in the feces, presumably through the biliary tract.

| Route | Onset | Peak | Duration |
|-------|-------|------|----------|
| I.V. | Rapid | 1-3 hr | 40-50 min after infusion ends |

## Contraindications and precautions
Argatroban is contraindicated in patients with overt major bleeding and in patients hypersensitive to argatroban or any of its constituents.

Caution should be used in patients with hepatic disease. Use with caution in disease states in which there is increased risk of hemorrhage, such as severe hypertension, in hematologic conditions with increased bleeding tendencies, such as congenital or acquired bleeding disorders, and in gastrointestinal lesions, such as ulcerations. Also use caution immediately following lumbar puncture, spinal anesthesia, and major surgery, especially involving the brain, spinal cord, or eye.

## Interactions
**Drug-drug.** *Oral anticoagulants:* May result in the prolongation of the PT and INR and may increase the risk of bleeding. Advise clinician to monitor patient closely.
*Thrombolytic agents:* Increased risk of intracranial bleeding. Avoid concomitant use.

## Adverse reactions
**CV:** *atrial fibrillation, cardiac arrest, cerebrovascular disorder,* hypotension, *ventricular tachycardia.*
**GI:** abdominal pain, diarrhea, *GI bleeding,* hemoptysis, nausea, vomiting.
**GU:** abnormal renal function, groin bleeding, *hematuria,* urinary tract infection.
**Hematologic:** *decreased hemoglobin and hematocrit.*
**Respiratory:** coughing, dyspnea, pneumonia.
**Other:** *allergic reactions,* brachial bleeding, fever, infection, pain, *sepsis.*

## Overdose and treatment
Excessive anticoagulation, with or without bleeding, may occur in argatroban overdose. No specific antidote to argatroban is available if life-threatening bleeding occurs. Recommend discontinuing argatroban therapy immediately and advise clinician to monitor the aPTT and other coagulation tests. Symptomatic and supportive therapy should be provided.

## Clinical considerations
■ Argatroban is intended for I.V. administration. All parenteral anticoagulants should be discontinued before administering argatroban. Coadministration of argatroban with antiplatelet drugs, thrombolytics, and other anticoagulants may increase the risk of bleeding.
■ Hemorrhage may occur at any site in the body in patients receiving argatroban. Any unexplained fall in hematocrit, fall in blood pressure, or any other unexplained symptoms should lead to consideration of a hemorrhagic event.
■ To convert to oral anticoagulant therapy, advise clinician to give warfarin with argatroban at doses up to 2 mcg/kg/minute until the INR is > 4 on combined therapy. After argatroban is discontinued, the INR should be repeated in 4 to 6 hours. If the repeat INR is below the desired therapeutic range, advise clinician to resume the argatroban infusion. The procedure should be repeated daily until the desired therapeutic range on warfarin alone is reached.
**H ALERT** Don't confuse Aggrastat (tirofiban) with Acova (argatroban).

## Therapeutic monitoring
■ Advise clinician to obtain baseline coagulation tests, platelets, hemoglobin, and hematocrit before therapy starts.

■ Argatroban is monitored by the aPTT. Recommend checking aPTT 2 hours after the administration of argatroban; dosage adjustments may be required to get a targeted aPTT (1.5 to 3 times the baseline, not to exceed 100 seconds). Steady state is achieved within 1 to 3 hours following start of argatroban.

### Special populations
**Breast-feeding patients.** It isn't known if argatroban appears in human milk. A decision should be made to discontinue nursing or to discontinue the drug, taking into account the importance of the drug to the mother.
**Pediatric patients.** The safety and efficacy of argatroban in patients younger than age 18 haven't been established.

## Patient counseling
■ Advise patient that this drug can cause bleeding and inform patient to report any unusual bruising or bleeding (nosebleeds, bleeding gums) or tarry stools to the prescriber immediately.
■ Advise patient to avoid activities that carry a risk of injury and instruct patient to use a soft toothbrush and electric razor while on argatroban.
■ Instruct patient to notify prescriber if wheezing, trouble breathing, or skin rash occurs.
■ Inform patient to notify prescriber if she is pregnant, breast-feeding, or has recently had a baby.
■ Inform patient to notify prescriber if he has stomach ulcers or liver disease, has had any type of surgery or radiation treatments, or has suffered a fall or other injury recently.

# arsenic trioxide
Trisenox

*Pharmacologic classification:* arsenic trioxide
*Therapeutic classification:* antineoplastic
*Pregnancy risk category D*

## Available forms
Available by prescription only
*Injection:* 1 mg/ml

## Indications and dosages
*Acute promyelocytic leukemia in patients who have relapsed from, or are refractory to, retinoid and anthracycline chemotherapy*
*Adults and children age 5 and older:*
**Induction phase**
0.15 mg/kg I.V. daily until bone marrow remission. Maximum 60 doses.
**Consolidation phase**

0.15 mg/kg I.V. daily for 25 doses over a period up to 5 weeks, beginning 3 to 6 weeks after completion of induction therapy.

## I.V. administration
■ Follow institutional policy regarding preparation and handling of antineoplastics. The active ingredient is a carcinogen.
■ Dilute with 100 to 250 ml of $D_5W$ or normal saline solution. After dilution, drug is stable at controlled room temperature for 24 hours and refrigerated for 48 hours.
■ Give I.V. over 1 to 2 hours. Infusion time may be extended up to 4 hours if vasomotor reactions occur.

### Incompatibilities
None reported.

## Mechanism of action
Arsenic trioxide causes morphologic changes and DNA fragmentation resulting in death of promyelocytic leukemic cells.

## Pharmacokinetics
*Absorption:* Administered I.V.
*Distribution:* Arsenic is stored mainly in the liver, kidney, heart, lung, hair, and nails.
*Metabolism:* Metabolized in the liver.
*Excretion:* Excreted in urine in the methylated form.

| Route | Onset | Peak | Duration |
|-------|-------|------|----------|
| I.V. | Unknown | Unknown | Unknown |

## Contraindications and precautions
Contraindicated in patients hypersensitive to arsenic.

Use cautiously in patients with heart failure, renal failure, a history of torsades de pointes, preexisting QT interval prolongation, or conditions that cause hypokalemia or hypomagnesemia.

## Interactions
**Drug-drug.** *Drugs that can lead to electrolyte abnormalities (amphotericin B or diuretics):* Increased risk of electrolyte abnormalities. Use cautiously.
*Drugs that can prolong the QT interval (antiarrhythmics or thioridazine):* May further prolong QT interval. Use cautiously.

## Adverse reactions
**CNS:** *headache, insomnia, parasthesia, dizziness,* tremor, **seizures,** somnolence, coma, *anxiety, depression,* agitation, confusion, *fatigue, weakness.*
**CV:** *tachycardia,* **PROLONGED QT INTERVAL,** *palpitations, edema, chest pain,* ECG abnormalities, *hypotension, flushing, hypertension.*
**EENT:** *eye irritation, epistaxis, blurred vision,* dry eye, earache, tinnitus, *sore throat, post*

*nasal drip,* eyelid edema, *sinusitis,* nasopharyngitis, painful red eye.
**GI:** *nausea, vomiting, diarrhea, anorexia, abdominal pain, constipation, loose stools, dyspepsia,* oral blistering, fecal incontinence, GI hemorrhage, dry mouth, abdominal tenderness or distension, bloody diarrhea, oral candidiasis.
**GU:** *renal failure,* renal impairment, oliguria, incontinence, *vaginal hemorrhage,* intermenstrual bleeding.
**Hematologic:** *leukocytosis, anemia,* **THROMBOCYTOPENIA, NEUTROPENIA,** *DIC, hemorrhage,* lymphadenopathy.
**Hepatic:** *increased ALT and AST.*
**Metabolic:** *hypokalemia, hypomagnesemia, hyperglycemia, hypocalcemia,* hypoglycemia, acidosis, *weight gain,* weight loss, *hyperkalemia.*
**Musculoskeletal:** *arthralgia, myalgia, bone pain, back pain, neck pain, limb pain.*
**Respiratory:** *cough, dyspnea, hypoxia, pleural effusion, wheezing, decreased breath sounds, crepitations, rales,* hemoptysis, tachypnea, rhonci, *upper respiratory tract infection.*
**Skin:** *dermatitis, pruritus, ecchymosis, dry skin, erythema, increased sweating,* night sweats, petechiae, hyperpigmentation, urticaria, skin lesions, local exfoliation, *pallor.*
**Other:** *fever,* drug hypersensitivity, *pain, erythema, or edema at injection site, rigors,* lymphadenopathy, facial edema, *herpes simplex infection,* bacterial infection, herpes zoster, *sepsis.*

## Overdose and treatment
Symptoms of acute arsenic toxicity include confusion, muscle weakness, and seizures.

If overdose occurs, advise clinician to immediately stop Trisenox. Advise clinician to consider treatment with dimercaprol 3 mg/kg I.M. q 4 hours until life-threatening toxicity has subsided, followed by penicillamine 250 mg P.O. up to q.i.d. (≤ 1 g per day).

## Clinical considerations
**Ⓗ ALERT** Arsenic trioxide may cause fatal arrhythmias and complete AV block.
**Ⓗ ALERT** Arsenic trioxide has been linked to acute promyelocytic leukemia differentiation syndrome, characterized by fever, dyspnea, weight gain, pulmonary infiltrates, and pleural or pericardial effusions, with or without leukocytosis. This syndrome can be fatal and requires treatment with high-dose steroids.
■ Advise clinician to perform ECG, and obtain potassium, calcium, magnesium, and creatinine levels before starting therapy. Electrolyte abnormalities should be corrected before beginning drug.

### Therapeutic monitoring
■ Advise clinician to monitor electrolytes and hematologic and coagulation profiles at least

twice weekly during treatment. Advise clinician to keep potassium levels above 4 mEq/dl and magnesium levels above 1.8 mg/dl.

■ Advise clinician to monitor patient for syncope and rapid or irregular heart rate. If these occur, advise clinician to stop drug, hospitalize patient, and monitor serum electrolytes and QTc interval. Drug may be restarted when electrolyte abnormalities are corrected and QTc interval falls below 460 msec.

■ Advise clinician to monitor ECG at least weekly during therapy. Prolonged QTc interval commonly occurs between 1 and 5 weeks after infusion, and returns to baseline about 8 weeks after infusion. If QTc interval is greater than 500 msec at any time during therapy, advise clinician to assess patient closely and consider discontinuing drug.

### Special populations

**Pregnant patients.** Caution women of child-bearing age to avoid becoming pregnant during therapy. Also recommend consulting with prescriber before becoming pregnant.

**Breast-feeding patients.** Arsenic appears in breast milk. Because of the potential for serious adverse reactions in nursing infants, breast-feeding should be discontinued.

**Pediatric patients.** Safety and efficacy have not been established in children younger than age 5.

### Patient counseling

■ Tell patient to report fever, shortness of breath, or weight gain immediately.

■ Teach patient or caregiver how to check radial pulse. Tell him to keep record of pulse rate and to notify prescriber of significant changes.

■ Instruct patient to notify prescriber of all the medications he is currently taking and to check with prescriber before staring any new drug.

■ Instruct diabetic patients that the drug may cause hyperglycemia or hypoglycemia and to monitor blood glucose level closely.

## ascorbic acid (vitamin C)

Ascorbicap, Cebid Timecelles, Cecon, Cevalin, Cevi-Bid, Ce-Vi-Sol, Dull-C, Flavorcee

*Pharmacologic classification:* water-soluble vitamin
*Therapeutic classification:* vitamin
*Pregnancy risk category A (C if exceeds RDA)*

### Available forms

Available by prescription only
*Injection:* 100 mg/ ml, 250 mg/ml in 2-ml ampules and 2-ml and 30-ml vials; 500 mg/ml in 2-ml and 5-ml ampules and 50-ml vials; 500 mg/ml (with monothioglycerol) in 1-ml ampules

Available without a prescription
*Tablets:* 25 mg, 50 mg, 100 mg, 250 mg, 500 mg, 1,000 mg
*Tablets (chewable):* 100 mg, 250 mg, 500 mg
*Tablets (extended-release):* 500 mg, 1,000 mg, 1,500 mg
*Capsules (extended-release):* 250 mg, 500 mg
*Crystals:* 100 g (4 g/tsp), 1,000 g (4 g/tsp, sugar-free)
*Lozenges:* 60 mg
*Powder:* 100 g (4 g/tsp), 500 g (4 g/tsp)
*Liquid:* 50 ml (35 mg/0.6 ml)
*Solution:* 50 ml (100 mg/ml)
*Syrup:* 20 mg/ml in 120 ml and 480 ml; 500 mg/5 ml in 5 ml, 10 ml, 120 ml, and 473 ml

### Indications and dosages

*Frank and subclinical scurvy*
*Adults:* 100 to 250 mg, depending on severity, P.O., S.C., I.M., or I.V. daily or b.i.d., then at least 50 mg/day for maintenance.
*Infants and children:* 100 to 300 mg, depending on severity, P.O., S.C., I.M., or I.V. daily, then at least 35 mg/day for maintenance.
*Prevention of ascorbic acid deficiency in those with poor nutritional habits or increased requirements*
*Adults:* 45 to 60 mg P.O., S.C., I.M., or I.V. daily.
*Pregnant or breast-feeding women:* At least 60 to 80 mg P.O., S.C., I.M., or I.V. daily.
*Children and infants over age 2 weeks:* At least 20 to 50 mg P.O., S.C., I.M., or I.V. daily.
*Potentiation of methenamine in urine acidification*
*Adults:* 4 to 12 g daily in divided doses.
*Adjunctive therapy in the treatment of idiopathic methemoglobinemia*
*Adults:* 300 to 600 mg P.O. daily in divided doses.
*Reduce tyrosinemia in premature infants on high-protein diets*
*Premature infants:* 100 mg P.O. or I.M. daily.
*To increase iron excretion caused by deferoxamine administration*
*Adults:* 100 to 200 mg P.O. q day.
*Prevent and treat the common cold*
*Adults:* 1 to 3 g or more P.O. per day.

### I.V. administration

■ Give I.V. solution slowly. Rapid infusion may cause dizziness.

### Incompatibilities

Incompatible with aminophylline, bleomycin, cefazolin, cephapirin, chlorothiazide, conjugated estrogens, erythromycin lactobionate, nafcillin and sodium bicarbonate. May be incompatible with chloramphenicol and hydrocortisone.

### Mechanism of action

*Nutritional action:* Ascorbic acid, an essential vitamin, is involved with the biologic oxidavitro inhibition of HMG-CoA reductase by or-thohydroxylated and parahydroxylated metabolites is equivalent to that of atorvastatin. About 70% of circulating inhibitory activity for HMG-CoA reductase is attributed to active metabolites. In vitro studies suggest the importance of atorvastatin metabolism by cytochrome P-450 CYP3A4.

*Excretion:* Eliminated primarily in bile following hepatic or extrahepatic metabolism; however, drug doesn't appear to undergo enterohepatic recirculation. Mean plasma elimination half-life of atorvastatin is about 14 hours, but the half-life of inhibitory activity for HMG-CoA reductase is 20 to 30 hours because of the contribution of active metabolites. Less than 2% of a dose of atorvastatin is recovered in urine following oral administration.

| Route | Onset | Peak | Duration |
|-------|-------|------|----------|
| P.O. | Unknown | 1-2 hr | Unknown |

## Contraindications and precautions
Contraindicated in patients hypersensitive to drug or with active hepatic disease or conditions related to unexplained persistent elevations of serum transaminase levels, in pregnant or breast-feeding women, and in women of child-bearing age (except in women not at risk for becoming pregnant).

Use cautiously in patients with history of hepatic disease or heavy alcohol use.

## Interactions
**Drug-drug.** *Antacids:* May cause decreased levels of atorvastatin. LDL-cholesterol reduction not affected. Advise clinician to monitor patient.

*Azole antifungals, cyclosporine, erythromycin, fibric acid derivatives, and niacin:* May increase risk of rhabdomyolysis. Avoid use together.

*Digoxin:* May increase plasma digoxin levels. Advise clinician to monitor serum digoxin levels.

*Erythromycin:* Increases plasma level of drug. Advise clinician to monitor patient.

*Oral contraceptives:* May increase levels of hormones. Consider when selecting an oral contraceptive.

## Adverse reactions
**CNS:** asthenia, *headache.*
**EENT:** pharyngitis, sinusitis.
**GI:** abdominal pain, constipation, diarrhea, dyspepsia, flatulence.
**Hepatic:** increased liver function test results.
**Musculoskeletal:** arthralgia, back pain, myalgia.
**Skin:** rash.
**Other:** accidental injury, *allergic reaction,* flu-like syndrome, *infection.*

## Overdose and treatment
There is no specific treatment for atorvastatin overdose. If overdose occurs, recommend treating patient symptomatically and providing supportive measures as required. Because of extensive drug binding to plasma proteins, hemodialysis isn't expected to significantly enhance drug clearance.

## Clinical considerations
■ Recommend withholding or discontinuing drug in patients with serious, acute conditions that suggest myopathy or those at risk for renal failure secondary to rhabdomyolysis as a result of trauma; major surgery; severe metabolic, endocrine, and electrolyte disorders; severe acute infection; hypotension; or uncontrolled seizures.

■ Drug should only be used after diet and other nonpharmacologic treatments prove ineffective. Patient should follow a standard low-cholesterol diet before and during therapy.

■ Drug may be given as a single dose at any time of day without regard for food.

### Therapeutic monitoring
■ Before treatment starts, recommend excluding secondary causes for hypercholesterolemia and performing a baseline lipid profile. Periodic liver function tests and lipid levels should be checked before starting treatment, at 6 and 12 weeks after therapy starts or changes, and periodically thereafter.

■ Recommend checking patient for signs of myositis.

### Special populations
**Breast-feeding patients.** Because of the potential for adverse reactions in breast-fed infants, women taking atorvastatin shouldn't breast-feed.

**Pediatric patients.** Experience in children is limited to drug doses up to 80 mg daily for 1 year in eight patients with homozygous familial hypercholesteremia. No clinical or biochemical abnormalities were reported in these patients. Safety and efficacy haven't been established in children under age 9.

**Geriatric patients.** Safety and efficacy in patients age 70 and older with drug doses up to 80 mg daily were similar to those of patients under age 70.

## Patient counseling
■ Teach patient proper dietary management, weight control, and exercise. Explain the importance of controlling elevated serum lipid levels.

■ Warn patient to avoid alcohol.

■ Tell patient to report adverse reactions, such as muscle pain, malaise, and fever.

■ Warn women that drug is contraindicated during pregnancy because of potential danger

---

to the fetus. Advise her to call prescriber immediately if pregnancy occurs.

---

# atovaquone and proguanil hydrochloride
Malarone

*Pharmacologic classification:* hydroxy-napthalenedione/biguanide hydrochloride
*Therapeutic classification:* antimalarial
*Pregnancy risk category C*

## Available forms
Available by prescription only
*Tablets:* 250 mg atovaquone and 100 mg proguanil hydrochloride; 62.5 mg atovaquone and 25 mg proguanil hydrochloride (HCl)

## Indications and dosages
*Prevention of Plasmodium falciparum malaria, including in areas where chloroquine resistance has been reported*
Adults and pediatric patients over 40 kg (88 lb): 1 adult-strength tablet (250 mg atovaquone/100 mg proguanil HCl) P.O. once daily with food or a milky drink. Begin 1 or 2 days before entering a malaria-endemic area. Continue prophylactic treatment during the stay and for 7 days after return.
*Children 31 to 40 kg (68 to 88 lb):* 3 pediatric-strength tablets P.O. once daily with food or milk, beginning 1 or 2 days before entering endemic area. Total daily dose is 187.5 mg atovaquone/75 mg proguanil. Treatment should continue during stay and for 7 days after return.
*Children 21 to 30 kg (46 to 68 lb):* 2 pediatric-strength tablets P.O. once daily with food or milk, beginning 1 or 2 days before entering endemic area. Total daily dose is 125 mg atovaquone/50 mg proguanil. Treatment should continue during stay and for 7 days after return.
*Children 11 to 20 kg (24 to 45 lb):* 1 pediatric-strength tablet P.O. daily with food or milk, beginning 1 or 2 days before entering endemic area. Continue treatment during stay and for 7 days after return.
*Treatment of acute, uncomplicated P. falciparum malaria*
Adults and pediatric patients over 40 kg (88 lb): 4 adult strength tablets (total daily dose 1 g atovaquone/400 mg proguanil) P.O. once daily for 3 consecutive days. Take with food or a milky drink.
*Children 31 to 40 kg (68 to 88 lb):* 3 adult-strength tablets P.O. once daily, with food or milk, for 3 consecutive days. Total daily dose is 750 mg atovaquone/300 mg proguanil.
*Children 21 to 30 kg (46 to 68 lb):* 2 adult-strength tablets P.O. once daily, with food or milk, for 3 consecutive days. Total daily dose is 500 mg atovaquone/200 mg proguanil.

*Children 11 to 20 kg (24 to 45 lb):* 1 adult-strength tablet P.O. once daily, with food or milk, for 3 consecutive days.

## Mechanism of action
*Antimalarial action:* Thought to interfere with nucleic acid replication in the malarial parasite by inhibiting the biosynthesis of pyrimidine compounds. Atovaquone selectively inhibits mitochondrial electron transport in the parasite. Cycloguanil, an active metabolite of proguanil HCl, disrupts deoxythymidilate synthesis through inhibition of dihydrofolate reductase. Atovaquone and cycloguanil are active against the erythrocytic and exoerythrocytic stages of *Plasmodium* spp.

## Pharmacokinetics
*Absorption:* Bioavailability of atovaquone is 23% when the tablet formulation is taken with food. Atovaquone bioavailability varies considerably among individuals. Dietary fat increases the rate and extent of atovaquone absorption compared with fasting. Proguanil is well absorbed without regard to food.
*Distribution:* Atovaquone is highly protein bound. Proguanil exhibits moderate (75%) protein binding.
*Metabolism:* Atovaquone undergoes virtually no metabolism. Proguanil is metabolized to cycloguanil (primarily via cytochrome P450 2C19) and 4-chlorophenylbiguanide.
*Excretion:* More than 94% of atovaquone is eliminated unchanged in the feces over 21 days. Proguanil (40% to 60%) and its metabolites are eliminated by the kidneys. The elimination half-life of atovaquone is 2 to 3 days in adults. In adults and children, proguanil exhibits an elimination half-life of 12 to 21 hours.

| Route | Onset | Peak | Duration |
|-------|-------|------|----------|
| P.O. | Unknown | Unknown | Unknown |

## Contraindications and precautions
Contraindicated in patients hypersensitive to atovaquone or proguanil HCl or any component of the formulation.

Use with caution in patients with severe renal failure because proguanil HCl is renally eliminated. Use cautiously in vomiting patients.

## Interactions
**Drug-drug.** *Metoclopramide:* May decrease the bioavailability of atovaquone. Recommend considering alternative antiemetics.
*Rifampin:* Reduces the plasma level of atovaquone by about 50%. Avoid concurrent use.
*Tetracycline:* Reduces plasma levels of atovaquone by about 40%. Parasitemia should be closely monitored in patients receiving concurrent tetracycline.

## Adverse reactions
**CNS:** asthenia, dizziness, *headache.*

---

**GI:** *abdominal pain*, diarrhea, anorexia, dyspepsia, gastritis, *nausea, vomiting*.
**Hepatic:** elevated transaminase levels.
**Musculoskeletal:** back pain, *myalgia*.
**Respiratory:** cough, upper respiratory tract infection.
**Skin:** pruritus.
**Other:** fever, flu syndrome.

## Overdose and treatment

There have been no reports of overdose of atovaquone and proguanil HCl. In the event of an overdose, recommend supportive measures.

## Clinical considerations

■ Atovaquone absorption may be decreased by persistent diarrhea or vomiting. Alternative antimalarial therapy may be needed in patients with persistent diarrhea or vomiting.
■ Atovaquone and proguanil HCl haven't been studied in the treatment of cerebral malaria or other forms of complicated malaria.
■ In the event of a treatment or prophylaxis failure, an alternative antimalarial is indicated.
■ Atovaquone and proguanil HCl should be given at the same time each day with food or a milky drink.
■ Store tablets at controlled room temperature 15° to 30° C (59° to 86° F).

### Therapeutic monitoring

■ Advise clinician to monitor intake and output closely.
■ Recommend watching patient for new or worsened symptoms.

### Special populations

**Breast-feeding patients.** It isn't known if atovaquone appears in human milk. Proguanil appears in breast milk in small amounts. Therefore, use caution when giving to breast-feeding patients.
**Pediatric patients.** Safety and efficacy haven't been established in pediatric patients weighing less than 11 kg.
**Geriatric patients.** It isn't known if geriatric patients respond differently than younger patients. Use with caution in geriatric patients because they have a greater frequency of decreased renal, hepatic, and cardiac function.

## Patient counseling

■ Tell patient to take dose at the same time each day.
■ Advise patient to take his drug with food or a milky drink.
■ If patient vomits within 1 hour after taking a dose, tell him to take a repeat dose.
■ Advise patient to contact his prescriber if he is unable to complete his course of therapy, as prescribed.
■ Instruct patient that, in addition to drug therapy, malaria prophylaxis should include the use of protective clothing, bednets, and insect repellents.

# atracurium besylate
Tracrium

*Pharmacologic classification:* nondepolarizing neuromuscular blocker
*Therapeutic classification:* skeletal muscle relaxant
*Pregnancy risk category C*

## Available forms

Available by prescription only
*Injection:* 10 mg/ml

## Indications and dosages

***Adjunct to general anesthesia, to facilitate endotracheal intubation, and to provide skeletal muscle relaxation during surgery or mechanical ventilation***
Dosage depends on anesthetic used, individual needs, and response. Doses are representative and must be adjusted.
*Adults and children over age 2:* Initially, 0.4 to 0.5 mg/kg by I.V. bolus. Maintenance dosage of 0.08 to 0.10 mg/kg within 20 to 45 minutes of initial dose should be given during prolonged surgical procedures. Maintenance dosages may be given q 15 to 25 minutes in patients receiving balanced anesthesia.
*Children ages 1 month to 2 years:* Initially, 0.3 to 0.4 mg/kg by I.V. bolus when under halothane anesthesia. Frequent maintenance dosages may be needed.

## I.V. administration

■ Dilute to desired level, usually 0.2 to 0.5 mg/ml.
■ Dilute drug in $D_5W$, 5% dextrose and normal saline sloution, or normal saline solution.
■ Drug is stable for 24 hours when diluted in most solutions.
■ If drug is used for prolonged surgical procedure, it may be given by continuous I.V. infusion following rapid I.V. administration of initial dose of drug.
■ Use of a controlled infusion device is recommended for continuous infusion.
■ Store in refrigerator at 36° to 46° F (2° to 8° C). Use within 14 days after removing from refrigerator, even if returned for storage.

### Incompatibilities

Incompatible with alkaline solutions (such as barbiturates) because of drug's acid pH. Incompatible with lactated Ringer's solution.

## Mechanism of action

*Skeletal muscle relaxant action:* Atracurium produces skeletal muscle paralysis by causing a decreased response to acetylcholine (ACh) at the neuromuscular junction. Because of its

---

* Canada only    ◇ Unlabeled clinical use

high affinity to ACh receptor sites, atracurium competitively blocks access of ACh to the motor end-plate, thus blocking depolarization. At usual doses (0.45 mg/kg), atracurium produces minimal CV effects and doesn't affect intraocular pressure, lower esophageal sphincter pressure, barrier pressure, heart rate or rhythm, mean arterial pressure, systemic vascular resistance, cardiac output, or central venous pressure. CV effects such as decreased peripheral vascular resistance, usually seen at doses greater than 0.5 mg/kg, are caused by histamine release.

## Pharmacokinetics

*Absorption:* Administered I.V.
*Distribution:* Distributed into the extracellular space after I.V. administration; about 82% protein-bound.
*Metabolism:* In plasma, is rapidly metabolized by Hofmann elimination and by nonspecific enzymatic ester hydrolysis. The liver doesn't appear to play a major role.
*Excretion:* Excreted in urine and feces by biliary elimination.

| Route | Onset | Peak | Duration |
|---|---|---|---|
| I.V. | 2 min | 3-5 min | 35-70 min |

## Contraindications and precautions

Contraindicated in patients hypersensitive to drug. Use cautiously in patients with CV disease; severe electrolyte disorder; bronchogenic carcinoma; hepatic, renal, or pulmonary impairment; neuromuscular disease; myasthenia gravis; and in geriatric or debilitated patients.

## Interactions

**Drug-drug.** *Aminoglycoside antibiotics, beta blockers, clindamycin, depolarizing neuromuscular blockers, enflurane and isoflurane, furosemide, lincomycin, lithium, other nondepolarizing neuromuscular blockers, parenteral magnesium salts, polymyxin antibiotics, potassium-depleting drugs, procainamide, quinidine, quinine, and thiazide diuretics:* The neuromuscular blockade caused by atracurium may be enhanced by use with many general anesthetics. Recommend carefully monitoring patient.
*Opioid analgesics:* May cause additive respiratory depression. Recommend using with extreme caution during surgery and immediately postoperatively.

## Adverse reactions

**CV:** *bradycardia,* hypotension, tachycardia.
**Respiratory:** *prolonged dose-related apnea,* wheezing, increased bronchial secretions, dyspnea, **bronchospasm, laryngospasm.**
**Skin:** *flushing,* erythema, pruritus, urticaria, rash.
**Other:** *anaphylaxis.*

## Overdose and treatment

Signs and symptoms of overdose include prolonged respiratory depression or apnea and CV collapse. A sudden release of histamine may also occur.

A peripheral nerve stimulator is recommended to monitor response and to determine the nature and degree of neuromuscular block. Recommend maintaining an adequate airway and manual or mechanical ventilation until patient can maintain respiration unassisted.

For treatment, advise clinician to give cholinesterase inhibitors, such as edrophonium, neostigmine, or pyridostigmine, to reverse neuromuscular blockade; and atropine or glycopyrrolate to counteract muscarinic adverse effects of cholinesterase inhibitors. Advise clinician to monitor vital signs at least every 15 minutes until patient is stable, then every 30 minutes for next 2 hours. Advise clinician to observe airway until patient has fully recovered from drug effects. Rate, depth, and pattern of respirations should be noted.

## Clinical considerations

■ Recommend I.V. injection because I.M. injection causes tissue irritation.
■ Recommend reducing dose and administration rate in patients for whom histamine release may be hazardous.
■ Prior administration of succinylcholine doesn't prolong duration of action of atracurium, but it quickens onset and may deepen neuromuscular blockade.
■ Atracurium has a longer duration of action than succinylcholine and a shorter duration than tubocurarine or pancuronium.
■ Drug has little or no effect on heart rate and doesn't counteract or reverse the bradycardia caused by anesthetics or vagal stimulation. Thus, bradycardia is seen more frequently with atracurium than with other neuromuscular blockers. Pretreatment with anticholinergics (atropine or glycopyrrolate) is advised.
■ Alkaline solutions, such as barbiturates, shouldn't be mixed in the same syringe or given through the same needle with atracurium.
■ Use drug only if endotracheal intubation, administration of oxygen under positive pressure, artificial respiration, and assisted or controlled ventilation are immediately available.
■ Until head and neck muscles recover from blockade effects, patient may find speech difficult.
■ If indicated, recommend assessment of need for pain medication or sedation. Drug doesn't affect consciousness or relieve pain.

### Therapeutic monitoring

■ Advise clinician to monitor patient for bradycardia during drug administration; patient may require I.V. atropine.
■ Advise clinician to use a peripheral nerve stimulator to monitor responses during inten-

---

Reactions may be *common,* uncommon, *life-threatening,* or COMMON AND LIFE-THREATENING.

sive care unit administration; it may be used to detect residual paralysis during recovery and to avoid atracurium overdose.

### Special populations

**Pregnant patients.** There are no adequate and controlled studies for use in this population.
**Breast-feeding patients.** It's unknown if drug appears in breast milk; therefore, use cautiously in breast-feeding women.
**Pediatric patients.** Safety and efficacy haven't been established for children under age 1 month.
**Geriatric patients.** Geriatric patients may be more sensitive to the effects of the drug.

### Patient counseling

Remind staff to explain all events and procedures to patient because he can still hear.

# atropine sulfate

*Pharmacologic classification:* anticholinergic, belladonna alkaloid
*Therapeutic classification:* antiarrhythmic, vagolytic
*Pregnancy risk category C*

## Available forms

Available by prescription only
*Tablets:* 0.4 mg
*Injection:* 0.05 mg/ml, 0.1 mg/ml, 0.3 mg/ml, 0.4 mg/ml, 0.5 mg/ml, 0.8 mg/ml, and 1 mg/ml
*Ophthalmic ointment:* 1%
*Ophthalmic solution:* 0.5%, 1%, 2%

## Indications and dosages

**Symptomatic bradycardia, bradyarrhythmia (junctional or escape rhythm)**
*Adults:* Usually 0.5 to 1 mg by I.V. push; repeat q 3 to 5 minutes, to maximum of 0.03 mg/kg in patients with mild bradycardia and 2.5 mg (0.4 mg/kg) in patients with severe bradycardia or ventricular asystole. Lower doses (less than 0.5 mg) may cause bradycardia.
*Children:* 0.02 mg/kg I.V. up to maximum 1 mg; or 0.3 mg/m$^2$; may repeat q 5 minutes.
   Note: Dose may be given at 2½ times the I.V. dose and diluted in 10 ml of normal saline solution (adults) or 1 to 2 ml of half-normal or normal saline solution (child) and given via the endotracheal tube during cardiopulmonary resuscitation if I.V. access unavailable.
**Preoperatively for diminishing secretions and blocking cardiac vagal reflexes**
*Adults and children weighing over 20 kg (44 lb):* 0.4 mg I.M. or S.C. 30 to 60 minutes before anesthesia.
*Children weighing less than 20 kg:* 0.1 mg I.M. for 3 kg, 0.2 mg I.M. for 4 to 9 kg, 0.3 mg I.M. for 10 to 20 kg 30 to 60 minutes before anesthesia.

**To block adverse muscarinic effects of anticholinesterase agents when these drugs are used to reverse neuromuscular blockade produced by curariform drugs**
*Adults:* 0.6 to 1.2 mg for each 0.5 to 2.5 mg of neostigmine or 10 to 20 mg of pyridostigmine given; give I.V. a few minutes before the anticholinesterase agent.
**Antidote for anticholinesterase insecticide poisoning**
*Adults:* 1 to 2 mg I.M. or I.V. repeated q 5 to 60 minutes until muscarinic symptoms disappear. In severe cases, 2 to 6 mg may be given initially, repeating doses every 5 to 60 minutes.
*Children:* 0.05 mg/kg I.V. or I.M. repeated every 10 to 30 minutes until muscarinic signs and symptoms disappear.
**Hypotonic radiograph of the GI tract**
*Adults:* 1 mg I.M.
**Short-term treatment or prevention of bronchospasm**
*Adults:* 0.025 mg/kg given via nebulizer t.i.d. or q.i.d. to maximum dose of 2.5 mg.
*Children:* 0.05 mg/kg t.i.d. or q.i.d.
**Acute iritis, uveitis**
*Adults:* 1 to 2 drops (0.5% or 1% solution) into the eye t.i.d. (in children use 0.5% solution) or a small amount of ointment in the conjunctival sac t.i.d.
**Cycloplegic refraction**
*Adults:* 1 drop (1% solution) 1 hour before refraction.
*Children:* 1 to 2 drops (0.5% solution) into each eye b.i.d. for 1 to 3 days before eye examination and 1 hour before examination.

## I.V. administration

■ With slow I.V. administration, drug may cause paradoxical bradycardia, which usually disappears within 2 minutes.
■ In situations such as cardiopulmonary resuscitation, atropine is usually given by rapid I.V. injection.

## Incompatibilities

Incompatible with alkalies, bromides, iodides, isoproterenol, metaraminol, methohexital, norepinephrine, pentobarbital sodium, and sodium bicarbonate.

## Mechanism of action

*Antiarrhythmic action:* An anticholinergic (parasympatholytic) with many uses, atropine remains the mainstay of pharmacologic treatment for bradyarrhythmias. It blocks the effects of acetylcholine on the SA and AV nodes, thereby increasing SA and AV node conduction velocity. It also increases sinus node discharge rate and decreases the effective refractory period of the AV node. These changes result in an increased heart rate (both atrial and ventricular).
   Atropine has variable—and clinically negligible—effects on the His-Purkinje system.

Doses below 0.5 mg and occasionally larger doses may lead to a paradoxical slowing of the heart rate, which may be followed by a more rapid rate.

*Anticholinergic action:* As a cholinergic blocker, atropine decreases the action of the parasympathetic nervous system on certain glands (bronchial, salivary, and sweat), resulting in decreased secretions. It also decreases cholinergic effects on the iris, ciliary body, and intestinal and bronchial smooth muscle.

*Antidote for cholinesterase poisoning:* As an antidote for cholinesterase poisoning, atropine blocks the cholinomimetic effects of these pesticides.

## Pharmacokinetics

*Absorption:* I.V. administration is the most common route for bradyarrhythmia treatment. With endotracheal administration, is well absorbed from the bronchial tree; drug has been used in 1-mg doses in acute bradyarrhythmia when an I.V. line hasn't been established.

*Distribution:* Well distributed throughout the body, including the CNS. Only 18% plasma protein–bound.

*Metabolism:* Metabolized in the liver to several metabolites. About 30% to 50% of a dose is excreted by the kidneys as unchanged drug.

*Excretion:* Excreted primarily through the kidneys; however, small amounts may be excreted in the feces and expired air. Elimination half-life is biphasic, with an initial 2-hour phase followed by a terminal half-life of about 12¼ hours.

| Route | Onset | Peak | Duration |
|-------|-------|------|----------|
| P.O. | ½-2 hr | 1-2 hr | 4 hr |
| I.V. | Immediate | 2-4 min | 4 hr |
| I.M. | 5-40 min | 20-60 min | 4 hr |
| S.C. | Unknown | Unknown | Unknown |
| Ophthalmic | Unknown | ½-3 hr | 7-10 days |

## Contraindications and precautions

Contraindicated in patients hypersensitive to drug or sodium metabisulfite, acute angle-closure glaucoma, obstructive uropathy, obstructive disease of GI tract, paralytic ileus, toxic megacolon, intestinal atony, unstable CV status in acute hemorrhage, asthma, and myasthenia gravis.

Ophthalmic form is contraindicated in patients with glaucoma or hypersensitivity to drug or belladonna alkaloids and in those who have adhesions between the iris and lens. Atropine shouldn't be used during the first 3 months of life because of the possible association between cycloplegia produced and development of amblyopia.

Use cautiously in patients with Down syndrome. Ophthalmic form should be used with caution in patients with increased intraocular pressure and the elderly.

## Interactions

**Drug-drug.** *Amantadine:* May result in an increase in anticholinergic adverse effects. Advise clinician to monitor patient carefully.

*Other anticholinergics or drugs with anticholinergic effects:* Additive effects. Advise clinician to monitor patient carefully.

**Drug-herb.** *Betel palm:* May cause reduced temperature elevating effects and enhanced CNS effects. Discourage use together.

*Jaborandi tree:* May reduce effects of atropine. Advise clinician to monitor patient closely.

*Jimsonweed:* May adversely affect CV function. Discourage use together.

*Pill-bearing spurge:* May decrease effects of atropine. Discourage use together.

*Squaw vine:* May decrease metabolic breakdown of atropine. Advise clinician to monitor patient.

## Adverse reactions

**CNS:** *headache, restlessness,* ataxia, disorientation, hallucinations, delirium, *insomnia, dizziness,* excitement, agitation, confusion, especially in geriatric patients (with systemic or oral form); confusion, somnolence, headache (with ophthalmic form).

**CV:** palpitations and bradycardia following low-dose atropine, tachycardia after higher doses (with systemic or oral form); tachycardia (with ophthalmic form).

**EENT:** photophobia, increased intraocular pressure, *blurred vision, mydriasis,* cycloplegia (with systemic or oral form), ocular congestion with long-term use, conjunctivitis, contact dermatitis of eye, ocular edema, eye dryness, transient stinging and burning, eye irritation, hyperemia (with ophthalmic form).

**GI:** *dry mouth,* thirst, *constipation,* nausea, vomiting (with systemic or oral form); dry mouth, abdominal distention in infants (with ophthalmic form).

**GU:** urine retention, impotence (with systemic or oral form).

**Hematologic:** leukocytosis (with systemic or oral form).

**Skin:** dryness (with ophthalmic form).

**Other:** severe allergic reactions, including *anaphylaxis* and urticaria (systemic or oral form).

## Overdose and treatment

Signs of overdose reflect excessive anticholinergic activity, especially CV and CNS stimulation.

Treatment includes physostigmine administration to reverse excessive anticholinergic activity and general supportive measures, p.r.n.

## Clinical considerations

■ High doses may cause hyperpyrexia, urinary retention, and CNS effects, including hallucinations and confusion (anticholinergic delirium). Other anticholinergic drugs may increase vagal blockage.

---

- Store drug at 59° to 86° F (15° to 30° C) and protect from heat, light, and air.

### Therapeutic monitoring
- Advise clinician to observe patient for tachycardia if he has cardiac disorder.
- Advise clinician to monitor patient's fluid intake and output; drug causes urine retention and hesitancy. If possible, patient should void before taking drug.

### Special populations
**Geriatric patients.** Advise clinician to monitor patient closely for urine retention in elderly men with BPH.

### Patient counseling
- Tell patient to report serious adverse reactions promptly.
- Teach patient how to instill eye medication.
- Warn patient to avoid hazardous activities until blurry vision subsides.
- Advise patient to ease photophobia by wearing dark glasses.

---

# attapulgite
Children's Kaopectate, Diasorb, Donnagel, Fowler's*, Kaopectate, Kaopectate Advanced Formula, Kaopectate Maximum Strength, K-Pek, Parepectolin, Rheaban, Rheaban Maximum Strength

*Pharmacologic classification:* hydrated magnesium aluminum silicate
*Therapeutic classification:* antidiarrheal
*Pregnancy risk category NR*

### Available forms
Available without a prescription
*Tablets:* 300 mg, 600 mg*, 630 mg*, 750 mg
*Tablets (chewable):* 600 mg
*Oral suspension:* 600 mg/15 ml, 750 mg/5 ml, 750 mg/15 ml*, 900 mg/15 ml*

### Indications and dosages
*Acute, nonspecific diarrhea*
*Adults and adolescents:* 1.2 to 1.5 g (if using Diasorb, dosage can be as high as 3 g) P.O. after each loose bowel movement; don't exceed 9 g within 24 hours.
*Children ages 6 to 12:* 600 mg (suspension) or 750 mg (tablet) P.O. after each loose bowel movement; don't exceed 4.2 g (suspension and chewable tablets) or 4.5 g (tablet) within 24 hours.
*Children ages 3 to 6:* 300 mg P.O. after each loose bowel movement; don't exceed 2.1 g within 24 hours.

### Mechanism of action
*Antidiarrheal action:* Although its exact action is unknown, it's believed that attapulgite ab-

sorbs large numbers of bacteria and toxins and reduces water loss in the GI tract.

### Pharmacokinetics
*Absorption:* Not absorbed.
*Distribution:* Not applicable.
*Metabolism:* Not applicable.
*Excretion:* Excreted unchanged in feces.

| Route | Onset | Peak | Duration |
|---|---|---|---|
| P.O. | Unknown | Unknown | Unknown |

### Contraindications and precautions
Contraindicated in patients with dysentery or suspected bowel obstruction. Should be used cautiously in dehydrated patients.

### Interactions
**Drug-drug.** *Other drugs:* Absorption of oral medications may be impaired if given with attapulgite. Attapulgite must be given not less than 2 hours before or 3 to 4 hours after these drugs; advise clinician to monitor patient for decreased effectiveness.

### Adverse reactions
**GI:** constipation.

### Overdose and treatment
Because attapulgite isn't absorbed, an overdose is unlikely to pose a significant health problem.

### Clinical considerations
- Ensure that patient achieves adequate fluid intake to compensate for fluid loss from diarrhea.
- Drug shouldn't be used if diarrhea is accompanied by fever or blood or mucus in the stool. Discontinue drug if any of these signs occur during treatment.

### Therapeutic monitoring
Advise clinician to monitor patient for signs and symptoms of dehydration.

### Special populations
**Pediatric patients.** Use only under medical supervision in children under age 3.
**Geriatric patients.** Use cautiously and only under medical supervision.

### Patient counseling
- Tell patient to take drug after each loose bowel movement until diarrhea is controlled.
- Instruct patient to call prescriber if diarrhea isn't controlled within 48 hours or if fever develops.

---

# auranofin
Ridaura

*Pharmacologic classification:* gold salt
*Therapeutic classification:* antiarthritic
*Pregnancy risk category C*

## Available forms
Available by prescription only
*Capsules:* 3 mg

## Indications and dosages
*Rheumatoid arthritis in patients whose symptoms progress despite an adequate NSAID regimen,* ◇ *psoriatic arthritis,* ◇ *active systemic lupus erythematosus,* ◇ *Felty's syndrome*
*Adults:* 6 mg P.O. daily, given either as 3 mg b.i.d. or 6 mg once daily. After 4 to 6 months, may be increased to 9 mg daily (3 mg t.i.d.). If response remains inadequate after 3 months at 9 mg daily, discontinue drug.

## Mechanism of action
*Antiarthritic action:* Auranofin suppresses or prevents, but doesn't cure, adult or juvenile arthritis and synovitis. It's anti-inflammatory in active arthritis. This drug is thought to reduce inflammation by altering the immune system. Auranofin has been shown to decrease high serum levels of immunoglobulins and rheumatoid factors in patients with arthritis. However, the exact mechanism of action remains unknown.

## Pharmacokinetics
*Absorption:* When given P.O., 25% of the gold in auranofin is absorbed through the GI tract.
*Distribution:* 60% protein-bound and is distributed widely in body tissues. Oral gold from auranofin is bound to a higher degree than gold from the injectable form. Synovial fluid levels are about 50% of blood levels. No correlation between blood-gold levels and safety or efficacy has been determined.
*Metabolism:* The metabolic fate of auranofin isn't known, but it's believed that drug isn't broken down into elemental gold.
*Excretion:* 60% of absorbed auranofin (15% of the given dose) is excreted in the urine and the remainder in the feces. Average plasma half-life is 26 days, compared with about 6 days for gold sodium thiomalate.

| Route | Onset | Peak | Duration |
|-------|-------|------|----------|
| P.O. | Unknown | 2 hr | Unknown |

## Contraindications and precautions
Contraindicated in patients with history of severe gold toxicity, necrotizing enterocolitis, pulmonary fibrosis, exfoliative dermatitis, bone marrow aplasia, severe hematologic disorders, or history of severe toxicity caused by previous exposure to other heavy metals.

Use cautiously with other drugs that cause blood dyscrasias or in patients with renal, hepatic, or inflammatory bowel disease; rash; or bone marrow depression. Use of drug in pregnant women isn't recommended.

## Interactions
**Drug-drug.** *Other drugs that may cause blood dyscrasias:* May produce additive hematologic toxicity. Advise clinician to monitor hematologic studies.

## Adverse reactions
**CNS:** confusion, hallucinations, *seizures.*
**EENT:** conjunctivitis.
**GI:** *diarrhea, abdominal pain, nausea, stomatitis,* glossitis, anorexia, metallic taste, dyspepsia, flatulence, constipation, dysgeusia, *ulcerative colitis.*
**GU:** proteinuria, hematuria, *nephrotic syndrome,* glomerulonephritis, **acute renal failure.**
**Hematologic:** *thrombocytopenia* (with or without purpura), **aplastic anemia, agranulocytosis, leukopenia,** eosinophilia, anemia.
**Hepatic:** jaundice, elevated liver enzyme levels.
**Respiratory:** interstitial pneumonitis.
**Skin:** *rash, pruritus, dermatitis,* exfoliative dermatitis, urticaria, erythema, alopecia.

## Overdose and treatment
In acute overdose, recommend emptying gastric contents by inducing emesis or performing gastric lavage. When severe reactions to gold occur, corticosteroids, dimercaprol (a chelating agent), or penicillamine may be given to aid recovery. Prednisone 40 to 100 mg daily in divided doses is recommended to manage severe renal, hematologic, pulmonary, or enterocolitic reactions to gold. Dimercaprol may be used with steroids to facilitate the removal of the gold when steroid treatment alone is ineffective. Use of chelating drugs is controversial, and caution is recommended. Appropriate supportive therapy is indicated p.r.n.

## Clinical considerations
■ When switching from injectable gold, initial dose is 6 mg P.O. daily.
■ To encourage patient compliance with follow up, initial prescription should be for 2 weeks and subsequent prescriptions for 1 month.
■ Serum protein-bound iodine test, especially when performed by the chloric acid digestion method, gives false readings during and for several weeks after gold therapy. TB skin test may have an enhanced response. This effect should be considered when results are interpreted.

## Therapeutic monitoring
■ Recommend discontinuing drug if platelet count decreases to below 100,000/mm³.
■ Advise clinician to monitor CBC, platelet count, urinalysis, and kidney and liver function test results before therapy for baseline and then monthly.
■ Patient should be monitored for signs of toxicity, which include leukocyte count less than 400/mm³, granulocyte count less than 1,500/mm³, decreased platelet count to 150,000/mm³, proteinuria, hematuria, pruritus, rash, stomatitis, and persistent diarrhea.
■ Advise clinician to monitor patient for uncontrolled diarrhea; dosage reduction or temporary discontinuance of drug may relieve diarrhea.

## Special populations
**Pregnant patients.** There are no adequate and controlled studies, but clinical experience doesn't indicate evidence of adverse effects on the fetus.
**Breast-feeding patients.** Drug isn't recommended for use during breast-feeding.
**Pediatric patients.** Controlled clinical trials for the treatment of juvenile rheumatoid arthritis in children ages 4 to 16 is ongoing. Safe dosage hasn't been established; use in children currently isn't recommended.
**Geriatric patients.** Give usual adult dose. Use cautiously in patients with decreased renal function.

## Patient counseling
■ Emphasize importance of monthly follow-up to monitor patient's platelet count.
■ Reassure patient that beneficial drug effect may be delayed for 3 months. However, if response is inadequate after 6 to 9 months, auranofin will probably be discontinued.
■ Encourage patient to take drug as prescribed and not to alter the dosage schedule.
■ Diarrhea is the most common adverse reaction. Tell patient to continue taking drug if he experiences mild diarrhea; however, tell him to call prescriber immediately if blood occurs in stool.
■ Tell patient to continue taking concomitant drug therapy, such as NSAIDs, if prescribed.
■ Dermatitis is a common adverse reaction. Advise patient to report rash or other skin problems immediately.
■ Stomatitis is another common adverse reaction. Tell patient that stomatitis is often preceded by a metallic taste and advise him to call his prescriber immediately.

# azathioprine
Imuran

# azathioprine sodium
Imuran

*Pharmacologic classification:* purine antagonist
*Therapeutic classification:* immunosuppressive
*Pregnancy risk category D*

## Available forms
Available by prescription only
*Tablets:* 50 mg
*Injection:* 100 mg per vial

## Indications and dosages
*Prevention of the rejection of kidney transplants*
*Adults and children:* Initially, 3 to 5 mg/kg P.O. daily beginning on day of (or 1 to 3 days before) transplantation. After transplantation, dosage may be given I.V., until patient is able to tolerate oral dosage. Usual maintenance dosage is 1 to 3 mg/kg daily. Dosage varies with patient response.
*Severe, refractory rheumatoid arthritis*
*Adults:* Initially, 1 mg/kg (about 50 to 100 mg) P.O. taken as a single dose or in divided doses. If patient response is unsatisfactory after 6 to 8 weeks, dose may be increased by 0.5 mg/kg daily (up to a maximum of 2.5 mg/kg daily) at 4-week intervals. If no response after 12 weeks, discontinue.

## I.V. administration
■ Reconstitute 100 mg vial with 10 ml of sterile water for injection. The resultant level is 10 mg/ml. Visually inspect for particles before use.
■ Drug may be given by direct I.V. injection or further diluted in normal saline for injection or D₅W and infused over 30 to 60 minutes.

## Incompatibilities
None Reported.

## Mechanism of action
*Immunosuppressant action:* The mechanism of immunosuppressive activity is unknown; however, drug may inhibit RNA and DNA synthesis, mitosis, or (in patients undergoing renal transplantation) coenzyme formation and functioning. Azathioprine suppresses cell-mediated hypersensitivity and alters antibody production.

## Pharmacokinetics
*Absorption:* Well absorbed when taken orally.
*Distribution:* Drug and its major metabolite, mercaptopurine, are distributed throughout the

body; both are 30% protein-bound. Azathioprine and its metabolites cross the placenta.

*Metabolism:* Metabolized primarily to mercaptopurine.

*Excretion:* Small amounts of azathioprine and mercaptopurine are excreted in urine intact; most of a given dose is excreted in urine as secondary metabolites.

| Route | Onset | Peak | Duration |
|-------|-------|------|----------|
| P.O., I.V. | 4-8 wk | 1-2 hr | Several days |

## Contraindications and precautions

Contraindicated in patients hypersensitive to drug and during pregnancy.

Use cautiously in patients with impaired renal or hepatic function.

## Interactions

**Drug-drug.** *ACE inhibitors:* Anemia and severe leukopenia have been reported with use of azathioprine. Use together cautiously.

*Allopurinol:* The major metabolic pathway of azathioprine is inhibited by allopurinol, which competes for the oxidative enzyme xanthine oxidase. Azathioprine with allopurinol is potentially hazardous and should be avoided. If use together is unavoidable, reduce dose by one-third to one-fourth the usual dose.

*Cyclosporine:* Plasma levels of cyclosporine may be decreased. Advise clinician to monitor patient for clinical effect.

*Methotrexate:* May increase plasma levels of the metabolite 6-MP. Advise clinician to monitor patient for toxicity.

*Pancuronium and tubocurarine:* Drug may reverse neuromuscular blockade resulting from use of the nondepolarizing muscle relaxants. Advise clinician to monitor patient for this effect.

## Adverse reactions

**GI:** *nausea, vomiting, **pancreatitis,** steatorrhea, diarrhea, abdominal pain.

**Hematologic:** LEUKOPENIA, *bone marrow suppression,* anemia, *pancytopenia, thrombocytopenia, immunosuppression* (possibly profound).

**Hepatic:** *hepatotoxicity,* jaundice.

**Musculoskeletal:** arthralgia, myalgia.

**Skin:** alopecia, rash.

**Other:** *infections,* fever, *increased risk of neoplasia.*

## Overdose and treatment

Signs and symptoms of overdose include nausea, vomiting, diarrhea, and extension of hematologic effects.

Supportive treatment may include treatment with blood products, if needed.

## Clinical considerations

■ If used to treat rheumatoid arthritis, advise clinician to continue NSAIDs when azathioprine therapy starts.

■ Chronic immunosuppression with azathioprine is linked to an increased risk of neoplasia.

■ Use only in patients who are unable to tolerate oral medications.

■ If infection occurs, recommend reducing drug dosage.

■ If nausea and vomiting occur, dose may be divided or given with or after meals.

### Therapeutic monitoring

■ Advise clinician to monitor patient for signs of hepatic damage: clay-colored stools, dark urine, jaundice, pruritus, and elevated liver enzyme levels.

■ Advise clinician to monitor patient for unusual bleeding or bruising, fever, or sore throat.

■ Advise clinician to monitor hematologic status while patient is receiving azathioprine. CBCs, including platelet counts, should be taken at least weekly during the first month, twice monthly for the second and third months, then monthly.

### Special populations

**Pregnant patients.** May cause fetal harm in pregnant women. Drug may also cause temporary depression of spermatogenesis.

### Patient counseling

■ Explain possible adverse effects of drug and importance of reporting them, especially unusual bleeding or bruising, fever, sore throat, mouth sores, abdominal pain, pale stools, or dark urine.

■ Encourage compliance with therapy and follow-up visits.

■ Advise patient to avoid pregnancy during therapy and for 4 months after stopping therapy.

■ Tell patient with rheumatoid arthritis that clinical response may not be apparent for up to 12 weeks.

■ Suggest taking drug with or after meals or in divided doses to prevent nausea.

# azelastine hydrochloride, ophthalmic solution

Optivar

# azelastine hydrochloride, nasal spray

Astelin

*Pharmacologic classification:* H$_1$-receptor antagonist
*Therapeutic classification:* ophthalmic and nasal antihistamine
*Pregnancy risk category C*

## Available forms
Available by prescription only
*Ophthalmic solution:* 0.05%
*Nasal solution:* 1 mg/ml

## Indications and dosages
*Treatment of itching of the eye associated with allergic conjunctivitis*
*Adults and children ages 3 and older:* One drop instilled into affected eye b.i.d.
*Treatment of the symptoms of seasonal allergic rhinitis such as rhinorrhea, sneezing, and nasal pruritus*
*Adults and children ages 12 and older:* 2 sprays (137 mcg/spray) per nostril b.i.d.
*Children ages 5 to 11:* 1 spray (137 mcg/spray) per nostril b.i.d.
*Treatment of the symptoms of vasomotor rhinitis, such as rhinorrhea, nasal congestion, and postnasal drip*
*Adults and children ages 12 and older:* 2 sprays (137 mcg/spray) per nostril b.i.d.

## Mechanism of action
*Antihistamine action:* Thought to be a relatively selective H$_1$ histamine antagonist. Azelastine inhibits the release of histamine and other mediators from cells, such as mast cells, involved in the allergic response. Also may decrease chemotaxis and activate eosinophils.

## Pharmacokinetics
*Absorption:* Relatively low after ocular administration. After nasal administration, 40% systemically bioavailable.
*Distribution:* Plasma protein–binding of azelastine and desmethylazelastine, an active metabolite, are approximately 88% and 97%, respectively.
*Metabolism:* Oxidatively metabolized by cytochrome P450 enzyme system to desmethylazelastine. The specific P450 isoforms haven't been identified; however, clinical interaction studies with erythromycin didn't inhibit CYP3A4.
*Excretion:* Unknown. Elimination half-life is 22 hours. Excreted in feces with 10% as unchanged drug.

| Route | Onset | Peak | Duration |
|---|---|---|---|
| Ophthalmic | ≤ 3 min | Unknown | About 8 hr |
| Nasal | Unknown | 2-3 hr | 12 hr |

## Contraindications and precautions
Contraindicated in patients hypersensitive to drug or any of its components.

## Interactions
**Drug-lifestyle.** *Alcohol use:* Concurrent use with alcohol or other CNS depressants may cause decreased alertness. Advise patient to avoid alcohol.

## Adverse reactions
**CNS:** fatigue, *headaches, somnolence,* dizziness.
**EENT:** transient eye burning, stinging, nasal burning, conjunctivitis, eye pain, pharyngitis, rhinitis, paroxysmal sneezing, temporary eye blurring, epistaxis, sinusitis.
**GI:** *bitter taste,* dry mouth, nausea.
**Metabolic:** weight increase.
**Respiratory:** asthma, dyspnea.
**Skin:** pruritus.
**Other:** influenza-like symptoms, dysesthesia.

## Overdose and treatment
No information available.

## Clinical considerations
■ Shouldn't be used to treat contact lens–related irritation.
■ The preservative in the eyedrop, benzalkonium, may be absorbed by soft contact lenses.

### Therapeutic monitoring
■ Recommend inspecting eyes and nasal passages for localized adverse reactions.
■ Advise clinician to monitor patient for adverse CNS effects.

### Special populations
**Breast-feeding patients.** It isn't known if azelastine appears in human milk. Use caution when giving to a breast-feeding woman.
**Pediatric patients.** Safety and effectiveness in pediatric patients younger than age 3 haven't been established.

## Patient counseling
■ Instruct patient to prevent contamination of the eyedrops by not touching any surface, the eyelids, or surrounding areas with the dropper tip.
■ Instruct patient to keep bottle tightly closed when not in use.
■ Advise patient not to wear a contact lens if his eye is red.
■ Warn patient that the preservative in the eyedrop, benzalkonium, may be absorbed by soft contact lenses.
■ Tell patient who wears soft contact lenses, and whose eyes aren't red, to wait at least 10 minutes after instilling eyedrop before inserting contact lenses.
■ Warn patient to use caution when driving a car or operating potentially dangerous machinery, or using alcohol or other CNS depressants.

---

* Canada only   ◇ Unlabeled clinical use

■ Instruct patient to prime the nasal pump before initial use and after storage for 3 or more days.
■ Advise against the concurrent use of the nasal spray with other antihistamines without consulting the prescriber.

---

# azithromycin
Zithromax

*Pharmacologic classification:* azalide macrolide
*Therapeutic classification:* antibiotic
*Pregnancy risk category B*

---

## Available forms
Available by prescription only
*Tablets:* 250 mg
*Powder for oral suspension:* 100 mg/5 ml, 200 mg/5 ml; 300 mg*, 600 mg*, 900 mg*, 1,000 mg/packet
*Injection:* 500 mg

## Indications and dosages
**Acute bacterial exacerbations of chronic obstructive pulmonary disease caused by** **Haemophilus influenzae, Moraxella catarrhalis,** *or* **Streptococcus pneumoniae;** *uncomplicated skin and skin-structure infections caused by* **Staphylococcus aureus, Streptococcus pyogenes,** *or* **Streptococcus agalactiae;** *and second-line therapy of pharyngitis or tonsillitis caused by* **S. pyogenes**
*Adults and adolescents age 16 and older:* Initially, 500 mg P.O. as a single dose on day 1, followed by 250 mg daily on days 2 through 5. Total cumulative dose is 1.5 g.
**Community-acquired pneumonia caused by** **Chlamydia pneumoniae, H. influenzae, Mycoplasma pneumoniae, S. pneumoniae;** *I.V. form can be used for above infections and those caused by* **Legionella pneumophila, M. catarrhalis,** *and* **S. aureus**
*Adults and adolescents age 16 and older:* 500 mg P.O. as a single dose on day 1, followed by 250 mg P.O. daily on days 2 to 5. Total dose is 1.5 g. For those who require initial I.V. therapy, 500 mg I.V. as a single daily dose for 2 days, followed by 500 mg P.O. as a single daily dose to complete a 7- to 10-day course of therapy. The timing of the change from I.V. to P.O. therapy should be based on patient's clinical response.
**Nongonococcal urethritis or cervicitis caused by** **Chlamydia trachomatis**
*Adults and adolescents age 16 and older:* 1 g P.O. as a single dose.
**Gonococcal urethritis or cervicitis caused by** **Neisseria gonorrhoeae**
*Adults:* 2 g P.O. given as a single dose.

**Pelvic inflammatory disease caused by** **Chlamydia trachomatis, N. gonorrhoeae,** *or* **Mycoplasma hominis** *in patients requiring initial I.V. therapy*
*Adults:* 500 mg I.V. as a single daily dose for 1 to 2 days, followed by 250 mg P.O. daily to complete a 7-day course of therapy. The timing of the change from I.V. to P.O. therapy should be directed by the prescriber based on patient's clinical response.
**Otitis media**
*Children over age 6 months:* 10 mg/kg dose P.O. on day 1; then 5 mg/kg (maximum dose 250 mg/day) once daily on days 2 to 5.
**Tonsillitis and pharyngitis**
*Children over age 2:* 12 mg/kg (maximum 500 mg/day) P.O. daily for 5 days.
**Chancroid**
*Adults:* 1 g P.O. as a single dose.
◊ *Infants and children:* 20 mg/kg (maximum of 1 g) as a single oral dose
**Prevention of disseminated Mycobacterium avium** *complex (MAC) in patients with advanced HIV infection*
*Adults:* 1.2 g P.O. once weekly alone or with rifabutin.
◊ *Children:* 20 mg/kg P.O. (maximum of 1.2 g) weekly or 5 mg/kg (maximum of 250 mg) can be given P.O. daily.
◊ **Prophylaxis of bacterial endocarditis in penicillin-allergic adults at moderate to high risk**
*Adults:* 500 mg 1 hour before the procedure.
◊ **Chlamydial ophthalmia neonatorum**
*Infants:* 20 mg/kg once daily P.O. for 3 days.

## I.V. administration
■ Use a standard 5-ml (nonautomated) syringe to ensure withdrawl of exact volume.
■ Reconstitute 500-mg vial with 4.8 ml of sterile water for injection. Shake well until drug is dissolved (yields a level of 100 mg/ml). Dilute solution further in at least 250 ml of normal saline, 0.45% saline, $D_5W$, or lactated Ringer's solution to yield a level range of 1 to 2 mg/ml.
**⛓ ALERT** Recommend infusion of 500-mg dose of azithromycin I.V. over 1 or more hours. Don't give as a bolus or I.M. injection.

### Incompatibilities
None reported.

## Mechanism of action
*Antibiotic action:* Azithromycin, a derivative of erythromycin, binds to the 50S subunit of bacterial ribosomes, blocking protein synthesis. It is bacteriostatic or bactericidal, depending on level. Azithromycin is effective against many gram-positive and gram-negative aerobic and anaerobic bacteria in addition to *Borrelia burgdorferi, Chlamydia pneumoniae, C. trachomatis, Mycoplasma pneumoniae,* and MAC.

---

## Pharmacokinetics

*Absorption:* Rapidly absorbed from the GI tract; food decreases both maximum plasma levels and amount of drug absorbed.

*Distribution:* Rapidly distributed throughout the body and readily penetrates cells; it doesn't readily enter the CNS. It concentrates in fibroblasts and phagocytes. Significantly higher levels of drug are reached in the tissues as compared with the plasma. Uptake and release of drug from tissues contributes to the long half-life. With a loading dose, peak and trough blood levels are stable within 48 hours. Without a loading dose, 5 to 7 days are required before steady state is reached.

*Metabolism:* Not metabolized.

*Excretion:* Excreted mostly in the feces after excretion into the bile. Less than 10% is excreted in the urine. Terminal elimination half-life is 68 hours.

| Route | Onset | Peak | Duration |
|---|---|---|---|
| P.O. | Unknown | 2½-4½ hr | Unknown |
| I.V. | Unknown | Unknown | Unknown |

## Contraindications and precautions

Contraindicated in patients hypersensitive to erythromycin or other macrolides.

Use cautiously in patients with impaired hepatic function.

## Interactions

**Drug-drug.** *Aluminum- and magnesium-containing antacids:* May result in lower peak plasma levels of azithromycin. Recommend separating administration times by at least 2 hours.

*Dihydroergotamine or ergotamine :* Acute ergot toxicity has been reported when macrolides have been given with dihydroergotamine or ergotamine. Use together cautiously.

*Drugs metabolized by the hepatic cytochrome P-450 system (such as barbiturates, carbamazepine, cyclosporine, and phenytoin):* May result in impaired metabolism of these drugs and increased risk of toxicity. Advise clinician to monitor patient for signs of drug toxicity.

*Theophylline:* Macrolides may increase plasma theophylline levels by decreasing theophylline clearance. Advise clinician to monitor theophylline levels carefully.

*Triazolam:* Clearance of triazolam may be decreased, increasing the risk of triazolam toxicity. Advise clinician to monitor patient for signs of drug toxicity.

*Warfarin:* Other macrolides may increase PT and INR; effect of azithromycin is unknown. Advise clinician to monitor PT and INR carefully.

## Adverse reactions

**CNS:** dizziness, vertigo, headache, fatigue, somnolence, anxiety, aggressive reaction.

**CV:** palpitations, chest pain.

**GI:** *nausea, vomiting, diarrhea, abdominal pain,* dyspepsia, flatulence, melena, cholestatic jaundice, pseudomembranous colitis.

**GU:** candidiasis, vaginitis, nephritis.

**Hepatic:** *hepatic necrosis, hepatic failure.*

**Skin:** rash, photosensitivity.

**Other:** *angioedema.*

## Overdose and treatment

No information available. Treat symptomatically.

## Clinical considerations

- Azithromycin has been used investigationally in *H. pylori* regimens, infections caused by *Bartonella,* Lyme disease caused by *Borrelia burgdorferi, Toxoplasma gondii* encephalitis, babesiosis, granuloma inguanale, and AIDS-related cryptosporidiosis.

- Advise clinician to obtain culture and sensitivity tests before giving first dose. Therapy can begin before results are obtained.

- Oral form shouldn't be used for moderate to severe pneumonia or when complicating risk factors exist.

### Therapeutic monitoring

- Advise clinician to monitor liver enzymes, especially in patients with impaired renal function.

- Recommend serologic tests for syphilis and cultures for gonorrhea in patients diagnosed with sexually transmitted urethritis or cervicitis. Drug shouldn't be used to treat gonorrhea or syphilis.

- Drug may cause overgrowth of nonsusceptible bacteria or fungi. Watch for signs and symptoms of superinfection.

### Special populations

**Pregnant patients.** Preliminary studies have proven drug to be safe for the treatment of chlamydial infection in pregnant women, but there are insufficient data for routine use.

**Breast-feeding patients.** It's unknown if drug appears in breast milk. Use cautiously in breast-feeding women.

**Pediatric patients.** Safety and efficacy in children age 16 and under for I.V. administration and 6 months and under for P.O. administration haven't been established.

**Geriatric patients.** In clinical trials of patients with normal hepatic and renal function, in using the 5-day dosage regimen, no significant pharmacokinetic differences were seen in those between ages 65 and 85.

## Patient counseling

- Tell patient to take all of drug prescribed, even if he's feeling better.

- Remind patient that drug should always be taken on an empty stomach because food or antacids decrease absorption. Patient should

---

take drug 1 hour before or 2 hours after a meal and shouldn't take antacids.
■ Instruct patient to promptly report adverse reactions.

# aztreonam
Azactam

*Pharmacologic classification:* monobactam
*Therapeutic classification:* antibiotic
*Pregnancy risk category B*

## Available forms
Available by prescription only
*Injection:* 500-mg, 1-g, 2-g vials

## Indications and dosages
***Urinary tract, respiratory tract, intra-abdominal, gynecologic, or skin infections; septicemia caused by gram-negative bacteria;*** ◇ *adjunct therapy in pelvic inflammatory disease;* ◇ *gonorrhea*
*Adults:* 500 mg to 2 g I.V. or I.M. q 8 to 12 hours. For severe systemic or life-threatening infections, 2 g q 6 to 8 hours may be given. Maximum dose is 8 g daily. For gonorrhea, give 1 g I.M. single dose.
**≡ *Dosage adjustment.*** In patients with a creatinine clearance of 10 to 30 ml/minute, reduce dose by one-half after an initial dose of 1 to 2 g. In patients with a creatinine clearance below 10 ml/minute, an initial dose of 500 mg to 2 g should be followed by one-fourth of the usual dose at the usual intervals; give one-eighth the initial dose after each session of hemodialysis.

## I.V. administration
■ To reconstitute for I.M. use, dilute with at least 3 ml of sterile water for injection, bacteriostatic water for injection, normal saline solution, or bacteriostatic normal saline solution for each gram of aztreonam (15-ml vial).
■ To reconstitute for I.V. use, add 6 to 10 ml of sterile water for injection to each 15-ml vial; for I.V. infusion, prepare as for I.M. solution. May be further diluted by adding to normal saline, Ringer's solution, lactated Ringer's solution, $D_5W$, $D_{10}W$, or other electrolyte-containing solutions. For I.V. piggyback (100-ml bottles), add at least 50 ml of diluent for each gram of aztreonam. Final level shouldn't exceed 20 mg/ml.
■ I.V. route is preferred for doses larger than 1 g or in patients with bacterial septicemia, localized parenchymal abscesses, peritonitis, or other life-threatening infections; give by direct I.V. push over 3 to 5 minutes or by intermittent infusion over 20 to 60 minutes.

## Incompatibilities
Incompatible with ampicillin sodium, amsacrine, cephradine, metronidazole, nafcillin, and vancomycin. Shouldn't be mixed with any drug.

## Mechanism of action
*Antibacterial action:* Aztreonam is a monobactam that inhibits mucopeptide synthesis of the bacterial cell wall. It preferentially binds to penicillin-binding protein 3 (PBP3) of susceptible organisms and often causes cell lysis and cell death.

Aztreonam has a narrow spectrum of activity and is usually bactericidal in action. Aztreonam is effective against *Escherichia coli, Enterobacter, Klebsiella pneumoniae, Proteus mirabilis,* and *Pseudomonas aeruginosa.* It has limited activity against *Citrobacter, Haemophilus influenzae, K. oxytoca, Hafnia, Serratia marcescens, E. aerogenes, Morganella morganii, Providencia, Moraxella catarrhalis, Proteus vulgaris,* and *Neisseria gonorrhoeae.*

## Pharmacokinetics
*Absorption:* Distributed rapidly and completely after I.M. or I.V. administration.
*Distribution:* Distributed widely to all body fluids and tissues, including bile, breast milk, and CSF. It crosses the placental barrier and is found in fetal circulation.
*Metabolism:* From 6% to 16% is metabolized to inactive metabolites by nonspecific hydrolysis of the beta-lactam ring; 56% to 60% is protein-bound, less if renal impairment is present.
*Excretion:* Excreted principally in urine as unchanged drug by glomerular filtration and tubular secretion; 1½% to 3½% is excreted in feces as unchanged drug. Half-life averages 1¾ hours. Drug appears in breast milk; it may be removed by hemodialysis and peritoneal dialysis.

| Route | Onset | Peak | Duration |
|---|---|---|---|
| I.V. | Unknown | Immediate | Unknown |
| I.M. | Unknown | < 1 hr | Unknown |

## Contraindications and precautions
Contraindicated in patients hypersensitive to drug.
Use cautiously in patients with impaired renal function and in the elderly.

## Interactions
**Drug-drug.** *Aminoglycosides, or other beta-lactam antibiotics, including cefoperazone, cefotaxime, clindamycin, metronidazole, or piperacillin:* Synergistic or additive effects occur. Avoid use together.
*Chloramphenicol:* Antagonistic reaction. Advise staff to give the two preparations several hours apart.

---

*Clavulanic acid:* May be synergistic or antagonistic, depending on organism involved. Avoid use together.

*Potent inducers of beta-lactamase production (cefoxitin, imipenem):* May inactivate aztreonam. Avoid use together.

*Probenecid:* May prolong the rate of tubular secretion of aztreonam. Avoid use together.

## Adverse reactions

**CNS:** *seizures,* headache, insomnia, confusion.
**CV:** hypotension.
**GI:** diarrhea, nausea, vomiting.
**GU:** transient elevation of creatinine.
**Hematologic:** *neutropenia,* anemia, *pancytopenia, thrombocytopenia,* leukocytosis, thrombocytosis.
**Hepatic:** transient elevation of LDH, ALT, and AST.
**Other:** hypersensitivity reactions (rash, *anaphylaxis*), thrombophlebitis (at I.V. site); discomfort, swelling (at I.M. injection site).

## Overdose and treatment

No information is available on the symptoms of overdose. Hemodialysis or peritoneal dialysis increases elimination of aztreonam.

## Clinical considerations

■ Drug has also been used to treat bone and joint infection caused by susceptible aerobic, gram-negative bacteria.
■ Solutions may be colorless or light straw yellow. On standing, they may develop a slight pink tint; potency isn't affected.
■ Drug may be stored at controlled room temperature for 48 hours or in refrigerator for 7 days.
■ Aztreonam therapy alters urinary glucose determinations using cupric sulfate (Clinitest or Benedict's solution) and gives false-positive Coombs' test results.

### Therapeutic monitoring

■ Advise clinician to monitor renal and hepatic function test results. Reduced dosage may be required in patients with impaired renal function, cirrhosis, or other hepatic impairment.
■ Recommend testing for *Clostridium difficile* in patients with prolonged diarrhea.

### Special populations

**Pregnant patients.** There are no adequate and controlled studies for use in pregnant women.
**Breast-feeding patients.** Although drug appears in breast milk, it isn't absorbed from infant's GI tract and is unlikely to cause any serious problems.
**Pediatric patients.** Manufacturer doesn't recommend use of drug in infants under age 1 month.
**Geriatric patients.** Studies in patients ages 65 to 75 have shown that the half-life of aztreonam may be prolonged in geriatric patients because of their diminished renal function.

## Patient counseling

Tell patient to call prescriber immediately if rash, redness, or itching develops.

**B**

# bacillus Calmette-Guérin (BCG), live
TheraCys, TICE BCG

*Pharmacologic classification:* biological response modifier
*Therapeutic classification:* antineoplastic
*Pregnancy risk category C*

## Available forms
Available by prescription only
*Suspension (powder form):* 50 mg/vial, 81 mg/vial

## Indications and dosages
*Treatment of in situ carcinoma of the urinary bladder (primary and relapsed)*
*Adults:* Consult published protocols, specialized references, and manufacturer's recommendations.

Typical dose is 1 to $8 \times 10^8$ colony-forming units (CFUs). Be aware that FDA has reported errors in some treatment protocols giving 10 times the recommended dose.

## Mechanism of action
*Antitumor action:* Exact mechanism unknown. Instillation of the live bacterial suspension causes a local inflammatory response. Local infiltration of histiocytes and leukocytes is followed by a decrease in the superficial tumors within the bladder.

*Antituberculotic action:* Mycobacterium bovis present in the vaccine is immunologically similar to *M. tuberculosis*; vaccination stimulates natural infection with *M. tuberculosis* and promotes cell-mediated immunity.

## Pharmacokinetics
No information available.

| Route | Onset | Peak | Duration |
|-------|-------|------|----------|
| Intravesical | Unknown | Unknown | Unknown |

## Contraindications and precautions
Contraindicated in immunocompromised patients, in those receiving immunosuppressive therapy, and in those with urinary tract infection or fever of unknown origin. If fever is caused by infection, drug should be withheld until patient recovers.

## Interactions
**Drug-drug.** *Antimicrobial therapy for other infections:* May attenuate the response to BCG live. Avoid use together.
*Drugs that depress the bone marrow; radiation therapy; and immunosuppressants:* May impair the response to BCG intravesical because these treatments can decrease the patient's immune response. These treatments may also increase the risk of osteomyelitis or disseminated BCG infection. Avoid use together.

## Adverse reactions
**CNS:** *malaise.*
**GI:** *nausea, vomiting, anorexia,* diarrhea.
**GU:** *dysuria, urinary frequency, hematuria, cystitis, urinary urgency,* nocturia, urinary incontinence, *urinary tract infection,* cramps, pain, decreased bladder capacity, renal toxicity, genital pain.
**Hematologic:** anemia, *leukopenia.*
**Hepatic:** elevated liver enzyme levels.
**Musculoskeletal:** myalgia, arthralgia.
**Other:** hypersensitivity reaction, *fever, chills, disseminated mycobacterial infection.*

## Overdose and treatment
Advise clinician to closely monitor the patient for signs of systemic BCG infection. Consult an infections disease specialist experienced in BCG complications.

## Clinical considerations
**⚠ ALERT** Drug isn't for I.V. use.
■ Reconstitute drug just before use, using only diluent provided. All persons handling drug should wear masks and gloves.
■ Handle drug and all material used for instillation of the drug as infectious material because it contains live attenuated mycobacteria. Dispose of all associated materials (syringes, catheters, and containers) as biohazardous waste.
■ The vial of TheraCys should be reconstituted with 3 ml of the supplied diluent. Don't remove the rubber stopper to prepare the solution. Further dilute in 50 ml of sterile, preservative-free saline (final volume, 53 ml). A urethral catheter is instilled into the bladder under aseptic conditions, the bladder is drained, and then the prepared solution is added by gravity feed. The catheter is then removed.
■ Advise clinician to use strict aseptic technique to give drug, to minimize the trauma to

the GU tract and prevent introduction of other contaminants to the area.

■ If there's evidence of traumatic catheterization, drug shouldn't be given, and treatment should be delayed for at least 1 week. Subsequent treatment may resume as if no interruption of the schedule has occurred.

■ Bladder irritation can be treated symptomatically with phenazopyridine, acetaminophen, and propantheline bromide. Systemic adverse reactions that are caused by hypersensitivity can be treated with diphenhydramine hydrochloride.

■ Protect drug from light and store at below 41° F (5° C). Drug expires 1 year after date of issue if stored at this temperature.

### Therapeutic monitoring
■ Advise clinician to monitor patient for cystitis and hematuria.

### Special populations
**Breast-feeding patients.** It isn't known if drug appears in breast milk. Use with caution in breast-feeding women.
**Pediatric patients.** Safety in children hasn't been established.

### Patient counseling
■ After instillation, patient should retain the fluid in bladder for 2 hours (if possible). For the first hour, patient should lie 15 minutes prone, 15 minutes supine, and 15 minutes on each side. Patient may be up for the second hour.

■ For safety, patient should be seated when voiding. Instruct patient to disinfect urine for 6 hours after instillation of drug. Tell patient to add undiluted household bleach (5% sodium hypochlorite solution) to the toilet in equal volume to voided urine; let stand for 15 minutes before flushing.

■ Tell patient to call prescriber if symptoms worsen or if any of the following occur: blood in the urine, fever and chills, frequent urge to urinate or painful urination, nausea, vomiting, joint pain, rash, or cough.

---

# bacitracin
AK-Tracin, Altracin, Baciguent, Baci-IM

*Pharmacologic classification:* polypeptide antibiotic
*Therapeutic classification:* antibiotic
*Pregnancy risk category C*

### Available forms
Available without a prescription
*Topical:* ointment form (500 units/g) and in combination products containing neomycin, polymyxin B, and bacitracin
Available by prescription only

*Injection:* 50,000-unit vials
*Ophthalmic ointment:* 500 units/g

## Indications and dosages
*Topical infections, impetigo, abrasions, cuts, and minor wounds*
*Adults and children:* Apply thin film to cleansed area once daily to t.i.d. for no longer than 7 days.
*Pneumonia and empyema caused by a staphylococcal infection*
*Children weighing under 2.5 kg (5.5 lb):* Give 900 units/kg I.M. daily in two or three divided doses.
*Children weighing over 2.5 kg:* Give 1,000 units/kg I.M. daily in two or three divided doses.
◊*Adults:* 10,000 to 25,000 units I.M. q 6 hours not to exceed 100,000 units per day.
◊ *Treatment of antibiotic-associated pseudomembranous colitis caused by* **Clostridium difficile**
*Adults:* 20,000 to 25,000 units P.O. q 6 hours for 7 to 10 days.
*Short-term topical treatment of superficial infections of the eye involving the conjunctiva and cornea caused by bacitracin-susceptible organisms*
*Adults and children:* Apply ophthalmic ointment to affected area 1 or more times daily.

## Mechanism of action
*Antibacterial action:* Bacitracin impairs bacterial cell wall synthesis, damaging the bacterial plasma membrane and making the cell more vulnerable to osmotic pressure. Drug is effective against many gram-positive organisms, such as staphylococci, streptococci, anaerobic cocci, corynebacteria, and *C. difficile.* The drug is also effective against gonococci, meningococci, fusobacteria, *Actinomyces israelii, Treponema pallidum,* and *Treponema vincenti.* Drug is only minimally active against gram-negative organisms.

## Pharmacokinetics
*Absorption:* With I.M. administration, drug is absorbed rapidly and completely; serum levels range from 0.2 to 2 mcg/ml. Drug isn't absorbed from the GI tract and isn't significantly absorbed from intact or denuded skin wounds or mucous membranes.
*Distribution:* Distributed widely throughout all body organs and fluids except CSF (unless meninges are inflamed). Binding to plasma protein is minimal.
*Metabolism:* Not significantly metabolized.
*Excretion:* When given I.M., the kidneys excrete 10% to 40% of dose.

| Route | Onset | Peak | Duration |
|---|---|---|---|
| I.M. | Unknown | 1-2 hr | Unknown |
| Ophthalmic, topical | Unknown | Unknown | Unknown |

---

## Contraindications and precautions
Contraindicated in patients hypersensitive to drug and in atopic patients.

Use cautiously in patients with myasthenia gravis and neuromuscular disease.

## Interactions
**Drug-drug.** *Anesthetics or neuromuscular blockers:* Prolonged or increased neuromuscular blockade. Advise clinician to carefully monitor patient.

*Other nephrotoxic drugs:* Systemically given bacitracin may induce additive damage when given with bacitracin. Give together cautiously.

## Adverse reactions
**CV:** tightness in chest, hypotension.
**EENT:** slowed corneal wound healing, temporary visual haze (with ophthalmic form), ototoxicity (when topical form is used over large areas for prolonged periods or with systemic use).
**GU:** *nephrotoxicity, renal failure.*
**Skin:** stinging, rash, other allergic reactions; pruritus, burning, swelling of lips or face (with topical form).
**Other:** hypersensitivity reactions; overgrowth of nonsusceptible organisms (with ophthalmic form).

## Overdose and treatment
With parenteral administration over several days, bacitracin may cause nephrotoxicity. Acute oral overdose may cause nausea, vomiting, and minor GI upset. Treatment is supportive.

## Clinical considerations
■ Bacitracin is used orally as an intestinal antiseptic. Sterile solutions have been injected intrathecally for the treatment of meningitis, intraperitoneally for peritoneal infections, intrapleurally for staphylococcal empyema, and intrasynovially after surgical treatment of chronic osteomyelitis.
■ Culture and sensitivity tests should be performed before starting treatment.
■ Patients allergic to neomycin may also be allergic to bacitracin.
■ Injectable forms of drug may be used for I.M. administration only; I.V. administration may cause severe thrombophlebitis. Dilute injectable drug in solution containing sodium chloride and 2% procaine hydrochloride (if hospital policy permits). After reconstitution, bacitracin level should range from 5,000 to 10,000 units/ml. Inject deeply into upper outer quadrant of buttocks (may be painful). Don't give if patient is sensitive to procaine or para-aminobenzoic acid derivatives.
■ Drug may be used orally with neomycin as bowel preparation or in solution as wound-irrigating drug.

## Therapeutic monitoring
■ Advise clinician to obtain baseline renal function test results before therapy starts and monitoring results daily for signs of deterioration.
■ Advise clinician to ensure adequate fluid intake and monitoring output closely.
■ Advise clinician to monitor patient's urine pH. It should be kept above 6 with good hydration; alkalinizing drugs (such as sodium bicarbonate) should be given, if needed, to limit nephrotoxicity.

## Special populations
**Pregnant patients.** Bacitracin shouldn't be used in pregnancy.

## Patient counseling
■ Advise patient to discontinue topical use of drug and to call prescriber promptly if condition worsens or doesn't respond to treatment.
■ Warn patient with a skin infection to avoid sharing washcloths and towels with family members.
■ Instruct patient to wash hands before and after applying ointment.
■ Advise patient using ophthalmic ointment to clean eye area of excess exudate before applying ointment. Warn him not to touch tip of tube to any part of eye or surrounding tissue.
■ Warn patient that ophthalmic ointment may cause blurred vision. Tell him to stop drug immediately and report symptoms of sensitivity, such as itchy eyelids or constant burning.
■ Instruct patient to store ophthalmic ointment in tightly closed, light-resistant container.
■ Caution patient not to share eye medications with other persons.

# baclofen
Atrophen, Lioresal

*Pharmacologic classification:* chlorophenyl derivative
*Therapeutic classification:* skeletal muscle relaxant
*Pregnancy risk category C*

## Available forms
Available by prescription only
*Tablets:* 10 mg, 20 mg
*Intrathecal kit:* 50 mcg/ml, 0.5 mg/ml, 2 mg/ml

## Indications and dosages
*Spasticity in multiple sclerosis and other spinal cord lesions*
*Adults:* Initially, 5 mg P.O. t.i.d. for 3 days. Dosage may be increased (based on response) at 3-day intervals by 15 mg (5 mg/dose) daily up to maximum of 80 mg daily. For geriatric patients, increase oral dose more gradually.
**Intrathecal administration**
Must be diluted with sterile, preservative-free normal saline injection.

*Adults:* Initial intrathecal bolus of 50 mcg in 1 ml over ≥ 1 minute. Observe patient for response over subsequent 4 to 8 hours. A positive response consists of a significant decrease in muscle tone or frequency or severity of spasm. If initial response is inadequate, repeat dose with 75 mcg in 1.5 ml 24 hours after last injection. Repeat observation of patient over 4 to 8 hours. If the response is still inadequate, repeat dosing at 100 mcg in 2 ml 24 hours later. If still no response, patient shouldn't be considered for an implantable pump for chronic baclofen administration. Ranges for chronic doses are 12 to 2,003 mcg/day.

*Children under age 12:* Test dose is the same as for adults (50 mcg); but for very small pediatric patients, an initial dose of 25 mcg may be given. Maintenance dosage averages 274 mcg daily (range 24 to 1,200 mcg daily).

**Postimplant dose titration**
If the screening dose produced the desired effect for over 8 hours, the initial intrathecal dose is the same as the test dose; this dose is infused intrathecally for 24 hours. If the screening dose produced the desired effect for less than 8 hours, the initial intrathecal dose is twice the test dose, followed slowly by 10% to 30% increments at 24-hour intervals.

## Mechanism of action

*Skeletal muscle relaxant action:* Precise mechanism of action is unknown, but drug appears to act at the spinal cord level to inhibit transmission of monosynaptic and polysynaptic reflexes, possibly through hyperpolarization of afferent fiber terminals. It may also act at supraspinal sites because baclofen at high doses produces generalized CNS depression. Baclofen decreases the number and severity of spasms and relieves associated pain, clonus, and muscle rigidity and therefore improves mobility.

## Pharmacokinetics

*Absorption:* Rapidly and extensively absorbed from the GI tract, but is subject to individual variation. As dose increases, rate and extent of absorption decrease. Onset of therapeutic effect may not be immediately evident, varying from hours to weeks. Peak effect is seen at 2 to 3 hours.

*Distribution:* Studies indicate that baclofen is widely distributed throughout body, with small amounts crossing the blood-brain barrier. About 30% is plasma protein–bound.

*Metabolism:* About 15% is metabolized in the liver via deamination.

*Excretion:* 70% to 80% appears in urine unchanged or as its metabolites; remainder, in feces.

| Route | Onset | Peak | Duration |
|---|---|---|---|
| P.O. | Hrs-wks | 2-3 hr | Unknown |
| Intrathecal | ½-1 hr | 4 hr | 4-8 hr |

## Contraindications and precautions

Contraindicated in patients hypersensitive to drug.

Use cautiously in patients with renal impairment or seizure disorders and when spasticity is used to maintain motor function.

## Interactions

**Drug-drug.** *Antidiabetics or insulin:* Baclofen may increase blood glucose levels and require dosage adjustments of antidiabetic or insulin. Advise clinician to monitor serum glucose levels.

*CNS depressant drugs, including antipsychotics, anxiolytics, general anesthetics, and narcotics:* May add to the CNS effects of drug. Use together cautiously.

*MAO inhibitors or tricyclic antidepressants:* May cause CNS depression, respiratory depression, and hypotension. Avoid use together.

**Drug-lifestyle.** *Alcohol use:* May add to the CNS effects of drug. Advise patient to avoid alcohol.

## Adverse reactions

**CNS:** CNS depression *(potentially life-threatening with intrathecal administration)*, drowsiness, dizziness, headache, *weakness, fatigue, hypotonia, confusion,* insomnia, dysarthria, *seizures.*

**CV:** *CV collapse* (secondary to CNS depression), hypotension, hypertension.

**EENT:** blurred vision, nasal congestion, slurred speech.

**GI:** *nausea,* constipation, *vomiting.*

**GU:** urinary frequency.

**Hepatic:** increased AST and alkaline phosphatase levels.

**Metabolic:** hyperglycemia, weight gain.

**Respiratory:** *respiratory failure,* dyspnea.

**Skin:** rash, pruritus, excessive perspiration.

## Overdose and treatment

Signs and symptoms of overdose include absence of reflexes, vomiting, muscular hypotonia, marked salivation, drowsiness, visual disorders, seizures, respiratory depression, and coma.

Treatment requires supportive measures, including endotracheal intubation and positive-pressure ventilation. If patient is conscious, advise removing drug by induced emesis followed by gastric lavage.

If patient is comatose, don't induce emesis. Gastric lavage may be performed after endotracheal tube is in place with cuff inflated. Don't use respiratory stimulants. Advise clinician to monitor vital signs closely.

## Clinical considerations

■ Intrathecal administration should be performed only by qualified individuals familiar with administration techniques and patient management problems.

**H ALERT** Risk of adverse reactions may be reduced by slowly decreasing the dosage. Abrupt withdrawal may cause hallucinations or seizures and acute exacerbation of spasticity.

■ Baclofen is used investigationally to reduce choreiform movements in Huntington's chorea; to reduce rigidity in Parkinson's disease; to reduce spasticity in CVA, cerebral lesions, cerebral palsy, and rheumatic disorders; to reduce pain in trigeminal neuralgia; and to treat unstable bladder.

■ In some patients, smoother response may be obtained by giving daily dose in four divided doses.

■ Patient may need supervision during walking. The initial loss of spasticity induced by baclofen may affect patient's ability to stand or walk. In some patients, spasticity helps patient to maintain upright posture and balance.

■ Drug should be stopped if signs of improvement don't occur within 1 to 2 months.

■ Implantable pump or catheter failure may result in sudden loss of effectiveness of intrathecal baclofen.

■ During prolonged intrathecal baclofen therapy for spasticity, about 10% of patients become refractory to baclofen therapy requiring a "drug holiday" to regain sensitivity to its effects.

■ Store tablets in a tight container.

■ Store baclofen at temperatures not exceeding 86° F (30° C). Don't freeze. Each vial is for individual use. Use only sterile, preservative-free normal saline for injection for dilution. Baclofen must be diluted to a level of 50 mcg/ml before it is injected into the subarachnoid space.

**Therapeutic monitoring**
■ Advise clinician to routinely monitor blood glucose levels in diabetic patients.

■ Patient's response to drug should be observed. Signs of effective therapy may appear in a few hours to 1 week and may include diminished frequency of spasms and severity of foot and ankle clonus, increased ease and range of joint motion, and enhanced performance of daily activities.

■ Patients with epilepsy may have increased risk of seizures. Advise clinician to closely monitor epileptic patients by EEG, clinical observation, and interview for possible loss of seizure control.

**Special populations**
**Pediatric patients.** Use of oral form isn't recommended for children younger than age 12. Safety of intrathecal administration in children younger than age 4 hasn't been established.
**Geriatric patients.** Geriatric patients are especially sensitive to drug. Advise clinician to carefully observe patient for adverse reactions,

such as mental confusion, depression, and hallucinations. Lower doses are usually indicated.

**Patient counseling**
■ Advise patient to report adverse reactions promptly. Most can be reduced by decreasing dosage. Reportedly, drowsiness, dizziness, and ataxia are more common in patients older than age 40.

■ Warn patient of additive effects with use of other CNS depressants, including alcohol.

■ Caution patient to avoid hazardous activities that require mental alertness.

■ Tell diabetic patient that baclofen may elevate blood glucose levels and may require adjustment of insulin dosage during treatment with baclofen. Urge patient to promptly report changes in urine or blood glucose tests.

■ Caution patient against taking OTC drugs without medical approval. Explain that hazardous drug interactions are possible.

■ Inform patient that drug should be withdrawn gradually over 1 to 2 weeks. Abrupt withdrawal after prolonged use of drug may cause anxiety, agitated behavior, auditory and visual hallucinations, severe tachycardia, and acute spasticity.

# balsalazide disodium
Colazal

*Pharmacologic classification:* gastrointestinal drug
*Therapeutic classification:* anti-inflammatory
*Pregnancy risk category B*

## Available forms
Available by prescription only
*Capsules:* 750 mg

## Indications and dosages
*Treatment of ulcerative colitis*
Adults: 2.25 grams P.O. t.i.d. (three 750-mg capsules) for a total of 6.75 g/day for 8 weeks.

## Mechanism of action
*Anti-inflammatory action:* Balsalazide is converted to mesalamine in the colon, which is then converted to 5-aminosalicylic acid. The mechanism of action is unknown, but it appears to be topical. It may decrease inflammation by blocking production of arachidonic acid metabolites in the colon.

## Pharmacokinetics
*Absorption:* Systemic absorption is very low and variable in healthy patients. Absorption is 60 times greater in patients with ulcerative colitis.
*Distribution:* Drug is plasma protein–bound.

*Metabolism:* Metabolized to mesalamine (5-aminosalicylic acid), the active component of the drug.
*Excretion:* Excreted by the kidneys. Less than 1% of dose recovered in the urine.

| Route | Onset | Peak | Duration |
|-------|-------|------|----------|
| P.O. | Unknown | Unknown | Unknown |

## Contraindications and precautions
Contraindicated in patients hypersensitive to salicylates or to any of the components of capsules or balsalazide metabolites.
    Use cautiously in patients with history of renal disease or renal dysfunction.

## Interactions
**Drug-drug.** *Oral antibiotics:* May interfere with the release of mesalamine in the colon. Advise clinician to monitor patient for effect.

## Adverse reactions
**CNS:** dizziness, fatigue, headache, insomnia.
**EENT:** pharyngitis, rhinitis, sinusitis.
**GI:** abdominal pain, anorexia, constipation, cramps, diarrhea, dyspepsia, flatulence, frequent stools, nausea, rectal bleeding, vomiting, dry mouth.
**GU:** urinary tract infection.
**Musculoskeletal:** arthralgia, back pain, myalgia.
**Respiratory:** cough, respiratory infection.
**Other:** fever, flulike disorder, pain.

## Overdose and treatment
No case of overdose has been reported. If an overdose occurs, treatment should be supportive, with monitoring and correction of electrolyte abnormalities.

## Clinical considerations
■ Safety and effectiveness for longer than 12 weeks haven't been established.
■ Patients with pyloric stenosis may have prolonged retention of drug.

### Therapeutic monitoring
Hepatotoxicity, including elevated liver function test results, jaundice, cirrhosis, liver necrosis, and liver failure, may occur with other products containing or metabolized to mesalamine. Although no signs of hepatotoxicity have been reported with Colazal, advise clinician to monitor patient closely for signs and symptoms of hepatic dysfunction.

### Special populations
**Breast-feeding patients.** It's unknown if balsalazide appears in breast milk. Use caution when giving drug to a breast-feeding woman.
**Pediatric patients.** The safety and effectiveness in pediatric patients haven't been established.

## Patient counseling
■ Advise patients allergic to aspirin not to take drug.
■ Instruct patient to swallow capsules whole.
■ Advise patient to report adverse reactions promptly.

# basiliximab
Simulect

*Pharmacologic classification:* recombinant chimeric human monoclonal antibody $IgG_{1K}$
*Therapeutic classification:* immunosuppressant
*Pregnancy risk category B*

## Available forms
Available by prescription only
*Injection:* 20-mg single-dose vials

## Indications and dosages
**Prophylaxis of acute organ rejection in patients receiving renal transplant when used as part of immunosuppressive regimen including cyclosporine and corticosteroids**
*Adults:* 20 mg I.V. given within 2 hours before transplant surgery and 20 mg I.V. given 4 days after transplantation.
*Children weighing under 35 kg (77 lb):* Two doses of 10 mg given by I.V. bolus on days 0 and 4 after transplant.
*Children weighing over 35 kg:* Two doses of 20 mg, given by I.V. bolus on days 0 and 4 after transplant.

## I.V. administration
■ Reconstitute with 5 ml sterile water for injection. Shake vial gently to dissolve powder. Dilute reconstituted solution to volume of 50 ml with normal saline solution or $D_5W$ for infusion. When mixing solution, gently invert bag to avoid foaming. Don't shake.
■ Drug should be infused over 20 to 30 minutes via a central or peripheral vein. Don't add or infuse other drugs simultaneously through same I.V. line.
■ Use reconstituted solution immediately; otherwise, refrigerate at 36° to 46° F (2° to 8° C) for up to 24 hours or at controlled room temperature for 4 hours.

### Incompatibilities
None reported.

## Mechanism of action
*Immunosuppressant action:* Basiliximab binds specifically to and blocks the interleukin-2 receptor alpha-chain (IL-2Rα) on the surface of activated T-lymphocytes. This inhibits interleukin-2 mediated activation of lympho-

cytes, a critical pathway in the cellular immune response involved in allograft rejection.

## Pharmacokinetics
*Absorption:* Administered I.V.
*Distribution:* Unknown.
*Metabolism:* Unknown.
*Excretion:* Half-life is about 7 days in adults, 11 days in children.

| Route | Onset | Peak | Duration |
|-------|-------|------|----------|
| I.V. | Unknown | Unknown | Unknown |

## Contraindications and precautions
Contraindicated in patients hypersensitive to drug or its components. Anaphylactoid reactions may result after administration of proteins. Make sure that drugs used to treat severe hypersensitivity reactions are available for immediate use.

## Interactions
None reported.

## Adverse reactions
**CNS:** agitation, anxiety, *asthenia,* depression, *dizziness, headache,* hypoesthesia, *insomnia,* neuropathy, paresthesia, *tremor,* fatigue, malaise.
**CV:** angina pectoris, ***arrhythmias,*** atrial fibrillation, ***cardiac failure,*** chest pain, abnormal heart sounds, aggravated hypertension, *hypertension,* hypotension, tachycardia.
**EENT:** abnormal vision, cataract, conjunctivitis, *rhinitis, pharyngitis,* sinusitis.
**GI:** *abdominal pain, candidiasis, constipation, diarrhea, dyspepsia,* esophagitis, enlarged abdomen, flatulence, gastroenteritis, GI disorder, ***GI hemorrhage,*** gum hyperplasia, melena, *nausea,* ulcerative stomatitis, *vomiting.*
**GU:** abnormal renal function, albuminuria, bladder disorder, *dysuria,* frequent micturition, hematuria, *increased nonprotein nitrogen,* oliguria, renal tubular necrosis, ureteral disorder, *urinary tract infection,* urine retention.
**Hematologic:** *anemia,* hematoma, hemorrhage, polycythemia, purpura, ***thrombocytopenia,*** thrombosis.
**Metabolic:** *acidosis,* dehydration, diabetes mellitus, fluid overload, hypercalcemia, *hypercholesterolemia, hyperglycemia, hyperkalemia,* hyperlipemia, *hyperuricemia, hypocalcemia, hypokalemia,* hypomagnesemia, hypoglycemia, *hypophosphatemia,* hypoproteinemia, *weight increase.*
**Musculoskeletal:** arthralgia, arthropathy, *back pain,* bone fracture, cramps, hernia, *leg pain,* myalgia.
**Respiratory:** abnormal chest sounds, bronchitis, ***bronchospasm,*** *cough, dyspnea,* pneumonia, pulmonary disorder, pulmonary edema, *upper respiratory tract infection.*
**Skin:** *acne,* cyst, hypertrichosis, pruritus, rash, skin disorder or ulceration.

**Other:** herpes simplex, herpes zoster, accidental trauma, *surgical wound complications, viral infection, leg or peripheral edema, pain,* general edema, infection, rigors, ***sepsis,*** fever, hypersensitivity reactions.

## Overdose and treatment
No overdose reported. Single doses up to 60 mg have been given without significant adverse effects.

## Clinical considerations
■ Drug should be used cautiously and only under the supervision of a prescriber experienced in immunosuppression therapy and management of organ transplantation.
**H ALERT** Severe acute hypersensitivity reactions may occur within 24 hours after initial exposure or reexposure to basiliximab. Drugs to treat hypersensitivity reactions should be available for immediate use and the second dose of basiliximab should be withheld if hypersensitivity reactions occur.
■ Basiliximab should be used only with cyclosporine and corticosteroids; data are lacking regarding use with other immunosuppressants.
■ It isn't known if the response to vaccines will be altered with drug administration.

### *Therapeutic monitoring*
■ Advise clinician to monitor patient for electrolyte imbalances and acidosis during drug therapy.
■ Advise clinician to monitor patient's intake and output, vital signs, hemoglobin, and hematocrit during therapy.
■ Advise clinician to monitor patient for signs of opportunistic infections during drug therapy.

### *Special populations*
**Breast-feeding patients.** It isn't known if drug appears in breast milk. A decision should be made to discontinue the drug or to stop breast-feeding, depending on the importance of the drug to the mother.
**Pediatric patients.** Basiliximab may be given to children as young as age 2.
**Geriatric patients.** No significant difference has been seen between geriatric and younger adults; however, caution should be used when prescribing immunosuppressive drugs to this population.

## Patient counseling
■ Inform patient of potential benefits and risks of immunosuppressive therapy, including a decreased risk of graft loss or acute rejection.
■ Advise patient that immunosuppressive therapy increases risk of developing lymphoproliferative disorders and opportunistic infections.

---

■ Advise women of childbearing age to use effective contraception before beginning therapy and for 2 months after therapy stops.
■ Instruct patient to report adverse effects or signs of infection immediately.

# becaplermin
Regranex Gel

*Pharmacologic classification:* recombinant human platelet-derived growth factor (rhPDGF-BB)
*Therapeutic classification:* wound repair drug
*Pregnancy risk category C*

## Available forms
Available by prescription only
*Gel:* 100 mcg/g in tubes of 2 g, 7.5 g, 15 g

## Indications and dosages
*Treatment of lower extremity diabetic neuropathic ulcers that extend into the subcutaneous tissue and beyond and have an adequate blood supply*
*Adults:* Apply daily in $\frac{1}{16}''$ even thickness to entire surface of wound. Cover site with a saline-moistened dressing. Remove after 12 hours. Rinse gel from wound with saline or water and cover wound with moist dressing. Continue treatment until complete healing occurs.

When squeezing gel from tube, length of gel to be applied varies with tube size and ulcer area.

| Tube size (g) | Ulcer area (inches) | Ulcer area (centimeters) |
|---|---|---|
| 2 | ulcer length × ulcer width × 1.3 | (ulcer length × ulcer width) ÷ 2 |
| 7.5, 15 | ulcer length × ulcer width × 0.6 | (ulcer length × ulcer width) ÷ 4 |

## Mechanism of action
*Wound repair action:* Recombinant of human platelet-derived growth factor that promotes the chemotactic recruitment and proliferation of cells involved in wound repair and enhances the formation of new granulation tissue.

## Pharmacokinetics
*Absorption:* Minimal systemic absorption.
*Distribution:* Unknown.
*Metabolism:* Unknown.
*Excretion:* Unknown.

| Route | Onset | Peak | Duration |
|---|---|---|---|
| Topical | Unknown | Unknown | Unknown |

## Contraindications and precautions
Contraindicated in patients hypersensitive to any component of product or in those with known neoplasms at site of application. Gel is for external use only. If an application site reaction occurs, consider possibility of sensitization or irritation caused by parabens or m-cresol.

## Interactions
None reported.

## Adverse reactions
**Skin:** erythematous rash.

## Overdose and treatment
No information available.

## Clinical considerations
■ When used as an adjunct to (not a substitute for) good ulcer care practices, including initial sharp debridement, pressure relief, and infection control, gel increases risk of complete healing of diabetic ulcers. Its efficacy in treating diabetic neuropathic ulcers that don't extend through the dermis into S.C. tissue or ischemic diabetic ulcers hasn't been evaluated.
■ Gel shouldn't be used in wounds that close by primary intention.
■ To apply gel, recommend squeezing the calculated length of gel onto a clean measuring surface, such as wax paper, then transferring the measured gel from the measuring surface using an application aid.
■ Gel should be used in addition to good ulcer care program, including a strict non–weight-bearing program.

### Therapeutic monitoring
■ Advise clinician to monitor patient for wound healing and application site reactions.
■ Advise clinician to recalculate amount of gel to be applied weekly. If ulcer doesn't decrease in size by about one-third after 10 weeks or complete healing hasn't occurred by 20 weeks, continued treatment should be reassessed.

### Special populations
**Breast-feeding patients.** It isn't known if drug appears in breast milk. Use drug with caution when giving to breast-feeding patients.
**Pediatric patients.** Safety and efficacy in patients younger than age 16 haven't been established.

## Patient counseling
■ Instruct patient to wash hands thoroughly before applying gel.
■ Advise patient not to touch tip of tube against ulcer or other surfaces.
■ Inform patient to use a cotton swab, tongue blade, or other application aid to apply gel evenly over the surface of the ulcer, producing a thin ($\frac{1}{16}''$) continuous layer.
■ Tell patient to apply drug once daily in a carefully measured quantity. Quantity will change on a weekly basis.

- Tell patient to store gel in the refrigerator, and never to freeze it.
- Inform patient not to use gel after expiration date on the bottom, crimped end of the tube.

---

# beclomethasone dipropionate

## beclomethasone dipropionate monohydrate

*Nasal inhalants*
Beconase, Vancenase

*Nasal sprays*
Beconase AQ, Vancenase AQ, Vancenase AQ Double Strength

*Oral inhalants*
Becloforte*, Beclovent, Vanceril, Vanceril Double Strength

*Pharmacologic classification:* glucocorticoid
*Therapeutic classification:* antiinflammatory, antiasthmatic
*Pregnancy risk category C*

## Available forms
Available by prescription only
*Nasal aerosol:* 42 mcg/metered spray
*Nasal spray:* 42 mcg/metered spray, 84 mcg/metered spray
*Oral inhalation aerosol:* 42 mcg/metered spray, 84 mcg/metered spray

## Indications and dosages
**Steroid-dependent asthma**
**Oral inhalation**
*Adults and children over age 12:* For regular strength formulation: Two inhalations t.i.d. or q.i.d. or four inhalations b.i.d. For severe asthma, start with 12 to 16 sprays per day and then reduce the dosage to the lowest effective level. Maximum of 20 inhalations daily. Double strength: 2 inhalations b.i.d.; in severe asthma start with 6 to 8 inhalations and adjust down. Don't exceed 10 inhalations/day.
*Children ages 6 to 12:* For regular strength formulation: One to two inhalations t.i.d. or q.i.d. Maximum of 10 inhalations daily. Double strength: Two inhalations b.i.d.; don't exceed five inhalations/day.
**Perennial or seasonal rhinitis; prevention of recurrence of nasal polyps after surgical removal**
**Nasal inhalation**
*Adults and children over age 12:* One spray (42 mcg) in each nostril b.i.d. to q.i.d. Usual total dose is 168 to 336 mcg daily.
*Children ages 6 to 12:* One spray in each nostril t.i.d. (252 mcg daily).

**Nasal spray**
*Adults and children over age 6:* One or two sprays of single strength (42 to 84 mcg) in each nostril b.i.d. If the double strength preparation is used, 1 or 2 sprays (84 to 168 mcg) into each nostril once daily (168 to 336 mcg). Maintenance dosage: 1 spray (42 mcg) into each nostril t.i.d.

## Mechanism of action
*Anti-inflammatory action:* Beclomethasone stimulates the synthesis of enzymes needed to decrease the inflammatory response. The antiinflammatory and vasoconstrictor potency of topically applied beclomethasone is, on a weight basis, about 5,000 times greater than that of hydrocortisone, 500 times greater than that of betamethasone or dexamethasone, and about 5 times greater than fluocinolone or triamcinolone.
*Antiasthmatic action:* Beclomethasone is used as a nasal inhalant to treat symptoms of seasonal or perennial rhinitis and to prevent the recurrence of nasal polyps after surgical removal, and as an oral inhalant to treat bronchial asthma in patients who require chronic administration of corticosteroids to control symptoms.

## Pharmacokinetics
*Absorption:* After nasal inhalation, absorbed primarily through the nasal mucosa, with minimal systemic absorption. After oral inhalation, absorbed rapidly from the lungs and GI tract. Greater systemic absorption is achieved with oral inhalation, but systemic effects don't occur at usual doses because of rapid metabolism in the liver and local metabolism of drug that reaches the lungs.
*Distribution:* Distribution after intranasal administration hasn't been described. There is no evidence of tissue storage of drug or its metabolites. About 10% to 25% of a nasal spray or orally inhaled dose is deposited in the respiratory tract. The remainder, deposited in the mouth and oropharynx, is swallowed. When absorbed, it is 87% plasma protein–bound.
*Metabolism:* Swallowed drug undergoes rapid metabolism in the liver or GI tract to several metabolites, some of which have minor glucocorticoid activity. The portion inhaled into the respiratory tract is partially metabolized before absorption into systemic circulation. Mostly metabolized in the liver.
*Excretion:* Excretion of inhaled drug hasn't been described; however, when drug is given systemically, its metabolites are excreted mainly in feces via biliary elimination and to a lesser extent in urine. Biological half-life of drug averages 15 hours.

| Route | Onset | Peak | Duration |
|---|---|---|---|
| Nasal | 5-7 days | 3 wk | Unknown |
| Inhalation | 1-4 wk | Unknown | Unknown |

---

*Haloperidol and phenothiazines:* May decrease their effect, possibly reflecting direct CNS antagonism. Advise clinician to monitor patient for clinical effect.

*Phenothiazines:* Increases the risk of adverse anticholinergic effects. Advise reduced phenothiazine dose.

**Drug-lifestyle.** *Alcohol use:* Increases the sedative effects of benztropine. Advise patient to avoid alcohol.

### Adverse reactions

**CNS:** disorientation, hallucinations, depression, toxic psychosis, confusion, memory impairment, nervousness.
**CV:** tachycardia.
**EENT:** dilated pupils, blurred vision.
**GI:** dry mouth, *constipation,* nausea, vomiting, paralytic ileus.
**GU:** urine retention, dysuria.

### Overdose and treatment

Signs and symptoms of overdose include central stimulation followed by depression and psychotic symptoms such as disorientation, confusion, hallucinations, delusions, anxiety, agitation, and restlessness. Peripheral effects may include dilated, nonreactive pupils; blurred vision; hot, flushed, dry skin; dryness of mucous membranes; dysphagia; advise decreased or absent bowel sounds; urine retention; hyperthermia; tachycardia; hypertension; and increased respiration.

Treatment is primarily symptomatic and supportive, p.r.n. Recommend maintaining a patent airway. If patient is alert, advise clinician to induce emesis (or use gastric lavage) and follow with a sodium chloride cathartic and activated charcoal to prevent further absorption. In severe cases, physostigmine may be given to block the antimuscarinic effects of benztropine. Advise clinician to give fluids, p.r.n., to treat shock, diazepam to control psychotic symptoms, and pilocarpine (instilled into the eyes) to relieve mydriasis. If urine retention occurs, catheterization may be needed.

### Clinical considerations

■ To help prevent gastric irritation, recommend giving drug after meals.
■ Drug should never be discontinued abruptly.
■ Some adverse reactions may result from atropine-like toxicity and are dose related.
■ Advise storing in well-sealed containers between 59° and 86° F (15° and 30° C). Avoid freezing injectable preparation.

### Therapeutic monitoring

■ Advise clinician to monitor patient for intermittent constipation and abdominal distention and pain, which may indicate paralytic ileus.

■ Recommend periodic monitoring of patient because effects are cumulative, especially if patient is prone to tachycardia and prostatic hypertrophy.
■ Advise clinician to observe patients with mental disorders for worsening symptoms or toxic psychoses, especially when therapy starts or changes.

### Special populations

**Pregnant patients.** Safe use during pregnancy hasn't been established.
**Breast-feeding patients.** Drug may appear in breast milk, possibly causing infant toxicity. Avoid use in breast-feeding women. Benztropine may decrease milk production.
**Pediatric patients.** Drug isn't recommended for use in children younger than age 3.

### Patient counseling

■ Explain to patient that the full effect of the drug may not occur for 2 to 3 days after therapy begins.
■ Caution patient not to discontinue drug suddenly; dosage should be reduced gradually.
■ Tell patient that drug may increase sensitivity of eyes to light.

---

# bepridil hydrochloride
Vascor

*Pharmacologic classification:* calcium channel blocker
*Therapeutic classification:* antianginal
*Pregnancy risk category C*

---

### Available forms

Available by prescription only
*Tablets:* 200 mg, 300 mg

### Indications and dosages

***Treatment of chronic stable angina (classic effort-associated angina) in patients who are unresponsive or inadequately responsive to other antianginals***
*Adults:* Initially, 200 mg P.O. daily; after 10 days, adjust dosage based on patient tolerance and response. Most common maintenance dosage is 300 mg daily. Maximum daily dose, 400 mg.

### Mechanism of action

*Antianginal action:* Precise mechanism of action is unknown. It inhibits calcium ion influx into cardiac and vascular smooth muscle and also inhibits the sodium inward influx, resulting in reductions in the maximal upstroke velocity and amplitude of the action potential. It's believed to reduce heart rate and arterial pressure by dilating peripheral arterioles and reducing total peripheral resistance (afterload). The effects are dose-dependent. Bepridil has dose-related class I antiarrhythmic properties affecting electrophysiologic changes, such as prolongation of QT and QTc intervals.

## Pharmacokinetics
*Absorption:* Rapidly and completely absorbed after oral administration.
*Distribution:* Drug is plasma protein–bound.
*Metabolism:* Metabolized in the liver.
*Excretion:* Elimination is biphasic. Bepridil has a distribution half-life of 2 hours. Over 10 days, 70% appears in urine, 22% in feces as metabolites. Terminal half-life after multiple dosing averaged 42 hours (range, 26 to 64 hours).

| Route | Onset | Peak  | Duration |
|-------|-------|-------|----------|
| P.O.  | 1 hr  | 2-3 hr | 24 hr   |

## Contraindications and precautions
Contraindicated in patients hypersensitive to drug; and those with uncompensated cardiac insufficiency, sick sinus syndrome, or second- or third-degree AV block unless pacemaker is present; or with hypotension (below 90 mm Hg systolic), congenital QT interval prolongation, or history of serious ventricular arrhythmias. Also contraindicated in those receiving other drugs that prolong QT interval.

Use cautiously in patients with left bundle-branch block, sinus bradycardia, impaired renal or hepatic function, or heart failure. Drug isn't recommended for use in patients within 3 months of an MI.

## Interactions
**Drug-drug.** *Beta blockers:* Excessive bradycardia and conduction abnormalities. Avoid use together.
*Digoxin:* Modest increases in steady-state serum digoxin level. Advise clinician to monitor serum digoxin level.
*Potassium-wasting diuretics:* Potential for causing hypokalemia, which increases risk of serious ventricular arrhythmias. Avoid use together.
*Procainamide, quinidine, or tricyclic antidepressants:* Additive prolongation of QT interval. Avoid use together.

## Adverse reactions
**CNS:** *dizziness,* drowsiness, *nervousness, headache,* insomnia, paresthesia, *asthenia,* tremor.
**CV:** edema, flushing, palpitations, tachycardia, *ventricular arrhythmias, including torsades de pointes, ventricular tachycardia, ventricular fibrillation.*
**EENT:** tinnitus.
**GI:** *nausea, diarrhea,* constipation, abdominal discomfort, dry mouth, anorexia.
**Hematologic:** *agranulocytosis.*
**Hepatic:** increased ALT levels and abnormal liver function test results.
**Respiratory:** dyspnea, shortness of breath.
**Skin:** rash.
**Other:** flu syndrome.

## Overdose and treatment
Exaggerated adverse reactions, especially clinically significant hypotension, high-degree AV block, and ventricular tachycardia, have been observed.

Advise clinician to treat with appropriate supportive measures, including gastric lavage, beta-adrenergic stimulation, parenteral calcium solutions, vasopressor drugs, and cardioversion, p.r.n. Close observation in a cardiac care facility for a minimum of 48 hours is recommended.

## Clinical considerations
**⚕ ALERT** Careful patient selection and monitoring are essential. Use the following selection criteria: diagnosis of chronic stable angina with failure to respond or inadequate response to other therapies, QTc interval less than 0.44 second, absence of hypokalemia, hypotension, severe left ventricular dysfunction, serious ventricular arrhythmias, unpacked sick sinus syndrome, second- or third-degree AV block, and no use of other drugs that prolong the QT interval.
■ Beta blockers, nitrates, digoxin, insulin, and oral antidiabetics may be used with bepridil.
■ Food doesn't interfere with absorption of bepridil. Food may alleviate or prevent nausea.
■ Drug should be used cautiously in patients with renal or hepatic disorders. No clinical data are available.

### Therapeutic monitoring
■ Advise clinician to monitor serum potassium level and correcting hypokalemia before therapy starts and to use potassium-sparing diuretics for patients who require diuretic therapy.
■ Advise clinician to monitor QTc interval before and during therapy. Reduced dosage is required if QTc prolongation is greater than 0.52 second or increases more than 25%. If prolongation of QTc interval persists, bepridil should be stopped.
■ Advise clinician to monitor patient for development of cough or dyspnea and consider pulmonary infiltrates or fibroses as a potential cause.

### Special populations
**Breast-feeding patients.** Drug appears in breast milk; risk-benefit ratio must be assessed.
**Pediatric patients.** Safety and efficacy in children younger than age 18 haven't been established.
**Geriatric patients.** Recommended starting dose is same as in adult patients; however, more frequent monitoring may be required.

## Patient counseling
■ Instruct patient to recognize signs and symptoms of hypokalemia and the importance of

compliance with prescribed potassium supplements.
- Tell patient to report signs or symptoms of infection, such as sore throat and fever.
- Instruct patient to take drug with food or at bedtime if nausea occurs.

---

# betamethasone (systemic)
Betnelan*, Celestone

# betamethasone sodium phosphate
Betnesol*, Celestone Phosphate

# betamethasone sodium phosphate and betamethasone acetate
Celestone Soluspan

*Pharmacologic classification:* glucocorticoid
*Therapeutic classification:* anti-inflammatory
*Pregnancy risk category NR*

## Available forms
Available by prescription only
**betamethasone**
*Tablets:* 0.6 mg
*Syrup:* 0.6 mg/5 ml
**betamethasone sodium phosphate**
*Tablets (effervescent):* 500 mcg*
*Injection:* 4 mg (3 mg base)/ml in 5-ml vials
*Enema*:* 5 mg (base)
**betamethasone sodium phosphate and betamethasone acetate suspension**
*Injection:* betamethasone acetate 3 mg and betamethasone sodium phosphate (equivalent to 3 mg base) per ml (not for I.V. use)

## Indications and dosages
**Severe inflammation or immunosuppression**
*Adults:* 0.6 to 7.2 mg P.O. daily; usually 2.4 to 4.8 mg daily divided into two to four doses.
*Children:* 0.0175 to 0.25 mg/kg P.O. daily or 0.5 to 7.5 mg/m$^2$ daily in three to four divided doses.
**betamethasone sodium phosphate**
*Adults:* 0.5 to 9 mg I.M., I.V., or into joint or soft tissue daily.
**betamethasone sodium phosphate and betamethasone acetate suspension**
*Adults:* 0.25 to 2 ml into joint or soft tissue q 1 to 2 weeks, p.r.n. Effects may last a few days or 1 to 2 weeks depending on the joint condition being treated.
◊ *Hyaline membrane disease*
*Adults:* Give 2 ml I.M. daily to expectant mothers for 2 to 3 days before delivery.

## I.V. administration
**◪ ALERT** Know the differences in forms and in the ways they are given.
- Betametasone suspension is not given I.V.
- Betamethasone sodium phosphate may be given I.V.
- Betamethasone sodium phosphate and betamethasone acetate suspension is not given I.V.

### Incompatibilities
Betamethasone sodium phosphate is incompatible with parenteral local diluents or anesthetics containing preservatives, such as parabens or phenols, because betamethasone may flocculate.

## Mechanism of action
*Anti-inflammatory action:* Stimulates the synthesis of enzymes needed to decrease the inflammatory response. It's a long-acting steroid with an anti-inflammatory potency 25 times that of an equal weight of hydrocortisone. It has essentially no mineralocorticoid activity. Betamethasone tablets and syrup are used as oral anti-inflammatory drugs.

Betamethasone sodium phosphate is highly soluble, has a prompt onset of action, and may be given I.V.

Betamethasone sodium phosphate and betamethasone acetate (Celestone Soluspan) combine the rapid-acting phosphate salt and the slightly soluble, slowly released acetate salt to provide rapid anti-inflammatory effects with a sustained duration of action. It's a suspension and isn't to be given I.V. It's particularly useful as an anti-inflammatory in intra-articular, intradermal, and intralesional injections.

## Pharmacokinetics
*Absorption:* Absorbed readily after oral administration. Systemic absorption occurs slowly after intra-articular injections.
*Distribution:* Removed rapidly from the blood and distributed to muscle, liver, skin, intestines, and kidneys. Betamethasone is bound weakly to plasma proteins (transcortin and albumin). Only the unbound portion is active. Adrenocorticoids appear in breast milk and through the placenta.
*Metabolism:* Metabolized in the liver to inactive glucuronide and sulfate metabolites.
*Excretion:* Inactive metabolites and small amounts of unmetabolized drug are excreted by the kidneys. Insignificant quantities of drug are also excreted in feces. Biological half-life of drug is 36 to 54 hours.

| Route | Onset | Peak | Duration |
|-------|--------|---------|-----------|
| P.O. | Prompt | Unknown | 3-25 days |
| I.M. | Unknown | Unknown | 7-14 days |

---

## Contraindications and precautions

Contraindicated in patients hypersensitive to drug and in those with viral or bacterial infections (except in life-threatening situations) or systemic fungal infections.

Use with caution in patients with renal disease, hypertension, osteoporosis, diabetes mellitus, hypothyroidism, cirrhosis, diverticulitis, nonspecific ulcerative colitis, recent intestinal anastomoses, thromboembolic disorders, seizures, myasthenia gravis, heart failure, tuberculosis, ocular herpes simplex, emotional instability, and psychotic tendencies.

## Interactions

**Drug-drug.** *Amphotericin B or diuretic therapy:* Betamethasone may enhance hypokalemia. Advise clinician to monitor serum potassium level and observe patient carefully.
*Antacids, cholestyramine, and colestipol:* Decreased effect of betamethasone by adsorbing the corticosteroid, decreasing the amount absorbed. Use together cautiously.
*Barbiturates, phenytoin, and rifampin:* Decreased corticosteroid effects because of increased hepatic metabolism. Advise clinician to monitor patient for clinical effect.
*Cardiac glycosides:* Increased risk of toxicity in patients concurrently receiving cardiac glycosides. Use together cautiously.
*Estrogens:* Reduced metabolism of corticosteroids by increasing transcortin levels. Advise clinician to monitor patient for adverse effects.
*Insulin or oral antidiabetics:* Hyperglycemia, requiring dosage adjustment in diabetic patients. Advise clinician to monitor serum glucose level.
*Isoniazid and salicylates:* Increased metabolism of these drugs. Advise clinician to monitor patient for clinical effect.
*Oral anticoagulants:* Decreased effects of oral anticoagulants (rarely). Advise clinician to monitor PT and INR.
*Ulcerogenic drugs such as NSAIDs:* May increase the risk of GI ulceration. Use together cautiously.

## Adverse reactions

Most adverse reactions to corticosteroids are dose- or duration-dependent.
**CNS:** *euphoria, insomnia,* psychotic behavior, pseudotumor cerebri, vertigo, headache, paresthesia, *seizures.*
**CV:** *heart failure,* hypertension, edema, *arrhythmias,* thrombophlebitis, *thromboembolism.*
**EENT:** cataracts, glaucoma.
**GI:** *peptic ulceration,* GI irritation, increased appetite, *pancreatitis,* nausea, vomiting.
**GU:** menstrual irregularities.
**Metabolic:** hypokalemia, hyperglycemia, and carbohydrate intolerance; increased $T_3$ and $T_4$ levels.

**Musculoskeletal:** muscle weakness, osteoporosis, growth suppression in children.
**Skin:** delayed wound healing, acne, various skin eruptions, hirsutism.
**Other:** cushingoid state (moonface, buffalo hump, central obesity), susceptibility to infections; *acute adrenal insufficiency may follow increased stress (infection, surgery, or trauma) or abrupt withdrawal after long-term therapy.*

## Overdose and treatment

Acute ingestion, even in massive doses, rarely occurs. Toxic signs and symptoms rarely occur if drug is used for less than 3 weeks, even at large doses. However, chronic use causes adverse physiologic effects, including suppression of the hypothalamic-pituitary-adrenal axis, cushingoid appearance, muscle weakness, and osteoporosis.

## Clinical considerations

**H ALERT** The correct form of drug should be used, in the correct route of administration.
■ Investigational use includes prevention of respiratory distress syndrome in premature infants (hyaline membrane disease). Advise giving 6 mg (2 ml) of Celestone Soluspan I.M. once daily 24 to 36 hours before induced delivery.
**H ALERT** Advise clinician to gradually reduce dose after long-term use. After abrupt withdrawal, patient may experience rebound inflammation, fatigue, weakness, arthralgia, fever, dizziness, lethargy, depression, fainting, orthostatic hypotension, dyspnea, anorexia, and hypoglycemia. After prolonged use, sudden withdrawal may be fatal.
■ Store tablets in a well-closed container and protected from light at temperatures of 36° to 86° F (2° to 30° C).
■ Protect betamethasone sodium phosphate injection from light and store between 59° and 86° F (15° and 30° C). Avoid freezing.
■ Protect betamethasone sodium phosphate and betamethasone acetate sterile solution from light and store at 36° to 77° F (2° to 25° C); avoid freezing. Don't mix the sterile solution with diluents or local anesthetics containing preservatives because flocculation of the suspension may occur.
■ Adrenocorticoid therapy suppresses reactions to skin tests and causes false-negative results in the nitroblue tetrazolium tests for systemic bacterial infections.

### Therapeutic monitoring

Recommend continuous monitoring for effect and dosage adjustment, remissions, exacerbations, and stress.

### Special populations
**Breast-feeding patients.** Information is incomplete. Risk versus benefits must be determined and reviewed with patient.
**Pediatric patients.** Chronic use of betamethasone in children and adolescents may delay growth and maturation.

### Patient counseling
- Warn patient not to stop drug abruptly.
- Instruct patient to take drug with food or milk.
- Tell patient to report symptoms associated with corticosteroid withdrawal, including fatigue, weakness, arthralgia, orthostatic hypotension, and dyspnea.
- Instruct patient to carry a card indicating his need for supplemental glucocorticoid therapy during stress.

# betamethasone dipropionate, augmented
Diprolene, Diprolene AF

# betamethasone dipropionate
Alphatrex, Diprosone, Maxivate

# betamethasone valerate
Betaderm\*, Betatrex, Beta-Val, Betnovate\*, Celestoderm-V\*, Ectosone\*, Luxig, Metaderm\*, Novobetamet\*, Valisone

*Pharmacologic classification:* topical glucocorticoid
*Therapeutic classification:* anti-inflammatory
*Pregnancy risk category C*

### Available forms
Available by prescription only
**betamethasone dipropionate, augmented**
*Cream, gel, lotion, ointment:* 0.05%
**betamethasone dipropionate**
*Lotion, ointment, cream:* 0.05%
*Aerosol:* 0.1%
**betamethasone valerate**
*Lotion, ointment:* 0.1%
*Cream:* 0.01%, 0.1%,
*Foam:* 0.12%

### Indications and dosages
*Inflammation of corticosteroid-responsive dermatoses*
**betamethasone valerate**
*Adults and children:* Apply cream, lotion, ointment, or gel in a thin layer once daily to q.i.d.

*Relief of inflammatory and pruritic manifestations of corticosteroid-responsive dermatoses of scalp*
*Adults:* Gently massage small amounts of foam into affected scalp areas b.i.d. (apply once in the morning and once at night) until control is achieved. If no improvement is seen within 2 weeks, reassess diagnosis.
**betamethasone dipropionate**
*Adults and children over age 12:* Apply cream, lotion, or ointment sparingly daily or b.i.d. Dosage of augmented 0.05% gels or lotions shouldn't exceed 50 g or 50 ml per week. Dosage of Diprolene ointments or creams 0.05% shouldn't exceed 45 g per week. To apply aerosol, direct spray onto affected area from a distance of 6 inches (15 cm) for only 3 seconds t.i.d. or q.i.d.

### Mechanism of action
*Anti-inflammatory action:* Stimulates the synthesis of enzymes needed to decrease the inflammatory response. Betamethasone, a fluorinated derivative, has the advantage of availability in various bases to vary the potency for individual conditions.

### Pharmacokinetics
*Absorption:* Amount absorbed depends on the potency of the preparation, amount applied, and nature of the skin at the application site. It ranges from about 1% in areas with a thick stratum corneum to as high as 36% in areas with a thin stratum corneum. Absorption increases in areas of skin damage, inflammation, or occlusion. Some systemic absorption of topical steroids occurs.
*Distribution:* After topical application, distributed throughout the local skin. Drug absorbed into circulation is removed rapidly from the blood and distributed into muscle, liver, skin, intestines, and kidneys.
*Metabolism:* After topical administration, metabolized primarily in the skin. The small amount that's absorbed into systemic circulation is metabolized primarily in the liver to inactive compounds.
*Excretion:* Inactive metabolites are excreted by the kidneys, primarily as glucuronides and sulfates, but also as unconjugated products. Small amounts of the metabolites are also excreted in feces.

| Route | Onset | Peak | Duration |
|---|---|---|---|
| Topical | Unknown | Unknown | Unknown |

### Contraindications and precautions
Contraindicated in patients hypersensitive to corticosteroids.

### Interactions
None significant.

## Adverse reactions

**Skin:** burning, pruritus, irritation, dryness, erythema, folliculitis, acneiform eruptions, perioral dermatitis, hypopigmentation, hypertrichosis, allergic contact dermatitis; *secondary infection, maceration, atrophy, striae, miliaria* (with occlusive dressings).
**Metabolic:** hyperglycemia, glycosuria (with betamethasone dipropionate).
**Other:** *hypothalamic-pituitary-adrenal axis suppression,* Cushing's syndrome.

## Overdose and treatment

No information available.

## Clinical considerations

■ Diprolene ointment may suppress the hypothalamic-pituitary-adrenal axis at doses as low as 7 g daily. Patient shouldn't use more than 45 g weekly and shouldn't use occlusive dressings.
■ Recommend gently washing skin before applying. To prevent skin damage, recommend rubbing drug in gently, leaving a thin coat. When treating hairy sites, advise clinician to part hair and apply directly to lesions.
■ For application to the scalp, advise clinician to invert the can containing the foam and dispense a small amount of drug onto a cool surface (but not directly to the hand because the drug will melt). Foam should be massaged into scalp until foam disappears.

### Therapeutic monitoring

Advise clinician to monitor patient for systemic adverse reactions if prolonged use or if used on a large body surface area.

### Special populations

**Pediatric patients.** Treatment with Diprolene ointment isn't recommended in children younger than age 12.

## Patient counseling

■ Teach patient how to apply drug.
■ Tell patient to stop drug and report signs of systemic absorption, skin irritation or ulceration, hypersensitivity, or infection.

---

# betaxolol hydrochloride

Betoptic, Betoptic S, Kerlone

*Pharmacologic classification:* beta blocker
*Therapeutic classification:* antiglaucoma, antihypertensive
*Pregnancy risk category C*

## Available forms

Available by prescription only
*Tablets:* 10 mg, 20 mg
*Ophthalmic solution:* 5 mg/ml (0.5%) in 2.5-ml, 5-ml, 10-ml, 15-ml dropper bottles

*Ophthalmic suspension:* 2.5 mg/ml (0.25%) in 2.5-ml, 5-ml, 10-ml, 15-ml dropper bottles

## Indications and dosages

*Chronic open-angle glaucoma and ocular hypertension*
*Adults:* Instill 1 to 2 drops in eyes b.i.d.
*Management of hypertension (used alone or with other antihypertensives)*
*Adults:* Initially, 10 mg P.O. once daily. After 7 to 14 days, full antihypertensive effect should be seen. If needed, double the dose to 20 mg P.O. once daily. Doses up to 40 mg daily have also been used.
≡*Dosage adjustment.* In patients with renal impairment and geriatic patients, initial dose is 5 mg P.O. daily. Increase by 5-mg/day increments q 2 weeks to maximum of 20 mg/day.

## Mechanism of action

*Antihypertensive action:* Cardioselective adrenergic blocking effects of betaxolol slow heart rate and decrease cardiac output.
*Ocular hypotensive action:* Betaxolol hydrochloride is a cardioselective beta$_1$ blocker that reduces intraocular pressure (IOP), possibly by reducing production of aqueous humor when given as an ophthalmic solution.

## Pharmacokinetics

*Absorption:* Essentially complete after oral administration; minimal after ophthalmic use. A small first-pass effect reduces bioavailability by about 10%. Absorption isn't affected by food or alcohol.
*Distribution:* About 50% plasma protein–bound.
*Metabolism:* Hepatic; about 85% of drug is recovered in the urine as metabolites. Elimination half-life is prolonged in patients with hepatic disease, but clearance isn't affected, so dosage adjustment is unnecessary.
*Excretion:* Primarily renal (about 80%). Plasma half-life is 14 to 22 hours.

| Route | Onset | Peak | Duration |
|-------|-------|------|----------|
| P.O. | 3 hr | 2-4 hr | 24-48 hr |
| Ophthalmic | ½-1 hr | 2 hr | > 12 hr |

## Contraindications and precautions

Contraindicated in patients hypersensitive to drug, and those with severe bradycardia, greater than first-degree heart block, cardiogenic shock, or uncontrolled heart failure.

## Interactions

**Drug-drug.** *Beta blockers:* Betaxolol may increase the effects of lidocaine. Advise clinician to monitor patient for clinical effect.
*Beta blockers:* Ophthalmic betaxolol may increase the systemic effect of oral beta blockers. Advise clinician to monitor patient closely.

---

*Calcium channel blockers:* Increases risk of hypotension, left-sided heart failure, and AV conduction disturbances. Advise clinician to use I.V. calcium antagonists with caution.

*Carbonic anhydrase inhibitors, epinephrine, and pilocarpine :* Ophthalmic betaxolol enhances the lowering of IOP with these drugs. Advise clinician to monitor patient for clinical effect.

*General anesthetics:* May cause increased hypotensive effects. Advise clinician to observe patient carefully for excessive hypotension, bradycardia, or orthostatic hypotension.

*Reserpine and catecholamine-depleting drugs:* Use of oral betaxolol with these drugs may have an additive effect when given with a beta blocker.

*Reserpine and catecholamine-depleting drugs:* Ophthalmic betaxolol enhances the hypotensive and bradycardiac effect of these drugs. Advise clinician to monitor patient closely.

## Adverse reactions
**Ophthalmic form**
**CNS:** insomnia, depressive neurosis.
**EENT:** *eye stinging on instillation causing brief discomfort,* photophobia, pharyngitis, erythema, itching, keratitis, occasional tearing.
**Systemic form**
**CNS:** dizziness, fatigue, headache, insomnia, lethargy, anxiety.
**CV:** *bradycardia,* chest pain, *heart failure,* edema.
**GI:** nausea, diarrhea, dyspepsia.
**GU:** impotence.
**Metabolic:** altered results of glucose tolerance tests.
**Musculoskeletal:** arthralgia.
**Respiratory:** dyspnea, *bronchospasm.*
**Skin:** rash.

## Overdose and treatment
Signs and symptoms of overdose, which are extremely rare with ophthalmic use, may include diplopia, bradycardia, heart block, hypotension, shock, increased airway resistance, cyanosis, fatigue, sleepiness, headache, sedation, coma, respiratory depression, seizures, nausea, vomiting, diarrhea, hypoglycemia, hallucinations, and nightmares.

Advise clinician to stop drug and flush eye with normal saline solution or water. For treatment of accidental substantial ingestion, emesis is most effective if started within 30 minutes, providing the patient isn't obtunded, comatose, or having seizures. Activated charcoal may be used. Bradycardia, conduction defects, and hypotension should be treated with I.V. fluids, glucagon, atropine, or isoproterenol; refractory bradycardia may require a transvenous pacemaker. Bronchoconstriction should be treated with I.V. aminophylline; seizures, with I.V. diazepam.

## Clinical considerations
**Ophthalmic use**
■ Betaxolol is a cardioselective beta blocker. Its pulmonary and systemic effects are considerably milder than those of timolol or levobunolol.
■ Ophthalmic betaxolol is intended for twice-daily dosage. Encourage patient to comply with this regimen.
**Systemic use**
■ Withdrawal of beta blocker therapy before surgery is controversial. Some clinicians advocate withdrawal to prevent any impairment of cardiac responsiveness to reflex stimuli and to prevent any decreased responsiveness to exogenous catecholamines.
■ To withdraw drug, dosage should be gradually reduced over at least 2 weeks.

### Therapeutic monitoring
■ In some patients, a few weeks' treatment may be required to stabilize pressure-lowering response. Determine IOP during the first 4 weeks of drug therapy.
■ Advise clinician to monitor blood pressure closely.
■ Advise clinician to monitor serum glucose level; signs of hypoglycemia may be masked in patients taking beta blockers.

### Special populations
**Breast-feeding patients.** Use with caution. After oral administration, betaxolol appears in breast milk in sufficient amounts to exert an effect on the breast-feeding infant.
**Pediatric patients.** The ophthalmic preparation shouldn't be used in patients younger than age 18.
**Geriatric patients.** Use with caution in geriatric patients with cardiac or pulmonary disease.

## Patient counseling
**Ophthalmic use**
■ Tell patient to shake suspension well before use.
■ Instruct patient to tilt head back and, while looking up, instill the drug into the lower lid.
■ Warn patient not to touch dropper to eye or surrounding tissue.
■ Instruct patient not to close eyes tightly or blink more than usual after instillation.
■ Remind patient to wait at least 5 minutes before using other eyedrops.
■ Advise patient to wear sunglasses or avoid exposure to bright lights.
**Systemic use**
■ Instruct patient to take drug exactly as prescribed and warn against discontinuing it suddenly.
■ Advise patient to report shortness of breath or difficulty breathing, unusually fast heartbeat, cough, or fatigue with exertion.

---

* Canada only    ◇ Unlabeled clinical use

# bethanechol chloride

Duvoid, Myotonachol, Urecholine

*Pharmacologic classification:* cholinergic agonist
*Therapeutic classification:* urinary tract and GI tract stimulant
*Pregnancy risk category C*

## Available forms
Available by prescription only
*Tablets:* 5 mg, 10 mg, 25 mg, 50 mg
*Injection:* 5 mg/ml

## Indications and dosages
*Acute postoperative and postpartum nonobstructive (functional) urine retention, neurogenic atony of urinary bladder with retention*
*Adults:* 10 to 50 mg P.O. b.i.d., t.i.d., or q.i.d. Or 2.5 to 5 mg S.C. Never give I.M. or I.V. When used for urine retention, some patients may require 50 to 100 mg P.O. per dose. Use such doses with extreme caution. Test dose: 2.5 mg S.C. repeated at 15- to 30-minute intervals to a maximum of four doses to determine the minimal effective dose, then use minimal effective dose three or four times daily. Adjust dosage to meet individual requirements.
*Restore bladder function in patients with chronic neurogenic bladder*
*Adults:* 7.5 to 10 mg S.C. q 4 hours around the clock. Dosage adjustments are made based on residual urine measurements.
◊ *Bladder dysfunction caused by phenothiazines*
*Adults:* 50 to 100 mg P.O. q.i.d.
◊ *Lessen the adverse effects of tricyclic antidepressants*
*Adults:* 25 mg P.O. t.i.d.
◊ *Chronic gastric reflux*
*Adults:* 25 mg P.O. q.i.d.
◊ *Familial dysautonomia*
*Children:* 0.2 to 0.4 mg/kg S.C. q.i.d. 30 minutes before meals with an oral antacid; then after 2 weeks, give 1 to 2 mg P.O. q.i.d.
◊ *To diagnose flaccid or atonic neurogenic bladder*
*Adults:* 2.5 mg S.C.
◊ *To diagnose cystic fibrosis*
Before administration, dilute 5 mg of drug in 3 ml of $D_5W$ to yield a concentration of 1.25 mg/ml.
*Children over age 1:* 1 mg intradermally.
*Children ages 2 months to 1 year:* 0.5 mg intradermally.
*Infants from birth to age 2 months:* 0.25 mg intradermally.

## Mechanism of action
*Urinary tract stimulant action:* Bethanechol directly binds to and stimulates muscarinic receptors of the parasympathetic nervous system. This increases tone of the bladder detrusor muscle, usually resulting in contraction, decreased bladder capacity, and subsequent urination.
*GI tract stimulant action:* Bethanechol directly stimulates cholinergic receptors, leading to increased gastric tone and motility and peristalsis. Drug improves lower esophageal sphincter tone by directly stimulating cholinergic receptors, thereby alleviating gastric reflux.

## Pharmacokinetics
*Absorption:* Poorly absorbed from the GI tract (absorption varies considerably among patients).
*Distribution:* Largely unknown; however, therapeutic doses don't penetrate the blood-brain barrier.
*Metabolism:* Unknown.
*Excretion:* Unknown.

| Route | Onset | Peak | Duration |
|-------|-------|------|----------|
| P.O. | 30-90 min | 1 hr | 6 hr |
| S.C. | 5-15 min | 15-30 min | 2 hr |

## Contraindications and precautions
Contraindicated for I.M. or I.V. use and in patients hypersensitive to drug or its components and in patients with uncertain strength or integrity of bladder wall; mechanical obstructions of GI or urinary tract; hyperthyroidism, peptic ulceration, latent or active bronchial asthma, pronounced bradycardia or hypotension, vasomotor instability, cardiac or coronary artery disease, seizure disorder, Parkinson's disease, spastic GI disturbances, acute inflammatory lesions of the GI tract, peritonitis, or marked vagotonia; or when increased muscular activity of GI or urinary tract is harmful.
   Use cautiously in pregnant women.

## Interactions
**Drug-drug.** *Cholinergics, especially cholinesterase inhibitors:* Additive effects may occur. Avoid use together.
*Ganglionic blockers such as mecamylamine:* May cause a critical blood pressure decrease; this effect is usually preceded by abdominal symptoms. Avoid use together.
*Procainamide and quinidine:* May reverse the cholinergic effect of bethanechol on muscle. Advise clinician to monitor patient for clinical effect.

## Adverse reactions
**CNS:** headache, malaise.
**CV:** hypotension, reflex tachycardia.
**EENT:** lacrimation, miosis.
**GI:** *abdominal cramps, diarrhea,* excessive salivation, nausea, belching, borborygmus.
**GU:** urinary urgency.

---

**Hepatic:** increased serum levels of amylase, lipase, bilirubin, and AST.
**Respiratory:** *bronchoconstriction,* increased bronchial secretions.
**Skin:** flushing, diaphoresis.

## Overdose and treatment
Clinical signs and symptoms of overdose include nausea, vomiting, abdominal cramps, diarrhea, involuntary defecation, urinary urgency, excessive salivation, miosis, excessive tearing, bronchospasm, increased bronchial secretions, hypotension, excessive sweating, bradycardia or reflex tachycardia, and substernal pain.

Treatment requires discontinuation of drug and administration of atropine by S.C., I.M., or I.V. route. (Atropine must be given cautiously; an overdose could cause bronchial plug formation.) Contact local or regional poison control center for more information.

## Clinical considerations
■ Atropine sulfate should be readily available to counteract toxic reactions that may occur during treatment with bethanechol.
**⋈ ALERT** Never give bethanechol I.M. or I.V. because that could cause circulatory collapse, hypotension, severe abdominal cramps, bloody diarrhea, shock, or cardiac arrest. Give only by S.C. route when giving parenterally.
■ For administration to treat urine retention, bedpan should be readily available.
■ Advise clinician to give drug on an empty stomach; eating soon after drug administration may cause nausea and vomiting.
■ Store drug in tight container between 59° and 86° F (15° and 30° C). Avoid freezing. The injection may be autoclaved at 248° F (120° C) for 20 minutes without discoloration or loss of potency.

### Therapeutic monitoring
Advise clinician to monitor blood pressure; patients with hypertension receiving bethanechol may experience a precipitous decrease in blood pressure.

### Special populations
**Pregnant patients.** Bethanechol shouldn't be used in pregnant women.
**Pediatric patients.** Safety and efficacy haven't been established in children.

## Patient counseling
Instruct patient to take oral form on an empty stomach and at regular intervals.

# bexarotene
Targretin

*Pharmacologic classification:* retinoid (selective retinoid X receptor activator)
*Therapeutic classification:* tumor cell growth inhibitor
*Pregnancy risk category* X

## Available forms
Available by prescription only
*Capsules:* 75 mg

## Indications and dosages
**Cutaneous manifestations of cutaneous T-cell lymphoma in patients refractory to at least one prior systemic therapy**
*Adults:* 300 mg/m$^2$/day P.O. as a single dose with a meal. If no response after 8 weeks, increase to 400 mg/m$^2$/day if initial dose was tolerated.
**≡Dosage adjustment.** For patients with hepatic insufficiency, lower doses may be needed. If toxicity occurs, dose may be adjusted to 200 mg/m$^2$/day, then to 100 mg/m$^2$/day, or drug may be temporarily suspended. When toxicity is controlled, doses may be carefully readjusted upward.

## Mechanism of action
*Tumor cell growth inhibition effect:* Bexarotene selectively binds and activates retinoid X receptor (RXR) subtypes. Once activated, these receptors function as transcription factors that regulate the expression of genes that control cellular differentiation and proliferation. Bexarotene inhibits the growth *in vitro* of some tumor cell lines of hematopoietic and squamous cell origin and it induces tumor cell regression *in vivo* in some animal models. The exact mechanism of action in the treatment of cutaneous T-cell lymphoma is unknown.

## Pharmacokinetics
**Absorption:** Absorbed from the GI tract. Absorption is increased if given with a fat-containing meal.
**Distribution:** Drug is plasma protein–bound.
**Metabolism:** Metabolized through oxidative pathways, primarily by the cytochrome P-450 3A4 system, to four metabolites. These metabolites may maintain retinoid receptor activity. The terminal half-life is 7 hours.
**Excretion:** Thought to be eliminated primarily through the hepatobiliary system.

| Route | Onset | Peak | Duration |
|-------|-------|------|----------|
| P.O. | Unknown | Unknown | Unknown |

## Contraindications and precautions
Contraindicated in patients hypersensitive to drug or its components and in pregnant women.

Drug isn't recommended for patients who have risk factors for pancreatitis, such as prior pancreatitis, uncontrolled hyperlipidemia, excessive alcohol consumption, uncontrolled diabetes mellitus, or biliary tract disease, or for those taking drugs known to increase triglyceride levels or that are associated with pancreatic toxicity.

Use cautiously in women of child-bearing potential, in patients with hepatic insufficiency, and in patients hypersensitive to retinoids.

## Interactions

**Drug-drug.** *Erythromycin, gemfibrozil, itraconazole, ketoconazole, other inhibitors of cytochrome P-450 3A4:* Increased plasma levels of bexarotene. Avoid use together.

*Insulin, sulfonylureas:* May enhance hypoglycemic action of these drugs, resulting in hypoglycemia in patients with diabetes mellitus. Use together cautiously.

*Phenobarbital, phenytoin, rifampin, other inducers of cytochrome P-450 3A4:* Decrease plasma levels of bexarotene. Avoid use together.

*Vitamin A preparations:* Increased potential for vitamin A toxicity. Avoid vitamin A supplements.

**Drug-food.** *Any food:* Recommend giving with food for better absorption.

*Grapefruit juice:* May inhibit cytochrome P-450 3A4. Avoid use together.

**Drug-lifestyle.** *Sun exposure:* Retinoids cause photosensitivity. Minimize exposure to sunlight and artificial ultraviolet light.

## Adverse reactions

**CNS:** *headache,* insomnia, *asthenia,* fatigue, syncope, depression, agitation, ataxia, *CVA,* confusion, dizziness, hyperesthesia, hypoesthesia, neuropathy.

**CV:** *peripheral edema,* chest pain, *hemorrhage,* hypertension, angina, *heart failure,* tachycardia.

**EENT:** cataracts, pharyngitis, rhinitis, dry eyes, conjunctivitis, ear pain, blepharitis, corneal lesion, keratitis, otitis externa, visual field defect.

**GI:** *nausea,* diarrhea, vomiting, anorexia, *pancreatitis, abdominal pain,* elevated amylase level, constipation, dry mouth, flatulence, colitis, dyspepsia, cheilitis, gastroenteritis, gingivitis, melena.

**GU:** elevated creatinine level, albuminuria, hematuria, incontinence, urinary tract infection, urinary urgency, dysuria, abnormal kidney function, breast pain.

**Hematologic:** *leukopenia,* anemia, eosinophilia, thrombocythemia, lymphocytosis, *thrombocytopenia.*

**Hepatic:** increased LD, aspartate transaminase, and alanine transaminase levels; bilirubinemia, *liver failure.*

**Metabolic:** *hyperlipemia, hypercholesteremia, hypothyroidism,* hyperglycemia, hypoproteinemia, hypocalcemia, hyponatremia, weight change.

**Musculoskeletal:** arthralgia, myalgia, back pain, bone pain, myasthenia, arthrosis.

**Respiratory:** pneumonia, dyspnea, hemoptysis, pleural effusion, bronchitis, cough, lung edema, *hypoxia.*

**Skin:** *rash, dry skin, exfoliative dermatitis, alopecia, photosensitivity,* pruritus, cellulitis, acne, skin ulcer, skin nodule.

**Other:** *infection,* chills, fever, flulike syndrome, *sepsis.*

## Overdose and treatment

Overdose doesn't appear to produce acute toxic effects. Any overdose with bexarotene should be treated with supportive care for the signs and symptoms exhibited by the patient.

## Clinical considerations

**✚ ALERT** Women of child-bearing potential should use effective contraception at least 1 month before therapy starts, during therapy, and for at least 1 month after therapy is stopped. While on therapy, two reliable forms of contraception used simultaneously are recommended, unless abstinence is the chosen method. A negative pregnancy test should be obtained within 1 week before therapy starts and monthly while on therapy.

■ Therapy should begin on the second or third day of a normal menstrual period.

■ Male patients with sexual partners who are pregnant, possibly pregnant, or who could become pregnant must use condoms during sexual intercourse during therapy and for at least 1 month after therapy.

■ No more than a 1-month supply of bexarotene should be given to patients with child-bearing potential so the results of pregnancy testing can be assessed and counseling regarding avoidance of pregnancy and birth defects can be reinforced.

■ Advise clinician to obtain total cholesterol, high-density lipoprotein cholesterol, and triglyceride levels when drug therapy starts, then weekly until the lipid response is established (2 to 4 weeks), and at 8-week intervals thereafter. Elevated triglycerides during treatment should be treated with antilipemic therapy; if needed, the dose of bexarotene should be reduced or suspended.

■ Advise clinician to obtain ophthalmologic evaluation for cataracts in patients who experience visual difficulties.

■ CA 125 assay values in patients with ovarian cancer may be increased by bexarotene therapy.

### Therapeutic monitoring

■ Advise clinician to monitor baseline thyroid function test results and monitor during treatment.

---

- Advise clinician to monitor WBC with differential at baseline and periodically during treatment.
- Advise clinician to monitor liver function test results at baseline and after 1, 2, and 4 weeks of treatment. If stable, advise clinician to monitor every 8 weeks during treatment. Advise clinician to consider suspending treatment if results are 3 times the upper limit of normal.

### Special populations
**Breast-feeding patients.** Bexarotene isn't recommended in breast-feeding women. A decision should be made whether to discontinue nursing or to discontinue the drug, taking into account the importance of the drug to the mother.
**Pediatric patients.** Safety and effectiveness in pediatric patients haven't been established.
**Geriatric patients.** Bexarotene has been used in geriatric patients without any overall differences in safety or efficacy, but greater sensitivity of some older individuals cannot be ruled out.

### Patient counseling
- Advise patient to minimize exposure to sunlight and artificial ultraviolet light and to take appropriate precautions.
- Tell patient that it may take several capsules to reach the needed dose and these capsules should all be taken at the same time and with a meal.
- Inform woman of child-bearing potential about the dangers of becoming pregnant while taking bexarotene and the need for monthly pregnancy tests.
- Explain the need for obtaining baseline laboratory tests and for periodic monitoring of these tests.
- Tell patient to report any visual changes.

# bimatoprost
Lumigan

*Pharmacologic classification:* prostaglandin analogue
*Therapeutic classification:* antiglaucoma drug, ocular antihypertensive
*Pregnancy risk category C*

### Available forms
Available by prescription only
*Ophthalmic solution:* 0.03%

### Indications and dosages
*Reduction of elevated intraocular pressure (IOP) in patients with open-angle glaucoma or ocular hypertension who are intolerant of, or unresponsive to, other IOP-lowering drugs*
*Adults:* Instill 1 drop in the conjunctival sac of the affected eye once daily in the evening.

## Mechanism of action
*Antiglaucoma action:* Bimatoprost is a prostamide, which is a synthetic analog of prostaglandin with ocular hypotensive activity. It selectively mimics the effects of naturally occurring prostaglandins. Bimatoprost is believed to lower IOP by increasing outflow of aqueous humor through both the trabecular meshwork and uveoscleral routes.

## Pharmacokinetics
*Absorption:* Absorbed through the cornea.
*Distribution:* Moderately distributed into body tissues. Bimatoprost resides mainly in the plasma, and approximately 12% remains unbound in human plasma.
*Metabolism:* Mainly metabolized by oxidation.
*Excretion:* Metabolites are 67% eliminated in the urine; 25% eliminated in the feces.

| Route | Onset | Peak | Duration |
|-------|-------|------|----------|
| Ophthalmic | Unknown | 10 min | 1.5 hr |

## Contraindications and precautions
Contraindicated in patients hypersensitive to bimatoprost, benzalkonium chloride, or any other ingredients in this product. Don't use in patients with angle-closure glaucoma or inflammatory or neovascular glaucoma.

Use cautiously in patients with renal or hepatic impairment. Use with caution in patients with active intraocular inflammation (iritis/uveitis), aphakic patients, pseudophakic patients with a torn posterior lens capsule, and in patients at risk for macular edema.

## Interactions
None significant

## Adverse reactions
**CNS:** headache, asthenia.
**EENT:** *conjunctival hyperemia, growth of eyelashes, ocular pruritus,* ocular dryness, visual disturbance, ocular burning, foreign body sensation, eye pain, pigmentation of the periocular skin, blepharitis, cataract, superficial punctate keratitis, eyelid erythema, ocular irritation, eyelash darkening, eye discharge, tearing, photophobia, allergic conjunctivitis, asthenopia, increase in iris pigmentation, conjunctival edema.
**Hepatic:** abnormal liver function test results.
**Respiratory:** upper respiratory tract infection.
**Skin:** hirsutism.
**Other:** infection.

## Overdose and treatment
No information is available on overdosage of bimatoprost. Treatment should be symptomatic if overdose occurs.

## Clinical considerations

■ Temporary or permanent increased pigmentation of the iris and eyelid may occur, as well as increased pigmentation and growth of the eyelashes.
■ Contact lenses should be removed before instillation of drug and may be reinserted 15 minutes after administration.
■ If more than one ophthalmic drug is being used, the drugs should be given at least 5 minutes apart.
■ Store in original container at between 59° to 77°F (15° and 25° C).

### Therapeutic monitoring

Advise clinician to monitor patient for excessive ocular irritation and evaluate the success of treatment.

### Special populations

**Breast-feeding patients.** It isn't known if drug appears in breast milk. Use caution when giving to a nursing woman.
**Pediatric patients.** Safety and efficacy in children haven't been established

## Patient counseling

■ Tell the patient about the potential for increased brown pigmentation of the iris and eyelid skin darkening, and increased length, thickness, pigmentation, and number of lashes in the treated eye.
■ Teach patient to instill drops and advise him to wash hands before and after instilling solution. Warn him not to touch dropper or tip to eye or surrounding tissue.
■ Tell patient that if eye trauma or infection occurs or if eye surgery is needed, he should seek medical advice before continuing to use the multidose container.
■ Advise patient to immediately report conjunctivitis or lid reactions.
■ Advise patient to apply light pressure on lacrimal sac for 1 minute after instillation to minimize systemic absorption of the drug.
■ Tell patient that contact lenses should be removed before administration of solution and may be reinserted 15 minutes after administration.
■ Advise patient that if more than one ophthalmic drug is being used, the drugs should be given at least 5 minutes apart.
■ Stress the importance of compliance with the recommended therapy.

# bisacodyl

Alophen, Bisac-Evac, Bisacodyl Uniserts, Bisco-Lax, Carter's Little Pills, Correctol, Dulcagen, Dulcolax, Feen-A-Mint, Fleet Laxative

*Pharmacologic classification:* diphenylmethane derivative
*Therapeutic classification:* stimulant laxative
*Pregnancy risk category B*

## Available forms

Available without a prescription
*Tablets:* 5 mg
*Suppositories:* 10 mg
*Rectal suspension:* 10 mg/30 ml

## Indications and dosages

*Constipation, preparation for delivery, surgery, or rectal or bowel examination*
*Adults and children over age 12:* 5 to 15 mg P.O. daily. In adults, up to 30 mg may be used for thorough evacuation needed for examinations or surgery. Alternatively, give one suppository (10 mg) or 30 ml of rectal suspension P.R. daily.
*Children ages 3 to 12:* 5 to 10 mg P.O. daily or 0.3 mg/kg daily.
*Children ages 2 to 11:* ½ to 1 suppository (5 to 10 mg) or 15 ml of rectal suspension P.R. daily.
*Children under age 2:* ½ suppository (5 mg) P.R. daily.

## Mechanism of action

*Laxative action:* Bisacodyl has a direct stimulant effect on the colon, increasing peristalsis and enhancing bowel evacuation.

## Pharmacokinetics

*Absorption:* Minimal.
*Distribution:* Distributed locally.
*Metabolism:* Absorbed minimally; metabolized in the liver.
*Excretion:* Excreted primarily in feces; some in urine.

| Route | Onset | Peak | Duration |
|-------|-------|------|----------|
| P.O. | 6-12 hr | Variable | Variable |
| P.R. | 15-60 min | Variable | Variable |

## Contraindications and precautions

Contraindicated in patients with hypersensitivity, abdominal pain, nausea, vomiting, or other symptoms of appendicitis or acute surgical abdomen and in those with rectal bleeding, gastroenteritis, or intestinal obstruction.

## Interactions

**Drug-drug.** *Antacids and drugs that increase gastric pH levels:* May cause premature dissolution of the enteric coating, resulting in intestinal or gastric irritation or cramping. Avoid use together.

**Drug-food.** *Milk:* May cause premature dissolution of the enteric coating, resulting in intestinal or gastric irritation or cramping. Avoid use together.

## Adverse reactions

**CNS:** muscle weakness with excessive use, dizziness, faintness.

**GI:** *nausea, vomiting, abdominal cramps,* diarrhea (with high doses), *burning sensation in rectum* (with suppositories), laxative dependence with long-term or excessive use.

**Metabolic:** alkalosis, hypokalemia, tetany, protein-losing enteropathy in excessive use, fluid and electrolyte imbalance.

## Overdose and treatment

No cases of overdose have been reported.

## Clinical considerations

Patient should swallow tablets whole rather than crushing or chewing them, to avoid GI irritation. Give with 8 ounces (240 ml) of fluid.

### Therapeutic monitoring

Advise clinician to monitor patient for diarrhea, electrolyte abnormalities (hypokalemia), dehydration (with chronic use); drug is meant for short-term therapy.

### Special populations

**Breast-feeding patients.** May be used by breast-feeding women.

## Patient counseling

■ Instruct patient not to take drug within 1 hour of milk or antacid consumption.

■ Tell patient to take only as directed to avoid laxative dependence.

# bismuth subsalicylate

Pepto-Bismol

*Pharmacologic classification:* adsorbent
*Therapeutic classification:* antidiarrheal
*Pregnancy risk category C (D in third trimester)*

## Available forms

Available without a prescription
*Tablets (chewable):* 262 mg
*Suspension:* 262 mg/15 ml, 524 mg/15 ml

## Indications and dosages

*Mild, nonspecific diarrhea*

Adults: 30 ml or 2 tablets P.O. q 30 minutes to 1 hour up to a maximum of eight doses and for no longer than 2 days.

*Children ages 9 to 12:* 15 ml or 1 tablet P.O.
*Children ages 6 to 9:* 10 ml or ⅔ tablet P.O.

*Children ages 3 to 6:* 5 ml or ⅓ tablet P.O.

Children's doses given q 30 minutes to 1 hour up to a maximum of eight doses in 24 hours and for no longer than 2 days.

## Mechanism of action

*Antidiarrheal action:* Bismuth adsorbs extra water in the bowel during diarrhea. It also adsorbs toxins and forms a protective coating for the intestinal mucosa.

## Pharmacokinetics

**Absorption:** Absorbed poorly; significant salicylate absorption may occur after using bismuth subsalicylate.

**Distribution:** Distributed locally in the gut.

**Metabolism:** Metabolized minimally.

**Excretion:** Excreted in urine.

| Route | Onset | Peak | Duration |
|-------|-------|------|----------|
| P.O. | 1 hr | Unknown | Unknown |

## Contraindications and precautions

Contraindicated in patients hypersensitive to salicylates. Use cautiously in patients already taking aspirin or aspirin-containing drugs.

## Interactions

**Drug-drug.** *Salicylates:* Increased risk of aspirin toxicity. Advise clinician to monitor patient closely.

*Sulfinpyrazone:* Impaired uricosuric effect. Advise clinician to monitor patient for clinical effect.

*Tetracycline:* Bismuth subsalicylate may impair tetracycline absorption. Separate administration times.

## Adverse reactions

**GI:** temporary darkening of tongue and stools.
**Other:** salicylism (with high doses).

## Overdose and treatment

Overdose hasn't been reported. However, overdose is more likely with bismuth subsalicylate; probable clinical effects include CNS effects, such as tinnitus and fever.

## Clinical considerations

■ Bismuth subsalicylate has been used investigationally to treat peptic ulcer. Doses of 600 mg P.O. t.i.d. may be as effective as cimetidine 800 mg P.O. once daily.

■ If giving drug by nasogastric tube, advise clinician to flush tube to clear it before administration to ensure drug delivery to stomach and to flush afterward.

■ If patient is also receiving tetracycline, bismuth should be given at least 1 hour apart; to avoid decreased drug absorption, dosages or schedules of other drugs may require adjustment.

■ Drug shouldn't be given to children or adolescents recovering from flu or chickenpox.

■ Drug should be stopped if tinnitus occurs.
■ Drug is useful for indigestion without causing constipation; for nausea; and for relief of flatulence and abdominal cramps.
■ Because bismuth is radiopaque, it may interfere with radiologic examination of the GI tract.

### Therapeutic monitoring

Advise clinician to monitor hydration status and serum electrolyte levels and record number and consistency of stools.

### Special populations

**Breast-feeding patients.** Small amounts of drug appear in breast milk. Patient should seek medical approval before use.

### Patient counseling

■ Advise patient taking anticoagulants or drugs for diabetes or gout to seek medical approval before taking drug.
■ Instruct patient to chew tablets well or to shake suspension well before using.
■ Tell patient to report persistent diarrhea.
■ Warn patient that bismuth may temporarily darken stools and tongue.

# bisoprolol fumarate

Zebeta

*Pharmacologic classification:* beta blocker
*Therapeutic classification:* antihypertensive
*Pregnancy risk category C*

### Available forms

Available by prescription only
*Tablets:* 5 mg, 10 mg

### Indications and dosages

*Hypertension (used alone or with other antihypertensives)*
*Adults:* Initially, 2.5 to 5 mg P.O. once daily. If response is inadequate, increase to 10 mg once daily. Maximum recommended dose, 20 mg daily.
≡ *Dosage adjustment.* In adults with renal impairment (creatinine clearance less than 40 ml/minute) or hepatic dysfunction, cirrhosis, or hepatitis, start at 2.5 mg P.O.; then increase with caution.
◇ *Heart failure*
*Adults:* 1.25 mg P.O. daily for 2 to 4 weeks. This low-dose strength is not available in the U.S. If dose is tolerated, increase to 2.5 mg daily for 2 to 4 weeks. Subsequent doses can be doubled every 2 to 4 weeks if tolerated. May be adjusted up to 5 to 10 mg daily.

### Mechanism of action

*Antihypertensive action:* Mechanism of action hasn't been completely established. Possible antihypertensive factors include decreased cardiac output, inhibition of renin release by the kidneys, and diminution of tonic sympathetic outflow from the vasomotor centers in the brain.

### Pharmacokinetics

*Absorption:* Bioavailability after a 10-mg oral dose is about 80%. Absorption isn't affected by the presence of food.
*Distribution:* About 30% serum protein–bound.
*Metabolism:* The first-pass metabolism is about 20%.
*Excretion:* Eliminated equally by renal and nonrenal pathways, with about 50% of dose appearing unchanged in the urine and the remainder appearing as inactive metabolites. Less than 2% of dose appears in the feces. The plasma elimination half-life of drug is 9 to 12 hours (slightly longer in geriatric patients, in part because of decreased renal function in that population).

| Route | Onset | Peak | Duration |
|-------|-------|------|----------|
| P.O. | Unknown | 1-4 hr | 24 hr |

### Contraindications and precautions

Contraindicated in patients hypersensitive to drug and in those with cardiogenic shock, overt cardiac failure, marked sinus bradycardia, or second- or third-degree AV block.
    Use cautiously in patients with bronchospastic disease.

### Interactions

**Drug-drug.** *Other beta blockers:* Bisoprolol shouldn't be used with other beta blockers.
*Catecholamine-depleting drugs, such as reserpine or guanethidine:* Excessively reduced sympathetic activity. Advise clinician to monitor patient closely.
*Concurrent therapy with clonidine:* Severe hypertensive episode may occur after stopping clonidine in patients currently using a beta blocker or when withdrawing both at the same time. Advise clinician to stop bisoprolol for several days before clonidine withdrawal. Advise clinician to monitor patient closely.

### Adverse reactions

**CNS:** asthenia, fatigue, dizziness, *headache,* hypesthesia, vivid dreams, depression, insomnia.
**CV:** *bradycardia,* peripheral edema, chest pain.
**EENT:** pharyngitis, rhinitis, sinusitis.
**GI:** nausea, vomiting, diarrhea, dry mouth.
**Metabolic:** hypoglycemia; interference with glucose or insulin tolerance tests.
**Musculoskeletal:** arthralgia.
**Respiratory:** cough, dyspnea.

---

## Overdose and treatment
The most common signs of overdose from a beta blocker such as bisoprolol are bradycardia, hypotension, heart failure, bronchospasm, and hypoglycemia. If overdose occurs, advise clinician to stop drug therapy and provide supportive and symptomatic treatment.

## Clinical considerations
- Patients with renal or hepatic dysfunction or bronchospastic disease unresponsive to, or intolerant of, other antihypertensives should start therapy at 2.5 mg P.O. daily. A beta₂-adrenergic agonist (bronchodilator) should be made available to patients with bronchospastic disease.

**H ALERT** Exacerbation of angina pectoris, MI, and ventricular arrhythmia has been observed in patients with coronary artery disease after abrupt cessation of therapy with beta blockers. It's advisable, even in patients without overt coronary artery disease, to taper therapy with bisoprolol over 1 week, with patient under careful observation. If withdrawal symptoms occur, bisoprolol therapy should be reinstituted, at least temporarily.

### Therapeutic monitoring
- Advise clinician to monitor blood pressure closely.
- Advise clinician to monitor serum glucose levels; signs of hypoglycemia may be masked in patients taking beta blockers.
- Advise clinician to monitor patients with hyperthyroidism carefully; beta blockers mask symptoms (tachycardia).

### Special populations
**Breast-feeding patients.** It isn't known if drug appears in breast milk. Use with caution when giving to breast-feeding women.
**Pediatric patients.** Safety and efficacy in children haven't been established.

## Patient counseling
- Inform diabetic patients prone to spontaneous hypoglycemia or those requiring insulin or oral hypoglycemics that bisoprolol may mask some manifestations of hypoglycemia, particularly tachycardia.
- Warn patient not to drive, operate machinery, or perform any other task requiring alertness until reaction to bisoprolol has been established.
- Stress importance of taking drug as prescribed, even when feeling well. Advise patient not to discontinue drug abruptly because serious consequences can occur.
- Instruct patient to call prescriber if adverse reactions occur.
- Tell patient to seek medical approval before taking OTC drugs.

# bivalirudin
Angiomax

*Pharmacologic classification:* direct thrombin inhibitor
*Therapeutic classification:* anticoagulant
*Pregnancy risk category B*

## Available forms
Available by prescription only
*Injection:* 250 mg vial

## Indications and dosages
***Unstable angina in patients undergoing percutaneous transluminal coronary angioplasty (PTCA)***
*Adults:* 1 mg/kg I.V. bolus just before PTCA, then begin 4-hour I.V. infusion at 2.5 mg/kg/hr. After the initial 4-hour infusion, an additional I.V. infusion at 0.2 mg/kg/hr for up to 20 hours may be given p.r.n. Give with 300 to 325 mg of aspirin.

≡*Dosage adjustment.* In patients with renal impairment, adjust dosage according to glomerular filtration rate (GFR). For moderate renal impairment (GFR 30-59 ml/min), reduce dosage by 20%. For severe renal impairment (GFR 10-29 ml/min), reduce dosage by 60%. For dialysis-dependent patients (off dialysis), reduce dose by 90%.

## I.V. administration
- Reconstitute with 5 ml of sterile water for injection. Each reconstituted vial should be further diluted in 50 ml of D₅W in water or 0.9% sodium chloride for injection to yield a final level of 5 mg/ml.
- To prepare the low-rate infusion, each reconstituted vial should be further diluted in 500 ml of D₅W or 0.9% sodium chloride for injection to yield a final level of 0.5 mg/ml.
- The prepared solution is stable for 24 hours at 36° to 46° F (2° to 8° C).

### Incompatibilities
No other drugs should be mixed with bivalirudin before or during administration.

## Mechanism of action
*Anticoagulant action:* Bivalirudin is highly specific for thrombin and directly inhibits both clot-bound and circulating thrombin. Therefore, bivalirudin prevents thrombin-induced generation of fibrin and further activation of the clotting cascade, and it inhibits thrombin-induced platelet activation, granule release, and aggregation. Bivalirudin doesn't require the presence of antithrombin to produce an anticoagulant effect.

## Pharmacokinetics

*Absorption:* Binds rapidly to thrombin and has a rapid onset of action.
*Distribution:* Doesn't bind to plasma proteins or red blood cells.
*Metabolism:* Rapidly cleared from plasma by a combination of renal mechanisms and proteolytic cleavage, with a half-life of 25 minutes in patients with normal renal function.
*Excretion:* Eliminated renally. Total body clearance is similar in patients with normal and mild renal impairment. Clearance is reduced approximately 20% in patients with moderate and severe renal impairment and is reduced approximately 80% in dialysis-dependent patients. Bivalirudin is hemodialyzable.

| Route | Onset | Peak | Duration |
|-------|-------|------|----------|
| I.V. | Rapid | Immediate | Duration of infusion |

## Contraindications and precautions

Bivalirudin is contraindicated in patients with active major bleeding and in patients hypersensitive to bivalirudin or any of its constituents. Don't use in patients with unstable angina who are not undergoing PTCA or in patients with other acute coronary syndromes.

Use cautiously in patients with heparin-induced thrombocytopenia or heparin-induced thrombocytopenia-thrombosis syndrome and in patients with diseases associated with increased risk of bleeding.

## Interactions

**Drug-drug.** *Heparin, warfarin, other oral anticoagulants:* Increased risk of bleeding. Use together cautiously. Discontinue heparin at least 8 hours before administration of bivalirudin.
*Glycoprotein IIb/IIIa inhibitors:* Safety and effectiveness haven't been established. Avoid use together.

## Adverse reactions

**CNS:** anxiety, *headache,* insomnia, nervousness.
**CV:** *bradycardia,* hypertension, *hypotension.*
**GI:** abdominal pain, dyspepsia, *nausea,* vomiting.
**GU:** urine retention.
**Musculoskeletal:** *back pain,* pelvic pain.
**Hematologic:** *severe, spontaneous bleeding.*
**Other:** fever, *pain,* pain at injection site.

## Overdose and treatment

There has been no experience of overdose with bivalirudin. In the event of overdose, advise discontinuing drug and monitoring patient for bleeding. There is no known antidote to bivalirudin. The anticoagulant effects will be gradually reduced. Symptomatic and supportive therapy should be provided. Bivalirudin is hemodialyzable.

## Clinical considerations

■ Don't give by I.M. route.
■ Hemorrhage may occur at any site in the body in patients receiving bivalirudin. Unexplained drop in hematocrit, fall in blood pressure, or any other unexplained symptom should lead to consideration of a hemorrhagic event.

### Therapeutic monitoring

■ Advise clinician to monitor baseline coagulation tests, hemoglobin, and hematocrit before start of therapy and periodically throughout.
■ Advise clinician to monitor venipuncture sites for bleeding, hematoma, or inflammation.

### Special populations

**Breast-feeding patients.** It isn't known if bivalirudin appears in human milk; therefore, caution should be used when bivalirudin is given to nursing women.
**Pediatric patients.** The safety and efficacy of bivalirudin in pediatric patients haven't been established.
**Geriatric patients.** No individual bleeding events with a difference of ≥ 5% between age groups have been observed. However, puncture site hemorrhage and catheterization site hematoma have been observed in a higher percentage of patients age 65 and older than in patients under age 65.

## Patient counseling

■ Advise patient that this drug can cause bleeding and inform patient to report any unusual bruising or bleeding (nosebleeds, bleeding gums) or tarry stools immediately.
■ Counsel patient that bivalirudin is given with aspirin and caution patient to avoid other aspirin-containing drugs or anti-inflammatory drugs (Motrin, Naprosyn, Aleve) while receiving bivalirudin.
■ Advise patient to avoid activities that carry a risk of injury and instruct patient to use a soft toothbrush and electric razor while on bivalirudin.

# bleomycin sulfate

Blenoxane

*Pharmacologic classification:* antibiotic, antineoplastic (cell cycle-phase specific, G2 and M phase)
*Therapeutic classification:* antineoplastic
*Pregnancy risk category D*

## Available forms

Available by prescription only
*Injection:* 15-unit, 30-unit vials

## Indications and dosages

Dosage and indications may vary. Check literature for current protocol.

***Hodgkin's disease, squamous cell carcinoma, malignant lymphoma, or testicular carcinoma***
*Adults:* 10 to 20 units/m² (0.25 to 0.5 units/kg) I.V., I.M., or S.C., one or two times weekly. After 50% response in regression of tumor size in Hodgkin's disease, maintenance dosage of 1 unit daily or 5 units weekly.

***Malignant pleural effusion; prevention of recurrent pleural effusions or ◇ to manage pneumothorax associated with AIDS and* Pneumocystis carinii *pneumonia***
*Adults:* 50 to 60 units in 50 to 100 ml of normal saline solution by intracavitary administration not to exceed 1 unit/kg.

≡ *Dosage adjustment.* For geriatric patients receiving intracavitary administration in the pleural space, don't exceed 40 units/m².

***Tumors of the head and neck***
*Adults:* 10 to 20 units/m² daily by I.V. or ◇ regional arterial administration for 5 to 14 days.

***◇ AIDS-related Kaposi's sarcoma***
*Adults:* 20 units/m² daily I.V. continuously over 72 hours every 3 weeks.

## I.V. administration

■ Dilute with a minimum of 5 ml (15-unit vial) or 10 ml (30-unit vial) of diluent (level shouldn't exceed 3 units/ml).

■ Give over 10 minutes as I.V. push injection.

### Incompatibilities

Incompatible with solutions containing divalent and trivalent cations, especially calcium salts and copper, because drug causes chelation. Also incompatible with amino acids, aminophylline, ascorbic acid injection, cephalosporins, diazepam, drugs containing sulfhydryl groups, furosemide, hydrocortisone, methotrexate, mitomycin, penicillin, riboflavin, and terbutaline sulfate. To maintain drug potency, avoid diluting with dextrose-containing fluids.

## Mechanism of action

*Antineoplastic action:* The exact mechanism of cytotoxicity of bleomycin is unknown. Its action may be through scission of single- and double-stranded DNA and inhibition of DNA, RNA, and protein synthesis. Bleomycin also appears to inhibit cell progression out of the G2 phase.

## Pharmacokinetics

*Absorption:* Poorly absorbed across the GI tract after oral administration. I.M. administration results in lower serum levels than those occurring after equivalent I.V. doses.

*Distribution:* Distributes widely into total body water, mainly in the skin, lungs, kidneys, peritoneum, and lymphatic tissue.

*Metabolism:* Metabolic fate of drug is undetermined; however, extensive tissue inactivation occurs in the liver and kidney and much less in the skin and lungs.

*Excretion:* Excreted primarily in urine. The terminal plasma elimination phase half-life is reported at 2 hours.

| Route | Onset | Peak | Duration |
|---|---|---|---|
| I.V., S.C. | Unknown | Unknown | Unknown |
| I.M. | Unknown | ½-1 hr | Unknown |

## Contraindications and precautions

Contraindicated in patients hypersensitive to drug.

Use cautiously in patients with renal or pulmonary impairment.

## Interactions

**Drug-drug.** *Digoxin and phenytoin:* Using together may decrease serum levels of these drugs. Advise clinician to monitor serum levels.

## Adverse reactions

**CNS:** malaise.

**GI:** stomatitis, anorexia, nausea, vomiting, diarrhea.

**Metabolic:** increased blood and urine concentrations of uric acid.

**Respiratory:** *pulmonary fibrosis,* pulmonary toxicity such as PNEUMONITIS.

**Skin:** *erythema, hyperpigmentation, acne, rash, reversible alopecia, striae, skin tenderness, pruritus,* scleroderma-like skin change.

**Other:** *chills,* fever, weight loss, *severe idiosyncratic reaction consisting of hypotension, mental confusion, fever, chills, and wheezing.*

## Overdose and treatment

Signs and symptoms of bleomycin overdose include pulmonary fibrosis, fever, chills, vesiculation, and hyperpigmentation.

Treatment is usually supportive and includes antipyretics for fever.

## Clinical considerations

■ To prepare solution for I.M. administration, reconstitute drug with 1 to 5 ml (15-unit vial) or 2 to 10 ml (30-unit vial) of normal saline solution, bacteriostatic water, or sterile water for injection. D₅W or dextrose-containing diluents shouldn't be used.

■ For intrapleural administration, dissolve 60 units of bleomycin in 50 to 100 ml of normal saline injection and give via thoracostomy tube.

■ Use precautions in preparing and handling drug; wear gloves and wash hands after preparing and giving.

■ Drug can be given by intracavitary route (see manufacturer's recommendation) or via intratumoral injection. It can also be instilled into bladder for bladder tumors.

---

* Canada only    ◇ Unlabeled clinical use

- Cumulative lifetime dosage shouldn't exceed 400 units.
- Response to bleomycin therapy may take 2 to 3 weeks.
- Recommend giving a 1- to 2-unit test dose to lymphoma patients for the first two doses to assess hypersensitivity to bleomycin. If no reaction occurs, recommend following the dosing schedule. The test dose can be incorporated as part of the total dose for the regimen.
- Epinephrine, diphenhydramine, I.V. corticosteroids, and oxygen should be available in case of anaphylactic reaction.
- Premedication with aspirin, steroids, and diphenhydramine may reduce drug fever and risk of anaphylaxis.
- Advise clinician to reduce dosage in patients with renal or pulmonary impairment.
- Lung damage may occur at lower oxygen levels than normal. This is an important consideration for patients undergoing surgery.
- Drug concentrates in keratin of squamous epithelium. To prevent linear streaking, adhesive dressings shouldn't be used on skin.
- Allergic reactions may be delayed, especially in patients with lymphoma.
- Investigational uses for the drug include treatment of AIDS-related Kaposi's sarcoma, renal carcinomas, soft tissue sarcomas, otorhinolaryngeal tumors, and mycosis fungoides.
- Bleomycin is stable for 24 hours at controlled room temperature and 48 hours under refrigeration. Refrigerate unopened vials containing dry powder.

### Therapeutic monitoring
- Pulmonary function tests may be useful in predicting fibrosis; they should be performed to establish a baseline and the results monitored periodically.
- Advise clinician to monitor chest X-rays and auscultate the lungs to monitor for pulmonary toxicity.

### Special populations
**Pregnant patients.** Drug may cause fetal toxicity in pregnant women.
**Breast-feeding patients.** It isn't known if drug occurs in breast milk. However, because of risk of serious adverse reactions, mutagenicity, and carcinogenicity in infants, breast-feeding isn't recommended.
**Geriatric patients.** Use with caution in patients older than age 70 because they're at increased risk for pulmonary toxicity.

### Patient counseling
Explain to patient that hair should grow back after treatment is discontinued.

# bretylium tosylate
Bretylate*, Bretylol

*Pharmacologic classification:* adrenergic blocker
*Therapeutic classification:* ventricular antiarrhythmic
*Pregnancy risk category C*

### Available forms
Available by prescription only
*Injection:* 50 mg/ml
*Injection in dextrose:* 500 mg, 1 g in D$_5$W; 2 mg/ml, 4 mg/ml

### Indications and dosages
*Ventricular fibrillation and hemodynamically unstable ventricular tachycardia*
*Adults:* 5 mg/kg undiluted by rapid I.V. injection. If ventricular fibrillation persists, increase dosage to 10 mg/kg and repeat, p.r.n. (usually 5- to 30-minute intervals) to total of 30 to 35 mg/kg. For continuous suppression, give diluted solution by continuous I.V. infusion at 1 to 2 mg/minute, or infuse diluted solution at 5 to 10 mg/kg over more than 8 to 10 minutes q 6 hours.
*Other ventricular arrhythmias*
*Adults:* Initially, 5 to 10 mg/kg I.M., undiluted, or I.V. diluted. Repeat in 1 to 2 hours if needed. Maintenance dosage is 5 to 10 mg/kg q 6 to 8 hours I.M. or I.V. or 1 to 2 mg/minute I.V. infusion.
◇ *Children:* For acute ventricular fibrillation, initially 5 mg/kg I.V., followed by 10 mg/kg q 15 to 30 minutes, with a maximum total dose of 30 mg/kg; maintenance dosage, 5 to 10 mg/kg q 6 hours. For other ventricular arrhythmias, 5 to 10 mg/kg q 6 hours or 2 to 5 mg/kg I.M. as a single dose.
≡ *Dosage adjustment.* In patients with renal impairment, dose interval should be increased because drug is primarily excreted by kidneys.

### I.V. administration
- Give I.V. infusion at appropriate rate to avoid or minimize adverse reactions.
- Drug is given undiluted by rapid I.V. injection over approximately 1 minute for the treatment of immediately life-threatening ventricular arrhythmias.

### Incompatibilities
None reported.

### Mechanism of action
*Ventricular antiarrhythmic action:* Bretylium is a class III antiarrhythmic used to treat ventricular fibrillation and tachycardia. Like other class III antiarrhythmics, it widens the action potential duration (repolarization inhibition) and increases the effective refractory period (ERP); it doesn't affect conduction

velocity. These actions follow a transient increase in conduction velocity and shortening of the action potential duration and ERP.

Initial effects stem from norepinephrine release from sympathetic ganglia and postganglionic adrenergic neurons immediately after drug administration. Norepinephrine release also accounts for an increased threshold for successful defibrillation, increased blood pressure, and increased heart rate. This initial phase of drug's action is brief (up to 1 hour).

Bretylium also alters the disparity in action potential duration between ischemic and nonischemic myocardial tissue; its antiarrhythmic action may result from this activity.

Hemodynamic drug effects include increased blood pressure, heart rate, and possible cardiac irritability (all resulting from initial norepinephrine release). Drug-induced adrenergic blockade ultimately predominates, leading to vasodilation and a subsequent blood pressure drop (primarily orthostatic). This effect has been referred to as chemical sympathectomy.

### Pharmacokinetics
*Absorption:* Incompletely and erratically absorbed from the GI tract; well absorbed after I.M. administration.
*Distribution:* Distributed widely throughout the body. Doesn't cross the blood-brain barrier. Only about 1% to 10% is plasma protein–bound.
*Metabolism:* No metabolites have been identified.
*Excretion:* Excreted in urine mostly as unchanged drug; half-life ranges from 5 to 10 hours (longer in patients with renal impairment).

| Route | Onset | Peak | Duration |
|-------|-------|------|----------|
| P.O. | Unknown | Unknown | Unknown |
| I.V. | Immediate | Immediate | 6-24 hr |
| I.M. | 5-40 min | 1 hr | 6-24 hr |

### Contraindications and precautions
Contraindicated in digitalized patients unless the arrhythmia is life-threatening, not caused by a cardiac glycoside, and unresponsive to other antiarrhythmics.

Use with caution in patients with aortic stenosis and pulmonary hypertension.

### Interactions
**Drug-drug.** *Cardiac glycosides:* May exacerbate ventricular tachycardia associated with digitalis toxicity. Use together cautiously.
*MAO inhibitors:* May potentiate the bretylium-induced release of catecholamines from nerve endings. Use together cautiously.

*Other antiarrhythmics:* Additive toxic effects and additive or antagonistic cardiac effects. Avoid use if possible.
*Pressor amines (sympathomimetics):* Bretylium may potentiate the action of these drugs. Advise clinician to monitor patient for the effects of these drugs.

### Adverse reactions
**CNS:** *vertigo, dizziness, light-headedness, syncope* (usually secondary to hypotension).
**CV:** SEVERE HYPOTENSION (especially orthostatic), *bradycardia,* anginal pain, transient *arrhythmias,* transient hypertension, increased PVCs.
**GI:** severe nausea, vomiting.
**Other:** hyperthermia.

### Overdose and treatment
Clinical effects of overdose primarily involve severe hypotension.

Treatment includes administration of vasopressors to support blood pressure, and general supportive measures. Volume expanders and positional changes also may be effective.

### Clinical considerations
■ For I.M. injection, don't exceed 5-ml volume in any one site and rotate sites.
■ Advise patient to remain supine and avoid sudden postural changes until tolerance to hypotension develops.
■ Avoid simultaneous initiation of therapy with a cardiac glycoside and bretylium.
■ Subtherapeutic doses (less than 5 mg/kg) may cause hypotension.
■ Drug isn't a first-line drug, according to American Heart Association advanced cardiac life-support (ACLS) guidelines.
■ Ventricular tachycardia and other ventricular arrhythmias respond to drug less rapidly than ventricular fibrillation.
■ Drug is ineffective against atrial arrhythmias.
■ Store bretylium between 59° and 86° F (15° and 30° C). Solutions in $D_5W$ should be protected from freezing and stored at controlled room temperature. After dilution of bretylium injection to 10 mg/ml, the drug is stable for 48 hours at controlled room temperature or 7 days at 40° F (4° C). Drug is compatible with most standard I.V. solutions.

*Therapeutic monitoring*
■ Advise clinician to monitor ECG and blood pressure throughout therapy.
■ Advise clinician to monitor patient closely if he is receiving pressor amines (sympathomimetics) to correct hypotension; bretylium potentiates the effects of these drugs.
■ Advise clinician to observe susceptible patients for increased anginal pain.

## Special populations
**Breast-feeding patients.** Safety in breast-feeding women hasn't been established.
**Pediatric patients.** Safety and efficacy in children haven't been established.
**Geriatric patients.** Dosing should be started at lower end of dosing range. Geriatric patients are at greater risk for adverse effects and orthostatic hypotension.

## Patient counseling
■ Instruct patient to report adverse reactions immediately.
■ Advise patient to avoid any sudden postural changes.

# bromocriptine mesylate
Parlodel

*Pharmacologic classification:* dopamine receptor agonist
*Therapeutic classification:* semisynthetic ergot alkaloid, dopaminergic agonist, antiparkinsonian, inhibitor of prolactin release, inhibitor of growth hormone release
*Pregnancy risk category B*

## Available forms
Available by prescription only
*Tablets:* 2.5 mg
*Capsules:* 5 mg

## Indications and dosages
*Amenorrhea and galactorrhea associated with hyperprolactinemia; female infertility*
*Adults:* 1.25 to 2.5 mg P.O. daily, increased by 2.5 mg daily at 3- to 7-day intervals as tolerated until optimal therapeutic effects are achieved. Maintenance dosage is usually 5 to 7.5 mg daily (range, 2.5 to 15 mg daily). Up to 40 mg daily has been used.
*Acromegaly*
*Adults:* Initially, 1.25 to 2.5 mg P.O. daily h.s. for 3 days. An additional 1.25 to 2.5 mg may be added q 3 to 7 days until patient receives therapeutic benefit. Therapeutic dose range varies from 20 to 30 mg daily in most patients. Maximum dose shouldn't exceed 100 mg daily. Dosages of 20 to 60 mg daily have been given as divided doses.
*Parkinson's disease*
*Adults:* Initially, 1.25 mg P.O. b.i.d. with meals. Dosage may be increased by 2.5 mg daily q 14 to 28 days, up to 100 mg daily or until a maximal therapeutic response is achieved. Safety in doses over 100 mg daily hasn't been established.
◊ *Premenstrual syndrome*
*Adults:* 2.5 to 7.5 mg P.O. b.i.d. from day 10 of menstrual cycle until onset of menstruation.
◊ *Cushing's syndrome*
*Adults:* 1.25 to 2.5 mg P.O. b.i.d. to q.i.d.

◊ *Hepatic encephalopathy*
*Adults:* 1.25 mg P.O. daily, increased by 1.25 mg q 3 days until 15 mg is reached.
◊ *Neuroleptic malignant syndrome associated with neuroleptic drug therapy*
*Adults:* 2.5 to 5 mg P.O. 2 to 6 times per day.

## Mechanism of action
*Prolactin-inhibiting action:* Reduces prolactin concentrations by inhibiting release of prolactin from the anterior pituitary gland, a direct action on the pituitary. It may also stimulate postsynaptic dopamine receptors in the hypothalamus to release prolactin-inhibitory factor via a complicated catecholamine pathway. Drug reduces high serum prolactin levels and restores ovulation and ovarian function in amenorrheic women and suppresses puerperal or nonpuerperal lactation in women with adequate gonadotropin levels and ovarian function. The average time for reversing amenorrhea is 6 to 8 weeks, but it may take up to 24 weeks.
*Antiparkinsonian action:* Activates dopaminergic receptors in the neostriatum of the CNS, which may produce its antiparkinsonism activity. Dysregulation of brain serotonin activity also may occur. The precise role of bromocriptine in treating parkinsonism syndrome requires further study of its safety and efficacy in long-term therapy.

## Pharmacokinetics
*Absorption:* 28% absorbed when given orally.
*Distribution:* About 90% to 96% is bound to serum albumin.
*Metabolism:* First-pass metabolism occurs with over 90% of the absorbed dose. Metabolized completely in the liver, principally by hydrolysis, before excretion. The metabolites aren't active or toxic.
*Excretion:* Primarily excreted in bile. Only 2.5% to 5.5% of dose appears in urine. Almost all (85%) of dose appears in feces within 5 days.

| Route | Onset | Peak | Duration |
|-------|-------|------|----------|
| P.O. | 2 hr | 8 hr | 24 hr |

## Contraindications and precautions
Contraindicated in patients hypersensitive to ergot derivatives, and those with uncontrolled hypertension or toxemia of pregnancy.
Use cautiously in patients with renal or hepatic impairment and history of MI with residual arrhythmias.

## Interactions
**Drug-drug.** *Amitriptyline, butyrophenones, imipramine, methyldopa, phenothiazines, and reserpine:* Increased prolactin levels. This may require increased dosage of bromocriptine.
*Antihypertensive drugs:* Potentiation of effects. Reduced dosage prevents hypotension.

**Drug-lifestyle.** *Alcohol use:* Intolerance may result when high doses of bromocriptine are given. Advise patient to limit ingestion of alcohol.

## Adverse reactions
**CNS:** *dizziness, headache,* fatigue, mania, lightheadedness, drowsiness, delusions, nervousness, insomnia, depression, *seizures.*
**CV:** *hypotension, stroke, acute MI.*
**EENT:** nasal congestion, blurred vision.
**GI:** *nausea,* vomiting, *abdominal cramps, constipation,* diarrhea, anorexia.
**GU:** urine retention, urinary frequency.
**Skin:** coolness and pallor of fingers and toes.

## Overdose and treatment
Overdose of bromocriptine may cause nausea, vomiting, and severe hypotension. Treatment includes emptying the stomach by aspiration and lavage, and giving I.V. fluids to treat hypotension.

## Clinical considerations
**⚠ ALERT** Patient must be examined carefully for pituitary tumor (Forbes-Albright syndrome). Bromocriptine doesn't affect tumor size, although it may alleviate amenorrhea or galactorrhea.
■ First-dose phenomenon occurs in 1% of patients. Sensitive patients may experience syncope for 15 to 60 minutes but can usually tolerate subsequent treatment without ill effects. Patient should begin therapy with lowest dosage, taken at bedtime.
■ Advise clinician to give drug with meals, milk, or snacks to diminish GI distress.
■ Alcohol intolerance may occur, especially when high doses of bromocriptine are given; advise patient to limit alcohol intake.
■ As an antiparkinsonian, drug is usually given with either levodopa alone or levodopa-carbidopa combination. In treatment of parkinsonism, if levodopa dosage must be decreased because of adverse effects, daily bromocriptine doses may be increased gradually in 2.5-mg increments.
■ Adverse reactions are more common when drug is given in high doses, as in the treatment of parkinsonism.

### Therapeutic monitoring
■ Advise clinician to monitor hepatic, hematopoietic, CV, and renal function in long-term use.
■ Advise clinician to monitor blood pressure, especially during first few days of therapy.
■ Advise clinician to monitor patient for pulmonary changes in long-term use.
■ Advise clinician to monitor patient with acromegaly for cold-induced digital vasospasm and signs and symptoms of peptic ulcer.

### Special populations
**Pregnant patients.** Drug should be stopped if pregnancy occurs. Recommend regular checks of the visual field in patients with underlying prolactin-secreting pituitary tumors.
**Breast-feeding patients.** Because drug inhibits lactation, it shouldn't be used in women who intend to breast-feed.
**Pediatric patients.** Drug isn't recommended for children younger than age 15.
**Geriatric patients.** Use with caution, particularly in patients receiving long-term, high-dose therapy. Regular physical assessment is recommended, with particular attention toward changes in pulmonary function and blood pressure. Safety isn't established for long-term use at the doses required to treat Parkinson's disease. Therapy should be started at the low end of the dosage range.

## Patient counseling
■ Advise patient that it may take 6 to 8 weeks or longer for menses to resume and for galactorrhea to be suppressed.
■ Tell patient to take first dose where and when she can lie down because drowsiness commonly occurs after therapy starts.
■ Instruct patient to report visual problems, severe nausea and vomiting, or acute headaches.
■ Tell patient to take drug with meals to avoid GI upset.
■ Warn patient that the CNS effects of drug may impair ability to perform tasks that require alertness and coordination.
■ Instruct patient to use a nonhormonal contraceptive during treatment because of potential amenorrheic adverse effects.
■ Advise patient to limit use of alcohol during treatment.

# budesonide
Pulmicort Respules, Pulmicort Turbuhaler, Rhinocort

*Pharmacologic classification:* corticosteroid
*Therapeutic classification:* anti-inflammatory
*Pregnancy risk category C*

## Available forms
Available by prescription only
*Nasal inhaler:* 32 mcg/metered dose (200 doses per container)
*Oral inhalation powder:* 200 mcg/dose (200 doses per container)
*Ampules:* 0.25 mg, 0.5 mg

---

## Indications and dosages

### Management of symptoms of seasonal or perennial allergic rhinitis or nonallergic perennial rhinitis

*Adults and children over age 6:* 2 sprays in each nostril in the morning and evening or 4 sprays in each nostril in the morning. Maintenance dosage should be the fewest number of sprays needed to control symptoms. Doses exceeding 256 mcg/day (4 sprays/nostril) aren't recommended. If improvement doesn't occur within 3 weeks, discontinue treatment.

### Chronic asthma

*Adults:* 200 to 400 mcg oral inhalation b.i.d. when previously used bronchodilators alone or inhaled corticosteroids; 400 to 800 mcg oral inhalation b.i.d. when previously used oral corticosteroids.

*Children age 6 or over:* Initially, 200 mcg oral inhalation b.i.d. Maximum dose is 400 mg b.i.d.

*Children ages 1 to 8:* (Respules) If previous therapy was bronchodilators alone, initiate therapy at 0.5 mg via jet nebulizer once daily or 0.25 mg b.i.d. Maximum recommended dose, 0.5 mg daily. If previous therapy was inhaled corticosteroids, initiate therapy at 0.5 mg daily or 0.25 mg b.i.d. Maximum recommended dose, 1 mg daily. If previous therapy was oral corticosteroids, initiate therapy at 1 mg daily or 0.5 mg b.i.d. Respules should be used with the patient's usual maintenance dose of systemic corticosteroids for approximately 1 week. After this, gradual withdrawal of the systemic corticosteroid may begin by reducing the daily or alternate daily dose. Further reductions may be made in intervals of 1 to 2 weeks.

## Mechanism of action

*Anti-inflammatory action:* Precise mechanism of action of corticosteroids like budesonide on allergic and nonallergic rhinitis isn't known. Corticosteroids show a wide range of inhibitory activities against multiple cell types (such as mast cells, eosinophils, neutrophils, macrophages, and lymphocytes) and mediators (such as histamine, eicosanoids, leukotrienes, and cytokines) involved in allergic and nonallergic, irritant-mediated inflammatory processes.

## Pharmacokinetics

*Absorption:* The amount of an intranasal dose that reaches systemic circulation is generally low (about 20%).

*Distribution:* 88% protein-bound in the plasma; volume of distribution is 200 L.

*Metabolism:* Rapidly and extensively metabolized in the liver.

*Excretion:* Eliminated in urine (about 67%) and feces (about 33%).

| Route | Onset | Peak | Duration |
|-------|-------|------|----------|
| Inhalation | 24 hr | 1-2 wk | Unknown |
| Nasal | Unknown | Unknown | Unknown |

## Contraindications and precautions

Contraindicated in patients hypersensitive to drug or its components and in those who have had recent septal ulcers, nasal surgery, or nasal trauma until total healing has occurred. Respules is contraindicated as the primary treatment of status asthmaticus or other acute episodes of asthma that warrant more intensive therapy.

Use cautiously in patients with tuberculosis infections; untreated fungal, bacterial, or systemic viral infections; or ocular herpes simplex.

## Interactions

**Drug-drug.** *Other inhaled corticosteroids or alternate-day prednisone therapy:* May increase the risk of hypothalamic-pituitary-adrenal suppression. Advise clinician to monitor patient closely.

*Ketoconazole:* May increase plasma levels of budesonide. Advise clinician to monitor patient.

## Adverse reactions

**CNS:** *headache,* nervousness.

**EENT:** *nasal irritation, epistaxis, pharyngitis, sinusitis,* reduced sense of smell, nasal pain, hoarseness.

**GI:** taste perversion, dry mouth, dyspepsia, nausea, vomiting.

**Respiratory:** *cough,* candidiasis, wheezing, dyspnea.

**Metabolic:** weight gain.

**Musculoskeletal:** myalgia.

**Skin:** facial edema, rash, pruritus, contact dermatitis.

**Other:** hypersensitivity reactions.

## Overdose and treatment

Acute overdose is unlikely as a result of the limited amount of product in each container. Chronic overdose may produce signs and symptoms of hyperadrenocorticism.

## Clinical considerations

■ Replacing a systemic corticosteroid with a topical corticosteroid may result in signs of adrenal insufficiency; in addition, some patients may experience symptoms of withdrawal, such as joint or muscular pain, lassitude, and depression.

**H ALERT** In patients with asthma or other clinical conditions requiring long-term systemic treatment, a too-rapid decrease in systemic corticosteroids may severely exacerbate symptoms.

■ Excessive doses of budesonide or use of drug with other inhaled corticosteroids may lead to signs or symptoms of hyperadrenocorticism.

■ Respules should be given via jet nebulizer with an adequate air flow, using a mouth piece or suitable face mask. Ultrasonic nebulizers

---

Reactions may be *common,* uncommon, *life-threatening,* or COMMON AND LIFE-THREATENING.

don't provide adequate delivery of drug and aren't recommended.

- Don't mix Respules in the nebulizer with other drugs.

### Therapeutic monitoring
- Advise clinician to carefully monitor patients previously treated for prolonged periods with systemic corticosteroids who are subsequently given topical glucocorticosteroids for acute adrenal insufficiency in response to stress.
- Because corticosteroids can affect growth, advise clinician to monitor children closely, weighing benefits of therapy against the possibility of growth suppression.
- Patients using budesonide for several months or longer should be examined for evidence of *Candida* infection or other signs of adverse effects on the nasal mucosa.

### Special populations
**Breast-feeding patients.** Use cautiously when giving drug to breast-feeding women.
**Pediatric patients.** Safety and efficacy of drug for treating seasonal or perennial allergic rhinitis in children younger than age 6 haven't been established. Drug isn't recommended for treatment of nonallergic rhinitis in children because adequate numbers of such children haven't been studied.

### Patient counseling
- Warn patient not to exceed prescribed dosage or to use for long periods because of risk of hypothalamic-pituitary-adrenal axis suppression.
- Tell patient to follow these instructions for the nasal inhaler: After opening aluminum pouch, use within 6 minutes. Shake canister well before using. Blow nose to clear nasal passages. Tilt head slightly forward; insert nozzle into nostril, pointing away from septum; hold other nostril closed; inspire gently; and spray. Shake canister again and repeat in other nostril. Store with valve downward. Don't store in area of high humidity. Don't break, incinerate, or store canister in extreme heat; contents under pressure.
- Instruct patient to hold the inhaler upright when loading Pulmicort Turbuhaler, not to blow or exhale into the inhaler nor shake it while loaded, and to hold inhaler upright while orally inhaling the dose. Place the mouthpiece between the lips and inhale forcefully and deeply.
- Assure patient that drug rarely causes nasal irritation or burning; advise patient to call prescriber if such symptoms recur.
- Warn patient to avoid exposure to chickenpox or measles, if at risk for contacting these diseases, and to consult prescriber immediately if exposed.
- Teach patient good nasal and oral hygiene.

- Tell patient to call prescriber if condition worsens or if symptoms don't improve within 3 weeks.
- Inform patient that effects aren't immediate; response requires regular use.
- Inform patient that with use of oral inhaler improvement in asthma control can occur within 24 hours, with maximum benefit anticipated between 1 to 2 weeks and possibly taking longer.
**◄ ALERT** Advise patient that Pulmicort Turbohaler and Pulmicort Respules aren't indicated for relief of acute bronchospasm.

## bumetanide
Bumex

*Pharmacologic classification:* loop diuretic
*Therapeutic classification:* diuretic
*Pregnancy risk category C*

### Available forms
Available by prescription only
*Tablets:* 0.5 mg, 1 mg, 2 mg
*Injection:* 0.25 mg/ml

### Indications and dosages
*Edema (heart failure, hepatic and renal disease); ◇ postoperative edema; ◇ premenstrual syndrome; ◇ disseminated cancer*
*Adults:* 0.5 to 2 mg P.O. once daily. If diuretic response isn't adequate, give a second or third dose at 4- to 5-hour intervals. Maximum dose is 10 mg/day. Give parenterally when oral route isn't feasible. Usual initial dose is 0.5 to 1 mg I.V. over 1 to 2 minutes or I.M. If response isn't adequate, give a second or third dose at 2- to 3-hour intervals. Maximum dose is 10 mg/day.
*◇ Pediatric heart failure*
*Children:* 0.015 mg/kg every other day to 0.1 mg/kg daily. Use with extreme caution in neonates.
*◇ Hypertension*
*Adults:* 0.5 mg P.O. daily. Oral maintenance of 1 to 4 mg daily; a maximum of 5 mg has been used in patients with normal renal function
**≡ Dosage adjustment.** In patients with impaired renal function, oral or I.V. dosages up to 20 mg have been given despite manufacturer recommendations for a maximum of 10 mg/day for the management of edema.

### I.V. administration
- Dilute bumetanide in $D_5W$, normal saline solution, or lactated Ringer's solution; use within 24 hours.
- Advise clinician to give I.V. bumetanide slowly, over 1 to 2 minutes, for I.V. infusion.

### Incompatibilities
Incompatible with dobutamine.

### Mechanism of action
*Diuretic action:* Loop diuretics inhibit sodium and chloride reabsorption in the proximal part of the ascending loop of Henle, promoting the excretion of sodium, water, chloride, and potassium; bumetanide produces renal and peripheral vasodilation and may temporarily increase glomerular filtration rate and decrease peripheral vascular resistance.

### Pharmacokinetics
*Absorption:* After oral administration, 85% to 95% of dose is absorbed; food delays oral absorption. I.M. bumetanide is completely absorbed.
*Distribution:* About 92% to 96% protein-bound; it's unknown if bumetanide enters CSF, crosses the placenta, or appears in breast milk.
*Metabolism:* Metabolized by the liver to at least five metabolites. Elimination is slower in neonates as compared to older pediatric and adult patients.
*Excretion:* Excreted in urine (80%) and feces (10% to 20%). Half-life ranges from 1 to 1½ hours.

| Route | Onset | Peak | Duration |
|-------|-------|------|----------|
| P.O. | ½-1 hr | 1-2 hr | 4-6 hr |
| I.V. | Within minutes | 15-30 min | ½-1 hr |
| I.M. | 40 min | Unknown | 5-6 hr |

### Contraindications and precautions
Contraindicated in patients hypersensitive to drug or sulfonamides (possible cross-sensitivity), in those with anuria or hepatic coma, and in patients in states of severe electrolyte depletion.

Use cautiously in patients with hepatic cirrhosis and ascites and in those with depressed renal function.

### Interactions
**Drug-drug.** *Other antihypertensives and diuretics:* Bumetanide potentiates the hypotensive effects. These actions are used to therapeutic advantage.
*Indomethacin and probenecid:* May reduce the diuretic effect of bumetanide. Their combined use isn't recommended; however, if there's no therapeutic alternative, an increased dose of bumetanide may be required.
*Lithium:* Reduced renal clearance of lithium and increased lithium levels. Lithium dosage may require adjustment.
*Ototoxic or nephrotoxic drugs:* May result in enhanced toxicity. Use together cautiously.
*Potassium-sparing diuretics (spironolactone, triamterene, amiloride):* May decrease bumetanide-induced potassium loss. Advise clinician to monitor serum potassium levels.

*Other potassium-depleting drugs such as steroids and amphotericin B:* May cause severe potassium loss. Use together cautiously.
**Drug-herb.** *Dandelion:* Possible interference with diuretic activity. Discourage use together.
*Licorice root:* May contribute to potassium depletion. Discourage use together.

### Adverse reactions
**CNS:** dizziness, headache, vertigo.
**CV:** volume depletion and dehydration, orthostatic hypotension, ECG changes, chest pain.
**EENT:** transient deafness, tinnitus.
**GI:** nausea, vomiting, upset stomach, dry mouth, diarrhea, pain.
**GU:** *renal failure,* premature ejaculation, difficulty maintaining erection, oliguria.
**Hematologic:** azotemia, *thrombocytopenia.*
**Metabolic:** hypokalemia; hypochloremic alkalosis; asymptomatic hyperuricemia; fluid and electrolyte imbalances, including dilutional hyponatremia, hypocalcemia, hyperglycemia, and glucose intolerance impairment.
**Musculoskeletal:** weakness; arthritic pain; muscle pain and tenderness.
**Skin:** rash, pruritus, diaphoresis.

### Overdose and treatment
Signs and symptoms of overdose include profound electrolyte and volume depletion, which may cause circulatory collapse.

Treatment of drug overdose is primarily supportive; advise clinician that fluid and electrolytes should be replaced p.r.n.

### Clinical considerations
■ To prevent nocturia, drug should be given in the morning. If second dose is needed, it should be given in early afternoon.
■ Safest and most effective dosage schedule for control of edema is intermittent dosage given on alternate days or 3 to 4 days with 1 or 2 days off between cycles.
■ Advise patient about a high-potassium diet. Foods rich in potassium include citrus fruits, tomatoes, bananas, dates, and apricots.
■ Bumetanide can lead to profound water and electrolyte depletion.
■ If oliguria or azotemia develops or increases, drug should be stopped.
■ Bumetanide can be safely used in patients allergic to furosemide; 1 mg of bumetanide equals 40 mg of furosemide.
**H ALERT** Don't confuse Bumex with Buprenex.

### Therapeutic monitoring
■ Advise clinician to monitor for clinical effect in renally and hepatically impaired patients.
■ With increased dosage, advise clinician to monitor patient for ototoxicity.
■ Advise clinician to monitor patient for electrolyte imbalance, especially hypokalemia.

---

Reactions may be *common,* uncommon, **life-threatening,** or COMMON AND LIFE-THREATENING.

## Special populations
**Breast-feeding patients.** Drug shouldn't be used in breast-feeding women.
**Pediatric patients.** Safety and efficacy in children younger than age 18 haven't been established. Use with caution in critically ill or jaundiced neonates who are at risk for kernicterus.
**Geriatric patients.** Geriatric and debilitated patients require close observation because they're more susceptible to drug-induced diuresis. Excessive diuresis promotes rapid dehydration, hypovolemia, hypokalemia, and hyponatremia in these patients, and may cause circulatory collapse. Reduced dosages may be indicated.

## Patient counseling
■ Tell patient to take drug in the morning to prevent nocturia, and if second dose is prescribed, to take it in early afternoon.
■ Instruct patient to take drug with food or milk.
■ Advise patient to stand up slowly to prevent dizziness, and to limit alcohol intake and strenuous exercise in hot weather to avoid exacerbating orthostatic hypertension.
■ Instruct patient to weigh himself daily to monitor fluid status.

# bupivacaine hydrochloride
Sensorcaine MPF, Sensorcaine, Sensorcaine MPF Spinal, Marcaine

*Pharmacologic classification:* amide local anesthetic
*Therapeutic classification:* local anesthetic
*Pregnancy risk category C*

## Available forms
Available by prescription only
*Injection:* 0.25%, 0.5%, 0.75%

## Indications and dosages
Dosages given are for the drug without epinephrine.
*Epidural block*
*Adults:* 25 to 50 mg (10 to 20 ml) 0.25% solution, 50 to 100 mg (10 to 20 ml) 0.5% solution, 75 to 100 mg (15 to 30 ml) 0.75% solution, single-dose only.
*Caudal block*
*Adults:* 37.5 to 75 mg (15 to 30 ml) 0.25% solution, 75 to 150 mg (15 to 30 ml) 0.5% solution.
*Spinal block*
*Adults:* 7.5 to 12 mg (1 to 1.6 ml) 0.75% solution (in dextrose 8.25%).
*Peripheral nerve block*
*Adults:* 12.5 mg (5 ml) 0.25% solution, 25 mg (5 ml) 0.5% solution.
*Retrobulbar block*
*Adults:* 15 to 30 mg (2 to 4 ml) 0.75% solution.

Note: Dose will differ depending on anesthetic procedure, area to be anesthetized, vascularity of area, number of neuronal segments to be blocked, degree of block, duration of anesthesia desired, and individual patient conditions and tolerance. Always use incremental doses.

## Mechanism of action
*Local anesthetic action:* Bupivacaine is thought to block the generation and conduction of nerve impulses by increasing the threshold for electrical excitation in the nerve, by slowing propagation of the nerve impulse, and by reducing the rate of the action potential.

## Pharmacokinetics
*Absorption:* Absorption from the site of administration is affected by vascularity of tissue and depends on dose, concentration, and route of administration. After injection for caudal, epidural, or peripheral nerve block, levels peak in 30 to 45 minutes.
*Distribution:* 95% protein-bound. Drug is distributed to some extent to all tissues.
*Metabolism:* Metabolized primarily in the liver.
*Excretion:* Mostly excreted by the kidney with only 5% of unchanged drug in the urine.

| Route | Onset | Peak | Duration |
|---|---|---|---|
| Epidural, caudal, peripheral nerve block | Unknown | 30-45 min | Unknown |

## Contraindications and precautions
Contraindicated in patients hypersensitive to bupivacaine or to any local anesthetic of the amide type. Avoid 0.75% bupivacaine in obstetric patients, and don't use solutions of bupivacaine for the production of obstetric paracervical block anesthesia. Also not recommended for intravenous regional anesthesia (Bier block). Solutions containing preservatives shouldn't be used for caudal or epidural anesthesia.
Use cautiously when giving to patients with hypotension, heart block, hepatic disease, or impaired CV function.

## Interactions
**Drug-drug.** *Beta blockers:* Enhanced sympathomimetic effects when used with bupivacaine and epinephrine. Use with caution.
*Butyrophenones, phenothiazines:* May reduce or reverse pressor effect of epinephrine. Advise clinician to monitor patient.
*Chloroprocaine:* May lessen bupivacaine's action. Don't use together.
*CNS depressants:* May cause additive CNS effects. Recommend reduced dosage of CNS depressants.
*Enflurane, halothane, isoflurane, related drugs:* Arrhythmias when used with bupivacaine and

epinephrine. Should be used with extreme caution.

*MAO inhibitors, tricyclic antidepressants:* Severe, sustained hypertension when used with bupivacaine and epinephrine. Avoid using together.

## Adverse reactions
**CNS:** anxiety, nervousness, *seizures,* dizziness, tremors.
**CV:** *arrhythmias, bradycardia, cardiac arrest,* hypotension, myocardial depression, *heart block.*
**EENT:** blurred vision, tinnitus.
**GI:** nausea, vomiting.
**Respiratory:** *respiratory arrest,* status asthmaticus.
**Skin:** urticaria, erythema, pruritus.
**Other:** *anaphylactoid reactions, anaphylaxis*, edema, angioneurotic edema.

## Overdose and treatment
Acute emergencies are generally related to high plasma levels. Toxic reactions usually involve the CNS and CV system.

To treat toxic reactions, advise clinician to immediately establish and maintain a patent airway or give controlled ventilation with 100% oxygen. If needed, drugs can be used to control convulsions. Supportive treatment of circulatory depression may require the administration of I.V. fluids and appropriate vasopressors. If difficulty is encountered in maintaining a patent airway, or if prolonged ventilatory support is needed, endotracheal intubation may be indicated. If maternal hypotension or fetal bradycardia occurs in the pregnant patient, advise clinician to maintain the patient in the left lateral decubitus position, if possible, or manually displace the uterus off the great vessels.

## Clinical considerations
**H ALERT** Local anesthetics should be given only by prescribers experienced in the diagnosis and management of drug-related toxicity and other acute emergencies that may occur.
■ Resuscitative equipment, drugs, and oxygen should be immediately available.
■ Advise clinician to check solution before giving. Don't use if there is particulate matter or if solution is a pinkish or slightly darker than yellow color.
■ Don't use disinfectants containing heavy metals for skin or mucous membrane disinfection because they may cause swelling and edema.
■ Advise clinician to use solutions with epinephrine cautiously in patients with CV disorders and in body areas with limited blood supply (such as ears, nose, fingers, toes).
■ A test dose of a local anesthetic with a fast onset, preferably a solution containing epinephrine, should be given before epidural anesthesia with bupivacaine, and the patient should be monitored for CNS and CV toxicity. Advise clinician to monitor patient for increased heart rate.
■ Aspiration for blood or CSF should be performed before any dose of bupivacaine is injected to avoid intravascular or intrathecal injection.
**H ALERT** An intravascular injection is still possible even if aspirations for blood are negative.
■ Advise clinician to give the smallest dose and concentration required to produce the desired result. Dosages should be reduced for young, geriatric, and debilitated patients and those with cardiac or liver disease.
■ During epidural administration, advise clinician to give in incremental volumes of 3 to 5 ml with sufficient time between doses to detect toxicity.
■ Small doses of local anesthetics injected into the head and neck area may produce adverse reactions similar to systemic toxicity seen with unintentional intravascular injections of larger doses. Advise clinician to monitor the patient's circulatory and respiratory status.
■ The 0.75% level is indicated for nonobstetric surgery patients requiring long duration of profound muscle relaxation.
■ Discard partially used bottles without preservatives.

### Therapeutic monitoring
■ Local anesthetics rapidly cross the placenta and can cause maternal, fetal, and neonatal toxicity. Adverse reactions may involve alterations in the CNS, peripheral vascular tone, and cardiac function.
■ Advise clinician to continuously monitor CV and respiratory status and patient's state of consciousness after each injection. Restlessness, anxiety, incoherent speech, light-headedness, numbness and tingling of mouth and lips, metallic taste, tinnitus, dizziness, blurred vision, tremors, twitching, depression, or drowsiness may be early signs of CNS toxicity.

### Special populations
**Breast-feeding patients.** It is unknown if drug appears in breast milk. Use cautiously in nursing women.
**Pediatric patients.** Administration to children younger than age 12 isn't recommended.
**Geriatric patients.** Dosage reductions are recommended.

## Patient counseling
■ Advise patient that temporary loss of sensation and motor activity in the anesthetized part of the body may occur.
■ Encourage patient to discuss concerns and ask questions regarding drug administration and use.

| Route | Onset | Peak | Duration |
|-------|-------|------|----------|
| I.V. | Immediate | 2 min | 6 hr |
| I.M. | 15 min | 1 hr | 6 hr |

# buprenorphine hydrochloride
Buprenex

*Pharmacologic classification:* narcotic agonist-antagonist, opioid partial agonist
*Therapeutic classification:* analgesic
*Pregnancy risk category C*
*Controlled substance schedule V*

## Available forms
Available by prescription only
*Injection:* 0.3 mg/ml in 1-ml ampules

## Indications and dosages
**Moderate to severe pain**
*Adults and children over age 13:* 0.3 mg I.M. or slow I.V. q 6 hours, p.r.n. May repeat 0.3 mg 30 to 60 minutes after initial dose or increase to 0.6 mg per dose if necessary. S.C. administration isn't recommended.
◊ *Adults:* 25 to 250 mcg/hour via I.V. infusion (over 48 hours for postoperative pain).
◊ *Adults:* 60 to 180 mcg via epidural injection.
◊ **Reverse fentanyl-induced anesthesia**
*Adults:* 0.3 to 0.8 mg, I.V. or I.M., 1 to 4 hours after the induction of anesthesia and about 30 minutes before the end of surgery.
◊ **Circumcision**
*Children ages 9 months to 9 years:* 3 mcg/kg I.M. along with surgical anesthesia.

## I.V. administration
■ Buprenorphine has been diluted to a concentration of 15 mcg/ml in normal saline solution for continuous I.V. infusion. For epidural injection, drug has been diluted to a level of 6 to 30 mcg/ml in 0.9% sodium chloride.
■ Store ampules between 59° and 86° F (15° and 30° C) and protect from light.

### Incompatibilities
Incompatible with diazepam, furosemide, and lorazepam.

## Mechanism of action
*Analgesic action:* Exact mechanisms of action of buprenorphine are unknown. It's believed to be a competitive antagonist at some opiate receptors and an agonist at others, thus relieving moderate to severe pain.

## Pharmacokinetics
*Absorption:* Absorbed rapidly after I.M. administration.
*Distribution:* About 96% protein–bound.
*Metabolism:* Metabolized in the liver.
*Excretion:* Duration of action is 6 hours. Excreted primarily in the feces as unchanged drug with about 30% excreted in urine.

## Contraindications and precautions
Contraindicated in patients hypersensitive to drug.
Use cautiously in geriatric or debilitated patients and in patients with head injuries, increased intracranial pressure, and intracranial lesions; respiratory, kidney, or hepatic impairment; CNS depression or coma; thyroid irregularities; adrenal insufficiency; prostatic hyperplasia; urethral stricture; acute alcoholism; delirium tremens; or kyphoscoliosis.

## Interactions
**Drug-drug.** *Barbiturate anesthetics such as thiopental:* Buprenorphine may produce additive CNS and respiratory depressant effects and, possibly, apnea. Use together cautiously.
*CNS depressants (antihistamines, narcotic analgesics; barbiturates, benzodiazepines, phenothiazines, sedative-hypnotics), muscle relaxants, and tricyclic antidepressants:* Potentiate the respiratory and CNS depression, sedation, and hypotensive effects. Reduced doses of buprenorphine are usually needed.
*Diazepam:* Potential for respiratory and CV collapse. Avoid use together.
*General anesthetics:* Severe CV depression. Use together cautiously.
*MAO inhibitors:* Additive effects. Use together cautiously.
**Drug-lifestyle.** *Alcohol use:* May potentiate the respiratory and CNS depression, sedation, and hypotensive effects of the drug. Advise patient to avoid alcohol.

## Adverse reactions
**CNS:** *dizziness, sedation, headache,* confusion, nervousness, euphoria, *vertigo,* **increased intracranial pressure.**
**CV:** *hypotension,* **bradycardia,** tachycardia, hypertension.
**EENT:** *miosis,* blurred vision.
**GI:** *nausea,* vomiting, constipation, dry mouth.
**GU:** urine retention.
**Respiratory:** *respiratory depression,* hypoventilation, dyspnea.
**Skin:** pruritus, *diaphoresis.*

## Overdose and treatment
Safety of buprenorphine in acute overdose is expected to be better than that of other opioid analgesics because of its antagonist properties at high doses. Overdose may cause CNS depression, respiratory depression, and miosis (pinpoint pupils). Other acute toxic effects might include hypotension, bradycardia, hypothermia, shock, apnea, cardiopulmonary arrest, circulatory collapse, pulmonary edema, and seizures.

To treat acute overdose, recommend first establishing adequate respiratory exchange via a patent airway and ventilation p.r.n.; recommend giving a narcotic antagonist (naloxone) to reverse buprenorphine's respiratory depression. Because the duration of buprenorphine is longer than that of naloxone, repeated naloxone dosing is needed. Naloxone shouldn't be given unless the patient has clinically significant respiratory or CV depression. Advise clinician to monitor vital signs closely.

Naloxone doesn't completely reverse buprenorphine-induced respiratory depression; mechanical ventilation and higher-than-usual doses of naloxone and doxaprane may be indicated.

Advise clinician to provide symptomatic and supportive treatment (continued respiratory support, correction of fluid or electrolyte imbalance). Advise clinician to closely monitor laboratory effects, vital signs, and neurologic status.

## Clinical considerations

■ Adverse effects of drug may not be as readily reversed by naloxone as are those of pure agonists.

■ Patients who become physically dependent on this drug may experience acute withdrawal syndrome if given an antagonist. Use with caution and advise clinician to monitor closely.

■ Buprenorphine 0.3 mg is equal to 10 mg morphine or 75 to 100 mg meperidine in analgesic potency; duration of analgesia is longer than either.

■ Use I.M. injection in adults not at risk for respiratory depression.

### Therapeutic monitoring

Advise clinician to monitor patient for respiratory depression. Avoid use in patients with pulmonary impairment or compromised respiratory function.

### Special populations

**Breast-feeding patients.** It's unknown if drug appears in breast milk; use with caution.
**Pediatric patients.** Buprenorphine has an unlabeled use as a supplement to anesthesia for children. Safety and efficacy hasn't been established in children younger than age 2.
**Geriatric patients.** Give with caution; lower doses are usually indicated for geriatric patients, who may be more sensitive to the therapeutic and adverse effects of these drugs.

## Patient counseling

■ Teach patient to avoid activities that require full alertness.

■ Instruct patient to avoid alcohol and other CNS depressants.

# bupropion hydrochloride
Wellbutrin, Wellbutrin SR

*Pharmacologic classification:* aminoketone
*Therapeutic classification:* antidepressant
*Pregnancy risk category B*

## Available forms

Available by prescription only
*Tablets:* 75 mg, 100 mg
*Tablets (sustained-release):* 100 mg, 150 mg

## Indications and dosages

*Depression*
*Adults:* Initially, 100 mg P.O. b.i.d. or 75 mg P.O. t.i.d. If needed, increase after 3 days to usual dosage of 100 mg P.O. t.i.d. (maximum dose). If no response occurs after several weeks of therapy, consider increasing dosage to 150 mg t.i.d. For sustained-release tablets, start with 150 mg P.O. q morning; increase to target dose of 150 mg P.O. b.i.d. as tolerated as early as day 4 of dosing. Maximum dose is 400 mg/day.
*Attention deficit hyperactivity disorder*
*Adults:* 150 mg P.O. daily with regular release tablets. Dosage may be titrated to maximum daily dose of 450 mg P.O.

## Mechanism of action

*Antidepressant action:* Mechanism of action is unknown. Bupropion doesn't inhibit MAO; it's a weak inhibitor of norepinephrine, dopamine, and serotonin reuptake.

## Pharmacokinetics

*Absorption:* Only 5% to 20% is bioavailable in animal studies.
*Distribution:* At plasma levels up to 200 mcg/ml, appears to be about 80% plasma protein-bound.
*Metabolism:* Metabolism is probably hepatic; several active metabolites have been identified. With prolonged use, the active metabolites are expected to accumulate in the plasma and their level may exceed that of the parent compound. Appears to induce its own metabolism.
*Excretion:* Excretion is primarily renal; elimination half-life of parent compound in single-dose studies ranged from 8 to 24 hours.

| Route | Onset | Peak | Duration |
|-------|-------|------|----------|
| P.O. | Unknown | 2 hr | Unknown |
| P.O. (sustained) | Unknown | 3 hr | Unknown |

## Contraindications and precautions

Contraindicated in patients hypersensitive to drug or those with seizure disorders and who have taken MAO inhibitors within previous 14 days. Also contraindicated in patients taking the smoking cessation drug Zyban, or those with history of bulimia or anorexia nervosa because of a higher risk of seizures.

Use cautiously in patients with recent MI, unstable heart disease, and renal or hepatic impairment.

## Interactions

**Drug-drug.** *Levodopa, MAO inhibitors, phenothiazines, or tricyclic antidepressants or recent and rapid withdrawal of benzodiazepines:* May increase the risk of adverse effects, including seizures. Advise clinician to monitor patient closely.

**Drug-lifestyle.** *Alcohol use:* Possibility for increased risk of seizures. Discourage patient use.

*Sun exposure:* Photosensitivity reactions may occur. Advise patient to avoid prolonged or unprotected sun exposure.

## Adverse reactions

**CNS:** *headache, seizures,* anxiety, *confusion,* delusions, euphoria, hostility, impaired sleep quality, *insomnia, sedation, tremor,* akinesia, akathisia, *agitation, dizziness,* fatigue.

**CV:** *arrhythmias,* hypertension, hypotension, palpitations, syncope, *tachycardia.*

**EENT:** *auditory disturbances,* blurred vision.

**GI:** *dry mouth,* taste disturbance, increased appetite, *constipation,* dyspepsia, *nausea, vomiting, anorexia,* diarrhea.

**GU:** impotence, menstrual complaints, urinary frequency, urine retention.

**Metabolic:** *weight loss, weight gain,* hyperglycemia.

**Musculoskeletal:** arthritis.

**Skin:** pruritus, rash, cutaneous temperature disturbance, *excessive diaphoresis.*

**Other:** fever, chills, decreased libido.

## Overdose and treatment

Signs of overdose include labored breathing, salivation, arched back, ptosis, ataxia, and seizures.

If ingestion was recent, advise clinician to empty the stomach using gastric lavage or induce emesis with ipecac, as appropriate; follow with activated charcoal. Treatment should be supportive. Recommend controlling seizures with I.V. benzodiazepines; stuporous, comatose, or convulsing patients may need intubation. There are no data to evaluate the benefits of dialysis, hemoperfusion, or diuresis.

## Clinical considerations

■ Consider the inherent risk of suicide until significant improvement of depressive state occurs. High-risk patients should have close supervision when drug therapy starts. To reduce risk of suicidal overdose, advise prescribing the smallest quantity of tablets consistent with good management.

■ Gradual increase of drug (no more than 75 mg/day to 100 mg/day q 2 to 3 days) reduces the risk of seizures and occurrences of agitation, motor restlessness, and insomnia.

■ Many patients experience a period of increased restlessness, especially when therapy starts. This may include agitation, insomnia, and anxiety. In clinical studies, these symptoms required sedative-hypnotic drugs in some patients; about 2% had to stop drug.

■ Antidepressants may cause manic episodes during the depressed phase in patients with bipolar disorder.

■ Investigational uses of drug include treatment of bipolar depression and attention deficit hyperactivity disorder in children.

### Therapeutic monitoring

Advise clinician to monitor renal and hepatic function during therapy.

### Special populations

**Pregnant patients.** Safety hasn't been established in pregnant women. Use drug only when absolutely needed, and use registry for monitoring outcomes: Bupropion Pregnancy Registry, 1-800-336-2176.

**Breast-feeding patients.** Because of the potential for serious adverse reactions in the infant, breast-feeding during therapy isn't recommended.

**Pediatric patients.** Safety in children younger than age 18 hasn't been established.

### Patient counseling

■ Advise patient to take drug regularly as scheduled, and to take each day's dosage in three divided doses, preferably at 6-hour intervals, to minimize risk of seizures.

■ Warn patient to avoid alcohol, which may contribute to the development of seizures.

■ Advise patient to avoid activities that require alertness and coordination until CNS effects of drug are known.

■ Tell patient not to chew, divide, or crush sustained-release tablets.

■ Instruct patient not to take Zyban with Wellbutrin; he shouldn't take other drugs, including OTC drugs, without medical approval.

# bupropion hydrochloride
Zyban

*Pharmacologic classification:* aminoketone
*Therapeutic classification:* nonnicotine aid to smoking cessation
*Pregnancy risk category B*

## Available forms
Available by prescription only
*Tablets (sustained-release):* 150 mg

## Indications and dosages
### Aid to smoking cessation treatment
*Adults:* 150 mg daily P.O. for 3 days; increased to maximum of 300 mg daily P.O. given as two doses of 150 mg taken at least 8 hours apart. Therapy is started while patient is still smoking; approximately 1 week is needed to achieve steady-state blood levels of drug. Patient should set target cessation date during second week of treatment. Course of treatment is usually 7 to 12 weeks.

## Mechanism of action
*Smoking cessation action:* Bupropion is a relatively weak inhibitor of the neuronal uptake of norepinephrine, serotonin, and dopamine, and doesn't inhibit MAO. The mechanism by which drug enhances the ability to abstain from smoking is unknown.

## Pharmacokinetics
*Absorption:* Well absorbed after oral administration.
*Distribution:* Volume of distribution from a single 150-mg dose is estimated to be 1,950 L. At levels up to 200 mcg/ml, drug is 84% plasma protein–bound.
*Metabolism:* Extensively metabolized in the liver mainly by the CYP-450 2B6 isoenzyme system to three active metabolites.
*Excretion:* Mean elimination half-life is thought to be about 21 hours. After oral administration, 87% of a dose is recovered in the urine and 10% in the feces. The fraction of a dose excreted unchanged is 0.5%.

| Route | Onset | Peak | Duration |
|-------|-------|------|----------|
| P.O. | Unknown | 3 hr | Unknown |

## Contraindications and precautions
Contraindicated in patients with seizure disorders or with a current or prior diagnosis of bulimia or anorexia nervosa because of potential for seizures.

Use with MAO inhibitors is contraindicated; at least 14 days must elapse between discontinuation of an MAO inhibitor and starting bupropion therapy. Use with Wellbutrin, Wellbutrin SR, or others drugs containing bupropion is contraindicated because of potential for seizures. Also contraindicated in patients allergic to drug or to its formulation.

## Interactions
**Drug-drug.** *Antidepressants, antipsychotics, theophylline, systemic steroids, or treatment regimens (abrupt withdrawal of benzodiazepines):* Lower seizure threshold. Use together cautiously.
*Carbamazepine, phenobarbital, and phenytoin:* Induced metabolism of bupropion. Advise clinician to closely monitor patient.
*Cimetidine:* Inhibited metabolism of bupropion. Advise clinician to closely monitor patient.

*Drugs that affect enzyme metabolism, such as orphenadrine and cyclophosphamide:* May cause an interaction because bupropion is metabolized to hydroxybupropion by the CYP2B6 isoenzyme. Advise clinician to closely monitor patient.
*Levodopa:* Higher risk of adverse reactions in patients receiving concurrent administration. If concurrent use is needed, advise giving small initial doses of bupropion and gradually increase dose.
*MAO inhibitors, phenelzine:* Enhanced acute toxicity of bupropion. Avoid use together.
**Drug-lifestyle.** *Alcohol use:* Possibility for increased risk of seizures. Advise patient to avoid alcohol.
*Sun exposure:* Photosensitivity reactions may occur. Advise patient to use sunblock.

## Adverse reactions
**CNS:** agitation, dizziness, hot flashes, *insomnia,* somnolence, tremor.
**CV:** *complete AV block,* hypertension, hypotension, tachycardia.
**EENT:** *dry mouth,* taste perversion.
**GI:** anorexia, dyspepsia, increased appetite.
**GU:** impotence, polyuria, urinary frequency and urgency.
**Metabolic:** edema, weight gain, weight loss, hyperglycemia.
**Musculoskeletal:** arthralgia, leg cramps and twitching, myalgia, neck pain.
**Respiratory:** bronchitis, *bronchospasm.*
**Skin:** dry skin, pruritus, rash, urticaria.
**Other:** *allergic reactions.*

## Overdose and treatment
Hospitalization is recommended for overdoses. If patient is conscious, advise inducing vomiting with syrup of ipecac. Activated charcoal may also be given every 6 hours for first 12 hours. Advise performing ECG and EEG monitoring for first 48 hours. Advise clinician to provide adequate fluid intake and obtain baseline tests.

If patient is stuporous, comatose, or experiencing seizures, airway intubation is recommended before undertaking gastric lavage. Gastric lavage may be beneficial within first 12 hours after ingestion because drug absorption may not be complete. Although diuresis, dialysis, or hemoperfusion is sometimes used to treat drug overdose, there is no experience with their use in managing bupropion overdose. Seizures may be treated with an I.V. benzodiazepine and other supportive measures.

## Clinical considerations
**H** *ALERT* Because drug use has a dose-dependent risk of seizures, 300 mg daily shouldn't be exceeded for smoking cessation. Make sure patient isn't currently taking (or has taken within the past 2 weeks of starting therapy) Wellbutrin, Wellbutrin SR, or other drugs

containing bupropion because of the risk of seizures.

■ If patient hasn't made progress toward abstinence by week 7 of therapy, stop therapy because it's unlikely that he'll quit smoking.

■ Dose doesn't have to be tapered when stopping treatment.

### Therapeutic monitoring

■ Advise clinician to monitor patient for development of hypertension when bupropion is used with transdermal nicotine.

■ Advise clinician to monitor renal and hepatic functions.

### Special populations

**Pregnant patients.** Drug isn't for use in pregnant women.

**Breast-feeding patients.** Drug and its metabolites appear in breast milk. Because of the potential for serious adverse reactions in the infant, a choice must be made between breast-feeding and drug therapy.

**Pediatric patients.** Safety and efficacy in children haven't been established. However, drug has been used in children ages 7 to 16 years for treatment of attention deficit hyperactivity disorder without unusual adverse effects.

**Geriatric patients.** Experience in patients age 60 and older was similar to that in younger patients. However, drug may be metabolized slower in this population.

### Patient counseling

■ Stress importance of combining behavioral interventions, counseling, and support services with drug therapy.

■ Explain to the patient that risk of seizures is increased if the patient has a seizure or eating disorder (bulimia or anorexia nervosa), exceeds the recommended dose, or takes other drugs containing bupropion.

■ Instruct patient to take doses at least 8 hours apart.

■ Inform patient that drug is usually taken for 7 to 12 weeks.

■ Advise patient that, although he may continue to smoke during drug therapy, it reduces his chance of breaking the smoking habit.

■ Tell patient that drug and nicotine patch should only be used together under medical supervision because his blood pressure may increase.

# buspirone hydrochloride
BuSpar

*Pharmacologic classification:* azaspirodecanedione derivative
*Therapeutic classification:* antianxiety
*Pregnancy risk category B*

## Available forms

Available by prescription only
*Tablets:* 5 mg, 10 mg, 15 mg, 30 mg

## Indications and dosages

*Management of anxiety disorders*
*Adults:* Initially, 5 mg P.O. t.i.d. Dosage may be increased at 3-day intervals. Usual maintenance dose is 20 to 30 mg daily in divided doses. Don't exceed 60 mg/day.
≡*Dosage adjustment.* When given with a CYP3A4 inhibitor, a lower dose (2.5 mg b.i.d.) should be used initially. Subsequent dosage adjustment of either drug may also be needed.

## Mechanism of action

*Anxiolytic action:* Buspirone is an azaspirodecanedione derivative with anxiolytic activity. It suppresses conflict and aggressive behavior and inhibits conditioned avoidance responses. Its precise mechanism of action hasn't been determined, but it appears to depend on simultaneous effects on several neurotransmitters and receptor sites: decreasing serotonin neuronal activity, increasing norepinephrine metabolism, and partial action as a presynaptic dopamine antagonist. Studies suggest an indirect effect on benzodiazepine gamma-aminobutyric acid (GABA)-chloride receptor complex or GABA receptors, or on other neurotransmitter systems.

Buspirone isn't pharmacologically related to benzodiazepines, barbiturates, or other sedatives and anxiolytics. It exhibits a nontraditional clinical profile and is uniquely anxiolytic. It has no anticonvulsant or muscle relaxant activity and doesn't appear to cause physical dependence or significant sedation.

## Pharmacokinetics

*Absorption:* Absorbed rapidly and completely after oral administration, but extensive first-pass metabolism limits absolute bioavailability to 1% to 13% of the oral dose. Food slows absorption but increases the amount of unchanged drug in systemic circulation. Increased area under the curve in patients with renal or hepatic impairment.
*Distribution:* 95% protein-bound; it doesn't displace other highly protein-bound drugs such as warfarin.
*Metabolism:* Metabolized in the liver by hydroxylation and oxidation, resulting in at least one pharmacologically active metabolite, 1, pyrimidinylpiperazine (1-PP).

*Excretion:* 29% to 63% appears in urine in 24 hours, primarily as metabolites; 18% to 38% appears in feces.

| Route | Onset | Peak | Duration |
|-------|-------|------|----------|
| P.O. | Unknown | 40-90 min | Unknown |

## Contraindications and precautions
Contraindicated in patients hypersensitive to drug or within 14 days of MAO inhibitor therapy.

Use cautiously in patients with renal or hepatic impairment.

## Interactions
**Drug-drug.** *CNS depressants:* Increased sedation. Avoid use together.
*Digoxin:* Buspirone may displace digoxin from serum-binding sites when the drugs are used together. Advise clinician to monitor digoxin levels.
*Haloperidol:* Increased serum haloperidol levels. Advise decreasing doses of haloperidol.
*MAO inhibitors:* Elevated blood pressure. Avoid use together.
**Drug-food.** *Grapefruit juice:* Elevates levels of buspirone, increasing the pharmacologic and adverse effects. Advise patient to take with liquid other than grapefruit juice.
**Drug-lifestyle.** *Alcohol use:* Increased sedation may result. Advise patient to avoid alcohol.

## Adverse reactions
**CNS:** *dizziness, drowsiness,* nervousness, insomnia, headache, light-headedness, fatigue, numbness.
**EENT:** blurred vision.
**GI:** dry mouth, nausea, diarrhea, abdominal distress.

## Overdose and treatment
Signs of overdose include severe dizziness, drowsiness, unusual constriction of pupils, and stomach upset, including nausea and vomiting.

Treatment of overdose is symptomatic and supportive; advise emptying stomach with immediate gastric lavage. Advise clinician to monitor respiration, pulse, and blood pressure. No specific antidote is known. Effect of dialysis is unknown.

## Clinical considerations
■ Buspirone has been used investigationally to treat nonmelancholic depression and parkinsonian syndrome.
■ Patients previously given benzodiazepines may not show good clinical response to this drug.
■ Although buspirone doesn't appear to cause tolerance or physical or psychological dependence, the possibility exists that a patient prone to drug abuse may experience these effects.
**H** *ALERT* Buspirone doesn't block the withdrawal syndrome caused by benzodiazepines

or other common sedative and hypnotic drugs; therefore, these drugs should be withdrawn gradually before replacement with buspirone therapy.
■ Store tablets in tight, light-resistant containers at temperatures less than 86° F (30° C).

### Therapeutic monitoring
Advise clinician to monitor hepatic and renal function. Hepatic and renal impairment impedes metabolism and excretion of drug and may lead to toxic accumulation; dosage reduction may be needed.

### Special populations
**Breast-feeding patients.** Buspirone and its metabolites appear in the breast milk of rats. The extent of excretion of buspirone in human milk is unknown. Avoid using buspirone in breast-feeding women.

## Patient counseling
■ Advise patient to take drug exactly as prescribed; explain that therapeutic effect may not occur for 2 weeks or longer. Warn patient not to double the dose if one is missed, but to take a missed dose as soon as possible, unless it's almost time for next dose.
■ Caution patient to avoid hazardous tasks requiring alertness until the effects of the drug are known. The effects of alcohol and other CNS depressants, such as antihistamines, sedatives, tranquilizers, sleeping aids, prescription pain medication, barbiturates, seizure drugs, muscle relaxants, anesthetics, and drugs for colds, coughs, hay fever, or allergies, may be enhanced by additive sedation and drowsiness caused by buspirone.
■ Tell patient to store drug away from heat and light and out of the reach of children.
■ Explain importance of regular follow-up visits to check progress. Urge patient to report adverse reactions immediately.
■ Inform patient that results may not be seen in 3 to 4 weeks; however, an improvement may be noted within 7 to 10 days.

# busulfan
Busulfex, Myleran

*Pharmacologic classification:* alkylating drug (cell cycle-phase nonspecific)
*Therapeutic classification:* antineoplastic
*Pregnancy risk category D*

## Available forms
Available by prescription only
*Tablets (scored):* 2 mg
*Injection for I.V. infusions:* 6 mg/ml

## Indications and dosages

Dosage and indications may vary. Check package insert for recommended protocol.

*Chronic myelogenous leukemia*
*Adults:* For remission induction, usual dosage is 4 to 8 mg P.O. daily; however, may range from 1 to 12 mg P.O. daily (0.06 mg/kg or 1.8 mg/m²). For maintenance therapy, 1 to 3 mg P.O. daily.
*Children:* 0.06 to 0.12 mg/kg or 1.8 to 4.6 mg/m² P.O. daily. Dosage should be adjusted to maintain WBC count of about 20,000/mm³.

◇ *Myelofibrosis*
*Adults:* Initially, 2 to 4 mg P.O. daily then followed by the same dose two to three times weekly.

*Allogenic hematopoietic stem cell transplantation*
*Adults:* 0.8 mg/kg of ideal body weight or actual body weight (whichever is lower) I.V. q 6 hours for 4 consecutive days for a total of 16 doses. Give phenytoin for seizure prophylaxis.

## I.V. administration

■ Busulfan injection is given by I.V. infusion.
■ Drug must be diluted before I.V. infusion.
■ Recommended dilutents are normal saline solution and D₅W.
■ A nylon filter (provided by manufacturer) should be used to withdraw bisulfan from ampule.
■ Apply a new needle to inject drug into I.V. bag.
■ Diluted solution should be given via a central venous catheter over 2 hours using a controlled infusion pump.

### Incompatibilities

None reported.

## Mechanism of action

*Antineoplastic action:* Busulfan is an alkylating drug that exerts its cytotoxic activity by interfering with DNA replication and RNA transcription, causing a disruption of nucleic acid function.

## Pharmacokinetics

*Absorption:* Well absorbed from the GI tract.
*Distribution:* Distribution into the brain and CSF is unknown.
*Metabolism:* Metabolized in the liver.
*Excretion:* Cleared rapidly from the plasma. Drug and its metabolites are excreted in urine.

| Route | Onset | Peak | Duration |
|-------|-------|------|----------|
| P.O. | 1-2 wk | Unknown | Unknown |
| I.V. | Unknown | Unknown | Unknown |

## Contraindications and precautions

Contraindicated in patients whose chronic myelogenous leukemia has shown prior resistance to drug. Also contraindicated in patients

with chronic lymphocytic leukemia or acute leukemia and in those in "blastic" crisis of chronic myelogenous leukemia.

Use cautiously in patients recently given other myelosuppressants or radiation treatment; in those with depressed neutrophil or platelet counts, head trauma, and seizures; or in patients taking other drugs that reduce seizure threshold.

## Interactions

None reported.

## Adverse reactions

**CNS:** unusual tiredness or weakness, fatigue.
**EENT:** cataracts.
**GI:** cheilosis, dry mouth, anorexia.
**GU:** profound hyperuricemia caused by increased cell lysis.
**Hematologic:** *leukopenia* (WBC count decreasing after about 10 days and continuing to decrease for 2 weeks after stopping drug), *thrombocytopenia, anemia, severe pancytopenia.*
**Respiratory:** *irreversible pulmonary fibrosis.*
**Skin:** alopecia, *transient hyperpigmentation,* rash, urticaria, anhidrosis, jaundice.
**Other:** gynecomastia, Addison-like wasting syndrome.

## Overdose and treatment

Signs and symptoms of overdose include hematologic manifestations, such as leukopenia and thrombocytopenia.

Treatment is supportive and includes transfusion of blood components and antibiotics for infections that may develop.

## Clinical considerations

■ Avoid all I.M. injections when platelets are less than 100,000/mm³.
■ Patient response (increased appetite, sense of well-being, decreased total leukocyte count, reduction in size of spleen) usually begins 1 to 2 weeks after starting the drug.
■ Pulmonary fibrosis may be delayed for 4 to 6 months.
■ Persistent cough and progressive dyspnea with alveolar exudate may result from drug toxicity, not pneumonia. Instruct patient to report symptoms so dosage adjustments can be made.
■ Minimize hyperuricemia by adequate hydration, alkalinization of urine, and administration of allopurinol.
■ Care needs to be taken when handling drug because of potential dematologic reactions.
■ Drug-induced cellular dysplasia may interfere with interpretation of cytologic studies.

### Therapeutic monitoring

■ Advise clinician to observe patient for signs or symptoms of infection, such as fever and sore throat.

---

■ Advise clinician to monitor uric acid, CBC, and kidney function.

■ Advise clinician to monitor serum alkaline phosphatase, bilirubin, and serum aminotransferase levels for potential hepatotoxicity.

■ Advise clinician to monitor leukocyte count; the manufacturer recommends discontinuing busulfan when the leukocyte count is 15,000/mm$^3$ or less.

### Special populations

**Pregnant patients.** Busulfan may cause fetal harm (malformations, bone marrow depression, fetal growth retardation, and fetal death). Also, drug may impair fertility. Avoid use.

**Breast-feeding patients.** It isn't known if drug appears in breast milk. However, potential for mutagenicity, carcinogenicity, and serious adverse reactions in the infant should be taken into consideration when a decision to breast-feed is made.

### Patient counseling

■ Advise patient to use caution when taking aspirin-containing products and to promptly report any signs of bleeding.

■ Tell patient to take drug at the same time each day.

■ Emphasize importance of continuing to take the drug despite nausea and vomiting.

■ Instruct patient about the signs and symptoms of infection and tell him to report them promptly if they occur.

■ Advise patient to use contraceptive methods during therapy.

---

# butorphanol tartrate

Stadol, Stadol NS

*Pharmacologic classification:* narcotic agonist-antagonist; opioid partial agonist
*Therapeutic classification:* analgesic, adjunct to anesthesia
*Pregnancy risk category C*
*Controlled substance schedule IV*

### Available forms

Available by prescription only
*Injection:* 1 mg/ml, 1-ml vials; 2 mg/ml, 1-ml, 2-ml, and 10-ml vials
*Nasal spray:* 10 mg/ml

### Indications and dosages

*Moderate to severe pain*
*Adults:* 1 to 4 mg I.M. q 3 to 4 hours, p.r.n.; or 0.5 to 2 mg I.V. q 3 to 4 hours, p.r.n., or around-the-clock. Alternatively, give 1 mg by nasal spray (1 spray in one nostril). Repeat if pain relief is inadequate after 60 to 90 minutes. Repeat q 3 to 4 hours, p.r.n. For severe pain, an initial 2 mg by nasal spray (1 spray in each

nostril). Repeat no more than q 3 to 4 hours, p.r.n.

*Pain during labor*
*Adults:* 1 to 2 mg I.M. or I.V. q 4 hours but not 4 hours before delivery.

*Preoperative anesthesia*
*Adults:* 2 mg I.M. 60 to 90 minutes before surgery or 2 mg I.V. shortly before induction.
≣*Dosage adjustment.* Patients with hepatic or renal impairment and geriatric patients should receive one-half of the usual parenteral adult dose at 6-hour intervals p.r.n. For nasal spray, the initial dose (1 spray in 1 nostril) is the same, but repeat dose is in 90 to 120 minutes, if needed. Repeat doses thereafter q 6 hours, p.r.n.

### I.V. administration

■ Give by direct injection into a vein or into the tubing of a free-forming I.V. solution. Compatible solutions include $D_5W$ and normal saline solution.

### Incompatibilities

Incompatible with pentobarbital sodium.

### Mechanism of action

*Analgesic action:* The exact mechanisms of action of butorphanol are unknown. Drug is believed to be a competitive antagonist at some, and an agonist at other, opiate receptors, thus relieving moderate to severe pain. Like narcotic agonists, it causes respiratory depression, sedation, and miosis.

### Pharmacokinetics

*Absorption:* Well absorbed after I.M. administration.
*Distribution:* Rapidly crosses the placenta; neonatal serum levels are 0.4 to 1.4 times maternal levels.
*Metabolism:* Metabolized extensively in the liver, primarily by hydroxylation, to inactive metabolites.
*Excretion:* Excreted in inactive form, mainly by the kidneys. About 11% to 14% of a parenteral dose appears in feces.

| Route | Onset | Peak | Duration |
|-------|-------|------|----------|
| I.V. | 2-3 min | 30-60 min | 3-4 hr |
| I.M. | 10-15 min | 30-60 min | 3-4 hr |
| Nasal | 15 min | 1-2 hr | 4-5 hr |

### Contraindications and precautions

Contraindicated in patients receiving repeated doses of narcotic drugs or with narcotic addiction; may precipitate withdrawal syndrome. Also contraindicated in patients hypersensitive to drug or to the preservative benzethonium chloride.

Use cautiously in emotionally unstable patients and in those with history of drug abuse, head injuries, increased intracranial pressure, acute MI, ventricular dysfunction, coronary insufficiency, respiratory disease or depression, and renal or hepatic dysfunction.

## Interactions

**Drug-drug.** *Barbiturate anesthetics such as thiopental:* Additive CNS and respiratory depressant effects and, possibly, apnea. Advise clinician to closely monitor patient.

*Cimetidine:* May potentiate butorphanol toxicity, causing disorientation, respiratory depression, apnea, and seizures. Advise using cautiously and be prepared to give a narcotic antagonist if toxicity occurs.

*Digitoxin, phenytoin, rifampin:* Drug accumulation and enhanced effects. Recommend reduced butorphanol dose.

*General anesthetics:* Severe CV depression. Avoid use together.

*Narcotic antagonists:* Patients who become physically dependent on opioids may experience acute withdrawal syndrome. Use with caution and advise clinician to monitor patient closely.

*Other CNS depressants (narcotic analgesics, antihistamines, phenothiazines, barbiturates, benzodiazepines, sedative-hypnotics, tricyclic antidepressants, muscle relaxants):* Potentiate respiratory and CNS depression, sedation, and hypotensive effects. Reduced doses of butorphanol are usually needed.

*Pancuronium:* May increase conjunctival changes. Advise clinician to monitor patient.

**Drug-lifestyle.** *Alcohol use:* May potentiate respiratory and CNS depression, sedation, and hypotensive effects of the drug. Advise patient to avoid alcohol.

## Adverse reactions

**CNS:** *confusion,* nervousness, lethargy, headache, *somnolence, dizziness, insomnia,* anxiety, paresthesia, euphoria, hallucinations, flushing, ***increased intracranial pressure.***
**CV:** palpitations, vasodilation, hypotension.
**EENT:** blurred vision, *nasal congestion* (with nasal spray), tinnitus.
**GI:** *nausea, vomiting, constipation,* taste perversion, anorexia.
**Respiratory:** *respiratory depression.*
**Skin:** rash, hives, *clamminess, excessive diaphoresis.*
**Other:** sensation of heat.

## Overdose and treatment

No information available.

## Clinical considerations

■ Patients using nasal formulation for severe pain may start therapy with 2 mg (one spray in each nostril) provided they remain recumbent. Dose isn't repeated for 3 to 4 hours.

### *Therapeutic monitoring*

■ Drug has the potential to be abused. Recommend close supervision in emotionally unstable patients and in those with history of drug abuse when long-term therapy is needed.

■ Advise clinician to monitor patient for respiratory depression.

### *Special populations*

**Pregnant patients.** Safe use during pregnancy (except during labor) hasn't been established.

**Breast-feeding patients.** Use of drug in breast-feeding women isn't recommended.

**Pediatric patients.** Safety and efficacy in children younger than age 18 haven't been established.

**Geriatric patients.** Lower doses are usually indicated for geriatric patients because they may be more sensitive to the therapeutic and adverse effects of the drug. Plasma half-life is increased by 25% in patients older than age 65.

## Patient counseling

■ Teach patient how to use nasal spray. Patient should use one spray in one nostril unless otherwise directed.

■ Tell patient that before initial use, the pump should be fully primed. The pump should be reprimed if not used for 48 hours or longer.

■ Inform patient that the pump delivery system is an open delivery system; he should aim the spray away from any people in close contact so they are not exposed to the drug.

# calcipotriene

Dovonex

*Pharmacologic classification:* synthetic vitamin $D_3$ analogue
*Therapeutic classification:* topical antipsoriatic
*Pregnancy risk category C*

## Available forms
Available by prescription only
*Cream, ointment, solution:* 0.005%

## Indications and dosages
*Moderate plaque psoriasis*
*Adults:* Cream—Apply a thin layer to affected skin b.i.d. Rub in gently and completely. Ointment—Apply a thin layer to affected skin once daily to b.i.d. Rub in gently and completely. Solution—Apply to affected area of scalp b.i.d. First remove scaly debris; then apply solution and rub in completely.

## Mechanism of action
*Antipsoriatic action:* Calcipotriene is a synthetic vitamin $D_3$ analogue that binds to vitamin $D_3$ receptors in skin cells (keratinocytes), regulating skin cell production and development.

## Pharmacokinetics
*Absorption:* About 6% of the applied dose of calcipotriene is absorbed systemically when the ointment is applied topically to psoriasis plaques or 5% when applied to normal skin.
*Distribution:* Vitamin D and its metabolites are transported in the blood (bound to specific plasma proteins) to many parts of the body containing keratinocytes. (The scaly red patches of psoriasis are caused by the abnormal growth and production of keratinocytes.)
*Metabolism:* Drug metabolism after systemic uptake is rapid and occurs via a pathway similar to the natural hormone. The primary metabolites are much less potent than the parent compound.
*Excretion:* The active form of the vitamin, 1,25-dihydroxy vitamin $D_3$ (calcitriol), is recycled via the liver and excreted in bile.

| Route | Onset | Peak | Duration |
|---|---|---|---|
| Topical | Unknown | Unknown | Unknown |

## Contraindications and precautions
Contraindicated in patients hypersensitive to drug or its components. Also contraindicated in patients with hypercalcemia or evidence of vitamin D toxicity. Use cautiously in breast-feeding and geriatric patients. Drug shouldn't be used on the face.

## Interactions
None reported.

## Adverse reactions
**Metabolic:** hypercalcemia.
**Skin:** *burning, pruritus, irritation,* atrophy, dermatitis, dry skin, erythema, folliculitis, hyperpigmentation, peeling, rash, worsening of psoriasis.

## Overdose and treatment
Topically applied calcipotriene can be absorbed in sufficient amounts to produce systemic effects. Serum calcium levels may increase with excessive use.

## Clinical considerations
■ Drug is for topical dermatologic use only. It isn't intended for ophthalmic, oral, or intra-vaginal use.
■ Improvement usually begins after 2 weeks of therapy and marked improvement occurs after 8 weeks; only about 10% of cases show complete clearing.
■ Safety and effectiveness of topical calcipotriene in dermatoses other than psoriasis haven't been established.
■ Use of calcipotriene may cause irritation of lesions and surrounding uninvolved skin. If irritation develops, drug should be stopped.

### *Therapeutic monitoring*
■ Transient, rapidly reversible elevation of serum calcium level may occur. If serum calcium level increases outside the normal range, treatment should be stopped until normal calcium levels are restored.

### *Special populations*
**Breast-feeding patients.** It isn't known if drug appears in breast milk. Use caution when giving calcipotriene ointment to a breast-feeding patient.
**Pediatric patients.** Safety and effectiveness in children haven't been established.

---

Reactions may be *common,* uncommon, *life-threatening,* or COMMON AND LIFE-THREATENING.

**Geriatric patients.** Adverse dermatologic effects of topical calcipotriene may be more severe in patients over age 65.

## Patient counseling
■ Tell patient that drug is for external use only, as directed, and to avoid contact with the face or eyes.
■ Instruct patient to wash hands thoroughly after application.
■ Tell patient to report signs of local adverse reactions.

# calcitonin
Miacalcin (salmon), Osteocalcin (salmon), Salmonine (salmon)

*Pharmacologic classification:* thyroid hormone
*Therapeutic classification:* hypocalcemic
*Pregnancy risk category C*

## Available forms
Available by prescription only
*Injection:* 200-IU/ml, 2-ml vials (salmon)
*Nasal spray:* 200 IU/activation

## Indications and dosages
*Paget's bone disease (osteitis deformans)*
*Adults:* Initially, 100 IU salmon calcitonin S.C. or I.M. daily. Maintenance dosage is 50 to 100 IU salmon calcitonin, three times weekly.
*Hypercalcemia*
*Adults:* 4 IU/kg calcitonin (salmon) I.M. or S.C. q 12 hours; increase by 8 IU/kg q 12 hours, or ◊ 2 to 16 IU/kg I.V. infusion q 12 hours.
*Postmenopausal osteoporosis*
*Adults:* 100 IU calcitonin (salmon) S.C. or I.M. daily, or 200 IU (one spray) daily in alternating nostril.
◊ *Osteogenesis imperfecta*
*Adults:* 2 IU/kg calcitonin (salmon) three times weekly, with daily calcium supplementation.

## I.V. administration
■ Follow standard I.V. technique. I.V. use is currently an unlabeled clinical use for emergency situations.
■ Use S.C. route when possible. Use I.M. route only when volume exceeds 2 ml.

### Incompatibilities
None reported.

## Mechanism of action
*Hypocalcemic action:* Calcitonin directly inhibits the bone resorption of calcium. This effect is mediated by drug-induced increase of cAMP concentration in bone cells, which alters transport of calcium and phosphate across the plasma membrane of the osteoclast. A secondary effect occurs in the kidneys, where calcitonin directly inhibits tubular resorption of calcium, phosphate, and sodium, thereby increasing their excretion. A clinical effect may not be seen for several months in patients with Paget's disease.

## Pharmacokinetics
*Absorption:* Drug can be given parenterally or nasally. Plasma levels of 0.1 to 0.4 mg/ml are achieved within 15 minutes of a 200-IU S.C. dose. The maximum effect is seen in 2 to 4 hours; duration of action may be 8 to 24 hours for S.C. or I.M. doses, and ½ to 12 hours for I.V. doses. Peak plasma levels appear 31 to 39 minutes after using the nasal form.
*Distribution:* It's unknown if drug enters the CNS or crosses the placenta.
*Metabolism:* Rapid metabolism occurs in the kidney, with additional activity in the blood and peripheral tissues.
*Excretion:* Excreted in urine as inactive metabolites.

| Route | Onset | Peak | Duration |
|---|---|---|---|
| I.V. | Immediate | 2-4 hr | ½-12 hr |
| I.M., S.C. | 15 min | 4 hr | 8-24 hr |
| Intranasal | Rapid | ½ hr | 1 hr |

## Contraindications and precautions
Contraindicated in patients hypersensitive to salmon calcitonin.

## Interactions
None reported.

## Adverse reactions
**CNS:** headache, weakness, dizziness, paresthesia.
**CV:** edema of feet, chest pressure.
**EENT:** eye pain, nasal congestion.
**GI:** *transient nausea,* unusual taste, diarrhea, anorexia, *vomiting,* epigastric discomfort, abdominal pain.
**GU:** *increased urinary frequency,* nocturia.
**Respiratory:** shortness of breath.
**Skin:** *facial flushing,* rash, pruritus of ear lobes, *inflammation at injection site.*
**Other:** chills, hypersensitivity reactions, *anaphylaxis,* tender palms and soles.

## Overdose and treatment
Signs and symptoms of overdose include hypocalcemia and hypocalcemic tetany, usually occurring in patients at higher risk during the first few doses. Parenteral calcium will correct the symptoms and should be readily available.

## Clinical considerations
■ S.C. is the preferred administration method.

### Therapeutic monitoring
■ A skin test using salmon calcitonin should be considered before calcitonin therapy starts. If patient has allergic reactions to foreign pro-

---

teins, recommend testing for hypersensitivity before therapy. Systemic allergic reactions are possible because hormone is a protein. Epinephrine should be kept readily available.

■ Advise clinician to keep parenteral calcium available during the first doses in case of hypocalcemic tetany.

■ Recommend periodic monitoring of serum calcium levels during therapy.

■ Advise clinician to observe patient for signs of hypocalcemic tetany during therapy (muscle twitching, tetanic spasms, and convulsions if hypocalcemia is severe).

■ Advise clinician to watch patient for the following signs of hypercalcemic relapse: bone pain, renal calculi, polyuria, anorexia, nausea, vomiting, thirst, constipation, lethargy, bradycardia, muscle hypotonicity, pathologic fracture, psychosis, and coma. Patient with good initial clinical response to calcitonin who suffers relapse should be evaluated for antibody formation response to the hormone protein.

■ Solution should be refrigerated. Once activated, store nasal spray upright at controlled room temperature.

### Special populations

**Pregnant patients.** Use with caution.
**Breast-feeding patients.** Use with caution.
**Pediatric patients.** There are inadequate data to support the use of calcitonin in children.

### Patient counseling

■ Instruct patient on self-administration of drug and assist him until proper technique is achieved.

■ Tell patient to handle missed doses as follows:
*Daily dosing:* Take as soon as possible; don't double the doses.

*Every-other-day dosing:* Take as soon as possible, then restart the alternate days from this dose.

■ Stress importance of regular follow-up to assess progress.

■ If given for postmenopausal osteoporosis, remind patient to take adequate calcium and vitamin D supplements.

■ Tell patient to report nasal irritation. Recommend performing periodic nasal examination.

---

# calcitriol

Calcijex, Rocaltrol

*Pharmacologic classification:* vitamin D analogue
*Therapeutic classification:* antihypocalcemic
*Pregnancy risk category C*

### Available forms

Available by prescription only
*Capsules:* 0.25 mcg, 0.5 mcg
*Injection:* 1 mcg/ml, 2 mcg/ml
*Oral solution:* 1 mcg/ml

## Indications and dosages

*Management of hypocalcemia in patients undergoing chronic dialysis*
**Oral**
*Adults:* Initially, 0.25 mcg P.O. daily. Dosage may be increased by 0.25 mcg daily at 4- to 8-week intervals. Maintenance dosage, 0.25 mcg every other day up to 0.5 to 1 mcg P.O. daily.
**Parenteral**
*Adults:* 0.5 mcg I.V. three times weekly, about every other day. Dosage may be increased by 0.25 to 0.5 mcg at 2- to 4-week intervals. Maintenance dosage, 0.5 to 3 mcg I.V. three times weekly.
*Management of hypoparathyroidism and pseudohypoparathyroidism*
*Adults and children ages 6 and older:* Initially, 0.25 mcg P.O. daily in the morning. Dosage may be increased at 2- to 4-week intervals. Maintenance dosage, 0.5 to 2 mcg daily.
*Children ages 1 to 5 (hypoparathyroidism only):* Initially, 0.25 mcg P.O. daily. Dosage may be increased at 2- to 4-week intervals. Maintenance dosage, 0.25 to 0.75 mcg P.O. daily.
*Prevention or management of secondary hyperparathyroidism and resultant metabolic bone disease in predialysis patients (moderate to severe chronic renal failure with creatinine clearance of 15 to 55 ml/minute)*
*Adults and children ages 3 and older:* Initially, 0.25 mcg P.O. daily. Dosage may be increased to 0.5 mcg/day, if needed.
*Children under age 3:* Initially, 10 to 15 ng/kg P.O. daily.
◊ *Psoriasis vulgaris*
*Adults:* 0.5 mcg/day P.O. for 6 months and topically (0.5 mcg/g petroleum) daily for 8 weeks.

## I.V. administration

■ Drug may be given by rapid I.V. injection through the dialysis catheter at the end of a period of hemodialysis.

■ Protect solution from heat and light.

### Incompatibilities

None reported.

## Mechanism of action

*Antihypocalcemic action:* Calcitriol is a vitamin D analogue (1,25-dihydroxycholecalciferol), or activated cholecalciferol. It promotes absorption of calcium from the intestine by forming a calcium-binding protein. It reverses the signs of rickets and osteomalacia in patients who can't activate or use ergocalciferol or cholecalciferol. In patients with renal failure, it reduces bone pain, muscle weakness, and parathyroid serum levels.

## Pharmacokinetics

*Absorption:* Absorbed readily after oral administration.

*Distribution:* Distributed widely and is protein-bound.
*Metabolism:* Metabolized in the liver and kidney, with a half-life of 3 to 8 hours. No activation step is required.
*Excretion:* Excreted primarily in the feces.

| Route | Onset | Peak | Duration |
|-------|-------|------|----------|
| P.O. | 2-6 hr | 3-6 hr | 3-5 days |
| I.V. | Immediate | Unknown | 3-5 days |

## Contraindications and precautions
Contraindicated in patients with hypercalcemia or vitamin D toxicity. Withhold all preparations containing vitamin D.

## Interactions
**Drug-drug.** *Antacids containing magnesium:* Possible induced hypermagnesemia, especially in patients with chronic renal failure. Avoid use together.
*Cardiac glycosides:* Increased risk of arrhythmias. Avoid use together.
*Cholestyramine, colestipol, and mineral oil:* Possible alteration of calcitriol absorption. Avoid use together.
*Corticosteroids:* May counteract the effects of vitamin D analogues. Don't use together.
*Orlistat:* Decreased absorption of vitamin D. Recommend giving at least 2 hours apart.

## Adverse reactions
**CNS:** headache, somnolence, weakness, irritability, psychosis.
**CV:** hypertension, *arrhythmias.*
**EENT:** conjunctivitis, photophobia, rhinorrhea.
**GI:** nausea, vomiting, constipation, polydipsia, *pancreatitis,* metallic taste, dry mouth, anorexia.
**GU:** polyuria, nocturia.
**Metabolic:** weight loss.
**Musculoskeletal:** bone and muscle pain.
**Skin:** pruritus.
**Other:** hyperthermia, nephrocalcinosis, decreased libido.

## Overdose and treatment
Treatment of hypercalcemia (a sign of overdose) requires discontinuation of drug, institution of a low-calcium diet, increased fluid intake, and supportive measures. Calcitonin administration may help reverse hypercalcemia. In severe cases, death has followed CV and renal failure.

## Clinical considerations
■ Vitamin D intoxication is linked to hypercalcemia.
■ Calcitriol therapy may falsely elevate cholesterol determinations made using the Zlatkis-Zak reaction. It also alters serum alkaline phosphatase levels and may alter electrolyte levels,

such as magnesium, phosphate, and calcium in serum and urine.
■ Protect drug from heat and light.

### Therapeutic monitoring
■ Advise clinician to monitor serum calcium levels several times weekly after therapy starts.
■ There is some evidence that monitoring urine calcium and urine creatinine is very helpful in screening for hypercalciuria. The ratio of urine calcium to urine creatinine should be less than or equal to 0.18. A value of more than 0.2 suggests hypercalciuria, and the dose should be decreased regardless of serum calcium level. The product of serum calcium times phosphate shouldn't be allowed to exceed 70.

### Special populations
**Breast-feeding patients.** Very little drug appears in breast milk; however, the effect of vitamin D levels exceeding the recommended daily allowance in infants isn't known. Therefore, large doses shouldn't be given to breast-feeding women.
**Pediatric patients.** Some infants may be hyperreactive to drug. Long-term treatment has been well-tolerated except for occasional episodes of electrolyte imbalance, which resolves with alteration of therapy.

### Patient counseling
■ Instruct patient on the importance of a calcium-rich diet.
■ Tell patient that drug must not be taken by anyone for whom it wasn't prescribed. It's the most potent form of vitamin D.
■ Advise patient to report adverse reactions immediately.
■ Tell patient to avoid antacids containing magnesium and other self-prescribed drugs.

# calcium salts
# calcium acetate
PhosLo

# calcium carbonate
Alka-Mints, Amitone, Calciday-667, Caltrate 600, Chooz, Os-Cal 500, Titralac, Tums, Tums E-X

# calcium chloride
# calcium citrate
Citracal

# calcium gluceptate
# calcium gluconate
# calcium lactate

---

# calcium phosphate, tribasic
Posture

*Pharmacologic classification:* calcium supplement
*Therapeutic classification:* therapeutic agent for electrolyte balance, cardiotonic
*Pregnancy risk category C*

## Available forms
Available by prescription only
**calcium chloride**
*Injection:* 10% solution (1 g/10 ml; each ml of solution provides 27.2 mg or 1.36 mEq of calcium) in 10-ml ampules, vials, and syringes
Available without a prescription
**calcium acetate**
*Tablets:* 250 mg (62.5 mg of calcium), 668 mg (167 mg of calcium), 1,000 mg (250 mg of calcium)
*Capsules:* 500 mg
**calcium carbonate**
*Tablets:* 500 mg, 650 mg, 667 mg, 1.25 g, 1.5 g
*Tablets (chewable):* 350 mg, 420 mg, 500 mg, 750 mg, 835 mg, 850 mg, 1.25 g
*Oral suspension:* 1.25 g (500 mg of calcium) per 5 ml
*Capsules:* 1.25 g (500 mg of calcium), 1.5 g (600 mg of calcium)
*Powder:* 6.5 g
**calcium citrate**
*Tablets:* 950 mg (contains 200 mg of elemental calcium/g)
*Tablets (effervescent):* 2,376 mg (500 mg of calcium)
**calcium gluceptate**
*Injection:* 1.1 g/5 ml ampules or 50-ml vials for preparation of I.V. admixtures (each ml of solution provides 18 mg or 0.9 mEq of calcium)
**calcium gluconate**
*Tablets:* 500 mg, 650 mg, 975 mg, 1 g (contains 90 mg of elemental calcium/g)
*Injection:* 10% solution (1 g/10 ml; each ml of solution provides 9.3 mg or 0.46 mEq of calcium) in 10-ml ampules and vials, or 20-ml vials
**calcium lactate**
*Tablets:* 325 mg, 650 mg (contains 130 mg of elemental calcium/g)
**calcium phosphate, tribasic**
*Tablets:* 600 mg

## Indications and dosages
*Emergency treatment of hypocalcemia*
**calcium chloride**
*Adults:* 500 mg to 1 g I.V. slowly (not to exceed 1 ml/minute).
*Children:* 0.2 ml/kg I.V. slowly (not to exceed 1 ml/minute).

**calcium gluconate**
*Adults:* 7 to 14 mEq I.V. slowly (not to exceed 0.7 to 1.8 mEq/minute).
*Children:* 1 to 7 mEq I.V. slowly (not to exceed 0.7 to 1.8 mEq/minute).
Repeat above dosage based on clinical laboratory value.
*Cardiotonic use*
**calcium chloride**
*Adults:* 500 mg to 1 g I.V. slowly (not to exceed 1 ml/minute); or 200 to 800 mg intraventricularly as a single dose during cardiac resuscitation.
*Hyperkalemia*
**calcium gluconate**
*Adults:* 2.25 to 14 mEq I.V. slowly. Adjust administration based on ECG response.
*Hypermagnesemia*
**calcium chloride**
*Adults:* 500 mg I.V. initially, repeated based on clinical response.
**calcium gluceptate**
*Adults:* 2 to 5 ml I.M., or 5 to 20 ml I.V.
**calcium gluconate**
*Adults:* 4.5 to 9 mEq I.V. slowly.
*During exchange transfusions*
*Adults:* 1.35 mEq I.V. concurrently with each 100-ml citrated blood exchange.
*Neonates:* 0.45 mEq I.V. after every 100 ml of citrated blood exchange.
*Hypocalcemia*
**calcium acetate**
*Adults:* 2 to 4 tablets P.O. with meals.
**calcium gluconate**
*Adults:* For hypocalcemic tetany, 4.5 to 16 mEq I.V. until therapeutic response is obtained.
*Children:* For hypocalcemic tetany, 0.5 to 0.7 mEq/kg I.V. t.i.d. or q.i.d. or until tetany is controlled.
*Neonates:* 2.4 mEq/kg/day in divided doses until therapeutic response is obtained.
**calcium lactate**
*Adults:* 325 mg to 1.3 g P.O. t.i.d. with meals.
*Osteoporosis prevention*
*Adults:* 1 to 1.5 g P.O. daily of elemental calcium.
*Hyperphosphatemia in end-stage renal failure*
**calcium acetate**
*Adults:* 2 to 4 tablets P.O. with each meal.

## I.V. administration
■ Calcium chloride should only be given I.V.
■ Recommend giving I.V. calcium slowly through a small-bore needle into a large vein to avoid extravasation and necrosis. Injection should be stopped if patient complains of discomfort.
■ If perivascular infiltration occurs, I.V. should be stopped immediately. Venospasm may be reduced by giving 1% procaine hydrochloride and hyaluronidase to the affected area.
■ After I.V. injection, keep patient recumbent for 15 minutes to prevent orthostasis.

**Other:** pain and irritation (with S.C. infiltration); *vein irritation* (with I.V. use).

## Overdose and treatment
Acute hypercalcemia syndrome is characterized by a markedly elevated plasma calcium level, lethargy, weakness, nausea and vomiting, and coma, and may lead to sudden death.

In case of overdose, calcium should be stopped immediately. After oral ingestion of calcium overdose, treatment includes removal by emesis or gastric lavage followed by supportive therapy, p.r.n.

## Clinical considerations
- I.M. route should only be used in emergencies when no I.V. route is available. Recommend giving I.M. injections in the gluteal region in adults, lateral thigh in infants.
- I.V. calcium may produce transient elevation of plasma 11-hydroxycorticosteroid levels (Glen-Nelson technique) and false-negative values for serum and urine magnesium as measured by the Titan yellow method.
- Hypercalcemia may result when large doses are given to patients with chronic renal failure.
- Severe necrosis and tissue sloughing may occur after extravasation. Calcium gluconate is less irritating to veins and tissue than calcium chloride.
- If GI upset occurs with oral calcium, give 2 to 3 hours after meals.
- With oral product, patient may need laxatives or stool softeners to manage constipation.
**⚠ ALERT** Current guidelines for ACLS and PALS state that calcium shouldn't be used during resuscitation except when hyperkalemia, hypocalcemia, or calcium-channel blocking drug toxicity is present and epinephrine and isoproterenol have failed.

### Therapeutic monitoring
- Advise clinician to monitor serum calcium levels frequently, especially in patients with renal impairment.
- Assess Chvostek's and Trousseau's signs periodically to check for tetany.
- Advise clinician to monitor patient for signs and symptoms of hypercalcemia (nausea, vomiting, headache, mental confusion, anorexia), and report them immediately. Calcium absorption of an oral dose is decreased in patients with certain disease states such as achlorhydria, renal osteodystrophy, steatorrhea, or uremia.

### Special populations
**Breast-feeding patients.** Calcium appears in breast milk, but not in quantities large enough to affect the breast-feeding infant.
**Pediatric patients.** Give calcium cautiously to children by I.V. route (usually not given I.M.).

**Geriatric patients.** Calcium absorption (after oral administration) may be decreased in geriatric patients.

## Patient counseling
- Tell patient not to exceed the manufacturer's recommended dosage of calcium.
- Warn patient not to use bone meal or dolomite as a source of calcium; they may contain lead.
- Advise patient to avoid tobacco and to limit intake of alcohol and caffeine-containing beverages.

# candesartan cilexetil
Atacand

*Pharmacologic classification:* selective angiotensin II receptor antagonist
*Therapeutic classification:* antihypertensive
*Pregnancy risk category C (D in second and third trimesters)*

## Available forms
Available by prescription only
*Tablets:* 4 mg, 8 mg, 16 mg, 32 mg

## Indications and dosages
*Treatment of hypertension (used alone or with other antihypertensives)*
*Adults:* Initially, 16 mg P.O. once daily when used as monotherapy; usual dosage range is 8 to 32 mg P.O. daily as a single dose or divided b.i.d.

## Mechanism of action
*Antihypertensive action:* Inhibits the vasoconstrictor and aldosterone-secreting effects of angiotensin II by selectively blocking the binding of angiotensin II to the $AT_1$ receptor in many tissues, such as vascular smooth muscle and the adrenal gland.

## Pharmacokinetics
*Absorption:* Rapidly and completely bioactivated during absorption from the GI tract.
*Distribution:* Highly plasma protein–bound.
*Metabolism:* Undergoes minor hepatic metabolism.
*Excretion:* Primarily recovered in the urine and feces. Elimination half life is about 9 hours.

| Route | Onset | Peak | Duration |
|-------|-------|------|----------|
| P.O. | Unknown | 3-4 hr | 24 hr |

## Contraindications and precautions
Contraindicated in patients hypersensitive to drug or its components.

Use cautiously in patients whose renal function depends on the renin-angiotensin-aldosterone system (such as patients with heart failure) because there's potential for oliguria and progressive azotemia with acute renal failure or death. Also use cautiously in patients who are volume- or salt-depleted because there is potential for symptomatic hypotension. Start therapy with a lower dosage range, as ordered, and monitor blood pressure carefully.

## Interactions
None reported.

## Adverse reactions
**CNS:** dizziness, fatigue, headache.
**CV:** chest pain, peripheral edema.
**EENT:** pharyngitis, rhinitis, sinusitis.
**GI:** abdominal pain, diarrhea, nausea, vomiting.
**GU:** albuminuria.
**Musculoskeletal:** arthralgia, back pain.
**Respiratory:** cough, bronchitis, upper respiratory tract infection.

## Overdose and treatment
The most likely signs and symptoms of overdose are hypotension, dizziness, and tachycardia; bradycardia could occur from parasympathetic (vagal) stimulation. Treatment should be supportive. Dialysis isn't effective.

## Clinical considerations
■ Drugs that act directly on the renin-angiotensin system (such as candesartan) can cause fetal and neonatal morbidity and death when given to pregnant women. These problems haven't been detected when exposure was limited to first trimester. If pregnancy is suspected, patient should stop drug immediately.

### Therapeutic monitoring
■ If hypotension occurs after a dose of candesartan, patient should be placed in the supine position and, if needed, given an I.V. infusion of normal saline.
■ Most of the antihypertensive effect is present within 2 weeks. Maximal antihypertensive effect is obtained within 4 to 6 weeks. Diuretic may be added if blood pressure isn't controlled by drug alone.

### Special populations
**Pregnant patients.** Inform woman of childbearing age of the consequences of second and third trimester exposure to drug. Advise her to notify prescriber immediately if pregnancy is suspected.
**Breast-feeding patients.** It isn't known if drug appears in breast milk; therefore, breast-feeding during drug therapy isn't recommended.
**Pediatric patients.** Safety and efficacy in children haven't been established.
**Geriatric patients.** Serum levels of drug are higher in these patients than in younger adults; however, the drug and its inactive metabolite don't accumulate in the serum of geriatric patients after repeated once-daily dosing.

## Patient counseling
■ Instruct patient to store drug at controlled room temperature and to keep container tightly sealed.
■ Inform patient to report adverse reactions without delay.
■ Tell patient that drug may be taken without regard to meals.

# capecitabine
Xeloda

*Pharmacologic classification:* fluoro-pyrimidine carbamate
*Therapeutic classification:* antineo-plastic
*Pregnancy risk category D*

## Available forms
Available by prescription only
*Tablets:* 150 mg, 500 mg

## Indications and dosages
*Treatment of patients with metastatic breast cancer resistant to both paclitaxel and an anthracycline-containing chemotherapy regimen or resistant to paclitaxel and for whom further anthracycline therapy isn't indicated; first-line treatment of patients with metastatic colorectal cancer when treatment with fluoropyrimidine therapy alone is preferred; treatment of patients with metastatic breast cancer with docetaxel, after failure of prior anthracycline-containing chemotherapy*
Adults: 2,500 mg/m² P.O. daily in two divided doses (about 12 hours apart) with food for 2 weeks, followed by a 1-week rest period and given as 3-week cycles.
≣*Dosage adjustment.* For patients with moderate renal impairment, reduce starting dose to 75% of the recommended starting dose.
≣*Dosage adjustment.* National Cancer Institute of Canada (NCIC) Common Toxicity Criteria:
  *NCIC grade 2:* First appearance, interrupt treatment until resolved to grade 0 to 1, then restart at 100% of starting dose for next cycle; second appearance, interrupt treatment until resolved to grade 0 to 1 and use 75% of starting dose for next cycle; third appearance, interrupt treatment until resolved to grade 0 to 1 and use 50% of starting dose for next cycle; fourth appearance, discontinue treatment permanently.
  *NCIC grade 3:* First appearance, interrupt treatment until resolved to grade 0 to 1 and use 75% of starting dose for next cycle; second appearance, interrupt treatment until resolved to grade 0 to 1 and use 50% of starting dose for next cycle; third appearance, discontinue treatment permanently.

*NCIC grade 4:* First appearance, discontinue treatment permanently or interrupt treatment until resolved to grade 0 to 1 and use 50% of starting dose for next cycle.

Note: Toxicity criteria relate to degrees of severity of diarrhea, nausea, vomiting, stomatitis, and hand-foot syndrome. Refer to capecitabine package insert for specific toxicity definitions.

## Mechanism of action

*Antineoplastic action:* Capecitabine is converted to the active drug 5-fluorouracil (5-FU). 5-FU is metabolized by both normal and tumor cells to metabolites that cause cellular injury by way of two different mechanisms: interference with DNA synthesis to inhibit cell division and interference with RNA processing and protein synthesis.

## Pharmacokinetics

*Absorption:* Readily absorbed from the GI tract. The rate and extent of absorption are decreased with food.
*Distribution:* About 60% is plasma protein–bound.
*Metabolism:* Extensively metabolized to 5-FU (an active metabolite).
*Excretion:* Elimination half-life of the parent drug and the active moiety is about 45 minutes with 70% excreted in the urine.

| Route | Onset | Peak | Duration |
|-------|-------|------|----------|
| P.O. | Unknown | 1½-2 hr | Unknown |

## Contraindications and precautions

Contraindicated in patients hypersensitive to 5-FU. Contraindicated in patients with severe renal impairment. Severe diarrhea can occur; advise clinician to monitor electrolytes and ensure proper hydration.

Use cautiously in geriatric patients and in patients with history of coronary artery disease, mild-to-moderate hepatic dysfunction resulting from liver metastases, hyperbilirubinemia, and renal insufficiency. Capecitabine therapy may need to be interrupted or decreased if hand-foot syndrome (characterized by numbness, paresthesia, tingling, painless or painful swelling, erythema, desquamation, blistering, and severe pain of hands or feet, hyperbilirubinemia, and severe nausea) occurs.

## Interactions

**Drug-drug.** *Antacids:* Increased rate of absorption of capecitabine. Dosage change may be needed.
*Coumadin:* Altered PT and bleeding with use together. Advise clinician to monitor anticoagulant response frequently.
*Leucovorin:* Increased concentration of 5-FU with enhanced toxicity. Advise clinician to monitor patient closely.

## Adverse reactions

**CNS:** dizziness, *fatigue,* headache, insomnia, *paresthesia.*
**CV:** edema.
**EENT:** eye irritation.
**GI:** *diarrhea, nausea, vomiting, stomatitis, abdominal pain, constipation, anorexia,* **intestinal obstruction,** *dyspepsia.*
**Hematologic:** NEUTROPENIA, THROMBOCYTOPENIA, *anemia, lymphopenia.*
**Hepatic:** *hyperbilirubinemia.*
**Musculoskeletal:** myalgia, pain in limb.
**Skin:** *hand-foot syndrome, dermatitis,* nail disorder.
**Other:** *pyrexia,* dehydration.

## Overdose and treatment

Overdose should be managed by supportive medical care aimed at correcting the signs and symptoms. Dialysis may be of benefit in drug removal.

## Clinical considerations

■ Store tablets at controlled room temperature. Keep container tightly closed.
■ Tablets should be taken within 30 minutes after a meal.
■ Inform prescriber if patient is taking folic acid or warfarin.

### Therapeutic monitoring

■ Altered coagulation parameters and bleeding may occur within several days up to several months after therapy starts and, rarely, within one month after stopping capecitabine therapy.
■ Fluid and electrolyte replacement may be needed for severe diarrhea.
■ Drug may need to be immediately interrupted until diarrhea resolves or decreases in intensity.
■ Hyperbilirubinemia may require discontinuing drug.
■ Advise clinician to monitor patient carefully for toxicity. Toxicity may be managed by symptomatic treatment, dose interruptions, and dosage adjustments.

### Special populations

**Pregnant patients.** Because of teratogenic effects, women of childbearing age should avoid becoming pregnant while taking capecitabine.
**Breast-feeding patients.** Patients should discontinue breast-feeding while on drug therapy.
**Pediatric patients.** Safety and efficacy in patients under age 18 haven't been established.
**Geriatric patients.** Patients over age 80 may experience a greater risk of GI adverse effects.

## Patient counseling

■ Inform patient and caregiver of expected adverse effects of drug, especially nausea, vomiting, diarrhea, and hand-foot syndrome (pain, swelling or redness of hands or feet). Tell them that patient-specific dose adaptations during therapy are expected and needed.

■ Instruct patient to stop taking drug and contact prescriber immediately if the following adverse effects occur: diarrhea (more than four bowel movements daily or diarrhea at night), vomiting (two to five episodes in a 24-hour period), nausea, appetite loss or decrease in amount of food taken each day, stomatitis (pain, redness, swelling, or sores in mouth), hand-foot syndrome, temperature of 100.5° F (38° C) or greater, or other evidence of infection.

■ Tell patient that most adverse effects improve within 2 to 3 days after stopping drug. If they don't improve, tell him to contact prescriber.

■ Tell patient how to take the drug. Drug is usually taken for 14 days followed by a 7-day rest period (no drug) given as a 21-day cycle. The prescriber determines the number of treatment cycles.

■ Instruct patient to take drug with water within 30 minutes after end of a meal (breakfast and dinner).

■ If a combination of tablets is prescribed, teach patient importance of correctly identifying the tablets to avoid possible misdosing.

■ For missed doses, instruct patient not to take the missed dose and not to double the next one. Instead, he should continue with regular dosing schedule and check with the prescriber.

■ Instruct patient to inform prescriber if he's taking the vitamin folic acid.

■ Advise women of childbearing age to avoid becoming pregnant while receiving treatment.

# captopril
Capoten

*Pharmacologic classification:* ACE inhibitor
*Therapeutic classification:* antihypertensive, adjunctive treatment of heart failure
*Pregnancy risk category C (D in second and third trimesters)*

## Available forms
Available by prescription only
*Tablets:* 12.5 mg, 25 mg, 50 mg, 100 mg

## Indications and dosages
*Mild to severe hypertension;* ◇ *idiopathic edema;* ◇ *Raynaud's phenomenon*
*Adults:* Initially, 25 mg P.O. b.i.d. or t.i.d.; if needed, dosage may be increased to 50 mg b.i.d. or t.i.d. after 1 to 2 weeks; if control is still inadequate after 1 to 2 weeks more, a diuretic may be added. Dosage may be increased to a maximum of 150 mg t.i.d. (450 mg/day) while continuing the diuretic. Daily dose may be given b.i.d.

*Heart failure*
*Adults:* 25 mg P.O. t.i.d. If patient is on a diuretic, is hyponatremic or hypovolemic, an initial dose of 6.25 to 12.5 mg t.i.d. should be given. Maintenance dosage is 50 to 100 mg t.i.d.
*Prevention of diabetic nephropathy*
*Adults:* 25 mg P.O. t.i.d.
*Left ventricular dysfunction after MI*
*Adults:* 6.25 mg P.O. as a single dose 3 days after an MI; then 12.5 mg t.i.d., increasing dose to 25 mg t.i.d. Target dose is 50 mg t.i.d.
≡ *Dosage adjustment.* For geriatric patients and patients with renal failure, use lower initial daily doses and smaller increments for adjustment.

## Mechanism of action
*Antihypertensive action:* Captopril inhibits ACE, preventing conversion of angiotensin I to angiotensin II, a potent vasoconstrictor. Reduced formation of angiotensin II decreases peripheral arterial resistance, which results in decreased aldosterone secretion, thus reducing sodium and water retention and lowering blood pressure.
*Cardiac load-reducing action:* Captopril decreases systemic vascular resistance (afterload) and pulmonary capillary wedge pressure (preload), thus increasing cardiac output in patients with heart failure.

## Pharmacokinetics
*Absorption:* 60% to 75% of an oral dose is absorbed through the GI tract; food may reduce absorption by up to 40%. Antihypertensive effect begins in 15 minutes. Maximum therapeutic effect may require several weeks.
*Distribution:* Distributed into most body tissues except CNS; drug is about 25% to 30% protein-bound.
*Metabolism:* About 50% is metabolized in the liver.
*Excretion:* Excreted primarily in urine; small amounts are excreted in feces. Duration of effect is usually 2 to 6 hours, increasing with higher doses. Elimination half-life is less than 3 hours. Duration of action may be increased in patients with renal dysfunction.

| Route | Onset | Peak | Duration |
|---|---|---|---|
| P.O. | ½-1 hr | 1-1½ hr | 6-12 hr |

## Contraindications and precautions
Contraindicated in patients hypersensitive to drug or other ACE inhibitors. Use cautiously in patients with impaired renal function, renal artery stenosis, or serious autoimmune diseases (especially lupus erythematosus) and in those taking drugs that affect WBC counts or immune response.

## Interactions

**Drug-drug.** *Antacids:* Decrease effects of captopril and should be given at different dose intervals.

*Digoxin:* May increase serum digoxin level by 15% to 30%. Advise clinician to monitor patient closely.

*Diuretics or other antihypertensives:* Risk of excessive hypotension. Diuretics may need to be discontinued or captopril dosage lowered.

*Insulin, oral antidiabetics:* Risk of hypoglycemia when captopril therapy starts. Advise clinician to monitor patient closely.

*Lithium:* Increased lithium levels and symptoms of toxicity may occur. Advise clinician to monitor patient closely.

*NSAIDs:* May decrease the antihypertensive effect of captopril. Advise clinician to monitor patient closely.

*Potassium-sparing diuretics, potassium supplements:* Increased risk of hyperkalemia. Avoid these drugs unless hypokalemic blood levels are confirmed.

**Drug-herb.** *Black catechu:* Possible additional hypotensive effects. Discourage use together.

*Capsaicin:* Increased risk of cough. Discourage use together.

*Licorice:* Possible sodium retention and increased blood pressure interfering with the therapeutic effects of ACE inhibitors. Discourage use together.

## Adverse reactions

**CNS:** dizziness, fainting, headache, malaise, fatigue.
**CV:** tachycardia, hypotension, angina pectoris.
**GI:** anorexia, *dysgeusia,* nausea, vomiting, abdominal pain, constipation, dry mouth.
**Hematologic:** *leukopenia, agranulocytosis, pancytopenia,* anemia, *thrombocytopenia.*
**Hepatic:** transient increase in hepatic enzymes.
**Metabolic:** hyperkalemia.
**Respiratory:** *dry, persistent, tickling, nonproductive cough;* dyspnea.
**Skin:** *urticarial rash, maculopapular rash,* pruritus, alopecia.
**Other:** fever, *angioedema.*

## Overdose and treatment

A sign of overdose is severe hypotension. After acute ingestion, stomach must be emptied by induced emesis or gastric lavage. Recommend following with activated charcoal to reduce absorption. Subsequent treatment is usually symptomatic and supportive. In severe cases, hemodialysis may be considered.

## Clinical considerations

■ Diuretic therapy is usually discontinued 2 to 3 days before beginning ACE inhibitor therapy, to reduce risk of hypotension; if drug doesn't adequately control blood pressure, diuretics may be reinstated.

■ Captopril may cause false-positive results for urinary acetone.

### Therapeutic monitoring

■ WBC and differential counts should be checked before treatment, every 2 weeks for 3 months, and periodically thereafter; serum potassium levels must be checked because of potassium retention.

■ Lowered dosage or reduced dosing frequency is needed in patients with impaired renal function. Recommend adjusting drug to effective levels over a 1- to 2-week interval, then reducing dosage to lowest effective level.

■ Several weeks of therapy may be required before the beneficial effects of captopril are seen.

■ Proteinuria and nephrotic syndrome may occur in patients.

### Special populations

**Pregnant patients.** Because ACE inhibitors can cause fetal harm or death, patient should stop drug as soon as pregnancy is detected.
**Breast-feeding patients.** Captopril appears in breast milk, but its effect on breast-feeding infants is unknown. Use drug with caution in breast-feeding women.
**Pediatric patients.** Safety and efficacy in children haven't been established; use only if potential benefit outweighs risk.
**Geriatric patients.** Geriatric patients may need lower doses because of impaired drug clearance. They also may be more sensitive to the hypotensive effects of captopril.

## Patient counseling

■ Instruct patient to call prescriber immediately if pregnancy occurs.

■ Tell patient to report feelings of lightheadedness, especially in first few days, so dosage can be adjusted; signs and symptoms of infection, such as sore throat or fever, because drug may decrease WBC count; facial swelling or difficulty breathing, because drug may cause angioedema; and loss of taste, which may necessitate discontinuing drug.

■ Instruct patient to take captopril 1 hour before meals to prevent decreased absorption.

■ Advise patient to avoid sudden position changes to minimize orthostatic hypotension.

■ Warn patient to seek medical approval before taking OTC cold preparations.

■ Tell patient that a persistent, dry cough may occur and usually doesn't subside until drug is stopped. He should call prescriber if this effect becomes bothersome.

# carbamazepine
Atretol, Carbatrol, Epitol, Tegretol

*Pharmacologic classification:* iminostilbene derivative; chemically related to tricyclic antidepressants
*Therapeutic classification:* anticonvulsant, analgesic
*Pregnancy risk category D*

## Available forms
Available by prescription only
*Tablets:* 200 mg
*Tablets (chewable):* 100 mg
*Tablets (extended-release):* 100 mg, 200 mg, 400 mg
*Capsules (extended-release):* 200 mg, 300 mg
*Oral suspension:* 100 mg/5 ml

## Indications and dosages
*Generalized tonic-clonic, complex-partial, mixed seizure patterns*
*Adults and children over age 12:* 200 mg P.O. b.i.d., or 100 mg P.O. q.i.d. of suspension, on day 1. May increase by 200 mg/day P.O. at weekly intervals, in divided doses at 6- to 8-hour intervals. Adjust to minimum effective level when control is achieved; don't exceed 1,000 mg/day in children ages 12 to 15, or 1,200 mg/day in those over age 15. In rare instances, doses up to 1,600 mg/day have been used in adults.

For extended-release capsules, initial dose, 200 mg P.O. b.i.d. Increase at weekly intervals by up to 200 mg/day until optimal response is obtained. Dose shouldn't exceed 1,000 mg/day in children ages 12 to 15 and 1,200 mg/day in patients over age 15. Some adult doses may be up to 1,600 mg/day. Maintenance dosage is usually 800 to 1,200 mg/day.
*Children ages 6 to 12:* Initially, 100 mg P.O. b.i.d., or 50 mg P.O. q.i.d. of suspension. Increase at weekly intervals by adding 100 mg P.O. daily, first using a t.i.d. schedule and then q.i.d., if needed. Adjust dosage based on patient response. Generally, dose shouldn't exceed 1,000 mg/day. Children taking total daily dose of immediate-release form of 400 mg or more may be converted to same total daily dose of extended-release capsules using a b.i.d. regimen.
*Children under age 6:* Initially, 10 to 20 mg/kg/day P.O. b.i.d. or t.i.d. as tablets or q.i.d. as suspension. Increase weekly to achieve optimal clinical response given t.i.d. or q.i.d. There is no recommendation for safe administration at doses of more than 35 mg/kg/day. If optimal clinical response hasn't been achieved at a dose less than 35 mg/kg/day, check plasma levels to determine whether they're within the therapeutic range.

*Oral loading dose for rapid seizure control*
*Adults and children over age 12:* 8 mg/kg P.O. of oral suspension.
◇ *Bipolar affective disorder, intermittent explosive disorder*
*Adults:* Initially, 200 mg P.O. b.i.d.; increase, p.r.n., q 3 to 4 days. Maintenance dosage may range from 600 to 1,600 mg/day.
*Trigeminal neuralgia*
*Adults:* 100 mg P.O. b.i.d. with meals on day 1. Increase by 100 mg q 12 hours until pain is relieved. Don't exceed 1.2 g daily. Maintenance dosage is 200 to 1,200 mg P.O. daily. For extended-release capsules, 200 mg P.O. day 1. Daily dose may be increased by up to 200 mg/day q 12 hours, p.r.n., to achieve freedom from pain. Maintenance dosage is usually 400 to 800 mg/day.
◇ *Chorea*
*Children:* 15 to 25 mg/kg P.O. per day.
◇ *Restless leg syndrome*
*Adults:* 100 to 300 mg P.O. h.s.

## Mechanism of action
*Anticonvulsant action:* Carbamazepine is chemically unrelated to other anticonvulsants and its mechanism of action is unknown. The anticonvulsant activity appears principally to involve limitations of seizure propagation by reduction of posttetanic potentiation (PTP) of synaptic transmissions.
*Analgesic action:* In trigeminal neuralgia, carbamazepine is a specific analgesic through its reduction of synaptic neurotransmission.

## Pharmacokinetics
*Absorption:* Absorbed slowly from the GI tract.
*Distribution:* Distributed widely throughout body; it crosses the placenta and accumulates in fetal tissue. About 75% is protein-bound. Therapeutic serum levels in adults are 4 to 12 mcg/ml; nystagmus can occur at serum levels of more than 4 mcg/ml, and ataxia, dizziness, and anorexia can occur at serum levels of 10 mcg/ml or more. Serum levels may be misleading because an unmeasured active metabolite also can cause toxicity. Carbamazepine levels in breast milk approach 60% of serum levels. There is poor correlation between plasma levels and dose in children.
*Metabolism:* Metabolized by the liver to an active metabolite. It may also induce its own metabolism; over time, higher doses are needed to maintain plasma levels. Half-life is initially 25 to 65 hours and 12 to 17 hours with multiple dosing.
*Excretion:* Excreted in urine (70%) and feces (30%).

| Route | Onset | Peak | Duration |
|-------|-------|------|----------|
| P.O. | Unknown | 1½-12 hr | Unknown |

## Contraindications and precautions

Contraindicated in patients with history of previous bone marrow suppression or hypersensitivity to drug or tricyclic antidepressants and in patients who have taken an MAO inhibitor within 14 days of therapy. Use cautiously in patients with mixed-type seizure disorders.

## Interactions

**Drug-drug.** *Cimetidine, danazol, diltiazem, fluoxetine, fluvoxamine, isoniazid, macrolides (such as erythromycin), propoxyphene, valproic acid, verapamil:* Possible increased carbamazepine blood levels. Use cautiously.
*Doxycycline, felbamate, haloperidol, oral contraceptives, phenytoin, theophylline, warfarin:* Possible decreased blood levels of these drugs. Advise clinician to monitor patient for decreased effect.
*Lithium:* Increased CNS toxicity of lithium. Avoid use together.
*MAO inhibitors:* Increased depressant and anticholinergic effects. Don't use together.
*Phenobarbital, phenytoin, primidone:* Possible decreased carbamazepine levels. Advise clinician to monitor patient for decreased effect.
**Drug-herb.** *Plantain:* Possible decreased carbamazepine absorption, decreasing the pharmacologic effect. Discourage use together.
*Psyllium seed:* Possible inhibited GI absorption; discourage use together.

## Adverse reactions

**CNS:** *dizziness, vertigo, drowsiness,* fatigue, *ataxia,* **worsening of seizures** (usually in patients with mixed-type seizure disorders, including atypical absence seizures), confusion, headache, syncope.
**CV:** *HF,* hypertension, hypotension, aggravation of coronary artery disease, ***arrhythmias, AV block.***
**EENT:** conjunctivitis, dry pharynx, blurred vision, diplopia, nystagmus.
**GI:** *nausea, vomiting,* abdominal pain, diarrhea, anorexia, stomatitis, glossitis, dry mouth.
**GU:** urinary frequency, urine retention, impotence, albuminuria, glycosuria, elevated BUN.
**Hematologic:** *aplastic anemia, agranulocytosis,* eosinophilia, leukocytosis, ***thrombocytopenia.***
**Hepatic:** abnormal liver function test results, ***hepatitis.***
**Respiratory:** pulmonary hypersensitivity.
**Skin:** rash, urticaria, excessive diaphoresis, ***erythema multiforme, Stevens-Johnson syndrome.***
**Other:** fever, chills, SIADH, decrease values of thyroid function tests results.

## Overdose and treatment

Signs and symptoms of overdose may include irregular breathing, respiratory depression, tachycardia, blood pressure changes, shock, arrhythmias, impaired consciousness (ranging to deep coma), seizures, restlessness, drowsiness, psychomotor disturbances, nausea, vomiting, anuria, or oliguria.

Recommend treating overdose with repeated gastric lavage, especially if patient ingested alcohol concurrently. Oral charcoal and laxatives may hasten excretion. Recommend carefully monitoring vital signs, ECG, and fluid and electrolyte balance. Diazepam may control seizures but can exacerbate respiratory depression.

## Clinical considerations

■ Adjust drug dosage based on individual response.
■ Chewable tablets are available for children.
■ Unlabeled uses of carbamazepine include hypophyseal diabetes insipidus, certain psychiatric disorders, and management of alcohol withdrawal.
■ For administering through a nasogastric tube, mix with an equal volume of diluent ($D_5W$ or normal saline solution) and administer; then flush with 100 ml of diluent.

### Therapeutic monitoring

■ Hematologic toxicity is rare but serious. Hematologic and liver function test results must be checked. Periodic eye examinations are recommended.

### Special populations

**Breast-feeding patients.** Significant amounts of drug appear in breast milk; alternative feeding method is recommended during therapy.
**Pediatric patients.** Safety and efficacy haven't been established for children under age 6 in doses higher than 35 mg/kg/day.
**Geriatric patients.** Drug may activate latent psychosis, confusion, or agitation in geriatric patients; patients should use with caution.

## Patient counseling

■ Remind patient to store drug in a cool, dry place, and not in the medicine cabinet. Reduced bioavailability has been reported with use of improperly stored tablets.
■ Tell patient that drug may cause GI distress. Patient should take drug with food at equally spaced intervals.
■ Warn patient not to stop drug abruptly.
■ Encourage patient to promptly report unusual bleeding, bruising, jaundice, dark urine, pale stools, abdominal pain, impotence, fever, chills, sore throat, mouth ulcers, edema, or disturbances in mood, alertness, or coordination.
■ Warn patient that drug may cause drowsiness, dizziness, and blurred vision. Patient should avoid hazardous activities that require alertness, especially during first week of therapy and when dosage is increased.
■ Remind patient to shake suspension well before using.

- Tell patient that, if needed, the Carbatrol capsule can be opened and its contents sprinkled over food (such as a teaspoon of applesauce), but the capsule or its contents should never be crushed or chewed.
- Emphasize importance of follow-up laboratory tests and continued medical supervision.

# carboplatin
Paraplatin

*Pharmacologic classification:* alkylating agent (cell cycle–phase nonspecific)
*Therapeutic classification:* antineoplastic
*Pregnancy risk category D*

## Available forms
Available by prescription only
*Injection:* 50-mg, 150-mg, 450-mg vials

## Indications and dosages
*Initial and secondary (palliative) treatment of ovarian carcinoma*
*Adults:* Initial recommended dose for single-agent therapy is 360 mg/m² I.V. on day 1. Dose is repeated q 4 weeks. In combination therapy (with cyclophosphamide), give 300 mg/m² I.V. on day 1 q 4 weeks for 6 cycles.
≡ *Dosage adjustment.* Dosage adjustments are based on the lowest posttreatment platelet or neutrophil value obtained in weekly blood counts.

For patients with impaired renal function, initial recommended dose is 250 mg/m² for creatinine clearance levels between 41 and 59 ml/minute; for creatinine clearance levels between 16 and 40 ml/minute, dose is 200 mg/m².

## I.V. administration
- Reconstitute with D₅W, normal saline solution, or sterile water for injection to make a concentration of 10 mg/ml.
- Drug can be further diluted to concentrations as low as 0.5 mg/ml using normal saline solution or D₅W.
- Infuse over at least 15 minutes.
- Store unopened vials at controlled room temperature. Once reconstituted and diluted, as directed, solution is stable at controlled room temperature for 8 hours. Because drug doesn't contain antibacterial preservatives, discard unused drug after 8 hours.

## Incompatibilities
Incompatible with aluminum, fluorouracil, mesna, and sodium bicarbonate. Needles or I.V. administration sets containing aluminum may precipitate drug and cause a loss of potency.

## Mechanism of action
*Antineoplastic action:* Carboplatin causes cross-linking of DNA strands.

## Pharmacokinetics
*Absorption:* Administered I.V.
*Distribution:* Volume of distribution is about equal to total body water. Drug isn't protein-bound but degraded to platinum-containing products, which are 87% protein-bound at 24 hours.
*Metabolism:* Hydrolyzed to form hydroxylated and aquated species. Half-life of drug is 2 to 3 hours; terminal half-life for platinum is 4 to 6 days.
*Excretion:* 65% is excreted by the kidneys within 12 hours, 71% within 24 hours. Enterohepatic recirculation may occur.

| Route | Onset | Peak | Duration |
|-------|-------|------|----------|
| I.V. | Unknown | Unknown | Unknown |

## Contraindications and precautions
Contraindicated in patients with history of hypersensitivity to cisplatin, platinum-containing compounds, or mannitol or in patients with severe bone marrow suppression or bleeding.

## Interactions
*Drug-drug. Aspirin:* Increased risk of bleeding. Avoid use together.
*Bone marrow suppressants (including radiation therapy):* Increased hematologic toxicity. Advise clinician to monitor patient closely.
*Myelosuppressants:* Concurrent use can cause additive myelosuppression. Advise clinician to monitor patient.
*Nephrotoxic drugs:* Produces additive nephrotoxicity of carboplatin. Patients should use cautiously.

## Adverse reactions
**CNS:** dizziness, confusion, peripheral neuropathy, central neurotoxicity, paresthesia, *CVA,* asthenia.
**CV:** *cardiac failure, embolism,* hypertension.
**EENT:** visual disturbances, ototoxicity.
**GI:** constipation, diarrhea, change in taste, *nausea, vomiting.*
**GU:** increased BUN and creatinine levels.
**Hematologic:** THROMBOCYTOPENIA, *leukopenia,* NEUTROPENIA, anemia, BONE MARROW SUPPRESSION.
**Hepatic:** increased AST or alkaline phosphatase levels.
**Metabolic:** decreased serum electrolyte levels.
**Skin:** alopecia.
**Other:** hypersensitivity reactions, pain, *anaphylaxis.*

## Overdose and treatment
Symptoms of overdose result from bone marrow suppression or hepatotoxicity. There is no known antidote for carboplatin overdose.

## Clinical considerations

- Administration of carboplatin requires the supervision of a prescriber experienced in the use of chemotherapeutic drugs.
- There is an increased risk of alergic reaction in patients with prior exposure to drug.

### Therapeutic monitoring

- Although drug is promoted as causing less nausea and vomiting than cisplatin, it may cause severe emesis. Antiemetic therapy may be needed; advise clinician to monitor electrolyte levels regularly.
- Advise clinician to monitor hematologic tests. Don't give repeat dose until patient's hematologic tests are within acceptable limits.

### Special populations

**Pregnant patients.** May cause fetal harm. Carboplatin may be used during pregnancy if it's decided that the benefit outweighs the risk, or in life-threatening situations. Advise patient to avoid becoming pregnant while on carboplatin therapy.
**Breast-feeding patients.** It's unknown if carboplatin appears in breast milk; however, because of the potential for toxicity to the infant, patient should discontinue breast-feeding.
**Pediatric patients.** Safety in children hasn't been established.
**Geriatric patients.** Patients over age 65 are at greater risk for neurotoxicity.

## Patient counseling

- Stress importance of adequate fluid intake and increase in urine output, to facilitate uric acid excretion.
- Tell patient to report tinnitus immediately, to prevent permanent hearing loss. Patient should have audiometric testing before initial and subsequent course.
- Advise patient to avoid exposure to people with infections.
- Instruct patient to promptly report unusual bleeding or bruising.

## carmustine (BCNU)

BiCNU, Gliadel

*Pharmacologic classification:* alkylating agent; nitrosourea (cell cycle–phase nonspecific)
*Therapeutic classification:* antineoplastic
*Pregnancy risk category D*

## Available forms

Available by prescription only
*Injection:* 100-mg vial (lyophilized), with a 3-ml vial of absolute alcohol supplied as a diluent
*Implant:* 7.7 mg wafer

## Indications and dosages

Dosage and indications may vary. Check current literature for recommended protocol.
◇ *Brain,* ◇ *breast,* ◇ *GI tract,* ◇ *lung,* ◇ *hepatic cancer; Hodgkin's disease; malignant lymphomas;* ◇ *malignant melanomas; multiple myeloma*
*Adults:* 75 to 100 mg/m$^2$ I.V. by slow infusion daily for 2 consecutive days, repeated q 6 weeks if platelet count is above 100,000/mm$^3$ and WBC count is above 4,000/mm$^3$.
≡ *Dosage adjustment.* Reduce dosage p.r.n., using the following guidelines.

| Nadir after prior dose | | Percentage of prior dose to be given |
|---|---|---|
| Leukocytes/ mm$^3$ | Platelets/ mm$^3$ | |
| > 4,000 | > 100,000 | 100% |
| 3,000-3,999 | 75,000-99,999 | 100% |
| 2,000-2,999 | 25,000-74,999 | 70% |
| < 2,000 | < 25,000 | 50% |

*Alternative therapy:* 150 to 200 mg/m$^2$ I.V. slow infusion as a single dose, repeated q 6 to 8 weeks.
***Recurrent glioblastoma and metastatic brain tumors (adjunct to surgery to prolong survival)***
*Adults:* Implant 8 wafers in the resection cavity, if allowed, by size and shape of cavity.

## I.V. administration

- Wear gloves to administer drug infusion and when changing I.V. tubing. Avoid contact with skin because carmustine causes a brown stain. If drug comes into contact with skin, wash off thoroughly.
- Solution is unstable in plastic I.V. bags. Give only in glass containers.
- Reconstitute 100-mg vial with the 3 ml of absolute alcohol provided by manufacturer, then dilute further with 27 ml sterile water for injection. Resultant solution contains 3.3 mg carmustine/ml in 10% ethanol. Dilute in D$_5$W for I.V. infusion. Give at least 250 ml over 1 to 2 hours. Discard excess drug.
- Reconstituted solution may be stored in refrigerator for 24 hours (48 hours if reconstituted to 0.2 mg/ml in D$_5$W or normal saline solution).
- Carmustine may decompose at temperatures of more than 80° F (27° C). If powder liquefies or appears oily, discard it because it's a sign of decomposition.
- To reduce pain on infusion, suggest further dilution or slow infusion rate.
- At first sign or symptom of extravasation, recommend stopping infusion and infiltrating area with liberal injections of 0.5 mEq/ml sodium bicarbonate solution.

- Intense flushing of skin may occur during an I.V. infusion, but usually disappears within 2 to 4 hours.

### Incompatibilities
Don't mix carmustine with other drugs during administration. Incompatible with sodium bicarbonate.

## Mechanism of action
*Antineoplastic action:* The cytotoxic action of carmustine is mediated through its metabolites, which inhibit several enzymes involved with DNA formation. This drug can also cause cross-linking of DNA. Cross-linking interferes with DNA, RNA, and protein synthesis. Cross-resistance between carmustine and lomustine has occurred.

## Pharmacokinetics
*Absorption:* Not absorbed across the GI tract. Implant wafers are biodegradable in the human brain when implanted into the tumor resection cavity.
*Distribution:* Cleared rapidly from plasma. After I.V. administration, carmustine and its metabolites are distributed rapidly into CSF.
*Metabolism:* Metabolized extensively in the liver.
*Excretion:* About 60% to 70% of drug and its metabolites are excreted in urine within 96 hours, 6% to 10% is excreted as carbon dioxide by the lungs, and 1% is excreted in feces. Enterohepatic circulation and protein-binding can occur and may cause delayed hematologic toxicity.
Note: Concerning implant wafer, the absorption, distribution, metabolism, and excretion of the copolymer are unknown.

| Route | Onset | Peak | Duration |
|-------|---------|---------|----------|
| I.V. | Unknown | Unknown | Unknown |

## Contraindications and precautions
Contraindicated in patients hypersensitive to drug.

## Interactions
**Drug-drug.** *Anticoagulants, aspirin:* Increased risk of bleeding. Avoid use together.
*Cimetidine:* Increased bone marrow toxicity of carmustine. Avoid use together.
*Myelosuppressants:* Concurrent use can cause additive myelosuppression. Advise clinician to monitor patient closely.

## Adverse reactions
**CNS:** ataxia, drowsiness.
**EENT:** ocular toxicities.
**GI:** *nausea beginning in 2 to 6 hours (can be severe),* vomiting.
**GU:** *nephrotoxicity,* azotemia, *renal failure.*
**Hematologic:** *cumulative bone marrow suppression* (delayed 4 to 6 weeks, lasting 1 to 2

weeks); *leukopenia; thrombocytopenia; acute leukemia, bone marrow dysplasia* (after long-term use); anemia.
**Hepatic:** *hepatotoxicity.*
**Respiratory:** *pulmonary fibrosis.*
**Skin:** facial flushing, hyperpigmentation.
**Other:** *intense pain at infusion site from venous spasm;* possible hyperuricemia (in lymphoma patients when rapid cell lysis occurs).

## Overdose and treatment
Signs and symptoms of overdose include leukopenia, thrombocytopenia, nausea, and vomiting. Treatment consists of supportive measures, including transfusion of blood components, antibiotics for infections that may develop, and antiemetics.

## Clinical considerations
- For wafers, use double gloves and surgical instruments dedicated to the handling of implant wafers.
- Pulmonary toxicity is more likely in patients who smoke.
- Drug has been applied topically in levels of 0.05% to 0.4% to treat mycosis fungoides.
- Because drug crosses the blood-brain barrier, it may be used to treat primary brain tumors.

### Therapeutic monitoring
- Avoid I.M. injections when platelet count is less than 50,000/mm$^3$.
- To reduce nausea, suggest giving antiemetic before administering.
- Advise clinician to monitor patient's CBC.

### Special populations
**Pregnant patients.** Advise women to avoid becoming pregnant and to report suspected pregnancy.
**Breast-feeding patients.** Active metabolites of drug appear in breast milk. Therefore, it isn't advisable for women receiving drug to breast-feed because of risk of serious adverse reactions, mutagenicity, and carcinogenicity in the infant.
**Pediatric patients.** Safety and effectiveness in children haven't been established.

## Patient counseling
- Warn patient to watch for signs and symptoms of infection and bone marrow toxicity (fever, sore throat, anemia, fatigue, easy bruising, nose or gum bleeds, melena). Patient should take temperature daily.
- Remind patient to return for follow-up blood work weekly, or p.r.n., and to watch for signs and symptoms of infection.
- Advise patient to avoid exposure to people with infections.
- Tell patient to avoid OTC products containing aspirin because they may precipitate bleeding. Advise patient to report signs of bleeding promptly.

# carteolol hydrochloride
Cartrol, Ocupress

*Pharmacologic classification:* beta
blocker
*Therapeutic classification:* antihypertensive
*Pregnancy risk category C*

## Available forms
Available by prescription only
*Tablets:* 2.5 mg, 5 mg
*Ophthalmic solution:* 1%

## Indications and dosages
**Hypertension**
*Adults:* Initially, 2.5 mg P.O. as a single daily
dose. Gradually increase the dose, p.r.n., to
5 mg daily or 10 mg daily as a single dose.
◇*Angina*
*Adults:* 10 mg/day P.O.
≡*Dosage adjustment.* Patients with substantial renal impairment should receive the usual
dose of carteolol scheduled at longer intervals
as shown.

| Creatinine clearance (ml/min) | Dosage interval (hr) |
| --- | --- |
| 20-60 | 48 |
| < 20 | 72 |

*Open-angle glaucoma*
*Adults:* 1 drop b.i.d. in eye.

## Mechanism of action
*Antihypertensive action:* Drug is a nonselective beta blocker with intrinsic sympathomimetic activity (ISA). Its antihypertensive
effects are probably caused by decreased sympathetic outflow from the brain and decreased
cardiac output. Carteolol doesn't have a consistent effect on renin output.

## Pharmacokinetics
*Absorption:* Absorbed rapidly. Bioavailability is about 85%.
*Distribution:* 20% to 30% plasma protein–
bound.
*Metabolism:* Only 30% to 50% is metabolized
in the liver to 8-hydroxycarteolol, an active
metabolite, and the inactive metabolite glucuronoside.
*Excretion:* Primarily renal. Plasma half-life is
about 6 hours.

| Route | Onset | Peak | Duration |
| --- | --- | --- | --- |
| P.O. | Unknown | 1-3 hr | 24 hr |
| Ophthalmic | Unknown | Unknown | Unknown |

## Contraindications and precautions
Contraindicated in patients hypersensitive to
any component of drug and in those with
bronchial asthma, severe COPD, sinus bradycardia, second- or third-degree AV block, overt
cardiac failure, or cardiogenic shock.

Use cautiously in breast-feeding women
and in patients with nonallergic bronchospastic disease, diabetes mellitus, hyperthyroidism,
or decreased pulmonary function.

## Interactions
**Drug-drug.** *Calcium channel blockers:* Increased risk of hypotension, left ventricular
failure, and AV conduction disturbances. I.V.
calcium antagonists should be used with caution.
*Cardiac glycosides:* May produce additive effects on slowing AV node conduction. Avoid
use together.
*Catecholamine-depleting drugs, such as reserpine, oral adrenergic blockers:* May have
an additive effect and contribute to the development of hypotension or bradycardia. Advise
clinician to monitor patients closely.
*General anesthetics:* Increased hypotensive effects. Carefully observe for hypotension, bradycardia, or orthostatic hypotension.
*Insulin and oral antidiabetics:* May alter hypoglycemic response. Dosage may need adjustment.
**Drug-lifestyle.** *Sun exposure:* Photophobia
may occur with ophthalmic form of drug. Advise patient to use sunblock.

## Adverse reactions
**CNS:** lassitude, fatigue, somnolence, *asthenia, paresthesia.*
**CV:** *conduction disturbances.*
**EENT:** transient irritation, conjunctival hyperemia, *edema.*
**GI:** diarrhea, nausea, abdominal pain.
**Musculoskeletal:** *muscle cramps,* arthralgia.
**Skin:** rash.

## Overdose and treatment
No information available. The likely symptoms are bradycardia, bronchospasm, heart failure, and hypotension.

Use atropine to treat symptomatic bradycardia. If no response is seen, cautiously use
isoproterenol. Treat bronchospasm with a beta$_2$-agonist such as isoproterenol, or theophylline.
Cardiac glycosides or diuretics may be useful
in treating heart failure. Give vasopressors (epinephrine, dopamine, or norepinephrine) to
combat hypotension.

## Clinical considerations
**H***ALERT* Discontinue drug at first sign of cardiac failure and notify prescriber.
■ Dosage of more than 10 mg/day doesn't produce a greater response; it may actually decrease response.

---

- Food may slow the rate, but not the extent, of carteolol absorption.
- Steady-state levels are reached rapidly (within 1 to 2 days) in patients with normal renal function.

### Therapeutic monitoring
- Advise clinician to monitor heart rate and blood pressure; slow heart rate must be reported to prescriber.

### Special populations
**Breast-feeding patients.** Drug may appear in breast milk. Use with caution in breast-feeding women.
**Pediatric patients.** Safety in children hasn't been established.
**Geriatric patients.** No specific age-related recommendations are available.

### Patient counseling
- Advise patient to take drug exactly as prescribed and not to discontinue drug suddenly.
- Tell patient to report shortness of breath or difficulty breathing, unusually fast heartbeat, cough, or fatigue with exertion.
- Inform patient that transient stinging or discomfort may occur with ophthalmic use; if reaction is severe, he should call prescriber immediately.
- Tell patient that if more than one topical ophthalmic drug is to be used, they should be given at least 10 minutes apart.

---

# carvedilol
Coreg

*Pharmacologic classification:* alpha-nonselective beta blocker
*Therapeutic classification:* antihypertensive, adjunct treatment for heart failure
*Pregnancy risk category C*

### Available forms
Available by prescription only
*Tablets:* 3.125 mg, 6.25 mg, 12.5 mg, 25 mg

### Indications and dosages
*Hypertension*
*Adults:* Dosage individualized. Initially, 6.25 mg P.O. b.i.d. with food; obtain standing systolic pressure 1 hour after initial dose. If tolerated, continue dosage for 7 to 14 days. Can increase to 12.5 mg P.O. b.i.d., repeating monitoring protocol as above. Maximum dose is 25 mg P.O. b.i.d., as tolerated.
*Heart failure*
*Adults:* Dosage individualized and adjusted carefully. Stabilize dosing of cardiac glycosides, diuretics, and ACE inhibitors before therapy starts. Initially, 3.125 mg P.O. b.i.d. with food for 2 weeks; if tolerated, possibly in-

creasing to 6.25 mg P.O. b.i.d. for 2 weeks. Dose can be doubled q 2 weeks to highest level tolerated by patient. At initiation of new dose, observe patient for dizziness or light-headedness for 1 hour. Maximum dosing for patients weighing less than 85 kg (187 lb) is 25 mg P.O. b.i.d.; for those weighing more than 85 kg, give 50 mg P.O. b.i.d.

### Mechanism of action
*Antihypertensive action:* Mechanism not established. Beta blockade reduces cardiac output and tachycardia. Alpha blockade is shown by the attenuated pressor effects of phenylephrine, vasodilation, and decreases in peripheral vascular resistance.
*Heart failure:* Not fully established. Drug has been shown to decrease systemic blood pressure, pulmonary artery pressure, right atrial pressure, systemic vascular resistance, and heart rate while increasing stroke volume index.

### Pharmacokinetics
*Absorption:* Rapidly and extensively metabolized following oral administration, with absolute bioavailability of 25% to 35% because of significant first-pass metabolism.
*Distribution:* Plasma levels are proportional to oral dose given. Absorption is slowed when given with food, as evidenced by a delay in the time to reach peak plasma levels with no significant difference in extent of bioavailability.
*Metabolism:* Extensively metabolized, primarily by aromatic ring oxidation and glucuronidation. The oxidative metabolites are further metabolized by conjugation via glucuronidation and sulfation. Demethylation and hydroxylation at the phenol ring produce three active metabolites with beta-blocking activity.
*Excretion:* Metabolites are primarily excreted via bile into the feces. Less than 2% of dose is excreted unchanged in urine.

| Route | Onset | Peak | Duration |
|-------|-------|------|----------|
| P.O. | Unknown | 1-2 hr | 7-10 hr |

### Contraindications and precautions
Contraindicated in patients with New York Heart Association (NYHA) class IV decompensated cardiac failure requiring I.V. inotropic therapy, bronchial asthma or related bronchospastic conditions, second- or third-degree AV block, sick sinus syndrome (unless a permanent pacemaker is in place), cardiogenic shock, severe bradycardia, or hypersensitivity to drug. Drug isn't recommended in patients with hepatic impairment.

Use cautiously in hypertensive patients with left ventricular failure, perioperative patients who receive anesthetics that depress myocardial function, such as ether, cyclopropane, trichloroethylene, or in diabetic patients receiving insulin or oral antidiabetics, or in persons subject to spontaneous hypoglycemia. Also use

---

* Canada only    ◇ Unlabeled clinical use

with caution in patients with thyroid disease (may mask hyperthyroidism and drug withdrawal may precipitate thyroid storm or an exacerbation of hyperthyroidism), pheochromocytoma, Prinzmetal's variant angina, or peripheral vascular disease (may precipitate or aggravate symptoms of arterial insufficiency).

## Interactions
**Drug-drug.** *Calcium channel blockers:* May cause isolated conduction disturbances; advise clinician to monitor ECG and blood pressure.
*Catecholamine-depleting drugs, such as MAO inhibitors, reserpine:* May cause severe bradycardia or hypotension. Advise clinician to monitor patient closely.
*Cimetidine:* Increases bioavailability of carvedilol. Advise clinician to monitor vital signs closely.
*Clonidine:* May potentiate blood pressure and heart rate lowering effects. Advise clinician to monitor patient carefully.
*Digoxin:* Increases levels by about 15% while on concurrent therapy. Evaluate digoxin levels.
*Insulin and oral antidiabetics:* May enhance hypoglycemic properties; advise clinician to monitor blood glucose levels.
*Rifampin:* Reduces plasma levels of carvedilol by 70%. Advise clinician to monitor vital signs.
**Drug-food.** *Any food:* Delays rate of absorption of carvedilol but doesn't alter extent of bioavailability. Advise patient to take drug with food to minimize orthostatic effects.

## Adverse reactions
**CNS:** malaise, *dizziness, fatigue,* headache, hypesthesia, insomnia, pain, paresthesia, somnolence, vertigo.
**CV:** aggravated angina pectoris, *AV block, bradycardia,* chest pain, fluid overload, hypertension, hypotension, postural hypertension, syncope, edema, peripheral edema, *sudden death.*
**EENT:** abnormal vision, pharyngitis, rhinitis, sinusitis.
**GI:** abdominal pain, *diarrhea,* melena, nausea, periodontitis, vomiting.
**GU:** abnormal renal function, albuminuria, hematuria, impotence, urinary tract infection, increased BUN.
**Hematologic:** decreased PT, purpura, *thrombocytopenia.*
**Hepatic:** increased ALT, AST levels.
**Metabolic:** dehydration, glycosuria, gout, hypercholesterolemia, *hyperglycemia,* hypertriglyceridemia, hyperuricemia, hypoglycemia, hyponatremia, weight gain, increased alkaline phosphatase or nonprotein nitrogen.
**Musculoskeletal:** arthralgia, back pain, myalgia.
**Respiratory:** bronchitis, dyspnea, *upper respiratory tract infection.*
**Other:** allergy, fever, hypovolemia, viral infection, hypervolemia.

## Overdose and treatment
Overdose may cause severe hypotension, bradycardia, cardiac insufficiency, cardiogenic shock, and cardiac arrest. Respiratory effects, bronchospasm, vomiting, lapses of consciousness, and generalized seizures may also occur.

Recommend placing patient in supine position. Gastric lavage or pharmacologically induced emesis may be effective shortly after ingestion. May use atropine 2 mg I.V. for bradycardia; glucagon 5 to 10 mg I.V. rapidly over 30 seconds, followed by continuous infusion at 5 mg/hour to support CV function; sympathomimetics (dobutamine, adrenaline) at doses based on body weight and effect. If peripheral vasodilation dominates, recommend giving epinephrine or norepinephrine, if needed, and continuously monitoring circulatory conditions. For therapy-resistant bradycardia, recommend performing pacemaker therapy. For bronchospasm, recommend giving betasympathomimetics by aerosol or I.V. or aminophylline I.V. If seizures occur, slow I.V. injection of diazepam or clonazepam may be effective. If severe intoxication and symptoms of shock occur, treatment should be continued with antidotes for a sufficiently long period of time consistent with the drug's 7- to 10-hour half-life.

## Clinical considerations
■ Drug should be stopped gradually over 1 to 2 weeks. Dosage should be decreased if heart rate is less than 55 beats/minute.
■ Patients with HF require monitoring for worsened condition, renal dysfunction, or fluid retention; diuretics may need to be increased; advise clinician to monitor diabetic patient for worsening of hyperglycemia.
■ Patients on beta blocker therapy with history of severe anaphylactic reaction to several allergens may be more reactive to repeated challenge, either accidental, diagnostic, or therapeutic. They may be unresponsive to the usual doses of epinephrine used to treat allergic reactions.

### Therapeutic monitoring
■ Mild hepatocellular injury may occur during therapy. At first sign of hepatic dysfunction, recommend performing tests for hepatic injury or jaundice; if present, drug should be stopped.

### Special populations
**Breast-feeding patients.** It's unknown if drug appears in breast milk. Use cautiously.
**Pediatric patients.** Safety of drug in patients under age 18 hasn't been established.
**Geriatric patients.** Plasma levels must be monitored carefully; drug occurs about 50% higher in geriatric patients compared with younger patients. No significant difference was found in adverse effects between older and younger

patients; dizziness was slightly more common in geriatric patients.

## Patient counseling
- Tell patient not to interrupt or discontinue drug without medical approval.
- Advise heart failure patient to call if weight gain or shortness of breath occurs.
- Inform patient that he may experience lowered blood pressure when standing. If dizziness occurs, advise him to sit or lie down.
- Caution patient against performing hazardous tasks when therapy starts. If dizziness or fatigue occurs, tell him to call for an adjustment in dosage.
- Advise diabetic patient to report changes in serum glucose level promptly.
- Inform patients who wear contact lenses that decreased lacrimation may occur.

---

## cascara sagrada

## cascara sagrada aromatic fluidextract

*Pharmacologic classification:* anthraquinone glycoside mixture
*Therapeutic classification:* laxative
*Pregnancy risk category C*

## Available forms
Available without a prescription
*Tablets:* 325 mg
*Aromatic fluidextract:* 1 g/ml with 19% alcohol

## Indications and dosages
**Acute constipation, preparation for bowel or rectal examination**
*Adults and children ages 12 and older:* 1 tablet P.O. h.s. or 2 to 6 ml of aromatic fluidextract P.O. once daily.
*Children ages 2 to 11:* 50% of adult dose.

## Mechanism of action
*Laxative action:* Cascara sagrada, obtained from the dried bark of the buckthorn tree *(Rhamnus purshianus),* contains cascarosides A and B (barbaloin glycosides) and cascarosides C and D (chrysaloin glycosides). Drug exerts a direct irritant action on the colon that promotes peristalsis and bowel motility. Cascara also enhances colonic fluid accumulation, increasing the laxative effect.

## Pharmacokinetics
*Absorption:* Minimal drug absorption occurs in the small intestine. Although onset of action usually occurs in about 6 to 12 hours, onset may not occur for 3 or 4 days.
*Distribution:* May be distributed in the bile, saliva, and colonic mucosa.
*Metabolism:* Metabolized in the liver.

*Excretion:* Excreted in feces via biliary elimination, in urine, or in both.

| Route | Onset | Peak | Duration |
|-------|-------|------|----------|
| P.O. | 6-10 hr | Variable | Variable |

## Contraindications and precautions
Contraindicated in patients with abdominal pain, nausea, vomiting, or other symptoms of appendicitis or acute surgical abdomen; acute surgical delirium; fecal impaction; and intestinal obstruction or perforation. Use cautiously in patients with rectal bleeding.

## Interactions
None reported.

## Adverse reactions
**GI:** *nausea;* vomiting; diarrhea; loss of normal bowel function with excessive use; *abdominal cramps,* especially in severe constipation; malabsorption of nutrients; "cathartic colon" (syndrome resembling ulcerative colitis radiologically and pathologically) with chronic misuse; discoloration of rectal mucosa after long-term use.
**Metabolic:** hypokalemia, protein enteropathy, electrolyte imbalance (with excessive use).
**Other:** laxative dependence (with long-term or excessive use).

## Overdose and treatment
No information available.

## Clinical considerations
- Prescribe doses carefully; fluidextract preparation is five times as potent as aromatic fluidextract.
- Cascara is a common ingredient in many natural laxatives available without a prescription.

### Therapeutic monitoring
- Cascara turns alkaline urine pink to red, red to violet, or red to brown and turns acidic urine yellow to brown in the phenolsulfonphthalein excretion test.

### Special populations
**Pregnant patients.** Bulk-forming or surfactant laxatives are preferred during pregnancy.
**Breast-feeding patients.** Cascara may appear in breast milk, which may cause increased risk of diarrhea in infant.
**Pediatric patients.** Use with caution in children.
**Geriatric patients.** Because many of these patients use laxatives, they're at particularly high risk for development of laxative dependence. Encourage them to use laxatives only for short periods.

## Patient counseling
- Warn patient that drug may turn urine reddish pink or brown.

- Tell patient to take with a full glass of water.

---

# caspofungin acetate
Cancidas

*Pharmacologic classification:* glucan synthesis inhibitor
*Therapeutic classification:* antifungal
*Pregnancy risk category C*

## Available forms
*Lyophilized powder for injection:* 50-mg and 70-mg single-use vials

## Indications and dosages
*Invasive aspergillosis in patients refractory to or intolerant of other therapies (such as amphotericin B, lipid formulations of amphotericin B, itraconazole)*
*Adults:* A single 70-mg loading dose on day 1, followed by 50 mg daily thereafter. Recommend giving by slow I.V. infusion over about 1 hour. Duration of treatment based on severity of patient's underlying disease, recovery from immunosuppression, and clinical response.
≡ *Dosage adjustment.* Patients with hepatic insufficiency may require dosage reduction. For patients with moderate hepatic insufficiency (Child-Pugh score 7 to 9), recommend giving 35 mg daily after the first 70-mg loading dose. There's no clinical experience in patients with severe hepatic insufficiency (Child-Pugh score above 9).

## I.V. administration
- Advise clinician to give drug by slow I.V. infusion over about 1 hour.
- Reconstituted vials should be used within 1 hour or discarded.
- Caspofungin generally should be diluted in 250 ml of normal saline solution for all (70-mg, 50-mg, 35-mg) doses. In patients with fluid restrictions, the 50-mg and 35-mg doses may be diluted in 100 ml of normal saline solution.
- Refer to manufacturer's instructions for specific reconstitution and I.V. dose preparation guidelines.
- Advise clinician to monitor I.V. site carefully for phlebitis.

### Incompatibilities
**⊫ALERT** Never mix or dilute caspofungin with dextrose solution. Don't mix or infuse it with other drugs.

## Mechanism of action
*Antifungal action:* Caspofungin inhibits synthesis of beta (1,3)-D-glucan, an integral component of the cell walls of susceptible filamentous fungi that isn't found in mammal cells. Caspofungin has in vitro activity against *Aspergillus fumigatus, A. flavus,* and *A. terreus.*

Development of resistance to caspofungin by *Aspergillus* species in vitro is unknown.

## Pharmacokinetics
*Absorption:* Administered I.V.
*Distribution:* Distribution, rather than excretion or biotransformation, is the dominant mechanism influencing plasma clearance. Caspofungin is about 97% albumin-bound and distribution into RBCs is minimal. There's little excretion or biotransformation of caspofungin during the first 30 hours after administration. There are three phases of decline in serum levels; the first is rapid, and the half-lives of the last two phases are 9 to 11 hours and 40 to 50 hours, respectively.
*Metabolism:* Slowly metabolized by hydrolysis and N-acetylation. It also undergoes spontaneous chemical degradation to an open-ring peptide compound.
*Excretion:* After single-dose I.V. administration, about 35% of drug and metabolites is excreted in feces and 41% in urine. Renal clearance of parent drug is very low.

| Route | Onset | Peak | Duration |
|-------|-------|------|----------|
| I.V. | Unknown | Unknown | Unknown |

## Contraindications and precautions
Contraindicated in patients hypersensitive to drug or its components.

## Interactions
**Drug-drug.** *Carbamazepine, dexamethasone, efavirenz, nelfinavir, nevirapine, phenytoin, rifampin:* Possible decreased caspofungin levels. Consider increasing caspofungin dosage if patient fails to respond.
*Cyclosporine:* Significantly increased caspofungin and ALT levels. Use together isn't recommended unless potential benefit outweighs potential risk.
*Tacrolimus:* Decreased tacrolimus levels. Advise clinician to monitor tacrolimus levels; dosage adjustment of tacrolimus may be needed.

## Adverse reactions
**CNS:** headache, *paresthesia.*
**CV:** *tachycardia.*
**GI:** nausea, vomiting, diarrhea, abdominal pain, *anorexia.*
**GU:** proteinuria, hematuria.
**Hematologic:** eosinophilia, *anemia.*
**Hepatic:** increased alkaline phosphatase level.
**Metabolic:** hypokalemia.
**Musculoskeletal:** *pain, myalgia.*
**Respiratory:** *tachypnea.*
**Skin:** histamine-mediated symptoms, including rash, facial swelling, pruritus, and sensation of warmth.
**Other:** fever, infused vein complications, phlebitis, *chills, sweating.*

---

## Overdose and treatment
In clinical studies, the highest dose was 100 mg, given as a single dose to five patients, and was generally well tolerated. No overdoses have been reported. Caspofungin isn't removed by dialysis.

## Clinical considerations
■ The efficacy of a 70-mg dose regimen in patients who don't respond to a 50-mg dose regimen isn't known, but the increase seems to be well tolerated. Safety of treatment lasting longer than 2 weeks is unclear, but longer courses seem to be well tolerated.
■ Duration of treatment should be based on the severity of the patient's underlying disease, recovery from immunosuppression, and response.
■ Advise clinician to observe patient for histamine-mediated reactions, such as rash, facial swelling, pruritis, and sensation of warmth.

### Therapeutic monitoring
■ Monitor CBC and liver enzyme levels during therapy. Patients also receiving cyclosporine may develop increased ALT and AST levels.

### Special populations
**Breast-feeding patients.** It isn't known if drug appears in breast milk. Because many drugs do appear in breast milk, use cautiously when giving caspofungin to a breast-feeding patient.
**Pediatric patients.** Safety and effectiveness in patients under age 18 are unknown.
**Geriatric patients.** No dosage adjustments are needed.

## Patient counseling
■ Instruct patient to report signs and symptoms of phlebitis.

# castor oil
Emulsoil, Neoloid, Purge

*Pharmacologic classification:* glyceride, *Ricinus communis* derivative
*Therapeutic classification:* stimulant laxative
*Pregnancy risk category X*

## Available forms
Available without a prescription
*Liquid:* 60 ml, 120 ml
*Liquid (95%):* 30 ml, 60 ml
*Liquid emulsion:* 60 ml (95%), 90 ml (67%)

## Indications and dosages
*Preparation for rectal or bowel examination or surgery; acute constipation*
**Liquid**
*Adults:* 15 to 60 ml (or 30 to 60 ml, 95%) P.O.
*Children ages 2 to 12:* 5 to 15 ml P.O.

**Liquid emulsion**
*Adults:* 45 ml (67%) or 15 to 60 ml (95%) P.O. mixed with ½ to 1 glass liquid.
*Children ages 2 to 12:* 15 ml (67%) or 5 to 15 ml (95%) P.O. mixed with ½ to 1 glass liquid.

## Mechanism of action
*Laxative action:* Castor oil acts primarily in the small intestine, where it's metabolized to ricinoleic acid, which stimulates the intestine, promoting peristalsis and bowel motility.

## Pharmacokinetics
*Absorption:* Unknown.
*Distribution:* Distributed locally, primarily in the small intestine.
*Metabolism:* Like other fatty acids, castor oil is metabolized by intestinal enzymes into its active form, ricinoleic acid.
*Excretion:* Excreted in feces.

| Route | Onset | Peak | Duration |
|-------|-------|------|----------|
| P.O. | 2-6 hr | Variable | Variable |

## Contraindications and precautions
Contraindicated in patients with ulcerative bowel lesions; abdominal pain, nausea, vomiting, or other symptoms of appendicitis or acute surgical abdomen.
    Also contraindicated in those with anal or rectal fissures, fecal impaction, or intestinal obstruction or perforation; and during menstruation or pregnancy. Use cautiously in patients with rectal bleeding.

## Interactions
**Drug-drug.** *Intestinally absorbed drugs:* Castor oil may decrease absorption of these drugs. Advise clinician to monitor patient closely.
**Drug-herb.** *Male fern:* May increase absorption and increase risk of toxicity. Discourage use together.

## Adverse reactions
**GI:** *nausea;* vomiting; diarrhea; loss of normal bowel function with excessive use; *abdominal cramps,* especially in severe constipation; malabsorption of nutrients; "cathartic colon" (syndrome resembling ulcerative colitis radiologically and pathologically) with chronic misuse; laxative dependence with longterm or excessive use. May cause constipation after catharsis.
**Metabolic:** hypokalemia, protein-losing enteropathy, other electrolyte imbalances (with excessive use).

## Overdose and treatment
No information available.

## Clinical considerations
■ Failure to respond to drug may indicate acute condition requiring surgery.

■ Castor oil isn't recommended for routine use in constipation; it's commonly used to evacuate the bowels before diagnostic or surgical procedures.
■ Because of rapid onset of action, drug shouldn't be given at bedtime.
■ Drug is most effective when taken on an empty stomach; shake well.
■ Flavored preparations are available.

### Therapeutic monitoring
■ Advise clinician to observe patient for signs and symptoms of dehydration.

### Special populations
**Pregnant patients.** Drug shouldn't be used in pregnant women because there's a possibility of fetal abnormalities.
**Breast-feeding patients.** Breast-feeding women should seek medical approval before using castor oil.
**Geriatric patients.** With long-term use, geriatric patients may experience electrolyte depletion, resulting in weakness, incoordination, and orthostatic hypotension.

### Patient counseling
■ Advise pregnant women against use of castor oil.
■ Recommend that drug be chilled or taken with juice or carbonated beverage for palatability.
■ Instruct patient to shake emulsion well before taking it.
■ Reassure patient that after response to drug, he may not need to move bowels again for 1 or 2 days.

---

# cefaclor
Ceclor, Ceclor CD

*Pharmacologic classification:* second-generation cephalosporin
*Therapeutic classification:* antibiotic
*Pregnancy risk category B*

## Available forms
Available by prescription only
*Tablets (extended-release):* 375 mg, 500 mg
*Capsules:* 250 mg, 500 mg
*Suspension:* 125 mg/5 ml, 187 mg/5 ml, 250 mg/5 ml, 375 mg/5 ml

## Indications and dosages
*Infections of respiratory or urinary tract and skin; otitis media caused by susceptible organisms*
*Adults:* 250 to 500 mg P.O. q 8 hours. Total daily dose shouldn't exceed 4 g. For extended-release tablets, 375 to 500 mg P.O. q 12 hours for 7 to 10 days.

*Children:* 20 mg/kg P.O. daily (40 mg/kg for severe infections and otitis media) in divided doses q 8 hours, not to exceed 1 g/day.
◇ *Acute uncomplicated urinary tract infection*
*Adults:* 2 g P.O. as single dose.
≡ *Dosage adjustment.* Because cefaclor is dialyzable, patients receiving treatment with hemodialysis or peritoneal dialysis may need dosage adjustment.
To prevent toxic accumulation, reduced dosage may be needed if patient's creatinine clearance is less than 40 ml/minute.

## Mechanism of action
*Antibacterial action:* Drug is primarily bactericidal; however, it may be bacteriostatic. Activity depends on the specific organism, extent of tissue penetration, drug dosage, and rate of organism multiplication. It acts by adhering to bacterial penicillin-binding proteins, thereby inhibiting cell-wall synthesis.

Cefaclor has the same bactericidal spectrum as other second-generation cephalosporins except that it has increased activity against ampicillin- or amoxicillin-resistant *Haemophilus influenzae* and *Moraxella catarrhalis.*

## Pharmacokinetics
*Absorption:* Well absorbed from the GI tract. Food will delay but not prevent complete GI tract absorption.
*Distribution:* Distributed widely into most body tissues and fluids; CSF penetration is poor. Cefaclor crosses the placenta; it's 25% protein-bound.
*Metabolism:* Not metabolized.
*Excretion:* Excreted primarily in urine by renal tubular secretion and glomerular filtration; small amounts of drug appear in breast milk. Elimination half-life is ½ to 1 hour in patients with normal renal function; end-stage renal disease prolongs half-life to 3 to 5½ hours. Hemodialysis removes cefaclor.

| Route | Onset | Peak | Duration |
|---|---|---|---|
| P.O. | Unknown | ½-1 hr | Unknown |
| P.O. (extended-release) | Unknown | ½-2½ hr | Unknown |

## Contraindications and precautions
Contraindicated in patients hypersensitive to other cephalosporins. Use cautiously in patients with impaired renal function or penicillin allergy and in breast-feeding women.

## Interactions
**Drug-drug.** *Antacids:* Absorption of extended-release cefaclor is decreased if taken within 1 hour. Separate administration by 1 hour.
*Chloramphenicol:* Antagonistic effect. Don't use together.

---

*Nephrotoxic drugs (aminoglycosides, colistin, polymyxin B, vancomycin) or loop diuretics:* May increase the risk of nephrotoxicity. Advise clinician to monitor patient.

*Probenecid:* Competitively inhibits renal tubular secretion of cephalosporins, resulting in higher, prolonged serum levels of these drugs. Advise clinician to monitor patient.

## Adverse reactions
**CNS:** dizziness, headache, somnolence, malaise.
**GI:** *nausea,* vomiting, *diarrhea,* anorexia, dyspepsia, abdominal cramps, pseudomembranous colitis, oral candidiasis.
**GU:** vaginal candidiasis, vaginitis.
**Hematologic:** *transient leukopenia,* anemia, eosinophilia, *thrombocytopenia,* lymphocytosis.
**Hepatic:** increased liver enzyme levels.
**Skin:** *maculopapular rash,* dermatitis, pruritus, *Stevens-Johnson syndrome.*
**Other:** hypersensitivity reactions, serum sickness, *anaphylaxis,* fever.

## Overdose and treatment
Signs and symptoms of overdose include neuromuscular hypersensitivity; seizure may follow high CNS levels. Remove cefaclor by hemodialysis or peritoneal dialysis.

## Clinical considerations
■ Total daily dose may be given b.i.d. rather than t.i.d. with similar therapeutic effect.
■ Stock oral suspension is stable for 14 days if refrigerated.
■ Cefaclor may cause false-positive Coombs' test results. Cefaclor also causes false-positive results in urine glucose tests using cupric sulfate (Benedict's reagent or Clinitest); use glucose oxidase tests (Chemstrip uG, Diastix, or glucose enzymatic test strip) instead.
■ Cefaclor causes false elevations in serum or urine creatinine levels in tests using Jaffé's reaction.

### Therapeutic monitoring
■ Monitor for signs and symptoms of superinfection.

### Special populations
**Breast-feeding patients.** Drug appears in breast milk; use with caution in breast-feeding women.
**Pediatric patients.** Drug can be used safely in children over age 1 month. Extended-release tablets should only be used in children ages 16 and older.
**Geriatric patients.** No dosage adjustments are needed.

## Patient counseling
■ Instruct patient to take extended-release tablets with food and not to cut, crush, or chew them.

■ Tell patient to take the entire amount of drug exactly as prescribed, even if he feels better.

# cefadroxil
Duricef

*Pharmacologic classification:* first-generation cephalosporin
*Therapeutic classification:* antibiotic
*Pregnancy risk category B*

## Available forms
Available by prescription only
*Tablets:* 1 g
*Capsules:* 500 mg
*Suspension:* 125 mg/5 ml, 250 mg/5 ml, 500 mg/5 ml

## Indications and dosages
***Urinary tract, skin, and soft-tissue infections caused by susceptible organisms; pharyngitis; tonsillitis***
*Adults:* 1 to 2 g P.O. daily, depending on the infection treated. Usually given once or twice daily.
*Children:* 30 mg/kg P.O. daily in two divided doses.
≡*Dosage adjustment.* For patients with creatinine clearance less than 10 ml/minute, extend dosing interval to q 36 hours; if creatinine clearance is between 10 and 25 ml/minute, administer q 24 hours; if it's between 25 and 50 ml/minute, give q 12 hours. Because drug is dialyzable, patients receiving treatment with hemodialysis may need dosage adjustment.

## Mechanism of action
*Antibacterial action:* Cefadroxil is primarily bactericidal; however, it may be bacteriostatic. Activity depends on the organism, tissue penetration, drug dosage, and rate of organism multiplication. It acts by adhering to bacterial penicillin-binding proteins, thereby inhibiting cell-wall synthesis.

Cefadroxil is active against many gram-positive cocci, including penicillinase-producing *Staphylococcus aureus* and *Staphylococcus epidermidis; Streptococcus pneumoniae,* group B streptococci, and group A beta-hemolytic streptococci; and susceptible gram-negative organisms, including *Klebsiella pneumoniae, Escherichia coli,* and *Proteus mirabilis.*

## Pharmacokinetics
*Absorption:* Absorbed rapidly and completely from the GI tract after oral administration.
*Distribution:* Distributed widely into most body tissues and fluids, including the gallbladder, liver, kidneys, bone, bile, sputum, and pleural and synovial fluids; CSF penetration is poor. Drug crosses the placenta; it's 20% protein-bound.
*Metabolism:* Not metabolized.

---

*Excretion:* Excreted primarily unchanged in the urine by way of glomerular filtration and renal tubular secretion; small amounts may appear in breast milk. End-stage renal disease prolongs half-life to 25 hours. Drug can be removed by hemodialysis.

| Route | Onset | Peak | Duration |
|-------|-------|------|----------|
| P.O. | Unknown | 1-2 hr | Unknown |

## Contraindications and precautions
Contraindicated in patients hypersensitive to drug or other cephalosporins. Use cautiously in patients with impaired renal function or penicillin allergy and in breast-feeding women.

## Interactions
**Drug-drug.** *Bacteriostatic drugs (chloramphenicol, erythromycin, tetracyclines):* May interfere with bactericidal activity. Use with caution.
*Nephrotoxic drugs (aminoglycosides, colistin, polymyxin B, vancomycin) or loop diuretics:* May increase the risk of nephrotoxicity. Advise clinician to monitor patient closely.
*Probenecid:* Competitively inhibits renal tubular secretion of cephalosporins, resulting in higher, prolonged serum levels of these drugs. Use together cautiously.

## Adverse reactions
**CNS:** *seizures.*
**GI:** pseudomembranous colitis, *nausea,* vomiting, *diarrhea,* glossitis, abdominal cramps, oral candidiasis.
**GU:** genital pruritus, candidiasis, vaginitis, renal dysfunction.
**Hematologic:** *transient neutropenia,* eosinophilia, *leukopenia,* anemia, *agranulocytosis, thrombocytopenia.*
**Hepatic:** increased liver enzyme levels.
**Respiratory:** dyspnea.
**Skin:** *maculopapular and erythematous rashes,* urticaria.
**Other:** hypersensitivity reactions, serum sickness, *anaphylaxis, angioedema,* fever.

## Overdose and treatment
Signs and symptoms of overdose include neuromuscular hypersensitivity; seizure may follow high CNS levels. Remove cefadroxil by hemodialysis. Other treatment is supportive.

## Clinical considerations
▪ Cefadroxil causes false-positive results in urine glucose tests using cupric sulfate (Benedict's reagent or Clinitest); use glucose oxidase test (Chemstrip uG, Diastix, or glucose enzymatic test strip) instead. Cefadroxil causes false elevations in serum or urine creatinine levels in tests using Jaffé's reaction. Positive Coomb's test results occur in about 3% of patients taking cephalosporins.

▪ Consider the recommendations relevant to all cephalosporins; longer half-life of drug permits once- or twice-daily dosing.

### Therapeutic monitoring
▪ With large doses or prolonged therapy, advise clinician to watch for superinfection, especially in high-risk patients.

### Special populations
**Breast-feeding patients.** Drug appears in breast milk; use with caution in breast-feeding women.
**Pediatric patients.** Serum half-life is prolonged in neonates and infants under age 1.
**Geriatric patients.** Reduce dosage in geriatric patients with diminished renal function.

## Patient counseling
▪ Inform patient of potential adverse reactions.
▪ Instruct patient to take drug with food to lessen GI discomfort.

# cefamandole nafate
Mandol

*Pharmacologic classification:* second-generation cephalosporin
*Therapeutic classification:* antibiotic
*Pregnancy risk category B*

## Available forms
Available by prescription only
*Injection:* 1 g, 2 g

## Indications and dosages
*Serious respiratory tract, GU, skin and soft-tissue, and bone and joint infections; septicemia; peritonitis from susceptible organisms*
*Adults:* 500 mg to 1 g I.M. or I.V. q 4 to 8 hours. In life-threatening infections, up to 2 g q 4 hours may be needed.
*Infants and children:* 50 to 100 mg/kg I.M. or I.V. daily in equally divided doses q 4 to 8 hours. May be increased to total daily dose of 150 mg/kg (not to exceed maximum adult dose) for severe infections.
    Total daily dose is same for I.M. or I.V. administration and depends on susceptibility of organism and severity of infection. Inject drug deep I.M. into a large muscle mass, such as the gluteus or the lateral aspect of the thigh.
≡*Dosage adjustment.* For patients with impaired renal function, doses or frequency of administration must be modified according to degree of renal impairment, severity of infection, and susceptibility of organism. The following table gives appropriate doses for adults.

| Creatinine clearance (ml/min) | Severe infections | Life-threatening infections (maximum) |
|---|---|---|
| > 80 | 1-2 g q 6 hr | 2 g q 4 hr |
| 50-80 | 750 mg-1.5 g q 6 hr | 1.5 g q 4 hr; or 2 g q 6 hr |
| 25-50 | 750 mg-1.5 g q 8 hr | 1.5 g q 6 hr; or 2 g q 8 hr |
| 10-25 | 500 mg-1 g q 8 hr | 1 g q 6 hr; or 1.25 g q 8 hr |
| 2-10 | 500-750 mg q 12 hr | 670 mg q 8 hr; or 1 g q 12 hr |
| < 2 | 250-500 mg q 12 hr | 500 mg q 8 hr; or 750 mg q 12 hr |

## I.V. administration
■ Reconstitute 1 g with 10 ml of sterile water for injection, $D_5W$, or normal saline injection. Give slowly, over 3 to 5 minutes, or by intermittent infusion or continuous infusion in compatible solutions. Check package insert.

### Incompatibilities
Don't mix with I.V. infusions containing magnesium or calcium ions, which are chemically incompatible and may cause irreversible effects. Incompatible with aminoglycosides, amiodarone, calcium gluceptate, calcium gluconate, cimetidine, hetastarch, Isolyte M, and magnesium and calcium ions, including Ringer's injection and lactated Ringer's injection.

## Mechanism of action
*Antibacterial action:* Cefamandole is primarily bactericidal; however, it may be bacteriostatic. Activity depends on the organism, tissue penetration, drug dosage, and rate of organism multiplication. It acts by adhering to bacterial penicillin-binding proteins, thereby inhibiting cell-wall synthesis.

Cefamandole is active against *Escherichia coli* and other coliform bacteria, *Staphylococcus aureus* (penicillinase- and nonpenicillinase-producing), *Staphylococcus epidermidis,* group A beta-hemolytic streptococci, *Klebsiella, Haemophilus influenzae, Proteus mirabilis,* and *Enterobacter* as the second-generation drugs. *Bacteroides fragilis* and *Acinetobacter* are resistant.

## Pharmacokinetics
*Absorption:* Not absorbed from the GI tract; must be given parenterally.
*Distribution:* Distributed widely into most body tissues and fluids, including the gallbladder, liver, kidneys, bone, sputum, bile, and pleural and synovial fluids; CSF penetration is poor.

Cefamandole crosses the placenta; it's 65% to 75% protein-bound.
*Metabolism:* Not metabolized.
*Excretion:* Excreted primarily in urine by renal tubular secretion and glomerular filtration; small amounts of drug appear in breast milk. Elimination half-life is about ½ to 1 hour in patients with normal renal function; severe renal disease prolongs half-life to 12 to 18 hours.

| Route | Onset | Peak | Duration |
|---|---|---|---|
| I.V., I.M. | Unknown | 1½-2 hr | Unknown |

## Contraindications and precautions
Contraindicated in patients hypersensitive to drug or other cephalosporins. Use cautiously in patients with impaired renal function or penicillin allergy and in breast-feeding women.

## Interactions
**Drug-drug.** *Anticoagulants:* May increase risk of bleeding. Avoid use together.
*Bacteriostatic drugs (chloramphenicol, erythromycin, tetracyclines):* May impair its bactericidal activity. Use with caution.
*Nephrotoxic drugs (aminoglycosides, colistin, polymyxin B, vancomycin) or loop diuretics:* May increase the risk of nephrotoxicity. Advise clinician to monitor patient closely.
*Probenecid:* Competitively inhibits renal tubular secretion of cephalosporins, resulting in higher, prolonged serum levels of these drugs. Advise clinician to monitor patient closely.
**Drug-lifestyle.** *Alcohol use:* May cause severe disulfiram-like reactions. Advise patient not to consume alcohol while on drug therapy.

## Adverse reactions
**GI:** pseudomembranous colitis, nausea, vomiting, *diarrhea,* oral candidiasis.
**Hematologic:** eosinophilia, coagulation abnormalities.
**Hepatic:** increased liver enzymes levels.
**Skin:** *maculopapular and erythematous rashes, urticaria, pain, induration, sterile abscesses,* temperature elevation, tissue sloughing (at injection site).
**Other:** hypersensitivity reactions, serum sickness, *anaphylaxis; phlebitis, thrombophlebitis* (with I.V. injection).

## Overdose and treatment
Signs and symptoms of overdose include neuromuscular hypersensitivity. Seizure may follow high CNS levels. Hypoprothrombinemia and bleeding may occur; they may be treated with vitamin K or blood products. Some drug may be removed by hemodialysis.

## Clinical considerations
■ For most cephalosporin-sensitive organisms, cefamandole offers little advantage over other cephalosporins; it's less effective than cefoxitin against anaerobic infections. Some clini-

cians consider it inappropriate for pediatric use, especially for serious infections such as *Haemophilus influenzae.*

■ For I.M. use, dilute 1 g of cefamandole in 3 ml of sterile water for injection, bacteriostatic water for injection, normal saline solution for injection, or 0.9% bacteriostatic saline for injection.

■ Recommend giving cefamandole deeply into large muscle mass to ensure maximum absorption. Injection sites should be rotated.

■ I.M. cefamandole is less painful than cefoxitin injection; it doesn't require addition of lidocaine.

■ After reconstitution, solution remains stable for 24 hours at controlled room temperature or 96 hours under refrigeration. Solution should be light yellow to amber. Don't use solution if it's discolored or contains a precipitate.

■ Cefamandole causes false-positive results in urine glucose tests using cupric sulfate (Benedict's reagent or Clinitest); use glucose oxidase tests (Chemstrip uG, Diastix, or glucose enzymatic test strip) instead. Cefamandole also causes false elevations in serum or urine creatinine levels in tests using Jaffé's reaction. Drug may cause positive Coombs' test results.

### Therapeutic monitoring

■ Advise clinician to monitor patient for signs or symptoms of bleeding, with evaluation of PT and platelet level. Patient may require prophylactic use of vitamin K to prevent bleeding.

■ Bleeding can be reversed by giving vitamin K or blood products.

### Special populations

**Breast-feeding patients.** Drug appears in breast milk; use with caution in breast-feeding women. Safety hasn't been established.

**Pediatric patients.** Safety in infants under age 1 month hasn't been established.

**Geriatric patients.** Dosage reduction may be required in patients with diminished renal function. Hypoprothrombinemia and bleeding have been reported most frequently in geriatric, malnourished, and debilitated patients.

### Patient counseling

■ Inform patient of potential adverse reactions.

## cefazolin sodium

Ancef, Kefzol

*Pharmacologic classification:* first-generation cephalosporin
*Therapeutic classification:* antibiotic
*Pregnancy risk category B*

### Available forms

Available by prescription only
*Injection (parenteral):* 500 mg, 1 g, 5 g, 10 g, 20 g

*Infusion:* 500-mg or 1-g Redi Vials, Faspaks, or ADD-Vantage vials

## Indications and dosages

*Serious respiratory tract, GU, skin and soft-tissue, and bone and joint infections; biliary tract infections; septicemia, endocarditis from susceptible organisms;* ◇ *perioperative prophylaxis; contaminated surgery*

*Adults:* 250 mg I.M. or I.V. q 8 hours to 1.5 g q 6 hours. Maximum dose is 12 g/day in life-threatening situations.

*Children over age 1 month:* 25 to 100 mg/kg/day I.M. or I.V. in divided doses q 6 to 8 hours.

Total daily dose is same for I.M. or I.V. administration and depends on the susceptibility of organism and severity of infection. Inject cefazolin deep I.M. into a large muscle mass, such as the gluteus or the lateral aspect of the thigh.

≡ *Dosage adjustment.* Dose or frequency of administration must be modified according to the degree of renal impairment, severity of infection, susceptibility of organism, and serum levels of drug. Because drug can be removed by hemodialysis, patients undergoing hemodialysis may require dosage adjustment.

| Creatinine clearance (ml/min) | Adult dosage |
|---|---|
| 35-54 | Full dose q 8 hr or less frequently |
| 11-34 | ½ usual dose q 12 hr |
| ≤ 10 | ½ usual dose q 18-24 hr |

| Creatinine clearance (ml/min) | Pediatric dosage |
|---|---|
| 40-70 | 60% of normal daily dose q 12 hr |
| 20-40 | 25% of normal daily dose q 12 hr |
| 5-20 | 10% of normal daily dose q 24 hr |

## I.V. administration

■ For direct I.V. injection, reconstitute 500-mg vial with 2-ml or 1-g vial with 2.5 ml of sterile water for injection. Further dilute in 5 ml of sterile water for injection; then inject over 3 to 5 minutes directly into vein or the tubing of a compatible free-flowing I.V. solution.

■ For intermittent I.V. administration, dilute in 50 to 100 ml of $D_5W$ or normal saline solution.

- Reconstituted solution is stable for 24 hours at controlled room temperature and for 10 days, if refrigerated.

### Incompatibilities
Incompatible with aminoglycosides, amiodarone, amobarbital, ascorbic acid injection, bleomycin, calcium gluceptate, calcium gluconate, cimetidine, colistimethate, erythromycin gluceptate, hydrocortisone, idarubicin, lidocaine, norepinephrine, oxytetracycline, pentobarbital sodium, polymyxin B, ranitidine, tetracycline, theophylline, and vitamin B complex with C.

### Mechanism of action
*Antibacterial action:* Cefazolin is primarily bactericidal; however, it may be bacteriostatic. Activity depends on the organism, tissue penetration, drug dosage, and rate of organism multiplication. It acts by adhering to bacterial penicillin-binding proteins, thereby inhibiting cell-wall synthesis.

Cefazolin is active against *Escherichia coli,* Enterobacteriaceae, *Haemophilus influenzae, Klebsiella, Proteus mirabilis, Staphylococcus aureus, Streptococcus pneumoniae,* and group A beta-hemolytic streptococci.

### Pharmacokinetics
*Absorption:* Not well absorbed from the GI tract; must be given parenterally.
*Distribution:* Distributed widely into most body tissues and fluids, including the gallbladder, liver, kidneys, bone, sputum, bile, and pleural and synovial fluids; CSF penetration is poor. It crosses the placenta; it's 74% to 86% protein-bound.
*Metabolism:* Not metabolized.
*Excretion:* Excreted primarily unchanged in urine by renal tubular secretion and glomerular filtration; small amounts of drug appear in breast milk. Elimination half-life is about 1 to 2 hours in patients with normal renal function; end-stage renal disease prolongs half-life to 12 to 50 hours. Hemodialysis or peritoneal dialysis removes cefazolin.

| Route | Onset | Peak | Duration |
|-------|-------|------|----------|
| I.V. | Immediate | Immediate | Unknown |
| I.M. | Unknown | 1-2 hr | Unknown |

### Contraindications and precautions
Contraindicated in patients hypersensitive to other cephalosporins. Use cautiously in patients with impaired renal function or penicillin allergy and in breast-feeding women.

### Interactions
**Drug-drug.** *Bacteriostatic drugs (chloramphenicol, erythromycin, tetracyclines):* Use together may interfere with bactericidal activity. Avoid use together.

*Nephrotoxic drugs (aminoglycosides, colistin, polymyxin B, vancomycin) or loop diuretics:* Use together may increase the risk of nephrotoxicity. Advise clinician to monitor patient closely.
*Probenecid:* Competitively inhibits renal tubular secretion of cephalosporins, resulting in higher, prolonged serum levels of these drugs. Advise clinician to monitor patient closely.

### Adverse reactions
**GI:** pseudomembranous colitis, nausea, anorexia, vomiting, *diarrhea,* glossitis, dyspepsia, abdominal cramps, anal pruritus, oral candidiasis.
**GU:** genital pruritus, candidiasis, vaginitis.
**Hematologic: *neutropenia, leukopenia,*** eosinophilia, ***thrombocytopenia.***
**Hepatic:** transient increases in liver enzymes.
**Skin:** *maculopapular and erythematous rashes, urticaria, pruritus,* **Stevens-Johnson syndrome,** *pain, induration, sterile abscesses, tissue sloughing* (at injection site); *phlebitis, thrombophlebitis* (with I.V. injection).
**Other:** hypersensitivity reactions, serum sickness, *anaphylaxis.*

### Overdose and treatment
Signs and symptoms of overdose include neuromuscular hypersensitivity; seizure may follow high CNS levels. Cefazolin may be removed by hemodialysis.

### Clinical considerations
- For I.M. use, reconstitute with sterile water, bacteriostatic water, or normal saline solution: 2 ml to a 500-mg vial, and 2.5 ml to a 1-g vial produces levels of 225 mg/ml, and 330 mg/ml respectively.
- I.M. cefazolin injection is less painful than that of other cephalosporins.
- Cephalosporins cause false-positive results in urine glucose tests utilizing cupric sulfate (Benedict's reagent or Clinitest); use glucose oxidase tests (Chemstrip uG, Diastix, or glucose enzymatic test strip) instead. Cefazolin causes false elevations in serum or urine creatinine levels in tests using Jaffé's reaction. Cefazolin also causes positive Coombs' test results.

### Therapeutic monitoring
- For patients on sodium restrictions, note that cefazolin injection contains 2 mEq of sodium per gram of drug.
- Electrolyte studies should be performed.

### Special populations
**Breast-feeding patients.** Safety hasn't been established. Use drug with caution in breast-feeding women.
**Pediatric patients.** Drug has been used in children. However, safety in infants under age 1 month hasn't been established.

## Patient counseling
■ Inform patient of potential adverse reactions.

# cefdinir
Omnicef

*Pharmacologic classification:* third-generation cephalosporin
*Therapeutic classification:* antibiotic
*Pregnancy risk category B*

## Available forms
Available by prescription only
*Capsules:* 300 mg
*Suspension:* 125 mg/5 ml

## Indications and dosages
*Treatment of mild to moderate infections caused by susceptible strains of microorganisms for conditions of community-acquired pneumonia, acute exacerbations of chronic bronchitis, acute maxillary sinusitis, acute bacterial otitis media, and uncomplicated skin and skin structure infections*
*Adults and adolescents ages 13 and older:* 300 mg P.O. q 12 hours or 600 mg P.O. q 24 hours for 10 days. (Use q-12-hour doses for pneumonia and skin infections; treat acute otitis media for 5 to 10 days.)
*Children ages 6 months to 12 years:* 7 mg/kg P.O. q 12 hours or 14 mg/kg P.O. q 24 hours for 10 days, up to maximum dose of 600 mg daily. (Use q-12-hour dosages for skin infections; treat acute otitis media for 5 to 10 days.)
*Treatment of pharyngitis and tonsillitis*
*Adults and adolescents ages 13 and older:* 300 mg P.O. q 12 hours for 5 to 10 days or 600 mg P.O. q 24 hours for 10 days.
*Children ages 6 months to 12 years:* 7 mg/kg P.O. q 12 hours for 5 to 10 days or 14 mg/kg P.O. q 24 hours for 10 days.
≡ *Dosage adjustment.* If creatinine clearance is less than 30 ml/minute, reduce dosage to 300 mg P.O. once daily for adults and 7 mg/kg P.O. (up to 300 mg) once daily for children.

For patients receiving chronic hemodialysis, 300 mg or 7 mg/kg P.O. at end of each dialysis session and subsequently every other day.

## Mechanism of action
*Antibiotic action:* The bactericidal activity of cefdinir results from inhibition of cell-wall synthesis. Drug is stable in the presence of some beta-lactamase enzymes, causing some microorganisms resistant to penicillins and cephalosporins to be susceptible to cefdinir. Excluding *Pseudomonas, Enterobacter, Enterococcus,* and methicillin-resistant *Staphylococcus* species, the spectrum of activity of cefdinir includes a broad range of gram-positive and gram-negative aerobic microorganisms.

## Pharmacokinetics
*Absorption:* Estimated bioavailability of drug is 21% following administration of a 300-mg capsule dose, 16% following a 600-mg capsule dose, and 25% for the suspension.
*Distribution:* Mean volume of distribution for adults and children is 0.35 and 0.67 L/kg, respectively, and distribution to tonsil, sinus, lung, and middle ear tissue and fluid ranges from 15% to 35% of corresponding plasma levels. 60% to 70% plasma protein–bound; binding is independent of level.
*Metabolism:* Not appreciably metabolized; its activity is primarily from parent drug.
*Excretion:* Excreted principally by renal excretion; mean plasma elimination half-life is 1.7 hours. Drug clearance is reduced in patients with renal dysfunction.

| Route | Onset | Peak | Duration |
|-------|-------|------|----------|
| P.O. | Unknown | 2-4 hr | Unknown |

## Contraindications and precautions
Contraindicated in patients with known allergy to cephalosporin class of antibiotics. Use cautiously in patients hypersensitive to penicillin because of the possibility of cross-sensitivity with other beta-lactam antibiotics. Also use with caution in patients with history of colitis.

## Interactions
**Drug-drug.** *Antacids containing magnesium and aluminum, iron supplements:* Decreased rate of absorption and bioavailability of cefdinir. Give these preparations 2 hours before or after cefdinir dose.
*Probenecid:* Inhibited renal secretion of cefdinir. Advise clinician to monitor patient.
**Drug-food.** *Foods fortified with iron, such as infant formula:* Decreased rate of absorption and bioavailability of cefdinir. Advise clinician to monitor patient.

## Adverse reactions
**CNS:** headache.
**GI:** abdominal pain, *diarrhea,* nausea, vomiting.
**GU:** vaginal candidiasis, vaginitis.
**Skin:** rash.

## Overdose and treatment
No information available. Toxic signs of overdose with other beta-lactam antibiotics include nausea, vomiting, epigastric distress, diarrhea, and seizures. Drug is removed by hemodialysis.

## Clinical considerations
■ Pseudomembranous colitis has been reported with many antibiotics, including cefdinir, and should be considered in patients whose symptoms include diarrhea subsequent to antibiotic therapy or in those with history of colitis.
■ False-positive reactions for ketones (tests using nitroprusside only) and glucose (Clinitest,

Benedict's solution, Fehling's solution) in the urine have been reported. Generally, cephalosporins can induce a positive direct Coombs' test.

### Therapeutic monitoring
■ As with many antibiotics, prolonged drug treatment may result in possible emergence and overgrowth of resistant organisms. Consider alternative therapy if superinfection occurs.

### Special populations
**Breast-feeding patients.** Drug doesn't appear in breast milk after 600-mg doses.
**Pediatric patients.** Safety and efficacy in infants under age 6 months haven't been established. Pharmacokinetic data for the pediatric population are comparable to data for adults.
**Geriatric patients.** Cefdinir is well tolerated in all age-groups. Safety and efficacy are comparable in geriatric patients and younger patients. Dosage adjustment isn't needed unless patient has renal impairment.

### Patient counseling
■ Instruct patient to take antacids, iron supplements, and iron-fortified foods 2 hours before or after a cefdinir dose.
■ Inform diabetic patient that each teaspoon of suspension contains 2.86 g of sucrose.
■ Advise patient to report severe diarrhea or diarrhea with abdominal pain.

# cefepime hydrochloride
Maxipime

*Pharmacologic classification:* semi-synthetic third- or fourth-generation cephalosporin
*Therapeutic classification:* antibiotic
*Pregnancy risk category B*

### Available forms
Available by prescription only
*Injection:* 500 mg/15 ml vial, 1 g/100 ml piggyback bottle, 1 g/ADD-Vantage vial, 1 g/15 ml vial, 2 g/100 ml piggyback bottle, 2 g/20 ml vial

### Indications and dosages
*Mild to moderate urinary tract infections caused by* **Escherichia coli, Klebsiella pneumoniae,** *or* **Proteus mirabilis,** *including cases caused by concurrent bacteremia with these microorganisms*
*Adults:* 0.5 to 1 g I.M. (use I.M. route only for infections caused by *E. coli*), or I.V. infused over 30 minutes q 12 hours for 7 to 10 days.

*Severe urinary tract infections including pyelonephritis caused by* **E. coli** *or* **K. pneumoniae**
*Adults:* 2 g I.V. infused over 30 minutes q 12 hours for 10 days.
*Moderate to severe pneumonia caused by* **Streptococcus pneumoniae, Pseudomonas aeruginosa, K. pneumoniae,** *or* **Enterobacter** *species*
*Adults:* 1 to 2 g I.V. infused over 30 minutes q 12 hours for 10 days.
*Moderate to severe uncomplicated skin and skin-structure infections from* **Staphylococcus aureus** *(methicillin-susceptible strains only) or* **Streptococcus pyogenes**
*Adults:* 2 g I.V. infused over 30 minutes q 12 hours for 10 days.
*Empiric therapy in febrile neutropenia*
*Adults:* 2 g I.V. q 8 hours for 7 days or until neutropenia resolves.
*Children weighing less than 40 kg (88 lb):* 50 mg/kg I.V. q 8 hours.
*Uncomplicated and complicated urinary tract infections, uncomplicated skin and skin-structure infections, or pneumonia*
*Children weighing less than 40 kg (88 lb):* 50 mg/kg I.V. q 12 hours.
◇ *Children over age 1 month:* 1 to 2 g daily, divided b.i.d., for mild to moderate infections; or 2 to 4 g daily, divided b.i.d., for severe infections.
   Pediatric dosages shouldn't exceed the recommended adult dosages.
≡*Dosage adjustment.* Adjust dosage in patients with impaired renal function. Consult manufacturer's recommendations. Patients receiving hemodialysis should receive a repeat dose at the end of dialysis. Patients undergoing continuous ambulatory peritoneal dialysis (CAPD) should receive the usual dose q 48 hours.

### I.V. administration
■ Follow manufacturer guidelines closely when reconstituting drug. Variations occur in constituting drug for administration and depend on level of drug needed and how drug is packaged (piggyback vial, ADD-Vantage vial, or regular vial). Type of diluent used for constitution varies, depending on product used. Use only solutions recommended by manufacturer. Give the resulting solution over 30 minutes.
■ Intermittent I.V. infusion with a Y-type administration set can be accomplished with compatible solutions. However, during infusion of a solution containing cefepime, discontinuing the other solution is recommended.

### Incompatibilities
Incompatible with aminophylline, gentamicin, metronidazole, netilmicin, tobramycin, and vancomycin.

## Mechanism of action
*Antibiotic action:* Cefepime exerts its bactericidal action by inhibition of cell-wall synthesis. It's usually active against gram-positive microorganisms such as *S. pneumoniae, S. aureus,* and *S. pyogenes* and gram-negative microorganisms such as *Enterobacter* species, *E. coli, K. pneumoniae, P. mirabilis,* and *P. aeruginosa.*

## Pharmacokinetics
*Absorption:* Completely absorbed after I.M. administration.
*Distribution:* Widely distributed; about 20% serum protein-bound.
*Metabolism:* Metabolized rapidly.
*Excretion:* About 85% is excreted in urine as unchanged drug; less than 1% as the metabolite, 6.8% as the metabolite oxide, and 2.5% as an epimer of cefepime.

| Route | Onset | Peak | Duration |
|-------|-------|------|----------|
| I.V., I.M. | ½ hr | 1-2 hr | Unknown |

## Contraindications and precautions
Contraindicated in patients hypersensitive to drug, other cephalosporins, penicillins, or other beta-lactam antibiotics. Use cautiously in patients with history of GI disease (especially colitis), impaired renal function, or poor nutritional status and in those receiving a protracted course of antimicrobial therapy.

## Interactions
**Drug-drug.** *Aminoglycosides:* Possible increased risk of nephrotoxicity and ototoxicity. Advise clinician to monitor renal and hearing functions.
*Potent diuretics such as furosemide:* Possible increased risk of nephrotoxicity. Advise clinician to monitor renal function.

## Adverse reactions
**CNS:** headache.
**GI:** colitis, diarrhea, nausea, vomiting, oral candidiasis.
**GU:** vaginitis.
**Skin:** rash, pruritus, urticaria.
**Other:** phlebitis, pain, inflammation, fever.

## Overdose and treatment
Overdose may result in the patient experiencing seizures, encephalopathy, and neuromuscular excitability. Patients who receive an overdose should be carefully observed and given supportive treatment. In the presence of renal insufficiency, hemodialysis, not peritoneal dialysis, is recommended to aid in the removal of cefepime from the body.

## Clinical considerations
**⊌ALERT** Names of some cephalosporins are similar. Use caution when dispensing.

■ Recommend culture and sensitivity tests before giving first dose. Therapy may begin pending results.
■ For I.M. administration, constitute drug using sterile water for injection, normal saline solution, $D_5W$, 5% or 1% lidocaine hydrochloride, or bacteriostatic water for injection with parabens or benzyl alcohol. Follow manufacturer guidelines for quantity of diluent to use.
■ Inspect solution visually for particulate matter before administration. The powder and its solutions tend to darken depending on storage conditions. However, product potency isn't adversely affected when stored as recommended.
■ Cefepime may result in a false-positive reaction for glucose in the urine when using Clinitest tablets. Use glucose tests based on enzymatic glucose oxidase reactions (such as Chemstrip uG, Diastix, or glucose enzymatic test strip) instead. A positive direct Coombs' test may occur during treatment with drug.

### Therapeutic monitoring
■ Many cephalosporins may cause a decrease in prothrombin activity; patients at risk include those with renal or hepatic impairment or poor nutritional status and those receiving prolonged cefepime therapy. PT must be checked. Exogenous vitamin K can be given, if needed.

### Special populations
**Pregnant patients.** Use drug only when clearly needed during pregnancy.
**Breast-feeding patients.** Drug appears in breast milk in very low levels; use cautiously.
**Pediatric patients.** Safety and effectiveness in children under age 2 months haven't been established.
**Geriatric patients.** Use caution when giving cefepime to geriatric patients. Dosage adjustment may be needed in patients with impaired renal function.

## Patient counseling
■ Warn patient receiving drug I.M. that pain may occur at injection site.
■ Instruct patient to report adverse reactions promptly.

# cefixime
Suprax

*Pharmacologic classification:* third-generation cephalosporin
*Therapeutic classification:* antibiotic
*Pregnancy risk category B*

## Available forms
Available by prescription only
*Tablets:* 200 mg, 400 mg
*Powder for oral suspension:* 100 mg/5 ml

---

## Indications and dosages

*Otitis media; acute bronchitis; acute exacerbations of chronic bronchitis, pharyngitis, tonsillitis; uncomplicated urinary tract infections caused by* Escherichia coli *and* Proteus mirabilis; *uncomplicated gonorrhea;* ◇ *disseminated gonococcal infections*

*Adults and children weighing more than 50 kg (110 lb) or over age 12:* 400 mg P.O. daily in one or two divided doses; for uncomplicated gonorrhea, 400 mg as a single dose.

*Children over age 6 months weighing less than 50 kg (110 lb) or under age 12:* 8 mg/kg P.O. daily in one or two divided doses.

≡ *Dosage adjustment.* For renally impaired patients, dosage must be adjusted based on degree of renal impairment, severity of infection, and susceptibility of organism. To prevent toxic accumulation in patients with creatinine clearance less than 60 ml/minute, reduced dosage may be needed.

| Creatinine clearance (ml/min) | Adult dosage |
|---|---|
| 20-60 | 75% of the usual dose |
| < 20 or patients receiving continuous ambulatory peritoneal dialysis | 50% of the usual dose |

## Mechanism of action

*Antibacterial action:* Cefixime is primarily bactericidal; it acts by binding to penicillin-binding proteins in the bacterial cell wall, thereby inhibiting cell-wall synthesis.

It's used in the treatment of otitis media caused by *Haemophilus influenzae* (penicillinase- and nonpenicillinase-producing), *Moraxella catarrhalis* (which is penicillinase-producing), and *Streptococcus pyogenes.* Substantial drug resistance has been noted. Cefixime is also active in the treatment of acute bronchitis and acute exacerbations of chronic bronchitis caused by *Streptococcus pneumoniae* and *H. influenzae* (penicillinase- and non-penicillinase-producing), pharyngitis and tonsillitis caused by *S. pyogenes,* and uncomplicated urinary tract infections caused by *E. coli* and *P. mirabilis.*

## Pharmacokinetics

*Absorption:* About 30% to 50% is absorbed following oral administration. The suspension form provides a higher serum level than the tablet form. Absorption is delayed by food, but the total amount absorbed isn't affected.

*Distribution:* Widely distributed; about 65% plasma protein–bound.

*Metabolism:* About 50% is metabolized.

*Excretion:* Excreted primarily in the urine. In patients with end-stage renal disease, half-life may be prolonged to 11½ hours.

| Route | Onset | Peak | Duration |
|---|---|---|---|
| P.O. | Unknown | 3-4½ hr | Unknown |

## Contraindications and precautions

Contraindicated in patients hypersensitive to drug or other cephalosporins. Use cautiously in patients with impaired renal function.

## Interactions

*Drug-drug. Carbamazepine:* Elevated carbamazepine levels reported when given together. Avoid use together.

*Probenecid:* May inhibit excretion and increase blood levels of cefixime. Use together cautiously.

*Salicylates:* May increase serum level of cefixime. Use together cautiously.

## Adverse reactions

**CNS:** headache, dizziness.

**GI:** *diarrhea,* loose stools, abdominal pain, nausea, vomiting, dyspepsia, flatulence, pseudomembranous colitis.

**GU:** genital pruritus, vaginitis, genital candidiasis, transient increases in BUN and serum creatinine levels.

**Hematologic:** *thrombocytopenia, leukopenia,* eosinophilia.

**Hepatic:** transient increases in liver enzymes.

**Skin:** pruritus, rash, urticaria, erythema multiforme, *Stevens-Johnson syndrome.*

**Other:** drug fever, hypersensitivity reactions, serum sickness, *anaphylaxis.*

## Overdose and treatment

No specific antidote available. Gastric lavage and supportive treatment are recommended. Peritoneal dialysis and hemodialysis will remove substantial quantities of drug.

## Clinical considerations

**⊌ ALERT** Names of some cephalosporins are similar. Use caution when dispensing.

■ Cefixime is the first orally active, third-generation cephalosporin that's effective with once-daily dosage.

■ The manufacturer suggests that tablets shouldn't be substituted for suspension when treating otitis media.

■ Treat acute hypersensitivity reactions immediately. Emergency measures, such as airway management, pressor amines, epinephrine, oxygen, antihistamines, and corticosteroids, may be needed.

■ Some cephalosporins may cause seizures, especially in patients with renal failure who receive full therapeutic dosages. If seizures occur, recommend stopping drug and starting anticonvulsant therapy.

■ Cefixime may cause false-positive results in urine glucose tests using cupric sulfate (Benedict's reagent or Clinitest); use glucose oxidase tests (Chemstrip uG, Diastix, or glucose enzymatic test strip) instead. Cefixime may cause false-positive results in tests for urine ketones that use nitroprusside (but not nitroferricyanide).

■ False-positive direct Coombs' test results have been seen with other cephalosporins.

### Therapeutic monitoring

■ Recommend evaluating patients with antibiotic-induced diarrhea for overgrowth of pseudomembranous colitis caused by *Clostridium difficile*. Mild cases usually respond to discontinuation of the drug; moderate to severe cases may require fluid, electrolyte, and protein supplementation. Oral vancomycin is the drug of choice for the treatment of *C. difficile* pseudomembranous colitis caused by antibiotics.

### Special populations

**Pregnant patients.** Use during pregnancy only when clearly needed.

**Breast-feeding patients.** It's not known if drug appears in breast milk. The manufacturer recommends stopping breast-feeding during cefixime therapy.

**Pediatric patients.** The risk of adverse GI effects in children receiving oral suspension is similar to those in adults receiving tablets.

### Patient counseling

■ Instruct patient to report rash, or signs and symptoms of superinfection.

■ Advise patient that oral suspension is stable for 14 days after reconstitution and doesn't require refrigeration.

■ Tell patient to take all of the drug exactly as prescribed, even if he feels better.

## cefoperazone sodium
Cefobid

*Pharmacologic classification:* third-generation cephalosporin
*Therapeutic classification:* antibiotic
*Pregnancy risk category B*

### Available forms

Available by prescription only
*Parenteral:* 1 g, 2 g, 10 g
*Infusion:* 1 g, 2 g piggyback

### Indications and dosages

*Serious respiratory tract, intra-abdominal, gynecologic, skin and structure, urinary tract, and enterococcal infections; bacteri-al septicemia caused by susceptible organisms; perioperative prophylaxis*
*Adults:* Usual dose is 1 to 2 g q 12 hours I.M. or I.V. In severe infections or infections caused by less sensitive organisms, the total daily dose or frequency may be increased up to 16 g/day in certain situations.

≡ *Dosage adjustment.* No dosage adjustment is usually needed in patients with renal impairment. However, give doses of 4 g/day cautiously to patients with hepatic disease. Adults with combined hepatic and renal function impairment shouldn't receive more than 1 g (base) daily without serum determinations. For patients receiving hemodialysis treatments, schedule a dose to follow hemodialysis.

### I.V. administration

■ Allow solution to stand after reconstituting to allow foam to dissipate and solution to clear. Solution can be shaken vigorously to ensure complete drug dissolution.

■ After reconstitution, solution is stable for 24 hours at a controlled room temperature or 3 days if refrigerated. Protecting drug from light is unnecessary.

■ Infuse over 15 to 30 minutes.

### Incompatibilities

Incompatible with aminoglycosides, doxapram hydrochloride, hetastarch, labetalol hydrochloride, meperidine hydrochloride, ondansetron hydrochloride, perphenazine, promethazine hydrochloride, and sargramostim.

### Mechanism of action

*Antibacterial action:* Cefoperazone is primarily bactericidal; however, it may be bacteriostatic. Activity depends on the organism, tissue penetration, drug dosage, and rate of organism multiplication. It acts by adhering to bacterial penicillin-binding proteins, thereby inhibiting cell-wall synthesis. Third-generation cephalosporins appear more active against some beta-lactamase-producing gram-negative organisms.

Cefoperazone is active against some gram-positive organisms and many enteric gram-negative bacilli, including *Streptococcus pneumoniae* and *Streptococcus pyogenes, Staphylococcus aureus* (penicillinase- and nonpenicillinase-producing), *Staphylococcus epidermidis, Escherichia coli, Klebsiella, Haemophilus influenzae, Enterobacter, Citrobacter, Proteus,* some *Pseudomonas* species (including *Pseudomonas aeruginosa*), and *Bacteroides fragilis. Acinetobacter* and *Listeria* usually are resistant. Cefoperazone is less effective than cefotaxime or ceftizoxime against Enterobacteriaceae but is slightly more active than those drugs against *Pseudomonas aeruginosa.*

# Pharmacokinetics

**Absorption:** Not absorbed from the GI tract; must be given parenterally.

**Distribution:** Distributed widely into most body tissues and fluids, including the gallbladder, liver, kidneys, bone, sputum, bile, and pleural and synovial fluids; CSF penetration is achieved in patients with inflamed meninges. It crosses the placenta. Protein binding is dose-dependent and decreases as serum levels rise; average is 82% to 93%.

**Metabolism:** Not substantially metabolized.

**Excretion:** Excreted primarily in bile; some drug is excreted in urine by renal tubular secretion and glomerular filtration; small amounts appear in breast milk. Elimination half-life is about 1½ to 2½ hours in patients with normal hepatorenal function; biliary obstruction or cirrhosis prolongs half-life to about 3½ to 7 hours. Hemodialysis removes cefoperazone.

| Route | Onset | Peak | Duration |
|-------|-------|------|----------|
| I.V. | Immediate | Immediate | Unknown |
| I.M. | Unknown | 1-2 hr | Unknown |

# Contraindications and precautions

Contraindicated in patients hypersensitive to drug or other cephalosporins. Use cautiously in patients with impaired renal or hepatic function or penicillin allergy and in breast-feeding women.

# Interactions

**Drug-drug.** *Aminoglycosides:* Concurrent use results in synergistic activity against *P. aeruginosa* and *Serratia marcescens;* such combined use slightly increases the risk of nephrotoxicity. Use together cautiously. Advise clinician to monitor serum creatinine and BUN.

*Anticoagulants:* May increase risk of bleeding. Use together cautiously.

*Clavulanic acid:* Concurrent use results in synergistic activity against many Enterobacteriaceae, *B. fragilis, P. aeruginosa,* and *S. aureus.* Use together cautiously.

*Probenecid:* Competitively inhibits renal tubular secretions of cephalosporins, causing prolonged serum levels of these drugs. Use together cautiously.

**Drug-lifestyle.** *Alcohol use:* Can cause disulfiram-like reaction. Discourage use.

# Adverse reactions

**GI:** pseudomembranous colitis, nausea, vomiting, *diarrhea.*

**Hematologic:** *transient neutropenia, eosinophilia,* anemia, hypoprothrombinemia, bleeding.

**Hepatic:** slightly elevated liver enzyme levels.

**Skin:** *maculopapular and erythematous rashes, urticaria, pain, induration, sterile abscesses, temperature elevation, tissue sloughing* (at injection site); *phlebitis, thrombophlebitis,* drug fever (with I.V. injection).

**Other:** hypersensitivity reactions, serum sickness, *anaphylaxis.*

# Overdose and treatment

Signs and symptoms of overdose include neuromuscular hypersensitivity. Seizure may follow high CNS levels. Hypoprothrombinemia and bleeding may occur and may require treatment with vitamin K or blood products. Hemodialysis removes cefoperazone.

# Clinical considerations

■ Diarrhea may be more common with drug than with other cephalosporins because of high degree of biliary excretion.

■ Patients with biliary disease may need lower doses.

■ For patients on sodium restriction, note that cefoperazone injection contains 1.5 mEq of sodium per gram of drug.

■ To prepare I.M. injection, use the appropriate diluent, including sterile water for injection or bacteriostatic water for injection. Follow manufacturer's recommendations for mixing drug with sterile water for injection and lidocaine 2% injection. Final solution for I.M. injection will contain 0.5% lidocaine and will be less painful upon administration (recommended for levels of 250 mg/ml or greater). Recommend injecting cefoperazone deep I.M. into a large muscle mass, such as the gluteus or the lateral aspect of the thigh.

■ Store drug in refrigerator and away from light before reconstituting.

■ Because cefoperazone is dialyzable, patients undergoing treatment with hemodialysis may require dosage adjustment.

■ Cephalosporins cause false-positive results in urine glucose tests using cupric sulfate (Benedict's reagent or Clinitest); use glucose oxidase (Chemstrip uG, Diastix, or glucose enzymatic test strip) instead. Cefoperazone may cause positive Coombs' test results.

## Therapeutic monitoring

■ Advise clinician to monitor INR regularly. Vitamin K promptly reverses bleeding if it occurs.

## Special populations

**Pregnant patients.** Use during pregnancy only when clearly needed.

**Breast-feeding patients.** Drug appears in breast milk; use with caution in breast-feeding women.

**Pediatric patients.** Safety and effectiveness in children under age 12 haven't been established.

**Geriatric patients.** Hypoprothrombinemia and bleeding have been reported more frequently in geriatric patients. Use with caution, and monitor PT and check for signs of abnormal bleeding.

## Patient counseling
■ Inform patient of potential adverse reactions.
■ Tell patient to report discomfort at I.V. site.

# cefotaxime sodium
Claforan

*Pharmacologic classification:* third-
generation cephalosporin
*Therapeutic classification:* antibiotic
*Pregnancy risk category B*

## Available forms
Available by prescription only
*Injection:* 500 mg, 1 g, 2 g
*Pharmacy bulk package:* 10-g vial
*Infusion:* 1 g, 2 g

## Indications and dosages
**Serious lower respiratory, urinary, CNS,
bone and joint, intra-abdominal, gynecologic, and skin infections; bacteremia; septicemia caused by susceptible organisms;**
◇ *pelvic inflammatory disease*
*Adults and children weighing more than 50 kg
(110 lb):* Usual dose is 1 g I.V. or I.M. q 6 to
12 hours. Up to 12 g daily can be given in life-
threatening infections.
*Children ages 1 month to 12 years weighing
less than 50 kg:* 50 to 180 mg/kg/day I.V. in
four or six equally divided doses. Higher doses are reserved for serious infections (such as
meningitis).
*Neonates ages 1 to 4 weeks:* 50 mg/kg I.V. q
8 hours.
*Neonates up to age 1 week:* 50 mg/kg I.V. q 12
hours.
   Total daily dose is same for I.M. or I.V. administration and depends on susceptibility of
organism and severity of infection. Inject cefotaxime deep I.M. into a large muscle mass,
such as the gluteus or the lateral aspect of the
thigh.
*Uncomplicated gonorrhea*
*Adults and adolescents:* 1 g I.M. as a single
dose.
*Perioperative prophylaxis*
*Adults:* 1 g I.V. or I.M. 30 to 90 minutes before surgery.
◇ *Disseminated gonococcal infection*
*Adults:* 1 g I.V. q 8 hours.
*Neonates and infants:* 25 to 50 mg/kg I.V. q 8
to 12 hours for 7 days or 50 to 100 mg/kg I.M.
or I.V. q 12 hours for 7 days.
◇ *Gonococcal ophthalmia*
*Adults:* 500 mg I.V. q.i.d.
*Neonates:* 100 mg I.V. or I.M. for one dose;
may continue until ocular cultures are nega-
tive at 48 to 72 hours.
◇ *Gonorrheal meningitis or arthritis*
*Neonates and infants:* 25 to 50 mg/kg I.V. q 8
to 12 hours for 10 to 14 days or 50 to 100 mg/kg
I.M. or I.V. q 12 hours for 10 to 14 days.

≡ *Dosage adjustment.* For patients with impaired renal function, recommend modifying
dose or frequency of administration based on
degree of renal impairment, severity of infection, and susceptibility of organism. To prevent toxic accumulation, reduced dosage may
be needed in patients with creatinine clearance
below 20 ml/minute.

## I.V. administration
■ For I.V. use, reconstitute all strengths of an
I.V. dose with 10 ml of sterile water for injection. For infusion bottles, add 50 to 100 ml of
normal saline solution injection or $D_5W$. Infuse over 20 to 30 minutes.
■ Once reconstituted, drug may also be given
by direct I.V. injection over 3 to 5 minutes into
the vein or tubing of a free flowing compatible I.V. solution.
■ Solution is stable for 24 hours at controlled
room temperature or at least 10 days under refrigeration in the original container. Cefotaxime
may be stored in disposable glass or plastic
syringes for 24 hours at controlled room temperature or 5 days in the refrigerator.

## Incompatibilities
Incompatible with aminoglycosides, aminophylline, doxapram, fluconazole, hetastarch,
sodium bicarbonate injection, and fluids with
a pH above 7.5.

## Mechanism of action
*Antibacterial action:* Cefotaxime is primarily
bactericidal; however, it may be bacteriostatic. Activity depends on the organism, tissue
penetration, drug dosage, and rate of organism
multiplication. It acts by adhering to bacterial
penicillin-binding proteins, thereby inhibiting
cell-wall synthesis.
   Third-generation cephalosporins appear
more active against some beta-lactamase producing gram-negative organisms.
   Cefotaxime is active against some gram-
positive organisms and many enteric gram-
negative bacilli, including streptococci
(*Streptococcus pneumoniae* and *pyogenes*),
*Staphylococcus aureus* (penicillinase- and
nonpenicillinase-producing), *Staphylococcus
epidermidis, Escherichia coli, Klebsiella*
species, *Haemophilus influenzae, Enterobacter* species, *Proteus* species, *Peptostreptococcus* species, and some strains of *Pseudomonas
aeruginosa. Listeria* and *Acinetobacter* are often resistant. The active metabolite of cefotaxime, desacetylcefotaxime, may act synergistically with the parent drug against some
bacterial strains.

## Pharmacokinetics
*Absorption:* Not absorbed from the GI tract;
must be given parenterally.
*Distribution:* Distributed widely into most body
tissues and fluids, including the gallbladder,

liver, kidneys, bone, sputum, bile, and pleural and synovial fluids. Unlike most other cephalosporins, drug has adequate CSF penetration when meninges are inflamed; it crosses the placenta; 13% to 38% is protein-bound.

*Metabolism:* Metabolized partially to an active metabolite, desacetylcefotaxime.

*Excretion:* Excreted primarily in urine by renal tubular secretion; some drug may appear in breast milk. About 25% of cefotaxime is excreted in urine as the active metabolite; elimination half-life in normal adults is about 1 to 1½ hours for cefotaxime and about 1½ to 2 hours for desacetylcefotaxime; severe renal impairment prolongs the half-life of cefotaxime to 11½ hours and that of the metabolite to as much as 56 hours. Hemodialysis removes both drug and its metabolites.

| Route | Onset | Peak | Duration |
|-------|-------|------|----------|
| I.V. | Immediate | Immediate | Unknown |
| I.M. | Unknown | ½ hr | Unknown |

## Contraindications and precautions
Contraindicated in patients hypersensitive to drug or other cephalosporins. Use cautiously in patients with impaired renal function or penicillin allergies and in breast-feeding women.

## Interactions
**Drug-drug.** *Aminoglycosides:* Concurrent use results in apparent synergistic activity against Enterobacteriaceae and some strains of *P. aeruginosa* and *Serratia marcescens;* such combined use may increase risk of nephrotoxicity. Advise clinician to monitor patient closely.
*Probenecid:* May block renal tubular secretion of cefotaxime and prolong its half-life. Use together carefully.

## Adverse reactions
**CNS:** headache.
**GI:** pseudomembranous colitis, nausea, vomiting, *diarrhea.*
**GU:** vaginitis, candidiasis, interstitial nephritis.
**Hematologic:** *transient neutropenia,* eosinophilia, hemolytic anemia, *thrombocytopenia, agranulocytosis.*
**Hepatic:** transient increases in liver enzymes.
**Skin:** *maculopapular and erythematous rashes, urticaria.*
**Other:** hypersensitivity reactions, serum sickness, *anaphylaxis;* elevated temperature; *pain, induration, sterile abscesses, temperature elevation, tissue sloughing* (at injection site); *phlebitis, thrombophlebitis* (with I.V. injection).

## Overdose and treatment
Signs and symptoms of overdose include neuromuscular hypersensitivity. Seizure may follow high CNS levels. Cefotaxime may be removed by hemodialysis.

## Clinical considerations
**⊩ALERT** Names of some cephalosporins are similar. Use caution when dispensing.
■ For patients on sodium restriction, note that cefotaxime contains 2.2 mEq of sodium per gram of drug.
■ For I.M. injection, add 2 ml, 3 ml, or 5 ml of sterile or bacteriostatic water for injection to each 500-mg, 1-g, or 2-g vial. Shake well to dissolve drug completely. Check solution for particles and discoloration. Color ranges from light yellow to amber.
■ Don't inject more than 1 g into a single I.M. site to prevent pain and tissue reaction.
■ Cephalosporins cause false-positive results in urine glucose tests using cupric sulfate (Benedict's reagent or Clinitest); use glucose oxidase (Chemstrip uG, Diastix, or glucose enzymatic test strip) instead. Cefotaxime also causes false elevations in urine creatinine levels in tests using Jaffé's reaction. Cefotaxime may cause positive Coombs' tests results.

### Therapeutic monitoring
■ With large doses or prolonged therapy, advise clinician to watch for superinfection, especially in high-risk patients.

### Special populations
**Breast-feeding patients.** Drug appears in breast milk and should be used with caution in breast-feeding women.
**Pediatric patients.** Cefotaxime may be used in neonates, infants, and children.
**Geriatric patients.** Use with caution in geriatric patients with diminished renal function.

## Patient counseling
■ Inform patient of potential adverse reactions.
■ Instruct patient to report discomfort at I.V. site.

# cefotetan disodium
Cefotan

*Pharmacologic classification:* second-generation cephalosporin, cephamycin
*Therapeutic classification:* antibiotic
*Pregnancy risk category B*

## Available forms
Available by prescription only
*Injection:* 1 g, 2 g
*Injection:* 10 g bulk package
*Infusion:* 1 g, 2 g piggyback vials; frozen, premixed solutions of 1 g, 2 g in 50 ml

## Indications and dosages
*Serious urinary, lower respiratory, gynecologic, skin, intra-abdominal, and bone*

*and joint infections caused by susceptible organisms*
*Adults:* 500 mg to 3 g I.V. or I.M. q 12 hours for 5 to 10 days. Up to 6 g daily in life-threatening infections.
◊ *Children:* 40 to 60 mg/kg daily I.V. divided in equally divided doses q 12 hours.
*Preoperative prophylaxis; ◊ use in contaminated surgery*
*Adults:* 1 to 2 g I.V. 30 to 60 minutes before surgery.
*Postcesarean*
*Adults:* 1 to 2 g I.V. as soon as umbilical cord is clamped.

Total daily dose is same for I.M. or I.V. administration and depends on the susceptibility of the organism and severity of infection. Recommend injecting cefotetan deep I.M. into a large muscle mass, such as the gluteus or the lateral aspect of the thigh.

≡ *Dosage adjustment.* For patients with impaired renal function, doses or frequency of administration must be modified based on degree of renal impairment, severity of infection, and susceptibility of organism. To prevent toxic accumulation, reduced dosage may be needed in patients with creatinine clearance less than 30 ml/minute. Because drug is hemodialyzable, hemodialysis patients may require dosage adjustment.

| Creatinine clearance (ml/min) | Adult dosage |
|---|---|
| 10-30 | Usual adult dose q 24 hours; or one-half the usual adult dose q 12 hours |
| < 10 | Usual adult dose q 48 hours; or one-fourth the usual adult dose q 12 hours |
| Hemodialysis patients | One-fourth the usual adult dose q 24 hours on the days between hemodialysis sessions; and one-half the usual adult dose on the day of hemodialysis |

## I.V. administration
▪ For I.V. use, reconstitute with sterile water for injection. Then it may be mixed with 50 to 100 ml D₅W or normal saline solution. Infuse intermittently over 30 to 60 minutes.
▪ Reconstituted solution remains stable for 24 hours at controlled room temperature or for 96 hours when refrigerated.

## Incompatibilities
Incompatible with aminoglycosides, doxapram, and heparin sodium.

## Mechanism of action
*Antibacterial action:* Cefotetan is primarily bactericidal; however, it may be bacteriostatic. Activity depends on the organism, tissue penetration, drug dosage, and rate of organism multiplication. It acts by adhering to bacterial penicillin-binding proteins, thereby inhibiting cell-wall synthesis.

Cefotetan is active against many gram-positive organisms and enteric gram-negative bacilli, including streptococci, *Staphylococcus aureus* (penicillinase- and nonpenicillinase-producing), *Staphylococcus epidermidis, Escherichia coli, Klebsiella* species, *Enterobacter* species, *Proteus* species, *Haemophilus influenzae, Neisseria gonorrhoeae,* and *Bacteroides* species (including some strains of *B. fragilis*); however, some *B. fragilis* strains, *Pseudomonas,* and *Acinetobacter* are resistant to cefotetan. Most Enterobacteriaceae are more susceptible to cefotetan than to other second-generation cephalosporins.

## Pharmacokinetics
*Absorption:* Not absorbed from the GI tract; must be given parenterally.
*Distribution:* Distributed widely into most body tissues and fluids, including the gallbladder, liver, kidneys, bone, sputum, bile, and pleural and synovial fluids; CSF penetration is poor. Biliary concentration levels of cefotetan can be up to 20 times higher than serum levels in patients with good gallbladder function. Cefotetan crosses the placenta, and is 75% to 90% protein-bound.
*Metabolism:* Not metabolized.
*Excretion:* Excreted primarily in urine by glomerular filtration and some renal tubular secretion; 20% is excreted in the bile. Small amounts of drug appear in breast milk. Elimination half-life is about 3 to 4½ hours in patients with normal renal function.

| Route | Onset | Peak | Duration |
|---|---|---|---|
| I.V. | Immediate | Immediate | Unknown |
| I.M. | Unknown | 1½-3 hr | Unknown |

## Contraindications and precautions
Contraindicated in patients hypersensitive to drug or other cephalosporins. Use cautiously in patients with impaired renal function or penicillin allergy and in breast-feeding women.

## Interactions
**Drug-drug.** *Anticoagulants:* May increase risk of bleeding. Patient needs close monitoring.
*Nephrotoxic drugs (aminoglycosides, colistin, polymyxin B, vancomycin) or loop diuretics:* May increase the risk of nephrotoxicity. Advise clinician to monitor patient closely.
*Probenecid:* May inhibit excretion and increase blood levels of cefotetan. Sometimes used for this effect. Advise clinician to monitor patient closely.

**Drug-lifestyle.** *Alcohol use:* May cause disulfiram-like reactions (flushing, sweating, tachycardia, headache, and abdominal cramping). Patient should avoid alcohol consumption while on therapy and shouldn't drink alcohol for several days after discontinuing cefotetan therapy.

## Adverse reactions

**GI:** pseudomembranous colitis, nausea, *diarrhea.*
**GU:** *nephrotoxicity.*
**Hematologic:** *transient neutropenia,* eosinophilia, hemolytic anemia, hypoprothrombinemia, bleeding, thrombocytosis, *agranulocytosis, thrombocytopenia.*
**Hepatic:** transient increases in liver enzymes.
**Skin:** *maculopapular and erythematous rashes, urticaria,* elevated temperature, *pain, induration, sterile abscesses, tissue sloughing* (at injection site); *phlebitis, thrombophlebitis* (with I.V. injection).
**Other:** hypersensitivity reactions, serum sickness, *anaphylaxis.*

## Overdose and treatment

Signs and symptoms of overdose include neuromuscular hypersensitivity. Seizure may follow high CNS levels. Hypoprothrombinemia and bleeding may occur; they may be treated with vitamin K or blood products. Cefotetan may be removed by hemodialysis.

## Clinical considerations

**ᗺALERT** Names of some cephalosporins are similar. Use caution when dispensing.
■ For I.M. injection, cefotetan may be reconstituted with sterile water or bacteriostatic water for injection or with normal saline or 0.5% or 1% lidocaine hydrochloride. Shake to dissolve and let solution stand until clear.
■ Cefotetan also causes false-positive results in urine glucose tests using cupric sulfate (Benedict's reagent or Clinitest); use glucose oxidase tests (Chemstrip uG, Diastix, or glucose enzymatic test strip) instead. Cefotetan causes false elevations in serum or urine creatinine levels in tests using Jaffé's reaction. It may cause positive Coombs' test results.

### Therapeutic monitoring

■ Patient should be assessed for signs and symptoms of overt and occult bleeding. Advise clinician to monitor vital signs and checking CBC with differential, platelet levels, and PT for abnormalities.
■ Bleeding can be reversed promptly by giving vitamin K.

### Special populations

**Pregnant patients.** Use only when clearly needed.
**Breast-feeding patients.** Cephalosporins appear in breast milk; use with caution in breast-feeding women. Safety in breast-feeding women hasn't been established.
**Pediatric patients.** Safety in children hasn't been established.
**Geriatric patients.** Hypoprothrombinemia and bleeding have been reported more frequently in geriatric and debilitated patients.

## Patient counseling

■ Inform patient of potential adverse reactions.
■ Tell patient to promptly report signs of bleeding and discomfort at I.V. site.

# cefoxitin sodium
Mefoxin

*Pharmacologic classification:* second-generation cephalosporin, cephamycin
*Therapeutic classification:* antibiotic
*Pregnancy risk category B*

## Available forms

Available by prescription only
*Injection:* 1 g, 2 g
*Pharmacy bulk package:* 10 g
*Infusion:* 1 g, 2 g in 50-ml containers

## Indications and dosages

*Serious respiratory, GU, gynecologic, skin, soft-tissue, bone and joint, blood, and intra-abdominal infections caused by susceptible organisms*
*Adults:* 1 to 2 g I.V. q 6 to 8 hours for uncomplicated forms of infection. Up to 12 g daily in life-threatening infections.
*Children over age 3 months:* 80 to 160 mg/kg I.V. daily given in four to six equally divided doses. Don't exceed 12 g/day.
 Total daily dose is same for I.M. and I.V. administration and depends on susceptibility of organism and severity of infection. Inject cefoxitin deep I.M. into a large muscle mass, such as the gluteus or lateral aspect of the thigh.
*Perioperative prophylaxis; ◇ use in contaminated surgery*
*Adults:* 2 g I.V. 30 to 60 minutes before surgery; then 2 g I.V. q 6 hours for 24 hours postoperatively.
*Children over age 3 months:* 30 to 40 mg/kg I.V. 30 to 60 minutes before surgery; then 30 mg/kg I.V. q 6 hours for 24 hours postoperatively. For contaminated surgery, 1 to 2 g I.V. q 6 hours with or without I.V. gentamicin (1.5 mg/kg q 8 hours) for 5 days.
*Uncomplicated gonorrhea*
*Adults:* Give 2 g I.M. as a single dose with 1 g probenecid P.O. at the same time or up to 30 minutes beforehand.
*Pelvic inflammatory disease*
*Adults:* 2 g I.V. q 6 hours. (If *Chlamydia trachomatis* is suspected, give additional antichlamydial coverage.)

≣*Dosage adjustment.* For patients with impaired renal function, doses or frequency of administration must be modified based on degree of renal impairment, severity of infection, and susceptibility of organism. To prevent toxic accumulation, reduced dosage may be needed in patients with creatinine clearance less than 50 ml/minute.

| Creatinine clearance (ml/min) | Adult dosage |
|---|---|
| 30-50 | 1-2 g q 8-12 hr |
| 10-29 | 1-2 g q 12-24 hr |
| 5-9 | 500 mg-1 g q 12-24 hr |
| < 5 | 500 mg-1 g q 24-48 hr |

## I.V. administration

■ For I.V. use, reconstitute 1 g of cefoxitin with at least 10 ml of sterile water for injection, or 2 g of cefoxitin with 10 to 20 ml. Solutions of D$_5$W and normal saline solution for injection can also be used.
■ After reconstituting, shake vial and then let stand until clear to ensure complete drug dissolution. Solution is stable for 24 hours at controlled room temperature, for 1 week if refrigerated, or 26 weeks if frozen.
■ Solution may range from colorless to light amber and may darken during storage. Slight color change doesn't indicate loss of potency.
■ Infuse slowly by intermittent I.V. infusion or drug can be given by direct injection into the vein over 3 to 5 minutes or into the tubing of a free flowing compatible I.V. solution.

### Incompatibilities

Incompatible with aminoglycosides and hetastarch.

## Mechanism of action

*Antibacterial action:* Cefoxitin is primarily bactericidal; however, it may be bacteriostatic. Activity depends on the organism, tissue penetration, drug dosage, and rate of organism multiplication. It acts by adhering to bacterial penicillin-binding proteins, thereby inhibiting cell-wall synthesis.

Cefoxitin is active against many gram-positive organisms and enteric gram-negative bacilli, including *Escherichia coli* and other coliform bacteria, *Staphylococcus aureus* (penicillinase- and nonpenicillinase-producing), *Staphylococcus epidermidis,* streptococci, *Klebsiella, Haemophilus influenzae,* and *Bacteroides* species (including *B. fragilis*). *Enterobacter, Pseudomonas,* and *Acinetobacter* are resistant to cefoxitin.

## Pharmacokinetics

*Absorption:* Not absorbed from the GI tract; must be given parenterally.
*Distribution:* Distributed widely into most body tissues and fluids, including the gallbladder, liver, kidneys, bone, sputum, bile, and pleural and synovial fluids; CSF penetration is poor. Cefoxitin crosses the placenta, and is 50% to 80% protein-bound.
*Metabolism:* About 2% of a cefoxitin dose is metabolized.
*Excretion:* Excreted primarily in urine by renal tubular secretion and glomerular filtration; small amounts of drug appear in breast milk. Elimination half-life is about 0.7 to 1.1 hours in patients with normal renal function; half-life is prolonged in patients with severe renal dysfunction to 6 to 21½ hours. Cefoxitin can be removed by hemodialysis but not by peritoneal dialysis.

| Route | Onset | Peak | Duration |
|---|---|---|---|
| I.V. | Immediate | Immediate | Unknown |
| I.M. | Unknown | 20-30 min | Unknown |

## Contraindications and precautions

Contraindicated in patients hypersensitive to drug or other cephalosporins. Use cautiously in patients with impaired renal function or penicillin allergy and in breast-feeding women.

## Interactions

**Drug-drug.** *Bacteriostatic drugs (chloramphenicol, erythromycin, tetracyclines):* May impair the bactericidal activity of cefoxitin. Avoid use together.
*Nephrotoxic agents (aminoglycosides, colistin, polymyxin B, vancomycin) or loop diuretics:* May increase the risk of nephrotoxicity. Advise clinician to monitor patient closely.
*Probenecid:* Competitively inhibits renal tubular secretion of cephalosporins, resulting in higher, prolonged serum levels of these drugs. Advise clinician to monitor patient closely.

## Adverse reactions

**CV:** hypotension.
**GI:** pseudomembranous colitis, nausea, vomiting, *diarrhea.*
**GU:** *acute renal failure.*
**Hematologic:** *transient neutropenia,* eosinophilia, *hemolytic anemia,* anemia, *thrombocytopenia.*
**Hepatic:** transient increases in liver enzymes.
**Respiratory:** dyspnea (with I.V. injection).
**Skin:** *maculopapular and erythematous rash,* urticaria, exfoliative dermatitis; elevated temperature, *pain, induration, sterile abscesses, tissue sloughing* (at injection site).
**Other:** hypersensitivity reactions, serum sickness, *anaphylaxis; phlebitis,* thrombophlebitis.

---

## Overdose and treatment

Signs and symptoms of overdose include neuromuscular hypersensitivity. Seizure may follow high CNS levels. Cefoxitin may be removed by hemodialysis.

## Clinical considerations

**⚠ALERT** Names of some cephalosporins are similar. Use caution when dispensing.

■ For I.M. injection, reconstitute with 0.5% to 1% lidocaine hydrochloride (without epinephrine) to minimize pain at injection site; or with sterile water for injection.

■ Recommend giving cefoxitin I.M. deep into a large muscle mass. Recommend aspiration before injecting to prevent inadvertent injection into a blood vessel, and rotation of sites to prevent tissue damage.

■ Cefoxitin injection contains 2.3 mEq of sodium per gram of drug.

■ Cefoxitin causes false-positive results in urine glucose tests using cupric sulfate (Benedict's reagent or Clinitest); use glucose oxidase tests (Chemstrip uG, Diastix, or glucose enzymatic test strip) instead. Cefoxitin also causes false elevations in serum or urine creatinine levels in tests using Jaffé's reaction. May cause positive Coombs' test results.

### Therapeutic monitoring

■ Cefoxitin has caused thrombophlebitis. Frequent assessment of I.V. site for signs of infiltration or phlebitis is recommended.

### Special populations

**Pregnant patients.** Use only when clearly needed.

**Breast-feeding patients.** Drug appears in breast milk; use with caution in breast-feeding women.

**Pediatric patients.** Dosage may need to be reduced in infants under age 3 months. Safety hasn't been established.

**Geriatric patients.** Dosage reduction may be needed in patients with diminished renal function.

## Patient counseling

■ Inform patient of potential adverse reactions.

---

# cefpodoxime proxetil
Vantin

*Pharmacologic classification:* third-generation cephalosporin
*Therapeutic classification:* antibiotic
*Pregnancy risk category B*

## Available forms

Available by prescription only
*Tablets (film-coated):* 100 mg, 200 mg
*Oral suspension:* 50 mg/5 ml, 100 mg/5 ml

## Indications and dosages

***Acute, community-acquired pneumonia caused by non-beta-lactamase-producing strains of* Haemophilus influenzae *or* Streptococcus pneumoniae**
*Adults:* 200 mg P.O. q 12 hours for 14 days.
***Acute bacterial exacerbations of chronic bronchitis caused by non–beta-lactamase-producing strains of* H. influenzae, S. pneumoniae, *or* Moraxella catarrhalis**
*Adults:* 200 mg P.O. q 12 hours for 10 days.
***Uncomplicated gonorrhea in men and women; rectal gonococcal infections in women***
*Adults:* 200 mg P.O. as a single dose. Follow with doxycycline 100 mg P.O. b.i.d. for 7 days.
***Uncomplicated skin and skin-structure infections caused by* Staphylococcus aureus *or* Streptococcus pyogenes**
*Adults:* 400 mg P.O. q 12 hours for 7 to 14 days.
***Acute otitis media caused by* S. pneumoniae, H. influenzae, *or* M. catarrhalis**
*Children ages 2 months to 12 years:* 5 mg/kg (not to exceed 200 mg) P.O. q 12 hours for 5 days.
***Pharyngitis or tonsillitis caused by* S. pyogenes**
*Adults:* 100 mg P.O. q 12 hours for 7 to 10 days.
*Children ages 2 months to 12 years:* 5 mg/kg (not to exceed 100 mg) P.O. q 12 hours for 5 to 10 days.
***Uncomplicated urinary tract infections caused by* Escherichia coli, Klebsiella pneumoniae, Proteus mirabilis, *or* Staphylococcus saprophyticus**
*Adults:* 100 mg P.O. q 12 hours for 7 days.
***Acute maxillary sinusitis***
*Children ages 2 months to 12 years:* 5 mg/kg (up to 200 mg) q 12 hours for 10 days.
≡*Dosage adjustment.* For patients with renal impairment when creatinine clearance is less than 30 ml/minute, increase dosage interval to q 24 hours. Patients receiving hemodialysis should get drug three times weekly, after dialysis.

## Mechanism of action

*Antibiotic action:* A second-generation cephalosporin, cefpodoxime proxetil is a bactericidal drug that inhibits cell-wall synthesis. It's usually active against gram-positive aerobes, such as *Staphylococcus aureus* (including penicillinase-producing strains), *S. saprophyticus, S. pneumoniae,* and *S. pyogenes,* and gram-negative aerobes, such as *Escherichia coli, Haemophilus influenzae* (including beta-lactamase-producing strains), *Klebsiella pneumoniae, Branhamella catarrhalis, Neisseria gonorrhoeae* (including penicillinase-producing strains), and *Proteus mirabilis.*

---

## Pharmacokinetics

*Absorption:* Absorbed via the GI tract. Absorption and mean peak plasma levels increase when drug is given with food.

*Distribution:* Widely distributed to most tissues and fluids. Second-generation cephalosporins don't enter CSF even when the meninges are inflamed. Protein-binding ranges from 22% to 33% in serum and from 21% to 29% in plasma.

*Metabolism:* De-esterified to its active metabolite, cefpodoxime.

*Excretion:* Excreted primarily in urine.

| Route | Onset | Peak | Duration |
|-------|-------|------|----------|
| P.O. | Unknown | 2-3 hr | Unknown |

## Contraindications and precautions

Contraindicated in patients hypersensitive to drug or other cephalosporins. Use cautiously in patients with impaired renal function or penicillin allergy and in breast-feeding women.

## Interactions

**Drug-drug.** *Antacids:* Decrease absorption of cefpodoxime proxetil. Give antibiotic 2 hours before or after antacids.

*H₂ antagonists:* Reduce serum levels of cefpodoxime. Don't give together.

*Probenecid:* Decreases the excretion of cefpodoxime proxetil by inhibiting renal tubular secretion. May be used together for this effect.

**Drug-food.** *Any food:* Increased absorption. Give drug with food.

## Adverse reactions

**CNS:** headache.

**GI:** *diarrhea,* nausea, vomiting, abdominal pain.

**GU:** candidiasis.

**Skin:** rash.

**Other:** hypersensitivity reactions, *anaphylaxis.*

## Overdose and treatment

No information available. Toxic symptoms after an overdose of beta-lactam antibiotics may include nausea, vomiting, epigastric distress, and diarrhea. In the event of serious toxic reaction from overdose, hemodialysis or peritoneal dialysis may aid in removing drug from the body, particularly if renal function is compromised.

## Clinical considerations

**❗ALERT** Names of some cephalosporins are similar. Use caution when dispensing.

■ Drug is highly stable in presence of beta-lactamase enzymes. As a result, many organisms resistant to penicillins and some cephalosporins, because of presence of beta-lactamases, may be susceptible to cefpodoxime proxetil.

■ Cefpodoxime is inactive against most strains of *Pseudomonas, Enterobacter,* and *Enterococcus.*

■ Specimens are obtained for culture and sensitivity tests before first dose. Therapy may begin pending test results.

■ Store suspension in refrigerator (36° to 46° F [2° to 8° C]). Shake well before using. Discard unused portion after 14 days.

■ Cefpodoxime proxetil may induce a positive direct Coombs' test.

### Therapeutic monitoring

■ As with other antibiotics, prolonged use of cefpodoxime proxetil may result in overgrowth of nonsusceptible organisms. Repeated evaluation of the patient's condition is essential, and appropriate measures should be taken if superinfection occurs during therapy.

### Special populations

**Pregnant patients.** Use only when clearly needed.

**Breast-feeding patients.** Drug appears in breast milk. Because of the potential for serious reactions in breast-fed infants, a decision must be made to discontinue breast-feeding or drug, taking into account the importance of drug to the woman.

**Pediatric patients.** Safety and efficacy in infants under age 6 months haven't been established.

**Geriatric patients.** No dosage adjustment is needed based on age. Any patient on dialysis, especially geriatric patient, should receive the dose after dialysis treatment.

### Patient counseling

■ Tell patient to report rash or signs and symptoms of superinfection.

■ Advise patient to continue taking drug for the prescribed course of therapy, even after feeling better.

# cefprozil

Cefzil

*Pharmacologic classification:* second-generation cephalosporin
*Therapeutic classification:* antibiotic
*Pregnancy risk category B*

## Available forms

Available by prescription only
*Tablets:* 250 mg, 500 mg
*Oral suspension:* 125 mg/5 ml, 250 mg/5 ml

## Indications and dosages

*Pharyngitis or tonsillitis caused by* **Streptococcus pyogenes**

*Adults and children ages 13 and older:* 500 mg P.O. daily for at least 10 days.

*Children ages 2 to 12:* 7.5 mg/kg P.O. q 12 hours for 10 days.
*Otitis media caused by* **Streptococcus pneumoniae, Haemophilus influenzae,** *and* **Moraxella catarrhalis**
*Infants and children ages 6 months to 12 years:* 15 mg/kg P.O. q 12 hours for 10 days.
*Secondary bacterial infections of acute bronchitis and acute bacterial exacerbation of chronic bronchitis caused by* **S. pneumoniae, H. influenzae,** *and* **M. catarrhalis**
*Adults:* 500 mg P.O. q 12 hours for 10 days.
*Uncomplicated skin and skin-structure infections caused by* **Staphylococcus aureus** *and* **S. pyogenes**
*Adults and children ages 13 and older:* 250 mg P.O. b.i.d. or 500 mg daily to b.i.d. for 10 days. *Children ages 2 to 12:* 20 mg/kg P.O. q 24 hours for 10 days.
≡*Dosage adjustment.* No adjustments are needed for patients with creatinine clearance of more than 30 ml/minute. For patients with creatinine clearance of 30 ml/minute or less, dose should be reduced by 50%; however, dosing interval remains unchanged. Because drug is partially removed by hemodialysis, recommend giving after the hemodialysis session.

## Mechanism of action
*Antibiotic action:* Cefprozil interferes with bacterial cell-wall synthesis during cell replication, leading to osmotic instability and cell lysis. Action is bactericidal or bacteriostatic, depending on concentration.

## Pharmacokinetics
Note: Pharmacokinetic data are derived from investigational studies that used an oral capsule formulation that isn't commercially available.
*Absorption:* About 95% absorbed from the GI tract.
*Distribution:* About 36% protein-bound.
*Metabolism:* Probably metabolized by the liver; plasma half-life increases only slightly in patients with impaired hepatic function.
*Excretion:* About 60% of a dose is recovered unchanged in the urine. Plasma half-life is 1½ hours in patients with normal renal function; 2 hours, impaired hepatic function; and 5½ to 6 hours, end-stage renal disease. Drug is removed by hemodialysis.

| Route | Onset | Peak | Duration |
|-------|-------|------|----------|
| P.O. | Unknown | 1½ hr | Unknown |

## Contraindications and precautions
Contraindicated in patients hypersensitive to drug or other cephalosporins. Use cautiously in patients with impaired renal function or penicillin allergy and in breast-feeding women.

## Interactions
**Drug-drug.** *Aminoglycosides:* May increase the risk of nephrotoxicity of cephalosporins. Advise clinician to monitor patient closely.
*Probenecid:* May decrease excretion and increase blood levels of cefprozil. Use together cautiously.

## Adverse reactions
**CNS:** dizziness, hyperactivity, headache, nervousness, insomnia, confusion, somnolence.
**GI:** *diarrhea, nausea,* vomiting, abdominal pain.
**GU:** elevated BUN level, elevated serum creatinine level, genital pruritus, vaginitis.
**Hematologic:** *leukopenia,* eosinophilia.
**Hepatic:** elevated liver enzyme levels, cholestatic jaundice.
**Skin:** rash, urticaria, diaper rash.
**Other:** superinfection, hypersensitivity reactions, serum sickness, *anaphylaxis.*

## Overdose and treatment
Because drug is eliminated primarily by the kidneys, the manufacturer states that hemodialysis may aid in removal of drug in cases of extreme overdose, especially in patients with decreased renal function.

## Clinical considerations
**⊞ALERT** Names of some cephalosporins are similar. Use caution when dispensing.
■ Obtain specimens for culture and sensitivity tests before first dose. Therapy may begin pending test results.
■ Drug may cause overgrowth of nonsusceptible bacteria or fungi, so patient will be observed for signs and symptoms of superinfection.
■ Advise patients with phenylketonuria that oral suspension contains 28 mg/5 ml phenylalanine.
■ Cephalosporins may produce a false-positive test for urine glucose with tests that use copper reduction method (Benedict's test, Fehling's solution, or Clinitest tablets). Instead, use enzymatic methods, such as glucose enzymatic test strip. A false-negative reaction may occur in the ferricyanide test for blood glucose.

### Therapeutic monitoring
■ Pseudomembranous colitis has been reported with nearly all antibacterial drugs. It may occur in patients for whom diarrhea develops secondary to antibiotic therapy. Although most patients respond to withdrawal of drug therapy alone, it may be necessary to institute treatment with an antibacterial drug effective against *Clostridium difficile,* an organism linked to this disorder.

### Special populations
**Pregnant patients.** Use during pregnancy or labor and delivery only when clearly needed.

**Breast-feeding patients.** It's unknown if drug appears in breast milk. Use with caution in breast-feeding women.

**Pediatric patients.** Oral suspensions contain drug in a bubble gum-flavored vehicle to improve palatability and compliance in children. Store reconstituted suspension in the refrigerator, and discard unused drug after 14 days. Shake suspension well before measuring dose.

**Geriatric patients.** People ages 65 and older exhibited a higher area under the plasma-concentration-versus-time curve and lower renal clearance compared with younger people.

## Patient counseling

■ Tell patient to take all of drug as prescribed, even if he feels better.

■ Instruct patient to notify prescriber if rash or symptoms of superinfection occur.

# ceftazidime

Ceptaz, Fortaz, Tazicef, Tazidime

*Pharmacologic classification:* third-generation cephalosporin
*Therapeutic classification:* antibiotic
*Pregnancy risk category B*

## Available forms

Available by prescription only
*Injection:* 500 mg, 1 g, 2 g
*Injection:* 6 g, 10 g bulk package
*Infusion:* 1 g, 2 g in 20-, 50-, and 100-ml vials and bags

## Indications and dosages

***Bacteremia, septicemia, and serious respiratory, urinary, gynecologic, bone and joint, intra-abdominal, CNS, and skin infections from susceptible organisms***
*Adults:* 1 g I.V. or I.M. q 8 to 12 hours; up to 6 g daily in life-threatening infections.
*Children ages 1 month to 12 years:* 30 to 50 mg/kg I.V. q 8 hours to a maximum of 6 g/day (Fortaz, Tazicef, and Tazidime only).
*Neonates up to 4 weeks:* 30 mg/kg I.V. q 12 hours (Fortaz, Tazicef, and Tazidime only).

Total daily dose is the same for I.M. or I.V. administration and depends on susceptibility of organism and severity of infection. Inject ceftazidime deep I.M. into a large muscle mass, such as the gluteus or lateral aspect of the thigh.

◊ *Empiric therapy in febrile neutropenic patients*
*Adults:* 100 mg/kg I.V. daily in 3 divided doses; or 2 g I.V. q 8 hours either alone or with an aminoglycoside such as amikacin.
*Children ages 2 and older:* 50 mg/kg (maximum 2 g) q 8 hours given I.V.

≡ *Dosage adjustment.* For patients with impaired renal function, doses or frequency of administration must be modified according to the degree of renal impairment, severity of in-

fection, and susceptibility of organism. To prevent toxic accumulation, reduced dosage may be needed in patients with creatinine clearance less than 50 ml/minute. For patients with creatinine clearance of 50 ml/minute or less, initially give 1 g loading dose then follow maintenance recommendations.

| Creatinine clearance (ml/min) | Adult dosage |
|---|---|
| 31-50 | 1 g q 12 hr |
| 16-30 | 1 g q 24 hr |
| 6-15 | 500 mg q 24 hr |
| ≤ 5 | 500 mg q 48 hr |
| Hemodialysis patients | 1 g after each hemodialysis period |
| Peritoneal dialysis patients | 500 mg q 24 hr |

## I.V. administration

■ Reconstitute solutions containing sodium carbonate with sterile water for injection. Add 5 ml to a 500-mg vial, or add 10 ml to a 1-g or 2-g vial. Shake well to dissolve drug. Carbon dioxide is released during dissolution, and positive pressure will develop in vial.

■ Reconstitute solutions containing arginine with 10 ml of sterile water for injection. This formulation won't release gas bubbles.

■ Each brand of ceftazidime includes specific instructions for reconstitution. Read and follow them carefully.

■ Infuse drug over 15 to 30 minutes.

■ Once reconstituted, drug may also be given by direct I.V. injection over 3 to 5 minutes directly into the vein or into the tubing of a compatible I.V. solution.

### Incompatibilities

Incompatible with aminoglycosides, fluconazole, idarubicin, sargramostim, sodium bicarbonate solutions, and vancomycin.

## Mechanism of action

*Antibacterial action:* Ceftazidime is primarily bactericidal; however, it may be bacteriostatic. Activity depends on the organism, tissue penetration, drug dosage, and rate of organism multiplication. It acts by adhering to bacterial penicillin-binding proteins, thereby inhibiting cell-wall synthesis. Third-generation cephalosporins appear more active against some beta-lactamase-producing gram-negative organisms.

Ceftazidime is active against some gram-positive organisms and many enteric gram-negative bacilli, as well as streptococci (*Streptococcus pneumoniae* and *S. pyogenes*); *Staphylococcus aureus* (penicillinase- and nonpenicillinase-producing); *Escherichia coli; Klebsiella* species; *Proteus* species; *Enter-*

*obacter* species; *Haemophilus influenzae; Pseudomonas* species; and some strains of *Bacteroides* species. It's more effective than any cephalosporin or penicillin derivative against *Pseudomonas*. Some other third-generation cephalosporins are more active against gram-positive organisms and anaerobes.

## Pharmacokinetics
*Absorption:* Not absorbed from the GI tract; must be given parenterally.
*Distribution:* Distributed widely into most body tissues and fluids, including the gallbladder, liver, kidneys, bone, sputum, bile, and pleural and synovial fluids; unlike most other cephalosporins, ceftazidime has good CSF penetration; it crosses the placenta. Ceftazidime is 5% to 24% protein-bound.
*Metabolism:* Not metabolized.
*Excretion:* Excreted primarily in urine by glomerular filtration; small amounts of drug appear in breast milk. Elimination half-life is about 1½ to 2 hours in patients with normal renal function; up to 35 hours in patients with severe renal disease. Hemodialysis or peritoneal dialysis removes ceftazidime.

| Route | Onset | Peak | Duration |
|-------|-------|------|----------|
| I.V. | Immediate | Immediate | Unknown |
| I.M. | Unknown | 1 hr | Unknown |

## Contraindications and precautions
Contraindicated in patients hypersensitive to drug or other cephalosporins. Use cautiously in breast-feeding women and in patients with poor renal function or penicillin allergy.

## Interactions
**Drug-drug.** *Aminoglycosides:* Concurrent use results in synergistic activity against some strains of *Pseudomonas aeruginosa* and Enterobacteriaceae. Advise clinician to monitor patient for effects.
*Chloramphenicol:* Antagonistic effect. Avoid use together.
*Probenicid:* May inhibit excretion and increase levels. May be used as a therapeutic effect. Advise clinician to monitor patient for adverse reactions.
*Quinolones:* In vitro studies show synergistic effect against *Burkholderia cepacia.* Advise clinician to monitor patient for efficacy.

## Adverse reactions
**CNS:** headache, dizziness, paresthesia, *seizures.*
**GI:** pseudomembranous colitis, nausea, vomiting, diarrhea, abdominal cramps.
**GU:** vaginitis, candidiasis.
**Hematologic:** eosinophilia, thrombocytosis, *leukopenia,* hemolytic anemia, *agranulocytosis, thrombocytopenia.*
**Hepatic:** elevated liver enzymes levels.

**Skin:** *maculopapular and erythematous rash, urticaria, pain, induration, sterile abscesses, tissue sloughing* (at injection site).
**Other:** hypersensitivity reactions, serum sickness, *anaphylaxis, phlebitis, thrombophlebitis* (with I.V. injection).

## Overdose and treatment
Signs and symptoms of overdose include neuromuscular hypersensitivity. Seizure may follow high CNS levels. Drug may be removed by hemodialysis or peritoneal dialysis.

## Clinical considerations
**ℍALERT** Names of some cephalosporins are similar. Use caution when dispensing.
■ For patients on sodium restriction, note that ceftazidime contains 2.3 mEq of sodium per gram of drug.
■ Ceftazidime powders (excluding Ceptaz) for injection contain 118 mg sodium carbonate per gram of drug; ceftazidime sodium is more water-soluble and is formed in situ on reconstitution.
■ Vials are supplied under reduced pressure. When antibiotic is dissolved, carbon dioxide is released and a positive pressure develops. Each brand of ceftazidime includes specific instructions for reconstitution. Read carefully.
■ Because drug is hemodialyzable, patients undergoing treatments with hemodialysis or peritoneal dialysis may require dosage adjustment.
■ Ceftazidime causes false-positive results in urine glucose tests using cupric sulfate (Benedict's reagent or Clinitest); use glucose oxidase (Chemstrip uG, Diastix, or glucose enzymatic test strip) instead. Ceftazidime also causes false elevations in urine creatinine levels in tests using Jaffé's reaction. Ceftazidime may cause positive Coombs' test results.

### Therapeutic monitoring
■ With large doses or prolonged therapy, watch for superinfection, especially in high-risk patients.

### Special populations
**Pregnant patients.** Use only when clearly needed.
**Breast-feeding patients.** Drug appears in breast milk; use with caution in breast-feeding women. Safety hasn't been established.
**Pediatric patients.** Only Fortaz, Tazicef, and Tazidime may be used in infants and children. Ceptaz shouldn't be used in children under age 12 because it contains arginine.
**Geriatric patients.** Reduced dosage may be needed in geriatric patients with diminished renal function.

## Patient counseling
■ Advise patient to report discomfort at I.V. site.

---

* Canada only   ◇ Unlabeled clinical use

■ Tell patient to report rash or symptoms of superinfection.

# ceftibuten
Cedax

*Pharmacologic classification:* third-generation cephalosporin
*Therapeutic classification:* antibiotic
*Pregnancy risk category B*

## Available forms
Available by prescription only
*Capsules:* 400 mg
*Oral suspension:* 90 mg/5 ml, 180 mg/5 ml

## Indications and dosages
***Acute bacterial exacerbations of chronic bronchitis caused by*** Haemophilus influenzae, Moraxella catarrhalis, *or* Streptococcus pneumoniae
*Adults and children ages 12 and older:* 400 mg P.O. daily for 10 days.
***Pharyngitis and tonsillitis caused by*** Streptococcus pyogenes; *acute bacterial otitis media caused by* H. influenzae, M. catarrhalis, *or* S. pyogenes
*Adults and children ages 12 and older:* 400 mg P.O. daily for 10 days.
*Children under age 12:* 9 mg/kg P.O. daily for 10 days. Children weighing more than 45 kg (99 lb) should receive the maximum daily dose of 400 mg.
≡*Dosage adjustment.* Give 4.5 mg/kg (or 200 mg) daily to patients with creatinine clearance between 30 and 49 ml/minute and 2.25 mg/kg (or 100 mg) daily for those with creatinine clearance of 5 to 29 ml/minute. For patients undergoing hemodialysis two or three times weekly, give a single 400-mg dose (capsule form) or give a single dose of 9 mg/kg (maximum dose, 400 mg) using oral suspension at the end of each hemodialysis session.

## Mechanism of action
*Antibiotic action:* Ceftibuten exerts its bactericidal action by binding to essential target proteins of the bacterial cell wall. This binding leads to inhibition of cell-wall synthesis. It's usually active against gram-positive aerobes (*S. pneumoniae, S. pyogenes*) and gram-negative aerobes (*H. influenzae, M. catarrhalis*).

## Pharmacokinetics
*Absorption:* Rapidly absorbed from GI tract. Food decreases the bioavailability of drug.
*Distribution:* 65% plasma protein–bound.
*Metabolism:* Metabolized to its predominant component, cis-ceftibuten. About 10% of ceftibuten is converted to the trans-isomer.

*Excretion:* Excreted in urine and feces.

| Route | Onset | Peak | Duration |
|-------|---------|--------|----------|
| P.O. | Unknown | 2-4 hr | Unknown |

## Contraindications and precautions
Contraindicated in patients hypersensitive to the cephalosporin group of antibiotics. Use cautiously if giving to patients with history of hypersensitivity to penicillin because up to 10% of these patients will exhibit cross-sensitivity to a cephalosporin. Also use cautiously in patients with impaired renal function and GI disease (especially colitis).

## Interactions
**Drug-food.** *Any food:* Decreased bioavailability of drug, which slows its absorption. Advise patient to take drug 2 hours before or 1 hour after a meal.

## Adverse reactions
**CNS:** headache, dizziness, fatigue, paresthesia, somnolence, agitation, hyperkinesia, insomnia, irritability.
**EENT:** nasal congestion.
**GI:** nausea, dyspepsia, abdominal pain, vomiting, anorexia, constipation, dry mouth, eructation, flatulence, loose stools, melena, taste perversion.
**GU:** dysuria, hematuria, elevated BUN and serum creatinine level, vaginitis, candidiasis.
**Hematologic:** eosinophila, decreased hemoglobin, altered platelet count, decreased leukocyte count.
**Hepatic:** elevated levels of liver enzymes, bilirubin, and alkaline phosphatase.
**Respiratory:** dyspnea.
**Skin:** rash, pruritus, diaper dermatitis, urticaria.
**Other:** dehydration, fever, rigors.

## Overdose and treatment
Overdose of cephalosporins may cause cerebral irritation leading to seizures. Ceftibuten is readily dialyzable and significant quantities (65% of plasma levels) can be removed from the circulation by a single hemodialysis session. Information regarding the removal of ceftibuten by peritoneal dialysis doesn't exist.

## Clinical considerations
■ Pseudomembranous colitis has been reported with nearly all antibacterial drugs; it may occur in patients for whom diarrhea develops secondary to antibiotic therapy. Although most patients respond to withdrawal of drug therapy alone, it may be necessary to institute treatment with an antibacterial drug effective against *Clostridium difficile,* an organism linked to this disorder.
■ Obtain specimens for culture and testing for sensitivity before first dose. Therapy may begin pending test results.

■ When preparing oral suspension, first tap the bottle to loosen powder. Follow chart supplied by manufacturer for amount of water to add to powder when mixing oral suspension form. Add water in two portions, shaking well after each aliquot. After mixing, the suspension may be kept for 14 days and must be stored in the refrigerator.

■ Although ceftibuten hasn't been known to affect the direct Coombs' test, other cephalosporins have caused a false-positive direct Coombs' test. Therefore, it should be recognized that a positive Coombs' test could be from the drug.

### Therapeutic monitoring

■ Drug may cause overgrowth of nonsusceptible bacteria or fungi. Patient requires observation for signs and symptoms of superinfection.

### Special populations

**Breast-feeding patients.** It isn't known if drug appears in breast milk. Use cautiously in breast-feeding women.

**Pediatric patients.** Safety and effectiveness in infants under age 6 months haven't been established.

**Geriatric patients.** Use with caution in geriatric patients. Dosage adjustment may be needed if patient has impaired renal function.

### Patient counseling

■ Tell patient to take all of drug as prescribed, even if he's feeling better.

■ Inform diabetic patient that oral suspension contains 1 g of sucrose per teaspoon of suspension.

■ Instruct patient using oral suspension to shake bottle well before measuring dose.

# ceftizoxime sodium
Cefizox

*Pharmacologic classification:* third-generation cephalosporin
*Therapeutic classification:* antibiotic
*Pregnancy risk category B*

### Available forms

Available by prescription only
*Injection:* 500 mg, 1 g, 2 g, 10 g bulk package
*Infusion:* 1 g, 2 g in 100-ml vials

### Indications and dosages

*Bacteremia, septicemia, meningitis, pelvic inflammatory disease, and serious respiratory, urinary, gynecologic, intra-abdominal, bone and joint, and skin infections from susceptible organisms*
*Adults:* Usual dosage is 500 mg to 2 g I.V. or I.M. q 8 to 12 hours. In life-threatening infections, 3 to 4 g I.V. q 8 hours.

*Children ages 6 months and older:* 50 mg/kg I.V. or I.M. q 6 to 8 hours.

Total daily dose is same for I.M. or I.V. administration and depends on susceptibility of organism and severity of infection. Inject ceftizoxime deep I.M. into a large muscle mass, such as the gluteus or lateral aspect of the thigh.

*Uncomplicated gonorrhea*
*Adults:* 1 g I.M. given as a single dose.
≡*Dosage adjustment.* For patients with impaired renal function, recommend modifying doses or frequency of administration according to degree of renal impairment, severity of infection, and susceptibility of organism. To prevent toxic accumulation, reduced dosage may be needed in patients with creatinine clearance less than 80 ml/minute. The following table gives appropriate doses for adults.

| Creatinine clearance (ml/min) | Less severe infections | Life-threatening infections |
|---|---|---|
| 50-79 | 500 mg q 8 hr | 750 mg-1.5 g q 8 hr |
| 5-49 | 250-500 mg q 12 hr | 500 mg-1 g q 12 hr |
| 0-4 | 500 mg q 48 hr; or 250 mg q 24 hr | 500 mg-1 g q 48 hr; or 500 mg q 24 hr |

### I.V. administration

■ Reconstitute I.V. dose with sterile water for injection. After it has been shaken well, solution should clear and range in color from yellow to amber. If particles are visible, discard solution. Reconstituted solution is stable for 24 hours at controlled room temperature or 96 hours if refrigerated.

■ Drug may be given as a direct injection slowly over 3 to 5 minutes directly in the vein, or through tubing of compatible infusion fluid. If given as intermittent infusion, the reconstituted drug is diluted in 50 to 100 ml of compatible fluid and given over 15 to 30 minutes.

### Incompatibilities

Incompatible with aminoglycosides.

### Mechanism of action

*Antibacterial action:* Ceftizoxime is primarily bactericidal; however, it may be bacteriostatic. Activity depends on the organism, tissue penetration, drug dosage, and rate of organism multiplication. It acts by adhering to bacterial penicillin-binding proteins, thereby inhibiting cell-wall synthesis. Third-generation cephalosporins appear more active against some beta-lactamase-producing gram-negative organisms.

Drug is active against some gram-positive organisms and many enteric gram-negative bacilli, as well as streptococci (*Streptococcus pneumoniae* and *pyogenes*); *Staphylococcus aureus* (penicillinase- and non–penicillinase-producing); *Staphylococcus epidermidis; Escherichia coli; Klebsiella* species; *Haemophilus influenzae; Enterobacter* species; *Proteus* species; *Bacteroides* species (including *Bacteroides fragilis*); *Peptostreptococcus* species; some strains of *Pseudomonas* and *Acinetobacter.* Cefotaxime and moxalactam are slightly more active than ceftizoxime against gram-positive organisms but are less active against gram-negative organisms.

## Pharmacokinetics
*Absorption:* Not absorbed from the GI tract; must be given parenterally.
*Distribution:* Distributed widely into most body tissues and fluids, including the gallbladder, liver, kidneys, bone, sputum, bile, and pleural and synovial fluids. Unlike most other cephalosporins, ceftizoxime has good CSF penetration and achieves adequate concentration in inflamed meninges; ceftizoxime crosses the placenta and is 30% protein-bound.
*Metabolism:* Not metabolized.
*Excretion:* Excreted primarily in urine by renal tubular secretion and glomerular filtration; small amounts of drug appear in breast milk. Elimination half-life is about 1½ to 2 hours in patients with normal renal function; severe renal disease prolongs half-life up to 30 hours. Hemodialysis or peritoneal dialysis removes minimal amounts of ceftizoxime.

| Route | Onset | Peak | Duration |
|-------|-------|------|----------|
| I.V. | Immediate | Immediate | Unknown |
| I.M. | Unknown | ½-1½ hr | Unknown |

## Contraindications and precautions
Contraindicated in patients hypersensitive to ceftizoxime or other cephalosporins. Use cautiously in breast-feeding women and in patients with impaired renal function or penicillin allergy.

## Interactions
**Drug-drug.** *Aminoglycosides:* May slightly increase the risk of nephrotoxicity. Avoid use.
*Probenecid:* Competitively inhibits renal tubular secretion of cephalosporins, causing higher, prolonged serum levels. May be used for this effect.

## Adverse reactions
**GI:** pseudomembranous colitis, nausea, anorexia, vomiting, *diarrhea.*
**GU:** vaginitis.
**Hematologic:** *transient neutropenia,* eosinophilia, hemolytic anemia, thrombocytosis, anemia, *thrombocytopenia.*
**Hepatic:** transient elevation in liver enzymes.
**Respiratory:** dyspnea.
**Skin:** *maculopapular and erythematous rash, urticaria pain, induration, sterile abscesses, tissue sloughing (at injected site).*

**Other:** hypersensitivity reactions, serum sickness, *anaphylaxis,* elevated temperature, *phlebitis, thrombophlebitis.*

## Overdose and treatment
Signs and symptoms of overdose include neuromuscular hypersensitivity. Seizure may follow high CNS levels. Ceftizoxime may be removed by hemodialysis.

## Clinical considerations
**⚠ALERT** Names of some cephalosporins are similar. Use caution when dispensing.
■ For patients on sodium restriction, note that ceftizoxime contains 2.6 mEq of sodium per gram of drug.
■ Drug may be supplied as frozen, sterile solution in plastic containers. Thaw at controlled room temperature. Thawed solution is stable for 24 hours at controlled room temperature or for 21 days if refrigerated. Don't refreeze.
■ For I.M. use, reconstitute with sterile water for injection. Shake vial well to ensure complete dissolution of drug. To administer a dose that exceeds 1 g, divide the dose and inject it into separate sites to prevent tissue injury.
■ Ceftizoxime causes false-positive results in urine glucose tests using cupric sulfate (Benedict's reagent or Clinitest); use glucose oxidase (Chemstrip uG, Diastix, or glucose enzymatic test strip) instead. Ceftizoxime also causes false elevations in urine creatinine levels using Jaffé's reaction. Ceftizoxime may cause positive Coombs' test results.

### Therapeutic monitoring
■ If a severe hypersensitivity reaction occurs during therapy, discontinue drug and institute appropriate therapy (such as epinephrine, I.V. fluids, oxygen).

### Special populations
**Breast-feeding patients.** Drug appears in breast milk; use with caution in breast-feeding women. Safety hasn't been established.
**Pediatric patients.** Safety and efficacy haven't been established in infants under age 6 months.
**Geriatric patients.** Reduced dosage may be needed in geriatric patients with diminished renal function.

## Patient counseling
■ Inform patient of potential adverse reactions.
■ Tell patient to report discomfort at I.V. site.

# ceftriaxone sodium
Rocephin

*Pharmacologic classification:* third-generation cephalosporin
*Therapeutic classification:* antibiotic
*Pregnancy risk category B*

---

## Available forms
Available by prescription only
*Injection:* 250 mg, 500 mg, 1 g, 2 g, 10-g bulk package
*Infusion:* 1 g, 2 g

## Indications and dosages
***Bacteremia, septicemia, and serious respiratory, bone, joint, urinary, gynecologic, intra-abdominal, and skin infections from susceptible organisms***
*Adults and children ages 12 and older:* 1 to 2 g I.M. or I.V. once daily or in equally divided doses b.i.d. Total daily dose shouldn't exceed 4 g.
*Children under age 12:* Total daily dose is 50 to 75 mg/kg I.M. or I.V., given in divided doses q 12 hours. Maximum daily dose is 2 g.
***Gonococcal meningitis, endocarditis***
*Adults:* 1 to 2 g I.V. q 12 hours for 10 to 14 days for meningitis and 3 to 4 weeks for endocarditis.
*Children:* 50 to 100 mg/kg (maximum daily dose, 4 g) I.M. or I.V. daily or divided q 12 hours for 7 to 14 days for meningitis and 28 days for endocarditis.
　　May give an initial dose of 100 mg/kg (not to exceed 4 g) I.M. or I.V. to begin therapy. Total daily dose is same for I.M. or I.V. administration and depends on susceptibility of organism and severity of infection. Inject ceftriaxone deep I.M. into a large muscle mass, such as the gluteus or lateral aspect of the thigh.
***Preoperative prophylaxis***
*Adults:* 1 g I.M. or I.V. 30 minutes to 2 hours before surgery.
***Uncomplicated gonorrhea***
*Adults:* 125 to 250 mg I.M. given as a single dose; ◇ 1 to 2 g I.M. or I.V. daily until improvement occurs.
◇ ***Haemophilus ducreyi infection***
*Adults:* 250 mg I.M. as a single dose.
◇ ***Sexually transmitted epididymitis, pelvic inflammatory disease***
*Adults:* 250 mg I.M. as a single dose; follow up with other antibiotics.
◇ ***Anti-infectives for sexual assault victims***
*Adults:* 125 mg I.M. as a single dose in conjunction with other antibiotics.
◇ ***Lyme disease***
*Adults:* 1 to 2 g I.M. or I.V. q 12 to 24 hours.
◇ ***Persisting or relapsing otitis media in children***
*Children ages 3 months and older:* 50 mg/kg I.M. once daily for 3 days.
≡ ***Dosage adjustment.*** For patients with impaired hepatic and renal function, dose shouldn't exceed 2 g/day without monitoring serum drug levels.

## I.V. administration
■ Reconstitute drug with sterile water for injection, normal saline solution for injection, $D_5W$ or $D_{10}W$ injection, or a combination of normal saline solution and dextrose injection and other compatible solutions.
■ Reconstitute by adding 2.4 ml of diluent to the 250-mg vial, 4.8 ml to the 500-mg vial, 9.6 ml to the 1-g vial, and 19.2 ml to the 2-g vial.
■ All reconstituted solutions yield a concentration that averages 100 mg/ml. After reconstitution, dilute further for intermittent infusion to desired concentration.
■ Infuse over 15 to 30 minutes.

### Incompatibilities
Incompatible with aminoglycosides. Don't mix with amsacrine, clindamycin phosphate, fluconazole, or vancomycin.

## Mechanism of action
*Antibacterial action:* Ceftriaxone is primarily bactericidal; however, it may be bacteriostatic. Activity depends on organism, tissue penetration, and drug dosage and on rate of organism multiplication. It acts by adhering to bacterial penicillin-binding proteins, thereby inhibiting cell-wall synthesis. Third-generation cephalosporins appear more active against some beta-lactamase-producing, gram-negative organisms.
　　Ceftriaxone is active against some gram-positive organisms and many enteric gram-negative bacilli, as well as streptococci; *Streptococcus pneumoniae* and *pyogenes; Staphylococcus aureus* (penicillinase and nonpenicillinase producing); *Staphylococcus epidermidis; Escherichia coli; Klebsiella* species; *Haemophilus influenzae, Enterobacter; Proteus;* some strains of *Pseudomonas* and *Peptostreptococcus* and spirochetes such as *Borrelia burgdorferi* (the causative organism of Lyme disease). Most strains of *Listeria, Pseudomonas,* and *Acinetobacter* are resistant. Generally, the activity of ceftriaxone is most like that of cefotaxime and ceftizoxime.

## Pharmacokinetics
*Absorption:* Not absorbed from the GI tract and must be given parenterally.
*Distribution:* Distributed widely into most body tissues and fluids, including the gallbladder, liver, kidneys, bone, sputum, bile, and pleural and synovial fluids; unlike most other cephalosporins, ceftriaxone has good CSF penetration. Ceftriaxone crosses the placenta. Protein binding is dose-dependent and decreases as serum levels rise; average is 84% to 96%.
*Metabolism:* Partially metabolized.
*Excretion:* Excreted principally in urine; some drug is excreted in bile by biliary mechanisms, and small amounts appear in breast milk. Elimination half-life is 5½ to 11 hours in adults with normal renal function; severe renal disease prolongs half-life only moderately. Neither hemodialysis nor peritoneal dialysis will remove ceftriaxone.

---

* Canada only    ◇ Unlabeled clinical use

| Route | Onset | Peak | Duration |
|-------|-------|------|----------|
| I.V. | Immediate | Immediate | Unknown |
| I.M. | Unknown | 1½-4 hr | Unknown |

## Contraindications and precautions
Contraindicated in patients hypersensitive to ceftriaxone or other cephalosporins. Use cautiously in breast-feeding women and in patients with penicillin allergy.

## Interactions
**Drug-drug.** *Aminoglycosides:* Synergistic antimicrobial activity against *Pseudomonas aeruginosa* and some strains of Enterobacteriaceae. Advise clinician to monitor patient closely.
*Probenecid:* May increase clearance by blocking biliary secretion and displacement of ceftriaxone from plasma proteins. Avoid use together.
*Quinolones:* In vitro synergism against *S. pneumoniae.*

## Adverse reactions
**CNS:** headache, dizziness.
**GI:** pseudomembranous colitis, nausea, vomiting, diarrhea, urolithiasis.
**GU:** genital pruritus, candidiasis, elevated BUN levels.
**Hematologic:** eosinophilia, thrombocytosis, *leukopenia.*
**Hepatic:** elevated liver function test results, jaundice.
**Skin:** pain, induration, tenderness (at injection site); phlebitis; *rash;* pruritus.
**Other:** hypersensitivity reactions, serum sickness, *anaphylaxis,* elevated temperature, chills.

## Overdose and treatment
Signs and symptoms of overdose include neuromuscular hypersensitivity. Seizure may follow high CNS levels. Treatment is supportive.

## Clinical considerations
**⚠ALERT** Names of some cephalosporins are similar. Use caution when dispensing.
■ For patients on sodium restriction, note that ceftriaxone injection contains 3.6 mEq of sodium per gram of drug.
■ Dosage adjustment usually isn't needed in patients with renal insufficiency because of partial biliary excretion.
■ Ceftriaxone causes false-positive results in urine glucose tests using cupric sulfate (Benedict's reagent or Clinitest); use glucose oxidase (Chemstrip uG, Diastix, or glucose enzymatic test strip) instead. Ceftriaxone also causes false elevations in urine creatinine levels in tests using Jaffé's reaction. Ceftriaxone may cause positive Coombs' test results.

### Therapeutic monitoring
■ With large doses or prolonged therapy, advise clinician to monitor high-risk patients for superinfection.

### Special populations
**Breast-feeding patients.** Drug appears in breast milk. Use with caution in breast-feeding women.
**Pediatric patients.** Ceftriaxone may be used in neonates and children. Use cautiously in hyperbilirubinemic neonates because of the ability of the drug to displace bilirubin.

### Patient counseling
■ Inform patient of potential adverse reactions.
■ Tell patient to report discomfort at I.V. site.

# cefuroxime axetil
Ceftin

# cefuroxime sodium
Kefurox, Zinacef

*Pharmacologic classification:* second-generation cephalosporin
*Therapeutic classification:* antibiotic
*Pregnancy risk category B*

## Available forms
Available by prescription only
**cefuroxime axetil**
*Tablets (film-coated):* 125 mg, 250 mg, 500 mg
*Suspension:* 125 mg/5 ml, 250 mg/5 ml
**cefuroxime sodium**
*Injection:* 750 mg, 1.5 g, 7.5 g
*Infusion:* 750 mg, 1.5-g infusion packets

## Indications and dosages
*Serious lower respiratory, urinary tract, skin and skin-structure infections; septicemia; meningitis caused by susceptible organisms*
*Adults:* Usual dosage is 750 mg to 1.5 g I.M. or I.V. q 8 hours, usually for 5 to 10 days. For life-threatening infections and infections caused by less susceptible organisms, 1.5 g I.M. or I.V. q 6 hours; for bacterial meningitis, up to 3 g I.V. q 8 hours.
*Children and infants over age 3 months:* 50 to 100 mg/kg/day I.M. or I.V. in divided doses q 6 to 8 hours. Some clinicians give 100 to 150 mg/kg/day. For meningitis, the usual starting dosage is 200 to 240 mg/kg/day I.V. in divided doses q 6 to 8 hours, reduced to 100 mg/kg/day when clinical improvement is seen. However, some clinicians prefer other drugs for meningitis.
    Total daily dose is the same for I.M. and I.V. administration, and depends on susceptibility of organism and severity of infection. Inject cefuroxime deep I.M. into a large muscle

mass, such as the gluteus or lateral aspect of the thigh.

*Pharyngitis, tonsillitis, lower respiratory infection, urinary tract infection*
*Adults and children over age 12:* 125 to 500 mg P.O. b.i.d. for 10 days.
*Children under age 12 who can swallow pills:* 125 to 250 mg P.O. b.i.d. (tablets) for 10 days.
*Children ages 3 months to 12 years:* 20 mg/kg/day P.O. in divided doses b.i.d. (oral suspension) to maximum dose of 500 mg for 10 days.

*Otitis media, impetigo*
*Children ages 3 months to 12 years:* 30 mg/kg/day P.O. oral suspension divided into two doses (maximum dose, 1 g) for 10 days.
*Children who can swallow pills:* 250 mg P.O. b.i.d. for 10 days.
   Note: Compliance may be a problem when treating otitis media in children. Use suspension form if child is unable to swallow pills.

*Perioperative prophylaxis*
*Adults:* 1.5 g I.V. 30 to 60 minutes before surgery; then 750 mg I.M. or I.V. q 8 hours intraoperatively for a prolonged procedure. Open-heart surgery patients can receive 1.5 g I.V. at induction, then q 12 hours for 3 doses.

◊ *Gonorrhea (urethral, endocervical, rectal)*
*Adults:* 1.5 g I.M. given as a single dose, alone or with other antibiotics.

*Lyme disease (erythema migrans) caused by* **Borrelia burgdorferi**
*Adults and children ages 13 and older:* 500 mg P.O. b.i.d. for 20 days.

≡*Dosage adjustment.* Safety of drug in renal patients hasn't been established. For patients with impaired renal function, dose or frequency of administration must be modified based on degree of renal impairment, severity of infection, and susceptibility of organism. To prevent toxic accumulation, reduced I.M. or I.V. dosage may be needed in patients with creatinine clearance of less than 20 ml/minute.

| Creatinine clearance (ml/min) | Adult dosage |
|---|---|
| 10-20 | 750 mg q 12 hr |
| < 10 | 750 mg q 24 hr |

◊ *Hemodialysis patients:* 750 mg at end of each dialysis period in addition to regular dose.

## I.V. administration
■ For each 750-mg vial of Kefurox, reconstitute with 7 ml of sterile water for injection. For each 1.5-g vial of Kefurox, reconstitute with 14 ml of sterile water for injection; withdraw entire contents of vial for a dose.

■ For each 750-ml vial of Zinacef, reconstitute with 8 ml of sterile water for injection; for each 1.5-g vial, reconstitute with 16 ml. In each case, withdraw entire contents of vial for a dose.
■ To give by direct injection, inject into a large vein or into the tubing of a free-flowing I.V. solution over 3 to 5 minutes.
■ For intermittent infusion, add reconstituted drug to 100 ml D₅W, normal saline solution for injection, or other compatible I.V. solution. Infuse over 15 to 60 minutes.

## Incompatibilities
Cefuroxime sodium is incompatible with aminoglycosides, doxapram, fluconazole, and sodium bicarbonate injection.

## Mechanism of action
*Antibacterial action:* Cefuroxime is primarily bactericidal; however, it may be bacteriostatic. Activity depends on the organism, tissue penetration, drug dosage, and rate of organism multiplication. It acts by adhering to bacterial penicillin-binding proteins, thereby inhibiting cell-wall synthesis.
   Cefuroxime is active against many gram-positive organisms and enteric gram-negative bacilli, including *Streptococcus pneumoniae* and *S. pyogenes, Haemophilus influenzae, Klebsiella* species, *Staphylococcus aureus, Escherichia coli, Enterobacter,* and *Neisseria gonorrhoeae; Bacteroides fragilis, Pseudomonas,* and *Acinetobacter* are resistant to cefuroxime.

## Pharmacokinetics
*Absorption:* Cefuroxime sodium isn't well absorbed from the GI tract and must be given parenterally. Cefuroxime axetil is better absorbed orally, with between 37% to 52% of an oral dose reaching the systemic circulation. Food appears to enhance absorption. Tablets and suspension aren't bioequivalent.
*Distribution:* Distributed widely into most body tissues and fluids, including the gallbladder, liver, kidneys, bone, bile, and pleural and synovial fluids; CSF penetration is greater than that of most first- and second-generation cephalosporins and achieves adequate therapeutic levels in inflamed meninges. Cefuroxime crosses the placenta, and is 33% to 50% protein-bound.
*Metabolism:* Not metabolized.
*Excretion:* Primarily excreted in urine by renal tubular secretion and glomerular filtration; elimination half-life is 1 to 2 hours in patients with normal renal function; end-stage renal disease prolongs half-life 15 to 22 hours. Some

drug appears in breast milk. Hemodialysis removes cefuroxime.

| Route | Onset | Peak | Duration |
|-------|-------|------|----------|
| P.O. | Unknown | 15-60 min | Unknown |
| I.V. | Immediate | Immediate | Unknown |
| I.M. | Unknown | 2 hr | Unknown |

## Contraindications and precautions

Contraindicated in patients hypersensitive to cefuroxime or other cephalosporins. Use cautiously in breast-feeding women and in those with impaired renal function or penicillin allergy.

## Interactions

**Drug-drug.** *Aminoglycosides:* Synergistic activity against some organisms; potential for increased nephrotoxicity. Advise clinician to monitor BUN and serum creatinine levels closely.
*Diuretics:* Increased risk of adverse effects. Advise clinician to monitor patient closely.
*Probenecid:* Competitively inhibits renal tubular secretion of cephalosporins, resulting in higher, prolonged serum levels of these drugs. Sometimes used for this effect.
**Drug-food.** *Any food:* Increased absorption. Advise patient to take drug with food.

## Adverse reactions

**GI:** pseudomembranous colitis, nausea, anorexia, vomiting, *diarrhea.*
**Hematologic:** *transient neutropenia,* eosinophilia, hemolytic anemia, *thrombocytopenia,* decreased hemoglobin and hematocrit.
**Hepatic:** transient increases in liver enzymes.
**Skin:** *maculopapular and erythematous rash, urticaria, pain, induration, sterile abscesses, temperature elevation, tissue sloughing* (at injection site).
**Other:** hypersensitivity reactions, serum sickness, *anaphylaxis; phlebitis, thrombophlebitis* (with I.V. injection).

## Overdose and treatment

Signs and symptoms of overdose include neuromuscular hypersensitivity. Seizure may follow high CNS levels. Hemodialysis or peritoneal dialysis will remove cefuroxime.

## Clinical considerations

**⚠ALERT** Names of some cephalosporins are similar. Use caution when dispensing.
■ Tablets and suspension are not bioequivalent and cannot be substituted on a milligram per milligram basis.
■ For patients on sodium restriction, note that cefuroxime sodium contains 2.4 mEq of sodium per gram of drug.
■ Check solutions for particulate matter and discoloration. Solution may range in color from light yellow to amber without affecting potency.
■ Recommend shaking I.M. solution gently before administration to ensure complete drug dissolution, and giving deep I.M. in a large muscle mass, preferably the gluteus area. Recommend aspiration before injecting to prevent inadvertent injection into a blood vessel. Rotate injection sites to prevent tissue damage. Ice to injection site may relieve pain.
■ Because drug is hemodialyzable, patients undergoing treatment with hemodialysis or peritoneal dialysis may need dosage adjustments.
■ Reconstituted suspension can be stored at controlled room temperature or in refrigerator. Discard unused portion after 10 days. Shake well before each dose.
■ Drug causes false-positive results in urine glucose tests using cupric sulfate (Benedict's reagent or Clinitest); use glucose oxidase tests (Chemstrip uG, Diastix, or glucose enzymatic test strip) instead. Cefuroxime also causes false elevations in serum or urine creatinine levels in tests using Jaffé's reaction. Cefuroxime may cause positive Coombs' test results.

### Therapeutic monitoring

■ With large doses or prolonged therapy, watch for superinfection, especially in high-risk patients.

### Special populations

**Breast-feeding patients.** Drug appears in breast milk; use with caution in breast-feeding women.
**Pediatric patients.** Safety in infants under age 3 months hasn't been established.
**Geriatric patients.** Use with caution in geriatric patients.

## Patient counseling

■ Inform patient of potential adverse reactions.
■ Patient should report discomfort at I.V. site.

---

# celecoxib

Celebrex

*Pharmacologic classification:* cyclooxygenase-2 (COX-2) inhibitor
*Therapeutic classification:* anti-inflammatory
*Pregnancy risk category C*

## Available forms

Available by prescription only
*Capsules:* 100 mg, 200 mg

## Indications and dosages

*Relief from signs and symptoms of osteoarthritis in adults*
*Adults:* 200 mg P.O. daily as a single dose or divided equally b.i.d.

***Relief from the signs and symptoms of rheumatoid arthritis in adults***
*Adults:* 100 to 200 mg P.O. b.i.d.
***Adjunct to treatment for familial adenomatous polyposis to reduce the number of adenomatous colorectal polyps***
*Adults:* 400 mg P.O. b.i.d. with food for up to 6 months.
≡ ***Dosage adjustment.*** For patients weighing less than 50 kg (110 lb), start at lowest recommended dosage. For patients with moderate hepatic impairment (Child-Pugh Class II), start therapy with reduced dosage.

## Mechanism of action
*Anti-inflammatory, analgesic, and antipyretic actions:* Celecoxib is thought to act by selective inhibition of cyclooxygenase-2 (COX-2) resulting in decreased prostaglandin synthesis. Because celecoxib doesn't inhibit COX-1 at therapeutic levels, the reduction in symptoms of osteoarthritis and rheumatoid arthritis may be related to a lower risk of peripheral side effects.

## Pharmacokinetics
***Absorption:*** Steady-state plasma levels can be expected within 5 days if celecoxib is given in multiple dosages.
***Distribution:*** Highly protein bound, primarily to albumin.
***Metabolism:*** Primarily metabolized by cytochrome P-450 2C9.
***Excretion:*** Eliminated primarily by hepatic metabolism; 27% is excreted into the urine. Elimination half-life under fasting conditions is about 11 hours.

| Route | Onset | Peak | Duration |
|-------|-------|------|----------|
| P.O. | Unknown | 3 hr | Unknown |

## Contraindications and precautions
Contraindicated in patients with severe hepatic impairment or hypersensitivity to celecoxib, sulfonamides, aspirin, or other NSAIDs and during the third trimester of pregnancy.

Use cautiously in patients with history of ulcers or GI bleeding, advanced renal disease, anemia, symptomatic liver disease, hypertension, edema, heart failure, or asthma. Also use cautiously in patients who smoke or use alcohol chronically, in those taking oral corticosteroids or anticoagulants, and in elderly or debilitated patients.

## Interactions
**Drug-drug.** *Aluminum and magnesium antacids:* Possible decreased plasma levels of celecoxib. Give at least 1 hour apart.
*Angiotensin-converting enzyme inhibitors:* Diminished antihypertensive effects. Advise clinician to monitor blood pressure.
*Aspirin:* Increased risk of ulcers; low aspirin dosages can be used safely for prevention of CV events. Advise clinician to monitor patient for signs and symptoms of GI bleeding.
*Fluconazole:* Possible increased level of celecoxib. May need adjustment of celecoxib to minimal effective dosage.
*Furosemide:* NSAIDs can reduce sodium excretion caused by diuretics, leading to sodium retention. Observe patient for swelling and increase in blood pressure.
*Lithium:* Increased level may occur. Advise clinician to monitor lithium plasma levels.
*Warfarin:* A direct interaction hasn't been reported; however, advise clinician to observe patient for signs and symptoms of bleeding.
**Drug-herb.** *Dong quai, feverfew, garlic, ginger, horse chestnut, red clover:* Possible increased risk of bleeding. Discourage use together.
*Dong quai, St. John's wort:* Increased risk of photosensitivity. Advise patient to avoid unprotected exposure to sunlight.
**Drug-lifestyle.** *Alcohol use:* Possible increased risk of GI irritation or bleeding if used long-term. Discourage alcohol consumption. Observe patient for signs of bleeding.

## Adverse reactions
**CNS:** dizziness, *headache,* insomnia.
**CV:** *peripheral edema.*
**EENT:** pharyngitis, rhinitis, sinusitis.
**GI:** abdominal pain, diarrhea, dyspepsia, flatulence, nausea.
**GU:** elevated BUN.
**Hepatic:** elevated liver enzyme levels.
**Metabolic:** hyperchloremia, hypophosphatemia.
**Musculoskeletal:** *back pain.*
**Respiratory:** upper respiratory tract infection.
**Skin:** rash.
**Other:** *accidental injury.*

## Overdose and treatment
Common signs and symptoms of overdose include lethargy, drowsiness, nausea, vomiting, epigastric pain, and GI bleeding. Other possible symptoms include hypertension, acute renal failure, respiratory depression, and coma. Although there is no antidote for treatment of overdose, symptomatic and supportive care is usually sufficient. If a patient is seen within 4 hours of the overdose, emesis, activated charcoal, an osmotic cathartic, or a combination of these can be used. Because of the high protein-binding, dialysis is unlikely to be effective.

## Clinical considerations
■ Patients may be allergic to celecoxib if they have an allergy to sulfonamides, aspirin, or other NSAIDs.
■ Patients will need assessment for signs and symptoms of hepatic and renal toxicity, especially if they are dehydrated.
■ Patients with a history of ulcers or GI bleeding are at higher risk for GI bleeding.

**H*ALERT*** Read label carefully: Potential name confusion with Celebrex, Cerebyx, Celexa.

## Therapeutic monitoring
■ Aluminum and magnesium antacids may decrease the effect of celecoxib and should be given at least an hour apart.

## Special populations
**Breast-feeding patients.** It's unknown if drug appears in breast milk. Risks and benefits must be determined before using celecoxib in breast-feeding women.
**Pediatric patients.** Drug hasn't been studied in patients under age 18.
**Geriatric patients.** Dosage adjustment isn't needed unless the patient weighs less than 110 lb; however, geriatric patients experience more adverse effects overall.

## Patient counseling
■ Inform the patient that it may take several days before feeling consistent pain relief and to notify prescriber if no relief is experienced.
■ Advise patient to immediately report any signs of swelling, excessive fatigue, yellowing of the skin, flulike symptoms, any signs of bleeding or difficulty breathing.
■ Instruct the patient to take drug with food if stomach upset occurs.

## cephalexin hydrochloride
Keftab

## cephalexin monohydrate
Biocef, Keflex, Novo-Lexin*

*Pharmacologic classification:* first-generation cephalosporin
*Therapeutic classification:* antibiotic
*Pregnancy risk category B*

## Available forms
Available by prescription only
**cephalexin hydrochloride**
*Tablets:* 500 mg
**cephalexin monohydrate**
*Tablets (film-coated):* 250 mg, 500 mg
*Capsules:* 250 mg, 500 mg
*Suspension:* 125 mg/5 ml, 250 mg/5 ml

## Indications and dosages
*Respiratory, GU, skin and soft-tissue, or bone and joint infections caused by susceptible organisms*
*Adults:* 250 mg to 1 g P.O. q 6 hours.
*Children:* 25 to 50 mg/kg/day P.O. divided into three to four doses. For patients over age 1 with streptococcal pharyngitis or skin and structure infections, dose may be given q 12 hours.

*Otitis media*
*Adults:* 250 mg to 1 g P.O. q 6 hours.
*Children:* 75 to 100 mg/kg/day P.O. divided into four doses.
≣*Dosage adjustment.* To prevent toxic accumulation in patients with impaired renal function and creatinine clearance less than 40 ml/minute, give reduced dosage. If creatinine clearance is less than 5 ml/minute, give 250 mg q 12 to 24 hours; if it ranges between 5 and 10 ml/minute, give 250 mg q 12 hours; and if it's 11 to 40 ml/minute, give 500 mg q 8 to 12 hours.

## Mechanism of action
*Antibacterial action:* Cephalexin is primarily bactericidal; however, it may be bacteriostatic. Activity depends on the organism, tissue penetration, drug dosage, and rate of organism multiplication. It acts by adhering to bacterial penicillin-binding proteins, thereby inhibiting cell-wall synthesis.
  Drug is active against many gram-positive organisms, including penicillinase-producing *Staphylococcus aureus* and *S. epidermidis, Streptococcus pneumoniae,* group B streptococci, and group A beta-hemolytic streptococci; susceptible gram-negative organisms include *Klebsiella pneumoniae, Escherichia coli, Proteus mirabilis,* and *Shigella.*

## Pharmacokinetics
*Absorption:* Absorbed rapidly and completely from the GI tract after oral administration. The base monohydrate is probably converted to the hydrochloride in the stomach before absorption. Food delays but doesn't prevent complete absorption.
*Distribution:* Distributed widely into most body tissues and fluids, including the gallbladder, liver, kidneys, bone, sputum, bile, and pleural and synovial fluids; CSF penetration is poor. Cephalexin crosses the placenta, and is 6% to 15% protein-bound.
*Metabolism:* Not metabolized.
*Excretion:* Excreted primarily unchanged in urine by glomerular filtration and renal tubular secretion; small amounts of drug may appear in breast milk. Elimination half-life is about ½ to 1 hour in patients with normal renal function; 7½ to 14 hours in patients with severe renal impairment. Hemodialysis or peritoneal dialysis removes cephalexin.

| Route | Onset | Peak | Duration |
|-------|-------|------|----------|
| P.O. | Unknown | 1 hr | Unknown |

## Contraindications and precautions
Contraindicated in patients hypersensitive to cephalosporins. Use cautiously in patients with impaired renal function or penicillin allergy and in breast-feeding women.

## Interactions

**Drug-drug.** *Loop diuretics, nephrotoxic drugs (aminoglycosides, colistin, polymyxin B, vancomycin):* May increase the risk of nephrotoxicity. Advise clinician to monitor patient closely.

*Probenecid:* Competitively inhibits renal tubular secretion of cephalosporins, resulting in higher, prolonged serum levels of these drugs. May be used for this effect.

## Adverse reactions

**CNS:** dizziness, headache, fatigue, agitation, confusion, hallucinations.
**GI:** pseudomembranous colitis, *nausea, anorexia,* vomiting, *diarrhea,* gastritis, glossitis, dyspepsia, abdominal pain, anal pruritus, tenesmus, oral candidiasis.
**GU:** genital pruritus and candidiasis, vaginitis, interstitial nephritis.
**Hematologic:** *neutropenia,* eosinophilia, anemia, *thrombocytopenia.*
**Hepatic:** transient increases in liver enzymes.
**Musculoskeletal:** arthritis, arthralgia, joint pain.
**Skin:** *maculopapular and erythematous rash, urticaria.*
**Other:** hypersensitivity reactions, serum sickness, *anaphylaxis.*

## Overdose and treatment

Signs and symptoms of overdose include neuromuscular hypersensitivity; seizure may follow high CNS levels. Remove cephalexin by hemodialysis or peritoneal dialysis. Other treatment is supportive.

## Clinical considerations

- To prepare the oral suspension, add the required amount of water to the powder in two portions. Shake well after each addition. After mixing, store in refrigerator. Suspension is stable for 14 days without significant loss of potency. Store mixture in tightly closed container. Shake well before using.
- Because cephalexin is dialyzable, patients undergoing treatment with hemodialysis or peritoneal dialysis may need dosage adjustment.
- Drug causes false-positive results in urine glucose tests using cupric sulfate (Benedict's reagent or Clinitest); use glucose oxidase test (Chemstrip uG, Diastix, or glucose enzymatic test strip) instead. Cephalexin also causes false elevations in serum or urine creatinine levels using Jaffé's reaction. Positive Coombs' test results occur in about 3% of patients taking cephalexin.

## Therapeutic monitoring

- With large doses or prolonged therapy, advise clinician to monitor patient for superinfection, especially in high-risk patients.

## Special populations

**Breast-feeding patients.** Drug appears in breast milk; use with caution in breast-feeding women.
**Pediatric patients.** Serum half-life is prolonged in neonates and in infants under age 1. Safety and effectiveness in children haven't been established.
**Geriatric patients.** Reduced dosage may be needed in geriatric patients with diminished renal function.

## Patient counseling

- Inform patient of potential adverse reactions.
- Instruct patient to take drug with food to avoid GI upset.

# cephradine
Velosef

*Pharmacologic classification:* first-generation cephalosporin
*Therapeutic classification:* antibiotic
*Pregnancy risk category B*

## Available forms

Available by prescription only
*Capsules:* 250 mg, 500 mg
*Suspension:* 125 mg/5 ml, 250 mg/5 ml

## Indications and dosages

***Serious respiratory, GU, skin and soft-tissue, bone and joint infections; septicemia; endocarditis; and otitis media***
*Adults:* 250 to 500 mg P.O. q 6 hours. Severe or chronic infections may need larger or more frequent doses (up to 1 g P.O. q 6 hours).
*Children over age 9 months:* 25 to 100 mg/kg P.O. daily in equally divided doses q 6 to 12 hours.

Larger doses (up to 1 g q.i.d.) may be given for severe or chronic infections in all patients regardless of age and weight.
≣*Dosage adjustment.* To prevent toxic accumulation, reduced dosage may be needed in patients with creatinine clearance below 20 ml/minute.

| Creatinine clearance (ml/min) | Adult dosage |
| --- | --- |
| 5-20 | 250 mg q 6 hr |
| < 5 | 250 mg q 12 hr |

For patients on chronic intermittent dialysis, give 250 mg initially; repeat in 12 hours and after 36 to 48 hours. Children may need dose modifications proportional to weight and severity of infection.

## Mechanism of action
*Antibacterial action:* Primarily bactericidal; however, it may be bacteriostatic. Activity depends on the organism, tissue penetration, drug dosage, and rate of organism multiplication. It acts by adhering to bacterial penicillin-binding proteins, inhibiting cell-wall synthesis.

Like other first-generation cephalosporins, cephradine is active against many gram-positive organisms and some gram-negative organisms. Susceptible organisms include *Escherichia coli* and other coliform bacteria, group A beta-hemolytic streptococci, *Haemophilus influenzae, Klebsiella, Proteus mirabilis, Staphylococcus aureus, Streptococcus pneumoniae,* staphylococci, and *Streptococcus viridans.*

## Pharmacokinetics
*Absorption:* Well absorbed from the GI tract.
*Distribution:* Distributed widely into most body tissues and fluids, including the gallbladder, liver, kidneys, bone, sputum, bile, and pleural and synovial fluids; CSF penetration is poor. Cephradine crosses the placenta, and is 6% to 20% protein-bound.
*Metabolism:* Not metabolized.
*Excretion:* Excreted primarily in urine by renal tubular and glomerular filtration; small amounts of drug appear in breast milk. Elimination half-life is about ½ to 2 hours in normal renal function; end-stage renal disease prolongs half-life to 8 to 15 hours. Hemodialysis or peritoneal dialysis removes drug.

| Route | Onset | Peak | Duration |
|-------|-------|------|----------|
| P.O. | Unknown | 1 hr | Unknown |

## Contraindications and precautions
Contraindicated in patients hypersensitive to drug and other cephalosporins. Use cautiously in patients with impaired renal function and penicillin allergy and in breast-feeding women.

## Interactions
**Drug-drug.** *Bacteriostatic drugs (chloramphenicol, erythromycin, tetracyclines):* May interfere with bactericidal activity. Avoid use together.
*Loop diuretics, nephrotoxic drugs (aminoglycosides, colistin, polymyxin B, vancomycin):* May increase the risk of nephrotoxicity. Advise clinician to monitor patient closely.
*Probenecid:* Competitively inhibits renal tubular secretion of cephalosporins, resulting in higher, prolonged serum levels of these drugs. Sometimes used for this effect.

## Adverse reactions
**CNS:** dizziness, headache, malaise, paresthesia.
**GI:** pseudomembranous colitis, *nausea, anorexia,* vomiting, heartburn, abdominal cramps, *diarrhea,* oral candidiasis.

**GU:** genital pruritus and candidiasis, vaginitis.
**Hematologic:** *transient neutropenia,* eosinophilia, *thrombocytopenia.*
**Hepatic:** transient increases in liver enzymes.
**Skin:** *maculopapular and erythematous rash, urticaria.*
**Other:** hypersensitivity reactions, serum sickness, *anaphylaxis.*

## Overdose and treatment
Signs and symptoms of overdose include neuromuscular hypersensitivity; seizure may follow high CNS levels. Cephradine should be removed by hemodialysis.

## Clinical considerations
**⚠ALERT** Names of some cephalosporins are similar. Use caution when dispensing.
■ Reconstituted oral suspension may be stored for 7 days at controlled room temperature or for 14 days in the refrigerator.
■ Because drug is dialyzable, patients undergoing treatment with hemodialysis may need dosage adjustments.
■ Drug causes false-positive results in urine glucose tests using cupric sulfate (Benedict's reagent or Clinitest); use glucose oxidase tests (Chemstrip uG, Diastix, or glucose enzymatic test strip) instead. Cephradine also causes false elevations in serum or urine creatinine levels in tests using Jaffé's reaction. Cephradine may cause positive Coombs' test results.

### Therapeutic monitoring
■ With large doses or prolonged therapy, watch for superinfection, especially in high-risk patients.

### Special populations
**Breast-feeding patients.** Drug appears in breast milk; use with caution in breast-feeding women. Safety hasn't been established.
**Pediatric patients.** Serum half-life is prolonged in neonates and infants under age 12 months. Safety hasn't been established.
**Geriatric patients.** Reduced dosage may be required in patients with reduced renal function. Use with caution.

## Patient counseling
■ Inform patient of potential adverse reactions.
■ Inform patient to take drug with food to lessen GI upset.
■ Inform patient to take all of the drug as prescribed, even if he feels better.

# cetirizine hydrochloride
Zyrtec

*Pharmacologic classification:* selective H₁-receptor antagonist
*Therapeutic classification:* antihistamine
*Pregnancy risk category B*

## Available forms
Available by prescription only
*Tablets (film-coated):* 5 mg, 10 mg
*Syrup:* 5 mg/5 ml

## Indications and dosages
*Seasonal allergic rhinitis, perennial allergic rhinitis, chronic urticaria*
Adults and children ages 6 and older: 5 or 10 mg P.O. daily.
≡*Dosage adjustment.* For hemodialysis patients or those with hepatic impairment or creatinine clearance less than 31 ml/minute, 5 mg P.O. daily.

## Mechanism of action
*Antihistaminic action:* Cetirizine's principal effects are mediated by way of selective inhibition of peripheral H₁ receptors.

## Pharmacokinetics
*Absorption:* Rapidly absorbed.
*Distribution:* About 93% plasma protein–bound.
*Metabolism:* Metabolized to a very limited extent by oxidative O-dealkylation to a metabolite with negligible antihistaminic activity.
*Excretion:* Primarily excreted in urine with 50% as unchanged drug. A small amount is excreted in feces.

| Route | Onset | Peak | Duration |
|-------|-------|------|----------|
| P.O. | 20-60 min | ½-1½ hr | 24 hr |

## Contraindications and precautions
Contraindicated in patients hypersensitive to drug or hydroxyzine. Use cautiously in patients with impaired renal function.

## Interactions
**Drug-drug.** *Anticholinergics, CNS depressants:* May cause a possible additive effect. Avoid use together.
*Theophylline:* May cause decreased clearance of cetirizine. Advise clinician to monitor patient closely.
**Drug-lifestyle.** *Alcohol use:* May cause a possible additive effect. Avoid use together.

## Adverse reactions
**CNS:** somnolence, fatigue, dizziness.
**EENT:** pharyngitis.
**GI:** dry mouth.

## Overdose and treatment
Overdose may result in somnolence. If overdose occurs, treatment should be symptomatic or supportive. There is no known specific antidote for cetirizine and the drug isn't effectively removed by dialysis.

## Clinical considerations
■ There is no information to indicate that abuse or dependency occurs with cetirizine use.
◨ *ALERT* Don't confuse Zantac (ranitidine) and Zyrtec (certirizine).

### Therapeutic monitoring
■ Discontinue drug 4 days before performing diagnostic skin tests; it can prevent, reduce, or mask positive skin test response.

### Special populations
**Breast-feeding patients.** Drug reportedly appears in breast milk. Avoid use in breast-feeding women.
**Pediatric patients.** Safety and efficacy in children under age 6 haven't been established.
**Geriatric patients.** Half-life of the drug may be prolonged, as may total body clearance. No dosage adjustments are needed, however.

## Patient counseling
■ Caution patient not to perform hazardous activities if somnolence occurs with drug use.
■ Tell patient that coffee or tea may help reduce drowsiness.

---

# cetrorelix acetate
Cetrotide

*Pharmacologic classification:* gonadotropin-releasing hormone (GnRH) analogue
*Therapeutic classification:* infertility drug
*Pregnancy risk category X*

## Available forms
Available by prescription only
*Powder for injection:* 0.25 mg, 3 mg

## Indications and dosages
*Inhibition of premature luteinizing hormone surges in women undergoing controlled ovarian stimulation*
Adults: 3 mg S.C. once during early to mid follicular phase given when the serum estradiol level is indicative of an appropriate stimulation response, usually on stimulation day 7 (range day 5 to 9). If human chorionic gonadotropin (hCG) hasn't been given within 4 days after injection, cetrorelix 0.25 mg should be given S.C. once daily until the day of hCG administration. Or, 0.25 mg S.C. multiple-dose regimen is given on either stimulation day 5 (morning or evening) or day 6 (morning) and

continued once daily until the day of hCG administration.

## Mechanism of action
*GnRH antagonist action:* Cetrorelix acetate competes with natural GnRH for binding to membrane receptors on pituitary cells, which controls the release of LH and follicle-stimulating hormone (FSH).

## Pharmacokinetics
*Absorption:* Rapidly absorbed following subcutaneous injection. Levels peak 1 to 2 hours after administration.
*Distribution:* 86% human plasma–bound.
*Metabolism:* After subcutaneous administration of 10 mg, small amounts of drug were found in bile samples over 24 hours.
*Excretion:* Excreted unchanged in urine and as metabolites in bile.

| Route | Onset  | Peak   | Duration |
|-------|--------|--------|----------|
| S.C.  | 1-2 hr | 1-2 hr | ≥ 4 days |

## Contraindications and precautions
Contraindicated in patients hypersensitive to cetrorelix acetate, extrinsic peptide hormones, mannitol, GnRH, or other GnRH analogues. Also contraindicated in women with known or suspected pregnancy and in breast-feeding women.

## Interactions
None reported.

## Adverse reactions
**CNS:** headache.
**GI:** nausea.
**GU:** ovarian hyperstimulation syndrome.
**Hepatic:** elevated ALT, AST, GGT, and alkaline phosphatase levels.

## Overdose and treatment
There have been no reported overdoses with cetrorelix acetate. Single doses up to 120 mg have been well tolerated in patients treated for other indications without signs of overdose.

## Clinical considerations
■ Only prescribers experienced in fertility treatment should prescribe drug.
■ Dosage is adjusted according to patient response.
■ When ultrasound shows a sufficient number or follicles of adequate size, hCG is given to induce ovulation and maturation of oocytes.
■ hCG shouldn't be given if ovaries show an excessive response to treatment to reduce the risk of ovarian hyperstimulation syndrome.
■ Drug can be given by the patient after proper instruction.

## Therapeutic monitoring
■ Pregnancy must be excluded before starting treatment.

## Special populations
**Pregnant patients.** Not for use during pregnancy.
**Breast-feeding patients.** It's not known if drug appears in breast milk. Don't give drug to breast-feeding women.
**Pediatric patients.** Not for use in children.

## Patient counseling
■ Instruct patient on proper administration technique and stress importance of strict compliance.
■ Instruct patient to store cetrorelix acetate 3 mg at controlled room temperature (77° F [25° C]) and to store cetrorelix acetate 0.25 mg in the refrigerator (36° to 46° F [2° to 8° C]).
■ Instruct patient to contact prescriber if side effect becomes bothersome.

# cevimeline hydrochloride
Evoxac

*Pharmacologic classification:* cholinergic agonist
*Therapeutic classification:* prosecretory
*Pregnancy risk category C*

## Available forms
Available by prescription only
*Tablets:* 30 mg

## Indications and dosages
*Symptoms of dry mouth in patients with Sjögren's syndrome*
*Adults:* 30 mg P.O. t.i.d.

## Mechanism of action
*Prosecretory action:* As a cholinergic agonist, cevimeline binds to and stimulates muscarinic receptors. This results in increased secretion of exocrine glands that causes salivation, sweating, and increases tone of smooth muscles in the GI and GU tracts.

## Pharmacokinetics
*Absorption:* Rapidly absorbed. Plasma levels peak between 1½ and 2 hours. Food decreases rate of absorption and peak level is reduced by 17.3%.
*Distribution:* Less than 20% protein-bound.
*Metabolism:* The liver enzymes CYP2D6, CYP3A3, and CYP3A4 are involved in the metabolism of cevimeline. Drug is metabolized to a number of metabolites.

*Excretion:* Excreted primarily in urine and has a half-life of about 5 hours.

| Route | Onset | Peak | Duration |
|-------|-------|------|----------|
| P.O. | Unknown | 1½-2 hr | Unknown |

## Contraindications and precautions

Contraindicated in patients hypersensitive to drug. Also contraindicated in patients with uncontrolled asthma, or when miosis is undesirable, such as in acute iritis or angle-closure glaucoma.

Use cautiously in patients with significant CV disease, evidenced by angina pectoris or MI, because it can alter cardiac conduction and heart rate. Use cautiously in patients with controlled asthma, chronic bronchitis or COPD because it can cause bronchial constriction and increase bronchial secretions. Use cautiously in patients with a history of nephrolithiasis because an increase in ureteral smooth-muscle tone could cause renal colic or ureteral reflux. Use cautiously in patients with cholelithiasis because contractions of the gallbladder or biliary smooth muscle could cause cholecystitis, cholangitis, and biliary obstruction.

## Interactions

**Drug-drug.** *Beta-adrenergic antagonists:* Possible conduction disturbances. Use cautiously.
*Drugs that inhibit CYP2D6, CYP3A4, CYP3A3:* Increased cevimeline levels. Advise clinician to monitor patient closely.
*Parasympathomimetics:* Additive effects. Use cautiously.

## Adverse reactions

**CNS:** anxiety, depression, dizziness, fatigue, *headache,* hypesthesia, insomnia, migraine, pain, tremor, vertigo.
**CV:** chest pain, palpitations, peripheral edema, edema.
**EENT:** abnormal vision, conjunctivitis, earache, epistaxis, eye infection, eye pain, otitis media, pharyngitis, *rhinitis, sinusitis,* xerophthalmia, eye abnormality.
**GI:** abdominal pain, anorexia, constipation, *diarrhea,* dry mouth, eructation, excessive salivation, flatulence, gastroesophageal reflux, *nausea,* salivary gland enlargement and pain, sialadenitis, ulcerative stomatitis, vomiting, dyspepsia, tooth disorder, toothache.
**GU:** cystitis, candidiasis, urinary tract infection, vaginitis.
**Hematologic:** anemia.
**Hepatic:** increased amylase levels.
**Musculoskeletal:** arthralgia, back pain, hypertonia, hyporeflexia, leg cramps, myalgia, rigors, skeletal pain.
**Respiratory:** *upper respiratory tract infection,* bronchitis, pneumonia, coughing, hiccups.
**Skin:** rash, pruritus, skin disorder, erythematous rash, *excessive sweating.*

**Other:** fever, fungal infections, flulike symptoms, injury, surgical intervention, hot flushes, postoperative pain, allergic reaction, infection, abscess.

## Overdose and treatment

Toxicity is characterized by exaggeration of parasympathomimetic effects, which may include headache, visual disturbance, lacrimation, sweating, respiratory distress, GI spasm, nausea, vomiting, diarrhea, AV block, tachycardia, bradycardia, hypotension, shock, mental confusion, cardiac arrhythmias, and tremors. General supportive treatment should be instituted. If medically indicated, atropine may be of value as an antidote. Epinephrine may be useful in the presence of severe CV depression or bronchconstriction. It's not known if cevimeline is dialyzable.

## Clinical considerations

■ Sweating is a common side effect of drug. Fluid intake is important to prevent dehydration.
■ Drug may cause visual disturbances, especially at night, that can impair driving ability.

### Therapeutic monitoring

■ Advise clinician to monitor patients with a history of asthma, COPD, or chronic bronchitis for an increase in such symptoms as wheezing, increased sputum production, or cough.
■ Advise clinician to monitor patients with a history of cardiac disease for increased frequency, severity, or duration of angina or changes in heart rate.

### Special populations

**Breast-feeding patients.** It's not known if drug appears in breast milk. A decision should be made to either continue breast-feeding or discontinue drug based on importance of drug to mother.
**Pediatric patients.** Safety and efficacy haven't been established.
**Geriatric patients.** Advise clinician to monitor these patients closely because of greater frequency of decreased renal, hepatic, and cardiac function and the likelihood of concomitant disease and the use of other drugs.

## Patient counseling

■ Tell patient not to interrupt or discontinue treatment without medical approval.
■ Instruct patient to avoid driving at night and to be alert to changes in visual acuity.

# chlorambucil
Leukeran

*Pharmacologic classification:* alkylating agent (cell cycle–phase nonspecific)
*Therapeutic classification:* antineoplastic
*Pregnancy risk category D*

## Available forms
Available by prescription only
*Tablets (sugar-coated):* 2 mg

## Indications and dosages
Dosage and indications may vary. Check current literature for recommended protocol.
*Chronic lymphocytic leukemia, malignant lymphomas including lymphosarcoma, giant follicular lymphomas, Hodgkin's disease, ◇autoimmune hemolytic anemias, ◇nephrotic syndrome, ◇polycythemia vera, ◇macroglobulinemia, ◇ovarian neoplasms*
*Adults:* 100 to 200 mcg/kg P.O. daily or 3 to 6 mg/m² P.O. daily as a single dose or in divided doses, for 3 to 6 weeks. Usual dose is 4 to 10 mg daily. Reduce dose if full course of radiation therapy is planned within 4 weeks.
*◇Macroglobulinemia*
*Adults:* 2 to 10 mg P.O. daily.
*◇Metastatic trophoblastic neoplasia*
*Adults:* 6 to 10 mg P.O. daily for 5 days; repeat q 1 to 2 weeks.
*◇Idiopathic uveitis*
*Adults:* 6 to 12 mg P.O. daily for 1 year.
*◇Rheumatoid arthritis*
*Adults:* 0.1 to 0.3 mg/kg P.O. daily.

## Mechanism of action
*Antineoplastic action:* Chlorambucil exerts its cytotoxic activity by cross-linking strands of cellular DNA and RNA, disrupting normal nucleic acid function.

## Pharmacokinetics
*Absorption:* Well absorbed from the GI tract.
*Distribution:* Not well understood. However, drug and its metabolites have been shown to be highly bound to plasma and tissue proteins.
*Metabolism:* Metabolized in the liver. Its primary metabolite, phenylacetic acid mustard, also possesses cytotoxic activity.
*Excretion:* Metabolites are excreted in urine. Half-life of parent compound is 2 hours; the phenylacetic acid metabolite, 2½ hours.

| Route | Onset | Peak | Duration |
|-------|-------|------|----------|
| P.O. | 3-4 wk | 1 hr | Unknown |

## Contraindications and precautions
Contraindicated in patients with hypersensitivity or resistance to previous therapy. Patients hypersensitive to other alkylating drugs also may be hypersensitive to drug. Use cautiously in patients with history of head trauma or seizures and in those receiving other drugs that lower seizure threshold.

## Interactions
*Drug-drug. Anticoagulants, aspirin:* Increased risk of bleeding. Avoid use together.
*Myelosuppressants:* Concurrent use can cause additive myelosuppression. Advise clinician to monitor patient closely.

## Adverse reactions
**CNS:** *seizures,* peripheral neuropathy, tremor, muscle twitching, confusion, agitation, ataxia, flaccid paresis.
**GI:** *nausea, vomiting, stomatitis,* diarrhea.
**GU:** *azoospermia, infertility.*
**Hematologic:** *neutropenia,* delayed up to 3 weeks, lasting up to 10 days after last dose; *bone marrow suppression; thrombocytopenia; anemia.*
**Hepatic:** *hepatotoxicity.*
**Respiratory:** interstitial pneumonitis, *pulmonary fibrosis.*
**Skin:** rash, hypersensitivity.
**Other:** allergic febrile reaction.

## Overdose and treatment
Signs and symptoms of overdose include reversible pancytopenia in adults, and vomiting, ataxia, abdominal pain, muscle twitching, and major motor seizures in children.

Treatment is usually supportive with transfusion of blood components, if needed, and appropriate anticonvulsant therapy if seizures occur. Induction of emesis, activated charcoal, and gastric lavage may be useful in removing unabsorbed drug. Drug is probably not dialyzable.

## Clinical considerations
■ Oral suspension can be prepared in the pharmacy by crushing tablets and mixing powder with a suspending agent and simple syrup.
■ I.M. injections shouldn't be given when platelets are below 100,000/mm³.
■ Store tablets in a tightly closed, light-resistant container.

### Therapeutic monitoring
■ Drug-induced pancytopenia generally lasts 1 to 2 weeks but may persist for 3 to 4 weeks. It's reversible up to a cumulative dose of 6.5 mg/kg in a single course.
■ To prevent hyperuricemia with resulting uric acid nephropathy, allopurinol may be used with adequate hydration.

### Special populations
**Pregnant patients.** Drug should be used only in life-threatening cases, or when safer drugs can't be used or are ineffective. Inform patient of potential hazards to fetus.

**Breast-feeding patients.** It's unknown if drug appears in breast milk. Consider risk of potential serious adverse reactions, mutagenicity, and carcinogenicity in breast-feeding infant and the woman's need for the drug in deciding whether to discontinue drug or breast-feeding.

**Pediatric patients.** Safety and efficacy in children haven't been established. The potential benefits versus risks must be evaluated.

## Patient counseling

- Emphasize importance of continuing drug despite nausea and vomiting, and of keeping appointments for periodic blood work.
- Advise patient to report if vomiting occurs shortly after taking dose or if symptoms of infection or bleeding are present.
- Tell patient to avoid exposure to people with infections.

---

## chloramphenicol
Ak-Chlor, Chloromycetin, Chloroptic, Fenicol*, Ocu-chlor, Pentamycetin*

## chloramphenicol sodium succinate
Chloromycetin Sodium Succinate, Pentamycetin*

*Pharmacologic classification:* dichloroacetic acid derivative
*Therapeutic classification:* antibiotic
*Pregnancy risk category C*

## Available forms
Available by prescription only
*Powder for solution:* 25 mg/vial
*Injection:* 1-g vial
*Ophthalmic solution:* 0.5%
*Ophthalmic ointment:* 1%
*Otic solution:* 0.5%

## Indications and dosages
*Severe meningitis, brain abscesses, bacteremia, or other serious infections*
*Adults and children:* 50 to 100 mg/kg I.V. daily, divided q 6 hours. Maximum dose, 100 mg/kg daily.
*Premature infants and neonates weighing less than 2 kg (4.4 lb) or under age 7 days:* 25 mg/kg I.V. daily.
*Neonates weighing more than 2 kg and ages 7 days and older:* 25 mg/kg I.V. q 12 hours. I.V. route must be used to treat meningitis.
*Superficial infections of the skin caused by susceptible bacteria*
*Adults and children:* Rub into affected area b.i.d. or t.i.d.
*External ear canal infection*
*Adults and children:* Instill 2 to 3 drops into ear canal t.i.d. or q.i.d.

*Surface bacterial infection involving conjunctiva or cornea*
*Adults and children:* Instill 2 drops of solution in eye q hour until condition improves, or instill q.i.d., depending on severity of infection. Apply small amount of ointment to lower conjunctival sac h.s. as supplement to drops. To use ointment alone, apply small amount to lower conjunctival sac q 3 to 6 hours or more frequently, p.r.n. Continue with treatment up to 48 hours after condition improves.

## I.V. administration
- Reconstitute 1-g vial of powder for injection with 10 ml of sterile water for injection; level will be 100 mg/ml.
- Solution remains stable for 30 days at controlled room temperature; however, refrigeration is recommended. Don't use cloudy solutions.
- Recommend giving I.V. infusion slowly, over at least 1 minute.

## Incompatibilities
Chloramphenicol sodium succinate is incompatible with many drugs, depending on the level of the drugs, specific diluents used, resulting pH, and temperature.

## Mechanism of action
*Antibacterial action:* Chloramphenicol and chloramphenicol sodium succinate must be hydrolyzed to chloramphenicol before antimicrobial activity can take place. The active compound then inhibits bacterial protein synthesis by binding to the 50S subunit of the ribosome, thus inhibiting peptide bond formation.

Drug usually produces bacteriostatic effects on susceptible bacteria, including *Rickettsia, Chlamydia, Mycoplasma,* and certain *Salmonella* strains, as well as most gram-positive and gram-negative organisms. Chloramphenicol is used to treat *Haemophilus influenzae* infection, Rocky Mountain spotted fever, meningitis, lymphogranuloma, psittacosis, severe meningitis, and bacteremia.

## Pharmacokinetics
*Absorption:* With I.V. administration, serum levels vary greatly, depending on patient's metabolism.
*Distribution:* Distributed widely to most body tissues and fluids, including CSF, liver, and kidneys; it readily crosses the placenta. About 50% to 60% plasma protein–bound.
*Metabolism:* Parent drug is metabolized primarily by hepatic glucuronyl transferase to inactive metabolites.
*Excretion:* About 8% to 12% of dose is excreted by the kidneys as unchanged drug; the remainder is excreted as inactive metabolites. (However, some drug may appear in breast milk.) Plasma half-life ranges from about 1½ to 4½ hours in adults with normal hepatic and

renal function. Plasma half-life of parent drug is prolonged in patients with hepatic dysfunction. Peritoneal hemodialysis doesn't remove significant drug amounts. Plasma chloramphenicol levels may be elevated in patients with renal impairment after I.V. chloramphenicol administration.

| Route | Onset | Peak | Duration |
|---|---|---|---|
| I.V. | Unknown | 1-3 hr | Unknown |
| Ophthalmic | Unknown | Unknown | Unknown |
| Otic | Unknown | Unknown | Unknown |

## Contraindications and precautions

Contraindicated in patients hypersensitive to chloramphenicol. Use cautiously in patients with impaired renal or hepatic function, acute intermittent porphyria, or G6PD deficiency and in those taking drugs that suppress bone marrow function.

## Interactions

**Drug-drug.** *Acetaminophen:* Elevated serum chloramphenicol level (by an unknown mechanism), possibly resulting in an enhanced pharmacologic effect. This may be useful. Advise clinician to monitor patient for adverse reactions.

*Chlorpropamide, cyclophosphamide, dicumarol, phenobarbital, phenytoin, and tolbutamide:* Chloramphenicol inhibits hepatic metabolism (by inhibiting microsomal enzyme activity); that leads to prolonged plasma half-life of these drugs and possible toxicity from increased serum drug levels. Avoid use together.

*Folic acid, iron salts,* and *vitamin $B_2$:* Reduced hematologic response to these substances. Advise clinician to monitor patient closely.

*Penicillin:* Chloramphenicol may antagonize the bactericidal activity. Give penicillin 1 hour or more before giving chloramphenicol.

## Adverse reactions

**CNS:** headache, mild depression, confusion, delirium, peripheral neuropathy with prolonged therapy.

**EENT:** optic neuritis (in patients with cystic fibrosis), decreased visual acuity, optic atrophy in children, stinging of eye after instillation, blurred vision (with ointment).

**GI:** nausea, vomiting, stomatitis, diarrhea, enterocolitis, glossitis.

**Hematologic:** *aplastic anemia, hypoplastic anemia, agranulocytosis, thrombocytopenia.*

**Hepatic:** jaundice.

**Skin:** possible contact sensitivity; burning, urticaria, pruritus, rash.

**Other:** fever, *anaphylaxis,* hemoglobinuria, lactic acidosis, *gray syndrome in neonates* (abdominal distention, gray cyanosis, vasomotor collapse, respiratory distress, death within a few hours of onset of symptoms), *angioedema* in hypersensitive patients.

## Overdose and treatment

Clinical effects of parenterally administered overdose include anemia and metabolic acidosis followed by hypotension, hypothermia, and abdominal distention, and possibly, death.

Initial treatment is symptomatic and supportive. Drug may be removed by charcoal hemoperfusion.

## Clinical considerations

■ Culture and sensitivity tests may be performed concurrently with first dose and repeated p.r.n.

■ Use drug only when clearly indicated for severe infection. Because of drug's potential for severe toxicity, it should be reserved for potentially life-threatening infections.

■ Refrigerate ophthalmic solution.

■ Therapeutic range is 10 to 20 mcg/ml for peak levels and 5 to 10 mcg/ml for trough levels.

■ False elevation of urinary para-aminobenzoic acid (PABA) levels will result if chloramphenicol is given during a bentiromide test for pancreatic function. Drug therapy will cause false-positive results on tests for urine glucose level using cupric sulfate (Clinitest).

## *Therapeutic monitoring*

■ CBC, platelet count, reticulocyte count, and serum iron level are needed before therapy begins and every 2 days during therapy. Discontinue drug immediately if test results indicate anemia, reticulocytopenia, leukopenia, or thrombocytopenia.

■ Advise clinician to observe patient for signs and symptoms of superinfection by nonsusceptible organisms.

■ Injection site should be checked daily for phlebitis and irritation.

## *Special populations*

**Breast-feeding patients.** Drug appears in breast milk in low levels, posing risk of bone marrow depression and slight risk of gray syndrome. Alternative feeding method is recommended during treatment with chloramphenicol.

**Pediatric patients.** Use drug cautiously in children under age 2 because of risk of gray syndrome (although most cases occur in first 48 hours after birth). Drug has prolonged half-life in neonates, necessitating reduced dose.

**Geriatric patients.** Give drug cautiously to geriatric patients with impaired liver function.

## Patient counseling

■ Instruct patient to report adverse reactions, especially nausea, vomiting, diarrhea, bleeding, fever, confusion, sore throat, or mouth sores.

■ Tell patient to take drug for prescribed period and to take it exactly as directed, even after he feels better.

■ Instruct patient to wash hands before and after applying topical ointment or solution.

---

- Warn patient using otic solution not to touch ear with dropper.
- Caution patient using topical cream to avoid sharing washcloths and towels with family members.
- Tell patient using ophthalmic drug to clean eye area of excess exudate before applying drug; show him how to instill drug in eye. Warn him not to touch applicator tip to eye or surrounding tissue. Instruct him to observe for signs and symptoms of sensitivity, such as itchy eyelids or constant burning, and to discontinue drug and call prescriber immediately should any occur.

# chlordiazepoxide
Libritabs

# chlordiazepoxide hydrochloride
Librium, Mitran, Reposans-10

*Pharmacologic classification:* benzodiazepine
*Therapeutic classification:* anxiolytic, anticonvulsant, sedative-hypnotic
*Pregnancy risk category D*
*Controlled substance schedule IV*

## Available forms
Available by prescription only
*Tablets:* 5 mg, 10 mg, 25 mg
*Capsules:* 5 mg, 10 mg, 25 mg
*Powder for injection:* 100 mg/ampule

## Indications and dosages
*Mild to moderate anxiety and tension*
*Adults:* 5 to 10 mg P.O. t.i.d. or q.i.d.
*Children over age 6 and elderly or debilitated patients:* 5 mg P.O. b.i.d. to q.i.d. Maximum dose, 10 mg P.O. b.i.d. or t.i.d.
*Severe anxiety and tension*
*Adults:* 20 to 25 mg P.O. t.i.d. or q.i.d.
*Withdrawal symptoms of acute alcoholism*
*Adults:* 50 to 100 mg P.O., I.M., or I.V. Maximum dose, 300 mg/day.
*Preoperative apprehension and anxiety*
*Adults:* 5 to 10 mg P.O. t.i.d. or q.i.d. on day before surgery; or 50 to 100 mg I.M. 1 hour before surgery.
   Note: Parenteral form isn't recommended in children under age 12.

## I.V. administration
- Prepare solutions immediately before administration. Discard unused portions.
- Reconstitute drug with sterile water or normal saline solution and infuse slowly, directly into a large vein, at a rate not exceeding 50 mg/minute for adults.
- Chlordiazepoxide shouldn't be infused into small veins. Avoid extravasation into S.C. tissue.

- Resuscitation equipment should be kept nearby in case of an emergency.

## Incompatibilities
Manufacturer recommends that chlordiazepoxide not be mixed with any drug.

## Mechanism of action
*Anticonvulsant action:* Drug suppresses the spread of seizure activity produced by the epileptogenic foci in the cortex, thalamus, and limbic structures by enhancing presynaptic inhibition.
*Anxiolytic:* Chlordiazepoxide depresses the CNS at the limbic and subcortical levels of the brain. It produces an anxiolytic effect by influencing the effect of the neurotransmitter gamma-aminobutyric acid (GABA) on its receptor in the ascending reticular activating system, which increases inhibition and blocks both cortical and limbic arousal after stimulation of the reticular formation.

## Pharmacokinetics
*Absorption:* When given orally, is absorbed well through the GI tract. I.M. administration results in erratic absorption.
*Distribution:* Distributed widely throughout the body; 90% to 98% is protein-bound.
*Metabolism:* Metabolized in the liver to several active metabolites.
*Excretion:* Most metabolites are excreted in urine as glucuronide conjugates. Half-life of drug is 5 to 30 hours.

| Route | Onset | Peak | Duration |
|-------|-------|------|----------|
| P.O. | Unknown | ½-4 hr | Unknown |
| I.V. | 1-5 min | Unknown | 15-60 min |
| I.M. | 15-30 min | Unknown | Unknown |

## Contraindications and precautions
Contraindicated in patients hypersensitive to drug. Use cautiously in patients with impaired renal or hepatic function, mental depression, or porphyria.

## Interactions
**Drug-drug.** *Antacids:* May delay the absorption of chlordiazepoxide. Advise clinician to monitor patient closely.
*Antidepressants, antihistamines, barbiturates, general anesthetics, MAO inhibitors, narcotics, phenothiazines:* Chlordiazepoxide potentiates the CNS depressant effects. Avoid use together.
*Cimetidine, possibly disulfiram:* Diminishes hepatic metabolism of chlordiazepoxide, which increases its plasma levels. Advise clinician to monitor patient carefully.
*Digoxin, phenytoin:* Levels may be increased. Avoid use together.
*Haloperidol:* May decrease serum levels. Avoid use together.

*Levodopa:* May decrease the therapeutic effects of levodopa. Avoid use together.

*Oral contraceptives:* May impair the metabolism of chlordiazepoxide. Avoid use together.

**Drug-herb.** *Catnip, kava, lady's slipper, lemon balm, passion flower, sassafras, skullcap, valerian:* Sedative effects may be enhanced. Discourage use together.

**Drug-lifestyle.** *Alcohol use:* Potentiates the CNS depressant effects. Discourage use together.

*Heavy smoking:* Accelerates chlordiazepoxide's metabolism, thus lowering clinical effectiveness. Discourage use together.

## Adverse reactions
**CNS:** *drowsiness, lethargy,* ataxia, confusion, extrapyramidal symptoms, EEG changes.
**GI:** nausea, constipation.
**GU:** menstrual irregularities.
**Hematologic:** *agranulocytosis.*
**Hepatic:** jaundice.
**Skin:** *swelling, pain at injection site,* skin eruptions, increased or decreased libido.

## Overdose and treatment
Signs and symptoms of overdose include somnolence, confusion, coma, hypoactive reflexes, dyspnea, labored breathing, hypotension, bradycardia, slurred speech, and unsteady gait or impaired coordination.

Support blood pressure and respiration until drug effects subside; advise clinician to monitor vital signs. Flumazenil, a specific benzodiazepine antagonist, may be useful. Mechanical ventilatory assistance via endotracheal tube may be required to maintain a patent airway and support adequate oxygenation. Recommend the use of I.V. fluids and vasopressors, such as dopamine and phenylephrine, to treat hypotension p.r.n. Recommend using gastric lavage if ingestion was recent, but only if an endotracheal tube is in place to prevent aspiration. Recommend inducing emesis if the patient is conscious. After emesis or lavage, recommend giving activated charcoal with a cathartic as a single dose. Barbiturates shouldn't be given if excitation occurs. Dialysis is of limited value.

## Clinical considerations
■ I.M. administration isn't recommended because of erratic and slow absorption. However, if I.M. route is used, reconstitute with special diluent only. Don't use diluent if hazy. Discard unused portion. Recommend injecting I.M. deep into large muscle mass.
■ Lower doses are effective in patients with renal or hepatic dysfunction. Advise clinician to closely monitor renal and hepatic studies for signs of dysfunction.
■ Prepare solutions for I.M. use immediately before administration. Discard unused portions.

■ Minor changes in EEG patterns, usually low-voltage, fast activity, may occur during and after chlordiazepoxide therapy.
■ Chlordiazepoxide may cause a false-positive pregnancy test, depending on method used. It may also alter urinary 17-ketosteroids (Zimmerman reaction), urine alkaloid determination (Frings thin layer chromatography method), and urinary glucose determinations (with Chemstrip uG and Diastix, but not glucose enzymatic test strip).

## Therapeutic monitoring
■ Patients should remain in bed under observation for at least 3 hours after parenteral administration of chlordiazepoxide.

## Special populations
**Breast-feeding patients.** The breast-fed infant of a woman who uses chlordiazepoxide may become sedated, have feeding difficulties, or lose weight. Don't give drug to breast-feeding women.

**Pediatric patients.** Safety of oral form hasn't been established in children under age 6. Safety of parenteral form hasn't been established in children under age 12.

**Geriatric patients.** Geriatric patients show a greater sensitivity to the CNS depressant effects of drug. Some may require supervision with ambulation and activities of daily living when therapy starts or changes. Lower doses are usually effective in geriatric patients because of decreased elimination. Parenteral administration of drug is more likely to cause apnea, hypotension, and bradycardia in geriatric patients.

## Patient counseling
■ Warn patient that sudden changes in position may cause dizziness. Advise patient to dangle legs a few minutes before getting out of bed to prevent falls and injury.
■ Warn patient not to abruptly stop using drug because withdrawal symptoms may occur.

---

# chloroquine hydrochloride
Aralen Hydrochloride

# chloroquine phosphate
Aralen Phosphate

*Pharmacologic classification:* 4-amino-quinoline
*Therapeutic classification:* antimalarial, amebicide, anti-inflammatory
*Pregnancy risk category C*

## Available forms
Available by prescription only
**chloroquine hydrochloride**
*Injection:* 50 mg/ml (40 mg/ml base)

---

**chloroquine phosphate**
*Tablets:* 500 mg (300-mg base)

# Indications and dosages
### Suppressive prophylaxis
*Adults:* Give 500 mg (300-mg base) P.O. on same day once weekly beginning 2 weeks before exposure.
*Children:* 5 mg (base)/kg P.O. on same day once weekly (not to exceed adult dosage) beginning 2 weeks before exposure.
### Treatment of acute attacks of malaria
*Adults:* 1 g (600-mg base) P.O. followed by 500 mg (300-mg base) P.O. after 6 to 8 hours; then a single dose of 500 mg (300-mg base) P.O. for next 2 days or 4 to 5 ml (160- to 200-mg base) I.M. and repeated in 6 hours if needed; change to P.O. as soon as possible.
*Children:* Initial dose is 10 mg (base)/kg P.O.; then 5 mg (base)/kg after 6 hours. Third dose is 5 mg (base)/kg 18 hours after second dose; fourth dose is 5 mg (base)/kg 24 hours after third dose; or 5 mg (base)/kg I.M. May repeat in 6 hours and change to P.O. as soon as possible.
### Extraintestinal amebiasis
*Adults:* 1 g (600-mg base) daily for 2 days, then 500 mg (300-mg base) daily for 2 to 3 weeks or 4 to 5 ml (160- to 200-mg base) I.M. for 10 to 12 days; change to P.O. as soon as possible. Give with an intestinal amebicide.
◊ *Rheumatoid arthritis*
*Adults:* 250 mg P.O. daily (chloroquine phosphate) with evening meal.
◊ *Lupus erythematosus*
*Adults:* 250 mg P.O. daily (chloroquine phosphate) with evening meal; reduce dosage gradually over several months when lesions regress.

# Mechanism of action
*Antimalarial action:* Chloroquine binds to DNA, interfering with protein synthesis. It also inhibits both DNA and RNA polymerases.
*Amebicidal action:* Mechanism of action is unknown.
*Anti-inflammatory action:* Mechanism of action is unknown. Drug may antagonize histamine and serotonin and inhibit prostaglandin effects by inhibiting conversion of arachidonic acid to prostaglandin $F_2$; it also may inhibit chemotaxis of polymorphonuclear leukocytes, macrophages, and eosinophils.
Chloroquine's spectrum of activity includes the asexual erythrocytic forms of *Plasmodium malariae, P. ovale, P. vivax,* many strains of *P. falciparum,* and *Entamoeba histolytica.*

# Pharmacokinetics
*Absorption:* Absorbed readily and almost completely.
*Distribution:* 55% plasma protein–bound. It concentrates in erythrocytes, liver, spleen, kidneys, heart, and brain and is strongly bound in melanin-containing cells.

*Metabolism:* About 30% of a given dose is metabolized by the liver to monodesethylchloroquine and bidesethylchloroquine.
*Excretion:* About 70% of an administered dose is excreted unchanged in urine; unabsorbed drug is excreted in feces. Small amounts of the drug may be present in urine for months after the drug is discontinued. Renal excretion is enhanced by urinary acidification. Drug appears in breast milk.

| Route | Onset | Peak | Duration |
|-------|-------|------|----------|
| P.O. | Unknown | 1-3 hr | Unknown |
| I.M. | Unknown | ½ hr | Unknown |

# Contraindications and precautions
Contraindicated in patients hypersensitive to drug and in those with retinal or visual field changes or porphyria. Use cautiously in patients with GI, neurologic, or blood disorders.

# Interactions
**Drug-drug.** *Cimetidine:* May reduce oral clearance and metabolism. Advise clinician to monitor patient for toxicity.
*Intradermal human diploid cell rabies vaccine:* May interfere with antibody response. Use together cautiously.
*Kaolin, magnesium and aluminum salts:* May decrease absorption of chloroquine. Separate administration times.
**Drug-lifestyle.** *Sun exposure:* May exacerbate drug-induced dermatoses. Advise patient to avoid excessive sun exposure.

# Adverse reactions
**CNS:** mild and transient headache, psychic stimulation, *seizures,* dizziness, neuropathy.
**CV:** hypotension, ECG changes, *AV block,* cardiomyopathy.
**EENT:** visual disturbances (blurred vision; difficulty in focusing; reversible corneal changes; typically irreversible, sometimes progressive or delayed retinal changes, such as narrowing of arterioles; macular lesions; pallor of optic disk; optic atrophy; patchy retinal pigmentation, typically leading to blindness); ototoxicity.
**GI:** anorexia, abdominal cramps, diarrhea, nausea, vomiting, stomatitis.
**Hematologic:** *agranulocytosis, aplastic anemia,* hemolytic anemia, *thrombocytopenia.*
**Skin:** pruritus, lichen planus eruptions, skin and mucosal pigmentary changes, pleomorphic skin eruptions.

# Overdose and treatment
Signs and symptoms of drug overdose may appear within 30 minutes after ingestion and may include headache, drowsiness, visual changes, CV collapse, and seizures followed by respiratory and cardiac arrest. Treatment is symptomatic. Stomach should be emptied by eme-

---

sis or lavage. After lavage, activated charcoal in an amount at least five times the estimated amount of drug ingested may be helpful if given within 30 minutes of ingestion.

Ultra–short-acting barbiturates may help control seizures. Intubation may be needed. Peritoneal dialysis and exchange transfusions also may be useful. Forced fluids and acidification of the urine are helpful after the acute phase.

## Clinical considerations

**ALERT** Drug dosage may be discussed in milligrams or milligrams base. Be aware of the difference.

■ Resistance of *P. falciparum* to chloroquine has spread to most areas with malaria except the Dominican Republic, Haiti, Central America west of the Panama Canal, and Egypt.

■ Some forms of drug contain the dye tartrazine (Yellow no. 5), which may cause allergic reactions.

■ It may also be advisable for traveler to take sulfadoxine and pyrimethamine (Fansidar) when traveling. Instruct patient to take drug if a febrile illness occurs when professional medical care isn't available. Emphasize that such self-treatment is a temporary measure and that he must seek medical care as soon as possible. He should continue prophylaxis after the treatment dose of Fansidar.

### Therapeutic monitoring

■ Baseline and periodic ophthalmologic examinations are needed in prolonged or high-dosage therapy.

■ Advise clinician to assist patient in obtaining audiometric examinations before, during, and after therapy, especially if therapy is long-term.

### Special populations

**Breast-feeding patients.** Safety hasn't been established. Use with caution in breast-feeding women.

**Pediatric patients.** Children are extremely susceptible to toxicity; advise clinician to monitor children closely for adverse effects.

## Patient counseling

■ Tell patient to report blurred vision, increased sensitivity to light, hearing loss, pronounced GI disturbances, or muscle weakness promptly.

■ Advise patient to take drug immediately before or after meals on the same day each week to minimize gastric distress. Patients who can't tolerate drug because of GI distress may tolerate hydroxychloroquine.

# chlorpheniramine maleate
Aller-Chlor, Chlo-Amine, Chlor-Trimeton

*Pharmacologic classification:* propylamine-derivative antihistamine
*Therapeutic classification:* antihistamine ($H_1$-receptor antagonist)
*Pregnancy risk category B*

## Available forms

Available with or without a prescription
*Tablets:* 4 mg
*Tablets (chewable):* 2 mg
*Tablets (extended-release):* 8 mg, 12 mg
*Capsules (extended-release):* 8 mg, 12 mg
*Syrup:* 2 mg/5 ml
*Injection:* 10 mg/ml

## Indications and dosages
*Rhinitis, allergy symptoms*

*Adults and children ages 12 and older:* 4 mg of tablets or syrup P.O. q 4 to 6 hours; or 8 to 12 mg of extended-release tablets b.i.d. or t.i.d. Maximum dose, 24 mg/day; 10 to 20 mg S.C., I.V., or I.M. also may be used.
*Children ages 6 to 11:* 2 mg of tablets or syrup P.O. q 4 to 6 hours; or one 8-mg extended-release tablet in 24 hours. Maximum dose, 12 mg/day.
*Children ages 2 to 5:* 1 mg of syrup P.O. q 4 to 6 hours. Maximum dose, 6 mg/day. Safety and efficacy of extended release preparations for children under age 6 haven't been established.

## I.V. administration

**ALERT** Drug is available in 10-mg/ml ampules for I.V. use. Don't give the 100-mg/ml strength I.V.

■ I.V. solution should be given slowly, over 1 minute.

### Incompatibilities

None reported.

## Mechanism of action

*Antihistamine action:* Antihistamines compete with histamine for $H_1$-receptor sites on smooth muscle of the bronchi, GI tract, uterus, and large blood vessels; they bind to cellular receptors, preventing access of histamine, thereby suppressing histamine-induced allergic symptoms. They don't directly alter histamine or its release.

## Pharmacokinetics

*Absorption:* Well absorbed from the GI tract. Food in the stomach delays absorption but doesn't affect bioavailability.
*Distribution:* Distributed extensively into the body; drug is about 72% protein-bound.

*Metabolism:* Metabolized largely in GI mucosal cells and liver (first-pass effect).

*Excretion:* Half-life is 12 to 43 hours in adults and 10 to 13 hours in children; drug and metabolites are excreted in urine.

| Route | Onset | Peak | Duration |
|---|---|---|---|
| P.O. | 15-60 min | 2-6 hr | 24 hr |
| I.V. | 15-60 min | Immediate | 24 hr |
| I.M., S.C. | 15-60 min | Unknown | 24 hr |

## Contraindications and precautions

Contraindicated in patients having acute asthmatic attacks. Antihistamines aren't recommended for breast-feeding women because small amounts of drug appear in breast milk.

Use cautiously in geriatric patients and in patients with increased intraocular pressure, hyperthyroidism, CV or renal disease, hypertension, bronchial asthma, urine retention, prostatic hyperplasia, bladder neck obstruction, or stenosing peptic ulcers.

## Interactions

**Drug-drug.** *CNS depressants:* Increased sedation. Use together cautiously.

*Epinephrine:* Chlorpheniramine enhances the effects. Advise clinician to monitor patient.

*Heparin:* Chlorpheniramine may partially counteract the anticoagulant action. Avoid use together.

*MAO inhibitors:* Increased anticholinergic effects. Use caution when using together.

*Sulfonylureas:* May diminish the effects. Advise patient to report effectiveness of treatment.

**Drug-lifestyle.** *Alcohol use:* Additive sedation may occur when antihistamines are given with chlorpheniramine. Discourage use together.

## Adverse reactions

**CNS:** *stimulation,* sedation, *drowsiness,* excitability in children.

**CV:** hypotension, palpitations, weak pulse.

**GI:** epigastric distress, *dry mouth.*

**GU:** urine retention.

**Respiratory:** thick bronchial secretions.

**Skin:** rash, urticaria, local stinging, burning sensation (after parenteral administration), pallor.

## Overdose and treatment

Signs and symptoms of overdose may include either CNS depression (sedation, reduced mental alertness, apnea, and CV collapse) or CNS stimulation (insomnia, hallucinations, tremors, and seizures). Atropine-like symptoms, such as dry mouth, flushed skin, fixed and dilated pupils, and GI symptoms are common, especially in children.

Advise clinician to treat overdose by inducing emesis with ipecac syrup (in conscious patient), followed by activated charcoal to reduce further drug absorption. Recommend using gastric lavage if patient is unconscious or

ipecac fails. Recommend treating hypotension with vasopressors, and control seizures with diazepam or phenytoin. Stimulants shouldn't be given. Administering ammonium chloride or vitamin C to acidify urine promotes drug excretion.

## Clinical considerations

- Don't use parenteral solutions intradermally.
- Injectable form contains benzyl alcohol. Avoid use in infants.
- Discontinue drug 4 days before diagnostic skin tests; antihistamines can prevent, reduce, or mask positive skin test response.

### Therapeutic monitoring

- If symptoms occur during or after parenteral dose, drug should be stopped and prescriber informed.

### Special populations

**Breast-feeding patients.** Antihistamines such as chlorpheniramine shouldn't be used during breast-feeding. Many of these drugs appear in breast milk, exposing the infant to risks of unusual excitability; premature infants are at particular risk for seizures.

**Pediatric patients.** Drug isn't indicated for use in premature or newborn infants. Children, especially those under age 6, may experience paradoxical hyperexcitability.

**Geriatric patients.** Geriatric patients are usually more sensitive to adverse effects of antihistamines and are especially likely to experience a greater degree of dizziness, sedation, hyperexcitability, dry mouth, and urine retention than younger patients. Symptoms usually respond to a decrease in drug dosage.

## Patient counseling

- Instruct patient to swallow extended-release tablets whole; they shouldn't be crushed or chewed.
- Inform patient to store syrup and parenteral solution away from light.

---

# chlorpromazine hydrochloride

Chlorpromanyl-5*, Chlorpromanyl-20*, Largactil*, Novo-Chlorpromazine*, Ormazine, Thorazine

*Pharmacologic classification:* aliphatic phenothiazine
*Therapeutic classification:* antipsychotic, antiemetic
*Pregnancy risk category C*

## Available forms

Available by prescription only
*Tablets:* 10 mg, 25 mg, 50 mg, 100 mg, 200 mg

*Capsules (sustained-release):* 30 mg, 75 mg, 150 mg
*Syrup:* 10 mg/5 ml
*Oral concentrate:* 30 mg/ml, 100 mg/ml
*Suppositories:* 25 mg, 100 mg
*Injection:* 25 mg/ml

## Indications and dosages
### Psychosis
*Adults:* 30 to 75 mg P.O. daily in two to four divided doses. Dosage may be increased twice weekly by 20 to 50 mg until symptoms are controlled. Most patients respond to 200 mg daily, but doses up to 800 mg may be needed. 25 to 50 mg may be given I.M., and may be repeated in 1 hour, if needed. Gradually increase subsequent I.M. doses over several days to a maximum of 400 mg q 4 to 6 hours. Switch to oral therapy as soon as possible.
*Children ages 6 months and older:* 0.55 mg/kg P.O. q 4 to 6 hours; or I.M. q 6 to 8 hours; or 1.1 mg/kg P.R. q 6 to 8 hours. Maximum I.M. dose is 40 mg in children under age 5 or weighing less than 22.7 kg (50 lb), and 75 mg in children ages 5 to 12 or weighing 22.7 to 45.4 kg (50 to 100 lb).
### Nausea, vomiting
*Adults:* 10 to 25 mg P.O. q 4 to 6 hours, p.r.n.; or 50 to 100 mg P.R. q 6 to 8 hours, p.r.n.; or 25 mg I.M. initially. If no hypotension occurs, 25 to 50 mg I.M. q 3 to 4 hours may be given, p.r.n., until vomiting stops.
*Children ages 6 months and older:* 0.55 mg/kg P.O. q 4 to 6 hours, p.r.n.; or I.M. q 6 to 8 hours, p.r.n.; or 1.1 mg/kg P.R. q 6 to 8 hours, p.r.n. Maximum I.M. dose in children under 5 or weighing less than 22.7 kg (50 lb) is 40 mg. Maximum I.M. dose in children ages 5 to 12 or weighing 22.7 to 45.4 kg (50 to 100 lb) is 75 mg.
### Intractable hiccups; acute intermittent porphyria
*Adults:* 25 to 50 mg P.O. or I.M. t.i.d. or q.i.d. For hiccups, if symptoms persist, 25 to 50 mg diluted in 500 to 1,000 ml of normal saline solution and infused I.V. slowly with patient in supine position.
### Tetanus
*Adults:* 25 mg to 50 mg I.M. or I.V. t.i.d. or q.i.d.
*Children ages 6 months and older:* 0.55 mg/kg I.M. or I.V. q 6 to 8 hours. Maximum parenteral dose in children weighing less than 22.7 kg (50 lb) is 40 mg daily; for children weighing 22.7 to 45.4 kg (50 to 100 lb), maximum parenteral dose is 75 mg daily, except in severe cases.
### Surgery
*Adults:* Preoperatively, 25 to 50 mg P.O. 2 to 3 hours before surgery or 12.5 to 25 mg I.M. 1 to 2 hours before surgery; during surgery, 12.5 mg I.M., repeated in 30 minutes, if needed, or fractional 2 mg doses I.V. at 2-minute intervals up to maximum of 25 mg; postoper-

atively, 10 to 25 mg P.O. q 4 to 6 hours or 12.5 to 25 mg I.M., repeated in 1 hour, if needed.
*Children ages 6 months and older:* Preoperatively, 0.55 mg/kg P.O. 2 to 3 hours before surgery or I.M. 1 to 2 hours before surgery; during surgery, 0.275 mg/kg I.M., repeated in 30 minutes, if needed, or fractional 1 mg doses I.V. at 2-minute intervals, up to maximum of 0.275 mg/kg; postoperatively, 0.55 mg/kg P.O. or I.M., oral dose repeated q 4 to 6 hours or I.M. dose repeated in 1 hour, if needed, and if hypotension doesn't occur.

## I.V. administration
**ℏALERT** I.V. form should be used only during surgery or for severe hiccups. Dilute injection to 1 mg/ml with normal saline solution and administer at 1 mg/2 minutes for children and 1 mg/minute for adults.

## Incompatibilities
Incompatible with aminophylline, amphotericin B, ampicillin, atropine, chloramphenicol sodium succinate, chlorothiazide, cimetidine, dimenhydrinate, heparin sodium, melphalan, methicillin, methohexital, paclitaxel, penicillin, pentobarbital, phenobarbital, thiopental, and solutions having a pH of 4 to 5.

## Mechanism of action
*Antipsychotic action:* Chlorpromazine is thought to exert its antipsychotic effects by postsynaptic blockade of CNS dopamine receptors, thereby inhibiting dopamine-mediated effects; antiemetic effects are attributed to dopamine receptor blockade in the medullary chemoreceptor trigger zone (CTZ). Drug has many other central and peripheral effects; it produces both alpha and ganglionic blockade and counteracts histamine- and serotonin-mediated activity. Its most prominent adverse reactions are antimuscarinic and sedative.

## Pharmacokinetics
*Absorption:* Rate and extent of absorption vary with route of administration. Oral tablet absorption is erratic; sustained-release preparations have similar absorption. Oral concentrates and syrups are much more predictable; I.M. drug is absorbed rapidly.
*Distribution:* Distributed widely into the body; appears in breast milk; level is usually higher in CNS than in plasma. Steady-state serum level is achieved within 4 to 7 days. Drug is 91% to 99% protein-bound.
*Metabolism:* Metabolized extensively by the liver and forms 10 to 12 metabolites; some are pharmacologically active.
*Excretion:* Mostly excreted as metabolites in urine; some is excreted in feces via the biliary tract. It may undergo enterohepatic circulation.

---

| Route | Onset | Peak | Duration |
|---|---|---|---|
| P.O. | ½-1 hr | Unknown | 4-6 hr |
| P.O. (extended) | ½-1 hr | Unknown | 10-12 hr |
| I.V., I.M. | Unknown | Unknown | Unknown |
| P.R. | > 1 hr | Unknown | 3-4 hr |

## Contraindications and precautions

Contraindicated in patients hypersensitive to drug or in patients experiencing CNS depression, bone marrow suppression, subcortical damage, and coma.

Use cautiously in acutely ill or dehydrated children; geriatric or debilitated patients; and in patients with impaired renal or hepatic function, severe CV disease, glaucoma, prostatic hyperplasia, respiratory or seizure disorders, hypocalcemia, reaction to insulin or electroconvulsive therapy, or exposure to heat, cold, or organophosphate insecticides.

## Interactions

**Drug-drug.** *Antiarrhythmics, disopyramide, procainamide, quinidine:* Increased risk of arrhythmias and conduction defects. Avoid use together.
*Anticholinergics:* Increased anticholinergic activity, aggravated parkinsonian symptoms. Use with caution.
*Beta blockers:* May inhibit chlorpromazine metabolism, increasing plasma levels and toxicity. Advise clinician to monitor patient closely.
*Centrally acting antihypertensives:* Chlorpromazine may decrease blood pressure. Advise clinician to monitor patient closely.
*CNS depressants, parenteral magnesium sulfate:* Additive effects are likely. Avoid use together.
*Epinephrine:* Chlorpromazine may cause epinephrine reversal. Avoid use together.
*Lithium:* May cause severe neurologic toxicity and a decreased therapeutic response to chlorpromazine. Avoid use together.
*Propylthiouracil:* Concurrent use increases risk of agranulocytosis. Avoid use together.
*Sympathomimetics:* Concurrent use may decrease their stimulatory and pressor effects. Avoid use together.
*Warfarin:* Decreased effect of oral anticoagulants. Advise clinician to monitor INR and PT.
**Drug-herb.** *Kava:* Possible increased risk or severity of dystonic reactions. Discourage use together.
**Drug-food.** *Caffeine:* Pharmacokinetic alterations and subsequent decreased therapeutic response. Avoid caffeinated foods and beverages.
**Drug-lifestyle.** *Alcohol use:* Additive effects likely after use. Discourage use.
*Heavy smoking:* May reduce therapeutic response to chlorpromazine. Discourage smoking.
*Sun exposure:* Photosensitivity reactions may result. Take precautions.

## Adverse reactions

**CNS:** extrapyramidal reactions, drowsiness, sedation, *seizures,* tardive dyskinesia, pseudoparkinsonism, dizziness, *neuroleptic malignant syndrome.*
**CV:** *orthostatic hypotension,* tachycardia, ECG changes.
**EENT:** ocular changes, blurred vision, nasal congestion.
**GI:** *dry mouth, constipation,* nausea.
**GU:** *urine retention,* menstrual irregularities, inhibited ejaculation, priapism.
**Hematologic:** *leukopenia, agranulocytosis,* eosinophilia, hemolytic anemia, *aplastic anemia, thrombocytopenia.*
**Hepatic:** jaundice, abnormal liver function test results.
**Skin:** *mild photosensitivity,* allergic reactions, *pain at I.M. injection site,* sterile abscess, skin pigmentation.
**Other:** gynecomastia.
**After abrupt withdrawal of long-term therapy:** gastritis, nausea, vomiting, dizziness, tremor.

## Overdose and treatment

CNS depression is characterized by deep, unarousable sleep and possible coma, hypotension, or hypertension, extrapyramidal symptoms, abnormal involuntary muscle movements, agitation, seizures, arrhythmias, ECG changes, hypothermia or hyperthermia, and autonomic nervous system dysfunction.

Treatment is symptomatic and supportive, including maintaining vital signs, airway, stable body temperature, and fluid and electrolyte balance.

Vomiting shouldn't be induced: drug inhibits cough reflex, and aspiration may occur. Advise clinician to use gastric lavage, then activated charcoal and sodium chloride cathartics; dialysis doesn't help. Body temperature should be regulated p.r.n. Recommend treating hypotension with I.V. fluids; epinephrine shouldn't be given. Seizures should be treated with parenteral diazepam or barbiturates; arrhythmias with parenteral phenytoin (1 mg/kg with rate adjusted to blood pressure); extrapyramidal reactions with benztropine 1 to 2 mg or parenteral diphenhydramine 10 to 50 mg.

## Clinical considerations

■ Sustained-release preparations shouldn't be crushed or opened, but swallowed whole.
■ Oral formulations may cause stomach upset and may be given with food or fluid.
■ Recommend diluting concentrate in 2 to 4 ounces of liquid, preferably water, carbonated drinks, fruit juice, tomato juice, milk, pudding, or applesauce.
■ Store suppository form in a cool place.
■ Recommend giving I.M. injection deep in the upper outer quadrant of the buttocks. In-

jection is usually painful; massaging the area after administration may prevent abscesses.

■ Liquid and injectable forms may cause a rash if skin contact occurs.

■ Solution for injection may be slightly discolored. Don't use if drug is excessively discolored or if a precipitate is evident.

■ Drug causes false-positive test results for urinary porphyrins, urobilinogen, amylase, and 5-hydroxyindoleacetic acid because of darkening of urine by metabolites; it also causes false-positive results in urine pregnancy tests using human chorionic gonadotropin.

### Therapeutic monitoring

■ If tissue irritation occurs, chlorpromazine injection may be diluted with normal saline solution or 2% procaine.

■ Advise clinician to monitor blood pressure before and after parenteral administration.

### Special populations

**Breast-feeding patients.** Drug appears in breast milk. Potential benefits to the woman should outweigh potential harm to the infant.

**Pediatric patients.** Drug isn't recommended for patients under age 6 months. Sudden infant death syndrome has been reported in children under age 1 receiving drug. Extrapyramidal effects may be more common in children.

**Geriatric patients.** Older patients tend to require lower doses, adjusted individually. Adverse reactions, especially tardive dyskinesia and other extrapyramidal effects, are more likely to develop in geriatric patients.

### Patient counseling

■ Explain what fluids are appropriate for diluting the concentrate and the dropper technique for measuring dose. Teach patient how to use suppository form.

■ Tell patient not to spill the liquid preparation on skin because rash and irritation may result.

■ Instruct patient to take drug exactly as prescribed and not to double dose to compensate for missed ones.

■ Explain risks of dystonic reactions and tardive dyskinesia, and tell patient to report abnormal involuntary body movements or painful muscle contractions.

■ Warn patient to avoid extremely hot or cold baths or exposure to temperature extremes, sunlamps, or tanning beds. Drug may cause thermoregulatory changes.

■ Explain that many drug interactions are possible. Patient should seek medical approval before taking any self-prescribed drugs.

■ Tell patient not to stop taking drug suddenly.

■ Encourage patient to report difficulty urinating, sore throat, dizziness, fever, or fainting.

■ Advise patient to avoid hazardous activities that require alertness until the effect of the drug

is established. Excessive sedative effects tend to subside after several weeks.

■ Inform patient that sugarless chewing gum or hard candy, ice chips, or artificial saliva may help to alleviate dry mouth.

---

# chlorpropamide

Diabinese, Novo-Propamide*

*Pharmacologic classification:* sulfonylurea
*Therapeutic classification:* antidiabetic
*Pregnancy risk category C*

## Available forms

Available by prescription only
*Tablets:* 100 mg, 250 mg

## Indications and dosages

*Adjunct to diet to lower blood glucose levels in patients with type 2 (non–insulin-dependent) diabetes*

*Adults ages 65 and younger:* 250 mg P.O. daily with breakfast or in divided doses if GI disturbances occur. First dosage increase may be made after 5 to 7 days because of extended duration of action; then dosage may be increased q 3 to 5 days by 50 to 125 mg, if needed, to a maximum of 750 mg daily.

*Adults over age 65:* Initial dose should be 100 to 125 mg daily.

*To change from insulin to oral therapy*

*Adults:* If insulin dosage is less than 40 units daily, insulin may be stopped and oral therapy started as above. If insulin dosage is 40 units or more daily, start oral therapy as above, with insulin dose reduced 50% the first few days. Further insulin reductions should be made based on patient response.

## Mechanism of action

*Antidiabetic action:* Chlorpropamide lowers blood glucose levels by stimulating insulin release from beta cells in the pancreas. After prolonged administration, it produces hypoglycemic effects through extrapancreatic mechanisms, including reduced basal hepatic glucose production and enhanced peripheral sensitivity to insulin; the latter may result either from an increased number of insulin receptors or from changes in events that follow insulin binding.

*Antidiuretic action:* Drug potentiates the effects of minimal levels of antidiuretic hormone.

## Pharmacokinetics

*Absorption:* Absorbed readily from the GI tract. Maximum decrease in serum glucose levels at 3 to 6 hours.

*Distribution:* Distribution isn't fully understood, but is probably similar to that of the other sulfonylureas. It's highly protein-bound.

---

*Metabolism:* About 80% of drug is metabolized by the liver. Whether the metabolites have hypoglycemic activity is unknown.

*Excretion:* Excreted in urine. Rate of excretion depends on urinary pH; it increases in alkaline urine and decreases in acidic urine. Duration of action is up to 60 hours; half-life is 36 hours.

| Route | Onset | Peak | Duration |
|-------|-------|------|----------|
| P.O. | 1 hr | 2-4 hr | 24 hr |

## Contraindications and precautions

Contraindicated for treating type 1 diabetes or diabetes that can be adequately controlled by diet. Also contraindicated in patients with type 2 diabetes complicated by ketosis, acidosis, diabetic coma, major surgery, severe infections, or severe trauma, or during pregnancy or breast-feeding, and in those hypersensitive to drug.

Use cautiously in geriatric, debilitated, or malnourished patients and in those with porphyria or impaired renal or hepatic function.

## Interactions

**Drug-drug.** *Anticoagulants:* May increase plasma levels of both drugs and, after continued therapy, may reduce plasma levels and anticoagulant effects. Advise clinician to monitor patient closely.

*Beta blockers:* May increase the risk of hypoglycemia. Advise clinician to monitor patient closely.

*Chloramphenicol, guanethidine, insulin, MAO inhibitors, probenecid, salicylates, sulfonamides:* May enhance hypoglycemic effects by displacing chlorpropamide from its protein-binding sites. Avoid use together.

**Drug-herb.** *Bitter melon, ginkgo biloba:* Possible increased risk of hypoglycemia. Discourage use together.

**Drug-lifestyle.** *Alcohol use:* May produce disulfiram-like reaction. Advise patient to avoid alcohol.

*Smoking:* Increased corticosteroid release. May require higher dosages of chlorpropamide.

## Adverse reactions

**CNS:** paresthesia, fatigue, dizziness, vertigo, malaise, headache.

**EENT:** tinnitus.

**GI:** nausea, heartburn, epigastric distress.

**GU:** tea-colored urine.

**Hematologic:** *leukopenia, thrombocytopenia, aplastic anemia, agranulocytosis,* hemolytic anemia.

**Hepatic:** elevated alkaline phosphatase and bilirubin levels.

**Metabolic:** prolonged hypoglycemia, dilutional hyponatremia, alterations in cholesterol, urine phenyl ketone, porphyrins, protein levels, and cephalin flocculation.

**Skin:** rash, pruritus, erythema, urticaria.

**Other:** hypersensitivity reactions.

## Overdose and treatment

Signs and symptoms of overdose include low blood glucose levels, tingling of lips and tongue, hunger, nausea, decreased cerebral function (lethargy, yawning, confusion, agitation, and nervousness), increased sympathetic activity (tachycardia, sweating, and tremor), and ultimately seizures, stupor, and coma.

Mild hypoglycemia (without loss of consciousness or neurologic findings) can be treated with oral glucose and dosage adjustments. If patient loses consciousness or experiences neurologic symptoms, he should receive rapid injection of dextrose 50%, followed by a continuous infusion of dextrose 10% at a rate to maintain blood glucose levels greater than 100 mg/dl. Because of chlorpropamide's long half-life, advise clinician to monitor patient for 3 to 5 days.

## Clinical considerations

- To avoid GI intolerance in those patients who require dosages of 250 mg/day or more and to improve control of hyperglycemia, divided doses are recommended. These are given before the morning and evening meals.
- Geriatric, debilitated, or malnourished patients and those with impaired renal or hepatic function usually require a lower initial dosage.
- Patients switching from chlorpropamide to another sulfonylurea should be monitored closely for 1 week because of chlorpropamide's prolonged retention in the body.
- Because of the long duration of action of the drug, adverse reactions, especially hypoglycemia, may be more frequent or severe than with some other sulfonylureas.
- Patients with severe diabetes who don't respond to 500 mg usually won't respond to higher doses.
- Oral hypoglycemic drugs have been linked to an increased risk of CV mortality compared with diet or diet and insulin treatments.

### Therapeutic monitoring

- Drug may accumulate in patients with renal insufficiency. Observe patient for signs such as dysuria, anuria, and hematuria.
- Chlorpropamide may potentiate antidiuretic effects of vasopressin. Advise clinician to monitor patient for drowsiness, muscle cramps, seizures, unconsciousness, water retention, and weakness.

### Special populations

**Breast-feeding patients.** Drug appears in breast milk and shouldn't be used in breast-feeding women.

**Pediatric patients.** Drug is ineffective in type 1 (insulin-dependent) diabetes.

**Geriatric patients.** Geriatric patients may be more sensitive to the effects of drug because of reduced metabolism and elimination. They're more likely to develop neurologic symptoms of hypoglycemia. Avoid drug in geriatric patients because of its longer duration of action. Geriatric patients usually require a lower initial dosage.

## Patient counseling
■ Emphasize importance of following prescribed diet, as well as the exercise and medical regimen.
■ Instruct patient to take drug at the same time each day. If a dose is missed, it should be taken immediately, unless it's almost time for the next dose. Patient should never double the dose.
■ Instruct patient to take drug with food if it causes GI upset.
■ Encourage patient to wear a medical identification bracelet or necklace.
■ Teach patient how to monitor blood glucose, urine glucose, and ketone levels p.r.n.
■ Teach patient to recognize the signs and symptoms of hypoglycemia and hyperglycemia and what to do if they occur.

---

# chlorzoxazone
Parafon Forte DSC, Remular-S

*Pharmacologic classification:* benzoxazole derivative
*Therapeutic classification:* skeletal muscle relaxant
*Pregnancy risk category C*

## Available forms
Available by prescription only
*Tablets:* 250 mg, 500 mg

## Indications and dosages
*Adjunct in acute, painful musculoskeletal conditions*
*Adults:* 250, 500, or 750 mg P.O. t.i.d. or q.i.d. Reduce to lowest effective dose after response is obtained.
*Children:* 20 mg/kg or 600 mg/m$^2$ P.O. daily divided t.i.d. or q.i.d. Or, 125 to 500 mg t.i.d. or q.i.d., depending on age and weight.

## Mechanism of action
*Skeletal muscle relaxant action:* Chlorzoxazone doesn't relax skeletal muscle directly, but apparently does so through its sedative effects. However, exact mechanism of action is unknown.

## Pharmacokinetics
*Absorption:* Rapidly and completely absorbed from the GI tract.
*Distribution:* Widely distributed in the body.
*Metabolism:* Metabolized in the liver to inactive metabolites. The half-life of chlorzoxazone is 66 minutes.

*Excretion:* Excreted in urine as glucuronide metabolite.

| Route | Onset | Peak | Duration |
|-------|-------|------|----------|
| P.O. | 1 hr | 1-2 hr | 3-4 hr |

## Contraindications and precautions
Contraindicated in patients hypersensitive to drug and in those with impaired hepatic function.

## Interactions
**Drug-drug.** *CNS depressants:* Further CNS depression. Avoid use together.
*MAO inhibitors, tricyclic antidepressants:* Possible increased CNS and respiratory depression and hypotensive effects. Reduce dosage of one or both drugs.
**Drug-herb.** *Watercress:* Elevated chlorzoxazone levels, increasing therapeutic effect and adverse reactions. Discourage use together.
**Drug-lifestyle.** *Alcohol use:* Further CNS depression. Discourage alcohol use.

## Adverse reactions
**CNS:** *drowsiness, dizziness, light-headedness,* malaise, headache, overstimulation, tremor.
**GI:** anorexia, nausea, vomiting, heartburn, abdominal distress, constipation, diarrhea.
**GU:** urine discoloration (orange or purple-red).
**Hepatic:** hepatic dysfunction.
**Skin:** urticaria, redness, pruritus, petechiae, bruising.
**Other:** *angioneurotic edema, anaphylaxis.*

## Overdose and treatment
Signs and symptoms of overdose include nausea, vomiting, diarrhea, drowsiness, dizziness, light-headedness, headache, malaise, and sluggishness, followed by loss of muscle tone, decreased or absent deep tendon reflexes, respiratory depression, and hypotension.

To treat overdose, induce emesis or perform gastric lavage followed by activated charcoal. Advise clinician to closely monitor vital signs and neurologic status, provide general supportive measures, including maintenance of adequate airway and assisted ventilation, and use caution if giving pressor drugs.

## Clinical considerations
■ Drug may cause drowsiness.
■ Urine may turn orange or reddish purple.

### Therapeutic monitoring
■ Advise clinician to monitor liver function test results in patients receiving long-term therapy. Watch for early signs of hepatic dysfunction or abnormal liver enzyme levels.

### Special populations
**Pregnant patients.** Safety hasn't been established. Use only when benefits outweigh risks.

---

**Breast-feeding patients.** It's unknown if drug appears in breast milk. No clinical problems have been reported.

**Pediatric patients.** Tablets may be crushed and mixed with food, milk, or fruit juice to aid administration in children.

**Geriatric patients.** Geriatric patients may be more sensitive to effects of drug.

## Patient counseling

- Caution patient to avoid hazardous activities that require alertness or physical coordination until CNS depression is determined.
- Advise patient to store drug away from heat or light.
- Tell patient to take missed dose only if remembered within 1 hour of scheduled time. If beyond 1 hour, tell patient to skip dose and go back to regular schedule. Caution patient not to double the dose.
- Advise patient not to stop taking drug without calling for specific instructions.

---

# cholestyramine

Locholest, Questran, Questran Light

*Pharmacologic classification:* anion exchange resin
*Therapeutic classification:* antilipemic, bile acid sequestrant
*Pregnancy risk category C*

## Available forms

Available by prescription only
*Powder:* 378-g cans, 9-g single-dose packets (Questran). 5-g single dose packets (Questran Light). Each scoop of powder or single-dose packet contains 4 g of cholestyramine resin.

## Indications and dosages

*Primary hyperlipidemia and hypercholesterolemia unresponsive to dietary measures alone; to reduce the risks of atherosclerotic coronary artery disease and MI; to relieve pruritus associated with partial biliary obstruction;* ◇ *cardiac glycoside toxicity*
Adults: 4 g P.O. before meals and h.s. not to exceed 32 g daily. Can be given in one to six divided doses.
*Children ages 6 to 12:* 80 mg/kg or 2.35 g/m$^2$ P.O. t.i.d.

## Mechanism of action

*Antilipemic action:* Bile is normally excreted into the intestine to facilitate absorption of fat and other lipid materials. Cholestyramine binds with bile acid, forming an insoluble compound that's excreted in feces. With less bile available in the digestive system, less fat and lipid materials in food are absorbed, more cholesterol is used by the liver to replace its supply of bile acids, and the serum cholesterol level

decreases. In partial biliary obstruction, excess bile acids accumulate in dermal tissue, resulting in pruritus; by reducing levels of dermal bile acids, cholestyramine combats pruritus.

Drug can also act as an antidiarrheal in postoperative diarrhea caused by bile acids in the colon.

## Pharmacokinetics

*Absorption:* Not absorbed. Cholesterol levels may begin to decrease 24 to 48 hours after the start of therapy and may continue to fall for up to 12 months. In some patients, the initial decrease is followed by a return to or above baseline cholesterol levels on continued therapy. Relief from pruritus caused by cholestasis occurs 1 to 3 weeks after therapy starts. Diarrhea caused by bile acids may cease in 24 hours.
*Distribution:* None.
*Metabolism:* None.
*Excretion:* Insoluble cholestyramine with bile acid complex is excreted in feces.

| Route | Onset | Peak | Duration |
|-------|-------|------|----------|
| P.O. | Unknown | Unknown | 2-4 wk |

## Contraindications and precautions

Contraindicated in patients hypersensitive to bile-acid sequestering resins and in those with complete biliary obstruction. Use cautiously in patients with coronary artery disease or a predisposition to constipation.

## Interactions

**Drug-drug.** *Acetaminophen, cardiac glycosides, corticosteroids, thiazide diuretics, thyroid hormones:* May reduce absorption of these drugs. Recommend giving other drugs 1 hour before or 4 to 6 hours after cholestyramine. Readjustment must also be made when cholestyramine is withdrawn, to prevent high-dose toxicity.
*Warfarin:* May decrease anticoagulant effects. Avoid use together. Careful monitoring of PT and INR is mandatory.

## Adverse reactions

**CNS:** headache, anxiety, vertigo, dizziness, insomnia, fatigue, syncope.
**EENT:** tinnitus.
**GI:** *constipation,* fecal impaction, hemorrhoids, *abdominal discomfort,* flatulence, *nausea,* vomiting, steatorrhea, GI bleeding, diarrhea, anorexia.
**GU:** hematuria, dysuria.
**Hematologic:** anemia, bleeding tendencies.
**Hepatic:** alters serum levels of ALT, AST.
**Metabolic:** alters serum concentrations of chloride, phosphorus, potassium, calcium, and sodium; hyperchloremic acidosis (with long-term use or very high doses).
**Musculoskeletal:** backache; muscle and joint pain; osteoporosis.

---

*\* Canada only*   ◇ Unlabeled clinical use

**Skin:** *rash;* ecchymoses; irritation of skin, tongue, and perianal area.
**Other:** *vitamin A, D, E, and K deficiencies from decreased absorption.*

## Overdose and treatment

Drug overdose hasn't been reported. Chief potential risk is intestinal obstruction; treatment would depend on location and degree of obstruction and on amount of gut motility.

## Clinical considerations

■ To mix, sprinkle powder on surface of preferred beverage or wet food, let stand a few minutes, and stir to obtain uniform suspension; avoid excess foaming by using large glass and mixing slowly. Use at least 90 ml of water or other fluid, soup, milk, or pulpy fruit; rinse container and have patient drink this liquid to be sure he ingests entire dose.
■ Drug has been used to treat cardiac glycoside overdose because it binds these agents and prevents enterohepatic recycling. When used as an adjunct to hyperlipidemia, advise clinician to monitor levels of cardiac glycosides and other drugs to ensure appropriate dosage during and after therapy with cholestyramine.
■ Antilipemic therapy, along with aspirin, nitrates, and beta blockers, is recommended by the American Heart Association and the American College of Cardiology for the management of chronic stable angina in patients with (or suspected of having) coronary heart disease whose low-density lipoprotein level is greater than 130 mg/dl.
■ Questran Light contains aspartame and provides 1.6 calories per packet or scoop.
■ Cholecystography using iopanoic acid will yield abnormal results because iopanoic acid is also bound by cholestyramine.

### Therapeutic monitoring

■ Advise clinician to monitor serum cholesterol level frequently during first few months of therapy and periodically thereafter.
■ Advise clinician to monitor bowel function and treat constipation promptly by decreasing dosage, adding a stool softener, or discontinuing drug.
■ Advise clinician to observe patient for signs of vitamin A, D, or K deficiency.

### Special populations

**Pregnant patients.** Use dietary management.
**Breast-feeding patients.** Safety in breast-feeding women hasn't been established.
**Pediatric patients.** Children may be at greater risk for hyperchloremic acidosis during cholestyramine therapy. Safe dosage hasn't been established for children under age 6.
**Geriatric patients.** Patients over age 60 are more likely to experience adverse GI effects as well as adverse nutritional effects.

## Patient counseling

■ Encourage patient to comply with continued blood testing and special diet; although therapy isn't curative, it helps control serum cholesterol level.
■ Encourage patient to control weight and to stop smoking as part of attempt to increase awareness of other cardiac risk factors.
■ Tell patient not to take the powder in dry form; teach him to mix drug with fluids or pulpy fruits.

# choline magnesium trisalicylate
Tricosal, Trilisate

# choline salicylate
Arthropan

*Pharmacologic classification:* salicylate
*Therapeutic classification:* nonnarcotic analgesic, anti-inflammatory, antipyretic
*Pregnancy risk category C*

## Available forms

Available by prescription only
*Tablets:* 500 mg, 750 mg, 1,000 mg of salicylate (as choline and magnesium salicylate)
*Solution:* 500 mg of salicylate/5 ml (as choline and magnesium salicylate); 870 mg/5 ml (as choline salicylate)

## Indications and dosages

**Rheumatoid arthritis, osteoarthritis**
*Adults:* 1,500 mg P.O. b.i.d. or 3,000 mg h.s.
*Elderly:* 750 mg t.i.d.
**Mild arthritis, antipyresis**
*Adults:* 2,000 to 3,000 mg P.O. daily in divided doses b.i.d.
**Mild to moderate pain and fever**
*Children:* Based on weight, and the doses should be divided b.i.d.
*Children weighing 12 to 13 kg (26 to 29 lb):* 500 mg P.O. daily.
*Children weighing 14 to 17 kg (30 to 38 lb):* 750 mg P.O. daily.
*Children weighing 18 to 22 kg (39 to 49 lb):* 1,000 mg P.O. daily.
*Children weighing 23 to 27 kg (50 to 60 lb):* 1,250 mg P.O. daily.
*Children weighing 28 to 32 kg (61 to 71 lb):* 1,500 mg P.O. daily.
*Children weighing 33 to 37 kg (72 to 82 lb):* 1,750 mg P.O. daily.

## Mechanism of action

*Analgesic action:* Choline salicylates produce analgesia by an ill-defined effect on the hypothalamus (central action) and by blocking generation of pain impulses (peripheral action).

The peripheral action may involve inhibition of prostaglandin synthesis.

*Anti-inflammatory action:* These drugs exert their anti-inflammatory effect by inhibiting prostaglandin synthesis; they may also inhibit the synthesis or action of other inflammation mediators.

*Antipyretic action:* Choline salicylates relieve fever by acting on the hypothalamic heat-regulating center to produce peripheral vasodilation. This increases peripheral blood supply and promotes sweating, which leads to loss of heat and to cooling by evaporation. These drugs don't affect platelet aggregation and shouldn't be used to prevent thrombosis.

## Pharmacokinetics
*Absorption:* Absorbed rapidly and completely from the GI tract.
*Distribution:* Protein binding depends on level and ranges from 75% to 90%, decreasing as serum level increases. Severe toxic effects may occur at serum levels greater than 400 mcg/ml.
*Metabolism:* Hydrolyzed to salicylate in the liver.
*Excretion:* Metabolites are excreted in urine.

| Route | Onset | Peak | Duration |
|-------|-------|------|----------|
| P.O. | Unknown | 1-2 hr | Unknown |

## Contraindications and precautions
Contraindicated in patients hypersensitive to drug. Also contraindicated in patients with hemophilia, bleeding ulcers, hemorrhagic states, and for patients who consume three or more alcoholic beverages per day. Use cautiously in patients with impaired renal or hepatic function, peptic ulcer disease, or gastritis. Don't give to children or teenagers with chickenpox or influenza-like illnesses.

## Interactions
**Drug-drug.** *Ammonium chloride, urine acidifiers:* Increase choline salicylate blood levels. Advise clinician to monitor choline salicylate blood levels and thus toxicity.
*Antacids:* Delay and decrease absorption of choline salicylates. Advise clinician to monitor patient closely.
*Antibiotics, corticosteroids, NSAIDs:* Enhanced risk of adverse GI effects. Use together with caution.
*Corticosteroids:* Enhance salicylate elimination. Observe for decreased effect.
*Lithium carbonate:* Choline salicylates decrease renal clearance, increasing serum lithium levels and the risk of adverse effects. Advise clinician to monitor patient closely.
*Methotrexate:* Concurrent use may cause displacement of bound methotrexate and inhibition of renal excretion. Avoid use together.
*Phenytoin, sulfonylureas, warfarin:* Concurrent use may cause displacement of either drug,

and adverse effects. Advise clinician to monitor therapy closely for both drugs.
*Warfarin:* Salicylates enhance the hypoprothrombinemic effects. Avoid use together.
**Drug-food.** *Any food:* Delays and decreases absorption of choline salicylates. Give on an empty stomach.
**Drug-lifestyle.** *Alcohol use:* Enhanced risk of adverse GI effects. Discourage use together.

## Adverse reactions
**EENT:** tinnitus, hearing loss.
**GI:** GI distress, nausea, vomiting.
**GU:** *acute tubular necrosis with renal failure.*
**Skin:** rash.
**Other:** elevated free $T_4$ levels, hypersensitivity reactions, *anaphylaxis, Reye's syndrome.*

## Overdose and treatment
Signs and symptoms of overdose include metabolic acidosis with respiratory alkalosis, hyperpnea, and tachypnea from increased carbon dioxide production and direct stimulation of the respiratory center.

To treat overdose of choline salicylates, advise clinician to empty stomach immediately by inducing emesis with ipecac syrup, if patient is conscious, or by gastric lavage. Recommend giving activated charcoal via nasogastric tube. Symptomatic and supportive measures (respiratory support and correction of fluid and electrolyte imbalances) should be provided. Advise clinician to monitor laboratory parameters and vital signs closely. Hemodialysis is effective in removing choline salicylates but is used only in severe poisoning. Forced diuresis with alkalinizing agent accelerates salicylate excretion.

## Clinical considerations
■ Choline salicylates shouldn't be mixed with antacids.
■ Recommend giving oral solution of choline salicylate mixed with fruit juice. Follow with a full 240-ml (8-ounce) glass of water to ensure passage into stomach.
■ Choline salicylates may interfere with urinary glucose analysis performed via Chemstrip uG, Diastix, glucose enzymatic test strip, Clinitest, and Benedict's solution. These drugs also interfere with urinary 5-hydroxyindole acetic acid and vanillymandelic acid.

### Therapeutic monitoring
■ Advise clinician to monitor serum magnesium levels to prevent possible magnesium toxicity.

### Special populations
**Pregnant patients.** Avoid use of choline salicylates in the third trimester of pregnancy.
**Breast-feeding patients.** Salicylates appear in breast milk. Avoid use in breast-feeding women.

**Pediatric patients.** Safety of long-term drug use in children under age 14 hasn't been established. Because of epidemiologic association with Reye's syndrome, the Centers for Disease Control and Prevention recommend that children with chickenpox or flulike symptoms not be given salicylates. Toxicity can develop rapidly in febrile, dehydrated children. Usually, they shouldn't receive more than five doses in 24 hours.

**Geriatric patients.** Patients over age 60 may be more susceptible to the toxic effects of these drugs.

## Patient counseling

- Warn patient not to take drug longer than prescribed or to increase dosage without consulting a prescriber.

# cidofovir
Vistide

*Pharmacologic classification:* nucleotide analogue
*Therapeutic classification:* antiviral
*Pregnancy risk category C*

## Available forms
Available by prescription only
*Injection:* 75 mg/ml

## Indications and dosages
***Cytomegalovirus (CMV) retinitis in patients with AIDS;*** ◇ *acyclovir-resistant herpes simplex infections in immunocompromised patients*
*Adults:* Give 5 mg/kg I.V. infused over 1 hour once weekly for 2 consecutive weeks followed by a maintenance dosage of 5 mg/kg I.V. infused over 1 hour once q 2 weeks. Probenecid must be given concomitantly.
≡ *Dosage adjustment.* For patients with creatinine clearance of 41 to 55 ml/minute, reduce induction and maintenance doses to 2 mg/kg; if creatinine clearance is 30 to 40 ml/minute, reduce induction and maintenance doses to 1.5 mg/kg; if creatinine clearance is 20 to 29 ml/minute, reduce induction and maintenance doses to 1 mg/kg; and if creatinine clearance is 19 ml/minute or less, reduce induction and maintenance doses to 0.5 mg/kg.

## I.V. administration
- Recommend giving probenecid, 2 g, P.O. 3 hours before the cidofovir dose and 1 g at 2 hours, and again at 8 hours after completion of the 1-hour infusion (total 4 g).
- Because of the mutagenic properties of cidofovir, prepare drug in a class II laminar flow biological safety cabinet. Personnel preparing drug should wear surgical gloves and a closed-front, surgical-type gown with knit cuffs.

- If drug contacts the skin, wash membranes and flush thoroughly with water. Place excess drug and all other materials used in the admixture preparation and administration in a leak-proof, puncture-proof container. The recommended method of disposal is high temperature incineration.
- To prepare infusion, extract the appropriate amount of cidofovir from the vial with a syringe and transfer the dose to an infusion bag containing 100 ml normal saline solution. The entire volume is infused I.V. at a constant rate over a 1-hour period. Use a standard infusion pump for administration.
- Administer cidofovir infusion admixtures within 24 hours of preparation; refrigerator or freezer storage shouldn't be used to extend this 24-hour period. If admixtures aren't to be used immediately, they may be refrigerated at 36° to 46° F (2° to 8° C) for no longer than 24 hours. Allow refrigerated admixtures to equilibrate to room temperature before use.
- Recommend giving normal saline solution, 1 L, over a 1- to 2-hour period immediately before each cidofovir infusion. Recommend giving a second liter in patients who can tolerate the additional fluid load. If the second liter is given, administer it either at the start of the cidofovir infusion or immediately afterward; infuse it over a 1- to 3-hour period.

### Incompatibilities
Don't mix with other drugs or supplements. Compatibility with Ringer's solution, lactated Ringer's solution, or bacteriostatic infusion fluids hasn't been evaluated.

## Mechanism of action
*Antiviral action:* Cidofovir suppresses CMV replication by selective inhibition of viral DNA synthesis.

## Pharmacokinetics
*Absorption:* Administered only I.V.
*Distribution:* Unknown.
*Metabolism:* Not metabolized.
*Excretion:* 80% to 100% is excreted unchanged in urine.

| Route | Onset | Peak | Duration |
|-------|-------|------|----------|
| I.V. | Unknown | Unknown | Unknown |

## Contraindications and precautions
Contraindicated in patients hypersensitive to drug or with a history of clinically severe hypersensitivity to probenecid or other sulfa-containing drugs. Don't administer as a direct intraocular injection (direct injection may be associated with significant decreases in intraocular pressure and vision impairment). Use cautiously in patients with impaired renal function.

---

## Interactions
**Drug-drug.** *Ganciclovir ocular implants:* May result in profound hypotony. Don't give cidofovir within 1 month before or after placement of implant.
*Nephrotoxic drugs (such as aminoglycosides, amphotericin B, foscarnet, I.V. pentamidine):* May increase nephrotoxicity. Avoid use together.

## Adverse reactions
**CNS:** malaise; *asthenia, headache,* amnesia, anxiety, confusion, *seizures,* depression, dizziness, abnormal gait, hallucinations, insomnia, neuropathy, paresthesia, somnolence, vasodilation.
**CV:** hypotension, orthostatic hypotension, pallor, syncope, tachycardia, chest pain.
**EENT:** amblyopia, conjunctivitis, eye disorders, ocular hypotony, iritis, retinal detachment, uveitis, abnormal vision, pharyngitis, rhinitis, sinusitis.
**GI:** *nausea, vomiting, diarrhea, anorexia, abdominal pain,* dry mouth, colitis, constipation, tongue discoloration, dyspepsia, dysphagia, flatulence, gastritis, melena, oral candidiasis, rectal disorders, stomatitis, aphthous stomatitis, mouth ulceration, taste perversion.
**GU:** *elevated creatinine levels, nephrotoxicity, proteinuria,* decreased creatinine clearance levels, glycosuria, hematuria, urinary incontinence, urinary tract infection.
**Hematologic:** NEUTROPENIA, *anemia, thrombocytopenia.*
**Hepatic:** hepatomegaly, abnormal liver function test results, increased alkaline phosphatase levels.
**Metabolic:** fluid imbalances, hyperglycemia, hyperlipemia, hypocalcemia, hypokalemia, weight loss.
**Musculoskeletal:** arthralgia, myasthenia, myalgia, pain in back or neck.
**Respiratory:** asthma, bronchitis, coughing, dyspnea, hiccups, increased sputum, lung disorders, pneumonia.
**Skin:** *rash, alopecia,* acne, skin discoloration, dry skin, pruritus, sweating, urticaria.
**Other:** *fever; infections; chills;* allergic reactions; facial edema; *sarcoma, sepsis,* herpes simplex.

## Overdose and treatment
No information available. However, hemodialysis and hydration may reduce drug plasma levels in patients who receive an overdose of the drug. Probenecid may reduce the potential for nephrotoxicity in patients who receive a drug overdose through reduction of active tubular secretion.

## Clinical considerations
■ Renal impairment is the major toxicity of cidofovir. To minimize possible nephrotoxicity, use I.V. prehydration with normal saline and administer probenecid with each cidofovir infusion.
■ Drug is indicated only for the treatment of CMV retinitis in patients with AIDS. Safety and efficacy of drug haven't been established for treating other CMV infections, congenital or neonatal CMV disease, and CMV disease in patients not infected with HIV.
■ Fanconi's syndrome and decreased serum bicarbonate levels with evidence of renal tubular damage have been reported in patients receiving cidofovir. Advise clinician to monitor patient closely.
■ Discontinue zidovudine therapy or reduce dosage by 50% in patients receiving zidovudine on the days cidofovir is given because probenecid reduces metabolic clearance of zidovudine.

## Therapeutic monitoring
■ WBC counts with differential should be monitored before each dose.
■ Advise clinician to monitor renal function (serum creatinine and urine protein) before each dose of the drug and modify the dosage for changes in renal function.
■ Granulocytopenia has been observed with cidofovir treatment; advise clinician to monitor neutrophil counts during therapy.
■ Intraocular pressure, visual acuity, and ocular symptoms should be monitored periodically.
■ Drug shouldn't be initiated in patients with baseline serum creatinine exceeding 1.5 mg/dl or calculated creatinine clearances of 55 ml/minute or less unless the potential benefits exceed the potential risks.

## Special populations
**Pregnant patients.** Instruct women of child-bearing potential to use effective contraception during and for 1 month after treatment with cidofovir. Tell men to practice barrier contraceptive methods during and for 3 months after drug treatment.
**Breast-feeding patients.** It isn't known if drug appears in breast milk. Drug shouldn't be given to breast-feeding women.
**Pediatric patients.** Safety and effectiveness in children haven't been established.
**Geriatric patients.** Use with caution when giving cidofovir to geriatric patients. Dosage adjustment will be needed if patient is renally impaired.

## Patient counseling
■ Inform patient that drug isn't a cure for CMV retinitis and that regular ophthalmologic follow-up examinations are needed.
■ Alert patient on zidovudine therapy that he'll need to obtain dosage guidelines on days that cidofovir is given.
■ Tell patient that close monitoring of renal function will be needed during cidofovir ther-

apy and that an abnormality may require a change in cidofovir therapy.

- Stress importance of completing a full course of probenecid with each cidofovir dose. Tell patient to take probenecid after a meal to decrease nausea.
- Advise patient that cidofovir is considered a potential carcinogen in humans.

# cilostazol
Pletal

*Pharmacologic classification:* quinolinone phosphodiesterase inhibitor
*Therapeutic classification:* antiplatelet agent
*Pregnancy risk category C*

## Available forms
Available by prescription only
*Tablets:* 50 mg, 100 mg

## Indications and dosages
*Intermittent claudication*
*Adults:* 100 mg P.O. b.i.d., taken ½ hour before or 2 hours after breakfast and dinner.

## Mechanism of action
*Antiplatelet action:* Mechanism of action not fully understood. Believed to be from inhibition of the enzyme phosphodiesterase (type III), causing an increase of cAMP in platelets and blood vessels, resulting in inhibition of platelet aggregation and vasodilation. Cilostazol reversibly inhibits platelet aggregation induced by various stimuli, such as thrombin, adenosine diphosphate, collagen, arachidonic acid, epinephrine, and stress.

## Pharmacokinetics
*Absorption:* Absorbed following oral administration. A high fat meal increases peak serum levels about 90% and bioavailability by 25%. Absolute bioavailability isn't known.
*Distribution:* 95% to 98% protein-bound, primarily to albumin.
*Metabolism:* Extensively metabolized by hepatic cytochrome P-450 enzyme system, primarily CYP3A4.
*Excretion:* Excreted primarily in urine, mostly of metabolites (about 74%). Remaining drug is eliminated in the feces (about 20%). Half-life of cilostazol and active metabolites is about 11 to 13 hours.

| Route | Onset | Peak | Duration |
|---|---|---|---|
| P.O. | Unknown | Unknown | Unknown |

## Contraindications and precautions
Contraindicated in patients with heart failure of any severity. It's also contraindicated in patients hypersensitive to any of its components. Use cautiously in patients with severe under-

lying heart disease and with other drugs having antiplatelet activity.

## Interactions
**Drug-drug.** *Diltiazem, erythromycin and other macrolides, omeprazole, strong inhibitors of CYP3A4, such as fluconazole, fluoxetine, fluvoxamine, itraconazole, ketoconazole, miconazole, nefazodone, sertraline:* Increased peak serum levels of cilostazol or one of its metabolites. Avoid use together.
**Drug-food.** *Grapefruit juice:* May increase cilostazol levels. Discourage use together.
**Drug-lifestyle.** *Smoking:* Decreases drug exposure by about 20%. Discourage smoking.

## Adverse reactions
**CNS:** *headache, dizziness,* vertigo.
**CV:** *palpitation,* tachycardia, peripheral edema.
**EENT:** *pharyngitis, rhinitis.*
**GI:** *abnormal stools, diarrhea,* dyspepsia, abdominal pain, flatulence, nausea.
**Musculoskeletal:** back pain, myalgia.
**Respiratory:** cough aggravation.
**Other:** *infection.*

## Overdose and treatment
Signs and symptoms of overdose include severe headache, diarrhea, hypotension, tachycardia, and, possibly, cardiac arrhythmias. Observe patient carefully and give supportive treatment. Because drug is highly protein-bound, it may not be efficiently removed by hemodialysis.

## Clinical considerations
- A thorough drug history must be obtained before therapy starts.
- Several drugs that inhibit the enzyme phosphodiesterase have caused decreased survival in patients with class III-IV heart failure. Therefore, cilostazol is contraindicated in patients with congestive heart failure.

### Therapeutic monitoring
- There's uncertainty concerning CV risk in long-term use or in patients with severe underlying heart disease.

### Special populations
**Breast-feeding patients.** Because drug appears in breast milk, a decision should be made to discontinue breast-feeding or drug.
**Pediatric patients.** Safety and effectiveness haven't been established.
**Geriatric patients.** No overall differences in safety, efficacy, or pharmacokinetics have been observed between geriatric and younger patients.

## Patient counseling
- Instruct patient that cilostazol should be taken at least ½ hour before or 2 hours after breakfast and dinner.

■ Tell patient that a beneficial effect won't be noticed before 2 to 4 weeks, and that it may take as long as 12 weeks before a beneficial effect is experienced.
■ To chart effects of drug therapy, advise patient to keep a log of how far he's able to walk without pain.

# cimetidine
Tagamet, Tagamet HB

*Pharmacologic classification:* $H_2$-receptor antagonist
*Therapeutic classification:* antiulcerative
*Pregnancy risk category B*

## Available forms
Available by prescription only
*Tablets:* 200 mg, 300 mg, 400 mg, 800 mg
*Injection:* 300 mg/2 ml, 300 mg/50 ml normal saline (premixed)
*Liquid:* 300 mg/5 ml
*Suspension:* 0 mg/ml, 200 mg/20 ml
Available without a prescription
*Tablets:* 200 mg

## Indications and dosages
*Duodenal ulcer (short-term treatment)*
*Adults:* 800 mg P.O. h.s. for maximum of 8 weeks. Alternatively, give 400 mg P.O. b.i.d. or 300 mg P.O. q.i.d. with meals and h.s. When healing occurs, stop treatment or give h.s. dose only to control nocturnal hypersecretion. Or, 300 mg I.M. or I.V. q 6 to 8 hours. To increase dose, give more frequently to maximum daily dose of 2,400 mg.
*Duodenal ulcer prophylaxis*
*Adults:* 400 mg P.O. h.s.
*Active benign gastric ulcer*
*Adults:* 800 mg P.O. h.s., or 300 mg P.O. q.i.d. with meals and h.s. for up to 8 weeks.
*Pathologic hypersecretory conditions (such as Zollinger-Ellison syndrome, systemic mastocytosis, and multiple endocrine adenomas);* ◊ *short-bowel syndrome*
*Adults:* 300 mg P.O. q.i.d. with meals and h.s.; adjust to patient needs. Maximum daily dose, 2,400 mg.
*Parenteral:* 300 mg diluted to 20 ml with normal saline solution or other compatible I.V. solution by I.V. push over 5 minutes q 6 to 8 hours. Or 300 mg diluted in 50 ml $D_5W$ solution or other compatible I.V. solution by I.V. infusion over 15 to 20 minutes q 6 to 8 hours. To increase dosage, give 300 mg doses more frequently to maximum daily dose of 2,400 mg.
*Symptomatic relief of gastroesophageal reflux*
*Adults:* 800 mg P.O. b.i.d. or 400 mg q.i.d., before meals and h.s.

◊ *Active upper GI bleeding, peptic esophagitis, stress ulcer*
*Adults:* 1 to 2 g I.V. or P.O. daily, in four divided doses.
*Continuous infusion for patients unable to tolerate oral drugs*
*Adults:* 37.5 mg/hour (900 mg/day) by continuous I.V. infusion. Use an infusion pump if total volume is below 250 ml/day.
*Heartburn, acid indigestion, sour stomach*
*Adults:* 200 mg P.O. up to a maximum of b.i.d. (400 mg).
≡ *Dosage adjustment.* For patients with renal failure, recommended dosage is 300 mg P.O. or I.V. q 8 to 12 hours at end of dialysis. Dosage may be decreased further if hepatic failure is also present.

## I.V. administration
**⊕ALERT** Cimetidine must be diluted before I.V. administration. Don't dilute drug with sterile water for injection; use normal saline solution or $D_5W$.
■ Dilute with 20 ml normal saline solution or other compatible I.V. solution and give by I.V. push over 5 minutes. Or, dilute in 50 ml $D_5W$ or other compatible I.V. solution and infuse over 15 to 20 minutes.

## Incompatibilities
Incompatible with aminophylline, amphotericin B, barbiturates, cefamandole, cefazolin, indomethacin sodium trihydrate, pentobarbital sodium, and a combination of atropine sulfate and pentobarbital sodium.

## Mechanism of action
*Antiulcer action:* Cimetidine competitively inhibits histamine's action at $H_2$ receptors in gastric parietal cells, inhibiting basal and nocturnal gastric acid secretion (such as from stimulation by food, caffeine, insulin, histamine, betazole, or pentagastrin). Cimetidine may also enhance gastromucosal defense and healing.
A 300-mg oral or parenteral dose inhibits about 80% of gastric acid secretion for 4 to 5 hours.

## Pharmacokinetics
*Absorption:* About 60% to 75% of oral dose is absorbed. Absorption rate (but not extent) may be affected by food.
*Distribution:* Distributed to many body tissues. About 15% to 20% of drug is protein-bound. Cimetidine apparently crosses the placenta and appears in breast milk.
*Metabolism:* About 30% to 40% of dose is metabolized in the liver. Drug has a half-life of 2 hours in patients with normal renal function; half-life increases with decreasing renal function.
*Excretion:* Excreted primarily in urine (48% of oral dose, 75% of parenteral dose); 10% of

oral dose is excreted in feces. Some drug appears in breast milk.

| Route | Onset | Peak | Duration |
|-------|-------|------|----------|
| P.O. | Unknown | 45-90 min | 4-5 hr |
| I.V. | Unknown | Immediate | Unknown |
| I.M. | Unknown | Unknown | Unknown |

## Contraindications and precautions
Contraindicated in patients hypersensitive to drug. Use with caution in elderly or debilitated patients.

## Interactions
**Drug-drug.** *Benzodiazepines, beta blockers (such as propranolol), carmustine, disulfiram, isoniazid, lidocaine, metronidazole, oral contraceptives, phenytoin, procainamide, quinidine, triamterene, tricyclic antidepressants, warfarin, xanthines:* Cimetidine decreases the metabolism of these drugs, increasing potential toxicity and possibly necessitating dosage reduction. Advise clinician to monitor patient closely.
*Digoxin:* Serum digoxin levels may be reduced. Advise clinician to monitor patient closely.
*Ferrous salts, indomethacin, ketoconazole, tetracyclines:* May affect the absorption of these drugs altering gastric pH. Avoid use together.
*Flecainide:* Serum levels of flecainide may be increased. Avoid use together.
**Drug-herb.** *Guarana:* May increase caffeine serum levels or prolong serum caffeine half-life. Advise clinician to monitor patient closely.
*Pennyroyal:* May change the rate of formation of toxic metabolites of pennyroyal. Discourage use together.
*Yerba maté:* May decrease clearance of yerba maté methylxanthines and cause toxicity. Discourage use together.
**Drug-lifestyle.** *Smoking:* May increase gastric acid secretion and worsen disease. Discourage use together.

## Adverse reactions
**CNS:** confusion, dizziness, headache, peripheral neuropathy, somnolence, hallucinations.
**GI:** *mild and transient diarrhea.*
**GU:** elevated serum creatinine levels, impotence, increased serum creatinine levels.
**Hematologic:** *agranulocytosis, neutropenia, thrombocytopenia, aplastic anemia.*
**Hepatic:** jaundice, increased serum alkaline phosphatase levels.
**Musculoskeletal:** muscle pain, arthralgia.
**Other:** hypersensitivity reactions, mild gynecomastia if used for over 1 month, increased prolactin levels.

## Overdose and treatment
Signs and symptoms of overdose include respiratory failure and tachycardia. Overdose is rare.

Advise clinician to support respiration and maintain a patent airway. Recommend inducing emesis or using gastric lavage, followed with activated charcoal to prevent further absorption. Tachycardia can be treated with propranolol, if needed. Hemodialysis removes drug.

## Clinical considerations
- For I.M. administration, drug may be given undiluted. Injection may be painful.
- After administration of the liquid via nasogastric tube, flush tube to clear it and ensure passage of drug to stomach.
- Because hemodialysis removes drug, schedule dose after dialysis session.
- Cimetidine may antagonize pentagastrin's effect during gastric acid secretion tests; it may cause false-negative results in skin tests using allergen extracts.
- FD&C blue dye #2 used in Tagamet tablets may impair interpretation of Hemoccult and Gastroccult tests on gastric content aspirate. Be sure to wait at least 15 minutes after tablet administration before drawing the sample, and follow test manufacturer's instructions closely.

### Therapeutic monitoring
- Advise clinician to assess patient for abdominal pain and note any blood in emesis, stool, or gastric aspirate.

### Special populations
**Breast-feeding patients.** Drug appears in breast milk. Avoid use in breast-feeding women.
**Geriatric patients.** Use caution when giving cimetidine to geriatric patients because of the potential for adverse reactions affecting the CNS.

## Patient counseling
- Instruct patient to take drug as directed and to continue taking it even after pain subsides, to allow for adequate healing.
- Urge patient to avoid smoking because it may worsen disease.

# ciprofloxacin (systemic)
Cipro

*Pharmacologic classification:* fluoroquinolone antibiotic
*Therapeutic classification:* antibiotic
*Pregnancy risk category C*

## Available forms
Available by prescription only
*Tablets (film-coated):* 100 mg, 250 mg, 500 mg, 750 mg
*Injection for infusion:* 200 mg/20-ml vial; 400 mg/40-ml vial; 200 mg in 100 ml $D_5W$; 400 mg in 200 ml $D_5W$
*Oral suspension:* 250 mg/5 ml, 500 mg/5 ml

---

## Indications and dosages

*Mild to moderate urinary tract infection caused by susceptible bacteria*
*Adults:* 250 mg P.O. or 200 mg I.V. q 12 hours.
*Infectious diarrhea, mild to moderate respiratory tract infections, bone and joint infections, severe or complicated urinary tract infections*
*Adults:* 500 mg P.O. q 12 hours or 400 mg I.V. q 12 hours.
*Severe or complicated infections of the respiratory tract, bones, joints, skin, or skin structures;* ◇ *mycobacterial infections*
*Adults:* 750 mg P.O. q 12 hours or 400 mg I.V. q 8 hours.
*Typhoid fever*
*Adults:* 500 mg P.O. q 12 hours.
*Intra-abdominal infections (with metronidazole)*
*Adults:* 500 mg P.O. q 12 hours.
*Treatment of mild to moderate acute sinusitis caused by* **Haemophilus influenzae, Streptococcus pneumoniae,** *or* **Moraxella catarrhalis;** *mild to moderate chronic bacterial prostatitis caused by* **Escherichia coli** *or* **Proteus mirabilis**
*Adults:* 400 mg I.V. infusion given over 60 minutes q 12 hours.
◇ *Uncomplicated gonorrhea*
*Adults:* 250 mg P.O. as a single dose.
◇ **Neisseria meningitidis** *in nasal passages*
*Adults:* 500 to 750 mg P.O. as a single dose, or 250 mg P.O. b.i.d. for 2 days, or 500 mg P.O. b.i.d. for 5 days.
*Anthrax caused by aerosolized* **Bacillus anthracis**
*Adults:* 500 mg P.O. q 12 hours for 60 days, beginning as soon as possible after suspected or confirmed exposure.
*Children:* 15 mg/kg/dose P.O. q 12 hours for 60 days, beginning as soon as possible after suspected or confirmed exposure. Maximum dose 500 mg.
≡ *Dosage adjustment.* For patients with renal impairment, refer to the table.

| ORAL CIPROFLOXACIN | |
|---|---|
| Creatinine clearance (ml/min) | Adult dosage |
| 30-50 | 250-500 mg q 12 hr |
| 5-29 | 250-500 mg q 18 hr |

| I.V. CIPROFLOXACIN | |
|---|---|
| Creatinine clearance (ml/min) | Adult dosage |
| 5 to 29 | 200-400 mg. I.V. q 18-24 hr |

*Hemodialysis patients:* 200 to 400 mg q 24 hours after dialysis period.

## I.V. administration

■ I.V. infusions should be administered over 60 minutes into a large vein to decrease potential adverse reactions.

### Incompatibilities

Incompatible with aminophylline and clindamycin phosphate.

## Mechanism of action

*Antibiotic action:* Ciprofloxacin inhibits DNA gyrase, preventing bacterial DNA replication. The following organisms have been reported to be susceptible (in vitro) to ciprofloxacin: *Campylobacter jejuni, Citrobacter diversus, Citrobacter freundii, Enterobacter cloacae, Escherichia coli* (including enterotoxigenic strains), *Haemophilus parainfluenzae, Klebsiella pneumoniae, Morganella morganii, Proteus mirabilis, Proteus vulgaris, Providencia rettgeri, Providencia stuartii, Pseudomonas aeruginosa, Serratia marcescens, Shigella flexneri, Shigella sonnei, Staphylococcus aureus* (penicillinase- and non–penicillinase-producing strains), *Staphylococcus epidermidis, Streptococcus faecalis,* and *Streptococcus pyogenes.*

## Pharmacokinetics

*Absorption:* About 70% is absorbed after oral tablet administration. Food delays rate of absorption but not extent.
*Distribution:* Serum levels peak within 1 to 2 hours after oral tablet dosing. Drug is 20% to 40% protein-bound; CSF levels are only about 10% of plasma levels.
*Metabolism:* Metabolism is probably hepatic. Four metabolites have been identified; each has less antimicrobial activity than the parent compound.
*Excretion:* Excretion is primarily renal. Serum half-life is about 4 hours in adults with normal renal function.

| Route | Onset | Peak | Duration |
|---|---|---|---|
| P.O. (tablet) | Unknown | ½-2⅓ hr | Unknown |
| P.O. (suspension) | Unknown | Unknown | Unknown |
| I.V. | Unknown | Immediate | Unknown |

## Contraindications and precautions
Contraindicated in patients sensitive to fluoroquinolone antibiotics. Use cautiously in patients with CNS disorders or those at risk for seizures.

## Interactions
**Drug-drug.** *Aminoglycosides, beta-lactams:* Synergistic effects have occurred with concurrent use. Avoid use together.
*Antacid supplements containing aluminum, calcium, magnesium:* May interfere with ciprofloxacin absorption. Ciprofloxacin may be safely given 2 hours before or 6 hours after antacids.
*Probenecid:* Concurrent use interferes with renal tubular secretion and results in higher plasma levels of ciprofloxacin. Avoid use together.
*Sucralfate:* Reduces absorption of ciprofloxacin by 50%. Avoid use together.
*Theophylline:* Increased risk of theophylline toxicity. Closer monitoring of theophylline levels may be needed.
*Warfarin:* Increased PT. Avoid use together.
**Drug-herb.** *Yerba maté:* May decrease clearance of yerba maté methylxanthine component and cause toxicity. Discourage use together.
**Drug-food.** *Caffeine:* Ciprofloxacin prolongs elimination half-life of caffeine. Discourage caffeine intake.
*Iron, minerals, vitamins:* May interfere with absorption of ciprofloxacin. Discourage use together.
**Drug-lifestyle.** *Sun exposure:* Photosensitivity reaction may occur from sun exposure. Advise patient to use sunblock.

## Adverse reactions
**CNS:** headache, restlessness, tremor, dizziness, fatigue, drowsiness, insomnia, depression, light-headedness, confusion, hallucinations, *seizures,* paresthesia.
**CV:** chest pain.
**GI:** *nausea, diarrhea,* vomiting, abdominal pain or discomfort, oral candidiasis, pseudomembranous colitis, dyspepsia, flatulence, constipation.
**GU:** crystalluria, increased serum creatinine and BUN levels, interstitial nephritis.
**Hepatic:** elevated liver enzyme levels.
**Musculoskeletal:** arthralgia, joint or back pain, joint inflammation and stiffness, aching, neck pain.
**Skin:** pruritus, erythema, *rash,* photosensitivity, *Stevens-Johnson syndrome,* toxic epidermal necrolysis, exfoliative dermatitis.
**Other:** photosensitivity, hypersensitivity; thrombophlebitis, burning, edema (with I.V. administration).

## Overdose and treatment
To treat drug overdose, empty the stomach by induced vomiting or lavage. Provide general supportive measures and maintain hydration. Peritoneal dialysis or hemodialysis may be helpful, particularly if patient's renal function is compromised.

## Clinical considerations
■ Duration of therapy depends on type and severity of infection. Therapy should continue for 2 days after symptoms have abated. Most infections are well controlled in 1 to 2 weeks, but bone or joint infections may require therapy for 4 weeks or longer.
■ Don't give oral suspension through feeding tube.

### Therapeutic monitoring
■ Patient's intake and output should be monitored; also advise clinician to observe patient for signs and symptoms of crystalluria.

### Special populations
**Breast-feeding patients.** Drug may appear in breast milk. Consider discontinuing breast-feeding or drug therapy to avoid serious toxicity in the infant.
**Pediatric patients.** Avoid use in children.
**Geriatric patients.** Use with caution.

## Patient counseling
■ Tell patient that drug may be taken without regard to meals. The preferred time is 2 hours after a meal.
■ Advise patient to avoid taking drug with antacids, iron, or calcium and to drink plenty of fluids during therapy.
■ Inform patient that because dizziness, light-headedness, or drowsiness may occur, he should avoid hazardous activities requiring mental alertness until CNS effects of drug are determined.

# ciprofloxacin hydrochloride (ophthalmic)
Ciloxan

*Pharmacologic classification:* fluoroquinolone
*Therapeutic classification:* antibacterial
*Pregnancy risk category C*

## Available forms
Available by prescription only
*Ophthalmic solution:* 0.3% in 2.5- and 5-ml containers

## Indications and dosages
*Corneal ulcers caused by* **Pseudomonas aeruginosa, Staphylococcus aureus, Staphylococcus epidermidis, Streptococcus pneumoniae,** *and possibly* **Serratia marcescens** *and* **Streptococcus viridans**
*Adults and children over age 12:* Instill 2 drops in the affected eye every 15 minutes for

first 6 hours, then 2 drops q 30 minutes for remainder of first day. On day 2, instill 2 drops hourly. On days 3 to 14, instill 2 drops q 4 hours.
*Bacterial conjunctivitis caused by* S. aureus *and* S. epidermidis *and possibly* S. pneumoniae
*Adults and children over age 12:* Instill 1 or 2 drops into the conjunctival sac of affected eye q 2 hours while awake, for first 2 days. Then 1 or 2 drops q 4 hours while awake, for next 5 days.

## Mechanism of action
*Antibacterial action:* Ciprofloxacin hydrochloride inhibits bacterial DNA gyrase, an enzyme needed for bacterial replication. Bacteriostatic or bactericidal, depending on level.

## Pharmacokinetics
*Absorption:* Systemic absorption is limited. The maximum plasma level is less than 5 ng/ml, and the mean plasma level is usually below 2.5 ng/ml.
*Distribution:* Unknown.
*Metabolism:* Unknown.
*Excretion:* Unknown.

| Route | Onset | Peak | Duration |
|-------|-------|------|----------|
| Ophthalmic | Unknown | Unknown | Unknown |

## Contraindications and precautions
Contraindicated in patients hypersensitive to drug or other fluoroquinolone antibiotics. Use with caution in breast-feeding women.

## Interactions
None reported.

## Adverse reactions
**EENT:** *local burning or discomfort, white crystalline* precipitate (in the superficial portion of the corneal defect in patients with corneal ulcers), *margin crusting, crystals or scales, foreign body sensation, itching, conjunctival hyperemia,* corneal staining, keratopathy, lid edema, tearing, photophobia, decreased vision.
**GI:** nausea, bad or bitter taste in mouth.
**Other:** allergic reactions.

## Overdose and treatment
A topical overdose of drug may be flushed from the eye with warm tap water.

## Clinical considerations
■ If corneal epithelium is still compromised after 14 days of treatment, advise clinician to continue therapy.

### Therapeutic monitoring
■ Drug should be stopped at first sign of hypersensitivity reactions, such as rash, itching

eyelids, redness or swelling, and prescriber should be notified.

### Special populations
**Breast-feeding patients.** It's unknown if drug appears in breast milk after application to the eye; however, systemically administered ciprofloxacin has been detected in breast milk. Use with caution.
**Pediatric patients.** Safety and efficacy in children under age 12 haven't been established.

## Patient counseling
■ Teach patient how to instill drug correctly. Remind him not to touch the tip of the bottle with his hands and to avoid contact of the tip with the eye or surrounding tissue.
■ Remind patient not to share washcloths or towels with other family members to avoid spreading infection.
■ Advise patient to wash hands before and after instilling solution.

# cisatracurium besylate
Nimbex

*Pharmacologic classification:* nondepolarizing neuromuscular blocker
*Therapeutic classification:* skeletal muscle relaxant
*Pregnancy risk category B*

## Available forms
Available by prescription only
*Injection:* 2 mg/ml, 10 mg/ml

## Indications and dosages
*Adjunct to general anesthesia, to facilitate tracheal intubation, and to provide skeletal muscle relaxation during surgery or mechanical ventilation in the intensive care unit*
*Adults and children ages 12 and older:* Initially, 150 or 200 mcg/kg I.V.; then after an initial dose of 150 mcg/kg, give 30 mcg/kg I.V. q 40 to 50 minutes, or q 50 to 60 minutes following an initial dose of 200 mcg/kg, for maintenance in prolonged surgical procedures. Alternatively, give 3 mcg/kg/minute maintenance infusion after initial dose and then decrease to 1 to 2 mcg/kg/minute, p.r.n.
*Children ages 2 to 12:* 100 mcg/kg I.V. over 5 to 10 seconds. Give 3 mcg/kg/minute maintenance I.V. infusion after initial dose and then decrease to 1 to 2 mcg/kg/minute, p.r.n., in prolonged surgical procedures.
*Maintenance of neuromuscular blockade in intensive care unit*
*Adults:* 3 mcg/kg/minute I.V. infusion.
　　Note: Dosage requirements among patients vary widely. Also, dosages may increase or decrease over time.

## I.V. administration

**◢ALERT** 20-ml vial is intended for use in the intensive care unit only.

**◢ALERT** Drug shouldn't be diluted in lactated Ringer's injection because of chemical instability.

### Incompatibilities

Incompatible with alkaline solutions with pH above 8.5, such as barbiturate solutions for Y-site administration. Also incompatible with lactated Ringer's injection and propofol or ketorolac injection for Y-site administration.

## Mechanism of action

*Skeletal muscle relaxation action:* Cisatracurium binds competitively to cholinergic receptors on the motor end-plate to antagonize the action of acetylcholine, resulting in blockage of neuromuscular transmission.

## Pharmacokinetics

*Absorption:* Only administered I.V.

*Distribution:* Volume of distribution is limited by its large molecular weight and high polarity. Drug binding to plasma proteins hasn't been successfully studied because of its rapid degradation at physiologic pH.

*Metabolism:* The degradation of cisatracurium is largely independent of liver metabolism. It's believed drug undergoes Hofmann elimination (a pH- and temperature-dependent chemical process) to form laudanosine and the monoquaternary acrylate metabolite.

*Excretion:* The metabolites of cisatracurium are excreted primarily in urine and feces. Elimination half-life is between 22 and 29 minutes.

| Route | Onset | Peak | Duration |
|-------|-------|------|----------|
| I.V. | 1-3 min | 2-5 min | 25-44 min |

## Contraindications and precautions

Contraindicated in patients hypersensitive to drug, other bis-benzylisoquinolinium drugs, or benzyl alcohol. Use cautiously in pregnant patients.

## Interactions

**Drug-drug.** *Aminoglycosides, bacitracin, clindamycin, colistimethate sodium, colistin, lincomycin, lithium, local anesthetics, magnesium salts, polymyxins, procainamide, quinidine, tetracyclines:* May enhance the neuromuscular blocking action of cisatracurium. Use together cautiously.

*Carbamazepine, phenytoin:* May cause slightly shorter duration of neuromuscular blockage, requiring higher infusion rate requirements. Advise clinician to monitor patient closely.

*Enflurane, isoflurane given with nitrous oxide or oxygen:* May prolong the clinically effective duration of action of initial and maintenance dosages of cisatracurium. In long surgical procedures, less frequent maintenance dosing, lower maintenance dosages, or reduced infusion rates of cisatracurium may be needed.

*Succinylcholine:* Shorter time to onset of maximum neuromuscular block. Advise clinician to monitor patient closely.

## Adverse reactions

**CV:** *bradycardia,* hypotension.
**Respiratory:** *bronchospasm.*
**Skin:** flushing, rash.

## Overdose and treatment

Overdose with neuromuscular blockers may result in neuromuscular block beyond the time needed for surgery and anesthesia. The primary treatment is maintenance of a patent airway and controlled ventilation until recovery of normal neuromuscular function is assured. Once recovery from neuromuscular block begins, further recovery may be facilitated by administration of an anticholinesterase drug (neostigmine, edrophonium) and an appropriate anticholinergic.

## Clinical considerations

■ Drug isn't recommended for rapid sequence endotracheal intubation because of its intermediate onset of action.

■ Cisatracurium has no known effect on consciousness, pain threshold, or cerebration. To avoid patient distress, neuromuscular block shouldn't be induced before patient is unconscious.

■ Drug is a colorless to slightly yellow or greenish-yellow solution. Inspect vial visually for particulate matter and discoloration before administration. Solutions that are not clear or that contain visible particulates shouldn't be used.

■ To avoid inaccurate dosing, advise clinician to perform neuromuscular monitoring on a nonparetic limb in patients with hemiparesis or paraparesis.

■ In patients with neuromuscular disease (myasthenia gravis and myasthenic syndrome), prolonged neuromuscular block may occur. The use of a peripheral nerve stimulator and a dose not exceeding 20 mcg/kg is recommended to assess the level of neuromuscular block and to monitor dosage requirements.

■ Because patients with burns have been shown to develop resistance to nondepolarizing neuromuscular blocking agents, these patients may require increased dosing requirements and exhibit shortened duration of action. Advise clinician to monitor closely.

### Therapeutic monitoring

■ Advise clinician to monitor neuromuscular function during drug administration with a nerve stimulator. Additional doses of drug shouldn't be given before there is a definite response to nerve stimulation. If no response oc-

curs, discontinue infusion until a response returns.
- Advise clinician to monitor patient's acid-base balance and electrolyte levels. Acid-base or serum electrolyte abnormalities may potentiate or antagonize the action of cisatracurium.
- Advise clinician to monitor patient for malignant hyperthermia.

### Special populations

**Breast-feeding patients.** It's not known if drug appears in breast milk. Use cautiously in breast-feeding women.

**Pediatric patients.** Safety and effectiveness in children under age 2 haven't been established.

**Geriatric patients.** Use with caution when giving to geriatric patients. The time to maximum block is about 1 minute slower in geriatric patients.

### Patient counseling

- Reassure patient and family that patient will be monitored continuously throughout drug use; explain reason for its use.
- All procedures and events must be explained to the patient because the drug doesn't interfere with patient's ability to hear.

# cisplatin (cis-platinum)

Platinol, Platinol-AQ

*Pharmacologic classification:* alkylating agent (cell cycle–phase nonspecific)
*Therapeutic classification:* antineoplastic
*Pregnancy risk category D*

## Available forms

Available by prescription only
*Injection:* 1 mg/ml (50-mg, or 100-mg vials)

## Indications and dosages

Indications and dosages may vary. Check current literature for recommended protocol.

*Adjunctive therapy in metastatic testicular cancer*
*Adults:* 20 mg/m² I.V. daily for 5 days. Repeat q 3 weeks for three cycles or more. Usually used in therapeutic regimen with bleomycin and vinblastine.

*Adjunctive therapy in metastatic ovarian cancer*
*Adults:* 75 to 100 mg/m² I.V. Repeat q 4 weeks or 50 mg/m² I.V. q 3 weeks with concurrent doxorubicin hydrochloride therapy.

*Treatment of invasive or advanced bladder cancer*
*Adults:* 50 to 70 mg/m² I.V. once q 3 to 4 weeks. Patients who have received other antineoplastics or radiation therapy should receive 50 mg/m² q 4 weeks.

◇ *Head and neck cancer*
*Adults:* 80 to 120 mg/m² I.V. once q 3 weeks.

◇ *Cervical cancer*
*Adults:* 50 mg/m² I.V. once q 3 weeks.

◇ *Non–small-cell lung cancer*
*Adults:* 75 to 100 mg/m² I.V. q 3 to 4 weeks with other drugs.

◇ *Brain tumor*
*Children:* 60 mg/m² I.V. for 2 days q 3 to 4 weeks.

◇ *Osteogenic sarcoma or neuroblastoma*
*Children:* 90 mg/m² I.V. q 3 weeks.

◇ *Advanced esophageal cancer*
*Adults:* 50 to 120 mg/m² I.V. once every 3 to 4 weeks when used alone or 75 to 100 mg/m² I.V. once every 3 to 4 weeks when used in combination chemotherapy regimens.

## I.V. administration

- Reconstitute 10-mg vial with 10 ml and 50-mg vial with 50 ml of sterile water for injection to yield a level of 1 mg/ml. The drug may be diluted further in a sodium chloride-containing solution for I.V. infusion.
- Don't use aluminum needles for reconstitution or administration of cisplatin; a black precipitate may form. Use stainless steel needles.
- Infusions are most stable in chloride-containing solutions, such as normal saline, 0.45% saline, or 0.225% saline.
- Mannitol may be given as a 12.5-g I.V. bolus before starting cisplatin infusion. Follow by infusion of mannitol at rate of up to 10 g per hour p.r.n. to maintain urine output during cisplatin infusion and for 6 to 24 hours after infusion.
- Drug is stable for 24 hours in normal saline solution at controlled room temperature. Don't refrigerate because precipitation may occur. Discard solution containing precipitate.

### Incompatibilities

Incompatible with aluminum, $D_5W$, sodium bicarbonate, 0.1% NaCl, and solutions with a chloride content under 2%, sodium thiosulfate, and sodium bisulfate.

## Mechanism of action

*Antineoplastic action:* Cisplatin exerts its cytotoxic effects by binding with DNA and inhibiting DNA synthesis and, to a lesser extent, by inhibition of protein and RNA synthesis. Cisplatin also acts as a bifunctional alkylating agent, causing intrastrand and interstrand cross-links of DNA. Interstrand cross-linking appears to correlate well with the cytotoxicity of drug.

## Pharmacokinetics

*Absorption:* Not given orally or intramuscularly.

*Distribution:* Distributed widely into tissues, with the highest levels found in the kidneys, liver, and prostate. Drug can accumulate in body tissues, with drug being detected up to 6

months after the last dose. Cisplatin doesn't readily cross the blood-brain barrier. Drug is extensively and irreversibly bound to plasma proteins and tissue proteins.
*Metabolism:* Unknown.
*Excretion:* Excreted primarily unchanged in urine. In patients with normal renal function, the half-life of the initial elimination phase is 25 to 79 minutes and the terminal phase 58 to 78 hours. The terminal half-life of total cisplatin is up to 10 days.

| Route | Onset | Peak | Duration |
|-------|-------|------|----------|
| I.V. | Unknown | Unknown | Several days |

## Contraindications and precautions

Contraindicated in patients hypersensitive to drug or to other platinum-containing compounds and in those with severe renal disease, hearing impairment, or myelosuppression.

## Interactions

**Drug-drug.** *Aminoglycosides:* Concurrent use potentiates the cumulative nephrotoxicity caused by cisplatin. Therefore, don't give aminoglycosides within 2 weeks of cisplatin therapy; advise clinician to monitor renal function studies carefully.
*Aspirin:* Increased risk of bleeding. Avoid use together.
*Loop diuretics:* Concurrent use increases the risk of ototoxicity. Advise clinician to closely monitor patient's audiologic status.
*Phenytoin:* May decrease serum level of phenytoin. Advise clinician to monitor phenytoin level.

## Adverse reactions

**CNS:** *peripheral neuritis, seizures,* neuropathy.
**EENT:** *tinnitus, hearing loss, ototoxicity,* vestibular toxicity.
**GI:** *nausea, vomiting* (beginning 1 to 4 hours after dose and lasting for 24 hours), loss of taste.
**GU:** more prolonged and SEVERE RENAL TOXICITY with repeated courses of therapy.
**Hematologic:** MYELOSUPPRESSION; *leukopenia, thrombocytopenia;* anemia; nadirs in circulating platelet and WBC counts on days 18 to 23, with recovery by day 39.
**Metabolic:** *hypomagnesemia,* hypokalemia, hypocalcemia, hyponatremia, hypophosphatemia, hyperuricemia.
**Other:** *anaphylactoid reaction.*

## Overdose and treatment

Signs and symptoms of overdose include leukopenia, thrombocytopenia, nausea, and vomiting.

Treatment is generally supportive and includes transfusion of blood components, antibiotics for possible infections, and antiemet-

ics. Cisplatin can be removed by dialysis, but only within 3 hours after administration.

## Clinical considerations

■ Advise clinician to review hematologic status and creatinine clearance before therapy.
■ Advise clinician to hydrate patient, with P.O. fluids if possible, or with normal saline solution before giving drug. A urine output of 100 ml/hour should be maintained for 4 consecutive hours before and 24 hours after infusion. Prehydration and mannitol diuresis may significantly reduce renal toxicity and ototoxicity.
■ Nausea and vomiting may be severe and protracted (up to 24 hours). Antiemetics can be started 24 hours before therapy. Advise clinician to monitor fluid intake and output and continue I.V. hydration until patient can tolerate adequate oral intake.
■ High-dose metoclopramide (2 mg/kg I.V.) has been used to prevent and treat nausea and vomiting. Dexamethasone 10 to 20 mg has been given I.V. with metoclopramide to help alleviate nausea and vomiting. Many patients respond favorably to treatment with ondansetron (Zofran). Pretreatment with this 5-$HT_3$ antagonist should begin 30 minutes before cisplatin therapy starts.
■ Treat extravasation with local injections of a 1/6 M sodium thiosulfate solution (prepared by mixing 4 ml of sodium thiosulfate 10% and 6 ml of sterile water for injection).
■ Anaphylactoid reaction usually responds to immediate treatment with epinephrine, corticosteroids, or antihistamines.
■ Avoid contact with skin and mucosa. If contact occurs, flush and wash drug off immediately.
■ I.V. sodium thiosulfate may be given with cisplatin infusion to decrease risk of nephrotoxicity.

## Therapeutic monitoring

■ Advise clinician to monitor CBC, platelet count, and renal function studies before initial and subsequent doses. Don't repeat dose unless platelet count is more than 100,000/mm³, WBC count is more than 4,000/mm³, serum creatinine level is less than 1.5 mg/dl, or BUN level is less than 25 mg/dl.
■ Renal toxicity becomes more severe with repeated doses. Renal function must return to normal before next dose can be given.
■ Advise clinician to monitor electrolyte levels extensively; aggressive supplementation is often required after a course of therapy.

## Special populations

**Pregnant patients.** Caution women of childbearing age not to become pregnant during therapy. Also advise them to consult with prescriber before becoming pregnant.

**Breast-feeding patients.** It's unknown if cisplatin appears in breast milk. However, because of risk to infant of serious adverse reactions, mutagenicity, and carcinogenicity, breast-feeding isn't recommended during therapy.

**Pediatric patients.** Pediatric dosages of cisplatin haven't been fully established. Unlabeled uses of cisplatin include osteogenic sarcoma and neuroblastoma. Ototoxicity appears to be more severe in children.

### Patient counseling
■ Stress importance of adequate fluid intake and increase in urine output, to facilitate uric acid excretion.

■ Tell patient to report tinnitus immediately, to prevent permanent hearing loss. Patient should have audiometric tests before initial and subsequent courses.

■ Advise patient to avoid exposure to people with infections.

■ Inform patient to promptly report unusual bleeding or bruising.

# citalopram hydrobromide
Celexa

*Pharmacologic classification:* SSRI
*Therapeutic classification:* antidepressant
*Pregnancy risk category C*

### Available forms
Available by prescription only
*Tablets:* 20 mg, 40 mg
*Solution:* 10 mg/5 ml

### Indications and dosages
*Depression*
*Adults:* Initially, 20 mg P.O. once daily, increasing to 40 mg daily after no less than 1 week. Maximum recommended dose is 40 mg daily.
*Elderly:* 20 mg/day P.O. with increase to 40 mg/day for nonresponding patients.
≡*Dosage adjustment.* For patients with hepatic impairment, use 20 mg/day P.O. Adjust dosage to 40 mg/day only for nonresponding patients.

### Mechanism of action
*Antidepressant action:* A selective serotonin reuptake inhibitor (SSRI) whose action is presumed to be linked to potentiation of serotonergic activity in the CNS resulting from inhibition of neuronal reuptake of serotonin.

### Pharmacokinetics
*Absorption:* Absolute bioavailability is 80% following oral administration.
*Distribution:* Highly plasma protein–bound (80%).

*Metabolism:* Extensively metabolized primarily by cytochrome P-4503A4 and cytochrome P-4502C19 to inactive metabolites.
*Excretion:* About 20% of drug is excreted in urine. Elimination half-life is about 35 hours. In geriatric patients over age 60, the half-life is increased up to 30%.

| Route | Onset | Peak | Duration |
|-------|-------|------|----------|
| P.O. | Unknown | 4 hr | Unknown |

### Contraindications and precautions
Contraindicated in patients also taking MAO inhibitors or within 14 days of MAO inhibitor therapy and in those hypersensitive to drug or its inactive ingredients.

### Interactions
**Drug-drug.** *Carbamazepine:* May increase citalopram clearance. Advise clinician to monitor patient for effects.
*CNS drugs:* Have additive effects. Use together cautiously.
*Drugs that inhibit cytochrome P-450 isoenzymes 3A4 and 2C19:* Decreased clearance of citalopram. Advise clinician to monitor patient closely.
*Imipramine, other tricyclic antidepressants:* Level of imipramine metabolite desipramine increased by about 50%. Use together cautiously.
*Lithium:* May enhance serotonergic effect of citalopram. Use with caution, and advise clinician to monitor lithium level.
*MAO inhibitors:* Serious, sometimes fatal, reactions may occur. Don't use drug within 14 days of MAO inhibitor.
*Sumatriptan:* Potential serotonergic interaction. Avoid concomitant use.
*Warfarin:* PT is increased by 5%. Advise clinician to monitor patient carefully.
**Drug-herb.** *St. John's wort:* Serotonin levels may rise too high, causing serotonin syndrome. Discourage use together.
**Drug-lifestyle.** *Alcohol use:* May increase CNS effects. Discourage use together.

### Adverse reactions
**CNS:** tremor, *somnolence, insomnia,* anxiety, agitation, dizziness, paresthesia, migraine, impaired concentration, amnesia, depression, apathy, *suicide attempt,* confusion, fatigue.
**CV:** tachycardia, orthostatic hypotension, hypotension.
**EENT:** rhinitis, sinusitis, abnormal accommodation.
**GI:** *dry mouth, nausea,* diarrhea, anorexia, dyspepsia, vomiting, abdominal pain, taste perversion, increased saliva, flatulence, increased appetite.
**GU:** dysmenorrhea, amenorrhea, ejaculation disorder, impotence, polyuria.
**Metabolic:** decreased and increased weight, hyponatremia.

---

**Musculoskeletal:** arthralgia, myalgia.
**Respiratory:** upper respiratory tract infection, coughing.
**Skin:** rash, pruritus, *increased sweating.*
**Other:** fever, yawning, decreased libido, SIADH.

## Overdose and treatment
Common clinical signs and symptoms of overdose include lethargy, drowsiness, nausea, vomiting, epigastric pain, and GI bleeding. Other symptoms may include hypertension, acute renal failure, respiratory depression, and coma. While there is no antidote for treatment of overdose, symptomatic and supportive care is usually sufficient. If a patient is seen within 4 hours of the overdose, emesis and activated charcoal, and an osmotic cathartic can be used. Because of the high protein binding, dialysis is unlikely to be effective.

## Clinical considerations
■ Use cautiously in patients with history of mania, seizures, suicidal ideation, or hepatic or renal impairment.
■ Although drug hasn't been shown to impair psychomotor performance, any psychoactive drug has the potential to impair judgment, thinking, or motor skills.
■ Taper dose gradually to reduce risk of withdrawal symptoms.

### Therapeutic monitoring
■ The possibility of a suicide attempt is inherent in depression and may persist until significant remission occurs. Advise clinician to closely observe high-risk patients when drug therapy starts. Reduce risk of overdose by limiting the amount of drug available per refill.

### Special populations
**Breast-feeding patients.** Drug appears in breast milk with subsequent effects in the infant; therefore, a decision to discontinue drug or breast-feeding should be made during drug therapy.
**Pediatric patients.** Safety and effectiveness haven't been established.
**Geriatric patients.** Use cautiously in geriatric patients because greater sensitivity to drug hasn't been ruled out.

## Patient counseling
**◄ ALERT** If a patient wishes to switch from an SSRI to St. John's wort, he may need to wait a few weeks for the SSRI to wash out of his system before it's safe to start taking the herb. The exact time required depends on which SSRI he's taking. He should consult his prescriber.
■ Inform patient that although improvement may occur within 1 to 4 weeks, he should continue therapy, as prescribed.
■ Instruct patient to exercise caution when operating hazardous machinery, including automobiles, because of the potential of psycho-active drugs to impair judgment, thinking, and motor skills.
■ Advise patient to consult prescriber before taking other prescription or OTC drugs or herbs.
■ Tell patient that drug may be taken in the morning or evening without regard to meals.

# cladribine
Leustatin

*Pharmacologic classification:* purine nucleoside analogue
*Therapeutic classification:* antineoplastic
*Pregnancy risk category D*

## Available forms
Available by prescription only
*Injection:* 1 mg/ml

## Indications and dosages
**Active hairy cell leukemia**
*Adults:* 0.09 mg/kg/day by continuous I.V. infusion for 7 days.
◇ *Advanced cutaneous T-cell lymphomas, chronic lymphocytic leukemia, malignant lymphomas, acute myeloid leukemias, autoimmune hemolytic anemia, mycosis fungoides, or Sézary syndrome*
*Adults:* Usually 0.1 mg/kg/day by continuous I.V. infusion for 7 days.

## I.V. administration
■ For a 24-hour infusion, add the calculated dose to a 500-ml infusion bag of normal saline solution. Once diluted, give promptly or store in the refrigerator for no longer than 8 hours before administration.
■ Don't use solutions that contain dextrose because studies have shown increased degradation of drug.
■ Because the product doesn't contain bacteriostatic agents, use strict aseptic technique to prepare the admixture.
■ Solutions containing cladribine shouldn't be mixed with other I.V. drugs or infused simultaneously via a common I.V. line.
■ Alternatively, prepare a 7-day infusion solution, using bacteriostatic sodium chloride injection, which contains 0.9% benzyl alcohol. First, pass the calculated amount of drug through a disposable 0.22-micron hydrophilic syringe filter into a sterile infusion reservoir. Next, add sufficient bacteriostatic sodium chloride injection to bring the total volume to 100 ml. Clamp off the line; then disconnect and discard the filter. If needed, aseptically aspirate air bubbles from the reservoir, using a new filter or sterile vent filter assembly.

### Incompatibilities
Limited incompatibility data are available. Don't mix with other I.V. drugs or additives.

---

Don't infuse simultaneously through a common I.V. line with other drugs. Dextrose solutions accelerate degradation of cladribine.

## Mechanism of action
*Antineoplastic action:* Cladribine enters tumor cells, where it's phosphorylated by deoxycytidine kinase and subsequently converted into an active triphosphate deoxynucleotide. This metabolite impairs synthesis of new DNA, inhibits repair of existing DNA, and disrupts cellular metabolism.

## Pharmacokinetics
*Absorption:* Administered I.V.
*Distribution:* About 20% of cladribine is plasma protein–bound.
*Metabolism:* Information not available.
*Excretion:* For patients with normal renal function, the mean terminal half-life of cladribine is 5½ hours.

| Route | Onset | Peak | Duration |
|-------|-------|------|----------|
| I.V. | 4 mo | Unknown | > 8 mo |

## Contraindications and precautions
Contraindicated in patients hypersensitive to drug. Use cautiously in patients with impaired renal or hepatic function.

## Interactions
**Drug-drug.** *Amphotericin B:* May increase the risk of nephrotoxicity, hypotension, and bronchospasm. Advise clinician to monitor patient closely.

## Adverse reactions
**CNS:** *malaise, headache, fatigue,* dizziness, insomnia, asthenia.
**CV:** tachycardia, edema.
**EENT:** epistaxis.
**GI:** *nausea, decreased appetite, vomiting, diarrhea,* constipation, abdominal pain.
**GU:** acute renal insufficiency.
**Hematologic:** NEUTROPENIA, anemia, *thrombocytopenia.*
**Metabolic:** hyperuricemia.
**Musculoskeletal:** *trunk pain, myalgia, arthralgia.*
**Respiratory:** *abnormal breath or chest sounds, cough,* shortness of breath.
**Skin:** *rash, pruritus, erythema, purpura,* petechiae, *local reaction at the injection site, diaphoresis.*
**Other:** *fever, infection, chills.*

## Overdose and treatment
High doses of cladribine have caused irreversible neurologic toxicity (paraparesis and quadriparesis), acute nephrotoxicity, and severe bone marrow suppression that results in neutropenia, anemia, and thrombocytopenia. No antidote specific to cladribine overdose is known. Besides discontinuation of cladribine, treatment consists of careful observation and appropriate supportive measures. It isn't known if drug can be removed from the circulation by dialysis or hemofiltration.

## Clinical considerations
- Fever is commonly observed during the first month of therapy and frequently requires antibiotic therapy.
- Because of risk of hyperuricemia from tumor lysis, recommend giving allopurinol during therapy.
- Physical and chemical stability are acceptable using Pharmacia Deltec drug cassettes.
- Refrigerate unopened vials at 36° to 46° F (2° to 8° C), and protect from light. Although freezing doesn't adversely affect the drug, a precipitate may form; this will disappear if the drug is allowed to warm to controlled room temperature gradually and the vial is vigorously shaken. Don't heat, microwave, or refreeze.

### Therapeutic monitoring
- Cladribine is a toxic drug, and some toxicity is expected during treatment. Advise clinician to monitor hematologic function closely, especially during the first 4 to 8 weeks of therapy. Severe bone marrow suppression, including neutropenia, anemia, and thrombocytopenia, has commonly been observed in patients treated with drug; many patients also have preexisting hematologic impairment from their disease.

### Special populations
**Pregnant patients.** Women of childbearing age should avoid pregnancy during drug therapy because of risk of fetal malformations.
**Breast-feeding patients.** It isn't known if drug appears in breast milk. A decision should be made whether to discontinue breast-feeding or drug, taking into account the importance of drug to the woman.
**Pediatric patients.** Safety and effectiveness in children haven't been established.

## Patient counseling
- Teach patient to watch for signs of infection and bleeding (easy bruising, nosebleeds).
- Tell patient to take his temperature daily.

---

# clarithromycin
Biaxin, Biaxin XL

*Pharmacologic classification:* macrolide
*Therapeutic classification:* antibiotic
*Pregnancy risk category C*

## Available forms
Available by prescription only
*Tablets:* 250 mg, 500 mg

---

*Tablets (extended-release):* 500 mg
*Suspension:* 125 mg/5 ml, 187.5 mg/5 ml,
250 mg/5 ml

## Indications and dosages
*Pharyngitis or tonsillitis caused by* **Strep-tococcus pyogenes**
*Adults:* 250 mg P.O. q 12 hours for 10 days.
*Children:* 15 mg/kg/day P.O. divided q 12 hours
for 10 days.
*Acute maxillary sinusitis caused by* **Strep-tococcus pneumoniae, Haemophilus in-fluenzae,** *or* **Moraxella catarrhalis**
*Adults:* 500 mg P.O. q 12 hours or two 500-mg
extended-release tablets P.O. once daily for 14
days.
*Children:* 15 mg/kg/day P.O. divided q 12 hours
for 10 days.
*Acute exacerbations of chronic bronchitis caused by* **M. catarrhalis** *or* **S. pneumoni-ae,** *pneumonia caused by* **S. pneumoniae** *or* **Mycoplasma pneumoniae**
*Adults:* 250 mg P.O. q 12 hours for 7 to 14 days.
*Acute exacerbations of chronic bronchitis caused by* **M. catarrhalis, S. pneumoniae; H. parainfluenzae,** *or* **H. influenzae**
*Adults:* Two 500-mg extended-release tablets
P.O. once daily for 7 days.
*Acute exacerbations of chronic bronchitis caused by* **H. influenzae**
*Adults:* 500 mg P.O. q 12 hours for 7 to 14 days.
*Uncomplicated skin and skin structure in-fections caused by* **Staphylococcus aureus** *or* **S. pyogenes**
*Adults:* 250 mg P.O. q 12 hours for 7 to 14 days.
*Prophylaxis and treatment of disseminated infection from* **Mycobacterium avium complex**
*Adults:* 500 mg P.O. b.i.d.
*Children:* 7.5 mg/kg P.O. b.i.d. up to 500 mg
b.i.d.
*Acute otitis media caused by* **H. influen-zae, M. catarrhalis,** *or* **S. pneumoniae**
*Children:* 7.5 mg/kg P.O. b.i.d. up to 500 mg
b.i.d.
**H. pylori** *eradication to reduce risk of duodenal ulcer recurrence*
*Adults:* 500 mg Biaxin with 30 mg lansopra-zole and 1 g amoxicilin, all given q 12 hours
for 10 to 14 days. Alternatively, dual therapy
with 500 mg Biaxin q 8 hours and 40 mg
omeprazole once daily for 14 days.
*Mild to moderate community-acquired pneumonia (CAP) caused by Haemophilis influenzae, H. parainfluenzae, Moraxella catarrhalis, Streptococcus pneumoniae, Chlamydia pneumoniae (TWAR), and My-coplasma pneumoniae*
*Adults:* Two 500-mg extended-release tablets
P.O. once daily for 7 days.
≡*Dosage adjustment.* For patients with cre-atinine clearance of less than 30 ml/minute, cut
dose in half or double frequency interval.

## Mechanism of action
*Antibiotic action:* Clarithromycin, a macrolide
antibiotic, binds to the 50S subunit of bacter-ial ribosomes, blocking protein synthesis. It's
bacteriostatic or bactericidal, depending on the
level.

## Pharmacokinetics
*Absorption:* Rapidly absorbed from the GI
tract; absolute bioavailability is about 50%. Al-though food slightly delays onset of absorp-tion, clarithromycin may be taken without re-gard to meals because food doesn't alter the
total amount of drug absorbed.
*Distribution:* Widely distributed; because it
readily penetrates cells, tissue levels are high-er than plasma levels. Plasma half-life is dose-dependent; half-life is 3 to 4 hours at doses of
250 mg q 12 hours and increases to 5 to 7 hours
at doses of 500 mg q 12 hours.
*Metabolism:* Clarithromycin's major metabo-lite, 14-hydroxy clarithromycin, has signifi-cant antimicrobial activity. It's about twice as
active against *H. influenzae* as the parent drug.
*Excretion:* In patients taking 250 mg q 12
hours, about 20% is eliminated in the urine un-changed; this increases to 30% in patients tak-ing 500 mg q 12 hours. The major metabolite
accounts for about 15% of drug in the urine.
Elimination half-life of the active metabolite
is dose-dependent: 5 to 6 hours with 250 mg
q 12 hours; 7 hours with 500 mg q 12 hours.

| Route | Onset | Peak | Duration |
|---|---|---|---|
| P.O. | Unknown | 2-4 hr | Unknown |
| P.O. (extended-release) | Unknown | 5-6 hr | Unknown |

## Contraindications and precautions
Contraindicated in patients hypersensitive to
erythromycin or other macrolides or patients
who have preexisting cardiac abnormalities or
electrolyte disturbances. Use cautiously in pa-tients with impaired renal or hepatic function.

## Interactions
**Drug-drug.** *Carbamazepine, theophylline:*
May increase serum levels. Advise clinician to
monitor plasma levels of these drugs carefully.
*Cyclosporine, phenytoin, triazolam:* Decreased
metabolism of these drugs. Advise clinician to
monitor patient closely.
*Digoxin:* Increased levels. Advise clinician to
monitor patient for signs of digoxin toxicity.
*Dihydroergotamine, ergotamine:* Acute ergot
toxicity. Avoid use together.
*Warfarin:* Increased INR with other macrolides,
and possibly with clarithromycin. Advise clin-ician to monitor patient closely.

## Adverse reactions
**CNS:** headache.
**GI:** *diarrhea, nausea, abnormal taste,* dys-pepsia, abdominal pain or discomfort.

---

**GU:** elevated BUN and creatinine levels.
**Hematologic:** increased PT; decreased WBCs.
**Hepatic:** elevated liver function tests results.

## Overdose and treatment
No information available.

## Clinical considerations
■ Obtain specimen for culture and sensitivity tests before giving first dose. Therapy may begin pending test results.
■ Reconstituted suspension shouldn't be refrigerated; discard any unused portion after 14 days.
■ Also used off-label for prophylaxis of bacterial endocarditis, treatment of Lyme disease and toxoplasmic encephalitis in patients with AIDS.
■ Patient shouldn't chew or crush the extended-release tablets.

### Therapeutic monitoring
■ Drug may cause overgrowth of nonsusceptible bacteria or fungi. Advise clinician to monitor patient for signs and symptoms of superinfection.

### Special populations
**Breast-feeding patients.** It's unknown if drug appears in breast milk; however, other macrolides have been found in breast milk. Use with caution.
**Pediatric patients.** Safety and efficacy in children under age 12 haven't been established.

## Patient counseling
■ Tell patient to take all of drug as prescribed, even if he feels better.
■ Inform patient that he may take drug without regard to meals.
■ Instruct patient to shake suspension well before use; don't refrigerate. Discard unused portion after 10 days.
■ Advise patient to not chew or crush the extended-release tablets.

---

# clemastine fumarate
Tavist, Tavist Allergy

*Pharmacologic classification:*
ethanolamine-derivative antihistamine
*Therapeutic classification:* antihistamine ($H_1$-receptor antagonist)
*Pregnancy risk category C*

## Available forms
Available without a prescription
*Tablets:* 1.34 mg (Tavist Allergy), 2.68 mg (Tavist)
*Syrup:* 0.5 mg /5 ml

## Indications and dosages
*Rhinitis, allergy symptoms*
*Adults and children ages 12 and older:* 1.34 to 2.68 mg P.O. b.i.d. or t.i.d. Maximum recommended daily dose is 8.04 mg.
*Children ages 6 to 11:* 0.67 mg P.O. b.i.d.; not to exceed 4.02 mg/day.
*Allergic skin manifestation of urticaria and angioedema*
*Adults and children ages 12 and older:* 2.68 mg P.O. up to t.i.d. maximum.
*Children ages 6 to 11:* 1.34 mg P.O. b.i.d.; not to exceed 4.02 mg/day.

## Mechanism of action
*Antihistamine action:* Antihistamines compete with histamine for histamine $H_1$-receptor sites on the smooth muscle of the bronchi, GI tract, uterus, and large blood vessels; by binding to cellular receptors, they prevent access of histamine and suppress histamine-induced allergic symptoms, even though they don't prevent its release.

## Pharmacokinetics
*Absorption:* Absorbed readily from the GI tract.
*Distribution:* Unknown.
*Metabolism:* Extensively metabolized.
*Excretion:* Excreted in urine

| Route | Onset | Peak | Duration |
|-------|-------|------|----------|
| P.O. | 15-60 min | 5-7 hr | 12 hr |

## Contraindications and precautions
Contraindicated in patients hypersensitive to drug or other antihistamines of similar chemical structure; in those with acute asthma; in neonates or premature infants; and in breast-feeding patients.

Use cautiously in geriatric patients and in patients with increased intraocular pressure, glaucoma, hyperthyroidism, CV or renal disease, hypertension, bronchial asthma, pyloroduodenal obstruction, prostatic hyperplasia, bladder neck obstruction, and stenosing peptic ulcers.

## Interactions
**Drug-drug.** *CNS depressants:* Increased sedation. Use together cautiously.
*Heparin:* May partially counteract the anticoagulant effect. Advise clinician to monitor patient closely.
*MAO inhibitors:* Prolong and intensify the central depressant and anticholinergic effects. Don't use together.
*Sulfonylureas:* May diminish the effects. Advise clinician to monitor patient closely.
**Drug-lifestyle.** *Alcohol use:* Additive CNS depression may occur. Discourage use together.
*Sun exposure:* Photosensitivity reactions may occur. Advise patient to take precautions.

---

## Adverse reactions

**CNS:** *sedation, drowsiness, **seizures**,* nervousness, tremor, confusion, restlessness, vertigo, headache, *sleepiness, dizziness, incoordination,* fatigue.
**CV:** hypotension, palpitations, tachycardia.
**GI:** *epigastric distress,* anorexia, diarrhea, nausea, vomiting, constipation, *dry mouth.*
**GU:** urine retention, urinary frequency.
**Hematologic:** hemolytic anemia, ***thrombocytopenia, agranulocytosis.***
**Respiratory:** *thick bronchial secretions.*
**Skin:** rash, urticaria, photosensitivity, diaphoresis.
**Other:** *anaphylactic shock.*

## Overdose and treatment

Signs and symptoms of overdose may include either CNS depression (sedation, reduced mental alertness, apnea, and CV collapse) or CNS stimulation (insomnia, hallucinations, tremors, or seizures). Anticholinergic symptoms, such as dry mouth, flushed skin, fixed and dilated pupils, and GI symptoms are common, especially in children.

Recommend treating overdose by inducing emesis with ipecac syrup (in conscious patient), followed by activated charcoal to reduce further drug absorption. Recommend using gastric lavage if patient is unconscious or if ipecac fails. Recommend treating hypotension with vasopressors, and controlling seizures with diazepam or phenytoin. Stimulants shouldn't be given.

## Clinical considerations

■ Consider the recommendations relevant to all antihistamines; drug is indicated for treatment of urticaria only at dosages of 2.68 mg up to t.i.d.
■ Discontinue clemastine 4 days before diagnostic skin tests; antihistamines can prevent, reduce, or mask positive skin test response.

### Therapeutic monitoring

■ Advise clinician to monitor blood counts during long-term therapy; advise clinician to observe patient for signs of blood dyscrasias.

### Special populations

**Breast-feeding patients.** Drug shouldn't be used during breast-feeding because it appears in breast milk, exposing infant to risks of unusual excitability; premature infants are at particular risk for seizures.
**Pediatric patients.** Drug isn't indicated for use in premature infants or neonates. Children, especially those under age 6, may experience paradoxical hyperexcitability.
**Geriatric patients.** Geriatric patients are more susceptible to the sedative effect of drug and may experience dizziness or hypotension more readily than younger people. Instruct

older patient to change positions slowly and gradually.

## Patient counseling

■ Inform patient of potential adverse reactions.
■ Tell patient to report if tolerance develops because a different antihistamine may need to be prescribed.

# clindamycin hydrochloride
Cleocin

# clindamycin palmitate hydrochloride
Cleocin Pediatric

# clindamycin phosphate
Cleocin Phosphate, Cleocin T

*Pharmacologic classification:* lincomycin derivative
*Therapeutic classification:* antibiotic
*Pregnancy risk category NR (B, vaginal and topical creams)*

## Available forms

Available by prescription only
*Capsules:* 75 mg, 150 mg, 300 mg
*Solution (granules):* 75 mg/5 ml
*Injection:* 150 mg/ml
*Infusion for I.V. use:* 150 mg/ml (300 mg, 600 mg, 900 mg)
*Gel, lotion, topical solution, pledgets:* 1%
*Vaginal cream:* 2%

## Indications and dosages

*Infections caused by sensitive organisms*
*Adults:* 150 to 450 mg P.O. q 6 hours; or 600 to 2,700 mg/day I.M. or I.V. divided into two to four equal doses.
*Children over age 1 month:* 8 to 20 mg/kg/day P.O. or 20 to 40 mg/kg/day I.V. divided into three or four equal doses.
*Children under age 1 month:* 15 to 20 mg/kg/day I.V. divided into three or four equal doses.
*Bacterial vaginosis*
*Adults:* 100 mg (1 applicatorful of clindamycin phosphate) intravaginally h.s. for 7 days.
*Acne vulgaris*
*Adults:* Apply thin film of topical solution, gel, or lotion to affected areas b.i.d.
◊ *Toxoplasmosis (cerebral or ocular) in immunocompromised patients*
*Adults and adolescents:* 300 to 450 mg P.O. q 6 to 8 hours with pyrimethamine (25 to 75 mg once daily) and leucovorin (10 to 25 mg once daily).
*Infants and children:* 20 to 30 mg/kg daily P.O. in four divided doses with oral pyrimethamine (1 mg/kg daily) and oral leucovorin (5 mg once every 3 days).

◇ **Pneumocystis carinii** *pneumonia*
*Adults:* 600 mg I.V. q 6 hours or 300 to 450 mg
P.O. q.i.d. With primaquine, give 15 to 30 mg
P.O. daily.

## I.V. administration
- For infusion, dilute each 300 mg in 50 ml of
$D_5W$, normal saline, or lactated Ringer's solution and give no faster than 30 mg/minute.
- Don't give more than 1.2 g/hour.

### Incompatibilities
Incompatible with aminophylline, ampicillin,
barbiturates, calcium gluconate, ciprofloxacin,
idarubicin magnesium sulfate, phenytoin sodium, and theophylline. Also incompatible with
rubber closures, such as those on I.V. tubing.

## Mechanism of action
*Antibacterial action:* Drug inhibits bacterial
protein synthesis by binding to ribosome's 50S
subunit. Clindamycin may produce bacteriostatic or bactericidal effects on susceptible bacteria, including most aerobic gram-positive
cocci and anaerobic gram-negative and gram-
positive organisms. It's considered a first-line
drug in the treatment of *Bacteroides fragilis*
and most other gram-positive and gram-
negative anaerobes. It's also effective against
*Mycoplasma pneumoniae, Leptotrichia buc-
calis,* and some gram-positive cocci and bacilli.

## Pharmacokinetics
*Absorption:* When given orally, drug is absorbed rapidly and almost completely from the
GI tract, regardless of formulation. Drug may
also be given I.M. with good absorption. With
300-mg dose, peak levels are about 6 mcg/ml;
with 600-mg dose, about 10 mcg/ml.
*Distribution:* Distributed widely to most body
tissues and fluids (except CSF) and crosses the
placental barrier. About 93% plasma protein–bound.
*Metabolism:* Metabolized partially to inactive
metabolites.
*Excretion:* About 10% of dose is excreted unchanged in urine; rest is excreted as inactive
metabolites (some drug appears in breast milk).
Plasma half-life is 2½ to 3 hours in patients
with normal renal function; 3½ to 5 hours in
anephric patients; and 7 to 14 hours in patients
with hepatic disease. Peritoneal dialysis and
hemodialysis don't remove drug.

| Route | Onset | Peak | Duration |
|---|---|---|---|
| P.O. | Unknown | 45-60 min | Unknown |
| I.V. | Unknown | Immediate | Unknown |
| I.M. | Unknown | 3 hr | Unknown |
| Topical, intravaginal | Unknown | Unknown | Unknown |

## Contraindications and precautions
Contraindicated in patients hypersensitive to
the antibiotic congener lincomycin; in those
with a history of ulcerative colitis, regional enteritis, or antibiotic-associated colitis; and in
those with a history of atopic reactions.
Use cautiously in patients with asthma, impaired renal or hepatic function, or history of
GI diseases or significant allergies.

## Interactions
**Drug-drug.** *Acne preparations:* Topical clindamycin may cause a cumulative irritant or
drying effect. Advise clinician to monitor patient carefully.
*Diphenoxylate, opiates:* May prolong or wors-
en clindamycin-induced diarrhea. Advise clinician to monitor patient closely.
*Erythromycin:* May block clindamycin from
reaching its site of action. Avoid use together.
*Kaolin:* May reduce GI absorption of clindamycin. Separate administration times.
*Neuromuscular blockers:* May potentiate the
neuromuscular blockade. Advise clinician to
monitor patient closely.
**Drug-food.** *Diet foods with sodium cyclamate:*
Decreased serum level of drug. Don't use together.

## Adverse reactions
**GI:** *nausea,* vomiting, abnormal liver function
test results, abdominal pain, diarrhea, pseudomembranous colitis.
**GU:** *cervicitis, vaginitis, Candida albicans*
overgrowth, *vulvar irritation.*
**Hematologic:** *transient leukopenia,* eosinophilia, *thrombocytopenia.*
**Hepatic:** jaundice.
**Skin:** maculopapular rash, urticaria, dryness,
*redness,* pruritus, swelling, irritation, contact
dermatitis, burning.
**Other:** *anaphylaxis.*

## Overdose and treatment
No information available.

## Clinical considerations
- Take culture and sensitivity tests before treatment starts; repeat, p.r.n.
- Don't refrigerate reconstituted oral solution because it will thicken. Drug remains stable for 2 weeks at controlled room temperature.
- I.M. preparation should be given deep I.M.
Rotate sites. Doses exceeding 600 mg aren't
recommended.
- I.M. injection may increase creatine kinase
levels because of muscle irritation.
- Topical form may produce adverse systemic
effects.

### Therapeutic monitoring

■ Advise clinician to monitor renal, hepatic, and hematopoietic functions during prolonged therapy.

### Special populations

**Breast-feeding patients.** Drug appears in breast milk. Advise breast-feeding women to use alternative feeding method during clindamycin therapy.
**Pediatric patients.** Give drug cautiously, if at all, to neonates and infants. Advise clinician to monitor closely, especially for diarrhea.
**Geriatric patients.** Geriatric patients may tolerate drug-induced diarrhea poorly. Advise clinician to monitor patient closely for change in bowel frequency and dehydration.

## Patient counseling

■ Warn patient that I.M. injection may be painful.
■ Advise patient to take capsules with 8 ounces (240 ml) of water to prevent dysphagia.
■ Instruct patient using topical solution to wash, rinse, and dry affected areas before application. Warn patient not to use topical solution near eyes, nose, mouth, or other mucous membranes, and caution about sharing washcloths and towels with family members.
■ Instruct patient to report adverse effects, especially diarrhea. Warn patient not to self-treat diarrhea.

---

## clobetasol propionate

Clobevate, Cormax, Dermovate*, Olux, Temovate

*Pharmacologic classification:* topical adrenocorticoid
*Therapeutic classification:* anti-inflammatory
*Pregnancy risk category C*

## Available forms

Available by prescription only
*Cream:* 0.05%
*Foam:* 0.05%
*Gel:* 0.05%
*Ointment:* 0.05%
*Solution:* 0.05%

## Indications and dosages

*Inflammation of corticosteroid-responsive dermatoses*
*Adults:* Apply a thin layer to affected areas b.i.d., once in the morning and once at night. Limit treatment to 14 days, with no more than 50 g of the cream, foam, or ointment or 50 ml of lotion (25 mg total) weekly.

## Mechanism of action

*Anti-inflammatory action:* Clobetasol is effective because of anti-inflammatory, antipruritic, and vasoconstrictive actions; however, exact mechanism of actions is unknown. Drug is a high-potency group I fluorinated corticosteroid that's usually reserved for the management of severe dermatoses that haven't responded satisfactorily to a less potent formulation.

## Pharmacokinetics

*Absorption:* Amount absorbed depends on potency of preparation, amount applied, and nature of skin at application site. It ranges from about 1% in areas with a thick stratum corneum (such as palms, soles, elbows, and knees) to 36% in areas with a thin stratum corneum (face, eyelids, and genitals). Absorption increases in areas of skin damage, inflammation, or occlusion. Some systemic absorption of topical steroids occurs, especially through the oral mucosa.
*Distribution:* After topical application, clobetasol is distributed throughout the local skin. Any drug absorbed into the circulation is rapidly removed from the blood and distributed into muscle, liver, skin, intestines, and kidneys.
*Metabolism:* After topical administration, drug is metabolized primarily in the skin. The small amount absorbed into systemic circulation is metabolized primarily in the liver to inactive compounds.
*Excretion:* Inactive metabolites are excreted by the kidneys, primarily as glucuronides and sulfates, but also as unconjugated products. Small amounts of the metabolites are also excreted in feces.

| Route | Onset | Peak | Duration |
|-------|-------|------|----------|
| Topical | Unknown | Unknown | Unknown |

## Contraindications and precautions

Contraindicated in patients hypersensitive to corticosteroids.

## Interactions

None reported.

## Adverse reactions

**Skin:** burning, pruritus, irritation, dryness, erythema, folliculitis, perioral dermatitis, allergic contact dermatitis, hypopigmentation, hypertrichosis, acneiform eruptions, numb fingers, skin atrophy and telangiectasia, stinging, cracking and fissuring of skin.
**Other:** *hypothalamic-pituitary-adrenal (HPA) axis suppression,* Cushing's syndrome, hyperglycemia, glycosuria.

## Overdose and treatment

No information available.

## Clinical considerations

■ Don't use occlusive dressings or bandages. Don't cover or wrap treated area unless instructed by prescriber.

---

- Apply sparingly in light film.
- "Pulse" therapy is sometimes used with topical corticosteroids of this potency; that is, twice a day for 3 days, then none for 3 days. Intermittent use prevents cumulative effects. Drug suppresses HPA axis at doses as low as 2 g/day.
- Foam contents under pressure. Don't puncture or incinerate container. Don't expose to heat or store at temperatures above 120° F (49° C).
- Foam contents are flammable. Avoid flame and smoking during and immediately following application.

### Therapeutic monitoring
- Recommend stopping drug and notifying prescriber if skin infection, striae, or atrophy occurs.

### Special populations
**Pregnant patients.** Because of the possibility of teratogenic effects; avoid use in pregnancy.
**Pediatric patients.** Drug isn't recommended for patients under age 12.

### Patient counseling
- Inform patient of potential adverse reactions.
- Advise patient to avoid contact with eyes.
- Warn patient not to use drug for longer than 14 days.
- Inform patient that foam contents are under pressure and not to puncture or incinerate container. Tell him not to expose to heat or store at temperatures above 120° F (49° C).
- Advise patient that foam contents are flammable. Tell him to avoid flame and smoking during and immediately following application.

---

# clofibrate
Atromid-S

*Pharmacologic classification:* fibric acid derivative
*Therapeutic classification:* antilipemic
*Pregnancy risk category C*

## Available forms
Available by prescription only
*Capsules:* 500 mg
*Powder:* 25 G

## Indications and dosages
*Hyperlipidemia and xanthoma tuberosum; type III hyperlipidemia that doesn't respond adequately to diet*
*Adults:* 2 g P.O. daily in two to four divided doses. Some patients may respond to lower doses as assessed by serum lipid monitoring.

◊ *Diabetes insipidus*
*Adults:* 1.5 to 2 g P.O. daily in divided doses.
≣ *Dosage adjustment.* For patients with decreased renal function, reduced dosage frequency (q 12 to 18 hours) may be needed.

## Mechanism of action
*Antilipemic action:* Clofibrate may lower serum triglyceride levels by accelerating catabolism of very low-density lipoproteins; drug lowers serum cholesterol levels (to a lesser degree) by inhibiting cholesterol biosynthesis. Both mechanisms are unknown. Drug is closely related to gemfibrozil.

## Pharmacokinetics
*Absorption:* Absorbed slowly but completely from GI tract. Serum triglyceride levels decrease in 2 to 5 days, with peak clinical effect at 21 days.
*Distribution:* Distributed into extracellular space as its active form, clofibric acid, which is up to 98% protein-bound. Animal studies suggest that fetal concentration levels may exceed maternal concentration levels.
*Metabolism:* Hydrolyzed by serum enzymes to clofibric acid, which is metabolized by the liver.
*Excretion:* 20% is excreted unchanged in urine; 70% is eliminated in urine as conjugated metabolite. Plasma half-life after a single dose ranges from 6 to 25 hours; in patients with renal impairment and cirrhosis, half-life can be as long as 113 hours.

| Route | Onset | Peak | Duration |
|-------|-------|------|----------|
| P.O. | Unknown | 2-6 hr | Unknown |

## Contraindications and precautions
Contraindicated in patients with significant hepatic or renal dysfunction, primary biliary cirrhosis, or hypersensitivity to drug and in pregnant or breast-feeding women. Use cautiously in patients with peptic ulcer or history of gallbladder disease.

## Interactions
**Drug-drug.** *Cholestyramine:* Concurrent use reduces absorption rate of clofibrate. Avoid use together.
*Furosemide:* Concurrent use may cause increased diuresis. Use cautiously.
*Oral anticoagulants:* Clofibrate potentiates the effects. If such a combination is needed, reduce oral anticoagulant dosage by 50%, and evaluate PT and INR frequently.
*Sulfonylureas:* Clofibrate may enhance the effects of sulfonylureas, causing hypoglycemia. Dosage adjustment may be needed.

## Adverse reactions
**CNS:** fatigue, weakness, drowsiness, dizziness, headache.

---

**CV:** *arrhythmias,* angina, *thromboembolic events,* intermittent claudication.
**GI:** *nausea, diarrhea, vomiting,* stomatitis, *dyspepsia,* flatulence.
**GU:** impotence, renal dysfunction (dysuria, hematuria, proteinuria, decreased urine output).
**Hematologic:** *leukopenia,* anemia, eosinophilia.
**Hepatic:** *transient and reversible elevations of liver function test results,* hepatomegaly, *cholelithiasis, cholecystitis.*
**Metabolic:** *weight gain.*
**Musculoskeletal:** myalgia and arthralgia.
**Skin:** rash, urticaria, pruritus, dry skin and hair.
**Other:** *polyphagia,* decreased libido.

## Overdose and treatment
No information available.

## Clinical considerations
- Clofibrate shouldn't be used indiscriminately; it may pose an increased risk of gallstones, heart disease, and cancer.
- Clofibrate may increase risk of death from cancer, postcholecystectomy complications, and pancreatitis.

### Therapeutic monitoring
- Advise clinician to monitor serum cholesterol and triglyceride levels regularly during clofibrate therapy.
- Advise clinician to observe patient for the following serious adverse reactions: thrombophlebitis, pulmonary embolism, angina, and dysrhythmias; advise clinician to monitor renal and hepatic function, blood counts, and serum electrolyte and blood glucose levels.

### Special populations
**Breast-feeding patients.** Clofibrate may appear in breast milk; an alternative feeding method is recommended during therapy.
**Pediatric patients.** Safety and efficacy haven't been established in children under age 14.

## Patient counseling
- Warn patient to report flulike symptoms immediately.
- Stress importance of close medical supervision and of reporting adverse reactions; encourage compliance with prescribed regimen and diet.
- Warn patient not to exceed prescribed dose.
- Advise patient to take drug with food to minimize GI discomfort.
- Emphasize that drug therapy won't replace diet, exercise, and weight reduction for the control of hyperlipidemia.

# clomiphene citrate
Clomid, Milophene, Serophene

*Pharmacologic classification:* chlorotrianisene derivative
*Therapeutic classification:* ovulation stimulant
*Pregnancy risk category X*

## Available forms
Available by prescription only
*Tablets:* 50 mg

## Indications and dosages
*To induce ovulation*
*Adults:* 50 mg P.O. daily for 5 days, starting any time in women who have had no recent uterine bleeding; or 50 mg P.O. daily starting on day 5 of menstrual cycle (first day of menstrual flow is day 1). Dose may be increased to 100 mg if ovulation doesn't occur. Repeat the 5-day course each ovulatory cycle until conception occurs or until 3 courses of therapy are completed.
◇ *Male infertility*
*Adults:* 50 to 400 mg P.O. daily for 2 to 12 months.

## Mechanism of action
*Ovulation stimulant action:* Mechanism of action for inducing ovulation in anovulatory females is unknown. Drug may stimulate release of pituitary gonadotropin, follicle-stimulating hormone (FSH), and luteinizing hormone (LH), which results in development and maturation of the ovarian follicle, ovulation, and subsequent development and function of corpus luteum.

## Pharmacokinetics
*Absorption:* Absorbed readily from the GI tract.
*Distribution:* May undergo enterohepatic recirculation or may be stored in body fat.
*Metabolism:* Metabolized by the liver.
*Excretion:* Half-life is about 5 days. Drug is excreted principally in feces via biliary elimination.

| Route | Onset | Peak | Duration |
|-------|-------|------|----------|
| P.O. | Unknown | Unknown | Unknown |

## Contraindications and precautions
Contraindicated during pregnancy and in patients with undiagnosed abnormal genital bleeding, ovarian cyst not caused by polycystic ovarian syndrome, hepatic disease or dysfunction, uncontrolled thyroid or adrenal dysfunction, or presence of organic intracranial lesion (such as a pituitary tumor).

## Interactions
None reported.

## Adverse reactions
**CNS:** headache, restlessness, insomnia, dizziness, light-headedness, depression, fatigue, aggressive behavior.
**EENT:** blurred vision, diplopia, scotoma, photophobia, epistaxis, pharyngitis, rhinitis, sinusitis.
**GI:** nausea, vomiting, bloating, distention, weight gain.
**GU:** urinary frequency and polyuria; abnormal uterine bleeding; *ovarian enlargement* and cyst formation, which regress spontaneously when drug is stopped.
**Hematologic:** *thrombocytopenia, leukopenia,* anemia.
**Respiratory:** coughing, dyspnea.
**Skin:** alopecia, urticaria, rash, dermatitis.
**Other:** *hot flashes,* reversible *breast discomfort;* increased levels of serum thyronine, thyroxine-binding globulin, sex hormone-binding globulin, sulfobromophthalein retention and FSH and LH secretion.

## Overdose and treatment
No information available.

## Clinical considerations
■ Advise patient to stop drug and notify prescriber immediately if abdominal symptoms or pain occur; these may indicate ovarian enlargement or ovarian cyst. Also, immediately report visual disturbances.
■ Human chorionic gonadotropin (5,000 to 10,000 units) may be given 5 to 7 days after the last dose of drug to stimulate ovulation.

### Therapeutic monitoring
■ Patient must be monitored closely because of risk of serious adverse effects.

### Special populations
**Pregnant patients.** Drug is contraindicated during pregnancy because of teratogenic possibilities. Advise patient to stop drug and contact her prescriber if she suspects she's pregnant.

## Patient counseling
■ Advise patient of possibility of multiple births, which increases with higher doses.
■ Patient should take basal body temperature every morning (starting on day 1 of menstrual period) and chart on a graph to detect ovulation.
■ Instruct patient on importance of properly timed coitus.
■ Warn patient to avoid hazardous tasks until response to drug is known because dizziness or visual disturbances may occur.

# clomipramine hydrochloride
Anafranil

*Pharmacologic classification:* tricyclic antidepressant (TCA)
*Therapeutic classification:* antiobsessional
*Pregnancy risk category C*

## Available forms
Available by prescription only
*Capsules:* 25 mg, 50 mg, 75 mg

## Indications and dosages
***Treatment of obsessive-compulsive disorder (OCD)***
*Adults:* Initially, 25 mg P.O. daily, gradually increasing to 100 mg P.O. daily (in divided doses, with meals) during the first 2 weeks. Maximum dosage, 250 mg daily. After adjustment, entire daily dose may be given h.s.
*Children and adolescents:* Initially, 25 mg P.O. daily, gradually increased to a maximum of 3 mg/kg or 100 mg P.O. daily, whichever is smaller (in divided doses, with meals) over the first 2 weeks. Maximum daily dose is 3 mg/kg or 200 mg, whichever is smaller. After adjustment, entire daily dose may be given h.s.

## Mechanism of action
*Antiobsessional action:* A selective inhibitor of serotonin (5-HT) reuptake into neurons within the CNS. It may also have some blocking activity at postsynaptic dopamine receptors. The exact mechanism by which clomipramine treats OCD is unknown.

## Pharmacokinetics
*Absorption:* Well absorbed from GI tract, but extensive first-pass metabolism limits bioavailability to about 50%.
*Distribution:* Distributed well into lipophilic tissues; the volume of distribution is about 12 L/kg; 98% plasma protein–bound.
*Metabolism:* Metabolism is primarily hepatic. Several metabolites have been identified; desmethylclomipramine is the primary active metabolite.
*Excretion:* About 66% is excreted in the urine and the remainder in the feces. Mean elimination half-life of the parent compound is about 36 hours; the elimination half-life of desmethyl-clomipramine has a mean of 69 hours. After multiple dosing, the half-life may increase.

| Route | Onset | Peak | Duration |
|-------|-------|------|----------|
| P.O. | ≥ 2 wk | 2-6 hr | Unknown |

## Contraindications and precautions
Contraindicated in patients hypersensitive to drug or other TCAs; in those who have taken MAO inhibitors within the previous 14 days;

and in patients during acute recovery period after MI.

Use cautiously in patients with urine retention, suicidal tendencies, glaucoma, increased intraocular pressure, brain damage, or seizure disorders and in those taking drugs that may lower the seizure threshold. Also use cautiously in patients with impaired renal or hepatic function, hyperthyroidism, or tumors of the adrenal medulla and in those undergoing elective surgery or receiving thyroid hormones or electroconvulsive treatment.

## Interactions
**Drug-drug.** *Barbiturates:* Decreased TCA blood levels. Advise clinician to monitor patient for decreased effectiveness.
*Barbiturates, CNS depressants:* May cause an exaggerated depressant effect when used with TCAs. Avoid use together.
*Epinephrine, norepinephrine:* May produce an increased hypertensive effect in patients taking TCAs. Avoid use together.
*MAO inhibitors:* May cause hyperpyretic crisis, seizures, coma, and death. Don't use together.
*Methylphenidate:* May increase TCA blood levels. Advise clinician to monitor patient closely.
**Drug-herb.** *Evening primrose:* Possible additive or synergistic effect resulting in lower seizure threshold and increasing the risk of seizure. Discourage use together.
*St. John's wort, SAMe, yohimbe:* Use with some TCAs may cause elevation of serotonin levels. Discourage use together.
**Drug-food.** *Grapefruit juice:* Elevated levels of clomiptamine and reduced levels of the metabolite, desmethylclomipramine. Discourage fluctuations in ingestion of grapefruit juice while taking the drug unless instructed by a prescriber to take clomipramine with grapefruit juice.
**Drug-lifestyle.** *Alcohol use:* Exaggerated depressant effect when used with TCAs. Discourage use together.
*Smoking:* Lower levels of clomipramine have been noted. Advise patient to avoid smoking.
*Sun exposure:* Increased risk of photosensitivity. Advise patient to take precautions.

## Adverse reactions
**CNS:** *somnolence, tremor, dizziness, headache, insomnia, nervousness, myoclonus, fatigue,* EEG changes, *seizures.*
**CV:** orthostatic hypotension, palpitations, tachycardia.
**EENT:** *pharyngitis, rhinitis, visual changes.*
**GI:** *dry mouth, constipation, nausea, dyspepsia, increased appetite,* diarrhea, *anorexia, abdominal pain.*
**GU:** *urinary hesitancy,* urinary tract infection, *dysmenorrhea, ejaculation failure, impotence.*
**Hematologic:** purpura, anemia.

**Metabolic:** *weight gain.*
**Skin:** *diaphoresis,* rash, pruritus, dry skin.
**Other:** *myalgia, altered libido.*

## Overdose and treatment
Signs and symptoms of clomipramine overdose are similar to those of other TCAs and have included sinus tachycardia, intraventricular block, hypotension, irritability, fixed and dilated pupils, drowsiness, delirium, stupor, hyperreflexia, and hyperpyrexia.

Treatment should include gastric lavage with large quantities of fluid. Continue lavage for 12 hours because the anticholinergic effects of the drug slow gastric emptying. Hemodialysis, peritoneal dialysis, and forced diuresis are ineffective because of the high degree of plasma protein–binding. Recommend supporting respirations and monitoring cardiac function. Recommend treating shock with plasma expanders or corticosteroids and treating seizures with diazepam.

## Clinical considerations
**⊞ALERT** To minimize risk of overdose, dispense drug in small quantities.
■ Don't withdraw drug abruptly.
■ Allow 2 weeks lapse between MAO inhibitor or SSRI therapy and clomipramine therapy.
■ Activation of mania or hypomania may occur with clomipramine therapy.

### Therapeutic monitoring
■ Patient needs observation for urine retention and constipation. Suggest stool softener or high-fiber diet p.r.n., and encourage adequate fluid intake.

### Special populations
**Breast-feeding patients.** It isn't known if drug appears in breast milk. Use with caution in breast-feeding women.

## Patient counseling
■ Warn patient to avoid hazardous activities that require alertness or good psychomotor coordination until adverse CNS effects are known. This is especially important during initial titration period when daytime sedation and dizziness may occur.
■ Suggest that dry mouth may be relieved with saliva substitutes or sugarless candy or gum.
■ Tell patient adverse GI effects may be minimized by taking drug with meals during the titration period. Later, the entire daily dose may be taken at bedtime to limit daytime drowsiness.
■ Inform patient to avoid using OTC drugs, particularly antihistamines and decongestants, unless recommended by prescriber.
■ Encourage patient to continue therapy, even if adverse reactions are troublesome. Advise patient not to stop taking it without notifying caregiver.

# clonazepam
Klonopin, Rivotril*

*Pharmacologic classification:* benzodiazepine
*Therapeutic classification:* anticonvulsant
*Pregnancy risk category C*
*Controlled substance schedule IV*

## Available forms
Available by prescription only
*Tablets:* 0.5 mg, 1 mg, 2 mg

## Indications and dosages
**Absence and atypical absence seizures, akinetic and myoclonic seizures, ◊ generalized tonic-clonic seizures**
*Adults:* Initial dosage shouldn't exceed 1.5 mg P.O. daily, divided into three doses. May be increased by 0.5 to 1 mg q 3 days until seizures are controlled. Maximum recommended daily dose, 20 mg.
*Children up to age 10 or weighing 30 kg (66 lb) or less:* 0.01 to 0.03 mg/kg P.O. daily (not to exceed 0.05 mg/kg daily), divided q 8 hours. Increase dosage by 0.25 to 0.5 mg q third day to a maximum maintenance dose of 0.1 to 0.2 mg/kg daily.
**◊ Leg movements during sleep; ◊ adjunct treatment in schizophrenia**
*Adults:* 0.5 to 2 mg P.O. h.s.
**◊ Parkinsonian dysarthria**
*Adults:* 0.25 to 0.5 mg P.O. daily.
**◊ Acute manic episodes**
*Adults:* 0.75 to 16 mg P.O. daily.
**◊ Multifocal tic disorders**
*Adults:* 1.5 to 12 mg P.O. daily.
**◊ Neuralgia**
*Adults:* 2 to 4 mg P.O. daily.

## Mechanism of action
*Anticonvulsant action:* Mechanism of anticonvulsant activity is unknown; clonazepam appears to act in the limbic system, thalamus, and hypothalamus. It's used to treat myoclonic, atonic, and absence seizures resistant to other anticonvulsants and to suppress or eliminate attacks of sleep-related nocturnal myoclonus (restless legs syndrome).

## Pharmacokinetics
*Absorption:* Well absorbed from the GI tract.
*Distribution:* Distributed widely throughout the body; about 85% protein-bound.
*Metabolism:* Metabolized by the liver to several metabolites. The half-life of drug is 18 to 39 hours.
*Excretion:* Excreted in urine.

| Route | Onset | Peak | Duration |
|-------|-------|------|----------|
| P.O. | 20-60 min | 1-2 hr | 6-12 hr |

## Contraindications and precautions
Contraindicated in patients with significant hepatic disease; in those with sensitivity to benzodiazepines; and in patients with acute angle-closure glaucoma. Use cautiously in children and in patients with mixed-type seizures, respiratory disease, or glaucoma.

## Interactions
**Drug-drug.** *Anticonvulsants, CNS depressants:* Additive CNS depressant effects. Avoid use together.
*Ritonavir:* May significantly increase levels of clonazepam. Advise clinician to monitor patient closely.
*Valproic acid:* May induce absence seizures. Don't use together.
**Drug-lifestyle.** *Alcohol use:* Additive CNS depressant effects. Advise patient to avoid alcohol.

## Adverse reactions
**CNS:** *drowsiness, ataxia, behavioral disturbances* (especially in children), slurred speech, tremor, confusion, psychosis, agitation.
**CV:** palpitations.
**EENT:** nystagmus, abnormal eye movements.
**GI:** constipation, gastritis, change in appetite, nausea, anorexia, diarrhea, sore gums.
**GU:** dysuria, enuresis, nocturia, urine retention.
**Hematologic:** *leukopenia, thrombocytopenia,* eosinophilia.
**Hepatic:** elevated liver function test results.
**Respiratory:** *respiratory depression,* chest congestion, shortness of breath.
**Skin:** rash.

## Overdose and treatment
Signs and symptoms of overdose may include ataxia, confusion, coma, decreased reflexes, and hypotension. Recommend treating overdose with gastric lavage and supportive therapy. Flumazenil, a specific benzodiazepine antagonist, may be useful. Vasopressors should be used to treat hypotension. Advise clinician to carefully monitor vital signs, ECG, and fluid and electrolyte balance. Clonazepam isn't dialyzable.

## Clinical considerations
■ Abrupt withdrawal may precipitate status epilepticus; after long-term use, lower dosage gradually.
■ Advise clinician to monitor patient for oversedation, especially in geriatric patients.

### Therapeutic monitoring
■ Advise clinician to monitor CBC and liver function test results periodically.

### Special populations
**Breast-feeding patients.** Alternative feeding method is recommended during clonazepam therapy.

---

*Canada only    ◊ Unlabeled clinical use

**Pediatric patients.** Long-term safety in children hasn't been established.

**Geriatric patients.** Geriatric patients may require lower doses because of diminished renal function; such patients also are at greater risk for oversedation from CNS depressants.

## Patient counseling

■ Explain reason for therapy and risks and benefits that may be anticipated.

■ Teach patient signs and symptoms of adverse reactions, and explain the need to report them promptly.

■ Warn patient not to discontinue drug or change dosage unless prescribed.

■ Advise patient to avoid tasks that require mental alertness until degree of sedative effect is determined.

# clonidine hydrochloride
Catapres, Catapres-TTS, Dixarit*

*Pharmacologic classification:* centrally acting alpha-adrenergic agonist
*Therapeutic classification:* antihypertensive
*Pregnancy risk category C*

## Available forms
Available by prescription only
*Tablets:* 0.1 mg, 0.2 mg, 0.3 mg
*Transdermal:* TTS-1 (releases 0.1 mg/24 hours); TTS-2 (releases 0.2 mg/24 hours); TTS-3 (releases 0.3 mg/24 hours)

## Indications and dosages
*Hypertension*
*Adults:* Initially, 0.1 mg P.O. b.i.d.; then increased by 0.1 to 0.2 mg daily or every few days until desired response is achieved. Usual dose range is 0.2 to 0.6 mg daily in divided doses. Maximum effective dose is 2.4 mg/day. If transdermal patch is used, apply to area of hairless intact skin once q 7 days.
◊ *Adjunctive therapy in nicotine withdrawal*
*Adults:* Initially, 0.1 mg P.O. b.i.d., gradually increased by 0.1 mg/day every week up to 0.75 mg P.O. daily as tolerated. Alternatively, apply transdermal patch (0.1 to 0.2 mg/24 hours) and replace weekly for the first 2 or 3 weeks after smoking cessation.
◊ *Prophylaxis for vascular headache*
*Adults:* 0.025 mg P.O. b.i.d. to q.i.d. up to 0.15 mg P.O. daily in divided doses.
◊ *Adjunctive treatment of menopausal symptoms*
*Adults:* 0.025 to 0.2 mg P.O. b.i.d. Alternatively, apply transdermal patch (0.1 mg/24 hours) and replace weekly.
◊ *Adjunctive therapy in opiate withdrawal*
*Adults:* 5 to 17 mcg/kg P.O. daily in divided doses for up to 10 days. Adjust dosage to avoid hypotension and excessive sedation, and slowly withdraw drug.
◊ *Dysmenorrhea*
*Adults:* 0.025 mg P.O. b.i.d. for 14 days before onset of menses and during menses.
◊ *Ulcerative colitis*
*Adults:* 0.3 mg P.O. t.i.d.
◊ *Neuralgia*
*Adults:* 0.2 mg P.O. daily.
◊ *Tourette syndrome*
*Adults:* 0.15 to 0.2 mg P.O. daily.
◊ *Diabetic diarrhea*
*Adults:* 0.15 to 1.2 mg/day P.O. or 1 to 2 patches/week (0.3 mg/24 hours).
◊ *Growth delay in children*
*Children:* 0.0375 to 0.15 mg/m$^2$ P.O. daily.
◊ *To diagnose pheochromocytoma*
*Adults:* 0.3 mg given as a single dose.
◊ *Attention deficit hyperactivity disorder (ADHD)*
*Children:* Initially, 0.05 mg P.O. daily h.s. Increase dose cautiously over 2 to 4 weeks. Maintenance dose ranges from 0.05 mg to 0.4 mg daily depending on patient's weight and tolerance.

## Mechanism of action
*Antihypertensive action:* Clonidine decreases peripheral vascular resistance by stimulating central alpha-adrenergic receptors, thus decreasing cerebral sympathetic outflow; drug may also inhibit renin release. Initially, clonidine may stimulate peripheral alpha-adrenergic receptors, producing transient vasoconstriction.

## Pharmacokinetics
*Absorption:* Absorbed well from the GI tract when given orally; absorbed well percutaneously after transdermal topical administration.
*Distribution:* Distributed widely into the body.
*Metabolism:* Metabolized in the liver, where nearly 50% is transformed to inactive metabolites.
*Excretion:* About 65% of a given dose is excreted in urine; 20% is excreted in feces. Half-life of clonidine ranges from 6 to 20 hours in patients with normal renal function. After oral administration, the antihypertensive effect lasts up to 8 hours; after transdermal application, the antihypertensive effect persists for up to 7 days.

| Route | Onset | Peak | Duration |
|---|---|---|---|
| P.O. | ½-1 hr | 2-4 hr | 12-24 hr |
| Transdermal | 2-3 days | 2-3 days | 7-8 days |

## Contraindications and precautions
Contraindicated in patients hypersensitive to drug. Transdermal form is contraindicated in patients hypersensitive to any component of the adhesive layer of the transdermal system. Use cautiously in patients with severe coro-

nary disease, recent MI, cerebrovascular disease, and impaired hepatic or renal function.

## Interactions

**Drug-drug.** *Barbiturates:* Clonidine may increase CNS depressant effects. Avoid use together.

*MAO inhibitors, tolazoline, tricyclic antidepressants:* May inhibit the antihypertensive effects of clonidine. Avoid use together.

*Propranolol, other beta blockers:* May have an additive effect, producing bradycardia. Avoid use together.

**Drug-herb.** *Capsicum:* May reduce antihypertensive effectiveness. Discourage use together.

**Drug-lifestyle.** *Alcohol use:* Increases CNS depressant effects. Advise patient to avoid alcohol.

## Adverse reactions

**CNS:** *drowsiness, dizziness,* fatigue, *sedation, weakness,* malaise, agitation, depression.
**CV:** orthostatic hypotension, ***bradycardia,*** *severe rebound hypertension.*
**GI:** *constipation, dry mouth,* nausea, vomiting, anorexia.
**GU:** urine retention, impotence.
**Metabolic:** possible slight increase in serum glucose levels, weight gain.
**Skin:** *pruritus, dermatitis* (with transdermal patch), rash.
**Other:** loss of libido.

## Overdose and treatment

Signs and symptoms of overdose include bradycardia, CNS depression, respiratory depression, hypothermia, apnea, seizures, lethargy, agitation, irritability, diarrhea, and hypotension; hypertension has also been reported.

After overdose with oral clonidine, emesis shouldn't be induced because rapid onset of CNS depression can lead to aspiration. After adequate airway is assured, recommend emptying stomach by gastric lavage followed by administration of activated charcoal. If overdose occurs in patients receiving transdermal therapy, recommend removing transdermal patch. Further treatment is usually symptomatic and supportive.

## Clinical considerations

**⊩ALERT** Remove transdermal systems when attempting defibrillation or synchronized cardioversion because of electrical conductivity.
■ Clonidine may be used to lower blood pressure quickly in some hypertensive emergencies.
■ Because rebound hypertension can occur when drug is discontinued, drug shouldn't be stopped abruptly; advise clinician to reduce dosage gradually over 2 to 4 days.
■ Optimal dosage for nicotine withdrawal hasn't been established.

■ Patients with renal impairment may respond to smaller doses of drug.
■ Give drug 4 to 6 hours before scheduled surgery.
■ Patient may need oral antihypertensive therapy when transdermal therapy starts.
■ Clonidine may decrease urinary excretion of vanillylmandelic acid and catecholamines; may cause a weakly positive Coombs' test.

### Therapeutic monitoring

■ Advise clinician to monitor pulse and blood pressure frequently; dosage is usually adjusted to patient's response and tolerance. Systolic blood pressure is considered the principal clinical endpoint for detecting and treating hypertension.
■ Advise clinician to record daily weight during initiation of therapy to monitor fluid retention.

### Special populations

**Breast-feeding patients.** Clonidine appears in breast milk. An alternative feeding method is recommended during treatment.
**Pediatric patients.** Efficacy and safety in children haven't been established; use drug only if potential benefit outweighs risk.
**Geriatric patients.** Geriatric patients may require lower doses because they may be more sensitive to the hypotensive effects of clonidine. Advise clinician to monitor renal function closely.

## Patient counseling

■ Explain disease and reason for therapy; emphasize importance of follow-up visits in establishing therapeutic regimen.
■ Teach patient signs and symptoms of adverse effects and the need to report them; patient should also report excessive weight gain (more than 5 lb weekly).
■ Warn patient to avoid hazardous activities that require mental alertness until tolerance develops to CNS effects.
■ Advise patient to avoid sudden position changes to minimize orthostatic hypotension.
■ Inform patient that ice chips, hard candy, or gum will relieve dry mouth.
■ Warn patient to call for specific instructions before taking OTC cold preparations.
■ Recommend taking last dose at bedtime to ensure night-time blood pressure control.
■ Tell patient not to discontinue drug suddenly because rebound hypertension may develop.
■ Teach patient to rotate transdermal patch site weekly.

# clopidogrel bisulfate
Plavix

*Pharmacologic classification:* inhibitor of ADP-induced platelet aggregation
*Therapeutic classification:* antiplatelet agent
*Pregnancy risk category B*

## Available forms
Available by prescription only
*Tablets:* 75 mg

## Indications and dosages
*To reduce atherosclerotic events (MI, CVA, vascular death) in patients with atherosclerosis documented by recent CVA, MI, or peripheral arterial disease*
Adults: 75 mg P.O. once daily with or without food.

## Mechanism of action
*Antiplatelet action:* Clopidogrel inhibits the binding of adenosine diphosphate (ADP) to its platelet receptor and the subsequent ADP-mediated activation of glycoprotein IIb/IIIa complex, thereby inhibiting platelet aggregation. Because clopidogrel acts by irreversibly modifying the platelet ADP receptor, platelets exposed to the drug are affected for their life span.

## Pharmacokinetics
*Absorption:* After repeated oral doses, plasma levels of parent compound, which has no platelet-inhibiting effect, are very low and generally below quantification limit. Pharmacokinetic evaluations are generally stated in terms of the main circulating metabolite. Rapidly absorbed after oral dosing. Following oral administration, about 50% of dose is absorbed.
*Distribution:* Clopidogrel and main circulating metabolite binds reversibly to human plasma proteins (98% and 94%, respectively).
*Metabolism:* Extensively metabolized by the liver. Main circulating metabolite is the carboxylic acid derivative that has no effect on platelet aggregation. It represents about 85% of circulating drug. Elimination half-life of main circulating metabolite is 8 hours after single and repeated doses.
*Excretion:* Following oral administration, about 50% is excreted in the urine and 46% in feces.

| Route | Onset | Peak | Duration |
|-------|-------|------|----------|
| P.O. | 2 hr | Unknown | 5 days |

## Contraindications and precautions
Contraindicated in patients with pathologic bleeding, such as peptic ulcer or intracranial hemorrhage, and in those hypersensitive to drug or its components.

Use with caution in patients at risk for increased bleeding from trauma, surgery, or other pathologic conditions and in those with hepatic impairment or severe hepatic disease.

## Interactions
**Drug-drug.** *Aspirin, NSAIDs:* May increase risk for GI bleeding. Use together cautiously.
*Heparin, warfarin:* Safety hasn't been established. Use together cautiously.
**Drug-herb.** *Red clover:* May cause increased bleeding if taken with drug. Use together cautiously.

## Adverse reactions
**CNS:** asthenia, depression, dizziness, fatigue, headache, paresthesia, syncope.
**CV:** chest pain, edema, hypertension, palpitation.
**EENT:** epistaxis, rhinitis.
**GI:** abdominal pain, constipation, diarrhea, dyspepsia, gastritis, *hemorrhage,* nausea, vomiting.
**GU:** urinary tract infection.
**Hematologic:** purpura.
**Musculoskeletal:** arthralgia.
**Respiratory:** bronchitis, coughing, dyspnea, upper respiratory infection.
**Skin:** rash, pruritus.
**Other:** flulike symptoms, pain.

## Overdose and treatment
No adverse effects were reported after single oral administration of 600 mg (equivalent to eight standard 75-mg tablets). The bleeding time was prolonged by a factor of 1.7, which is similar to that observed with the therapeutic dosage of 75 mg daily.

Based on biological plausibility, platelet transfusion may be appropriate to reverse the pharmacologic effects of clopidogrel if quick reversal is needed.

## Clinical considerations
■ Drug is usually used in patients who are hypersensitive or intolerant to aspirin.
■ If patient is to undergo surgery and an antiplatelet effect isn't desired, drug should be stopped 7 days before surgery.

### Therapeutic monitoring
■ If patient shows signs and symptoms of thrombotic thrombocytopenic purpura, prompt treatment is required.

### Special populations
**Breast-feeding patients.** It isn't known if drug or its metabolites appear in breast milk. Assess risks and benefits before continuing drug in breast-feeding women.
**Pediatric patients.** Safety and efficacy in children haven't been established.

## Patient counseling
- Inform patient it may take longer than usual to stop bleeding; therefore, advise him to refrain from activities in which trauma and bleeding may occur. Encourage use of seat belts.
- Tell patient to inform prescriber or dentist of clopidogrel use before scheduling surgery or taking new drugs.
- Inform patient that drug may be taken without regard to meals.
- Instruct patient to report unusual bleeding or bruising.

# clorazepate dipotassium
Novo-Clopate*, Tranxene*, Tranxene-SD, Tranxene-SD Half Strength

*Pharmacologic classification:* benzodiazepine
*Therapeutic classification:* anxiolytic, sedative-hypnotic, anticonvulsant
*Pregnancy risk category NR*
*Controlled substance schedule IV*

## Available forms
Available by prescription only
*Tablets:* 3.75 mg, 7.5 mg, 11.25 mg, 15 mg, 22.5 mg
*Capsules:* 3.75 mg, 7.5 mg, 15 mg

## Indications and dosages
*Acute alcohol withdrawal*
Adults: Day 1—initially, 30 mg P.O., followed by 30 to 60 mg P.O. in divided doses; day 2—45 to 90 mg P.O. in divided doses; day 3—22.5 to 45 mg P.O. in divided doses; day 4—15 to 30 mg P.O. in divided doses; gradually reduce daily dose to 7.5 to 15 mg.
*Anxiety*
Adults: 15 to 60 mg P.O. daily.
*As an adjunct in treatment of partial seizures*
Adults and children over age 12: Maximum recommended initial dose is 7.5 mg P.O. t.i.d. Dosage increases shouldn't exceed 7.5 mg/week. Maximum daily dose shouldn't exceed 90 mg.
Children ages 9 to 12: Maximum recommended initial dose is 7.5 mg P.O. b.i.d. Dosage increases shouldn't exceed 7.5 mg/week. Maximum daily dose shouldn't exceed 60 mg.

## Mechanism of action
*Anticonvulsant action:* Drug suppresses spread of seizure activity produced by epileptogenic foci in the cortex, thalamus, and limbic structures by enhancing presynaptic inhibition.
*Anxiolytic and sedative actions:* Clorazepate depresses the CNS at the limbic and subcortical levels of the brain. It produces an antianxiety effect by enhancing the effect of the neurotransmitter gamma-aminobutyric acid (GABA) on its receptor in the ascending reticular activating system, which increases inhibition and blocks both cortical and limbic arousal.

## Pharmacokinetics
*Absorption:* After oral administration, clorazepate is hydrolyzed in the stomach to desmethyldiazepam, which is absorbed completely and rapidly.
*Distribution:* Distributed widely throughout the body. About 80% to 95% of an administered dose is plasma protein–bound.
*Metabolism:* Metabolized in the liver to conjugated oxazepam.
*Excretion:* Inactive glucuronide metabolites are excreted in urine. The half-life of desmethyldiazepam ranges from 30 to 100 hours.

| Route | Onset | Peak | Duration |
|---|---|---|---|
| P.O. | Unknown | ½-2 hr | Unknown |

## Contraindications and precautions
Contraindicated in patients hypersensitive to drug or other benzodiazepines and those with acute angle-closure glaucoma. Avoid use in pregnant patients, especially during the first trimester.
Use cautiously in patients with impaired renal or hepatic function, suicidal tendencies, or history of drug abuse.

## Interactions
**Drug-drug.** *Antidepressants, antihistamines, barbiturates, general anesthetics, MAO inhibitors, narcotics, phenothiazines:* Potentiate the CNS depressant effects. Avoid use together.
*Cimetidine, disulfiram:* Increased plasma level. Avoid use together.
*Haloperidol:* Reduces serum levels. Advise clinician to monitor patient closely.
*Levodopa:* Decreased therapeutic effectiveness of levodopa. Avoid use together.
**Drug-herb.** *Catnip, kava, lady's slipper, lemon balm, passion flower, sassafras, skullcap, valerian:* Sedative effects may be enhanced. Discourage use together.
**Drug-lifestyle.** *Alcohol use:* Potentiates CNS-depressant effects. Advise patient to avoid alcohol.
*Heavy smoking:* Accelerates clorazepate's metabolism, thus lowering clinical effectiveness. Discourage smoking.

## Adverse reactions
**CNS:** *drowsiness,* dizziness, nervousness, confusion, headache, insomnia, depression, irritability, tremor.
**CV:** hypotension, minor changes in EEG patterns.
**EENT:** blurred vision, diplopia.
**GI:** nausea, vomiting, abdominal discomfort, dry mouth.
**GU:** urine retention, incontinence.

**Hepatic:** elevated liver function test results.
**Skin:** rash.

## Overdose and treatment

Signs and symptoms of overdose include somnolence, confusion, coma, hypoactive reflexes, dyspnea, labored breathing, hypotension,
bradycardia, slurred speech, and unsteady gait
or impaired coordination.

Recommend supporting blood pressure and
respiration until drug effects subside and monitoring vital signs. Flumazenil, a specific benzodiazepine antagonist, may be useful. Mechanical ventilatory assistance via endotracheal
tube may be required to maintain a patent airway and support adequate oxygenation. Treat
hypotension with I.V. fluids and vasopressors
such as dopamine and phenylephrine p.r.n. Recommend inducing emesis if patient is conscious. Recommend using gastric lavage if ingestion was recent, but only if an endotracheal
tube is present to prevent aspiration. After emesis or lavage, activated charcoal may be given
with a cathartic as a single dose. Dialysis is of
limited value. Don't use barbiturates because
they may worsen CNS adverse effects.

## Clinical considerations

■ Lower doses are effective in geriatric patients
and patients with renal or hepatic dysfunction.
■ Store in a cool, dry place away from direct
light.

### Therapeutic monitoring

■ Advise clinician to monitor liver, renal, and
hematopoietic function test results periodically in patients receiving repeated or prolonged
therapy.

### Special populations

**Breast-feeding patients.** The breast-fed infant
of a woman who uses clorazepate may become
sedated, have feeding difficulties, or lose
weight. Avoid use in breast-feeding women.
**Pediatric patients.** Safety hasn't been established in children under age 9.
**Geriatric patients.** Lower doses are usually
effective in geriatric patients because of decreased elimination. Use with caution. Geriatric patients who receive this drug require supervision with ambulation and activities of
daily living when therapy starts or changes.

## Patient counseling

■ Advise patient of potential for physical and
psychological dependence with chronic use of
clorazepate.
■ Instruct patient not to alter drug regimen
without medical approval.
■ Warn patient that sudden position changes
may cause dizziness. Advise patient to dangle
legs for a few minutes before getting out of bed
to prevent falls and injury.

■ Advise patient to take antacids 1 hour before
or after clorazepate.
■ Advise patient not to suddenly stop taking
drug.

# clotrimazole

FemCare, Gyne-Lotrimin, Lotrimin,
Lotrimin AF, Mycelex, Mycelex-G,
Mycelex-7

*Pharmacologic classification:* synthetic
imidazole derivative
*Therapeutic classification:* antifungal
*Pregnancy risk category B (C, oral
form)*

## Available forms

Available by prescription only
*Vaginal tablets:* 100 mg, 200 mg, 500 mg
*Topical cream:* 1%
*Topical lotion:* 1%
*Topical solution:* 1%
*Oral lozenges:* 10 mg
Available without a prescription
*Vaginal tablets:* 100 mg
*Vaginal cream:* 1%
*Combination pack:* Vaginal tablets 500 mg/top-
ical cream 1% 7 g

## Indications and dosages

*Tinea pedis, tinea cruris, tinea versicolor,
tinea corporis, cutaneous candidiasis*
*Adults and children:* Apply thinly and massage
into cleansed affected and surrounding area,
morning and evening, for prescribed period
(usually 1 to 4 weeks; however, therapy may
take up to 8 weeks).
*Vulvovaginal candidiasis*
*Adults:* Insert one tablet intravaginally h.s. for
7 consecutive days. If vaginal cream is used,
insert one applicatorful intravaginally, h.s. for
7 to 14 consecutive days.
*Treatment of oropharyngeal candidiasis*
*Adults and children:* Usual dosage is one
lozenge P.O. five times daily for 14 consecutive days.
*Prophylaxis of oropharyngeal candidiasis
in immunocompromised patients*
*Adults:* 1 lozenge t.i.d. for duration of chemotherapy.
◇ *Keratitis*
*Adults:* 1% ointment in sterile peanut oil q 2
to 4 hours for up to 6 weeks.

## Mechanism of action

*Antifungal action:* Clotrimazole alters cell
membrane permeability by binding with phospholipids in the fungal cell membrane. Clotrimazole inhibits or kills many fungi, including
yeast and dermatophytes, and also is active
against various species of gram-positive bacteria.

---

## Pharmacokinetics

*Absorption:* Absorption is limited with topical administration. Absorption following dissolution of a lozenge in the mouth isn't determined.
*Distribution:* Distributed minimally with local application.
*Metabolism:* Unknown.
*Excretion:* Unknown.

| Route | Onset | Peak | Duration |
|-------|-------|------|----------|
| P.O. | Unknown | Unknown | 3 hr |
| Topical, intravaginal | Unknown | Unknown | Unknown |

## Contraindications and precautions

Contraindicated in patients hypersensitive to drug. Also contraindicated for ophthalmic use.

## Interactions

None reported.

## Adverse reactions

**GI:** nausea, vomiting, unpleasant mouth sensation (with lozenges); lower abdominal cramps.
**GU:** *mild vaginal burning or irritation* (with vaginal use), cramping, urinary frequency.
**Hepatic:** abnormal liver function test results.
**Skin:** blistering, *erythema,* edema, pruritus, burning, stinging, peeling, urticaria, skin fissures, general irritation.

## Overdose and treatment

Acute overdose is unlikely and not expected to be life threatening.

## Clinical considerations

■ Improvement is usually seen within 1 week; if no improvement occurs in 4 weeks, review diagnosis.

### Therapeutic monitoring

■ Patients given clotrimazole oral lozenges, especially those who have preexisting liver dysfunction, should have periodic liver function tests.

### Special populations

**Pregnant patients.** Use lozenges only when potential benefits outweigh the risks.
**Breast-feeding patients.** It's unknown if drug appears in breast milk. Use drug with caution in breast-feeding women.
**Pediatric patients.** Drug isn't recommended for use in children under age 3.

## Patient counseling

■ Advise patient that lozenges must dissolve slowly (15 to 30 minutes) in the mouth to achieve maximum effect. Tell patient not to chew lozenges.
■ Instruct patient using intravaginal application to insert drug high into the vagina and to refrain from sexual contact during treatment period to avoid reinfection. Also tell patient to use a sanitary napkin to prevent staining of clothing and to absorb discharge.
■ Tell patient to complete the full course of therapy. Improvement usually will be noted within 1 week. Patient should call if no improvement occurs in 4 weeks or if condition worsens.
■ Advise patient to watch for and report irritation or sensitivity and, if this occurs, to discontinue use.

# cloxacillin sodium

Cloxapen

*Pharmacologic classification:* penicillinase-resistant penicillin
*Therapeutic classification:* antibiotic
*Pregnancy risk category B*

## Available forms

Available by prescription only
*Capsules:* 250 mg, 500 mg
*Oral solution:* 125 mg/5 ml (after reconstitution)

## Indications and dosages

*Systemic infections caused by penicillinase-producing staphylococci organisms*
*Adults:* 250 to 500 mg P.O. q 6 hours.
*Children:* 50 to 100 mg/kg P.O. daily, divided into doses given q 6 hours.

## Mechanism of action

*Antibiotic action:* Cloxacillin is bactericidal; it adheres to bacterial penicillin-binding proteins, thereby inhibiting bacterial cell-wall synthesis.

Cloxacillin resists the effects of penicillinases—enzymes that inactivate penicillin—and therefore is active against many strains of penicillinase-producing bacteria; this activity is most pronounced against penicillinase-producing staphylococci; some strains may remain resistant. Cloxacillin is also active against gram-positive aerobic and anaerobic bacilli but has no significant effect on gram-negative bacilli.

## Pharmacokinetics

*Absorption:* Absorbed rapidly but incompletely (37% to 60%) from the GI tract; it's relatively acid stable. Food may decrease both rate and extent of absorption.
*Distribution:* Distributed widely. CSF penetration is poor but enhanced in meningeal inflammation. Cloxacillin crosses the placenta, and is 90% to 96% protein-bound.
*Metabolism:* Only partially metabolized.
*Excretion:* Excreted in urine by renal tubular secretion and glomerular filtration; also appears in breast milk. Elimination half-life

in adults is ½ to 1 hour, extended minimally to 2½ hours in patients with renal impairment.

| Route | Onset | Peak | Duration |
|-------|-------|------|----------|
| P.O. | Unknown | 2 hr | 6 hr |

## Contraindications and precautions
Contraindicated in patients hypersensitive to drug or other penicillins.

## Interactions
**Drug-drug.** *Aminoglycosides:* Produce synergistic bactericidal effects against *Staphylococcus aureus.* However, the drugs are physically and chemically incompatible and are inactivated when mixed or given together. Don't use together.
*Probenecid:* Increases serum levels of cloxacillin. Probenecid may be used for this purpose.
**Drug-food.** *Any food:* Decrease drug absorption. Advise patient to take drug on an empty stomach.
*Carbonated beverages, fruit juices:* May inactivate drug. Don't give together.

## Adverse reactions
**CNS:** lethargy, hallucinations, *seizures,* anxiety, confusion, agitation, depression, dizziness, fatigue.
**EENT:** sneezing.
**GI:** *nausea,* vomiting, *epigastric distress, diarrhea,* enterocolitis, pseudomembranous colitis, black "hairy" tongue, abdominal pain.
**GU:** interstitial nephritis, nephropathy.
**Hematologic:** eosinophilia, anemia, ***thrombocytopenia, leukopenia,*** hemolytic anemia, ***agranulocytosis.***
**Hepatic:** intrahepatic cholestasis, transient elevations in liver function test results.
**Repiratory:** wheezing.
**Skin:** rash, urticaria.
**Other:** chills, fever, *anaphylaxis,* overgrowth of nonsusceptible organisms.

## Overdose and treatment
Signs and symptoms of overdose include neuromuscular irritability or seizures. No specific recommendation is available. Treatment is symptomatic. After recent ingestion (within 4 hours), recommend emptying the stomach by induced emesis or gastric lavage and following with activated charcoal to reduce absorption. Cloxacillin isn't appreciably removed by hemodialysis or peritoneal dialysis.

## Clinical considerations
■ Give dose on empty stomach with water only.
■ Refrigerate oral suspension and discard any unused drug after 14 days. Unrefrigerated suspension is stable for 3 days.
■ Cloxacillin alters test results for urine and serum proteins; it produces false-positive or elevated results in turbidimetric urine and serum protein tests using sulfosalicylic acid or trichloroacetic acid; it also reportedly produces false results on the Bradshaw screening test for Bence Jones protein.
■ Cloxacillin may falsely decrease serum aminoglycoside levels.

### Therapeutic monitoring
■ Periodically assess renal, hepatic, and hematopoietic function in patients receiving long-term therapy.

### Special populations
**Breast-feeding patients.** Drug appears in breast milk; use cautiously in breast-feeding women.
**Pediatric patients.** Elimination of cloxacillin is reduced in neonates; safety of drug in neonates hasn't been established.

## Patient counseling
■ Inform patient of potential adverse reactions (such as fever, chills, or rash); advise him to report adverse reactions promptly.
■ Instruct patient to take drug on an empty stomach and take with water only.
■ Tell patient to refrigerate oral suspension and to discard any unused suspension after the course of treatment.

# clozapine
Clozaril

*Pharmacologic classification:* tricyclic dibenzodiazepine derivative
*Therapeutic classification:* antipsychotic
*Pregnancy risk category B*

## Available forms
Available by prescription only
*Tablets:* 25 mg, 100 mg

## Indications and dosages
*Treatment of schizophrenia in severely ill patients unresponsive to other therapies*
*Adults:* Initially, 12.5 mg P.O. once or twice daily, adjusted upward at 25 to 50 mg daily (if tolerated) to a daily dose of 300 to 450 mg by end of 2 weeks. Individual dosage is based on clinical response, patient tolerance, and adverse reactions. Subsequent increases of dosage should occur no more than once or twice weekly and shouldn't exceed 100 mg. Many patients respond to doses of 300 to 600 mg daily, but some patients require as much as 900 mg daily. Don't exceed 900 mg/day.

## Mechanism of action
*Antipsychotic action:* Clozapine binds to dopamine receptors (D-1, D-2, D-3, D-4, and D-5) within the limbic system of the CNS. It also may interfere with adrenergic, choliner-

gic, histaminergic, and serotoninergic receptors.

## Pharmacokinetics
*Absorption:* Food doesn't appear to interfere with bioavailability. Only 27% to 50% of the dose reaches systemic circulation.
*Distribution:* About 95% serum protein–bound.
*Metabolism:* Metabolism is nearly complete; very little unchanged drug appears in the urine.
*Excretion:* About 50% appears in the urine and 30% in the feces, mostly as metabolites. Elimination half-life appears proportional to dose and may range from 4 to 66 hours.

| Route | Onset | Peak | Duration |
|-------|-------|------|----------|
| P.O. | Unknown | 2½ hr | 4-12 hr |

## Contraindications and precautions
Contraindicated in patients with uncontrolled epilepsy or history of clozapine-induced agranulocytosis; in patients with a WBC count below 3,500/mm³; in patients with severe CNS depression or coma; in patients taking other drugs that suppress bone marrow function; and in those with myelosuppressive disorders.

Use cautiously in patients with renal, hepatic, or cardiac disease, prostatic hyperplasia, or angle-closure glaucoma and in those receiving general anesthesia.

Use cautiously with other drugs metabolized by cytochrome P-450 2D6, including antidepressants, phenothiazines, carbamazepine, and type IC antiarrhythmics (propafenone, flecainide), or drugs that inhibit this enzyme, such as quinidine.

## Interactions
**Drug-drug.** *Anticholinergics:* May potentiate the anticholinergic effects of clozapine. Avoid use together.
*Anticonvulsants:* Clozapine may lower seizure threshold. Avoid use together.
*Antihypertensives:* May potentiate the hypotensive effects. Check blood pressure frequently.
*Benzodiazepines:* Concurrent use may pose a risk of respiratory arrest and severe hypotension. Avoid use together.
*Bone marrow suppressants:* Increased bone marrow toxicity. Use together cautiously.
*Carbamazepine:* Potential for neuroleptic malignant syndrome; decreased clozapine serum level by up to 50%. Use together isn't recommended.
*Cimetidine, erythromycin, phenothiazines, quinidine, SSRIs, type IC antiarrhythmics:* Increased levels of clozapine. Avoid use together.
*CNS-active drugs:* Potential for additive effects. Use together cautiously.
*Digoxin, highly protein-bound drugs, warfarin:* Increased serum levels. Advise clinician to monitor patient closely for adverse reactions.

*Phenytoin:* Substantial decrease in clozapine levels. Monitor patient for reemergence of psychotic symptoms and adjust clozapine dosage accordingly.
**Drug-herb.** *Catnip, kava, lady's slipper, lemon balm, passion flower, sassafras, skullcap, valerian:* Sedative effects may be enhanced. Discourage use together.
*Nutmeg:* May reduce effectiveness of drug. Avoid use together.
**Drug-food.** *Beverages containing caffeine:* May inhibit antipsychotic effects of clozapine. Advise clinician to monitor patient closely.
**Drug-lifestyle.** *Alcohol use:* Increased CNS depression. Advise patient to avoid alcohol.
*Smoking:* May reduce plasma clozapine levels. Discourage smoking.

## Adverse reactions
**CNS:** *drowsiness, sedation, seizures,* dizziness, syncope, vertigo, headache, tremor, disturbed sleep or nightmares, restlessness, hypokinesia or akinesia, agitation, rigidity, akathisia, confusion, fatigue, insomnia, hyperkinesia, weakness, lethargy, ataxia, slurred speech, depression, myoclonus, anxiety, *neuroleptic malignant syndrome.*
**CV:** *tachycardia, hypotension,* hypertension, chest pain, ECG changes, orthostatic hypotension.
**EENT:** visual disturbances.
**GI:** *dry mouth, constipation,* nausea, vomiting, *excessive salivation,* heartburn, constipation, diarrhea.
**GU:** urinary frequency or urgency, urine retention, incontinence, abnormal ejaculation.
**Hematologic:** *leukopenia, agranulocytosis.*
**Metabolic:** weight gain.
**Musculoskeletal:** muscle pain or spasm, muscle weakness.
**Skin:** rash, diaphoresis.
**Other:** fever.
**After abrupt withdrawal of long-term therapy:** Possible abrupt recurrence of psychotic symptoms. Advise clinician to monitor patient closely.

## Overdose and treatment
Fatalities have occurred at doses exceeding 2.5 g. Signs and symptoms include drowsiness, delirium, coma, hypotension, hypersalivation, tachycardia, respiratory depression and, rarely, seizures.

Treat symptomatically. Establish an airway and ensure adequate ventilation. Gastric lavage with activated charcoal and sorbitol may be effective. Advise clinician to monitor vital signs. Avoid epinephrine (and derivatives), quinidine, and procainamide when treating hypotension and arrhythmias.

## Clinical considerations
■ When discontinuing clozapine therapy, drug must be withdrawn gradually (over a 1- to 2-

week period). However, changes in the patient's clinical status (including the development of leukopenia) may require abrupt discontinuation of the drug. If so, advise clinician to monitor patient closely for recurrence of psychotic symptoms.

■ To reinstate therapy in patients withdrawn from drug, follow usual guidelines for dosage buildup. However, reexposure of the patient may increase the risk and severity of adverse reactions. If therapy was terminated for WBC counts of less than 2,000/mm$^3$ or granulocyte counts of less than 1,000/mm$^3$, drug shouldn't be reinstated.

■ Some patients experience transient fevers (temperature of more than 100.4° F [38° C]), especially in the first 3 weeks of therapy. Advise clinician to monitor patient closely.

### Therapeutic monitoring

■ For the first 6 months, clozapine therapy must be given with a monitoring program that ensures weekly testing of WBC counts. Blood tests must be performed weekly, and no more than a 1-week supply of drug can be distributed. Blood testing then can be performed every other week.

■ Patient needs periodic assessment for abnormal body movement.

### Special populations

**Breast-feeding patients.** Drug appears in breast milk. Women taking clozapine shouldn't breast-feed.

**Pediatric patients.** Safety in children hasn't been established.

**Geriatric patients.** Geriatric patients may require reduced dosages, because they may be more sensitive to adverse reactions, especially orthostatic hypotension, dry mouth, and constipation. Advise clinician to monitor these patients closely.

### Patient counseling

■ Warn patient about risk of developing agranulocytosis. Safe use of drug requires blood tests weekly for the first 6 months, then every other week to monitor for agranulocytosis.

■ Advise patient to promptly report flulike symptoms, fever, sore throat, lethargy, malaise, or other signs of infection.

■ Advise patient to call prescriber before taking OTC drugs or alcohol.

■ Tell patient that ice chips or sugarless candy or gum may help to relieve dry mouth.

■ Warn patient to rise slowly to upright position to avoid orthostatic hypotension.

# codeine phosphate
# codeine sulfate

*Pharmacologic classification:* opioid
*Therapeutic classification:* analgesic, antitussive
*Pregnancy risk category C*
*Controlled substance schedule II*

## Available forms

Available by prescription only
*Tablets:* 15 mg, 30 mg, 60 mg; 30 mg, 60 mg (soluble)
*Oral solution:* 15 mg/5 ml codeine phosphate
*Injection:* 15 mg/ml, 30 mg/ml, 60 mg/ml codeine phosphate

## Indications and dosages

*Mild to moderate pain*
*Adults:* 15 to 60 mg P.O. or 15 to 60 mg (phosphate) S.C. or I.M. q 4 to 6 hours, p.r.n., or around-the-clock.
*Children:* 0.5 mg/kg (or 15 mg/m$^2$) P.O. q 4 to 6 hours, or 0.5 mg/kg (or 15 mg/m$^2$) (phosphate) S.C. or I.M.
*Nonproductive cough*
*Adults and children ages 12 and older:* 10 to 20 mg P.O. q 4 to 6 hours. Maximum dose is 120 mg/24 hours.
*Children ages 6 to 11:* 5 to 10 mg P.O. q 4 to 6 hours, not to exceed 60 mg daily.
*Children ages 2 to 6:* 1 mg/kg P.O. daily divided into four equal doses, given q 4 to 6 hours, not to exceed 30 mg in 24 hours.

## Mechanism of action

*Analgesic action:* Codeine has analgesic properties that result from its agonist activity at the opiate receptors.
*Antitussive action:* Codeine has a direct suppressant action on the cough reflex center.

## Pharmacokinetics

*Absorption:* Well absorbed after oral or parenteral administration. It's about two-thirds as potent orally as parenterally.
*Distribution:* Distributed widely throughout the body; it crosses the placenta and appears in breast milk.
*Metabolism:* Metabolized mainly in the liver, by demethylation or by conjugation with glucuronic acid.
*Excretion:* Excreted mainly in the urine as norcodeine and free and conjugated morphine.

| Route | Onset | Peak | Duration |
|-------|-------|------|----------|
| P.O. | 30-45 min | 1-2 hr | 4-6 hr |
| I.M. | 10-30 min | ½-1 hr | 4-6 hr |
| S.C. | 10-30 min | Unknown | 4-6 hr |

## Contraindications and precautions

Contraindicated in patients hypersensitive to drug. Use cautiously in patients with impaired renal or hepatic function, head injuries, increased intracranial pressure, increased CSF pressure, hypothyroidism, Addison's disease, acute alcoholism, CNS depression, bronchial asthma, COPD, respiratory depression, or shock, and in geriatric or debilitated patients.

## Interactions

**Drug-drug.** *Anticholinergics:* Concurrent use may cause paralytic ileus. Advise clinician to monitor patient closely.

*Antihistamines, barbiturates, benzodiazepines, CNS depressants, general anesthetics, MAO inhibitors, muscle relaxants, narcotic analgesics, phenothiazines, sedative-hypnotics, tricyclic antidepressants:* Potentiate drug's respiratory and CNS depression, sedation, and hypotensive effects. Use together with extreme caution.

*Cimetidine:* Increases respiratory and CNS depression. Avoid use together.

*Digitoxin (Canadian), phenytoin, rifampin:* Drug accumulation and enhanced effects may result. Advise clinician to monitor patient closely.

**Drug-lifestyle.** *Alcohol use:* Potentiates respiratory and CNS depression, sedation, and hypotensive effects of drug. Discourage alcohol use.

## Adverse reactions

**CNS:** *sedation, clouded sensorium, euphoria, dizziness, light-headedness,* physical dependence.
**CV:** *hypotension, **bradycardia.***
**GI:** *nausea, vomiting, constipation, dry mouth,* ileus.
**GU:** *urine retention.*
**Respiratory:** ***respiratory depression.***
**Skin:** pruritus, flushing, *diaphoresis.*

## Overdose and treatment

The most common signs and symptoms of overdose are CNS depression, respiratory depression, and miosis (pinpoint pupils). Other acute toxic effects include hypotension, bradycardia, hypothermia, shock, apnea, cardiopulmonary arrest, circulatory collapse, pulmonary edema, and seizures.

To treat acute overdose, recommend first establishing adequate respiratory exchange via a patent airway and ventilation p.r.n.; narcotic antagonist (naloxone) may be given to reverse respiratory depression. (Because the duration of action of codeine is longer than that of naloxone, repeated naloxone dosing is needed.) Naloxone shouldn't be given unless the patient has clinically significant respiratory or CV depression. Advise clinician to monitor vital signs closely.

If patient shows signs and symptoms within 2 hours of ingestion of an oral overdose, recommend emptying the stomach immediately by inducing emesis (ipecac syrup) or using gastric lavage. Use caution to avoid risk of aspiration. Recommend giving activated charcoal via nasogastric tube for further removal of drug in an oral overdose.

Recommend providing symptomatic and supportive treatment (continued respiratory support, correction of fluid or electrolyte imbalance). Advise clinician to monitor laboratory effects, vital signs, and neurologic status closely.

## Clinical considerations

■ Codeine and aspirin have additive analgesic effects. Give together for maximum pain relief.
■ Codeine has much less abuse potential than morphine.
■ Patients who become physically dependent on drug may experience acute withdrawal syndrome if given a narcotic antagonist.
■ Drug may increase plasma amylase and lipase levels, delay gastric emptying, increase biliary tract pressure caused by contraction of the sphincter of Oddi, and may interfere with hepatobiliary imaging studies.

### Therapeutic monitoring

■ Advise clinician to monitor cough type and frequency.
■ Advise clinician to monitor respiratory and circulatory status.

### Special populations

**Breast-feeding patients.** Drug appears in breast milk; assess risk-to-benefit ratio before administering.
**Pediatric patients.** Give cautiously to children. Codeine-containing cough preparations may be hazardous in young children. Use a calibrated measuring device and don't exceed the recommended daily dose.
**Geriatric patients.** Lower doses are usually indicated for geriatric patients, who may be more sensitive to the therapeutic and adverse effects of drug.

## Patient counseling

■ Inform patient that codeine may cause drowsiness, dizziness, or blurring of vision; tell him to use caution while driving or performing tasks that require mental alertness.
■ Instruct patient to ask for or to take drug before pain is intense.
■ Advise patient that GI distress from oral drug can be lessened when drug is taken with milk.

---

* Canada only    ◇ Unlabeled clinical use

# colchicine

*Pharmacologic classification:*
*Colchicum autumnale* alkaloid
*Therapeutic classification:* antigout
drug
*Pregnancy risk category C (oral), D
(parenteral)*

## Available forms

Available by prescription only
*Tablets:* 0.5 mg, 0.6 mg
*Injection:* 0.5 mg/ml

## Indications and dosages

*To prevent acute attacks of gout as prophy-
lactic or maintenance therapy*
*Adults:* 0.5 or 0.6 mg P.O. one to four times
weekly.
*To prevent attacks of gout in patients un-
dergoing surgery*
*Adults:* 0.5 to 0.6 mg P.O. t.i.d. 3 days before
and 3 days after surgery.
*Acute gout, acute gouty arthritis*
*Adults:* Initially, 0.5 to 1.2 mg P.O., followed
by 0.5 to 1.2 mg P.O. q 1 to 2 hours; total dai-
ly dose is usually 4 to 8 mg P.O.; give until pain
is relieved or until nausea, vomiting, or diar-
rhea ensues. Or 2 mg I.V. followed by 0.5 mg
I.V. q 6 hours, if needed. Total I.V. dose over
24 hours (one course of treatment) not to ex-
ceed 4 mg.
◊ *Familial Mediterranean fever*
*Adults:* 1 to 2 mg/day P.O. in divided doses.
◊ *Amyloidosis suppressant*
*Adults:* 0.5 to 0.6 mg P.O. once daily to b.i.d.
◊ *Dermatitis herpetiformis suppressant*
*Adults:* 0.6 mg P.O. b.i.d. or t.i.d.
◊ *Hepatic cirrhosis*
*Adults:* 1 mg P.O. 5 days weekly.
◊ *Primary biliary cirrhosis*
*Adults:* 0.6 mg b.i.d.

## I.V. administration

■ Give colchicine by slow I.V. push over 2 to
5 minutes by direct I.V. injection or into tubing of a free-flowing I.V. with compatible I.V.
fluid. Avoid extravasation.
■ If lower concentration of colchicine injection is needed, dilute with sterile water or normal saline solution. However, if diluted solution becomes turbid, don't inject.

## Incompatibilities

Incompatible with $D_5W$ and bacteriostatic normal saline injection or other fluids that might
change the pH of colchicine solution.

## Mechanism of action

*Antigout action:* Colchicine's exact mechanism of action is unknown, but it's involved in
leukocyte migration inhibition; reduction of
lactic acid production by leukocytes, resulting

in decreased deposits of uric acid; and interference with kinin formation.
*Anti-inflammatory action:* Colchicine reduces
the inflammatory response to deposited uric
acid crystals and diminishes phagocytosis.

## Pharmacokinetics

*Absorption:* When given P.O., rapidly absorbed
from the GI tract. Unchanged drug may be
reabsorbed from the intestine by biliary
processes.
*Distribution:* Distributed rapidly into various
tissues after reabsorption from the intestine.
It's concentrated in leukocytes and distributed
into the kidneys, liver, spleen, and intestinal
tract, but is absent in the heart, skeletal muscle,
and brain.
*Metabolism:* Metabolized partially in the liver and also slowly metabolized in other tissues.
*Excretion:* Excreted primarily in the feces,
with lesser amounts excreted in urine.

| Route | Onset | Peak | Duration |
|-------|-------|------|----------|
| P.O. | < 12 hr | ½-2 hr | Unknown |
| I.V. | 6-12 hr | Unknown | Unknown |

## Contraindications and precautions

Contraindicated in patients hypersensitive to
drug; blood dyscrasias; or serious CV, renal,
or GI disease. Use cautiously in geriatric or debilitated patients and in those with early signs
of CV, renal, or GI disease.

## Interactions

**Drug-drug.** *Cyclosporine:* Increased GI toxicity with concurrent use. Dosage may require
adjustment.
*Erythromycin:* Increased serum colchicine levels. May need to reduce colchicine dosage.
*Loop diuretics:* May decrease efficacy of
colchicine prophylaxis. Avoid use together.
*Phenylbutazone:* May increase risk of leukopenia or thrombocytopenia. Avoid use together.
*Vitamin B:* Impaired absorption. Avoid use together.
**Drug-lifestyle.** *Alcohol use:* May inhibit drug
action. Discourage alcohol use.

## Adverse reactions

**CNS:** peripheral neuritis.
**GI:** *nausea, vomiting, abdominal pain, diar-
rhea.*
**GU:** reversible azoospermia.
**Hematologic:** *aplastic anemia, thrombocy-
topenia, and agranulocytosis* (with long-term
use); nonthrombocytopenic purpura.
**Hepatic:** increased alkaline phosphatase, AST,
and ALT levels.
**Musculoskeletal:** myopathy.
**Skin:** alopecia, urticaria, dermatitis, severe lo-
cal irritation if extravasation occurs.
**Other:** hypersensitivity reactions.

## Overdose and treatment

Signs and symptoms of overdose include nausea, vomiting, abdominal pain, and diarrhea. Diarrhea may be severe and bloody from hemorrhagic gastroenteritis. Burning sensations in the throat, stomach, and skin also may occur. Extensive vascular damage may result in shock, hematuria, and oliguria, indicating kidney damage. Patient develops severe dehydration, hypotension, and muscle weakness with an ascending paralysis of the CNS. Patient usually remains conscious, but delirium and convulsions may occur. Death may result from respiratory depression.

There is no known specific antidote. Treatment begins with gastric lavage and preventive measures for shock. Recent studies support the use of hemodialysis and peritoneal dialysis; atropine and morphine may relieve abdominal pain; paregoric usually is given to control diarrhea and cramps. Respiratory assistance may be needed.

## Clinical considerations

■ To avoid cumulative toxicity, a course of oral colchicine shouldn't be repeated for at least 3 days; a course of I.V. colchicine shouldn't be repeated for several weeks.
■ Don't administer I.M. or S.C.; severe local irritation occurs.
■ Drug should be stopped if weakness, anorexia, nausea, vomiting, or diarrhea occurs. First sign of acute overdose may be GI symptoms, followed by vascular damage, muscle weakness, and ascending paralysis. Delirium and convulsions may occur without loss of consciousness.
■ Store drug in a tightly closed, light-resistant container, away from moisture and high temperatures.

### Therapeutic monitoring

■ Advise clinician to obtain baseline laboratory studies, including CBC, before therapy starts and periodically thereafter.

### Special populations

**Breast-feeding patients.** Safety hasn't been established in breast-feeding women. It isn't known if drug appears in breast milk.
**Pediatric patients.** Safety and efficacy in children haven't been established.
**Geriatric patients.** Give with caution to geriatric or debilitated patients, especially those with renal, GI, or heart disease or hematologic disorders. Reduce dosage if weakness, anorexia, nausea, vomiting, or diarrhea occurs.

## Patient counseling

■ Advise patient to report rash, sore throat, fever, unusual bleeding, bruising, tiredness, weakness, numbness, or tingling.
■ Tell patient to discontinue drug as soon as gout pain is relieved or at the first sign of nausea, vomiting, stomach pain, or diarrhea, and to report persistent symptoms.

# colesevelam hydrochloride
Welchol

*Pharmacologic classification:* polymeric bile acid sequestrant
*Therapeutic classification:* antilipemic
*Pregnancy risk category B*

## Available forms

Available by prescription only
*Tablets:* 625 mg

## Indications and dosages

*Adjunct to diet and exercise, either alone or with an HMG-CoA reductase inhibitor, for the reduction of elevated low-density lipoprotein (LDL) cholesterol in patients with primary hypercholesterolemia (Frederickson Type IIa)*
*Adults:* Three tablets (1,875 mg) P.O. b.i.d. with meals and liquid or six tablets (3,750 mg) once daily with a meal and liquid. Daily dose can be increased to seven tablets (4,375 mg) for added effect.

## Mechanism of action

*Antilipemic action:* Colesevelam binds bile acids in the intestinal tract, impeding their absorption and resulting in their elimination via the feces. Cholesterol is needed for the repletion of bile acid stores. The liver utilizes LDL cholesterol from the serum in order to manufacture bile acids. As a result of bile acid depletion, serum LDL cholesterol level decreases.

## Pharmacokinetics

*Absorption:* Not absorbed.
*Distribution:* None.
*Metabolism:* None.
*Excretion:* Excreted in feces as a complex bound to bile acids.

| Route | Onset | Peak | Duration |
|-------|-------|------|----------|
| P.O. | Unknown | About 2 wk | Unknown |

## Contraindications and precautions

Contraindicated in patients with bowel obstruction and in patients hypersensitive to drug or its components.

Use cautiously in patients with dysphagia, swallowing disorders, severe GI motility disorders, or major GI tract surgery and in patients with susceptibility to vitamin K or fat-soluble vitamin deficiencies. Also use cautiously in patients with serum triglyceride levels exceeding 300 mg/dl.

## Interactions

None reported.

## Adverse reactions
**CNS:** headache, pain, asthenia.
**EENT:** pharyngitis, rhinitis, sinusitis.
**GI:** abdominal pain, *constipation,* diarrhea, dyspepsia, *flatulence,* nausea.
**Musculoskeletal:** myalgia, back pain.
**Respiratory:** increased cough.
**Other:** accidental injury, *infection,* flu syndrome.

## Overdose and treatment
Risk of systemic toxicity is low because drug isn't systemically absorbed. Doses as high as 4.5 g/day have been well tolerated. There is no experience with higher doses.

## Clinical considerations
- Rule out secondary causes of hypercholesterolemia, such as poorly controlled diabetes, hypothyroidism, nephrotic syndrome, dysproteinemias, obstructive liver disease, other drug therapy, or alcoholism before starting drug.
- Give drug with a meal, including a liquid.
- Store tablets at controlled room temperature and protect from moisture.

### Therapeutic monitoring
- Advise clinician to monitor patient's bowel habits. If severe constipation occurs, advise clinician to decrease dosage, add a stool softener, or discontinue drug.
- Advise clinician to monitor clinical effects of concurrent drug therapy to identify potential drug interactions.
- Advise clinician to monitor total cholesterol, low-density lipoprotein cholesterol, and triglyceride levels periodically during therapy.

### Special populations
**Breast-feeding patients.** No information available. Use in breast-feeding women only when needed.
**Pediatric patients.** Safety and efficacy haven't been established.

## Patient counseling
- Instruct patient to take drug with a meal, including a liquid.
- Teach patient to monitor bowel habits. Encourage a diet high in fiber and fluids. Instruct patient to notify prescriber promptly if severe constipation occurs.
- Encourage patient to adhere to prescribed regimen of diet, exercise, and monitoring of serum lipid levels.
- Tell a woman to notify prescriber if she is pregnant or breast-feeding.

# colestipol hydrochloride
Colestid

*Pharmacologic classification:* anion exchange resin
*Therapeutic classification:* antilipemic
*Pregnancy risk category C*

## Available forms
Available by prescription only
*Tablets:* 1 g
*Granules for oral suspension:* 5 g/packet, 300 g and 500 g multidose with calibrated scoop

## Indications and dosages
*Primary hypercholesterolemia and xanthomas*
*Adults:* Tablets—Initially, 2 g P.O. once daily or b.i.d., then increase in 2-g increments at 1- to 2-month intervals. Usual dosage is 2 to 16 g P.O. daily given as a single dose or in divided doses.
Granules—Initially, 5 g P.O. once daily or b.i.d., then increase in 5-g increments at 1- to 2-month intervals. Usual dosage is 5 to 30 g P.O. daily given as a single dose or in divided doses.
◊ *Children:* 10 to 20 g or 500 mg/kg P.O. daily in two to four divided doses (lower doses of 125 to 250 mg/kg used when serum cholesterol levels were 15% to 20% above normal after only dietary management).
◊ *Digitoxin overdose*
*Adults:* Initially, 10 g P.O. followed by 5 g P.O. q 6 to 8 hours.

## Mechanism of action
*Antilipemic action:* Bile is normally excreted into the intestine to facilitate absorption of fat and other lipid materials. Colestipol binds with bile acid, forming an insoluble compound that is excreted in feces. With less bile available in the digestive system, less fat and lipid materials in food are absorbed, more cholesterol is used by the liver to replace its supply of bile acids, and the serum cholesterol level decreases.

## Pharmacokinetics
*Absorption:* Not absorbed. Cholesterol levels may decrease in 24 to 48 hours, with peak effect occurring at 1 month. In some patients, the initial decrease is followed by a return to or above baseline cholesterol levels on continued therapy.
*Distribution:* None.
*Metabolism:* None.
*Excretion:* Excreted in feces; cholesterol levels return to baseline within 1 month after therapy stops.

| Route | Onset | Peak | Duration |
|-------|-------|------|----------|
| P.O. | 1 mo | Unknown | 1 mo |

## Contraindications and precautions

Contraindicated in patients hypersensitive to bile-acid sequestering resins. Use cautiously in patients prone to constipation and in those with conditions aggravated by constipation, such as symptomatic coronary artery disease.

## Interactions

**Drug-drug.** *Cardiac glycosides, chenodiol, digitoxin, digoxin, penicillin G, tetracycline, thiazide diuretics:* Colestipol impairs absorption, thus decreasing their therapeutic effect. Give other drugs 1 hour before or 4 hours after colestipol.
*Any oral drug:* Possible binding with colestipol. Dosage adjustment may be needed; readjustment must be made when colestipol is withdrawn to prevent high-dose toxicity.

## Adverse reactions

**CNS:** headache, dizziness, anxiety, vertigo, insomnia, fatigue, syncope.
**EENT:** tinnitus.
**GI:** *constipation,* fecal impaction, hemorrhoids, abdominal discomfort, flatulence, nausea, vomiting, steatorrhea, GI bleeding, diarrhea, anorexia, difficulty swallowing, transient esophageal obstruction.
**GU:** dysuria, hematuria.
**Hematologic:** anemia, ecchymoses, bleeding tendencies.
**Hepatic:** alterations in serum levels of alkaline phosphatase, ALT, and AST.
**Metabolic:** alterations in serum levels of chloride, phosphorus, potassium, and sodium.
**Musculoskeletal:** backache, muscle and joint pain, osteoporosis.
**Skin:** rash, irritation of tongue and perianal area.
**Other:** vitamin A, D, E, and K deficiencies from decreased absorption; hyperchloremic acidosis with long-term use or high dosage.

## Overdose and treatment

Overdose of colestipol hasn't been reported. Chief potential risk is intestinal obstruction; treatment would depend on location and degree of obstruction and on amount of gut motility.

## Clinical considerations

■ To mix, sprinkle granules on surface of preferred beverage or wet food, let stand a few minutes, and stir to obtain uniform suspension; avoid excess foaming by using large glass and mixing slowly. Use at least 90 ml of water or other fluid, soups, milk, or pulpy fruit; rinse container and have patient drink this to be sure he ingests entire dose. Tablets should be swallowed whole.
■ Antilipemic therapy along with aspirin, nitrates, and beta blockers are recommended by the American Heart Association and the American College of Cardiology for the management of chronic stable angina in patients with (or suspected of having) coronary heart disease whose low-density lipoprotein levels are greater than 130 mg/dl.
■ Drug effects are most successful if used together with a diet and exercise program.

### Therapeutic monitoring

■ Advise clinician to monitor levels of cardiac glycosides and other drugs to ensure appropriate dosage during and after therapy with colestipol.
■ Check serum cholesterol levels frequently during first few months of therapy and periodically thereafter.
■ Observe patient for signs of vitamin A, D, or K deficiency.
■ Advise clinician to monitor patient's bowel habits. Constipation should be treated promptly by decreasing dosage, increasing fluid intake, adding a stool softener, or discontinuing drug.

### Special populations

**Breast-feeding patients.** Safety in breast-feeding women hasn't been established.
**Pediatric patients.** Safety in children hasn't been established. Drug isn't usually recommended; however, it's been used in a limited number of children with hypercholesteremia.
**Geriatric patients.** Geriatric patients are more likely to experience adverse GI and nutritional effects.

## Patient counseling

■ Explain disease process and reason for therapy and encourage patient to comply with continued blood testing and special diet; although therapy isn't curative, it helps control serum cholesterol levels.
■ Teach patient how to administer drug. To enhance palatability, tell patient to mix and refrigerate the next daily dose the previous evening.

# corticotropin (adrenocorticotropic hormone, ACTH)

ACTH, Acthar, Cortrophin-Zinc, H.P. Acthar Gel

*Pharmacologic classification:* anterior pituitary hormone
*Therapeutic classification:* diagnostic aid, replacement hormone, multiple sclerosis and nonsuppurative thyroiditis treatment
*Pregnancy risk category C*

## Available forms

Available by prescription only
*Injection:* 25-unit/vial, 40-unit/vial
*Repository injection:* 40-unit/ml, 80-unit/ml

## Indications and dosages
*Diagnostic test of adrenocortical function*
*Adults:* Up to 80 units I.M. or S.C. in divided doses; or a single dose of repository form; or 10 to 25 unit (aqueous form) in 500 ml of $D_5W$ I.V. over 8 hours, between blood samplings.

Individual dosages vary with adrenal glands' sensitivity to stimulation and with the specific disease. Infants and younger children require larger doses per kilogram than do older children and adults.
*Replacement hormone*
*Adults:* 20 units S.C. or I.M. q.i.d.
*Exacerbations of multiple sclerosis*
*Adults:* 80 to 120 units I.M. daily for 2 to 3 weeks.
*Severe allergic reactions, collagen disorders, dermatologic disorders, inflammation*
*Adults:* 40 to 80 units/day I.M. or S.C. Adjust dosage based upon patient response.
*Infantile spasms*
*Infants:* 20 to 40 units I.M. (of repository injection) daily or 80 units I.M. every other day for 3 months or 1 month after spasm ceases.

## Mechanism of action
*Diagnostic action:* Corticotropin is used to test adrenocortical function. Corticotropin binds with a specific receptor in the adrenal cell plasma membrane, stimulating the synthesis of the entire spectrum of adrenal steroids, one of which is cortisol. The effect of corticotropin is measured by analyzing plasma cortisol before and after drug administration. In patients with primary adrenocortical insufficiency, corticotropin doesn't increase plasma cortisol levels significantly.
*Anti-inflammatory action:* In nonsuppurative thyroiditis and acute exacerbations of multiple sclerosis, corticotropin stimulates release of adrenal cortex hormones, which combat tissue responses to inflammatory processes.

## Pharmacokinetics
*Absorption:* Absorbed rapidly after I.M. administration.
*Distribution:* Exact distribution of corticotropin is unknown, but it's removed rapidly from plasma by many tissues.
*Metabolism:* Unknown.
*Excretion:* Probably excreted by the kidneys. Half-life is about 15 minutes.

| Route | Onset | Peak | Duration |
|---|---|---|---|
| I.V., I.M. | Rapid | 1 hr | 2-4 hr |
| I.M. (repository) | Unknown | Unknown | 3 days |
| S.C. | Unknown | Unknown | Unknown |

## Contraindications and precautions
Contraindicated in patients with peptic ulcer, scleroderma, osteoporosis, systemic fungal infections, ocular herpes simplex, peptic ulceration, heart failure, hypertension, sensitivity to pork and pork products, adrenocortical hyperfunction or primary insufficiency, or Cushing's syndrome. Also contraindicated in those who've had recent surgery.

Use cautiously in pregnant patients and in women of childbearing age. Also use cautiously in patients being immunized and in those with latent tuberculosis, hypothyroidism, cirrhosis, acute gouty arthritis, psychotic tendencies, renal insufficiency, diverticulitis, ulcerative colitis, thromboembolic disorders, seizures, uncontrolled hypertension, or myasthenia gravis.

Use with caution if surgery or emergency treatment is needed.

## Interactions
**Drug-drug.** *Amphotericin B, carbonic anhydrase inhibitors, diuretics:* Accentuate the electrolyte loss caused by diuretic therapy. Advise clinician to monitor serum blood levels, especially potassium.
*Cardiac glycosides:* May increase the risk of arrhythmias or digitalis toxicity associated with hypokalemia. Advise clinician to monitor patient closely.
*Cortisone, estrogens, hydrocortisone:* May abnormally elevate plasma cortisol levels. Use with caution.
*Hepatic enzyme-inducing drugs:* May increase corticotropin metabolism. Advise clinician to monitor patient closely.
*Insulin, oral antidiabetics:* May require increased dosage of the antidiabetic. Advise clinician to monitor blood glucose levels closely.
*NSAIDs, salicylates:* Increased risk of GI bleeding. Avoid use together.

## Adverse reactions
**CNS:** *seizures, dizziness,* vertigo, ***increased intracranial pressure with papilledema,*** pseudotumor cerebri.
**CV:** hypertension, ***HF,*** necrotizing vasculitis, ***shock.***
**EENT:** cataracts, glaucoma.
**GI:** ***peptic ulceration with perforation and hemorrhage, pancreatitis,*** abdominal distention, ulcerative esophagitis, nausea, vomiting.
**GU:** menstrual irregularities.
**Metabolic:** activation of latent diabetes mellitus, *sodium and fluid retention,* calcium and potassium loss, hypokalemic alkalosis, negative nitrogen balance.
**Musculoskeletal:** muscle weakness, steroid myopathy, loss of muscle mass, osteoporosis, suppression of growth in children, vertebral compression fractures.
**Respiratory:** pneumonia, ***bronchospasm.***
**Skin:** impaired wound healing; thin, fragile skin; petechiae; ecchymoses; facial erythema; diaphoresis; acne; hyperpigmentation; allergic reactions; hirsutism, rash.

---

Reactions may be *common,* uncommon, *life-threatening,* or COMMON AND LIFE-THREATENING.

**Other:** abscess and septic infection, cushingoid symptoms, progressive increase in antibodies, loss of corticotropin stimulatory effect.

## Overdose and treatment
Specific information unavailable. Treatment is supportive, as appropriate.

## Clinical considerations
■ Cosyntropin is less antigenic and less likely to cause allergic reactions than corticotropin. However, allergic reactions occur rarely with corticotropin.
■ In patient with suspected sensitivity to porcine proteins, advise clinician to perform skin testing. To decrease the risk of anaphylactic reaction in patient with limited adrenal reserves, 1 mg of dexamethasone may be given at midnight before the corticotropin test and 0.5 mg at start of test.
■ Advise clinician to observe neonates of corticotropin-treated women for signs of hypoadrenalism.
■ Edema may be counteracted by low-sodium, high-potassium intake; nitrogen loss by high-protein diet; and psychotic symptoms by reducing corticotropin dosage or giving sedatives.
■ Drug may mask signs of chronic disease and decrease host resistance and ability to localize infection.
■ Refrigerate reconstituted product and use within 24 hours.
■ If administering gel, it must be warmed to controlled room temperature, drawn into a large needle, and given slowly, deep I.M. with a 22G needle.
■ Drug shouldn't be stopped abruptly, especially after prolonged therapy. An addisonian crisis may occur.
■ Corticotropin therapy alters protein-bound iodine levels; radioactive iodine ($^{131}$I) uptake and $T_3$ uptake; total protein values; serum amylase, urine amino acid, serotonin, uric acid and 17-ketosteroid levels; and leukocyte counts.

### Therapeutic monitoring
■ Advise clinician to monitor weight, fluid exchange, and resting blood pressure levels until minimal effective dosage is achieved.

### Special populations
**Breast-feeding patients.** Safety hasn't been established. Because the potential for severe adverse reactions exists, benefits and risks must be weighed.
**Pediatric patients.** Use with caution because prolonged use of drug inhibits skeletal growth. Intermittent administration is recommended.

## Patient counseling
■ Warn patient that injection is painful.

■ Tell patient to report marked fluid retention, muscle weakness, abdominal pain, seizures, or headache.
■ Instruct patient not to be vaccinated during corticotropin therapy.
■ Teach patient how to monitor for edema, and tell him about the need for fluid and salt restriction, as appropriate.
■ Warn patient not to stop drug except as prescribed. Tell him that abrupt discontinuation may provoke severe adverse reactions.

# cortisone acetate
Cortone

*Pharmacologic classification:* glucocorticoid, mineralocorticoid
*Therapeutic classification:* anti-inflammatory, replacement therapy
*Pregnancy risk category NR*

## Available forms
Available by prescription only
*Tablets:* 5 mg, 10 mg, 25 mg
*Injection (I.M. use):* 50 mg/ml suspension

## Indications and dosages
*Adrenal insufficiency, allergy, inflammation*
*Adults:* 25 to 300 mg P.O. or 20 to 300 mg I.M. daily or on alternate days. Dosage highly individualized, depending on severity of disease.
*Children:* 20 to 300 mg/m$^2$ P.O. daily in four divided doses or 7 to 37.5 mg/m$^2$ I.M. once daily or b.i.d. Dosage must be highly individualized.

## Mechanism of action
*Adrenocorticoid replacement:* Cortisone acetate is an adrenocorticoid with both glucocorticoid and mineralocorticoid properties. A weak anti-inflammatory, drug has only about 80% of the anti-inflammatory activity of an equal weight of hydrocortisone. It's a potent mineralocorticoid, however, having twice the potency of prednisone. Cortisone (or hydrocortisone) is usually the drug of choice for replacement therapy in patients with adrenal insufficiency. It's usually not used for inflammatory or immunosuppressant activity because of the extremely large doses that must be used and because of the unwanted mineralocorticoid effects. Injectable form has a slow onset but a long duration of action. It's usually used only when the oral dosage form can't be used.

## Pharmacokinetics
*Absorption:* Absorbed readily after oral administration.
*Distribution:* Distributed rapidly to muscle, liver, skin, intestines, and kidneys. Cortisone is extensively bound to plasma proteins (transcortin and albumin). Only the unbound por-

tion is active. Cortisone appears in breast milk and through the placenta.

*Metabolism:* Metabolized in the liver to the active metabolite hydrocortisone, which in turn is metabolized to inactive glucuronide and sulfate metabolites. Duration of hypothalamic-pituitary-adrenal (HPA) axis suppression is 1¼ to 1½ days.

*Excretion:* Inactive metabolites and small amounts of unmetabolized drug are excreted by the kidneys. Insignificant quantities of the drug are also excreted in feces. Biological half-life of cortisone is 8 to 12 hours.

| Route | Onset | Peak | Duration |
|-------|-------|------|----------|
| P.O. | Variable | 1-2 hr | Variable |
| I.M. | 24-48 hr | Variable | Variable |

## Contraindications and precautions
Contraindicated in patients hypersensitive to drug or its ingredients or systemic fungal infections. Use cautiously in patients with renal disease, recent MI, GI ulcer, hypertension, osteoporosis, diabetes mellitus, hypothyroidism, cirrhosis, diverticulitis, ulcerative colitis, recent intestinal anastomosis, thromboembolic disorders, seizures, myasthenia gravis, heart failure, tuberculosis, ocular herpes, emotional instability, or psychotic tendencies.

## Interactions
**Drug-drug.** *Antacids, cholestyramine, colestipol:* Decrease cortisone's effect by adsorbing the corticosteroid, decreasing the amount absorbed. Advise clinician to monitor patient carefully.

*Barbiturates, phenytoin, rifampin:* Decreased corticosteroid effects. Advise clinician to monitor patient closely.

*Cardiac glycosides:* Hypokalemia may increase the risk of toxicity in patients also receiving cardiac glycosides. Avoid use together.

*Diuretic or amphotericin B therapy:* Cortisone may enhance hypokalemia associated with diuretic or amphotericin B therapy. Advise clinician to monitor serum blood levels closely, especially potassium.

*Estrogens:* May reduce the metabolism of cortisone. The half-life of cortisone is then prolonged. Avoid use together.

*Insulin, oral antidiabetics:* Cause hyperglycemia. Dosage adjustment may be needed.

*Isoniazid, salicylates:* When used together, cortisone increases the metabolism of isoniazid and salicylates. Use together cautiously.

*NSAIDs:* May increase the risk of GI ulceration. Avoid use together.

*Oral anticoagulants:* When used together, cortisone may decrease the effects. Advise clinician to monitor PT.

*Toxoids, inactivated vaccines:* Cortisone may have a diminished response to toxoids or inactivated vaccines. Avoid use together.

**Drug-lifestyle.** *Alcohol use:* Increased risk of gastric irritation and GI ulceration. Advise patient to avoid alcohol.

## Adverse reactions
Most adverse reactions to corticosteroids are dose- or duration-dependent.

**CNS:** euphoria, insomnia, psychotic behavior, pseudotumor cerebri, vertigo, headache, paresthesia, *seizures.*

**CV:** *HF,* hypertension, edema, *arrhythmias,* thrombophlebitis, *thromboembolism.*

**EENT:** cataracts, glaucoma.

**GI:** *peptic ulcer,* GI irritation, increased appetite, *pancreatitis,* nausea, vomiting.

**GU:** menstrual irregularities, increased urine glucose and calcium levels.

**Metabolic:** hypokalemia, hyperglycemia, hypocalcemia, hypercholesterolemia; decreased serum thyroxine and triiodothyronine levels.

**Musculoskeletal:** muscle weakness, osteoporosis, growth suppression in children.

**Skin:** delayed wound healing, acne, various skin eruptions, atrophy at I.M. injection sites, hirsutism.

**Other:** susceptibility to infections; *acute adrenal insufficiency may follow increased stress (infection, surgery, trauma) or abrupt withdrawal after long-term therapy,* cushingoid symptoms (moonface, buffalo hump, central obesity).

**After abrupt withdrawal:** rebound inflammation, fatigue, weakness, arthralgia, fever, dizziness, lethargy, depression, fainting, orthostatic hypotension, dyspnea, anorexia, hypoglycemia. **After prolonged use**, sudden withdrawal may be fatal.

## Overdose and treatment
Acute ingestion, even in massive doses, is rarely a clinical problem. Toxic signs and symptoms rarely occur if the drug is used for less than 3 weeks, even at large dosage ranges. However, chronic use causes adverse physiologic effects.

## Clinical considerations
**◀ALERT** Check for sensitivity to any other corticosteroid. Drug isn't for I.V. use. For better results and less toxicity, give a once-daily dose in the morning.

■ Drug therapy suppresses reactions to skin tests; causes false-negative results in the nitroblue tetrazolium test for systemic bacterial infections; and decreases [131]I uptake and protein-bound iodine levels in thyroid function test results.

### Therapeutic monitoring
■ Advise clinician to monitor serum electrolyte and blood glucose levels.
■ Advise clinician to monitor patient for fluid and electrolyte imbalance.

### Special populations
**Pediatric patients.** Long-term use of cortisone in children and adolescents may delay growth and maturation.
**Geriatric patients.** Use with caution in geriatric patients because osteoporosis is more likely to develop in this group.

### Patient counseling
■ Inform patient of potential adverse reactions.
■ Tell patient not to discontinue drug abruptly or without prescriber's consent.
■ Advise patient to avoid exposure to infections (such as measles and chickenpox) and to notify prescriber if such exposure occurs.
■ Instruct patient to carry a card indicating his need for supplemental glucocorticoids during stress. This card should contain prescriber's name, drug, and dose taken.

# cosyntropin
Cortrosyn

*Pharmacologic classification:* anterior pituitary hormone
*Therapeutic classification:* diagnostic
*Pregnancy risk category C*

### Available forms
Available by prescription only
*Injection:* 0.25 mg

### Indications and dosages
*Diagnostic test of adrenocortical function*
*Adults and children ages 2 and older:* 0.25 to 0.75 mg I.M. or I.V. (unless label prohibits I.V. administration) between blood samplings. To administer as I.V. infusion, dilute 0.25 mg in $D_5W$ or normal saline solution, and infuse over 6 hours (40 mcg/hour).
*Children under age 2:* 0.125 mg I.M. or I.V.

### I.V. administration
■ Reconstitute powder by adding 1 ml of normal saline solution to 0.25-mg vial to yield a solution containing 0.25 mg/ml.
■ For rapid screening, plasma cortisol level is determined before and 30 minutes after administration of 0.25 mg I.M. or I.V. injection over 2 minutes. Some clinicians prefer plasma cortisol level determinations at 60 minutes after injection of cosyntropin.
■ Reconstituted solution remains stable at controlled room temperature for 24 hours or for 21 days at 36° to 46° F (2° to 8° C).
■ More cortisol is secreted if dose is given slowly, not rapidly I.V.

### Incompatibilities
Incompatible with both blood and plasma because enzymes inactivate drug.

### Mechanism of action
*Diagnostic action:* Cosyntropin is used to test adrenal function. Drug binds with a specific receptor in the adrenal cell plasma membrane to initiate synthesis of its entire spectrum of hormones, one of which is cortisol. In patients with primary adrenocortical insufficiency, cosyntropin doesn't increase plasma cortisol levels significantly.

### Pharmacokinetics
*Absorption:* Inactivated by the proteolytic enzymes in the GI tract. After I.M. administration, cosyntropin is absorbed rapidly. After rapid I.V. administration in patients with normal adrenocortical function, plasma cortisol levels begin to increase within 5 minutes and double within 15 to 30 minutes. Peak levels begin to decrease in 2 to 4 hours.
*Distribution:* Not fully understood, but drug is removed rapidly from plasma by many tissues.
*Metabolism:* Unknown.
*Excretion:* Probably excreted by the kidneys.

| Route | Onset | Peak | Duration |
|---|---|---|---|
| I.V. | Rapid | 45-60 min | Unknown |
| I.M., S.C. | Unknown | 45-60 min | Unknown |

### Contraindications and precautions
Contraindicated in patients hypersensitive to drug.

### Interactions
**Drug-drug.** *Blood, plasma products:* Inactivate cosyntropin. Avoid administration together.
*Cortisone, estrogens, hydrocortisone:* May cause abnormally elevated plasma cortisol levels. Avoid use together.

### Adverse reactions
**CNS:** *seizures,* dizziness, vertigo, *increased intracranial pressure with papilledema,* pseudotumor cerebri.
**EENT:** cataracts, glaucoma.
**GI:** peptic ulcer, *pancreatitis,* abdominal distension, ulcerative esophagitis, nausea, vomiting.
**GU:** menstrual irregularities.
**Metabolic:** alterations in blood glucose levels.
**Musculoskeletal:** fractures, muscle weakness, steroid myopathy, loss of muscle mass, osteoporosis, vertebral compression.
**Skin:** pruritus; impaired wound healing; thin, fragile skin; petechiae; ecchymoses; facial erythema; diaphoresis; acne; hyperpigmentation; hirsutism, flushing.
**Other:** hypersensitivity reactions, cushingoid symptoms.

### Overdose and treatment
Acute overdose requires no therapy other than symptomatic treatment and supportive care.

## Clinical considerations
■ Cosyntropin is less antigenic than corticotropin and less likely to produce allergic reactions.
■ High plasma cortisol levels may be reported erroneously in patients receiving spironolactone, cortisone, or hydrocortisone when fluorometric analysis is used. This doesn't occur with the radioimmunoassay or competitive protein-binding method. However, therapy can be maintained with prednisone, dexamethasone, or betamethasone because these aren't detectable by the fluorometric method.

### Therapeutic monitoring
■ A normal response to cosyntropin includes: The control plasma cortisol level should exceed 5 mcg/100 ml plasma; 30 minutes after the injection, cortisol levels increase by 7 mcg/100 ml above control; 30-minute cortisol levels exceed 18 mcg/100 ml.

### Special populations
**Pregnant patients.** Since effects of drug on fetus aren't known, drug should be used during pregnancy only if clearly needed.
**Breast-feeding patients.** It's unknown if drug appears in breast milk. Use cautiously in breast-feeding mothers.

## Patient counseling
■ Inform patient taking spironolactone, cortisone, hydrocortisone, or estrogen that these drugs may interfere with test results.
■ Tell patient to report adverse effects immediately.

## co-trimoxazole (trimethoprim-sulfamethoxazole)
Apo-Sulfatrim*, Bactrim, Bactrim DS, Bactrim IV, Cotrim, Cotrim D.S., Novo-Trimel*, Roubac*, Septra, Septra DS, Septra IV, SMZ-TMP, Sulfatrim

*Pharmacologic classification:* sulfonamide and folate antagonist
*Therapeutic classification:* antibiotic
*Pregnancy risk category C*

## Available forms
Available by prescription only
*Tablets:* trimethoprim 80 mg and sulfamethoxazole 400 mg; trimethoprim 160 mg and sulfamethoxazole 800 mg
*Suspension:* trimethoprim 40 mg and sulfamethoxazole 200 mg/5 ml
*Injectable:* trimethoprim 16 mg/ml and sulfamethoxazole 80 mg/ml

## Indications and dosages
*Urinary tract infections and shigellosis*
*Adults:* One double-strength or two regular-strength tablets P.O. q 12 hours for 10 to 14 days or 5 days for shigellosis. Or, 8 to 10 mg/kg (based on trimethoprim) I.V. daily given in two to four equally divided doses for up to 14 days (5 days for shigellosis). Maximum daily dose, 960 mg.
*Children over age 2 months:* 8 mg/kg trimethoprim and 40 mg/kg sulfamethoxazole P.O. daily in two divided doses q 12 hours (10 days for urinary tract infections; 5 days for shigellosis).
*Primary prophylaxis against toxoplasmosis in HIV-infected patients*
*Adults and adolescents:* 160 mg (based on trimethoprim) daily P.O.
*Children:* 150 mg/m$^2$ (based on trimethoprim) P.O. daily in two divided doses.
*Otitis media*
*Children over age 2 months:* 8 mg/kg trimethoprim and 40 mg/kg sulfamethoxazole P.O. daily, in two divided doses q 12 hours for 10 days.
*Pneumocystis carinii pneumonitis*
*Adults and children over age 2 months:* 15 to 20 mg/kg trimethoprim and 75 to 100 mg/kg sulfamethoxazole P.O. daily, in equally divided doses, q 6 to 8 hours for 14 to 21 days.
*Prophylaxis of* P. carinii *pneumonia*
*Adults:* 160 mg (based on trimethoprim) daily.
*Children:* 150 mg/m$^2$ (based on trimethoprim) daily in two divided doses for 3 consecutive days each week.
*Chronic bronchitis*
*Adults:* One double-strength or two regular-strength tablets P.O. q 12 hours for 14 days.
*Traveler's diarrhea*
*Adults:* One double-strength or two regular-strength tablets P.O. q 12 hours for 5 days.
   Note: For the following unlabeled uses, dosages refer to oral trimethoprim (as co-trimoxazole).
◇ *Septic agranulocytosis*
*Adults:* 2.5 mg/kg I.V. q.i.d.; for prophylaxis, 80 to 160 mg b.i.d.
◇ *Nocardia infection*
*Adults:* 640 mg P.O. daily for 7 months.
◇ *Pharyngeal gonococcal infections*
*Adults:* 720 mg P.O. daily for 5 days.
◇ *Chancroid*
*Adults:* 160 mg P.O. b.i.d. for 7 days.
◇ *Pertussis*
*Adults:* 320 mg P.O. daily in two divided doses.
*Children:* 40 mg/kg/day P.O. in two divided doses.
◇ *Cholera*
*Adults:* 160 mg P.O. b.i.d. for 3 days.
*Children:* 4 to 5 mg/kg P.O. b.i.d. for 3 days.
◇ *Isosporiasis*
*Adults:* 160 mg P.O. q.i.d. for 10 days, followed by 160 mg b.i.d. for 3 weeks.
≡ *Dosage adjustment.* For patients with impaired renal function, adjust dosage or fre-

quency of administration of parenteral form according to degree of renal impairment, severity of infection, and susceptibility of organism.

## I.V. administration
■ Dilute infusion in D₅W. Don't mix with other drugs. Don't administer by rapid infusion or bolus injection. Infuse slowly over 60 to 90 minutes.
■ Infusion must be diluted before use. Each 5 ml should be added to 125 ml $D_5W$. Don't refrigerate solution; diluted solutions must be used within 6 hours. A dilution of 5 ml per 75 ml $D_5W$ may be prepared for patients requiring fluid restriction, but these solutions should be used within 2 hours.
■ Check solution carefully for precipitate before starting infusion. Don't use solution containing a precipitate.
■ Assess I.V. site for signs of phlebitis or infiltration.

### Incompatibilities
Avoid diluting with any solution but $D_5W$ because drug components lose potency. Manufacturer recommends mixing no other drugs with co-trimoxazole.

## Mechanism of action
*Antibacterial action:* Co-trimoxazole is generally bactericidal; it acts by sequential blockade of folic acid enzymes in the synthesis pathway. The sulfamethoxazole component inhibits formation of dihydrofolic acid from para-aminobenzoic (PABA), whereas trimethoprim inhibits dihydrofolate reductase. Both drugs block folic acid synthesis, preventing bacterial cell synthesis of essential nucleic acids.

Co-trimoxazole is effective against *E. coli, Klebsiella, Enterobacter, P. mirabilis, H. influenzae, S. pneumoniae, S. aureus, Acinetobacter, Salmonella, Shigella,* and *P. carinii.*

## Pharmacokinetics
*Absorption:* Well absorbed from the GI tract after oral administration.
*Distribution:* Distributed widely into body tissues and fluids, including middle ear fluid, prostatic fluid, bile, aqueous humor, and CSF. Protein binding is 44% for trimethoprim, 70% for sulfamethoxazole. Drug crosses the placenta.
*Metabolism:* Metabolized by the liver.
*Excretion:* Both components of co-trimoxazole are excreted primarily in urine by glomerular filtration and renal tubular secretion; some appears in breast milk. Trimethoprim's plasma half-life in patients with normal renal function is 8 to 11 hours, extended to 26 hours in severe renal dysfunction; sulfamethoxazole's plasma half-life is normally 10 to 13 hours, extended to 30 to 40 hours in severe renal

dysfunction. Hemodialysis removes some co-trimoxazole.

| Route | Onset | Peak | Duration |
|-------|-------|------|----------|
| P.O. | Unknown | 1-4 hr | Unknown |
| I.V. | Immediate | Immediate | Unknown |

## Contraindications and precautions
Contraindicated in patients hypersensitive to trimethoprim or sulfonamides, severe renal impairment (creatinine clearance of less than 15 ml/minute), or porphyria; in those with megaloblastic anemia caused by folate deficiency; in pregnant women at term; in breast-feeding women; and in children under age 2 months.

Use cautiously in patients with impaired renal or hepatic function, severe allergies, severe bronchial asthma, G6PD deficiency, or blood dyscrasia.

## Interactions
**Drug-drug.** *Cyclosporine:* Decreased therapeutic effect and an increased risk of nephrotoxicity. Avoid use together.
*Digoxin:* Increased serum digoxin levels. Advise clinician to monitor serum levels closely.
*Indomethacin:* May increase plasma levels of sulfamethoxazole. Dosage adjustment may be needed.
*Methotrexate:* Concurrent use can increase levels. Use together cautiously.
*Oral anticoagulants:* Co-trimoxazole may inhibit hepatic metabolism, enhancing anticoagulant effects. Observe patient for signs of bleeding.
*Oral sulfonylureas:* Concurrent use enhances their hypoglycemic effects. Advise clinician to monitor glucose levels.
*PABA:* Concurrent use antagonizes sulfonamide effects. Advise clinician to monitor patient closely.
*Phenytoin:* Co-trimoxazole may inhibit metabolism of phenytoin. Dosage adjustment may be needed.
*Pyrimethamine:* May cause megaloblastic anemia in pyrimethamine doses greater than 25 mg weekly. Avoid use together.
*Tricyclic antidepressants:* May decrease antidepressant effect. Advise clinician to monitor patient closely.
*Zidovudine:* Serum levels of zidovudine may be increased. Advise clinician to monitor patient carefully.
**Drug-herb.** *Dong quai, St. John's wort:* Additive photosensitivity risk. Advise patient to use take precautions.
**Drug-lifestyle.** *Sun exposure:* Photosensitivity reaction may occur. Advise patient to use sunblock.

## Adverse reactions
**CNS:** headache, mental depression, aseptic meningitis, apathy, *seizures,* hallucinations, ataxia, nervousness, fatigue, vertigo, insomnia.

**EENT:** tinnitus.
**GI:** *nausea, vomiting, diarrhea,* abdominal pain, anorexia, stomatitis, *pancreatitis,* pseudomembranous colitis.
**GU:** *toxic nephrosis with oliguria and anuria,* crystalluria, hematuria, interstitial nephritis.
**Hematologic:** *agranulocytosis, aplastic anemia,* megaloblastic anemia, *thrombocytopenia, leukopenia,* hemolytic anemia, *pancytopenia.*
**Hepatic:** jaundice, *hepatic necrosis.*
**Musculoskeletal:** muscle weakness, arthralgia, myalgia, rhabdomyolysis.
**Respiratory:** pulmonary infiltrates.
**Skin:** *erythema multiforme (Stevens-Johnson syndrome),* generalized skin eruptions, epidermal necrolysis, exfoliative dermatitis, photosensitivity, urticaria, pruritus.
**Other:** hypersensitivity reactions (*serum sickness, drug fever, anaphylaxis*), thrombophlebitis.

## Overdose and treatment

Signs and symptoms of overdose include mental depression, drowsiness, anorexia, jaundice, confusion, headache, nausea, vomiting, diarrhea, facial swelling, slight elevations in liver function test results, and bone marrow depression.

Recommend treating by emesis or gastric lavage, followed by supportive care (correction of acidosis, forced oral fluid, and I.V. fluids). Treatment of renal failure may be required; transfuse appropriate blood products in severe hematologic toxicity; use folinic acid to rescue bone marrow. Hemodialysis has limited ability to remove co-trimoxazole. Peritoneal dialysis isn't effective.

## Clinical considerations

**ℍALERT** DS means double-strength.
**ℍALERT** Occasionally, dosage is written as trimethoprim component; check it carefully.
■ Drug isn't for I.M. use.
■ Co-trimoxazole has been used effectively to treat chronic bacterial prostatitis and as prophylaxis against recurrent urinary tract infection in women and traveler's diarrhea.
■ Shake oral suspension thoroughly before administering.
■ Trimethoprim can interfere with serum methotrexate assay as determined by the competitive binding protein technique. No interference occurs if radioimmunoassay is used.

### Therapeutic monitoring
■ Advise clinician to monitor renal and liver function test results.

### Special populations
**Pregnant patients.** Use only when needed in pregnant women.

**Breast-feeding patients.** Drug isn't recommended in breast-feeding women.
**Pediatric patients.** Drug isn't recommended for infants under age 2 months.
**Geriatric patients.** In geriatric patients, diminished renal function may prolong half-life. Such patients also have an increased risk of adverse reactions.

## Patient counseling
■ Inform patient of potential adverse reactions.
■ Tell patient to take drug as prescribed, even if he feels better.
■ Instruct patient to take oral dose with 8 ounces (240 ml) of water on an empty stomach.

# cromolyn sodium
Crolom, Gastrocrom, Intal Aerosol Spray, Intal Nebulizer Solution, Nasalcrom, Opticrom

*Pharmacologic classification:* chromone derivative
*Therapeutic classification:* mast cell stabilizer, antasthmatic
*Pregnancy risk category B*

## Available forms
Available by prescription only
*Aerosol:* 800 mcg/metered spray
*Solution:* 20 mg/2 ml for nebulization
*Ophthalmic solution:* 4%
*Oral concentrate:* 100 mg/5ml
Available without a prescription
*Nasal solution:* 5.2 mg/metered spray (40 mg/ml)

## Indications and dosages
*Adjunct in treatment of severe perennial bronchial asthma*
*Adults and children over age 5:* Two inhalations q.i.d. at regular intervals; aqueous solution given through a nebulizer, one ampule q.i.d.
*Prevention and treatment of allergic rhinitis*
*Adults and children ages 2 and older:* One spray (5.2 mg) of nasal solution in each nostril t.i.d. or q.i.d. May give up to six times daily.
*Prevention of exercise-induced bronchospasm*
*Adults and children over age 5:* Two metered sprays using inhaler no longer than 1 hour before anticipated exercise.

Inhalation of 20 mg of oral inhalation solution may be used in adults or children ages 2 and older. Repeat inhalation p.r.n. for protection during long exercise.
*Allergic ocular disorders (giant papillary conjunctivitis, vernal keratoconjunctivitis, vernal keratitis, allergic keratoconjunctivitis)*
*Adults and children over age 4:* Instill 1 to 2 drops in each eye four to six times daily at reg-

ular intervals. One drop contains about 1.6 mg cromolyn sodium.

*Systemic mastocytosis*
*Adults:* 200 mg P.O. q.i.d.
*Children ages 2 to 12:* 100 mg P.O. q.i.d.
*Children under age 2:* 20 mg/kg daily P.O. divided in four equal doses.

◊ *Food allergy, inflammatory bowel disease*
*Adults:* 200 mg P.O. q.i.d. 15 to 20 minutes before meals.

## Mechanism of action

*Antasthmatic action:* Cromolyn prevents release of mediators of type I allergic reactions, including histamine and slow-reacting substance of anaphylaxis (SRS-A), from sensitized mast cells after the antigen-antibody union has taken place. Cromolyn doesn't inhibit binding of IgE to mast cells nor the interaction between cell-bound IgE and the specific antigen. It does inhibit the release of substances (such as histamine and SRS-A) in response to IgE binding to mast cells. Main site of action occurs locally on the lung mucosa, nasal mucosa, and eyes.

*Bronchodilating action:* Besides mast cell stabilization, recent evidence suggests that drug may have a bronchodilating effect by an unknown mechanism. Comparative studies have shown cromolyn and theophylline to be equally efficacious but less effective than orally inhaled beta₂-adrenergic agonists in preventing this bronchospasm.

*Ocular antiallergy action:* Cromolyn inhibits degranulation of sensitized mast cells that occurs after exposure to specific antigens, preventing release of histamine and SRS-A.

Cromolyn has no direct anti-inflammatory, vasoconstrictor, antihistamine, antiserotonin, or corticosteroid-like properties.

Cromolyn dissolved in water and given orally has been found to be effective in managing food allergy, inflammatory bowel disease (Crohn's disease, ulcerative colitis), and systemic mastocytosis.

## Pharmacokinetics

*Absorption:* Only 0.5% to 2% of an oral dose is absorbed. The amount reaching the lungs depends on patient's ability to use inhaler correctly, amount of bronchoconstriction, and size or presence of mucus plugs. The degree of absorption depends on method of administration; most absorption occurs with the aerosol via metered-dose inhaler, and least occurs with the administration of the solution via power-operated nebulizer. Less than 7% of an intranasal dose of cromolyn as a solution is absorbed systemically. Only minimal absorption (0.03%) of an ophthalmic dose occurs after instillation into the eye. Absorption half-life from the lung is 1 hour. A plasma level of 9 ng/ml

can be achieved 15 minutes following a 20-mg dose.

*Distribution:* Cromolyn doesn't cross most biological membranes because it's ionized and lipid-insoluble at the body's pH. Less than 0.1% of a dose crosses to the placenta; it isn't known if drug appears in breast milk.

*Metabolism:* None significant.

*Excretion:* Excreted unchanged in urine (50%) and bile (about 50%). Small amounts may be excreted in the feces or exhaled. Elimination half-life is 81 minutes.

| Route | Onset | Peak | Duration |
|---|---|---|---|
| P.O., inhalation, intranasal, ophthalmic | Unknown | Unknown | Unknown |

## Contraindications and precautions

Contraindicated in patients experiencing acute asthma attacks or status asthmaticus and in patients hypersensitive to drug. Use inhalation form cautiously in patients with cardiac disease or arrhythmias.

## Interactions

None reported.

## Adverse reactions

**CNS:** dizziness, headache.
**EENT:** *irritated throat and trachea,* nasal congestion, pharyngeal irritation, *sneezing,* nasal burning and irritation, epistaxis, lacrimation, swollen parotid gland.
**GI:** nausea, esophagitis, abdominal pain, bad taste in mouth.
**GU:** dysuria, urinary frequency.
**Musculoskeletal:** joint swelling and pain.
**Respiratory:** *bronchospasm* (after inhalation of dry powder), *cough,* wheezing, *eosinophilic pneumonia.*
**Skin:** rash, urticaria.
**Other:** *angioedema.*

## Overdose and treatment

No information available.

## Clinical considerations

■ Bronchospasm or cough occasionally occur after inhalation and may require stopping therapy. Prior bronchodilation may help but it may still be necessary to stop the cromolyn therapy.
■ Asthma symptoms may recur if cromolyn dosage is reduced below recommended dosage.
■ Use reduced dosage in patients with impaired renal or hepatic function.
■ Eosinophilic pneumonia or pulmonary infiltrates with eosinophilia requires stopping drug.
■ Nasal solution may cause nasal stinging or sneezing immediately after instillation of drug but this reaction rarely requires discontinuation of drug.

■ Watch for recurrence of asthmatic symptoms when corticosteroids are also used. Use only when acute episode has been controlled, airway is cleared, and patient is able to inhale.
■ Protect oral solution and ophthalmic solution from direct sunlight.
■ Therapeutic effects may not be seen for 2 to 4 weeks after therapy starts.

### Therapeutic monitoring
■ Advise clinician to monitor pulmonary status before and immediately after therapy.
■ Pulmonary function tests are needed to confirm significant bronchodilator-reversible component of airway obstruction in patients considered for cromolyn therapy.

### Special populations
**Pregnant patients.** Animal studies have shown adverse fetal effects when cromolyn sodium is given parenterally in high doses with high-dose isoproterenol.
**Pediatric patients.** Cromolyn use in children under age 5 is limited to the inhalation route of administration. The safety of the nebulizer solution in children under age 2 hasn't been established. Safety of nasal solution in children under age 6 hasn't been established.

### Patient counseling
■ Teach correct use of metered-dose inhaler: exhale completely before placing mouthpiece between lips, then inhale deeply and slowly with steady, even breath; remove inhaler from mouth, hold breath for 5 to 10 seconds, and exhale.
■ Urge patient to call prescriber if drug causes wheezing or coughing.
■ Instruct patient with asthma or seasonal or perennial allergic rhinitis to administer drug at regular intervals to ensure clinical effectiveness.
■ Advise patient that gargling and rinsing mouth after administration can help reduce mouth dryness.
■ Tell patient taking prescribed adrenocorticoids to continue taking them during therapy, if appropriate.
■ Instruct patient who uses a bronchodilator inhaler to administer dose about 5 minutes before taking cromolyn (unless otherwise indicated); explain that this step helps reduce adverse reactions.

# cyanocobalamin (vitamin B$_{12}$)
Bedoz,* Cobex, Crystamine, Cyanoject, Cyomin, Rubesol-1000, Rubramin PC, Vibal

# hydroxocobalamin (vitamin B$_{12}$)
Hydrobexan, Hydro-Cobex, LA-12

*Pharmacologic classification:* water-soluble vitamin
*Therapeutic classification:* vitamin, nutrition supplement
*Pregnancy risk category C (parenteral)*

## Available forms
Available by prescription only
*Tablets:* 25 mcg, 50 mcg, 100 mcg, 250 mcg, 500 mcg, 1,000 mcg
*Injection:* 100 mcg/ml, 1,000 mcg/ml

## Indications and dosages
### RDA for vitamin B$_{12}$
*Neonates and infants up to age 6 months:* 0.4 mcg
*Infants ages 6 months to 1 year:* 0.5 mcg
*Children ages 1 to 3 years:* 0.9 mcg
*Children ages 4 to 8 years:* 1.2 mcg
*Children ages 9 to 13 years:* 1.8 mcg
*Adults and children ages 14 and older:* 2.4 mcg
*Pregnant women:* 2.6 mcg
*Breast-feeding women:* 2.8 mcg
### Vitamin B$_{12}$ deficiency from any cause except malabsorption related to pernicious anemia or other GI disease
*Adults:* 30 mcg S.C. or I.M. daily for 5 to 10 days, depending on severity of deficiency. Maintenance dose is 100 to 200 mcg I.M. once monthly. For subsequent prophylaxis, recommend adequate nutrition and daily RDA vitamin B$_{12}$ supplements.
*Children:* 1 to 5 mg given in single doses of 100 mcg I.M. or S.C. over the course of 2 or more weeks. Maintenance dose is 60 mcg/month I.M. or S.C.
### Schilling test flushing dose
*Adults and children:* 1,000 mcg I.M. in a single dose.

## Mechanism of action
*Nutritional action:* Vitamin B$_{12}$ can be converted to coenzyme B$_{12}$ in tissues and, as such, is essential for conversion of methyl-malonate to succinate and synthesis of methionine from homocystine, a reaction that also requires folate. Without coenzyme B$_{12}$ folate deficiency occurs. Vitamin B$_{12}$ is also associated with fat and carbohydrate metabolism and protein synthesis. Cells characterized by rapid division (epithelial cells, bone marrow, and myeloid

cells) appear to have the greatest requirement for vitamin $B_{12}$.

Vitamin $B_{12}$ deficiency may cause megaloblastic anemia, GI lesions, and neurologic damage; it begins with an inability to produce myelin followed by gradual degeneration of the axon and nerve. Parenteral administration of vitamin $B_{12}$ completely reverses the megaloblastic anemia and GI symptoms of vitamin $B_{12}$ deficiency.

## Pharmacokinetics

*Absorption:* After oral administration, vitamin $B_{12}$ is absorbed irregularly from the distal small intestine. Vitamin $B_{12}$ is protein-bound, and this bond must be split by proteolysis and gastric acid before absorption. Absorption depends on sufficient intrinsic factor and calcium. Vitamin $B_{12}$ is inadequate in malabsorptive states and in pernicious anemia. After oral administration of doses of less than 3 mcg, peak plasma levels aren't reached for 8 to 12 hours.

*Distribution:* Distributed into the liver, bone marrow, and other tissues, including the placenta. At birth, the vitamin $B_{12}$ level in neonates is three to five times that in the mother. Vitamin $B_{12}$ appears in breast milk in levels about equal to the maternal vitamin $B_{12}$ level. Unlike cyanocobalamin, hydroxocobalamin is absorbed more slowly parenterally and may be taken up by the liver in larger quantities; it also produces a greater increase in serum cobalamin levels and less urinary excretion.

*Metabolism:* Cyanocobalamin and hydroxocobalamin are metabolized in the liver.

*Excretion:* In healthy persons receiving only dietary vitamin $B_{12}$, about 3 to 8 mcg of the vitamin is secreted into the GI tract daily, mainly from bile, and all but about 1 mcg is reabsorbed; less than 0.25 mcg is usually excreted in the urine daily. When vitamin $B_{12}$ is given in amounts that exceed the binding capacity of plasma, the liver, and other tissues, it's free in the blood for urinary excretion.

| Route | Onset | Peak | Duration |
|---|---|---|---|
| P.O. | Unknown | 8-12 hr | Unknown |
| I.M., S.C. | Unknown | 1 hr | Unknown |

## Contraindications and precautions

Contraindicated in patients hypersensitive to vitamin $B_{12}$ or cobalt and in patients with early Leber's disease. Use cautiously in anemic patients with coexisting cardiac, pulmonary, or hypertensive disease and in those with severe vitamin $B_{12}$-dependent deficiencies.

## Interactions

**Drug-drug.** *Aminoglycosides, aminosalicylic acid and its salts, anticonvulsants, cobalt irradiation of the small bowel, colchicine, extended-release potassium preparations:* Concurrent use decreases vitamin $B_{12}$ absorption from the GI tract. Don't use together.

*Ascorbic acid:* May destroy vitamin $B_{12}$; shouldn't be given within 1 hour of taking vitamin $B_{12}$.

*Chloramphenicol:* Antagonized hematopoietic response. Don't give together.

*Colchicine:* Concurrent use may increase neomycin-induced malabsorption of vitamin $B_{12}$. Don't use together.

**Drug-lifestyle.** *Alcohol use:* Decreases vitamin $B_{12}$ absorption from the GI tract. Advise patient to avoid alcohol.

*Smoking:* Appears to increase requirement for vitamin $B_{12}$. Discourage smoking.

## Adverse reactions

**CV:** peripheral vascular thrombosis, *HF.*
**GI:** transient diarrhea.
**Respiratory:** pulmonary edema.
**Skin:** itching, transitory exanthema, urticaria, pain, burning (at S.C. or I.M. injection sites).
**Other:** *anaphylaxis, anaphylactoid reactions* (with parenteral administration).

## Overdose and treatment

Not applicable. Even in large doses, vitamin $B_{12}$ isn't usually toxic.

## Clinical considerations

■ Recommended RDA for vitamin $B_{12}$ is 0.3 mcg in infants to 2 mcg in adults, as follows:

*Infants up to age 6 months:* 0.3 mcg
*Children ages 6 months to 1 year:* 0.5 mcg
*Children ages 1 to 3:* 0.7 mcg
*Children ages 4 to 6:* 1 mcg
*Children ages 7 to 10:* 1.4 mcg
*Children ages 11 to adult:* 2 mcg
*Pregnant women:* 2.2 mcg
*Breast-feeding women:* 2.6 mcg

■ Determine patient's diet and drug history, including patterns of alcohol use, to identify poor nutritional habits.

■ Oral solution should be given promptly after mixing with fruit juice. Ascorbic acid causes instability of vitamin $B_{12}$. Protect oral solution from light.

■ Oral vitamin $B_{12}$ should be given with meals to increase absorption.

■ Advise clinician to monitor patient's bowel function because regularity is essential for consistent absorption of oral preparations.

■ Don't mix the parenteral form with dextrose solutions, alkaline or strongly acidic solutions, or oxidizing and reducing agents, because anaphylactic reactions may occur with I.V. use.

■ Parenteral therapy is preferred for patients with pernicious anemia because oral administration may be unreliable. In patients with neurologic complications, prolonged inadequate oral therapy may lead to permanent spinal cord damage. Oral therapy is appropriate for mild

conditions without neurologic signs and for those patients who refuse or are sensitive to the parenteral form.
- Patients with a history of sensitivities and those suspected of being sensitive to vitamin $B_{12}$ should receive an intradermal test dose before therapy begins. Sensitization to vitamin $B_{12}$ may develop after as many as 8 years of treatment.
- Expect therapeutic response to occur within 48 hours; it's measured by laboratory values and effect on fatigue, GI symptoms, anorexia, pallid or yellow complexion, glossitis, distaste for meat, dyspnea on exertion, palpitation, neurologic degeneration (paresthesia, loss of vibratory and position sense and deep reflexes, incoordination), psychotic behavior, anosmia, and visual disturbances.
- Therapeutic response to vitamin $B_{12}$ may be impaired by concurrent infection, uremia, folic acid or iron deficiency, or drugs having bone marrow suppressant effects. Large doses of vitamin $B_{12}$ may improve folate-deficient megaloblastic anemia.
- Patients with mild peripheral neurologic defects may respond to concomitant physical therapy. Usually, neurologic damage that doesn't improve after 12 to 18 months of therapy is considered irreversible. Severe vitamin $B_{12}$ deficiency that persists for 3 months or longer may cause permanent spinal cord degeneration.
- Vitamin $B_{12}$ therapy may cause false-positive results for intrinsic factor antibodies, which are present in the blood of half of all patients with pernicious anemia. Methotrexate, pyrimethamine, and most anti-infectives invalidate diagnostic blood assays for vitamin $B_{12}$.

### Therapeutic monitoring
- Advise clinician to monitor vital signs in patients with cardiac disease and those receiving parenteral vitamin $B_{12}$. Advise clinician to watch for signs and symptoms of pulmonary edema, which tend to develop early in therapy.
- Expect reticulocyte level to rise in 3 to 4 days, peak in 5 to 8 days, and then gradually decline as erythrocyte count and hemoglobin rise to normal levels (in 4 to 6 weeks).
- Advise clinician to monitor potassium levels during the first 48 hours, especially in patients with pernicious anemia or megaloblastic anemia. Potassium supplements may be required. Conversion to normal erythropoiesis increases erythrocyte potassium requirement and may result in fatal hypokalemia in these patients.
- Periodic hematologic evaluations should be continued throughout patient's lifetime.

### Special populations
**Breast-feeding patients.** Vitamin $B_{12}$ appears in breast milk in levels that approximate the maternal vitamin $B_{12}$ level. The Food and Nutrition Board of the National Academy of Sciences-National Research Council recommends that breast-feeding women consume 2.6 mcg/day of vitamin $B_{12}$.
**Pediatric patients.** Safety and efficacy of vitamin $B_{12}$ for use in children haven't been established. Intake for children should be 0.5 to 2 mcg daily, as recommended by the Food and Nutrition Board of the National Academy of Sciences-National Research Council.
   Some of these products contain benzyl alcohol, which has caused a fatal "gasping syndrome" in premature infants.

### Patient counseling
- Emphasize importance of a well-balanced diet. To prevent progression of subacute combined degeneration, don't use folic acid instead of vitamin $B_{12}$ to prevent anemia.
- Instruct patient to report infection or disease in case his condition requires increased dosage of vitamin $B_{12}$.
- Tell patient with pernicious anemia that he must have lifelong treatment with vitamin $B_{12}$ to prevent recurring symptoms and the risk of incapacitating and irreversible spinal cord damage.
- Instruct patient to store tablets in a tightly closed container at controlled room temperature.

## cyclobenzaprine hydrochloride
Flexeril

*Pharmacologic classification:* tricyclic antidepressant derivative
*Therapeutic classification:* skeletal muscle relaxant
*Pregnancy risk category B*

### Available forms
Available by prescription only
*Tablets:* 10 mg

### Indications and dosages
*Adjunct in acute, painful musculoskeletal conditions*
*Adults:* 20 to 40 mg P.O. divided b.i.d. to q.i.d.; maximum dose, 60 mg daily. Drug shouldn't be given for longer than 3 weeks.
◊ *Fibrositis*
*Adults:* 10 to 40 mg P.O. daily.

### Mechanism of action
*Skeletal muscle relaxant action:* Cyclobenzaprine relaxes skeletal muscles through an unknown mechanism of action. Cyclobenzaprine is a CNS depressant.
   Drug also potentiates the effects of norepinephrine and exhibits anticholinergic effects similar to those of tricyclic antidepressants, in-

cluding central and peripheral antimuscarinic actions, sedation, and an increase in heart rate.

## Pharmacokinetics

*Absorption:* Almost completely absorbed during first pass through GI tract.

*Distribution:* About 93% is plasma protein–bound.

*Metabolism:* During first pass through GI tract and liver, drug and metabolites undergo enterohepatic recycling. The half-life of cyclobenzaprine is 1 to 3 days.

*Excretion:* Excreted primarily in urine as conjugated metabolites; also in feces via bile as unchanged drug.

| Route | Onset | Peak | Duration |
|-------|-------|------|----------|
| P.O. | 1 hr | 3-8 hr | 12-24 hr |

## Contraindications and precautions

Contraindicated in patients who have received MAO inhibitors within 14 days; during acute recovery phase of MI; and in patients with hyperthyroidism, hypersensitivity to drug, heart block, arrhythmias, conduction disturbances, or heart failure. Use cautiously in geriatric or debilitated patients and in those with increased intraocular pressure, glaucoma, or urine retention.

## Interactions

**Drug-drug.** *Antidyskinetics, antimuscarinics:* Antimuscarinic effects may be potentiated when used together. Use together cautiously.

*CNS depressants:* May potentiate the CNS depression. Avoid use together.

*Guanadrel, guanethidine:* Cyclobenzaprine may decrease or block the antihypertensive effects. Avoid use together.

*MAO inhibitors:* Hyperpyretic crisis, seizures, and death have occurred with concomitant use of MAO inhibitors and tricyclics; the potential for this interaction with cyclobenzaprine also exists. Allow 14 days to elapse after stopping MAO inhibitor therapy before starting cyclobenzaprine, and allow 5 to 7 days after stopping cyclobenzaprine therapy and starting MAO inhibitor.

**Drug-lifestyle.** *Alcohol use:* May potentiate CNS depressant effects when used together. Advise patient to avoid alcohol.

## Adverse reactions

**CNS:** *drowsiness,* headache, insomnia, fatigue, asthenia, nervousness, confusion, paresthesia, *dizziness,* depression, *seizures.*

**CV:** tachycardia, syncope, *arrhythmias,* palpitations, hypotension, vasodilation.

**EENT:** blurred vision, visual disturbances.

**GI:** dyspepsia, abnormal taste, constipation, nausea, *dry mouth.*

**GU:** urine retention, urinary frequency.

**Skin:** rash, urticaria, pruritus.

**Other:** with high doses, watch for adverse reactions similar to those of other tricyclic antidepressants.

## Overdose and treatment

Signs and symptoms of overdose include severe drowsiness, troubled breathing, syncope, seizures, tachycardia, arrhythmias, hallucinations, increase or decrease in body temperature, and vomiting.

To treat overdose, advise clinician to induce emesis or perform gastric lavage. Recommend giving 20 to 30 g activated charcoal every 4 to 6 hours for 24 to 48 hours p.r.n. Recommend taking ECG and monitoring cardiac functions for arrhythmias. Advise clinician to monitor vital signs, especially body temperature and ECG. Adequate airway and fluid intake should be maintained. If needed, 1 to 3 mg I.V. physostigmine may be given to combat severe life-threatening antimuscarinic effects. Supportive therapy for arrhythmias, cardiac failure, circulatory shock, seizures, and metabolic acidosis should be provided p.r.n.

## Clinical considerations

■ Drug may cause effects and adverse reactions similar to those of other tricyclic antidepressants.

■ The antimuscarinic effect of the drug may inhibit salivary flow, causing development of dental caries, periodontal disease, oral candidiasis, and mouth discomfort.

■ Drug is intended for short-term (2 or 3 weeks) treatment, because risk-benefit ratio with prolonged use isn't known. Additionally, muscle spasm accompanying acute musculoskeletal conditions is usually transient.

■ Spasmolytic effect usually begins within 1 or 2 days and may be manifested by lessening of pain and tenderness and an increase in range of motion and ability to perform activities of daily living.

### Therapeutic monitoring

■ Advise clinician to monitor patient for GI problems.

■ Clinician should be alert for nausea, headache, and malaise, which may occur if drug is stopped abruptly after long-term therapy.

### Special populations

**Pediatric patients.** Drug isn't recommended for children under age 15.

**Geriatric patients.** Geriatric patients are more sensitive to the effects of the drug.

## Patient counseling

■ Warn patient about possible drowsiness and dizziness. Tell him to avoid hazardous activities that require alertness until reaction to drug is known.

■ Advise patient to relieve dry mouth (anticholinergic effect) with frequent clear water

rinses, extra fluid intake, or with sugarless gum or candy.
- Tell patient to report discomfort immediately.
- Advise patient to use cough and cold preparations cautiously because some products contain alcohol.
- Instruct patient to check with dentist to minimize risk of dental disease (tooth decay, fungal infections, or gum disease) if treatment lasts longer than 2 weeks.

# cyclopentolate hydrochloride

AK-Pentolate, Cyclogyl, Minims Cyclopentolate*, Pentolair

*Pharmacologic classification:* anticholinergic
*Therapeutic classification:* cycloplegic, mydriatic
*Pregnancy risk category C*

## Available forms

Available by prescription only
*Ophthalmic solution:* 0.5%, 1%, 2%

## Indications and dosages

*Diagnostic procedures requiring mydriasis and cycloplegia*
*Adults:* Instill one drop of 1% solution in eye, followed by another drop in 5 minutes, 40 to 50 minutes before procedure. Use 2% solution in heavily pigmented irises.
*Children:* Instill one drop of 0.5%, 1%, or 2% solution in each eye, followed by one drop of 0.5% or 1% solution in 5 minutes, if needed, 40 to 50 minutes before procedure.

## Mechanism of action

*Cycloplegic and mydriatic action:* Anticholinergic action prevents the sphincter muscle of the iris and the muscle of the ciliary body from responding to cholinergic stimulation. This results in unopposed adrenergic influence, producing pupillary dilation (mydriasis) and paralysis of accommodation (cycloplegia).

## Pharmacokinetics

*Absorption:* Rapid onset of action and shorter duration of action than atropine or homatropine.
*Distribution:* Unknown.
*Metabolism:* Unknown.
*Excretion:* Recovery from mydriasis usually occurs in about 24 hours; recovery from cycloplegia may occur in 6 to 24 hours.

| Route | Onset | Peak | Duration |
|-------|-------|------|----------|
| Ophthalmic | Rapid | ¼-1¼ hr | 6-24 hr |

## Contraindications and precautions

Contraindicated in patients with glaucoma, hypersensitivity to drug or belladonna alkaloids, or adhesions between the iris and lens. Use cautiously in children, geriatric patients, and in patients with increased intraocular pressure.

## Interactions

**Drug-drug.** *Carbachol, cholinesterase inhibitors, pilocarpine:* Cyclopentolate may interfere with the antiglaucoma action of these drugs. Avoid use together.
**Drug-lifestyle.** *Sun exposure:* Photophobia may occur. Advise patient to use sunblock.

## Adverse reactions

**CNS:** irritability, confusion, somnolence, hallucinations, ataxia, *seizures,* behavioral disturbances in children.
**CV:** tachycardia.
**EENT:** eye burning on instillation, blurred vision, eye dryness, *photophobia,* ocular congestion, contact dermatitis in eye, conjunctivitis, increased intraocular pressure, transient stinging and burning, irritation, hyperemia.
**GU:** urine retention.
**Skin:** dryness.

## Overdose and treatment

Signs and symptoms of overdose include flushing, warm dry skin, dry mouth, dilated pupils, delirium, hallucinations, tachycardia, bladder distention, ataxia, hypotension, respiratory depression, coma, and death. Advise clinician to induce emesis or give activated charcoal. Recommend using physostigmine to antagonize cyclopentolate's anticholinergic activity, and in severe toxicity; propranolol may be used to treat symptomatic tachyarrhythmias unresponsive to physostigmine.

## Clinical considerations

- Superior to homatropine hydrobromide, cyclopentolate has a shorter duration of action.
- Recovery usually occurs within 24 hours; however, 1 to 2 drops of a 1% or 2% pilocarpine solution instilled into the eye may reduce recovery time to 3 to 6 hours.
- To minimize systemic absorption, prescriber should apply light finger-pressure to lacrimal sac during and for 1 to 2 minutes following topical instillation especially in children and when the 2% solution is used.

### Therapeutic monitoring

- Patient's CNS status should be assessed.

### Special populations

**Breast-feeding patients.** No data are available; however, use drug with extreme caution in breast-feeding women because of potential for CNS and cardiopulmonary effects in infants.

---

**Pediatric patients.** Avoid getting preparation in child's mouth while administering. Infants and young children may experience an increased sensitivity to the cardiopulmonary and CNS effects of drug. Young infants shouldn't be given a solution more concentrated than 0.5%.

**Geriatric patients.** Use drug with caution in geriatric patients because undiagnosed angle-closure glaucoma may be present.

### Patient counseling
■ Warn patient that drug will cause burning sensation when instilled.
■ Advise patient to protect eyes from bright illumination; dark glasses may reduce sensitivity.
■ Teach patient to instill drug. Warn him not to touch tip of dropper to eye or surrounding tissue.

# cyclophosphamide
Cytoxan, Neosar

*Pharmacologic classification:* alkylating drug (cell cycle–phase nonspecific)
*Therapeutic classification:* antineoplastic
*Pregnancy risk category D*

### Available forms
Available by prescription only
*Tablets:* 25 mg, 50 mg
*Injection:* 100-mg, 200-mg, 500-mg, 1-g, 2-g vials

### Indications and dosages
Dosage and indications may vary. Check literature for recommended protocols.
*Breast, head, neck, lung, and ovarian carcinoma; Hodgkin's disease; chronic lymphocytic or myelocytic and acute lymphoblastic leukemia; neuroblastoma; retinoblastoma; malignant lymphomas; multiple myeloma; mycosis fungoides; sarcomas; severe rheumatoid disorders; glomerular and nephrotic syndrome (in children); immunosuppression after transplants*
*Adults:* 40 to 50 mg/kg I.V. in divided doses over 2 to 5 days. Oral dosing for initial and maintenance dosage is 1 to 5 mg/kg P.O. daily.
◇ *Polymyositis*
*Adults:* 1 to 2 mg/kg P.O. daily.
◇ *Rheumatoid arthritis*
*Adults:* 1.5 to 3 mg/kg P.O. daily.
◇ *Wegener's granulomatosis*
*Adults:* 1 to 2 mg/kg P.O. daily (usually given with prednisone).
◇ *Nephrotic syndrome in children*
*Children:* 2.5 to 3 mg/kg P.O. daily for 60 to 90 days.

≡ *Dosage adjustment.* For patients with renal impairment, adjust dosage of cyclophosphamide.

### I.V. administration
■ Follow institutional guidelines for safe preparation, administration, and disposal of chemotherapeutic drugs.
■ Reconstitute vials with appropriate volume of bacteriostatic or sterile water for injection to give a level of 20 mg/ml.
■ Drug can be given by direct I.V. push into a running I.V. line or by infusion in normal saline solution or $D_5W$.
■ Reconstituted solution is stable for 6 days if refrigerated or 24 hours at controlled room temperature.

*Incompatibilities*
None reported.

### Mechanism of action
*Antineoplastic action:* Cytotoxic action of cyclophosphamide is mediated by its two active metabolites. These metabolites function as alkylating agents, preventing cell division by cross-linking DNA strands. This results in an imbalance of growth within the cell, leading to cell death. Cyclophosphamide also has significant immunosuppressive activity.

### Pharmacokinetics
*Absorption:* Almost completely absorbed from the GI tract at doses of 100 mg or less. Higher doses (300 mg) are about 75% absorbed.
*Distribution:* Distributed throughout the body, although only minimal amounts have been found in saliva, sweat, and synovial fluid. The level in the CSF is too low for treatment of meningeal leukemia. The active metabolites are about 50% plasma protein–bound.
*Metabolism:* Metabolized to its active form by hepatic microsomal enzymes. The activity of these metabolites is terminated by metabolism to inactive forms.
*Excretion:* Eliminated primarily in urine, with 15% to 30% excreted as unchanged drug. The elimination half-life ranges from 3 to 12 hours.

| Route | Onset | Peak | Duration |
|---|---|---|---|
| P.O., I.V. | Unknown | Unknown | Unknown |

### Contraindications and precautions
Contraindicated in patients hypersensitive to drug or with severe bone marrow suppression. Use cautiously in patients with impaired renal or hepatic function, leukopenia, thrombocytopenia, or malignant cell infiltration of bone marrow and in those who have recently undergone radiation therapy or chemotherapy.

### Interactions
**Drug-drug.** *Allopurinol, chloramphenicol, chloroquine, imipramine, phenothiazines,*

*potassium iodide, vitamin A:* May inhibit cyclophosphamide metabolism. Advise clinician to monitor patient closely.

*Barbiturates, chloral hydrate, phenytoin:* Increase rate of cyclophosphamide metabolism. Use cautiously.

*Corticosteroids:* Inhibit cyclophosphamide metabolism, reducing its effect. Eventual reduction of dose or discontinuation of steroids may increase cyclophosphamide metabolism to a toxic level. Use with extreme caution.

*Doxorubicin:* Use of cyclophosphamide may potentiate the cardiotoxic effects. Avoid use together.

*Succinylcholine:* Prolonged respiratory distress and apnea. Use succinylcholine with caution or not at all.

## Adverse reactions

**CV:** *cardiotoxicity* (with very high doses and with doxorubicin).
**GI:** anorexia, *nausea, vomiting* (within 6 hours); abdominal pain; stomatitis; mucositis.
**GU:** HEMORRHAGIC CYSTITIS, fertility impairment.
**Hematologic:** *leukopenia,* nadir between days 8 to 15, recovery in 17 to 28 days; *thrombocytopenia; anemia.*
**Hepatic:** *hepatotoxicity.*
**Respiratory:** *pulmonary fibrosis* (with high doses).
**Skin:** *reversible alopecia.*
**Other:** *secondary malignant disease, anaphylaxis,* hypersensitivity reactions; increased serum uric acid levels and decreased serum pseudocholinesterase levels.

## Overdose and treatment

Signs and symptoms of overdose include myelosuppression, alopecia, nausea, vomiting, and anorexia. Treatment is generally supportive and includes transfusion of blood components and antiemetics. Drug is dialyzable.

## Clinical considerations

■ Don't give I.M. injections when platelet count is less than 50,000 mm³.
■ Oral medication should be taken with or after a meal. Higher oral doses (400 mg) may be tolerated better if divided into smaller doses.
■ Administration with cold foods such as ice cream may improve toleration of oral dose.
■ Push fluid (3 L daily) to prevent hemorrhagic cystitis. Some clinicians use uroprotectant agents such as mesna. Drug shouldn't be given at bedtime, because voiding afterward is too infrequent to avoid cystitis. If hemorrhagic cystitis occurs, discontinue drug. Cystitis can occur months after therapy has been discontinued.
■ Reduced drug dosage is warranted if patient is also receiving corticosteroid therapy and develops viral or bacterial infections.

■ Used off-label for treatment of endometrial cancer and Wilms' tumor.
■ Advise clinician to monitor patient for cyclophosphamide toxicity if patient's corticosteroid therapy is discontinued.
■ Nausea and vomiting are most common with high doses of I.V. cyclophosphamide.
■ Drug has been used successfully to treat many nonmalignant conditions, for example, multiple sclerosis, because of its immunosuppressive activity.
■ Drug may suppress positive reaction to *Candida,* mumps, trichophytin, and tuberculin TB skin tests. A false-positive result for the Papanicolaou test may occur.

### Therapeutic monitoring

■ Advise clinician to monitor uric acid, CBC, and renal and hepatic functions.
■ Advise clinician to observe patient for hematuria and dysuria.

### Special populations

**Pregnant patients.** Advise both men and women to use contraception while taking drug and for 4 months after because drug has teratogenic properties.

**Breast-feeding patients.** Drug appears in breast milk; therefore, discontinue breast-feeding because of risk of serious adverse reactions, mutagenicity, and carcinogenicity in the infant.

### Patient counseling

■ Emphasize importance of continuing drug despite nausea and vomiting.
■ Advise patient to report vomiting that occurs shortly after an oral dose.
■ Warn patient that alopecia is likely to occur, but that it's reversible.
■ Encourage adequate fluid intake to prevent hemorrhagic cystitis and to facilitate uric acid excretion.
■ Tell patient to promptly report unusual bleeding or bruising.
■ Advise patient to avoid individuals with infections and to call prescriber immediately if fever, chills, or signs of infection occur.

# cycloserine

Seromycin

*Pharmacologic classification:* isoxizolidone, d-alanine analogue
*Therapeutic classification:* antituberculotic
*Pregnancy risk category C*

## Available forms

Available by prescription only
*Capsules:* 250 mg

## Indications and dosages

*Adjunctive treatment in pulmonary or extrapulmonary tuberculosis*

*Adults:* Initially, 250 mg P.O. q 12 hours for 2 weeks; then, if blood levels are below 25 to 30 mcg/ml and there are no signs of toxicity, dosage is increased to 250 mg P.O. q 8 hours for 2 weeks. If optimum blood levels are still not achieved, and there are no signs of clinical toxicity, then dosage is increased to 250 mg P.O. q 6 hours. Maximum dose is 1 g/day. If CNS toxicity occurs, drug is discontinued for 1 week, then resumed at 250 mg/day for 2 weeks. If no serious toxic effects occur, dosage is increased by 250-mg increments q 10 days until blood levels reach 25 to 30 mcg/ml.
◊ *Children:* 10 to 20 mg/kg (maximum, 750 to 1,000 mg) P.O. daily administered in two equally divided doses.

*Urinary tract infections*

*Adults:* 250 mg P.O. q 12 hours for 2 weeks.

## Mechanism of action

*Antibiotic action:* Cycloserine inhibits bacterial cell utilization of amino acids, thereby inhibiting cell-wall synthesis. Its action is bacteriostatic or bactericidal, depending on organism susceptibility and drug level at infection site. Cycloserine is active against *Mycobacterium tuberculosis, M. bovis,* and some strains of *M. kansasii, M. marinum, M. ulcerans, M. avium, M. smegmatis,* and *M. intracellulare.* It's also active against some gramnegative and gram-positive bacteria, including *Staphylococcus aureus, Enterobacter,* and *Escherichia coli.* Cycloserine is considered adjunctive therapy in tuberculosis and is combined with other antitubercular agents to prevent or delay development of drug resistance by *M. tuberculosis.*

## Pharmacokinetics

*Absorption:* About 80% of oral dose is absorbed from the GI tract.
*Distribution:* Distributed widely into body tissues and fluids, including CSF. Drug crosses the placenta; it isn't plasma protein–bound.
*Metabolism:* May be metabolized partially.
*Excretion:* Excreted primarily in urine by glomerular filtration. Small amounts of drug are excreted in feces and appear in breast milk. Elimination plasma half-life in adults is 10 hours. Drug is hemodialyzable.

| Route | Onset | Peak | Duration |
|-------|-------|------|----------|
| P.O. | Unknown | 4-8 hr | Unknown |

## Contraindications and precautions

Contraindicated in patients hypersensitive to drug and in those with seizure disorders, depression or severe anxiety, psychosis, severe renal insufficiency, or excessive concurrent use of alcohol. Use cautiously in patients with impaired renal function.

## Interactions

**Drug-drug.** *Ethionamide, isoniazid:* Increase hazard of CNS toxicity, drowsiness, and dizziness. Use with extreme caution.
*Phenytoin:* Cycloserine may inhibit metabolism of phenytoin, producing toxic blood levels. Dosage adjustment may be required.
**Drug-lifestyle.** *Alcohol use:* May increase risk of seizures. Advise patient to avoid alcohol.

## Adverse reactions

**CNS:** *seizures,* drowsiness, somnolence, headache, tremor, dysarthria, vertigo, confusion, loss of memory, *suicidal tendencies,* psychosis, hyperirritability, character changes, aggression, paresthesia, paresis, hyperreflexia, *coma.*
**CV:** *sudden-onset HF.*
**Hepatic:** elevated transaminase level.
**Skin:** allergic dermatitis, skin rash.

## Overdose and treatment

Signs and symptoms of overdose include CNS depression with dizziness, hyperreflexia, confusion, or seizures.

Advise clinician to treat with gastric lavage and supportive care, including oxygen, I.V. fluids, pressor agents (for circulatory shock), and body temperature stabilization. Recommend treating seizures with anticonvulsants and pyridoxine.

## Clinical considerations

■ Drug should be taken after meals to avoid gastric irritation.
■ Advise clinician to take specimens for culture and perform sensitivity testing before first dose. Therapy can begin pending test results; advise clinician to repeat periodically to detect drug resistance.
■ Pyridoxine (200 to 300 mg daily) may be used to treat or prevent neurotoxic effects.
■ Anticonvulsants, tranquilizers, or sedatives may be prescribed to relieve adverse reactions.

### Therapeutic monitoring

■ Advise clinician to monitor hematologic, renal, and liver function test results before and periodically during therapy to minimize toxicity; toxic reactions may occur at blood levels in excess of 30 mcg/ml.
■ Advise clinician to assess level of consciousness and neurologic function and monitor patient for personality changes and other early signs of CNS toxicity.

### Special populations

**Breast-feeding patients.** Drug appears in breast milk; use cautiously in breast-feeding women.
**Geriatric patients.** Because geriatric patients commonly have renal impairment, which decreases excretion of drugs, use drug with caution.

## Patient counseling

- Explain reason for long-term therapy.
- Teach signs and symptoms of hypersensitivity and other adverse reactions, and emphasize the need to report any unusual effects and rash promptly.
- Warn patient to avoid hazardous tasks that require mental alertness because drug may cause patient to become drowsy or dizzy.
- Advise patient to take drug after meals to avoid gastric irritation.
- Urge patient to complete entire prescribed regimen, to comply with instructions for around-the-clock dosage, and not to stop drug without medical approval.
- Explain importance of follow-up appointments.

---

# cyclosporine

Gengraf, Neoral, Sandimmune

*Pharmacologic classification:* polypeptide antibiotic
*Therapeutic classification:* immunosuppressant
*Pregnancy risk category C*

## Available forms

Available by prescription only
*Capsules:* 25 mg, 50 mg, 100 mg
*Oral solution:* 100 mg/ml
*Emulsion solution:* 100 mg
*Injection:* 50 mg/ml
*Capsules for microemulsion:* 25 mg, 100 mg

## Indications and dosages

*Prophylaxis of organ rejection in kidney, liver, heart, bone marrow, ◊pancreas, ◊cornea transplants*
*Adults and children:* 15 mg/kg P.O. daily 4 to 12 hours before transplantation. Continue daily dose postoperatively for 1 to 2 weeks. Then, gradually reduce dosage by 5% weekly to maintenance level of 5 to 10 mg/kg/day. Alternatively, recommend giving an I.V. concentrate of 5 to 6 mg/kg 4 to 12 hours before transplantation.

Postoperatively, recommend giving 5 to 6 mg/kg daily as an I.V. dilute solution infusion (50 mg per 20 to 100 ml infused over 2 to 6 hours) until patient can tolerate oral forms.

Note: Sandimmune and Neoral aren't bioequivalent and can't be used interchangeably without prescriber supervision. When converting to Neoral from Sandimmune, start with same daily dose (1:1) and follow serum trough levels frequently. Gengraf is bioequivalent to and interchangeable with Neoral capsules.
*Treatment of severe, active rheumatoid arthritis that hasn't adequately responded to methotrexate*
*Adults and children ages 18 and older:* 2.5 mg/kg/day taken b.i.d. Dosage may be increased by 0.5 to 0.75 mg/kg/day after 8 weeks and again after 12 weeks to a maximum of 4 mg/kg/day.
*Nonimmunocompromised patients with severe, recalcitrant plaque psoriasis who have failed to respond to at least one systemic therapy; patients for whom other systemic therapies are contraindicated or can't be tolerated*
*Adults and children ages 18 and older:* 2.5 mg/kg/day given b.i.d for at least 4 weeks. If no improvement, increase dosage at 2-week intervals by 0.5 mg/kg/day to a maximum of 4 mg/kg/day.

## I.V. administration

- Administer cyclosporine I.V. concentrate at ⅓ oral dose. Dilute each ml of concentrate in 20 to 100 ml of $D_5W$ or normal saline solution for injection.
- Dilute immediately before use; infuse over 2 to 6 hours. I.V. administration is usually reserved for patients who can't tolerate oral drugs.
- Protect I.V. solution from light.

## Incompatibilities

Incompatible with amphotericin B cholesteryl sulfate complex.

## Mechanism of action

*Immunosuppressant action:* Exact mechanism unknown; its action may be related to the inhibition of induction of interleukin-2, which plays a role in both cellular and humoral immune responses.

## Pharmacokinetics

*Absorption:* Absorption after oral administration varies widely between patients and in the same individual. Only 30% of an oral dose reaches systemic circulation. Neoral has a greater bioavailability than Sandimmune.
*Distribution:* Distributed widely outside the blood volume. About 33% to 47% is found in plasma; 4% to 9%, in leukocytes; 5% to 12%, in granulocytes; and 41% to 58%, in erythrocytes. In plasma, about 90% is bound to proteins, primarily lipoproteins. Cyclosporine crosses the placenta; cord blood levels are about 60% those of maternal blood. Cyclosporine appears in breast milk.
*Metabolism:* Metabolized extensively in the liver.
*Excretion:* Primarily excreted in the feces (biliary excretion) with only 6% of drug found in urine.

| Route | Onset | Peak | Duration |
|-------|-------|------|----------|
| P.O. | Unknown | 3½ hr | Unknown |
| P.O. (Gengraf) | Unknown | 1½-2 hr | Unknown |
| I.V. | Unknown | Unknown | Unknown |

## Contraindications and precautions

Contraindicated in patients hypersensitive to drug or to polyoxyethylated castor oil (found in injectable form). Also contraindicated in patients with rheumatoid arthritis or psoriasis with abnormal renal function, uncontrolled hypertension, or malignancies. Psoriasis patients shouldn't receive PUVA or UVB therapy, methotrexate, other immunosuppressants, coal tar, or radiation.

## Interactions

**Drug-drug.** *Aminoglycosides, amphotericin B:* Increase nephrotoxicity and amphotericin B may increase cyclosporine blood levels. Avoid use together.

*Co-trimoxazole phenobarbital, phenytoin, rifampin:* Lower plasma levels of cyclosporine. Advise clinician to monitor patient closely.

*Diltiazem, erythromycin, fluconazole, itraconazole, ketoconazole, verapamil, possibly corticosteroids:* Increase plasma cyclosporine levels. Reduced dosage of cyclosporine may be needed.

*Immunosuppressants (except corticosteroids):* Increased risk of malignancy (lymphoma) and susceptibility to infection. Avoid use together.

**Drug-herb.** *Alfalfa sprouts, atragulus, echinacea, licorice:* Possible interference with immunosuppressive effect of the drug. Discourage use together.

*Pill-bearing spurge:* May inhibit CYPSA enzyme affecting drug metabolism. Discourage use together.

*St. John's wort:* May reduce cyclosporine levels, resulting in decrease in efficacy. Discourage use together.

**Drug-food.** *Grapefruit juice:* Can increase trough concentrations. Discourage use together.

## Adverse reactions

**CNS:** *tremor, headache, **seizures,*** confusion, paresthesia.

**CV:** hypertension.

**EENT:** *gum hyperplasia,* oral candidiasis, sinusitis.

**GI:** *nausea, vomiting,* diarrhea, abdominal discomfort.

**GU:** *nephrotoxicity.*

**Hematologic:** anemia, ***leukopenia, thrombocytopenia,*** hemolytic anemia.

**Hepatic:** *hepatotoxicity.*

**Metabolic:** increased low-density lipoprotein levels.

**Skin:** acne, flushing, hirsutism.

**Other:** *infections, **anaphylaxis,*** gynecomastia.

## Overdose and treatment

Signs and symptoms of overdose include extensions of common adverse effects. Hepatotoxicity and nephrotoxicity often accompany nausea and vomiting; tremor and seizures may occur. Up to 2 hours after ingestion, stomach may be emptied by induced emesis or lavage; thereafter, treatment is supportive. Advise clinician to monitor vital signs and fluid and electrolyte levels closely. Drug isn't removed by hemodialysis or charcoal hemoperfusion.

## Clinical considerations

- Cyclosporine usually is prescribed with corticosteroids.
- Consider possible kidney rejection before discontinuation of drug for suspected nephrotoxicity.
- Give dose at the same time each day. Measure oral solution carefully in oral syringe and mix with plain or chocolate milk or fruit juice to increase palatability; serve in a glass to minimize drug adherence to container walls. Drug can be taken with food to minimize nausea.
- Neoral capsules and oral solution are bioequivalent. Sandimmune capsules and oral solution have decreased bioavailability compared with Neoral. Gengraf is bioequivalent to and interchangeable with Neoral capsules.
- Psoriasis patients previously treated with PUVA, methotrexate, immunosuppressants, UVB, coal tar or radiation therapy are at increased risk for developing skin malignancies when taking Gengraf.
- Warn patient to wear protection when in the sun and to avoid excessive sun exposure.
- Explain to patient the importance of frequent laboratory monitoring while receiving therapy.
- Advise patient of the potential risk during pregnancy and the increased risk of neoplasia, hypertension, and renal dysfunction.
- Warn patient that during the use of cyclosporine, vaccination may be less effective.

### Therapeutic monitoring

- Advise clinician to monitor hepatic and renal function test results routinely; hepatotoxicity may occur in first month after transplantation, but renal toxicity may be delayed for 2 to 3 months.
- For patient with rheumatoid arthritis, evaluate blood pressure and serum creatinine level every 2 weeks during initial 3 months and then monthly if patient is stable. Advise clinician to monitor blood pressure and serum creatinine level after an increase in dosage of NSAIDs or introduction of a new NSAID. Advise clinician to monitor CBCs and liver function test results monthly if patient is also receiving methotrexate. If hypertension occurs, decrease dosage of Gengraf by 25% to 50%. If hypertension persists, decrease dosage further or control blood pressure with antihypertensives.
- For patient with psoriasis, evaluate patient for occult infection and tumors initially and throughout treatment. Determine CBC and baseline serum creatinine, BUN, serum magnesium, uric acid, potassium and lipid levels. Evaluate serum creatinine and BUN levels every 2 weeks during initial 3 months and then monthly thereafter if patient is stable. If serum crea-

tinine level is greater than or equal to 25% above pretreatment, evaluate serum creatinine level within 2 weeks. If level remains greater than or equal to 25% to 50% above baseline, reduce dosage by 25% to 50%. If serum creatinine level is ever greater than or equal to 50% above baseline, reduce dosage by 25% to 50%. Discontinue drug if reversibility of serum creatine level isn't achieved after two dosage modifications. Advise clinician to monitor serum creatinine level after dosage increase of NSAID or after initiation of new NSAID.

■ Advise clinician to evaluate blood pressure, CBC, and uric acid, potassium, lipid, and magnesium levels every 2 weeks for the first 3 months, then monthly if patient is stable or more frequently when dosage adjustments are made. Dosage should be reduced by 25% to 50% for an abnormality of clinical concern.

### Special populations
**Breast-feeding patients.** Safety hasn't been established; avoid use in breast-feeding women.
**Pediatric patients.** Safety and efficacy haven't been established; however, drug has been used in children as young as age 6 months. Use with caution.

### Patient counseling
■ Teach patient reason for therapy; explain possible adverse effects and importance of reporting them, especially fever, sore throat, mouth sores, abdominal pain, unusual bleeding or bruising, pale stools, or dark urine.
■ Encourage compliance with therapy and follow-up visits.
■ Teach patient how and when to take drug for optimal benefit and minimal discomfort; caution against stopping drug without medical approval.
■ Advise patient to make oral solution more palatable by diluting with room temperature milk, chocolate milk, or orange juice. Don't use grapefruit juice or food when taking Neoral.
■ Tell patient not to rinse syringe with water.

---

# cyproheptadine hydrochloride
Periactin

*Pharmacologic classification:* piperidine-derivative antihistamine
*Therapeutic classification:* antihistamine ($H_1$-receptor antagonist), antipruritic
*Pregnancy risk category B*

### Available forms
Available by prescription only
*Tablets:* 4 mg
*Syrup:* 2 mg/5 ml

### Indications and dosages
*Allergy symptoms, pruritus, cold urticaria, allergic conjunctivitis, appetite stimulant, vascular cluster headaches*
*Adults:* 4 mg P.O. t.i.d. or q.i.d. Maximum dose, 0.5 mg/kg daily.
*Children ages 7 to 14:* 4 mg P.O. b.i.d. or t.i.d. Maximum dose, 16 mg daily.
*Children ages 2 to 6:* 2 mg P.O. b.i.d. or t.i.d. Maximum dose, 12 mg daily.
◊ *Cushing's syndrome*
*Adults:* 8 to 24 mg P.O. daily in divided doses.

### Mechanism of action
*Antihistamine action:* Antihistamines compete with histamine for $H_1$-receptor sites on smooth muscle of the bronchi, GI tract, uterus, and large blood vessels; they bind to cellular receptors, preventing access of histamine, thereby suppressing histamine-induced allergic symptoms. They don't directly alter histamine or its release.
Drug also displays significant anticholinergic and antiserotonin activity.

### Pharmacokinetics
*Absorption:* Well absorbed from the GI tract.
*Distribution:* Unknown.
*Metabolism:* Appears to be almost completely metabolized in the liver.
*Excretion:* Drug's metabolites are excreted primarily in urine; unchanged drug isn't excreted in urine. Small amounts of unchanged cyproheptadine and metabolites are excreted in feces.

| Route | Onset | Peak | Duration |
|-------|-------|------|----------|
| P.O. | 15-60 min | 6-9 hr | Unknown |

### Contraindications and precautions
Contraindicated in patients hypersensitive to drug or other drugs of similar chemical structure; in those with acute asthma, angle-closure glaucoma, stenosing peptic ulcer, symptomatic prostatic hyperplasia, bladder neck obstruction, and pyloroduodenal obstruction; in concurrent therapy with MAO inhibitors; in neonates or premature infants; in geriatric or debilitated patients; and in breast-feeding patients.
Use cautiously in patients with increased intraocular pressure, hyperthyroidism, CV disease, hypertension, or bronchial asthma.

### Interactions
**Drug-drug.** *CNS depressants:* Additive sedative effects result when cyproheptadine is used. Avoid use together.
*MAO inhibitors:* Prolong and intensify their central depressant and anticholinergic effects. Avoid use together.
*Thyrotropin-releasing hormone:* Serum amylase and prolactin levels may be increased. Advise clinician to monitor patient closely.

---

**Drug-lifestyle.** *Alcohol use:* Additive sedative effects result when cyproheptadine is used with alcohol. Discourage alcohol use.
*Sun exposure:* Photosensitivity reactions may occur. Advise patient to use sunblock.

## Adverse reactions

**CNS:** *drowsiness,* dizziness, headache, fatigue, sedation, sleepiness, incoordination, confusion, restlessness, insomnia, nervousness, tremor, *seizures,* toxic psychosis.
**CV:** hypotension, palpitations, tachycardia.
**GI:** nausea, vomiting, epigastric distress, *dry mouth,* diarrhea, constipation.
**GU:** urine retention, urinary frequency.
**Hematologic:** hemolytic anemia, *leukopenia, agranulocytosis, thrombocytopenia.*
**Metabolic:** weight gain.
**Skin:** rash, urticaria, photosensitivity.
**Other:** *anaphylactic shock.*

## Overdose and treatment

Signs and symptoms of overdose may include either CNS depression (sedation, reduced mental alertness, apnea, and CV collapse) or CNS stimulation (insomnia, hallucinations, tremors, or seizures). Anticholinergic symptoms, such as dry mouth, flushed skin, fixed and dilated pupils, and GI symptoms, are common, especially in children.

Advise clinician to treat overdose by inducing emesis with ipecac syrup (in conscious patient), followed by activated charcoal to reduce further drug absorption. Recommend using gastric lavage if patient is unconscious or ipecac fails. Recommend treating hypotension with vasopressors, and controlling seizures with diazepam or phenytoin. Stimulants shouldn't be given.

## Clinical considerations

■ Drug can cause weight gain. Advise clinician to monitor patient's weight.
■ Drug also has been used experimentally to stimulate appetite and increase weight gain in children.
■ In some patients, sedative effect disappears within 3 or 4 days.
■ Discontinue drug 4 days before diagnostic skin tests. Antihistamines can prevent, reduce, or mask positive skin test response.

### Therapeutic monitoring
■ Assess patient's CNS status.

### Special populations
**Breast-feeding patients.** Antihistamines such as cyproheptadine shouldn't be used during breast-feeding. Many of these drugs appear in breast milk, exposing the infant to risks of unusual excitability; premature infants are at particular risk for seizures.
**Pediatric patients.** CNS stimulation (agitation, confusion, tremors, hallucinations) is more common in children and may require dosage reduction. Drug isn't indicated for use in newborn or premature infants.
**Geriatric patients.** Geriatric patients are more susceptible to the sedative effect of drug. Instruct patient to change positions slowly and gradually. Geriatric patients may experience dizziness or hypotension more readily than younger patients.

## Patient counseling

■ Inform patient about potential adverse reactions.
■ Tell patient that GI distress can be reduced by taking drug with food or milk.
■ Instruct patient to report to prescriber if tolerance to drug develops, because a different antihistamine may need to be prescribed.

# cytarabine (ara-C, cytosine arabinoside)
Cytosar-U

*Pharmacologic classification:* antimetabolite (cell cycle–phase specific, S phase)
*Therapeutic classification:* antineoplastic
*Pregnancy risk category D*

## Available forms

Available by prescription only
*Injection:* 100-mg, 500-mg, 1-g, 2-g vials
*Injection:* 20 mg/ml (100 mg); 20 mg/ml pharmacy bulk package (1 g)

## Indications and dosages

Dosage and indications may vary. Check literature for recommended protocols.
*Acute myelocytic and other acute leukemias*
*Adults and children:* 200 mg/m$^2$ I.V. daily by continuous I.V. infusion for 5 days at approximately 2-week intervals for remission induction; or 30 mg/m$^2$ intrathecally (range, 5 to 75 mg/m$^2$) q 4 days until CSF findings are normal, then followed by one additional dose.
◇ Dosages up to 3 g/m$^2$ q 12 hours for up to 12 doses have been given by continuous infusion for refractory acute leukemias.

## I.V. administration

■ To reconstitute the 100-mg vial, use 5 ml bacteriostatic water for injection (20 mg/ml). For the 500-mg vial, use 10 ml bacteriostatic water for injection (50 mg/ml).
■ Drug may be further diluted with D$_5$W or normal saline solution for continuous I.V. infusion.
■ For intrathecal injection, dilute drug in 5 to 15 ml of lactated Ringer's solution, Elliot's B solution, or normal saline solution with no

preservative, and administer after withdrawing an equivalent volume of CSF.

■ Don't reconstitute drug with bacteriostatic diluent for intrathecal administration because the preservative, benzyl alcohol, has been associated with a higher risk of neurologic toxicity.

■ Reconstituted solutions are stable for 48 hours at controlled room temperature. Infusion solutions up to a level of 5 mg/ml are stable for 7 days at controlled room temperature. Discard cloudy reconstituted solution.

### Incompatibilities
Incompatible with cephalothin, flurouracil, heparin sodium, methylprednisolone sodium succinate, nafcillin, oxacillin, and penicillin.

### Mechanism of action
*Antineoplastic action:* Cytarabine requires conversion to its active metabolite within the cell. This metabolite acts as a competitive inhibitor of the enzyme DNA polymerase, disrupting the normal synthesis of DNA.

### Pharmacokinetics
*Absorption:* Poorly absorbed (less than 20%) across the GI tract because of rapid deactivation in the gut lumen. After I.M. or subcutaneous administration, peak plasma levels are less than after I.V. administration.
*Distribution:* Rapidly distributed widely through the body. About 13% is plasma protein–bound. Drug penetrates the blood-brain barrier only slightly after a rapid I.V. dose; however, when given by continuous I.V. infusion, CSF levels achieve a level 40% to 60% of that of plasma levels.
*Metabolism:* Metabolized primarily in the liver but also in the kidneys, GI mucosa, and granulocytes.
*Excretion:* Biphasic elimination of drug, with an initial half-life of 8 minutes and a terminal phase half-life of 1 to 3 hours. Cytarabine and its metabolites are excreted in urine. Less than 10% of a dose is excreted as unchanged drug in urine.

| Route | Onset | Peak | Duration |
|---|---|---|---|
| I.V., intrathecal | Unknown | Unknown | Unknown |
| S.C. | Unknown | 20-60 min | Unknown |

### Contraindications and precautions
Contraindicated in patients hypersensitive to drug. Use cautiously in patients with impaired hepatic function.

### Interactions
**Drug-drug.** *Digoxin:* Combination chemotherapy (including cytarabine) may decrease digoxin absorption even several days after stopping chemotherapy. Digoxin capsules and dig-

itoxin don't appear to be affected. Evaluate patient effect and serum digoxin levels.
*Gentamicin:* Cytarabine may antagonize the activity of gentamicin. Use cautiously.
*Methotrexate:* When used together, cytarabine decreases the cellular uptake of methotrexate, reducing its effectiveness. Avoid use together.

### Adverse reactions
**CNS:** neurotoxicity, malaise, dizziness, headache.
**CV:** edema.
**EENT:** conjunctivitis.
**GI:** *nausea; vomiting;* diarrhea; anorexia; anal ulcer; abdominal pain; oral ulcers in 5 to 10 days; high dose given rapidly I.V. may cause projectile vomiting.
**GU:** renal dysfunction.
**Hematologic:** *leukopenia,* with initial WBC count nadir 7 to 9 days after drug is stopped and a second (more severe) nadir 15 to 24 days after drug is stopped; anemia; reticulocytopenia; *thrombocytopenia,* with platelet count nadir occurring between days 12 to 15; *megaloblastosis.*
**Hepatic:** *hepatotoxicity* (usually mild and reversible), jaundice.
**Metabolic:** hyperuricemia.
**Musculoskeletal:** myalgia, bone pain.
**Skin:** rash, pruritus.
**Other:** flulike syndrome, infection, fever, thrombophlebitis, *anaphylaxis.*

### Overdose and treatment
Signs and symptoms of overdose include myelosuppression, nausea, vomiting, and megaloblastosis. Treatment is usually supportive and includes transfusion of blood components and antiemetics.

### Clinical considerations
■ Dose modification may be needed in thrombocytopenia, leukopenia, renal or hepatic disease, and after other chemotherapy or radiation therapy.

■ Excellent mouth care can help prevent adverse oral reactions.

■ Nausea and vomiting are more frequent when large doses are given rapidly by I.V. push. These reactions are less frequent with infusion. To reduce nausea, recommend giving antiemetic before administering.

■ Steroid eyedrops (dexamethasone) may be prescribed to prevent drug-induced keratitis.

■ Avoid I.M. injections of any drugs in patient with severely depressed platelet count (thrombocytopenia) to prevent bleeding.

■ Pyridoxine supplements may be given to prevent neuropathies; reportedly, however, prophylactic use of pyridoxine doesn't prevent cytarabine neurotoxicity.

---

## Therapeutic monitoring

■ Advise clinician to watch for signs and symptoms of infection (cough, fever, sore throat) and monitor CBC.

■ Advise clinician to monitor intake and output carefully. Recommend maintaining high fluid intake and giving allopurinol, if ordered, to avoid urate nephropathy in leukemia induction therapy. Advise clinician to monitor uric acid and plasma digoxin levels.

■ Advise clinician to monitor hepatic function.

■ Advise clinician to monitor patients receiving high doses for cerebellar dysfunction.

## Special populations

**Breast-feeding patients.** It isn't known if drug appears in breast milk. However, because of the risk of serious adverse reactions, mutagenicity, and carcinogenicity in the infant, breast-feeding isn't recommended.

**Pregnant patients.** Caution women of childbearing age to avoid becoming pregnant during therapy. Also, advise them to consult with prescriber before becoming pregnant. Drug may harm fetus.

## Patient counseling

■ Encourage adequate fluid intake to increase urine output and facilitate excretion of uric acid.

■ Advise patient to avoid exposure to people with infections. Tell him to call prescriber immediately if signs or symptoms of infection or unusual bleeding occurs.

# dacarbazine (DTIC)
DTIC-Dome

*Pharmacologic classification:* alkylating agent (cell cycle–phase nonspecific)
*Therapeutic classification:* antineoplastic
*Pregnancy risk category C*

## Available forms
Available by prescription only
*Injection:* 200 mg

## Indications and dosages
Dosage and indications may vary. Check current literature for recommended protocols.
**Metastatic malignant melanoma**
*Adults:* 2 to 4.5 mg/kg I.V. daily for 10 days, then repeat q 4 weeks as tolerated; or 250 mg/m² I.V. daily for 5 days, repeated at 3-week intervals.
**Hodgkin's disease**
*Adults:* 150 mg/m² I.V. (with other drugs) for 5 days, repeat q 4 weeks; or 375 mg/m² on day 1 of a combination regimen, repeated q 15 days.
≡ *Dosage adjustment.* Recommend reducing dosage when giving repeated doses to patients with severely impaired renal function. Use lower dose if renal function or bone marrow is impaired.

## I.V. administration
■ Follow all procedures for safe handling, administration, and disposal of chemotherapeutic drugs.
■ To reconstitute drug, use a volume of sterile water for injection that gives a concentration of 10 mg/ml (19.7 ml for 200-mg vial).
■ Drug may be diluted further with D₅W or normal saline solution to a volume of 100 to 200 ml for I.V. infusion over 30 minutes. Increase volume or slow the rate of infusion to decrease pain at infusion site.
■ Drug may be given by I.V. push over 1 to 2 minutes.
■ A change in solution color from ivory to pink indicates some drug degradation. During infusion, protect solution from light to avoid possible drug breakdown.

## Incompatibilities
Incompatible with cefepime, hydrocortisone sodium succinate, piperacillin, and tazobactam.

## Mechanism of action
*Antineoplastic action:* Three mechanisms have been proposed to explain the cytotoxicity of dacarbazine: alkylation, in which DNA and RNA synthesis is inhibited; antimetabolite activity as a false precursor for purine synthesis; and binding with protein sulfhydryl groups.

## Pharmacokinetics
*Absorption:* Because of poor absorption from the GI tract, dacarbazine isn't given orally.
*Distribution:* Believed to localize in body tissues, especially the liver. It crosses the blood-brain barrier to a limited extent and is minimally bound to plasma proteins.
*Metabolism:* Rapidly metabolized in the liver to several compounds, some of which may be active.
*Excretion:* Eliminated in a biphasic manner, with an initial phase half-life of 19 minutes and terminal phase of 5 hours in patients with normal renal and hepatic function. About 30% to 45% of a dose is excreted unchanged in urine.

| Route | Onset | Peak | Duration |
|-------|-------|------|----------|
| I.V. | Unknown | Unknown | Unknown |

## Contraindications and precautions
Contraindicated in patients hypersensitive to drug. Use cautiously in patients with impaired bone marrow function.

## Interactions
**Drug-drug.** *Amphotericin B:* Increased risk of nephrotoxicity. Advise clinician to monitor BUN and serum creatinine levels carefully.
*Anticoagulants, aspirin:* Increased risk of bleeding. Avoid use together.
*Bone marrow suppressants:* Additive toxicity. Advise clinician to monitor patient carefully.
*Phenobarbitol, phenytoin:* Increased risk of toxicity. Advise clinician to monitor patient carefully.
**Drug-lifestyle.** *Sun exposure:* Photosensitivity reactions may occur, especially during the first 2 days of therapy. Advise patient to take precautions.

## Adverse reactions
**CNS:** facial paresthesia.
**GI:** *severe nausea and vomiting, anorexia,* diarrhea.
**GU:** increased serum BUN.
**Hematologic:** *leukopenia, thrombocytopenia.*
**Hepatic:** transient increase in liver enzyme levels, *hepatotoxicity.*
**Skin:** phototoxicity, rash, facial flushing, alopecia, tissue damage.
**Other:** *flulike syndrome* (fever, malaise; myalgia, beginning 7 days after treatment ends and lasting possibly 7 to 21 days), *anaphylaxis;* severe pain (if I.V. solution infiltrates or if solution is too concentrated).

## Overdose and treatment
Signs and symptoms of overdose include myelosuppression and diarrhea. Treatment is supportive and includes transfusion of blood components and monitoring of hematologic parameters.

## Clinical considerations
■ Treatment of extravasation with application of hot packs may relieve burning sensation, local pain, and irritation.
■ Discard refrigerated solution after 72 hours; room temperature solution after 8 hours.
■ Nausea and vomiting may be minimized by giving dacarbazine by I.V. infusion and by hydrating patient 4 to 6 hours before therapy.

### Therapeutic monitoring
■ Advise clinician to monitor uric acid levels.
■ Drug should be stopped if the WBC count goes to 3,000/mm³ or the platelet count goes to 100,000/mm³. Advise clinician to monitor CBC.
■ Advise clinician to monitor daily temperature. Observe for signs and symptoms of infection.

### Special populations
**Pregnant patients.** Counsel patient to avoid pregnancy. Advise her to inform prescriber immediately if she suspects she's pregnant.
**Breast-feeding patients.** It isn't known if drug appears in breast milk. However, because of risk of serious adverse reactions, mutagenicity, and carcinogenicity in the infant, breast-feeding isn't recommended during therapy.

## Patient counseling
■ Instruct patient to avoid contact with people who have infections and to report signs or symptoms of infection or unusual bleeding immediately.
■ Reassure patient that growth of hair should return 4 to 8 weeks after treatment has ended, but hair is usually of a different texture and color as therapy continues.

■ Reassure patient that flulike syndrome may be treated with mild antipyretics such as acetaminophen.
■ Teach the patient the signs and symptoms of bleeding, and instruct him to report them promptly.

# dactinomycin (actinomycin D)
Cosmegen

*Pharmacologic classification:* antibiotic antineoplastic (cell cycle–phase nonspecific)
*Therapeutic classification:* antineoplastic
*Pregnancy risk category C*

## Available forms
Available by prescription only
*Injectable:* 500-mcg vial

## Indications and dosages
Dosage and indications may vary. Check current literature for recommended protocols.
*Uterine cancer, testicular cancer, Wilms' tumor, rhabdomyosarcoma, Ewing's sarcoma, sarcoma botryoides, ◇ Kaposi's sarcoma, ◇ acute organ (kidney or heart) rejection, ◇ malignant melanoma, ◇ acute lymphocytic leukemia, ◇ Paget's disease of bone*
*Adults:* 500 mcg I.V. daily for a maximum of 5 days. Maximum dose is 15 mcg/kg/day or 400 to 600 mcg/m²/day for 5 days. After bone marrow recovery, course may be repeated.
*Children:* 15 mcg/kg I.V. daily for a maximum of 5 days. Alternatively, give a total dosage of 2,500 mcg/m² I.V. over a 1-week period. Maximum dose is 15 mcg/kg/day or 400 to 600 mcg/m²/day. After bone marrow recovery, course may be repeated.
For isolation-perfusion, use 50 mcg/kg for legs or pelvis; 35 mcg/kg for arms.
Base dose on body surface area in obese or edematous patients.

## I.V. administration
■ Use gloves when preparing and administering this drug.
■ To reconstitute, add 1.1 ml of preservative-free sterile water for injection to drug to give a concentration of 0.5 mg/ml. Don't use a preserved diluent because precipitation may occur.
■ Drug may be diluted further with $D_5W$ or normal saline solution for administration by I.V. infusion.
■ Drug may be given by I.V. push injection into the tubing of a freely flowing I.V. infusion. Don't administer through an in-line I.V. filter.
■ Protect from light and excessive heat.

■ Discard unused solution because it doesn't contain preservatives.

### Incompatibilities
Incompatible with filgrastim and diluents containing preservatives because of precipitation.

### Mechanism of action
*Antineoplastic action:* Dactinomycin exerts its cytotoxic activity by intercalating between DNA base pairs and uncoiling the DNA helix. The result is inhibition of DNA synthesis and DNA-dependent RNA synthesis.

### Pharmacokinetics
*Absorption:* Because of its vesicant properties, dactinomycin must be given I.V.
*Distribution:* Widely distributed into body tissues, with highest levels found in the bone marrow and nucleated cells. Drug doesn't significantly cross the blood-brain barrier.
*Metabolism:* Only minimally metabolized in the liver.
*Excretion:* Excreted in the urine and bile. Plasma elimination half-life of drug is 36 hours.

| Route | Onset | Peak | Duration |
|---|---|---|---|
| I.V. | Unknown | Unknown | Unknown |

### Contraindications and precautions
Contraindicated in patients with chickenpox or herpes zoster.

### Interactions
**Drug-drug.** *Bone marrow suppressants:* May cause additive toxicity. Advise clinician to monitor patient closely.
*Vitamin K derivatives:* Decrease effectiveness of drug. Advise clinician to monitor patient closely.

### Adverse reactions
**CNS:** malaise, fatigue, lethargy.
**GI:** *anorexia, nausea, vomiting,* abdominal pain, diarrhea, *stomatitis,* ulceration, proctitis.
**Hematologic:** anemia, *leukopenia, thrombocytopenia, pancytopenia, aplastic anemia, agranulocytosis.*
**Hepatic:** *hepatotoxicity.*
**Metabolic:** increased blood and urine levels of uric acid, hypocalcemia.
**Musculoskeletal:** myalgia.
**Skin:** *erythema;* desquamation; *hyperpigmentation of skin, especially in previously irradiated areas; acnelike eruptions* (reversible), severe damage to soft tissue at injection site, reversible alopecia.
**Other:** phlebitis, fever.

### Overdose and treatment
Signs and symptoms of overdose include myelosuppression, nausea, vomiting, glossitis, and oral ulceration. Treatment is general-

ly supportive and includes antiemetics and transfusion of blood components.

### Clinical considerations
■ Recommend using body surface area calculation in obese or edematous patients.
■ Treatment of extravasation includes topical administration of dimethyl sulfoxide and cold compresses.
■ To reduce nausea, recommend giving an antiemetic before administering. Nausea usually occurs within 30 minutes of a dose.
■ Patients who have received other cytotoxic drugs or radiation within 6 weeks of dactinomycin may exhibit erythema, followed by hyperpigmentation or edema, or both; desquamation; vesiculation; and, rarely, necrosis.

### Therapeutic monitoring
■ Advise clinician to monitor CBC daily and platelet counts every third day. Leukocyte and platelet nadirs usually occur 14 to 21 days after completion of course of therapy. Advise clinician to observe patient for signs of bleeding.
■ Advise clinician to monitor renal and hepatic functions.

### Special populations
**Breast-feeding patients.** It isn't known if drug appears in breast milk. However, because of risks of serious adverse reactions, mutagenicity, and carcinogenicity in infants, breast-feeding isn't recommended.
**Pediatric patients.** Restrict use of drug in infants ages 6 months and older; adverse reactions are more frequent in infants under age 6 months.

### Patient counseling
■ Advise patient to avoid exposure to people with infections.
■ Warn patient that alopecia may occur but is usually reversible.
■ Tell patient to report sore throat, fever, or signs of bleeding promptly.

# dalteparin sodium
Fragmin

*Pharmacologic classification:* low-molecular-weight heparin derivative
*Therapeutic classification:* anticoagulant
*Pregnancy risk category B*

### Available forms
Available by prescription only
*Injection:* 2,500 anti-factor Xa IU/0.2 ml, 5,000 anti-factor Xa IU/0.2 ml, 95,000 anti-factor Xa IU/9.5 ml

## Indications and dosages

*Prophylaxis against deep vein thrombosis (DVT) in patients undergoing abdominal surgery who are at risk for thromboembolic complications (including those who are over age 40, obese, undergoing general anesthesia lasting longer than 30 minutes, and with history of DVT or pulmonary embolism)*

*Adults:* 2,500 IU S.C. daily, starting 1 to 2 hours before surgery and repeated once daily for 5 to 10 days postoperatively. In abdominal surgery patients at high risk for thromboembolic complications (such as those with malignant disease), 5,000 IU S.C. daily starting on the evening before surgery and repeated once daily for 5 to 10 days postoperatively. Alternatively, 2500 IU S.C. within 1 to 2 hours before surgery, followed 12 hours later by a second dose of 2,500 IU S.C., then 5,000 IU S.C. once daily for 5 to 10 days postoperatively.

*Prophylaxis against DVT in patients undergoing hip replacement surgery*

*Adults:* 2,500 IU S.C. within 2 hours before surgery and second dose 2,500 IU S.C. in the evening of surgery (at least 6 hours after first dose). If surgery is performed in the evening, omit second dose on day of surgery. Starting on first postoperative day, 5,000 IU S.C. once daily for 5 to 10 days. Alternatively, 5,000 IU S.C. on the evening before surgery, followed by 5,000 IU S.C. once daily starting in the evening of surgery for 5 to 10 days postoperatively.

## Mechanism of action

*Anticoagulant action:* Dalteparin sodium acts by enhancing the inhibition of factor Xa and thrombin by antithrombin.

## Pharmacokinetics

*Absorption:* Absolute bioavailability measured in anti-factor Xa activity is about 87%.
*Distribution:* Volume of distribution for dalteparin anti-factor Xa activity is 40 to 60 ml/kg.
*Metabolism:* Unknown.
*Excretion:* Unknown.

| Route | Onset | Peak | Duration |
|-------|-------|------|----------|
| S.C. | Unknown | 4 hr | Unknown |

## Contraindications and precautions

Contraindicated in patients hypersensitive to drug, heparin, or pork products; those with active major bleeding; or thrombocytopenia with positive in vitro tests for antiplatelet antibody in the presence of drug.

Use with extreme caution in patients with history of heparin-induced thrombocytopenia or in those with increased risk of hemorrhage, such as those with severe uncontrolled hypertension, bacterial endocarditis, congenital or acquired bleeding disorders, active ulceration and angiodysplastic GI disease, hemorrhagic CVA; or shortly after brain, spinal, or ophthalmic surgery. Use cautiously in patients with bleeding diathesis, thrombocytopenia, or platelet defects; severe liver or kidney insufficiency; hypertensive or diabetic retinopathy; and recent GI bleeding.

## Interactions

**Drug-drug.** *Oral anticoagulants, platelet inhibitors:* May increase risk of bleeding. Use together with caution.

## Adverse reactions

**Hematologic:** *thrombocytopenia, hemorrhage,* ecchymoses, bleeding complications.
**Hepatic:** elevated AST and ALT levels.
**Skin:** pruritus, rash, *hematoma,* pain or skin necrosis (at injection site).
**Other:** fever, *anaphylactoid reactions.*

## Overdose and treatment

Overdose may cause hemorrhagic complications. These may generally be stopped by the slow I.V. injection of protamine sulfate (1% solution), at a dose of 1 mg protamine for every 100 anti-factor Xa IU of dalteparin given. A second infusion of 0.5 mg protamine sulfate per 100 anti-factor Xa IU of dalteparin may be given if the aPTT measured 2 to 4 hours after the first infusion remains prolonged. Even with these additional doses of protamine sulfate, the aPTT may remain more prolonged than would usually be found following administration of conventional heparin.

## Clinical considerations

**ALERT** Dalteparin should never be given I.M.

**ALERT** Drug isn't interchangeable (unit for unit) with unfractionated heparin or other low-molecular-weight heparins.

■ Patients receiving dalteparin who require neuraxial anesthesia or spinal puncture may be at increased risk for development of an epidural or spinal hematoma, which can cause long-term or permanent paralysis.

■ Patient should assume a sitting or supine position when drug is given. Recommend injecting dalteparin S.C. deeply. Injection sites include a U-shaped area around the navel, the upper outer side of the thigh, or the upper outer quadrangle of the buttock. Recommend rotating sites daily. The thumb and forefinger should be used to lift a fold of skin while the injection is being given around the navel or thigh. Insertion of the entire length of the needle should be at a 45- to 90-degree angle.

■ Don't mix drug with other injections or infusions unless specific compatibility data are available that support such mixing.

### Therapeutic monitoring

■ Periodic routine CBC, including platelet count, and stool occult blood tests are recommended in patients receiving treatment with dalteparin. Patients don't require regular monitoring of PT, INR, or PTT.

■ Advise clinician to monitor patient closely for thrombocytopenia.

■ Drug should be stopped if a thromboembolic event occurs despite dalteparin prophylaxis.

### Special populations

**Breast-feeding patients.** It isn't known if drug appears in breast milk; use with caution in breast-feeding women.

**Pediatric patients.** Safety and effectiveness in children haven't been established.

### Patient counseling

■ Instruct patient and his family to watch for signs of bleeding and report them to his prescriber immediately.

■ Tell patient to avoid OTC drugs containing aspirin or other salicylates.

---

# danaparoid sodium

Orgaran

*Pharmacologic classification:* glycosaminoglycan
*Therapeutic classification:* antithrombotic
*Pregnancy risk category B*

### Available forms

Available by prescription only
*Ampule:* 750 anti-Xa units/0.6 ml
*Syringe:* 750 anti-Xa units/0.6 ml

### Indications and dosages

*Prophylaxis against postoperative deep vein thrombosis (DVT), which may lead to pulmonary embolism in patients undergoing elective hip replacement surgery*
*Adults:* 750 anti-Xa units S.C. b.i.d. beginning 1 to 4 hours preoperatively; then no sooner than 2 hours after surgery. Continue treatment for 7 to 10 days postoperatively or until risk of DVT has diminished (up to 14 days).

### Mechanism of action

*Antithrombotic action:* Danaparoid sodium prevents fibrin formation by inhibiting generation of thrombin by anti-Xa and anti-IIa. Because of its predominant anti-Xa activity, danaparoid injection has little effect on clotting assays such as PT, INR, and PTT. Drug has only minor effect on platelet function and platelet aggregability.

### Pharmacokinetics

Drug pharmacokinetics have been described by monitoring its biologic activity (plasma anti-Xa activity) because no specific chemical assay methods are currently available.

*Absorption:* S.C. administration is about 100% bioavailable, compared with same dose given I.V. Onset and duration are unknown.

*Distribution:* Not reported.

*Metabolism:* Not reported.

*Excretion:* Mainly eliminated through the kidneys. Mean value for the terminal half-life is about 24 hours. In patients with severely impaired renal function, elimination half-life of plasma anti-Xa activity may be prolonged.

| Route | Onset | Peak | Duration |
|-------|-------|------|----------|
| S.C. | Unknown | 2-5 hr | Unknown |

### Contraindications and precautions

Contraindicated in patients hypersensitive to drug or to pork products, or patients with severe hemorrhagic diathesis (such as hemophilia or idiopathic thrombocytopenic purpura), active major bleeding (including hemorrhagic CVA in the acute phase), or type II thrombocytopenia with positive in vitro tests for antiplatelet antibody in the presence of the drug.

Use with extreme caution in patients at increased risk of hemorrhage, such as in severe uncontrolled hypertension, acute bacterial endocarditis, congenital or acquired bleeding disorders, active ulcerative and angiodysplastic GI disease, nonhemorrhagic CVA, or postoperative use of indwelling epidural catheter; or shortly after brain, spinal, or ophthalmic surgery.

Use cautiously in patients with impaired renal function and in those receiving oral anticoagulants or platelet inhibitors.

### Interactions

**Drug-drug.** *Oral anticoagulants, platelet inhibitors:* May increase the risk of bleeding; use together cautiously.

### Adverse reactions

**CNS:** insomnia, headache, asthenia, dizziness.
**CV:** peripheral edema, *hemorrhage.*
**GI:** *nausea, constipation,* vomiting.
**GU:** urinary tract infection, urine retention.
**Hematologic:** anemia.
**Musculoskeletal:** joint disorder, pain.
**Skin:** rash, pruritus.
**Other:** *fever,* pain at injection site, infection.

### Overdose and treatment

Overdose of danaparoid injection may lead to bleeding complications. The effects of danaparoid on anti-Xa activity can't be currently antagonized with other known drugs. Although protamine sulfate partially neutralizes the anti-Xa activity of danaparoid and can be safely coadministered, there's no evidence that protamine sulfate is capable of reducing severe nonsurgical bleeding during treatment with

---

danaparoid. If serious bleeding occurs, stop drug and give blood or blood products, p.r.n.

Symptoms of acute toxicity after I.V. dosing are respiratory depression, prostration, and twitching.

## Clinical considerations

**ℍ *ALERT*** Drug isn't interchangeable (unit for unit) with heparin or low-molecular-weight heparin.

**ℍ *ALERT*** Don't give drug I.M.

■ Drug contains sodium sulfite, which may cause allergic-type reactions, including anaphylactic symptoms and life-threatening or less severe asthmatic episodes in certain patients. The overall prevalence of sulfite allergy in the general population is unknown and probably low. Sulfite sensitivity is seen more frequently in asthmatic than in nonasthmatic patients.

■ Risks and benefits of danaparoid injection should be carefully considered before use in patients with severely impaired renal function or hemorrhagic disorders.

■ To administer drug, have patient lie down. Recommend giving S.C. injection deeply, using a 25G to 26G needle. Injection sites should be alternated between the left and right anterolateral and posterolateral abdominal wall. Recommend gently pulling up a skin fold with thumb and forefinger and inserting entire length of the needle into tissue. Advise clinician not to rub or pinch afterward.

■ Monitoring of anticoagulant activity of oral anticoagulants by PT and Thrombotest is unreliable within 5 hours after danaparoid administration.

### Therapeutic monitoring

■ Periodic, routine CBCs (including platelet count) and fecal occult blood tests are recommended during therapy. Patients don't require regular monitoring of PT, INR, or PTT.

■ Drug has little effect on PT, INR, PTT, fibrinolytic activity, and bleeding time.

■ Advise clinician to monitor patient's hematocrit and blood pressure closely; a decrease in either may signal hemorrhage. If serious bleeding occurs, advise clinician to stop drug and transfuse blood products, if needed.

### Special populations

**Breast-feeding patients.** It isn't known if drug appears in breast milk; use cautiously in breast-feeding women.

**Pediatric patients.** Safety and effectiveness in children haven't been established.

## Patient counseling

■ Instruct patient and family to watch for and report signs of bleeding.

■ Tell patient to avoid OTC drugs containing aspirin or other salicylates.

# dantrolene sodium
Dantrium

*Pharmacologic classification:* hydantoin derivative
*Therapeutic classification:* skeletal muscle relaxant
*Pregnancy risk category C*

## Available forms

Available by prescription only
*Capsules:* 25 mg, 50 mg, 100 mg
*Injection:* 20 mg parenteral (contains 3 g mannitol)

## Indications and dosages

*Spasticity resulting from upper motor neuron disorders*

*Adults:* 25 mg P.O. daily, increased gradually in increments of 25 mg at 4- to 7-day intervals, up to 100 mg b.i.d. to q.i.d., to maximum of 400 mg daily.

*Children over age 5:* 0.5 mg/kg P.O. b.i.d., increased to t.i.d., then q.i.d. Increase dosage further, p.r.n., by 0.5 mg/kg up to 3 mg/kg b.i.d. to q.i.d. Maximum dose is 100 mg q.i.d.

*Prevention of malignant hyperthermia in susceptible patients who require surgery*

*Adults:* 4 to 8 mg/kg/day P.O. given in three to four divided doses for 1 to 2 days before procedure; give last dose 3 to 4 hours before procedure. Alternatively, give 2.5 mg/kg I.V. over 1 hour about 75 minutes before anesthesia.

*Management of malignant hyperthermia crisis*

*Adults and children:* Initially, 1 mg/kg I.V.; then continue until symptoms subside or maximum cumulative dose of 10 mg/kg has been reached.

*Prevention of recurrence of malignant hyperthermia after crisis*

*Adults:* 4 to 8 mg/kg/day P.O. given in four divided doses for up to 3 days after crisis. Alternatively, give 1 mg/kg or more I.V. based on clinical situation.

◇ *To reduce succinylcholine-induced muscle fasciculations and postoperative muscle pain*

*Adults weighing less than 45 kg (99 lb):* 100 mg P.O. 2 hours before succinylcholine.

*Adults weighing more than 45 kg:* 150 mg P.O. 2 hours before succinylcholine.

## I.V. administration

■ In malignant hyperthermia crisis, recommend giving drug by rapid I.V. injection as soon as reaction is recognized.

■ To reconstitute, add 60 ml sterile water for injection to 20-mg vial. Don't use bacteriostatic water, $D_5W$, or normal saline for injection. Store reconstituted solution away from direct sunlight at controlled room temperature, and discard after 6 hours.

### Incompatibilities

Incompatible with D₅W or normal saline. Don't mix with other drugs in a syringe.

## Mechanism of action

*Skeletal muscle relaxant action:* A hydantoin derivative, dantrolene is chemically and pharmacologically unrelated to other skeletal muscle relaxants. It directly affects skeletal muscle, reducing muscle tension. It interferes with the release of calcium ions from the sarcoplasmic reticulum, resulting in decreased muscle contraction. This mechanism is of particular importance in malignant hyperthermia when increased myoplasmic calcium ion levels activate acute catabolism in the skeletal muscle cell. Dantrolene prevents or reduces the increase in myoplasmic calcium levels caused by malignant hyperthermia crises.

## Pharmacokinetics

*Absorption:* 35% of oral dose is absorbed through GI tract, with serum half-life reached within 8 to 9 hours after oral administration. Therapeutic effect in patients with upper motor neuron disorders may take 1 week or longer.
*Distribution:* Substantially plasma protein–bound, mainly to albumin.
*Metabolism:* Metabolized in the liver to its less active 5-hydroxy derivatives, and to its amino derivative by reductive pathways.
*Excretion:* Excreted in urine as metabolites.

| Route | Onset | Peak | Duration |
|-------|-------|------|----------|
| P.O. | Unknown | 5 hr | Unknown |
| I.V. | Unknown | Unknown | 3 hr after infusion ends |

## Contraindications and precautions

Contraindicated in patients when spasticity is used to maintain motor function, for those with upper motor neuron disorders, for spasms in rheumatic disorders, in patients with active hepatic disease, and in breast-feeding women. Contraindicated with verapamil in management of malignant hyperthermia. Use cautiously in women (especially those taking estrogen), in patients over age 35, and in patients with severely impaired cardiac or pulmonary function or preexisting hepatic disease.

## Interactions

**Drug-drug.** *CNS depressants:* Increase CNS depression. Avoid use together.
*Estrogen:* Increases risk of hepatotoxicity. Use together cautiously.
*Verapamil:* Has resulted in cardiac collapse. Don't use together.
**Drug-lifestyle.** *Alcohol use:* Increases CNS depression. Advise patient to avoid alcohol.

## Adverse reactions

**CNS:** *drowsiness, dizziness, light-headedness, malaise, fatigue, headache, confusion, nervousness, insomnia,* **seizures.**
**CV:** tachycardia, blood pressure changes.
**EENT:** excessive lacrimation, speech disturbance, diplopia, visual disturbances.
**GI:** anorexia, constipation, cramping, dysphagia, metallic taste, severe diarrhea, *GI bleeding,* altered taste.
**GU:** urinary frequency, hematuria, incontinence, nocturia, dysuria, crystalluria, difficult erection, urine retention.
**Hepatic:** altered liver function test results; *hepatitis.*
**Musculoskeletal:** myalgia, back pain, *muscle weakness.*
**Respiratory:** pleural effusion with pericarditis.
**Skin:** eczematous eruption, pruritus, urticaria, abnormal hair growth, diaphoresis.
**Other:** chills, fever.

## Overdose and treatment

Signs and symptoms of overdose include exaggeration of adverse reactions, particularly CNS depression, and nausea and vomiting.

Treatment includes supportive measures, gastric lavage, and observation of symptoms. Recommend maintaining adequate airway, having emergency ventilation equipment on hand, monitoring ECG, and giving large quantities of I.V. solutions to prevent crystalluria. Advise clinician to monitor vital signs closely. The benefit of dialysis isn't known.

## Clinical considerations

■ To prepare suspension for single oral dose, recommend dissolving contents of appropriate number of capsules in fruit juice or other suitable liquid.
■ Before therapy begins, patient's baseline neuromuscular functions—posture, gait, coordination, range of motion, muscle strength and tone, presence of abnormal muscle movements, and reflexes—should be checked and documented for later comparisons.
■ Drug may cause muscle weakness and impaired walking ability. Use with caution; patients receiving drug for prophylactic treatment should be carefully supervised for malignant hyperthermia.
■ Because of the risk of hepatic injury, drug should be stopped if improvement isn't evident within 45 days.
■ Risk of hepatotoxicity may be greater in women, patients over age 35, and in those taking other drugs (especially estrogen) or high dantrolene doses (400 mg or more daily) for prolonged periods.
■ Signs of malignant hyperthermia include skeletal muscle rigidity (often the first sign), sudden tachycardia, cardiac arrhythmias, cyanosis, tachypnea, severe hypercarbia, un-

stable blood pressure, rapidly rising temperature, acidosis, and shock.

### Therapeutic monitoring

■ Advise clinician to perform baseline and regularly scheduled liver function tests (alkaline
phosphatase, ALT, AST, and total bilirubin),
blood cell counts, and renal function tests.

### Special populations

**Breast-feeding patients.** Contraindicated for
use in breast-feeding women.
**Pediatric patients.** Drug isn't recommended
for long-term use in children under age 5.
**Geriatric patients.** Use drug with extreme caution in geriatric patients.

### Patient counseling

■ Instruct patient to report promptly the onset
of jaundice: yellow skin or sclerae, dark urine,
clay-colored stools, itching, and abdominal discomfort. Hepatotoxicity occurs more frequently between the third and twelfth month of therapy.
■ Advise patient susceptible to malignant hyperthermia to wear medical identification (e.g.,
Medic Alert) indicating diagnosis, prescriber's
name and telephone number, drug causing reaction, and treatment used.
■ Advise patient to avoid excessive or unnecessary exposure to sunlight and to use protective clothing and a sunscreen because photosensitivity reactions may occur.
■ Warn patient to avoid hazardous activities
that require alertness until CNS depressant
effects are determined. Drug may cause drowsiness.
■ Advise patient to report adverse reactions
immediately.
■ Tell patient to store drug away from heat and
direct light (not in bathroom medicine cabinet)
and to keep drug away from children.
■ If patient misses a dose, tell him to take it
within 1 hour; otherwise, he should omit the
dose and return to regular dosing schedule. Tell
him not to double the dose.

---

# dapsone

Avlosulfon*

*Pharmacologic classification:* synthetic
sulfone
*Therapeutic classification:* antileprotic,
antimalarial
*Pregnancy risk category C*

### Available forms

Available by prescription only
*Tablets:* 25 mg, 100 mg

## Indications and dosages

### Treatment of multibacillary leprosy

*Adults:* 100 mg P.O. daily plus rifampin and
clofazimine given for 12 months.
*Children ages 10 to 14:* 50 mg daily P.O. plus
rifampin and clofazimine given for 12 months.
*Children under age 10:* Give appropriately adjusted dosage plus rifampin and clofazimine
for 12 months.

### Treatment of paucibacillary leprosy

*Adults:* 100 mg P.O. daily plus rifampin given
for 6 months.
*Children ages 10 to 14:* 50 mg daily P.O. plus
rifampin given for 6 months.
*Children under age 10:* Give appropriately adjusted dosage plus rifampin for 6 months.

### Prophylaxis for leprosy patient's close contacts

*Adults and children ages 12 and older:* 50 mg
P.O. daily.
*Children ages 6 to 12:* 25 mg P.O. daily.
*Children ages 2 to 5:* 25 mg P.O. three times
weekly.
*Infants ages 6 to 23 months:* 12 mg P.O. three
times weekly.
*Infants under age 6 months:* 6 mg P.O. three
times weekly.

### Dermatitis herpetiformis

*Adults:* Initially, 50 mg P.O. daily; dose may
be increased p.r.n., to obtain full control.
**≡ Dosage adjustment.** Dapsone levels are influenced by acetylation rates. Patients with high
acetylation rates may need dosage adjustments.

### ◊ Malaria suppression or prophylaxis

*Adults:* 100 mg P.O. weekly, with pyrimethamine 12.5 mg P.O. weekly.
*Children:* 2 mg/kg P.O. weekly, with pyrimethamine 0.25 mg/kg weekly.
    Continue prophylaxis throughout exposure
and 6 months after exposure.

### ◊ Treatment of Pneumocystis carinii pneumonia

*Adults:* 100 mg P.O. daily. Usually given with
trimethoprim, 20 mg/kg daily, for 21 days.

### ◊ Prophylaxis of P. carinii pneumonia

*Adults:* 50 mg b.i.d or 100 mg daily P.O.

### ◊ Prophylaxis against toxoplasmosis in HIV-infected patients

*Adults and adolescents:* 50 mg daily with
pyrimethamine 50 mg once weekly and leucovorin 25 mg once weekly, P.O.
*Children ages 1 month and older:* 2 mg/kg or
15 mg/m² (maximum 25 mg) P.O. once daily
plus pyrimethamine and leucovorin.

## Mechanism of action

*Antibiotic action:* Drug is bacteriostatic and
bactericidal; like sulfonamides, it's thought to
act principally by inhibition of folic acid. It
acts against *Mycobacterium leprae* and *Mycobacterium tuberculosis* and has some activity against *P. carinii* and *Plasmodium.*

---

## Pharmacokinetics

*Absorption:* When given orally, drug is rapidly and almost completely absorbed.
*Distribution:* Distributed widely into most body tissues and fluids; 50% to 90% is protein-bound.
*Metabolism:* Undergoes acetylation by liver enzymes; rate varies and is genetically determined. Almost 50% of blacks and whites are slow acetylators, and more than 80% of Chinese, Japanese, and Inuits are fast acetylators.
*Excretion:* Excreted primarily in urine; small amounts of drug are excreted in feces; and substantial amounts appear in breast milk. Dapsone undergoes enterohepatic circulation; half-life in adults ranges between 10 and 50 hours (average 28 hours). Orally administered charcoal may enhance excretion. Dapsone is dialyzable.

| Route | Onset | Peak | Duration |
|-------|-------|------|----------|
| P.O. | Unknown | 4-8 hr | Unknown |

## Contraindications and precautions

Contraindicated in patients hypersensitive to drug. Use cautiously in patients with impaired renal, hepatic, or CV disease; refractory types of anemia; and G6PD deficiency.

## Interactions

**Drug-drug.** *Activated charcoal:* Decreases GI absorption of dapsone. Advise clinician to monitor patient carefully.
*Didanosine:* May produce a possible therapeutic failure of dapsone, leading to an increase in infection. Avoid use together.
*Folic acid antagonists such as methotrexate:* Increased risk of adverse hematologic reactions. Avoid use together.
*PABA:* May antagonize the effect of dapsone by interfering with the primary mechanism of action. Advise clinician to monitor patient for lack of efficacy.
*Probenecid:* Reduces urinary excretion of dapsone metabolites, increasing plasma levels. Advise clinician to monitor patient closely.
*Rifampin:* Increased hepatic metabolism of dapsone. Advise clinician to monitor patient for lack of efficacy.
*Trimethoprim:* Increased serum levels of both drugs may occur, possibly increasing the pharmacologic and toxic effects of each drug. Advise clinician to monitor patient carefully.
**Drug-lifestyle.** *Sun exposure:* Photosensitivity reactions may occur. Tell patient to take precautions.

## Adverse reactions

**CNS:** insomnia, psychosis, headache, paresthesia, peripheral neuropathy, vertigo.
**CV:** tachycardia.
**EENT:** tinnitus, blurred vision.
**GI:** anorexia, *pancreatitis,* abdominal pain, nausea, vomiting.

**GU:** albuminuria, nephrotic syndrome, renal papillary necrosis, male infertility.
**Hematologic:** hemolytic anemia, *agranulocytosis, aplastic anemia.*
**Respiratory:** *pulmonary eosinophilia.*
**Skin:** lupus erythematosus, phototoxicity, *exfoliative dermatitis, toxic erythema, erythema multiforme, toxic epidermal necrolysis, morbilliform and scarlatiniform reactions, urticaria, erythema nodosum.*
**Other:** fever, tachycardia, infectious mononucleosis-like syndrome, *sulfone syndrome (fever, malaise, jaundice [with hepatic necrosis],* exfoliative dermatitis, lymphadenopathy, methemoglobinemia, hemolytic anemia).
*Leprosy reactional states*
During therapy for leprosy, two types of reactions related to the effectiveness of dapsone therapy may occur.

Type I, reversal reaction, includes erythema, followed by swelling of skin and nerve lesions in tuberculoid patients; skin lesions may ulcerate and multiply, and acute neuritis may cause neural dysfunction. Severe cases require hospitalization, analgesics, corticosteroids, and nerve trunk decompression while dapsone therapy is continued.

Type II, erythema nodosum leprosum, occurs primarily in lepromatous leprosy, with an incidence of about 50% during the first year of therapy. Signs and symptoms include tender erythematous skin nodules, fever, malaise, orchitis, neuritis, albuminuria, iritis, joint swelling, epistaxis, and depression; skin lesions may ulcerate. Treatment includes one or more of the following drugs while dapsone is continued: corticosteroids, analgesics, and thalidomide.

Additional treatment guidelines are available from National Hansen's Disease Programs at the U.S. Public Health Service in Baton Rouge, LA, 1-800-642-2477.

## Overdose and treatment

Signs and symptoms of overdose include nausea, vomiting, and hyperexcitability, occurring within minutes or up to 24 hours after ingestion; methemoglobin-induced depression, cyanosis, and seizures may occur. Hemolysis is a late complication (up to 14 days after ingestion).

Treatment is by gastric lavage, followed by activated charcoal; dapsone-induced methemoglobinemia (in patients without G6PD deficiency) can be given methylene blue. Hemodialysis may also be used to enhance elimination.

## Clinical considerations

■ Recommend giving drug with or after meals to avoid gastric irritation. Advise clinician to ensure adequate fluid intake.
■ Specimens for culture and sensitivity testing should be taken before first dose, but therapy may begin before test results are complete; repeat periodically to detect drug resistance.

■ Isolation of patient with inactive leprosy isn't required; however, recommend disinfecting surfaces in contact with discharge from nose or skin lesions.

■ Therapeutic effect on leprosy may not be evident until 3 to 6 months after start of therapy.

■ Because drug is dialyzable, patients undergoing hemodialysis may require dosage adjustments.

### Therapeutic monitoring
■ Advise clinician to monitor dapsone serum levels periodically to maintain effective levels. Levels of 0.1 to 7 mcg/ml (average 2.3 mcg/ml) are usually effective and safe.

■ Advise clinician to monitor vital signs frequently during early weeks of drug therapy. Frequent or high fever may require reduced dosage or discontinuation of drug.

■ Patient requires observation for adverse effects and monitoring of hematologic and liver function test results to minimize toxicity.

■ Watch skin and mucous membranes for early signs of allergic reactions or leprosy reactional states.

### Special populations
**Breast-feeding patients.** Dapsone appears in breast milk. An alternative feeding method is recommended during therapy with dapsone.
**Pediatric patients.** Use drug with caution in children.
**Geriatric patients.** Geriatric patients often have decreased renal function, which decreases drug excretion. Use with caution.

### Patient counseling
■ Explain disease process and rationale for long-term therapy to patient and family; emphasize that improvement may not occur for 3 to 6 months and that treatment must continue for at least 1 to 2 years.

■ Teach signs and symptoms of hypersensitivity and other adverse reactions, and emphasize need to report these promptly; explain possibility of cumulative effects; urge patient to report any unusual effects or reactions and to report loss of appetite, nausea, or vomiting promptly.

■ Teach patient how to take drug and of the need to comply with prescribed regimen. Encourage patient to report no improvement or worsening of symptoms after 3 months of drug treatment. Urge patient not to stop drug without medical approval.

■ Explain importance of follow-up visits and need to monitor close contacts at 6- to 12-month intervals for 10 years.

■ Teach sanitary disposal of secretions from nose or skin lesions.

■ Assure patient and family that inactive leprosy is no barrier to employment or school attendance.

■ New mothers need not be separated from infant during therapy; teach signs and symptoms of cyanosis and methemoglobinemia.

# daunorubicin citrate liposomal
DaunoXome

*Pharmacologic classification:* anthracycline
*Therapeutic classification:* antineoplastic
*Pregnancy risk category D*

## Available forms
Available by prescription only
*Injection:* 2 mg/ml (equivalent to 50 mg daunorubicin base)

## Indications and dosages
*First-line cytotoxic therapy for advanced HIV-associated Kaposi's sarcoma*
*Adults:* 40 mg/m² I.V. over 60 minutes once every 2 weeks. Continue treatment until there is evidence of progressive disease or until other complications of HIV preclude continuation of therapy.

≡*Dosage adjustment.* For patients with impaired hepatic and renal function, reduce dosage as follows: If serum bilirubin is 1.2 to 3 mg/dl, give three-fourths the normal dose; if serum bilirubin or creatinine is greater than 3 mg/dl, give one-half the normal dose.

## I.V. administration
■ Dilute drug with D₅W before administration. Withdraw the calculated volume of drug from the vial and transfer it into an equivalent amount of D₅W. The recommended level after dilution should be 1 mg/ml.

■ After dilution, recommend immediately giving I.V. over 60 minutes. If unable to use immediately, refrigerate at 36° to 46° F (2° to 8° C) for a maximum of 6 hours.

■ Don't use in-line filters for the I.V. infusion.

### Incompatibilities
Don't mix daunorubicin citrate liposomal with other drugs, saline, bacteriostatic drugs, or other solutions.

## Mechanism of action
*Antineoplastic action:* Daunorubicin exerts its cytotoxic activity by intercalating between DNA base pairs and uncoiling the DNA helix. This results in the inhibition of DNA synthesis and DNA-dependent RNA synthesis. The drug may also inhibit polymerase activity. The liposomal preparation of daunorubicin maximizes the selectivity of daunorubicin for solid tumors in situ. After penetrating the tumor,

---

daunorubicin is released over time to exert its antineoplastic activity.

## Pharmacokinetics

*Absorption:* Must be given I.V. because of its vesicant nature.

*Distribution:* Thought to be distributed primarily in the vascular fluid volume.

*Metabolism:* Metabolized by the liver into active metabolites.

*Excretion:* Apparent elimination half-life is 4½ hours.

| Route | Onset | Peak | Duration |
|-------|-------|------|----------|
| I.V. | Unknown | Unknown | Unknown |

## Contraindications and precautions

Contraindicated in patients hypersensitive to daunorubicin citrate liposomal or any constituents of this product. Use cautiously in patients with myelosuppression, preexisting cardiac disease, previous radiotherapy encompassing the heart, prior anthracycline use (doxorubicin more than 300 mg/m$^2$ or equivalent), hepatic or renal dysfunction.

## Interactions

None reported.

## Adverse reactions

**CNS:** *headache, neuropathy,* depression, dizziness, insomnia, amnesia, anxiety, ataxia, confusion, *seizures,* hallucination, tremor, hypertonia, meningitis, *fatigue,* malaise, emotional lability, abnormal gait, hyperkinesia, somnolence, abnormal thinking.

**CV:** *cardiomyopathy,* chest pain, hypertension, palpitation, syncope, *arrhythmias, pericardial effusion, pericardial tamponade, cardiac arrest,* angina pectoris, *pulmonary hypertension,* flushing, edema, tachycardia, *MI.*

**EENT:** *rhinitis,* stomatitis, sinusitis, abnormal vision, conjunctivitis, tinnitus, eye pain, deafness, earache.

**GI:** *nausea, diarrhea, abdominal pain, vomiting, anorexia,* constipation, *GI hemorrhage,* gastritis, dysphagia, stomatitis, increased appetite, melena, hemorrhoids, tenesmus, taste disturbances, gingival bleeding, dry mouth.

**GU:** dysuria, nocturia, polyuria.

**Hematologic:** NEUTROPENIA.

**Hepatic:** hepatomegaly.

**Musculoskeletal:** *back pain,* arthralgia, myalgia.

**Respiratory:** *cough, dyspnea,* hemoptysis, hiccups, pulmonary infiltration, increased sputum.

**Skin:** alopecia, pruritus, *increased sweating,* dry skin, seborrhea, folliculitis, injection site inflammation.

**Other:** *fever,* splenomegaly, lymphadenopathy, *opportunistic infections, allergic reactions,* influenzalike symptoms, dehydration, tooth caries, thirst, *rigors.*

## Overdose and treatment

The signs and symptoms of acute overdose are an increased severity of adverse effects, such as myelosuppression, fatigue, nausea, and vomiting. Treatment is usually supportive.

## Clinical considerations

■ Give only under the supervision of clinicians specializing in cancer chemotherapy.

**⊞ ALERT** Daunorubicin citrate liposomal exhibits unique pharmacokinetic properties compared with conventional daunorubicin hydrochloride and shouldn't be substituted on a milligram per milligram basis.

■ A triad of back pain, flushing, and chest tightness may occur within the first 5 minutes of the infusion. This triad subsides after stopping the infusion and generally doesn't recur when the infusion is given at a slower rate.

■ Because extravasation can cause local tissue necrosis, advise clinician to monitor I.V. site closely.

■ Follow procedures for proper handling and disposal of antineoplastics.

### Therapeutic monitoring

■ Advise clinician to monitor and assess cardiac function regularly before giving each dose because of the potential risk for cardiac toxicity and heart failure. Recommend performing determination of left ventricular ejection fraction at total cumulative doses of 320 mg/m$^2$ and every 160 mg/m$^2$ thereafter.

■ Careful hematologic monitoring is required because severe myelosuppression may occur. Recommend repeated blood counts before each dose and withholding treatment if absolute granulocyte count is less than 750 cells/mm$^3$.

■ Advise clinician to monitor patient closely for signs of opportunistic infections especially because patients with HIV infection are immunocompromised.

### Special populations

**Pregnant patients.** Drug causes severe maternal toxicity and embryolethality; advise patient to avoid becoming pregnant during treatment.

**Breast-feeding patients.** Safety during breast-feeding hasn't been established. Because of the potential for serious adverse effects occurring in the breast-feeding infant, tell patient to avoid breast-feeding.

**Pediatric patients.** Safety and efficacy haven't been established in pediatric patients.

**Geriatric patients.** Safety and efficacy haven't been established in geriatric patients.

## Patient counseling

■ Inform patient that alopecia may occur, but is usually reversible.

■ Instruct patient to report sore throat, fever, or any other signs of infection; tell patient to avoid exposure to people with infections.

---

Reactions may be *common,* uncommon, *life-threatening,* or COMMON AND LIFE-THREATENING.

- Advise patient to report suspected or confirmed pregnancy while receiving the drug.
- Tell patient to report back pain, flushing, and chest tightness during the infusion.

# daunorubicin hydrochloride
Cerubidine

*Pharmacologic classification:* antibiotic antineoplastic (cell cycle–phase nonspecific)
*Therapeutic classification:* antineoplastic
*Pregnancy risk category D*

## Available forms
Available by prescription only
*Injection:* 20-mg vials (with 100 mg of mannitol)

## Indications and dosages
Dosage and indications may vary. Check current literature for recommended protocols.
*Remission induction in acute nonlymphocytic leukemia (myelogenous, monocytic, erythroid)*
*Adults under age 60:* 45 mg/m² I.V. daily on days 1 to 3 of first course and on days 1 and 2 of subsequent courses. Give all courses with cytosine arabinoside infusions.
*Adults ages 60 and older:* 30 mg/m² I.V. daily on days 1 to 3 of first course and on days 1 and 2 of subsequent courses. Give all courses with cytosine arabinoside infusions.
*Remission induction in acute lymphocytic leukemia*
*Adults:* 45 mg/m²/day I.V. on days 1 to 3; give with vincristine, prednisone, and l-asparaginase.
*Children ages 2 and older:* 25 mg/m² I.V. on day 1 weekly for up to 6 weeks, if needed; give with vincristine and prednisone.
*Children under age 2 or with a body surface area of less than 0.5 m²:* Calculate dose based on body weight (1 mg/kg), rather than body surface area.
≡ *Dosage adjustment.* Use reduced dosage if patient has hepatic or renal impairment. For patients with serum bilirubin of 1.2 to 3 mg/dl, reduce dosage by 25%; with serum bilirubin or creatinine levels of more than 3 mg/dl, reduce dosage by 50%.

## I.V. administration
- To reconstitute, add 4 ml of sterile water for injection to a 20-mg vial to give a concentration of 5 mg/ml.
- Drug may be diluted further into 100 ml of D₅W or normal saline solution and infused over 30 to 45 minutes.
- For I.V. push administration, reconstituted drug is withdrawn into a syringe containing 10 to 15 ml of normal saline or D₅W and injected over 2 to 3 minutes into the tubing of a freely

flowing I.V. infusion. Reconstituted solution is stable for 24 hours at controlled room temperature and 48 hours in refrigeration.

### Incompatibilities
Incompatible with heparin and dexamethasone. Don't mix with other drugs.

## Mechanism of action
*Antineoplastic action:* Drug exerts its cytotoxic activity by intercalating between DNA base pairs and uncoiling the DNA helix. The result is inhibition of DNA synthesis and DNA-dependent RNA synthesis. Drug may also inhibit polymerase activity.

## Pharmacokinetics
*Absorption:* Administered I.V.
*Distribution:* Widely distributed into body tissues, with the highest levels being found in the spleen, kidneys, liver, lungs, and heart. It doesn't cross the blood-brain barrier.
*Metabolism:* Extensively metabolized in the liver by microsomal enzymes. One of the metabolites has cytotoxic activity.
*Excretion:* Primarily excreted in bile, with a small portion excreted in urine. Plasma elimination has been described as biphasic, with an initial phase half-life of 45 minutes and a terminal phase half-life of 18½ hours.

| Route | Onset | Peak | Duration |
|-------|-------|------|----------|
| I.V. | Unknown | Unknown | Unknown |

## Contraindications and precautions
No known contraindications. Use cautiously in patients with myelosuppression or impaired cardiac, renal, or hepatic function.

## Interactions
*Drug-drug.* *Dexamethasone phosphate, heparin sodium:* Admixture of these drugs causes the formation of a precipitate. Don't mix daunorubicin with either heparin sodium or dexamethasone phosphate.
*Doxorubicin:* Additive cardiotoxicity. Advise clinician to monitor patient closely.
*Hepatotoxic drugs:* Increase the risk of hepatotoxicity. Advise clinician to monitor patient closely.

## Adverse reactions
**CV:** *irreversible cardiomyopathy,* ECG changes.
**GI:** *nausea, vomiting,* diarrhea, *mucositis* (may occur 3 to 7 days after administration).
**GU:** red urine (transient).
**Hematologic:** *bone marrow suppression* (lowest blood counts 10 to 14 days after administration).
**Hepatic:** *hepatotoxicity.*
**Metabolic:** hyperuricemia.
**Skin:** rash; *severe cellulitis, tissue sloughing with extravasation; alopecia.*
**Other:** fever, chills.

## Overdose and treatment
Signs and symptoms of overdose include myelosuppression, nausea, vomiting, and stomatitis. Treatment is usually supportive and includes transfusion of blood components and antiemetics.

## Clinical considerations
**H ALERT** Reddish color of drug looks similar to that of doxorubicin (Adriamycin). Don't confuse the two drugs.
- Erythematous streaking along the vein or flushing in the face indicates that the drug is being given too rapidly.
- Extravasation may be treated with topical application of dimethyl sulfoxide and ice packs to the site.
- Antiemetics may be used to prevent or treat nausea and vomiting.
- Darkening or redness of the skin may occur in prior radiation fields.
- ECG monitoring or monitoring of systolic injection fraction may help to identify early changes associated with drug-induced cardiomyopathy. An ECG or determination of systolic injection fraction should be performed before each course of therapy.
- To prevent cardiomyopathy, advise clinician to limit cumulative dose in adults to 500 to 600 mg/m$^2$ (400 to 450 mg/m$^2$ when patient has been receiving other cardiotoxic drugs, such as cyclophosphamide, or radiation therapy that encompasses the heart).

### Therapeutic monitoring
- Advise clinician to monitor CBC and hepatic function.
- A high resting pulse rate must be reported to prescriber (a sign of cardiac adverse reactions).
- Advise clinician against the use of a scalp tourniquet or ice to prevent alopecia, which may compromise effectiveness of drug.

### Special populations
**Breast-feeding patients.** It isn't known if drug appears in breast milk. However, because of potential for serious adverse reactions, mutagenicity, and carcinogenicity in the infant, breast-feeding isn't recommended.
**Pediatric patients.** Children have an increased risk of drug-induced cardiotoxicity, which may occur at lower doses. Total lifetime dosage for children over age 2 is 300 mg/m$^2$; for children under age 2, it is 10 mg/kg.
**Geriatric patients.** Geriatric patients have an increased risk of drug-induced cardiotoxicity. Advise clinician to monitor patient for hematologic toxicity because some geriatric patients have poor bone marrow reserve.

## Patient counseling
- Warn patient that urine may be red for 1 to 2 days and that this is a drug effect, not bleeding.
- Advise patient that alopecia may occur, but that it's usually reversible.
- Tell patient to avoid exposure to people with infections.
- Encourage adequate fluid intake to increase urine output and facilitate excretion of uric acid.
- Warn patient that nausea and vomiting may be severe and may last for 24 to 48 hours.
- Instruct patient to call prescriber if a sore throat, fever, or signs of bleeding occurs.

# delavirdine mesylate
Rescriptor

*Pharmacologic classification:* nonnucleoside reverse-transcriptase inhibitor of HIV-1
*Therapeutic classification:* antiviral
*Pregnancy risk category C*

## Available forms
Available by prescription only
*Tablets:* 100 mg, 200 mg

## Indications and dosages
**HIV infection**
*Adults:* 400 mg P.O. t.i.d.; use with other antiretrovirals as appropriate.

## Mechanism of action
*Antiviral action:* Delavirdine is a nonnucleoside reverse transcriptase (RT) inhibitor of HIV-1. It binds directly to RT and blocks RNA- and DNA-dependent DNA polymerase activities.

## Pharmacokinetics
*Absorption:* Rapidly absorbed following oral administration.
*Distribution:* 98% plasma protein–bound, primarily albumin. Distribution into CSF, saliva, and semen is about 0.4%, 6%, and 2%, respectively, of the corresponding plasma levels.
*Metabolism:* Converted to several inactive metabolites; primarily metabolized in liver by cytochrome P-450 3A (CYP3A) enzyme system; however, CYP2D6 may also be involved. Delavirdine can reduce CYP3A activity and can inhibit its own metabolism; this is usually reversed within 1 week after discontinuation of the drug. CYP2C9 and CYP2C19 activity may also be reduced by delavirdine.
*Excretion:* After many doses, 44% of the dose was recovered in feces and 51% was excreted in urine. Less than 5% of the dose was recovered unchanged in urine. Mean elimination half-life was 5¾ hours.

| Route | Onset | Peak | Duration |
|-------|-------|------|----------|
| P.O. | Unknown | 1 hr | Unknown |

## Contraindications and precautions

Contraindicated in patients hypersensitive to formulation of drug. Use caution when giving to patients with impaired hepatic function. Nonnucleoside RT inhibitors, when used alone or in combination, may confer cross-resistance to other drugs in that class.

## Interactions

**Drug-drug.** *Amphetamines, benzodiazepines, calcium channel blockers, clarithromycin, dapsone, ergot alkaloid preparations, indinavir, nonsedating antihistamines, quinidine, rifabutin, saquinavir, sedative hypnotics, warfarin:* Increase or prolong both therapeutic and adverse effects. Avoid use together; however, reduced doses of indinavir with delavirdine may be used.

*Antacids:* Reduced absorption of delavirdine. Separate doses by at least 1 hour.

*Carbamazepine, phenobarbital, phenytoin, rifabutin, rifampin:* Decrease plasma delavirdine levels. Use with caution.

*Clarithromycin, fluoxetine, ketoconazole:* Cause a 50% increase in delavirdine bioavailability. Advise clinician to monitor patient.

*Didanosine:* Coadministration with delavirdine results in 20% decrease in absorption of both drugs. Recommend separating doses by at least 1 hour.

*H$_2$-receptor antagonists:* Increased gastric pH reduces absorption of delavirdine. Long-term use of these drugs with delavirdine isn't recommended.

*Indinavir:* Increased plasma levels. Consider a lower dose of indinavir when given with delavirdine.

*Saquinavir:* Five-fold increase in bioavailability. Advise clinician to monitor AST and ALT levels frequently when used together.

**Drug-herb.** *St. John's wort:* Decreased delavirdine levels. Discourage use together.

## Adverse reactions

**CNS:** asthenia, *fatigue,* headache, abnormal coordination, agitation, amnesia, anxiety, change in dreams, lethargy, malaise, cognitive impairment, confusion, depression, disorientation, emotional lability, hallucinations, hyperesthesia, hyperreflexia, hypesthesia, impaired concentration, insomnia, manic symptoms, muscle cramps, nervousness, neuropathy, nightmares, nystagmus, paralysis, paranoid symptoms, paresthesia, restlessness, somnolence, tingling, tremor, vertigo, weakness, pallor.
**CV:** *bradycardia,* palpitation, orthostatic hypotension, syncope, tachycardia, vasodilation, chest pain, peripheral edema.
**EENT:** blepharitis, conjunctivitis, diplopia, dry eyes, ear pain, photophobia, tinnitus, laryngismus, pharyngitis, rhinitis, sinusitis.
**GI:** *nausea,* vomiting, diarrhea, anorexia, aphthous stomatitis, bloody stools, colitis, constipation, decreased appetite, diverticulitis, duo-

denitis, dry mouth, dyspepsia, dysphagia, enteritis, esophagitis, fecal incontinence, flatulence, gagging, gastritis, gastroesophageal reflux, *GI bleeding,* gingivitis, gum hemorrhage, increased thirst and appetite, increased saliva, mouth ulcer, nonspecific *hepatitis, pancreatitis,* sialadenitis, stomatitis, tongue edema or ulceration, abdominal cramps, distention, pain (generalized or localized), taste perversion.
**GU:** renal calculi, epididymitis, hematuria, hemospermia, impotence, renal pain, metrorrhagia, nocturia, polyuria, proteinuria, vaginal candidiasis.
**Hematologic:** bruises, anemia, ecchymosis, eosinophilia, *granulocytosis, neutropenia, pancytopenia,* petechia, prolonged PTT, purpura, spleen disorder, *thrombocytopenia.*
**Hepatic:** *increased ALT and AST levels.*
**Metabolic:** alcohol intolerance; bilirubinemia; hyperkalemia; hyperuricemia; hypocalcemia; hyponatremia; hypophosphatemia; increased GGT, lipase, serum alkaline phosphatase, serum amylase, and serum CK; weight gain or loss.
**Musculoskeletal:** flank pain, back pain, pain (generalized or localized), neck rigidity, arthralgia or arthritis of single and many joints, bone pain, leg cramps, muscular weakness, myalgia, tendon disorder, tenosynovitis, tetany.
**Respiratory:** upper respiratory infection, bronchitis, chest congestion, cough, dyspnea, epistaxis.
**Skin:** epidermal cyst, *rash, pruritus,* dermal leukocytoblastic vasculitis, dermatitis, desquamation, diaphoresis, dry skin, erythema multiforme, folliculitis, fungal dermatitis, alopecia, nail disorder, petechial rash, seborrhea, skin nodule, *Stevens-Johnson syndrome,* urticaria.
**Other:** allergic reaction, chills, edema (generalized or localized), fever, flu syndrome, lip edema, *angioedema,* sebaceous cyst, trauma, breast enlargement, decreased libido.

## Overdose and treatment

Although no information is available, advise clinician to provide supportive treatment and remove drug by gastric lavage or emesis, if needed. Dialysis is unlikely to be effective because drug is highly protein-bound.

## Clinical considerations

■ Rash is more common in patients with lower CD4+ cell counts and usually occurs within the first 3 weeks of treatment. Severe rash occurs in 3.6% of patients. In most cases, rash lasts less than 2 weeks and doesn't require dose reduction or drug discontinuation. Most patients are able to resume therapy after treatment interruption caused by rash.

■ Rash occurs mainly on the upper body and proximal arms, with decreasing lesion intensity on the neck and face and less on the rest of the trunk and limbs. Erythema multiforme and Stevens-Johnson syndrome are rarely seen,

and resolve after drug is stopped. Occurrence of drug-related rash after 1 month of therapy is uncommon unless prolonged interruption of drug treatment occurs.
■ Symptomatic relief may be obtained by using diphenhydramine, hydroxyzine, or topical corticosteroids.

### Therapeutic monitoring
■ Neutropenia (absolute neutrophil count less than 750/mm$^3$), anemia (hemoglobin less than 7 g/dl), thrombocytopenia (platelet count less than 50,000/mm$^3$), ALT and AST (more than five times upper limit of normal), bilirubin (more than 2½ times upper limit of normal) and amylase (more than twice upper limit of normal) may occur while on delavirdine. Advise clinician to monitor patient carefully.
■ Advise clinician to monitor patients with hepatic or renal impairment because effect of drug hasn't been studied.

### Special populations
**Breast-feeding patients.** Women infected with HIV are advised not to breast-feed.
**Pediatric patients.** Safety and effectiveness haven't been studied in patients under age 16.
**Geriatric patients.** Safety and effectiveness haven't been studied in patients over age 65.

### Patient counseling
■ Instruct patient to discontinue drug and call prescriber if severe rash or signs and symptoms such as fever, blistering, oral lesions, conjunctivitis, swelling, or muscle or joint aches occurs.
■ Tell patient that drug isn't a cure for HIV-1 infection. He may continue to acquire illnesses caused by HIV-1 infection, including opportunistic infections. Therapy doesn't reduce the risk or frequency of such illnesses.
■ Advise patient to remain under medical supervision when taking drug because long-term effects aren't known.
■ Inform patient to take drug as prescribed and not to alter doses without medical approval. If a dose is missed, tell him to take the next dose as soon as possible; he shouldn't double the next dose.
■ Inform patient that drug may be dispersed in water before ingestion. Add tablets to at least 3 ounces (90 ml) of water, allow to stand for a few minutes, and stir until a uniform dispersion occurs. Tell patient to drink dispersion promptly, rinse glass, and swallow the rinse to ensure that entire dose is consumed.
■ Advise patient with achlorhydria to take drug with an acidic beverage such as orange or cranberry juice.
■ Advise patient to report the use of other prescription or OTC drugs to prescriber.

# desipramine hydrochloride
Norpramin

*Pharmacologic classification:* dibenzazepine tricyclic antidepressant
*Therapeutic classification:* antidepressant
*Pregnancy risk category NR*

## Available forms
Available by prescription only
*Tablets:* 10 mg, 25 mg, 50 mg, 75 mg, 100 mg, 150 mg
*Tablets (film-coated):* 10 mg, 25 mg, 50 mg, 75 mg, 100 mg, 150 mg

## Indications and dosages
*Depression*
*Adults:* 100 to 200 mg P.O. daily in divided doses, increasing to maximum of 300 mg daily. Alternatively, the entire dose can be given once daily, usually h.s.
*Geriatric patients and adolescents:* 25 to 100 mg P.O. daily, increasing gradually to a maximum of 100 mg daily (maximum 150 mg/daily only for the severely ill in these age groups).

## Mechanism of action
*Antidepressant action:* Drug is thought to exert its antidepressant effects by inhibiting reuptake of norepinephrine and serotonin in CNS nerve terminals (presynaptic neurons), which results in increased levels and enhanced activity of these neurotransmitters in the synaptic cleft. Desipramine more strongly inhibits reuptake of norepinephrine than serotonin; it has a lesser risk of sedative effects and less anticholinergic and hypotensive activity than its parent compound, imipramine.

## Pharmacokinetics
*Absorption:* Absorbed rapidly from the GI tract after oral administration.
*Distribution:* Distributed widely into the body, including the CNS and breast milk. Drug is 90% protein-bound. Proposed therapeutic plasma levels (parent drug and metabolite) range from 125 to 300 ng/ml.
*Metabolism:* Metabolized by the liver; a significant first-pass effect may explain variability of serum levels in different patients taking the same dosage.
*Excretion:* Excreted primarily in urine.

| Route | Onset | Peak | Duration |
|-------|-------|------|----------|
| P.O. | Unknown | 4-6 hr | 2-4 wk |

## Contraindications and precautions
Contraindicated in patients hypersensitive to drug, in those who have taken MAO inhibitors within the previous 14 days, and in patients during acute recovery phase of MI.

---

Use with extreme caution in patients with history of seizure disorders or urine retention, CV or thyroid disease, or glaucoma, and in those taking thyroid hormones.

## Interactions

**Drug-drug.** *Antiarrhythmics, pimozide, thyroid hormones:* May increase risk of cardiac arrhythmias and conduction defects. Avoid use together.

*Barbiturates:* Induce desipramine metabolism and decrease therapeutic efficacy. Advise clinician to monitor patient carefully.

*Beta blockers, cimetidine, methylphenidate, oral contraceptives, propoxyphene:* May inhibit desipramine metabolism, increasing plasma levels and toxicity. Avoid use together.

*Cimetidine, fluoxetine, fluvoxamine, paroxetine, sertraline:* May increase serum desipramine levels. Advise clinician to monitor patient carefully.

*Clonidine:* May cause dangerous increase in blood pressure or hypertensive crisis. Avoid use together.

*Ephedrine, epinephrine, norepinephrine, phenylephrine:* May increase blood pressure. Use with caution.

*Guanabenz, guanadrel, guanethidine, methyldopa, reserpine:* Desipramine may decrease hypotensive effects. Avoid use together.

*CNS depressants:* Additive effects. Avoid use together.

*Disulfiram, ethchlorvynol:* May cause delirium and tachycardia. Avoid use together.

*Haloperidol, phenothiazines:* Decrease its metabolism, decreasing therapeutic efficacy. Advise clinician to monitor patient carefully.

*MAO inhibitors:* May cause severe excitation, hyperpyrexia, or seizures, usually with high dosage. Avoid use together.

*SSRIs:* Patient may become toxic to tricyclic antidepressant at much lower dosages. Dosage reduction may be needed.

*Warfarin:* May increase PT and cause bleeding. Advise clinician to monitor PT and INR.

**Drug-herb.** *Evening primrose:* Possible additive or synergistic effect resulting in lower seizure threshold and increased risk of seizure. Discourage use together.

*St. John's wort, SAMe, yohimbe:* Use with some tricyclic antidepressants may cause elevation of serotonin levels. Discourage use together.

**Drug-lifestyle.** *Alcohol use:* May enhance CNS depression. Encourage patient to avoid alcohol use.

*Heavy smoking:* May lower plasma levels of desipramine. Discourage smoking.

*Sun exposure:* May increase risk of photosensitivity. Advise patient to take precautions.

## Adverse reactions

**CNS:** *drowsiness, dizziness,* excitation, tremor, weakness, confusion, anxiety, restlessness, agitation, headache, nervousness, EEG changes, *seizures,* extrapyramidal reactions.

**CV:** orthostatic hypotension, *tachycardia, ECG changes,* hypertension.

**EENT:** *blurred vision,* tinnitus, mydriasis.

**GI:** *dry mouth, constipation,* nausea, vomiting, anorexia, paralytic ileus.

**GU:** *urine retention.*

**Hematologic:** decreased WBC counts.

**Hepatic:** elevated liver function test results.

**Metabolic:** hyperglycemia, hypoglycemia.

**Skin:** rash, urticaria, photosensitivity, *diaphoresis.*

**Other:** hypersensitivity reaction, *sudden death* (in children).

**After abrupt withdrawal of long-term therapy:** nausea, headache, malaise (doesn't indicate addiction).

## Overdose and treatment

The first 12 hours after acute ingestion are a stimulatory phase characterized by excessive anticholinergic activity (agitation, irritation, confusion, hallucinations, parkinsonian symptoms, hyperthermia, seizures, urine retention, dry mucous membranes, pupillary dilatation, constipation, and ileus). This is followed by CNS-depressant effects, including hypothermia, decreased or absent reflexes, sedation, hypotension, cyanosis; and cardiac irregularities, including tachycardia, conduction disturbances, and quinidine-like effects on the ECG.

Severity of overdose is best indicated by widening of the QRS complex, which usually represents a serum level in excess of 1,000 ng/ml; serum levels are generally not helpful. Metabolic acidosis may follow hypotension, hypoventilation, and seizures.

Treatment is symptomatic and supportive, including maintaining airway, stable body temperature, and fluid and electrolyte balance. Recommend inducing emesis with ipecac if patient is conscious; followed with gastric lavage and activated charcoal to prevent further absorption. Dialysis is of little use. Physostigmine may be used with caution to reverse CV abnormalities or coma; too rapid administration may cause seizures. Recommend treating seizures with parenteral diazepam or phenytoin; arrhythmias, with parenteral phenytoin or lidocaine; and acidosis, with sodium bicarbonate. Barbiturates shouldn't be given; these may enhance CNS and respiratory depressant effects.

## Clinical considerations

■ Dispense drug in the smallest possible quantities to depressed outpatients, as suicide has been accomplished with drug.

■ Drug has a lesser risk of sedative effects and fewer anticholinergic and hypotensive effects than its parent compound imipramine.

■ Tolerance usually develops to the sedative effects of the drug during initial weeks of therapy.

- Drug shouldn't be withdrawn abruptly; rather, it should be tapered gradually over 3 to 6 weeks.
- Discontinue drug at least 48 hours before surgical procedures.
- Drug therapy in patients with bipolar illness may induce a hypomanic state.

### Therapeutic monitoring
- Advise clinician to check standing and sitting blood pressure to assess orthostasis before administration of desipramine.

### Special populations
**Breast-feeding patients.** Drug appears in breast milk in levels equal to those in maternal serum. The potential benefit to the woman should outweigh the possible adverse reactions in the infant.
**Pediatric patients.** Drug isn't recommended for patients under age 12. Sudden death has been reported in children given the drug.
**Geriatric patients.** Geriatric patients may be more susceptible to adverse CV and anticholinergic effects.

### Patient counseling
- Tell patient to take the full dose at bedtime to alleviate daytime sedation.
- Explain that full effects of drug may not become apparent for 4 weeks or longer after therapy starts.
- Tell patient to take drug exactly as prescribed and not to double the dose for missed ones.
- To prevent dizziness, advise patient to lie down for about 30 minutes after each dose at start of therapy and to avoid sudden postural changes, especially when rising to upright position.
- Warn patient not to stop taking drug suddenly.
- Encourage patient to report unusual or troublesome effects, especially confusion, movement disorders, rapid heartbeat, dizziness, fainting, or difficulty urinating.
- Tell patient sugarless chewing gum or hard candy or ice may alleviate dry mouth.
- Stress importance of regular dental hygiene to avoid caries.

## desmopressin acetate
DDAVP, Stimate

*Pharmacologic classification:* posterior pituitary hormone
*Therapeutic classification:* antidiuretic, hemostatic
*Pregnancy risk category B*

### Available forms
Available by prescription only
*Tablets:* 0.1 mg
*Nasal solution:* 0.1 mg/ml, 1.5 mg/ml

*Injection:* 4 mcg/ml in 1-ml single-dose ampules and 10-ml multiple-dose vials

### Indications and dosages
***Central cranial diabetes insipidus, temporary polyuria, polydipsia associated with pituitary trauma***
*Adults:* 0.1 to 0.4 ml (10 to 40 mcg) intranasally in one to three divided doses daily. Adjust morning and evening doses separately for adequate diurnal rhythm of water turnover. Use the lowest effective dosage.
    Alternatively, 50 mcg P.O. b.i.d. initially. Adjust individual dosage in increments of 100 to 1,200 mcg daily, divided into two or three doses. Optimal dosage range is 100 to 800 mcg daily in divided doses. Or give 0.5 ml (2 mcg) to 1 ml (4 mcg) I.V. or S.C. daily, usually in two divided doses.
*Children ages 3 months to 12 years:* 0.05 to 0.3 ml (5 to 30 mcg) intranasally daily in one or two doses.
***Hemophilia A, von Willebrand's disease***
*Adults and children:* 0.3 mcg/kg diluted in normal saline solution and infused I.V. slowly over 15 to 30 minutes. May repeat dosage, p.r.n., as indicated by laboratory response and patient's condition. Alternatively, recommend giving one spray per nostril.
***Primary nocturnal enuresis***
*Children ages 6 and older:* 20 mcg (two to four metered sprays), intranasally h.s. Dosage adjusted according to response. Maximum recommended dose is 40 mcg daily.

### I.V. administration
- Recommend giving slow I.V. infusion over 15 to 30 minutes.
- Advise clinician to monitor blood pressure and pulse rate during infusion.
- For patients who weigh more than 10 kg (22 lbs), dilute with 50 ml normal saline solution. For children who weigh less than 10 kg, dilute with 10 ml of normal saline solution.

### Incompatibilities
None reported.

### Mechanism of action
*Antidiuretic action:* Desmopressin is used to control or prevent signs and complications of neurogenic diabetes insipidus. The site of action is primarily at the renal tubular level. Desmopressin increases water permeability at the renal tubule and collecting duct, resulting in increased urine osmolality and decreased urinary flow rate.
*Hemostatic action:* Desmopressin increases factor VIII activity by releasing endogenous factor VIII from plasma storage sites.

## Pharmacokinetics

*Absorption:* Destroyed in the GI tract. After intranasal administration, 10% to 20% of dose is absorbed through nasal mucosa.
*Distribution:* Not fully understood.
*Metabolism:* Unknown.
*Excretion:* Plasma levels decline in two phases: the half-life of the fast phase is about 8 minutes; the slow phase, 75 minutes. Duration of action after intranasal administration is 8 to 20 hours; after I.V. administration, 12 to 24 hours for mild hemophilia and about 3 hours for von Willebrand's disease.

| Route | Onset | Peak | Duration |
|-------|-------|------|----------|
| P.O. | 1 hr | 1-1½ hr | 8-12 hr |
| I.V. | 15-30 min | Unknown | 4-12 hr |
| Nasal | 1 hr | 1-5 hr | 8-12 hr |

## Contraindications and precautions

Contraindicated in patients hypersensitive to drug and in patients with type IIB von Willebrand's disease. Use cautiously in patients with coronary artery insufficiency or hypertensive CV disease and in those with conditions associated with fluid and electrolyte imbalances, such as cystic fibrosis, because these patients are susceptible to hyponatremia.

## Interactions

**Drug-drug.** *Carbamazepine, chlorpropamide, clofibrate:* May potentiate the antidiuretic action of desmopressin action. Avoid use together. *Demeclocycline, epinephrine, heparin, lithium, norepinephrine:* May decrease the antidiuretic effect. Use together cautiously.
**Drug-lifestyle.** *Alcohol use:* May increase risk of adverse effects. Avoid use together.

## Adverse reactions

**CNS:** headache.
**CV:** slight rise in blood pressure (at high dosage).
**EENT:** rhinitis, epistaxis, sore throat.
**GI:** nausea, abdominal cramps.
**GU:** vulval pain.
**Respiratory:** cough.
**Other:** flushing, local erythema, swelling, burning (after injection).

## Overdose and treatment

Signs and symptoms of overdose include drowsiness, listlessness, headache, confusion, anuria, and weight gain (water intoxication). Treatment requires water restriction and temporary withdrawal of desmopressin until polyuria occurs. Severe water intoxication may require osmotic diuresis with mannitol, hypertonic dextrose, or urea—alone or with furosemide.

## Clinical considerations

- Desmopressin may be given intranasally through a flexible catheter called a rhinyle. A measured quantity is drawn up into the catheter, one end is inserted into patient's nose, and patient blows on the other end to deposit drug into nasal cavity. Alternatively, drug is newly available in nasal spray, which may be easier for some patients.
- Desmopressin isn't indicated for hemophilia A patients with factor VIII levels up to 5% or in patients with severe von Willebrand's disease.
- Drug therapy may enable some patients to avoid the hazards of contaminated blood products.

### Therapeutic monitoring

- Advise clinician to watch for early signs and symptoms of water intoxication—drowsiness, listlessness, headache, confusion, anuria, and weight gain—to prevent seizures, coma, and death.
- Advise clinician to monitor patient's fluid intake, which may require adjustment to reduce risk of water intoxication and sodium depletion, especially in young or elderly patients.
- Advise clinician to weigh patient daily and observe for edema.

### Special populations

**Pediatric patients.** Drug isn't recommended in infants under age 3 months because of their increased tendency to develop fluid imbalance. Use with caution in infants because of risk of hyponatremia and water intoxication. Safety and efficacy of parenteral desmopressin haven't been established for management of diabetes insipidus in children under age 12.
**Geriatric patients.** Geriatric patients have an increased risk of hyponatremia and water intoxication; therefore, restriction of their fluid intake is recommended. Because geriatric patients are more sensitive to effects of drug, they may need a lower dosage.

## Patient counseling

- Teach patient correct administration technique, then evaluate his proficiency at drug administration and accurate measurement on return visits; some patients may have difficulty measuring and inhaling drug into nostrils.
- Emphasize that patient shouldn't increase or decrease dosage unless it's prescribed.
- Assist patient in planning a schedule for fluid intake if oral fluids must be reduced to decrease the possibility of water intoxication and hyponatremia. A diuretic may be given if excessive fluid retention occurs.
- Tell patient to store drug away from heat and direct light, not in bathroom, where heat and moisture can cause drug to deteriorate.

# dexamethasone
# (ophthalmic suspension)
Maxidex

# dexamethasone sodium phosphate
AK-Dex, Decadron, Ocu-Dex

*Pharmacologic classification:* cortico-steroid
*Therapeutic classification:* ophthalmic anti-inflammatory
*Pregnancy risk category C*

## Available forms
Available by prescription only
**dexamethasone**
*Ophthalmic suspension:* 0.1%
**dexamethasone sodium phosphate**
*Ophthalmic ointment:* 0.05%
*Ophthalmic solution:* 0.1%

## Indications and dosages
*Uveitis; iridocyclitis; inflammation of eyelids, conjunctiva, cornea, anterior segment of globe; corneal injury from burns or penetration by foreign bodies; allergic conjunctivitis; suppression of graft rejection after keratoplasty*
Adults and children: Instill 1 to 2 drops of suspension or solution or apply 1.25 to 2.5 cm of ointment into conjunctival sac. For initial therapy of severe cases, instill the solution or suspension into the conjunctival sac every hour, gradually discontinue dose as patient's condition improves. In mild condition, use drops up to four to six times daily or apply ointment t.i.d. or q.i.d. As patient's condition improves, taper dose to b.i.d. then once daily. Treatment may extend from a few days to several weeks.

## Mechanism of action
*Anti-inflammatory action:* Corticosteroids stimulate the synthesis of enzymes needed to decrease the inflammatory response. Dexamethasone, a long-acting fluorinated synthetic adrenocorticoid with strong anti-inflammatory activity and minimal mineralocorticoid activity, is 25 to 30 times more potent than an equal weight of hydrocortisone.

Drug is poorly soluble and therefore has a slower onset of action but a longer duration of action when applied in a liquid suspension. The sodium phosphate salt is highly soluble and has a rapid onset but short duration of action.

## Pharmacokinetics
*Absorption:* After ophthalmic administration, drug is absorbed through the aqueous humor. Because only low doses are given, little if any systemic absorption occurs.

*Distribution:* Distributed throughout the local tissue layers. Drug absorbed into circulation is rapidly removed from the blood and distributed into muscle, liver, skin, intestines, and kidneys.
*Metabolism:* Primarily metabolized locally. The small amount absorbed into systemic circulation is metabolized primarily in the liver to inactive compounds.
*Excretion:* Inactive metabolites are excreted by the kidneys, primarily as glucuronides and sulfates, but also as unconjugated products. Small amounts of the metabolites are also excreted in feces.

| Route | Onset | Peak | Duration |
|-------|-------|------|----------|
| Ophthalmic | Unknown | Unknown | Unknown |

## Contraindications and precautions
Contraindicated in patients with acute superficial herpes simplex (dendritic keratitis), vaccinia, varicella, or other fungal or viral diseases of cornea and conjunctiva; ocular tuberculosis; or acute, purulent, untreated infections of the eye.

Use cautiously in patients with corneal abrasions that may be infected (especially with herpes). Also use cautiously in patients with glaucoma because intraocular pressure may increase. Glaucoma drugs may need to be increased to compensate.

## Interactions
None reported.

## Adverse reactions
**EENT:** increased intraocular pressure; thinning of cornea, interference with corneal wound healing, increased susceptibility to viral or fungal corneal infection, corneal ulceration; glaucoma exacerbation, cataracts, defects in visual acuity and visual field, optic nerve damage; mild blurred vision; burning, stinging, or redness of eyes; watery eyes, discharge, discomfort, ocular pain, foreign body sensation (with excessive or long-term use).
**Other:** systemic effects and adrenal suppression (with excessive or long-term use).

## Overdose and treatment
None reported.

## Clinical considerations
**⚠ ALERT** Warn patient to call prescriber immediately and stop drug if visual acuity changes or visual field diminishes.
■ Shake suspension well before use.
■ Drug isn't recommended for long-term use.

### Therapeutic monitoring
■ Advise clinician to monitor patient for signs of corneal ulceration. The presence of corneal ulceration may require stopping drug.

---

## Patient counseling

- Teach patient how to instill eyedrops or ointment. Advise him to wash hands before and after administration, and warn him not to touch tip of dropper to eye or surrounding tissue.
- Tell patient to apply light finger pressure on lacrimal sac for 1 minute after installation.
- Warn patient not to share drug.

# dexamethasone (systemic)
Decadron, Deronil*, Dexasone*, Dexone, Hexadrol

## dexamethasone acetate
Dalalone D.P., Decadron-LA, Decaject-L.A., Dexasone-L.A., Dexpak

## dexamethasone sodium phosphate
Dalalone, Decadron Phosphate, Decaject, Dexameth, Dexasone, Dexone, Hexadrol Phosphate, Solurex

*Pharmacologic classification:* glucocorticoid
*Therapeutic classification:* anti-inflammatory, immunosuppressant
*Pregnancy risk category NR*

## Available forms
Available by prescription only
**dexamethasone**
*Tablets:* 0.25 mg, 0.5 mg, 0.75 mg, 1 mg, 1.5 mg, 2 mg, 4 mg, 6 mg
*Elixir:* 0.5 mg/5 ml
*Oral solution:* 0.5 mg/0.5 ml, 0.5 mg/5 ml
**dexamethasone acetate**
*Injection:* 8 mg/ml, 16 mg/ml suspension
**dexamethasone sodium phosphate**
*Injection:* 4 mg/ml, 10 mg/ml
*Injection (I.V. use only):* 24 mg/ml

## Indications and dosages
### Cerebral edema
**dexamethasone sodium phosphate**
*Adults:* Initially, 10 mg I.V., then 4 mg I.M. q 6 hours for 2 to 4 days, then taper over 5 to 7 days.
### Inflammatory conditions, allergic reactions, neoplasias
*Adults:* 0.75 to 9 mg P.O. daily divided b.i.d., t.i.d., or q.i.d.
*Children:* 0.024 to 0.34 mg/kg P.O. daily in four divided doses.
**dexamethasone acetate**
*Adults:* 4 to 16 mg intra-articularly or into soft tissue q 1 to 3 weeks; 0.8 to 1.6 mg into lesions q 1 to 3 weeks; or 8 to 16 mg I.M. q 1 to 3 weeks, p.r.n.
**dexamethasone sodium phosphate**
*Adults:* 0.2 to 6 mg intra-articularly, intralesionally, or into soft tissue; or 0.5 to 9 mg I.M.

*Shock (other than adrenal crisis)*
**dexamethasone sodium phosphate**
*Adults:* 1 to 6 mg/kg I.V. daily as a single dose; or 40 mg I.V. q 2 to 6 hours, p.r.n.
***Dexamethasone suppression test***
*Adults:* 0.5 mg P.O. q 6 hours for 48 hours.
***Adrenal insufficiency***
*Adults:* 0.75 to 9 mg P.O. daily in divided doses.
*Children:* 0.024 to 0.34 mg/kg P.O. daily in four divided doses.
**dexamethasone sodium phosphate**
*Adults:* 0.5 to 9 mg I.M. or I.V. daily.
*Children:* 0.235 to 1.25 mg/m² I.M. or I.V. once daily or b.i.d.
***Tuberculous meningitis***
*Adults:* 8 to 12 mg daily tapered over 6 to 8 weeks.
◊ *Prevention of hyaline membrane disease in premature infants*
*Adults:* 5 mg (phosphate) I.M. t.i.d. to mother for 2 days before delivery.
◊ *Prevention of chemotherapy-induced nausea and vomiting*
*Adults:* 10 to 20 mg I.V. before giving chemotherapy. Additional doses (individualized for each patient and usually lower than initial dose) may be given I.V. or P.O. for 24 to 72 hours following cancer chemotherapy, if needed.

## I.V. administration
- If giving by direct injection, inject undiluted over at least 1 minute.
- When giving an intermittent or continuous infusion, drug may be diluted in $D_5W$ or normal saline and infused over prescribed interval.

### Incompatibilities
Dexamethasone sodium phosphate is incompatible with daunorubicin, doxorubicin, and vancomycin.

## Mechanism of action
*Anti-inflammatory action:* Dexamethasone stimulates the synthesis of enzymes needed to decrease the inflammatory response. It causes suppression of the immune system by reducing activity and volume of the lymphatic system, producing lymphocytopenia (primarily T-lymphocytes), decreasing passage of immune complexes through basement membranes, and possibly by depressing reactivity of tissue to antigen-antibody interactions.

Drug is a long-acting synthetic adrenocorticoid with strong anti-inflammatory activity and minimal mineralocorticoid properties. It's 25 to 30 times more potent than an equal weight of hydrocortisone.

The acetate salt is a suspension and shouldn't be used I.V. It's particularly useful as an anti-inflammatory in intra-articular, intradermal, and intralesional injections.

The sodium phosphate salt is highly soluble and has a more rapid onset and a shorter duration of action than does the acetate salt.

It's most commonly used for cerebral edema and unresponsive shock. It can also be used in intra-articular, intralesional, or soft tissue inflammation. Other uses for dexamethasone are symptomatic treatment of bronchial asthma, chemotherapy-induced nausea, and as a diagnostic test for Cushing's syndrome.

## Pharmacokinetics

*Absorption:* After oral administration, drug is absorbed readily. The suspension for injection has a variable onset and duration of action, depending on whether it's injected into an intra-articular space, a muscle, or the blood supply to the muscle. After I.V. injection, dexamethasone is rapidly and completely absorbed into the tissues.

*Distribution:* Removed rapidly from the blood and distributed to muscle, liver, skin, intestines, and kidneys. Dexamethasone is bound weakly to plasma proteins (transcortin and albumin). Only the unbound portion is active. Adrenocorticoids appear in breast milk and the placenta.

*Metabolism:* Metabolized in the liver to inactive glucuronide and sulfate metabolites.

*Excretion:* Inactive metabolites and small amounts of unmetabolized drug are excreted by the kidneys. Insignificant quantities of drug are also excreted in feces; biologic half-life is 36 to 54 hours.

| Route | Onset | Peak | Duration |
|---|---|---|---|
| P.O. | 1-2 hr | 1-2 hr | 2½ days |
| I.V. | 1 hr | 1 hr | Variable |
| I.M. | 1 hr | 1 hr | 6 days |
| I.M. (acetate) | 1 hr | 8 hr | Unknown |

## Contraindications and precautions

Contraindicated in patients hypersensitive to drug or its components and in those with systemic fungal infections.

Use cautiously in patients with recent MI, GI ulcer, renal disease, hypertension, osteoporosis, diabetes mellitus, hypothyroidism, cirrhosis, diverticulitis, nonspecific ulcerative colitis, recent intestinal anastomoses, thromboembolic disorders, seizures, myasthenia gravis, heart failure, tuberculosis, ocular herpes simplex, emotional instability, and psychotic tendencies. Because some formulations contain sulfite preservatives, also use cautiously in patients sensitive to sulfites.

## Interactions

**Drug-drug.** *Antacids, cholestyramine, colestipol:* Decrease the corticosteroid effect. Advise clinician to monitor patient closely; patient may need dosage adjustment.

*Aspirin, NSAIDs:* May increase the risk of GI ulceration. Use together cautiously.

*Barbiturates, phenytoin, rifampin:* May cause decreased corticosteroid effects. Dosage adjustment may be needed.

*Cardiac glycosides:* Hypokalemia may increase the risk of toxicity. Advise clinician to monitor potassium levels and adjust dosage p.r.n.

*Diuretic or amphotericin B therapy:* May cause hypokalemia. Advise clinician to monitor serum potassium levels.

*Estrogens:* May reduce metabolism of dexamethasone by increasing the level of transcortin. Advise clinician to monitor patient closely.

*Insulin, oral antidiabetics:* Cause hyperglycemia. May require dosage adjustment.

*Isoniazid, salicylates:* Dexamethasone increases the metabolism of isoniazid and salicylates. Advise clinician to monitor patient carefully.

*Oral anticoagulants:* Decrease the effects. Advise clinician to monitor PT and INR closely.

*Skin-test antigens:* Decrease response. Defer skin testing until therapy is completed.

*Toxoids, vaccines:* Decrease antibody response and increase risk of neurologic complications. Avoid use together.

**Drug-lifestyle.** *Alcohol use:* Increases risk of gastric irritation and GI ulceration. Advise patient to avoid alcohol.

## Adverse reactions

Most adverse reactions to corticosteroids are dose-dependent or duration-dependent.

**CNS:** *euphoria, insomnia,* psychotic behavior, *pseudotumor cerebri,* vertigo, headache, paresthesia, *seizures.*

**CV:** *HF,* hypertension, edema, ***arrhythmias,*** thrombophlebitis, ***thromboembolism.***

**EENT:** cataracts, glaucoma.

**GI:** *peptic ulceration,* GI irritation, increased appetite, ***pancreatitis,*** nausea, vomiting.

**GU:** menstrual irregularities, increased urine glucose and calcium levels.

**Metabolic:** hypokalemia, hypocalcemia, hyperglycemia, carbohydrate intolerance, decreased levels of thyroxine, and triiodothyronine.

**Musculoskeletal:** muscle weakness, osteoporosis, growth suppression in children.

**Skin:** delayed wound healing, acne, various skin eruptions; atrophy (at I.M. injection sites), hirsutism.

**Other:** susceptibility to infections; *acute adrenal insufficiency may follow increased stress (infection, surgery, or trauma) or abrupt withdrawal after long-term therapy,* cushingoid state (moonface, buffalo hump, central obesity). **After abrupt withdrawal:** rebound inflammation, fatigue, weakness, arthralgia, fever, dizziness, lethargy, depression, fainting, orthostatic hypotension, dyspnea, anorexia, hypoglycemia. *After prolonged use, sudden withdrawal may be fatal.*

## Overdose and treatment

Acute ingestion, even in massive doses, rarely poses a clinical problem. Toxic signs and symp-

---

toms rarely occur if drug is used for less than 3 weeks, even at large dosage ranges. However, long-term use causes adverse physiologic effects, including suppression of the hypothalamic-pituitary-adrenal axis, cushingoid appearance, muscle weakness, and osteoporosis.

## Clinical considerations
■ Determine whether patient is sensitive to other corticosteroids.
■ For better results and less toxicity, a once-daily dose in the morning is recommended.
■ Recommend giving drug by I.M. injection deep into gluteal muscle, rotating sites, and avoiding S.C. injection.
■ Drug is being used investigationally to prevent hyaline membrane disease (respiratory distress syndrome) in premature infants. The suspension (phosphate salt) is given I.M. to the mother two or three times daily for 2 days before delivery.
■ Dexamethasone causes false-negative results in the nitroblue tetrazolium test for systemic bacterial infections and decreases [131]I uptake and protein-bound iodine levels in thyroid function test results.

### Therapeutic monitoring
■ Advise clinician to check patient's weight, blood pressure, and electrolyte levels frequently.
■ Advise clinician to monitor patient for depression or psychotic episodes.

### Special populations
**Pediatric patients.** Long-term use of drug in children and adolescents may delay growth and maturation.

## Patient counseling
■ Tell patient not to discontinue drug abruptly or without prescriber's consent.
■ Instruct patient to take drug with food or milk.
■ Teach patient signs and symptoms of early adrenal insufficiency: fatigue, muscular weakness, joint pain, fever, anorexia, nausea, dyspnea, dizziness, and fainting.

# dexamethasone sodium phosphate (topical)
Decadron Phosphate

*Pharmacologic classification:* corticosteroid
*Therapeutic classification:* anti-inflammatory
*Pregnancy risk category C*

## Available forms
Available by prescription only
*Aerosol:* 0.01%, 0.04%

## Indications and dosages
*Inflammation of corticosteroid-responsive dermatoses*
*Adults and children:* Apply sparingly t.i.d. or q.i.d. For aerosol use on scalp, shake can well and apply to dry scalp after shampooing. Hold can upright. Slide applicator tube under hair so that it touches scalp. Spray while moving tube to all affected areas, keeping tube under hair and in contact with scalp throughout spraying, which should take about 2 seconds. Inadequately covered areas may be spot sprayed. Slide applicator tube through hair to touch scalp; press and immediately release spray button. Don't massage medication into scalp or spray forehead or eyes.

## Mechanism of action
*Anti-inflammatory action:* Dexamethasone is a synthetic fluorinated corticosteroid. It's usually classed as a group VII potency anti-inflammatory. Occlusive dressings may be used in severe cases. The aerosol spray is usually used for dermatologic conditions of the scalp.

## Pharmacokinetics
*Absorption:* Absorption depends on the potency of the preparation, the amount applied, the vehicle used, and the nature of the skin at the application site. It ranges from about 1% in areas with a thick stratum corneum (such as the palms, soles, elbows, and knees) to 25% in areas of the thinnest stratum corneum (face, eyelids, and genitals). Inflamed or damaged skin may absorb more than 33%. Absorption increases in areas of skin damage, inflammation, or occlusion. Some systemic absorption occurs, especially through the oral mucosa.
*Distribution:* After topical administration, dexamethasone is distributed throughout the local skin layer. If absorbed into circulation, drug is distributed rapidly into muscle, liver, skin, intestines, and kidneys.
*Metabolism:* After topical administration, dexamethasone is metabolized primarily in the skin. The small amount that's absorbed into systemic circulation is primarily metabolized in the liver to inactive compounds.
*Excretion:* Inactive metabolites are excreted by the kidneys, primarily as glucuronides and sulfates, but also as unconjugated products. Small amounts of the metabolites are also excreted in feces.

| Route | Onset | Peak | Duration |
|-------|-------|------|----------|
| Topical | Unknown | Unknown | Unknown |

## Contraindications and precautions
Contraindicated in patients hypersensitive to drug.

## Interactions
None significant.

## Adverse reactions
**GU:** glycosuria.
**Metabolic:** hyperglycemia.
**Skin:** burning, pruritus, irritation, dryness, erythema, folliculitis, hypertrichosis, acneiform eruptions, perioral dermatitis, hypopigmentation, allergic contact dermatitis; *maceration, secondary infection, atrophy, striae, miliaria* (with occlusive dressings).
**Other:** *hypothalamic-pituitary-adrenal axis suppression,* Cushing's syndrome.

## Overdose and treatment
Topical corticosteroids can be absorbed in sufficient amounts to produce systemic effects.

## Clinical considerations
- Recommend gently washing skin before applying.
- To prevent skin damage, recommend rubbing cream in gently, leaving a thin coat.
- When treating hairy sites, recommend parting hair and applying directly to lesions.
- Treatment should be continued for a few days after lesions clear, p.r.n.

### Therapeutic monitoring
- Advise patient to stop drug and contact prescriber if skin infection, striae, or atrophy occurs.

### Special populations
The same considerations apply to all patients.

## Patient counseling
- Teach patient and family how to apply drug.
- Inform patient that if occlusive dressings are ordered and a fever develops, he should notify prescriber and remove dressing.
- Advise patient not to leave occlusive dressing on longer than 12 hours each day.
- Tell patient not to use occlusive dressing on infected or exudative lesions.

---

# dexmedetomidine hydrochloride
Precedex

*Pharmacologic classification:* selective alpha₂-adrenoceptor agonist with sedative properties
*Therapeutic classification:* sedative
*Pregnancy risk category C*

## Available forms
Available by prescription only
*Injection:* 100 mcg/ml in 2-ml vials and 2-ml ampules

## Indications and dosages
*Sedation of initially intubated and mechanically ventilated patients in intensive care setting*
*Adults:* Loading infusion of 1 mcg/kg I.V. over 10 minutes; then maintenance infusion of 0.2 to 0.7 mcg/kg/hr for up to 24 hours, adjusted to achieve the desired level of sedation.
≡ *Dosage adjustment.* Patients with renal or hepatic failure and geriatric patients may need dosage adjustment.

## I.V. administration
- Only persons skilled in the management of patients in an intensive care setting, where the patient's cardiac status can be continuously monitored, should give this drug.
- Dexmedetomidine must be diluted in normal saline solution before administration. To prepare the infusion, withdraw 2 ml of dexmedetomidine and add to 48 ml of normal saline injection to a total of 50 ml. Shake gently to mix well.
- Dexmedetomidine infusion has been shown to be compatible with lactated Ringer's, $D_5W$, normal saline in water, and 20% mannitol.
- Administer using a controlled infusion device at the rate calculated for body weight. Don't give infusion for longer than 24 hours.

### Incompatibilities
Don't coadminister dexmedetomidine through the same I.V. catheter with blood or plasma because physical compatibility hasn't been established.

## Mechanism of action
*Sedative action:* Thought to produce sedation by selective stimulation of alpha₂-adrenoceptor in the CNS. Dexmedetomidine is thought to produce sedation by selective stimulation of alpha₂-adrenoceptors in the CNS.

## Pharmacokinetics
*Absorption:* Given parenterally.
*Distribution:* After I.V. administration, rapidly and widely distributed. Drug is 94% protein-bound.
*Metabolism:* Almost completely hepatically metabolized to inactive metabolites.
*Excretion:* 95% of inactive metabolites are eliminated in the kidneys and 4% in feces. Elimination half-life is about 2 hours.

| Route | Onset | Peak | Duration |
|-------|-------|------|----------|
| I.V. | Unknown | Unknown | Unknown |

## Contraindications and precautions
Use cautiously in patients with advanced heart block or renal or hepatic impairment and in geriatric patients.

---

## Interactions
**Drug-drug.** *Anesthetics, hypnotics, opioids, sedatives:* Possible enhanced effects. A reduction of dexmedetomidine dosage may be needed.

## Adverse reactions
**CV:** *hypotension, bradycardia, arrhythmias.*
**GI:** nausea, thirst.
**GU:** oliguria.
**Hematologic:** anemia, leukocytosis.
**Respiratory:** *hypoxia,* pleural effusion, pulmonary edema.
**Other:** pain, infection.

## Overdose and treatment
Bradycardia, hypotension, and first- and second-degree AV block have occurred in patients receiving doses of dexmedetomidine substantially higher than the recommended dosage. These conditions resolved spontaneously. Stopping the infusion, supportive care, and resuscitation, if needed, are the primary treatments for overdose.

## Clinical considerations
■ Drug has been continuously infused in mechanically ventilated patients before extubation, during extubation, and after extubation. It isn't necessary to discontinue drug before extubation.
■ Some patients receiving dexmedetomidine are arousable and alert when stimulated. This alone shouldn't be considered evidence of lack of efficacy in the absence of other clinical signs and symptoms.

### Therapeutic monitoring
■ Advise clinician to continuously monitor cardiac status.
■ Renal and hepatic function should be determined before giving drug, particularly in geriatric patients.

### Special populations
**Breast-feeding patients.** It's unknown if drug appears in breast milk. Because many drugs appear in breast milk, use caution when giving drug to breast-feeding women.
**Pediatric patients.** Safety and effectiveness haven't been established in patients under age 18.
**Geriatric patients.** Bradycardia and hypotension have occurred after giving drug to patients over age 65. Dosage reduction may be considered in this group.

## Patient counseling
■ Tell patient he will be sedated while drug is given, but that he may awaken when stimulated.
■ Tell patient he will be closely monitored while sedated.

# dextroamphetamine sulfate
Dexedrine, DextroStat

*Pharmacologic classification:* amphetamine
*Therapeutic classification:* CNS stimulant, short-term adjunctive anorexigenic agent, sympathomimetic amine
*Pregnancy risk category C*
*Controlled substance schedule II*

## Available forms
Available by prescription only
*Tablets:* 5 mg, 10 mg
*Capsules (sustained-release):* 5 mg, 10 mg, 15 mg

## Indications and dosages
*Narcolepsy*
*Adults:* 5 to 60 mg P.O. daily in divided doses. Long-acting dosage forms allow once-daily dosing.
*Children over age 12:* 10 mg P.O. daily, with 10-mg increments weekly, as indicated.
*Children ages 6 to 12:* 5 mg P.O. daily, with 5-mg increments weekly, as indicated.
◇ *Short-term adjunct in exogenous obesity*
*Adults:* 5 to 30 mg P.O. daily 30 to 60 minutes before meals in divided doses of 5 to 10 mg. Alternatively, give one 10- or 15-mg sustained-release capsule daily as a single dose in the morning.
*Attention deficit hyperactivity disorder*
*Children ages 6 and older:* 5 mg P.O. once daily or b.i.d., with 5-mg increments weekly, p.r.n. Total daily dose should rarely exceed 40 mg.
*Children ages 3 to 5:* 2.5 mg P.O. daily, with 2.5-mg increments weekly p.r.n.; not recommended for children under age 3.

## Mechanism of action
*CNS stimulant action:* Amphetamines are sympathomimetic amines with CNS stimulant activity; in hyperactive children, they have a paradoxical calming effect.
*Anorexigenic action:* Anorexigenic effects are thought to occur in the hypothalamus, where decreased smell and taste acuity decreases appetite. They may be tried for short-term control of refractory obesity, with caloric restriction and behavior modification.

The cerebral cortex and reticular activating system appear to be the primary sites of activity; amphetamines release nerve terminal stores of norepinephrine, promoting nerve impulse transmission. At high dosages, effects are mediated by dopamine.

Amphetamines are used to treat narcolepsy and as adjuncts to psychosocial measures in attention deficit disorder in children. Their precise mechanism of action in these conditions is unknown.

## Pharmacokinetics
*Absorption:* Rapidly absorbed from the GI tract.
*Distribution:* Distributed widely throughout the body.
*Metabolism:* Unknown.
*Excretion:* Excreted in urine.

| Route | Onset | Peak | Duration |
|---|---|---|---|
| P.O. | Unknown | 2 hr | Unknown |
| P.O. (extended) | Unknown | 8-10 hr | Unknown |

## Contraindications and precautions
Contraindicated in patients with hypersensitivity or idiosyncrasy to the sympathomimetic amines, within 14 days of MAO inhibitor therapy, and in those with hyperthyroidism, moderate to severe hypertension, symptomatic CV disease, glaucoma, advanced arteriosclerosis, and history of drug abuse. Use cautiously in patients with motor and phonic tics, Tourette syndrome, and agitated states.

## Interactions
**Drug-drug.** *Acetazolamide, alkalizing drugs, antacids, sodium bicarbonate:* Enhance renal reabsorption. Advise clinician to monitor patient for enhanced amphetamine effects.
*Acidifying agents, ammonium chloride, ascorbic acid:* Enhance dextroamphetamine excretion and shorten duration of action. Advise clinician to monitor patient for decreased amphetamine effects.
*Adrenergic blockers:* Inhibited by amphetamines. Avoid use together.
*Antihypertensives:* May antagonize antihypertensive effects. Avoid use together.
*Barbiturates:* Antagonize dextroamphetamine by CNS depression. Avoid use together.
*Chlorpromazine:* Inhibits the central stimulant effects of amphetamines. May be used to treat amphetamine poisoning.
*CNS stimulants, haloperidol, phenothiazines, theophylline, tricyclic antidepressants:* Increase CNS effects. Avoid use together.
*Insulin, oral antidiabetics:* Dextroamphetamine may alter requirements. Advise clinician to monitor blood glucose levels.
*Lithium carbonate:* May inhibit antiobesity and stimulating effects of amphetamines. Advise clinician to monitor patient closely.
*MAO inhibitors:* May cause hypertensive crisis. Don't use together or within 14 days after MAO inhibitor has been discontinued.
*Meperidine:* Amphetamines potentiate the analgesic effect. Use together cautiously.
*Methenamine:* Increases urinary excretion of amphetamines and reduces efficacy. Advise clinician to monitor patient closely.
*Norepinephrine:* Amphetamines enhance the adrenergic effect. Advise clinician to monitor patient closely.

*Phenobarbital, phenytoin:* May produce a synergistic anticonvulsant action. Advise clinician to monitor patient closely.
**Drug-food.** *Caffeine:* May increase amphetamine and related amine effects. Advise patient to use cautiously.

## Adverse reactions
**CNS:** *restlessness,* tremor, *insomnia,* dizziness, headache, chills, overstimulation, dysphoria, euphoria.
**CV:** *tachycardia, palpitations,* hypertension, *arrhythmias.*
**GI:** dry mouth, unpleasant taste, diarrhea, constipation, anorexia, weight loss, other GI disturbances.
**GU:** impotence.
**Skin:** urticaria.
**Other:** altered libido.

## Overdose and treatment
Individual responses to overdose vary widely. Toxic symptoms may occur at 15 and 30 mg and can cause severe reactions; however, doses of 400 mg or more have not always proved fatal.

Signs and symptoms of overdose include restlessness, tremor, hyperreflexia, tachypnea, confusion, aggressiveness, hallucinations, and panic; fatigue and depression usually follow excitement stage. Other signs and symptoms may include arrhythmias, shock, alterations in blood pressure, nausea, vomiting, diarrhea, and abdominal cramps; death is usually preceded by seizures and coma.

Treat overdose symptomatically and supportively: if ingestion is recent (within 4 hours), use gastric lavage or emesis and sedate with a barbiturate; advise clinician to monitor vital signs and fluid and electrolyte balance. Urinary acidification may enhance excretion. Saline catharsis (magnesium citrate) may hasten GI evacuation of unabsorbed sustained-release drug.

## Clinical considerations
■ Drug may elevate plasma corticosteroid levels and may interfere with urinary steroid determinations.
■ Give dextroamphetamine 30 to 60 minutes before meals when using as an anorexigenic drug. To minimize insomnia, avoid giving within 6 hours of bedtime.
■ For narcolepsy, patient should take first dose on awakening.

### Therapeutic monitoring
■ Advise clinician to take vital signs regularly, and observe patient for signs of excessive stimulation.
■ When tolerance to anorexigenic effect develops, dosage should be discontinued, not increased.

■ Advise clinician to monitor blood and urine glucose levels. Drug may alter daily insulin requirement in patients with diabetes.

### Special populations
**Breast-feeding patients.** Safety hasn't been established. Alternative feeding method is recommended during therapy with dextroamphetamine sulfate.
**Pediatric patients.** Drug isn't recommended for treatment of obesity in children under age 12.
**Geriatric patients.** Use lower doses in geriatric patients. Avoid using drug in geriatric patients with CV, CNS, or GI disturbances.

### Patient counseling
■ Teach parents to provide drug-free periods for children with attention deficit disorder, especially during periods of reduced stress.
■ Warn patient to avoid hazardous activities that require alertness until CNS response is determined.
■ Instruct patient to take drug early in the day to minimize insomnia.
■ Tell patient not to crush sustained-release forms or to increase dosage.

# dextromethorphan hydrobromide
Balminil D.M.*, Benylin DM, Broncho-Grippol-DM*, Delsym, Dimetapp, Koffex*, Neo-DM*, Robidex*, Robitussin Nighttime, Sedatuss*, St. Joseph Cold Tablets for Children, Sucrets Cough Control, Suppress, Thera-Flu, Trocal, Vicks Formula 44

*Pharmacologic classification:* levorphanol derivative (dextrorotatory methyl ether)
*Therapeutic classification:* antitussive (nonnarcotic)
*Pregnancy risk category C*

### Available forms
Available without a prescription
*Syrup:* 10 mg/5 ml, 15 mg/15 ml
*Solution:* 3.5 mg/5 ml, 5 mg/5 ml, 7.5 mg/5 ml, 10 mg/5 ml, 12.5 mg/5 ml, 15 mg/5 ml
*Lozenges:* 5 mg, 7.5 mg, 15 mg
*Tablets:* 200 mg
*Capsules (liquid-filled):* 30 mg

### Indications and dosages
*Nonproductive cough (chronic)*
*Adults and children ages 12 and older:* 10 to 20 mg P.O. q 4 hours; or 30 mg q 6 to 8 hours; or controlled-release liquid b.i.d. (60 mg b.i.d.). Maximum dose is 120 mg daily.

*Children ages 6 to 12:* 5 to 10 mg P.O. q 4 hours; or 15 mg q 6 to 8 hours; or controlled-release liquid b.i.d. (30 mg b.i.d.). Maximum dose is 60 mg daily.
*Children ages 2 to 6:* 2.5 to 5 mg P.O. q 4 hours; or 7.5 mg q 6 to 8 hours; or sustained-action liquid 15 mg b.i.d. Maximum dose is 30 mg daily.

### Mechanism of action
*Antitussive action:* Dextromethorphan suppresses the cough reflex by direct action on the cough center in the medulla. Dextromethorphan is almost equal in antitussive potency to codeine but causes no analgesia or addiction and little or no CNS depression and has no expectorant action; it also produces fewer subjective and GI adverse effects than codeine. Treatment is intended to relieve cough frequency without abolishing protective cough reflex. In therapeutic doses, drug doesn't inhibit ciliary activity.

### Pharmacokinetics
*Absorption:* Absorbed readily from the GI tract.
*Distribution:* Unknown.
*Metabolism:* Metabolized extensively by the liver. Plasma half-life is about 11 hours.
*Excretion:* Little is excreted unchanged. Metabolites are excreted primarily in urine; about 7% to 10% is excreted in feces.

| Route | Onset | Peak | Duration |
|-------|-------|------|----------|
| P.O. | < ½ hr | Unknown | 3-6 hr |

### Contraindications and precautions
Contraindicated during or within 2 weeks of MAO inhibitor therapy. Use cautiously in atopic children, sedated or debilitated patients, and those patients confined to the supine position. Also use cautiously in patients sensitive to aspirin.

### Interactions
**Drug-drug.** *MAO inhibitors:* May cause nausea, hypotension, excitation, hyperpyrexia, and coma. Don't give dextromethorphan to patients at any interval less than 2 weeks after MAO inhibitors are discontinued.
*Selegiline:* May cause confusion, coma, or hyperpyrexia. Avoid use together.
**Drug-herb.** *Parsley:* May promote or produce serotonin syndrome. Advise patient not to use together.

### Adverse reactions
**CNS:** drowsiness, dizziness.
**GI:** nausea, vomiting, stomach pain.

### Overdose and treatment
Signs and symptoms of overdose may include nausea, vomiting, drowsiness, dizziness, blurred vision, nystagmus, shallow respirations, urine retention, toxic psychosis, stupor, and coma.

Treatment of overdose involves giving activated charcoal to reduce drug absorption and I.V. naloxone to support respiration. Other symptoms are treated supportively.

## Clinical considerations
- Treatment is intended to relieve cough intensity and frequency, without completely abolishing the protective cough reflex.
- May be used with percussion and chest vibration.

### Therapeutic monitoring
- Nature and frequency of coughing should be noted.

### Special populations
**Breast-feeding patients.** Safety hasn't been established.
**Pediatric patients.** Don't use syrup, tablets, or lozenges in children under age 2. Sustained-action liquid may be used in children under age 2, but dosage must be individualized.

## Patient counseling
- Tell patient to report persistent cough of longer than 7 days.
- Instruct patient to use sugarless throat lozenges for throat irritation and resulting cough.
- Recommend a humidifier to filter out dust, smoke, and air pollutants.

---

# diazepam
Apo-Diazepam*, Diastat, Novodipam*, Valium, Vivol*

*Pharmacologic classification:* benzodiazepine
*Therapeutic classification:* anxiolytic; skeletal muscle relaxant; amnesic; anticonvulsant; sedative-hypnotic
*Pregnancy risk category D*
*Controlled substance schedule IV*

## Available forms
Available by prescription only
*Tablets:* 2 mg, 5 mg, 10 mg
*Capsules (extended-release):* 15 mg
*Oral solution:* 5 mg/ml; 5 mg/5 ml, 10 mg/10 ml
*Injection:* 5 mg/ml in ampules, vials, and disposable syringes
*Rectal gel:* 2.5 mg, 5 mg, 10 mg, 15 mg, 20 mg twin packs

## Indications and dosages
### Anxiety
*Adults:* Depending on severity, 2 to 10 mg P.O. b.i.d. to q.i.d. or 15 to 30 mg extended-release capsules P.O. once daily. Alternatively, 2 to 10 mg I.M. or I.V. q 3 to 4 hours, p.r.n.

*Children ages 6 months and older:* 1 to 2.5 mg P.O. t.i.d. or q.i.d.; increase dose gradually, as needed and tolerated.
### Acute alcohol withdrawal
*Adults:* 10 mg P.O. t.i.d. or q.i.d. for the first 24 hours; reduce to 5 mg t.i.d. or q.i.d., p.r.n.; or 10 mg I.M. or I.V. initially, followed by 5 to 10 mg q 3 to 4 hours, p.r.n.
### Muscle spasm
*Adults:* 2 to 10 mg P.O. b.i.d. to q.i.d.; or 15 to 30 mg extended-release capsules once daily. Alternatively, 5 to 10 mg I.M. or I.V. q 3 to 4 hours, p.r.n.
### Tetanus
*Infants over age 30 days to children age 5:* 1 to 2 mg I.M. or I.V. slowly, repeated q 3 to 4 hours.
*Children ages 5 and older:* 5 to 10 mg I.M. or I.V. slowly q 3 to 4 hours, p.r.n.
### Adjunct to convulsive disorders
*Adults:* 2 to 10 mg P.O. b.i.d. to q.i.d.
*Children ages 6 months and older:* Initially, 1 to 2.5 mg P.O. t.i.d. or q.i.d.; increase dose as tolerated and needed.
### Adjunct to anesthesia, endoscopic procedures
*Adults:* 5 to 10 mg I.M. before surgery; or give I.V. slowly just before procedure, titrating dose to effect. Usually, less than 10 mg is used, but up to 20 mg may be given.
### Cardioversion
*Adults:* Give 5 to 15 mg I.V. 5 to 10 minutes before procedure.
### Status epilepticus
*Adults:* 5 to 10 mg I.V. (preferred) or I.M. initially, repeated at 10- to 15-minute intervals up to a maximum dose of 30 mg. Repeat q 2 to 4 hours, p.r.n.
*Children ages 5 and older:* 1 mg I.V. q 2 to 5 minutes up to a maximum dose of 10 mg; repeat in 2 to 4 hours, p.r.n.
*Infants over age 30 days to children age 5:* 0.2 to 0.5 mg I.V. q 2 to 5 minutes up to a maximum dose of 5 mg.
### Control of acute repetitive seizure activity in patients already taking antiepileptics
*Children ages 12 and older:* 0.2 mg/kg P.R. using applicator. A second dose may be given 4 to 12 hours after the first dose, if needed.
*Children ages 6 to 11:* 0.3 mg/kg P.R. using applicator. A second dose may be given 4 to 12 hours after the first dose, if needed.
*Children ages 2 to 5:* 0.5 mg/kg P.R. using applicator. A second dose may be given 4 to 12 hours after the first dose, if needed.

## I.V. administration
- I.V. route provides rapid and more uniform absorption.
- Don't mix diazepam with other drugs.
- Parenteral forms of diazepam may be diluted in normal saline solution; a slight precipitate may form, but the solution can still be used.

---

■ Recommend infusing drug slowly, directly into a large vein, not exceeding 5 mg/minute for adults or 0.25 mg/kg of body weight over 3 minutes for children. To avoid extravasation into S.C. tissue, diazepam shouldn't be injected into small veins. Infusion site should be observed for phlebitis. If direct I.V. administration isn't possible, recommend injecting diazepam directly into I.V. tubing at point closest to vein insertion site to prevent extravasation.

■ Administration by continuous I.V. infusion isn't recommended.

■ Patient should remain in bed under observation for at least 3 hours after parenteral administration of diazepam to prevent potential hazards; keep resuscitation equipment nearby.

### Incompatibilities
Incompatible with all other drugs and most I.V. solutions.

### Mechanism of action
*Amnesic action:* The exact mechanism of action is unknown.
*Anticonvulsant action:* Diazepam suppresses the spread of seizure activity produced by epileptogenic foci in the cortex, thalamus, and limbic structures by enhancing presynaptic inhibition.
*Anxiolytic and sedative-hypnotic actions:* Diazepam depresses the CNS at the limbic and subcortical levels of the brain. It produces an antianxiety effect by influencing the effect of the neurotransmitter gamma-aminobutyric acid on its receptor in the ascending reticular activating system, which increases inhibition and blocks cortical and limbic arousal.
*Skeletal muscle relaxant action:* The exact mechanism is unknown, but it's believed to inhibit polysynaptic afferent pathways.

### Pharmacokinetics
*Absorption:* When given orally, drug is absorbed through the GI tract. I.M. administration results in erratic absorption of the drug. Drug is well absorbed rectally and reaches peak plasma levels in 1½ hours.
*Distribution:* Distributed widely throughout the body. About 85% to 95% of a given dose is plasma protein–bound.
*Metabolism:* Metabolized in the liver to the active metabolite desmethyldiazepam.
*Excretion:* Most metabolites of diazepam are excreted in urine, with only small amounts excreted in feces. Half-life of desmethyldiazepam is 30 to 200 hours. Duration of sedative effect is 3 hours; this may be prolonged up to 90 hours in elderly patients and in patients with hepatic or renal dysfunction. Anti-convulsant effect is 30 to 60 minutes after I.V. administration.

| Route | Onset | Peak | Duration |
|-------|-------|------|----------|
| P.O. | ½ | 2 hr | 3-8 hr |
| I.V. | 1-5 min | Immediate | 15-60 min |
| I.M. | Unknown | 2 hr | Unknown |
| P.R. | Unknown | 1-5 hr | Unknown |

### Contraindications and precautions
Contraindicated in patients hypersensitive to drug and in those with angle-closure glaucoma. Also contraindicated in patients experiencing shock, coma, or acute alcohol intoxication (parenteral form); and in children under age 6 months (oral form).

Use cautiously in geriatric and debilitated patients, and in those with impaired hepatic or renal function, depression, or chronic open-angle glaucoma. Avoid use in pregnant women, especially during the first trimester.

### Interactions
**Drug-drug.** *Antacids:* Decrease the rate of absorption of diazepam. Avoid use together.
*Antidepressants, antihistamines, barbiturates, general anesthetics, MAO inhibitors, narcotics, phenothiazines:* Diazepam potentiates the CNS depressant effects. Avoid use together.
*Cimetidine, possibly disulfiram:* Diminished hepatic metabolism of diazepam, which increases its plasma level. Advise clinician to monitor patient closely.
*Digoxin:* Diazepam may decrease digoxin clearance. Advise clinician to monitor patient for digoxin toxicity.
*Haloperidol:* May change the seizure patterns; benzodiazepines also may reduce the serum levels of haloperidol. Avoid use together.
*Levodopa:* Diazepam may inhibit the therapeutic effect of levodopa. Advise clinician to monitor patient carefully.
*Nondepolarizing neuromuscular blockers, such as pancuronium and succinylcholine:* Intensified and prolonged respiratory depression. Don't use together.
*Oral contraceptives:* May impair the metabolism of diazepam. Advise clinician to monitor patient closely.
**Drug-herb.** *Catnip, kava, lady's slipper, lemon balm, passion flower, sassafras, skullcap, valerian:* Sedative effects may be enhanced. Discourage use together.
**Drug-lifestyle.** *Alcohol use:* Diazepam potentiates the CNS depressant effects of alcohol. Advise patient to avoid use together.
*Heavy smoking:* Accelerates metabolism of diazepam, lowering clinical effectiveness. Advise patient to avoid use together.

### Adverse reactions
**CNS:** *drowsiness,* slurred speech, tremor, transient amnesia, fatigue, ataxia, headache, insom-

nia, paradoxical anxiety, hallucinations, changes in EEG patterns.
**CV:** hypotension, *CV collapse, bradycardia.*
**EENT:** diplopia, blurred vision, nystagmus.
**GI:** nausea, constipation.
**GU:** incontinence, urine retention.
**Hematologic:** *neutropenia.*
**Hepatic:** elevated liver function test results, *jaundice.*
**Musculoskeletal:** *dysarthria.*
**Respiratory:** *respiratory depression.*
**Skin:** rash, *pain, phlebitis* (at injection site).
**Other:** physical or psychological dependence, *acute withdrawal syndrome* after sudden discontinuation in physically dependent persons, altered libido.

## Overdose and treatment

Signs and symptoms of overdose include somnolence, confusion, coma, hypoactive reflexes, dyspnea, labored breathing, hypotension, bradycardia, slurred speech, and unsteady gait or impaired coordination.

Recommend supporting blood pressure and respiration until drug effects subside and monitoring vital signs. Mechanical ventilatory assistance via endotracheal tube may be required to maintain a patent airway and support adequate oxygenation. Flumazenil, a specific benzodiazepine antagonist, may be useful, but shouldn't be given during status epilepticus. Use I.V. fluids and vasopressors such as dopamine and phenylephrine to treat hypotension, p.r.n. If patient is conscious, recommend inducing emesis; use gastric lavage if ingestion was recent, but only if an endotracheal tube is present to prevent aspiration. After emesis or lavage, recommend giving activated charcoal with a cathartic as a single dose. Dialysis is of limited value.

## Clinical considerations

■ Don't discontinue drug suddenly; decrease dosage slowly over 8 to 12 weeks after long-term therapy.
■ To enhance taste, oral solution can be mixed with liquids or semisolid foods, such as applesauce or pudding, immediately before administration.
■ Extended-release capsule should be swallowed whole; don't let patient crush or chew it.
■ Shake oral suspension well before administering.
■ When prescribing with opiates for endoscopic procedures, reduce opiate dose by at least one-third.
■ Inject I.M. dose deep into deltoid muscle. Aspirate for backflow to prevent inadvertent intra-arterial administration. Use I.M. route only if I.V. or oral routes are unavailable.
■ Diazepam interacts with plastic. Don't store diazepam in plastic syringes or give it in plastic administration sets, which decreases availability of the infused drug.

■ Lower doses are effective in patients with renal or hepatic dysfunction.
■ Anticipate possible transient increase in frequency or severity of seizures when diazepam is used as adjunctive treatment of convulsive disorders. Impose seizure precautions.
■ Don't mix diazepam with other drugs in a syringe or infusion container.
■ Use Diastat rectal gel to treat no more than five episodes per month and no more than one episode every 5 days.

### Therapeutic monitoring

■ During prolonged therapy, advise clinician to periodically monitor blood counts and liver function test results.
■ Advise clinician to assess gag reflex postendoscopy and before resuming oral intake to prevent aspiration.

### Special populations

**Pregnant patients.** Warn patient to call her prescriber immediately if she becomes pregnant.
**Breast-feeding patients.** Diazepam appears in breast milk. The breast-fed infant of a woman who uses diazepam may become sedated, have feeding difficulties, or lose weight. Avoid use of drug in breast-feeding women.
**Pediatric patients.** Safe use of oral diazepam in infants under age 6 months hasn't been established. Safe use of parenteral diazepam in infants under age 30 days hasn't been established. Closely observe neonates whose mothers took diazepam for a prolonged period during pregnancy; the infants may show withdrawal symptoms. Use of rectal diazepam during labor may cause neonatal flaccidity. Safety and efficacy of rectal diazepam haven't been established in children under age 2.
**Geriatric patients.** Geriatric patients are more sensitive to the CNS depressant effects of diazepam. Use with caution. Lower doses are usually effective in geriatric patients because of decreased elimination. Geriatric patients who receive this drug require assistance with walking and activities of daily living when therapy starts or changes. Parenteral administration of this drug is more likely to cause apnea, hypotension, and bradycardia in geriatric patients.

### Patient counseling

■ Advise patient of the potential for physical and psychological dependence with long-term use.
■ Warn patient that sudden changes of position can cause dizziness. Advise patient to dangle legs for a few minutes before getting out of bed to prevent falls and injury.
■ Caution patient to avoid alcohol while taking diazepam.
■ Advise patient not to stop drug abruptly.

---

- Teach patient's caregiver when to use rectal gel (to control bouts of increased seizure activity) and how to monitor and record patient's clinical response.
- Teach patient's caregiver how to administer rectal gel.

# diazoxide
Hyperstat IV, Proglycem

*Pharmacologic classification:* peripheral vasodilator
*Therapeutic classification:* antihypertensive, antihypoglycemic
*Pregnancy risk category C*

## Available forms
Available by prescription only
*Capsules:* 50 mg
*Oral suspension:* 50 mg/ml in 30-ml bottle
*Injection:* 15 mg/ml in 20-ml ampule

## Indications and dosages
**Hypertensive crisis**
*Adults and children:* 1 to 3 mg/kg I.V. (up to a maximum of 150 mg) q 5 to 15 minutes until an adequate reduction in blood pressure is achieved.
**Hypoglycemia from hyperinsulinism**
*Adults and children:* Usual daily dose is 3 to 8 mg/kg/day P.O. divided in two or three equal doses.
*Infants and newborns:* Usual daily dose is 8 to 15 mg/kg/day P.O. divided in two or three equal doses.

## I.V. administration
- Drug may be given by constant I.V. infusion (7.5 to 30 mg/minute) until adequate blood pressure reduction occurs.
- I.V. use of diazoxide is rarely needed for longer than 4 or 5 days.
- After I.V. injection, advise clinician to monitor blood pressure every 5 minutes for 15 to 30 minutes, then hourly when patient is stable. Drug should be stopped if severe hypotension develops or if blood pressure continues to decrease 30 minutes after drug infusion; advise clinician to keep patient recumbent during this time and have norepinephrine available. Advise clinician to monitor I.V. site for infiltration or extravasation.
- The use of 300-mg I.V. bolus push is no longer recommended. Switch to therapy with oral antihypertensives as soon as possible.

### Incompatibilities
Incompatible with hydralazine and propranolol.

## Mechanism of action
*Antihypertensive action:* Diazoxide directly relaxes arteriolar smooth muscle, causing vasodilation and reducing peripheral vascular resistance, thus reducing blood pressure.
*Antihypoglycemic action:* Diazoxide increases blood glucose levels by inhibiting pancreatic secretion of insulin, by stimulating catecholamine release, or by increasing hepatic release of glucose.

Diazoxide is a nondiuretic congener of thiazide diuretics.

## Pharmacokinetics
*Absorption:* After I.V. administration, blood pressure should decrease promptly, with maximum decrease in under 5 minutes. After oral administration, hyperglycemic effect begins in 1 hour.
*Distribution:* Distributed throughout the body; highest level is found in kidneys, liver, and adrenal glands; diazoxide crosses placenta and blood-brain barrier. Drug is about 90% protein-bound.
*Metabolism:* Metabolized partially in the liver.
*Excretion:* Excreted slowly by the kidneys. Duration of antihypertensive effect varies widely, ranging from 30 minutes to 72 hours (average 3 to 12 hours) after I.V. administration; after oral administration, antihypoglycemic effect persists for about 8 hours. Antihypertensive and antihypoglycemic effects may be prolonged in patients with renal dysfunction.

| Route | Onset | Peak | Duration |
|-------|-------|------|----------|
| P.O. | Unknown | Unknown | Unknown |
| I.V. | 1 min | 2-5 min | 2-12 hr |

## Contraindications and precautions
Parenteral form is contraindicated in patients hypersensitive to drug, other thiazides, or sulfonamide-derived drugs, and in the treatment of compensatory hypertension (such as that with coarctation of the aorta or arteriovenous shunt). Oral form is contraindicated in patients with functional hypoglycemia.

Use cautiously in patients with uremia or impaired cerebral or cardiac function.

## Interactions
**Drug-drug.** *Antihypertensives:* Diazoxide may potentiate antihypertensive effects; especially if I.V. diazoxide is given within 6 hours after patient has received another antihypertensive. Use together cautiously.
*Diuretics:* May potentiate antihypoglycemic, hyperuricemic, or antihypertensive effects of diazoxide. Advise clinician to monitor patient closely.
*Insulin, oral antidiabetics:* Diazoxide may alter insulin and oral antidiabetic requirements in previously stable diabetic patients. Advise clinician to monitor blood glucose levels.
*Phenytoin:* May increase metabolism and decrease the plasma protein–binding of phenytoin. Advise clinician to monitor patient closely.

*Thiazides:* May enhance effects of diazoxide. Use together cautiously.
*Warfarin:* Diazoxide may displace warfarin, bilirubin, or other highly protein-bound substances from protein-binding sites. Avoid use together.

## Adverse reactions
**CNS:** dizziness, weakness; headache, malaise, anxiety, insomnia, paresthesia (with oral form); headache, *seizures, paralysis, cerebral ischemia,* light-headedness, euphoria (with parenteral form).
**CV:** *arrhythmias,* tachycardia, hypotension, hypertension (with oral form); *sodium and water retention, orthostatic hypotension,* angina, myocardial ischemia, ECG changes, *shock, MI* (with parenteral form).
**EENT:** diplopia, transient cataracts, blurred vision, lacrimation (with oral administration), optic nerve infarction (with parenteral form).
**GI:** abdominal discomfort, diarrhea; nausea, vomiting, anorexia, taste alteration (with oral form); *nausea, vomiting,* dry mouth, constipation (with parenteral form).
**GU:** azotemia, reversible nephrotic syndrome, decreased urine output, hematuria, albuminuria (with oral administration).
**Hematologic:** *leukopenia, thrombocytopenia,* anemia, eosinophilia, excessive bleeding (with oral administration).
**Metabolic:** *sodium and fluid retention, ketoacidosis and hyperosmolar nonketotic syndrome, hyperuricemia, hyperglycemia.*
**Skin:** rash, pruritus (with oral administration), diaphoresis, flushing, warmth, hirsutism, inflammation and pain resulting from extravasation.
**Other:** fever (with oral administration).

## Overdose and treatment
Overdose is manifested primarily by hyperglycemia; ketoacidosis and hypotension may occur.
  Treatment of acute overdose is supportive and symptomatic. If hyperglycemia develops, recommend giving insulin and replacing fluid and electrolyte losses; use vasopressors if hypotension fails to respond to conservative treatment. Prolonged monitoring may be needed because of the long half-life of diazoxide.

## Clinical considerations
■ Diazoxide is used to treat only hypoglycemia resulting from hyperinsulinism; it isn't used to treat functional hypoglycemia. It may be used temporarily to control preoperative or postoperative hypoglycemia in patients with hyperinsulinism.
■ Significant hypotension doesn't occur after oral administration in doses used to treat hypoglycemia.

■ Diazoxide inhibits glucose-stimulated insulin release and may cause false-negative insulin response to glucagon.

### Therapeutic monitoring
■ Advise clinician to monitor blood pressure and ECG continuously and keep norepinephrine available.
■ Advise clinician to monitor intake and output carefully. If fluid or sodium retention develops, diuretics may be given 30 to 60 minutes after diazoxide. Patient must be recumbent for 8 to 10 hours after diuretic administration.
■ Advise clinician to monitor daily blood glucose and electrolyte levels, watching diabetic patients closely for severe hyperglycemia or hyperglycemic hyperosmolar nonketotic coma; also advise clinician to monitor daily urine glucose and ketone levels, intake and output, and weight and check serum uric acid levels frequently.

### Special populations
**Breast-feeding patients.** It isn't known if drug appears in breast milk; an alternative feeding method is recommended during therapy.
**Pediatric patients.** Use with caution in children.
**Geriatric patients.** Geriatric patients may have a more pronounced hypotensive response.

## Patient counseling
■ Explain that orthostatic hypotension can be minimized by rising slowly and avoiding sudden position changes.
■ Tell patient to report adverse effects immediately, including pain and redness at injection site, which may indicate infiltration.
■ Instruct patient to check weight daily and report gains of more than 5 lb/week; diazoxide causes sodium and water retention.
■ Reassure patient that excessive hair growth is a common reaction that subsides when drug treatment is completed.

# dibucaine
Nupercainal

*Pharmacologic classification:* local anesthetic (amine)
*Therapeutic classification:* local amide anesthetic
*Pregnancy risk category B*

## Available forms
Available without a prescription
*Ointment (rectal or topical):* 1%
*Cream (topical):* 0.5%

## Indications and dosages
*Temporary relief from pain and itching associated with abrasions, sunburn, minor*

*burns, insect bites, and other minor skin conditions*
*Adults and children:* Apply to affected areas, p.r.n. Maximum daily dose of 1% ointment is 30 g for adults and 7.5 g for children.
*Temporary relief from pain, itching, and burning caused by hemorrhoids*
*Adults:* Instill 1% ointment into rectum using a rectal applicator each morning and evening and after each bowel movement, p.r.n. Apply additional ointment topically to anal tissues. Maximum daily dose is 30 g.

## Mechanism of action
*Anesthetic action:* Dibucaine inhibits conduction of nerve impulses and decreases cell membrane permeability to ions, anesthetizing local nerve endings.

## Pharmacokinetics
*Absorption:* Dibucaine has limited absorption.
*Distribution:* None.
*Metabolism:* None.
*Excretion:* None.

| Route | Onset | Peak | Duration |
|---|---|---|---|
| Topical, P.R. | Unknown | Unknown | Unknown |

## Contraindications and precautions
Contraindicated in patients hypersensitive to drug, sulfites, or other amide-type local anesthetics and for use on large skin areas, on broken skin or mucous membranes, and in eyes.

## Interactions
None reported.

## Adverse reactions
**Skin:** irritation, inflammation, contact dermatitis, cutaneous lesions.
**Other:** hypersensitivity reactions (urticaria, edema, burning, stinging, tenderness).

## Overdose and treatment
If overdose occurs, area should be cleaned thoroughly with mild soap and water.

## Clinical considerations
■ Use dibucaine topically only for short periods.
■ Don't use in or near the eye.
■ Discontinue drug if sensitization occurs or if condition worsens.

### Therapeutic monitoring
■ If rectal bleeding, rash, pain, swelling, or other symptoms develop, notify prescriber immediately and discontinue use of drug.

### Special populations
**Breast-feeding patients.** Drug shouldn't be used in breast-feeding women.
**Pediatric patients.** Dosage may be adjusted to patient's age, size, and physical condition.

**Geriatric patients.** Dosage may be adjusted to patient's age, size, and physical condition.

## Patient counseling
■ Advise patient to call prescriber if condition worsens or if symptoms persist for longer than 7 days after use.
■ Explain correct use of drug.
■ Emphasize need to wash hands thoroughly after use.
■ Caution patient to apply drug sparingly to minimize untoward effects.
■ Tell patient to keep drug out of reach of children.

# diclofenac potassium
Cataflam
# diclofenac sodium
Voltaren, Voltaren-XR

*Pharmacologic classification:* NSAID
*Therapeutic classification:* antarthritic, anti-inflammatory
*Pregnancy risk category B*

## Available forms
Available by prescription only
**diclofenac potassium**
*Tablets:* 50 mg
**diclofenac sodium**
*Tablets (delayed-release):* 25 mg, 50 mg, 75 mg
*Tablets (extended-release):* 100 mg
*Ophthalmic drops:* 0.1%

## Indications and dosages
*Osteoarthritis*
*Adults:* 50 mg P.O. b.i.d. or t.i.d., or 75 mg P.O. b.i.d. (diclofenac sodium only).
*Ankylosing spondylitis*
*Adults:* 25 mg P.O. q.i.d. An additional 25 mg dose may be needed h.s.
*Rheumatoid arthritis*
*Adults:* 50 mg P.O. t.i.d. or q.i.d. Alternatively, 75 mg P.O. b.i.d. (diclofenac sodium only).
*Analgesia and primary dysmenorrhea*
*Adults:* 50 mg (diclofenac potassium only) P.O. t.i.d. Alternatively, 100 mg (diclofenac potassium only) P.O. initially, followed by 50 mg doses, up to a maximum dose of 200 mg in first 24 hours; subsequent dosing should follow 50 mg t.i.d. regimen.

## Mechanism of action
*Anti-inflammatory action:* Diclofenac exerts its anti-inflammatory and antipyretic actions through an unknown mechanism that may involve inhibition of prostaglandin synthesis.

## Pharmacokinetics

**Absorption:** After oral administration, diclofenac is rapidly and almost completely absorbed. Absorption is delayed by food.

**Distribution:** Highly protein-bound.

**Metabolism:** Undergoes first-pass metabolism, with 60% of unchanged drug reaching systemic circulation. The principal active metabolite, 48-hydroxydiclofenac, has about 3% of the activity of the parent compound. Mean terminal half-life is about $1\frac{1}{4}$ to $1\frac{3}{4}$ hours after an oral dose.

**Excretion:** About 40% to 60% is excreted in the urine; the balance is excreted in the bile. The 4'-hydroxy metabolite accounts for 20% to 30% of the dose excreted in the urine; the other metabolites account for 10% to 20%; 5% to 10% is excreted unchanged in the urine. More than 90% is excreted within 72 hours. Moderate renal impairment doesn't alter the elimination rate of unchanged diclofenac but may reduce the elimination rate of the metabolites. Hepatic impairment doesn't appear to affect the pharmacokinetics of diclofenac.

| Route | Onset | Peak | Duration |
|---|---|---|---|
| P.O. | 10 min | 1 hr | 8 hr |
| P.O. (enteric) | 30 min | 2-3 hr | 8 hr |
| P.O. (extended-release) | Unknown | Unknown | Unknown |

## Contraindications and precautions

Oral form is contraindicated in patients hypersensitive to drug and in those with hepatic porphyria or a history of asthma, urticaria, or other allergic reactions after taking aspirin or other NSAIDs. Avoid use during late pregnancy or while breast-feeding. Ophthalmic solution is contraindicated in patients hypersensitive to any component of the drug and in those wearing soft contact lenses; also avoid use during late pregnancy.

Use oral form cautiously in patients with history of peptic ulcer disease, hepatic or renal dysfunction, cardiac disease, hypertension, or conditions with fluid retention.

Use ophthalmic solution cautiously in patients hypersensitive to aspirin, phenyl-acetic acid derivatives, and other NSAIDs and in surgical patients with known bleeding tendencies or in those receiving drugs that may prolong bleeding time.

## Interactions

**Drug-drug.** *Aspirin:* Lowers plasma levels of diclofenac. Use together isn't recommended.

*Beta blockers:* May blunt antihypertensive effects. Don't use together.

*Cyclosporine, digoxin, methotrexate:* Increases the toxicity of these drugs. Advise clinician to monitor patient and serum levels closely.

*Diuretics:* Concurrent use of diclofenac may inhibit the action of diuretics. Advise clinician to monitor patient closely.

*Insulin, oral antidiabetics:* May alter the patient's response to these drugs. Advise clinician to monitor blood glucose levels closely.

*Lithium:* Decreases renal clearance of lithium and increases plasma levels; may lead to lithium toxicity. Advise clinician to monitor serum levels closely.

*Phenytoin:* May increase serum levels. Advise clinician to monitor patient for toxicity.

*Potassium-sparing diuretics:* May increase serum potassium levels. Advise clinician to monitor serum potassium levels closely.

*Warfarin:* Affects platelet function. Requires close monitoring of anticoagulant dosage.

**Drug-herb.** *Dong quai, feverfew, garlic, ginger, horse chestnut, red clover:* Possible increased risk of bleeding. Discourage use together.

*Dong quai, St. John's wort:* Increased risk of photosensitivity. Advise patient to avoid unprotected exposure to sunlight.

**Drug-lifestyle.** *Sun exposure:* May cause photosensitivity reactions. Advise patient to take precautions.

## Adverse reactions

Unless otherwise noted, the following adverse reactions refer to oral administration of drug:

**CNS:** anxiety, depression, dizziness, drowsiness, insomnia, irritability, headache.

**CV:** *HF,* hypertension, edema, fluid retention.

**EENT:** *tinnitus,* laryngeal edema, swelling of the lips and tongue, blurred vision, eye pain, night blindness, epistaxis, reversible hearing loss; *transient stinging and burning, increased intraocular pressure, keratitis,* anterior chamber reaction, ocular allergy (with ophthalmic solution).

**GI:** *abdominal pain or cramps, constipation, diarrhea, indigestion, nausea,* vomiting, abdominal distention, flatulence, peptic ulceration, *bleeding,* melena, bloody diarrhea, appetite change, colitis, taste disorder.

**GU:** proteinuria, *acute renal failure,* oliguria, interstitial nephritis, papillary necrosis, nephrotic syndrome.

**Hematologic:** increased platelet aggregation time.

**Hepatic:** elevated liver enzyme levels, jaundice, *hepatitis, hepatotoxicity.*

**Metabolic:** hypoglycemia; hyperglycemia.

**Musculoskeletal:** back, leg, or joint pain.

**Respiratory:** asthma.

**Skin:** rash, pruritus, urticaria, eczema, dermatitis, alopecia, photosensitivity, bullous eruption, *Stevens-Johnson syndrome,* allergic purpura.

**Other:** *anaphylaxis; anaphylactoid reactions; angioedema;* viral infection (with ophthalmic solution).

---

## Overdose and treatment
No information available. There is no special antidote. Supportive and symptomatic treatment may include induction of vomiting or gastric lavage. Treatment with activated charcoal or dialysis may also be appropriate.

## Clinical considerations
■ Administration with other drugs that produce adverse GI effects, such as glucocorticoids, may aggravate such effects.
■ Because the anti-inflammatory, antipyretic, and analgesic effects of diclofenac may mask the usual signs of infection, advise clinician to monitor patient carefully for infection. Consider disease-modifying antirheumatic drugs in patients with inadequate response to NSAIDs.

### Therapeutic monitoring
■ Advise clinician to monitor renal function during treatment. Use with caution and at reduced dosage in patients with renal impairment.
■ Periodic ophthalmologic examinations are recommended during prolonged therapy.
■ Advise clinician to monitor liver function during therapy. Abnormal liver function test results and severe hepatic reactions may occur.
■ Periodic evaluation of hematopoietic function is recommended because bone marrow abnormalities have occurred. Regular check of hemoglobin level is important to detect toxic effects on the GI tract.

### Special populations
**Breast-feeding patients.** Low levels of diclofenac appear in breast milk. Risk-to-benefit ratio must be considered.
**Pediatric patients.** Drug isn't recommended for use in children.
**Geriatric patients.** Use with caution in geriatric patients; they may be more susceptible to adverse reactions, especially GI toxicity and nephrotoxicity. Reduce dosage to lowest level that controls symptoms.

## Patient counseling
■ Advise patient to take drug with meals or milk to avoid GI upset.
■ Teach patient to restrict salt intake, as diclofenac may cause edema, especially if patient is hypertensive.
■ Instruct patient to report symptoms that may be related to GI ulceration, such as epigastric pain and black or tarry stools, as well as other unusual symptoms, such as skin rash, pruritus or significant edema or weight gain.

# dicloxacillin sodium
Dycill, Dynapen, Pathocil

*Pharmacologic classification:* penicillinase-resistant penicillin
*Therapeutic classification:* antibiotic
*Pregnancy risk category NR*

## Available forms
Available by prescription only
*Capsules:* 125 mg, 250 mg, 500 mg
*Oral suspension:* 62.5 mg/5 ml (after reconstitution)

## Indications and dosages
**Systemic infections caused by penicillinase-producing staphylococci**
*Adults and children weighing 40 kg (88 lb) or more:* 125 to 250 mg P.O. q 6 hours.
*Infants and children over age 1 month weighing less than 40 kg:* 12.5 to 50 mg/kg P.O. daily, divided into doses given q 6 hours. Serious infection may require higher dosage (75 to 100 mg/kg/day in divided doses q 6 hours).

## Mechanism of action
*Antibiotic action:* Dicloxacillin is bactericidal; it adheres to bacterial penicillin-binding proteins, thus inhibiting bacterial cell wall synthesis. Dicloxacillin resists the effects of penicillinases—enzymes that inactivate penicillin—and is thus active against many strains of penicillinase-producing bacteria; this activity is most important against penicillinase-producing staphylococci; some strains may remain resistant. Dicloxacillin is also active against a few gram-positive aerobic and anaerobic bacilli but has no significant effect on gram-negative bacilli.

## Pharmacokinetics
*Absorption:* Absorbed rapidly but incompletely (35% to 76%) from the GI tract; it's relatively acid stable. Food may decrease both rate and extent of absorption.
*Distribution:* Distributed widely into bone, bile, and pleural and synovial fluids. CSF penetration is poor but is enhanced by meningeal inflammation. Drug crosses the placenta and is 95% to 99% protein-bound.
*Metabolism:* Metabolized only partially.
*Excretion:* Excreted in urine by renal tubular secretion and glomerular filtration. The drug also appears in breast milk. Elimination half-life in adults is ½ to 1 hour, extended minimally to 2¼ hours in patients with renal impairment.

| Route | Onset | Peak | Duration |
|-------|-------|------|----------|
| P.O. | Unknown | 2 hr | 6 hr |

## Contraindications and precautions

Contraindicated in patients hypersensitive to drug or other penicillins. Use cautiously in patients with other drug allergies, especially to cephalosporins, or in those with mononucleosis.

## Interactions

**Drug-drug.** *Aminoglycosides:* Dicloxacillin may falsely decrease serum aminoglycoside levels. Advise clinician to monitor patient carefully.

*Oral contraceptives:* May decrease their efficacy. Recommend additional form of contraceptive during penicillin therapy.

*Probenecid:* Blocks renal tubular secretion of dicloxacillin, raising its serum levels. Probenecid may be used for this purpose.

## Adverse reactions

**CNS:** neuromuscular irritability, *seizures,* lethargy, hallucinations, anxiety, confusion, agitation, depression, dizziness, fatigue.

**GI:** *nausea,* vomiting, *epigastric distress,* flatulence, *diarrhea,* enterocolitis, pseudomembranous colitis, black "hairy" tongue, abdominal pain.

**GU:** interstitial nephritis, nephropathy.

**Hematologic:** eosinophilia, anemia, *thrombocytopenia, leukopenia,* hemolytic anemia, *agranulocytosis.*

**Hepatic:** transient elevations in liver function study results, cholestasis, *hepatitis.*

**Other:** hypersensitivity reactions (pruritus, urticaria, rash, *anaphylaxis*), overgrowth of nonsusceptible organisms.

## Overdose and treatment

Clinical signs and symptoms of overdose include neuromuscular irritability or seizures. No specific recommendations. Treatment is supportive. After recent ingestion (4 hours or less), recommend emptying the stomach by induced emesis or gastric lavage, followed by activated charcoal to reduce absorption. Drug isn't appreciably dialyzable.

## Clinical considerations

■ Aminoglycosides produce synergistic bactericidal effects against *Staphylococcus aureus.* However, the drugs are physically and chemically incompatible and are inactivated when mixed or given together. Dicloxacillin may falsely decrease serum aminoglycoside levels.

■ Give drug with water only; acid in fruit juice or carbonated beverage may inactivate drug.

■ Give dose on empty stomach; food decreases absorption.

■ Dicloxacillin alters test results for urine and serum proteins; it produces false-positive or elevated results in turbidimetric urine and serum protein tests using sulfosalicylic acid or trichloroacetic acid; it also reportedly produces false results on the Bradshaw screening test for Bence Jones protein.

### Therapeutic monitoring

■ Recommend regular assessment of renal, hepatic, and hematopoietic function during prolonged therapy.

### Special populations

**Breast-feeding patients.** Dicloxacillin appears in breast milk; use drug cautiously in breast-feeding women.

**Pediatric patients.** Elimination of dicloxacillin is reduced in neonates; safety in neonates hasn't been established.

**Geriatric patients.** Half-life may be prolonged in geriatric patients because of impaired renal function.

## Patient counseling

■ Tell patient to report severe diarrhea promptly and to also report rash or itching.

■ Instruct patient to complete full course of therapy as prescribed, even if feeling better.

# dicyclomine hydrochloride

Antispas, A-Spas, Bentyl, Bentylol*, Byclomine, Dibent, Formulex*, Lomine*, Neoquess, Or-Tyl, Spasmoban*, Spasmoject

*Pharmacologic classification:* anticholinergic
*Therapeutic classification:* antimuscarinic, GI antispasmodic
*Pregnancy risk category B*

## Available forms

Available by prescription only
*Tablets:* 20 mg
*Capsules:* 10 mg
*Syrup:* 10 mg/5 ml
*Injection:* 10 mg/ml in 2-ml vials, 10-ml vials, 2-ml ampules

## Indications and dosages

*Irritable bowel syndrome and other functional GI disorders*
*Adults:* Initially, 20 mg P.O. q.i.d., then increase to 40 mg P.O. q.i.d. during first week of therapy unless precluded by adverse reactions. Alternatively, give 20 mg I.M. q 4 to 6 hours.
*Children ages 2 and older:* 10 mg P.O. t.i.d. or q.i.d.
*Infants ages 6 to 23 months:* 5 to 10 mg P.O. t.i.d. or q.i.d.
◊ *Infant colic*
*Infants ages 6 months and older:* 5 to 10 mg P.O. t.i.d. or q.i.d. Adjust dosage according to patient's needs and response.
Note: High environmental temperatures may induce heatstroke during drug use. If symptoms occur, drug should be discontinued.

## Mechanism of action

*Antispasmodic action:* Dicyclomine exerts a nonspecific, direct spasmolytic action on smooth muscle. It also has some local anesthetic properties that may contribute to spasmolysis in the GI and biliary tracts.

## Pharmacokinetics

*Absorption:* About 67% of an oral dose is absorbed from the GI tract.
*Distribution:* Largely unknown.
*Metabolism:* Unknown.
*Excretion:* After oral administration, 80% of a dose is excreted in urine and 10% in feces.

| Route | Onset | Peak | Duration |
|-------|-------|------|----------|
| P.O., I.M. | Unknown | 1-1½ hr | Unknown |

## Contraindications and precautions

Contraindicated in patients with obstructive uropathy, obstructive disease of the GI tract, reflux esophagitis, severe ulcerative colitis, myasthenia gravis, hypersensitivity to anticholinergics, unstable CV status in acute hemorrhage, or glaucoma. Also contraindicated in breast-feeding patients and in children under age 6 months.

Use cautiously in patients with autonomic neuropathy, hyperthyroidism, coronary artery disease, arrhythmias, HF, hypertension, hiatal hernia, hepatic or renal disease, prostatic hyperplasia, and ulcerative colitis.

## Interactions

**Drug-drug.** *Amantadine, antihistamines, antiparkinsonians, disopyramide, glutethimide, meperidine, phenothiazines, procainamide, quinidine, tricyclic antidepressants:* May cause additive adverse effects. Avoid use together.
*Antacids:* Decrease oral absorption of anticholinergics. Give dicyclomine at least 1 hour before antacids.
*Digoxin (slowly dissolving tablets):* Higher serum digoxin levels when given with anticholinergics. Advise clinician to monitor digoxin levels closely.
*Ketoconazole, levodopa:* Decreased GI absorption. Avoid use together.
*Methotrimeprazine:* May enhance risk of extrapyramidal reactions. Avoid use together.
*Oral potassium supplements (especially wax-matrix formulations):* Potassium-induced GI ulcerations may be increased. Use together cautiously.

## Adverse reactions

**CNS:** *headache; dizziness;* insomnia; lightheadedness; drowsiness; nervousness, confusion, excitement (in elderly patients).
**CV:** *palpitations,* tachycardia.
**EENT:** blurred vision, increased intraocular pressure, mydriasis.
**GI:** nausea, vomiting, *constipation, dry mouth,* abdominal distention, heartburn, paralytic ileus.

**GU:** *urinary hesitancy, urine retention,* impotence.
**Skin:** urticaria, decreased sweating or possible anhidrosis, other dermal manifestations, local irritation.
**Other:** fever, allergic reactions, dependence.

Dicyclomine is a synthetic tertiary derivative that may have atropine-like adverse reactions.

## Overdose and treatment

Signs and symptoms of overdose include curare-like symptoms of CNS stimulation followed by depression, and such psychotic symptoms as disorientation, confusion, hallucinations, delusions, anxiety, agitation, and restlessness. Peripheral effects may include dilated, nonreactive pupils; hot, flushed, dry skin; tachycardia; hypertension; and increased respiration.

Treatment is primarily symptomatic and supportive p.r.n. Advise clinician to maintain patent airway. If patient is alert, recommend inducing emesis (or using gastric lavage) and following with a saline cathartic and activated charcoal to prevent further drug absorption. In severe cases, physostigmine may be given to block the antimuscarinic effects of dicyclomine. Recommend giving fluids p.r.n. to treat shock; diazepam to control psychotic symptoms; and pilocarpine (instilled into the eyes) to relieve mydriasis. If urine retention occurs, catheterization may be needed.

## Clinical considerations

**⊞ ALERT** Dicyclomine should never be given I.V. or S.C.
■ Advise clinician to be prepared to adjust dosage, based on patient's needs and response.

### Therapeutic monitoring

■ Advise clinician to monitor vital signs and urine output carefully.

### Special populations

**Breast-feeding patients.** Dicyclomine may appear in breast milk; it may also decrease milk production. Avoid use in breast-feeding women.
**Pediatric patients.** Safety and effectiveness in children haven't been established. Administer cautiously to infants ages 6 months and older; seizures have been reported. Drug is contraindicated in infants under age 6 months.
**Geriatric patients.** Administer drug cautiously to geriatric patients. Lower doses are indicated.

## Patient counseling

■ Tell patient that syrup formulation may be diluted with water.
■ Warn patient that high environmental temperatures may induce heatstroke while drug is being used; tell patient to avoid exposure to such temperatures.

■ Advise patient to avoid driving and other hazardous activities if drowsiness or blurred vision occurs and to report rash or other skin eruption.

## didanosine (ddl)
Videx, Videx EC

*Pharmacologic classification:* purine analogue
*Therapeutic classification:* antiviral
*Pregnancy risk category B*

### Available forms
Available by prescription only
*Capsules (extended-release):* 125 mg, 200 mg, 250 mg, 400 mg
*Tablets (chewable):* 25 mg, 50 mg, 100 mg, 150 mg
*Powder for oral solution (buffered):* 100 mg/packet, 167 mg/packet, 250 mg/packet
*Powder for oral solution (pediatric):* 2 g and 4 g in 4- and 8-ounce bottles, respectively

### Indications and dosages
*Treatment of HIV infection when antiretroviral therapy is warranted*
*Adults weighing 60 kg (132 lb) or more:* 200 mg (tablets) P.O. b.i.d., or 400 mg once daily, or 250 mg buffered powder P.O. b.i.d. or 400 mg (capsules) P.O. once daily.
*Adults weighing less than 60 kg:* 125 mg (tablets) P.O. b.i.d. or 250 mg once daily, or 167 mg buffered powder P.O. b.i.d. or 250 mg (capsules) P.O. once daily.
*Children:* 120 mg/m² P.O. b.i.d. To prevent gastric acid degradation, children over age 1 should receive a two-tablet dose, and children under age 1 should receive a one-tablet dose.
≡ *Dosage adjustment.* Patients with renal or hepatic impairment may need their dosage adjusted.

### Mechanism of action
*Antiviral action:* Didanosine is a synthetic purine analogue of deoxyadenosine. After didanosine enters the cell, it's converted to its active form dideoxyadenosine triphosphate (ddATP), which inhibits replication of HIV by preventing DNA replication. In addition, ddATP inhibits the enzyme HIV-RNA dependent DNA polymerase (reverse transcriptase).

### Pharmacokinetics
*Absorption:* Degrades rapidly in gastric acid. Commercially available preparations contain buffers to raise stomach pH. Bioavailability averages about 33%; tablets may exhibit better bioavailability than buffered powder for oral solution. Food can decrease absorption by 50%.
*Distribution:* Widely distributed; drug penetration into the CNS varies, but CSF levels average 46% of concurrent plasma levels.

*Metabolism:* Metabolism isn't fully understood, but is probably similar to that of endogenous purines.
*Excretion:* Excreted in urine as allantoin, hypoxanthine, xanthine, and uric acid. Serum half-life averages 0.8 hours.

| Route | Onset | Peak | Duration |
|---|---|---|---|
| P.O. | Unknown | ½-1 hr | Unknown |

### Contraindications and precautions
Contraindicated in patients hypersensitive to drug or its components. Use very cautiously in patients with history of pancreatitis. Also use cautiously in patients with peripheral neuropathy, impaired renal or hepatic function, or hyperuricemia.

### Interactions
**Drug-drug.** *Antacids containing magnesium or aluminum hydroxides:* May produce enhanced adverse effects, such as diarrhea or constipation. Avoid use together.
*Co-trimoxazole, pentamidine, and other drugs associated with pancreatitis:* Increased risk of pancreatitis. Avoid use together.
*Dapsone, drugs that require gastric acid for adequate absorption, ketoconazole:* Decreased buffering action of didanosine. Give such drugs 2 hours before didanosine.
*Fluoroquinolones, tetracyclines:* Decreased absorption from buffering agents in didanosine tablets or antacids in pediatric suspension. Avoid use together.
*Itraconazole:* May decrease serum levels of itraconazole. Avoid use together.
**Drug-food.** *Any food:* Decreased rate of absorption. Give drug on an empty stomach at least 30 minutes before a meal.

### Adverse reactions
**CNS:** *headache, seizures,* confusion, anxiety, nervousness, asthenia, abnormal thinking, twitching, depression, *peripheral neuropathy.*
**GI:** *diarrhea, nausea, vomiting, abdominal pain, pancreatitis,* dry mouth, anorexia.
**Hematologic:** *leukopenia,* granulocytosis, *thrombocytopenia,* anemia.
**Hepatic:** *hepatic failure,* elevated liver enzyme levels, hepatomegaly.
**Metabolic:** increased serum uric acid levels. lactic acidosis.
**Musculoskeletal:** myopathy.
**Respiratory:** pneumonia, dyspnea.
**Skin:** rash, pruritus, sarcoma.
**Other:** pain, infection, allergic reactions, *chills, fever.*

### Overdose and treatment
No specific information exists regarding the treatment of overdose; however, possible effects of overdose include diarrhea, pancreatitis, peripheral neuropathy, hyperuricemia,

and hepatic dysfunction. Treatment is supportive. No specific antidote is known, and it's unknown if drug is dialyzable.

## Clinical considerations

**⚠ ALERT** Didanosine shouldn't be used as monotherapy.

**⚠ ALERT** Pediatric powder for oral solution must be prepared by the pharmacist before dispensing. It must be constituted with water, then diluted with antacid (manufacturer recommends either Mylanta Double Strength Liquid or Maalox TC) to a final level of 10 mg/ml. The admixture is stable for 30 days if refrigerated at 36° to 46° F (2° to 8° C). Be sure to shake well before measuring the dose.

**⚠ ALERT** Don't confuse drug with other antivirals that use abbreviations for identification.

■ Recommend giving didanosine on an empty stomach for full absorption.

■ Most patients over age 1 should receive two tablets per dose. Tablets contain buffers that raise stomach pH to levels that prevent degradation of the active drug. Tablets should be thoroughly chewed before swallowing, and the patient should drink at least 1 ounce of water with each dose. If tablets are manually crushed, mix drug in 30 ml (1 ounce) water; stir to disperse uniformly, then have patient drink it immediately. Single-dose packets containing buffered powder for oral solution are available.

■ To give buffered powder for oral solution, recommend carefully opening the packet and pouring the contents into 120 ml (4 ounces) water. Don't use fruit juice or other acidic beverages. Recommend stirring for 2 or 3 minutes until the powder dissolves completely and giving it immediately.

■ The chewable tablets can be substituted if diarrhea occurs.

■ When preparing powder or crushing tablets, avoid excessive dispersal of drug particles into the air.

### Therapeutic monitoring

■ The major toxicity of drug use is pancreatitis, which has been fatal in some cases. It must be considered when abdominal pain, nausea, and vomiting develop or biochemical markers are elevated. Drug should be stopped until pancreatitis is excluded. If pancreatitis is confirmed, the drug shouldn't be used again.

### Special populations

**Pregnant patients.** Inadequate information for evaluation of the benefits must be evaluated against the risk to the fetus. An antiretroviral pregnancy registry has been established to enroll women known to have exposure during pregnancy (1-800-258-4263).

**Breast-feeding patients.** It's unknown if drug appears in breast milk. Because of risk of serious adverse effects in the infant, breast-feeding isn't recommended.

**Pediatric patients.** Retinal depigmentation has occurred in some children receiving drug. Children should receive dilated retinal examinations at least every 6 months or if a change in vision occurs.

## Patient counseling

■ Tell patient to take drug on an empty stomach to ensure adequate absorption, to chew tablets thoroughly before swallowing, and to drink at least 30 ml (1 ounce) water with each dose.

■ Remind patient not to crush or break the capsule form.

■ Remind patient using buffered powder for oral solution not to use fruit juice or other acidic beverages, to allow 3 minutes for powder to dissolve completely, and to take immediately. Be sure he understands how to mix the solution.

# diflunisal
Dolobid

*Pharmacologic classification:* NSAID, salicylic acid derivative
*Therapeutic classification:* nonnarcotic analgesic, antipyretic, anti-inflammatory
*Pregnancy risk category C*

## Available forms
Available by prescription only
*Tablets (film-coated):* 250 mg, 500 mg

## Indications and dosages
*Mild to moderate pain*
*Adults ages 65 and younger:* Start therapy with 1 g, then 500 mg P.O. daily in two or three divided doses, usually q 8 to 12 hours. Maximum dose is 1,500 mg daily.
*Adults over age 65:* Initially, one-half the usual adult dose.
*Rheumatoid arthritis and osteoarthritis*
*Adults:* 500 to 1,000 mg P.O. daily in two divided doses, usually q 12 hours. Maximum dose is 1,500 mg daily.

## Mechanism of action
*Analgesic, antipyretic, and anti-inflammatory actions:* Mechanisms of action are unknown, but are probably related to inhibition of prostaglandin synthesis. Diflunisal is a salicylic acid derivative, but isn't hydrolyzed to free salicylate in vivo.

## Pharmacokinetics
*Absorption:* Absorbed rapidly and completely via the GI tract.
*Distribution:* Highly protein-bound.
*Metabolism:* Metabolized in the liver; it isn't metabolized to salicylic acid.

*Excretion:* Excreted in urine. Half-life is 8 to 12 hours.

| Route | Onset | Peak | Duration |
|-------|-------|------|----------|
| P.O. | 1 hr | 2-3 hr | 8-12 hr |

## Contraindications and precautions

Contraindicated in patients hypersensitive to the drug or for whom acute asthmatic attacks, urticaria, or rhinitis are precipitated by aspirin or other NSAIDs. Use cautiously in patients with GI bleeding, history of peptic ulcer disease, renal impairment, and compromised cardiac function, hypertension, or other conditions predisposing patient to fluid retention.

Because of the epidemiologic association with Reye's syndrome, the Centers for Disease Control and Prevention recommends not giving salicylates to children and teenagers with chickenpox or influenza-like illness.

## Interactions

**Drug-drug.** *Acetaminophen:* May increase serum acetaminophen levels by as much as 50%, leading to potential hepatotoxicity. This interaction may also be nephrotoxic. Avoid use together.

*Antacids, aspirin:* Delay and decrease the absorption of diflunisal. Advise clinician to monitor patient for decreased therapeutic effect.

*Antibiotics, NSAIDs, steroids:* May potentiate the adverse GI effects of diflunisal. Use together cautiously.

*Anticoagulants, thrombolytics:* Potentiate their anticoagulant effects. Use together cautiously.

*Antihypertensives:* Decrease their effect on blood pressure. Advise clinician to monitor blood pressure closely.

*Cyclosporine, diuretics, gold compounds:* May increase nephrotoxic potential. Avoid use together.

*Furosemide:* Decreases the hyperuricemic effect of furosemide. Advise clinician to monitor patient carefully.

*Highly protein-bound drugs, such as phenytoin, sulfonylureas, warfarin:* May cause displacement of either drug and adverse effects. Advise clinician to monitor patient closely for both drugs.

*Hydrochlorothiazide:* Increased plasma level of hydrochlorothiazide; decreased hyperuricemic, diuretic, antihypertensive, and natriuretic effects. Avoid use together.

*Indomethacin:* Decreased renal clearance of indomethacin. Fatal GI hemorrhage has also been reported. Avoid use together.

*Lithium:* May result in increased lithium serum levels. Advise clinician to monitor lithium levels closely.

*Methotrexate, nifedipine, verapamil:* Diflunisal may decrease the renal excretion of these drugs. Advise clinician to monitor patient carefully.

*Probenecid:* May decrease renal clearance of diflunisal. Advise clinician to monitor patient closely.

*Sulindac:* Diflunisal decreases blood levels of sulindac's active metabolite. Advise clinician to monitor patient carefully for reduced effect.

**Drug-herb.** *Dong quai, feverfew, garlic, ginger, horse chestnut, red clover:* Possible increased risk of bleeding. Discourage use together.

*Dong quai, St. John's wort:* Increased risk of photosensitivity. Advise patient to avoid unprotected exposure to sunlight.

**Drug-lifestyle.** *Alcohol use:* May potentiate adverse GI effects of diflunisal. Advise patient to avoid alcohol consumption.

## Adverse reactions

**CNS:** *dizziness,* somnolence, insomnia, *headache,* fatigue.

**EENT:** *tinnitus, visual disturbances.*

**GI:** *nausea, dyspepsia, GI pain, diarrhea,* vomiting, constipation, flatulence, stomatitis.

**GU:** increased serum BUN and creatinine, renal impairment, hematuria, interstitial nephritis.

**Hematologic:** prolonged bleeding time.

**Hepatic:** elevated liver function test results.

**Metabolic:** hyperkalemia, hypouricemia.

**Skin:** *rash,* pruritus, sweating, ***erythema multiforme, Stevens-Johnson syndrome.***

## Overdose and treatment

Signs and symptoms of overdose include drowsiness, nausea, vomiting, hyperventilation, tachycardia, sweating, tinnitus, disorientation, stupor, and coma.

To treat overdose of diflunisal, empty stomach immediately by inducing emesis with ipecac syrup if patient is conscious, or by gastric lavage. Recommend giving activated charcoal via nasogastric tube. Recommend providing symptomatic and supportive measures (respiratory support and correction of fluid and electrolyte imbalances). Advise clinician to monitor laboratory parameters and vital signs closely. Hemodialysis has little effect.

## Clinical considerations

**⊞ ALERT** Don't give salicylates to children and teenagers with chickenpox or flulike symptoms because of the epidemiologic association with Reye's syndrome.

■ Diflunisal is recommended for twice-daily dosing for added patient convenience and compliance.

■ Don't break, crush, or allow patient to chew diflunisal. Patient should swallow drug whole.

■ Diflunisal should be given with water, milk, or meals to minimize GI upset.

■ Drug shouldn't be given with aspirin or acetaminophen.

■ Advise clinician to evaluate patient's response to diflunisal therapy as evidenced by a reduction in pain or inflammation. Advise clinician

to monitor vital signs frequently, especially temperature.
■ If patient experiences CNS effects, recommend instituting safety measures to prevent injury.

### Therapeutic monitoring
■ Advise clinician to monitor results of laboratory tests, especially renal and liver function test results. Recommend assessing presence and amount of peripheral edema. Recommend monitoring weight frequently.
■ Patient should be assessed for signs and symptoms of potential hemorrhage, such as bruising, petechiae, coffee ground emesis, and black, tarry stools.

### Special populations
**Breast-feeding patients.** Because drug appears in breast milk, breast-feeding isn't recommended.
**Pediatric patients.** Don't use long-term diflunisal therapy in children under age 14; safety hasn't been established.
**Geriatric patients.** Patients over age 65 may be more susceptible to the toxic effects (particularly GI toxicity) of this drug. The effects of this drug on renal prostaglandins may cause fluid retention and edema, a significant drawback for geriatric patients, especially those with heart failure or hypertension.

### Patient counseling
■ Instruct patient in diflunisal regimen and need for compliance. Advise him to report adverse reactions.
■ Tell patient to take diflunisal with foods to minimize GI upset and to swallow capsule whole.
■ Caution patient to avoid activities requiring alertness or concentration, such as driving, until CNS effects are known.
■ Instruct patient in safety measures to prevent injury.

# digoxin
Digitek, Lanoxicaps, Lanoxin, Novodigoxin*

*Pharmacologic classification:* cardiac glycoside
*Therapeutic classification:* inotropic, antiarrhythmic
*Pregnancy risk category C*

### Available forms
Available by prescription only
*Tablets:* 0.125 mg, 0.25 mg
*Capsules:* 0.05 mg, 0.10 mg, 0.20 mg
*Elixir:* 0.05 mg/ml
*Injection:* 0.1 mg/ml (pediatric), 0.25 mg/ml, 0.5 mg/2 ml

## Indications and dosages
*Heart failure, atrial fibrillation and flutter, paroxysmal atrial tachycardia*
**Tablets, elixir**
*Adults:* For rapid digitalization, give 0.75 to 1.25 mg P.O. over 24 hours in two or more divided doses q 6 to 8 hours. For slow digitalization, give 0.125 to 0.5 mg daily for 5 to 7 days. Maintenance dosage is 0.125 to 0.5 mg daily.
*Children ages 10 and older:* 10 to 15 mcg/kg P.O. over 24 hours in two or more divided doses q 6 to 8 hours. Maintenance dosage is 25% to 35% of total digitalizing dose.
*Children ages 5 to 10:* 20 to 35 mcg/kg P.O. over 24 hours in two or more divided doses q 6 to 8 hours. Maintenance dosage is 25% to 35% of total digitalizing dose.
*Children ages 2 to 5:* 30 to 40 mcg/kg P.O. over 24 hours in two or more divided doses q 6 to 8 hours. Maintenance dosage is 25% to 35% of total digitalizing dose.
*Infants ages 1 month to 2 years:* 35 to 60 mcg/kg P.O. over 24 hours in two or more divided doses q 6 to 8 hours. Maintenance dosage is 25% to 35% of total digitalizing dose.
*Neonates:* 25 to 35 mcg/kg P.O. over 24 hours in two or more divided doses q 6 to 8 hours. Maintenance dosage is 25% to 35% of total digitalizing dose.
*Premature infants:* 20 to 30 mcg/kg P.O. over 24 hours in two or more divided doses q 6 to 8 hours. Maintenance dosage is 20% to 30% of total digitalizing dose.
**Capsules**
*Adults:* For rapid digitalization, give 0.4 to 0.6 mg P.O. initially, followed by 0.1 to 0.3 mg q 6 to 8 hours, as needed and tolerated, for 24 hours. For slow digitalization, give 0.05 to 0.35 mg daily in two divided doses for 7 to 22 days, p.r.n., until therapeutic serum levels are reached. Maintenance dosage is 0.05 to 0.35 mg daily in one or two divided doses.
*Children:* Digitalizing dose is based on child's age and is given in three or more divided doses over the first 24 hours. Initial dose should be 50% of the total dose; subsequent doses are given q 4 to 8 hours, as needed and tolerated.
*Children ages 10 and older:* For rapid digitalization, give 8 to 12 mcg/kg P.O. over 24 hours, divided as above. Maintenance dosage is 25% to 35% of total digitalizing dose, given daily as a single dose.
*Children ages 5 to 10:* For rapid digitalization, give 15 to 30 mcg/kg P.O. over 24 hours, divided as above. Maintenance dosage is 25% to 35% of total digitalizing dose, divided and given in two or three equal portions daily.
*Children ages 2 to 5:* For rapid digitalization, give 25 to 35 mcg/kg P.O. over 24 hours, divided as above. Maintenance dosage is 25% to 35% of total digitalizing dose, divided and given in two or three equal portions daily.

### Injection

*Adults:* For rapid digitalization, give 0.4 to 0.6 mg I.V. initially, followed by 0.1 to 0.3 mg I.V. q 4 to 8 hours, as needed and tolerated, for 24 hours. For slow digitalization, give appropriate daily maintenance dosage for 7 to 22 days, p.r.n., until therapeutic serum levels are reached. Maintenance dosage is 0.125 to 0.5 mg I.V. daily in one or two divided doses.

*Children:* Digitalizing dose is based on child's age and is given in three or more divided doses over the first 24 hours. Initial dose should be 50% of total dose; subsequent doses are given q 4 to 8 hours, as needed and tolerated.

*Children ages 10 and older:* For rapid digitalization, give 8 to 12 mcg/kg I.V. over 24 hours, divided as above. Maintenance dosage is 25% to 35% of total digitalizing dose, given daily as a single dose.

*Children ages 5 to 10:* For rapid digitalization, give 15 to 30 mcg/kg I.V. over 24 hours, divided as above. Maintenance dosage is 25% to 35% of total digitalizing dose, divided and given in two or three equal portions daily.

*Children ages 2 to 5:* For rapid digitalization, give 25 to 35 mcg/kg I.V. over 24 hours, divided as above. Maintenance dosage is 25% to 35% of total digitalizing dose, divided and given in two or three equal portions daily.

*Infants ages 1 month to 2 years:* For rapid digitalization, give 30 to 50 mcg/kg I.V. over 24 hours, divided as above. Maintenance dosage is 25% to 35% of total digitalizing dose, divided and given in two or three equal portions daily.

*Neonates:* For rapid digitalization, give 20 to 30 mcg/kg I.V. over 24 hours, divided as above. Maintenance dosage is 25% to 35% of the total digitalizing dose, divided and given in two or three equal portions daily.

*Premature infants:* For rapid digitalization, give 15 to 25 mcg/kg I.V. over 24 hours, divided as above. Maintenance dosage is 20% to 30% of the total digitalizing dose, divided and given in two or three equal portions daily.

≡ *Dosage adjustment.* Dosage adjustment may be needed in patients with impaired renal function. Hypothyroid patients are highly sensitive to glycosides; hyperthyroid patients may need larger doses.

### I.V. administration

■ Obtain baseline heart rate and rhythm, blood pressure, and serum electrolyte levels before giving first dose.

■ Advise clinician to monitor clinical status, taking apical-radial pulse for a full minute, and watch for significant changes (sudden rate increase or decrease, pulse deficit, irregular beats, and especially regularization of a previously irregular rhythm).

■ Give slowly by direct I.V. administration over a minimum of 5 minutes.

■ Drug may be given undiluted or diluted with $D_5W$ or normal saline solution to 4-fold volume.

■ Closely follow administration schedule (see above).

### Incompatibilities

Incompatible with dobutamine, doxapram, fluconazole, and foscarnet. Manufacturer recommends not mixing digoxin with other drugs or giving them in the same I.V. line.

## Mechanism of action

Digoxin is the most widely used cardiac glycoside. Many oral forms and a parenteral form are available, facilitating use of the drug in both acute and long-term clinical settings.

*Inotropic action:* The effect of digoxin on the myocardium is dose-related and involves both direct and indirect mechanisms. It directly increases the force and velocity of myocardial contraction, AV node refractory period, and total peripheral resistance; at higher doses, it also increases sympathetic outflow. It indirectly depresses the SA node and prolongs conduction to the AV node. In patients with heart failure, increased contractile force boosts cardiac output, improves systolic emptying, and decreases diastolic heart size. It also reduces ventricular end-diastolic pressure and, consequently, pulmonary and systemic venous pressures. Increased myocardial contractility and cardiac output reflexively reduce sympathetic tone in patients with heart failure. This compensates for the direct vasoconstrictive action of the drug, thereby reducing total peripheral resistance. It also slows increased heart rate and causes diuresis in edematous patients.

*Antiarrhythmic action:* Digoxin-induced heart-rate slowing in patients without heart failure is negligible and stems mainly from vagal (cholinergic) and sympatholytic effects on the SA node; however, with toxic doses, heart-rate slowing results from direct depression of SA node automaticity. Therapeutic doses produce little effect on the action potential, but toxic doses increase the automaticity (spontaneous diastolic depolarization) of all cardiac regions except the SA node.

## Pharmacokinetics

*Absorption:* With tablet or elixir administration, 60% to 85% of dose is absorbed. With capsule form, bioavailability increases. About 90% to 100% of a dose is absorbed. With I.M. administration, about 80% of dose is absorbed.

*Distribution:* Distributed widely in body tissues; highest levels occur in the heart, kidneys, intestine, stomach, liver, and skeletal muscle; lowest levels are in the plasma and brain. Digoxin crosses both the blood-brain barrier and the placenta; fetal and maternal digoxin levels are equivalent at birth. About 20% to 30% of drug is plasma protein–bound. Usual therapeutic range for steady-state serum levels is 0.5 to 2 ng/ml. In treatment of atrial tachyarrhythmias, higher serum levels (such as 2 to 4 ng/ml) may be needed. Because of long half-life of drug, achievement of steady-state levels may take 7 days or longer, depending on patient's renal function. Toxic symptoms may appear within the usual therapeutic range; however, these are more frequent and serious with levels above 2.5 ng/ml.

*Metabolism:* In most patients, a small amount of digoxin apparently is metabolized in the liver and gut by bacteria. This metabolism varies and may be substantial in some patients. Drug undergoes some enterohepatic recirculation (also variable). Metabolites have minimal cardiac activity.

*Excretion:* Most of dose is excreted by the kidneys as unchanged drug. Some patients excrete a substantial amount of metabolized or reduced drug. In patients with renal failure, biliary excretion is a more important excretion route. In healthy patients, terminal half-life is 30 to 40 hours. In patients without functioning kidneys, half-life increases to at least 4 days.

| Route | Onset | Peak | Duration |
|-------|-------|------|----------|
| P.O. | 1½-2 hr | 2-6 hr | 3-4 days |
| I.M. | 30 min | 4-6 hr | Unknown |
| I.V. | 5-30 min | 1-4 hr | 3-4 days |

## Contraindications and precautions

Contraindicated in patients hypersensitive to drug, or those with digitalis-induced toxicity, ventricular fibrillation, or ventricular tachycardia unless caused by heart failure.

Use very cautiously in geriatric patients and in patients with acute MI, incomplete AV block, sinus bradycardia, PVCs, chronic constrictive pericarditis, hypertrophic cardiomyopathy, renal insufficiency, severe pulmonary disease, or hypothyroidism.

## Interactions

**Drug-drug.** *Amiloride:* Inhibits digoxin effect and increases digoxin excretion. Advise clinician to monitor patient for altered digoxin effect.

*Aminosalicylic acid, antacids, kaolin-pectin, magnesium trisilicate, sulfasalazine:* Decrease absorption of orally administered digoxin. Advise clinician to monitor patient for altered digoxin effect. Separate administration times as far as possible from each other.

*Amiodarone, diltiazem, nifedipine, quinidine, verapamil:* Increase serum digoxin levels, predisposing the patient to toxicity. Avoid use together.

*Amphotericin B, carbenicillin, corticosteroids, corticotropin, edetate disodium, laxatives, sodium polystyrene sulfonate, ticarcillin:* Possible digoxin toxicity. Advise clinician to monitor digoxin levels closely.

*Antibiotics:* Increase digoxin bioavailability and, consequently, increase serum digoxin levels. Advise clinician to monitor digoxin levels closely and separate administration times.

*Anticholinergics:* May increase digoxin absorption of oral digoxin tablets. Advise clinician to monitor blood levels and observe patient for toxicity.

*Cholestyramine, colestipol, metoclopramide:* Impair absorption. Advise clinician to monitor digoxin levels closely. Space doses by giving digoxin 1½ hours before or 2 hours after other drugs.

*Cytotoxic drugs, radiation therapy:* Decrease digoxin absorption if the intestinal mucosa is damaged. Use of digoxin elixir or capsules is recommended in this situation.

*Diuretics, such as bumetanide, ethacrynic acid, furosemide:* May cause hypokalemia and hypomagnesemia. Advise clinician to monitor blood levels closely.

*Glucagon, large dextrose doses, and dextrose-insulin infusions:* Digitalis toxicity. Avoid use together.

*I.V. calcium:* Synergistic effects that precipitate arrhythmias. Avoid use together.

*Parenteral calcium, thiazides:* May cause hypercalcemia. Advise clinician to monitor serum calcium levels.

*Procainamide, propranolol, verapamil:* Additive cardiac effects. Avoid use together.

*Succinylcholine:* May precipitate cardiac arrhythmias by potentiating effects of digoxin. Avoid use together.

*Sympathomimetics, such as ephedrine, epinephrine, isoproterenol, rauwolfia alkaloids:* May increase the risk of arrhythmias. Avoid use together.

**Drug-herb.** *Betel palm, fumitory, goldenseal, lily-of-the-valley, motherwort, rue, shepherd's purse:* Enhance cardiac effects. Advise clinician to monitor patient closely.

*Gossypol, hawthorn, licorice, oleander, Siberian ginseng, squill:* May enhance toxicity. Discourage use together.

*Licorice:* Licorice-induced potassium loss may cause hypokalemia, increasing risk of digoxin toxicity. Discourage use together.

*Plantain:* Possible decrease in digoxin absorption, decreasing the pharmacologic effect. Discourage use together.

*St. John's wort:* Decreases digoxin levels and therapeutic efficacy. Discourage use together.

## Adverse reactions

**CNS:** *fatigue, generalized muscle weakness, agitation, hallucinations,* headache, malaise, dizziness, vertigo, stupor, paresthesia.

**CV:** *arrhythmias* (most commonly, conduction disturbances with or without AV block,

PVCs, and supraventricular arrhythmias), *worsening HF,* hypotension.

**EENT:** *yellow-green halos around visual images, blurred vision,* light flashes, photophobia, diplopia.

**GI:** *anorexia, nausea,* vomiting, diarrhea.

## Overdose and treatment

Clinical effects of overdose are primarily GI, CNS, and cardiac reactions.

Severe intoxication may cause hyperkalemia, which may develop rapidly and result in life-threatening cardiac manifestations. Cardiac signs of digoxin toxicity may occur with or without other toxicity signs and commonly precede other toxic effects. Because toxic cardiac effects also can occur as manifestations of heart disease, determining whether these effects result from underlying heart disease or digoxin toxicity may be difficult. Digoxin has caused almost every kind of arrhythmia; various combinations of arrhythmias may occur in the same patient. Patients with chronic digoxin toxicity commonly have ventricular arrhythmias or AV conduction disturbances. Patients with digoxin-induced ventricular tachycardia have a high mortality because ventricular fibrillation or asystole may result.

If toxicity is suspected, recommend stopping drug and obtaining serum drug level measurements. Usually, drug takes at least 6 hours to distribute between plasma and tissue and reach equilibrium; plasma levels drawn earlier may show higher digoxin levels than those present after drug is distributed into the tissues.

Other treatment measures include immediate emesis induction, gastric lavage, and administration of activated charcoal to reduce absorption of drug remaining in the gut. Repeated doses of activated charcoal (such as 50 g q 6 hours) may help reduce further absorption, especially of any drug undergoing enterohepatic recirculation. Some clinicians advocate cholestyramine administration if digoxin was recently ingested; however, it may not be useful if the ingestion is life threatening. Interacting drugs probably should be discontinued. Ventricular arrhythmias may be treated with I.V. potassium (replacement dose; but not in patients with significant AV block), I.V. phenytoin, I.V. lidocaine, or I.V. propranolol. Refractory ventricular tachyarrhythmias may be controlled with overdrive pacing. Procainamide may be used for ventricular arrhythmias that don't respond to the above treatments. In severe AV block, asystole, and hemodynamically significant sinus bradycardia, atropine restores a normal rate.

Administration of digoxin-specific antibody fragments (digoxin immune Fab, or Digibind) is a treatment for life-threatening digoxin toxicity. Each 40 mg of digoxin immune Fab binds about 0.6 mg of digoxin in the bloodstream.

The complex is then excreted in the urine, rapidly decreasing serum levels and therefore cardiac drug levels.

## Clinical considerations

**H ALERT** Beware of soundalikes: digoxin and doxepin, or digitoxin.

**H ALERT** Excessive slowing of heart rate (60 beats/minute or less) may be a sign of digitalis toxicity. Withhold drug and notify prescriber.

■ Advise clinician to obtain baseline heart rate and rhythm, blood pressure, and serum electrolyte levels before giving first dose.

■ Advise clinician to monitor clinical status. Apical-radial pulse should be taken for a full minute. Advise clinician to watch for significant changes (sudden rate increase or decrease, pulse deficit, irregular beats, and especially regularization of a previously irregular rhythm). Advise clinician to check blood pressure and obtain 12-lead ECG if these changes occur.

■ Patient should be questioned about use of cardiac glycosides within the previous 2 to 3 weeks before giving a loading dose. Recommend always dividing loading dose over first 24 hours unless clinical situation indicates otherwise.

■ GI absorption may be reduced in patients with HF, especially right HF.

■ Because digoxin may predispose patients to postcardioversion asystole, most clinicians withhold digoxin 1 or 2 days before elective cardioversion in patients with atrial fibrillation. (However, consider consequences of increased ventricular response to atrial fibrillation if drug is withheld.)

■ Calcium must not be given rapidly I.V. to patient receiving digoxin. Calcium affects cardiac contractility and excitability in much the same way that digoxin does and may lead to serious arrhythmias.

■ Digoxin solution is enclosed in a soft capsule (Lanoxicaps). Because these capsules are better absorbed than tablets, dose is usually slightly less.

### Therapeutic monitoring

■ Dosage is adjusted to patient's clinical condition and renal function; advise clinician to monitor ECG and serum levels of digoxin, calcium, potassium, and magnesium as well as serum creatinine levels. Therapeutic serum digoxin levels range from 0.5 to 2 ng/ml. Recommend taking corrective action before hypokalemia occurs.

### Special populations

**Pediatric patients.** Children have a poorly defined range of serum levels; however, toxicity apparently doesn't occur at same levels considered toxic in adults. Divided daily dosing is recommended for infants and children under

---

age 10; older children require adult doses proportional to body weight.
**Geriatric patients.** Use with caution (especially if renally compromised); adjust dosage to prevent systemic accumulation.

## Patient counseling
■ Inform patient and responsible family member about drug action, drug regimen, how to take pulse, reportable signs, and follow-up plans. Patient must understand importance of follow-up laboratory tests and have access to outpatient laboratory facilities.
■ Instruct patient not to take an extra dose of digoxin if dose is missed.
■ Tell patient to call prescriber if severe nausea, vomiting, or diarrhea occurs because these conditions may make patient more susceptible to toxicity.
■ Advise patient to use the same brand consistently.
■ Tell patient to call prescriber before using OTC preparations, especially those high in sodium.

# digoxin immune FAB (ovine)
Digibind

*Pharmacologic classification:* antibody fragment
*Therapeutic classification:* cardiac glycoside antidote
*Pregnancy risk category C*

## Available forms
Available by prescription only
*Injection:* 38-mg vial

## Indications and dosages
*Potentially life-threatening digoxin or digitoxin intoxication*
*Adults and children:* Administered I.V. over 30 minutes or as a bolus if cardiac arrest is imminent. Dosage varies based on amount of drug to be neutralized; average dose for adults is 6 vials (228 mg). However, if toxicity resulted from acute digoxin ingestion and neither a serum digoxin level nor an estimated ingestion amount is known, 10 to 20 vials (380 to 760 mg) should be given. See package insert for complete, specific dosage instructions.

## I.V. administration
■ Reconstitute vial with 4 ml of sterile water for injection, mix gently, and use immediately.
■ Recommend giving I.V. using a 0.22-micron filter needle over 30 minutes or as a bolus injection when cardiac arrest is imminent.
■ May be stored in refrigerator up to 4 hours.

### Incompatibilities
None reported.

## Mechanism of action
*Cardiac glycoside antidote:* Specific antigen-binding fragments bind to free digoxin in extracellular fluid and intravascularly to prevent and reverse pharmacologic and toxic effects of the cardiac glycoside. This binding is preferential for digoxin and digitoxin; preliminary evidence suggests some binding to other digoxin derivatives and cardioactive metabolites.

Once free digoxin is bound and removed from serum, tissue-bound digoxin is released into the serum to maintain efflux-influx balance. As digoxin is released, it's bound and removed by digoxin immune Fab, resulting in a reduction of serum and tissue digoxin. Cardiac glycoside toxicity begins to subside within 30 minutes after completion of a 15- to 30-minute I.V. infusion of digoxin immune Fab. The onset of action and response is variable and appears to depend on rate of infusion, dose given relative to body load of glycoside, and possibly other, as yet unidentified, factors. Reversal of toxicity, including hyperkalemia, is usually complete within 2 to 6 hours after administration of digoxin immune Fab.

## Pharmacokinetics
*Absorption:* Serum levels peak at the completion of I.V. infusion. Digoxin immune Fab has a serum half-life of 15 to 20 hours. The association reaction between Fab fragments and glycoside molecules appears to occur rapidly; data are limited.
*Distribution:* Distribution isn't fully characterized. After I.V. administration, drug appears to be distributed rapidly throughout extracellular space, into both plasma and interstitial fluid. It isn't known if digoxin immune Fab crosses the placental barrier or appears in breast milk.
*Metabolism:* Unknown.
*Excretion:* Excreted in urine via glomerular filtration.

| Route | Onset | Peak | Duration |
|-------|-------|------|----------|
| I.V. | 30 min | End of infusion | 15-20 hr |

## Contraindications and precautions
No known contraindications. Use cautiously in patients known to be allergic to ovine proteins. In these high-risk patients, skin testing is recommended because drug is derived from digoxin-specific antibody fragments obtained from immunized sheep.

## Interactions
**Drug-drug.** *Cardiac glycosides, including digitoxin and digoxin:* When used together, digoxin immune Fab binds cardiac glycosides. This also occurs if redigitalization is attempted before elimination of digoxin immune Fab is complete (several days with normal renal function;

1 week or longer with renal impairment). Drug is used for this effect.

## Adverse reactions
**CV:** *HF,* rapid ventricular rate (both caused by reversal of cardiac glycoside's therapeutic effects).
**Metabolic:** hypokalemia.
**Other:** hypersensitivity reactions, *anaphylaxis.*

## Overdose and treatment
Limited information is available; however, administration of doses larger than needed for neutralizing the cardiac glycoside may subject the patient to increased risk of allergic or febrile reaction or delayed serum sickness. Large doses may also prolong the time span required before redigitalization.

## Clinical considerations
■ Recommend measuring serum digoxin or digitoxin levels before giving antidote because serum levels may be difficult to interpret after therapy with antidote.
■ To determine appropriate dose, recommend dividing the total digitalis body load by 0.5; the resultant number estimates the number of vials required for appropriate dose. Alternatively, in cases of acute ingestion of known quantity of digitalis, multiply the amount of digitalis ingested in milligrams by 0.80 (to account for incomplete absorption).
■ Skin testing may be appropriate for high-risk patients. One of two methods may be used:
*Intradermal test*—dilute 0.1 ml of reconstituted solution in 9.9 ml of sterile saline for injection; then withdraw and inject 0.1 ml of this solution intradermally. Inspect site after 20 minutes for signs of erythema or urticaria.
*Scratch test*—dilute as for intradermal test. Place one drop of diluted solution on skin and make a ¼″ scratch through the drop with a sterile needle. Inspect site after 20 minutes for signs of erythema or urticaria. If results are positive, avoid use of digoxin immune Fab unless needed. If systemic reaction occurs, treat symptomatically.
■ Advise clinician to pretreat patients with sensitivity or allergy to sheep or ovine products, or when skin test results are positive, with an antihistamine, such as diphenhydramine, and a corticosteroid before giving digoxin immune Fab.
■ Keep drugs and equipment for cardiopulmonary resuscitation readily available during administration of digoxin immune Fab for patients who respond poorly to withdrawal of inotropic effects of digoxin. Dopamine or dobutamine, or other cardiac load-reducing drugs, may be used. Catecholamines may aggravate arrhythmias induced by digitalis toxicity; use with caution.

■ Digoxin immune Fab therapy alters standard cardiac glycoside determinations by radioimmunoassay procedures. Results may be falsely increased or decreased, depending on separation method used. Serum potassium levels may decrease rapidly.

### Therapeutic monitoring
■ Advise clinician to closely monitor temperature, blood pressure, ECG, and potassium level before, during, and after administration of antidote.
■ Advise clinician to check potassium levels repeatedly because severe digitalis intoxication can cause life-threatening hyperkalemia, and reversal by digoxin immune Fab may lead to rapid hypokalemia.

### Special populations
**Breast-feeding patients.** It's unknown if digoxin immune Fab appears in breast milk; use cautiously in breast-feeding women.
**Pediatric patients.** Consider the risk-to-benefit ratio. Adverse effects haven't occurred in infants and small children. Advise clinician to monitor patient for volume overload in small children. Very small doses may require diluting reconstituted solution with 36 ml of sterile saline for injection to produce a 1 mg/ml solution.
  Infants may require smaller doses; manufacturer recommends reconstituting, as directed, and administering with a tuberculin syringe.

## Patient counseling
■ Explain use and administration to patient and family.
■ Instruct patient to report adverse effects immediately.

# diltiazem hydrochloride
Cardizem, Cardizem CD, Cardizem SR, CartiaXT, Dilacor XR, Diltia XT, Tiazac

*Pharmacologic classification:* calcium channel blocker
*Therapeutic classification:* antianginal, antiarrythmic, antihypertensive
*Pregnancy risk category C*

## Available forms
Available by prescription only
*Tablets:* 30 mg, 60 mg, 90 mg, 120 mg
*Capsules (extended-release):* 120 mg, 180 mg, 240 mg, 300 mg, 360 mg
*Capsules (extended-release, containing multiple 60-mg beads):* 120 mg, 180 mg, 240 mg
*Capsules (sustained-release):* 60 mg, 90 mg, 120 mg, 180 mg, 240 mg, 300 mg, 360 mg, 420 mg
*Injection:* 5 mg/ml (25 mg and 50 mg)

*Injection:* 25 mg
*Injection (for I.V. infusion only):* 100 mg

## Indications and dosages

**Management of Prinzmetal's or variant angina or chronic stable angina pectoris**
*Adults:* 30 mg P.O. q.i.d. before meals and h.s. Increase dose gradually to maximum of 360 mg/day divided into three to four doses, as indicated. Alternatively, give 120 or 180 mg (extended-release) P.O. once daily. Adjust over a 7- to 14-day period as needed and tolerated up to a maximum dose of 480 mg daily.

**Hypertension**
*Adults:* 60 to 120 mg P.O. b.i.d. (sustained-release). Adjust up to maximum recommended dose of 360 mg/day p.r.n. Alternatively, give 180 to 240 mg (extended-release) P.O. once daily. Adjust dose based on patient response to a maximum dose of 480 mg/day.

**Atrial fibrillation or flutter; paroxysmal supraventricular tachycardia**
*Adults:* 0.25 mg/kg I.V. as a bolus injection over 2 minutes. Repeat after 15 minutes if response isn't adequate with a dose of 0.35 mg/kg I.V. over 2 minutes. Follow bolus with continuous I.V. infusion at 5 to 15 mg/hour (for up to 24 hours).

## I.V. administration

- For direct I.V. injection, no dilution of 5-mg/ml injection is necessary. Give over 2 minutes.
- For continous infusion, 5-mg/ml injection should be added to 100, 200, or 500 ml of normal saline solution, $D_5W$, or 5% dextrose and half-normal saline solution to produce a final concentration of 0.45 mg/ml.
- Infusions lasting longer than 24 hours aren't recommended.
- Monitor continous ECG and blood pressure during administration.

### Incompatibilities
Incompatible when mixed directly with diazepam, furosemide, heparin, phenytoin, or rifampin.

## Mechanism of action

*Antianginal or antihypertensive action:* By dilating systemic arteries, diltiazem decreases total peripheral resistance and afterload, slightly reduces blood pressure, and increases cardiac index when given in high doses (more than 200 mg). Afterload reduction, which occurs at rest and with exercise, and the resulting decrease in myocardial oxygen consumption account for the effectiveness of diltiazem in controlling chronic stable angina.

Diltiazem also decreases myocardial oxygen demand and cardiac work by reducing heart rate, relieving coronary artery spasm (through coronary artery vasodilation), and dilating peripheral vessels. These effects relieve ischemia and pain. In patients with Prinzmetal's angina, diltiazem inhibits coronary artery spasm, increasing myocardial oxygen delivery.

*Antiarrhythmic action:* By impeding the slow inward influx of calcium at the AV node, diltiazem decreases conduction velocity and increases refractory period, thereby decreasing the impulses transmitted to the ventricles in atrial fibrillation or flutter. The end result is a decreased ventricular rate.

## Pharmacokinetics

*Absorption:* About 80% of a dose is absorbed rapidly from the GI tract. However, only about 40% of drug enters systemic circulation because of a significant first-pass effect in the liver.
*Distribution:* About 70% to 85% of circulating drug is plasma protein–bound.
*Metabolism:* Metabolized in the liver.
*Excretion:* About 35% is excreted in the urine and about 65% in the bile as unchanged drug and inactive and active metabolites. Elimination half-life is 3 to 9 hours. Half-life may increase in geriatric patients; however, renal dysfunction doesn't appear to affect half-life.

| Route | Onset | Peak | Duration |
|---|---|---|---|
| P.O. | ½-1 hr | 2-3 hr | 6-8 hr |
| P.O. (extended) | 2-3 hr | 10-14 hr | 12-24 hr |
| P.O. (sustained) | 2-3 hr | 6-11 hr | Unknown |
| P.O., Diltia XT (extended) | Unknown | 4-6 hr | 24 hr |
| I.V. | 3 min | Immediate | 1-10 hr |

## Contraindications and precautions

Contraindicated in patients with sick sinus syndrome or second- or third-degree AV block in the absence of an artificial pacemaker; in supraventricular tachycardias associated with a bypass tract such as in Wolff-Parkinson-White syndrome or Lown-Ganong-Levine syndrome; and in patients with left ventricular failure, hypotension (systolic blood pressure less than 90 mm Hg), hypersensitivity to the drug, acute MI, and pulmonary congestion (documented by X-ray). Use cautiously in geriatric patients and in patients with HF or impaired hepatic or renal function.

## Interactions

**Drug-drug.** *Anesthetics:* Effects may be potentiated. Advise clinician to monitor patient.
*Benzodiazepine, carbamazepine, lovastatin:* Toxicity of concomitant drug. Advise clinician to monitor closely. Use together cautiously.
*Beta blockers:* Combined effects that result in HF, conduction disturbances, arrhythmias, and hypotension. Use together cautiously.

*Cimetidine:* May increase plasma level of diltiazem. Advise clinician to monitor patient carefully.

*Cyclosporine:* Increased serum cyclosporine levels and subsequent cyclosporine-induced nephrotoxicity. If used together, advise clinician to monitor cyclosporine, BUN, and serum creatinine levels.

*Digoxin:* Diltiazem may increase serum levels of digoxin. Advise clinician to monitor patient for toxicity.

*Furosemide:* Forms a precipitate when mixed with diltiazem injection. Drug needs to be given through separate I.V. lines.

*Rifampin:* Decreased therapeutic effect. Avoid use together.

## Adverse reactions

**CNS:** *headache,* dizziness, asthenia, somnolence.
**CV:** *edema, **arrhythmias, bradycardia,** hypo*tension, conduction abnormalities, *HF, AV block,* abnormal ECG.
**GI:** *nausea, constipation,* abdominal discomfort.
**Hepatic:** acute hepatic injury.
**Skin:** *rash,* flushing.

## Overdose and treatment

Clinical effects of overdose primarily are extensions of adverse reactions of drug. Heart block, asystole, and hypotension are the most serious effects and require immediate attention.

Treatment may involve I.V. isoproterenol, norepinephrine, epinephrine, atropine, or calcium gluconate given in usual doses. Adequate hydration must be ensured. Inotropic agents, including dobutamine and dopamine, may be used, if needed. If patient develops severe conduction disturbances (such as heart block and asystole) with hypotension that doesn't respond to drug therapy, advise clinician to start cardiac pacing immediately with cardiopulmonary resuscitation measures, as indicated.

## Clinical considerations

■ S.L. nitroglycerin may be given concomitantly p.r.n. if patient has acute angina symptoms.
■ Diltiazem has been used investigationally to prevent reinfarction after non–Q-wave MI; as an adjunct in the treatment of peripheral vascular disorders; and in the treatment of several spastic smooth-muscle disorders, including esophageal spasm.

## *Therapeutic monitoring*

■ Advise clinician to monitor blood pressure and heart rate when therapy starts or changes.
■ If systolic blood pressure is less than 90 mm Hg or heart rate is less than 60 beats/minute, withhold dose and notify prescriber.

### Special populations

**Breast-feeding patients.** Drug appears in breast milk; therefore, patients should discontinue breast-feeding during diltiazem therapy.
**Geriatric patients.** Use drug with caution in geriatric patients because the half-life may be prolonged.

## Patient counseling

■ Tell patient that nitrate therapy prescribed during titration of diltiazem dosage may cause dizziness. Urge patient to continue compliance.
■ Inform patient of proper use, dose, and adverse effects of diltiazem use.
■ Instruct patient to continue taking drug even when feeling better.
■ Tell patient to report feelings of lightheadedness or dizziness and to avoid sudden position changes.

# dimenhydrinate

Apo-Dimenhydrinate*, Calm-X, Dimetabs, Dinate, DMH Syrup, Dramamine, Dymenate, PMS-Dimenhydrinate*, TripTone

*Pharmacologic classification:* ethanolamine-derivative antihistamine
*Therapeutic classification:* antihistamine (H$_1$-receptor antagonist), antiemetic, antivertigo drug
*Pregnancy risk category B*

## Available forms

Available with or without a prescription
*Tablets:* 50 mg
*Tablets (chewable):* 50 mg
*Tablets (film-coated):* 50 mg
*Solution:* 12.5 mg/5 ml
*Injection:* 50 mg/ml

## Indications and dosages

***Prophylaxis and treatment of nausea, vomiting, dizziness associated with motion sickness***
*Adults and children ages 12 and older:* 50 to 100 mg q 4 to 6 hours P.O., I.V., or I.M.
*Children:* 1.25 mg/kg/day or 37.5 mg/m$^2$/day P.O. or I.M. q.i.d. not to exceed 300 mg/day, or according to the following schedule:
*Children ages 6 to 12:* 25 to 50 mg P.O. q 6 to 8 hours; maximum dose is 150 mg/day.
*Children ages 2 to 6:* 12.5 to 25 mg P.O. q 6 to 8 hours; maximum dose is 75 mg/day.
◇ *Meniere's disease*
*Adults:* 50 mg I.M. for acute attack; maintenance dosage is 25 to 50 mg P.O. t.i.d.

## I.V. administration

■ Dilute each 50-mg dose in 10 ml of normal saline solution and inject slowly over 2 minutes.

**H ALERT** I.V. products that contain benzyl alcohol are linked to a fatal gasping syndrome in premature infants and low–birth-weight infants.
■ Incorrectly administered or undiluted I.V. solution is irritating to veins and may cause sclerosis.

### Incompatibilities
Incompatible with aminophylline, ammonium chloride, amobarbital, butorphanol, chlorpromazine, glycopyrrolate, heparin, hydrocortisone sodium succinate, hydroxyzine hydrochloride, midazolam, pentobarbital sodium, phenobarbital sodium, phenytoin, prochlorperazine, promazine, and thiopental.

### Mechanism of action
*Antiemetic and antivertigo actions:* Dimenhydrinate probably inhibits nausea and vomiting by centrally depressing sensitivity of the labyrinth apparatus that relays stimuli to the chemoreceptor trigger zone and stimulates the vomiting center in the brain.

### Pharmacokinetics
*Absorption:* Well absorbed.
*Distribution:* Well distributed throughout the body and crosses the placenta.
*Metabolism:* Metabolized in the liver.
*Excretion:* Metabolites are excreted in urine.

| Route | Onset | Peak | Duration |
|-------|-------|------|----------|
| P.O. | 15-30 min | Unknown | 3-6 hr |
| I.V. | Immediate | Unknown | 3-6 hr |
| I.M. | 20-30 min | Unknown | 3-6 hr |

### Contraindications and precautions
Contraindicated in patients hypersensitive to drug or its components. I.V. product contains benzyl alcohol, which is linked to a fatal "gasping syndrome" in premature infants and low-birth-weight infants.

Use cautiously in patients with seizures, acute angle-closure glaucoma, or enlarged prostate gland and in those receiving ototoxic drugs.

### Interactions
**Drug-drug.** *Aminoglycosides, cisplatin, loop diuretics, salicylates, vancomycin:* Dimenhydrinate may mask the signs of ototoxicity, which can be caused by these drugs. Advise clinician to monitor patient closely.

*Other CNS depressants, such as anxiolytics, barbiturates, sleeping aids, tranquilizers:* Additive CNS sedation and depression. Avoid use together.

**Drug-lifestyle.** *Alcohol use:* May cause additive CNS depression. Advise patient to avoid alcohol use.

### Adverse reactions
**CNS:** *drowsiness,* headache, dizziness, confusion, nervousness, insomnia (especially in children), vertigo, tingling and weakness of hands, lassitude, excitation.
**CV:** palpitations, hypotension, tachycardia, tightness of chest.
**EENT:** blurred vision, diplopia, nasal congestion.
**GI:** dry mouth, nausea, vomiting, diarrhea, epigastric distress, constipation, anorexia.
**Respiratory:** wheezing, thickened bronchial secretions, dry respiratory passages.
**Skin:** photosensitivity, urticaria, rash.
**Other:** *anaphylaxis.*

### Overdose and treatment
Signs and symptoms of overdose may include either CNS depression (sedation, reduced mental alertness, apnea, and CV collapse) or CNS stimulation (insomnia, hallucinations, tremors, or seizures). Anticholinergic symptoms, such as dry mouth, flushed skin, fixed and dilated pupils, and GI symptoms, are likely to occur, especially in children.

Recommend using gastric lavage to empty stomach contents; emetics may be ineffective. Diazepam or phenytoin may be used to control seizures. Supportive treatment should be provided.

### Clinical considerations
■ Parenteral solution is incompatible with many drugs; don't mix other drugs in the same syringe.
■ To prevent motion sickness, patient should take drug 30 minutes before traveling and again before meals and at bedtime.
■ Antiemetic effect may diminish with prolonged use.
■ Dimenhydrinate may alter or confuse test results for xanthines (caffeine, aminophylline) because of its 8-chlorotheophylline content; discontinue dimenhydrinate 4 days before diagnostic skin tests to avoid preventing, reducing, or masking test response.

### Therapeutic monitoring
■ Recommend safety measures for all patients; dimenhydrinate has a high incidence of drowsiness. Tolerance to CNS depressant effects usually develops within a few days.

### Special populations
**Breast-feeding patients.** Avoid use of antihistamines during breast-feeding. Many of these drugs, including dimenhydrinate, appear in breast milk, exposing the infant to risks of unusual excitability; premature infants are at particular risk for seizures.
**Pediatric patients.** Safety in neonates hasn't been established. Infants and children under age 6 may experience paradoxical hyperex-

citability. I.V. dosage for children hasn't been established.

**Geriatric patients.** Geriatric patients are usually more sensitive to adverse effects of antihistamines than younger patients and are especially likely to experience a greater degree of dizziness, sedation, hyperexcitability, dry mouth, and urine retention.

## Patient counseling
■ Tell patient to avoid hazardous activities, such as driving or operating heavy machinery, until adverse CNS effects of drug are known.
■ Tell patient to take drug for motion sickness 30 minutes before exposure.

# dimercaprol
BAL in Oil

*Pharmacologic classification:* chelate
*Therapeutic classification:* heavy metal antagonist
*Pregnancy risk category NR*

## Available forms
Available by prescription only
*Injection:* 100 mg/ml

## Indications and dosages
*Severe arsenic or gold poisoning*
*Adults and children:* 3 mg/kg deep I.M. q 4 hours for 2 days, then q.i.d. on day 3; then b.i.d. for 10 days.
*Mild arsenic or gold poisoning*
*Adults and children:* 2.5 mg/kg deep I.M. q.i.d. for 2 days, then b.i.d. on day 3; then once daily for 10 days.
*Severe gold dermatitis*
*Adults and children:* 2.5 mg/kg deep I.M. q 4 hours for 2 days, then b.i.d. for 7 days.
*Gold-induced thrombocytopenia*
*Adults and children:* 100 mg deep I.M. b.i.d. for 15 days.
*Mercury poisoning*
*Adults and children:* Initially, 5 mg/kg deep I.M., then 2.5 mg/kg daily or b.i.d. for 10 days.
*Acute lead encephalopathy or blood lead level greater than 100 mcg/dl*
*Adults and children:* 4 mg/kg (or 75 to 83 mg/m²) deep I.M. injection, then give simultaneously with edetate calcium disodium (250 mg/m²) q 4 hours for 3 to 5 days. Use separate injection sites.

## Mechanism of action
*Chelating action:* The sulfhydryl groups of dimercaprol form heterocyclic ring complexes with heavy metals, particularly arsenic, mercury, and gold, preventing or reversing their binding to body ligands.

## Pharmacokinetics
*Absorption:* Absorbed slowly through the skin.

*Distribution:* Distributed to all tissues, mainly the intracellular space, with the highest levels of dimercaprol occurring in the liver and kidneys.
*Metabolism:* Uncomplexed dimercaprol is metabolized rapidly to inactive products.
*Excretion:* Most dimercaprol-metal complexes and inactive metabolites are excreted in urine and feces.

| Route | Onset | Peak | Duration |
|-------|-------|------|----------|
| I.M. | Unknown | 30-60 min | 4 hr |

## Contraindications and precautions
Contraindicated in patients with hepatic dysfunction (except postarsenical jaundice). Use cautiously in patients with hypertension or oliguria. Avoid use in pregnant women unless required to treat a life-threatening acute poisoning.

## Interactions
**Drug-drug.** *Cadmium, iron, selenium, uranium:* Form toxic complexes with dimercaprol. Delay iron therapy for 24 hours after stopping dimercaprol.

## Adverse reactions
**CNS:** headache; paresthesia; anxiety.
**CV:** *transient increase in blood pressure* (returns to normal in 2 hours), *tachycardia,* pain or tightness in chest.
**EENT:** blepharospasm, conjunctivitis, lacrimation, rhinorrhea, excessive salivation, pain or tightness in throat.
**GI:** *nausea; vomiting; burning sensation in lips, mouth, and throat; abdominal pain.*
**Musculoskeletal:** muscle pain or weakness.
**Other:** *fever* (especially in children), pain or tightness hands.

## Overdose and treatment
Signs and symptoms of overdose include vomiting, seizures, stupor, coma, hypertension, and tachycardia; effects subside in 1 to 6 hours. Recommend supporting CV and respiratory status and controlling seizures with diazepam.

## Clinical considerations
**⚠ ALERT** Administer drug by deep I.M. injection only.
■ Advise clinician to treat patient as soon as possible after poisoning for optimal therapeutic effect.
■ Adverse effects of dimercaprol are usually mild and transitory and occur in about one half of patients who receive an I.M. dose of 5 mg/kg. In patients who receive doses in excess of 5 mg/kg, adverse effects usually occur within 30 minutes after injection and subside in 1 to 6 hours.
■ Drug has strong garlic odor.
■ Dimercaprol therapy blocks thyroid uptake of ¹³¹I, causing decreased values.

# diphenoxylate hydrochloride and atropine sulfate

Logen, Lomanate, Lomotil, Lonox

*Pharmacologic classification:* opiate
*Therapeutic classification:* antidiarrheal
*Pregnancy risk category C*
*Controlled substance schedule V*

## Available forms

Available by prescription only
*Tablets:* 2.5 mg diphenoxylate hydrochloride and 0.025 mg atropine sulfate per tablet
*Liquid:* 2.5 mg diphenoxylate hydrochloride and 0.025 mg atropine sulfate/5 ml

## Indications and dosages

*Acute, nonspecific diarrhea*
*Adults:* 5 mg diphenoxylate component P.O. q.i.d., then adjust, p.r.n.
*Children ages 2 and older:* 0.3 to 0.4 mg/kg diphenoxylate component P.O. daily in four divided doses using the liquid form; or administer according to diphenoxylate component, as follows:
*Children ages 8 to 12:* 2 mg P.O. five times daily.
*Children ages 5 to 8:* 2 mg P.O. q.i.d.
*Children ages 2 to 5:* 2 mg P.O. t.i.d.

## Mechanism of action

*Antidiarrheal action:* Diphenoxylate is a meperidine analogue that inhibits GI motility locally and centrally. In high doses, it may produce an opiate effect. Atropine is added in subtherapeutic doses to prevent abuse by deliberate overdose.

## Pharmacokinetics

*Absorption:* About 90% of an oral dose is absorbed.
*Distribution:* Appears in breast milk.
*Metabolism:* Metabolized extensively by the liver.
*Excretion:* Metabolites are excreted mainly in feces via the biliary tract, with lesser amounts excreted in urine.

| Route | Onset | Peak | Duration |
|-------|-------|------|----------|
| P.O. | 45-60 min | 3 hr | 3-4 hr |

## Contraindications and precautions

Contraindicated in patients hypersensitive to diphenoxylate or atropine, and those with acute diarrhea resulting from poison until toxic material is eliminated from GI tract, acute diarrhea caused by organisms that penetrate intestinal mucosa, or diarrhea resulting from antibiotic-induced pseudomembranous enterocolitis or enterotoxin-producing bacteria.

Also contraindicated in patients with obstructive jaundice and in children under age 2.
Use cautiously in children ages 2 and older; in patients with hepatic disease, narcotic dependence, or acute ulcerative colitis; and in pregnant women. Stop therapy immediately if abdominal distention or other signs of toxic megacolon develop.

## Interactions

**Drug-drug.** *CNS depressants, such as barbiturates, narcotic drugs, tranquilizers:* May result in an increased depressant effect. Avoid use together.
*MAO inhibitors:* May precipitate hypertensive crisis. Avoid use together.
**Drug-lifestyle.** *Alcohol use:* May enhance CNS depression. Advise patient to avoid alcohol.

## Adverse reactions

**CNS:** *sedation, dizziness,* headache, drowsiness, lethargy, restlessness, depression, euphoria, malaise, confusion, numbness in limbs, possible physical dependence with long-term use.
**CV:** tachycardia.
**EENT:** mydriasis.
**GI:** *dry mouth,* nausea, vomiting, abdominal discomfort or distention, *paralytic ileus,* anorexia, fluid retention in bowel or megacolon (may mask depletion of extracellular fluid and electrolytes, especially in young children treated for acute gastroenteritis), increased serum amylase, *pancreatitis,* swollen gums.
**GU:** urine retention.
**Respiratory:** *respiratory depression.*
**Skin:** pruritus, rash, dry skin.
**Other:** *angioedema, anaphylaxis.*

## Overdose and treatment

Signs and symptoms of overdose include drowsiness, low blood pressure, marked seizures, apnea, blurred vision, miosis, flushing, dry mouth and mucous membranes, and psychotic episodes.
Treatment is supportive; advise clinician to maintain airway and support vital functions. A narcotic antagonist, such as naloxone, may be given. Gastric lavage may be performed. Advise clinician to monitor patient for 48 to 72 hours.

## Clinical considerations

■ Drug is usually ineffective in treating antibiotic-induced diarrhea.
■ Reduce dosage as soon as symptoms are controlled.
■ Diphenoxylate may decrease urinary excretion of phenolsulfonphthalein (PSP) during the PSP excretion test.

## Therapeutic monitoring

■ Advise clinician to monitor vital signs and intake and output; recommend observing pa-

---

* Canada only    ◇ Unlabeled clinical use

tient for adverse reactions, especially CNS reactions.
- Recommend monitoring bowel function.

### Special populations
**Breast-feeding patients.** Drug appears in breast milk; drug effects have been reported in breast-fed infants of women taking drug.
**Pediatric patients.** Drug is contraindicated in children under age 2; some children may experience respiratory depression. Children, especially those with Down syndrome, appear to be particularly sensitive to atropine content of drug.
**Geriatric patients.** Geriatric patients may be more susceptible to respiratory depression and to exacerbation of preexisting glaucoma.

## Patient counseling
- Warn patient to take drug exactly as ordered and not to exceed recommended dose.
- Advise patient to maintain adequate fluid intake during course of diarrhea and teach him about diet and fluid replacement.
- Caution patient to avoid driving during drug therapy because drowsiness and dizziness may occur.
- Advise patient to call prescriber if drug isn't effective within 48 hours.
- Warn patient that prolonged use may result in tolerance and that use of larger-than-recommended doses may result in drug dependence.

---

# diphtheria and tetanus toxoids and acellular pertussis vaccine, adsorbed (DTaP)
Certiva, Infanrix, Tripedia

*Pharmacologic classification:* combination toxoid and vaccine
*Therapeutic classification:* diphtheria, tetanus, and pertussis prophylaxis
*Pregnancy risk category C*

## Available forms
Available by prescription only
*Injection:* 6.7 Lf units diphtheria, 5 Lf units tetanus, and 46.8 mcg pertussis antigens per 0.5 ml in single-dose and 7.5-ml vials; 15 Lf units of diphtheria toxoid, 6 Lf units tetanus toxoid, and 40 mcg pertussis toxoid per 0.5 ml in 7.5-ml vials; 25 Lf units of diphtheria toxoid, 10 Lf units tetanus toxoid, 25 mcg pertussis toxin, 25 mcg FHA, 8 mcg peractin per 0.5 ml in 0.5-ml vials

## Indications and dosages
*Primary immunization*
*Children ages 6 weeks to 7 years:* Give 0.5 ml I.M. 4 to 8 weeks apart for three doses and a

fourth dose at least 6 months after the third dose.
*Booster immunization*
If Tripedia was used for the first four doses, a fifth dose is recommended at 4 to 6 years of age before entering school. If the fourth dose was given after age 4, a fifth dose isn't needed.
Certiva as a fourth dose is recommended at 15 to 20 months of age in children who received their first three doses as whole-cell DTP vaccine. A fifth dose is recommended at 4 to 6 years of age in children who received four doses of whole-cell DTP vaccine or three doses of whole-cell vaccine followed by one dose of DTaP unless the fourth dose was given after the fourth birthday.
Infanrix is recommended as a fifth dose in children 4 to 6 years of age before entering school in those who received one dose or more of whole-cell DTP unless the fourth dose was given after the fourth birthday.

## Mechanism of action
*Diphtheria, tetanus, and pertussis (whooping cough) prophylaxis:* Vaccine promotes active immunity to diphtheria, tetanus, and pertussis by inducing production of antitoxin and antibodies.

## Pharmacokinetics
No information available.

| Route | Onset | Peak | Duration |
|-------|-------|------|----------|
| I.M. | 2 wk after last dose | Unknown | 10 yr |

## Contraindications and precautions
Contraindicated in immunosuppressed patients and in those on corticosteroid therapy or with history of seizures. Children whose seizures are well controlled or those with an explained single episode seizure may receive the acellular vaccine. Defer vaccination in patients with acute febrile illness. Children with preexisting neurologic disorders shouldn't receive pertussis component. Also, children who exhibit neurologic signs after injection shouldn't receive pertussis component in any succeeding injections. Give diphtheria and tetanus toxoids (called DT) instead. Not recommended for adults or children over 7 years of age.

## Interactions
**Drug-drug.** *Corticosteroids, immunosuppressants:* May impair the immune response to the toxoids and vaccine. Patient shouldn't have elective immunization under these circumstances.

## Adverse reactions
**CNS:** *encephalopathy, seizures,* peripheral neuropathy.
**Hematologic:** *thrombocytopenic purpura.*

**Skin:** soreness, redness, expected nodule remaining several weeks at injection site, urticaria.
**Other:** *anaphylaxis, fever,* hypersensitivity reactions, *shock.*

## Overdose and treatment
No information available.

## Clinical considerations
**◪ ALERT** Vaccine isn't routinely given to individuals ages 7 and older; it may be used only in special circumstances.
■ Obtain history of allergies and reactions to immunizations, especially to pertussis vaccine.
■ Epinephrine solution 1:1,000 should be available to treat allergic reactions.
■ Vaccine may be given at same time as trivalent oral polio vaccine and, if indicated, when the patient receives vaccines against *Haemophilus influenzae* type b, measles, mumps, and rubella.
**◪ ALERT** DTaP preparations are generally not interchangeable. It's recommended to use the vaccine from the same manufacturer, if possible, for at least the first three doses.

### Therapeutic monitoring
■ Acellular vaccine may have a lower incidence of local pain and fever.

## Patient counseling
■ Explain to parents that child may experience discomfort at the injection site after immunization and that a nodule may develop there and persist for several weeks. Fever, upset stomach, or general malaise may also develop. Recommend acetaminophen liquid to relieve such discomfort.
■ Tell parents to report worrisome or intolerable reactions promptly.
■ Stress importance of keeping scheduled appointments for subsequent doses. Full immunization requires a series of injections.

---

# dipyridamole
Persantine

*Pharmacologic classification:* pyrimidine analogue
*Therapeutic classification:* coronary vasodilator, platelet aggregation inhibitor
*Pregnancy risk category B*

## Available forms
Available by prescription only
*Tablets:* 25 mg, 50 mg, 75 mg
*Injection:* 10 mg/2 ml

## Indications and dosages
***Alternative to exercise in thallium myocardial perfusion imaging***
*Adults:* 0.142 mg/kg/minute I.V. infused over 4 minutes (0.57 mg/kg total).

***Inhibition of platelet adhesion in patients with prosthetic heart valves, with warfarin or aspirin***
*Adults:* 75 to 100 mg P.O. q.i.d.
◇ *Chronic angina pectoris*
*Adults:* 50 mg P.O. t.i.d. at least 1 hour before meals; 2 to 3 months of therapy may be required to achieve a clinical response.
◇ *Prevention of thromboembolic complications in patients with various thromboembolic disorders other than prosthetic heart valves*
*Adults:* 150 to 400 mg P.O. daily (with warfarin or aspirin).

## I.V. administration
■ Dilute I.V. form to at least a 1:2 ratio with 0.45% saline injection, normal saline injection, or $D_5W$ to a total volume of 20 to 50 ml.
■ Thallium should be injected within 5 minutes of dipyridamole.

### Incompatibilities
None reported.

## Mechanism of action
*Coronary vasodilating action:* Dipyridamole increases coronary blood flow by selectively dilating the coronary arteries. Coronary vasodilator effect follows inhibition of serum adenosine deaminase, which allows accumulation of adenosine, a potent vasodilator. Dipyridamole inhibits platelet adhesion by increasing effects of prostacyclin or by inhibiting phosphodiesterase.

## Pharmacokinetics
*Absorption:* Absorption is variable and slow; bioavailability ranges from 27% to 59%.
*Distribution:* Distributed widely in body tissues; small amounts cross the placenta. Protein-binding ranges from 91% to 97%.
*Metabolism:* Metabolized by the liver.
*Excretion:* Elimination occurs via biliary excretion of glucuronide conjugates. Some dipyridamole and conjugates may undergo enterohepatic circulation and fecal excretion; a small amount is excreted in urine. Half-life varies from 1 to 12 hours.

| Route | Onset | Peak | Duration |
|-------|-------|------|----------|
| P.O. | Unknown | 75 min | Unknown |

## Contraindications and precautions
Contraindicated in patients hypersensitive to drug or its components. Use cautiously in patients with hypotension or serious coronary artery disease.

## Interactions
**Drug-drug.** *Aminophylline:* Inhibits the action of dipyridamole. Avoid use together.

---

*Heparin, oral anticoagulants:* Can enhance the effects of oral anticoagulants and heparin. Advise clinician to monitor patient closely.

## Adverse reactions
**CNS:** *headache, dizziness.*
**CV:** flushing, fainting, *hypotension;* angina, chest pain, *blood pressure lability, hypertension* (with I.V. infusion).
**GI:** *nausea,* vomiting, diarrhea, abdominal distress.
**Hematologic:** increased bleeding time.
**Skin:** rash, irritation (with undiluted injection), pruritus.

## Overdose and treatment
Signs and symptoms of overdose include peripheral vasodilation and hypotension. Advise clinician to maintain blood pressure and treat symptomatically.

## Clinical considerations
■ Recommend giving drug at least 1 hour before meals.
■ When used as a pharmacologic "stress test," total doses beyond 60 mg aren't needed.

### Therapeutic monitoring
■ Advise clinician to monitor blood pressure.
■ Be alert for adverse reactions, including symptoms of bleeding and prolonged bleeding time, especially at high doses and during long-term therapy.

### Special populations
**Breast-feeding patients.** Safety in breast-feeding women hasn't been established.
**Pediatric patients.** Dosage hasn't been established in children.

## Patient counseling
■ Explain that clinical response may require 2 to 3 months of continuous therapy; encourage patient compliance.
■ Discuss adverse reactions and how to manage therapy.

# dirithromycin
Dynabac

*Pharmacologic classification:* macrolide
*Therapeutic classification:* antibiotic
*Pregnancy risk category C*

## Available forms
Available by prescription only
*Tablets:* 250 mg

## Indications and dosages
*Acute bacterial exacerbations of chronic bronchitis caused by* **Moraxella catarrhalis** *or* **Streptococcus pneumoniae;** *sec-*

*ondary bacterial infection of acute bronchitis caused by* **M. catarrhalis** *or* **S. pneumoniae;** *uncomplicated skin and skin structure infections caused by* **Staphylococcus aureus** *(methicillin susceptible)*
*Adults and children ages 12 and older:* 500 mg P.O. daily with food for 7 days.
*Community-acquired pneumonia caused by* **Legionella pneumophila, Mycoplasma pneumoniae,** *or* **S. pneumoniae**
*Adults and children ages 12 and older:* 500 mg P.O. daily with food for 14 days.
*Pharyngitis or tonsillitis caused by* **Streptococcus pyogenes**
*Adults and children ages 12 and older:* 500 mg P.O. daily with food for 10 days.

## Mechanism of action
*Antibiotic action:* Dirithromycin inhibits bacterial RNA-dependent protein synthesis by binding to the 5OS subunit of the ribosome. Its spectrum of activity includes gram-positive aerobes such as *S. aureus* (methicillin-susceptible strains only), *S. pneumoniae, S. pyogenes;* gram-negative aerobes such as *L. pneumophila* and *M. catarrhalis;* and other bacteria such as *M. pneumoniae.*

## Pharmacokinetics
*Absorption:* Rapidly absorbed from GI tract and converted by nonenzymatic hydrolysis to the microbiologically active compound erythromycylamine. Food slightly increases bioavailability of drug.
*Distribution:* Widely distributed throughout the body. The protein binding of erythromycylamine ranges from 15% to 30%.
*Metabolism:* Undergoes little to no hepatic metabolism.
*Excretion:* Primarily eliminated in bile or feces with a small amount in urine. Mean half-life of erythromycylamine is about 8 hours.

| Route | Onset | Peak | Duration |
|-------|---------|------|----------|
| P.O. | Unknown | 4 hr | Unknown |

## Contraindications and precautions
Contraindicated in patients hypersensitive to dirithromycin, erythromycin, or other macrolide antibiotics. Use cautiously in pregnant patients and those with hepatic insufficiency.

## Interactions
**Drug-drug.** *Alfentanil, anticoagulants, bromocriptine, carbamazepine, cyclosporine, digoxin, disopyramide, ergotamine, hexobarbital, lovastatin, phenytoin, triazolam, valproate:* These drugs interact with erythromycin products; it isn't known if these same drug interactions occur with dirithromycin. Use caution during coadministration.
*Antacids, H₂ antagonists:* Absorption may be slightly enhanced when dirithromycin is giv-

en immediately after these drugs. Monitor patient.

*Theophylline:* Dirithromycin may alter steady-state plasma level of theophylline. Advise clinician to monitor theophylline plasma levels. Dosage adjustments may be needed.

**Drug-food.** *Any food:* Increases absorption. Give drug with food.

### Adverse reactions
**CNS:** headache, dizziness, vertigo, insomnia, asthenia.
**GI:** abdominal pain, nausea, diarrhea, vomiting, dyspepsia, GI disorder, flatulence.
**Hematologic:** increased platelet, eosinophil, and neutrophil counts.
**Metabolic:** hyperkalemia, decreased bicarbonate levels, increased CK levels.
**Respiratory:** increased cough, dyspnea.
**Skin:** rash, pruritus, urticaria.
**Other:** pain (nonspecific).

### Overdose and treatment
Signs and symptoms of a macrolide antibiotic overdose may include nausea, vomiting, epigastric distress, and diarrhea. Treatment should be supportive because forced diuresis, dialysis, and hemoperfusion haven't been established to be helpful for an overdose of dirithromycin.

### Clinical considerations
■ Culture and sensitivity tests should be obtained before drug treatment starts. Therapy may begin pending results.
■ Drug shouldn't be used in patients with known, suspected, or potential bacteremias because serum levels are inadequate to provide antibacterial coverage of the bloodstream.

#### Therapeutic monitoring
■ Advise clinician to monitor patient for superinfection. Drug may cause overgrowth of nonsusceptible bacteria or fungi.

#### Special populations
**Breast-feeding patients.** It isn't known if dirithromycin appears in breast milk. Give cautiously to breast-feeding women.
**Pediatric patients.** Safety and effectiveness in children under age 12 haven't been established.

### Patient counseling
■ Tell patient to take all of drug as prescribed, even after he feels better.
■ Instruct patient to take drug with food or within 1 hour of having eaten. Tell him not to cut, chew, or crush the tablet.

# disopyramide phosphate
Norpace, Norpace CR, Rythmodan*, Rythmodan-LA*

*Pharmacologic classification:* pyridine derivative antiarrhythmic, group IA antiarrhythmic
*Therapeutic classification:* ventricular antiarrhythmic, supraventricular antiarrhythmic, atrial antitachyarrhythmic
*Pregnancy risk category C*

### Available forms
Available by prescription only
*Capsules:* 100 mg, 150 mg
*Capsules (extended-release):* 100 mg, 150 mg

### Indications and dosages
*PVCs (unifocal, multifocal, or coupled); ventricular tachycardia;* ◇ *conversion of atrial fibrillation, atrial flutter, and paroxysmal atrial tachycardia to normal sinus rhythm*
*Adults:* Initially, 200 to 300 mg loading dose. Usual maintenance dosage is 150 mg P.O. q 6 hours or 300 mg (extended-release) P.O. q 12 hours; for patients weighing less than 50 kg (110 lb), give 100 mg P.O. q 6 hours or 200 mg (extended-release) P.O. q 12 hours; and for patients with cardiomyopathy or possible cardiac decompensation, give 100 mg P.O. q 6 to 8 hours initially and then adjust, as indicated.
*Children ages 12 to 18:* 6 to 15 mg/kg/day P.O.
*Children ages 4 to 12:* 10 to 15 mg/kg/day P.O.
*Children ages 1 to 4:* 10 to 20 mg/kg/day P.O.
*Children under age 1:* 10 to 30 mg/kg/day P.O.

All children's doses should be divided equally and given q 6 hours. Extended-release capsules aren't recommended for use in children.
≡ *Dosage adjustment.* Geriatric patients may need dosage reduction. Adults with hepatic insufficiency or moderately impaired renal function should receive 100 mg P.O. q 6 hours or 200 mg (extended-release) q 12 hours. Patients with severely impaired renal function should receive only 100 mg (regular-release) at the following intervals.

| Creatinine clearance (ml/min) | Dosage interval |
| --- | --- |
| 30-40 | q 8 hr |
| 15-30 | q 12 hr |
| < 15 | q 24 hr |

### Mechanism of action
*Antiarrhythmic action:* A class IA antiarrhythmic, disopyramide depresses phase O of the action potential. It's considered a myocardial depressant because it decreases myocar-

dial excitability and conduction velocity and may depress myocardial contractility. It also possesses anticholinergic activity that may modify the direct myocardial effects of the drug. In therapeutic doses, disopyramide reduces conduction velocity in the atria, ventricles, and His-Purkinje system. By prolonging the effective refractory period (ERP), it helps control atrial tachyarrhythmias (however, this indication is unapproved in the United States). Its anticholinergic action, which is much greater than quinidine's, may increase AV node conductivity.

Disopyramide also has a greater myocardial depressant (negative inotropic) effect than quinidine. It helps manage premature ventricular beats by suppressing automaticity in the His-Purkinje system and ectopic pacemakers. At therapeutic doses, it usually doesn't prolong the QRS segment duration and PR interval but may prolong the QT interval.

## Pharmacokinetics
*Absorption:* Rapidly and well absorbed from the GI tract; about 60% to 80% of drug reaches systemic circulation.
*Distribution:* Well distributed throughout extracellular fluid but isn't extensively tissue-bound. Plasma protein–binding varies, depending on drug levels, but generally ranges from about 50% to 65%. Usual therapeutic serum level ranges from 2 to 4 mcg/ml, although some patients may require up to 7 mcg/ml. Levels above 9 mcg/ml generally are considered toxic.
*Metabolism:* Metabolized in the liver to one major metabolite that possesses little antiarrhythmic activity but greater anticholinergic activity than the parent compound.
*Excretion:* About 90% of an orally administered dose is excreted in the urine as unchanged drug and metabolites; 40% to 60% is excreted as unchanged drug. Usual elimination half-life is about 7 hours but lengthens in patients with renal or hepatic insufficiency. Duration of effect is usually 6 to 7 hours.

| Route | Onset | Peak | Duration |
|-------|-------|------|----------|
| P.O. | ½-3½ hr | 2-2½ hr | 1½-8½ hr |

## Contraindications and precautions
Contraindicated in patients hypersensitive to drug, or those with cardiogenic shock, or second- or third-degree heart block in the absence of an artificial pacemaker.

Use very cautiously or, if possible, avoid in patients with heart failure. Use cautiously in patients with underlying conduction abnormalities, urinary tract diseases (especially prostatic hyperplasia), hepatic or renal impairment, myasthenia gravis, or acute angle-closure glaucoma.

## Interactions
**Drug-drug.** *Antiarrhythmics:* May cause additive or antagonistic cardiac effects and additive toxicity. Advise clinician to monitor patient closely.
*Anticholinergics:* May cause additive anticholinergic effects. Advise clinician to monitor patient closely.
*Erythromycin:* Increases disopyramide levels, causing arrhythmias and increased QT intervals. Avoid use together.
*Insulin, oral antidiabetics:* Additive hypoglycemia. Advise clinician to monitor blood glucose levels.
*Rifampin:* May impair antiarrhythmic activity of disopyramide. Advise clinician to monitor patient closely.
*Warfarin:* May potentiate anticoagulant effects. Advise clinician to monitor PT and INR closely.
**Drug-herb.** *Jimsonweed:* May adversely affect the function of the CV system. Discourage use together.

## Adverse reactions
**CNS:** dizziness, agitation, depression, fatigue, muscle weakness, syncope.
**CV:** *hypotension, HF, heart block,* edema, *arrhythmias,* chest pain.
**EENT:** *blurred vision, dry eyes or nose.*
**GI:** nausea, vomiting, anorexia, bloating, abdominal pain, diarrhea.
**Hepatic:** cholestatic jaundice.
**Metabolic:** hypoglycemia, weight gain.
**Musculoskeletal:** aches, pain, muscle weakness.
**Respiratory:** shortness of breath.
**Skin:** rash, pruritus, dermatosis.

## Overdose and treatment
Signs and symptoms of overdose include anticholinergic effects, severe hypotension, widening of QRS complex and QT interval, ventricular arrhythmias, cardiac conduction disturbances, bradycardia, HF, asystole, loss of consciousness, seizures, apnea episodes, and respiratory arrest.

Treatment involves general supportive measures (including respiratory and CV support) and hemodynamic and ECG monitoring. If ingestion was recent, gastric lavage, emesis induction, and administration of activated charcoal may decrease absorption. Isoproterenol or dopamine may be given to correct hypotension after adequate hydration has been ensured. Digoxin and diuretics may be given to treat HF. Hemodialysis and charcoal hemoperfusion may effectively remove disopyramide. Some patients may require intra-aortic balloon counterpulsation, mechanically assisted respiration, or endocardial pacing.

## Clinical considerations
**H ALERT** Patients with atrial flutter or fibrillation should be digitalized before disopyra-

mide administration to ensure that enhanced AV conduction doesn't lead to ventricular tachycardia.

**ALERT** Anticoagulation therapy may be needed, especially for arrhythmia lasting longer than 48 hours.

■ Recommend correcting underlying electrolyte abnormalities, especially hypokalemia, before giving drug because disopyramide may be ineffective in patients with these problems.

■ Don't give sustained-release capsules for rapid control of ventricular arrhythmias if therapeutic blood drug levels must be attained rapidly, or if patient has cardiomyopathy, possible cardiac decompensation, or severe renal impairment.

■ If drug causes constipation, recommend giving laxatives and ensuring proper diet.

■ Drug is commonly prescribed for patients who can't tolerate quinidine or procainamide.

■ Pharmacist may prepare disopyramide suspension; 100-mg capsules are used with cherry syrup to prepare suspension (this may be best form for young children).

■ Drug is removed by hemodialysis. Dosage adjustments may be needed in patients undergoing dialysis.

### Therapeutic monitoring
■ Advise clinician to monitor patient for symptoms of developing heart block, such as QRS complex widening by more than 25% or QT interval lengthening by more than 25% above baseline.

### Special populations
**Breast-feeding patients.** Drug appears in breast milk; recommend alternative infant feeding methods during drug therapy.
**Pediatric patients.** Although safety and effectiveness of drug in children haven't been established, current recommendations call for total daily dose given in equally divided doses every 6 hours or at intervals based on individual requirements. Advise clinician to monitor patient during initial adjustment period; dosage adjustment should begin at lower end of recommended ranges. Advise clinician to monitor serum drug levels and therapeutic response carefully.
**Geriatric patients.** Advise clinician to monitor patients in this group closely for toxicity signs; also advise clinician to monitor serum electrolyte and drug levels.

### Patient counseling
■ When changing from immediate-release to sustained-release capsules, advise patient to begin taking sustained-release capsule 6 hours after last immediate-release capsule.

■ Teach patient importance of taking drug on time, exactly as prescribed. To do this, he may have to use an alarm clock for night doses.

■ Advise patient to use sugarless gum or hard candy to relieve dry mouth.

# disulfiram
Antabuse

*Pharmacologic classification:* aldehyde dehydrogenase inhibitor
*Therapeutic classification:* alcohol deterrent
*Pregnancy risk category C*

## Available forms
Available by prescription only
*Tablets:* 250 mg, 500 mg

## Indications and dosages
*Adjunct in management of chronic alcoholism*
*Adults:* Give maximum dose of 500 mg P.O. as a single dose in the morning for 1 to 2 weeks. Can be taken in evening if drowsiness occurs. Maintenance dosage is 125 to 500 mg daily (average dose 250 mg) until permanent self-control is established. Treatment may continue for months or years.

## Mechanism of action
*Antialcoholic action:* Disulfiram irreversibly inhibits aldehyde dehydrogenase, which prevents the oxidation of alcohol after the acetaldehyde stage. It interacts with ingested alcohol to produce acetaldehyde levels five to ten times higher than are produced by normal alcohol metabolism. Excess acetaldehyde produces a highly unpleasant reaction (nausea and vomiting) to even a small quantity of alcohol. Tolerance to disulfiram doesn't occur; rather, sensitivity to alcohol increases with longer duration of therapy.

## Pharmacokinetics
*Absorption:* Absorbed completely after oral administration, but 3 to 12 hours may be required before effects occur.
*Distribution:* Highly lipid-soluble and initially localized in adipose tissue.
*Metabolism:* Mostly oxidized in the liver and excreted in urine as free drug and metabolites (for example, diethyldithiocarbamate, diethylamine, and carbon disulfide).
*Excretion:* 5% to 20% is unabsorbed and is eliminated in feces. A small amount is eliminated through the lungs, but most is excreted in the urine. Several days may be required for total elimination of drug.

| Route | Onset | Peak | Duration |
|-------|-------|------|----------|
| P.O. | 1-2 hr | Unknown | 14 days |

## Contraindications and precautions
Contraindicated in patients intoxicated by alcohol and within 12 hours of alcohol inges-

tion; in those with psychoses, myocardial disease, coronary occlusion; those hypersensitive to disulfiram or other thiuram derivatives used in pesticides and rubber vulcanization; and in patients receiving metronidazole, paraldehyde, alcohol, or alcohol-containing preparations.

Use with extreme caution in patients with diabetes mellitus, hypothyroidism, seizure disorder, cerebral damage, or nephritis or hepatic cirrhosis or insufficiency and with concurrent phenytoin therapy. Drug shouldn't be given during pregnancy.

## Interactions
**Drug-drug.** *Alfentanil:* May prolong duration of effect. Advise clinician to closely monitor patient.
*Bacampicillin:* May precipitate disulfiram-like reaction. Don't use together.
*Barbiturates, chlordiazepoxide, CNS depressants, coumarin anticoagulants, diazepam, midazolam, paraldehyde, phenytoin:* Disulfiram may increase the blood level of these drugs. Use together cautiously.
*Isoniazid:* Ataxia, unsteady gait, or marked behavioral changes. Don't use together.
*Metronidazole:* Psychosis or confusion. Avoid use together.
*Tricyclic antidepressants, especially amitriptyline:* May cause transient delirium. Advise clinician to closely monitor patient.
**Drug-herb.** *Passion flower, pill-bearing spurge, pokeweed, squaw vine, squill, sundew, sweet flag, tormentil, valerian, yarrow:* Disulfiram-like reaction if herbal form contains alcohol. Warn patient not to use together.
**Drug-food.** *Caffeine:* Exaggerated or prolonged effects of caffeine may occur. Advise patient to avoid caffeine.
**Drug-lifestyle.** *Alcohol use (all sources including back-rub preparations, cough syrups, liniments, shaving lotions):* May precipitate disulfiram-like reaction. Alcohol reaction may occur as long as 2 weeks after single disulfiram dose; the longer patient remains on drug, the more sensitive he becomes to alcohol. Advise patient to be alert for and avoid use of these products.
*Marijuana:* Disulfiram produces a synergistic CNS stimulation when used with marijuana. Inform patient of this interaction.

## Adverse reactions
**CNS:** drowsiness, headache, fatigue, delirium, depression, neuritis, peripheral neuritis, polyneuritis, restlessness, psychotic reactions.
**EENT:** optic neuritis.
**GI:** metallic or garlic aftertaste.
**GU:** impotence.
**Metabolic:** elevated serum cholesterol.
**Skin:** acneiform or allergic dermatitis, occasional eruptions.
**Other:** *disulfiram-like reaction* (precipitated by ethanol use), which may include flushing, throbbing headache, dyspnea, nausea, copious vomiting, diaphoresis, thirst, chest pain, palpitations, hyperventilation, hypotension, syncope, anxiety, weakness, blurred vision, confusion, and arthropathy.

In severe reactions: respiratory depression, CV collapse, arrhythmias, MI, acute heart failure, seizures, unconsciousness, or death.

## Overdose and treatment
Overdose signs and symptoms include GI upset and vomiting, abnormal EEG findings, drowsiness, altered consciousness, hallucinations, speech impairment, incoordination, and coma. Treat overdose by gastric aspiration or lavage along with supportive therapy.

Treatment of alcohol-induced disulfiram-like reaction is supportive and symptomatic. These reactions aren't usually life-threatening. Emergency equipment and drugs should be available because arrhythmias and severe hypotension may occur. Treat severe reactions like shock by giving plasma or electrolyte solutions p.r.n. Large I.V. doses of ascorbic acid, iron, and antihistamines have been used but are of questionable value. Hypokalemia has been reported; it requires careful monitoring and potassium supplements.

## Clinical considerations
**H ALERT** Caution patient's family that disulfiram should never be given to the patient without his knowledge; severe reaction or death could result if patient ingests alcohol.
■ Disulfiram shouldn't be given for at least 12 hours after the last alcohol ingestion.
■ Drug use requires close medical supervision. Patients should clearly understand consequences of disulfiram therapy and give informed consent before use.
■ Use drug only in patients who are cooperative and well motivated, and who are receiving supportive psychiatric therapy.
■ Disulfiram may decrease urinary vanillylmandelic acid excretion and increase urinary levels of homovanillic acid.

### Therapeutic monitoring
■ Complete physical examination and laboratory studies (CBC, electrolytes, transaminases) should precede therapy and be repeated regularly.

### Special populations
**Pregnant patients.** Drug shouldn't be given during pregnancy.

## Patient counseling
■ Explain that, although disulfiram can help discourage use of alcohol, it isn't a cure for alcoholism.
■ Warn patient to avoid all sources of alcohol: sauces or soups made with sherry or other wines or alcohol (even "cooking alcohol"), some

herbal preparations, and cough syrups. External applications of after-shave lotion, liniments, or other topical preparations may cause disulfiram-like reaction.

■ Warn patient that drug may cause drowsiness.

■ Instruct patient to carry identification card stating that disulfiram is being used, including the telephone number of the prescriber or clinic to contact if a reaction occurs.

# dobutamine hydrochloride
Dobutrex

*Pharmacologic classification:* adrenergic, beta₁ agonist
*Therapeutic classification:* inotropic
*Pregnancy risk category B*

## Available forms
Available by prescription only
*Injection:* 12.5 mg/ml in 20-ml vials (parenteral)
*Premixed:* 0.5 mg/ml (125 or 250 mg) in $D_5W$; 1 mg/ml (250 or 500 mg) in $D_5W$; 2 mg/ml (500 mg) in $D_5W$; 4 mg/ml (1,000 mg) in $D_5W$

## Indications and dosages
*To increase cardiac output in short-term treatment of cardiac decompensation caused by depressed contractility*
Adults: 2 to 20 mcg/kg/minute as an I.V. infusion. Rarely, infusion rates up to 40 mcg/kg/minute may be needed. Adjust dosage carefully to patient response.

## I.V. administration
■ Dilute concentrate for injection before giving it. Compatible solutions include $D_5W$, half-normal or normal saline solution for injection, and lactated Ringer's injection. Contents of one vial (250 mg) diluted with 1,000 ml of solution yields 250 mcg/ml. Diluting with 500 ml yields 500 mcg/ml. Diluting with 250 ml yields 1,000 mcg/ml. Don't exceed maximum of 5 mg/ml.

■ Oxidation of drug may slightly discolor admixtures containing dobutamine. This doesn't indicate a significant loss of potency provided drug is used within 24 hours of reconstitution.

■ Administer through a central venous catheter or large peripheral vein. Titrate infusion according to prescriber's orders and patient's condition. Use an infusion pump. Infusions for up to 72 hours produce no more adverse effects than shorter infusions.

■ Extravasation may cause an inflammatory response. Change I.V. sites regularly to avoid phlebitis.

■ Use the solution within 24 hours.

## Incompatibilities
�024 ALERT Dobutamine is incompatible with alkaline solution (sodium bicarbonate). Also, don't mix with or give through same I.V. line as heparin, hydrocortisone, cefazolin, or penicillin.

Also incompatible with acyclovir, alkaline solutions, alteplase, aminophylline, bretylium, bumetanide, calcium chloride, calcium gluconate, cefamandole, cefazolin, cephalothin (neutral), diazepam, doxapram, foscarnet, hydrocortisone, indomethacin sodium trihydrate, insulin (regular), magnesium sulfate, penicillin, phenytoin, phytonadione, sodium bicarbonate, sodium ethacrynate, and verapamil.

## Mechanism of action
*Inotropic action:* Dobutamine selectively stimulates beta₁-adrenergic receptors to increase myocardial contractility and CVA volume, resulting in increased cardiac output (a positive inotropic effect in patients with normal hearts or in HF). At therapeutic doses, dobutamine decreases peripheral resistance (afterload), reduces ventricular filling pressure (preload), and may facilitate AV node conduction. Systolic blood pressure and pulse pressure may remain unchanged or increased from increased cardiac output. Increased myocardial contractility results in increased coronary blood flow and myocardial oxygen consumption. Heart rate usually remains unchanged; however, excessive doses do have chronotropic effects. Dobutamine doesn't appear to affect dopaminergic receptors, nor does it cause renal or mesenteric vasodilation; however, urine flow may increase because of increased cardiac output.

## Pharmacokinetics
*Absorption:* Rapid.
*Distribution:* Widely distributed throughout the body.
*Metabolism:* Metabolized by the liver and by conjugation to inactive metabolites.
*Excretion:* Excreted mainly in urine, with minor amounts in feces, as its metabolites and conjugates.

| Route | Onset | Peak | Duration |
|---|---|---|---|
| I.V. | 1-2 min | 10 min | < 5 min after infusion ends |

## Contraindications and precautions
Contraindicated in patients hypersensitive to drug or its formulation and in those with idiopathic hypertrophic subaortic stenosis. Use cautiously in patients with a history of hypertension or those who have had a recent MI. Drug may precipitate an exaggerated pressor response.

## Interactions
**Drug-drug.** *Beta blockers:* May antagonize the cardiac effects of dobutamine. Don't use together.
*Bretylium:* May potentiate actions of vasopressors on adrenergic receptors. Advise clinician to monitor patient closely for arrhythmias.
*Guanadrel, guanethidine:* May potentiate the pressor effects of dobutamine, possibly resulting in hypertension and cardiac arrhythmias. Advise clinician to monitor patient closely.
*Inhalation hydrocarbon anesthetics:* May trigger ventricular arrhythmias. Advise clinician to monitor ECG carefully.
*Nitroprusside:* May cause higher cardiac output and lower pulmonary wedge pressure. Advise clinician to monitor patient closely.
*Rauwolfia alkaloids:* May prolong the actions of dobutamine (a denervation supersensitivity response). Advise clinician to monitor patient closely.
*Tricyclic antidepressants:* May potentiate pressor response. Use with caution.
**Drug-herb.** *Rue:* May increase inotropic potential. Discourage use together.

## Adverse reactions
**CNS:** headache.
**CV:** *increased heart rate, hypertension*, PVCs, angina, nonspecific chest pain, palpitations, hypotension.
**GI:** nausea, vomiting.
**Respiratory:** shortness of breath, *asthmatic episodes.*
**Other:** phlebitis, hypersensitivity reactions, *anaphylaxis.*

## Overdose and treatment
Signs and symptoms of overdose include nervousness and fatigue. No treatment is needed beyond dosage reduction or withdrawal of drug.

## Clinical considerations
■ Before administration of dobutamine, correct hypovolemia with appropriate plasma volume expanders.
■ Before giving dobutamine, administer a cardiac glycoside if patient has atrial fibrillation (dobutamine increases AV conduction).
■ Response to drug varies widely in geriatric, pediatric, and critically ill patients.

## *Therapeutic monitoring*
■ Advise clinician to monitor ECG, blood pressure, cardiac output, and pulmonary wedge pressure. Advise clinician to monitor serum electrolytes, especially potassium.
■ Most patients experience an increase of 10 to 20 mm Hg in systolic blood pressure; some show an increase of 50 mm Hg or more. Most also experience an increase in heart rate of 5 to 15 beats per minute; some show increases

of 30 or more beats per minute. Premature ventricular arrhythmias may occur in about 5% of patients.

## *Special populations*
**Breast-feeding patients.** It's unknown if dobutamine appears in breast milk. Give cautiously to breast-feeding women.
**Pediatric patients.** Increases cardiac output and systemic pressure in children. Use with caution in pediatric patients.
**Geriatric patients.** Geriatric patients require lower doses because they may be more sensitive to the effects of the drug. Use with caution in geriatric patients.

## Patient counseling
■ Advise patient to report adverse reactions, especially dyspnea and drug-induced headache.
■ Instruct patient to report pain at I.V. site.

# docetaxel
Taxotere

*Pharmacologic classification:* taxoid
*Therapeutic classification:* antineoplastic
*Pregnancy risk category D*

## Available forms
Available by prescription only
*Injection:* 20 mg, 80 mg

## Indications and dosages
*Treatment of patients with locally advanced or metastatic breast cancer who have progressed during anthracycline-based therapy or have relapsed during anthracycline-based adjuvant therapy*
*Adults:* 60 to 100 mg/m$^2$ I.V. over 1 hour q 3 weeks.
*Non–small-cell lung carcinoma*
*Adults:* 75 mg/m$^2$ I.V. over 1 hour q 3 weeks.
**≡***Dosage adjustment.* Patients who initially receive 100 mg/m$^2$ and who experience either febrile neutropenia, a neutrophil count less than 500 cells/mm$^3$ for longer than 1 week, severe or cumulative cutaneous reactions, or severe peripheral neuropathy during docetaxel therapy should have dosage adjusted from 100 to 75 mg/m$^2$. If patients continue to experience these reactions, either the dosage should be decreased from 75 to 55 mg/m$^2$ or the treatment should be stopped.
   Patients who initially receive 60 mg/m$^2$ and who don't experience febrile neutropenia, a neutrophil count less than 500 cells/mm$^3$ for longer than 1 week, severe or cumulative cutaneous reactions, or severe peripheral neuropathy during docetaxel therapy may tolerate higher doses.

## I.V. administration

- Use caution during preparation and administration of docetaxel. Use gloves. If solution contacts skin, wash skin immediately and thoroughly with soap and water. If docetaxel contacts mucous membranes, flush membranes thoroughly with water. Mark all waste materials with CHEMOTHERAPY HAZARD labels.
- Prepare and store infusion solutions in bottles (glass, polypropylene) or plastic bags (polypropylene, polyolefin) and give through polyethylene-lined administration sets.
- Docetaxel requires dilution before administration using the diluent supplied with drug. Allow drug and diluent to stand at room temperature for about 5 minutes before mixing. After adding the entire contents of diluent to the vial of docetaxel, gently rotate the vial for about 15 seconds. Then allow solution to stand for a few minutes to allow any foam to dissipate.
- Aseptically withdraw the required amount of premix solution from the vial and inject into a 250-ml infusion bag or bottle of normal saline solution or D$_5$W solution to produce a final level of 0.3 to 0.9 mg/ml. Doses exceeding 240 mg require a larger volume of infusion solution so a level of 0.9 mg/ml of docetaxel isn't exceeded. Thoroughly mix the infusion by manual rotation.
- Discard solution if it isn't clear or if it contains precipitates.

### Incompatibilities
None reported.

### Mechanism of action
*Antineoplastic action:* Docetaxel acts by disrupting the microtubular network in cells that's essential for mitotic and interphase cellular functions.

### Pharmacokinetics
*Absorption:* Given I.V.
*Distribution:* About 94% protein-bound.
*Metabolism:* Undergoes oxidative metabolism.
*Excretion:* Eliminated primarily in feces with a small amount being eliminated in urine.

| Route | Onset | Peak | Duration |
|-------|-------|------|----------|
| I.V. | Rapid | Unknown | Unknown |

### Contraindications and precautions
Contraindicated in patients hypersensitive to drug or other drugs formulated with polysorbate 80. Don't use docetaxel in patients with neutrophil counts of less than 1,500 cells/mm$^3$.

### Interactions
**Drug-drug.** *Compounds that induce, inhibit, or are metabolized by cytochrome P-450 3A4, such as cyclosporine, erythromycin, ketoconazole, troleandomycin:* Metabolism of docetaxel may be modified by concomitant administration. Use together cautiously.

### Adverse reactions
**CNS:** paresthesia, dysesthesia, pain (including burning sensation), weakness.
**CV:** fluid retention, hypotension, chest tightness.
**GI:** *stomatitis,* nausea, vomiting, diarrhea.
**Hematologic:** *anemia,* NEUTROPENIA, FEBRILE NEUTROPENIA, MYELOSUPPRESSION, LEUKOPENIA, THROMBOCYTOPENIA.
**Hepatic:** *elevated liver function test results.*
**Musculoskeletal:** *myalgia,* arthralgia, back pain.
**Respiratory:** dyspnea.
**Skin:** *alopecia,* maculopapular eruptions, desquamation, nail pigmentation alteration, onycholysis, nail pain, flushing, rash.
**Other:** hypersensitivity reactions, *anaphylaxis, infections,* drug fever, chills.

### Overdose and treatment
Signs and symptoms of overdose may include bone marrow suppression, peripheral neurotoxicity, and mucositis. There's no known antidote for docetaxel. Advise clinician to closely monitor patient's vital functions.

### Clinical considerations
- Patients with bilirubin values greater than the upper limits of normal (ULN) should generally not receive docetaxel. Also, patients with ALT or AST that exceeds 1.5 times ULN concomitant with alkaline phosphatase greater than 2.5 times ULN should generally not receive drug.
- Patient should be premedicated with oral corticosteroids such as dexamethasone 16 mg daily for 5 days starting 1 day before docetaxel administration, to reduce the incidence and severity of fluid retention and hypersensitivity reactions.
- ▌*ALERT* Don't confuse Taxotere (docetaxel) with Taxol (paclitaxel).

### Therapeutic monitoring
- Advise clinician to monitor patient closely for hypersensitivity reactions, especially during the first and second infusions. If minor reactions such as flushing or localized skin reactions occur, interruption of therapy isn't required. More severe reactions require the immediate discontinuation of docetaxel and aggressive treatment.
- Bone marrow toxicity is the most frequent and dose-limiting toxicity. Frequent blood count monitoring is needed during therapy.

### Special populations
**Pregnant patients.** Advise patient of childbearing age to avoid becoming pregnant during therapy with docetaxel because of the potential harm to the fetus.
**Breast-feeding patients.** Because of potential for serious adverse reactions in breast-fed in-

fants, it's recommended that breast-feeding be stopped during docetaxel therapy.
**Pediatric patients.** Safety and effectiveness in children under age 16 haven't been established.

## Patient counseling
- Warn patient that alopecia occurs in almost 80% of all patients.
- Tell patient to promptly report a sore throat, fever, unusual bruising, or bleeding.

# docosanol
Abreva

*Pharmacologic classification:* antiviral
*Therapeutic classification:* antiviral
*Pregnancy risk category* B

## Available forms
Available without a prescription
*Cream:* 10%

## Indications and dosages
***Treatment of recurrent oral-facial herpes simplex***
*Adults and children ages 12 and older:* Apply topically five times daily starting with first indication of an episode and continuing until lesion is healed. Rub in gently but completely.

## Mechanism of action
*Antiviral action:* The predominant mechanism for the antiherpes simplex virus activity appears to be inhibition of fusion between the cell's plasma membrane and the herpes simplex virus envelope, thus blocking the entry and subsequent replication of the virus.

## Pharmacokinetics
*Absorption:* Not absorbed.
*Distribution:* Not applicable.
*Metabolism:* Not applicable.
*Excretion:* Not applicable.

| Route | Onset | Peak | Duration |
|---|---|---|---|
| Topical | Unknown | Unknown | Unknown |

## Contraindications and precautions
Contraindicated in patients hypersensitive to docosanol or its components.

## Interactions
None reported.

## Adverse reactions
**CNS:** *headache.*
**Skin:** reaction at application site.

## Overdose and treatment
Adverse reactions related to overdose by topical application are unlikely because of limited absorption. Poor oral absorption makes the occurrence of significant adverse reactions following ingestion unlikely.

## Clinical considerations
- Use drug to treat oral-facial herpes simplex only.
- Start treatment as early as possible after onset of symptoms.
- Continue treatment until lesion has healed.
- Avoid application in or near the eyes.

### *Therapeutic monitoring*
- Advise clinician to monitor lesions for therapeutic response and adjust therapy duration p.r.n.

### *Special populations*
**Breast-feeding patients.** It's not known if drug appears in breast milk. Because many drugs appear in breast milk, use cautiously in breast-feeding women.
**Pediatric patients.** Safety and efficacy in children under age 12 haven't been established.

## Patient counseling
- Tell patient that cream should be used on the lips or face only.
- Caution patient to avoid application in or near the eyes because it may cause irritation.
- Advise patient to begin treatment as soon as symptoms appear and to continue treatment until the lesion has healed.
- Advise patient that lesions are considered contagious until completely healed.
- Inform patient to notify prescriber if the condition gets worse.
- Caution patient that drug should be used during pregnancy only if clearly needed.
- Advise patient to store drug at controlled room temperature and not to freeze drug.

# docusate calcium
Surfak

# docusate sodium
Colace, Correctol, Diocto, Docu, Docusoft, DOK, DOS, DSS, Ex-Lax, Fleet, Genasoft, Modane Soft, Phillips, Regulax SS, Regulex*, Silace, Soft-Lax

*Pharmacologic classification:* surfactant
*Therapeutic classification:* emollient laxative
*Pregnancy risk category* C

## Available forms
Available without a prescription
*Tablets:* 100 mg
*Capsules:* 50 mg, 100 mg, 240 mg, 250 mg
*Syrup:* 16.7 mg/5 ml, 20 mg/5 ml
*Solution:* 10 mg/ml

## Indications and dosages
*Stool softener*
**docusate calcium**
*Adults:* 240 mg P.O. daily until bowel movements are normal. Higher doses are for initial therapy. Adjust dosage to individual response.
*Children ages 6 and older:* 50 to 150 mg P.O. daily.
**docusate sodium**
*Adults and children ages 12 and older:* 50 to 200 mg P.O. daily until bowel movements are normal. Alternatively, add 50 to 100 mg to saline or oil retention enema to treat fecal impaction.
*Children ages 6 to 12:* 40 to 120 mg P.O. daily.
*Children ages 3 to 6:* 20 to 60 mg P.O. daily.
*Children under age 3:* 10 to 40 mg P.O. daily.

## Mechanism of action
*Laxative action:* Docusate salts act as detergents in the intestine, reducing surface tension of interfacing liquids; this promotes incorporation of fat and additional liquid, softening the stool.

## Pharmacokinetics
*Absorption:* Absorbed minimally in the duodenum and jejunum.
*Distribution:* Distributed primarily locally, in the gut.
*Metabolism:* None.
*Excretion:* Excreted in feces.

| Route | Onset | Peak | Duration |
|---|---|---|---|
| P.O. | 24-72 hr | 24-72 hr | 24-72 hr |

## Contraindications and precautions
Contraindicated in patients hypersensitive to drug and in those with intestinal obstruction, undiagnosed abdominal pain, vomiting or other signs of appendicitis, fecal impaction, or acute surgical abdomen.

## Interactions
**Drug-drug.** *Mineral oil:* Docusate salts may increase absorption of mineral oil and cause toxicity. Separate administration times.

## Adverse reactions
**GI:** bitter taste, mild abdominal cramping, diarrhea, laxative dependence (with long-term or excessive use).

## Overdose and treatment
No information available.

## Clinical considerations
■ Liquid or syrup must be given in 180 to 240 ml (6 to 8 ounces) of milk or fruit juice or in infant's formula to prevent throat irritation.
■ Avoid using docusate sodium in sodium-restricted patients.

■ Docusate salts are available with casanthranol (Peri-Colace), senna (Senokot), and phenolphthalein (Ex-Lax, Feen-a-mint, Correctol).
■ Docusate salts are the preferred laxative for most patients who must avoid straining at stool, such as those recovering from MI or rectal surgery. They also are used commonly to treat patients with postpartum constipation.

### Therapeutic monitoring
■ Before giving for constipation, determine whether patient has adequate fluid intake, exercise, and diet.
■ Discontinue drug if severe cramping occurs; notify prescriber.

### Special populations
**Breast-feeding patients.** Because absorption of docusate salts is minimal, they presumably pose no risk to breast-feeding infants.
**Geriatric patients.** Docusate salts are good choices for geriatric patients because they rarely cause laxative dependence, cause fewer adverse effects, and are gentler than some other laxatives.

### Patient counseling
■ Docusate salts lose their effectiveness over time; advise patient to report failure of drug.
■ Teach patient about dietary sources of bulk, which include bran and other cereals, fresh fruit, and vegetables.

---

# dofetilide
Tikosyn

*Pharmacologic classification:* antiarrhythmic
*Therapeutic classification:* class III antiarrhythmic
*Pregnancy risk category C*

## Available forms
Available by prescription only
*Capsules:* 125 mcg, 250 mcg, 500 mcg

## Indications and dosages
*Maintenance of normal sinus rhythm in patients with symptomatic atrial fibrillation or atrial flutter for longer than 1 week; conversion of atrial fibrillation and atrial flutter to normal sinus rhythm*
*Adults:* Dosage is individualized and is based on creatinine clearance and QT interval, which must be determined before first dose. Usual recommended dose is 500 mcg P.O. b.i.d. for patients with creatinine clearance greater than 60 ml/minute.
≡*Dosage adjustment.* If creatinine clearance is 40 to 60 ml/minute, starting dose is 250 mcg P.O. b.i.d. If it's 20 to 39 ml/minute, starting dose is 125 mcg P.O. b.i.d.

At 2 to 3 hours after first dose, determine QT interval. If it has increased by more than 15% over baseline or if it's more than 500 msec (550 msec in patients with ventricular conduction abnormalities), adjust dosage as follows: If starting dose based on creatinine clearance was 500 mcg P.O. b.i.d., give 250 mcg P.O. b.i.d. If starting dose based on creatinine clearance was 250 mcg P.O. b.i.d., give 125 mcg P.O. b.i.d. If starting dose based on creatinine clearance was 125 mcg P.O. b.i.d., give 125 mcg P.O. once daily.

Determine QT interval 2 to 3 hours after each subsequent dose while patient is in hospital. If at any time after second dose QT interval is more than 500 msec (550 msec in patients with ventricular conduction abnormalities), stop drug.

## Mechanism of action
*Antiarrhythmic action:* Dofetilide prolongs repolarization without affecting conduction velocity by blocking the cardiac ion channel carrying potassium current. No effect is seen on sodium channels or alpha-adrenergic and beta-adrenergic receptors.

## Pharmacokinetics
*Absorption:* Bioavailability after oral administration is greater than 90% with plasma levels peaking in 2 to 3 hours. Steady-state plasma levels are achieved in 2 to 3 days. Absorption unaffected by food or antacid.
*Distribution:* Widely distributed throughout the body; has a distribution volume of 3 L/kg. 60% to 70% plasma protein–bound.
*Metabolism:* Metabolized to a small extent by CYP3A4 isoenzyme of cytochrome P-450 system of the liver.
*Excretion:* About 80% is excreted in urine, of which 80% is excreted as unchanged drug with remaining 20% as inactive or minimally active metabolites.

| Route | Onset | Peak | Duration |
|-------|-------|------|----------|
| P.O. | Unknown | 2-3 hr | Unknown |

## Contraindications and precautions
Contraindicated in patients with creatinine clearance less than 20 ml/minute and in those with congenital or acquired long QT interval syndrome. Contraindicated in patients with baseline QT interval greater than 440 msec (500 msec in patients with ventricular conduction abnormalities). Use with caution in patients with severe hepatic impairment.

Drug is distributed only to hospitals and other institutions confirmed to have received applicable dosing and treatment initiation programs. Such confirmation is also needed for inpatient and subsequent outpatient discharge and refill prescriptions.

## Interactions
**Drug-drug.** *Amiloride, amiodarone, diltiazem, macrolide antibiotics, metformin, nefazodone, norfloxacin, protease inhibitors, quinine, serotonin reuptake inhibitors, triamterene, zafirlukast:* Possible increased plasma dofetilide levels. Use together cautiously.
*Class I, Class III antiarrhythmics:* Effects unknown; use together isn't recommended. Hold antiarrhythmics for at least three half-lives before giving dofetilide.
*Drugs that prolong QT interval (bepridil, oral macrolides, phenothiazines, tricyclic antidepressants):* Avoid use together. Possible enhanced QT interval prolongation. Avoid use together.
*Potassium-wasting diuretics:* Increased risk of torsades de pointes. Maintain potassium levels within normal range before and throughout drug therapy.
*Verapamil, drugs that inhibit renal cation transport system (cimetidine, ketoconazole, megestrol, prochlorperazine, sulfamethoxazole, trimethoprim):* Decreased dofetilide metabolism and excretion and increased plasma levels with concomitant use. Don't use together.
**Drug-food.** *Grapefruit juice:* Possible decreased hepatic metabolism and increased plasma levels. Don't give together.

## Adverse reactions
**CNS:** *headache,* dizziness, syncope, paresthesia, insomnia, anxiety, migraine, cerebral ischemia, facial paralysis, *CVA.*
**CV:** *ventricular fibrillation, ventricular tachycardia, torsades de pointes, AV block,* chest pain, **bradycardia,** edema, *cardiac arrest, sudden death, MI.*
**GI:** nausea, diarrhea, abdominal pain.
**GU:** urinary tract infection.
**Hepatic:** liver damage.
**Musculoskeletal:** back pain, arthralgia, flaccid paralysis.
**Respiratory:** respiratory tract infection, dyspnea, increased cough.
**Skin:** rash.
**Other:** flulike syndrome, accidental injury, *angioedema.*

## Overdose and treatment
The most prominent symptom of overdose is excessive prolongation of QT interval. There is no known antidote. Treatment is symptomatic and supportive. Recommend cardiac monitoring. Charcoal slurry may be given and is useful especially within first 15 minutes after administration. Treatment of torsades de pointes or overdose may include isoproterenol, with or without cardiac pacing. Magnesium sulfate also may be effective.

## Clinical considerations
■ Patients in atrial fibrillation should be anticoagulated according to usual practice before electrical or pharmacologic cardioversion. Anti-

coagulation therapy may be continued after cardioversion according to usual medical practice.

- Dofetilide can be taken without regard to meals because food won't interfere with absorption.
- If a dose is missed, patient shouldn't double next dose. Instead, patient should skip that dose and wait until the next administration time for regularly scheduled dose.

### Therapeutic monitoring

- Advise clinician to monitor patient for prolonged diarrhea, sweating, or vomiting. These symptoms may indicate an electrolyte imbalance that may increase potential for arrhythmia.
- Advise clinician to monitor renal function routinely (at least every 3 months) and creatinine clearance.
- Withhold Class I or III antiarrhythmics for at least 3 half-lives before starting drug.

### Special populations

**Breast-feeding patients.** It's not known if drug appears in breast milk; advise women not to breast-feed while taking drug.
**Pediatric patients.** Safety and effectiveness in patients under age 18 haven't been established.
**Geriatric patients.** There is no change in elimination based on age when dosage is adjusted for renal function.

### Patient counseling

- Inform patient to report any change in OTC, prescription, or supplement or herb use.
- Tell patient not to use OTC Tagamet-HB for ulcers or heartburn. Antacids, Zantac 75 mg, and other acid-reduction drugs, such as Pepcid, Prilosec, Axid, Pilosec, and Prevacid, can be used.
- Inform patient that drug can be taken without regard to meals or antacid administration.
- Inform patient that grapefruit juice can decrease metabolism of drug and lead to toxicity.
- Instruct woman to call prescriber if she becomes pregnant.
- Advise woman not to breast-feed while taking drug.

# dolasetron mesylate

Anzemet

*Pharmacologic classification:* selective serotonin 5-HT$_3$ receptor antagonist
*Therapeutic classification:* antinauseant, antiemetic
*Pregnancy risk category B*

### Available forms

Available by prescription only
*Tablets:* 50 mg, 100 mg

*Injection:* 20 mg/ml as 12.5-mg/0.625 ml ampules or 100-mg/5 ml vials

## Indications and dosages

*Prevention of nausea and vomiting associated with cancer chemotherapy*
*Adults:* 100 mg P.O. given as a single dose 1 hour before chemotherapy; or 1.8 mg/kg as a single I.V. dose given 30 minutes before chemotherapy; or a fixed dose of 100 mg I.V. given 30 minutes before chemotherapy.
*Children ages 2 to 16:* 1.8 mg/kg P.O. given 1 hour before chemotherapy; or 1.8 mg/kg as a single I.V. dose given 30 minutes before chemotherapy. Injectable form can be mixed with apple or apple-grape juice and given P.O. 1 hour before chemotherapy. Maximum daily dose of 100 mg.
*Prevention of postoperative nausea and vomiting*
*Adults:* 100 mg P.O. within 2 hours before surgery; 12.5 mg as a single I.V. dose about 15 minutes before cessation of anesthesia.
*Children ages 2 to 16:* 1.2 mg/kg P.O. given within 2 hours before surgery, up to maximum of 100 mg; or 0.35 mg/kg (up to 12.5 mg) given as a single I.V. dose about 15 minutes before the cessation of anesthesia. Injectable form (1.2 mg/kg up to 100-mg dose) can be mixed with apple or apple-grape juice and given P.O. 2 hours before surgery.
*Treatment of postoperative nausea and vomiting (I.V. form only)*
*Adults:* 12.5 mg as a single I.V. dose as soon as nausea or vomiting occurs.
*Children ages 2 to 16:* 0.35 mg/kg, up to a maximum dose of 12.5 mg, given as a single I.V. dose as soon as nausea or vomiting occurs.

## I.V. administration

Drug can be infused as rapidly as 100 mg over 30 seconds or diluted in 50 ml compatible solution and infused over 15 minutes.

### Incompatibilities

Don't mix injection with other drugs.

## Mechanism of action

*Antinauseant and antiemetic actions:* Dolasetron is a selective serotonin 5-HT$_3$ receptor antagonist that blocks the action of serotonin. 5-HT$_3$ receptors are located on the nerve terminals of the vagus nerve in the periphery and in the central chemoreceptor trigger zone. Blocking the activity of the serotonin receptors prevents serotonin from stimulating the vomiting reflex.

## Pharmacokinetics

*Absorption:* Orally administered dolasetron, injection, the I.V. solution, and tablets are bioequivalent. Oral dolasetron is well absorbed, although parent drug is rarely detected in plasma because of rapid and complete metabolism

---

to the most clinically relevant metabolite, hydrodolasetron.

*Distribution:* Widely distributed in the body, with a mean apparent volume of distribution of 5.8 L/kg; 69% to 77% of hydrodolasetron is plasma protein–bound.

*Metabolism:* A ubiquitous enzyme, carbonyl reductase, mediates the reduction of dolasetron to hydrodolasetron. CYP2D6 and CYP3A are responsible for subsequent hydroxylation and N-oxidation of hydrodolasetron, respectively.

*Excretion:* Two-thirds of dose is excreted in the urine and one-third in the feces. Mean elimination half-life of hydrodolasetron is 8 hours.

| Route | Onset | Peak | Duration |
|-------|-------|------|----------|
| P.O. | Rapid | 1 hr | 8 hr |
| I.V. | Rapid | 36 min | 7 hr |

## Contraindications and precautions
Contraindicated in patients hypersensitive to drug.

Use drug cautiously in patients with or at risk for development of prolonged cardiac conduction intervals, particularly QTc. These include patients taking antiarrhythmic drugs or other drugs that lead to QT interval prolongation; hypokalemia or hypomagnesemia; patients with a potential for electrolyte abnormalities, including those receiving diuretics; patients with congenital prolonged QT interval syndrome; and those who have received cumulative high-dose anthracycline therapy.

## Interactions
**Drug-drug.** *Drugs that prolong ECG intervals, such as antiarrhythmics:* Can increase the risk of arrhythmias. Advise clinician to monitor patient closely.

*Drugs that inhibit the P-450 enzymes, such as cimetidine:* Can increase hydrodolasetron levels. Advise clinician to monitor patient for adverse effects.

*Drugs that induce the P-450 enzyme, such as rifampin:* May decrease hydrodolasetron levels. Advise clinician to monitor patient for decreased efficacy of antiemetic.

## Adverse reactions
**CNS:** *headache,* dizziness, drowsiness, fatigue.
**CV:** *arrhythmias,* ECG changes, hypotension, hypertension, tachycardia, **bradycardia.**
**GI:** *diarrhea,* dyspepsia, abdominal pain, constipation, anorexia.
**GU:** oliguria, urinary retention.
**Hepatic:** elevated liver function test results.
**Skin:** pruritus, rash.
**Other:** fever, chills, pain at injection site.

## Overdose and treatment
There is no specific antidote for dolasetron overdose; supportive care should be provided.

It isn't known if drug is removed by hemodialysis or peritoneal dialysis.

## Clinical considerations
**H ALERT** Safety and efficacy of several drug doses haven't been evaluated. Efficacy studies have all been conducted with single doses of drug.
■ Injection for oral administration is stable in apple or apple-grape juice for 2 hours at controlled room temperature.

### Therapeutic monitoring
■ Advise clinician to monitor ECG and blood pressure carefully.

### Special populations
**Breast-feeding patients.** It isn't known if drug appears in breast milk. Use caution when giving drug to breast-feeding women.
**Pediatric patients.** There are no studies in pediatric patients under age 2. Efficacy in pediatric patients ages 2 to 17 receiving cancer chemotherapy is consistent with that in adults. No efficacy information has been collected in pediatric postoperative nausea and vomiting studies.
**Geriatric patients.** Dosage adjustment isn't needed in patients over age 65. Effectiveness in prevention of nausea and vomiting in geriatric patients is no different from that in younger age groups.

## Patient counseling
■ Inform patient that oral doses of drug must be taken 1 to 2 hours before surgery or 1 hour before chemotherapy to be effective.
■ Instruct patient not to mix injection in juice for oral administration until just before dosing.
■ Tell patient to report nausea or vomiting.

# donepezil hydrochloride
Aricept

*Pharmacologic classification:* acetylcholinesterase inhibitor
*Therapeutic classification:* cholinomimetic
*Pregnancy risk category C*

## Available forms
Available by prescription only
*Tablets:* 5 mg, 10 mg

## Indications and dosages
*Mild to moderate dementia of the Alzheimer's type*
*Adults:* Initially, 5 mg P.O. daily h.s. After 4 to 6 weeks, dosage may be increased to 10 mg daily.

## Mechanism of action

*Anticholinesterase action:* Drug is believed to inhibit the enzyme acetylcholinesterase in the CNS, increasing the level of acetylcholine and temporarily improving cognitive function in patients with Alzheimer's disease. Drug doesn't alter the course of the underlying disease process.

## Pharmacokinetics

*Absorption:* Well absorbed with a relative bioavailability of 100%. Steady state is reached within 15 days.

*Distribution:* Steady-state volume of distribution is 12 L/kg. Donepezil is about 96% plasma protein–bound, mainly to albumins (about 75%) and alpha$_1$-acid glycoprotein (about 21%) over the concentration range of 2 to 1,000 ng/ml.

*Metabolism:* Extensively metabolized to four major metabolites (two are known to be active) and several minor metabolites (not all have been identified). Donepezil is metabolized by CYP 450 isoenzymes 2D6 and 3A4 and undergoes glucuronidation.

*Excretion:* Excreted in the urine intact and extensively metabolized by the liver. Elimination half-life is about 70 hours and mean apparent plasma clearance is 0.13 L/hr/kg. About 17% of drug is eliminated by the kidneys as unchanged drug.

| Route | Onset | Peak | Duration |
|-------|-------|------|----------|
| P.O. | Unknown | 3-4 hr | Unknown |

## Contraindications and precautions

Contraindicated in patients hypersensitive to drug or to piperidine derivatives. Use very cautiously in patients with "sick sinus syndrome" or other supraventricular cardiac conduction conditions because drug may cause bradycardia. Use cautiously in patients with CV disease, asthma, or history of ulcer disease and in those taking NSAIDs.

## Interactions

**Drug-drug.** *Anticholinergics:* May interfere with anticholinergic activity. Advise clinician to monitor patient.

*Bethanechol, succinylcholine:* May produce additive effects. Advise clinician to monitor patient closely.

*Carbamazepine, dexamethasone, phenobarbital, phenytoin, rifampin:* May increase rate of elimination of donepezil. Advise clinician to monitor patient.

*Cholinomimetics, cholinesterase inhibitors:* May produce synergistic effect. Advise clinician to monitor patient closely.

**Drug-herb.** *Jaborandi, pill-bearing spurge:* Additive effect may occur when used together, and the risk of toxicity may be increased. Discourage use together.

## Adverse reactions

**CNS:** abnormal dreams or crying, aggression, aphasia, ataxia, dizziness, fatigue, drowsiness, *headache, insomnia,* irritability, nervousness, paresthesia, restlessness, somnolence, *seizures,* tremor, vertigo.

**CV:** atrial fibrillation, chest pain, hypertension, vasodilation, hypotension, syncope.

**EENT:** blurred vision, cataract, eye irritation, sore throat.

**GI:** anorexia, bloating, *diarrhea,* epigastric pain, fecal incontinence, *GI bleeding, nausea,* vomiting, toothache.

**GU:** frequent urination, hot flashes, nocturia.

**Hematologic:** ecchymosis.

**Metabolic:** dehydration, weight loss.

**Musculoskeletal:** arthritis, bone fracture, muscle cramps.

**Respiratory:** bronchitis, dyspnea.

**Skin:** diaphoresis, pruritus, urticaria.

**Other:** influenza, pain, increased libido.

## Overdose and treatment

Overdose can result in cholinergic crisis characterized by severe nausea, vomiting, salivation, sweating, bradycardia, hypotension, respiratory depression, collapse, and seizures. Increasing muscle weakness may also occur and may cause death if respiratory muscles are involved. Tertiary anticholinergics such as atropine may be used as an antidote for drug overdose. I.V. atropine sulfate titrated to effect is recommended; recommend giving an initial dose of 1 to 2 mg I.V. and basing subsequent doses on response. Atypical responses in blood pressure and heart rate have been reported with other cholinomimetics when given with quaternary anticholinergics such as glycopyrrolate. It isn't known if donepezil or its metabolites can be removed by dialysis.

## Clinical considerations

■ Diarrhea, nausea, and vomiting occur more frequently with the 10-mg dose than with the 5-mg dose. These effects are mostly mild and transient, sometimes lasting 1 to 3 weeks, and resolve during continued drug therapy.

■ Drug has potential to cause bladder outflow obstruction.

■ Cholinomimetics have potential to cause generalized seizures. However, seizure activity also may be from Alzheimer's disease.

### Therapeutic monitoring

■ Drug may increase gastric acid secretion. Advise clinician to closely monitor patients at increased risk for development of ulcers for symptoms of active or occult GI bleeding.

### Special populations

**Breast-feeding patients.** It isn't known if donepezil appears in breast milk. Avoid use of donepezil in breast-feeding women.

---

**Pediatric patients.** Safety and efficacy in children haven't been established.
**Geriatric patients.** Mean plasma drug levels of geriatric patients with Alzheimer's disease are comparable with those observed in young healthy volunteers.

## Patient counseling

■ Explain to patient and caregiver that drug doesn't alter disease but can stabilize or alleviate symptoms. Effects of therapy depend on drug administration at regular intervals.
■ Tell caregiver to give drug in the evening, just before bedtime.
■ Advise patient and caregiver to immediately report significant adverse effects or changes in overall health status.
■ Tell patient to inform his prescriber that he's using this drug before he receives anesthesia.

## dopamine hydrochloride
Intropin

*Pharmacologic classification:* adrenergic
*Therapeutic classification:* inotropic, vasopressor
*Pregnancy risk category C*

## Available forms

Available by prescription only
*Injection:* 40 mg/ml, 80 mg/ml, and 160 mg/ml parenteral concentrate for injection for I.V. infusion; 0.8 mg/ml (200 or 400 mg) in $D_5W$, 1.6 mg/ml (400 or 800 mg) in $D_5W$, and 3.2 mg/ml (800 mg) in $D_5W$ parenteral injection for I.V. infusion

## Indications and dosages

*Adjunct in shock to increase cardiac output, blood pressure, and urine flow*
*Adults and children:* 2 to 5 mcg/kg/minute I.V. infusion, up to 20 to 50 mcg/kg/minute. Infusion rate may be increased by 1 to 4 mcg/kg/minute at 10- to 30-minute intervals until optimum response is achieved. In severely ill patient, infusion may begin at 5 mcg/kg/minute and be gradually increased by increments of 5 to 10 mcg/kg/minute until optimum response is achieved, up to 20-50 mcg/kg/minute.
*Short-term treatment of severe, refractory, chronic heart failure*
*Adults:* Initially, 0.5 to 2 mcg/kg/minute I.V. infusion. Dosage may be increased until desired renal response occurs. Average dosage, 1 to 3 mcg/kg/minute.

## I.V. administration

■ Use a central line or large vein, as in the antecubital fossa, to minimize risk of extravasation. Watch infusion site carefully for signs of extravasation; if it occurs, stop infusion immediately and call prescriber. Extravasation

may require treatment by infiltration of the area with 5 to 10 mg phentolamine in 10 to 15 ml normal saline solution.
■ Don't mix with alkaline solutions, oxidizing drugs, or iron salts. Use $D_5W$, normal saline solution, or a combination of $D_5W$ and normal saline solution. Mix just before use.
■ Use a continuous infusion pump to regulate flow rate. Patient response depends on dosage and pharmacologic effects. Dosages of 0.5 to 2 mcg/kg/minute predominantly stimulate dopamine receptors and produce vasodilation of the renal vasculature. Dosages of 2 to 10 mcg/kg/minute stimulate beta receptors for a positive inotropic effect. Higher dosages also stimulate alpha receptors, causing vasoconstriction and increased blood pressure. Most patients are satisfactorily maintained on dosages of less than 20 mcg/kg/minute.

### Incompatibilities

Incompatible with acyclovir sodium, alteplase, amphotericin B, ampicillin sodium, cephalothin, gentamicin, indomethacin sodium trihydrate, iron salts, oxidizing agents, penicillin G potassium, and sodium bicarbonate or other alkaline solutions.
Don't mix additives with a dopamine and dextrose solution because of the risk of incompatibility.

## Mechanism of action

*Vasopressor action:* An immediate precursor of norepinephrine, dopamine stimulates dopaminergic, beta-adrenergic, and alpha-adrenergic receptors of the sympathetic nervous system. The main effects produced are dose dependent. It has a direct stimulating effect on $beta_1$ receptors (in I.V. doses of 2 to 10 mcg/kg/minute) and little or no effect on $beta_2$ receptors. In I.V. doses of 0.5 to 2 mcg/kg/minute it acts on dopaminergic receptors, causing vasodilation in the renal, mesenteric, coronary, and intracerebral vascular beds; in I.V. doses of more than 10 mcg/kg/minute, it stimulates alpha receptors.

Low to moderate doses result in cardiac stimulation (positive inotropic effects) and renal and mesenteric vasodilation (dopaminergic response). High doses result in increased peripheral resistance and renal vasoconstriction.

## Pharmacokinetics

*Absorption:* Rapid onset of action, with a short duration.
*Distribution:* Widely distributed throughout the body; however, it doesn't cross the blood-brain barrier.
*Metabolism:* Metabolized to inactive compounds in the liver, kidneys, and plasma by MAO and catechol-O-methyltransferase. About 25% is metabolized to norepinephrine within adrenergic nerve terminals.

*Excretion:* Excreted in urine, mainly as its metabolites.

| Route | Onset | Peak | Duration |
|-------|-------|------|----------|
| I.V. | 5 min | Unknown | < 10 min after infusion ends |

## Contraindications and precautions
Contraindicated in patients with uncorrected tachyarrhythmias, pheochromocytoma, or ventricular fibrillation.

Use cautiously in patients with occlusive vascular disease, cold injuries, diabetic endarteritis, and arterial embolism; in those taking MAO inhibitors; and in pregnant women.

## Interactions
**Drug-drug.** *Alpha adrenergic blockers:* Antagonize the peripheral vasoconstriction caused by high doses of dopamine. Don't use together.
*Beta blockers:* Antagonize the cardiac effects of dopamine. Don't use together.
*Diuretics:* Increases diuretic effects of both drugs. Don't use together.
*Ergot alkaloids:* Extreme elevations in blood pressure. Don't use together.
*General anesthetics, especially halothane and other halogenated hydrocarbons:* Ventricular arrhythmias and hypertension. Don't use together.
*MAO inhibitors:* May prolong and intensify the effects of dopamine. Avoid use together.
*Oxytocics:* Advanced vasoconstriction. Dosage adjustments may be needed.
*Phenytoin:* Hypotension and bradycardia. Advise clinician to monitor blood pressure and heart rate closely.

## Adverse reactions
**CNS:** headache.
**CV:** ectopic beats, tachycardia, anginal pain, palpitations, *hypotension; bradycardia,* conduction disturbances, hypertension, vasoconstriction, widening of QRS complex.
**GI:** nausea, vomiting.
**GU:** azotemia, piloerection.
**Metabolic:** hyperglycemia, decreased TSH.
**Respiratory:** dyspnea, *asthmatic episodes.*
**Skin:** necrosis and tissue sloughing with extravasation.
**Other:** *anaphylactic reactions,* decreased growth hormone and prolactin.

## Overdose and treatment
Signs and symptoms of overdose include excessive, severe hypertension. No treatment is needed beyond dosage reduction or withdrawal of drug. If that fails to lower blood pressure, a short-acting alpha blocker may be helpful.

## Clinical considerations
**◾ ALERT** Severe hypotension may result with abrupt withdrawal of infusion; therefore, re-duce dose gradually. Expand blood volume with I.V. fluids, if needed.
◾ Correct hypovolemia with plasma volume expanders before administration of dopamine.
◾ Dosage may require adjustment to meet individual needs of patient and to achieve desired clinical response. If dose required to obtain desired systolic blood pressure exceeds optimum rate of renal response, reduce dosage as soon as hemodynamic condition is stabilized.
◾ Dopamine may cause elevated urinary catecholamine levels.

### Therapeutic monitoring
◾ During infusion, advise clinician to monitor ECG, blood pressure, cardiac output, central venous pressure, pulmonary artery wedge pressure, pulse rate, urine output, and color and temperature of limbs.

### Special populations
**Pregnant patients.** Use only when potential benefits outweigh the risks to the fetus.
**Breast-feeding patients.** It isn't known if drug appears in breast milk; use drug with caution in breast-feeding women.
**Pediatric patients.** No increase in adverse effects has been noted in children.
**Geriatric patients.** Lower doses are indicated because geriatric patients may be more sensitive to effects of the drug.

## Patient counseling
◾ Advise patient to report adverse reactions.
◾ Inform patient of need for frequent monitoring of his vital signs and condition.

# dorzolamide hydrochloride
Trusopt

*Pharmacologic classification:* sulfonamide
*Therapeutic classification:* antiglaucoma drug
*Pregnancy risk category C*

## Available forms
Available by prescription only
*Ophthalmic solution:* 2%

## Indications and dosages
*Treatment of increased intraocular pressure in patients with ocular hypertension or open-angle glaucoma*
*Adults:* Instill one drop in the conjunctival sac of affected eye t.i.d.

## Mechanism of action
*Antiglaucoma action:* Dorzolamide inhibits carbonic anhydrase in the ciliary processes of the eye, which decreases aqueous humor secretion, presumably by slowing the formation of bicarbonate ions with subsequent reduction

in sodium and fluid transport. The result is a reduction in intraocular pressure.

## Pharmacokinetics
*Absorption:* Reaches the systemic circulation when applied topically.
*Distribution:* Accumulates in RBCs during chronic dosing as a result of binding to carbonic anhydrase II.
*Metabolism:* Unknown.
*Excretion:* Primarily excreted unchanged in urine.

| Route | Onset | Peak | Duration |
|---|---|---|---|
| Ophthalmic | Unknown | Unknown | Unknown |

## Contraindications and precautions
Contraindicated in patients hypersensitive to drug or its components and in those with impaired renal function. Use cautiously in patients with impaired hepatic function.

## Interactions
**Drug-drug.** *Oral carbonic anhydrase inhibitors:* Possible additive effects. Don't give together.

## Adverse reactions
**CNS:** asthenia, headache, fatigue.
**EENT:** *ocular burning, stinging, discomfort; superficial punctate keratitis; ocular allergic reactions; blurred vision; lacrimation; dryness; photophobia;* iridocyclitis, redness, eyelid crusting, ocular pain.
**GI:** *bitter taste,* nausea.
**GU:** urolithiasis.
**Skin:** rash.

## Overdose and treatment
Overdose may result in electrolyte imbalance, acidosis, and possible CNS effects. Advise clinician to monitor serum electrolyte levels (especially potassium) and blood pH levels. Treatment is supportive.

## Clinical considerations
■ Because dorzolamide is a sulfonamide and is absorbed systemically, the same types of adverse reactions that are attributable to sulfonamides may occur with topical administration of dorzolamide.
■ If more than one topical ophthalmic drug is being used, give drugs at least 10 minutes apart.

## Therapeutic monitoring
■ Monitor patient for signs of conjunctivitis, lid reactions, or other ocular adverse effects if patient is using a multiuse container.

## Special populations
**Breast-feeding patients.** It isn't known if drug appears in breast milk. Because of the risk of serious adverse reactions in the breast-fed in-

fant, use in breast-feeding women isn't recommended.
**Pediatric patients.** Safety and effectiveness haven't been established.
**Geriatric patients.** Use with caution because greater sensitivity to drug may occur in this group.

## Patient counseling
■ Teach patient how to instill drops. Advise him to wash hands before and after instilling solution, and warn him not to touch dropper or tip to eye or surrounding tissue.
■ Advise patient to apply light finger pressure on lacrimal sac for 1 minute after instillation to minimize systemic absorption of drug.
■ Tell patient not to wear soft contact lenses while using drug.
■ Stress importance of compliance with recommended therapy.
■ Inform patient to report ocular reactions, particularly conjunctivitis and lid reactions. Tell him to discontinue drug if these occur.

# doxacurium chloride
Nuromax

*Pharmacologic classification:* nondepolarizing neuromuscular blocker
*Therapeutic classification:* skeletal muscle relaxant
*Pregnancy risk category C*

## Available forms
Available by prescription only
*Injection:* 1 mg/ml

## Indications and dosages
*To provide skeletal muscle relaxation for endotracheal intubation and during surgery as an adjunct to general anesthesia*
*Adults:* Dosage is highly individualized; 0.05 mg/kg rapid I.V. produces adequate conditions for endotracheal intubation in 5 minutes in about 90% of patients when used as part of a thiopental-narcotic induction technique. Lower doses may require longer delay before intubation is possible. Neuromuscular blockade at this dose lasts an average of 100 minutes.
*Children over age 2:* Dosage is highly individualized; an initial dose of 0.03 mg/kg I.V. given during halothane anesthesia produces effective blockade in 7 minutes and has a duration of 30 minutes. Under the same conditions, 0.05 mg/kg produces a blockade in 4 minutes and lasts 45 minutes.
*Maintenance of neuromuscular blockade during long procedures*
*Adults and children over age 2:* After initial dose of 0.05 mg/kg I.V., maintenance doses of 0.005 and 0.01 mg/kg prolong neuromuscular blockade for an average of 30 minutes and 45

minutes, respectively. Children usually require more frequent administration of maintenance doses.

≡ *Dosage adjustment.* Adjust dosage to ideal body weight in obese patients (patients whose weight is 30% or more above their ideal weight) to avoid prolonged neuromuscular blockade.

## I.V. administration

■ Use doxacurium only under direct supervision by medical staff skilled in using neuromuscular blockers and maintaining patent airway. Don't use unless an antagonist and resources for mechanical ventilation, oxygen therapy, and intubation are within reach.

■ To avoid patient distress, don't give drug until patient's consciousness is obtunded by general anesthetic. Drug has no effect on consciousness or pain threshold.

■ Prepare drug for I.V. use with $D_5W$, normal saline solution for injection, dextrose 5% in normal saline solution for injection, lactated Ringer's injection, or dextrose 5% in lactated Ringer's injection.

■ Administer product immediately after reconstitution. Diluted solutions are stable for 24 hours at room temperature; however, because reconstitution dilutes the preservative, risk of contamination increases. Discard unused solutions after 8 hours.

■ When diluted as directed, drug is compatible with alfentanil, fentanyl, and sufentanil.

### Incompatibilities

Incompatible with alkaline solutions, such as barbiturate solutions. Don't administer through the same I.V. line because a precipitate may form.

## Mechanism of action

*Skeletal muscle relaxant action:* Doxacurium binds competitively to cholinergic receptors on the motor end-plate to antagonize the action of acetylcholine, resulting in a block of neuromuscular transmission.

## Pharmacokinetics

*Absorption:* Effects are rapid after I.V. administration.

*Distribution:* About 30% human plasma protein–bound.

*Metabolism:* Not metabolized.

*Excretion:* Primarily eliminated as unchanged drug in urine and bile.

| Route | Onset | Peak | Duration |
|-------|-------|------|----------|
| I.V. | 2 min | 3-6 min | Variable |

## Contraindications and precautions

Contraindicated in patients hypersensitive to drug and in neonates. Drug contains benzyl ethanol, which has been linked to death in newborns.

Use cautiously, perhaps at a reduced dosage, in debilitated patients; in patients with metastatic cancer, severe electrolyte disturbances, or neuromuscular diseases; and in those for whom potentiation or difficulty in reversal of neuromuscular blockade is anticipated. Patients with myasthenia gravis or myasthenic syndrome (Eaton-Lambert syndrome) are particularly sensitive to the effects of nondepolarizing relaxants. Shorter-acting drugs are recommended for use in such patients.

## Interactions

**Drug-drug.** *Alkaline solutions:* Drug is physically incompatible with alkaline solutions; precipitate may form. Don't give these drugs through same I.V. line.

*Antibiotics (aminoglycosides [such as gentamicin, kanamycin, neomycin, streptomycin], bacitracin, clindamycin, colistimethate sodium, colistin, lincomycin, polymyxins, tetracyclines) lithium, local anesthetics, magnesium salts, procainamide, quinidine:* Neuromuscular blocking action of doxacurium may be enhanced. Use together cautiously. Advise clinician to monitor patient for excessive weakness.

*Carbamazepine, phenytoin:* Delay onset of neuromuscular blockade induced by doxacurium and shorten its duration. Advise clinician to monitor patient.

*Enflurane, isoflurane, halothane:* Decrease the effective dose required to produce a 50% suppression of the response to ulnar nerve stimulation of doxacurium by 30% to 45%. May also prolong the clinically effective duration of action of doxacurium by up to 25%. Don't use together.

## Adverse reactions

**Musculoskeletal:** prolonged muscle weakness.

**Respiratory:** dyspnea, *respiratory depression, respiratory insufficiency or apnea.*

## Overdose and treatment

Overdose with neuromuscular blockers such as doxacurium may result in neuromuscular block beyond the time needed for surgery and anesthesia. The primary treatment is maintenance of a patent airway and controlled ventilation until recovery of normal neuromuscular function is assured. Once initial evidence of recovery is observed, further recovery may be facilitated by administration of an anticholinesterase drug (such as neostigmine or edrophonium) with an appropriate anticholinergic.

## Clinical considerations

■ All times of onset and duration of neuromuscular blockade are averages; considerable individual variation in dosages is normal.

■ As with other nondepolarizing neuromuscular blockers, a reduction in dosage of doxacurium must be considered in cachectic or debilitated patients; in patients with neuromuscular diseases, severe electrolyte abnormalities, or carcinomatosis; and in other patients for whom potentiation of neuromuscular block or difficulty with reversal is anticipated. Increased doses of doxacurium may be required in burn patients.

■ Drug has no effect on consciousness or pain threshold. To avoid distress to the patient, it shouldn't be given until patient's consciousness is obtunded by general anesthetic.

■ Drug may prolong neuromuscular block in patients undergoing renal transplantation, and onset and duration of the block may vary with patients undergoing liver transplantation.

■ Use drug only under direct medical supervision by caregivers familiar with use of neuromuscular blockers and in airway management. Don't use unless facilities and equipment for mechanical ventilation, oxygen therapy, and intubation and an antagonist are within reach.

■ Use of a peripheral nerve stimulator will permit the most advantageous use of doxacurium, minimize the possibility of overdose or underdose, and assist in the evaluation of recovery.

### Therapeutic monitoring
■ Advise clinician to monitor ECG, especially for bradycardia.
■ Advise clinician to monitor respirations until patient is fully recovered from neuromuscular blockade, as evidenced by tests of muscle strength (such as hand grips, head lift, and ability to cough).

### Special populations
**Breast-feeding patients.** It isn't known if drug appears in breast milk. Use cautiously when giving to breast-feeding women.
**Pediatric patients.** Drug use hasn't been studied in children under age 2.
**Geriatric patients.** Geriatric patients may be more sensitive to the effects of the drug. They may experience a slower onset of the blockade and a longer duration.

### Patient counseling
■ Reassure patient and family that he will be monitored at all times.

---

# doxapram hydrochloride
Dopram

*Pharmacologic classification:* analeptic
*Therapeutic classification:* CNS and respiratory stimulant
*Pregnancy risk category B*

### Available forms
Available by prescription only
*Injection:* 20 mg/ml (benzyl alcohol 0.9%)

### Indications and dosages
*Postanesthesia respiratory stimulation*
*Adults:* 0.5 to 1 mg/kg of body weight as a single I.V. injection (not to exceed 1.5 mg/kg) or as several injections q 5 minutes, not to exceed 2 mg/kg total dosage. Alternatively, 250 mg in 250 ml of normal saline solution or $D_5W$ infused at an initial rate of 5 mg/minute I.V. until a satisfactory response is achieved. Maintain at 1 to 3 mg/minute. Recommended total dose for infusion shouldn't exceed 4 mg/kg.
*Drug-induced CNS depression*
*Adults:* For injection, priming dose of 2 mg/kg I.V. repeated in 5 minutes and again q 1 to 2 hours until patient awakens (and if relapse occurs). Maximum daily dose is 3 g.

For infusion, priming dose of 2 mg/kg I.V., repeated in 5 minutes and again in 1 to 2 hours, if needed. If response occurs, give I.V. infusion (1 mg/ml) at 1 to 3 mg/minute until patient awakens. Don't infuse for longer than 2 hours or administer more than 3 g/day. May resume I.V. infusion after a rest period of 30 minutes to 2 hours, if needed.
*Chronic pulmonary disease with acute hypercapnia*
*Adults:* Infusion of 1 to 2 mg/minute (using 2 mg/ml solution). Maximum dose is 3 mg/minute for a maximum duration of 2 hours. Don't use drug with mechanical ventilation. Use infusion pump to regulate rate.

### I.V. administration
■ For I.V. infusion, dilute with $D_5W$ or normal saline solution to 1 or 2 mg/ml. Infuse slowly to avoid hemolysis. Use only on an intermittent basis; maximum infusion period is 2 hours.
■ Avoid repeated injections in the site for long periods because of risk of thrombophlebitis or local skin irritation.

### Incompatibilities
Incompatible with aminophylline, ascorbic acid, cefoperazone, cefotaxime, cefotetan, cefuroxime sodium, dexamethasone sodium phosphate, diazepam, digoxin, dobutamine, folic acid, furosemide, hydrocortisone sodium phosphate, hydrocortisone sodium succinate, ketamine, methylprednisolone sodium succinate, minocycline, and ticarcillin disodium or alkaline solutions.

### Mechanism of action
*Respiratory stimulant action:* Doxapram increases respiratory rate by direct stimulation of the medullary respiratory center and possibly by indirect action on chemoreceptors in the carotid artery and aortic arch. Doxapram causes increased release of catecholamines.

### Pharmacokinetics
*Absorption:* Rapid.
*Distribution:* Distributed throughout the body.
*Metabolism:* 99% metabolized by the liver.

---

*Excretion:* Metabolites are excreted in urine.

| Route | Onset | Peak | Duration |
|-------|-------|------|----------|
| I.V. | 20-40 sec | 1-2 min | 5-12 min |

## Contraindications and precautions

Contraindicated in patients with seizure disorders; head injury; CV disorders; frank, uncompensated HF; severe hypertension; CVA; respiratory failure or incompetence secondary to neuromuscular disorders; muscle paresis; flail chest; obstructed airway; pulmonary embolism; pneumothorax; restrictive respiratory disease; acute bronchial asthma or extreme dyspnea; or hypoxia without hypercapnia. Drug also contraindicated in neonates because product contains benzyl alcohol.

Use cautiously in patients with bronchial asthma, severe tachycardia or arrhythmias, cerebral edema or increased CSF pressure, hyperthyroidism, pheochromocytoma, or metabolic disorders.

## Interactions

**Drug-drug.** *Anesthetics such as cyclopropane, enflurane, halothane:* Sensitize the myocardium to catecholamines. Discontinue at least 10 minutes before giving doxapram.
*MAO inhibitors, sympathomimetics:* Added pressor effects. Use together cautiously.
*Neuromuscular blockers:* Doxapram temporarily may mask residual effects of neuromuscular blockers used after anesthesia. Advise clinician to monitor patient closely.

## Adverse reactions

**CNS:** *seizures, headache,* dizziness, apprehension, disorientation, hyperactivity, bilateral Babinski's signs, paresthesia.
**CV:** *chest pain and tightness, variations in heart rate, hypertension,* lowered T waves, *arrhythmias.*
**EENT:** sneezing, *laryngospasm.*
**GI:** nausea, vomiting, diarrhea.
**GU:** urine retention, bladder stimulation with incontinence, increased BUN levels, albuminuria.
**Hematologic:** decreased erythrocyte and leukocyte counts, reduced hemoglobin and hematocrit levels.
**Musculoskeletal:** muscle spasms.
**Respiratory:** cough, *bronchospasm,* dyspnea, rebound hypoventilation, hiccups.
**Skin:** pruritus, diaphoresis, flushing.

## Overdose and treatment

Signs and symptoms of overdose include hypertension, tachycardia, arrhythmias, skeletal muscle hyperactivity, and dyspnea.

Treatment is supportive. Recommend keeping oxygen and resuscitative equipment available, but use oxygen with caution because rapid increase in partial pressure of oxygen can suppress carotid chemoreceptor activity.

I.V. anticonvulsants should be available to treat seizures.

## Clinical considerations

■ Use of doxapram as an analeptic is strongly discouraged; use only in surgery or emergency room.
■ Recommend establishing adequate airway before administering drug and preventing aspiration of vomitus by placing patient on his side.
■ Oxygen should be given cautiously to patients with COPD who are narcotized or those who have just undergone surgery; doxapram-stimulated respiration increases oxygen demand.

### *Therapeutic monitoring*

■ Advise clinician to monitor blood pressure, heart rate, deep tendon reflexes, and arterial blood gas (ABG) values before giving drug and every 30 minutes afterward. Discontinue drug if ABG values deteriorate or mechanical ventilation is started.

### *Special populations*

**Breast-feeding patients.** Safety in breast-feeding women hasn't been established. Distribution into breast milk is unknown.
**Pediatric patients.** Safety in children under age 12 hasn't been established.

## Patient counseling

■ Inform patient, if alert, and family of need for drug; answer questions and address concerns.

# doxazosin mesylate
Cardura

*Pharmacologic classification:* alpha adrenergic blocker
*Therapeutic classification:* antihypertensive
*Pregnancy risk category C*

## Available forms

Available by prescription only
*Tablets:* 1 mg, 2 mg, 4 mg, 8 mg

## Indications and dosages

*Essential hypertension*
*Adult:* Dosage must be individualized. Initially, administer 1 mg P.O. daily and determine effect on standing and supine blood pressure at 2 to 6 hours and 24 hours after dosing. If needed, increase dose to 2 mg daily. To minimize adverse reactions, adjust dosage slowly (dosage typically increased only q 2 weeks). If needed, increase dose to 4 mg daily, then 8 mg. Maximum daily dose is 16 mg, but doses exceeding 4 mg daily cause a greater risk of adverse reactions.

*BPH*
*Adults:* Initially, 1 mg P.O. once daily in the morning or evening; increase to 2 mg and, thereafter, to 4 mg and 8 mg once daily. Recommended adjustment interval is 1 to 2 weeks.

## Mechanism of action
*Hypotensive action:* Doxazosin selectively blocks postsynaptic alpha$_1$-adrenergic receptors, dilating both resistance (arterioles) and capacitance (veins) vessels. It lowers both supine and standing blood pressure, producing more pronounced effects on diastolic pressure. Maximum reductions occur 2 to 6 hours after dosing and may cause a small increase in standing heart rate. Doxazosin has a greater effect on blood pressure and heart rate in the standing position.
*BPH:* Doxazosin improves urine flow related to relaxation of smooth muscles produced by blockade of alpha adrenoreceptors in the bladder neck and prostate.

## Pharmacokinetics
*Absorption:* Readily absorbed from the GI tract after oral administration.
*Distribution:* 98% protein-bound. It appears in breast milk in levels about 20 times greater than in maternal plasma.
*Metabolism:* Extensively metabolized in the liver by *O*-demethylation or hydroxylation. Secondary peaking of plasma levels suggests enterohepatic recycling.
*Excretion:* 63% is excreted in bile and feces (4.8% as unchanged drug); 9% is excreted in urine.

| Route | Onset | Peak | Duration |
|-------|-------|------|----------|
| P.O. | 1-2 hr | 2-3 hr | 24 hr |

## Contraindications and precautions
Contraindicated in patients hypersensitive to drug and quinazoline derivatives (including prazosin and terazosin). Use cautiously in patients with impaired hepatic function.

## Interactions
**Drug-drug.** *Clonidine:* Antihypertensive effects of clonidine may be decreased. Advise clinician to monitor patient closely.
**Drug-herb.** *Butcher's broom:* Possibly reduce effects of doxazosin. Discourage use together.

## Adverse reactions
**CNS:** *dizziness,* vertigo, somnolence, drowsiness, *asthenia, headache.*
**CV:** *orthostatic hypotension,* hypotension, edema, palpitations, ***arrhythmias,*** tachycardia.
**EENT:** rhinitis, pharyngitis, abnormal vision.
**GI:** nausea, vomiting, diarrhea, constipation.
**Hematologic:** mean WBC and neutrophil counts may be decreased.
**Musculoskeletal:** arthralgia, myalgia, pain.
**Respiratory:** dyspnea.

**Skin:** rash, pruritus.

## Overdose and treatment
Patient should be kept supine to restore blood pressure and heart rate. If needed, recommend treating shock with volume expanders. Advise clinician to give vasopressors and monitor and support renal function.

## Clinical considerations
■ Tolerance to antihypertensive effects of doxazosin hasn't been observed.
■ No apparent differences exist in the hypotensive response of whites and blacks or of geriatric patients.
■ First-dose effect (orthostatic hypotension) occurs with doxazosin but is less pronounced than with prazosin or terazosin.

### Therapeutic monitoring
■ Orthostatic effects are most likely to occur 2 to 6 hours after dose. Advise clinician to monitor blood pressure during this time after the first dose and after subsequent increases in dosage.
■ Daily doses above 4 mg increase the potential of excessive orthostatic effects.

### Special populations
**Breast-feeding patients.** Drug appears in breast milk at levels about 20 times greater than in maternal plasma.
**Pediatric patients.** Safety and efficacy in children haven't been established.
**Geriatric patients.** Use drug with caution in geriatric patients with underlying autonomic dysfunction or arrhythmias.

## Patient counseling
■ Tell patient that orthostatic hypotension and syncope may occur, especially after first few doses and with dosage changes. Patient should rise slowly to prevent orthostatic hypotension.
■ Caution patient that drug may cause drowsiness and somnolence. Patient should avoid driving and other hazardous tasks that require alertness for 12 to 24 hours after first dose, after dosage increases, and after resumption of interrupted therapy.
■ Tell patient to report bothersome palpitations or dizziness.
■ Inform patient that drug may be taken with food if nausea occurs. Tell patient that nausea should improve as therapy continues.

---

Reactions may be *common,* uncommon, *life-threatening,* or COMMON AND LIFE-THREATENING.

# doxepin hydrochloride
Sinequan, Triadapin*

*Pharmacologic classification:* tricyclic antidepressant
*Therapeutic classification:* antidepressant
*Pregnancy risk category NR*

## Available forms
Available by prescription only
*Capsules:* 10 mg, 25 mg, 50 mg, 75 mg, 100 mg, 150 mg
*Oral concentrate:* 10 mg/ml

## Indications and dosages
*Depression or anxiety*
*Adults:* Initially, 25 to 75 mg P.O. daily in divided doses, to a maximum of 300 mg daily. Alternatively, give entire maintenance dose once daily with a maximum dose of 150 mg P.O.
≡ *Dosage adjustment.* Reduce dosage in geriatric, debilitated, or adolescent patients and in those receiving other drugs (especially anticholinergics).

## Mechanism of action
*Antidepressant action:* Doxepin is thought to exert its antidepressant effects by inhibiting reuptake of norepinephrine and serotonin in CNS nerve terminals (presynaptic neurons), which results in increased levels and enhanced activity of these neurotransmitters in the synaptic cleft. Doxepin more actively inhibits reuptake of serotonin than norepinephrine. Anxiolytic effects of this drug usually precede antidepressant effects. Doxepin also may be used as an anxiolytic. Doxepin has the greatest sedative effect of all tricyclic antidepressants; tolerance to this effect usually develops in a few weeks.

## Pharmacokinetics
*Absorption:* Absorbed rapidly from the GI tract after oral administration.
*Distribution:* Distributed widely into the body, including the CNS and breast milk. Drug is 90% protein-bound. Steady-state is achieved within 7 days. Therapeutic levels (parent drug and metabolite) are thought to range from 150 to 250 ng/ml.
*Metabolism:* Metabolized by the liver to the active metabolite desmethyldoxepin. A significant first-pass effect may explain variability of serum levels in different patients taking the same dosage.
*Excretion:* Mostly excreted in urine.

| Route | Onset | Peak | Duration |
|-------|-------|------|----------|
| P.O. | Unknown | 2 hr | Unknown |

## Contraindications and precautions
Contraindicated in patients hypersensitive to drug and in those with glaucoma or tendency to retain urine.

## Interactions
**Drug-drug.** *Antiarrhythmics, such as disopyramide, procainamide, quinidine; pimozide; thyroid hormones:* May increase risk of cardiac arrhythmias and conduction defects. Advise clinician to monitor ECG closely.
*Atropine, other anticholinergics:* Oversedation, paralytic ileus, visual changes, and severe constipation. Advise clinician to monitor patient closely.
*Barbiturates:* Induce doxepin metabolism and decrease therapeutic efficacy. Advise clinician to monitor patient closely; dosage adjustment may be needed.
*Beta blockers, cimetidine, fluoxetine, methylphenidate, oral contraceptives, propoxyphene, sertraline:* May inhibit doxepin metabolism, increasing plasma levels and toxicity. Advise clinician to monitor serum level closely.
*Centrally acting antihypertensives:* Doxepin may decrease hypotensive effects. Advise clinician to monitor blood pressure closely.
*Clonidine:* Increases hypertensive effect. Advise clinician to monitor blood pressure closely.
*CNS depressants:* Additive effects are likely after use of doxepin. Avoid use together.
*Disulfiram, ethchlorvynol:* Cause delirium and tachycardia. Advise clinician to monitor patient closely.
*Haloperidol, phenothiazines:* Decrease its metabolism, decreasing therapeutic efficacy. Avoid use together.
*MAO inhibitors:* May cause severe excitation, hyperpyrexia, or seizures, usually with high dose. Advise clinician to monitor patient closely.
*Metrizamide:* Increased risk of seizures. Avoid use together.
*Sympathomimetics, such as ephedrine, epinephrine, norepinephrine, phenylephrine:* May increase blood pressure. Use with caution.
*Warfarin:* May increase PT and INR and cause bleeding. Advise clinician to monitor PT and INR.
**Drug-herb.** *Evening primrose:* Possible additive or synergistic effect resulting in lower seizure threshold and increasing the risk of seizure. Discourage use together.
*St. John's wort, SAMe, yohimbe:* Use with some tricyclic antidepressants may cause elevation of serotonin levels. Discourage use together.
**Drug-food.** *Carbonated beverages, grape juice:* Incompatible. Don't give together.
**Drug-lifestyle.** *Alcohol use:* Enhanced CNS depression. Advise patient to avoid alcohol.
*Heavy smoking:* Induces doxepin metabolism and decreases therapeutic efficacy. Discourage smoking.

---

* Canada only    ◇ Unlabeled clinical use

*Sun exposure:* Increases risk of photosensitivity reactions. Advise patient to take precautions.

## Adverse reactions
**CNS:** *drowsiness, dizziness,* confusion, numbness, hallucinations, paresthesia, ataxia, weakness, headache, *seizures,* extrapyramidal reactions.
**CV:** *orthostatic hypotension, tachycardia,* ECG changes.
**EENT:** *blurred vision,* tinnitus.
**GI:** *dry mouth, constipation,* nausea, vomiting, anorexia.
**GU:** urine retention.
**Hematologic:** eosinophilia, *bone marrow depression.*
**Hepatic:** elevated liver function test results.
**Metabolic:** hyperglycemia, hypoglycemia.
**Skin:** *diaphoresis,* rash, urticaria, photosensitivity.
**Other:** *hypersensitivity reaction.*
**After abrupt withdrawal of long-term therapy:** nausea, headache, malaise (doesn't indicate addiction).

## Overdose and treatment
The first 12 hours after acute ingestion are a stimulatory phase characterized by excessive anticholinergic activity (agitation, irritation, confusion, hallucinations, hyperthermia, parkinsonian symptoms, seizures, urine retention, dry mucous membranes, pupillary dilatation, constipation, and ileus). This is followed by CNS depressant effects, including hypothermia, decreased or absent reflexes, sedation, hypotension, cyanosis, and cardiac irregularities, including tachycardia, conduction disturbances, and quinidine-like effects on the ECG.

Severity of overdose is best indicated by widening of QRS complex. Usually, this represents a serum level in excess of 1,000 ng/ml. Serum levels are usually not helpful. Metabolic acidosis may follow hypotension, hypoventilation, and seizures.

Treatment is symptomatic and supportive, including maintaining airway, stable body temperature, and fluid and electrolyte balance. Advise clinician to induce emesis with ipecac if patient is conscious and follow with gastric lavage and activated charcoal to prevent further absorption. Dialysis is of little use. Physostigmine may be cautiously used to reverse central anticholinergic effects. Recommend treating seizures with parenteral diazepam or phenytoin; arrhythmias with parenteral phenytoin or lidocaine; and acidosis with sodium bicarbonate. Barbiturates shouldn't be given; these may enhance CNS and respiratory depressant effects.

## Clinical considerations
**H** *ALERT* Because hypertensive episodes have occurred during surgery in patients receiving TCAs, drug should be gradually discontinued several days before surgery.
■ Recommendations for administration of doxepin, care of patients during therapy, and use in children are the same as those for all tricyclic antidepressants.

### Therapeutic monitoring
■ If signs of psychosis occur or increase, expect dosage to be reduced.
■ Mood changes should be recorded. Advise clinician to monitor patient for suicidal tendencies, and allow only a minimum supply of the drug.

### Special populations
**Breast-feeding patients.** Drug appears in breast milk. Avoid use of drug in breast-feeding women, especially if high doses are used.
**Pediatric patients.** Not recommended for use in children under 12 years.
**Geriatric patients.** Adverse CNS reactions, orthostatic hypotension, and GI and GU disturbances are more likely to develop in geriatric patients.

## Patient counseling
■ Teach patient to dilute oral concentrate with 120 ml (4 ounces) of water, milk, or juice (orange, pineapple, prune, or tomato). Drug is incompatible with carbonated beverages and grapefruit juice.
■ Tell patient to use ice chips, sugarless gum or hard candy, or saliva substitutes to treat dry mouth.
■ Warn patient to avoid taking other drugs while taking doxepin unless they've been prescribed.
■ Instruct patient to take full dose at bedtime.

# doxercalciferol
Hectorol

*Pharmacologic classification:* synthetic vitamin D analogue
*Therapeutic classification:* parathyroid hormone antagonist
*Pregnancy risk category B*

## Available forms
Available by prescription only
*Capsules:* 2.5 mcg

## Indications and dosages
*Reduction of elevated intact parathyroid hormone (PTH) levels in the management of secondary hyperparathyroidism in patients undergoing long-term renal dialysis*
*Adults:* Initially, 10 mcg P.O. three times weekly at dialysis. Adjust dosage, p.r.n., to lower

intact PTH levels to 150 to 300 pg/ml. Dosage may be increased by 2.5 mcg at 8-week intervals if the intact PTH level isn't decreased by 50% and fails to reach target range. Maximum dose is 20 mcg P.O. three times weekly. If intact PTH levels go below 100 pg/ml, suspend drug for 1 week, then resume at a dose that's at least 2.5 mcg lower than the last given dose.

## Mechanism of action
*PTH antagonist action:* Once activated, doxercalciferol and other biologically active vitamin D metabolites regulate blood calcium levels required for essential body functions. Doxercalciferol acts directly on the parathyroid glands to suppress PTH synthesis and secretion.

## Pharmacokinetics
*Absorption:* Absorbed from the GI tract.
*Distribution:* No information available.
*Metabolism:* Metabolized to its active forms in the liver.
*Excretion:* The major metabolite of doxercalciferol attains peak blood levels at 11 to 12 hours after repeated oral doses. Elimination half-life is 32 to 37 hours, with a range of up to 96 hours.

| Route | Onset | Peak | Duration |
|-------|-------|------|----------|
| P.O. | Unknown | 11-12 hr | Unknown |

## Contraindications and precautions
Contraindicated in patients with a recent history of hypercalcemia, hyperphosphatemia, or vitamin D toxicity. Use cautiously in patients with hepatic insufficiency and advise clinician to frequently monitor calcium, phosphorus, and intact PTH levels in these patients.

## Interactions
**Drug-drug.** *Antacids containing magnesium:* May cause hypermagnesemia. Avoid use together.
*Cholestyramine, mineral oil:* Reduce intestinal absorption of doxercalciferol. Avoid use together.
*Glutethimide, phenobarbital, other enzyme inducers; phenytoin, other enzyme inhibitors:* May affect the metabolism of doxercalciferol. Adjust dosage as appropriate.
*Orlistat:* May interfere with intestinal absorption of vitamin D analogues. Avoid use together.
*Phosphate binders containing calcium or nonaluminum:* May cause hypercalcemia or hyperphosphatemia and decrease effectiveness of doxercalciferol. Use cautiously together and adjust dosage of phosphate binders as appropriate.
*Vitamin D supplements:* May cause additive effects and hypercalcemia. Avoid use together.

## Adverse reactions
**CNS:** *dizziness, headache, malaise,* sleep disorder.
**CV:** *bradycardia, edema.*
**GI:** anorexia, dyspepsia, *nausea, vomiting,* constipation.
**Metabolic:** weight gain.
**Musculoskeletal:** arthralgia.
**Respiratory:** *dyspnea.*
**Skin:** pruritus.
**Other:** abscess.

## Overdose and treatment
Excessive doses of doxercalciferol can cause hypercalcemia, hypercalciuria, hyperphosphatemia, and oversuppression of PTH secretion. For hypercalcemia of greater than 1 mg/dl above the upper limit of normal, recommend suspending doxercalciferol therapy immediately, instituting a low-calcium diet, and withdrawing calcium supplements. Check serum calcium levels weekly until levels return to normal, usually in 2 to 7 days. Dialysis, using a low-calcium or calcium-free dialysate, may correct persistently or markedly elevated serum calcium levels. When serum calcium levels have returned to within normal limits, drug can be restarted at a dose that's at least 2.5 mcg lower than prior therapy.

For acute overdose, treatment should consist of general supportive measures. Within 10 minutes of ingestion, recommend inducing vomiting or performing gastric lavage to prevent further absorption. If postingestion time is longer than 10 minutes, administer mineral oil to promote fecal elimination. Advise clinician to monitor serum calcium levels, the rate of urinary calcium excretion, and ECG findings. If serum calcium levels are persistently and markedly elevated, consider drugs, such as corticosteroids or phosphates, or therapeutic measures, such as dialysis or forced diuresis.

## Clinical considerations
■ Management of secondary hyperparathyroidism may prevent bone disease in patients with renal failure.
■ Doxercalciferol is given with dialysis (about every other day). Dosing must be individualized and based on intact PTH levels, with monitoring of serum calcium and phosphorus levels before doxercalciferol therapy and weekly thereafter.
■ Calcium-based or nonaluminum-containing phosphate binders and a low-phosphate diet are used to control serum phosphorus levels in dialysis patients. Expect adjustments in doses of doxercalciferol and therapies such as dietary phosphate binders to sustain PTH suppression and maintain serum calcium and phosphorus levels within acceptable ranges.
■ Progressive hypercalcemia secondary to vitamin D overdose may require emergency at-

tention. Acute hypercalcemia may exacerbate arrhythmias and seizures and affect the action of digoxin. Chronic hypercalcemia can lead to vascular and soft-tissue calcification.

### Therapeutic monitoring

- If hypercalcemia, hyperphosphatemia, or a product of serum calcium times serum phosphorus ($Ca \times P$) greater than 70 is noted, stop doxercalciferol, as ordered, until these parameters are lowered.

### Special populations

**Breast-feeding patients.** It's unknown if drug appears in breast milk. However, because other vitamin D derivatives appear in breast milk, the potential for serious adverse reactions in breast-feeding infants exists. Based on importance of drug to the woman, it should be decided whether to discontinue breast-feeding or drug.
**Pediatric patients.** Safety and efficacy in pediatric patients haven't been established.

### Patient counseling

- Inform patient that dosage must be adjusted over several months to achieve satisfactory PTH suppression.
- Instruct patient to adhere to a low-phosphorus diet and to follow instructions regarding calcium supplementation.
- Tell patient to obtain his prescriber's approval before using OTC drugs, including antacids and vitamin preparations containing calcium or vitamin D.
- Inform patient that early signs and symptoms of hypercalcemia include weakness, headache, somnolence, nausea, vomiting, dry mouth, constipation, muscle pain, bone pain, and metallic taste. Late signs and symptoms include polyuria, polydipsia, anorexia, weight loss, nocturia, conjunctivitis, pancreatitis, photophobia.

---

# doxorubicin hydrochloride

Adriamycin PFS, Adriamycin RDF, Rubex

*Pharmacologic classification:* antineoplastic antibiotic (cell cycle–phase nonspecific)
*Therapeutic classification:* antineoplastic
*Pregnancy risk category D*

### Available forms

Available by prescription only
*Injection:* 10 mg, 20 mg, 50 mg, 100 mg, 150 mg vials
*Injection (preservative-free):* 2 mg/ml (10 mg, 20 mg, 50 mg, 75 mg, and 200 mg)

## Indications and dosages

Dosage and indications may vary. Check current literature for recommended protocol or for information on liposomal doxorubicin.
***Bladder, breast, lung, stomach, and thyroid cancers; Hodgkin's disease; acute lymphoblastic and myeloblastic leukemia; Wilms' tumor; neuroblastoma; lymphoma; sarcoma***
*Adults:* 60 to 75 mg/m² I.V. as a single dose q 21 days; or 25 to 30 mg/m² I.V. as a single daily dose on days 1 to 3 of 4-week cycle. Alternatively, 20 mg/m² I.V. once weekly. Maximum cumulative dosage is 550 mg/m² (450 mg/m² in patients who have received chest irradiation).

## I.V. administration

- To reconstitute, add 5 ml of normal saline injection, USP, to the 10-mg vial, 10 ml to the 20-mg vial, and 25 ml to the 50-mg vial, to yield a level of 2 mg/ml.
- Drug may be further diluted with normal saline solution or $D_5W$ and given by I.V. infusion.
- Drug may be given by I.V. push injection over 5 to 10 minutes into the tubing of a freely flowing I.V. infusion.
- Advise clinician to stop drug or slow rate of infusion if tachycardia develops. Recommend treating extravasation with topical application of dimethyl sulfoxide and ice packs.

### Incompatibilities

Incompatible with aluminum, aminophylline, bacteriostatic diluents, cephalothin, dexamethasone sodium phosphate, diazepam, fluorouracil, furosemide, heparin sodium, and hydrocortisone sodium succinate.

## Mechanism of action

*Antineoplastic action:* Doxorubicin is believed to exert its cytotoxic activity by intercalating between DNA base pairs and uncoiling the DNA helix. The result is inhibition of DNA synthesis and DNA-dependent RNA synthesis. Doxorubicin also inhibits protein synthesis.

## Pharmacokinetics

*Absorption:* Because of its vesicant effects, doxorubicin must be given I.V.
*Distribution:* Distributed widely into body tissues, with the highest levels found in the liver, heart, and kidneys. It doesn't cross the blood-brain barrier.
*Metabolism:* Extensively metabolized by hepatic microsomal enzymes to several metabolites, one of which possesses cytotoxic activity.
*Excretion:* Excreted primarily in bile. A minute amount is eliminated in urine. The plasma elimination of doxorubicin is described as biphasic with a half-life of about 15 to 30 minutes

in the initial phase and 16½ hours in the terminal phase.

| Route | Onset | Peak | Duration |
|-------|-------|------|----------|
| I.V. | Unknown | Unknown | Unknown |

## Contraindications and precautions
Contraindicated in patients with marked myelosuppression induced by previous treatment with other antitumor agents or by radiotherapy and in those who have received lifetime cumulative dosage of 550 mg/m$^2$.

## Interactions
**Drug-drug.** *Aminophylline, cephalosporins, fluorouracil, heparin sodium, hydrocortisone sodium phosphate:* Result in a precipitate when mixed with doxorubicin. Give through separate I.V. lines.
*Cyclophosphamide:* Doxorubicin may worsen induced hemorrhagic cystitis. Advise clinician to monitor patient closely.
*Cyclophosphamide, daunorubicin, idarubicin or mitoxantrone:* Potentiate the cardiotoxicity of doxorubicin through additive effects on the heart. Avoid use together.
*Cyclosporine, progesterone:* Potential toxicity for both. Advise clinician to monitor patient closely for signs of toxicity.
*Digoxin:* Levels may be decreased if used with doxorubicin. Advise clinician to monitor serum digoxin levels closely.
*Mercaptopurine:* Hepatotoxicity. Don't use together.
*Streptozocin:* Increases the plasma half-life of doxorubicin, increasing the activity of doxorubicin. Dosage may have to be adjusted.
**Drug-herb.** *Green tea:* May enhance the antitumor activity of doxorubicin. Discourage use together.

## Adverse reactions
**CV:** cardiac depression, seen in such ECG changes as sinus tachycardia, T-wave flattening, ST-segment depression, voltage reduction; *arrhythmias; acute left ventricular failure; irreversible cardiomyopathy.*
**EENT:** conjunctivitis.
**GI:** *nausea, vomiting,* diarrhea, *stomatitis,* esophagitis, anorexia.
**GU:** red urine (transient).
**Hematologic:** *leukopenia during days 10 to 15 with recovery by day 21; thrombocytopenia;* MYELOSUPPRESSION.
**Metabolic:** hyperuricemia.
**Skin:** urticaria, facial flushing, *severe cellulitis or tissue sloughing* (if drug extravasates); *complete alopecia within 3 to 4 weeks* (hair may regrow 2 to 5 months after drug is stopped).
**Other:** fever; chills, *anaphylaxis.*

## Overdose and treatment
Signs and symptoms of overdose include myelosuppression, nausea, vomiting, mucositis, and irreversible myocardial toxicity.
Treatment is usually supportive and includes transfusion of blood components, antiemetics, antibiotics for infections which may develop, symptomatic treatment of mucositis, and cardiac glycoside preparations.

## Clinical considerations
**⋈ ALERT** Reddish color is similar to that of daunorubicin. Don't confuse the two drugs.
■ If signs of HF occur, drug should be stopped and prescriber notified.
■ The alternative dosage schedule (once-weekly dosing) has been found to cause a lower risk of cardiomyopathy.
■ If cumulative dose exceeds 550 mg/m$^2$ body surface area, cardiac adverse reactions, which begin 2 weeks to 6 months after stopping drug, develop in 30% of patients. With high doses of doxorubicin, consider concomitant dosing with the cardioprotective drug dexrazoxane.
■ The occurrence of streaking along a vein or facial flushing indicates that drug is being given too rapidly.
■ Applying a scalp tourniquet or ice may decrease alopecia. However, don't use these if treating leukemias or other neoplasms in which stem cells may be present in scalp.
■ Toxicity from altered clearance can occur in patients with hepatic impairment, and in obese women (greather than 130% ideal body weight).
■ Esophagitis is very common in patients who have also received radiation therapy.

### Therapeutic monitoring
■ Advise clinician to monitor CBC and hepatic function.
■ Decrease dosage as follows if serum bilirubin level increases: 50% of dose when bilirubin level is 1.2 to 3 mg/100 ml; 25% of dose when bilirubin level exceeds 3 mg/100 ml.

### Special populations
**Breast-feeding patients.** It isn't known if doxorubicin appears in breast milk. However, because of the risk of serious adverse reactions, mutagenicity, and carcinogenicity in the infant, breast-feeding isn't recommended.
**Pediatric patients.** Children under age 2 have a higher risk of drug-induced cardiotoxicity.
**Geriatric patients.** Patients over age 70 have an increased risk of drug-induced cardiotoxicity. Take caution in geriatric patients with low bone marrow reserve to prevent serious hematologic toxicity.

## Patient counseling
■ Encourage adequate fluid intake to increase urine output and facilitate excretion of uric acid.

- Advise patient to avoid exposure to people with infections.
- Warn patient that alopecia will occur. Explain that hair growth should resume 2 to 5 months after drug is stopped.
- Advise patient that urine will appear red for 1 to 2 days after the dose and doesn't indicate bleeding. The urine may stain clothes.
- Instruct patient not to receive immunizations during therapy and for several weeks after. Other members of the patient's household should also not receive immunizations during the same period.
- Tell patient to call prescriber if unusual bruising or bleeding or signs of an infection occur.

# doxorubicin hydrochloride liposomal
Doxil

*Pharmacologic classification:* anthracycline
*Therapeutic classification:* antineoplastic
*Pregnancy risk category D*

## Available forms
Available by prescription only
*Injection:* 2 mg/ml

## Indications and dosages
*Metastatic carcinoma of the ovary in patients with disease that is refractory to both paclitaxel- and platinum-based chemotherapy regimens*
*Adults:* 50 mg/m² (doxorubicin hydrochloride equivalent) I.V. at an initial infusion rate of 1 mg/minute once every 4 weeks for a minimum of four courses. Continue treatment as long as the patient doesn't progress, shows no evidence of cardiotoxicity, and continues to tolerate treatment. If no infusion-related adverse events are observed, increase infusion rate to complete administration over 1 hour.
*AIDS-related Kaposi's sarcoma in patients with disease that has progressed on prior combination chemotherapy or in patients who are intolerant to such therapy*
*Adults:* 20 mg/m² (doxorubicin hydrochloride equivalent) I.V. over 30 minutes, once every 3 weeks, for as long as patient responds satisfactorily and tolerates treatment.
≡ *Dosage adjustment.* For patients with impaired hepatic function, reduce dosage as follows: If serum bilirubin is 1.2 to 3 mg/dl give one-half normal dose; if serum bilirubin is over 3 mg/dl give one-quarter normal dose.

The dosage modifications shown in the tables on page 441 are recommended for managing palmar-plantar erythrodysesthesia, hematologic toxicity, and stomatitis.

## I.V. administration
- Follow procedures for proper handling and disposal of antineoplastic drugs.
- Dilute appropriate dose (up to a maximum of 90 mg) in 250 ml of D₅W using aseptic technique. Refrigerate diluted solution at 36° to 46° F (2° to 8° C) and give within 24 hours.
**H ALERT** Carefully check the label on the I.V. bag before giving drug. Accidental substitution of doxorubicin hydrochloride liposomal for conventional doxorubicin hydrochloride has caused severe side effects.
- Don't use with in-line filters.
- Infuse drug I.V. over 30 to 60 minutes depending on the dose; advise clinician to carefully monitor patient during infusion. Acute infusion-associated reactions (flushing, shortness of breath, facial swelling, headache, chills, back pain, tightness in the chest or throat, or hypotension) may occur. These reactions resolve over several hours to a day once the infusion is stopped. The reaction may resolve by slowing the infusion rate.
- Don't give I.M. or S.C. Avoid extravasation. If signs or symptoms of extravasation occur, stop the I.V. infusion immediately and restart in another vein. Applying ice over the site of extravasation for about 30 minutes may be helpful in alleviating the local reaction.

### *Incompatibilities*
Don't mix with other drugs.

## Mechanism of action
*Antineoplastic action:* Doxorubicin hydrochloride liposomal is doxorubicin hydrochloride encapsulated in liposomes which, because of their small size and persistence in the circulation, are able to penetrate the altered vasculature of tumors. The mechanism of action of doxorubicin hydrochloride is thought to be related to its ability to bind DNA and inhibit nucleic acid synthesis.

## Pharmacokinetics
*Absorption:* Unknown.
*Distribution:* Distributed mostly to vascular fluid. Plasma protein–binding hasn't been determined; however, doxorubicin is about 70% plasma protein–bound.
*Metabolism:* Doxorubicinol, the major metabolite of doxorubicin, is detected at very low levels in the plasma.
*Excretion:* Plasma elimination is slow and is described as biphasic, with a half-life of about 5 hours in the first phase and 55 hours in the second phase at doses of 10 to 20 mg/m².

| Route | Onset | Peak | Duration |
|-------|-------|------|----------|
| I.V. | Unknown | Unknown | Unknown |

## PALMAR-PLANTAR ERYTHRODYSESTHESIA

| Grade | Symptoms | Dosage adjustment |
|---|---|---|
| 1 | Mild erythema, swelling, or desquamation not interfering with daily activities | Redose unless patient has experienced a previous grade 3 or 4 skin toxicity. If so, delay up to 2 weeks and decrease dosage by 25%. Return to original dose interval. |
| 2 | Erythema, desquamation, or swelling interfering with, but not precluding, normal physical activities; small blisters or ulcerations less than 2 cm in diameter | Delay dosing up to 2 weeks or until resolved to grade 0-1. If after 2 weeks there's no resolution, discontinue drug. |
| 3 | Blistering, ulceration, or swelling interfering with walking or normal daily activities; can't wear regular clothing | Delay dosing up to 2 weeks or until resolved to grade 0-1. Decrease dosage by 25% and return to original dose interval. If after 2 weeks there's no resolution, discontinue drug. |
| 4 | Diffuse or local process causing infectious complications, or a bedridden state or hospitalization | Delay dosing up to 2 weeks or until resolved to grade 0-1. Decrease dosage by 25% and return to original dose interval. If after 2 weeks there's no resolution, discontinue drug. |

## HEMATOLOGIC TOXICITY

| Grade | Absolute neutrophil count (ANC) (cells/mm$^3$) | Platelets (cells/mm$^3$) | Dosage adjustment |
|---|---|---|---|
| 1 | 1500-1900 | 75,000-150,000 | Resume treatment with no dosage reduction. |
| 2 | 1000-< 1500 | 50,000-< 75,000 | Wait until ANC > 1,500 and platelets > 75,000; redose with no dosage reduction. |
| 3 | 500-999 | 25,000-< 50,000 | Wait until ANC ≥ 1,500 and platelets ≥ 75,000; redose with no dosage reduction. |
| 4 | < 500 | < 25,000 | Wait until ANC ≥ 1,500 and platelets ≥ 75,000; redose at 25% dosage reduction or continue full dose with cytokine support. |

## STOMATITIS

| Grade | Symptoms | Dosage adjustment |
|---|---|---|
| 1 | Painless ulcers, erythema, or mild soreness | Redose unless patient has experienced previous grade 3 or 4 toxicity. If so, delay up to 2 weeks and decrease dosage by 25%. Return to original dosage interval. |
| 2 | Painful erythema, edema, or ulcers, but can eat | Delay dosing up to 2 weeks or until resolved to grade 0-1. If after 2 weeks there's no resolution, discontinue drug. |
| 3 | Painful erythema, edema, or ulcers, and can't eat | Delay dosing up to 2 weeks or until resolved to grade 0-1. Decrease dosage by 25% and return to original dosage interval. If after 2 weeks there's no resolution, discontinue drug. |
| 4 | Requires parenteral or enteral support | Delay dosing up to 2 weeks or until resolved to grade 0-1. Decrease dosage by 25% and return to original dosage interval. If after 2 weeks there's no resolution, discontinue drug. |

## Contraindications and precautions

Contraindicated in patients hypersensitive to the conventional formulation of doxorubicin hydrochloride or to any component in the liposomal formulation. Use with extreme caution in patients with marked myelosuppression or those who have received a lifetime cumulative dosage of 550 mg/m$^2$ or patients who received 400 mg/m$^2$ who have also received radiotherapy to the mediastinal area or concomitant therapy with other cardiotoxic drugs, such as cyclophosphamide. Use in patients with a history of CV disease only when the benefit of the drug outweighs the risk to the patient.

Use cautiously in patients who have received other anthracyclines. The total dose of doxorubicin hydrochloride given to the individual patient should also take into account any previous or concomitant therapy with related compounds such as daunorubicin. Cardiomyopathy and HF may be encountered after discontinuation of therapy.

## Interactions

None reported. However, doxorubicin hydrochloride liposomal may interact with drugs known to interact with the conventional formulation of doxorubicin hydrochloride.

## Adverse reactions

**CNS:** *asthenia*, paresthesia, headache, somnolence, dizziness, depression, insomnia, anxiety, malaise, emotional lability, fatigue.
**CV:** chest pain, hypotension, tachycardia, peripheral edema, cardiomyopathy, *HF, arrhythmias,* pericardial effusion.
**EENT:** *mucous membrane disorder,* mouth ulceration, pharyngitis, rhinitis, conjunctivitis, retinitis, optic neuritis.
**GI:** *nausea, vomiting, constipation, anorexia, diarrhea,* abdominal pain, dyspepsia, oral candidiasis, enlarged abdomen, esophagitis, dysphagia, *stomatitis,* taste perversion, glossitis.
**GU:** albuminuria.
**Hematologic:** LEUKOPENIA, NEUTROPENIA, THROMBOCYTOPENIA, *anemia,* increased PT.
**Hepatic:** hyperbilirubinemia.
**Metabolic:** dehydration, weight loss, hypocalcemia, hyperglycemia.
**Musculoskeletal:** myalgia, back pain.
**Respiratory:** dyspnea, increased cough, pneumonia.
**Skin:** *rash, alopecia,* dry skin, pruritus, skin discoloration, skin disorder, exfoliative dermatitis, sweating, *palmar-plantar erythrodysesthesia.*
**Other:** fever, allergic reaction, chills, infection, infusion-related reactions, herpes zoster.

## Overdose and treatment

Acute overdose with doxorubicin hydrochloride causes increases in mucositis, leukopenia, and thrombocytopenia. Treatment of acute overdose consists of treatment of the severely myelosuppressed patient with hospitalization, antibiotics, platelet and granulocyte transfusions, and symptomatic treatment of mucositis.

## Clinical considerations

■ Patient's hepatic function must be evaluated before therapy, and dosage adjusted accordingly.
**◄ ALERT** Doxorubicin hydrochloride liposomal exhibits unique pharmacokinetic properties compared with conventional doxorubicin hydrochloride and shouldn't be substituted on a mg-per-mg basis.

### Therapeutic monitoring

■ Drug may potentiate the toxicity of other antineoplastic therapies.
■ Advise clinician to monitor cardiac function closely by endomyocardial biopsy, echocardiography, or gated radionuclide scans. If results indicate possible cardiac injury, the benefit of continued therapy must be weighed against the risk of myocardial injury.
■ Advise clinician to monitor CBC, including platelets, before each dose and frequently throughout therapy. Leukopenia is usually transient. Hematologic toxicity may require dosage reduction or suspension or delay of therapy. Persistent, severe myelosuppression may result in superinfection or hemorrhage. Patient may require G-CSF (or GM-CSF) to support blood counts.

### Special populations

**Breast-feeding patients.** It isn't known if drug appears in breast milk. Because many drugs appear in breast milk and because of the potential for serious adverse reactions in breast-feeding infants, women should discontinue breast-feeding before taking this drug.
**Pediatric patients.** Safety and effectiveness in children haven't been established.
**Geriatric patients.** No overall differences were observed between geriatric and younger subjects, but greater sensitivity in some older individuals can't be ruled out.

## Patient counseling

■ Tell patient to notify his prescriber if he experiences symptoms of hand-foot syndrome, such as tingling or burning, redness, flaking, bothersome swelling, small blisters, or small sores on the palms of hands or soles of feet.
■ Advise patient to report symptoms of stomatitis such as painful redness, swelling, or sores in the mouth.
■ Advise patient to avoid exposure to people with infections. Tell patient to report temperature of 100.5° F (38° C) or higher.
■ Inform patient to report nausea, vomiting, tiredness, weakness, rash, or mild hair loss.
■ Advise women of childbearing age to avoid pregnancy during therapy.

---

# doxycycline
Vibramycin

# doxycycline calcium
Vibramycin

# doxycycline hyclate
Doryx, Doxy 100, Doxy 200, Doxy Caps, Vibramycin, Vibra-Tabs

# doxycycline monohydrate
Monodox, Vibramycin

*Pharmacologic classification:* tetracycline
*Therapeutic classification:* antibiotic
*Pregnancy risk category D*

## Available forms
Available by prescription only
**doxycycline calcium**
*Oral suspension:* 50 mg/5 ml
**doxycycline hyclate**
*Tablets (film-coated):* 100 mg
*Capsules:* 50 mg
*Capsules (delayed-release):* 100 mg
*Injection:* 100 mg, 200 mg
**doxycycline monohydrate**
*Capsules:* 50 mg, 100 mg
*Oral suspension:* 25 mg/5 ml

## Indications and dosages
*Infections caused by sensitive organisms*
*Adults and children weighing 45 kg (99 lb) and more:* 100 mg P.O. q 12 hours on day 1, then 100 mg P.O. daily; or 200 mg I.V. on day 1 in one or two infusions, then 100 to 200 mg I.V. daily.
*Children over age 8 weighing less than 45 kg:* 4.4 mg/kg P.O. or I.V. daily, divided q 12 hours day 1, then 2.2 to 4.4 mg/kg daily.
*Gonorrhea in patients allergic to penicillin*
*Adults:* 100 mg P.O. b.i.d. for 7 days; or 300 mg P.O. initially and repeat dose in 1 hour.
◊ *Syphilis in patients allergic to penicillin*
*Adults:* 100 mg P.O. b.i.d. for 2 weeks (early detection) or 4 weeks (if longer than 1 year's duration).
**Chlamydia trachomatis, nongonococcal urethritis, and uncomplicated urethral, endocervical, or rectal infections**
*Adults:* 100 mg P.O. b.i.d. for at least 7 days.
*Acute pelvic inflammatory disease (PID)*
*Adults:* 250 mg I.M. ceftriaxone, followed by 100 mg doxycycline P.O. b.i.d. for 10 to 14 days.
*Acute epididymoorchitis caused by* C. trachomatis *or* Neisseria gonorrhoeae
*Adults:* 100 mg P.O. b.i.d. for at least 10 days.
◊ *Prevention of traveler's diarrhea commonly caused by enterotoxigenic* E. coli
*Adults:* 100 mg P.O. daily for up to 3 days.

◊ *Prophylaxis for rape victims*
*Adults and adolescents:* 100 mg P.O. b.i.d. for 7 days after a single 2-g oral dose of metronidazole is given in conjunction with a single 125-mg I.M. dose of ceftriaxone.
◊ *Anthrax*
*Adults and children weighing more than 45 kg (99 lbs):* 200 mg loading dose I.V., followed by 50 to 100 mg every 12 hours. Continue for at least 14 days after symptoms abate.
*Children weighing 45 kg or less:* 2.5 mg/kg I.V. every 12 hours. Continue for at least 14 days after symptoms abate.
◊ *Prevention of anthrax when fluoroquinolones aren't available or are contraindicated*
*Adults:* 100 mg P.O. b.i.d. Continue until exposure is excluded. If confirmed exposure, continue for 4 weeks and until three vaccinations of anthrax have been given; or continue 8 weeks, if the vaccination is unavailable.
*Children ages 8 and older:* 5 mg/kg daily P.O. in divided doses every 12 hours. Continue until exposure is excluded. If confirmed exposure, continue for 4 weeks and until three vaccinations of anthrax have been given, or 8 weeks, if the vaccination is unavailable.
*Children under age 8:* 5 mg/kg daily P.O. in divided doses every 12 hours. Continue until exposure is excluded. If confirmed exposure, switch to amoxicillin 40 mg/kg daily P.O. in divided doses every 8 hours (maximum dose 500 mg P.O. t.i.d.) if organism is sensitive to penicillin.
*Chemoprophylaxis for malaria in travelers to areas where chloroquine-resistant* **Plasmodium falciparum** *is endemic and mefloquine is contraindicated*
*Adults:* 100 mg P.O. once daily. Begin prophylaxis 1 to 2 days before travel to malarious area; continue daily while in affected area, and continue for 4 weeks after return from malarious area.
*Children over age 8:* Give 2 mg/kg P.O. daily as a single dose; don't exceed 100 mg daily. Use the same dosage schedule as for adults.
◊ *Lyme disease*
*Adults and children ages 9 and older:* 100 mg P.O. b.i.d. or t.i.d. for 10 to 30 days.
◊ *Pleural effusions associated with cancer*
*Adults:* 500 mg of doxycycline diluted in 250 ml of normal saline and instilled into pleural space via chest tube.
*Trachoma*
*Adults:* 2.5 to 4 mg/kg P.O. once daily for 36 to 40 days.

## I.V. administration
**H** *ALERT* Check expiration date. Outdated or deteriorated tetracyclines have caused reversible nephrotoxicity (Fanconi's syndrome).
■ Reconstitute powder for injection with sterile water for injection. Use 10 ml in a 100-mg vial and 20 ml in a 200-mg vial. Dilute solu-

tion to 100 to 1,000 ml for I.V. infusion. Don't infuse solutions more concentrated than 1 mg/ml.
■ Give I.V. infusion slowly (minimum 1 hour). Infusion must be completed within 12 hours (within 6 hours in lactated Ringer's solution or D₅W in lactated Ringer's solution).
■ Reconstituted solution is stable for 72 hours if refrigerated and protected from light.

### Incompatibilities
Incompatible with drugs that aren't stable in acidic solutions, such as barbiturates, erythromycin, methicillin, nafcillin, oxacillin, penicillin G potassium, and sulfonamides. Also incompatible with riboflavin.

## Mechanism of action
*Antibacterial action:* Doxycycline is bacteriostatic; it binds reversibly to ribosomal units, thereby inhibiting bacterial protein synthesis.

Spectrum of activity of the drug includes many gram-negative and gram-positive organisms, *Mycoplasma, Rickettsia, Chlamydia,* and spirochetes.

## Pharmacokinetics
*Absorption:* About 90% to 100% is absorbed after oral administration. Doxycycline has the least affinity for calcium of all tetracyclines; its absorption is insignificantly altered by milk or other dairy products.
*Distribution:* Distributed widely into body tissues and fluids, including synovial, pleural, prostatic, and seminal fluids; bronchial secretions; saliva; and aqueous humor. CSF penetration is poor. Doxycycline readily crosses the placenta, and is 25% to 93% protein-bound.
*Metabolism:* Insignificantly metabolized; some hepatic degradation occurs.
*Excretion:* Excreted primarily unchanged in urine by glomerular filtration; some drug may appear in breast milk. Plasma half-life is 22 to 24 hours after multiple dosing in adults with normal renal function; 20 to 30 hours in patients with severe renal impairment. Some drug is excreted in feces.

| Route | Onset | Peak | Duration |
|-------|-------|------|----------|
| P.O. | Unknown | 1½ hr | Unknown |
| I.V. | Immediate | Unknown | Unknown |

## Contraindications and precautions
Contraindicated in patients hypersensitive to drug or other tetracyclines. Use cautiously in patients with impaired renal or hepatic function. Use during last half of pregnancy and in children under age 8 may cause permanent discoloration of teeth, enamel defects, and bone growth retardation.

## Interactions
**Drug-drug.** *Antacids containing aluminum, calcium, or magnesium; laxatives containing*

*magnesium; oral iron products, sodium bicarbonate, zinc:* Decrease oral absorption of doxycycline. Give antibiotic 1 hour before or 2 hours after any of these drugs.
*Carbamazepine, phenobarbital:* May cause decreased antibiotic effect. Avoid use together.
*Digoxin:* Increased bioavailability. Advise clinician to monitor serum digoxin levels. Lowered dosages of digoxin may be needed.
*Methoxyflurane:* Causes nephrotoxicity with tetracyclines. Advise clinician to monitor serum levels carefully.
*Oral anticoagulants:* Increased anticoagulant effect. Advise clinician to monitor PT and INR; dosage adjustment may be needed.
*Oral contraceptives:* Decrease contraceptive effectiveness and increase risk of breakthrough bleeding. Use a nonhormonal form of birth control.
*Penicillin:* May antagonize bactericidal effects. Administer penicillin 2 to 3 hours before tetracycline.
**Drug-lifestyle.** *Alcohol use:* May decrease antibiotic effect. Discourage use together.
*Sun exposure:* May cause photosensitivity reactions. Advise patient to take precautions.

## Adverse reactions
**CNS:** *intracranial hypertension (pseudotumor cerebri).*
**CV:** pericarditis.
**EENT:** glossitis, dysphagia.
**GI:** anorexia, *epigastric distress, nausea,* vomiting, *diarrhea,* oral candidiasis, enterocolitis, anogenital inflammation.
**Hematologic:** *neutropenia,* eosinophilia, *thrombocytopenia,* hemolytic anemia.
**Hepatic:** elevated liver enzymes.
**Musculoskeletal:** bone growth retardation if used in children under age 8.
**Skin:** *maculopapular and erythematous rashes, photosensitivity, increased pigmentation, urticaria.*
**Other:** hypersensitivity reactions *(anaphylaxis);* permanent discoloration of teeth, enamel defects, superinfection; thrombophlebitis.

## Overdose and treatment
Signs and symptoms of overdose are usually limited to the GI tract; advise clinician to give antacids or empty stomach by gastric lavage if ingestion occurred within the preceding 4 hours.

## Clinical considerations
**⚠ ALERT** Don't confuse sound-alike drugs: doxycycline, doxylamine, and dicyclomine.
■ Drug may not be given S.C. or I.M.
■ Drug may be used in patients with impaired renal function; it doesn't accumulate or cause a significant rise in BUN levels.
■ Doxycycline causes false-negative results in urine tests using glucose oxidase reagent (Diastix, Chemstrip uG, or glucose enzymatic test

---

Reactions may be *common,* uncommon, *life-threatening,* or COMMON AND LIFE-THREATENING.

strip); parenteral dosage form may cause false-negative Clinitest results.

■ Doxycycline also causes false elevations in fluorometric tests for urinary catecholamines.

### Therapeutic monitoring

■ With larger doses or prolonged therapy, advise clinician to watch for superinfection, especially in high-risk patients.

■ Tell patient to check tongue for fungal infection. Stress good oral hygiene.

### Special populations

**Pregnant patients.** Use caution in pregnant women. Consider benefits of treating infection versus risk of fetal damage and toxic effects to woman's liver. Advise clinician to carefully monitor results of sensitivity tests and periodic liver function test results.

**Breast-feeding patients.** Avoid use in breast-feeding women.

**Pediatric patients.** Avoid use of drug in children under age 8 unless other drugs prove ineffective or are contraindicated.

### Patient counseling

■ Instruct patient to take entire amount of drug as prescribed, even if he feels better.

■ Tell patient to take oral form of drug with food or milk if GI upset occurs.

# droperidol

Inapsine

*Pharmacologic classification:* butyrophenone derivative
*Therapeutic classification:* tranquilizer
*Pregnancy risk category C*

### Available forms

Available by prescription only
*Injection:* 2.5 mg/ml

### Indications and dosages

*Delirium*
*Adults:* 5 mg I.M., p.r.n. It's given for its quick onset and sedative quality.

*Anesthetic premedication*
*Adults:* 2.5 to 10 mg I.M. 30 to 60 minutes before induction of general anesthesia.
*Children ages 2 to 12:* 0.088 to 0.165 mg/kg I.V. or I.M.

*Adjunct for induction of general anesthesia*
*Adults:* 0.22 to 0.275 mg/kg I.V. (preferably) or I.M. with an analgesic or general anesthetic.
*Children:* 0.088 to 0.165 mg/kg I.V. or I.M.

*Adjunct for maintenance of general anesthesia*
*Adults:* 1.25 to 2.5 mg I.V.

*For use without a general anesthetic during diagnostic procedures*
*Adults:* 2.5 to 10 mg I.M. 30 to 60 minutes before the procedure. Additional doses of 1.25 to 2.5 mg I.V. are given, p.r.n.

*Adjunct to regional anesthesia*
*Adults:* 2.5 to 5 mg I.M. or slow I.V. injection.

◇ *Antiemetic in conjunction with cancer chemotherapy*
*Adults:* 6.25 mg I.M. or by slow I.V. injection.

### I.V. administration

■ Follow standard I.V. preparation technique.

■ Administration rate is determined by recommended use.

### Incompatibilities

Incompatible with barbiturates, fluorouracil, foscarnet, furosemide, heparin, leucovorin, methotrexate sodium, and nafcillin.

### Mechanism of action

*Tranquilizer action:* Droperidol produces marked sedation by directly blocking subcortical receptors. Droperidol also blocks CNS receptors at the chemoreceptor trigger zone, producing an antiemetic effect.

### Pharmacokinetics

*Absorption:* Well absorbed after I.M. injection. Some alteration of consciousness may persist for 12 hours.

*Distribution:* Not well understood; drug crosses the blood-brain barrier and is distributed in the CSF. It also crosses the placenta.

*Metabolism:* Metabolized by the liver to *p*-fluoro-phenylacetic acid and *p*-hydroxy-piperidine.

*Excretion:* Excreted in urine and feces.

| Route | Onset | Peak | Duration |
|---|---|---|---|
| I.V., I.M. | 3-10 min | ½ hr | 2-4 hr |

### Contraindications and precautions

Contraindicated in patients with known hypersensitivity or intolerance to drug. Use cautiously in patients with hypotension and other CV disease because of its vasodilatory effects, in patients with hepatic or renal disease for whom drug clearance may be impaired, and in patients taking other CNS depressants, including alcohol, opiates, and sedatives, because droperidol may potentiate the effects of these drugs.

### Interactions

**Drug-drug.** *Fentanyl citrate:* May cause hypertension and respiratory depression. Avoid use together, if possible.

*Opiates, other analgesics, other CNS depressants, such as barbiturates, sedative-hypnotics, tranquilizers:* Additive CNS depression. When used together, reduce dosage of both drugs.

**Drug-lifestyle.** *Alcohol use:* Drug potentiates CNS depressant effects. Advise patient to avoid alcohol.

## Adverse reactions
**CNS:** *sedation,* altered consciousness, postoperative hallucinations, extrapyramidal reactions, temporarily altered EEG pattern.
**CV:** *hypotension* with rebound tachycardia, *bradycardia,* hypertension when combined with fentanyl or other parenteral analgesics, decreased pulmonary artery pressure.
**Respiratory:** *respiratory depression.*

## Overdose and treatment
Signs and symptoms of overdose include extension of the pharmacologic actions of the drug. Treatment of overdose is symptomatic and supportive.

## Clinical considerations
**H** *ALERT* Recommend having fluids and other measures to manage hypotension readily available.
■ Droperidol has been used for its antiemetic effects in preventing or treating chemotherapy-induced nausea and vomiting, especially that produced by cisplatin.
■ Drug should be stopped if patient shows signs of hypersensitivity, severe persistent hypotension, respiratory depression, paradoxical hypertension, or dystonia.

### Therapeutic monitoring
■ Advise clinician to monitor vital signs and observe patient for extrapyramidal reactions. Droperidol is related to haloperidol and is more likely than other antipsychotics to cause extrapyramidal symptoms.
■ Observe patient for postoperative hallucinations or emergence delirium and drowsiness.

### Special populations
**Breast-feeding patients.** It's unknown if droperidol appears in breast milk.
**Pediatric patients.** Safety and efficacy in children under age 2 haven't been established.
**Geriatric patients.** Use drug with caution. Geriatric patients are more prone to extrapyramidal reactions, CNS disturbances, and CV side effects.

## Patient counseling
■ Advise patient of possible postoperative effects.
■ Warn patient to rise slowly to prevent orthostatic hypotension.

## econazole nitrate
Spectazole

*Pharmacologic classification:* synthetic imidazole derivative
*Therapeutic classification:* antifungal
*Pregnancy risk category C*

### Available forms
Available by prescription only
*Cream:* 1% (water-soluble base)

### Indications and dosages
**Cutaneous candidiasis**
*Adults and children:* Gently rub sufficient quantity into affected areas b.i.d. in the morning and evening.
**Tinea pedis, tinea cruris, tinea corporis, and tinea versicolor**
*Adults and children:* Gently rub into affected area once daily.

### Mechanism of action
*Antifungal action:* Although exact mechanism of action is unknown, drug may exert its effects by altering cellular membranes and interfering with intracellular enzymes. Econazole is active against many fungi, including dermatophytes and yeasts, as well as some gram-positive bacteria.

### Pharmacokinetics
*Absorption:* Minimal but rapid percutaneous absorption.
*Distribution:* Minimal.
*Metabolism:* Unknown.
*Excretion:* Unknown.

| Route | Onset | Peak | Duration |
|-------|-------|------|----------|
| Topical | Unknown | Unknown | Unknown |

### Contraindications and precautions
Contraindicated in patients hypersensitive to drug.

### Interactions
**Drug-drug.** *Corticosteroids:* Can inhibit the antifungal activity of econazole nitrate, in a level-dependent manner, in the treatment of *Saccharomyces cerevisiae* and *Candida albicans.* Avoid use together.

### Adverse reactions
**Skin:** burning, pruritus, stinging, erythema.

### Overdose and treatment
No overdose information available. If a reaction suggesting sensitivity or chemical irritation occurs, therapy should be stopped.

### Clinical considerations
■ Recommend washing affected area with soap and water and drying thoroughly before applying drug.

#### Therapeutic monitoring
■ Relief of symptoms usually occurs within 1 to 2 weeks of initiation of therapy.

#### Special populations
**Breast-feeding patients.** It's unknown if drug appears in breast milk. Use with caution in breast-feeding women.

### Patient counseling
■ Tell patient to wash hands well after application.
■ Caution patient to use drug as directed for the entire period of treatment, even though symptoms may lessen.
■ Instruct patient with tinea pedis (athlete's foot) to wear well-fitting, well-ventilated shoes, and to change all-cotton socks daily.

## edrophonium chloride
Enlon, Enlon-Plus, Reversol, Tensilon

*Pharmacologic classification:* cholinesterase inhibitor
*Therapeutic classification:* cholinergic agonist, diagnostic
*Pregnancy risk category NR*

### Available forms
Available by prescription only
*Injection:* 10 mg/ml in 1-ml ampule, 10-ml vial, 15-ml vial
*Enlon-Plus:* 10 mg/ml with atropine sulfate 0.14 mg/ml

### Indications and dosages
**Curare antagonist (to reverse neuromuscular blocking action)**
*Adults:* 10 mg I.V. given over 30 to 45 seconds, repeated every 5 to 10 minutes, p.r.n., to 40 mg

maximum dose. If large doses of edrophonium chloride (15 mg) are needed, they should be preceded by 0.4 to 1.6 mg of atropine sulfate I.V., depending on the patient's age and weight. Or, 0.05 to 0.1 ml/kg of the combination of edrophonium chloride (10 mg/ml) and atropine sulfate (0.14 mg/ml) may be given I.V. over 45 seconds to 1 minute.

*Diagnostic aid in myasthenia gravis*
*Adults:* 2 mg I.V. within 15 to 30 seconds, then 8 mg if no response (increase in muscular strength) occurs. Alternatively, 10 mg I.M. If cholinergic reaction occurs, 2 mg I.M. 30 minutes later to rule out false-negative response.
*Children weighing over 34 kg (75 lb):* 2 mg I.V. If no response within 45 seconds, give 1 mg q 45 seconds to maximum dose of 10 mg; alternatively, 5 mg I.M.
*Children weighing 34 kg or less:* 1 mg I.V. If no response within 45 seconds, give 1 mg q 45 seconds to maximum dose of 5 mg; alternatively, 2 mg I.M.
*Infants:* 0.5 mg I.V.

*To differentiate myasthenic crisis from cholinergic crisis*
*Adults:* 1 mg I.V. If no response occurs in 1 minute, repeat dose once. Increased muscular strength confirms myasthenic crisis; no increase or exaggerated weakness confirms cholinergic crisis. Tensilon test is used for evaluating treatment requirements in myasthenia gravis.
*Adults:* 1 to 2 mg I.V. given 1 hour after oral intake of drug being used in treatment. Response will be myasthenic in the undertreated patient, adequate in the controlled patient, and cholinergic in the overtreated patient.
◇ *To terminate paroxysmal atrial tachycardia or as an aid in diagnosing supraventricular tachyarrhythmias and evaluating the function of demand pacemakers*
*Adults:* 10 mg I.V. over 5 minutes.
≡ *Dosage adjustment.* In geriatric or digitalized adults, 5 to 7 mg I.V. over 5 minutes.
*To slow supraventricular tachyarrhythmias unresponsive to a cardiac glycoside*
*Adults:* 2 mg/minute I.V. test dose, followed by 2 mg q minute until a total dose of 10 mg is given. If heart rate decreases in response to this dose, infusion of 0.25 mg/minute may be started; rate of infusion may be increased to 2 mg/minute if needed.

## I.V. administration
■ For easier administration, use a tuberculin syringe with an I.V. needle.
■ Atropine sulfate injection should always be readily available as an antagonist for the muscarinic effects of edrophonium.

### Incompatibilities
None reported.

## Mechanism of action
*Cholinergic action:* Edrophonium blocks hydrolysis of acetylcholine by cholinesterase, resulting in acetylcholine accumulation at cholinergic synapses. This leads to increased cholinergic receptor stimulation at the neuromuscular junction and vagal sites. Edrophonium is a short-acting drug, which makes it particularly useful for the diagnosis of myasthenia gravis.

## Pharmacokinetics
*Absorption:* No information available.
*Distribution:* Not clearly identified.
*Metabolism:* Exact metabolic fate is unknown; drug isn't hydrolyzed by cholinesterases.
*Excretion:* Exact excretion mode is unknown.

| Route | Onset | Peak | Duration |
|-------|-------|------|----------|
| I.V. | < 1 min | Unknown | 5-20 min |
| I.M. | 2-10 min | Unknown | 10-30 min |

## Contraindications and precautions
Contraindicated in patients hypersensitive to anticholinesterase drugs and in those with mechanical obstruction of the intestine or urinary tract.

Use cautiously in patients with bronchial asthma or arrhythmias. When used with atropine, be aware that atropine is contraindicated in patients hypersensitive to drug and in those with acute angle-closure glaucoma, obstructive uropathy, obstructive disease of GI tract, paralytic ileus, toxic megacolon, intestinal atony, unstable CV status in acute hemorrhage, tachycardia, myocardial ischemia, asthma, and myasthenia gravis.

## Interactions
**Drug-drug.** *Aminoglycosides and anesthetics:* May potentiate prolonged or enhanced muscle weakness. Use together cautiously.
*Cardiac glycosides:* May increase the heart's sensitivity to edrophonium. Use together cautiously.
*Cholinergic drugs:* May lead to additive toxicity. Avoid use together.
*Corticosteroids:* May decrease the cholinergic effects of edrophonium; when corticosteroids are stopped, however, cholinergic effects may increase, possibly affecting muscle strength. Observe for lack of drug effect.
*Ganglionic blockers, such as mecamylamine:* May lead to a critical blood pressure decrease. Avoid use together.
*Magnesium:* Administration has a direct depressant effect on skeletal muscle. Avoid use together.
*Procainamide and quinidine:* May reverse the cholinergic effect of edrophonium on muscle. Use together cautiously.
*Succinylcholine:* May cause prolonged respiratory depression from plasma esterase inhibition. Avoid use together.

**Drug-herb.** *Jaborandi tree and pill-bearing spurge:* May cause an additive effect and increased risk of toxicity. Discourage use together.

## Adverse reactions
**CNS:** *seizures,* weakness.
**CV:** hypotension, bradycardia, *AV block, cardiac arrest.*
**EENT:** excessive lacrimation, diplopia, miosis, conjunctival hyperemia.
**GI:** nausea, vomiting, *diarrhea, abdominal cramps,* dysphagia, excessive salivation.
**GU:** urinary frequency, incontinence.
**Musculoskeletal:** dysarthria, muscle cramps, muscle fasciculation.
**Respiratory:** *paralysis of muscles of respiration, central respiratory paralysis, bronchospasm, laryngospasm,* increased bronchial secretions.
**Skin:** diaphoresis.

## Overdose and treatment
Signs and symptoms of overdose include muscle weakness, nausea, vomiting, diarrhea, blurred vision, miosis, excessive tearing, bronchospasm, increased bronchial secretions, hypotension, incoordination, excessive sweating, cramps, fasciculations, paralysis, bradycardia or tachycardia, excessive salivation, and restlessness or agitation. Muscles first weakened by overdose include neck, jaw, and pharyngeal muscles, followed by muscle weakening of the shoulders, arms, pelvis, outer eye, and legs.

Recommend discontinuing drug immediately. Recommend supporting respiration; bronchial suctioning may be performed. Atropine may be given to block the muscarinic effects of edrophonium but won't counter the paralytic effects of the drug on skeletal muscle. Atropine overdose should be avoided because it may lead to bronchial plug formation.

## Clinical considerations
■ When edrophonium is given to differentiate myasthenic crisis from cholinergic crisis, recommend evaluating patient's muscle strength closely.

### Therapeutic monitoring
■ Advise clinician to monitor patient for adverse reactions and for therapeutic effects.

### Special populations
**Pregnant patients.** Drug may cause uterine irritability and induce premature labor when given I.V. to patients near term.
**Breast-feeding patients.** Safety hasn't been established. Breast-feeding women should avoid edrophonium.
**Pediatric patients.** Children may require I.M. administration; with this route, drug effects may be delayed for 2 to 10 minutes.

**Geriatric patients.** Geriatric patients may be more sensitive to effects of this drug. Use with caution.

## Patient counseling
■ Tell patient that the adverse effects of the drug will be transient because of its short duration of effect.

# efavirenz
Sustiva

*Pharmacologic classification:* nonnucleoside, reverse transcriptase inhibitor (NNRTI)
*Therapeutic classification:* antiretroviral
*Pregnancy risk category C*

## Available forms
Available by prescription only
*Capsules:* 50 mg, 100 mg, 200 mg, 600 mg

## Indications and dosages
*Treatment of HIV-1 infection*
*Adults:* 600 mg P.O. once daily with a protease inhibitor or nucleoside analogue reverse transcriptase inhibitors.
*Children ages 3 and older weighing 40 kg (88 lb) or more:* 600 mg P.O. once daily with a protease inhibitor or nucleoside analogue reverse transcriptase inhibitors.
*Children ages 3 and older weighing 10 to 40 kg (22 to 88 lb):* Give the following doses with a protease inhibitor or nucleoside analogue reverse transcriptase inhibitors.
*Children weighing 10 to < 15 kg (22 to < 33 lb):* 200 mg P.O. once daily.
*Children weighing 15 to < 20 kg (33 to < 44 lb):* 250 mg P.O. once daily.
*Children weighing 20 to < 25 kg (44 to < 55 lb):* 300 mg P.O. once daily.
*Children weighing 25 to < 32.5 kg (55 to < 71.5 lb):* 350 mg P.O. once daily.
*Children weighing 32.5 to < 40 kg (71.5 to < 88 lb):* 400 mg P.O. once daily.

## Mechanism of action
*Antiretroviral action:* Efavirenz inhibits the transcription of HIV-1 RNA to DNA, a critical step in the viral replication process. Therefore, drug lowers the amount of HIV in the blood (the viral load) and increases CD4 lymphocytes.

## Pharmacokinetics
*Absorption:* Relative bioavailability increased by about 50% when taken with a high-fat meal.
*Distribution:* Highly plasma protein–bound; also distributed into the CSF.
*Metabolism:* Metabolized primarily by cytochrome P-450 3A4 and cytochrome P-450 2B6 to hydroxylated inactive metabolites.

*Excretion:* 14% to 34% is excreted in urine (less than 1% is excreted unchanged), and 16% to 61% is excreted in feces. Terminal elimination half-life is 52 to 76 hours.

| Route | Onset | Peak | Duration |
|-------|-------|------|----------|
| P.O. | Unknown | 3-5 hr | Unknown |

## Contraindications and precautions

Contraindicated in patients hypersensitive to efavirenz or its components.

Use cautiously in patients with hepatic impairment or in those concurrently receiving hepatotoxic drugs.

## Interactions

**Drug-drug.** *Clarithromycin and indinavir:* May decrease plasma levels. Consider alternative therapy or dosage adjustment.

*Drugs that induce the cytochrome P-450 enzyme system (such as phenobarbital and rifampin):* Increase clearance of efavirenz, resulting in lower plasma levels. Avoid use together.

*Ergot derivatives, midazolam, and triazolam:* Competition for cytochrome P-450 enzyme system may result in inhibition of the metabolism of these drugs and cause serious or life-threatening adverse events (such as arrhythmias, prolonged sedation, or respiratory depression). Avoid use together.

*Estrogens:* Increase plasma levels. Advise clinician to monitor patient.

*NNRTIs:* Concomitant use with efavirenz is not recommended.

*Oral contraceptives:* Potential interaction of efavirenz with oral contraceptives hasn't been determined. Advise use of a reliable method of barrier contraception in addition to use of oral contraceptives.

*Psychoactive drugs:* May cause additive CNS effects. Avoid use together.

*Rifabutin:* Decreased plasma levels of rifabutin. Dosage adjustment may be needed.

*Ritonavir:* Increased adverse effects of efavirenz. Don't use together.

*Saquinavir:* Plasma levels of saquinavir decrease significantly. Don't use with saquinavir as sole protease inhibitor. Use of saquinavir also decreases AUC of efavirenz by 12% to 13%.

*Warfarin:* Plasma levels and effects of warfarin are potentially increased or decreased. Advise clinician to monitor INR.

**Drug-herb.** *St. John's wort:* May decrease plasma levels. Discourage use together.

**Drug-food.** *High-fat meals:* May increase absorption of drug. Instruct patient to maintain a proper low-fat diet.

**Drug-lifestyle.** *Alcohol use:* Enhances CNS effects. Advise patient to avoid alcohol use.

## Adverse reactions

**CNS:** *abnormal dreams or thinking, agitation, amnesia, confusion, depersonalization,* depression, *dizziness, euphoria,* fatigue, *hallucinations,* headache, hypoesthesia, *impaired concentration, insomnia, somnolence,* nervousness, *stupor,* anxiety, pain.

**CV:** lipodystrophy, hypercholesterolemia.

**GI:** abdominal pain, anorexia, *diarrhea,* dyspepsia, flatulence, *nausea,* vomiting, pancreatitis.

**GU:** hematuria, kidney stones.

**Hepatic:** increased AST and ALT.

**Skin:** increased sweating, *erythema multiforme, Stevens-Johnson syndrome, toxic epidermal necrolysis, rash,* pruritus.

**Other:** fever.

## Overdose and treatment

Overdose has resulted in increased symptoms of the nervous system and involuntary muscle contractions.

Treatment should involve supportive care, including frequent monitoring of vital signs and observation of clinical status. Activated charcoal may be given to aid in the removal of unabsorbed drug. Efavirenz is unlikely to be removed by hemodialysis.

## Clinical considerations

■ Use drug with other antiretrovirals because resistant viruses emerge rapidly when used alone. Drug shouldn't be used as monotherapy, or added on as a single drug to a failing regimen.

■ Combination with ritonavir is linked to a higher frequency of adverse effects (such as dizziness, nausea, paresthesia) and laboratory abnormalities (elevated liver enzymes).

■ Pharmacokinetics of efavirenz are not affected by hemodialysis.

■ Drug therapy may cause false-positive urine cannabinoid test results.

### Therapeutic monitoring

■ Advise clinician to monitor liver function test results and cholesterol levels.

■ Advise clinician to monitor patient for adverse reactions.

### Special populations

**Pregnant patients.** Pregnancy must be ruled out before therapy is started in women of child-bearing age. To register pregnant women to monitor outcomes, call the antiretroviral pregnancy registry at 1-800-258-4263.

**Breast-feeding patients.** HIV-infected women shouldn't breast-feed their infants to avoid risking transmitting the disease. The drug appears in breast milk of animals. Instruct women not to nurse their infants.

**Pediatric patients.** Children may be more prone to adverse reactions, especially diarrhea, nausea, vomiting, and rash.

**Geriatric patients.** Geriatric patients may be more susceptible to the CNS effects of the drug.

## Patient counseling

■ Instruct patient to take drug with water, juice, milk, or soda. It may be taken without regard to meals.

■ Inform patient that drug isn't a cure for HIV infection and that it won't affect the development of opportunistic infections and other complications caused by HIV disease or transmission of HIV to others through sexual contact or blood contamination.

■ Instruct patient to take drug at the same time daily and always with other antiretrovirals.

■ Tell patient to take drug exactly as prescribed and not to discontinue it without medical approval.

■ Instruct patient to report adverse reactions.

■ Inform patient that rash is the most common adverse effect. If this occurs, tell patient to report it immediately, because it may be serious in rare cases.

■ Advise patient that dizziness, difficulty sleeping or concentrating, drowsiness, or unusual dreams may occur during the first few days of therapy. Reassure him that these symptoms generally resolve after 2 to 4 weeks and may be less problematic if drug is taken at bedtime.

■ Tell patient to avoid alcoholic beverages, driving, or operating machinery until the effects of the drug are known.

# eflornithine hydrochloride

Vaniqa

*Pharmacologic classification:* ornithine decarboxylase (ODC) inhibitor
*Therapeutic classification:* hair growth retardant
*Pregnancy risk category C*

## Available forms

Available by prescription only
*Cream:* 13.9 %

## Indications and dosages

*Reduction of unwanted facial hair in women*

*Adults and children over age 12:* Thin layer applied to affected areas of the face and adjacent areas under the chin and rubbed in thoroughly. Applied b.i.d. at least 8 hours apart.

## Mechanism of action

*Hair growth retardant action:* Thought to irreversibly inhibit skin ornithine decarboxylase (ODC) activity. This enzyme is needed in the synthesis of polyamines. Animal data indicate that inhibition of ODC affects cell division and synthetic functions, which affect the rate of hair growth. Drug retards the rate of hair growth in nonclinical and clinical studies.

## Pharmacokinetics

*Absorption:* Less than 1% of the radioactive dose is absorbed after single or multiple doses under conditions of clinical use that include shaving within 2 hours before radiolabeled dose application and other forms of cutting, plucking, and tweezing to remove facial hair.
*Distribution:* Time to reach steady state is 4 days of twice-daily application. The steady-state plasma half-life of eflornithine is about 8 hours.
*Metabolism:* Not known to be metabolized.
*Excretion:* Unchanged in urine.

| Route | Onset | Peak | Duration |
|-------|-------|------|----------|
| Topical | Unknown | 8 hr | Unknown |

## Contraindications and precautions

Contraindicated in patients sensitive to any component of the preparation.

## Interactions

No known interactions.

## Adverse reactions

**CNS:** headache, dizziness, asthenia, vertigo.
**GI:** dyspepsia, anorexia, nausea.
**Skin:** *acne, pseudofolliculitis barbae,* stinging or burning sensation, dry skin, pruritus, erythema, skin irritation, rash, alopecia, folliculitis, ingrown hair, facial edema.

## Overdose and treatment

Information unavailable. Given the low percutaneous penetration of this drug, overdosage through the topical route isn't expected. However, with very high topical doses (such as multiple tubes per day) or oral ingestion, recommend monitoring patient and providing appropriate supportive measures p.r.n.

## Clinical considerations

■ Drug has been studied only on the face and adjacent involved areas under the chin. Application of the cream should be limited to these areas.

■ Drug isn't expected to cause contact sensitization, phototoxicity, or photosensitization reactions.

■ Drug is available as a cream in a 30-g tube or two 30-g tubes for a total of 60 g. Drug should be stored at controlled room temperature of 59° to 86° F (15° to 30° C).

### Therapeutic monitoring

■ If adverse effects become bothersome, instruct the patient to limit use to once a day. If adverse effects persist, tell patient to consult prescriber.

### Special populations

**Breast-feeding patients.** It isn't known if drug appears in human milk. Drug should be used cautiously when given to nursing women.

**Pediatric patients.** Drug shouldn't be used in children under age 12.

## Patient counseling

- Tell patient that drug is intended to reduce unwanted facial and chin hair in women. Urge patient to limit use to these areas.
- Advise patient that drug isn't a depilatory, but rather is believed to slow hair growth. Patient will likely need to continue using a hair removal method with the drug.
- Tell patient that improvement may occur in 4 to 8 weeks and that the condition may return to pretreatment levels 8 weeks after drug is stopped.
- Instruct patient to apply drug in a thin layer to affected areas b.i.d., at least 8 hours apart. If skin irritation or intolerance develops, tell patient to temporarily reduce the frequency of application to once a day. If irritation continues, patient should stop using drug.
- Tell patient to store drug at controlled room temperature of 59° to 86° F (15° to 30° C) and not to freeze it.

---

## enalaprilat
Vasotec I.V.

## enalapril maleate
Vasotec

*Pharmacologic classification:* ACE inhibitor
*Therapeutic classification:* antihypertensive
*Pregnancy risk category C (D in second and third trimesters)*

## Available forms

Available by prescription only
*Tablets:* 2.5 mg, 5 mg, 10 mg, 20 mg
*Injection:* 1.25 mg/ml in 2-ml vials

## Indications and dosages

*Hypertension*
*Adults:* For patient not receiving diuretics, initially 5 mg P.O. once daily, then adjusted according to response. Usual dosage range is 10 to 40 mg daily as a single dose or two divided doses. Alternatively, 1.25 mg I.V. infusion q 6 hours over 5 minutes. For patient on diuretics, initially 2.5 mg P.O. once daily. Alternatively, give 0.625 mg I.V. over 5 minutes; repeat in 1 hour, if needed, then follow with 1.25 mg I.V. q 6 hours.
*To convert from I.V. therapy to oral therapy*
*Adults:* If patient wasn't given diuretics and was receiving 1.25 mg I.V. q 6 hours, then initially, 5 mg P.O. once daily. If patient was being given diuretics and was receiving 0.625 mg I.V. q 6 hours, then 2.5 mg P.O. once daily. Adjust dosage according to response.

*To convert from oral therapy to I.V. therapy*
*Adults:* 1.25 mg I.V. over 5 minutes q 6 hours.
≡ *Dosage adjustment.* In hypertensive patients with renal failure who have a creatinine clearance less than 30 ml/minute, begin therapy at 2.5 mg/day. Gradually adjust dosage according to response. Patients undergoing hemodialysis should receive a supplemental dose of 2.5 mg on days of dialysis.
*Heart failure*
*Adults:* Initially, 2.5 mg P.O. once or twice daily. Usual maintenance dose is 5 to 20 mg P.O. daily, given in two divided doses. Maximum daily dose is 40 mg P.O. in two divided doses.
*Asymptomatic left ventricular dysfunction*
*Adults:* Initially, 2.5 mg P.O. b.i.d.; adjust to targeted daily dose of 20 mg (in divided doses) as tolerated.
≡ *Dosage adjustment.* In patients with HF and renal impairment or hyponatremia (serum sodium less than 130 mEq/L or serum creatinine of more than 1.6 mg/dl), begin therapy with 2.5 mg P.O. daily. Increase dosage to 2.5 mg b.i.d., then 5 mg b.i.d. and higher as indicated, usually at intervals of 4 days or longer.

## I. V. administration

- Enalapril may be given by slow, direct I.V. injection over 5 minutes, or it can be diluted in up to 50 ml of $D_5W$; normal saline solution; 5% dextrose in normal saline solution; 5% dextrose in lactated Ringer's; or Isolyte E.
- Solutions are stable for 24 hours at room temperature.

## Incompatibilities

Incompatible with amphotericin B and phenytoin sodium.

## Mechanism of action

*Antihypertensive action:* Enalapril inhibits ACE, preventing conversion of angiotensin I to angiotensin II, a potent vasoconstrictor. Reduced angiotensin II levels decrease peripheral arterial resistance, thus lowering blood pressure, and decrease aldosterone secretion, thus reducing sodium and water retention.

## Pharmacokinetics

*Absorption:* About 60% of a given dose is absorbed from the GI tract.
*Distribution:* Full distribution pattern is unknown; drug doesn't appear to cross the blood-brain barrier.
*Metabolism:* Metabolized extensively to the active metabolite enalaprilat.
*Excretion:* About 94% of a dose is excreted in urine and feces as enalaprilat and enalapril.

| Route | Onset | Peak | Duration |
|-------|-------|------|----------|
| P.O. | 1 hr | 4-6 hr | 24 hr |
| I.V. | 15 min | 1-4 hr | 6 hr |

## Contraindications and precautions

Contraindicated in patients hypersensitive to drug, and those with a history of angioedema related to previous treatment with an ACE inhibitor, or with hereditary or idiopathic angioedema. Avoid use in patients at high risk for cardiogenic shock.

Use cautiously in patients with impaired renal function. Also use with caution in patients with obstruction in the outflow tract of the left ventricle (such as aortic stenosis, hypertrophic cardiomyopathy).

## Interactions

**Drug-drug.** *Diuretics, phenothiazines, or other antihypertensives:* Increase antihypertensive effects. Use together cautiously.
*Insulin, oral antidiabetics:* Increased risk of hypoglycemia, especially when enalapril therapy starts. Recommend close monitoring of glucose level.
*Lithium:* Decreased renal clearance of lithium. Advise clinician to monitor lithium level.
*NSAIDs and aspirin:* May decrease the antihypertensive effect of enalapril and may attenuate the hemodynamics of ACE inhibitors in patients with HF. Use together cautiously.
*Potassium-sparing diuretics and potassium supplements:* Enhanced diuretic effects and possibly hyperkalemia. Use together cautiously.
*Rifampin:* Decreased pharmacologic effects of rifampin. Advise clinician to closely monitor patient.
**Drug-herb.** *Licorice:* May cause sodium retention and increase blood pressure, interfering with the therapeutic effects of ACE inhibitors. Discourage use together.
*Capsaicin:* Increased risk of cough. Discourage use together.
**Drug-food.** *Salt substitutes:* May enhance effects, thereby causing hyperkalemia.

## Adverse reactions

**CNS:** *headache, dizziness, fatigue,* vertigo, asthenia, syncope.
**CV:** *hypotension,* chest pain, ***bradycardia.***
**GI:** diarrhea, nausea, abdominal pain, vomiting.
**GU:** elevated BUN and serum creatinine levels, decreased renal function (in patients with bilateral renal artery stenosis or heart failure).
**Hematologic:** *neutropenia, thrombocytopenia, agranulocytosis.*
**Hepatic:** increased liver enzyme and bilirubin levels.
**Respiratory:** *dry, persistent, tickling, nonproductive cough;* dyspnea.
**Skin:** rash.
**Other:** *angioedema.*

## Overdose and treatment

The most likely clinical sign is hypotension.

After acute ingestion, recommend emptying stomach by induced emesis or gastric lavage and following with activated charcoal to reduce absorption. Hemodialysis should be considered in severe cases. Subsequent treatment is usually symptomatic and supportive.

## Clinical considerations

■ Diuretic therapy should be discontinued 2 to 3 days before enalapril therapy is begun to reduce risk of hypotension; if drug doesn't adequately control blood pressure, diuretics should be reinstated.
■ Drug should be given without regard to meals; food doesn't appear to affect absorption.

### Therapeutic monitoring

■ WBC and differential counts should be checked before treatment, every 2 weeks for 3 months, and periodically thereafter.
■ Proteinuria and nephrotic syndrome may occur in patients on enalapril therapy.
■ Systolic blood pressure should be followed as primary clinical endpoint.

### Special populations

**Pregnant patients.** Neonatal and fetal death may occur when drug is given during second and third trimesters.
**Breast-feeding patients.** It's unknown if drug appears in breast milk; an alternative feeding method is recommended during therapy.
**Pediatric patients.** Safety and efficacy of enalapril in children haven't been established; drug should be used only if potential benefit outweighs risk.
**Geriatric patients.** Geriatric patients may need lower doses because of impaired drug clearance.

## Patient counseling

■ Tell patient to report light-headedness, especially during first few days, so dosage can be adjusted; signs of infection, such as sore throat and fever, because drug may decrease WBC count; facial swelling or difficulty breathing, because drug may cause angioedema; and loss of taste, which may necessitate discontinuing drug.
■ Advise patient not to change position suddenly to minimize orthostatic hypotension.
■ Warn patient to seek medical approval before taking OTC cold preparations, particularly cough medications.

# enoxaparin sodium
Lovenox

*Pharmacologic classification:*
low–molecular-weight heparin
*Therapeutic classification:* anticoagulant
*Pregnancy risk category B*

## Available forms
Available by prescription only
*Ampules, syringes (prefilled), and EasyInjector devices:* 30 mg/0.3 ml, 40 mg/0.4 ml, 60 mg/0.6 ml, 80 mg/0.8 ml, 100 mg/1 ml

## Indications and dosages
*Prevention of deep vein thrombosis (DVT), which may lead to pulmonary embolism, after hip or knee replacement surgery*
Adults: 30 mg S.C. q 12 hours for 7 to 10 days. Give initial dose between 12 and 24 hours postoperatively, provided hemostasis has been established. Or, in patients undergoing hip replacement surgery, 40 mg once daily.
*Prevention of DVT, which may lead to pulmonary embolism, after abdominal surgery*
Adults: 40 mg S.C. once daily for 7 to 10 days. Give initial dose 2 hours before surgery.
*Prevention of ischemic complications of unstable angina and non–Q-wave MI, when concurrently given with aspirin*
Adults: 1 mg/kg S.C. q 12 hours for 2 to 8 days in conjunction with oral aspirin therapy (75 to 325 mg once daily).
    Note: To minimize risk of bleeding following vascular instrumentation during the treatment of unstable angina, adhere precisely to the intervals recommended between enoxaparin doses.
*Inpatient treatment of acute DVT with and without pulmonary embolism when given in conjunction with warfarin sodium*
Adults: 1 mg/kg S.C. every 12 hours; alternatively, 1.5 mg/kg S.C. once daily (at the same time every day) for 5 to 7 days until therapeutic oral anticoagulant effect (INR 2 to 3) has been achieved. Warfarin sodium therapy is usually started within 72 hours of enoxaparin injection.
*Outpatient treatment of acute DVT without pulmonary embolism when given in conjunction with warfarin sodium*
Adults: 1 mg/kg S.C. every 12 hours for 5 to 7 days until therapeutic oral anticoagulant effect (INR 2 to 3) has been achieved. Warfarin sodium therapy is usually initiated within 72 hours of enoxaparin injection.
*Acutely ill patients who are at risk of embolism from decreased mobility*
Adults: 40 mg S.C. once daily for 6 to 11 days. Up to 14 days has been well tolerated.

## Mechanism of action
*Anticoagulant action:* Enoxaparin is a low–molecular-weight heparin that accelerates formation of antithrombin III-thrombin complex and deactivates thrombin, preventing conversion of fibrinogen to fibrin. It has a higher anti-factor Xa to anti-factor IIa activity than unfractionated heparin.

## Pharmacokinetics
*Absorption:* Bioavailability is 92%.
*Distribution:* Volume of distribution of anti-factor Xa activity is about 6 L.
*Metabolism:* Information not available.
*Excretion:* Elimination half-life based on anti-factor Xa activity is about 4½ hours after S.C. administration.

| Route | Onset | Peak | Duration |
|-------|-------|------|----------|
| S.C. | Unknown | 3-5 hr | 24 hr |

## Contraindications and precautions
Contraindicated in patients hypersensitive to drug or heparin or pork products; in patients with active, major bleeding or thrombocytopenia; and in those who have antiplatelet antibodies in the presence of drug.
    Use with extreme caution in patients with history of heparin-induced thrombocytopenia. Use cautiously in patients with conditions that put them at increased risk for hemorrhage, such as bacterial endocarditis; congenital or acquired bleeding disorders; ulcer disease; angiodysplastic GI disease; hemorrhagic CVA; or recent spinal, eye, or brain surgery; or in those treated concomitantly with NSAIDs, platelet inhibitors, or other anticoagulants that affect hemostasis.
    Use with extreme caution in patients with postoperative indwelling epidural catheters. Cases of epidural or spinal hematomas have been reported with the use of enoxaparin and spinal or epidural anesthesia or spinal puncture, resulting in long-term or permanent paralysis.
    Also use cautiously in patients with a bleeding diathesis, uncontrolled arterial hypertension, or history of recent GI ulceration, diabetic retinopathy, and hemorrhage.
    Use with care in geriatric patients and patients with renal insufficiency who may show delayed elimination of enoxaparin.

## Interactions
**Drug-drug.** *Other anticoagulants, antiplatelet drugs, and NSAIDs:* Increased risk of bleeding. May also lead to spinal or epidural hematomas in patients with spinal punctures or epidural or spinal anesthesia. Advise clinician to monitor patient for signs and symptoms of bleeding.
*Plicamycin and valproic acid:* May cause hypoprothrombinemia and inhibit platelet ag-

gregation. Advise clinician to monitor patient closely.

## Adverse reactions

**CNS:** confusion, *neurologic injury* when used with spinal or epidural puncture.
**CV:** edema, peripheral edema, CV toxicity (chest pain, dizziness, irregular heartbeat).
**GI:** nausea.
**Hematologic:** hypochromic anemia, *thrombocytopenia, hemorrhage,* ecchymoses, bleeding complications.
**Hepatic:** elevated liver enzyme levels.
**Skin:** *rash, hives,* irritation, pain, hematoma, erythema (at injection site).
**Other:** fever, pain, *angioedema.*

## Overdose and treatment

Accidental overdose after drug administration may lead to hemorrhagic complications. This may be largely neutralized by the slow I.V. injection of protamine sulfate (1%) solution. The dose of protamine sulfate should be equal to the dose of enoxaparin injection (1 mg of protamine neutralizes 1 mg of enoxaparin).

## Clinical considerations

**◨ ALERT** Drug can't be used interchangeably (unit for unit) with unfractionated heparin or other low–molecular-weight heparins.
■ Enoxaparin isn't intended for I.M. administration.
■ Drug shouldn't be mixed with other injections or infusions.
■ All patients should be screened before prophylactic administration of enoxaparin to rule out a bleeding disorder.
**◨ ALERT** Air bubble shouldn't be expelled from syringe before injection because some of the drug may be lost.

### Therapeutic monitoring

■ Advise clinician to monitor patient for adverse reactions, including angioedema.

### Special populations

**Breast-feeding patients.** It isn't known if drug appears in breast milk. Drug should be used cautiously when given to breast-feeding women.
**Pediatric patients.** Safety and efficacy of enoxaparin in children haven't been established.

## Patient counseling

■ Explain risk of adverse reactions.
■ Instruct patient to watch for signs of bleeding.
■ Caution patient against use of aspirin or other salicylates.

# entacapone
Comtan

*Pharmacologic classification:* catechol-O-methyltransferase (COMT) inhibitor
*Therapeutic classification:* antiparkinsonian
*Pregnancy risk category C*

## Available forms

Available by prescription only
*Tablets:* 200 mg

## Indications and dosages

***Adjunct to levodopa and carbidopa for treatment of idiopathic Parkinson's disease in patients with signs and symptoms of end-of-dose wearing off***
*Adults:* 200 mg P.O. with each dose of levodopa and carbidopa to maximum of eight times daily. Maximum recommended daily dose of entacapone is 1,600 mg/day. Reducing daily levodopa dose or extending the interval between doses may be needed to optimize patient's response.

## Mechanism of action

*Antiparkinsonian action:* A reversible inhibitor of peripheral COMT, which is responsible for elimination of various catecholamines, including dopamine. Blocking this pathway when giving levodopa and carbidopa should increase serum levodopa levels, thereby allowing greater dopaminergic stimulation in the CNS and a greater effect in treating parkinsonian symptoms.

## Pharmacokinetics

*Absorption:* Rapid, with serum levels peaking in about 1 hour. Food doesn't affect absorption.
*Distribution:* About 98% protein-bound, mainly to albumin; isn't distributed widely into tissues. Duration is about 6 hours.
*Metabolism:* Almost completely metabolized by glucuronidation before elimination. No active metabolites identified.
*Excretion:* About 10% excreted in urine; remainder excreted in bile and feces. Biphasic half-life: 0.4 to 0.7 hour for first phase; 2.4 hours for second phase.

| Route | Onset | Peak | Duration |
|-------|-------|------|----------|
| P.O. | 1 hr | 1 hr | 6 hr |

## Contraindications and precautions

Contraindicated in patients hypersensitive to drug.
    Use cautiously in patients with hepatic impairment, biliary obstruction, or orthostatic hypotension.

## Interactions
**Drug-drug.** *Ampicillin, chloramphenicol, cholestyramine, erythromycin, probenecid:* May block biliary excretion, resulting in higher serum levels of entacapone. Use cautiously.
*CNS depressants:* Additive effect. Use together cautiously.
*Drugs metabolized by COMT (bitolterol, dobutamine, dopamine, epinephrine, isoetharine, isoproterenol, norepinephrine):* May cause higher serum levels of these drugs, resulting in increased heart rate, changes in blood pressure, or, possibly, arrhythmias. Advise clinician to monitor vital signs and cardiac rhythm.
*Nonselective MAO inhibitors (such as phenelzine, tranylcypromine):* May inhibit normal catecholamine metabolism. Avoid use together.
**Drug-lifestyle.** *Alcohol use:* May cause additive CNS effects. Advise patient to avoid alcohol.

## Adverse reactions
**CNS:** *dyskinesia, hyperkinesia,* hypokinesia, dizziness, anxiety, somnolence, agitation, fatigue, asthenia, hallucinations.
**GI:** *nausea, diarrhea,* abdominal pain, constipation, vomiting, dry mouth, dyspepsia, flatulence, gastritis, taste perversion.
**GU:** *urine discoloration.*
**Hematologic:** purpura.
**Musculoskeletal:** back pain.
**Respiratory:** dyspnea.
**Skin:** sweating.
**Other:** bacterial infection.

## Overdose and treatment
Management of overdose is symptomatic; hemodialysis isn't effective because of high protein-binding. In acute stages of overdose, gastric lavage or activated charcoal may be helpful to limit GI absorption.

## Clinical considerations
■ Drug should be used only with levodopa and carbidopa; no antiparkinsonian effects will occur when drug is given as monotherapy.
■ Levodopa and carbidopa dosage requirements are usually lower when given with entacapone; the levodopa and carbidopa dose should be lowered or dosing interval increased to avoid adverse effects.
■ Drug may cause or worsen dyskinesia despite reduction of levodopa dose.
■ Hallucinations may occur or worsen when taking this drug.
■ Diarrhea most commonly begins within 4 to 12 weeks, but may begin as early as the first week or as late as many months after starting treatment.
■ Drug may discolor urine.
■ Rarely, rhabdomyolysis has occurred with drug use.
**⊌ ALERT** Rapid withdrawal or abrupt reduction in drug dose could lead to signs and symp-

toms of Parkinson's disease; it may also lead to hyperpyrexia and confusion, a symptom complex resembling neuroleptic malignant syndrome. Recommend stopping drug slowly and monitoring patient closely. Other dopaminergic treatment may need to be adjusted.
■ Drug can be given with immediate or sustained-release levodopa and carbidopa and can be taken with or without food.

### Therapeutic monitoring
■ Advise clinician to monitor blood pressure closely and observe for orthostatic hypotension.
■ Advise clinician to monitor patient for adverse effects.

### Special populations
**Breast-feeding patients.** It isn't known if drug appears in breast milk. Because many drugs do, it should be used cautiously when given to breast-feeding women.

### Patient counseling
■ Instruct patient not to crush or break tablet and to take it at the same time as levodopa and carbidopa.
■ Warn patient to avoid potentially hazardous activities, such as driving or operating heavy machinery, until CNS effects of drug are known.
■ Advise patient to avoid alcohol during treatment.
■ Instruct patient to be careful when standing after prolonged period of sitting or lying down because dizziness may occur. This effect is more common during initial therapy.
■ Warn patient that hallucinations, increased dyskinesia, nausea, and diarrhea may occur.
■ Inform patient that drug may cause urine to turn brownish orange.
■ Advise patient to report if she is pregnant or breast-feeding or if she plans to become pregnant.

# ephedrine
# ephedrine hydrochloride
# ephedrine sulfate
Pretz-D

*Pharmacologic classification:* adrenergic
*Therapeutic classification:* bronchodilator, vasopressor (parenteral form), nasal decongestant
*Pregnancy risk category C*

## Available forms
Available with and without a prescription
*Capsules:* 25 mg, 50 mg
*Nasal spray:* 0.25%
*Injection:* 25 mg/ml, 50 mg/ml

## Indications and dosages

*To correct hypotensive states*
*Adults:* 25 to 50 mg I.M. or S.C., or 10 to 25 mg via slow I.V. bolus. If needed, a second I.M. dose of 50 mg or I.V. dose of 25 mg may be given. Additional I.V. doses may be given in 5 to 10 minutes. Maximum dose is 150 mg daily.
*Children:* 3 mg/kg or 100 mg/m² S.C. or I.V. daily, divided into four to six doses.
*Orthostatic hypotension*
*Adults:* 25 mg P.O. once daily to q.i.d.
*Children:* 3 mg/kg P.O. daily, divided into four to six doses.
*Bronchodilator or nasal decongestant*
*Adults and children over age 12:* 12.5 to 50 mg P.O. q 3 to 4 hours, p.r.n., not to exceed 150 mg in 24 hours. As nasal decongestant: 2 to 3 sprays in each nostril not more often than q 4 hours.
*Children ages 6 to 12:* 6.25 to 12.5 mg P.O. q 4 hours, not to exceed 75 mg in 24 hours. As nasal decongestant: 1 to 2 sprays in each nostril, not more often than q 4 hours.
*Children ages 2 and older:* 2 to 3 mg/kg or 100 mg/m² P.O. daily in four to six divided doses.
*Severe, acute bronchospasm*
*Adults:* 12.5 to 25 mg I.M., S.C., or I.V.
*Enuresis*
*Adults:* 25 to 50 mg P.O. h.s.
*Myasthenia gravis*
*Adults:* 25 mg P.O. t.i.d. or q.i.d.

## I.V. administration
■ Ephedrine should be given slowly by direct I.V. injection. Additional I.V. doses may be given after 5 to 10 minutes.

## Incompatibilities
Incompatible with fructose; hydrocortisone sodium succinate; Ionosol B, D-CM, and D solutions; meperidine; pentobarbital sodium; phenobarbital sodium; secobarbital; and thiopental.

## Mechanism of action
*Bronchodilator action:* Ephedrine relaxes bronchial smooth muscle by stimulating beta₂-adrenergic receptors, resulting in increased vital capacity, relief of mild bronchospasm, improved air exchange, and decreased residual volume.
*Direct- and indirect-acting sympathomimetic action:* Ephedrine stimulates both alpha- and beta-adrenergic receptors. Release of norepinephrine from its storage sites is one of its indirect effects. In therapeutic doses, ephedrine relaxes bronchial smooth muscle and produces cardiac stimulation with increased systolic and diastolic blood pressure when norepinephrine stores aren't depleted.
*Nasal decongestant action:* Ephedrine stimulates alpha-adrenergic receptors in blood vessels of nasal mucosa, producing vasoconstriction and nasal decongestion.
*Vasopressor action:* Drug produces positive inotropic effects with low doses by action on beta₁-receptors in the heart. Vasodilation results from its effect on beta₂-adrenergic receptors; vasoconstriction results from its alpha-adrenergic effects. Pressor effects may result from vasoconstriction or cardiac stimulation; however, when peripheral vascular resistance is decreased, increased cardiac output causes blood pressure elevation.

## Pharmacokinetics
*Absorption:* Rapidly and completely absorbed after oral, S.C., or I.M. administration.
*Distribution:* Widely distributed throughout the body.
*Metabolism:* Slowly metabolized in the liver by oxidative deamination, demethylation, aromatic hydroxylation, and conjugation.
*Excretion:* Dose is mostly excreted unchanged in urine; rate of excretion depends on urine pH.

| Route | Onset | Peak | Duration |
|---|---|---|---|
| P.O. | 15-60 min | Unknown | 3-5 hr |
| I.V. | 5 min | Unknown | 1 hr |
| I.M., S.C. | 10-20 min | Unknown | ½-1 hr |
| Nasal spray | Unknown | Unknown | Unknown |

## Contraindications and precautions
Contraindicated in patients hypersensitive to drug and other sympathomimetics; in those with porphyria, severe coronary artery disease, arrhythmias, angle-closure glaucoma, psychoneurosis, angina pectoris, substantial organic heart disease, CV disease; and in those taking MAO inhibitors.
Nasal solution is contraindicated in patients with angle-closure glaucoma, psychoneurosis, angina pectoris, substantial organic heart disease, CV disease, and hypersensitivity to drug or other sympathomimetics.
Use with extreme caution in geriatric men and in those with hypertension, hyperthyroidism, nervous or excitable states, diabetes, and prostatic hyperplasia. Use nasal solution cautiously in patients with hyperthyroidism, hypertension, diabetes mellitus, or prostatic hyperplasia.
Use with ephedrine alkaloid–containing dietary supplements has been linked to serious nervous system and CV system adverse effects and death.

## Interactions
**Drug-drug.** *Acetazolamide:* May increase serum ephedrine levels. Advise clinician to monitor patient for toxicity.
*Alpha adrenergic blockers:* Unopposed beta-adrenergic effects, resulting in hypotension. Avoid use together.

---

*Antihypertensives:* Decreased effects of antihypertensives. Blood pressure must be monitored.

*Atropine:* Blocks reflex bradycardia and enhances pressor effects. Advise clinician to monitor patient carefully.

*Beta blockers:* Unopposed alpha-adrenergic effects, resulting in hypertension. Blood pressure must be monitored.

*Diuretics, methyldopa, reserpine:* Decreased pressor effects of ephedrine. Advise clinician to monitor patient carefully.

*Ergot alkaloids:* May enhance vasoconstrictor activity. Advise clinician to monitor patient cautiously.

*General anesthetics (especially cyclopropane, halothane) and cardiac glycosides:* May sensitize myocardium to effects of ephedrine, causing arrhythmias. Advise clinician to monitor patient closely.

*Guanadrel, guanethidine:* Enhanced pressor effects of ephedrine. Advise clinician to monitor patient and blood pressure closely.

*Levodopa:* Enhanced risk of ventricular arrhythmias. Advise clinician to monitor patient closely.

*MAO inhibitors and tricyclic antidepressants:* Enhanced pressor effects; may cause hypertensive crisis. Allow 14 days to lapse after withdrawal of MAO inhibitor before using ephedrine.

*Sympathomimetics:* Increased effects and toxicity. Avoid use together.

*Theophylline:* Causes more adverse reactions than either drug used alone. Use together cautiously.

## Adverse reactions

**CNS:** *insomnia, nervousness,* dizziness, headache, euphoria, confusion, delirium; nervousness, excitation (with nasal solution).

**CV:** *palpitations,* tachycardia, hypertension, precordial pain; *tachycardia* (with nasal solution), **arrhythmias**.

**EENT:** dry nose and throat; rebound nasal congestion with long-term or excessive use, mucosal irritation (with nasal solution).

**GI:** nausea, vomiting, anorexia.

**GU:** urine retention, painful urination caused by visceral sphincter spasm.

**Musculoskeletal:** muscle weakness.

**Skin:** diaphoresis.

## Overdose and treatment

Signs and symptoms of overdose include exaggeration of common adverse reactions, especially arrhythmias, extreme tremor or seizures, nausea and vomiting, fever, and CNS and respiratory depression.

Treatment requires supportive and symptomatic measures. If patient is conscious, recommend inducing emesis with ipecac followed by activated charcoal. If patient is depressed or hyperactive, recommend performing gastric lavage. Recommend maintaining airway and blood pressure. Vasopressors shouldn't be given. Advise clinician to monitor vital signs closely.

A beta blocker (such as propranolol) may be used to treat arrhythmias. A cardioselective beta blocker is recommended in asthmatic patients. Phentolamine may be used for hypertension, paraldehyde or diazepam for seizures, and dexamethasone for pyrexia.

## Clinical considerations

■ Consider the recommendations relevant to all adrenergics. As a pressor agent, ephedrine isn't a substitute for blood, plasma, fluids, or electrolytes. Fluid volume depletion should be corrected before administration.

### Therapeutic monitoring

■ Tolerance may develop after prolonged or excessive use; increased dosage may be needed. Also, if drug is discontinued for a few days and readministered, effectiveness may be restored.

■ With parenteral dosing, recommend monitoring vital signs closely during infusion. Tachycardia is common.

### Special populations

**Pregnant patients.** It isn't known if drug is safe for use during pregnancy. Drug should be used during pregnancy only when clearly indicated.

**Breast-feeding patients.** Use should be avoided in breast-feeding women.

**Pediatric patients.** Give drug cautiously.

**Geriatric patients.** Drug should be given cautiously because geriatric patients may be more sensitive to effects of the drug. Lower doses may be recommended.

## Patient counseling

■ Instruct patient to clear nose before instilling nasal solutions.

■ Tell patient using OTC product to follow directions on label, to take last dose a few hours before bedtime to reduce possibility of insomnia, to take only as directed, and not to increase dosage or frequency.

■ Advise patient to store drug away from heat and light (not in bathroom medicine cabinet) and to keep out of reach of children.

■ Instruct patient who misses a dose to take it as soon as remembered if within 1 hour. If beyond 1 hour, patient should skip dose and return to regular schedule.

■ Teach patient to be aware of palpitations and significant pulse rate changes.

# epinephrine
Bronkaid Mist, Bronkaid Mistometer*,
EpiPen, EpiPen Jr., Primatene Mist,
Sus-Phrine

# epinephrine bitartrate
AsthmaHaler

# epinephrine hydrochloride
Adrenalin Chloride, AsthmaNefrin,
Epifrin, Glaucon, microNefrin,
Vaponefrin

# epinephryl borate
Epinal

*Pharmacologic classification:* adrenergic
*Therapeutic classification:* bronchodilator, vasopressor, cardiac stimulant,
local anesthetic (adjunct), topical anti-
hemorrhagic, antiglaucoma
*Pregnancy risk category C*

## Available forms
Available by prescription only
*Injection:* 0.01 mg/ml (1:100,000), 0.1 mg/ml
(1:10,000), 0.5 mg/ml (1:2,000), 1 mg/ml
(1:1,000) parenteral; 5 mg/ml (1:200) parenteral
suspension
*Ophthalmic:* 0.1%, 0.25%, 0.5%, 1%, 2% so-
lution
Available without a prescription
*Nebulizer inhaler:* 1% (1:100), 1.25%, 2.25%
*Aerosol inhaler:* 160 mcg, 200 mcg, 250 mcg/
metered spray
*Nasal solution:* 0.1%

## Indications and dosages
*Bronchospasm, hypersensitivity reactions,
anaphylaxis*
*Adults:* Initially, 0.1 to 0.5 mg (0.1 to 0.5 ml
of a 1:1,000 solution) S.C. or I.M.; may be repeated at 5- to 15-minute intervals, p.r.n. for
patients with anaphylactic shock. In patients
with asthma, S.C. doses may be given at 20-
minute to 4-hour intervals depending on the
severity and the response of the patient. Alternatively, 0.1 to 0.25 mg (1 to 2.5 ml of a
1:10,000 solution) I.V. slowly over 5 to 10 minutes. May be repeated q 5 to 15 minutes if needed or followed by a 1- to 4-mcg/minute I.V. infusion.
*Children:* 0.01 mg/kg (0.01 ml/kg of a 1:1,000
solution) or 0.3 mg/m² (0.3 ml/ m² of a 1:1,000
solution) S.C. Dose not to exceed 0.5 mg. May
be repeated at 20-minute to 4-hour intervals,
p.r.n. Alternatively, 0.1 mg (10 ml of a 1:100,000
dilution) I.V. slowly over 5 to 10 minutes followed by a 0.1- to 1.5-mcg/kg/minute I.V. infusion.

*Bronchodilator*
*Adults and children:* 1 inhalation via metered
aerosol, repeated once if needed after 1 minute;
subsequent doses shouldn't be repeated for at
least 3 hours. Alternatively, 1 to 3 deep inhalations via hand-bulb nebulizer of a 1%
(1:100) solution; should not be repeated more
often than every 3 hours.
*Cardiopulmonary resuscitation and car-
diac arrhythmias*
*Adults:* Initially, 0.5 to 1 mg (range, 0.1 to
1 mg), usually as 1 to 10 ml of a 1:10,000 solution) I.V. bolus; may be repeated q 3 to 5
minutes, p.r.n. Alternatively, initial dose followed by 0.3 mg S.C. or 1 to 4 mcg/minute
I.V. infusion. Doses administered by the endotracheal route should be 2 to 2.5 times those
administered I.V. and should be diluted in 10 ml
of normal saline solution or sterile water. Intracardiac doses of 0.1 to 1 mg (1 to 10 ml of
a 1:10,000 solution) have been recommended.
For symptomatic bradycardia in patients who
are not in cardiac arrest, the drug may be given
by I.V. infusion at an initial rate of 1 mcg/min,
and may be increased to 2 to 10 mcg/min.
*Children:* Initially, 0.01 mg/kg (0.1 ml/kg of a
1:10,000 solution) I.V. bolus or intraosseous,
or 0.1 mg/kg (0.1 ml/kg of a 1:1,000 injection)
endotracheally; subsequent doses by these
routes range from 0.1 to 0.2 mg/kg (0.1 to
0.2 ml/kg of a 1:1,000 solution) q 3 to 5 min.
   Alternatively, initially, 0.1 mcg/kg/minute;
may increase in increments of 0.1 mcg/kg/
minute to a maximum of 1 mcg/kg/minute. Alternatively, 0.005 to 0.01 mg/kg (0.05 to
0.1 ml/kg of a 1:10,000 solution) by intracardiac injection.
*Infants:* Initially, 0.01 to 0.03 mg/kg (0.1 to
0.3 ml/kg of a 1:10,000 solution) I.V. bolus or
by intratracheal injection. May be repeated q
3 to 5 minutes, p.r.n.
*Hemostatic use*
*Adults:* 1:50,000 to 1:1,000, applied topically.
*To prolong local anesthetic effect*
*Adults and children:* 1:500,000 to 1:50,000
mixed with local anesthetic.
*Open-angle glaucoma*
*Adults:* 1 or 2 drops of 1% to 2% solution instilled daily or b.i.d.
*Nasal congestion, local superficial bleed-
ing*
*Adults and children:* 0.1% solution applied topically as 1 or 2 drops or sprays to mucosa, as
required.

## I.V. administration
■ In emergency situations, epinephrine may
be injected very slowly as a dilute injection or
infused slowly I.V.
■ If given via a peripheral vein, it is recommended that each dose be followed by a 20-ml
flush of I.V. fluid, and the limb should be elevated for 10 to 20 seconds.

■ When possible, I.V. epinephrine should be infused via central venous access to reduce the risk of extravasation and ensure good bioavailability.

■ Infusion solutions containing 2 or 4 mg/ml may be prepared by adding 1 mg of drug to 250 or 500 ml of compatible I.V. solution, such as normal saline solution.

## Incompatibilities

Rapidly destroyed by alkalies or oxidizing drugs, including halogens, nitrates, nitrites permanganates, sodium bicarbonate, and salts of easily reducible metals, such as iron, copper, and zinc. Incompatible with aminophylline; ampicillin sodium; cephapirin; furosemide; hyaluronidase; Ionosol D-CM, Ionosol PSL, and Ionosol T with dextrose 5%; and mephentermine.

## Mechanism of action

Epinephrine acts directly by stimulating alpha- and beta-adrenergic receptors in the sympathetic nervous system. Its main therapeutic effects include relaxation of bronchial smooth muscle, cardiac stimulation, and dilation of skeletal muscle vasculature.

*Antiglaucoma action:* Epinephrine's exact mechanism of lowering intraocular pressure is unknown. When applied topically to the conjunctiva or injected into the interior chamber of the eye, epinephrine constricts conjunctival blood vessels, contracts the dilator muscle of the pupil, and may dilate the pupil.

*Bronchodilator action:* Epinephrine relaxes bronchial smooth muscle by stimulating beta$_2$-adrenergic receptors. Epinephrine constricts bronchial arterioles by stimulating alpha-adrenergic receptors, resulting in relief of bronchospasm, reduced congestion and edema, and increased tidal volume and vital capacity. By inhibiting histamine release, it may reverse bronchiolar constriction, vasodilation, and edema.

*CV and vasopressor actions:* As a cardiac stimulant, epinephrine produces positive chronotropic and inotropic effects by action on beta$_1$ receptors in the heart, increasing cardiac output, myocardial oxygen consumption, and force of contraction and decreasing cardiac efficiency. Vasodilation results from its effect on beta$_2$ receptors; vasoconstriction results from alpha-adrenergic effects.

*Local anesthetic (adjunct) action:* Epinephrine acts on alpha receptors in skin, mucous membranes, and viscera; it produces vasoconstriction, which reduces absorption of local anesthetic, thus prolonging its duration of action, localizing anesthesia, and decreasing risk of anesthetic's toxicity.

*Local vasoconstrictive action:* Epinephrine's effect results from action on alpha receptors in skin, mucous membranes, and viscera, which produces vasoconstriction and hemostasis in small vessels.

## Pharmacokinetics

*Absorption:* Well absorbed after S.C. or I.M. injection; epinephrine has a rapid onset of action and a short duration of action.

*Distribution:* Distributed widely throughout the body.

*Metabolism:* Metabolized at sympathetic nerve endings, liver, and other tissues to inactive metabolites.

*Excretion:* Excreted in urine, mainly as its metabolites and conjugates.

| Route | Onset | Peak | Duration |
|-------|-------|------|----------|
| I.V. | Immediate | 5 min | Short |
| I.M. | Variable | Unknown | 1-4 hr |
| S.C. | 5-15 min | ½ hr | 1-4 hr |
| Inhalation | 1-5 min | Unknown | 1-3 hr |

## Contraindications and precautions

Contraindicated in patients with angle-closure glaucoma, shock (other than anaphylactic shock), organic brain damage, cardiac dilation, arrhythmias, coronary insufficiency, or cerebral arteriosclerosis. Also contraindicated in patients during general anesthesia with halogenated hydrocarbons or cyclopropane and in patients in labor (may delay second stage).

Some commercial products contain sulfites; contraindicated in patients with sulfite allergies except when epinephrine is being used for treatment of serious allergic reactions or other emergencies.

In conjunction with local anesthetics, epinephrine is contraindicated for use on fingers, toes, ears, nose, and genitalia.

Ophthalmic preparation is contraindicated in patients with angle-closure glaucoma or when nature of the glaucoma hasn't been established and in patients with hypersensitivity to the drug, organic mental syndrome, or cardiac dilation and coronary insufficiency. Nasal solution is contraindicated in patients hypersensitive to drug.

Use with extreme caution in patients with longstanding bronchial asthma and emphysema in whom degenerative heart disease has developed. Also use cautiously in geriatric patients and in those with hyperthyroidism, CV disease, hypertension, psychoneurosis, and diabetes.

Use ophthalmic preparation cautiously in geriatric patients and in patients with diabetes, hypertension, Parkinson's disease, hyperthyroidism, aphakia (eye without lens), cardiac disease, cerebral arteriosclerosis, or bronchial asthma.

## Interactions

**Drug-drug.** *Alpha adrenergic blockers:* Antagonize vasoconstriction and hypertension. Avoid use together.

*Antidiabetics:* May decrease blood sugar effects. Dosage adjustments may be needed.

*Beta blockers such as propranolol:* Antagonize cardiac and bronchodilating effects of epinephrine. Advise clinician to monitor patient carefully.

*Doxapram, mazindol, and methylphenidate:* May enhance CNS stimulation or pressor effects. Advise clinician to monitor patient closely.

*General anesthetics (especially cyclopropane and halothane) and cardiac glycosides:* May sensitize the myocardium to effects of epinephrine, causing arrhythmias. Patient requires ECG monitoring.

*Guanadrel and guanethidine:* Decreased hypotensive effects while potentiating effects of epinephrine, resulting in hypertension and arrhythmias. Patient and blood pressure require close monitoring.

*Levodopa:* Enhances risk of cardiac arrhythmias. Advise clinician to monitor patient carefully.

*MAO inhibitors:* Increased risk of hypertensive crisis. Advise clinician to monitor blood pressure closely.

*Miotics:* Reduce the ciliary spasm, mydriasis, blurred vision, and increased intraocular pressure that may occur with miotics or epinephrine alone. May be used for this reason concomitantly.

*Other sympathomimetics:* Additive effects and toxicity. Avoid use together.

*Oxytocics or ergot alkaloids:* May cause severe hypertension. Avoid use together.

*Phenothiazines:* Reversal of pressor effects. Avoid use together.

*Topical miotics, topical beta blockers, osmotic drugs, and carbonic anhydrase inhibitors:* May cause additive lowering of intraocular pressure. Avoid use together.

*Tricyclic antidepressants, antihistamines, and thyroid hormones:* May potentiate adverse cardiac effects of epinephrine. Avoid use together.

## Adverse reactions

**CNS:** *CVA, nervousness, tremor,* vertigo, *headache,* disorientation, agitation, *drowsiness,* fear, pallor, dizziness, weakness, *cerebral hemorrhage.* In patients with Parkinson's disease, drug increases rigidity, tremor; brow ache, headache, light-headedness (with ophthalmic preparation); nervousness, excitation (with nasal solution).

**CV:** *palpitations;* widened pulse pressure; *hypertension; tachycardia; ventricular fibrillation; shock;* anginal pain; ECG changes, including a decreased T-wave amplitude; palpitations, tachycardia, *arrhythmias,* hyperten-

sion (with ophthalmic preparation); *tachycardia* (with nasal solution).

**EENT:** corneal or conjunctival pigmentation or corneal edema in long-term use; follicular hypertrophy; chemosis; conjunctivitis; iritis; hyperemic conjunctiva; maculopapular rash; eye pain; allergic lid reaction; ocular irritation; eye stinging, burning, and tearing on instillation (with ophthalmic preparation); rebound nasal congestion; slight sting upon application (with nasal solution).

**GI:** *nausea, vomiting.*

**GU:** increased BUN levels.

**Metabolic:** increased glucose and lactic acid levels.

**Respiratory:** dyspnea.

**Skin:** urticaria, pain, hemorrhage (at injection site).

## Overdose and treatment

Signs and symptoms of overdose may include a sharp increase in systolic and diastolic blood pressure, increase in venous pressure, severe anxiety, irregular heartbeat, severe nausea or vomiting, severe respiratory distress, unusually large pupils, unusual paleness and coldness of skin, pulmonary edema, renal failure, and metabolic acidosis.

Treatment includes symptomatic and supportive measures, because epinephrine is rapidly inactivated in the body. Advise clinician to monitor vital signs closely. Phentolamine may be needed for hypotension; beta blockers (such as propranolol) may be needed for arrhythmias.

## Clinical considerations

■ After S.C. or I.M. injection, massaging the site may hasten absorption.

■ For the treatment of reactions caused by drugs given S.C. or I.M., epinephrine may be given at the same site to reduce further absorption.

■ Epinephrine is destroyed by oxidizing agents, alkalis (including sodium bicarbonate), halogens, permanganates, chromates, nitrates, and salts of easily reducible metals such as iron, copper, and zinc.

■ Avoid I.M. injection into buttocks. Epinephrine-induced vasoconstriction favors growth of the anaerobe *Clostridium perfringens.*

■ Intracardiac administration requires external cardiac massage to move drug into coronary circulation.

■ Breathing treatment should start with first symptoms of bronchospasm. Patient should use the fewest number of inhalations that provide relief. To prevent excessive dosage, at least 1 or 2 minutes should elapse before additional inhalations of epinephrine are taken. Dosage requirements vary.

■ Ophthalmic preparation may cause mydriasis with blurred vision and sensitivity to light in some patients being treated for glaucoma.

---

* Canada only    ◇ Unlabeled clinical use

Drug is usually given at bedtime or after prescribed miotic to minimize these symptoms.
■ When separate solutions of epinephrine and a topical miotic are used, the miotic should be instilled 2 to 10 minutes before epinephrine.
■ Epinephrine interferes with tests for urinary catecholamines.

### Therapeutic monitoring
■ Blood pressure, pulse, respirations, and urine output must be monitored, and the patient observed closely. Epinephrine may widen pulse pressure. If arrhythmias occur, epinephrine should be stopped immediately. Recommend watching for changes in intake and output ratio.
■ Patients, especially geriatric patients, should have regular tonometer readings during continuous therapy.

### Special populations
**Pregnant patients.** Drug inhibits spontaneous or oxytocin-induced labor. With dose sufficient to reduce uterine contractions, drug may cause a prolonged period of uterine atony with hemorrhage. Drug should be used during pregnancy only if the potential benefits justify the possible risks to the fetus.
**Breast-feeding patients.** Drug appears in breast milk. Patient should avoid breast-feeding during therapy with epinephrine.
**Pediatric patients.** Safety and efficacy of ophthalmic epinephrine in children haven't been established. Use with caution.
**Geriatric patients.** Geriatric patients may be more sensitive to effects of epinephrine; lower doses are indicated.

### Patient counseling
■ Urge patient to report diminishing effect. Repeated or prolonged use of epinephrine can cause tolerance to effects of drug. Continuing to take epinephrine despite tolerance can be hazardous. Interrupting drug therapy for 12 hours to several days may restore responsiveness to drug.
**Inhalation therapy**
■ Instruct patient in correct use of inhaler.
■ Warn patient that overuse or too-frequent use can cause severe adverse reactions.
■ Tell patient to save applicator; refills may be available.
■ Advise patient to contact prescriber immediately if he receives no relief within 20 minutes or if condition worsens.
**Nasal therapy**
■ Tell patient to contact prescriber if symptoms aren't relieved in 20 minutes or if they become worse, and to report bronchial irritation, nervousness, or sleeplessness, which require dosage reduction.
■ Warn patient that intranasal applications may sting slightly and cause rebound congestion or drug-induced rhinitis after prolonged use. Nose

drops should be used for 3 or 4 days only. Encourage patient to use drug exactly as prescribed.
■ Tell patient to rinse nose dropper or spray tip with hot water after each use to avoid contaminating the solution.
■ Instruct patient to gently press finger against nasolacrimal duct for at least 1 or 2 minutes immediately after drug instillation to avoid excessive systemic absorption.
**Ophthalmic therapy**
■ To minimize systemic absorption, tell patient to press finger during and for 1 to 2 minutes after instillation of eyedrops.
■ To prevent contamination, tell patient not to touch applicator tip to any surface and to keep container tightly closed.
■ Tell patient not to use epinephrine solution if it's discolored or contains a precipitate.
■ Advise patient to remove soft contact lenses before instilling eyedrops to avoid staining or damaging them.
■ Tell patient to apply a missed dose as soon as possible. If it's close to time for next dose, the patient should wait and apply at regularly scheduled time.
■ Tell patient to store drug away from heat and light (not in bathroom medicine cabinet where heat and moisture can cause drug to deteriorate) and out of reach of children.

# epirubicin hydrochloride
Ellence

*Pharmacologic classification:* anthracycline
*Therapeutic classification:* antineoplastic
*Pregnancy risk category D*

### Available forms
Available by prescription only
*Injection:* 2 mg/ml

### Indications and dosages
*Adjuvant therapy in patients with evidence of axillary node tumor involvement after resection of primary breast cancer*
*Adults:* 100 to 120 mg/m$^2$ I.V. infusion over 3 to 5 minutes via a free-flowing I.V. solution on day 1 of each cycle q 3 to 4 weeks, or divided equally into two doses on days 1 and 8 of each cycle. Maximum cumulative (lifetime) dose is 900 mg/m$^2$.

   Dosage modification after the first cycle is based on toxicity. For patients experiencing platelet counts less than 50,000/mm$^3$, absolute neutrophil count (ANC) less than 250/mm$^3$, neutropenic fever, or grade 3 or 4 nonhematologic toxicity, reduce the day-1 dose in subsequent cycles to 75% of the day-1 dose given in the current cycle. Delay day-1 therapy in subsequent cycles until platelets are at least 100,000/mm³, ANC is at least 1,500/mm³, and nonhematologic toxicities recover to grade 1.

For patients receiving divided doses (days 1 and 8), the day-8 dose should be 75% of the day-1 dose if platelet counts are 75,000 to 100,000/mm³ and ANC is 1,000 to 1,499/mm³. If day-8 platelet counts are less than 75,000/mm³, ANC is less than 1,000/mm³, or grade 3 or 4 nonhematologic toxicity has occurred, the day-8 dose should be omitted.

≡ *Dosage adjustment.* In patients with bone marrow dysfunction (heavily pretreated patients, patients with bone marrow depression, or those with neoplastic bone marrow infiltration), start at lower doses of 75 to 90 mg/m². In hepatic dysfunction, if bilirubin is 1.2 to 3 mg/dl or AST is two to four times upper limit of normal, give one-half the recommended starting dose. If bilirubin is greater than 3 mg/dl or AST is greater than four times upper limit of normal, give one-fourth the recommended starting dose. Effects in patients with severe hepatic impairment haven't been evaluated, so epirubicin shouldn't be used in these patients. In patients with severe renal dysfunction (serum creatinine over 5 mg/dl), consider lower dosages.

## I.V. administration

■ Administer drug slowly into the tubing of a freely running I.V. infusion of normal saline solution or D₅W.
■ Veins over joints or in limbs with compromised venous or lymphatic drainage should be avoided.
■ The rate of injection should not be faster than over 3 to 5 minutes.
■ Facial flushing and local erythematous streaking along the vein may indicate the injection rate is too fast.
■ Epirubicin is extremely irritating to tissues; if there is any sign of extravasation, the infusion should be immediately stopped and restarted at another site.

### Incompatibilities
Don't mix drug with heparin or fluorouracil because precipitation may result. Don't mix in same syringe with other drugs.

## Mechanism of action
*Antineoplastic action:* The precise mechanisms of cytotoxic effects of epirubicin aren't completely known. Epirubicin is thought to form a complex with DNA by intercalation between nucleotide base pairs, thereby inhibiting DNA, RNA, and protein synthesis; DNA cleavage occurs, resulting in cytocidal activity. The drug may also generate cytotoxic free radicals, as well as interfere with replication and transcription of DNA.

## Pharmacokinetics
*Absorption:* Administered I.V.
*Distribution:* Rapidly and widely distributed into tissues. It binds to plasma proteins, predominantly albumin, and appears to concentrate in red blood cells.
*Metabolism:* Extensively and rapidly metabolized by the liver. Several metabolites form with little to no cytotoxic activity.
*Excretion:* Eliminated mostly by biliary excretion and, to a lesser extent, urinary excretion.

| Route | Onset | Peak | Duration |
|-------|-------|------|----------|
| I.V. | Unknown | Unknown | Unknown |

## Contraindications and precautions
Contraindicated in patients hypersensitive to this drug, other anthracyclines, or anthracenediones. Also contraindicated in patients with baseline neutrophil counts of less than 1,500 cells/mm³, in patients with severe myocardial insufficiency or recent MI, in patients whose previous treatment with anthracyclines has reached total cumulative doses, and in patients with severe hepatic dysfunction.

Use cautiously in patients with active or dormant cardiac disease, patients with prior or concomitant radiotherapy to the mediastinal and pericardial area, and previous therapy with other anthracyclines or anthracenediones or other cardiotoxic drugs.

## Interactions
**Drug-drug.** *Calcium channel blockers, other cardioactive compounds:* May increase risk of HF. Advise clinician to monitor cardiac function closely.
*Cimetidine:* Increased levels of epirubicin by 50%. Avoid use together.
*Cytotoxic drugs:* Additive toxicities (especially hematologic and GI) may occur. Recommend monitoring patient closely.
*Radiation therapy:* Effects may be enhanced. Advise clinician to monitor patient carefully.

## Adverse reactions
**CNS:** lethargy.
**CV:** cardiomyopathy, *HF, cardiotoxicity,* sinus tachycardia, ECG changes, *AV block, ventricular tachycardia.*
**EENT:** conjunctivitis, keratitis.
**GI:** nausea, vomiting, diarrhea, anorexia, mucositis.
**GU:** *amenorrhea.*
**Hematologic:** LEUKOPENIA, NEUTROPENIA, *febrile neutropenia,* anemia, THROMBOCYTOPENIA.
**Skin:** alopecia, rash, itch, skin changes, urticaria, photosensitivity.
**Other:** infection, fever, hot flashes, local toxicity, *anaphylaxis.*

---

## Overdose and treatment

Signs and symptoms of overdose are similar to known toxicities of drug.

Recommend providing supportive treatment p.r.n. until recovery of toxicities. Advise clinician to monitor patient for signs of HF, which may occur months after therapy, and provide supportive therapy as appropriate.

## Clinical considerations

- Drug shouldn't be given I.M. or S.C.
- Patients receiving 120 mg/m$^2$ of epirubicin should also receive prophylactic antibiotic therapy with co-trimoxazole or a fluoroquinolone.
- Use of antiemetics before epirubicin may be needed to reduce nausea and vomiting.
- Anthracycline-induced leukemia may occur.
- Administration of drug after previous radiation therapy may induce an inflammatory cell reaction at the site of irradiation.
- Epirubicin should be given under the supervision of a prescriber who is experienced in the use of cancer chemotherapy.
- Pregnant prescribers shouldn't handle this drug.
- Contraceptive methods should be used by both men and women.

### Therapeutic monitoring

- Advise clinician to monitor left ventricular ejection fraction (LVEF) regularly during therapy and stop drug at the first sign of impaired cardiac function. Early signs of cardiac toxicity may include sinus tachycardia, ECG abnormalities, tachyarrhythmias, bradycardia, AV block, and bundle branch block.
- Advise clinician to obtain baseline total bilirubin, AST, creatinine, and CBC including ANC, and evaluate cardiac function by measuring LVEF before therapy.
- Advise clinician to obtain total and differential WBC, RBC, and platelet counts before and during each cycle of therapy.
- WBC nadir is usually reached 10 to 14 days after drug administration, and returns to normal by day 21.
- Advise clinician to monitor serum uric acid, potassium, calcium phosphate, and creatinine immediately after initial chemotherapy administration in patients susceptible to tumor lysis syndrome. Hydration, urine alkalinization, and prophylaxis with allopurinol may prevent hyperuricemia and minimize potential complications of tumor lysis syndrome.
- Delayed cardiac toxicity may occur 2 to 3 months after completion of treatment and depends on the cumulative dose of epirubicin. Don't exceed a cumulative dose of 900 mg/m$^2$.

### Special populations

**Pregnant patients.** Inform patient of potential hazard to the fetus if used during pregnancy.
**Breast-feeding patients.** It isn't known if drug appears in breast milk. Because many drugs, including anthracyclines, appear in breast milk and because of the potential for serious adverse reactions in nursing infants from epirubicin, women should discontinue nursing before taking this drug.
**Pediatric patients.** Safety and efficacy haven't been established in pediatric patients. They may be at greater risk for anthracycline-induced cardiotoxicity and HF.
**Geriatric patients.** Plasma clearance is decreased in geriatric women. Advise clinician to monitor geriatric patient closely for toxicity, especially women older than age 70.

## Patient counseling

- Advise patient to report nausea, vomiting, stomatitis, dehydration, fever, evidence of infection, or symptoms of HF (such as tachycardia, dyspnea, edema).
- Inform patient of the risks of cardiac damage and treatment-related leukemia with use of drug.
- Advise all patients to use effective contraception during treatment.
- Advise women that irreversible amenorrhea or premature menopause may occur.
- Tell patient that hair regrowth usually occurs within 2 to 3 months after therapy is discontinued.

# epoetin alfa (erythropoietin)
Epogen, Procrit

*Pharmacologic classification:* glycoprotein
*Therapeutic classification:* antianemic
*Pregnancy risk category C*

## Available forms

Available by prescription only
*Injection:* 2,000 units, 3,000 units, 4,000 units, 10,000 units, 20,000 units, 40,000 units

## Indications and dosages

*Anemia associated with chronic renal failure*
*Adults:* Begin therapy at 50 to 100 units/kg I.V. or S.C. three times weekly. Patients receiving dialysis should receive drug I.V.; patients with chronic renal failure who aren't on dialysis may receive drug S.C. or I.V.

Reduce dosage when target hematocrit is reached or if hematocrit increases by more than 4 points within a 2-week period. Increase dosage if hematocrit doesn't increase by 5 to 6 points after 8 weeks of therapy and hematocrit is below target range. Maintenance dose is highly individualized.
*Anemia related to zidovudine therapy in patients infected with HIV*
*Adults:* Before therapy, determine endogenous serum epoetin alfa levels. Patients with levels

of 500 or more milliunits/ml are unlikely to respond to therapy.

Initial dosage for patients with levels of less than 500 milliunits/ml who are receiving 4,200 mg weekly or less of zidovudine is 100 units/kg I.V. or S.C. three times weekly for 8 weeks. If response is inadequate after 8 weeks, increase dosage by increments of 50 to 100 units/kg three times weekly and reevaluate response q 4 to 8 weeks. Individualize maintenance dose to maintain response, which may be influenced by zidovudine dose or infection or inflammation.

***Anemia secondary to cancer chemotherapy***
*Adults:* 150 units/kg S.C. three times weekly for 8 weeks or until target hemoglobin level is reached. If response isn't satisfactory after 8 weeks, increase dosage up to 300 units/kg S.C. three times weekly.

***Reduction of need for allogeneic blood transfusion in anemic patients scheduled to undergo elective, noncardiac, nonvascular surgery***
*Adults:* 300 units/kg/day S.C. daily for 10 days before surgery, on day of surgery, and for 4 days after surgery. Alternatively, 600 units/kg S.C. in once-weekly doses (21, 14, and 7 days before surgery), plus a fourth dose on day of surgery. Before treatment starts, establish that hemoglobin level is above 10 g/dl and less than or equal to 13 g/dl.

◇ ***Anemia from rheumatoid arthritis and rheumatic disease***
*Adults:* 50 to 200 units/kg three times weekly.

◇ ***Anemia of prematurity***
*Neonates:* 25 to 100 units/kg S.C. three times weekly.

## I.V. administration
- Don't shake before use.
- Recommend giving by direct I.V. injection without dilution.
- Drug may be given via the venous return line of dialysis tubing after dialysis.
- Single-dose vials do not contain preservatives and should be used only once. Discard remaining contents after use.
- To prevent adherence to tubing, recommend injecting while blood is still in I.V. line, and follow with normal saline flush.

### *Incompatibilities*
Don't mix with other drugs.

## Mechanism of action
*Antianemic action:* Epoetin alfa is a glycoprotein consisting of 165 amino acids synthesized using recombinant DNA technology. It mimics naturally occurring erythropoietin, which is produced by the kidneys. It stimulates the division and differentiation of cells within bone marrow to produce RBCs.

## Pharmacokinetics
*Absorption:* Administered S.C. or I.V.
*Distribution:* Unknown.
*Metabolism:* Unknown.
*Excretion:* Unknown.

| Route | Onset | Peak | Duration |
|-------|-------|------|----------|
| I.V. | Unknown | Immediate | Unknown |
| S.C. | Unknown | 5-24 hr | Unknown |

## Contraindications and precautions
Contraindicated in patients with uncontrolled hypertension and those hypersensitive to mammalian cell–derived products or albumin (human).

## Interactions
None reported.

## Adverse reactions
**CNS:** *headache,* **seizures,** *paresthesia, fatigue, asthenia,* dizziness.
**CV:** *hypertension, edema.*
**GI:** *nausea, vomiting, diarrhea.*
**GU:** increased BUN and creatinine.
**Metabolic:** increased uric acid, phosphorus, and potassium levels.
**Musculoskeletal:** *arthralgia.*
**Respiratory:** *cough, shortness of breath.*
**Skin:** *rash,* urticaria.
**Other:** increased clotting of arteriovenous grafts, *pyrexia, injection site reactions.*

## Overdose and treatment
Maximum safe dose hasn't been established. Doses up to 1,500 units/kg have been given three times weekly for 3 weeks without direct toxic effects.

The drug can cause polycythemia; phlebotomy may be used to bring hematocrit to within appropriate levels.

## Clinical considerations
- For HIV-infected patients treated with zidovudine, hematocrit should be measured once weekly until stabilized and then periodically.
- Most patients eventually require supplemental iron therapy. Before and during therapy, recommend monitoring patient's iron stores, including serum ferritin and transferrin saturation.

### *Therapeutic monitoring*
- Routine monitoring of CBC with differential and platelet counts is recommended.
- Recommend measuring hematocrit twice weekly until it has stabilized and during adjustment to a maintenance dose in patients with chronic renal failure. An interval of 2 to 6 weeks may elapse before a dose change is reflected in the hematocrit level.
- Close monitoring of blood pressure is also recommended.
- If a patient fails to respond to epoetin alfa therapy, consider the following possible caus-

es: vitamin deficiency, iron deficiency, under-lying infection, occult blood loss, underlying hematologic disease, hemolysis, aluminum intoxication, osteitis fibrosa cystica, or increased dosage of zidovudine.

### Special populations
**Pregnant patients.** Drug should be used during pregnancy only when benefits outweigh risks to fetus.
**Breast-feeding patients.** It's unknown if drug appears in breast milk. Drug should be used with caution in breast-feeding women.
**Pediatric patients.** Safety and efficacy in children haven't been established.

### Patient counseling
■ Explain importance of regularly monitoring blood pressure in light of potential drug effects.
■ Advise patient to adhere to dietary restrictions during therapy. Make sure he understands that drug won't influence disease process.

## epoprostenol sodium
Flolan

*Pharmacologic classification:* naturally occurring prostaglandin
*Therapeutic classification:* vasodilator, antiplatelet aggregator
*Pregnancy risk category B*

### Available forms
Available by prescription only
*Injection:* 0.5 mg/17-ml vial, 1.5 mg/17-ml vial

### Indications and dosages
*Long-term I.V. treatment of primary pulmonary hypertension in New York Heart Association (NYHA) class III and class IV patients*
*Adults:* Initially for acute dose ranging, 2 ng/kg/minute as an I.V. infusion; increase in increments of 2 ng/kg/minute q 15 minutes or longer until dose-limiting pharmacologic effects are elicited. Begin maintenance dosing with 4 ng/kg/minute less than the maximum tolerated infusion rate as determined during acute dose ranging. If the maximum tolerated infusion rate is less than 5 ng/kg/minute, begin maintenance infusion at one-half the maximum tolerated infusion rate. Base subsequent dosage adjustments on persistence, recurrence, or worsening of patient's symptoms of primary pulmonary hypertension and the occurrence of adverse events because of excessive doses of drug. Increases in dose from the initial maintenance dose can generally be expected and are done in increments of 1 to 2 ng/kg/minute at intervals of at least 15 minutes.

### I.V. administration
■ Before use, protect reconstituted solutions of the drug from light and refrigerate at 36° to 46° F (2° to 8° C) if not used immediately.
■ Reconstitute drug only as directed, using sterile diluent for Flolan. Don't reconstitute or mix drug with other parenteral solutions before or during administration.
■ Don't freeze reconstituted solutions of drug.
■ Drug should be prepared in a drug delivery reservoir appropriate for the infusion pump, with a total reservoir volume of at least 100 ml.
■ Maintenance dosing should be given by continuous I.V. infusion via a permanent indwelling central venous catheter using an ambulatory infusion pump.
■ Discard reconstituted solution if it's been refrigerated for longer than 48 hours.

### Incompatibilities
Don't infuse drug with other drugs or I.V. solutions.

### Mechanism of action
*Vasodilator and antiplatelet actions:* Epoprostenol causes direct vasodilation of pulmonary and systemic arterial vascular beds and inhibits platelet aggregation.

### Pharmacokinetics
*Absorption:* Administered I.V.
*Distribution:* Unknown.
*Metabolism:* Extensively metabolized.
*Excretion:* Excreted primarily in urine with a small amount excreted in feces.

| Route | Onset | Peak | Duration |
|-------|-------|------|----------|
| I.V. | Unknown | Unknown | Unknown |

### Contraindications and precautions
Contraindicated in patients hypersensitive to drug or structurally related compounds. Long-term use of drug is also contraindicated in patients with HF because of severe left ventricular systolic dysfunction or in those for whom pulmonary edema develops during initial dose ranging.

### Interactions
**Drug-drug.** *Anticoagulants, antiplatelet drugs:* May increase risk of bleeding. Advise clinician to monitor patient closely for bleeding.
*Antihypertensives, diuretics, or other vasodilators:* May cause additional reduction in blood pressure. Advise clinician to monitor blood pressure closely.

### Adverse reactions
**CNS:** *headache, anxiety, nervousness, agitation, dizziness, hyperesthesia, paresthesia.*

**CV:** *tachycardia; hypotension, chest pain, bradycardia* (during initial dose ranging).
**GI:** *nausea, vomiting;* abdominal pain, dyspepsia (during initial dose ranging); *diarrhea* (during maintenance dosing).
**Hematologic:** *thrombocytopenia.*
**Musculoskeletal:** back pain, *jaw pain, myalgia, nonspecific musculoskeletal pain* (during maintenance dosing).
**Respiratory:** dyspnea.
**Skin:** *flushing,* sweating (during initial dose ranging).
**Other:** *flulike symptoms, chills, fever, sepsis.*

### Overdose and treatment
Overdose may result in flushing, headache, hypotension, tachycardia, nausea, vomiting, and diarrhea.

Treatment usually requires dosage reduction of epoprostenol.

### Clinical considerations
▪ Drug should be used only by staff experienced in the diagnosis and treatment of primary pulmonary hypertension. Determining the appropriate dose for the patient must be done in a setting with adequate personnel and equipment for physiologic monitoring and emergency care.
**H ALERT** Avoid abrupt withdrawal or sudden large reductions in infusion rates.
▪ Recommend giving anticoagulant therapy during long-term use of drug, unless contraindicated. Advise clinician to monitor PT and INR closely.

#### Therapeutic monitoring
▪ Advise clinician to observe patient closely and monitor standing and supine blood pressure and heart rate.
▪ During maintenance infusion, the occurrence of dose-related pharmacologic events similar to those observed during initial dosing may require a decrease in infusion rate, but the adverse event may occasionally resolve without dosage adjustment.
▪ Advise clinician to monitor patient for adverse reactions.

#### Special populations
**Breast-feeding patients.** It isn't known if drug appears in breast milk. Use drug cautiously in breast-feeding women.
**Pediatric patients.** Safety and efficacy in children haven't been established.
**Geriatric patients.** In general, dose selection for a geriatric patient should be cautious, reflecting the greater frequency of decreased hepatic, renal, or cardiac function and of concomitant disease or other drug therapy.

### Patient counseling
▪ Ensure that patient and family understand before therapy is begun that there's a high like-

lihood that I.V. therapy with epoprostenol will be needed for prolonged periods, possibly years, and that the patient or family has the ability to accept and care for a permanent I.V. catheter and infusion pump.
▪ Instruct patient and family how to reconstitute drug and give drug via infusion pump using sterile technique. Explain how to use infusion pump. Stress importance of maintaining continuous drug therapy. Provide patient and family with instructions on how to switch to a new infusion pump in the event of pump failure. Also instruct patient and family on how to store drug.
▪ Instruct patient to immediately report adverse reactions regarding drug therapy because dosage adjustments may be needed.
▪ Provide patient with telephone number to obtain assistance for 24-hour support.

# eprosartan mesylate
Teveten

*Pharmacologic classification:* angiotensin II receptor antagonist
*Therapeutic classification:* antihypertensive
*Pregnancy risk category C (D in second and third trimesters)*

### Available forms
Available by prescription only
*Tablets:* 400 mg, 600 mg

### Indications and dosages
*Hypertension, alone or with other antihypertensives*
*Adults:* Initially, 600 mg P.O. daily. Daily dose ranges from 400 to 800 mg given as single daily dose or in two divided doses.

### Mechanism of action
*Antihypertensive action:* Eproszartan is an angiotensin II receptor antagonist that blocks vasoconstrictor and aldosterone-secreting effects of angiotensin II by selectively blocking binding of angiotensin II to its receptor sites found in many tissues, such as vascular smooth muscle and the adrenal gland.

### Pharmacokinetics
*Absorption:* Absolute bioavailability of single oral dose is about 13%. Onset of action occurs in about 1 to 2 hours, with plasma levels peaking in 1 to 3 hours.
*Distribution:* About 98% plasma protein–bound. Duration about 24 hours.
*Metabolism:* No active metabolites.
*Excretion:* Eliminated by biliary and renal excretion, primarily as unchanged drug. Following oral administration, about 90% recovered

in feces and about 7% in urine. Terminal elimination half-life typically 5 to 9 hours.

| Route | Onset | Peak | Duration |
|-------|-------|------|----------|
| P.O. | 1-2 hr | 1-3 hr | 24 hr |

## Contraindications and precautions

Contraindicated in patients hypersensitive to drug or its components.

Use cautiously in patients with an activated renin-angiotensin system, such as volume- or salt-depleted patients, and patients whose renal function may depend on the activity of the renin-angiotensin-aldosterone system, such as patients with severe HF. Also use cautiously in patients with renal artery stenosis.

## Interactions

None reported.

## Adverse reactions

**CNS:** depression, fatigue, headache, dizziness.
**CV:** chest pain.
**EENT:** pharyngitis, rhinitis, sinusitis.
**GI:** abdominal pain, dyspepsia, diarrhea.
**GU:** urinary tract infection, increased BUN level.
**Hematologic:** *neutropenia.*
**Metabolic:** hypertriglyceridemia.
**Musculoskeletal:** arthralgia, myalgia.
**Respiratory:** cough, upper respiratory tract infection, bronchitis.
**Other:** injury, viral infection, dependent edema, facial edema, *angioedema.*

## Overdose and treatment

In case of overdose, symptomatic and supportive therapy should be given. Drug is poorly removed by hemodialysis.

## Clinical considerations

■ Hypovolemia and hyponatremia should be corrected before therapy to reduce risk of symptomatic hypotension.
■ A transient episode of hypotension isn't a contraindication to continued treatment. Drug may be restarted once patient's blood pressure has stabilized.
■ Drug should be used alone or with other antihypertensives, such as diuretics and calcium channel blockers. Maximal blood pressure response may take 2 to 3 weeks.

### Therapeutic monitoring

■ Advise clinician to monitor blood pressure closely for 2 hours during start of therapy. If hypotension occurs, recommend placing patient in supine position and, if needed, giving I.V. infusion of normal saline.
■ Advise clinician to monitor patient for facial or lip swelling; angioedema has occurred with other angiotensin II antagonists.

■ Advise clinician to closely observe neonates exposed to eprosartan in utero for hypotension, oliguria, and hyperkalemia.
■ Advise clinician to monitor renal function before treatment and periodically throughout.

### Special populations

**Pregnant patients.** Drugs that act directly on the renin-angiotensin system can cause fetal and neonatal morbidity and death when given to pregnant women. If pregnancy is detected, drug should be stopped as soon as possible. These adverse effects haven't occurred when intrauterine drug exposure has been limited to first trimester.
**Breast-feeding patients.** It isn't known if drug appears in breast milk. Because of potential for serious adverse reactions in breast-feeding infants, a decision should be made to stop drug or breast-feeding.
**Pediatric patients.** Safety and effectiveness in children haven't been established.
**Geriatric patients.** There is a slightly decreased response to drug in geriatric patients. No initial dosage adjustment is needed.

## Patient counseling

■ Advise woman of childbearing age to use reliable form of contraception and to call prescriber immediately if pregnancy is suspected. Drug may need to be stopped under medical supervision.
■ Advise patient to report facial or lip swelling and signs and symptoms of infection, such as fever or sore throat.
■ Tell patient to obtain medical approval before taking OTC product for dry cough.
■ Inform patient that drug may be taken without regard to meals.
■ Tell patient to store drug at a controlled room temperature of 68° to 77° F (20° to 25° C).

# eptifibatide
Integrilin

*Pharmacologic classification:* glycoprotein IIb/IIIa (GP IIb/IIIa) inhibitor
*Therapeutic classification:* antiplatelet drug
*Pregnancy risk category B*

## Available forms

Available by prescription only
*Injection:* 2 mg/ml, 10-ml vial, 0.75 mg/ml, 100-ml vial

## Indications and dosages

*Acute coronary syndrome (unstable angina or non–Q-wave MI) in patients being managed medically and in those undergoing percutaneous coronary intervention*
*Adults:* 180 mcg/kg (up to maximum dose of 22.6 mg) I.V. bolus as soon as possible fol-

lowing diagnosis, followed by a continuous I.V. infusion of 2 mcg/kg/minute (up to maximum infusion rate of 15 mg/hour) for up to 72 hours. Infusion rate may be decreased to 0.5 mcg/kg/minute during percutaneous coronary intervention. Infusion should then be continued for an additional 20 to 24 hours after the procedure for up to 96 hours of therapy.
*Treatment in patients without signs and symptoms of acute coronary syndrome who are undergoing percutaneous coronary intervention*
*Adults:* I.V. bolus of 135 mcg/kg given immediately before procedure, followed by a continuous infusion of 0.5 mcg/kg/minute for 20 to 24 hours.

## I.V. administration

■ Drug should be refrigerated at a temperature of 35° to 47° F (2° to 8° C) and protected from light until administration. The drug may be transferred to a controlled room temperature storage 59° to 86° F (15° to 30° C) for a period no longer than 2 months.
■ Drug may be administered in same I.V. line as alteplase, atropine, dobutamine, heparin, lidocaine, meperidine, metoprolol, midazolam, morphine, nitroglycerin, or verapamil.
■ Drug may be administered in same I.V. line with normal saline or normal saline solution and 5% dextrose, and solution may contain up to 60 mEq/L of potassium chloride.

### *Incompatibilities*
Don't administer drug in same I.V. line as furosemide.

## Mechanism of action
*Antiplatelet action:* Reversibly inhibits platelet aggregation by preventing the binding of fibrinogen, von Willebrand factor, and other adhesion molecules to the GP IIb/IIIa receptor on human platelets.

## Pharmacokinetics
*Absorption:* Administered I.V.
*Distribution:* 25% plasma protein–bound.
*Metabolism:* Not reported. No major metabolites have been detected in human plasma.
*Excretion:* Elimination half-life is 2½ hours. Most of drug is excreted in urine.

| Route | Onset | Peak | Duration |
|-------|-------|------|----------|
| I.V. | Immediate | Immediate | 4-6 hr after infusion |

## Contraindications and precautions
Contraindicated in patients hypersensitive to drug or its ingredients.
   Contraindicated in patients with a history of bleeding diathesis or evidence of active abnormal bleeding within previous 30 days; severe hypertension (systolic blood pressure exceeding 200 mm Hg or diastolic blood pressure of more than 110 mm Hg) not adequately controlled on antihypertensive therapy; major surgery within previous 6 weeks; history of CVA within 30 days; history of hemorrhagic CVA; current or planned use of another parenteral GP IIb/IIIa inhibitor; or a platelet count of less than 100,000/mm³.
   Contraindicated in patients whose serum creatinine is 2 mg/dl and higher (for the 180-mcg/kg bolus and 2-mcg/kg/minute infusion) or 4 mg/dl or higher (for the 135-mcg/kg bolus and 0.5-mcg/kg/minute infusion); or in patients who are dependent on renal dialysis.
   Use cautiously in patients at increased risk of bleeding and patients weighing over 143 kg (315 lb).

## Interactions
**Drug-drug.** *Clopidogrel, dipyridamole, NSAIDs, oral anticoagulants (warfarin), thrombolytics, and ticlopidine:* Increased risk of bleeding. Advise clinician to monitor patient closely.
*Other inhibitors of platelet receptor GP IIb/IIIa:* May potentiate serious bleeding. Don't give together.

## Adverse reactions
**CV:** hypotension.
**GU:** hematuria.
**Hematologic: *bleeding, thrombocytopenia.***
**Other:** bleeding at femoral artery access site.

## Overdose and treatment
Limited data exist. Few patients received doses greater than or equal to two times the recommended dose.

## Clinical considerations
■ Recommend using drug in conjunction with heparin and aspirin. The efficacy and safety of low–molecular-weight heparin with aspirin are still under evaluation.
■ Recommend stopping eptifibatide and heparin and achieving sheath hemostasis by standard compressive techniques at least 4 hours before hospital discharge. The arterial access site is the most common site of bleeding.
■ If patient is to undergo coronary artery bypass graft surgery, infusion should be stopped before surgery.
■ Recommend minimizing use of arterial and venous punctures, I.M. injections, urinary catheters, nasotracheal tubes, and nasogastric tubes.

### *Therapeutic monitoring*
■ Recommend performing baseline laboratory tests before drug therapy starts: hematocrit, hemoglobin, platelet count, serum creatinine level, PT, INR, and PTT.
■ Advise clinician to monitor patient for bleeding.

■ If patient's platelet count is less than 100,000/mm³, recommend stopping eptifibatide and heparin.

### Special populations
**Breast-feeding patients.** It isn't known if drug appears in breast milk. It should be given cautiously to breast-feeding women.
**Pediatric patients.** Safety in children hasn't been established.
**Geriatric patients.** Drug has been used in patients as old as age 94. No significant difference has been shown compared with younger population.

### Patient counseling
■ Advise patient of potential adverse reactions.
■ Instruct patient to immediately report chest discomfort or other adverse events.
■ Caution patient to avoid activities that might cause bleeding or bruising.

# ergocalciferol (vitamin D₂)
Calciferol, Drisdol, Vitamin D

*Pharmacologic classification:* vitamin
*Therapeutic classification:* antihypocalcemic
*Pregnancy risk category C*

### Available forms
Available by prescription only
*Capsules:* 1.25 mg (50,000 units)
*Injection:* 12.5 mg (500,000 units)/ml
Available without a prescription
*Liquid:* 8,000 units/ml in 60-ml dropper bottle

### Indications and dosages
**Nutritional rickets or osteomalacia**
*Adults:* 25 to 125 mcg P.O. daily if patient has normal GI absorption. With severe malabsorption, 250 mcg to 7.5 mg P.O. or 250 mcg I.M. daily.
*Children:* 25 to 125 mcg P.O. daily if patient has normal GI absorption. With malabsorption, 250 to 625 mcg P.O. daily.
**Familial hypophosphatemia**
*Adults:* 250 mcg to 1.5 mg P.O. daily with phosphate supplements.
*Children:* 1 to 2 mg P.O. daily with phosphate supplements. Increase daily dose in 250- to 500-mcg increments at 3- to 4-month intervals until adequate response is obtained.
**Vitamin D-dependent rickets**
*Adults:* 250 mcg to 1.5 mg P.O. daily.
*Children:* 75 to 125 mcg P.O. daily.
**Anticonvulsant-induced rickets and osteomalacia**
*Adults:* 50 mcg to 1.25 mg P.O. daily.

**Hypoparathyroidism and pseudohypoparathyroidism**
*Adults:* 625 mcg to 5 mg P.O. daily with calcium supplements.
*Children:* 1.25 to 5 mg P.O. daily with calcium supplements.
◇ **Fanconi's syndrome**
*Adults:* 1.25 to 5 mg P.O. daily.
*Children:* 625 mcg to 1.25 mg P.O. daily.
◇ **Osteoporosis**
*Adults:* 25 to 250 mcg P.O. daily or 1.25 mg P.O. weekly with calcium and fluoride supplements.

### Mechanism of action
*Antihypocalcemic action:* Once activated, ergocalciferol acts to regulate the serum levels of calcium by regulating absorption from the GI tract and resorption from bone.

### Pharmacokinetics
*Absorption:* Absorbed readily from the small intestine.
*Distribution:* Distributed widely and bound to proteins stored in the liver.
*Metabolism:* Metabolized in the liver and kidneys. It has an average half-life of 24 hours and a duration of up to 6 months.
*Excretion:* Bile (feces) is the primary excretion route. A small percentage is excreted in urine.

| Route | Onset | Peak | Duration |
|-------|-------|------|----------|
| P.O., I.M. | 2-24 hr | 4-12 hr | 2 days-6 mo |

### Contraindications and precautions
Contraindicated in patients with hypercalcemia, hypervitaminosis A, or renal osteodystrophy with hyperphosphatemia.
    Use with extreme caution, if at all, in patients with impaired renal function, heart disease, renal stones, or arteriosclerosis.

### Interactions
**Drug-drug.** *Cardiac glycosides:* May result in arrhythmias. Patient requires close monitoring.
*Cholestyramine, colestipol, and excessive use of mineral oil:* Interfere with absorption of ergocalciferol. Avoid use together.
*Corticosteroids:* Counteract effects of drug. Advise clinician to monitor patient carefully.
*Magnesium-containing antacids:* May lead to hypermagnesemia. Advise clinician to monitor magnesium level.
*Orlistat:* May decrease absorption of vitamin D analogues. Separate drugs by 2 hours.
*Phenobarbital or phenytoin:* May increase metabolism of drug to inactive metabolites. Use together cautiously.
*Thiazide diuretics:* May cause hypercalcemia in patients with hypoparathyroidism. Advise clinician to monitor patient closely.

*Verapamil:* Atrial fibrillation may occur when supplemental calcium and calciferol have induced hypercalcemia. Patient requires careful monitoring.

### Adverse reactions
Adverse reactions listed usually occur only in vitamin D toxicity.

**CNS:** headache, weakness, somnolence, overt psychosis, irritability.
**CV:** *calcifications of soft tissues, including the heart,* hypertension, ***arrhythmias.***
**EENT:** rhinorrhea, conjunctivitis (calcific), photophobia.
**GI:** anorexia, nausea, vomiting, constipation, dry mouth, metallic taste, polydipsia.
**GU:** polyuria, albuminuria, hypercalciuria, nocturia, impaired renal function, reversible azotemia.
**Hepatic:** elevated liver enzyme levels (falsely or actually).
**Metabolic:** *hypercalcemia,* hyperthermia, increased serum cholesterol levels, weight loss.
**Musculoskeletal:** bone and muscle pain, bone demineralization.
**Skin:** pruritus.
**Other:** decreased libido.

### Overdose and treatment
Signs and symptoms of overdose include hypercalcemia, hypercalciuria, and hyperphosphatemia, which may be treated by stopping therapy, starting a low-calcium diet, and increasing fluid intake. A loop diuretic, such as furosemide, may be given with I.V. saline infusion to increase calcium excretion. Supportive measures should be provided. In severe cases, death from cardiac or renal failure may occur. Calcitonin may decrease hypercalcemia.

### Clinical considerations
■ I.M. injection of ergocalciferol dispersed in oil is preferable in patients who are unable to absorb the oral form.
■ Patients with hyperphosphatemia require dietary phosphate restrictions and binding agents to avoid metastatic calcifications and renal calculi.

#### Therapeutic monitoring
■ Recommend monitoring eating and bowel habits; dry mouth, nausea, vomiting, metallic taste, and constipation may be early signs of toxicity.
■ When high therapeutic doses are used, frequent serum and urine calcium, potassium, and urea determinations should be made.
■ Malabsorption caused by inadequate bile or hepatic dysfunction may require addition of exogenous bile salts.

#### Special populations
**Breast-feeding patients.** Very little drug appears in breast milk; however, effect on infants of amounts exceeding RDA levels of vitamin D isn't known.
**Pediatric patients.** Some infants may be hyperreactive to drug.

### Patient counseling
■ Caution patient not to increase daily dose.
■ Tell patient to avoid magnesium-containing antacids and mineral oil.
■ Instruct patient to swallow tablets whole without crushing or chewing.

## ergonovine maleate
Ergotrate Maleate

*Pharmacologic classification:* ergot alkaloid
*Therapeutic classification:* oxytocic
*Pregnancy risk category NR*

### Available forms
Available by prescription only
*Injection:* 0.2-mg/ml ampules

### Indications and dosages
***Prevent or treat postpartum and postabortion hemorrhage caused by uterine atony or subinvolution***
*Adults:* 0.2 mg I.M. p.r.n. q 2 to 4 hours, maximum five doses; or 0.2 mg I.V. (only for severe uterine bleeding or other life-threatening emergency) over 1 minute. After initial I.M. or I.V. dose, 0.2 to 0.4 mg may be given P.O. q 6 to 12 hours for 2 to 7 days to reduce postpartum bleeding and puerperal uterine atony and subinvolution.
◇ *To diagnose coronary artery spasm (Prinzmetal's angina)*
*Adults:* 0.1 to 0.4 mg I.V. for one dose.

### I.V. administration
■ Tablets and injections should be stored in light-resistant containers.
■ I.V. dose may be diluted to 5 ml with normal saline injection.
■ Contractions begin immediately after I.V. injection. May continue for 45 minutes after I.V. injection.
■ Blood pressure and uterine contractions should be carefully monitored during I.V. dose.
■ I.V. doses should be given in a period of no less than 1 minute.

#### Incompatibilities
Don't mix drug with any I.V. infusions.

### Mechanism of action
*Oxytocic action:* Ergonovine maleate stimulates contractions of uterine and vascular smooth muscle. This produces intense uterine

contractions, followed by periods of relaxation. The drug produces vasoconstriction of primarily capacitance blood vessels, causing an increased CVP and elevated blood pressure.

The clinical effect is secondary to contraction of the uterine wall around bleeding vessels, producing hemostasis.

## Pharmacokinetics
*Absorption:* Absorption is rapid after I.M. administration.
*Distribution:* Unknown.
*Metabolism:* Metabolized in the liver.
*Excretion:* Primarily nonrenal elimination in feces has been suggested.

| Route | Onset | Peak | Duration |
|-------|-------|------|----------|
| I.V. | Immediate | Unknown | Unknown |
| I.M. | 2-5 min | Unknown | Unknown |

## Contraindications and precautions
Contraindicated in patients sensitive to ergot preparations; in threatened spontaneous abortion, induction of labor, or before delivery of placenta because captivation of placenta may occur; and in those with history of allergic or idiosyncratic reactions to drug.

Because of the potential for adverse CV effects, use cautiously in patients with hypertension, toxemia, sepsis, occlusive vascular disease, and hepatic, renal, and cardiac disease.

## Interactions
**Drug-drug.** *Cardiac glycosides:* Enhanced vasoconstriction. Avoid use together.
*Local anesthetics with vasoconstrictors (lidocaine with epinephrine):* Enhanced vasoconstriction. Use cautiously.
*Other ergot alkaloids and sympathomimetic amines:* Enhanced vasoconstrictor potential. Advise clinician to monitor patient carefully.
**Drug-lifestyle.** *Smoking:* Enhances vasoconstriction. Advise patient not to smoke.

## Adverse reactions
**CNS:** headache, confusion, dizziness, ringing in ears.
**CV:** chest pain, weakness in legs (peripheral vasospasm), hypertension, thrombophlebitis.
**GI:** nausea, vomiting, diarrhea, cramping.
**Metabolic:** decreased serum prolactin.
**Musculoskeletal:** pain in arms, legs, or lower back.
**Respiratory:** shortness of breath.
**Other:** itching; sweating; hypersensitivity reactions, *signs of shock.*

## Overdose and treatment
Signs and symptoms of overdose include seizures with nausea, vomiting, diarrhea, dizziness, fluctuations in blood pressure, weak pulse, chest pain, tingling, and numbness and coldness in the limbs. Rarely, gangrene has occurred.

Recommend treating seizures with anticonvulsants and hypercoagulability with heparin and giving vasodilators to improve blood flow. Gangrene may require amputation.

## Clinical considerations
■ Hypocalcemia may decrease patient response; I.V. administration of calcium salts is needed.
■ High doses during delivery may cause uterine tetany and possible infant hypoxia or intracranial hemorrhage.
■ Drug has been used as a diagnostic agent for angina pectoris.
■ Discontinue drug if hypertension or allergic reactions occur.

### Therapeutic monitoring
■ Advise clinician to monitor blood pressure, pulse rate, uterine response, and character and amount of vaginal bleeding. Watch for sudden changes in vital signs and frequent periods of uterine relaxation.

### Special populations
**Pregnant patients.** High doses during delivery may cause uterine tetany and possible infant hypoxia or intracranial hemorrhage.
**Breast-feeding patients.** Ergot alkaloids inhibit lactation. Drug appears in breast milk, and ergotism has been reported in breast-fed infants of women given other ergot alkaloids. Use with caution.

## Patient counseling
■ Tell patient not to smoke while taking drug.
■ Advise patient of possible adverse reactions.

# ergotamine tartrate
Bellamine, Bellamine-S, Bellergal-S, Bel-Phen-Ergot S, Cafergot, Duragal-S, Ercaf, Ergomar, Ergostat, Gynergen, Medihaler Ergotamine, Migergot, Mycomp-PB, Phenerbel-S, Wigraine

*Pharmacologic classification:* ergot alkaloid
*Therapeutic classification:* vasoconstrictor
*Pregnancy risk category X*

## Available forms
Available by prescription only
*Tablets (S.L.):* 2 mg
*Tablets:* 0.6 mg with levoratatory belladonna alkaloids 0.2 mg and phenobarbital 40 mg; 1 mg with caffeine 100 mg; 1 mg with levoratatory belladonna alkaloids 0.125 mg, caffeine 100 mg, and pentobarbital sodium 30 mg
*Suppositories:* 2 mg (with caffeine 100 mg)

---

## Indications and dosages

**To prevent or abort vascular headache, including migraine and cluster headaches**

*Adults:* Initially, 2 mg S.L. or P.O., then 1 to 2 mg S.L. q 30 minutes, or P.O. q hour, to maximum 6 mg per 24 hours, and 10 mg weekly. A single oral dose should not exceed 4 to 5 mg. In patients with daily attacks of cluster headaches, 1 to 2 mg P.O. at bedtime for 10 to 14 days. Patient may also use rectal suppositories. Initially, 2 mg P.R. at onset of attack; repeat in 1 hour, p.r.n. Maximum dose is 2 suppositories per attack or 5 suppositories weekly. In patients with cluster headaches in the morning, 2 to 4 mg may be given P.R. at bedtime on a short-term basis.

◇ *Children:* 1 mg S.L. or P.O. in older children and adolescents; if no improvement, additional 1-mg dose may be given in 30 minutes.

## Mechanism of action

*Vasoconstricting action:* By stimulating alpha-adrenergic receptors, ergotamine in therapeutic doses causes peripheral vasoconstriction (if vascular tone is low); however, if vascular tone is high, it produces vasodilation. In high doses, it's a competitive alpha blocker. In therapeutic doses, it inhibits the reuptake of norepinephrine, which increases the vasoconstricting activity of ergotamine. A weaker serotonin antagonist, it reduces the increased rate of platelet aggregation caused by serotonin.

In the treatment of vascular headaches, ergotamine probably causes direct vasoconstriction of dilated carotid artery beds while decreasing the amplitude of pulsations. Its serotoninergic and catecholamine effects also seem to be involved.

## Pharmacokinetics

*Absorption:* Rapidly absorbed after inhalation and variably absorbed after oral administration. Peak levels occur in ½ to 3 hours. Caffeine may increase rate and extent of absorption. Drug undergoes first-pass metabolism after oral administration.

*Distribution:* Widely distributed throughout the body.

*Metabolism:* Extensively metabolized in the liver.

*Excretion:* Part of dose (4%) is excreted in urine within 96 hours; remainder is presumed to be excreted in feces. Ergotamine is dialyzable. Onset of action depends on how promptly drug is given after onset of headache.

| Route | Onset | Peak | Duration |
|---|---|---|---|
| P.O. | Variable | ½-3 hr | Variable |
| S.L., inhalation | Variable | Unknown | Variable |
| P.R. | Unknown | Unknown | Unknown |

## Contraindications and precautions

Contraindicated in patients with peripheral and occlusive vascular diseases, coronary artery disease, hypertension, hepatic or renal dysfunction, severe pruritus, sepsis, or hypersensitivity to ergot alkaloids and during pregnancy.

## Interactions

**Drug-drug.** *Erythromycin and other macrolides:* May cause symptoms of ergot toxicity. Vasodilators (nifedipine, nitroprusside, or prazosin) may be ordered to treat ergot toxicity.

*Propranolol or other beta blockers:* Increased vasoconstrictor effects. Advise clinician to monitor patient carefully.

**Drug-food.** *Caffeine:* May increase rate and extent of absorption. Advise patient to avoid caffeine.

**Drug-lifestyle.** *Alcohol use:* May worsen headache. Advise patient to avoid alcohol.

*Smoking:* May increase adverse effects. Caution patient to avoid smoking.

## Adverse reactions

**CNS:** numbness and tingling in fingers and toes.

**CV:** transient tachycardia or bradycardia, precordial distress and pain, increased arterial pressure, angina, peripheral vasoconstriction.

**GI:** nausea, vomiting.

**Musculoskeletal:** weakness in legs, muscle pain in limbs.

**Skin:** pruritus, localized edema.

## Overdose and treatment

Signs and symptoms of overdose include adverse vasospastic effects, nausea, vomiting, lassitude, impaired mental function, delirium, severe dyspnea, hypotension or hypertension, rapid pulse, weak pulse, unconsciousness, spasms of the limbs, seizures, and shock.

Treatment is supportive and symptomatic, with prolonged and careful monitoring. If patient is conscious and ingestion is recent, recommend emptying stomach by emesis or gastric lavage; if comatose, recommend performing gastric lavage after placement of endotracheal tube with cuff inflated. Activated charcoal and a saline (magnesium sulfate) cathartic may be used. Recommend providing respiratory support. Warmth (not direct heat) should be applied to ischemic limbs if vasospasm occurs. As needed, recommend giving vasodilators (nitroprusside, prazosin, or tolazoline) and, if needed, I.V. diazepam to treat convulsions. Dialysis may be helpful.

## Clinical considerations

■ Drug is most effective when used in prodromal stage of headache or as soon as possible after onset. Recommend providing quiet, low-light environment to relax patient after dose is given.

■ S.L. tablet is preferred during early stage of attack because of its rapid absorption.
■ Drug isn't effective for muscle contraction headaches.

### Therapeutic monitoring
■ Rebound headache or increased duration or frequency of headache may occur when drug is stopped.
■ If patient experiences severe vasoconstriction with tissue necrosis, recommend giving I.V. sodium nitroprusside or intra-arterial tolazoline. I.V. heparin and 10% dextran 40 in $D_5W$ injection also may be given to prevent vascular stasis and thrombosis.

### Special populations
**Pregnant patients.** Drug is contraindicated in women who are or may become pregnant.
**Breast-feeding patients.** Drug appears in breast milk; therefore, it should be used with caution in breast-feeding women. Excessive drug use may inhibit lactation.
**Pediatric patients.** Safety and efficacy of ergotamine in children haven't been established.
**Geriatric patients.** Drug should be given cautiously to geriatric patients.

### Patient counseling
■ Instruct patient in correct use of drug.
■ Urge patient to immediately report feelings of numbness or tingling in fingers or toes or red or violet blisters on hands or feet.
■ Caution patient to avoid alcoholic beverages and smoking.
■ Warn patient to avoid prolonged exposure to very cold temperatures, which may increase adverse effects of drug.
■ Advise patient who uses an inhaler to call prescriber promptly if mouth, throat, or lung infection occurs or if condition worsens. Cough, hoarseness, or throat irritation may occur. Patient should gargle and rinse mouth after each dose to help prevent hoarseness and irritation.
■ Advise patient not to exceed recommended dosage.

---

## erythromycin base
E-Base, E-Mycin, ERYC, ERYC Sprinkle*, Ery-Tab, Erythromycin Base/Filmtabs, Ilotycin, PCE, Robimycin

## erythromycin estolate
erythromycin ethylsuccinate, E.E.S., EryPed, Pediazole

## erythromycin gluceptate
Ilotycin Gluceptate

## erythromycin lactobionate
Erythrocin Lactobionate

## erythromycin stearate
Apo-Erythro-S*, Erythrocin Stearate Filmtab, Novo-Rythro*

## erythromycin (topical)
Akne-Mycin, A/T/S, Benzamycin, Del-Mycin, Erycette, EryDerm, Erymax, Ery-Sol, Erythra-Derm, Staticin, Theramycin Z, T-Stat

## erythromycin (ophthalmic)
Ilotycin

*Pharmacologic classification:* erythromycin
*Therapeutic classification:* antibiotic
*Pregnancy risk category B*

### Available forms
Available by prescription only
**erythromycin base**
*Tablets (enteric-coated):* 250 mg, 333 mg, 500 mg
*Pellets (enteric-coated):* 250 mg
**erythromycin estolate**
*Capsules:* 250 mg
*Suspension:* 125 mg/5 ml, 250 mg/5 ml
**erythromycin ethylsuccinate**
*Tablets (chewable):* 200 mg
*Tablets:* 400 mg
*Oral suspension:* 200 mg/5 ml, 400 mg/5 ml
*Powder for oral suspension:* 100 mg/2.5 ml, 200 mg/5 ml, 400 mg/5 ml (after reconstitution)
*Granules for oral suspension:* 200 mg/5 ml (after reconstitution)
**erythromycin gluceptate**
*Injection:* 500-mg, 1-g vials
**erythromycin lactobionate**
*Injection:* 500-mg, 1-g vials
**erythromycin stearate**
*Tablets (film-coated):* 250 mg, 500 mg
**erythromycin (ophthalmic)**
*Ointment:* 5 mg/g
**erythromycin (topical)**
*Pledgets:* 2%
*Topical gel:* 2%
*Topical ointment:* 2%
*Topical solution:* 2%

### Indications and dosages
*Acute pelvic inflammatory disease caused by Neisseria gonorrhoeae*
*Adults:* 500 mg I.V. (gluceptate, lactobionate) q 6 hours for 3 days, then 250 mg (base, estolate, stearate) or 400 mg (ethylsuccinate) P.O. q 6 hours for 7 days.
*Endocarditis prophylaxis for dental procedures in patients allergic to penicillin*
*Adults:* Initially, 800 mg (ethylsuccinate) or 1 g (stearate) P.O. 2 hours before procedure; then 400 mg (ethylsuccinate) or 500 mg (stearate) P.O. 6 hours later.

---

*Children:* Initially, 20 mg/kg (ethylsuccinate or stearate) P.O. 2 hours before procedure, then 10 mg/kg 6 hours later.

***Intestinal amebiasis in patients who can't receive metronidazole***
*Adults:* 250 mg (base, estolate, stearate) or 400 mg (ethylsuccinate) P.O. q 6 hours for 10 to 14 days.
*Children:* 30 to 50 mg/kg (base, estolate, ethylsuccinate, stearate) P.O. daily, divided q 6 hours for 10 to 14 days.
Note: Base and stearate forms not available in liquid form.

***Mild to moderately severe respiratory tract, skin, and soft-tissue infections caused by susceptible organisms***
*Adults:* 250 to 500 mg (base, estolate, stearate) P.O. q 6 hours; or 400 to 800 mg (ethylsuccinate) P.O. q 6 hours; or 15 to 20 mg/kg (gluceptate, lactobionate) I.V. daily, in divided doses q 6 hours.
*Children:* 30 mg/kg to 50 mg/kg (oral erythromycin salts) P.O. daily, in divided doses q 6 hours; or 15 to 20 mg/kg I.V. daily, in divided doses q 4 to 6 hours.

***Syphilis***
*Adults:* 500 mg (base, estolate, stearate) P.O. q.i.d. for 14 days.

***Legionnaire's disease***
*Adults:* 1 to 4 g I.V. or P.O. (base, estolate, stearate) or 1.6 to 4 g (ethylsuccinate) P.O. in divided doses for 10 to 21 days. Some clinicians recommend 14 days for patients with mild disease and 21 days for those who are immunocompromised or have severe disease. A parenteral regimen is usually needed for initial treatment or severe disease, with the addition of rifampin for the first 3 to 5 days of therapy.

***Uncomplicated urethral, endocervical, or rectal infections when tetracyclines are contraindicated***
*Adults:* 500 mg (base, estolate, stearate) or 800 mg (ethylsuccinate) P.O. q.i.d. for at least 7 days.

***Urogenital Chlamydia trachomatis infections during pregnancy***
*Adults:* 500 mg (base, estolate, stearate) P.O. q.i.d. for at least 7 days or 250 mg (base, estolate, stearate) or 400 mg (ethylsuccinate) P.O. q.i.d. for at least 14 days.

***Conjunctivitis caused by C. trachomatis in neonates***
*Neonates:* 50 mg/kg/day P.O. in four divided doses for at least 2 weeks.

***Pneumonia of infancy caused by C. trachomatis***
*Infants:* 50 mg/kg/day P.O. in four divided doses for at least 3 weeks.

***Topical treatment of acne vulgaris***
*Adults and children:* Apply to the affected area b.i.d.

***Prophylaxis of ophthalmia neonatorum***
*Neonates:* Apply 1-cm-long ribbon ointment in the lower conjunctival sac of each eye no later than 1 hour after birth. Use new tube for each infant and don't flush after instillation.

***Acute and chronic conjunctivitis, trachoma, other eye infections***
*Adults and children:* Apply 1-cm-long ribbon ointment directly into infected eye up to six times daily, depending on severity of infection.

***Treatment or prevention of pertussis***
*Adults:* 1 g (base) P.O. daily or 40 to 50 mg/kg (estolate, ethylsuccinate, stearate) P.O. daily (maximum 2 g daily) in divided doses for 14 days.
*Children:* 40 to 50 mg/kg (base) P.O. daily (maximum 2 g daily) in divided doses for 14 days.

***Pharyngitis and tonsillitis caused by Streptococcus pyogenes***
*Adults:* 20 to 50 mg/kg (estolate) P.O. in 2 to 4 divided doses (maximum 1 g daily) for 10 days or longer. Or, 40 mg/kg (ethylsuccinate) P.O. in 2 to 4 divided doses for 10 days.

◊ ***Early form of Lyme disease in persons allergic to penicillins and cephalosporins and in whom tetracyclines are contraindicated***
*Adults:* 250 to 500 mg (base) P.O. t.i.d. to q.i.d., or 30 to 40 mg/kg daily in divided doses for 10 to 30 days.
*Children under age 8:* 30 to 40 mg/kg (base) P.O. daily in divided doses (not to exceed adult dose) for 10 to 30 days.

◊ ***Early Lyme disease manifested as erythema migrans***
*Adults:* 500 mg (base) P.O. q.i.d. for 14 to 21 days.
*Children:* 12.5 mg/kg (base) P.O. q.i.d. (maximum 500 mg/dose) for 14 to 21 days.

## I.V. administration

■ Erythromycin lactobionate is given by continuous or intermittent I.V. infusion.
■ Drug should not be given by direct I.V. injection.
■ Vials containing 500 mg or 1 g of drug are initially reconstituted with 10 or 20 ml, respectively, of sterile water for injection.
■ Before administration, drug should be diluted further with normal saline solution, lactated Ringer's, or Normosol-R.
■ For continuous infusion, dilute to 1 mg/ml.
■ For intermittent infusion, appropriate dose should be diluted to concentration of 1 to 5 mg/ml (no less than 100 ml) and given over 20 to 60 minutes.
■ Don't give erythromycin lactobionate with other drugs because of chemical instability. Reconstituted solutions are acidic and should be completely given within 8 hours of preparation.

### Incompatibilities

Incompatible with ampicillin sodium, ascorbic acid injection, colistimethate, dextrose 2.5% in half-strength Ringer's lactate, dextrose 5% in Ringer's lactate, dextrose 5% in normal saline, dextrose 5% and 10% in water, heparin sodium, metaraminol, Normosol-M in dextrose 5%, Ringer's injection, and vitamin B complex with C.

## Mechanism of action

*Antibacterial action:* Erythromycin inhibits bacterial protein synthesis by binding to the ribosomal 50S subunit. It's used in the treatment of infection with *Haemophilus influenzae, Entamoeba histolytica, Mycoplasma pneumoniae, Corynebacterium diphtheriae, Corynebacterium minutissimum, Legionella pneumophila,* and *Bordetella pertussis.* It may be used as an alternative to penicillins or tetracycline in the treatment of infection with *Streptococcus pneumoniae, Streptococcus viridans, Listeria monocytogenes, Staphylococcus aureus, C. trachomatis, N. gonorrhoeae,* and *Treponema pallidum.*

## Pharmacokinetics

*Absorption:* Because base salt is acid-sensitive, it must be buffered or have enteric coating to prevent destruction by gastric acids. Acid salts and esters (estolate, ethylsuccinate, and stearate) aren't affected by gastric acidity and therefore are well absorbed. Recommend giving base and stearate preparations on an empty stomach. Absorption of estolate and ethylsuccinate preparations is unaffected or possibly even enhanced by presence of food. When given topically, drug is absorbed minimally.

*Distribution:* Distributed widely to most body tissues and fluids except CSF, where it's distributed only in low levels. Drug crosses the placenta. About 80% of base and 96% of erythromycin estolate are protein-bound.

*Metabolism:* Metabolized partially in the liver to inactive metabolites.

*Excretion:* Excreted mainly unchanged in bile. Only small drug amounts (less than 5%) are excreted in urine; some drug appears in breast milk. In patients with normal renal function, plasma half-life is about 1½ hours. Drug isn't dialyzable.

| Route | Onset | Peak | Duration |
|---|---|---|---|
| P.O. | Unknown | 1-4 hr | Unknown |
| I.V. | Unknown | Immediate | Unknown |
| Topical | Unknown | Unknown | Unknown |

## Contraindications and precautions

Contraindicated in patients hypersensitive to drug or other macrolides. Erythromycin estolate is contraindicated in patients with hepatic disease.

Use erythromycin salts cautiously in patients with impaired hepatic function.

## Interactions

**Drug-drug.** *Carbamazepine:* Increased carbamazepine blood levels and increased risk of toxicity. Advise clinician to monitor patient and carbamazepine levels closely.

*Clindamycin and lincomycin:* May be antagonistic. Avoid use together.

*Cyclosporine:* Increased serum cyclosporine levels and possible nephrotoxicity. Patient requires close monitoring.

*Digoxin:* Increased serum digoxin levels. Advise clinician to monitor patient for digoxin toxicity.

*Disopyramide:* Increased disopyramide plasma levels, possibly causing arrhythmias and increased QT intervals. Patient requires ECG monitoring.

*Isotretinoin:* May cause cumulative dryness, resulting in excessive skin irritation. Advise clinician to monitor patient carefully.

*Midazolam and triazolam:* Increased effects of these drugs. Use together cautiously.

*Oral anticoagulants:* Excessive anticoagulant effect. Advise clinician to monitor PT and INR closely.

*Theophylline:* Increased serum theophylline levels and decreased erythromycin blood level. Use together cautiously.

**Drug-herb.** *Pill-bearing spurge:* Inhibition of CYP3A enzymes affecting drug metabolism. Discourage use together.

**Drug-lifestyle.** *Abrasive or medicated soaps or cleansers; acne preparations or other preparations containing peeling agents (benzoyl peroxide, resorcinol, salicylic acid, sulfur, tretinoin); alcohol-containing products (aftershave, perfumed toiletries, cosmetics, shaving creams or lotions); astringent soaps or cosmetics; medicated cosmetics or cover-ups:* May cause cumulative dryness, resulting in excessive dryness. Use together cautiously.

## Adverse reactions

**CV:** *ventricular arrhythmias.*

**EENT:** bilateral reversible hearing loss (with high systemic or oral doses in patients with renal or hepatic insufficiency); slowed corneal wound healing, blurred vision (with ophthalmic administration).

**GI:** *abdominal pain, cramping, nausea, vomiting, diarrhea* (with oral or systemic administration).

**Hepatic:** cholestatic jaundice (with estolate).

**Skin:** urticaria, rash, eczema (with oral or systemic administration); urticaria, dermatitis (with ophthalmic administration); sensitivity reactions, erythema, burning, *dryness, pruritus,* irritation, peeling, oily skin (with topical application).

**Other:** overgrowth of nonsusceptible bacteria or fungi; *anaphylaxis;* fever (with oral or systemic administration); *venous irritation, throm-bophlebitis* (after I.V. injection); overgrowth of nonsusceptible organisms (with long-term use); hypersensitivity reactions, including itching and burning eyes (with ophthalmic administration).

## Overdose and treatment
No information available.

## Clinical considerations
- Absorption of estolate and ethylsuccinate preparations is unaffected or possibly even enhanced by presence of food.
- Erythromycin estolate may cause serious hepatotoxicity (reversible cholestatic jaundice) in adults.
- Drug may cause overgrowth of nonsusceptible bacteria or fungi.
- Although drug is bacteriostatic, it may be bactericidal in high levels or against highly susceptible organisms.
- Erythromycin may interfere with fluorometric determination of urinary catecholamines. False elevation of liver function test results using colorimetric assays may occur (rare).

### Therapeutic monitoring
- Advise clinician to perform culture and sensitivity tests before treatment starts and then p.r.n.
- Advise clinician to monitor liver function test results for increased serum bilirubin, AST, and alkaline phosphatase levels. Other erythromycin salts can cause less severe hepatotoxicity. (Patients in whom hepatotoxicity develops from erythromycin estolate may react in a similar fashion to any erythromycin preparation.)

### Special populations
**Pregnant patients.** Use drug during pregnancy only when clearly indicated.
**Breast-feeding patients.** Although drug appears in breast milk, no adverse reactions have been reported. Give cautiously to breast-feeding women.

## Patient counseling
- Instruct patient to take oral form with full glass of water 1 hour before or 2 hours after meals; enteric-coated tablets may be taken with meals.
- Advise patient not to take drug with fruit juice. If patient takes chewable tablets, tell him not to swallow them whole.
- If patient uses topical solution, instruct patient to wash, rinse, and dry affected areas before applying it. Warn patient not to apply solution near eyes, nose, mouth, or other mucous membranes.
- Instruct patient to wash hands before and after applying ophthalmic ointment. Instruct him to cleanse eye area of excess exudate before applying ointment. Warn him not to allow tube to touch the eye or surrounding tissue. Instruct him to promptly report signs of sensitivity, such as itching eyelids and constant burning.
- Tell patient to take drug exactly as directed and to continue taking it for prescribed period, even after he feels better.
- Instruct patient to report adverse reactions promptly.

# esmolol hydrochloride
Brevibloc

*Pharmacologic classification:* beta blocker
*Therapeutic classification:* anti-arrhythmic
*Pregnancy risk category C*

## Available forms
Available by prescription only
*Injection:* 10 mg/ml in 10-ml vials; 250 mg/ml in 10-ml ampules

## Indications and dosages
### Supraventricular tachycardia
*Adults:* Dosage range is 50 to 200 mcg/kg/minute; average dose is 100 mcg/kg/minute. Individual dosage adjustment requires stepwise titration in which each step consists of a loading dose followed by a maintenance infusion.

To begin treatment, give a loading infusion of 500 mcg/kg/minute for 1 minute followed by a 4-minute maintenance infusion of 50 mcg/kg/minute. If tachycardia doesn't subside within 5 minutes, repeat loading dose and follow with maintenance infusion increased to 100 mcg/kg/minute for 4 minutes. Continue titration, repeating loading infusion and increasing each maintenance infusion by 50 mcg/kg/minute, up to a maximum of 200 mcg/kg/minute. Once the desired heart rate or a patient tolerance end-point has been nearly achieved, loading doses should be omitted and maintenance infusion can be titrated upward (maximum, 300 mcg/kg/minute) or downward as appropriate, every 5 to 10 minutes.
### Intraoperative and postoperative tachycardia and hypertension
*Adults: For immediate control,* 80 mg (about 1 mg/kg) I.V. bolus dose over 30 seconds followed by a 150-mcg/kg/minute infusion, if needed, up to a maximum dose of 300 mcg/kg/minute; *for gradual control,* a loading I.V. infusion of 500 mcg/kg/minute for 1 minute, followed by a 4-minute maintenance infusion of 50 mcg/kg/minute. If an adequate therapeutic effect isn't observed within 5 minutes, repeat the same loading dose and follow with a maintenance infusion increased to 100 mcg/kg/minute.

## I.V. administration
■ Drug shouldn't be given as I.V. push; use with an infusion control device. The 10 mg/ml single-dose vial may be used without diluting, but the injection concentrate (250 mg/ml) must be diluted to a maximum of 10 mg/ml before infusion.
■ I.V. infusion levels exceeding 10 mg of esmolol hydrochloride per ml may produce irritation.
■ Diluted solutions of esmolol hydrochloride are stable for at least 24 hours at room temperature.

### Incompatibilities
Incompatible with diazepam, furosemide, procainamide, sodium bicarbonate, and thiopental. Drug isn't compatible with 5% sodium bicarbonate injection USP.

## Mechanism of action
*Antiarrhythmic action:* Esmolol, a beta blocker with rapid onset and very short duration of action, decreases blood pressure and heart rate in a dose-related, titratable manner. Its hemodynamic effects are similar to those of propranolol, but it doesn't increase vascular resistance.

## Pharmacokinetics
*Absorption:* Administered I.V.
*Distribution:* Distributed rapidly throughout the plasma. Distribution half-life is about 2 minutes. Esmolol is 55% protein-bound.
*Metabolism:* Hydrolyzed rapidly by plasma esterases.
*Excretion:* Excreted by the kidneys as metabolites. Elimination half-life is about 9 minutes.

| Route | Onset | Peak | Duration |
|-------|-------|------|----------|
| I.V. | Immediate | 30 min | 30 min after infusion |

## Contraindications and precautions
Contraindicated in patients with sinus bradycardia, heart block greater than first-degree, cardiogenic shock, or overt HF.

Use cautiously in patients with impaired renal function, diabetes, or bronchospasm.

## Interactions
**Drug-drug.** *Antihypertensives:* May potentiate their hypotensive effects. Dosage adjustments may be needed.
*Insulin or oral antidiabetics:* May mask symptoms of developing hypoglycemia. Patient requires close observation.
*I.V. digoxin:* Increased digoxin blood levels 10% to 20%. Dosage adjustments may be needed.
*I.V. morphine:* Increases esmolol steady-state levels by 46%. Patient requires careful monitoring.

*I.V. phenytoin:* Additive cardiac depressant effects. Patient requires close monitoring.
*Nondepolarizing neuromuscular blockers, such as gallamine, metocurine, pancuronium, succinylcholine, or tubocurarine:* May potentiate and prolong their action; careful postoperative monitoring of patient is needed after concurrent or sequential use, especially if there's a possibility of incomplete reversal of neuromuscular blockade.
*Reserpine and other catecholamine-depleting drugs:* Additive and possibly excessive beta-adrenergic blockade with bradycardia and hypotension. Close observation is recommended.
*Sympathomimetic amines having beta-adrenergic stimulant activity:* Mutual but transient inhibition of therapeutic effects. Use together cautiously.
*Xanthines, especially aminophylline or theophylline:* Mutual inhibition of therapeutic effects (except for dyphylline) may decrease theophylline clearance, especially in patients with increased theophylline clearance induced by smoking; concurrent use requires careful monitoring to prevent toxic accumulation of theophylline.

## Adverse reactions
**CNS:** dizziness, somnolence, headache, agitation, fatigue, confusion.
**CV: HYPOTENSION** (sometimes with diaphoresis), peripheral ischemia.
**EENT:** nasal congestion.
**GI:** *nausea*, vomiting.
**Respiratory: bronchospasm,** wheezing, dyspnea.
**Skin:** inflammation, induration (at infusion site).

## Overdose and treatment
Limited information is available. Hypotension would be the most likely symptom.

Symptoms of esmolol overdose usually disappear quickly after esmolol is withdrawn. In addition to immediate discontinuation of esmolol infusion, treatment is supportive and symptomatic.

Glucagon has been reported to effectively combat the CV effects (bradycardia, hypotension) of overdose with beta blockers. An I.V. dose of 2 to 3 mg is given over 30 seconds and repeated if needed, followed by infusion at 5 mg per hour until patient's condition has stabilized.

## Clinical considerations
■ To convert to other antiarrhythmic therapy after control has been achieved with esmolol, recommend reducing infusion rate of esmolol by 50% 30 minutes after administration of first dose of the alternative drug. If after the second dose of the alternative drug a satisfactory re-

sponse is maintained for 1 hour, esmolol should be stopped.

### Therapeutic monitoring
■ Advise clinician to monitor patient's ECG and blood pressure continuously during infusion.

### Special populations
**Pregnant patients.** Use in third trimester may cause fetal bradycardia. Use drug during pregnancy only when benefits to patient outweigh potential risk to fetus.
**Breast-feeding patients.** It isn't known if drug appears in breast milk; however, no problems have been reported in breast-feeding women.
**Pediatric patients.** Adequate and well-controlled studies haven't been performed. Safety and efficacy in children haven't been established.
**Geriatric patients.** Geriatric patients may be less sensitive to some effects of beta blockers. However, reduced metabolic and excretory capabilities in many geriatric patients may cause increased myocardial depression and require dosage reduction of beta blockers. Base dosage adjustment on clinical response.

### Patient counseling
■ Advise patient to report adverse events including pain at I.V. site.

# esomeprazole magnesium
Nexium

*Pharmacologic classification:* proton pump inhibitor, s-isomer of omeprazole
*Therapeutic classification:* gastroesophageal drug
*Pregnancy risk category B*

### Available forms
Available by prescription only
*Capsules (delayed-release containing enteric-coated pellets):* 20 mg or 40 mg (supplied as 22.3 or 44.5 mg esomeprazole magnesium)

### Indications and dosages
**Gastroesopageal reflux disease (GERD), healing of erosive esophagitis**
*Adults:* 20 or 40 mg P.O. daily for 4 to 8 weeks.
**Maintenance of healing in erosive esophagitis**
*Adults:* 20 mg P.O. daily for no longer than 6 months.
**Symptomatic GERD**
*Adults:* 20 mg P.O. daily for 4 weeks. If symptoms continue, treatment may continue 4 more weeks.

**Eradication of Helicobacter pylori (with other drugs) to reduce duodenal ulcer recurrence**
*Adults:* Esomeprazole magnesium 40 mg P.O. daily plus amoxicillin 1,000 mg P.O. b.i.d. plus clarithromycin 500 mg P.O. b.i.d., all for 10 days.
≡ *Dosage adjustment.* In patients with severe hepatic failure, the maximum daily dose is 20 mg.

### Mechanism of action
*Gastric secretion inhibitor action:* Suppresses gastric secretion through proton pump inhibition. Inhibits the $H^+$-$K^+$-ATPase pump in gastric parietal cells, reducing gastric acidity by blocking the final step in acid production. Esomeprazole magnesium is the s-isomer of omeperazole.

### Pharmacokinetics
*Absorption:* Formulated as enteric-coated pellets in a gelatin capsule. Plasma levels peak 1½ hours after oral administration. The plasma level after a 40-mg dose is three-fold higher than after a 20-mg dose. Repeated once-daily dosing of 40 mg yields systemic bioavailability of 90% compared to a single 40-mg dose, which yields 64%. This may result from reduced hepatic metabolism and clearance with continued dosing. Giving esomeprazole with food reduces mean plasma level by 33% to 53%. Drug should be given at least 1 hour before meals.
*Distribution:* About 97% protein-bound. The volume of distribution in healthy patients at steady state is 16 L.
*Metabolism:* Extensively metabolized by cytochrome P-450 2C19 to form hydroxy and desmethyl metabolites that have no secretory activity. CYP2C19 exhibits polymorphism, and people who are poor metabolizers have increased esomeprazole plasma levels. About 3% of Whites and 15% to 20% of Asians lack cytochrome P-450 2C19. Cytochrome P-450 3A4 metabolizes the remaining amount of esomeprazole.
*Excretion:* Plasma elimination half-life is about 1 to 1½ hours. Less than 1% of active parent drug is excreted in urine. About 80% of an oral dose is excreted as inactive metabolites in urine. Remaining inactive metabolites are excreted in feces. Systemic clearance of esomeprazole decreases with multiple dose administration.

| Route | Onset | Peak | Duration |
|---|---|---|---|
| P.O. | Unknown | 1½ hours | 13-17 hr |

### Contraindications and precautions
Contraindicated in patients hypersensitive to any component of esomeprazole or omeprazole.

Use cautiously in pregnant patients, breast-feeding patients, or patients with hepatic insufficiency. Dosage adjustments are needed in patients with severe disease.

## Interactions
**Drug-drug.** *Amoxicillin, clarithromycin:* Increased esomeprazole levels. Advise clinician to monitor patient closely.
*Diazepam:* Decreased diazepam clearance. Recommend adjusting diazepam dosage, p.r.n.
*Other drugs metabolized by cytochrome P-450 2C19:* Altered esomeprazole clearance. Advise clinician to monitor patient closely, especially geriatric patients and patients with hepatic insufficiency.
**Drug-food.** *Any food:* Reduced bioavailability. Advise patient to take drug 1 hour before eating.

## Adverse reactions
**CNS:** headache.
**GI:** diarrhea, abdominal pain, nausea, flatulence, dry mouth, vomiting, constipation.

## Overdose and treatment
No antidote is known. Drug is highly protein-bound and therefore probably is not removed by dialysis. Supportive care is recommended.

## Clinical considerations
■ Symptomatic response to esomeprazole doesn't rule out the presence of a gastric malignancy.
■ Food decreases the extent of absorption; give esomeprazole at least 1 hour before meals.
■ Enteric-coated pellets can be removed from the capsule and given in applesauce as long as the enteric coating remains intact.
■ Antacids don't interfere with the absorption of esomeprazole.

### Therapeutic monitoring
■ Advise clinician to monitor liver function test results because drug is extensively metabolized by cytochrome P-450 2C19. Patients with hepatic insufficiency have a risk of elevated liver function test results.

### Special populations
**Breast-feeding patients.** It isn't known if drug appears in breast milk. It should be used cautiously, however, because omeprazole does appear in breast milk.

## Patient counseling
■ Tell patient to take drug exactly as prescribed and at least 1 hour before meals.
■ Inform patient that antacids may be used while taking this drug.
■ If patient has trouble swallowing the capsule, suggest that he open it, sprinkle contents into applesauce, and swallow applesauce immediately. Warn against crushing or chewing the drug pellets.

■ Urge patient to store capsules at room temperature in a tight container.
■ Tell patient to report continued or worsened symptoms; rash or other allergy symptoms; intended, suspected, or confirmed pregnancy; and breast-feeding or the intention to breast-feed.

# estazolam
ProSom

*Pharmacologic classification:* benzodiazepine
*Therapeutic classification:* hypnotic
*Pregnancy risk category X*
*Controlled substance schedule IV*

## Available forms
Available by prescription only
*Tablets:* 1 mg, 2 mg

## Indications and dosages
*Short-term management of insomnia characterized by difficulty falling asleep, frequent nocturnal awakenings, or early-morning awakenings*
*Adults:* Initially, 1 mg P.O. h.s.; may increase to 2 mg as needed and tolerated.
≡*Dosage adjustment.* In small or debilitated older adults, initially, 0.5 mg P.O. h.s.; may increase with care to 1 mg if needed.

## Mechanism of action
*Hypnotic action:* Estazolam depresses the CNS at the limbic and subcortical levels of the brain. It produces a sedative-hypnotic effect by potentiating the effect of the neurotransmitter gamma-aminobutyric acid on its receptor in the ascending reticular activating system, which increases inhibition and blocks both cortical and limbic arousal.

## Pharmacokinetics
*Absorption:* Rapidly and completely absorbed through the GI tract.
*Distribution:* 93% protein-bound.
*Metabolism:* Extensively metabolized in the liver.
*Excretion:* Metabolites are excreted primarily in the urine. Less than 5% is excreted in urine as unchanged drug; 4% of a 2-mg dose is excreted in feces. Elimination half-life ranges from 10 to 24 hours; clearance is accelerated in smokers.

| Route | Onset | Peak | Duration |
|-------|-------|------|----------|
| P.O. | Unknown | 1-3 hr | Unknown |

## Contraindications and precautions
Contraindicated in pregnant women or patients hypersensitive to drug.

---

Use cautiously in patients with depression, suicidal tendencies, and hepatic, renal, or pulmonary disease.

## Interactions

**Drug-drug.** *Cimetidine, disulfiram, isoniazid, and oral contraceptives:* May diminish hepatic metabolism, resulting in increased plasma levels of estazolam. Advise clinician to monitor patient for increased CNS depressant effects.

*Antihistamines, barbiturates, general anesthetics, MAO inhibitors, narcotics, phenothiazines, and tricyclic antidepressants:* Increased CNS effects. Avoid use together.

*Phenytoin and digoxin:* Increased level of these drugs, with possible toxicity. Advise clinician to monitor patient closely.

*Probenecid:* Increased benzodiazepine effect. Advise clinician to monitor patient carefully.

*Rifampin:* Increases clearance and decreases half-life of estazolam. Advise clinician to monitor patient for decrease in drug effect.

*Theophylline:* Antagonizes pharmacologic effects of estazolam. Advise clinician to monitor patient for drug effectiveness.

**Drug-herb.** *Catnip, kava, lady's slipper, lemon balm, passion flower, sassafras, skullcap, valerian:* Sedative effects may be enhanced. Discourage use together.

**Drug-lifestyle.** *Alcohol use:* May cause excessive respiratory and CNS depression. Advise patient to avoid alcohol.

*Caffeine:* May enhance CNS effects. Discourage use together.

*Smoking:* Accelerates metabolism of estazolam, resulting in diminished clinical efficacy. Advise patient to avoid smoking.

## Adverse reactions

**CNS:** fatigue, dizziness, *daytime drowsiness, somnolence, asthenia, hypokinesia, abnormal thinking.*
**GI:** dyspepsia, abdominal pain.
**Hepatic:** increased AST levels.
**Musculoskeletal:** back pain, stiffness.

## Overdose and treatment

Somnolence, confusion with reduced or absent reflexes, respiratory depression, apnea, hypotension, impaired coordination, slurred speech, seizures, or coma can occur from benzodiazepine overdose. If excitation occurs, don't use barbiturates. Several drugs may have been ingested.

Perform gastric evacuation and lavage immediately. Advise clinician to monitor respiration, pulse rate, and blood pressure. Use symptomatic and supportive measures. Maintain airway and give fluids. Flumazenil, a specific benzodiazepine antagonist, may be useful.

## Clinical considerations

■ Consider the recommendations relevant to all benzodiazepines; recommend withdrawing drug slowly after prolonged use.

### Therapeutic monitoring

■ Recommend regularly performing blood counts, urinalysis, and blood chemistry analyses.

### Special populations

**Pregnant patients.** Drug can cause harm to fetus when given during pregnancy. Safety during labor and delivery hasn't been established.
**Breast-feeding patients.** Drug appears in breast milk. Avoid use in breast-feeding women.
**Pediatric patients.** Safety and efficacy in children haven't been established.
**Geriatric patients.** Geriatric patients may be more susceptible to CNS depressant effects of estazolam. It should be used with caution. Lower dosage may be needed. To prevent injury from dizziness and falls, recommend supervising geriatric patients during daily living activities, especially when treatment starts or changes.

## Patient counseling

■ Advise the patient to avoid caffeine or other stimulants.
■ Tell patient to avoid alcohol and other CNS depressants.
■ Advise patient to immediately report if she suspects pregnancy or plans to become pregnant during therapy.
■ Warn patient that drug may cause drowsiness. Advise special caution and avoidance of driving or operating hazardous machinery until adverse CNS effects of the drug are known.
■ Caution patient not to discontinue drug abruptly after taking it daily for prolonged period and not to vary dosage or increase dosage unless prescribed. Drug should be taken until sleep pattern is established and then slowly tapered as prescribed.
■ Inform patient that nocturnal sleep may be disturbed for 1 or 2 nights after drug is stopped.

---

# esterified estrogens
Estratab, Menest

*Pharmacologic classification:* estrogen
*Therapeutic classification:* estrogen replacement, antineoplastic
*Pregnancy risk category X*

## Available forms

Available by prescription only
*Tablets:* 0.3 mg, 0.625 mg, 1.25 mg, 2.5 mg

## Indications and dosages

*Palliative treatment of advanced inoperable prostatic cancer*
*Adults:* 1.25 to 2.5 mg P.O. t.i.d.
*Breast cancer*
*Men and postmenopausal women:* 10 mg P.O. t.i.d. for 3 or more months.
*Female hypogonadism*
*Adults:* 2.5 mg P.O. daily to t.i.d. in cycles of 20 days on, 10 days off.
*Castration, primary ovarian failure*
*Adults:* 2.5 mg P.O. daily to t.i.d. in cycles of 3 weeks on, 1 week off.
*Vasomotor menopausal symptoms*
*Adults:* 0.3 to 1.25 mg P.O. daily in cycles of 3 weeks on, 1 week off; dosage may be increased to 2.5 or 3.75 mg P.O. daily, if needed.
*Atrophic vaginitis and atrophic urethritis*
*Adults:* 0.3 to 1.25 mg P.O. daily in cycles of 3 weeks on, 1 week off.

## Mechanism of action

*Estrogenic action:* Esterified estrogen mimics the action of endogenous estrogen in treating female hypogonadism, menopausal symptoms, and atrophic vaginitis. It inhibits growth of hormone-sensitive tissue in advanced, inoperable prostatic cancer and in certain carefully selected cases of breast cancer in men and postmenopausal women.

## Pharmacokinetics

*Absorption:* After oral administration, esterified estrogens are well absorbed from the GI tract.
*Distribution:* About 50% to 80% plasma protein–bound, particularly the estradiol-binding globulin. Distribution occurs throughout the body with highest levels appearing in fat.
*Metabolism:* Metabolized primarily in the liver, where estrogens are conjugated with sulfate and glucuronide.
*Excretion:* Eliminated through the kidneys in the form of sulfate or glucuronide conjugates.

| Route | Onset | Peak | Duration |
|---|---|---|---|
| P.O. | Unknown | Unknown | Unknown |

## Contraindications and precautions

Contraindicated in patients with breast cancer (except metastatic disease), estrogen-dependent neoplasia, active thrombophlebitis or thromboembolic disorders, undiagnosed abnormal genital bleeding, hypersensitivity to drug and history of thromboembolic disease, and during pregnancy or breast-feeding.

Use cautiously in patients with history of hypertension, mental depression, liver impairment, or cardiac or renal dysfunction and in those with bone disease, migraine, seizures, or diabetes mellitus.

## Interactions

**Drug-drug.** *Anticoagulants:* Decreased effects of warfarin-type anticoagulants. Advise clinician to monitor PT and INR closely.
*Corticosteroids:* Enhanced effects. Advise clinician to monitor patient's fluid and electrolyte status.
*Cyclosporine:* Increased risk of toxicity. Advise clinician to monitor patient closely.
*Dantrolene and other hepatotoxic drugs:* Increased risk of hepatotoxicity. Advise clinician to monitor patient carefully.
*Drugs that induce hepatic metabolism, such as rifampin, barbiturates, primidone, carbamazepine, and phenytoin:* Decreased estrogenic effects. Use together cautiously.
*Insulin or oral antidiabetics:* May require adjustment because estradiol may increase blood glucose levels.
*Tamoxifen:* Decreased effectiveness of tamoxifen. Advise clinician to monitor patient for drug effects.
**Drug-food.** *Caffeine:* Increased serum caffeine levels. Advise patient to avoid caffeine.
**Drug-lifestyle.** *Smoking:* Increased risk of adverse CV effects. Advise patient to avoid smoking.

## Adverse reactions

**CNS:** *increased risk of CVA,* headache, dizziness, chorea, depression, *seizures.*
**CV:** thrombophlebitis; *thromboembolism;* hypertension; edema; *pulmonary embolism, MI.*
**EENT:** worsening of myopia or astigmatism, intolerance of contact lenses.
**GI:** *nausea,* vomiting, abdominal cramps, bloating, anorexia, increased appetite, weight changes, *pancreatitis,* gallbladder disease.
**GU:** breakthrough bleeding, altered menstrual flow, dysmenorrhea, amenorrhea, *increased risk of endometrial cancer,* cervical erosion, altered cervical secretions, enlargement of uterine fibromas, vaginal candidiasis; testicular atrophy, impotence.
**Hematologic:** increased PT and INR and clotting factors VII to X and norepinephrine-induced platelet aggregability.
**Hepatic:** cholestatic jaundice, *hepatic adenoma.*
**Metabolic:** decreased serum folate, pyridoxine, and antithrombin III levels; increased triglyceride, glucose, and phospholipid levels; hypercalcemia.
**Skin:** melasma, rash, hirsutism or hair loss, erythema nodosum, dermatitis.
**Other:** in women, *possibility of increased risk of breast cancer,* breast changes (tenderness, enlargement, secretion); gynecomastia.

## Overdose and treatment

Serious toxicity after overdose of these drugs hasn't been reported. Nausea may occur. Provide appropriate supportive care.

## Clinical considerations
■ Clinical considerations are the same as for all estrogens.

### Therapeutic monitoring
■ Therapeutic monitoring is the same as for all estrogens.

### Special populations
**Pregnant patients.** Drug is contraindicated during pregnancy.
**Breast-feeding patients.** Esterified estrogens are contraindicated in breast-feeding women.

### Patient counseling
■ Patient counseling is the same as for all estrogens.

## estradiol
Alora, Climara, Estrace, Estrace Vaginal Cream, Estraderm, Estring, Vivelle

## estradiol cypionate
depGynogen, Depo-Estradiol Cypionate, Depogen, Estro-Cyp, Estrofem

## estradiol valerate
Delestrogen*, Dioval 40, Dioval XX, Estra-L 40, Gynogen L.A. 10, Gynogen L.A. 20, Valergen-20

## polyestradiol phosphate
Estradurin

*Pharmacologic classification:* estrogen
*Therapeutic classification:* estrogen replacement, antineoplastic
*Pregnancy risk category X*

### Available forms
Available by prescription only
**estradiol**
*Tablets:* 0.5 mg, 1 mg, 2 mg
*Vaginal:* 0.1 mg/g cream (in nonliquefying base)
*Transdermal:* 4 mg/10 cm² (delivers 0.05 mg/24 hours); 8 mg/20 cm² (delivers 0.1 mg/24 hours)
*Ring:* 2 mg (0.0075 mg/24 hours)
**estradiol cypionate**
*Injection:* 5 mg/ml (in oil)
**estradiol valerate**
*Injection:* 10 mg/ml, 20 mg/ml, 40 mg/ml (in oil)
**polyestradiol phosphate**
*Injection:* 40 mg/2 ml

### Indications and dosages
*Atrophic vaginitis, atrophic dystrophy of the vulva, vasomotor menopausal symp-*
*toms, hypogonadism, female castration, primary ovarian failure*
**estradiol (tablets)**
*Adults:* 1 to 2 mg P.O. daily, in cycles of 21 days on and 7 days off or cycles of 5 days on and 2 days off.
**estradiol (transdermal)**
*Adults:* Place one transdermal patch delivering 0.05 mg/24hours on trunk of the body, preferably the abdomen, twice weekly. Give on an intermittent cyclic schedule (3 weeks on and 1 week off). Subsequent dosage should be adjusted according to the patient's therapeutic response.
**estradiol cypionate**
*Adults:* 1 to 5 mg I.M. every 3 to 4 weeks.
**estradiol valerate**
*Adults:* 10 to 20 mg I.M. once a month.
*Atrophic vaginitis*
**estradiol (vaginal ring)**
*Adults:* Insert ring as deeply as possible into the upper third of the vaginal vault. The ring should remain in place for 3 months.
**estradiol (vaginal cream)**
*Adults:* 2 to 4 g daily for 1 to 2 weeks. When vaginal mucosa is restored, begin maintenance dose of 1 g one to three times weekly.
*Female hypogonadism*
**estradiol cypionate**
*Adults:* 1.5 to 2 mg I.M. at monthly intervals.
**estradiol valerate**
*Adults:* 10 to 20 mg I.M. q 4 weeks p.r.n.
*Inoperable breast cancer*
**estradiol (tablets)**
*Adults:* 10 mg P.O. t.i.d. for 3 months.
*Inoperable prostatic cancer*
**estradiol valerate**
*Adults:* 30 mg I.M. q 1 to 2 weeks.
**estradiol (tablets)**
*Adults:* 1 to 2 mg P.O. t.i.d.
**polyestradiol phosphate**
*Adults:* 40 mg I.M. q 2 to 4 weeks.
*Prevention of postmenopausal osteoporosis*
**estradiol (tablets)**
*Adults:* 0.5 mg P.O. daily in a cyclic regimen (21 days on and 7 days off).
**estradiol (transdermal)**
*Adults:* One system (Estraderm) 0.05 mg/24 hours or Vivelle (0.025 mg/24 hours) twice weekly in a cyclic regimen for a woman with an intact uterus, in a continuous regimen for a woman who has undergone a hysterectomy. Or one Climara (0.025 mg/24 hours) applied once weekly.

### Mechanism of action
*Estrogenic action:* Estradiol mimics the action of endogenous estrogen in treating female hypogonadism, menopausal symptoms, and atrophic vaginitis. It inhibits growth of hormone-sensitive tissue in advanced, inoperable prostatic cancer and in certain carefully selected cases

of breast cancer in men and postmenopausal women.

## Pharmacokinetics

*Absorption:* After oral administration, estradiol and other natural, unconjugated estrogens are well absorbed but substantially inactivated by the liver. Therefore, unconjugated estrogens are usually given parenterally.

After I.M. administration, absorption begins rapidly and continues for days. The cypionate and valerate esters administered in oil have prolonged durations of action because of their slow absorption characteristics.

Topically applied estradiol is absorbed readily into the systemic circulation.

*Distribution:* Estradiol and other natural estrogens are about 50% to 80% plasma protein–bound, particularly the estradiol-binding globulin. Distribution occurs throughout the body, with highest levels appearing in fat.

*Metabolism:* Steroidal estrogens, including estradiol, are metabolized primarily in the liver, where they are conjugated with sulfate and glucuronide. Because of the rapid rate of metabolism, nonesterified forms of estrogen, including estradiol, must usually be given daily.

*Excretion:* The majority of estrogen elimination occurs through the kidneys in the form of sulfate or glucuronide conjugates.

| Route | Onset | Peak | Duration |
|---|---|---|---|
| P.O., I.M., transdermal, intravaginal | Unknown | Unknown | Unknown |

## Contraindications and precautions

Contraindicated in patients with thrombophlebitis or thromboembolic disorders, estrogen-dependent neoplasia, breast or reproductive organ cancer (except for palliative treatment), or undiagnosed abnormal genital bleeding and during pregnancy. Also contraindicated in patients with history of thrombophlebitis or thromboembolic disorders from previous estrogen use (except for palliative treatment of breast and prostate cancer).

Use cautiously in patients with cerebrovascular or coronary artery disease, asthma, bone diseases, migraine, seizures, or cardiac, hepatic, or renal dysfunction and in women with a strong family history of breast cancer or who have breast nodules, fibrocystic disease, or abnormal mammographic findings.

## Interactions

**Drug-drug.** *Corticosteroids:* May cause enhanced effects. Advise clinician to monitor patient closely.

*Cyclosporine:* May increase risk of toxicity. Advise clinician to monitor patient and cyclosprine levels frequently.

*Dantrolene, other hepatotoxic medications:* May increase risk of hepatotoxicity. Advise clinician to monitor patient closely.

*Drugs that induce hepatic metabolism, such as barbiturates, carbamazepine, phenytoin, primidone, and rifampin:* Decreased estrogenic effects from a given dose. These drugs are known to accelerate the rate of metabolism of certain other drugs. Advise clinician to monitor patient closely.

*Insulin or oral antidiabetic agents:* May require adjustment because drug affects blood glucose.

*Tamoxifen:* Decreased effects of tamoxifen. Advise clinician to monitor patient closely.

*Warfarin-type anticoagulants:* Decreased anticoagulant effect. Dosage adjustment may be needed.

**Drug-food.** *Caffeine:* May increase serum caffeine levels. Advise patient to avoid caffeine.

*Grapefruit juice:* Elevated estrogen levels. Take with liquid other than grapefruit juice.

**Drug-lifestyle.** *Smoking:* Increases risk of adverse CV effects. Advise patient to avoid smoking.

## Adverse reactions

**CNS:** *CVA,* headache, dizziness, chorea, depression, *seizures.*

**CV:** thrombophlebitis, *thromboembolism,* hypertension, edema, *pulmonary embolism, MI.*

**EENT:** worsening of myopia or astigmatism, intolerance of contact lenses.

**GI:** *nausea,* vomiting, abdominal cramps, bloating, anorexia, increased appetite, weight changes, *pancreatitis,* gallbladder disease.

**GU:** in women, breakthrough bleeding, altered menstrual flow, dysmenorrhea, amenorrhea, *increased risk of endometrial cancer,* cervical erosion, altered cervical secretions, enlargement of uterine fibromas, vaginal candidiasis; in men, testicular atrophy, impotence.

**Hematologic:** increased PT and INR and clotting factors VII to X and norepinephrine-induced platelet aggregability.

**Hepatic:** cholestatic jaundice, *hepatic adenoma.*

**Metabolic:** decreased serum folate, pyridoxine, and antithrombin III levels; increased triglyceride, glucose, and phospholipid levels; hypercalcemia.

**Skin:** melasma, rash, hirsutism or hair loss, erythema nodosum, dermatitis.

**Other:** *possibility of increased risk of breast cancer,* breast changes (tenderness, enlargement, secretion); gynecomastia.

## Overdose and treatment

Serious toxicity after overdose of drug hasn't been reported. Nausea may occur. Recommend providing appropriate supportive care.

---

## Clinical considerations
- Clinical considerations are the same as for all other estrogen products.

### Therapeutic monitoring
- Consider the recommendations for all estrogen products; recommend monitoring patch site for skin reactions when using transdermal form of drug administration.

### Special populations
**Pregnant patients.** Drug is contraindicated in pregnant women.
**Breast-feeding patients.** Drug is contraindicated in breast-feeding women.
**Geriatric patients.** Frequent physical examinations are recommended in postmenopausal women taking estrogen.

## Patient counseling
- Tell patient not to apply patch to breast area.
- Remind patient not to use the same skin site for at least 1 week after removal of the transdermal system.

---

# estradiol/norethindrone acetate transdermal system
CombiPatch

*Pharmacologic classification:* estrogen/progestin
*Therapeutic classification:* postmenopausal drug
*Pregnancy risk category X*

## Available forms
Available by prescription only
*Transdermal:* 9-cm$^2$ system (0.05 mg estradiol and 0.14 mg norethindrone); 16-cm$^2$ system (0.05 mg estradiol and 0.25 mg norethindrone)

## Indications and dosages
*Moderate-to-severe vasomotor symptoms associated with menopause, vulvar and vaginal atrophy, and hypoestrogenemia caused by hypogonadism, castration, or primary ovarian failure in women with an intact uterus*
*Adults: Continuous combined regimen*—9-cm$^2$ patch worn continuously on the lower abdomen. Remove old system and apply new system twice weekly during a 28-day cycle. May increase to 16-cm$^2$ patch if more progestin is desired.
*Continuous sequential regimen*—patch can be applied as a sequential regimen with an estradiol-only transdermal system (such as Alora, Esclim, Estraderm, Vivelle). A 0.05-mg estradiol-only transdermal patch is worn for first 14 days of a 28-day cycle; replace system twice weekly according to product directions.

For remainder of 28-day cycle, apply the 9-cm$^2$ patch system to the lower abdomen and replace twice weekly. May increase to 16-cm$^2$ patch if more progestin is desired.

Women not currently receiving continuous estrogen or estrogen/progestin therapy may start therapy at any time.

Women currently receiving continuous hormone replacement therapy should complete the current cycle of therapy before starting new therapy. Women often experience withdrawal bleeding at the completion of the cycle; the first day of withdrawal bleeding would be an appropriate time to start therapy.

## Mechanism of action
*Hormone action:* Estrogen replacement therapy can reduce the frequency of menopausal symptoms by replacing the naturally declining levels that occur in postmenopausal women.

## Pharmacokinetics
*Absorption:* Estradiol and norethindrone are well absorbed transdermally.
*Distribution:* Estradiol is primarily bound to sex hormone–binding protein (SHBG) and norethindrone is primarily bound to albumin and SHBG.
*Metabolism:* Estradiol is minimally metabolized. Norethindrone is metabolized primarily by the liver.
*Excretion:* Elimination half-life of estradiol is 2 to 3 hours; of norethindrone, 6 to 8 hours.

| Route | Onset | Peak | Duration |
|-------|-------|------|----------|
| Transdermal | 12-24 hr | Unknown | Unknown |

## Contraindications and precautions
Contraindicated in women who may be pregnant; have known or suspected breast cancer, known or suspected estrogen-dependent neoplasia, undiagnosed abnormal genital bleeding, active thrombophlebitis, thromboembolic disorders, or CVA; or those hypersensitive to estrogen, progestin, or any component of the patch.

Use cautiously in patients with impaired liver function, asthma, epilepsy, migraine, and cardiac or renal dysfunction.

## Interactions
None reported.

## Adverse reactions
**CNS:** *asthenia,* depression, insomnia, nervousness, dizziness, *headache.*
**CV:** peripheral edema.
**EENT:** *pharyngitis, rhinitis, sinusitis.*
**GI:** *abdominal pain, diarrhea,* dyspepsia, flatulence, *nausea,* constipation.
**GU:** *dysmenorrhea, leukorrhea, menstrual disorder,* suspicious Papanicolaou test, *vaginitis,* menorrhagia, vaginal hemorrhage.

---

**Hematologic:** INR, aPTT, and platelet aggregation times may be altered; platelet count and fibrinogen activity may increase.
**Musculoskeletal:** arthralgia, *back pain*.
**Respiratory:** *respiratory disorder*, bronchitis.
**Skin:** application site reactions, acne.
**Other:** *accidental injury, flu syndrome, pain, breast pain*, breast enlargement, infection, tooth disorder.

## Overdose and treatment
Nausea and withdrawal bleeding are the most common consequences of overdose.

Treatment should involve discontinuation or removal of the patch. Medical treatment may be initiated.

## Clinical considerations
■ Store norethindrone patches in refrigerator before dispensing. Once dispensed, system may be stored at a temperature below 77° F (25° C) for up to 3 months.
■ Combination estrogen/progestin regimens are indicated for women with an intact uterus.
■ Progestins taken with estrogen drugs significantly reduce, but don't eliminate, the risk of endometrial cancer from the use of estrogen.
■ Drug may cause a reduced response to the metyrapone test and sulfobromophthalein retention. Increased thyroid-binding globulin may lead to increased total $T_3$ and $T_4$ levels and decreased $T_3$ resin uptake. Free $T_4$ and $T_3$ levels are unaffected.

### Therapeutic monitoring
■ Hormonal therapy should be reevaluated every 3 to 6 months.
■ Estrogen use may cause BP increases. Advise clinician to monitor patient's blood pressure regularly.

### Special populations
**Pregnant patients.** Contraindicated during pregnancy.
**Breast-feeding patients.** Estrogen and progestin appear in breast milk. The patch shouldn't be used during breast-feeding.

## Patient counseling
■ Instruct patient to apply patch system to a smooth (fold-free), clean, dry, nonirritated area of skin on the lower abdomen, avoiding the waistline. Application sites should be rotated, with an interval of at least 1 week between applications to the same site.
■ Don't apply patch on or near the breasts.
■ Advise patient of potential for adverse events.
■ Tell patient she may store patches at room temperature for up to 3 months.

# estramustine phosphate sodium
Emcyt

*Pharmacologic classification:* estrogen, alkylating agent
*Therapeutic classification:* antineoplastic
*Pregnancy risk category NR*

## Available forms
Available by prescription only
*Capsules:* 140 mg

## Indications and dosages
Dosage and indications may vary. Check literature for recommended protocols.
*Palliative treatment of metastatic or progressive cancer of the prostate*
*Adults:* 10 to 16 mg/kg P.O. in three or four divided doses. Usual dose is 14 mg/kg daily. Therapy should continue for up to 3 months and, if successful, be maintained as long as patient responds.

## Mechanism of action
*Antineoplastic action:* Exact mechanism of action is unclear. However, the estrogenic portion of the molecule may act as a carrier of the drug to facilitate selective uptake by tumor cells with estradiol hormone receptors, such as those in the prostate gland. At that point, the nitrogen mustard portion of the drug acts as an alkylating agent.

## Pharmacokinetics
*Absorption:* After oral administration, about 75% of a dose is absorbed across the GI tract.
*Distribution:* Estramustine is distributed widely into body tissues.
*Metabolism:* Extensively metabolized in the liver.
*Excretion:* Drug and its metabolites are eliminated primarily in feces, with a small amount excreted in urine. Terminal phase of plasma elimination has a half-life of 20 hours.

| Route | Onset | Peak | Duration |
|-------|-------|------|----------|
| P.O. | Unknown | Unknown | Unknown |

## Contraindications and precautions
Contraindicated in patients hypersensitive to estradiol and nitrogen mustard and in those with active thrombophlebitis or thromboembolic disorders, except when the actual tumor mass is the cause of the thromboembolic phenomenon. Contraindicated in pregnant and breast-feeding women.

Use cautiously in patients with history of thrombophlebitis or thromboembolic disorders and cerebrovascular or coronary artery disease.

## Interactions
**Drug-drug.** *Anticoagulants:* Decreased anticoagulant effect. May require increased dosage of anticoagulants.
*Calcium-containing drugs, such as antacids:* Impaired absorption of estramustine. They shouldn't be taken together.
**Drug-food.** *Calcium-rich foods, such as milk and dairy products:* May impair absorption of estramustine. Drug shouldn't be taken with these foods.

## Adverse reactions
**CNS:** *CVA,* lethargy, insomnia, headache, anxiety.
**CV:** chest pain, *MI,* sodium and fluid retention, thrombophlebitis, *HF, edema.*
**GI:** *nausea, vomiting,* diarrhea, anorexia, flatulence, GI bleeding, thirst.
**Hematologic:** *leukopenia, thrombocytopenia,* increased norepinephrine-induced platelet aggregability.
**Hepatic:** elevated liver enzyme levels.
**Metabolic:** decreased serum folate, pyridoxine, phosphate, and pregnanediol levels; increased ceruloplasmin, cortisol, prolactin PT, sodium, triglyceride, and phospholipid levels.
**Musculoskeletal:** leg cramps.
**Respiratory:** *pulmonary embolism,* dyspnea.
**Skin:** rash, pruritus, dry skin, flushing, thinning of hair.
**Other:** *painful gynecomastia and breast tenderness.*

## Overdose and treatment
Signs and symptoms of overdose include headache, nausea, vomiting, and myelosuppression.
Treatment is usually supportive and includes induction of emesis, gastric lavage, transfusion of blood components, and appropriate symptomatic therapy. Hematologic monitoring should continue for at least 6 weeks after the ingestion.

## Clinical considerations
- Store capsules in refrigerator.
- Phenothiazines can be used to treat nausea and vomiting.
- Estramustine may cause hypertension.
- Drug may exaggerate preexisting peripheral edema or HF.
- Estramustine therapy may cause a reduced response to the metyrapone test. Glucose tolerance may be decreased.

### Therapeutic monitoring
- Advise clinician to monitor blood pressure at baseline and routinely during therapy.
- Advise clinician to monitor glucose tolerance periodically during therapy.
- Patients may continue estramustine as long as they're responding favorably. Some patients have taken drug for longer than 3 years.

- Advise clinician to monitor weight gain regularly in these patients.

### Special populations
**Pregnant patients.** Drug is contraindicated during pregnancy.
**Breast-feeding patients.** Drug is contraindicated in breast-feeding women.
**Geriatric patients.** Use with caution in geriatric patients, who are more likely to have vascular disorders, because the use of estrogen is associated with vascular complications.

## Patient counseling
- Emphasize importance of continuing drug despite nausea and vomiting.
- Advise patient to call immediately if vomiting occurs shortly after a dose is taken.
- Because of possibility of mutagenic effects, advise patients of childbearing age to use contraceptive measures.

# estrogen and progestin
Alesse-28, Apri, Avaine, Brevicon, Cyclessa, Demulen 1/35, Demulen 1/50, Desogen, Enpresse, Estrostep, Loestrin 21 1/20, Loestrin 21 1.5/30, Loestrin Fe 1/20, Loestrin Fe 1.5/30, Lo/Ovral, Lo/Ovral-28, Modicon 21, Modicon 28, Nordette-21, Nordette-28, Norinyl 1+35 21-Day, Norinyl 1+35 28-Day, Norinyl 1+50 21-Day, Norinyl 1+50 28-Day, Norinyl 1+80 28-Day, Ortho-Novum 1/35 21, Ortho-Novum 1/35 28, Ortho-Novum 1/50 21, Ortho-Novum 1/50 28, Ortho-Novum 7/7/7-21, Ortho-Novum 7/7/7-28, Ortho-Novum 10/11-21, Ortho-Novum 10/11-28, Ovcon-35, Ovcon-50, Ovral, Ovral-28, Tri-Norinyl-21, Tri-Norinyl-28, Triphasil-21, Triphasil-28, Yasmin

*Pharmacologic classification:* estrogen with progestin
*Therapeutic classification:* contraceptive (hormonal)
*Pregnancy risk category X*

## Available forms
Available by prescription only
**Tablets—monophasic type**
Ethinyl estradiol 0.03 mg and desogestrel 0.15 mg
Ethinyl estradiol 0.03 mg and drosperinone 3 mg
Ethinyl estradiol 0.035 mg and ethynodiol diacetate 1 mg
Ethinyl estradiol 0.05 mg and ethynodiol diacetate 1 mg
Ethinyl estradiol 0.02 mg and levonorgestrel 0.1 mg
Ethinyl estradiol 0.03 mg and levonorgestrel 0.15 mg

Ethinyl estradiol 0.02 mg and norethindrone 1 mg
Ethinyl estradiol 0.035 mg and norethindrone 0.4 mg
Ethinyl estradiol 0.035 mg and norethindrone 0.5 mg
Ethinyl estradiol 0.035 mg and norethindrone 1 mg
Ethinyl estradiol 0.05 mg and norethindrone 1 mg
Ethinyl estradiol 0.05 mg and norethindrone acetate 1 mg
Ethinyl estradiol 0.03 mg and norethindrone acetate 1.5 mg
Ethinyl estradiol 0.05 mg and norethindrone acetate 2.5 mg
Ethinyl estradiol 0.03 mg and norgestrel 0.3 mg
Ethinyl estradiol 0.05 mg and norgestrel 0.5 mg
Mestranol 0.1 mg and ethynodiol diacetate 1 mg
Mestranol 0.1 mg and norethindrone 2 mg
Mestranol 0.05 mg and norethindrone 1 mg
Mestranol 0.08 mg and norethindrone 1 mg
Mestranol 0.1 mg and norethynodrel 2.5 mg
**Tablets—biphasic type**
10 tablets ethinyl estradiol 0.035 mg and norethindrone 0.5 mg; 11 tablets ethinyl estradiol 0.035 mg and norethindrone 1 mg
**Tablets—triphasic type**
7 tablets ethinyl estradiol 0.035 mg and norethindrone 0.5 mg; 9 tablets ethinyl estradiol 0.035 mg and norethindrone 1 mg; 5 tablets ethinyl estradiol 0.035 mg and norethindrone 0.5 mg
7 tablets ethinyl estradiol 0.035 mg and norethindrone 0.5 mg; 7 tablets ethinyl estradiol 0.035 mg and norethindrone 0.75 mg; 7 tablets ethinyl estradiol 0.035 mg and norethindrone 1 mg
6 tablets ethinyl estradiol 0.03 and levonorgestrel 0.05 mg; 5 tablets ethinyl estradiol 0.04 mg and levonorgestrel 0.075 mg; 10 tablets ethinyl estradiol 0.03 mg and levonorgestrel 0.125 mg
0.1 mg desogestrel with 25 mcg ethinyl estradiol (7 tablets); 0.125 mg desogestrel with 25 mcg ethinyl estradiol (7 tablets); 0.15 mg desogestrel with 25 mcg ethinyl estradiol (7 tablets)
0.02 mg ethinyl estradiol and 1 mg norethindrone acetate (5 tablets), 0.03 mg ethinyl estradiol and 1 mg norethindrone acetate (7 tablets), 0.035 mg ethinyl estradiol and 1 mg norethindrone acetate (9 tablets)

## Indications and dosages
*Contraception*
**Monophasic**
*Adults:* One tablet P.O. daily, beginning on day 5 of menstrual cycle (first day of menstrual flow is day 1), or on the first Sunday after onset of menstruation, or on day 1 of menstrual cycle depending on specific contraceptive. With 20- and 21-tablet packages, new dosing cycle

begins 7 days after last tablet was taken. With 28-tablet packages, dosage is one tablet daily without interruption; extra tablets are placebos or contain iron. If next menstrual period doesn't begin on schedule, rule out pregnancy before starting new dosing cycle. If menstrual period begins, start new dosing cycle 7 days after last tablet was taken. If all doses have been taken on schedule and one menstrual period is missed, continue dosing cycle. If two consecutive menstrual periods are missed, pregnancy test is required before new dosing cycle is started.
**Biphasic**
*Adults:* One color tablet P.O. daily (Ortho-Novum 10/11) for 10 days, then next color tablet for 11 days.
**Triphasic**
*Adults:* One tablet P.O. daily (Ortho-Novum 7/7/7, Tri-Norinyl, Triphasil, Estrostep, Cyclessa, Enpresse) in the sequence specified by the manufacturer.
*Hypermenorrhea*
*Adults:* Use high-dose combinations only. Dosage is same as for contraception.
*Endometriosis*
*Adults: Cyclic therapy:* One 10-mg tablet P.O. daily (Ortho-Novum) for 20 days from day 5 to day 24 of menstrual cycle. *Suppressive therapy:* One 5- or 10-mg tablet P.O. daily (Enovid) for 2 weeks, starting on day 5 of menstrual cycle. Continue without interruption for 6 to 9 months, increasing dose by 5 to 10 mg q 2 weeks, up to 20 mg daily. Up to 40 mg daily may be needed if breakthrough bleeding occurs.
*Treatment of women with moderate acne vulgaris with no contraindications to oral contraceptives, who desire oral contraception, have achieved menarche, and don't respond to topical antiacne drug*
*Women ages 15 and older:* 1 tablet P.O. daily (Estrostep).

## Mechanism of action
*Contraceptive action:* Estrogen components of oral contraceptives inhibit the release of follicle-stimulating hormone, thereby stopping follicular development and suppressing ovulation.
   Progestin components of oral contraceptives inhibit the release of luteinizing hormone, preventing ovulation even in the event of incomplete suppression of follicular development. Progestins also change the endometrial environment to inhibit nidation (implantation of the fertilized egg into the endometrium) and cause thickening of the cervical mucus, blocking the upward migration of sperm.

## Pharmacokinetics
*Absorption:* Most components of oral contraceptives are absorbed relatively well from the GI tract. Bioavailabilities range from 40% to

70%; considerable individual variation exists in extent of absorption.

*Distribution:* Protein-binding of the various drugs used in oral contraceptives is high, ranging from 80% to 98%. These drugs are distributed extensively into virtually all body tissues.

*Metabolism:* These drugs undergo metabolic transformation before excretion; their rates of metabolism may thus be affected by drugs that induce or inhibit metabolism.

*Excretion:* Very little, if any, is excreted unchanged in urine or feces. They appear primarily as sulfate and glucuronide conjugates.

| Route | Onset | Peak | Duration |
|-------|-------|------|----------|
| P.O. | Unknown | 1-2 hr | Unknown |

## Contraindications and precautions

Oral contraceptives are contraindicated in patients with thromboembolic disorders, cerebrovascular or coronary artery disease, or MI because of their association with thromboembolic disease; in patients with known or suspected cancer of the breast or reproductive organs or with benign or malignant liver tumors because of their association with tumorigenesis; in patients with undiagnosed abnormal vaginal bleeding; in women known or believed to be pregnant or breast-feeding; in adolescents with incomplete epiphyseal closure; and in women smokers older than age 35.

Use oral contraceptives cautiously in patients with systemic lupus erythematosus, hypertension, mental depression, migraine, epilepsy, asthma, diabetes mellitus, amenorrhea, scanty or irregular periods, fibrocystic breast disease, family history (mother, grandmother, sister) of breast or genital tract cancer, or renal or gallbladder disease. Advise patient to report development or worsening of any of these conditions. Prolonged therapy may be inadvisable in women who plan to become pregnant.

## Interactions

**Drug-drug.** *Aminoglutethimide, ampicillin, antihistamines, barbiturates, carbamazepine, chloramphenicol, griseofulvin, isoniazid, neomycin, nitrofurantoin, penicillin V, phenylbutazone, phenytoin, primidone, rifampin, sulfonamides, and tetracycline:* Increased metabolism of oral contraceptives, resulting in reduced efficacy, breakthrough bleeding, and occasionally contraceptive failure. Advise clinician to monitor patient for drug effects and encourage use of alternative contraceptive.

*Insulin or oral antidiabetic agents:* Serum glucose may be affected; dosage adjustment may be needed.

*Oral warfarin-type anticoagulants and anticonvulsants, antihypertensives, and tricyclic antidepressants:* Adverse effects may occur. Avoid use together.

**Drug-herb.** *Red clover:* May interfere with hormonal therapies. Avoid use together.

*St. John's wort:* Possible decreased efficacy of the oral contraceptive, caused by increased hepatic metabolism. Avoid use together, if possible. If concurrent use cannot be avoided, consider an additional method of contraception.

**Drug-food.** *Caffeine:* May increase serum caffeine levels. Advise patient to avoid caffeine.

**Drug-lifestyle.** *Smoking:* Increases risk of CV effects. Advise patient not to smoke.

## Adverse reactions

**CNS:** headache, dizziness, depression, lethargy, migraine.

**CV:** ***thromboembolism,*** hypertension, edema, increase in varicosities.

**EENT:** worsening of myopia or astigmatism, intolerance of contact lenses, unexplained loss of vision, optic neuritis, diplopia, retinal thrombosis, papilledema.

**GI:** *nausea, vomiting,* abdominal cramps, bloating, diarrhea, constipation, changes in appetite, bowel ischemia, granulomatous colitis.

**GU:** breakthrough bleeding, dysmenorrhea, amenorrhea, cervical erosion or abnormal secretions, enlargement of uterine fibromas, vaginal candidiasis, urinary tract infections.

**Hematologic:** increased prothrombin and clotting factors VII to X, plasminogen, norepinephrine-induced platelet aggregation, fibrinogen; decreased antithrombin III.

**Hepatic:** gallbladder disease, cholestatic jaundice, *liver tumors.*

**Metabolic:** hyperglycemia, hypercalcemia, folic acid deficiency; increased sulfobromophthalein retention, thyroid-binding globulin, triglycerides, phospholipids, transcortin and corticosteroids, transferrin, prolactin, renin, and vitamin A; decreased metyrapone, pregnanediol excretion, free $T_3$ resin uptake, glucose tolerance, zinc, and vitamin $B_{12}$; weight gain.

**Skin:** rash, acne, seborrhea, oily skin, erythema multiforme, hyperpigmentation.

**Other:** libido changes, possible increased risk of congenital anomalies, breast tenderness, enlargement, or secretion.

Note: Adverse effects may be more serious, frequent, and rapid in onset with high-dose than with low-dose combinations.

## Overdose and treatment

Serious toxicity after drug overdose hasn't been reported. Nausea and vomiting, as well as withdrawal bleeding, may occur.

## Clinical considerations

■ Astigmatic error and myopic refractive error may be increased twofold to threefold, usually after 6 months of oral contraceptive therapy.

■ If patient becomes hypersensitive, recommend stopping the drug.

■ Changes in ocular contour and lubricant quality of tears may necessitate change in size and shape of contact lenses.

### Therapeutic monitoring

■ Therapeutic monitoring considerations are the same as those relevant to all estrogens and progestins.

■ Breakthrough bleeding in patients taking high-dose estrogen-progestin combinations for menstrual disorders may necessitate dosage adjustment.

### Special populations

**Pregnant patients.** Drug is contraindicated during pregnancy.

**Breast-feeding patients.** Oral contraceptives are contraindicated in breast-feeding women.

**Pediatric patients.** To avoid later fertility and menstrual problems, hormonal contraception isn't advised for the adolescent until after at least 2 years of well-established menstrual cycles and completion of physiologic maturation. An estrogen-dominant drug is the best choice for the adolescent with scanty menses, moderate or severe acne, or candidiasis. A progestin-dominant drug is the best choice for the adolescent with dysmenorrhea, hypermenorrhea, fibrocystic breast disease, or cyclic premenstrual weight gain.

### Patient counseling

■ Advise patient of potential adverse reactions and inform her that these should diminish after 3 to 6 dosing cycles (months).

■ Advise patient to use an additional method of birth control for the first week of the initial cycle (unless using day-1 start).

■ Instruct patient to take drug at the same time each day at 24-hour intervals for efficacy of drug, to keep tablets in original container, and to take them in correct (color-coded) sequence.

■ Tell patient that night-time dosing may reduce risk of nausea and headaches.

■ Suggest taking drug with or immediately after food to reduce nausea.

■ Stress importance of annual Papanicolaou smears and gynecologic examinations while taking estrogen-progestin combinations.

■ Advise patient of increased risk of serious CV adverse effects from simultaneous use of cigarettes and oral contraceptives. Strongly advise women who use oral contraceptives not to smoke.

■ Instruct patient as follows regarding missed doses:

**Monophasic or biphasic cycles**

For 20-, 21-, or 24-day dosing schedule:

■ If one regular dose is missed, take tablet as soon as possible; if remembered on the next day, take two tablets, then continue regular dosing schedule.

■ If two consecutive days are missed, take two tablets a day for next 2 days, then resume regular dosing schedule.

■ If 3 consecutive days are missed, discontinue drug and substitute other contraceptive method until period begins or pregnancy is ruled out. Then start new cycle of tablets.

For 28-day dosing schedule:

■ Follow instructions for 21-day dosing schedule; if one of the last seven tablets is missed, be sure to take first tablet of next month's cycle on regularly scheduled day.

**Triphasic cycle**

For 21-day dosing schedule:

■ If 1 day is missed, take dose as soon as possible; if remembered on the next day, take two tablets, then continue regular dosing schedule while using additional method of contraception for remainder of cycle.

■ If 2 consecutive days are missed, take two tablets daily for next 2 days, then continue regular schedule while using additional contraceptive method for remainder of cycle.

■ If 3 consecutive days are missed, discontinue drug and use other contraceptive method until period begins or pregnancy is ruled out. Then start new cycle of tablets.

For 28-day dosing schedule:

■ Follow instructions for 21-day dosing schedule; if one of the last seven tablets was missed, be sure to take first tablet of next month's cycle on regularly scheduled day.

---

## estrogenic substances, conjugated

Cenestin, Premarin

*Pharmacologic classification:* estrogen
*Therapeutic classification:* estrogen replacement, antineoplastic, antiosteoporotic
*Pregnancy risk category X*

### Available forms

Available by prescription only
*Tablets:* 0.3 mg, 0.625 mg, 0.9 mg, 1.25 mg, 2.5 mg
*Injection:* 25 mg/5 ml
*Vaginal cream:* 0.0625%

### Indications and dosages

*Abnormal uterine bleeding (hormonal imbalance)*
*Adults:* 25 mg I.V. or I.M. Repeat dose in 6 to 12 hours, if needed.

*Castration and primary ovarian failure*
*Adults:* Initially, 1.25 mg P.O. daily in cycles of 3 weeks on, 1 week off. Adjust dosage p.r.n.

*Prevention of osteoporosis*
*Adults:* 0.625 mg P.O. daily given continuously, or cyclically, 25 days on, 5 days off.

*Female hypogonadism*
*Adults:* 0.3 to 0.625 mg P.O. daily, given cyclically 3 weeks on, 1 week off.
*Vasomotor menopausal symptoms*
*Adults:* 0.625 mg P.O. daily, or cyclically 25 days on, 5 days off. Or, synthetic conjugated estrogens A 0.625 mg P.O. daily in a continuous regimen, up to 1.25 mg daily if needed.
*Atrophic vaginitis or kraurosis vulvae*
*Adults:* 0.3 to 1.25 mg or more P.O. daily. Alternatively, 0.5 to 2 g intravaginally or topically once daily in cycles of 3 weeks on, 1 week off.
*Palliative treatment of inoperable prostatic cancer*
*Adults:* 1.25 to 2.5 mg P.O. t.i.d.
*Palliative treatment of breast cancer*
*Adults:* 10 mg P.O. t.i.d. for 3 months or longer.

## I.V. administration
■ Refrigerate before reconstitution.
■ Reconstituted drug may be safely stored in refrigeration for up to 60 days.
■ Administer slowly to avoid the occurrence of a flushing reaction.

### Incompatibilities
Incompatible with ascorbic acid, protein hydrolysate, or any solution with an acidic pH.

## Mechanism of action
*Estrogenic action:* Conjugated estrogenic substances mimic the action of endogenous estrogen in treating female hypogonadism, menopausal symptoms, and atrophic vaginitis. They inhibit growth of hormone-sensitive tissue in advanced, inoperable prostatic cancer and in certain carefully selected cases of breast cancer in men and postmenopausal women; they also retard progression of osteoporosis by enhancing calcium and phosphate retention and limiting bone decalcification.

## Pharmacokinetics
*Absorption:* Not well characterized. After I.M. administration, absorption begins rapidly and continues for days.
*Distribution:* Conjugated estrogens are about 50% to 80% plasma protein–bound and distributed throughout the body, with highest levels appearing in fat.
*Metabolism:* Conjugated estrogens are metabolized primarily in the liver, where they are conjugated with sulfate and glucuronide. Because of the rapid rate of metabolism, nonesterified forms of estrogen, including estradiol, must usually be given daily.
*Excretion:* The majority of estrogen elimination occurs through the kidneys, in the form of sulfate or glucuronide conjugates, or both.

| Route | Onset | Peak | Duration |
|---|---|---|---|
| P.O., I.V., I.M., intravaginal | Unknown | Unknown | Unknown |

## Contraindications and precautions
Contraindicated in patients with thrombophlebitis or thromboembolic disorders, estrogen-dependent neoplasia, breast or reproductive organ cancer (except for palliative treatment), or undiagnosed abnormal genital bleeding and during pregnancy.

Use cautiously in patients with cerebrovascular or coronary artery disease, asthma, bone disease, migraine, seizures, or cardiac, hepatic, or renal dysfunction or in women with family history (mother, grandmother, sister) of breast or genital tract cancer or who have breast nodules, fibrocystic disease, or abnormal mammographic findings.

## Interactions
**Drug-drug.** *Corticosteroids:* Enhanced effects. Use together cautiously.
*Cyclosporine:* Increased risk of toxicity. Advise clinician to monitor patient carefully.
*Dantrolene, other hepatotoxic drugs:* May increase risk of hepatotoxicity.
*Drugs that induce hepatic metabolism (such as barbiturates, carbamazepine, phenytoin, primidone, and rifampin):* May cause decreased estrogenic effects from a given dose. These drugs are known to accelerate the rate of metabolism of certain other drugs. Use together cautiously.
*Insulin or oral antidiabetics:* May require dosage adjustment as a result of effects of blood glucose level.
*Tamoxifen:* Decreased effects of tamoxifen. Advise clinician to monitor patient closely.
*Warfarin-type anticoagulants:* Decreased anticoagulant effect. Dosage adjustment may be needed.
**Drug-herb.** *Red clover:* May interfere with hormonal therapies. Avoid use together.
**Drug-food.** *Caffeine:* May increase serum caffeine levels. Advise patient to avoid caffeine.
**Drug-lifestyle.** *Smoking:* Increases risk of adverse CV effects. Advise patient to avoid smoking.

## Adverse reactions
**CNS:** *CVA,* headache, dizziness, chorea, depression, *seizures.*
**CV:** thrombophlebitis, *thromboembolism,* hypertension, edema, *pulmonary embolism, MI.*
**EENT:** worsening of myopia or astigmatism, intolerance of contact lenses.
**GI:** *nausea,* vomiting, abdominal cramps, bloating, anorexia, increased appetite, *pancreatitis,* gallbladder disease.
**GU:** breakthrough bleeding, altered menstrual flow, dysmenorrhea, amenorrhea, *increased risk of endometrial cancer,* cervical erosion, altered cervical secretions, enlargement of uterine fibromas, vaginal candidiasis; testicular atrophy, impotence.

---

**Hematologic:** increased PT and INR and clotting factors VII to X and norepinephrine-induced platelet aggregability.
**Hepatic:** cholestatic jaundice, *hepatic adenoma.*
**Metabolic:** decreased serum folate, pyridoxine, and antithrombin III levels; increased triglyceride, glucose, and phospholipid levels; hypercalcemia, weight changes.
**Skin:** melasma, urticaria, flushing (with rapid I.V. administration), hirsutism or hair loss, erythema nodosum, dermatitis.
**Other:** *possibility of increased risk of breast cancer,* breast changes (tenderness, enlargement, secretion); gynecomastia.

## Overdose and treatment

Serious toxicity after drug overdose hasn't been reported. Nausea may occur. Appropriate supportive care should be provided.

## Clinical considerations

■ For the rapid treatment of dysfunctional uterine bleeding or reduction of surgical bleeding, parenteral administration is preferred.
■ Therapy with estrogens increases sulfobromophthalein retention. Increases in the thyroid-binding globulin level may occur, resulting in increased total thyroid levels (measured by protein-bound iodine or total $T_4$) and decreased uptake of free $T_3$ resin. Glucose tolerance may be impaired. Pregnanediol excretion may decrease.

### Therapeutic monitoring

■ Therapeutic monitoring is the same as for all other estrogens.

### Special populations

**Pregnant patients.** Drug is contraindicated during pregnancy.
**Breast-feeding patients.** Estrogens are contraindicated in breast-feeding women.
**Geriatric patients.** Long-term use for menopausal symptoms may cause an increased risk of certain types of cancer. Frequent physical examinations are recommended.

## Patient counseling

■ Advise patient to report adverse experiences.

---

# estropipate
Ogen, Ortho-Est

*Pharmacologic classification:* estrogen
*Therapeutic classification:* estrogen replacement
*Pregnancy risk category X*

## Available forms

Estropipate is available as estrone sodium sulfate. Available by prescription only.
*Tablets:* 0.625 mg, 1.25 mg, 2.5 mg

*Vaginal cream:* 0.15%

## Indications and dosages

*Atrophic vaginitis, kraurosis vulvae, and vasomotor menopausal symptoms*
*Adults:* 0.75 to 6 mg P.O. daily for 21 days, followed by 7 days off therapy. Or, atrophic vaginitis or kraurosis vulvae, 2 to 4 g of 0.15% vaginal cream once daily in the cyclic regimen.
*Female hypogonadism, primary ovarian failure, or after castration*
*Adults:* 1.5 to 9 mg P.O. daily for 3 weeks, followed by 8 to 10 days off therapy. Cycle may be repeated if no withdrawal bleeding occurs within 10 days of therapy discontinuation.
*Prevention of osteoporosis*
*Adults:* 0.625 mg P.O. daily for 25 days of a 31-day cycle.

## Mechanism of action

*Estrogenic action:* Estropipate mimics the action of endogenous estrogen in treating female hypogonadism, menopausal symptoms, and atrophic vaginitis.

## Pharmacokinetics

*Absorption:* After oral administration, estropipate and other synthetic derivatives of the natural estrogens are rapidly absorbed after oral administration.
*Distribution:* About 50% to 80% plasma protein–bound. Distribution occurs throughout the body, with highest levels appearing in fat.
*Metabolism:* Steroidal estrogens are metabolized primarily in the liver, where they are conjugated with sulfate and glucuronide. Usually, because of the rapid rate of metabolism, many forms of estrogen must be given daily.
*Excretion:* Mostly eliminated through the kidneys in the form of sulfate or glucuronide conjugates.

| Route | Onset | Peak | Duration |
|-------|-------|------|----------|
| P.O. | Unknown | Unknown | Unknown |

## Contraindications and precautions

Contraindicated in patients with thrombophlebitis or thromboembolic disorders, estrogen-dependent neoplasia, breast or reproductive organ cancer (except for palliative treatment), or undiagnosed abnormal genital bleeding and during pregnancy.

Use cautiously in patients with cerebrovascular or coronary artery disease, asthma, bone diseases, mental depression, migraine, seizures, or cardiac, hepatic, or renal dysfunction or in women with family history (mother, grandmother, sister) of breast or genital tract cancer or who have breast nodules, fibrocystic disease, or abnormal mammographic findings.

---

## Interactions
**Drug-drug.** *Cyclosporine:* Increased risk of toxicity. Advise clinician to monitor cyclosporine levels.

*Dantrolene, other hepatotoxic drugs:* May increase risk of hepatotoxicity.

*Drugs that induce hepatic metabolism, such as rifampin, barbiturates, primidone, carbamazepine, phenytoin:* May result in decreased estrogenic effects from a given dose. These drugs are known to accelerate the rate of metabolism of certain other drugs. Use together cautiously.

*Insulin or oral antidiabetics:* May require dosage adjustment because of effects of blood glucose level.

*Tamoxifen:* Decreased effects of tamoxifen. Advise clinician to monitor patient closely.

*Warfarin-type anticoagulants:* Decreased anticoagulant effect. Dosage adjustment may be needed.

**Drug-herb.** *Red clover:* May interfere with hormonal therapies. Discourage use together.

**Drug-food.** *Caffeine:* May increase serum caffeine levels. Advise patient to avoid caffeine.

**Drug-lifestyle.** *Smoking:* Increases risk of adverse CV effects. Advise patient to avoid smoking.

## Adverse reactions
**CNS:** *CVA,* headache, dizziness, depression, migraine, *seizures.*

**CV:** *pulmonary embolism, MI, thromboembolism,* thrombophlebitis, edema.

**EENT:** worsening of myopia or astigmatism, intolerance of contact lenses.

**GI:** vomiting, abdominal cramps, bloating, gallbladder disease.

**GU:** breakthrough bleeding, increased size of uterine fibromas, dysmenorrhea, amenorrhea, vaginal candidiasis, *increased risk of endometrial cancer,* altered menstrual flow, cervical erosion, altered cervical secretions; testicular atrophy, cystitis-like syndrome, premenstrual-like syndrome.

**Hematologic:** increased PT and clotting factors VII to X and norepinephrine-induced platelet aggregability.

**Hepatic:** cholestatic jaundice, *hepatic adenoma.*

**Metabolic:** decreased serum folate, pyridoxine, and antithrombin III levels; increased triglyceride, glucose, and phospholipid levels; hypercalcemia, weight changes.

**Skin:** *erythema multiforme,* erythema nodosum, hair loss, hemorrhagic eruption, hirsutism, melasma.

**Other:** in women, aggravation of porphyria, breast changes (tenderness, enlargement, secretion), *possibility of increased risk of breast cancer;* in men, libido changes, gynecomastia.

## Overdose and treatment
Serious toxicity after overdose of this drug hasn't been reported. Nausea may occur. Provide appropriate supportive care.

## Clinical considerations
■ When used for progressive, inoperable prostate cancer, remission should be apparent within 3 weeks of therapy.

■ When specimens are submitted to pathologist for evaluation, it must be noted that patient is taking estrogens.

■ Therapy with estrogens increases sulfobromophthalein retention. Increases in the thyroid-binding globulin level may occur, resulting in increased total thyroid levels (measured by protein-bound iodine or total $T_4$) and decreased uptake of free $T_3$ resin. Glucose tolerance may be impaired. Pregnanediol excretion may decrease.

### Therapeutic monitoring
■ Therapeutic monitoring is the same as for all estrogens.

### Special populations
**Pregnant patients.** Drug is contraindicated during pregnancy.

**Breast-feeding patients.** Drug is contraindicated in breast-feeding women.

**Geriatric patients.** Frequent physical examinations are recommended for postmenopausal women taking estrogens.

## Patient counseling
■ Patient counseling is the same as for all estrogens.

# etanercept
Enbrel

*Pharmacologic classification:* tumor necrosis factor (TNF) blocker
*Therapeutic classification:* antirheumatic
*Pregnancy risk category B*

## Available forms
Available by prescription only
*Injection:* 25-mg single-use vial

## Indications and dosages
*Reduction in signs and symptoms of moderately to severely active rheumatoid arthritis in patients with inadequate response to one or more disease-modifying antirheumatic drugs; or with methotrexate in patients who don't respond adequately to methotrexate alone*
*Adults:* 25 mg S.C. twice weekly, 72 to 96 hours apart.

*Children ages 4 to 17:* 0.4 mg/kg (maximum dose 25 mg) S.C. twice weekly, 72 to 96 hours apart. Concomitant use with methotrexate has not been studied in children.

### Incompatibilities
Don't add other drugs or diluents to reconstituted solution.

## Mechanism of action
*Antirheumatic action:* Binds specifically to tumor necrosis factor (TNF) and blocks its action with cell-surface TNF receptors, reducing inflammatory and immune responses found in rheumatoid arthritis.

## Pharmacokinetics
*Absorption:* Not reported.
*Distribution:* Not reported.
*Metabolism:* Not reported.
*Excretion:* Elimination half-life is 115 hours.

| Route | Onset | Peak | Duration |
|-------|-------|------|----------|
| S.C. | Unknown | 72 hr | Unknown |

## Contraindications and precautions
Contraindicated in patients with sepsis and hypersensitivity to etanercept or any of its components.

Live vaccines are contraindicated during drug therapy.

Use drug cautiously in patients with underlying diseases that predispose them to infection, such as diabetes, HF, or history of active or chronic infections.

Caution should be used when treating rheumatoid arthritis patients with preexisting or recent onset of demyelinating disorders, including multiple sclerosis, myelitis, and optic neuritis.

## Interactions
None reported.

## Adverse reactions
**CNS:** asthenia, *headache,* dizziness.
**EENT:** *rhinitis,* pharyngitis, sinusitis.
**GI:** abdominal pain, dyspepsia.
**Respiratory:** *upper respiratory tract infections,* cough, respiratory disorder.
**Skin:** *injection site reaction,* rash.
**Other:** *infections, malignancies.*

## Clinical considerations
■ Drug is for S.C. injection only.
■ Anti-TNF therapies, including etanercept, may affect defenses against infection.
■ Live vaccines shouldn't be given concurrently during drug therapy.
■ Juvenile rheumatoid arthritis patients should, if possible, be brought up-to-date with all immunizations in compliance with current immunization guidelines before treatment starts.

■ Injection sites should be at least 1″ apart; areas where skin is tender, bruised, red, or hard should never be used. Recommended sites include the thigh, abdomen, or upper arm. Recommend rotating sites regularly.
■ Reconstitute aseptically with 1 ml of supplied sterile bacteriostatic water for injection (0.9% benzyl alcohol).
■ Don't filter reconstituted solution during preparation or administration.
■ Minimize foaming by gently swirling rather than shaking.
■ Use reconstituted solution as soon as possible; may be refrigerated in vial for up to 6 hours at 36° to 46° F (2° to 8° C).

### Therapeutic monitoring
■ Positive antinuclear antibodies or positive anti-double-stranded DNA antibodies may develop as measured by radioimmunoassay and *Crithidia lucilae* assay.
■ Advise clinician to monitor patient for infections.

### Special populations
**Breast-feeding patients.** Advise breast-feeding women to discontinue nursing during drug therapy.
**Pediatric patients.** Safety and efficacy haven't been studied in children under age 4. Children with juvenile rheumatoid arthritis are more susceptible to the adverse effects of abdominal pain and vomiting than adults with rheumatoid arthritis.
**Geriatric patients.** No overall differences in safety and efficacy have been noted between geriatric and younger adults; however, greater sensitivity to drug effects by geriatric patients can't be ruled out.

## Patient counseling
■ Instruct patient who will be self-administering drug about mixing and injection techniques, including rotation of injection sites.
■ Tell patient that injection site reactions generally occur within first month of therapy and decrease thereafter.
■ Inform patient of importance of avoiding live vaccine administration while receiving drug. Stress importance of alerting prescribers of drug use.
■ Instruct patient to promptly report signs and symptoms of infection.
■ Teach patient the signs and symptoms of pancytopenia.

# ethacrynate sodium

# ethacrynic acid

Edecrin

*Pharmacologic classification:* loop diuretic
*Therapeutic classification:* diuretic
*Pregnancy risk category B*

## Available forms

Available by prescription only
*Tablets:* 25 mg, 50 mg
*Injectable:* 50 mg (with 62.5 mg of mannitol and 0.1 mg of thimerosal)

## Indications and dosages

*Acute pulmonary edema*
*Adults:* 50 mg or 0.5 to 1 mg/kg I.V. to a maximum dose of 100 mg of ethacrynate sodium I.V. slowly over several minutes.
*Edema*
*Adults:* 50 to 200 mg P.O. daily. Refractory cases may require up to 200 mg b.i.d.
*Children:* Initially, 25 mg P.O., given cautiously and increased in 25-mg increments daily until desired effect is achieved.
◊*Hypertension*
*Adults:* Initially, 25 mg P.O. daily. Adjust dosage p.r.n. Maximum maintenance dose is 200 mg P.O. daily in two divided doses.

## I.V. administration

■ Add to vial 50 ml of D₅W or saline solution.
■ Don't use cloudy or opalescent solutions.
■ Recommend giving slowly through tubing of running infusion over 20 to 30 minutes or by direct I.V. injection over several minutes.
■ Discard unused solution after 24 hours.

*Incompatibilities*
Incompatible with hydralazine, Normosol-M, procainamide, reserpine, tolazoline, triflupromazine, whole blood and its derivatives, and any solution or drug with pH below 5.

## Mechanism of action

*Diuretic action:* Ethacrynic acid inhibits sodium and chloride reabsorption in the proximal part of the ascending loop of Henle, promoting the excretion of sodium, water, chloride, and potassium.

## Pharmacokinetics

*Absorption:* Absorbed rapidly from the GI tract.
*Distribution:* Ethacrynic acid accumulates in the liver of animals. Ethacrynic acid doesn't enter the CSF, and its distribution into breast milk or the placenta is unknown.
*Metabolism:* Metabolized by the liver to a potentially active metabolite.
*Excretion:* 30% to 65% is excreted in urine and 35% to 40% is excreted in bile as the

metabolite. Duration of action is 6 to 8 hours after oral administration and about 2 hours after I.V. administration.

| Route | Onset | Peak | Duration |
|-------|-------|------|----------|
| P.O. | 30 min | 2 hr | 6-8 hr |
| I.V. | 5 min | 15-30 min | 2 hr |

## Contraindications and precautions

Contraindicated in infants and in patients with anuria or those hypersensitive to drug.
Use cautiously in patients with electrolyte abnormalities or impaired hepatic function.

## Interactions

**Drug-drug.** *Aminoglycosides, some cephalosporins, or other ototoxic drugs, such as cisplatin:* May increase the risk of deafness; avoid use of such combinations.
*Antihypertensive agents:* Increased antihypertensive effect. Patients may require dosage reduction.
*Cardiac glycosides:* Increased risk of digoxin toxicity from ethacrynate-induced hypokalemia. Advise clinician to monitor digoxin and potassium levels.
*Diuretics, such as metolazone:* May enhance the diuretic effect of the other drugs; dosage should be reduced when adding ethacrynic acid to a diuretic regimen.
*Insulin or oral antidiabetics:* Elevated blood glucose; dosages may need to be increased.
*Lithium:* Reduced renal clearance of lithium; recommend monitoring lithium levels. Dosage adjustment may be needed.
*NSAIDs:* Decreased diuretic effectiveness; possible risk of renal failure. Drugs should be used together cautiously.
*Other potassium-depleting drugs, such as steroids and amphotericin B:* Severe potassium loss may occur. Advise clinician to monitor patient closely.
*Potassium-sparing diuretics, such as amiloride, spironolactone, and triamterene:* Decreased potassium loss induced by ethacrynic acid. May be used as a therapeutic advantage.
*Warfarin:* May potentiate anticoagulant effects. Use together cautiously.
**Drug-herb.** *Dandelion:* Possible interference with diuretic activity. Discourage use together.

## Adverse reactions

**CNS:** confusion, fatigue, vertigo, headache, malaise.
**CV:** volume depletion and dehydration, orthostatic hypotension.
**EENT:** transient deafness (with too-rapid I.V. injection), blurred vision, tinnitus, hearing loss.
**GI:** diarrhea, anorexia, nausea, vomiting, GI bleeding, *pancreatitis.*
**GU:** oliguria, hematuria, nocturia, polyuria, frequent urination, azotemia.
**Hematologic:** *agranulocytosis, neutropenia, thrombocytopenia.*

**Metabolic:** hypokalemia; hypochloremic alkalosis; asymptomatic hyperuricemia; fluid and electrolyte imbalances, including dilutional hyponatremia, hypocalcemia, hypomagnesemia; hyperglycemia; impaired glucose tolerance.
**Other:** fever, chills.

## Overdose and treatment
Signs and symptoms of overdose include profound electrolyte and volume depletion, which may precipitate circulatory collapse.

Treatment of ethacrynic acid overdose is primarily supportive; recommend emptying stomach by inducing emesis or gastric lavage. Recommend replacing fluid and electrolytes p.r.n.

## Clinical considerations
■ Drug shouldn't be given simultaneously with whole blood or blood products; hemolysis may occur.
■ I.V. ethacrynate sodium has been used to treat hypercalcemia and to manage ethylene glycol poisoning and bromide intoxication.

### Therapeutic monitoring
■ Recommend periodic assessment of hearing function in patients receiving high-dose therapy. Ethacrynic acid may potentiate ototoxicity of other drugs.

### Special populations
**Pregnant patients.** Use drug during pregnancy only when clearly indicated.
**Breast-feeding patients.** Don't use drug in breast-feeding women.
**Pediatric patients.** Ethacrynate sodium and ethacrynic acid shouldn't be given to infants. Safety in children hasn't been established.
**Geriatric patients.** Geriatric and debilitated patients require close observation because they're more susceptible to drug-induced diuresis. Excessive diuresis promotes rapid dehydration, leading to hypovolemia, hypokalemia, hyponatremia, and circulatory collapse. Reduced dosages may be indicated.

## Patient counseling
■ Advise patient receiving I.V. form of drug to report pain or irritation at I.V. site immediately.
■ Notify diabetic patient that antidiabetic dosage may need to be increased.

# ethambutol hydrochloride
Myambutol

*Pharmacologic classification:* semisynthetic antitubercular
*Therapeutic classification:* antitubercular
*Pregnancy risk category NR*

## Available forms
Available by prescription only
*Tablets:* 100 mg, 400 mg

## Indications and dosages
*Adjunctive treatment in pulmonary tuberculosis*
*Adults:* Initial treatment for patients who haven't received previous antitubercular therapy: 15 mg/kg P.O. once daily. *Retreatment:* 25 mg/kg P.O. daily for 60 days or until bacteriologic smears and cultures come back negative, followed by 15 mg/kg P.O. daily. *ATS/CDC short course regimen:* 15 to 25 mg/kg (up to 2.5 g) P.O. daily until drug susceptibility to rifampin and isoniazid is confirmed. *Or, with other antitubercular agents:* 50 mg/kg (up to 2.5 g) P.O. daily twice weekly, or 25 to 30 mg/kg (up to 2.5 g) three times weekly.
*Children ages 6 and older:* 10 to 15 mg/kg (up to 2.5 g) P.O. daily. *American Thoracic Society and U.S. Centers for Disease Control and Prevention (ATS/CDC) short-course regimen:* 15 to 25 mg/kg (up to 2.5 g) P.O. daily in children whose visual acuity can be monitored, or 50 mg/kg (up to 2.5 g) P.O. twice weekly, or 25 to 30 mg/kg (up to 2.5 g) three times per week. In children whose visual acuity cannot be closely monitored (very young children), I.M streptomycin 20 to 40 mg/kg daily until drug susceptibility to rifampin and isoniazid is confirmed.
≡*Dosage adjustment.* In patients with renal impairment, if creatinine clearance is 70 to 100 ml/minute, drug dose should not exceed 15 mg/kg daily. If creatinine clearance is less than 70 ml/minute, dosage should be further reduced. If creatinine clearance is 10 to 50 ml/minute, give drug every 24 to 36 hours. If creatinine clearance is less than 10 ml/minute, dose should be given every 48 hours.
◇*Adjunctive treatment for pulmonary Mycobacterium avium complex infections in patients without HIV*
*Adults:* 25 mg/kg P.O. daily for 2 months followed by 15 mg/kg P.O. daily until cultures negative for 1 year.
◇*Adjunctive treatment for disseminated Mycobacterium avium complex infections*
*Adults:* 15 mg/kg P.O. daily for patient's lifetime.

## Mechanism of action

*Antitubercular action:* Ethambutol is bacteriostatic; it interferes with mycolic acid incorporation into the mycobacterial cell wall. Ethambutol is active against *Mycobacterium tuberculosis, M. bovis,* and *M. marinum,* some strains of *M. kansasii, M. avium, M. fortuitum,* and *M. intracellulare,* and the combined strain of *M. avium* and *M. intracellulare* (MAC). Ethambutol is considered adjunctive therapy in tuberculosis and is combined with other antitubercular agents to prevent or delay development of drug resistance by *M. tuberculosis.*

## Pharmacokinetics

*Absorption:* Absorbed rapidly from the GI tract.
*Distribution:* Distributed widely into body tissues and fluids, especially into lungs, erythrocytes, saliva, and kidneys; lesser amounts distribute into brain, ascitic, pleural, and cerebrospinal fluids. Ethambutol is 8% to 22% protein-bound.
*Metabolism:* Undergoes partial hepatic metabolism.
*Excretion:* After 24 hours, about 50% of unchanged ethambutol and 8% to 15% of its metabolites are excreted in urine; 20% to 25% is excreted in feces. Small amounts of drug may appear in breast milk. Plasma half-life in adults is about 3¼ hours; half-life is prolonged in decreased renal or hepatic function. Ethambutol can be removed by peritoneal dialysis and, to a lesser extent, by hemodialysis.

| Route | Onset | Peak | Duration |
|-------|-------|------|----------|
| P.O. | Unknown | 2-4 hr | Unknown |

## Contraindications and precautions

Contraindicated in children under age 6 and in patients with optic neuritis or hypersensitivity to drug.
    Use cautiously in patients with impaired renal function, cataracts, recurrent eye inflammations, gout, and diabetic retinopathy.

## Interactions

**Drug-drug.** *Drugs that produce neurotoxicity:* Increased neurotoxic effects. Avoid use together.
*Aluminum salts:* May delay and reduce the absorption of ethambutol. Separate administration times by several hours.

## Adverse reactions

**CNS:** headache, malaise, dizziness, mental confusion, possible hallucinations, peripheral neuritis (numbness and tingling of limbs).
**EENT:** optic neuritis (related to dose and duration of treatment).
**GI:** anorexia, nausea, vomiting, abdominal pain, GI upset.
**Hematologic:** *thrombocytopenia.*
**Hepatic:** abnormal liver function test results.
**Metabolic:** elevated uric acid level.

**Musculoskeletal:** joint pain.
**Respiratory:** bloody sputum.
**Skin:** dermatitis, pruritus, toxic epidermal necrolysis.
**Other:** *anaphylactoid reactions,* fever, precipitation of acute gout.

## Overdose and treatment

No specific recommendation is available. Treatment is supportive. After recent ingestion (4 hours or less), recommend emptying stomach by induced emesis or gastric lavage. Recommend following with activated charcoal to decrease absorption.

## Clinical considerations

■ Drug can be given with food if needed to prevent gastric irritation; food doesn't interfere with absorption.
■ Specimens for culture and sensitivity testing should be collected before first dose, but therapy can begin before test results are complete; testing should be repeated periodically to detect drug resistance.

### Therapeutic monitoring

■ Recommend assessing visual status before therapy and testing visual acuity and color discrimination monthly in patients taking more than 15 mg/kg/day. Visual disturbances are dose-related and reversible if detected in time.
■ Advise clinician to monitor blood (including serum uric acid), renal, and liver function test results before and periodically during therapy to minimize toxicity.
■ Advise clinician to monitor patient for change in renal function. Dosage reduction may be needed.

### Special populations

**Pregnant patients.** Use drug during pregnancy only when benefits justify risk to the fetus.
**Breast-feeding patients.** Drug appears in breast milk. Use cautiously in breast-feeding women.
**Pediatric patients.** Although drug isn't recommended by the manufacturer for use in children under age 13, some clinicians have recommended using drug in children 6 years of age or older.

## Patient counseling

■ Inform patient of the potential for hypersensitivity and other adverse reactions, and emphasize need to report these reactions. Urge patient to report any unusual effects, especially blurred vision, red-green color blindness, or changes in urine elimination.
■ Assure patient that visual alterations will disappear within several weeks or months after drug is discontinued.
■ Urge patient to complete the prescribed regimen, to comply with instructions for daily dosage, to avoid missing doses, and not to discontinue drug without medical approval. Ex-

plain importance of keeping follow-up appointments.

# ethinyl estradiol
Estinyl

*Pharmacologic classification:* estrogen
*Therapeutic classification:* estrogen replacement, antineoplastic
*Pregnancy risk category X*

## Available forms
Available by prescription only
*Tablets:* 0.02 mg, 0.05 mg

## Indications and dosages
*Palliative treatment of metastatic breast cancer (at least 5 years after menopause)*
Adults: 1 mg P.O. t.i.d. for at least 3 months.
*Female hypogonadism*
Adults: 0.05 mg P.O. daily to t.i.d. for 2 weeks monthly, followed by 2 weeks progesterone therapy; continue for three to six monthly dosing cycles, followed by 2 months off.
*Vasomotor menopausal symptoms*
Adults: 0.02 to 0.05 mg P.O. daily for cycles of 3 weeks on, 1 week off.
*Palliative treatment of metastatic inoperable prostatic cancer*
Adults: 0.15 to 2 mg P.O. daily.

## Mechanism of action
*Estrogenic action:* Ethinyl estradiol mimics the action of endogenous estrogen in treating female hypogonadism and menopausal symptoms. It inhibits growth of hormone-sensitive tissue in advanced, inoperable prostatic cancer and in certain carefully selected cases of breast cancer in men and postmenopausal women.

## Pharmacokinetics
*Absorption:* After oral administration, estradiol is well absorbed but substantially inactivated by the liver.
*Distribution:* About 50% to 80% plasma protein–bound, particularly estradiol-binding globulin. Distribution occurs throughout the body, with highest levels appearing in fat.
*Metabolism:* Steroidal estrogens, including estradiol, are metabolized primarily in the liver, where they are conjugated with sulfate and glucuronide. Because of the rapid rate of metabolism, nonesterified forms of estrogen, including estradiol, must usually be given daily.
*Excretion:* The majority of estrogen elimination occurs through the kidneys in the form of sulfate or glucuronide conjugates.

| Route | Onset | Peak | Duration |
|-------|-------|------|----------|
| P.O. | Unknown | Unknown | Unknown |

## Contraindications and precautions
Contraindicated in patients with thrombophlebitis or thromboembolic disorders, estrogen-dependent neoplasia, breast or reproductive organ cancer (except for palliative treatment), and undiagnosed abnormal genital bleeding and during pregnancy.

Use cautiously in patients with cerebrovascular or coronary artery disease, asthma, mental depression, bone disease, or cardiac, hepatic, or renal dysfunction and in women with a family history (mother, grandmother, sister) of breast or genital tract cancer or who have breast nodules, fibrocystic disease, or abnormal mammographic findings.

## Interactions
**Drug-drug.** *Cyclosporine:* Increased risk of toxicity. Advise clinician to monitor cyclosporine levels.
*Dantrolene, other hepatotoxic medications:* May increase risk of hepatotoxicity. Advise clinician to monitor patient closely.
*Drugs that induce hepatic metabolism (such as barbiturates, carbamazepine, primidone, and rifampin):* May result in decreased estrogenic effects from a given dose. These drugs are known to accelerate the rate of metabolism of certain other drugs. Use together cautiously.
*Insulin or oral antidiabetics:* May require dosage adjustment as a result of effects of blood glucose level.
*Tamoxifen:* Decreased effects of tamoxifen. Advise clinician to monitor patient closely.
*Warfarin-type anticoagulants:* Decreased anticoagulant effect. Dosage adjustment may be needed.
**Drug-food.** *Caffeine:* May increase serum caffeine levels. Advise patient to avoid caffeine.
*Grapefruit juice:* Elevated estrogen levels. Take with liquid other than grapefruit juice.
**Drug-lifestyle.** *Smoking:* Increases risk of adverse CV effects. Advise patient to avoid smoking.

## Adverse reactions
**CNS:** *CVA,* headache, dizziness, chorea, depression, *seizures.*
**CV:** thrombophlebitis; *thromboembolism;* hypertension; edema; *pulmonary embolism, MI.*
**EENT:** worsening of myopia or astigmatism, intolerance of contact lenses.
**GI:** *nausea,* vomiting, abdominal cramps, bloating, anorexia, increased appetite, gallbladder disease.
**GU:** breakthrough bleeding, altered menstrual flow, dysmenorrhea, amenorrhea, *increased risk of endometrial cancer,* cervical erosion, altered cervical secretions, enlargement of uterine fibromas, vaginal candidiasis; testicular atrophy, impotence.

---

Hematologic: increased PT and INR and clotting factors VII to X, and norepinephrine-induced platelet aggregability.
Hepatic: cholestatic jaundice, *hepatic adenoma.*
Metabolic: decreased serum folate, pyridoxine, and antithrombin III levels; increased triglyceride, glucose, and phospholipid levels; hypercalcemia, weight changes.
Skin: melasma, urticaria, flushing (with rapid I.V. administration), hirsutism or hair loss, erythema nodosum, dermatitis.
Other: *possibility of increased risk of breast cancer,* breast changes (tenderness, enlargement, secretion); gynecomastia.

## Overdose and treatment
Serious toxicity after overdose of this drug hasn't been reported. Nausea may occur. Provide appropriate supportive care.

## Clinical considerations
■ Consider the recommendations relevant to all other estrogens. Because of risk of thromboembolism, discontinue drug therapy at least 1 month before procedures that may cause prolonged immobilization or thromboembolism.

### Therapeutic monitoring
■ Advise clinician to monitor patient for adverse reactions.
■ Recommend periodically monitoring serum lipid levels, blood pressure, body weight, and hepatic function p.r.n.

### Special populations
Pregnant patients. Drug is contraindicated for use during pregnancy.
Breast-feeding patients. Drug is contraindicated in breast-feeding women.
Geriatric patients. Use with caution in patients whose condition may be aggravated by fluid retention.

## Patient counseling
■ Provide patient with a package insert describing adverse reactions of estrogen as well as a verbal explanation.
■ Emphasize importance of regular physical examinations.
■ Warn patient to immediately report abdominal pain; pain, numbness, or stiffness in legs or buttocks; pressure or pain in chest; shortness of breath; severe headaches; visual disturbances such as blind spots, flashing lights, or blurriness; vaginal bleeding or discharge; breast lumps; swelling of hands or feet; yellow skin or sclera; dark urine; or light-colored stools.
■ Tell diabetic patient to report elevated blood glucose test results; antidiabetic dosage may be adjusted.

# ethosuximide
Zarontin

*Pharmacologic classification:* succinimide derivative
*Therapeutic classification:* anticonvulsant
*Pregnancy risk category C*

## Available forms
Available by prescription only
*Capsules:* 250 mg
*Syrup:* 250 mg/5 ml

## Indications and dosages
*Absence seizures*
*Adults and children ages 6 and older:* Initially, 250 mg P.O. b.i.d. May increase by 250 mg q 4 to 7 days up to 1.5 g daily.
*Children ages 3 to 6:* 250 mg P.O. daily. Optimal dose is 20 mg/kg/day.

## Mechanism of action
*Anticonvulsant action:* Ethosuximide raises the seizure threshold; it suppresses characteristic spike-and-wave pattern by depressing neuronal transmission in the motor cortex and basal ganglia. It's indicated for absence seizures refractory to other drugs.

## Pharmacokinetics
*Absorption:* Absorbed from the GI tract; steady-state plasma levels occur in 4 to 7 days.
*Distribution:* Distributed widely throughout the body; protein-binding is minimal.
*Metabolism:* Metabolized extensively in the liver to several inactive metabolites.
*Excretion:* Excreted in urine, with small amounts in bile and feces. Plasma half-life is about 60 hours in adults and about 30 hours in children.

| Route | Onset | Peak | Duration |
|-------|-------|------|----------|
| P.O. | Unknown | 3-7 hr | Unknown |

## Contraindications and precautions
Contraindicated in patients hypersensitive to succinimide derivatives.
    Use with extreme caution in patients with hepatic or renal disease.

## Interactions
Drug-drug. *Other CNS depressants (antidepressants, antipsychotics, anxiolytics, other anticonvulsants, narcotics):* Additive CNS depression and sedation. Advise clinician to monitor patient closely.
*Phenytoin:* Increased serum phenytoin levels. Advise clinician to monitor patient carefully.
*Valproic acid:* Increased or decreased serum levels of ethosuximide. Advise clinician to monitor patient closely.

**Drug-lifestyle.** *Alcohol use:* Additive CNS depression and sedation. Advise patient to avoid alcohol.

## Adverse reactions

**CNS:** *drowsiness, headache, fatigue, dizziness, ataxia, irritability, euphoria, lethargy, depression, psychosis.*
**EENT:** myopia, tongue swelling, gingival hyperplasia.
**GI:** *nausea, vomiting, diarrhea, cramps, anorexia, epigastric and abdominal pain.*
**GU:** vaginal bleeding, urinary frequency, abnormal renal function tests results.
**Hematologic:** *leukopenia,* eosinophilia, *agranulocytosis,* pancytopenia.
**Hepatic:** elevated liver enzyme levels.
**Metabolic:** *weight loss.*
**Respiratory:** *hiccups.*
**Skin:** urticaria, pruritic and erythematous rash, hirsutism, *Stevens-Johnson syndrome.*

## Overdose and treatment

Symptoms of ethosuximide overdose, when used alone or with other anticonvulsants, include CNS depression, ataxia, stupor, and coma.

Treatment is symptomatic and supportive. Recommend carefully monitoring vital signs and fluid and electrolyte balance.

## Clinical considerations

■ Recommend giving ethosuximide with food to minimize GI distress.
■ Abrupt discontinuation of drug may precipitate petit mal seizures.
■ Ethosuximide may cause false-positive Coombs' test results. May also cause abnormal renal function test results.

### Therapeutic monitoring

■ Recommend observing patient for dermatologic reactions, joint pain, unexplained fever, or unusual bruising or bleeding (which may signal hematologic or other severe adverse reactions).
■ Recommend performing CBC, liver function tests, and urinalysis periodically.
■ Therapeutic plasma levels range from 40 to 100 mcg/ml.

### Special populations

**Pregnant patients.** Safety hasn't been established.
**Breast-feeding patients.** Safety hasn't been established. Advise nursing women to use alternative feeding method during therapy with ethosuximide.
**Pediatric patients.** Don't use drug in children under age 3.
**Geriatric patients.** Use with caution in geriatric patients.

## Patient counseling

■ Advise patient to take drug with food or milk to prevent GI distress, to avoid use with alcoholic beverages, and to avoid hazardous tasks that require alertness if drug causes drowsiness, dizziness, or blurred vision.
■ Inform patient that drug may color urine pink to reddish-brown.
■ Tell patient to report to prescriber the following effects: rash, joint pain, fever, sore throat, or unusual bleeding or bruising.
■ Advise patient to contact prescriber immediately if pregnancy is suspected.

# etodolac

Lodine, Lodine XL

*Pharmacologic classification:* NSAID
*Therapeutic classification:* antiarthritic
*Pregnancy risk category C*

## Available forms

Available by prescription only
*Capsules:* 200 mg, 300 mg
*Tablets:* 400 mg, 500 mg
*Tablets (extended-release):* 400 mg, 500 mg, 600 mg

## Indications and dosages

*Acute and chronic management of osteoarthritis, rheumatoid arthritis, and pain*
*Adults:* For acute pain, give 200 to 400 mg P.O. q 6 to 8 hours, p.r.n., not to exceed 1,000 mg daily.

For osteoarthritis or rheumatoid arthritis, give 600 to 1,000 mg P.O. daily in 2 to 3 divided doses, or 400 to 1,000 mg of extended-release tablets P.O. daily. Daily doses should not exceed 1 g of conventional tablets or capsules or 1.2 g of extended-release tablets.

## Mechanism of action

*Antiarthritic action:* Mechanism of action is unknown but is presumed to be related to the inhibition of prostaglandin biosynthesis.

## Pharmacokinetics

*Absorption:* Well-absorbed from GI tract. Antacids don't appear to affect absorption of etodolac; however, they can decrease peak levels reached by 15% to 20% but have no effect when peak levels are reached.
*Distribution:* Found in liver, lungs, heart, and kidneys.
*Metabolism:* Extensively metabolized in the liver.
*Excretion:* Excreted in urine primarily as metabolites; 16% is excreted in feces.

| Route | Onset | Peak | Duration |
|-------|-------|------|----------|
| P.O. | 30 min | 1-2 hr | 4-12 hr |
| P.O. (extended) | Unknown | 3-12 hr | 6-12 hr |

## Contraindications and precautions

Contraindicated in patients hypersensitive to drug and in those with history of aspirin- or NSAID-induced asthma, rhinitis, urticaria, or other allergic reactions.

Use cautiously in patients with impaired renal or hepatic function, history of peptic ulcer disease, cardiac disease, hypertension, or conditions related to fluid retention.

## Interactions

**Drug-drug.** *Antacids:* Decreased peak levels of the drug. Advise clinician to monitor patient for decreased effects of etodolac.
*Aspirin:* Reduces protein-binding of etodolac without altering its clearance and may increase GI toxicity. Avoid use together.
*Cyclosporine:* Impaired elimination and increased risk of nephrotoxicity. Avoid use together.
*Digoxin, lithium, and methotrexate:* Increased levels of these drugs. Advise clinician to monitor drug levels.
*Diuretics and beta blockers:* May blunt effects of drug. Advise clinician to monitor patient carefully.
*Phenytoin:* Increased serum levels of phenytoin. Advise clinician to monitor patient for signs of toxicity.
*Warfarin:* Decreased protein-binding of warfarin but doesn't change its clearance. No dosage adjustment is needed, but recommend monitoring INR and watching for bleeding.
**Drug-lifestyle.** *Alcohol use:* Increases risk of adverse effects. Advise patient to avoid alcohol.
*Sun exposure:* Photosensitivity reactions may result from sun exposure. Advise patient to take precautions.

## Adverse reactions

**CNS:** *asthenia, malaise, dizziness,* depression, drowsiness, nervousness, insomnia.
**CV:** hypertension, *HF,* syncope, flushing, palpitations, edema, fluid retention.
**EENT:** blurred vision, tinnitus, photophobia.
**GI:** *dyspepsia, flatulence, abdominal pain, diarrhea, nausea,* constipation, gastritis, melena, vomiting, anorexia, peptic ulceration with or without *GI bleeding* or perforation, ulcerative stomatitis, thirst, dry mouth.
**GU:** dysuria, urinary frequency, *renal failure.*
**Hematologic:** anemia, *leukopenia, thrombocytopenia,* hemolytic anemia, *agranulocytosis.*
**Hepatic:** elevated liver function test results, *hepatitis.*
**Metabolic:** decreased serum uric acid levels, weight gain.
**Respiratory:** asthma.
**Skin:** pruritus, rash, *Stevens-Johnson syndrome.*
**Other:** chills, fever.

## Overdose and treatment

Signs of overdose include lethargy, drowsiness, nausea, vomiting, and epigastric pain. Rare symptoms include GI bleeding, coma, renal failure, hypertension, and anaphylaxis. Treatment is symptomatic and supportive, including stomach decontamination.

## Clinical considerations

■ Caution should be advised with concurrent use of diuretics in patients with cardiac, renal, or hepatic failure.
■ Etodolac 1,200 mg was shown to cause less GI bleeding than ibuprofen 2,400 mg daily, indomethacin 200 mg daily, naproxen 750 mg daily, or piroxicam 20 mg daily.
■ A false-positive test for urinary bilirubin may be caused by phenolic metabolites.

### Therapeutic monitoring

■ Advise clinician to monitor patient for signs and symptoms of GI ulceration and bleeding.
■ In chronic conditions, a therapeutic response to therapy is most often seen within 2 weeks.

### Special populations

**Pregnant patients.** Avoid drug during third trimester.
**Breast-feeding patients.** It's unknown if drug appears in breast milk. Use cautiously.
**Pediatric patients.** Safety and efficacy haven't been established in children under age 18.
**Geriatric patients.** Drug is well tolerated in older and younger adults and generally doesn't require age-related dosage adjustments. No age-related differences have been reported.

## Patient counseling

■ Advise patient of the potential for adverse events and instruct him to report to prescriber any GI effects of drug.
■ Tell patient that drug may be taken with food.

# etoposide
Toposar, VePesid

*Pharmacologic classification:* podophyllotoxin (cell cycle–phase specific, G2 and late S phases)
*Therapeutic classification:* antineoplastic
*Pregnancy risk category D*

## Available forms

Available by prescription only
*Capsules:* 50 mg
*Injection:* 20-mg/ml multiple-dose vials

## Indications and dosages

Dosage and indications may vary. Check literature for current protocol.

### Small-cell carcinoma of the lung
*Adults:* 70 mg/m² P.O. (rounded to the nearest 50 mg) for 4 days; or 100 mg/m² P.O. (rounded to the nearest 50 mg) daily for 5 days. Repeat q 3 to 4 weeks. Alternatively, 35 mg/m² I.V. daily for 4 days or 50 mg/m² I.V. daily for 5 days. Repeat q 3 to 4 weeks.

### Testicular carcinoma
*Adults:* 50 to 100 mg/m² I.V. daily on days 1 to 5; or 100 mg/m² I.V. daily on days 1, 3, and 5 of a regimen repeated q 3 or 4 weeks.

◇ *AIDS-related Kaposi's sarcoma*
*Adults:* 150 mg/m² daily I.V. for 3 consecutive days every 4 weeks. Repeat cycles p.r.n.
≡ *Dosage adjustment.* Dosage reduction may be needed in patients with impaired renal function.

## I.V. administration
■ Wear protective gloves during handling and preparation of drug.
■ Wash skin that comes in contact with drug immediately and thoroughly with soap and water.
■ Dilute drug to final level of 0.2 or 0.4 mg/ml in normal saline solution or D₅W.
■ Give drug by slow I.V. infusion over at least 30 to 60 minutes.
**⚠ ALERT** Drug should not be administered by rapid I.V. injection.
■ Observe patient for hypotension and anaphylaxis.

### Incompatibilities
Incompatible with idarubicin.

## Mechanism of action
*Antineoplastic action:* Etoposide exerts its cytotoxic action by arresting cells in the metaphase portion of cell division. Drug also inhibits cells from entering mitosis and depresses DNA and RNA synthesis.

## Pharmacokinetics
*Absorption:* Only moderately absorbed across the GI tract after oral administration. Etoposide's bioavailability ranges from 25% to 75%, with an average of 50% of the dose being absorbed.
*Distribution:* Distributed widely into body tissues; the highest levels are found in the liver, spleen, kidneys, healthy brain tissue, and brain tumor tissue. It crosses the blood-brain barrier to a limited and variable extent. Etoposide is about 94% bound to serum albumin.
*Metabolism:* Only a small portion of a dose of etoposide is metabolized. Metabolism occurs in the liver.
*Excretion:* Excreted primarily in the urine as unchanged drug. A smaller portion of a dose is excreted in the feces. The plasma elimination of etoposide is described as biphasic, with an initial phase half-life of about to ½ to 2 hours and a terminal phase of about 5¼ to 11 hours.

| Route | Onset | Peak | Duration |
|-------|-------|------|----------|
| P.O., I.V. | Unknown | Unknown | Unknown |

## Contraindications and precautions
Contraindicated in patients hypersensitive to drug.
Use cautiously in patients who have had cytotoxic or radiation therapy.

## Interactions
*Drug-drug. Cisplatin:* Etoposide increases cytotoxicity of cisplatin against certain tumors. May be used for this purpose.
*Warfarin:* Concurrent administration may cause elongation of PT and INR. Advise clinician to monitor patient closely.

## Adverse reactions
**CNS:** peripheral neuropathy.
**CV:** hypotension (from too-rapid infusion).
**GI:** *nausea and vomiting, anorexia, diarrhea,* abdominal pain, *stomatitis.*
**Hematologic:** *anemia, myelosuppression* (dose-limiting), LEUKOPENIA, THROMBOCYTOPENIA.
**Skin:** *reversible alopecia.*
**Other:** *anaphylaxis,* phlebitis at injection site.

## Overdose and treatment
Signs and symptoms of overdose include myelosuppression, nausea, and vomiting. Treatment is usually supportive and includes transfusion of blood components, antiemetics, and appropriate symptomatic therapy.

## Clinical considerations
■ Have diphenhydramine, hydrocortisone, epinephrine, and airway available in case of an anaphylactic reaction.
■ Pretreatment with antiemetics may reduce frequency and duration of nausea and vomiting.
■ At doses below 200 mg, extent of absorption after oral administration isn't affected by food.
■ Etoposide has produced complete remissions in small-cell lung cancer and testicular cancer.

### Therapeutic monitoring
■ Advise clinician to monitor blood pressure before infusion and at 30-minute intervals during infusion. If systolic blood pressure goes below 90 mm Hg, stop infusion.
■ Advise clinician to monitor CBC. Drug shouldn't be given if platelet count is less than 50,000/mm³ or absolute neutrophil count is less than 500/mm³.
■ GI toxicity occurs more frequently after oral administration.

## Special populations

**Pregnant patients.** High risk for fetal harm. During pregnancy, use drug only for life-threatening conditions or severe disease when much safer drugs aren't available or are ineffective.

**Breast-feeding patients.** Because drug appears in breast milk, its use in breast-feeding women isn't recommended.

**Pediatric patients.** Safety and effectiveness in children haven't been established.

**Geriatric patients.** Geriatric patients may be particularly susceptible to the hypotensive effects of etoposide.

## Patient counseling

■ Advise patient of potential adverse reactions and instruct to contact prescriber immediately if vomiting occurs shortly after dose.

■ Advise patient to report to prescriber sore throat, fever, or unusual bruising or bleeding.

■ Advise patient to avoid exposure to people with infections.

■ Tell patient not to receive immunizations during therapy with etoposide and that other family members also shouldn't receive immunizations during duration of therapy.

■ Advise patient to use contraceptive measures during therapy.

# etoposide phosphate

Etopophos

*Pharmacologic classification:* semisynthetic derivative of podophyllotoxin
*Therapeutic classification:* antineoplastic
*Pregnancy risk category D*

## Available forms

Available by prescription only
*Capsules:* 50 mg
*Injection:* Vials containing etoposide phosphate equivalent to 100 mg etoposide/5 ml

## Indications and dosages

*Adjunct treatment of refractory testicular cancer*

*Adults:* Etoposide phosphate doses equivalent to 50 to 100 mg/m²/day of etoposide I.V. on days 1 through 5 of each cycle and given in conjunction with other approved chemotherapeutic drugs. Cycle is repeated when adequate recovery from drug toxicity has occurred (usually at 3- to 4-week intervals). Alternatively, etoposide phosphate doses equivalent to 100 mg/m²/day of etoposide I.V. on days 1, 3, and 5 of each cycle and given in conjunction with other approved chemotherapeutic drugs. Cycle is repeated at 3- to 4-week intervals if adequate recovery from drug toxicity has occurred. Infusion rate may range from 5 minutes to 210 minutes, or VePesid may be given

P.O. Recommended dose is two times the I.V. dose rounded to the nearest 50 mg.

*Adjunct treatment of small-cell lung cancer*

*Adults:* Dosage is individualized but may range from etoposide phosphate doses equivalent to 35 mg/m²/day etoposide I.V. for 4 days to etoposide phosphate doses equivalent to 50 mg/m²/day etoposide I.V. for 5 days and given in conjunction with other approved chemotherapeutic agents. Cycle is repeated when adequate recovery from drug toxicity has occurred (usually at 3- to 4-week intervals). Infusion rate may range from 5 minutes to 210 minutes.

◇*AIDS-related Kaposi's sarcoma*

*Adults:* 150 mg/m² daily I.V. for 3 consecutive days every 4 weeks. Repeat cycles p.r.n.

≡*Dosage adjustment.* In patients with renal impairment with creatinine clearance above 50 ml/minute, give usual dosage; for creatinine clearance between 15 and 50 ml/minute, give 75% of usual dosage.

## I.V. administration

■ Wear protective gloves during handling and preparation of drug.

■ Wash skin that comes in contact with drug immediately and thoroughly with soap and water.

■ Reconstitute with 5 or 10 ml of sterile water for injection, normal saline solution, D₅W, bacteriostatic water for injection, or bacteriostatic sodium chloride for injection, resulting in level of 20 or 10 mg per ml, respectively. Drug may be given without further dilution, or diluted further to concentration as low as 0.1 mg/ml with $D_5W$ or normal saline solution.

■ Give drug by slow I.V. infusion over 5 to 210 minutes.

**⚠ ALERT** Drug should not be administered by rapid I.V. injection.

■ Observe patient for hypotension and anaphylaxis.

■ Etoposide diluted to 0.2 mg/ml is stable for 96 hours at room temperature in plastic or glass unprotected from light; solutions diluted to 0.4 mg/ml are stable for 48 hours under same conditions.

## Incompatibilities

Incompatible with idarubicin.

## Mechanism of action

*Antineoplastic action:* Although action of drug is unknown, it's believed to exert cytotoxicity by arresting cells in the metaphase portion of cell division. Drug may also inhibit cells from entering mitosis and depressing DNA and RNA synthesis.

## Pharmacokinetics

*Absorption:* Administered I.V.

*Distribution:* Distribution is believed to be similar to etoposide. Etoposide crosses the blood-brain barrier to a limited and variable extent and is about 97% bound to serum albumin.

*Metabolism:* Rapidly and completely converted to etoposide in plasma.

*Excretion:* After etoposide phosphate is converted to etoposide, etoposide is excreted primarily in the urine as unchanged drug. A smaller portion of a dose is excreted in the feces. The plasma elimination of etoposide is described as biphasic, with an initial phase half-life of about ½ to 2 hours and a terminal phase of about 5¼ to 11 hours.

| Route | Onset | Peak | Duration |
|-------|-------|------|----------|
| P.O., I.V. | Unknown | Unknown | Unknown |

## Contraindications and precautions

Contraindicated in patients hypersensitive to etoposide phosphate, etoposide, or other components of the formulation.

## Interactions

**Drug-drug.** *High-dose cyclosporine:* May increase the toxic effects of etoposide phosphate because of delayed excretion of the drug. Advise clinician to monitor patient closely for drug effects.

*Levamisole hydrochloride:* Known to inhibit phosphatase activities. Avoid using any drug that inhibits phosphatase activities.

*Warfarin:* Prolonged PT and INR. Advise clinician to monitor patient carefully.

## Adverse reactions

**CNS:** *asthenia, malaise,* dizziness, ***peripheral neurotoxicity.***

**CV:** hypertension, hypotension.

**GI:** *nausea, vomiting, anorexia, mucositis,* constipation, abdominal pain, diarrhea, taste alteration.

**Hematologic:** *anemia, myelosuppression* (dose-limiting)**, LEUKOPENIA, THROMBOCYTOPENIA, NEUTROPENIA.**

**Skin:** facial flushing, rash, *reversible alopecia.*

**Other:** *chills, fever,* phlebitis, ***anaphylaxis.***

## Overdose and treatment

Because etoposide phosphate is rapidly converted to etoposide, signs and symptoms of overdose would be expected to be similar. Signs of overdose of etoposide include myelosuppression, nausea, and vomiting.

Treatment is usually supportive and includes transfusion of blood components, antiemetics, and appropriate symptomatic therapy.

## Clinical considerations

■ Use of gloves is recommended when handling etoposide phosphate. If etoposide phosphate solution comes into contact with the skin or mucosa, recommend immediately and thoroughly washing the skin with soap and water and flushing the mucosa with water.

■ Patients with low serum albumin may be at increased risk for etoposide-associated toxicities.

### Therapeutic monitoring

■ Advise clinician to monitor CBC. Recommend observing patient for signs of bone marrow depression. Withhold drug if platelet count is less than 50,000/mm³ or absolute neutrophil count is less than 500/mm³ until the blood counts have sufficiently recovered.

■ Advise clinician that if an anaphylactic reaction occurs, infusion should be terminated immediately and pressor agents, corticosteroids, antihistamines, or volume expanders given p.r.n.

### Special populations

**Pregnant patients.** High risk for fetal harm. During pregnancy, drug should be used only for life-threatening conditions or severe disease when much safer drugs aren't available or are ineffective.

**Breast-feeding patients.** Drug isn't contraindicated in breast-feeding women.

**Pediatric patients.** Safety and efficacy in children haven't been established. Anaphylactic reactions have been reported in pediatric patients who received etoposide.

**Geriatric patients.** Geriatric patients may be particularly susceptible to the hypotensive effects of etoposide.

## Patient counseling

■ Advise patient to avoid exposure to people with infections.

■ Tell patient to promptly report a sore throat, fever, unusual bruising, or bleeding.

■ Reassure patient that hair should grow back after treatment has ended.

■ Tell patient to store capsules in refrigerator.

---

Reactions may be *common,* uncommon, *life-threatening,* or **COMMON AND LIFE-THREATENING.**

# famciclovir
Famvir

*Pharmacologic classification:* synthetic acyclic guanine derivative
*Therapeutic classification:* antiviral
*Pregnancy risk category B*

## Available forms
Available by prescription only
*Tablets:* 125 mg, 250 mg, 500 mg

## Indications and dosages
***Management of acute herpes zoster in immunocompetent patients***
*Adults:* 500 mg P.O. q 8 hours for 7 days.
≡ *Dosage adjustment.* In adults with renal impairment, adjust dosage using this table.

| Creatinine clearance (ml/min) | Dosage |
| --- | --- |
| 40-59 | 500 mg q 12 hr |
| 20-39 | 500 mg q 24 hr |
| < 20 | 250 mg q 48 hr |

***Recurrent genital herpes in immunocompetent patients***
*Adults:* 125 mg P.O. b.i.d. for 5 days.
≡ *Dosage adjustment.* In adults with renal impairment, adjust dosage using this table.

| Creatinine clearance (ml/min) | Dosage |
| --- | --- |
| 20-39 | 125 mg q 24 hr |
| < 20 | 125 mg q 24 hr |

◊ *Chronic suppression or maintenance prophylaxis of HSV infection in HIV-infected patients*
*Adults:* 500 mg P.O. b.i.d.

## Mechanism of action
*Antiviral action:* Famciclovir, a prodrug, changes to an active antiviral compound, penciclovir. It enters viral cells (herpes simplex types 1 and 2, varicella zoster), where it inhibits DNA polymerase, viral DNA synthesis, and, thus, viral replication.

## Pharmacokinetics
*Absorption:* Absolute bioavailability of famciclovir is 77%. Because bioavailability isn't affected by food intake, the drug can be taken without regard to meals.
*Distribution:* Less than 20% protein-bound.
*Metabolism:* Extensively metabolized in the liver to the active drug penciclovir (98.5%) and other inactive metabolites.
*Excretion:* Primarily eliminated in the urine.

| Route | Onset | Peak | Duration |
| --- | --- | --- | --- |
| P.O. | Unknown | 1 hr | Unknown |

## Contraindications and precautions
Contraindicated in patients hypersensitive to drug.
   Use cautiously in patients with impaired renal or hepatic function.

## Interactions
**Drug-drug.** *Probenecid or other drugs significantly eliminated by active renal tubular secretion:* May cause increased plasma levels of penciclovir. Advise clinician to monitor patient for increased adverse effects.

## Adverse reactions
**CNS:** headache, fatigue, dizziness, paresthesia, somnolence.
**EENT:** pharyngitis, sinusitis.
**GI:** diarrhea, nausea, vomiting, constipation, anorexia, abdominal pain.
**Musculoskeletal:** back pain, arthralgia.
**Skin:** pruritus.
**Other:** fever, injury, pain, rigors, zoster-related signs, symptoms, and complications.

## Overdose and treatment
No acute overdose reported. Therapy should be symptomatic and supportive. It isn't known if hemodialysis removes famciclovir from the blood. However, hemodialysis enhances elimination of acyclovir, a related nucleoside analogue.

## Clinical considerations
■ Drug may be given without regard to meals.
■ May interfere with cross-matching studies or hematologic studies.

### Therapeutic monitoring
- Advise clinician to monitor renal and liver function test results.

### Special populations
**Pregnant patients.** Drug should be used during pregnancy only when clearly indicated.
**Breast-feeding patients.** It isn't known if drug appears in breast milk. Drug should be used with caution in breast-feeding women.
**Pediatric patients.** Safety and effectiveness haven't been established in children under age 18.

## Patient counseling
- Explain that treatment is more effective when started within 48 hours of rash onset.
- Inform patient that drug isn't a cure for genital herpes but can decrease the duration and severity of symptoms.
- Advise patient of potential adverse reactions.

## famotidine
Pepcid, Pepcid AC

*Pharmacologic classification:* $H_2$-receptor antagonist
*Therapeutic classification:* antiulcer
*Pregnancy risk category B*

## Available forms
Available by prescription only
*Tablets:* 20 mg, 40 mg
*Injection:* 10 mg/ml
*Injection, premixed:* 20 mg/50 ml normal saline solution
*Suspension:* 40 mg/5 ml
Available without a prescription (Pepcid AC)
*Tablets:* 10 mg

## Indications and dosages
*Duodenal and gastric ulcer*
*Adults:* For acute therapy, 40 mg P.O. h.s. for 4 to 8 weeks; for maintenance therapy, 20 mg P.O. h.s.
*Pathologic hypersecretory conditions (such as Zollinger-Ellison syndrome)*
*Adults:* 20 mg P.O. q 6 hours. As much as 160 mg q 6 hours may be given.
*Short-term treatment of gastroesophageal reflux disease (GERD)*
*Adults:* 20 to 40 mg P.O. b.i.d. for up to 12 weeks.
◇ *Hospitalized patients with intractable ulcers or hypersecretory conditions or patients who can't take oral medication, patients with GI bleeding; to control gastric pH in critically ill patients*
*Adults:* 20 mg I.V. q 12 hours.
*Prevention or treatment of heartburn*
*Adults:* 10 mg P.O. (Pepcid AC) when symptoms occur; or 10 mg P.O. 1 hour before meals for prevention of symptoms. Drug can be used b.i.d. if needed.
≡ *Dosage adjustment.* In patients with moderate renal insufficiency (creatinine clearance less than 50 ml/minute) or severe renal insufficiency (creatinine clearance less than 10 ml/minute), dosage may be reduced to half the dose or the dosing interval may be prolonged to 36 to 48 hours to avoid excess accumulation of drug.

## I.V. administration
- For I.V. injection, dilute 20 mg of drug to a total of 5 or 10 ml of normal saline solution injection or another comparable diluent to provide a solution of 4 or 2 mg/ml, respectively. Recommend administering no faster than 10 mg/min.
- For intermittent I.V. infusion, add 20 mg of drug to 100 ml of injection or another $D_5W$ comparable I.V. solution to provide a concentration of 0.2 mg/ml. Recommend administering over 15 to 30 minutes. Or, recommend giving commercially prepared solution of 0.4 mg/ml over 15 to 30 minutes.
- After dilution, solution is stable for 48 hours at room temperature.
- Store I.V. injection in refrigerator at 36° to 46° F (2° to 8° C).

## Incompatibilities
Incompatible with cefepime, piperacillin, and tazobactam.

## Mechanism of action
*Antiulcer action:* Famotidine competitively inhibits action of histamine at $H_2$-receptors in gastric parietal cells. This inhibits basal and nocturnal gastric acid secretion from stimulation by such factors as caffeine, food, and pentagastrin.

## Pharmacokinetics
*Absorption:* When given orally, about 40% to 45% of dose is absorbed.
*Distribution:* Distributed widely to many body tissues.
*Metabolism:* About 30% to 35% of a given dose is metabolized by the liver.
*Excretion:* Most is excreted unchanged in urine. Famotidine has a longer duration of effect than its 2½- to 4-hour half-life suggests.

| Route | Onset | Peak | Duration |
|-------|-------|------|----------|
| P.O. | 1 hr | 1-3 hr | 12 hr |
| I.V. | Unknown | 30 min | 12 hr |

## Contraindications and precautions
Contraindicated in patients hypersensitive to drug.

## Interactions
**Drug-drug.** *Enteric-coated drugs:* Enteric coatings may dissolve too rapidly because of increased gastric pH. Use together cautiously.
*Ketoconazole:* Decreased absorption of ketoconazole. Increased dose of ketoconazole may be needed.

## Adverse reactions
**CNS:** *headache,* dizziness, vertigo, malaise, paresthesia.
**CV:** palpitations.
**EENT:** tinnitus, orbital edema.
**GI:** diarrhea, constipation, anorexia, dry mouth, taste disorder.
**GU:** increased BUN and creatinine levels.
**Hepatic:** elevated liver enzyme levels.
**Musculoskeletal:** musculoskeletal pain.
**Skin:** acne, dry skin, flushing, transient irritation (at I.V. site).
**Other:** fever.

## Overdose and treatment
Overdose hasn't been reported. Treatment should include gastric lavage or induced emesis, followed by activated charcoal to prevent further absorption and supportive and symptomatic therapy. Hemodialysis doesn't remove famotidine.

## Clinical considerations
■ Drug isn't recommended for use longer than 8 weeks in patients with uncomplicated duodenal ulcer.
■ After administration via nasogastric tube, flush tube to clear it and ensure passage of drug to stomach.
■ Antacids may be given concurrently.
■ Drug appears to cause fewer adverse reactions and drug interactions than cimetidine.
■ Drug may antagonize pentagastrin during gastric acid secretion tests. In skin tests using allergen extracts, drug may cause false-negative results.
**◄ALERT** Don't confuse drug with drugs of similar names, such as felodipine.

### Therapeutic monitoring
■ Therapeutic monitoring is the same for all H$_2$-receptor antagonists.

### Special populations
**Pregnant patients.** Drug should be used during pregnancy only when clearly indicated.
**Breast-feeding patients.** Drug may appear in breast milk. Drug should be used with caution in breast-feeding women.
**Geriatric patients.** Use cautiously in geriatric patients because of increased risk of adverse reactions, particularly those affecting the CNS.

## Patient counseling
■ Caution patient to take drug only as directed and to continue taking doses, even after pain subsides, to ensure adequate healing.
■ Instruct patient to take dose at bedtime.

# felodipine
Plendil

*Pharmacologic classification:* calcium channel blocker
*Therapeutic classification:* antihypertensive
*Pregnancy risk category C*

## Available forms
Available by prescription only
*Tablets (extended-release):* 2.5 mg, 5 mg, 10 mg

## Indications and dosages
*Hypertension*
*Adults:* 5 mg P.O. daily. Adjust dosage based on patient response, generally at intervals not less than 2 weeks. Usual dose is 2.5 to 10 mg P.O. daily; doses exceeding 10 mg daily increase rate of peripheral edema and vasodilatory adverse effects.

≡*Dosage adjustment.* Geriatric patients or patients with impaired hepatic function should receive a starting dose of 2.5 mg daily. Doses of more than 10 mg shouldn't be considered.

## Mechanism of action
*Antihypertensive action:* A dihydropyridine-derivative calcium channel blocker, felodipine blocks the entry of calcium ions into vascular smooth muscle and cardiac cells. This type of calcium channel blocker shows some selectivity for smooth muscle as compared with cardiac muscle. Effects on vascular smooth muscle are relaxation and vasodilation.

## Pharmacokinetics
*Absorption:* Almost completely absorbed, but extensive first-pass metabolism reduces absolute bioavailability to about 20%.
*Distribution:* Highly plasma protein–bound.
*Metabolism:* Metabolism mediated by the P-450 (CYP) isoenzyme 3A4.
*Excretion:* Over 70% of a dose appears in urine, and 10% appears in feces as metabolites.

| Route | Onset | Peak | Duration |
|-------|-------|------|----------|
| P.O. | 2-5 hr | 2½-5 hr | 24 hr |

## Contraindications and precautions
Contraindicated in patients hypersensitive to drug.
Use cautiously in patients with impaired hepatic function or HF, especially those receiving beta blockers.

## Interactions

**Drug-drug.** *Anticonvulsants:* May decrease plasma level of felodipine. Use together cautiously.

*Digoxin:* Decreased peak serum levels of digoxin, but total absorbed drug is unchanged. Clinical significance is unknown.

*Drugs that inhibit isoenzyme 3A4 (cimetidine, erythromycin, itraconazole, ketoconazole):* May increase plasma felodipine levels. Caution should be exercised with concomitant administration.

*Metoprolol:* Concurrent use may alter the pharmacokinetics of metoprolol. No dosage adjustment appears needed; however, recommend monitoring patient for adverse effects.

*Theophylline:* May slightly decrease theophylline levels. Advise clinician to monitor patient for drug effects.

**Drug-food.** *Grapefruit juice:* May increase bioavailability and effect of drug when taken together. Discourage use together.

## Adverse reactions

**CNS:** *headache,* dizziness, paresthesia, asthenia.

**CV:** *flushing, peripheral edema,* chest pain, palpitations.

**EENT:** rhinorrhea, pharyngitis.

**GI:** abdominal pain, nausea, constipation, diarrhea, gingival hyperplasia.

**Musculoskeletal:** muscle cramps, back pain.

**Respiratory:** upper respiratory infection, cough.

**Skin:** rash.

## Overdose and treatment

Expected symptoms include peripheral vasodilation, bradycardia, and hypotension.

Recommend providing supportive care. I.V. fluids or sympathomimetics may be useful in treating hypotension, and atropine (0.5 to 1 mg I.V.) may treat bradycardia. It isn't known if drug may be removed by dialysis.

## Clinical considerations

■ Peripheral edema appears to be both dose- and age-dependent. It's more common in patients taking higher doses, especially those ages 60 and older.

■ Drug may be given without regard to meals. However, a small study reported a more than twofold increase of bioavailability when drug was taken with doubly concentrated grapefruit juice compared with water or orange juice.

## Therapeutic monitoring

■ Advise clinician to monitor as for all calcium channel blockers.

## Special populations

**Pregnant patients.** Drug should be used in pregnancy only when benefits justify risk to fetus.

**Breast-feeding patients.** It's unknown if drug appears in breast milk. Because of risk of serious adverse effects to the infant, breast-feeding isn't recommended.

**Pediatric patients.** Safety and efficacy in children haven't been established.

**Geriatric patients.** Higher blood levels of drug are seen in geriatric patients. Mean clearance of drug from geriatric hypertensive patients (average age 74) was less than half of that observed in young patients (average age 26). Recommend checking blood pressure closely during dosage adjustment. Maximum daily dose is 10 mg.

## Patient counseling

■ Tell patient to observe good oral hygiene and to see a dentist regularly because drug has been associated with mild gingival hyperplasia.

■ Remind patient to swallow tablet whole and not to crush or chew it.

■ Inform patient that he should continue taking drug, even when feeling better. He should watch his diet and call his prescriber before taking other drugs, including OTC drugs.

# fenofibrate (micronized)
Tricor

*Pharmacologic classification:* fibric acid derivative
*Therapeutic classification:* antihyperlipidemic
*Pregnancy risk category C*

## Available forms

Available by prescription only
*Capsules:* 67 mg, 134 mg, 200 mg
*Tablets:* 54 mg, 160 mg

## Indications and dosages

*Adjunct to diet for treatment of patients with very high serum triglyceride levels (type IV and V hyperlipidemia) who are at high risk of pancreatitis and who don't respond adequately to diet alone*

*Adults:* 67- to 200-mg capsule or 54- to 160-mg tablet P.O. daily. Based on response, increase dosage if needed after repeat triglyceride levels at 4- to 8-week intervals to maximum dose of 200-mg capsule or 160-mg tablet daily.

*Adjunct to diet for the reduction of LDL cholesterol, total cholesterol, triglycerides, and apolipoprotein B, and to increase HDL-C in patients with primary hypercholesterolemia or mixed dyslipidemia (Fredrickson types IIa and IIb)*

*Adults:* 200-mg capsule or 160-mg tablet P.O. daily.

≡*Dosage adjustment.* Minimize dosage in geriatric patients or renally impaired patients (creatinine clearance < 50 ml/min). Initiate therapy at dose of 67-mg capsule or 54-mg tablet daily and increase only after effects on

---

Reactions may be *common,* uncommon, *life-threatening,* or COMMON AND LIFE-THREATENING.

renal function and triglyceride levels have been evaluated at this dose.

## Mechanism of action

*Antihyperlipidemic action:* Exact mechanism of action isn't known; drug is thought to lower triglyceride levels by inhibiting triglyceride synthesis, resulting in a decrease in the amount of very-low-density lipoprotein released into the circulation. Fenofibrate may stimulate the breakdown of triglyceride-rich protein.

## Pharmacokinetics

*Absorption:* Well absorbed. Food increases the absorption of drug by 35%.
*Distribution:* Steady-state plasma levels are achieved within 5 days after therapy starts. Drug is almost entirely plasma protein–bound.
*Metabolism:* Rapidly hydrolyzed by esterases to fenofibric acid, an active metabolite. Fenofibric acid is primarily conjugated with glucuronic acid and excreted in urine.
*Excretion:* Primarily excreted in the urine; 25% is excreted in the feces; elimination half-life is 20 hours.

| Route | Onset | Peak | Duration |
|-------|-------|------|----------|
| P.O. | Unknown | 6-8 hr | Unknown |

## Contraindications and precautions

Contraindicated in patients with preexisting gallbladder disease, hepatic dysfunction (including primary biliary cirrhosis), severe renal dysfunction, unexplained persistent liver function abnormalities, or hypersensitivity to drug.

## Interactions

**Drug-drug.** *Bile acid resins:* May bind and inhibit absorption of fenofibrate. Fenofibrate should be taken 1 hour before or 4 to 6 hours after taking these drugs.
*Coumarin-type anticoagulants:* Protein-binding displacement of the anticoagulant and potentiation of its effects. Use extreme caution; reduce dosage of anticoagulant to maintain PT and INR within desired range.
*Cyclosporine:* Cyclosporine-induced renal dysfunction may compromise the elimination of fenofibrate. Cyclosporine and fenofibrate should be used together cautiously.
*HMG-CoA inhibitors (statins):* No data are available on use of statins with fenofibrate; however, because of risk of myopathy, rhabdomyolysis, and acute renal failure reported with the combination use of statins with gemfibrozil (another fibrate derivative), these drugs shouldn't be given together.

## Adverse reactions

**CNS:** dizziness, miscellaneous pain, asthenia, fatigue, paresthesia, insomnia, headache.
**CV:** *arrhythmias*.
**EENT:** eye irritation, eye floaters, earache, conjunctivitis, blurred vision, rhinitis, sinusitis.
**GI:** dyspepsia, eructation, flatulence, increased appetite, nausea, vomiting, abdominal pain, constipation, diarrhea.
**GU:** polyuria, vaginitis, increased creatinine and BUN levels.
**Hematologic:** decreased hemoglobin.
**Hepatic:** elevated liver enzyme levels.
**Metabolic:** decreased uric acid levels.
**Musculoskeletal:** arthralgia.
**Respiratory:** cough.
**Skin:** urticaria, pruritis, rash.
**Other:** *infections,* decreased libido, flu syndrome.

## Overdose and treatment

No cases of overdose have been reported. If overdose does occur, supportive measures should be initiated. Because drug is highly protein-bound, hemodialysis is unlikely to be of value.

## Clinical considerations

■ Fenofibrate lowers serum uric acid levels in normal patients as well as hyperuricemic patients by increasing uric acid excretion.
■ Drug shouldn't be used for primary or secondary prevention of coronary artery disease.
■ Recommend changing or discontinuing the use of beta blockers, estrogens, and thiazide diuretics, if possible, because they may increase plasma triglyceride levels.
■ Therapy should be withdrawn in patients who don't have an adequate response after 2 months of treatment with maximum dose.
■ Pancreatitis may occur in patients receiving fenofibrate; myositis and rhabdomyolysis may occur in those with renal failure. Recommend assessing CK levels in patients with myalgia, muscle tenderness, or weakness.

### Therapeutic monitoring

■ Advise prescriber to withdraw therapy in patients who don't achieve an adequate response after 2 months of treatment with the maximum daily dose.
■ Drug may cause excretion of cholesterol into the bile, leading to cholelithiasis. If suspected, recommend performing appropriate tests and stopping drug.
■ Mild to moderate decreases in hemoglobin, hematocrit, and WBC count may occur when therapy starts but stabilize on long-term administration.

### Special populations

**Breast-feeding patients.** Don't use drug in breast-feeding patients; either the drug or breast-feeding should be discontinued.
**Pediatric patients.** Drug isn't indicated for use in children. Safety and efficacy haven't been established.
**Geriatric patients.** Drug acts similarly in geriatric patients (ages 77 to 87) as in young adults; similar dosing regimens can be used.

## Patient counseling
■ Advise patient to promptly report symptoms of unexplained muscle weakness, pain, or tenderness, especially if accompanied by malaise or fever.
■ Instruct patient to take tablets with meals to optimize drug absorption.

# fenoldopam mesylate
Corlopam

*Pharmacologic classification:*
dopamine $D_1$-like receptor agonist
*Therapeutic classification:* antihypertensive
*Pregnancy risk category B*

## Available forms
Available by prescription only
*Ampules:* 10 mg/ml in single-dose 1-ml, 2-ml, 5-ml ampules

## Indications and dosages
*Short-term (up to 48 hours) in-hospital management of severe hypertension when rapid but quickly reversible reduction of blood pressure is indicated, including malignant hypertension with deteriorating end-organ function*
*Adults:* Administer by continuous I.V. infusion. Infusion rate is initiated at 0.025 to 0.3 mcg/kg/minute and titrated upward or downward at a frequency not exceeding q 15 minutes to achieve desired blood pressure.

## I.V. administration
■ Dilute contents of single-dose ampules before use.
■ Dilute with $D_5W$ or normal saline solution to a final concentration of 40 mcg/ml by adding 40 mg of concentrate to 1,000 ml, 20 mg to 500 ml, or 10 mg to 250 ml of compatible solution.
■ Recommended increments for titration are 0.05 to 0.1 mcg/kg/minute.
■ Diluted solution is stable at room temperature for at least 24 hours.

### Incompatibilities
None reported.

## Mechanism of action
*Antihypertensive action:* Rapid-acting vasodilator. Fenoldopam is an agonist for $D_1$-like dopamine receptors and binds with moderate affinity to $alpha_2$ adrenoreceptors. No significant affinity for $D_2$-like receptors, $alpha_1$ or beta adrenoreceptors, 5HT, $5HT_2$, or muscarinic receptors has been noted. In addition, fenoldopam has no effect on ACE activity, although it may increase norepinephrine plasma levels.

## Pharmacokinetics
*Absorption:* Administered I.V.
*Distribution:* Not reported. Steady-state plasma levels of 3.2 to 4 ng/ml were reported with infusion rates of 0.1 mcg/kg/minute.
*Metabolism:* Principal routes of conjugation are methylation, glucuronidation, and sulfation.
*Excretion:* Elimination is largely by conjugation, without participation of cytochrome P-450 enzymes. Elimination half-life is reported to be about 5 minutes. After I.V. administration, 90% of drug is excreted in urine and 10% in the feces. Only 4% of drug is excreted unchanged.

| Route | Onset | Peak | Duration |
|-------|-------|------|----------|
| I.V. | 15 min | 20 min | Unknown |

## Contraindications and precautions
No contraindications are known. Use cautiously because drug is a rapid-acting, potent vasodilator that may precipitate severe hypotension.

Drug should be used with caution in patients with glaucoma or ocular hypertension because dose-dependent increases in intraocular pressure may occur. Drug may cause symptomatic hypotension; particular caution should be used when giving to patients who have sustained an acute cerebral infarction or hemorrhage.

Fenoldopam contains sodium metabisulfite, which may cause allergic-type reactions (including anaphylactic symptoms and severe asthmatic episodes in certain susceptible individuals). Sulfite sensitivity is more frequent in asthmatic than in nonasthmatic people.

## Interactions
*Drug-drug. Beta blockers:* Unexpected hypotension could result from beta-blocker inhibition of the reflex response to fenoldopam. Avoid use together.

## Adverse reactions
**CNS:** dizziness, headache, insomnia.
**CV:** hypotension, orthostatic hypotension, palpitations, *bradycardia,* tachycardia, angina, *MI, HF,* T-wave inversion, nonspecific chest pain.
**EENT:** nasal congestion.
**GI:** nausea, vomiting, abdominal pain, constipation, diarrhea.
**GU:** oliguria, urinary tract infection.
**Hematologic:** leukocytosis, bleeding.
**Metabolic:** increased BUN and creatinine, serum glucose, LDH, transaminases; hypokalemia.
**Musculoskeletal:** limb cramp, back pain.
**Respiratory:** dyspnea.
**Skin:** flushing, injection site reaction.
**Other:** pyrexia.

## Overdose and treatment
Intentional overdose hasn't been reported. The most likely reaction would be excessive hypotension, which should be treated with drug discontinuation and appropriate supportive measures.

## Clinical considerations
■ Drug causes a dose-related tachycardia, which diminishes over time but remains substantial at higher doses.
■ Drug may be abruptly discontinued or infusion gradually tapered. Oral antihypertensives can be added once blood pressure is stable during infusion or after its discontinuation.

### Therapeutic monitoring
■ Advise clinician to monitor blood pressure frequently during infusions and blood pressure and heart rate every 15 minutes until patient is stable.
■ Advise clinician to monitor serum electrolytes and watch for hypokalemia.

### Special populations
**Pregnant patients.** Use during pregnancy only if clearly needed.
**Breast-feeding patients.** Drug may appear in breast milk; caution should be used when giving to breast-feeding women.
**Pediatric patients.** Safety and efficacy in children haven't been established.

## Patient counseling
■ Advise patient that drug causes dose-related decreases in blood pressure and increases in heart rate.
■ Encourage patient to report adverse reactions promptly.

# fenoprofen calcium
Nalfon

*Pharmacologic classification:* NSAID
*Therapeutic classification:* nonnarcotic analgesic, anti-inflammatory, antipyretic
*Pregnancy risk category NR*

## Available forms
Available by prescription only
*Tablets:* 600 mg
*Capsules:* 200 mg, 300 mg

## Indications and dosages
**Rheumatoid arthritis and osteoarthritis**
*Adults:* 300 to 600 mg P.O. t.i.d. or q.i.d. Maximum dose is 3.2 g daily.
**Mild to moderate pain**
*Adults:* 200 mg P.O. q 4 to 6 hours, p.r.n.
◊ *Fever*
*Adults:* Single oral doses up to 400 mg P.O.

◊ *Acute gouty arthritis*
*Adults:* 800 mg P.O. q 6 hours; decrease dosage based on patient response.

## Mechanism of action
*Analgesic, anti-inflammatory, and antipyretic actions:* Mechanisms of action unknown, but drug is thought to inhibit prostaglandin synthesis. Fenoprofen decreases platelet aggregation and may prolong bleeding time.

## Pharmacokinetics
*Absorption:* Absorbed rapidly and completely from the GI tract.
*Distribution:* About 99% is protein-bound.
*Metabolism:* Metabolized in the liver.
*Excretion:* Excreted chiefly in urine with a serum half-life of 2½ to 3 hours. A small amount is excreted in feces.

| Route | Onset | Peak | Duration |
|-------|-------|------|----------|
| P.O. | 15-30 min | 2 hr | 4-6 hr |

## Contraindications and precautions
Contraindicated during pregnancy and in patients hypersensitive to drug, or those with significantly impaired renal function, or history of aspirin- or NSAID-induced asthma, rhinitis, or urticaria.

Use cautiously in geriatric patients and in patients with history of GI events, peptic ulcer disease, compromised cardiac function, or hypertension.

## Interactions
**Drug-drug.** *Anticoagulants and thrombolytics (coumarin derivatives, heparin, streptokinase, urokinase):* May potentiate anticoagulant effects. Drugs should be used together cautiously.
*Antihypertensives or diuretics:* Decreased effectiveness. Advise clinician to monitor patient for effects.
*Aspirin:* May decrease the bioavailability of fenoprofen. Avoid use together.
*Coumarin derivatives, nifedipine, phenytoin, or verapamil:* Toxicity may occur. Drugs should be used together cautiously.
*Diuretics:* Increased nephrotoxic potential. Drugs should be used together with caution.
*Drugs that inhibit platelet aggregation (such as dextran, dipyridamole, mezlocillin, piperacillin, sulfinpyrazone, ticarcillin, valproic acid) or cefamandole, cefoperazone, plicamycin, aspirin, salicylates, or other anti-inflammatory drugs:* Bleeding problems may occur. Avoid use together.
*Gold compounds, other anti-inflammatory drugs, or acetaminophen:* Increased nephrotoxicity may occur. Drugs should be used together cautiously.
*Insulin or oral antidiabetics:* Increased hypoglycemic effects. Dosage may require adjustment.

*Methotrexate and lithium:* May decrease the renal clearance of fenoprofen.

*Salicylates, anti-inflammatory drugs, corticotropin, or corticosteroids:* May cause increased GI adverse reactions, including ulceration and hemorrhage. Avoid use together.

**Drug-herb.** *Dong quai, feverfew, garlic, ginger, horse chestnut, red clover:* Possible increased risk of bleeding. Discourage use together.

*St. John's wort, dong quai:* Increased risk of photosensitivity. Advise patient to avoid unprotected exposure to sunlight.

**Drug-lifestyle.** *Alcohol use:* May increase risk of adverse GI reactions. Avoid use together.

## Adverse reactions

**CNS:** *headache,* dizziness, *somnolence,* fatigue, nervousness, asthenia, tremor, confusion.
**CV:** peripheral edema, palpitations.
**EENT:** tinnitus, blurred vision, decreased hearing, nasopharyngitis.
**GI:** *epigastric distress, nausea, GI bleeding,* vomiting, occult blood loss, peptic ulceration, constipation, anorexia, *dyspepsia,* flatulence.
**GU:** oliguria, interstitial nephritis, proteinuria, *reversible renal failure,* papillary necrosis, cystitis, hematuria, increased BUN and creatinine.
**Hematologic:** prolonged bleeding time, anemia, *aplastic anemia, agranulocytosis, thrombocytopenia, hemorrhage,* bruising, hemolytic anemia.
**Hepatic:** elevated liver enzyme levels, *hepatitis.*
**Metabolic:** hyperkalemia.
**Respiratory:** dyspnea, upper respiratory tract infections.
**Skin:** *pruritus,* rash, urticaria, increased diaphoresis.
**Other:** *anaphylaxis, angioedema.*

## Overdose and treatment

Little is known about the acute toxicity of fenoprofen. Nonoliguric renal failure, tachycardia, and hypotension have been observed. Other symptoms include drowsiness, dizziness, confusion and lethargy, nausea, vomiting, headache, tinnitus, and blurred vision. Elevations in serum creatinine and BUN levels may occur.

To treat an overdose of fenoprofen, recommend emptying stomach immediately by inducing emesis with ipecac syrup or by gastric lavage. Recommend giving activated charcoal via nasogastric tube. Recommend providing symptomatic and supportive measures (respiratory support and correction of fluid and electrolyte imbalances). Advise clinician to monitor laboratory effects and vital signs closely. Dialysis is of little value.

## Clinical considerations

■ Consider the recommendations relevant to all NSAIDs. Fenoprofen has been used to treat fever, acute gouty arthritis, and juvenile arthritis.

■ For patients at high risk for complications from NSAID-induced ulceration, misoprostol, a proton pump inhibitor, or an $H_2$ antagonist may be considered for prevention.

■ Drug may cause false elevations in both free and total serum $T_3$, but thyroid-stimulating hormone and $T_4$ are unaffected.

### Therapeutic monitoring

■ Advise clinician to monitor patient for potential CNS effects. Recommend instituting safety measures to prevent injury.

■ Advise clinician to monitor renal, hepatic, and auditory function in patients on long-term therapy. Drug should be stopped if abnormalities occur.

### Special populations

**Breast-feeding patients.** Because drug appears in breast milk, use should be avoided in breast-feeding women.

**Pediatric patients.** Safe use hasn't been established. Drug isn't recommended for use in children under age 14.

**Geriatric patients.** Patients over age 60 may be more susceptible to the toxic effects of fenoprofen, especially adverse GI reactions. Use with caution. The effects of drug on renal prostaglandins may cause fluid retention and edema, a significant drawback for geriatric patients and those with HF.

## Patient counseling

■ Tell patient to avoid activities that require alertness or concentration until CNS effects of drug are known.

■ Advise patient to call prescriber for specific instruction before taking OTC analgesics.

# fentanyl citrate
Sublimaze

# fentanyl transdermal system
Duragesic-25, Duragesic-50, Duragesic-75, Duragesic-100

# fentanyl transmucosal
Actiq, Fentanyl Oralet

*Pharmacologic classification:* opioid agonist
*Therapeutic classification:* analgesic, adjunct to anesthesia, anesthetic
*Pregnancy risk category C*
*Controlled substance schedule II*

## Available forms
Available by prescription only
*Injection:* 50 mcg/ml

*Transdermal system:* Patches designed to release 25 mcg, 50 mcg, 75 mcg, or 100 mcg of fentanyl/hour.
*Transmucosal (Oralet):* 100 mcg, 200 mcg, 300 mcg, 400 mcg
*Transmucosal (Actiq):* 200 mcg, 400 mcg, 600 mcg, 800 mcg, 1,200 mcg, 1,600 mcg

## Indications and dosages
*Preoperatively (Oralet)*
*Adults:* 50 to 100 mcg I.M. 30 to 60 minutes before surgery or 5 mcg/kg as lozenge P.O. for patient to suck until dissolved, 20 to 40 minutes before surgery.
*Children weighing over 10 kg (22 lb) but less than 40 kg (88 lb):* 10 to 15 mcg/kg as lozenge P.O. for patient to suck until dissolved, 20 to 40 minutes before surgery.
*Adjunct to general anesthetic*
**Low-dose regimen for minor procedures**
*Adults:* 2 mcg/kg I.V.
**Moderate-dose regimen for major procedures**
*Adults:* Initial dose is 2 to 20 mcg/kg I.V.; may give additional doses of 25 to 100 mcg I.V. or I.M., p.r.n.
**High-dose regimen for complicated procedures**
*Adults:* Initial dose is 20 to 50 mcg/kg I.V.; additional doses of 25 mcg to one-half the initial dose may be given, p.r.n.
*Adjunct to anesthesia (Oralet)*
*Adults and children 2 years and older:* 5-mcg/kg lozenge P.O.
*Adults over age 65:* 2.5- to 5-mcg/kg lozenge P.O.
*Adjunct to regional anesthesia*
*Adults:* 50 to 100 mcg I.M. or slow I.V. over 1 to 2 minutes.
*Induction and maintenance of anesthesia*
*Children ages 2 to 12:* Reduce dosage as low as 1.7 to 3.3 mcg/kg.
*Postoperative analgesic*
*Adults:* 50 to 100 mcg I.M. q 1 to 2 hours, p.r.n.
*Management of chronic pain in patients who can't be managed by lesser means*
*Adults:* Apply one transdermal system to a portion of the upper torso on an area of skin that isn't irritated and hasn't been irradiated. Start therapy with the 25-mcg/hour system; adjust dosage as needed and tolerated. Each system may be worn for 72 hours.
*Management of breakthrough cancer pain (Actiq only)*
*Adults:* Initial dose is 200 mcg. Give a second dose 15 minutes after the previous dose (unit) has been completed. Don't give more than 2 units for each breakthrough pain episode while the patient is in the titration phase. Evaluate each new dose used in the titration period over 1 to 2 days. Once an effective dose is established, limit patient to 4 units/day or less. Discontinue Actiq via gradual downward titration.

≡*Dosage adjustment.* Lower doses are usually indicated for geriatric patients who may be more sensitive to therapeutic and adverse effects of the drug.

## I.V. administration
■ Injections should be protected from light and stored at controlled room temperatures of 59° to 86° F (15° to 30° C).
■ Keep narcotic agonist (naloxone) and resuscitation equipment available when giving drug I.V.

### Incompatibilities
Incompatible with methohexital, pentobarbital sodium, and thiopental.

## Mechanism of action
*Analgesic action:* Fentanyl binds to the opiate receptors as an agonist to alter the patient's perception of painful stimuli, thus providing analgesia for moderate to severe pain. Its CNS and respiratory depressant effects are similar to those of morphine. Drug has little hypnotic activity and rarely causes histamine release.

## Pharmacokinetics
*Absorption:* Varies with form administered.
*Distribution:* Redistribution has been suggested as the main cause of the brief analgesic effect of fentanyl.
*Metabolism:* Metabolized in the liver.
*Excretion:* Excreted in the urine as metabolites and unchanged drug. Elimination half-life is about 7 hours after parenteral use, 5 to 15 hours after transmucosal use, and 18 hours after transdermal use.

| Route | Onset | Peak | Duration |
|---|---|---|---|
| I.V. | 1-2 min | 3-5 min | ½-1 hr |
| I.M. | 7-15 min | 20-30 min | 1-2 hr |
| Transdermal | 12-24 hr | 1-3 days | Variable |
| Transmucosal | 5-15 min | 20-50 min | Unknown |

## Contraindications and precautions
Contraindicated in patients with known intolerance of drug.
Use cautiously in geriatric or debilitated patients and in those with head injuries, increased CSF pressure, COPD, decreased respiratory reserve, compromised respirations, arrhythmias, or hepatic, renal, or cardiac disease.

## Interactions
**Drug-drug.** *Anticholinergics:* Avoid use together.
*Cimetidine:* May increase respiratory and CNS depression; such use requires that dosage of fentanyl be reduced by one-quarter to one-third.
*CNS depressants (antihistamines, barbiturates, benzodiazepines, general anesthetics, muscle relaxants, narcotic analgesics, phenothiazines, sedative-hypnotics, tricyclic antidepressants):*

Potentiated respiratory and CNS depression, sedation, and hypotensive effects of drug. Drugs should be used together cautiously.

*Droperidol:* Hypotension and a decrease in pulmonary artery pressure. Drugs should be used together cautiously.

*Drugs that are extensively metabolized in the liver (digitoxin, phenytoin, rifampin):* Drug accumulation and enhanced effects may result from use together. Drugs should be used together cautiously.

*General anesthetics, diazepam:* Severe CV depression may result. Avoid use together.

*MAO inhibitors:* Increased CNS effects. The manufacturer warns that fentanyl shouldn't be given to a patient who has received an MAO inhibitor within the past 14 days.

*Narcotic antagonists:* May cause acute withdrawal syndrome. Drugs should be used with caution.

*Spinal anesthesia and some peridural anesthetics:* When used together, fentanyl can alter respiration by blocking intercostal nerves. Avoid use together.

**Drug-lifestyle.** *Alcohol use:* May cause additive effects. Advise patient to avoid alcohol.

## Adverse reactions

**CNS:** *sedation, somnolence, clouded sensorium, euphoria,* dizziness, headache, *confusion, asthenia,* nervousness, hallucinations, anxiety, depression.

**CV:** *hypotension,* hypertension, ***arrhythmias,*** chest pain.

**GI:** *nausea, vomiting, constipation,* ileus, abdominal pain, *dry mouth,* anorexia, diarrhea, dyspepsia, increased plasma amylase and lipase levels.

**GU:** *urine retention.*

**Respiratory:** *respiratory depression,* hypoventilation, dyspnea, ***apnea.***

**Skin:** reaction at application site (erythema, papules, edema), *pruritus, diaphoresis.*

**Other:** physical dependence.

## Overdose and treatment

The most common signs and symptoms are extensions of its actions. They include CNS depression, respiratory depression, and miosis. Other acute toxic effects include hypotension, bradycardia, hypothermia, shock, apnea, cardiopulmonary arrest, circulatory collapse, pulmonary edema, and seizures.

To treat acute overdose, recommend first establishing adequate respiratory exchange via a patent airway and ventilation p.r.n.; a narcotic antagonist (naloxone) should be given to reverse respiratory depression. (Because the duration of action of fentanyl is longer than that of naloxone, repeated dosing may be needed.) Naloxone shouldn't be given unless the patient has clinically significant respiratory or CV depression. Advise clinician to monitor vital signs closely.

Recommend providing symptomatic and supportive treatment. Advise clinician to monitor laboratory values, vital signs, and neurologic status closely.

## Clinical considerations

■ The high lipid solubility of fentanyl may contribute to this potential adverse effect.

■ Fentanyl may cause bradycardia. Pretreatment with an anticholinergic (such as atropine or glycopyrrolate) may minimize this effect.

■ High doses can produce muscle rigidity. This effect can be reversed by naloxone.

■ Many anesthesiologists use epidural and intrathecal fentanyl as a potent adjunct to epidural anesthesia.

**Transdermal form**

■ Transdermal fentanyl isn't recommended for postoperative pain.

■ Dosage adjustments in patients using the transdermal system should be made gradually. Reaching steady-state levels of a new dose may take up to 6 days; dosage adjustment should be delayed until after at least two applications.

■ Most patients experience good control of pain for 3 days while wearing the transdermal system, although a few may need a new application after 48 hours. Because serum fentanyl level increases for the first 24 hours after application, analgesic effect can't be evaluated for the first day.

■ When reducing opiate therapy or switching to a different analgesic, the transdermal system should be withdrawn gradually. Because the serum level of fentanyl decreases very gradually after removal, recommend giving half of the equianalgesic dose of the new analgesic 12 to 18 hours after removal.

### Therapeutic monitoring

■ Recommend observing patient for delayed onset of respiratory depression.

■ Advise clinician to monitor patient's heart rate.

■ Advise clinician to monitor patient for at least 12 hours for adverse reactions to the transdermal system. Serum levels of fentanyl decrease very gradually and may take as long as 17 hours to decline by 50%.

### Special populations

**Pregnant patients.** Drug use is contraindicated during pregnancy unless benefits outweigh risks to fetus.

**Breast-feeding patients.** Drug appears in breast milk and shouldn't be given to breast-feeding women.

**Pediatric patients.** Safe use in children under age 2 hasn't been established for parenteral or transmucosal (buccal) use. Safe use in children under age 12 for transdermal system hasn't been established. Transdermal system also should not be used in children under age 18 weighing under 50 kg (110 lb), and the buccal form should not be used in any child weighing under 15 kg (33 lb).

**Geriatric patients.** Use with caution in geriatric patients.

## Patient counseling
- Advise patient of proper application of the transdermal patch.
- Tell patient to apply to a new site if another patch is needed after 72 hours.
- Warn patient to keep lozenges out of reach of children.
- Advise patient on proper disposal of lozenges.

# ferrous fumarate
Femiron, Feostat, Fumasorb, Fumerin, Hemocyte, Ircon, Ircon-FA, Neo-Fer*, Nephro-Fer, Novofumar*, Palafer*, Span-FF

*Pharmacologic classification:* oral iron supplement
*Therapeutic classification:* hematinic
*Pregnancy risk category A*

## Available forms
Available without a prescription. Ferrous fumarate is 33% elemental iron.
*Tablets:* 63 mg, 195 mg, 200 mg, 324 mg, 325 mg, 350 mg
*Tablets (chewable):* 100 mg
*Capsules (extended-release):* 325 mg
*Suspension:* 100 mg/5 ml
*Drops:* 45 mg/0.6 ml

## Indications and dosages
*Iron-deficiency states*
*Adults:* 50 to 100 mg P.O. of elemental iron, t.i.d. Adjust dosage gradually, as needed and tolerated. Geriatric patients may need higher doses because reduced gastric secretions and achlorhydria may lower capacity for iron absorption.
*Children:* 3 to 6 mg/kg P.O. of elemental iron daily divided into three doses.
≡ *Dosage adjustment.* For patients with chronic renal failure undergoing hemodialysis and epoetin alfa therapy, at least 200 mg of elemental iron daily for adults, and 2 to 3 mg/kg of elemental iron in 2 to 3 divided doses daily for children.
*Prevention of iron deficiency*
*Pregnant women:* Provide supplementation to maintain daily iron intake at 30 mg of elemental iron.
*Normal full-term infants who are not breast-fed or are partially breast-fed:* 1 mg/kg P.O. of elemental iron daily for first year of life (maximum 15 mg).

*Premature or low–birth-weight infants:* 2 to 4 mg/kg of elemental iron starting at ages 1 to 2 months (maximum 15 mg).
*Children 10 years and older who have begun pubertal growth spurt:* Males: 2 mg P.O. of elemental iron daily; females: 5 mg P.O. daily.

## Mechanism of action
*Hematinic action:* Ferrous fumarate replaces iron, an essential component in the formation of hemoglobin.

## Pharmacokinetics
*Absorption:* Absorbed from the entire length of the GI tract, but primary absorption sites are the duodenum and proximal jejunum. Up to 10% of iron is absorbed by healthy individuals; patients with iron-deficiency anemia may absorb up to 60%. Enteric coating and some extended-release formulas have decreased absorption because they're designed to release iron past the points of highest absorption; food may decrease absorption by 33% to 50%.
*Distribution:* Transported through GI mucosal cells directly into the blood, where it's immediately bound to a carrier protein, transferrin, and transported to the bone marrow for incorporation into hemoglobin. Iron is highly protein-bound.
*Metabolism:* Liberated by the destruction of hemoglobin, but is conserved and reused by the body.
*Excretion:* Healthy individuals lose only small amounts of iron daily. Men and postmenopausal women lose about 1 mg/day, and premenopausal women about 1.5 mg/day. The loss usually occurs in nails, hair, feces, and urine; trace amounts are lost in bile and sweat.

| Route | Onset | Peak | Duration |
|-------|-------|------|----------|
| P.O. | 4 days | 7-10 days | 2-4 mo |

## Contraindications and precautions
Contraindicated in patients with primary hemochromatosis or hemosiderosis, hemolytic anemia unless iron-deficiency anemia is also present, peptic ulcer disease, regional enteritis, or ulcerative colitis and in those receiving repeated blood transfusions.

Use cautiously on long-term basis.

## Interactions
**Drug-drug.** *Antacids, aluminum-containing phosphate binders, cholestyramine, cimetidine, and vitamin E:* Decrease ferrous fumarate absorption. Recommend separating doses by 1- to 2-hour intervals.
*Chloramphenicol:* Delays response to iron therapy. Advise clinician to monitor patient carefully.
*Doxycycline:* May interfere with ferrous fumarate absorption even when doses are separated. Avoid use together.

*L-thyroxine:* May decrease L-thyroxine absorption. Doses should be separated by at least 2 hours. Advise clinician to monitor thyroid function.

*Levodopa and methyldopa:* May decrease absorption of these drugs. Advise clinician to monitor patient carefully.

*Penicillamine:* Decreased penicillamine absorption; recommend separating doses by at least 2 hours.

*Quinolones:* Drug may decrease absorption of quinolones. Advise clinician to monitor patient closely.

*Tetracycline:* Inhibits absorption of both drugs; tetracycline should be given 3 hours after or 2 hours before iron supplement.

*Vitamin C:* Increases iron absorption. May be used as a beneficial drug interaction.

**Drug-herb.** *Black cohosh, chamomile, feverfew, gossypol, hawthorn, nettle, plantain, St. John's wort:* Decreased iron absorption. Use together should be discouraged.

**Drug-food.** *Cereals, cheese, coffee, eggs, milk, tea, whole-grain breads, yogurt:* May impair oral iron absorption. Shouldn't be used together.

### Adverse reactions
**GI:** *nausea,* epigastric pain, vomiting, *constipation,* diarrhea, black stools, anorexia.
**Other:** temporary staining of teeth (with suspension and drops).

### Overdose and treatment
The lethal dose of iron is between 200 and 250 mg/kg; fatalities have occurred with lower doses. Signs and symptoms may follow ingestion of 20 to 60 mg/kg.

Between 30 minutes and 8 hours after ingestion, patient may experience lethargy, nausea and vomiting, green then tarry stools, weak and rapid pulse, hypotension, dehydration, acidosis, and coma. If death doesn't immediately ensue, symptoms may clear for about 24 hours.

At 12 to 48 hours, symptoms may return, accompanied by diffuse vascular congestion, pulmonary edema, shock, seizures, anuria, and hyperthermia. Death may follow.

Treatment requires immediate support of airway, respiration, and circulation. In conscious patient with intact gag reflex, recommend inducing emesis with ipecac; if not, emptying stomach by gastric lavage. Recommend following emesis with lavage, using a 1% sodium bicarbonate solution, to convert iron to the less irritating, poorly absorbed form (phosphate solutions have been used, but carry hazard of other adverse effects). An X-ray of the abdomen should be taken to determine continued presence of excess iron; if serum iron levels exceed 350 mg/dl, deferoxamine may be used for systemic chelation.

Survivors are likely to sustain organ damage, including pyloric or antral stenosis, hepatic cirrhosis, CNS damage, and intestinal obstruction.

### Clinical considerations
■ Drug may cause dark-colored stools.
■ Liquid drug may stain teeth.
■ Drug may be taken with meals to minimize GI effects; maximum absorption will occur if drug is taken between meals.
■ Ferrous fumarate blackens feces and may interfere with tests for occult blood in the stool; the guaiac test and orthotoluidine test may yield false-positive results, but the benzidine test is usually not affected.
■ Iron overload may decrease uptake of technetium 99m and thus interfere with skeletal imaging.

### Therapeutic monitoring
■ Advise clinician to monitor patient for adverse reactions and for evidence of therapeutic results.

### Special populations
**Breast-feeding patients.** Iron supplements are often recommended for breast-feeding women; no adverse effects of such use have been documented.
**Pediatric patients.** Iron overdose may be fatal in children; recommend treating immediately.
**Geriatric patients.** Because iron-induced constipation is common in geriatric patients, stress proper diet to these patients.

### Patient counseling
■ Instruct patient to take tablets with orange juice or water, but not with milk or antacids.
■ Tell patient to take suspension with straw and place drops at back of throat.
**◖ ALERT** Inform parents that as few as three or four tablets can cause serious iron poisoning in children.

## ferrous gluconate
Apo-Ferrous Gluconate*, Fergon, Ferralet, Fertinic*, Novoferrogluc*, Simron

*Pharmacologic classification:* oral iron supplement
*Therapeutic classification:* hematinic
*Pregnancy risk category A*

### Available forms
Available without a prescription. Ferrous gluconate is 11.6% elemental iron.
*Tablets:* 300 mg (contains 35 mg Fe+), 320 mg, 325 mg (320-mg tablet contains 37 mg Fe+)
*Capsules:* 86 mg (contains 10 mg Fe+), 325 mg (contains 38 mg Fe+)
*Elixir:* 300 mg/5 ml (contains 35 mg Fe+)

## Indications and dosages
### Iron deficiency
*Adults:* 325 mg P.O. q.i.d., dosage increased as needed and tolerated, up to 650 mg q.i.d. Geriatric patients may need higher doses because reduced gastric secretions and achlorhydria may lower capacity for iron absorption.
*Children ages 2 to 12:* 3 mg/kg/day P.O. in three or four divided doses.
*Children ages 6 months to 2 years:* Up to 6 mg/kg/day P.O. in three or four divided doses.
*Infants:* 10 to 25 mg/day P.O. divided into three or four doses.

## Mechanism of action
*Hematinic action:* Ferrous gluconate replaces iron, an essential component in the formation of hemoglobin.

## Pharmacokinetics
*Absorption:* Absorbed from the entire length of the GI tract, but primary absorption sites are the duodenum and proximal jejunum. Up to 10% of iron is absorbed by healthy individuals; patients with iron-deficiency anemia may absorb up to 60%. Food may decrease absorption by 33% to 50%.
*Distribution:* Transported through GI mucosal cells directly into the blood, where it's immediately bound to a carrier protein, transferrin, and transported to the bone marrow for incorporation into hemoglobin. Iron is highly protein-bound.
*Metabolism:* Liberated by the destruction of hemoglobin, but is conserved and reused by the body.
*Excretion:* Healthy individuals lose only small amounts of iron daily. Men and postmenopausal women lose about 1 mg/day, premenopausal women about 1.5 mg/day. Loss usually occurs in nails, hair, feces, and urine; trace amounts are lost in bile and sweat.

| Route | Onset | Peak | Duration |
|---|---|---|---|
| P.O. | 4 days | 7-10 days | 2-4 mo |

## Contraindications and precautions
Contraindicated in patients with peptic ulceration, regional enteritis, ulcerative colitis, hemosiderosis, primary hemochromatosis, or hemolytic anemia unless iron-deficiency anemia is also present and in those receiving repeated blood transfusions.

Use cautiously on long-term basis.

## Interactions
**Drug-drug.** *Antacids, aluminum-containing phosphate binders, cholestyramine, cimetidine, vitamin E:* Decrease ferrous fumarate absorption. Recommend separating doses by 1- to 2-hour intervals.
*Chloramphenicol:* Delays response to iron therapy. Advise clinician to monitor patient carefully.

*Doxycycline:* May interfere with ferrous fumarate absorption even when doses are separated. Avoid use together.
*L-thyroxine:* May decrease L-thyroxine absorption. Recommend separating doses by at least 2 hours. Advise clinician to monitor thyroid function.
*Levodopa and methyldopa:* May decrease absorption of these drugs. Advise clinician to monitor patient carefully.
*Penicillamine:* Decreased penicillamine absorption; recommend separating doses by at least 2 hours.
*Quinolones:* May decrease absorption of quinolones. Advise clinician to monitor patient closely.
*Tetracycline:* Inhibits absorption of both drugs; tetracycline should be given 3 hours after or 2 hours before iron supplement.
*Vitamin C:* Increased iron absorption. May be used as a beneficial drug interaction.
**Drug-herb.** *Black cohosh, chamomile, feverfew, gossypol, hawthorn, nettle, plantain, St. John's wort:* Decreased iron absorption. Discourage use together.
**Drug-food.** *Cereals, cheese, coffee, eggs, milk, tea, whole-grain breads, yogurt:* May impair oral iron absorption. Avoid use together.

## Adverse reactions
**GI:** *nausea,* epigastric pain, vomiting, *constipation,* diarrhea, *black stools,* anorexia.
**Other:** temporary staining of teeth (with elixir).

## Overdose and treatment
The lethal dose of iron is between 200 and 250 mg/kg; fatalities have occurred with lower doses. Signs and symptoms may follow ingestion of 20 to 60 mg/kg.

Between 30 minutes and 8 hours after ingestion, patient may experience lethargy, nausea and vomiting, green then tarry stools, weak and rapid pulse, hypotension, dehydration, acidosis, and coma. If death doesn't immediately ensue, symptoms may clear for about 24 hours.

At 12 to 48 hours, symptoms may return, accompanied by diffuse vascular congestion, pulmonary edema, shock, seizures, anuria, and hyperthermia. Death may follow.

Treatment requires immediate support of airway, respiration, and circulation. In conscious patient with intact gag reflex, recommend inducing emesis with ipecac; if not, emptying stomach by gastric lavage. Recommend following emesis with lavage, using a 1% sodium bicarbonate solution, to convert iron to less irritating, poorly absorbed form (phosphate solutions have been used, but carry hazard of other adverse effects). An abdominal X-ray should be taken to determine continued presence of excess iron; if serum iron levels exceed 350 mg/dl, deferoxamine may be used for systemic chelation.

Survivors are likely to sustain organ damage, including pyloric or antral stenosis, hepatic cirrhosis, CNS damage, and intestinal obstruction.

## Clinical considerations

- Drug may cause dark-colored stools.
- Liquid drug may stain teeth.
- Drug may be taken with meals to minimize GI effects; maximum absorption will occur if drug is taken between meals.
- Ferrous gluconate blackens feces and may interfere with test for occult blood in the stools; the guaiac test and orthotoluidine test may yield false-positive results, but the benzidine test usually is not affected.
- Iron overload may decrease uptake of technetium 99m and thus interfere with skeletal imaging.

### Therapeutic monitoring

- Advise clinician to monitor patient for adverse reactions and for evidence of therapeutic effect.

### Special populations

**Breast-feeding patients.** Iron supplements are often recommended for breast-feeding women; no adverse effects of such use have been documented.
**Pediatric patients.** Overdose may be fatal in children; recommend treating immediately.
**Geriatric patients.** Iron-induced constipation is common in geriatric patients; stress proper diet to these patients.

## Patient counseling

- Instruct patient to take tablets with orange juice or water, but not with milk or antacids.
- Tell patient to take suspension with straw and place drops at back of throat.
**◆ ALERT** Inform parents that as few as three or four tablets can cause serious iron poisoning in children.

---

## ferrous sulfate

Apo-Ferrous Sulfate*, Feosol, Feratab, Fer-In-Sol, Fer-Iron, Fero-Grad-500*, Fero-Gradumet, Ferospace, Ferralyn Lanacaps, Ferra-TD, Mol-Iron, Novoferrosulfa*, PMS Ferrous Sulfate*, Slow FE

*Pharmacologic classification:* oral iron supplement
*Therapeutic classification:* hematinic
*Pregnancy risk category A*

## Available forms

Available without a prescription. Ferrous sulfate is 20% elemental iron; dried and powdered (exsiccated), it is about 32% elemental iron.

*Tablets:* 195 mg, 300 mg, 324 mg, 325 mg; 200 mg (exsiccated); 160 mg (exsiccated, extended-release); 525 mg (timed-release)
*Capsules:* 150 mg, 190 mg, 250 mg
*Capsules (extended-release):* 150 mg, 159 mg, 250 mg
*Syrup:* 90 mg/5 ml
*Elixir:* 220 mg/5 ml
*Liquid:* 75 mg/0.6 ml, 125 mg/ml

## Indications and dosages

### Iron deficiency

*Adults:* 300 mg P.O. b.i.d.; dosage gradually increased to 300 mg q.i.d. as needed and tolerated. For extended-release capsule, 150 to 250 mg P.O. once daily or b.i.d.; for extended-release tablets, 160 to 525 mg once daily or b.i.d. Geriatric patients may need higher doses because reduced gastric secretions and achlorhydria may lower capacity for iron absorption.
*Children ages 2 to 12:* 3 mg/kg/day P.O. in three or four divided doses.
*Children ages 6 months to 2 years:* Up to 6 mg/kg/day P.O. in three or four divided doses.
*Infants:* 10 to 25 mg/day P.O. in three or four divided doses.

## Mechanism of action

*Hematinic action:* Ferrous sulfate replaces iron, an essential component in the formation of hemoglobin.

## Pharmacokinetics

*Absorption:* Absorbed from the entire length of the GI tract, but primary absorption sites are the duodenum and proximal jejunum. Up to 10% of iron is absorbed by healthy individuals; patients with iron-deficiency anemia may absorb up to 60%. Enteric coating and some extended-release formulas have decreased absorption because they're designed to release iron past the points of highest absorption; food may decrease absorption by 33% to 50%.
*Distribution:* Transported through GI mucosal cells directly into the blood, where it's immediately bound to a carrier protein, transferrin, and transported to the bone marrow for incorporation into hemoglobin. Iron is highly protein-bound.
*Metabolism:* Liberated by the destruction of hemoglobin, but is conserved and reused by the body.
*Excretion:* Healthy individuals lose very little iron each day. Men and postmenopausal women lose about 1 mg/day, and premenopausal women about 1.5 mg/day. The loss usually occurs in nails, hair, feces, and urine; trace amounts are lost in bile and sweat.

| Route | Onset | Peak | Duration |
|-------|-------|------|----------|
| P.O. | 4 days | 7-10 days | 2-4 mo |

---

## Contraindications and precautions
Contraindicated in patients with hemosiderosis, primary hemochromatosis, hemolytic anemia unless iron deficiency anemia is also present, peptic ulceration, ulcerative colitis, or regional enteritis and in those receiving repeated blood transfusions.

Use cautiously on long-term basis.

## Interactions
**Drug-drug.** *Antacids, aluminum-containing phosphate binders, cholestyramine, cimetidine, and vitamin E:* Decrease ferrous fumarate absorption. Recommend separating doses by 1- to 2-hour intervals.

*Chloramphenicol:* Delays response to iron therapy. Advise clinician to monitor patient carefully.

*Doxycycline:* May interfere with ferrous fumarate absorption even when doses are separated. Avoid use together.

*L-thyroxine:* May decrease L-thyroxine absorption. Recommend separating doses by at least 2 hours. Advise clinician to monitor thyroid function.

*Levodopa and methyldopa:* May decrease absorption of these drugs. Advise clinician to monitor carefully.

*Penicillamine:* Decreased penicillamine absorption; recommend separating doses by at least 2 hours.

*Quinolones:* Drug may decrease absorption of quinolones. Advise clinician to monitor patient closely.

*Tetracycline:* Inhibits absorption of both drugs; tetracycline should be given 3 hours after or 2 hours before iron supplement.

*Vitamin C:* Increases iron absorption. May be used as a beneficial drug interaction.

**Drug-herb.** *Black cohosh, chamomile, feverfew, gossypol, hawthorn, nettle, plantain, St. John's wort:* Decreased iron absorption. Discourage use together.

**Drug-food.** *Cereals, cheese, coffee, eggs, milk, tea, whole-grain breads, yogurt:* May impair oral iron absorption. Avoid use together.

## Adverse reactions
**GI:** *nausea,* epigastric pain, vomiting, *constipation, black stools,* diarrhea, anorexia.

**Other:** temporary staining of teeth (with liquid forms).

## Overdose and treatment
The lethal dose of iron is 200 to 250 mg/kg; fatalities have occurred with lower doses. Signs and symptoms may follow ingestion of 20 to 60 mg/kg.

Between 30 minutes and 8 hours after ingestion, patient may experience lethargy, nausea and vomiting, green then tarry stools, weak and rapid pulse, hypotension, dehydration, acidosis, and coma. If death doesn't immediately ensue, symptoms may clear for about 24 hours.

At 12 to 48 hours, symptoms may return, accompanied by diffuse vascular congestion, pulmonary edema, shock, seizures, anuria, and hyperthermia. Death may follow.

Treatment requires immediate support of airway, respiration, and circulation. In conscious patient with intact gag reflex, recommend inducing emesis with ipecac; if not, emptying stomach by gastric lavage. Recommend following emesis with lavage, using a 1% sodium bicarbonate solution, to convert iron to less irritating, poorly absorbed form (phosphate solutions have been used, but carry hazard of other adverse effects). An abdominal X-ray should be taken to determine continued presence of excess iron; if serum iron levels exceed 350 mg/dl, deferoxamine may be used for systemic chelation.

Survivors are likely to sustain organ damage, including pyloric or antral stenosis, hepatic cirrhosis, CNS damage, and intestinal obstruction.

## Clinical considerations
■ Drug may be taken with meals to minimize GI effects; maximum absorption will occur if drug is taken between meals.

■ Drug may cause dark-colored stools.

■ Liquid drug may stain teeth.

■ Ferrous sulfate blackens feces and may interfere with tests for occult blood in the stool; the guaiac test and orthotoluidine test may yield false-positive results, but the benzidine test is usually not affected.

■ Iron overload may decrease uptake of technetium 99m and thus interfere with skeletal imaging.

### Therapeutic monitoring
■ Advise clinician to monitor patient for adverse reactions and for evidence of therapeutic effects.

### Special populations
**Breast-feeding patients.** Iron supplements often are recommended for breast-feeding women; no adverse effects have been documented.

**Pediatric patients.** Extended-release iron capsules or tablets are usually not recommended for children. Overdose may be fatal; recommend treating immediately.

**Geriatric patients.** Iron-induced constipation is common in geriatric patients; stress proper diet to minimize this adverse effect.

## Patient counseling
■ Instruct patient not to crush or chew extended-release forms.

**⊌ ALERT** Inform parents that three or four tablets can cause serious iron poisoning in children.

# fexofenadine hydrochloride
Allegra

*Pharmacologic classification:* $H_1$-receptor antagonist
*Therapeutic classification:* antihistamine
*Pregnancy risk category C*

## Available forms
Available by prescription only
*Capsules:* 60 mg
*Tablets:* 30 mg, 60 mg, 180 mg

## Indications and dosages
**Seasonal allergic rhinitis**
*Adults and children ages 12 and older:* 60 mg P.O. b.i.d. or 180 mg P.O. once daily.
*Children ages 6 to 11:* 30 mg P.O. b.i.d.
**Chronic idiopathic urticaria**
*Adults and children ages 12 and older:* 60 mg P.O. b.i.d.
*Children ages 6 to 11:* 30 mg P.O. b.i.d.
≡ *Dosage adjustment.* In patients with creatinine clearance of less than 80 ml/min, increase the dosage interval to every 24 hours.

## Mechanism of action
*Antihistaminic action:* Principal effects of fexofenadine are mediated through a selective inhibition of peripheral $H_1$ receptors.

## Pharmacokinetics
*Absorption:* Rapidly absorbed.
*Distribution:* 60% to 70% bound to plasma protein.
*Metabolism:* About 5% of drug is metabolized.
*Excretion:* Mainly excreted in feces, less so in urine. Mean elimination half-life of drug is 14½ hours.

| Route | Onset | Peak | Duration |
|-------|-------|------|----------|
| P.O. | Unknown | 3 hr | 14 hr |

## Contraindications and precautions
Contraindicated in patients hypersensitive to drug or its components.
    Use cautiously in patients with impaired renal function.

## Interactions
**Drug-drug.** *Antacids containing aluminum and magnesium:* Decreased plasma levels of fexofenadine. Recommend separating administration times.
*Erythromycin, ketoconazole:* Decreased oral clearance and urinary excretion of fexofenadine. Use together is permitted.
*MAO inhibitors:* Increased pressor effects of fixed-combination extended-release tablets. Avoid use during or within 2 weeks of MAO inhibitor therapy.

## Adverse reactions
**CNS:** fatigue, drowsiness, headache.
**EENT:** otitis media.
**GI:** nausea, dyspepsia.
**GU:** dysmenorrhea.
**Musculoskeletal:** back pain.
**Respiratory:** upper respiratory tract infection, sinusitis, cough, otitis media.
**Other:** viral infection.

## Overdose and treatment
Overdose of up to 800 mg doesn't result in significant clinical adverse reactions. If overdose occurs, treatment should be symptomatic or supportive. Fexofenadine isn't effectively removed by hemodialysis.

## Clinical considerations
■ No information indicates that abuse or dependency occurs with fexofenadine use.
■ Possible interference with antigen skin-testing procedures. Recommend discontinuing drug 24 to 48 hours before test.

### Therapeutic monitoring
■ Advise clinician to monitor patient for adverse reactions.

### Special populations
**Pregnant patients.** Drug should be used only during pregnancy only when potential benefit outweighs risk to fetus.
**Breast-feeding patients.** It isn't known if drug appears in breast milk. Caution is recommended when giving fexofenadine to breast-feeding women.
**Pediatric patients.** Safety and efficacy of fexofenadine in children under age 6 haven't been established.

## Patient counseling
■ Caution patient not to perform hazardous activities if drowsiness is experienced with drug use.
■ Instruct patient not to exceed prescribed dosage and to take drug only when needed.

# filgrastim (granulocyte colony-stimulating factor, G-CSF)
Neupogen

*Pharmacologic classification:* biologic response modifier
*Therapeutic classification:* colony-stimulating factor
*Pregnancy risk category C*

## Available forms
Available by prescription only
*Injection:* 300 mcg/ml in 1-ml and 1.6-ml single-dose vials

---

## Indications and dosages

*To decrease risk of infection after cancer chemotherapy for nonmyeloid malignancies, chronic severe neutropenia; to treat* ◇*agranulocytosis,* ◇*pancytopenia with colchicine overdose,* ◇*acute leukemia,* ◇*hematologic toxicity with zidovudine antiviral therapy*

*Adults:* Initially, 5 mcg/kg S.C. or I.V. as a single daily dose; may increase dose incrementally by 5 mcg/kg for each course of chemotherapy according to duration and severity of absolute neutrophil count (ANC) nadir. Give filgrastim daily for up to 2 weeks until ANC nadir reaches 10,000/mm³ after the anticipated chemotherapy-induced ANC nadir. Duration of treatment depends on the myelosuppressive potential of the chemotherapy used. Discontinue if ANC nadir surpasses 10,000/mm³.

*Bone marrow transplantation*

*Adults:* Initially, 10 mcg/kg/day I.V. over 4 or 24 hours or S.C. over 24 hours. When ANC is greater than 1,000/mm³ for 3 consecutive days, reduce dosage to 5 mcg/kg/day. If ANC remains greater than 1,000/mm³ for an additional 3 consecutive days, discontinue treatment. If discontinuance results in ANC less than 1,000/mm³, reinitiate at 5 mcg/kg/day. If ANC decreases to less than 1,000/mm³ at any time when the dose is 5 mcg/kg/day, increase the dosage to 10 mcg/kg/day, and repeat the preceding steps.

◇*Acquired immune deficiency syndrome (AIDS)*

*Adults:* 0.3 to 3.6 mcg/kg/day S.C. or I.V.

◇*Aplastic anemia*

*Adults:* 800 to 1,200 mcg/m²/day S.C. or I.V.

◇*Hairy cell leukemia, myelodysplasia*

*Adults:* 15 to 500 mcg/m²/day S.C. or I.V. Alternatively for myelodysplasia, 0.3 to 10 mcg/kg/day S.C.

◇*Neutropenia from HIV infection*

*Adults and adolescents:* 5 to 10 mcg/kg S.C. daily for 2 to 4 weeks.

## I.V. administration

- Drug may be stored at room temperature for up to 24 hours before administration. Drug should be refrigerated at 35° to 47° F (2° to 8° C), not frozen.
- Do not shake vial.
- For infusion over 15 to 60 minutes or continuous infusion for 24 hours, drug can be diluted in 50 to 100 ml $D_5W$.
- Dilution to a final concentration of less than 5 mcg/ml is not recommended.

### Incompatibilities

Incompatible with sodium solutions.

## Mechanism of action

*Immunostimulant action:* Filgrastim is a naturally occurring cytokine glycoprotein that stimulates proliferation, differentiation, and functional activity of neutrophils, causing a rapid increase in WBC count within 2 to 3 days in patients with normal bone marrow function or 7 to 14 days in patients with bone marrow suppression. Blood counts return to pretreatment levels, usually within 1 week after therapy ends.

## Pharmacokinetics

*Absorption:* After S.C. bolus dose, blood levels suggest rapid absorption.
*Distribution:* Unknown.
*Metabolism:* Unknown.
*Excretion:* Elimination half-life is about 3½ hours.

| Route | Onset | Peak | Duration |
|---|---|---|---|
| I.V. | 5-60 min | 24 hr | 1-7 days |
| S.C. | 5-60 min | 2-8 hr | 1-7 days |

## Contraindications and precautions

Contraindicated in patients hypersensitive to proteins derived from *Escherichia coli* or to drug or its components.

## Interactions

**Drug-drug.** *Chemotherapeutic drugs:* Cause rapidly dividing myeloid cells to be potentially sensitive to cytotoxic drugs. Drug shouldn't be used within 24 hours before or after a dose of one of these drugs.
*Lithium:* Use with caution in patients taking lithium.

## Adverse reactions

**CNS:** headache, weakness, *fatigue.*
**CV:** *MI, arrhythmias,* chest pain, transient hypotension.
**GI:** *nausea, vomiting, diarrhea, mucositis,* stomatitis, constipation.
**GU:** increased serum creatinine.
**Hematologic:** *thrombocytopenia,* leukocytosis, transient increases in neutrophils.
**Hepatic:** elevated liver enzyme levels.
**Metabolic:** elevations in uric acid.
**Musculoskeletal:** *skeletal pain.*
**Respiratory:** dyspnea, cough.
**Skin:** *alopecia,* rash, cutaneous vasculitis.
**Other:** *fever,* hypersensitivity reactions.

## Overdose and treatment

Maximum tolerated dose hasn't been determined. There have been no reports of overdose.

## Clinical considerations

- Don't give earlier than 24 hours after or within 24 hours before chemotherapy.

### Therapeutic monitoring

- Advise clinician to obtain CBC and platelet counts before and twice weekly during therapy.
- Regular monitoring of hematocrit and platelet counts is recommended.

---

* Canada only   ◇ Unlabeled clinical use

■ Adult respiratory distress syndrome may occur in septic patients because of the influx of neutrophils at the site of inflammation.

■ MI and arrhythmias have occurred; recommend closely monitoring patients with preexisting cardiac conditions.

■ Bone pain is the most frequent adverse reaction and may be controlled with nonnarcotic analgesics if mild to moderate, or may require narcotic analgesics if severe.

### Special populations
**Breast-feeding patients.** It's unknown if drug appears in breast milk. Risk-to-benefit ratio must be assessed.
**Pediatric patients.** Efficacy hasn't been established, but there's no evidence of greater toxicity in children than in adults.
**Geriatric patients.** No age-related problems have been reported.

### Patient counseling
■ Review "Information for Patients" section of package insert with patient. Thorough instruction is essential if home use is prescribed.

# finasteride
Propecia, Proscar

*Pharmacologic classification:* steroid (synthetic 4-azasteroid) derivative
*Therapeutic classification:* androgen synthesis inhibitor
*Pregnancy risk category X*

### Available forms
Available by prescription only
*Tablets:* 1 mg, 5 mg

### Indications and dosages
**Symptomatic BPH,** ◇ *adjuvant therapy after radical prostatectomy,* ◇ *first-stage prostate cancer,* ◇ *acne,* ◇ *hirsutism*
*Adults (men only):* 5 mg P.O. daily, usually for 6 to 12 months.
◇ *Male pattern baldness (androgenetic alopecia)*
*Adults:* 1 mg P.O. daily, usually for 3 months or more. Continued use is recommended to sustain benefit. Withdrawal of treatment leads to reversal of effect within 12 months.

### Mechanism of action
*Androgen synthesis inhibition action:* Finasteride competitively inhibits steroid $5\mu$, an enzyme responsible for formation of the potent androgen $5\mu$-dihydrotestosterone (DHT) from testosterone. Because DHT influences development of the prostate gland, decreasing levels of this hormone in adult men should relieve the symptoms associated with BPH. In men with male pattern baldness, the balding scalp contains miniaturized hair follicles and increased amounts of DHT. Finasteride decreases scalp and serum DHT levels in these men.

### Pharmacokinetics
*Absorption:* Average bioavailability of drug was 63% in one study.
*Distribution:* About 90% plasma protein–bound. Drug crosses the blood-brain barrier.
*Metabolism:* Extensively metabolized by the liver; at least 2 metabolites have been identified. Metabolites are responsible for less than 20% of total activity of the drug.
*Excretion:* Part of oral dose (39%) is excreted in urine as metabolites; 57% is excreted in feces. No unchanged drug is found in urine.

| Route | Onset | Peak | Duration |
|-------|-------|------|----------|
| P.O. | Unknown | 1-2 hr | 24 hr |

### Contraindications and precautions
Drug should be used with caution in patients with liver dysfunction. Contraindicated in patients hypersensitive to drug. Although drug isn't used in women, manufacturer indicates pregnancy as a contraindication.

### Interactions
**Drug-drug.** *Theophylline:* Clinically insignificant increases in theophylline clearance and decreased half-life (10%) have been observed. Use together with caution.

### Adverse reactions
**CV:** Nonbeneficial decreased prostate-specific antigen (PSA) serum levels.
**GU:** impotence, decreased volume of ejaculate.
**Other:** decreased libido.

### Overdose and treatment
Experience with overdose is limited. Patients have received single doses of 400 mg and doses of up to 80 mg daily for 3 months without adverse effects.

### Clinical considerations
■ Recommend closely evaluating patient for conditions that might mimic BPH before therapy, including hypotonic bladder, prostate cancer, infection, stricture, or other neurologic conditions.
**⛌ ALERT** All women of childbearing age should avoid exposure to drug and semen of patient receiving this drug. Exposure to semen of patient taking drug or to broken or crushed tablet presents hazard to male fetus.
■ Because it's not possible to identify prospectively which patients will respond to finasteride, a minimum of 6 months of therapy may be needed.
■ Long-term effects of drug on the complications of BPH, including acute urinary ob-

---

*Reactions may be* common, uncommon, *life-threatening,* or COMMON AND LIFE-THREATENING.

struction, or on the incidence of surgery aren't known.
■ Current investigations aim to determine effectiveness of drug as adjuvant therapy after radical prostatectomy; as adjunctive treatment of prostate cancer; and as treatment for acne and hirsutism.

### Therapeutic monitoring
■ Recommend carefully monitoring patients who have large residual urine volumes or severely diminished urine flows. Not all patients respond to drug, and these patients may not be candidates for finasteride therapy.
■ Recommend carefully evaluating sustained increases in serum PSA. In patients receiving finasteride therapy, this could indicate noncompliance with therapy.

### Special populations
**Pregnant patients.** Not indicated for use in women; potential hazard to male fetus when pregnant women come in contact with broken or crushed tablet or semen of male patient receiving drug.
**Breast-feeding patients.** It's unknown if drug appears in breast milk; however, it isn't indicated for use in women.
**Pediatric patients.** Drug isn't indicated for use in children.
**Geriatric patients.** Although elimination rate of drug is decreased in geriatric patients, dosage adjustments aren't needed.

### Patient counseling
■ Advise patient that anyone who is or may become pregnant must not handle crushed tablets or have contact with patient's semen because of risk of adverse effects on a male fetus.
■ Explain that drug may decrease the volume of ejaculate but doesn't appear to impair normal sexual function. However, impotence and decreased libido have occurred in less than 4% of patients treated with drug.

---

# flecainide acetate
Tambocor

*Pharmacologic classification:* benzamide derivative local anesthetic (amide)
*Therapeutic classification:* ventricular antiarrhythmic
*Pregnancy risk category C*

### Available forms
Available by prescription only
*Tablets:* 50 mg, 100 mg, 150 mg

## Indications and dosages
*Life-threatening ventricular tachycardia and PVCs*
*Adults:* 100 mg P.O. q 12 hours; may increase in increments of 50 mg b.i.d. q 4 days until efficacy is achieved. Maximum dose is 400 mg daily.
*Paroxysmal supraventricular tachycardia, paroxysmal atrial fibrillation or flutter in patients without structural heart disease*
*Adults:* 50 mg P.O. q 12 hours; may increase in increments of 50 mg b.i.d. q 4 days until efficacy is achieved. Maximum dose is 300 mg/day.
≡*Dosage adjustment.* Reduce dosage in patients with renal impairment (creatinine clearance of less than 35 ml/minute/1.73 m$^2$) beginning at 100 mg/day (50 mg b.i.d.); increase dosage cautiously at intervals longer than 4 days. For patients with less severe renal failure, initial dose is 100 mg q 12 hours, increasing cautiously at intervals longer than 4 days.

## Mechanism of action
*Antiarrhythmic action:* A class IC antiarrhythmic, flecainide suppresses SA node automaticity and prolongs conduction in the atria, AV node, ventricles, accessory pathways, and His-Purkinje system. It has the most pronounced effect on the His-Purkinje system, as shown by QRS complex widening; this leads to a prolonged QT interval. The drug has relatively little effect on action potential duration except in Purkinje's fibers, where it shortens it. A proarrhythmic (arrhythmogenic) effect may result from the potent effects of the drug on the conduction system. Effects on the sinus node are strongest in patients with sinus node disease (sick sinus syndrome). Flecainide also exerts a moderate negative inotropic effect.

## Pharmacokinetics
*Absorption:* Rapidly and almost completely absorbed from the GI tract; bioavailability of commercially available tablets is 85% to 90%.
*Distribution:* Apparently well distributed throughout the body. Only about 40% plasma protein–bound. Trough serum levels ranging from 0.2 to 1 mcg/ml provide the greatest therapeutic benefit. Trough serum levels higher than 0.7 mcg/ml have caused increased adverse effects.
*Metabolism:* Metabolized in the liver to inactive metabolites. About 30% of an orally given dose escapes metabolism and is excreted in the urine unchanged.
*Excretion:* Elimination half-life averages about 20 hours. Plasma half-life may be prolonged in patients with HF and renal disease.

| Route | Onset | Peak | Duration |
|-------|-------|------|----------|
| P.O. | Immediate | 2-3 hr | Unknown |

---

## Contraindications and precautions

Contraindicated in patients hypersensitive to drug or cardiogenic shock and in those with preexisting second- or third-degree AV block or right bundle branch block when associated with a left hemiblock (in the absence of an artificial pacemaker).

Use cautiously in patients with HF, cardiomyopathy, severe renal or hepatic disease, prolonged QT interval, sick sinus syndrome, or blood dyscrasia.

Tambocor has shown proarrhythmic effects in patients with atrial fibrillation or flutter; therefore, it isn't recommended for use in these patients.

## Interactions

**Drug-drug.** *Acidifying and alkalizing drugs:* Alkalization decreases renal flecainide excretion, and acidification increases it. Advise clinician to monitor patient carefully.

*Beta blockers:* May cause additive negative inotropic effects. Advise clinician to monitor patient carefully.

*Cimetidine:* May decrease both the renal and nonrenal clearance of flecainide. Advise clinician to monitor patient carefully.

*Digoxin:* May cause increased serum digoxin levels. Advise clinician to monitor digoxin levels.

*High-dose antacids, carbonic anhydrase inhibitors, sodium bicarbonate:* Marked effect on urine acidity; recommend monitoring patient for possible subtherapeutic or toxic levels and effects.

*Other antiarrhythmic drugs:* May cause additive, synergistic, or antagonistic cardiac effects and may cause additive adverse effects. Drugs should be used together cautiously; recommend monitoring patient.

**Drug-lifestyle.** *Smoking:* May lower flecainide serum levels. Discourage patient from smoking.

## Adverse reactions

**CNS:** dizziness, *headache,* fatigue, tremor, anxiety, insomnia, depression, malaise, paresthesia, ataxia, vertigo, *light-headedness, syncope,* asthenia.

**CV:** *new or worsened arrhythmias,* chest pain, edema, *HF, cardiac arrest,* palpitations.

**EENT:** *blurred vision and other visual disturbances.*

**GI:** nausea, constipation, abdominal pain, dyspepsia, vomiting, diarrhea, anorexia.

**Respiratory:** *dyspnea.*

**Skin:** rash, flushing.

**Other:** fever.

## Overdose and treatment

Clinical effects of overdose include increased PR and QT intervals, increased QRS complex duration, decreased myocardial contractility, conduction disturbances, and hypotension.

Treatment generally involves symptomatic and supportive measures along with ECG, blood pressure, and respiratory monitoring. Inotropic drugs, including dopamine and dobutamine, may be used. Hemodynamic support, including use of an intra-aortic balloon pump and transvenous pacing, may be needed. Because of long half-life of drug, supportive measures may need to be continued for extended periods. Hemodialysis is ineffective in reducing serum drug levels.

## Clinical considerations

**⚠ALERT** Tambocor has caused an excessive mortality or nonfatal cardiac arrest rate in national multicenter trials. Its use should be restricted to those patients for whom the benefits outweigh the risks.

■ Tambocor is a strong negative inotrope and may cause or worsen HF, especially in those with cardiomyopathy, preexisting HF, or low ejection fraction.

■ Hypokalemia or hyperkalemia may alter drug effects and should be corrected before drug therapy begins.

■ Therapy should be started in the hospital with careful monitoring of patient with symptomatic HF, sinus node dysfunction, sustained ventricular tachycardia, or underlying structural heart disease and in patient changing from another antiarrhythmic in whom discontinuation of current antiarrhythmic is likely to cause life-threatening arrhythmias.

■ Loading doses may exacerbate arrhythmias and therefore aren't recommended. Dosage adjustments should be made at intervals of at least 4 days because of long half-life of drug.

■ Most patients can be adequately maintained on an every-12-hour dosage schedule, but some need to receive drug every 8 hours.

■ Twice-daily dosing improves patient compliance.

■ Full therapeutic effect of drug may take 3 to 5 days. I.V. lidocaine may be given while awaiting full effect.

■ Flecainide is a first class IC antiarrhythmic. Incidence of adverse effects increases when trough serum drug levels exceed 0.7 mcg/ml. Recommend periodically monitoring blood levels, especially in patients with renal failure or HF. Therapeutic levels range from 0.2 to 1 mcg/ml.

■ Drug may increase acute and chronic endocardial pacing thresholds and may suppress ventricular escape rhythms. Recommend determining pacing threshold before drug is given, after 1 week of therapy, and regularly thereafter. It shouldn't be given to patients with preexisting poor thresholds or nonprogrammable artificial pacemakers unless pacing rescue is available.

■ In HF and myocardial dysfunction, initial dose shouldn't exceed 100 mg every 12 hours; common initial dose is 50 mg every 12 hours.

---

■ Use in hepatic impairment hasn't been fully evaluated; however, because flecainide is metabolized extensively (probably in the liver), it should be used in patients with significant hepatic impairment only when benefits clearly outweigh risks. Dosage reduction may be needed; recommend monitoring patient carefully for signs of toxicity. Serum levels also must be monitored.

### Therapeutic monitoring
■ Advise clinician to monitor patient for signs of toxicity.
■ Advise clinician to monitor cardiac status.
■ Advise clinician to monitor drug compliance.

### Special populations
**Breast-feeding patients.** Limited data indicate that drug appears in breast milk. Breast-feeding isn't recommended during flecainide therapy because of the risk of adverse effects on the infant.
**Pediatric patients.** Safety and efficacy haven't been established in children under age 18. Limited data suggest usefulness in management of paroxysmal reentrant supraventricular tachycardia.
**Geriatric patients.** Geriatric patients are more susceptible to adverse effects. Advise clinician to monitor patient carefully.

### Patient counseling
■ Advise patient to closely follow administration instruction.
■ Warn patient of potential adverse drug effects.

# floxuridine
FUDR

*Pharmacologic classification:* antimetabolite (cell cycle–phase specific, S phase)
*Therapeutic classification:* antineoplastic
*Pregnancy risk category D*

### Available forms
Available by prescription only
*Injection:* 500-mg vials

### Indications and dosages
Dosage and indications may vary. Check current literature for recommended protocol.
***Palliative management of GI adenocarcinoma metastatic to the liver; brain, head, neck, gallbladder, bile duct cancer***
*Adults:* 0.1 to 0.6 mg/kg daily by intra-arterial infusion; or 0.4 to 0.6 mg/kg daily into hepatic artery.
◇ ***Solid tumors***
*Adults:* 0.5 to 1 mg/kg daily by I.V. infusion for 6 to 15 days or until toxicity occurs; or 30 mg/kg daily by single injection for 5 days, then 15 mg/kg every other day for up to 11 days or until toxicity occurs.

### I.V. administration
■ Follow facility policy to reduce risks. Preparation and administration of parenteral form of drug are linked to carcinogenic, mutagenic, and teratogenic risks for staff.
■ Drug can be diluted with $D_5W$ or normal saline solution.
■ Refrigerated solution is stable for up to 2 weeks.
■ Floxuridine sterile powder should be protected from light and stored at 59° to 86° F (15° to 30° C).

### Incompatibilities
None reported.

### Mechanism of action
*Antineoplastic action:* Floxuridine exerts its cytotoxic activity after conversion to its active form, by competitively inhibiting the enzyme thymidylate synthetase; this halts DNA synthesis and leads to cell death.

### Pharmacokinetics
*Absorption:* Not given orally.
*Distribution:* Crosses the blood-brain barrier to a limited extent.
*Metabolism:* Metabolized to fluorouracil in the liver after intra-arterial infusions and rapid I.V. injections.
*Excretion:* About 60% of a dose is excreted through the lungs as carbon dioxide. A small amount is excreted by the kidneys as unchanged drug and metabolites.

| Route | Onset | Peak | Duration |
|---|---|---|---|
| Intra-arterial | Unknown | Unknown | Unknown |

### Contraindications and precautions
Contraindicated in patients with poor nutritional state, bone marrow suppression, or serious infection. Drug should be used in pregnancy only if the potential benefits justify the potential risk to the fetus.
Use cautiously in patients after high-dose pelvic radiation therapy or use of alkylating drugs and in those with impaired renal or hepatic function.

### Interactions
**Drug-lifestyle.** *Sun exposure:* May increase skin reaction. Advise patient to use sunblock.

### Adverse reactions
**CNS:** cerebellar ataxia, malaise, weakness, headache, lethargy, disorientation, confusion, euphoria.
**CV:** myocardial ischemia, angina.
**EENT:** blurred vision, nystagmus, photophobia, epistaxis.

**GI:** *anorexia, stomatitis, nausea, vomiting, diarrhea, bleeding, enteritis,* GI ulceration.
**Hematologic:** *leukopenia, anemia, thrombocytopenia, agranulocytosis.*
**Hepatic:** elevated liver enzyme levels, increased bilirubin, *drug-induced hepatotoxicity.*
**Skin:** *erythema,* dermatitis, pruritus, rash, alopecia, photosensitivity.
**Other:** thrombophlebitis, *anaphylaxis,* fever.

## Overdose and treatment

Signs and symptoms of overdose include myelosuppression, diarrhea, alopecia, dermatitis, and hyperpigmentation.

Treatment is usually supportive and includes transfusion of blood components and antidiarrheal drugs.

## Clinical considerations

■ Reconstituted drug solutions are stable for 14 days when refrigerated.
■ Drug is often given via hepatic arterial infusion in treating hepatic metastases.

### Therapeutic monitoring

■ Instruct prescriber to discontinue drug if severe skin and GI adverse reactions occur.
■ Advise clinician to monitor patient's intake and output, CBC, and renal and hepatic function.
■ Therapeutic effect may be delayed 1 to 6 weeks.

### Special populations

**Pregnant patients.** To avoid toxicity to the fetus, women of childbearing age shouldn't use this drug. Use only when potential benefits to pregnant woman justify risks to fetus.
**Breast-feeding patients.** It isn't known if drug appears in breast milk. However, because of risk of serious adverse reactions, mutagenicity, and carcinogenicity in the infant, breast-feeding isn't recommended.

## Patient counseling

■ Advise patient to report nausea, vomiting, stomach pain, signs of infection, or unusual bruising or bleeding.

## fluconazole

Diflucan

*Pharmacologic classification:* bistriazole derivative
*Therapeutic classification:* antifungal
*Pregnancy risk category C*

## Available forms

Available by prescription only
*Tablets:* 50 mg, 100 mg, 150 mg, 200 mg
*Injection:* 200 mg/100 ml, 400 mg/200 ml
*Suspension:* 350 mg/35 ml, 1,400 mg/35 ml

## Indications and dosages

*Oropharyngeal and esophageal candidiasis*
*Adults:* 200 mg P.O. or I.V. on day 1 followed by 100 mg P.O. or I.V. once daily. As much as 400 mg daily has been used for esophageal disease. Treatment should continue for at least 2 weeks after resolution of symptoms.
*Children:* 6 mg/kg on day 1, followed by 3 mg/kg for at least 2 weeks.
*Systemic candidiasis*
*Adults:* Up to 400 mg P.O. or I.V. once daily. Treatment should be continued for at least 2 weeks after resolution of symptoms.
*Cryptococcal meningitis*
*Adults:* 400 mg I.V. or P.O. on day 1, followed by 200 mg once daily. Continue treatment for 10 to 12 weeks after CSF culture becomes negative. For suppression of relapse in patients with AIDS, give 200 mg once daily.
*Vaginal candidiasis*
*Adults:* 150 mg P.O. as a single dose.
*Urinary tract infection or peritonitis*
*Adults:* 50 to 200 mg P.O. or I.V. daily.
*Prophylaxis in patients undergoing bone marrow transplantation*
*Adults:* 400 mg P.O. or I.V. daily for several days before transplantation and 7 days after neutrophil count rises above 1,000 cells/ mm³.
◇ *Candidal infection, long-term suppression in patients with HIV infection*
*Adults:* 100 to 200 mg P.O. or I.V. daily.
◇ *Prophylaxis against mucocutaneous candidiasis, cryptococcosis, coccidioidomycosis, or histoplasmosis in patients with HIV infection*
*Adults:* 200 to 400 mg P.O. or I.V. daily.
*Children and infants:* 2 to 8 mg/kg P.O. daily.
≡ *Dosage adjustment.* Patients with renal impairment should have their dosages adjusted based on this table.

| Creatinine clearance (ml/min) | Percentage of usual adult dosage |
|---|---|
| 21-49 | 50 |
| 11-20 | 25 |

Patients receiving hemodialysis should receive one full dose after each session.

## I.V. administration

■ Give drug once daily at a rate not greater than 200 mg/hour.
■ Don't remove protective overwrap from I.V. bags until just prior to use to ensure product sterility.
■ Don't add other drugs to I.V. bag.

### Incompatibilities

Incompatible with amphotericin B, ampicillin sodium, calcium gluconate, cefotaxime sodium, ceftazidime, ceftriaxone, cefuroxime sodi-

um, chloramphenicol sodium succinate, clindamycin phosphate, co-trimoxazole, diazepam,
digoxin, erythromycin lactobionate, furosemide,
haloperidol lactate, hydroxyzine hydrochloride, imipenem and cilastatin sodium, pentamidine, piperacillin sodium, and ticarcillin
disodium. Manufacturer recommends that drug
not be mixed with other drugs.

## Mechanism of action
*Antifungal action:* Fluconazole exerts its
fungistatic effects by inhibiting fungal cytochrome P-450. The spectrum of activity includes *Cryptococcus neoformans, Candida* (including systemic *C. albicans), Aspergillus
flavus, Aspergillus fumigatus, Coccidioides immitis,* and *Histoplasma capsulatum.*

## Pharmacokinetics
*Absorption:* After oral administration, absorption is rapid and complete.
*Distribution:* Well distributed to various sites,
including CNS, saliva, sputum, blister fluid,
urine, normal skin, nails, and blister skin. CNS
levels approach 50% to 90% of that of serum.
Fluconazole is 12% protein-bound.
*Metabolism:* Partially metabolized.
*Elimination:* Primarily excreted via the kidneys. More than 80% of a given dose is excreted unchanged in the urine. Excretion rate
diminishes as renal function decreases.

| Route | Onset | Peak | Duration |
|-------|-------|------|----------|
| P.O. | Unknown | 1-2 hr | 30 hr |
| I.V. | Immediate | Unknown | Unknown |

## Contraindications and precautions
Contraindicated in patients hypersensitive to
drug and other drugs in same class.

## Interactions
**Drug-drug.** *Cimetidine:* May reduce serum
levels of fluconazole. Advise clinician to monitor patient carefully.
*Cyclosporine:* Increased cyclosporine levels.
Advise clinician to monitor cyclosporine levels.
*Glipizide, glyburide, sulfonylureas, and tolbu-
tamide:* Concurrent use increases hypoglycemic
effects. Drugs should be used together cautiously; recommend monitoring glucose levels.
*Hydrochlorothiazide:* Decreased fluconazole
clearance, elevating serum levels of the drug.
Drugs should be used together cautiously.
*Isoniazid, phenytoin, rifampin, sulfonylureas,
valproic acid:* Elevated hepatic transaminase
levels. Advise clinician to monitor patient carefully.
*Phenytoin:* May significantly increase phenytoin serum levels. Advise clinician to monitor
phenytoin levels.

*Rifampin:* May lower fluconazole levels. Advise clinician to monitor patient for drug effects.
*Tacrolimus:* Increased level of tacrolimus. Advise clinician to monitor patient carefully.
*Theophylline:* Increased theophylline levels.
Advise clinician to monitor theophylline levels.
*Warfarin:* Enhanced hypoprothrombinemic effects. Advise clinician to monitor PT and INR
closely.
*Zidovudine:* Increased activity of zidovine may
occur. Advise clinician to monitor patient carefully.
**Drug-food.** *Caffeine:* May increase plasma
caffeine levels. Advise patient to avoid caffeine.

## Adverse reactions
**CNS:** headache.
**GI:** *nausea,* vomiting, abdominal pain, diar-
rhea.
**Hepatic:** *hepatotoxicity,* elevated liver enzyme
levels.
**Skin:** rash, *Stevens-Johnson syndrome,* alope-
cia.
**Other:** *anaphylaxis.*

## Overdose and treatment
Treatment is largely supportive.

## Clinical considerations
■ Recommend adjusting dosage in those with
renal dysfunction.
■ Bioavailability of oral drug is comparable
with I.V. dosing.
■ Adverse reactions (including transaminase
elevations) are more frequent and more severe
in patients with severe underlying illness (including AIDS and malignancies).

### Therapeutic monitoring
■ Advise clinician to monitor patient for anaphylaxis and other adverse reactions.

### Special populations
**Pregnant patients.** Fluconazole shouldn't be
given to pregnant HIV-infected women and
should be discontinued if pregnancy occurs.
Use in pregnancy only if potential benefits outweigh the risk to the fetus.
**Breast-feeding patients.** Drug appears in breast
milk at levels similar to those of plasma. Therefore, use in breast-feeding women isn't recommended.
**Pediatric patients.** Safety and efficacy in children under age 6 months aren't established.

## Patient counseling
■ Warn patient of potential adverse reactions
and advise to promptly report any adverse drug
events to prescriber.

# flucytosine (5-FC)

Ancobon

*Pharmacologic classification:* fluori-
nated pyrimidine
*Therapeutic classification:* antifungal
*Pregnancy risk category C*

## Available forms

Available by prescription only
*Capsules:* 250 mg, 500 mg

## Indications and dosages

**Severe fungal infections caused by suscep-
tible strains of Candida and Cryptococcus**
*Adults:* 50 to 150 mg/kg/day P.O., given in divided doses q 6 hours.
◇ *Chromomycosis*
*Adults:* 150 mg/kg P.O. daily.
≡ *Dosage adjustment.* In patients with renal
failure who have a creatinine clearance of
50 ml/minute or less, reduce dosage by 20%
to 80%. Alternatively, in patients with creatinine clearance of 20 to 40 ml/minute, increase
dosage interval to q 12 hours; creatinine clearance of 10 to 20 ml/minute, increase dosage
interval to q 24 hours; and for those with creatinine clearance of less than 10 ml/minute, increase dosage interval to q 24 to 48 hours. Advise clinician to monitor serum levels.
Flucytosine is removed by hemodialysis and
peritoneal dialysis.
   Dosage of 20 to 50 mg/kg P.O. immediately after hemodialysis q 2 to 3 days ensures therapeutic blood levels.

## Mechanism of action

*Antifungal action:* Flucytosine penetrates fungal cells, where it's converted to fluorouracil,
which interferes with pyrimidine metabolism;
it also may be converted to fluorodeoxyuredylic
acid, which interferes with DNA synthesis. Because human cells lack the enzymes needed to
convert drug to these toxic metabolites, flucytosine is selectively toxic to fungal, not host
cells. It's active against some strains of *Cryptococcus* and *Candida.*

## Pharmacokinetics

*Absorption:* About 75% to 90% of an oral dose
is absorbed. Food decreases rate of absorption.
*Distribution:* Distributed widely into the liver, kidneys, spleen, heart, bronchial secretions,
joints, peritoneal fluid, and aqueous humor.
CSF levels vary from 60% to 100% of serum
levels. It's 2% to 4% plasma protein–bound.
*Metabolism:* Only small amounts are metabolized.
*Excretion:* About 75% to 95% of a dose is excreted unchanged in urine; less than 10% is excreted unchanged in feces. Serum half-life is
2½ to 6 hours with normal renal function; as

long as 1,160 hours with creatinine clearance
less than 2 ml/minute.

| Route | Onset | Peak | Duration |
|-------|-------|------|----------|
| P.O. | Unknown | 2-6 hr | Unknown |

## Contraindications and precautions

Contraindicated in patients hypersensitive to
drug.
   Use cautiously in patients with impaired renal or hepatic function and bone marrow suppression.

## Interactions

**Drug-drug.** *Amphotericin B:* Synergistic effects and possible enhanced toxicity. Advise
clinician to monitor patient carefully.

## Adverse reactions

**CNS:** headache, vertigo, sedation, fatigue,
weakness, confusion, hallucinations, psychosis,
ataxia, hearing loss, paresthesia, parkinsonism,
peripheral neuropathy.
**CV:** *cardiac arrest, myocardial toxicity, ventricular dysfunction.*
**GI:** nausea, vomiting, diarrhea, abdominal pain,
emesis, dry mouth, duodenal ulcer, *hemorrhage,* ulcerative colitis.
**GU:** azotemia, elevated creatinine and BUN
levels, crystalluria, *renal failure.*
**Hematologic:** anemia, *leukopenia, bone marrow suppression, thrombocytopenia, eosinophilia, agranulocytosis, aplastic anemia.*
**Hepatic:** elevated liver enzyme levels, elevated serum alkaline phosphatase, jaundice.
**Metabolic:** hypoglycemia, hypokalemia.
**Respiratory:** *respiratory arrest,* chest pain,
dyspnea.
**Skin:** occasional rash, pruritus, urticaria, photosensitivity, allergic reactions, *toxic epidermal necrolysis.*

## Overdose and treatment

Flucytosine overdose may affect CV and pulmonary function. Treatment is largely supportive. Induced emesis or lavage may be useful within 4 hours after ingestion. Activated
charcoal and osmotic cathartics also may be
helpful. Flucytosine is readily removed by either hemodialysis or peritoneal dialysis.

## Clinical considerations

■ Hematologic studies and renal and hepatic
function test results should precede therapy
and should be repeated frequently thereafter.
■ Giving capsules over 15-minute period helps
reduce nausea, vomiting, and GI distress.
■ Flucytosine causes falsely elevated creatinine values on iminohydrolase enzymatic assay.

### Therapeutic monitoring

■ Advise clinician to monitor intake and output to ensure adequate renal function.

---

■ Prolonged serum levels in excess of 100 mcg/ml may cause toxicity; recommend monitoring serum levels, especially in patients with renal insufficiency.

### Special populations
**Pregnant patients.** Drug should be used only when potential benefits justify risk to fetus.
**Breast-feeding patients.** Safety hasn't been established in breast-feeding women.
**Pediatric patients.** Safety and efficacy in children haven't been established.

### Patient counseling
■ Advise patient of adverse reactions and the need to report them.
■ Tell patient to call prescriber promptly if urine output decreases or signs of bleeding or bruising occur.
■ Explain that adequate response may require several weeks or months of therapy.
■ Advise patient to adhere to medical regimen and to return as instructed for follow-up visits.

# fludarabine phosphate
Fludara

*Pharmacologic classification:* antimetabolite
*Therapeutic classification:* antineoplastic
*Pregnancy risk category D*

### Available forms
Available by prescription only
*Injection:* 50 mg as lyophilized powder

### Indications and dosages
***Treatment of B-cell chronic lymphocytic leukemia (CLL) in patients who haven't responded or have responded inadequately to at least one standard alkylating drug regimen,*** ◇*mycosis fungoides,* ◇*hairy cell leukemia,* ◇*Hodgkin's and malignant lymphoma*
*Adults:* Usually, 25 mg/m² I.V. over 30 minutes (◇ rapid I.V. injection or continuous I.V. infusion) for 5 consecutive days q 28 days. Therapy based on patient response and tolerance.
◇*Chronic lymphocytic leukemia*
*Adults:* Usually, 18 to 30 mg/m² I.V. over 30 minutes (◇ rapid I.V. injection or continuous I.V. infusion) for 5 consecutive days q 28 days. Therapy based on patient response and tolerance.

### I.V. administration
■ Because of the carcinogenic potential of the drug, wear gloves and protective eyewear to avoid exposure. If exposure occurs, wash skin and mucosa immediately with soap and water and flush eyes thoroughly with water or saline.
■ To reconstitute drug, add 2 ml of sterile water for injection to vial of 50 mg to provide solution of 25 mg/ml. The appropriate dose can then be further diluted in $D_5W$ or normal saline solution.
■ Administer drug by I.V. infusion over 30 minutes.
■ Drug should be used within 8 hours after reconstitution.

### Incompatibilities
Physically incompatible with acyclovir sodium, amphotericin B, chlorpromazine, daunorubicin, ganciclovir, hydroxyzine hydrochloride, miconazole, and prochlorperazine edisylate. Compatibility may depend on concentration of drugs, specific diluents, resulting pH of solution, and temperature. Consult specialized references.

### Mechanism of action
*Antineoplastic action:* After rapid conversion of fludarabine to its active metabolite, the metabolite appears to inhibit DNA synthesis by inhibiting DNA polymerase alpha, ribonucleotide reductase, and DNA primase. The exact mechanism of action isn't fully established.

### Pharmacokinetics
*Absorption:* Administered I.V.
*Distribution:* Widely distributed with a volume of distribution of 96 to 98 L/m² at steady state.
*Metabolism:* Rapidly dephosphorylated and then phosphorylated intracellularly to its active metabolite.
*Excretion:* 23% is excreted in urine as unchanged active metabolite. Half-life is about 10 hours.

| Route | Onset | Peak | Duration |
|-------|-------|------|----------|
| I.V. | 7-12 wk | Unknown | Unknown |

### Contraindications and precautions
Contraindicated in patients hypersensitive to drug or its components.
Use cautiously in patients with renal insufficiency.

### Interactions
**Drug-drug.** *Other myelosuppressive drugs:* Concurrent use may cause additive toxicity. Drug shouldn't be used with other myelosuppresive drugs.
*Pentostatin:* Increased risk of pulmonary toxicity. Avoid use together.

### Adverse reactions
**CNS:** *CVA, fatigue, malaise, weakness, paresthesia,* peripheral neuropathy, headache, sleep disorder, depression, cerebellar syndrome, agitation, *confusion,* **coma.**

**CV:** *edema,* angina, transient ischemic attack, phlebitis, ***arrhythmias, HF,*** supraventricular tachycardia, deep venous thrombosis, ***aneurysm, hemorrhage.***
**EENT:** *visual disturbances,* hearing loss, delayed blindness (with high doses), sinusitis, pharyngitis, epistaxis.
**GI:** *nausea, vomiting, diarrhea,* constipation, *anorexia,* stomatitis, ***GI bleeding,*** esophagitis, mucositis.
**GU:** dysuria, *urinary infection* or hesitancy, proteinuria, hematuria, ***renal failure.***
**Hematologic:** ***hemolytic anemia,*** MYELO-SUPPRESSION.
**Hepatic:** *liver failure,* cholelithiasis.
**Metabolic:** hypocalcemia, hyperkalemia, hyperglycemia, dehydration, hyperuricemia, hyperphosphatemia.
**Musculoskeletal:** *myalgia.*
**Respiratory:** *cough, pneumonia, dyspnea, upper respiratory tract infection,* allergic pneumonitis, hemoptysis, hypoxia, bronchitis.
**Skin:** alopecia, diaphoresis, *rash,* pruritus, seborrhea.
**Other:** *fever, chills, infection, pain,* tumor lysis syndrome, ***anaphylaxis.***

## Overdose and treatment
Irreversible CNS toxicity characterized by delayed blindness, coma, and death may result from high doses. Severe thrombocytopenia and neutropenia secondary to bone marrow suppression may also occur. There's no specific antidote, and treatment consists of discontinuing therapy and taking supportive measures.

## Clinical considerations
■ Drug has been used investigationally in the treatment of malignant lymphoma, macroglobulinemic lymphoma, prolymphocytic leukemia or prolymphocytoid variant of CLL, mycosis fungoides, hairy cell leukemia, cutaneous T-cell lymphoma, and Hodgkin's disease.
■ Drug should be given under the direct supervision of a prescriber experienced in antineoplastic therapy.
■ Tumor lysis syndrome (hyperuricemia, hyperphosphatemia, hypocalcemia, metabolic acidosis, hyperkalemia, hematuria, urate crystalluria, and renal failure) has occurred in CLL patients with large tumors.
■ Severe neurologic effects, including blindness, are seen when high doses are used to treat acute leukemia.
■ Advanced age, renal insufficiency, and bone marrow impairment may predispose patient to severe toxicity; toxic effects are dose-dependent.
■ Optimal duration of therapy hasn't been established; three additional cycles after achieving maximal response are recommended before stopping drug.

■ Consider using irradiated blood products in patients requiring transfusions to reduce risk of transfusion-associated graft-versus-host disease.

### Therapeutic monitoring
■ Careful hematologic monitoring is required, especially of neutrophil and platelet counts.

### Special populations
**Breast-feeding patients.** It's unknown if drug appears in breast milk. Risk-benefit ratio must be determined.
**Pediatric patients.** Safety and efficacy in children haven't been established.
**Geriatric patients.** Advanced age may increase toxicity potential.

## Patient counseling
■ Tell patient to avoid contact with infected persons and to report signs of infection or unusual bleeding immediately.

# fludrocortisone acetate
Florinef

*Pharmacologic classification:* mineralocorticoid, glucocorticoid
*Therapeutic classification:* mineralocorticoid replacement therapy
*Pregnancy risk category C*

## Available forms
Available by prescription only
*Tablets:* 0.1 mg

## Indications and dosages
***Adrenal insufficiency (partial replacement), salt-losing adrenogenital syndrome***
*Adults:* 0.1 to 0.2 mg P.O. daily.
*Children:* 0.05 to 0.1 mg P.O. daily.
***Postural hypotension in diabetic patients, ◇ orthostatic hypotension***
*Adults:* 0.1 to 0.4 mg P.O. daily.
***Postural hypotension caused by levodopa therapy***
*Adults:* 0.05 to 0.2 mg P.O. daily.

## Mechanism of action
*Adrenal hormone replacement:* Fludrocortisone, a synthetic glucocorticoid with potent mineralocorticoid activity, is used for partial replacement of steroid hormones in adrenocortical insufficiency and in salt-losing forms of congenital adrenogenital syndrome. In treating adrenocortical insufficiency, an exogenous glucocorticoid must also be given for adequate control. (Cortisone and hydrocortisone are usually the drugs of choice for replacement because they produce both mineralocorticoid and glucocorticoid activity.) Fludrocortisone is given on a variable schedule ranging from three

---

times weekly to b.i.d., depending on individual requirements.

## Pharmacokinetics

*Absorption:* Absorbed readily from the GI tract.
*Distribution:* Removed rapidly from blood and distributed to muscle, liver, skin, intestines, and kidneys. It has a plasma half-life of about 30 minutes. It's extensively bound to plasma proteins (transcortin and albumin). Only the unbound portion is active. Adrenocorticoids appear in breast milk and also can be transmitted through the placenta.
*Metabolism:* Metabolized in the liver to inactive glucuronide and sulfate metabolites.
*Excretion:* Inactive metabolites and small amounts of unmetabolized drug are excreted by the kidneys. Insignificant quantities of drug are also excreted in feces. Biologic half-life is 18 to 36 hours; plasma half-life is 3½ hours or longer.

| Route | Onset | Peak | Duration |
|-------|-------|------|----------|
| P.O. | Variable | 2 hr | 1-2 days |

## Contraindications and precautions

Contraindicated in patients with systemic fungal infections or hypersensitivity to drug.

Use cautiously in patients with hypothyroidism, cirrhosis, ocular herpes simplex, emotional instability, psychotic tendencies, nonspecific ulcerative colitis, diverticulitis, fresh intestinal anastomoses, peptic ulcer, renal insufficiency, hypertension, osteoporosis, and myasthenia gravis.

## Interactions

**Drug-drug.** *Barbiturates, phenytoin, rifampin:* May cause decreased corticosteroid effects. Advise clinician to monitor patient carefully.
*Cardiac glycosides:* If hypokalemia occurs, risk of toxicity is increased. Advise clinician to monitor patient closely.
*Isoniazid and salicylates:* Increased metabolism of these drugs. Advise clinician to monitor patient for drug effects.
*Thiazide diuretics or amphotericin B:* Concurrent use may enhance hypokalemia. Advise clinician to monitor electrolytes.
**Drug-food.** *Sodium-containing drugs or foods:* May increase blood pressure. Sodium intake may need to be adjusted.

## Adverse reactions

**CV:** *sodium and water retention,* hypertension, cardiac hypertrophy, edema, *HF.*
**Metabolic:** increased serum sodium levels, hypokalemia.
**Skin:** bruising, diaphoresis, urticaria, allergic rash.

## Overdose and treatment

Acute toxicity is manifested as an extension of the therapeutic effect, such as by disturbances in fluid and electrolyte balance, hypokalemia, edema, hypertension, and cardiac insufficiency. In acute toxicity, recommend giving symptomatic treatment and correcting fluid and electrolyte imbalance.

## Clinical considerations

■ Use only with other supplemental measures, such as administration of glucocorticoids, control of electrolytes, and control of infection.
■ Supplemental dosages may be needed in times of physiologic stress from serious illness, trauma, or surgery.
■ Recommend performing glucose tolerance tests only if needed, because severe hypoglycemia tends to develop in addisonian patients within 3 hours of the test.

### Therapeutic monitoring

■ Advise clinician to monitor patient for significant weight gain, edema, hypertension, or severe headaches.

### Special populations

**Pediatric patients.** Long-term use in children and adolescents may delay growth and maturation.

## Patient counseling

■ Teach patient to recognize signs of electrolyte imbalance: muscle weakness, paresthesia, numbness, fatigue, anorexia, nausea, altered mental status, increased urination, altered heart rhythm, severe or continuing headaches, unusual weight gain, or swelling of the feet.
■ Tell patient to take missed doses as soon as possible, unless it's almost time for the next dose, and not to double the dose.

---

# flumazenil
Romazicon

*Pharmacologic classification:* benzodiazepine antagonist
*Therapeutic classification:* antidote
*Pregnancy risk category C*

## Available forms

Available by prescription only
*Injection:* 0.1 mg/ml in 5-ml and 10-ml multiple-dose vials

## Indications and dosages

***Complete or partial reversal of sedative effects of benzodiazepines after anesthesia or short diagnostic procedures (conscious sedation)***
*Adults:* Initially, 0.2 mg I.V. over 15 seconds. If patient doesn't reach desired level of consciousness after 45 seconds, repeat dose. Repeat at 1-minute intervals until a cumulative dose of 1 mg has been given (initial dose plus four additional doses). Most patients respond

after 0.6 to 1 mg of drug. If resedation occurs, dose may be repeated after 20 minutes, but no more than 1 mg should be given at one time, and patient shouldn't receive more than 3 mg/hour.

*Management of suspected benzodiazepine overdose*
*Adults:* Initially, 0.2 mg I.V. over 30 seconds. If patient doesn't reach desired level of consciousness after 30 seconds, give 0.3 mg over 30 seconds. If patient still doesn't respond adequately, give 0.5 mg over 30 seconds, then repeat 0.5-mg doses at 1-minute intervals until a cumulative dose of 3 mg has been given. Most patients with benzodiazepine overdose respond to cumulative doses between 1 and 3 mg; rarely, patients who respond partially after 3 mg may require additional doses. Don't give more than 5 mg over 5 minutes initially; sedation that persists after this dose is unlikely to be caused by benzodiazepines. If resedation occurs, dose may be repeated after 20 minutes, but no more than 1 mg should be given at one time, and patient shouldn't receive more than 3 mg/hour.

## I.V. administration
▪ A secure airway and I.V. access should be established before administration of flumazenil.
▪ Flumazenil can be given by direct injection or diluted with a compatible solution. Compatible solutions include $D_5W$, lactated Ringer's solution, and normal saline solution.
▪ Drug is given by rapid I.V. injection over 15 to 30 seconds.
▪ Drug should be given through a free-flowing I.V. infusion into a large vein.
▪ Drug is stable in a syringe for maximum of 24 hours.

## Incompatibilities
None reported.

## Mechanism of action
*Antidote action:* Flumazenil competitively inhibits the actions of benzodiazepines on the gamma-aminobutyric acid–benzodiazepine receptor complex.

## Pharmacokinetics
*Absorption:* Administered I.V.
*Distribution:* After administration, drug redistributes rapidly (initial distribution half-life is 7 to 15 minutes). It's about 50% plasma protein–bound.
*Metabolism:* Rapidly extracted from the blood and metabolized by the liver. Metabolites that have been identified are inactive. Ingestion of food during an I.V. infusion enhances extraction of drug from plasma, probably by increasing hepatic blood flow.
*Excretion:* About 90% to 95% is excreted in the urine as metabolites; the remainder is ex-

creted in feces. Plasma half-life is about 54 minutes.

| Route | Onset | Peak | Duration |
|-------|-------|------|----------|
| I.V. | 1-2 min | 6-10 min | Variable |

## Contraindications and precautions
Contraindicated in patients hypersensitive to drug or benzodiazepines; in patients who show evidence of serious tricyclic antidepressant overdose; and in those who have received a benzodiazepine to treat a potentially life-threatening condition such as status epilepticus.

Use cautiously in alcohol-dependent or psychiatric patients, in those at high risk for seizures, or in those with head injuries, signs of seizures, or recent high intake of benzodiazepines, such as patients in the intensive care unit.

## Interactions
**Drug-drug.** *Antidepressants and drugs that can cause seizures or arrhythmias:* May cause seizures or arrhythmias after flumazenil removes the effects of the benzodiazepine overdose. Flumazenil shouldn't be used in mixed overdose, especially when seizures (from any cause) are likely to occur.

## Adverse reactions
**CNS:** *dizziness, abnormal or blurred vision, headache, seizures,* agitation, emotional lability, tremor, insomnia.
**CV:** *arrhythmias,* cutaneous vasodilation, palpitations.
**GI:** nausea, vomiting.
**Respiratory:** dyspnea, hyperventilation.
**Skin:** *diaphoresis.*
**Other:** *pain* (at injection site).

## Overdose and treatment
Large doses of flumazenil don't appear to cause serious adverse reactions.

In patients with benzodiazepine overdose, large doses of flumazenil may produce agitation or anxiety, hyperesthesia, increased muscle tone, or seizures. Seizures may be treated with barbiturates, phenytoin, or benzodiazepines.

## Clinical considerations
▪ Because duration of action of flumazenil is shorter than that of benzodiazepines, advise prescriber to monitor patient carefully and give additional drug p.r.n. Duration and degree of effect depend on plasma levels of the sedating benzodiazepine and the dose of flumazenil.
▪ Resedation may occur after reversal of benzodiazepine effect.

---

Reactions may be *common,* uncommon, *life-threatening,* or COMMON AND LIFE-THREATENING.

### Therapeutic monitoring
■ Advise clinician to monitor patient for resedation according to duration of drug being reversed. Usually, serious resedation is unlikely in patient who fails to show signs of resedation 2 hours after a 1-mg dose of flumazenil.

### Special populations
**Breast-feeding patients.** It's unknown if drug appears in breast milk. Use cautiously in breast-feeding women.
**Pediatric patients.** Because no clinical data exist regarding risks, benefits, or dosage range in children, manufacturer doesn't recommend its use.

### Patient counseling
■ Because of risk of resedation, advise patient to avoid hazardous activities (such as driving a car), alcohol, CNS depressants, and OTC drugs within 24 hours of the procedure.

---

# flunisolide
*Nasal inhalant*
Nasalide, Nasarel

*Oral inhalant*
AeroBid, AeroBid-M

*Pharmacologic classification:* glucocorticoid
*Therapeutic classification:* anti-inflammatory, antiasthmatic
*Pregnancy risk category C*

### Available forms
Available by prescription only
*Nasal inhalant:* 25 mcg/metered spray; 200 doses/bottle
*Oral inhalant:* 250 mcg/metered spray; at least 100 doses/inhaler

### Indications and dosages
*Corticosteroid-dependent asthma*
*Adults:* Two inhalations b.i.d. for a total daily dose of 1 mg. Don't exceed 8 inhalations (2 mg daily).
*Children ages 6 and older:* Two inhalations b.i.d. Don't exceed 4 inhalations daily.
*Seasonal or perennial rhinitis*
*Adults:* 2 sprays (50 mcg) in each nostril b.i.d. (total dose 200 mcg/day). If needed, increase to 2 sprays in each nostril t.i.d. (total dose 300 mcg/day).
*Children ages 6 to 14:* 1 spray (25 mcg) in each nostril t.i.d. or 2 sprays (50 mcg) in each nostril b.i.d. (total dose 150 to 200 mcg/day).

### Mechanism of action
*Anti-inflammatory action:* Flunisolide stimulates the synthesis of enzymes needed to decrease the inflammatory response. The anti-inflammatory and vasoconstrictor potency of topically applied flunisolide is several hundred times greater than that of hydrocortisone and about equal to that of an equal weight of triamcinolone; the metabolite, 6-beta-hydroxyflunisolide, has about three times the activity of hydrocortisone.
*Antiasthmatic action:* The nasal inhalant form is used in the symptomatic treatment of seasonal or perennial rhinitis. In patients who require corticosteroids to control symptoms, the oral inhalant form is used to treat bronchial asthma.

### Pharmacokinetics
*Absorption:* About 50% of a nasally inhaled dose is absorbed systemically. After oral inhalation, about 40% of dose is absorbed from the lungs and GI tract; only about 20% of an orally inhaled dose reaches systemic circulation unmetabolized because of extensive metabolism in the liver. Onset of action usually occurs in a few days but may take as long as 4 weeks.
*Distribution:* Distribution after intranasal administration or oral inhalation hasn't been described. No evidence exists of tissue storage of flunisolide or its metabolites.
*Metabolism:* When swallowed, undergoes rapid metabolism in the liver or GI tract to several metabolites, one of which has glucocorticoid activity. Flunisolide and its 6-beta-hydroxy metabolite are eventually conjugated in the liver, by glucuronic acid or surface sulfate, to inactive metabolites.
*Excretion:* Excretion pathway is unknown when drug is given as inhalant; however, when it's given systemically, metabolites are excreted in roughly equal portions in feces and urine. Biologic half-life of drug averages about 2 hours.

| Route | Onset | Peak | Duration |
|-------|-------|------|----------|
| Inhalation | Variable | 10-30 min | Unknown |

### Contraindications and precautions
Contraindicated in patients hypersensitive to drug. Use of nasal inhalant is contraindicated in the presence of untreated localized infection involving nasal mucosa; oral inhalant shouldn't be used in patients with status asthmaticus or respiratory infections.

Nasal inhalant should be used cautiously in patients with tuberculosis; untreated fungal, bacterial, or systemic viral or ocular herpes simplex infections; or septal ulcers, trauma, or surgery in the nasal region. Oral inhalant isn't recommended for patients with asthma controlled by bronchodilators or other noncorticosteroids alone or for those patients with nonasthma bronchial diseases.

---

* Canada only    ◇ Unlabeled clinical use

## Interactions
None reported.

## Adverse reactions
**CNS:** headache (with nasal inhalant); dizziness, irritability, nervousness (with oral inhalant).
**CV:** chest pain, edema (with oral inhalant).
**EENT:** nasopharyngeal fungal infection; *mild, transient nasal burning and stinging,* stinging, dryness, sneezing, epistaxis, watery eyes (with nasal inhalant); *aftertaste* (Nasarel); *epistaxis* (Nasarel).
**GI:** nausea, vomiting (with nasal inhalant), dry mouth, abdominal pain, decreased appetite, *nausea, vomiting, diarrhea, upset stomach* (with oral inhalant).
**Respiratory:** *upper respiratory tract infection* (with oral inhalant).
**Skin:** rash, pruritus (with oral inhalant).
**Other:** *cold symptoms, flu,* fever (with oral inhalant).

## Overdose and treatment
No information available.

## Clinical considerations
▪ If no benefit is seen after 3 weeks, use of intranasal product should be stopped.
▪ Nasarel is not the bioequivalent of Nasalide.
▪ Recommendations for use of flunisolide and for care and teaching of the patient during therapy are the same as those for all inhalant adrenocorticoids.

### Therapeutic monitoring
▪ Advise clinician to monitor patient for adverse reactions
▪ Advise clinician to monitor patient for development of oral fungal infections.

### Special populations
**Pregnant patients.** Drug should be used during pregnancy only when potential benefits justify risk to fetus.
**Breast-feeding patients.** Drug should be used with caution in breast-feeding patients.
**Pediatric patients.** Safety and efficacy haven't been established in children under age 6 months.

## Patient counseling
▪ Tell patient that effects are not immediate; full benefit requires regular use and can be achieved in several days.
▪ Inform patient that drug doesn't relieve emergency asthma attacks.
▪ Advise patient of proper administration.

# fluocinonide
Lidemol*, Lidex, Lidex-E, Lyderm*

*Pharmacologic classification:* topical adrenocorticoid
*Therapeutic classification:* anti-inflammatory
*Pregnancy risk category C*

## Available forms
Available by prescription only
*Cream, gel, ointment, solution:* 0.05%

## Indications and dosages
*Inflammation of corticosteroid-responsive dermatoses*
*Adults and children:* Apply sparingly b.i.d. or t.i.d. Occlusive dressings may be used for severe or resistant dermatoses.

## Mechanism of action
*Anti-inflammatory action:* Fluocinonide stimulates the synthesis of enzymes needed to decrease the inflammatory response. Fluocinonide is a high-potency fluorinated glucocorticoid categorized as a group II topical corticosteroid.

## Pharmacokinetics
*Absorption:* Amount absorbed depends on amount applied and on nature of skin at application site. It ranges from about 1% in areas of thick stratum corneum (such as the palms, soles, elbows, and knees) to as high as 36% in areas of thin stratum corneum (face, eyelids, and genitals). Absorption increases in areas of skin damage, inflammation, or occlusion. Some systemic absorption of corticosteroids occurs, especially through the oral mucosa.
*Distribution:* After topical application, drug is distributed throughout the local skin. Any drug absorbed into circulation is removed rapidly from the blood and distributed into muscle, liver, skin, intestines, and kidneys.
*Metabolism:* After topical administration, drug is metabolized primarily in the skin. The small amount absorbed into systemic circulation is metabolized primarily in the liver to inactive compounds.
*Excretion:* Inactive metabolites are excreted by the kidneys, primarily as glucuronides and sulfates, but also as unconjugated products. Small amounts of metabolites are excreted in feces.

| Route | Onset | Peak | Duration |
|-------|-------|------|----------|
| Topical | Unknown | Unknown | Unknown |

## Contraindications and precautions
Contraindicated in patients hypersensitive to drug.

## Interactions
None significant.

---

## Adverse reactions

**Metabolic:** hyperglycemia, glucosuria.
**Skin:** burning, pruritus, irritation, dryness, erythema, folliculitis, hypertrichosis, hypopigmentation, acneiform eruptions, perioral dermatitis, allergic contact dermatitis; *maceration, secondary infection, atrophy, striae, miliaria* (with occlusive dressings).
**Other:** *hypothalamic-pituitary-adrenal axis suppression,* Cushing's syndrome.

## Overdose and treatment

No information available.

## Clinical considerations

■ Gently wash skin before applying drug. Rub in gently, leaving a thin coat. When treating hairy sites, part hair and apply directly to lesion. Avoid applying near eyes or mucous membranes or in ear canal.
■ For patients whose skin may be irritated by tape, hold dressing in place with gauze, elastic bandages, or stockinette.
■ Remove occlusive dressing if fever develops.
■ If antifungals or antibiotics are used concurrently, stop drug until infection is controlled.
■ Continue treatment for a few days after lesions clear.
**⧏ ALERT** Don't confuse fluocinolone with fluocinonide.

### Therapeutic monitoring

■ Recommend monitoring patient for skin infection, striae, and atrophy. Stop drug if they occur.
■ Systemic absorption is likely with use of occlusive dressings, prolonged treatment, or extensive body surface treatment. Advise clinician to watch for symptoms.

### Special populations

**Pregnant patients.** Use hasn't been established.
**Breast-feeding patients.** Topical corticosteroids should be used with caution.
**Pediatric patients.** Children may be more prone to HPA-axis suppression and Cushing's syndrome than adults. Parents shouldn't use plastic pants or tight-fitting diapers on a child being treated in their diaper area.

## Patient counseling

■ Teach patient how to apply drug using gloves, sterile applicator, or careful hand washing.
■ Advise patient to leave occlusive dressing in place no longer than 12 hours each day and not to use occlusive dressings on infected or exudative lesions.
■ Tell patient to stop drug and report signs of systemic absorption, skin irritation or ulceration, hypersensitivity, or infection.

# fluorouracil (5-FU)

Adrucil, Carac, Efudex, Fluoroplex

*Pharmacologic classification:* antimetabolite (cell cycle–phase specific, S phase)
*Therapeutic classification:* antineoplastic
*Pregnancy risk category D (injection), X (cream)*

## Available forms

Available by prescription only
*Injection:* 50 mg/ml in 10-ml, 20-ml, 50-ml, 100-ml vials
*Cream:* 1%, 5%
*Topical solution:* 1%, 2%, 5%

## Indications and dosages

Dosage and indications may vary. Check current literature for recommended protocol.
*Palliative management of colon, rectal, breast, ◇ovarian, ◇cervical, gastric, ◇bladder, ◇liver, pancreatic cancers*
*Adults and children:* 12 mg/kg I.V. for 4 days; then if no toxicity occurs, give 6 mg/kg I.V. on days 6, 8, 10, and 12. Maintenance therapy is a repeated course q 30 days. Don't exceed 800 mg/day (400 mg/day in severely ill patients).
*Actinic or solar keratoses*
*Adults:* Sufficient cream or lotion to cover lesions b.i.d. for 2 to 4 weeks. Usually, 1% preparations are used on head, neck, and chest; 2% and 5% on hands. For Carac cream, wash and dry area; wait 10 minutes. Apply a thin layer of drug to skin where lesions appear, once daily for up to 4 weeks.
*Superficial basal cell carcinomas*
*Adults:* 5% solution or cream in a sufficient amount to cover lesion b.i.d. for 3 to 6 weeks, up to 12 weeks.

## I.V. administration

■ Follow facility policy to reduce risks. Preparation and administration of parenteral form of drug are linked to carcinogenic, mutagenic, and teratogenic risks for staff.
■ Don't refrigerate drug or expose to light.
■ Solution is more stable in plastic I.V. bags than in glass bottles.
■ Drug may be further diluted in $D_5W$ or normal saline solution for infusions up to 24 hours in duration.
■ Drug need not be further diluted and may be administered I.V. push over 1 to 2 minutes.

### Incompatibilities

Incompatible with carboplatin, cisplatin, cytarabine, diazepam, doxorubicin, droperidol, epirubicin, filgrastim, methotrexate, and ondansetron.

## Mechanism of action
*Antineoplastic action:* Fluorouracil acts as an antimetabolite, competing for the enzyme that's important in the synthesis of thymidine, an essential substrate for DNA synthesis. Therefore, DNA synthesis is inhibited. Drug also inhibits RNA synthesis to a lesser extent.

## Pharmacokinetics
*Absorption:* Given parenterally because it's absorbed poorly after oral administration.
*Distribution:* Distributes widely into all areas, including tumors, bone marrow, liver, and intestinal mucosa. Fluorouracil crosses the blood-brain barrier to a significant extent.
*Metabolism:* A small amount is converted in the tissues to the active metabolite, with most of drug degraded in the liver.
*Excretion:* Metabolites are primarily excreted through the lungs as carbon dioxide. A small portion of a dose is excreted in urine as unchanged drug.

| Route | Onset | Peak | Duration |
|---|---|---|---|
| I.V., topical | Unknown | Unknown | Unknown |

## Contraindications and precautions
Contraindicated in patients hypersensitive to drug; patients in a poor nutritional state; patients with bone marrow suppression (WBC counts of 5,000/mm³ or less, or platelet counts of 100,000/ mm³ or less); patients with potentially serious infections; and in those who have had major surgery within the previous month.

Drug should be used cautiously in patients after high-dose pelvic radiation therapy or use of alkylating drugs. Also use with caution in patients with widespread neoplastic infiltration of bone marrow and impaired renal or hepatic function.

## Interactions
**Drug-drug.** *Leucovorin calcium and prior treatment with alkylating drugs:* May enhance toxicity. Use with extreme caution.
**Drug-lifestyle.** *Sun exposure:* May cause photosensitivity reactions. Advise patient to take precautions.

## Adverse reactions
**CNS:** acute cerebellar syndrome, confusion, disorientation, euphoria, ataxia, headache, *weakness, malaise.*
**CV:** *myocardial ischemia,* angina.
**EENT:** nystagmus.
**GI:** *stomatitis, GI ulcer* (may precede leukopenia), *nausea, vomiting, diarrhea, anorexia,* GI bleeding.
**Hematologic:** *leukopenia, thrombocytopenia, agranulocytosis,* anemia; WBC count nadir 9 to 14 days after first dose; platelet count nadir in 7 to 14 days.
**Metabolic:** hypoalbuminemia because of drug-induced protein malabsorption.

**Skin:** *reversible alopecia; dermatitis; erythema; scaling; pruritus;* nail changes; pigmented palmar creases; erythematous contact dermatitis; desquamative rash of hands and feet with long-term use ("hand-foot syndrome"), swelling (with topical use).
**Other:** *pain, burning,* soreness, suppuration, *anaphylaxis,* thrombophlebitis.

## Overdose and treatment
Signs and symptoms of overdose include myelosuppression, diarrhea, alopecia, dermatitis, hyperpigmentation, nausea, and vomiting. Treatment is usually supportive and includes transfusion of blood components, antiemetics, and antidiarrheals.

## Clinical considerations
■ Fluorouracil shouldn't be refrigerated.
■ Drug can be diluted in 120 ml of water and given orally; however, this isn't an FDA-approved method of administration, and absorption is erratic.
■ Topical application to larger ulcerated areas may cause systemic toxicity.
■ With Carac cream, affected area shouldn't be occluded.

### Therapeutic monitoring
■ General photosensitivity occurs for 2 to 3 months after a dose.
■ Advise clinician to monitor intake and output, CBC, and renal and hepatic function.

### Special populations
**Pregnant patients.** During pregnancy, drug should be used only for life-threatening or serious situations when no other safe alternatives are available.
**Breast-feeding patients.** It isn't known if drug appears in breast milk; breast-feeding isn't recommended.

## Patient counseling
■ Warn patient to avoid strong sunlight or ultraviolet light. Encourage use of sunscreens.
■ Tell patient to avoid exposure to people with infections. Advise patient to promptly report signs of infection or unusual bleeding.
■ Advise patient to apply topical fluorouracil with gloves and to wash hands thoroughly after application.
■ Warn patient that treated area may be unsightly during therapy and for several weeks after therapy is stopped. Complete healing may not occur until 1 or 2 months after treatment is stopped.
■ Inform patient that sunscreen and moisturizer may be applied 2 hours after topical application.
■ Local irritation is not markedly increased by extending treatment from 2 to 4 weeks, and is

generally resolved within 2 weeks of cessation of topical treatment.

# fluoxetine
Prozac, Prozac Pulvules, Prozac Weekly, Sarafem Pulvules

*Pharmacologic classification:* selective serotonin reuptake inhibitor (SSRI)
*Therapeutic classification:* antidepressant
*Pregnancy risk category C*

## Available forms
Available by prescription only
*Tablets:* 10 mg
*Capsules:* 10 mg, 20 mg, 90 mg
*Oral solution:* 20 mg/5 ml

## Indications and dosages
**Major depressive disorder**
*Adults:* 20 mg P.O. daily. If no improvement after at least 4 weeks, dose can be increased. Don't exceed 80 mg daily. Alternatively, Prozac Weekly 90 mg P.O. once weekly.
◊ *Children ages 7 to 18:* 10 mg P.O. daily. Maximum dose is 20 mg daily.
**Obsessive-compulsive disorder**
*Adults:* 20 to 60 mg P.O. daily. Don't exceed 80 mg daily.
**Premenstrual dysphoric disorder (Sarafem)**
*Adults:* 20 mg P.O. daily. Don't exceed 80 mg daily.
**Bulimia nervosa**
*Adults:* 60 mg P.O. daily in the morning.
◊ *Anorexia nervosa*
*Adults:* 40 mg P.O. daily in weight-restored patients.
◊ *Depression associated with bipolar disorder*
*Adults:* 20 to 60 mg P.O. daily.
◊ *Panic disorder*
*Adults:* 10 to 20 mg P.O. daily. May increase in 10-mg increments at intervals of no less than 1 week to maximum dose of 80 mg.
◊ *Cataplexy*
*Adults:* 20 mg P.O. once daily or b.i.d. in conjunction with CNS stimulant therapy.
◊ *Alcohol dependence*
*Adults:* 60 mg P.O. daily.
≡ *Dosage adjustment.* For patients with hepatic impairment or concurrent disease and in those taking multiple drugs concomitantly, use reduced or less frequent dose.

## Mechanism of action
*Antidepressant action:* The antidepressant action of fluoxetine is purportedly related to its inhibition of CNS neuronal uptake of serotonin. Fluoxetine blocks uptake of serotonin, but not of norepinephrine, into human platelets. Animal studies suggest that it's a much more potent uptake inhibitor of serotonin than of norepinephrine.

## Pharmacokinetics
*Absorption:* Well absorbed after oral administration. Absorption isn't altered by food.
*Distribution:* Apparently highly protein-bound (about 95%).
*Metabolism:* Metabolized primarily in the liver to active metabolites.
*Excretion:* Excreted by the kidneys. Elimination half-life is 2 to 3 days. Norfluoxetine (the primary active metabolite) has an elimination half-life of 7 to 9 days.

| Route | Onset | Peak | Duration |
|-------|-------|------|----------|
| P.O. | Unknown | Unknown | Unknown |

## Contraindications and precautions
Contraindicated in patients hypersensitive to drug and in patients taking MAO inhibitors within 14 days of starting therapy. Use cautiously in patients at high risk of suicide or in those with a history of seizures, diabetes mellitus, or renal, hepatic, or CV disease.

Thioridazine is contraindicated in any patient who has used fluoxetine during previous 5 weeks.

## Interactions
**Drug-drug.** *Beta blockers:* Possible cardiac toxicity. Recommend closely monitoring patient.
*Clozapine:* Increased plasma level of clozapine. Advise clinician to monitor patient and considering reduction of clozapine dose.
*Cyproheptadine:* May reverse or decrease pharmacologic effect. Advise clinician to monitor patient closely.
*Drugs metabolized by cytochrome P-450 (CYP) 2D6 or cytochrome P-450 (CYP) 3A4:* May increase plasma levels of these drugs. Caution should be recommended with concomitant use.
*Flecainide, carbamazepine, and vinblastine:* Increased serum levels of these drugs. Advise clinician to monitor serum levels and the patient for adverse effects.
*Haloperidol:* Increased extrapyramidal symptoms. Recommend monitoring patient closely.
*Insulin, oral antidiabetics:* Altered glucose levels. May alter requirements for antidiabetic.
*Lithium and tricyclic antidepressants:* Increased adverse CNS effects. Avoid use together.
*Other serotonergic drugs, MAO inhibitors, buspirone:* Increased risk of serotonin syndrome. Avoid use together.
*Phenytoin:* Increased plasma phenytoin levels and risk of toxicity. Phenytoin level must be monitored; dosage adjustment may be needed.
*Sumatriptan:* Increase in frequency of migraine attacks. Patient should be observed closely.
*Thioridazine:* Elevated plasma levels of thioridazine, leading to an increased risk of serious ventricular arrhythmias and sudden death.

---

* Canada only   ◊ Unlabeled clinical use

Thioridazine should not be given with fluoxetine or within a minimum of 5 weeks after fluoxetine has been discontinued.

*Tryptophan:* Increased adverse CNS effects (agitation, restlessness) and GI distress. Drug should be used with caution.

*Warfarin and other highly protein-bound drugs:* Increased plasma levels of fluoxetine or other highly protein-bound drugs. Advise clinician to monitor patient closely.

**Drug-herb.** *St. John's wort:* Possible additive serotonin reuptake inhibition. Discourage use together.

**Drug-lifestyle.** *Alcohol use:* May increase CNS depression. Advise patient to avoid alcohol.

## Adverse reactions

**CNS:** *nervousness, anxiety, insomnia, headache, drowsiness, tremor, dizziness, asthenia,* fatigue.
**CV:** palpitations, hot flashes.
**EENT:** nasal congestion, pharyngitis, sinusitis.
**GI:** *nausea, diarrhea, dry mouth, anorexia, dyspepsia,* constipation, abdominal pain, vomiting, flatulence, increased appetite.
**GU:** sexual dysfunction, painful menstruation, frequent micturition, urinary tract infection.
**Metabolic:** *weight loss.*
**Musculoskeletal:** muscle pain.
**Respiratory:** upper respiratory tract infection, respiratory distress, cough.
**Skin:** *rash, pruritus,* diaphoresis.
**Other:** flulike syndrome, fever.

## Overdose and treatment

Symptoms of overdose include agitation, restlessness, hypomania, and other signs of CNS excitation; and, in patients who took higher doses of fluoxetine, nausea and vomiting.

To treat fluoxetine overdose, recommend establishing and maintaining an airway and ensuring adequate oxygenation and ventilation. Activated charcoal, which may be used with sorbitol, may be as effective as emesis or lavage.

Advise clinician to monitor cardiac and vital signs and provide usual supportive measures. Fluoxetine-induced seizures that don't subside spontaneously may respond to diazepam. Forced diuresis, dialysis, hemoperfusion, and exchange transfusion are unlikely to be of benefit.

## Clinical considerations

■ Advise prescriber to consider the inherent risk of suicide until significant improvement of depressive state occurs. High-risk patients should have close supervision when drug therapy starts. To reduce risk of suicidal overdose, the smallest quantity of pulvules consistent with good management should be used.
■ Full antidepressant effect may be delayed until after 4 weeks of treatment or longer.

■ Treatment of acute depression usually requires at least several months of continuous drug therapy; optimal duration of therapy hasn't been established.
■ Because of its long elimination half-life, changes in fluoxetine dosage won't be reflected in plasma for several weeks, affecting titration to final dose and withdrawal from treatment.
■ Fluoxetine therapy may activate mania or hypomania.
■ Recommend prescribing lower or less frequent dosages in patients with renal or hepatic impairment. Advise prescriber to consider lower or less frequent dosages in geriatric patients and others with concurrent disease or multiple drug therapy.
**⊞ ALERT** Initiate once-weekly dosing (Prozac Weekly) 7 days after the last daily dose of Prozac 20 mg.
■ Prozac Weekly is not for newly diagnosed depression.
**⊞ ALERT** If patient wishes to switch from an SSRI to St. John's wort, it may be necessary to wait a few weeks for the SSRI to wash out of his system before it is safe to start taking the herb. The exact time required depends on which SSRI he is taking.
**⊞ ALERT** Don't confuse Sarafem (fluoxetine) and Serophene (Clomid).

### Therapeutic monitoring

■ Patient must be closely monitored for improvement of depressive state and inherent risk of suicide.

### Special populations

**Pregnant patients.** Avoid using drug during pregnancy. Because of the long half-life of the drug, patient planning to become pregnant should consult prescriber to ascertain when risk to fetus has passed.
**Breast-feeding patients.** Drug appears in breast milk and shouldn't be used by breast-feeding patients.
**Pediatric patients.** Safety and efficacy in children haven't been established.
**Geriatric patients.** No overall differences in safety and efficacy in geriatric patients were observed; however, they may exhibit increased sensitivity to the drug.

## Patient counseling

■ Inform patient that drug may cause dizziness or drowsiness. Advise patient to avoid hazardous tasks that require alertness until CNS response to drug is established.
■ Caution patient to avoid ingestion of alcohol and to seek medical approval before taking other drugs.
■ Tell patient to promptly report rash or hives, anxiety, nervousness, anorexia (especially in underweight patients), suspicion of pregnancy, or intent to become pregnant.

■ Full antidepressant effect may be delayed until after 4 weeks of treatment or longer.

# fluphenazine decanoate
Modecate*, Prolixin Decanoate

# fluphenazine enanthate
Moditen Enanthate*, Prolixin Enanthate

# fluphenazine hydrochloride
Permitil, Prolixin

*Pharmacologic classification:* phenothiazine (piperazine derivative)
*Therapeutic classification:* antipsychotic
*Pregnancy risk category NR*

## Available forms
Available by prescription only
**fluphenazine decanoate**
*Depot injection:* 25 mg/ml
**fluphenazine enanthate**
*Depot injection:* 25 mg/ml
**fluphenazine hydrochloride**
*Tablets:* 1 mg, 2.5 mg, 5 mg, 10 mg
*Oral concentrate:* 5 mg/ml (Prolixin contains 14% alcohol and Permitil contains 1% alcohol)
*Elixir:* 2.5 mg/5 ml (with 14% alcohol)
*I.M. injection:* 2.5 mg/ml

## Indications and dosages
**Psychotic disorders**
*Adults:* Initially, 0.5 to 10 mg fluphenazine hydrochloride P.O. daily in divided doses q 6 to 8 hours; may increase cautiously to 20 mg. Maintenance dose is 1 to 5 mg P.O. daily. I.M. doses are one-third to one-half amounts of oral doses (starting dose is 1.25 mg I.M.). Use lower doses for geriatric patients (1 to 2.5 mg daily).

## Mechanism of action
*Antipsychotic action:* Fluphenazine is thought to exert its antipsychotic effects by postsynaptic blockade of CNS dopamine receptors, thereby inhibiting dopamine-mediated effects.

Fluphenazine has many other central and peripheral effects; it produces both alpha and ganglionic blockade and counteracts histamine- and serotonin-mediated activity. Its most prominent adverse reactions are extrapyramidal.

## Pharmacokinetics
*Absorption:* Rate and extent of absorption vary with route of administration; oral tablet absorption is erratic and variable.
*Distribution:* Distributed widely into the body; appears in breast milk. CNS levels are usually higher than those in plasma. Drug is 91% to 99% protein-bound.

*Metabolism:* Metabolized extensively by the liver, but no active metabolites are formed; duration of action is about 6 to 8 hours after oral administration; 1 to 6 weeks (average, 2 weeks) after I.M. depot administration.
*Excretion:* Mostly excreted in urine via the kidneys; some is excreted in feces via the biliary tract.

| Route | Onset | Peak | Duration |
|---|---|---|---|
| P.O. | < 1 hr | ½ hr | 6-8 hr |
| I.M. (HCl) | < 1 hr | 1½-2 hr | 6-8 hr |
| I.M. | 24-72 hr | Unknown | 1-6 wk |
| S.C. | Unknown | Unknown | Unknown |

## Contraindications and precautions
Contraindicated in patients hypersensitive to drug or in patients experiencing coma, CNS depression, bone marrow suppression or other blood dyscrasia, subcortical damage, or liver damage.

Use cautiously in geriatric or debilitated patients and in those with pheochromocytoma, severe CV disease, peptic ulcer disease, exposure to extreme hot or cold (including antipyretic therapy), exposure to phosphorous insecticides, respiratory or seizure disorders, hypocalcemia, severe reaction to insulin or electroconvulsive therapy, mitral insufficiency, glaucoma, or prostatic hyperplasia. Parenteral form should be used cautiously in patients with asthma and those allergic to sulfites.

## Interactions
**Drug-drug.** *Aluminum- and magnesium-containing antacids and antidiarrheals:* Decreased absorption of oral fluphenazine. Advise clinician to monitor patient.
*Antiarrhythmics, disopyramide, procainamide, and quinidine:* Increased risk of arrhythmias and conduction defects. Avoid use together.
*Atropine or other anticholinergics, including antidepressants, antihistamines, antiparkinsonians, MAO inhibitors, meperidine, and phenothiazines:* Oversedation, paralytic ileus, visual changes, and severe constipation. Avoid use together.
*Beta blockers:* Increased plasma levels and toxicity. Advise clinician to monitor patient closely.
*Bromocriptine:* Antagonized therapeutic effect of bromocriptine on prolactin secretion. Advise clinician to monitor patient for drug effect.
*Centrally acting antihypertensives such as clonidine, guanabenz, guanadrel, guanethidine, methyldopa, and reserpine:* Inhibition of blood pressure response; patient requires close monitoring.
*CNS depressants, including analgesics, barbiturates, narcotics, tranquilizers, and general, spinal, or epidural anesthetics, or parenteral magnesium sulfate:* Additive effects of overse-

---

dation, respiratory depression, and hypotension are likely. Avoid use together.

*Dopamine:* Decreased vasoconstricting effects. Advise clinician to monitor patient carefully.

*Levodopa:* Decreased effectiveness of levodopa. Advise clinician to monitor patient carefully.

*Lithium:* May result in severe neurologic toxicity with an encephalitis-like syndrome and a decreased therapeutic response to fluphenazine. Advise clinician to monitor patient closely.

*Metrizamide:* Increased risk of seizures. Patient requires close observation.

*Nitrates:* May result in hypotension. Recommend checking blood pressure frequently.

*Phenobarbital:* Enhanced renal excretion. Advise clinician to monitor patient closely.

*Phenytoin and tricyclic antidepressants:* Inhibited metabolism and increased toxicity of these drugs. Advise clinician to monitor patient closely.

*Propylthiouracil:* Increased risk of agranulocytosis. Advise clinician to monitor patient carefully.

*Sympathomimetics including epinephrine, phenylephrine, and ephedrine (often found in nasal sprays) and appetite suppressants:* May decrease their stimulatory and pressor effects. Drug should be used with caution.

**Drug-herb.** *Kava:* Increased risk for severity of dystonic reactions. Discourage use together.

*Yohimbe:* Increased risk of toxicity. Discourage use together.

**Drug-food.** *Caffeine:* May increase metabolism of fluphenazine. Advise patient to avoid caffeine.

**Drug-lifestyle.** *Alcohol use:* May increase CNS depression. Advise patient to avoid alcohol.

*Smoking:* Increased metabolism of fluphenazine. Discourage smoking.

*Sun exposure:* May increase risk of photosensitivity. Advise patient to use sunblock.

## Adverse reactions

**CNS:** *extrapyramidal reactions, tardive dyskinesia, sedation, pseudoparkinsonism, EEG changes, drowsiness, seizures, neuroleptic malignant syndrome,* dizziness.

**CV:** *orthostatic hypotension,* tachycardia, ECG changes.

**EENT:** ocular changes, *blurred vision,* nasal congestion.

**GI:** *dry mouth, constipation.*

**GU:** *urine retention,* dark urine, menstrual irregularities, inhibited ejaculation.

**Hematologic:** *leukopenia, agranulocytosis,* eosinophilia, hemolytic anemia, *aplastic anemia, thrombocytopenia.*

**Hepatic:** cholestatic jaundice, abnormal liver function test results.

**Metabolic:** elevated protein-bound iodine, weight gain, increased appetite.

**Skin:** mild photosensitivity, allergic reactions.

**Other:** gynecomastia.

After abrupt withdrawal of long-term therapy: gastritis, nausea, vomiting, dizziness, tremor, feeling of warmth or cold, diaphoresis, tachycardia, headache, insomnia.

## Overdose and treatment

CNS depression is characterized by deep, unarousable sleep and possible coma, hypotension or hypertension, extrapyramidal symptoms, dystonia, abnormal involuntary muscle movements, agitation, seizures, arrhythmias, ECG changes, hypothermia or hyperthermia, and autonomic nervous system dysfunction.

Treatment is symptomatic and supportive, including maintaining vital signs, airway, stable body temperature, and fluid and electrolyte balance.

Vomiting shouldn't be induced: drug inhibits cough reflex, and aspiration may occur. Recommend using gastric lavage, then activated charcoal and saline cathartics; dialysis doesn't help. Recommend regulating body temperature p.r.n. Recommend treating hypotension with I.V. fluids: epinephrine shouldn't be given. Recommend treating seizures with parenteral diazepam or barbiturates; arrhythmias with parenteral phenytoin (1 mg/kg with rate titrated to blood pressure); and extrapyramidal reactions with benztropine 1 to 2 mg or parenteral diphenhydramine at 10 to 50 mg.

## Clinical considerations

■ Note that depot injection (25 mg/ml) and I.M. injection (2.5 mg/ml) aren't interchangeable.

■ Depot injection isn't recommended for patients who aren't stabilized on a phenothiazine. This form has a prolonged elimination; its action couldn't be terminated in case of adverse reactions.

■ Fluphenazine causes false-positive test results for urinary porphyrins, urobilinogen, amylase, and 5-hydroxyindoleacetic acid, because of darkening of urine by metabolites; it also causes false-positive urine pregnancy test results using human chorionic gonadotropin.

■ Fluphenazine elevates test results for liver enzymes and causes quinidine-like ECG effects.

### Therapeutic monitoring

■ Recommendations are the same as for all phenothiazines.

### Special populations

**Pregnant patients.** Recommendations are the same as for all phenothiazines.

**Breast-feeding patients.** Drug appears in breast milk. Drug should be used with caution; potential benefits to the woman should outweigh the potential harm to the infant.

**Pediatric patients.** Safety and efficacy in children under age 12 haven't been established.

---

**Geriatric patients.** Recommendations are the same as for all phenothiazines.

## Patient counseling
■ Inform patient that drug may cause dizziness or drowsiness. Advise patient to avoid hazardous tasks that require alertness until CNS response to drug is established.
■ Tell patient to avoid alcohol and to seek medical approval before taking other drugs.
■ Instruct patient to promptly report rash or hives, anxiety, nervousness, anorexia (especially in underweight patients), suspicion of pregnancy, or intent to become pregnant.

# flurazepam hydrochloride
Apo-Flurazepam*, Dalmane, Novoflupam*

*Pharmacologic classification:* benzodiazepine
*Therapeutic classification:* sedative-hypnotic
*Pregnancy risk category X*
*Controlled substance schedule IV*

## Available forms
Available by prescription only
*Capsules:* 15 mg, 30 mg

## Indications and dosages
**Insomnia**
*Adults:* 15 to 30 mg P.O. h.s. In patients over age 65, 15 mg P.O. h.s.

## Mechanism of action
*Sedative action:* Flurazepam depresses the CNS at the limbic and subcortical levels of the brain. It produces a sedative effect by potentiating the effect of the neurotransmitter gamma-aminobutyric acid on its receptor in the ascending reticular activating system, which increases inhibition and blocks both cortical and limbic arousal.

## Pharmacokinetics
*Absorption:* When given orally, flurazepam is absorbed rapidly through the GI tract.
*Distribution:* Distributed widely throughout the body. About 97% of given dose is plasma protein–bound.
*Metabolism:* Metabolized in the liver to the active metabolite desalkylflurazepam.
*Excretion:* Desalkylflurazepam is excreted in urine; half-life is 50 to 100 hours.

| Route | Onset | Peak | Duration |
|---|---|---|---|
| P.O. | < 20 min | 1-2 hr | 7-10 hr |

## Contraindications and precautions
Contraindicated in patients hypersensitive to drug and during pregnancy.

Use cautiously in patients with impaired renal or hepatic function, chronic pulmonary insufficiency, mental depression, suicidal tendencies, or history of drug abuse.

## Interactions
**Drug-drug.** *General anesthetics, antidepressants, antihistamines, barbiturates, MAO inhibitors, narcotics, and phenothiazines:* Increased CNS depressant effects of these drugs. Use together cautiously.
*Cimetidine, disulfiram, isoniazid, oral contraceptives, and ritonavir:* May decrease metabolism of benzodiazepines, leading to toxicity. Advise clinician to monitor patient carefully.
*Digoxin:* Serum levels may increase resulting in toxicity. Advise clinician to monitor patient closely.
*Levodopa:* Decreased therapeutic effect of levodopa. Advise clinician to monitor patient for drug effects.
*Phenytoin:* Increased phenytoin levels. Advise clinician to monitor serum levels of phenytoin.
*Rifampin:* Enhanced metabolism of benzodiazepines. Advise clinician to monitor patient closely.
*Theophylline:* May act as an antagonist with flurazepam. Advise clinician to monitor patient closely.
**Drug-herb.** *Catnip, kava, lady's slipper, lemon balm, passion flower, sassafras, skullcap, valerian:* Sedative effects may be enhanced. Discourage use together.
**Drug-lifestyle.** *Alcohol use:* Excessive CNS and respiratory depression. Advise patient to avoid alcohol.
*Heavy smoking:* Accelerates metabolism of flurazepam. Advise clinician to monitor patient for drug effect.

## Adverse reactions
**CNS:** *daytime sedation, dizziness, drowsiness, disturbed coordination,* lethargy, confusion, *headache,* light-headedness, nervousness, hallucinations, staggering, ataxia, disorientation, changes in EEG patterns, *coma.*
**GI:** nausea, vomiting, heartburn, diarrhea, abdominal pain.
**Hepatic:** elevated liver enzyme levels.
**Other:** physical or psychological dependence.

## Overdose and treatment
Signs and symptoms of overdose include somnolence, confusion, hypoactive reflexes, dyspnea, labored breathing, hypotension, bradycardia, slurred speech, unsteady gait or impaired coordination, and, eventually, coma.

Recommend supporting blood pressure and respiration until drug effects subside; recommend monitoring vital signs. Mechanical ventilatory assistance via endotracheal (ET) tube may be required to maintain a patent airway and support adequate oxygenation. I.V. fluids should be used to promote diuresis, and vaso-

---

pressors such as dopamine and phenylephrine to treat hypotension p.r.n. Flumazenil, a specific benzodiazepine antagonist, may be useful as an adjunct to supportive therapy.

If patient is conscious, recommend inducing emesis. Recommend using gastric lavage if ingestion was recent, but only if an ET tube is present to prevent aspiration. After emesis or lavage, recommend giving activated charcoal with a cathartic as a single dose. Dialysis is of limited value. If excitation occurs, barbiturates shouldn't be given to avoid exacerbation of excitatory state or potentiation of CNS-depressant effects.

## Clinical considerations
■ Studies have shown a "carryover effect." Drug is most effective after 3 or 4 nights of use because of long half-life. Dose shouldn't be increased more frequently than every 5 days.
■ Drug is useful for patients who have trouble falling asleep and who awaken frequently at night and early in the morning.
■ Although prolonged use isn't recommended, this drug has proven effective for up to 4 weeks of continuous use.
■ Rapid withdrawal after prolonged use can cause withdrawal symptoms.
■ Lower doses are effective in patients with renal or hepatic dysfunction.

### Therapeutic monitoring
■ Advise clinician to monitor hepatic function and AST, ALT, bilirubin, and alkaline phosphatase levels for changes.

### Special populations
**Pregnant patients.** Drug is contraindicated during pregnancy.
**Breast-feeding patients.** Drug appears in breast milk. A breast-fed infant may become sedated, have feeding difficulties, or lose weight. Avoid use in breast-feeding women.
**Pediatric patients.** Closely observe a neonate for withdrawal symptoms if the mother took flurazepam during pregnancy. Use of flurazepam during labor may cause neonatal flaccidity. Drug isn't for use in children under age 15. Neonates are more sensitive to flurazepam because of slower metabolism. The possibility of toxicity is greatly increased.
**Geriatric patients.** Geriatric patients are more susceptible to CNS depressant effects of flurazepam. They may require assistance and supervision with walking and daily activities when therapy starts or changes. Lower doses usually are effective in geriatric patients because of decreased elimination.

## Patient counseling
■ Warn patient to avoid alcohol while taking drug.
■ Emphasize the potential for excessive CNS depression if drug is taken with alcohol, even if it's taken the evening before ingestion of alcohol.
■ Advise patient that rebound insomnia may occur after stopping drug, not to discontinue drug abruptly after prolonged therapy, and not to exceed prescribed dosage.

# flurbiprofen
Ansaid

*Pharmacologic classification:* NSAID, phenylalkanoic acid derivative
*Therapeutic classification:* antiarthritic
*Pregnancy risk category B*

## Available forms
Available by prescription only
*Tablets:* 50 mg, 100 mg

## Indications and dosages
**Rheumatoid arthritis and osteoarthritis**
*Adults:* 200 to 300 mg P.O. daily, divided b.i.d., t.i.d., or q.i.d.
≡*Dosage adjustment.* Patients with end-stage renal disease may accumulate flurbiprofen metabolites, but half-life of parent compound is unchanged. Advise clinician to monitor patient closely and adjust dosage accordingly.

## Mechanism of action
*Anti-inflammatory action:* Flurbiprofen interferes with the synthesis of prostaglandins.

## Pharmacokinetics
*Absorption:* Well absorbed after oral administration. Giving with food alters rate, but not extent, of absorption.
*Distribution:* Highly plasma protein–bound.
*Metabolism:* Metabolized primarily in the liver. The major metabolite shows little anti-inflammatory activity.
*Excretion:* Excreted primarily in urine. Average elimination half-life is 6 to 10 hours.

| Route | Onset | Peak | Duration |
|-------|-------|------|----------|
| P.O. | Unknown | 1½ hr | Unknown |

## Contraindications and precautions
Contraindicated in patients hypersensitive to drug, or in those with history of aspirin- or NSAID-induced asthma, urticaria, or other allergic-type reactions.

Use cautiously in geriatric or debilitated patients and in those with history of peptic ulcer disease, herpes simplex keratitis, impaired renal or hepatic function, cardiac disease, or conditions related to fluid retention.

## Interactions
**Drug-drug.** *Oral anticoagulants:* Increased bleeding tendencies. Avoid use together.
*Aspirin:* May decrease flurbiprofen levels and increase GI toxicity. Avoid use together.

*Beta blockers:* Antihypertensive effect of beta blockers may be impaired. Advise clinician to monitor patient carefully.

*Cyclosporine:* Increased risk of nephrotoxicity. Use together with extreme caution.

*Diuretics:* Decreased diuretic effect. Advise clinician to monitor patient carefully.

*Lithium:* Lithium levels may be increased. Advise clinician to monitor serum levels.

*Methotrexate:* May cause increased risk of methotrexate toxicity. Avoid use together.

**Drug-herb.** *Dong quai, feverfew, garlic, ginger, horse chestnut, red clover:* Possible increased risk of bleeding. Discourage use together.

*St. John's wort, dong quai:* Increased risk of photosensitivity. Advise patient to avoid unprotected exposure to sunlight.

**Drug-lifestyle.** *Alcohol use:* Increased risk of adverse GI reactions. Advise patient to avoid alcohol.

*Sun exposure:* May potentiate photosensitivity reactions. Advise patient to take precautions.

### Adverse reactions

**CNS:** *headache,* anxiety, insomnia, dizziness, increased reflexes, tremors, amnesia, asthenia, drowsiness, malaise, depression.

**CV:** *edema,* **HF,** hypertension, vasodilation.

**EENT:** rhinitis, tinnitus, visual changes, epistaxis.

**GI:** *dyspepsia, diarrhea, abdominal pain, nausea,* constipation, *bleeding,* flatulence, vomiting.

**GU:** *symptoms suggesting urinary tract infection,* hematuria, interstitial nephritis, ***renal failure.***

**Hematologic:** ***thrombocytopenia, neutropenia,*** anemia, ***aplastic anemia.***

**Hepatic:** *elevated liver enzyme levels, jaundice.*

**Metabolic:** weight changes.

**Respiratory:** asthma.

**Skin:** rash, photosensitivity, urticaria.

**Other:** *angioedema.*

### Overdose and treatment

Overdose has caused lethargy, coma, respiratory depression, epigastric pain, and distress.

Treatment should be supportive. Emptying the stomach by emesis or lavage would be of little use if the ingestion took place more than an hour before treatment, but is still recommended.

### Clinical considerations

■ Advise prescriber to closely monitor patient with impaired hepatic or renal function and geriatric or debilitated patients; they may need lower doses. These patients may be at risk for renal toxicity.

### Therapeutic monitoring

■ Patients receiving long-term therapy should have periodic liver function studies, ophthalmologic and auditory examinations, and hematocrit determinations.

### Special populations

**Pregnant patients.** Recommendations are the same as for all NSAIDs.

**Breast-feeding patients.** A breast-feeding woman taking 200 mg of flurbiprofen daily could deliver as much as 0.1 mg to the infant daily. Breast-feeding isn't recommended while using the drug.

**Pediatric patients.** Safety in children hasn't been established.

### Patient counseling

■ Advise patient to discontinue the drug and to contact prescriber promptly if GI bleeding occurs.

■ Tell patient to take drug with food, milk, or antacid to minimize GI upset.

■ Advise patient to avoid hazardous activities that require alertness until the adverse CNS effects of the drug are known.

■ Tell patient to immediately report to prescriber edema, substantial weight gain, black stools, rash, itching, or visual disturbances.

# flutamide
Eulexin

*Pharmacologic classification:* nonsteroidal antiandrogen
*Therapeutic classification:* antineoplastic
*Pregnancy risk category D*

### Available forms

Available by prescription only
*Capsules:* 125 mg

### Indications and dosages

***Treatment of metastatic prostatic carcinoma (stage D2) with luteinizing hormone-releasing hormone analogues, such as leuprolide acetate***
*Adults:* 250 mg P.O. q 8 hours.

### Mechanism of action

*Antitumor action:* Flutamide inhibits androgen uptake or prevents binding of androgens in nuclei of cells within target tissues. Prostatic carcinoma is known to be androgen-sensitive.

### Pharmacokinetics

*Absorption:* Rapidly and completely absorbed after oral administration.

*Distribution:* Concentrates in the prostate in animals. Drug and its active metabolite are about 95% protein-bound.

*Metabolism:* Metabolism is rapid, with at least six metabolites identified. More than 97% of drug is metabolized within 1 hour of administration.
*Excretion:* More than 95% is excreted in urine.

| Route | Onset | Peak | Duration |
|-------|-------|------|----------|
| P.O. | Unknown | 2 hr | Unknown |

## Contraindications and precautions
Contraindicated in patients hypersensitive to drug and in patients with severe hepatic impairment.

## Interactions
None reported.

## Adverse reactions
**CNS:** *drowsiness, confusion, depression, anxiety, nervousness.*
**CV:** *peripheral edema, hypertension.*
**GI:** *diarrhea, nausea, vomiting.*
**GU:** *impotence.*
**Hematologic:** anemia, *leukopenia, thrombocytopenia,* hemolytic anemia.
**Hepatic:** elevated liver enzyme levels, *hepatitis.*
**Skin:** rash, photosensitivity.
**Other:** *hot flashes,* gynecomastia, *loss of libido.*

## Overdose and treatment
No experience with overdose in humans has been reported. Dosage as high as 1,500 mg daily for 36 weeks has been reported without serious adverse effects.

## Clinical considerations
■ Flutamide must be taken continuously with drug used for medical castration (such as leuprolide acetate) to produce full benefit of therapy. Leuprolide suppresses testosterone production, and flutamide inhibits testosterone action at the cellular level. Together they can impair the growth of androgen-responsive tumors.
■ Elevation of plasma testosterone and estradiol levels has been reported. Serum ALT, AST, bilirubin, and creatinine levels may be increased.

### Therapeutic monitoring
■ Advise clinician to monitor patient for adverse reactions.
■ Advise clinician to monitor liver function test results and CBC.

### Special populations
**Pediatric patients.** Safety in children hasn't been established.

## Patient counseling
■ Tell patient not to discontinue either leuprolide or flutamide without medical approval.

■ Explain that some symptoms may worsen initially before they improve.

# fluticasone propionate
Cutivate, Flonase, Flovent, Flovent Rotadisk

*Pharmacologic classification:* corticosteroid
*Therapeutic classification:* topical/inhalation anti-inflammatory
*Pregnancy risk category C*

## Available forms
Available by prescription only
*Cream:* 0.05%
*Ointment:* 0.005%
*Metered nasal spray:* 50 mcg/actuation
*Inhalation aerosol:* 44 mcg/actuation, 110 mcg/actuation, 220 mcg/actuation
*Inhalation powder:* 50-mcg, 100-mcg, 250-mcg rotadisk

## Indications and dosages
*Relief of inflammation and pruritus of corticosteroid-responsive dermatoses*
*Adults:* Apply sparingly to affected area b.i.d. and rub in gently and completely.
*Allergic rhinitis*
*Adults:* 2 sprays in each nostril once daily or 1 spray b.i.d.
*Management of nasal symptoms of seasonal and perennial allergic rhinitis in children*
*Adolescents and children ages 4 and older:* Initially, 1 spray (50 mcg) in each nostril once daily. If patient doesn't respond or symptoms are severe, increase to 2 sprays in each nostril daily. Once adequate control is achieved, decrease dose to 1 spray in each nostril daily. Maximum dose is 2 sprays in each nostril daily.
*Maintenance treatment of asthma as prophylactic therapy*
*Adults and children ages 12 and older:* 88 to 220 mcg inhalation aerosol b.i.d., adjusting to maximum 440 mcg inhalation aerosol b.i.d.
*Adults and adolescents:* 100 mcg inhalation powder b.i.d., adjusting to maximum 500 mcg inhalation powder b.i.d.
*Children ages 4 to 11:* 50 mcg inhalation powder b.i.d., adjusting to maximum 100 mcg inhalation powder b.i.d.
See also package insert for dosing considerations with oral corticosteroids.

## Mechanism of action
*Anti-inflammatory action:* Fluticasone stimulates synthesis of enzymes needed to decrease inflammation.

## Pharmacokinetics
*Absorption:* Amount absorbed depends on amount applied, application site, vehicle used,

use of occlusive dressing, and integrity of epidermal barrier. Some systemic absorption does occur.

**Distribution:** Distributed throughout the local skin.

**Metabolism:** Metabolized primarily by the skin. Absorbed drug is extensively metabolized by the liver.

**Excretion:** Less than 5% is excreted in urine as metabolites; rest is excreted in feces as parent drug and metabolites.

| Route | Onset | Peak | Duration |
|---|---|---|---|
| Topical, inhalation | Unknown | Unknown | Unknown |

## Contraindications and precautions

Contraindicated in patients hypersensitive to drug or its components and in patients with viral, fungal, herpetic, or tubercular skin lesions.

Flovent inhalation aerosol and powder are contraindicated as the primary treatment in status asthmaticus or other acute episodes of asthma where intensive measures are required.

Care should be used when transferring patients from systemically active corticosteroids to Flovent inhalation aerosol or powder; deaths have occurred in asthmatic patients during and after transfer from systemic corticosteroids to less systemically available inhalation corticosteroids. During periods of stress or severe asthma attack, instruct patients who have been withdrawn from systemic corticosteroids to resume oral corticosteroids in large doses immediately and contact their prescribers for further assistance.

## Interactions

**Drug-drug.** *Ketoconazole:* May result in increased mean fluticasone levels. Use caution when fluticasone is coadministered with long-term ketoconazole and other known cytochrome P-450 3A4 inhibitors.

## Adverse reactions

**CNS:** dizziness, giddiness.
**GU:** dysmenorrhea.
**Metabolic:** hyperglycemia, glucosuria.
**Musculoskeletal:** pain in joints, sprain or strain aches and pains, pain in limbs.
**Respiratory:** bronchitis, chest congestion.
**Skin:** stinging, burning, pruritus, irritation, dryness, erythema, folliculitis, skin atrophy, leukoderma, vesicles, numbness of fingers, rash, hypertrichosis, acneiform eruptions, hypopigmentation, perioral dermatitis, allergic contact dermatitis, secondary infection, striae, miliaria.
**Other:** *hypothalamic-pituitary-adrenal axis suppression,* Cushing's syndrome, fever.

## Clinical considerations

■ Not used for treatment of rosacea, perioral dermatitis, or acne.

■ Mixing with other bases or vehicles may affect potency far beyond expectations.
■ Flovent inhalation aerosol and powder aren't indicated for the relief of acute bronchospasm.

## Therapeutic monitoring

■ During withdrawal from oral corticosteroids, some patients may experience symptoms of systemically active corticosteroid withdrawal, such as joint or musculoskeletal pain, malaise, and depression, despite maintenance or improvement of respiratory function.
■ Because of the possibility of systemic absorption of inhalation corticosteroids, recommend carefully observing patients treated with these drugs for any evidence of systemic corticosteroid effects. Take special care during periods of stress or postoperatively to note adrenal insufficiency.

## Special populations

**Pregnant patients.** Drug should be used during pregnancy only when potential benefits justify risks to fetus.

**Breast-feeding patients.** Use with caution in breast-feeding women because it's unknown if topical or inhalation corticosteroids undergo sufficient absorption to produce systemic effects in the infant.

**Pediatric patients.** Safety and efficacy of topical form haven't been established in children. Safety and efficacy of nasal form haven't been established in children under age 12; use of drug isn't recommended in these patients. A reduction of growth velocity in children or teenagers may occur as a result of the use of corticosteroids for treatment or because of inadequate control of chronic disease such as asthma. The benefits of asthma control from corticosteroid therapy must be weighed against the possibility of growth suppression in these patients.

## Patient counseling

■ Advise patient that proper application includes washing area before application and applying drug sparingly and rubbing it in lightly.
■ Instruct patient to report burning, irritation, or persistent or worsened condition.
■ Tell patient to avoid prolonged use, contact with eyes, or use around genital area, rectal area, on face, and in skin creases.
■ Inform patient to rinse mouth well after corticosteroid inhalation.
■ Inform patient on inhalation corticosteroids to avoid exposure and to consult prescriber immediately if he has been exposed to chickenpox or measles.
■ Instruct patient about proper administration using the nasal spray pump, including the need to prime the pump.

# fluticasone propionate and salmeterol inhalation powder

Advair Diskus 100/50, Advair Diskus 250/50, Advair Diskus 500/50

*Pharmacologic classification:* corticosteroid, long-acting beta₂ agonist
*Therapeutic classification:* anti-inflammatory, bronchodilator
*Pregnancy risk category C*

## Available forms

Available by prescription only
*Inhalation powder:* 100 mcg fluticasone/50 mcg salmeterol, 250 mcg fluticasone/50 mcg salmeterol, 500 mcg fluticasone/50 mcg salmeterol

## Indications and dosages

*Long-term maintenance of asthma*
*Adults and children over age 12:* One oral inhalation b.i.d., morning and evening, at least 12 hours apart.
*Adults and children over age 12 not currently taking an inhaled corticosteroid:* One oral inhalation of Advair Diskus 100/50 b.i.d.
*Adults and children over age 12 currently taking beclomethasone dipropionate:* If daily dose of beclomethasone dipropionate is 420 mcg or less, start with one oral inhalation of Advair Diskus 100/50 b.i.d. If beclomethasone dipropionate daily dose is 462 to 840 mcg, start with one oral inhalation of Advair Diskus 250/50 b.i.d.
*Adults and children over age 12 currently taking budesonide:* If daily dose of budesonide is 400 mcg or less, start with one oral inhalation of Advair Diskus 100/50 b.i.d. If budesonide daily dose is 800 to 1,200 mcg, start with one oral inhalation of Advair Diskus 250/50 b.i.d. If budesonide daily dose is 1,600 mcg, start with one oral inhalation of Advair Diskus 500/50 b.i.d.
*Adults and children over age 12 currently taking flunisolide:* If daily dose of flunisolide is 1,000 mcg or less, start with one oral inhalation of Advair Diskus 100/50 b.i.d. If flunisolide daily dose is 1,250 to 2,000 mcg, start with one oral inhalation of Advair Diskus 250/50 b.i.d.
*Adults and children over age 12 currently taking fluticasone propionate inhalation aerosol:* If daily dose of fluticasone propionate inhalation aerosol is 176 mcg or less, start with one oral inhalation of Advair Diskus 100/50 b.i.d. If fluticasone propionate inhalation aerosol daily dose is 440 mcg, start with one oral inhalation of Advair Diskus 250/50 b.i.d. If fluticasone propionate inhalation aerosol daily dose is 660 to 880 mcg, start with one oral inhalation of Advair Diskus 500/50 b.i.d.
*Adults and children over age 12 currently taking fluticasone propionate inhalation powder:* If fluticasone propionate inhalation powder daily dose is 200 mcg or less, start with one oral inhalation of Advair Diskus 100/50 b.i.d. If fluticasone propionate inhalation powder daily dose is 500 mcg, start with one oral inhalation of Advair Diskus 250/50 b.i.d. If fluticasone propionate inhalation powder daily dose is 1,000 mcg, start with one oral inhalation of Advair Diskus 500/50 b.i.d.
*Adults and children over age 12 currently taking triamcinolone acetonide:* If triamcinolone acetonide daily dose is 1,000 mcg or less, start with one oral inhalation of Advair Diskus 100/50 b.i.d. If triamcinolone acetonide daily dose is 1,100 to 1,600 mcg, start with one oral inhalation of Advair Diskus 250/50 b.i.d.
Maximum oral inhalation of Advair Diskus is 500/50 b.i.d.

## Mechanism of action

*Anti-inflammatory action:* Fluticasone is a synthetic corticosteroid with potent anti-inflammatory activity, although precise mechanisms of action in asthma are unknown. Corticosteroids inhibit mast cells, eosinophils, basophils, lymphocytes, macrophages, and neutrophils, and they inhibit production or secretion of histamine, eicosanoids, leukotrienes, and cytokines, which are involved in the asthmatic response.

Salmeterol xinafoate is a long-acting beta agonist selective for beta₂-adrenoceptors. Pharmacologic effects are at least in part attributable to stimulation of intracellular adenyl cyclase, the enzyme that catalyzes conversion of adenosine triphosphate (ATP) to cAMP. Increased cAMP levels relax bronchial smooth muscle and inhibit release of mediators of immediate hypersensitivity from cells, especially mast cells. In vitro tests show that salmeterol is a potent and long-lasting inhibitor of the release of mast cell mediators, such as histamine, leukotrienes, and prostaglandin D₂, from human lung.

## Pharmacokinetics

*Absorption:* Most of the fluticasone propionate delivered to the lung is systemically absorbed. Salmeterol xinafoate acts locally in the lung; therefore, plasma levels do not predict therapeutic effect. Because of the small therapeutic dose, systemic levels of salmeterol are low and undetectable after inhalation of recommended doses. After long-term administration of an inhaled dose of 50 mcg of salmeterol inhalation b.i.d., salmeterol was detected in plasma within 5 to 45 minutes and peaked at 20 minutes.
*Distribution:* Drug is 91% plasma protein-bound, is weakly and reversibly bound to erythrocytes, and is not significantly bound to human transcortin. Binding of salmeterol to human plasma proteins averages 96%.

*Metabolism:* The total clearance of fluticasone propionate is high, with renal clearance accounting for less than 0.02% of the total. The only circulating metabolite is the 17 beta-carboxylic acid derivative, which is formed via the cytochrome P-450 3A4 pathway. Salmeterol base is extensively metabolized by hydroxylation, with subsequent elimination predominantly in the feces. No significant amount of unchanged salmeterol base was detected in either urine or feces.

*Excretion:* After I.V. dosing, fluticasone had a terminal elimination half-life of about 7.8 hours. Less than 5% of a dose is excreted in urine as metabolites, with the remainder excreted in feces as parent drug and metabolite. Salmeterol xinafoate is about 25% to 60% eliminated in urine and feces, respectively, over a period of 7 days. Terminal elimination half-life is about 5½ hours.

| Route | Onset | Peak | Duration |
|---|---|---|---|
| Inhalation | Unknown | salmeterol 5 min<br>fluticasone 1-2 hr | Unknown |

## Contraindications and precautions

Contraindicated in patients hypersensitive to any component of the drug. Also contraindicated as primary treatment of status asthmaticus or other acute asthmatic episodes.

Drug should be used extremely cautiously, if at all, in patients with active or quiescent respiratory tuberculosis infection; untreated systemic fungal, bacterial, viral, or parasitic infection; or ocular herpes simplex. Use cautiously in patients with CV disorders, especially coronary insufficiency, cardiac arrhythmias, and hypertension; in patients with seizure disorders or thyrotoxicosis; in patients unusually responsive to sympathomimetic amines; and in patients with hepatic impairment (because salmeterol is metabolized mainly in the liver).

## Interactions

**Drug-drug.** *Beta blockers:* Blocked pulmonary effect of salmeterol may produce severe bronchospasm in patients with asthma. Avoid use together. If needed, a cardioselective beta blocker should be used extremely cautiously.

*Ketoconazole, other inhibitors of cytochrome P-450:* May increase fluticasone levels and adverse effects. Use together cautiously.

*Loop diuretics, thiazide diuretics:* ECG changes or hypokalemia may result from or be worsened by potassium-wasting diuretics. Use together cautiously.

*MAO inhibitors, tricyclic antidepressants:* May potentiate the action of salmeterol on the vascular system. Use within 2 weeks of taking these drugs should be avoided.

## Adverse reactions

**CNS:** sleep disorders, tremors, hypnagogic effects, compressed nerve syndromes, *headache.*

**CV:** palpitations, chest symptoms, fluid retention.

**EENT:** *pharyngitis,* sinusitis, hoarseness, dysphonia, rhinorrhea, rhinitis, sneezing, nasal irritation, blood in nasal mucosa, keratitis, conjunctivitis, eye redness, viral eye infections, congestion.

**GI:** nausea, vomiting, abdominal pain and discomfort, diarrhea, gastroenteritis, oral discomfort and pain, constipation, oral ulcerations, oral erythema and rashes, appendicitis, dental discomfort and pain, unusual taste, oral candidiasis.

**Musculoskeletal:** muscle pain, arthralgia, articular rheumatism, muscle stiffness, tightness, rigidity, bone and cartilage disorders.

**Hepatic:** abnormal liver function test results.

**Respiratory:** *upper respiratory tract infection,* upper respiratory inflammation, lower viral respiratory infections, bronchitis, cough, pneumonia.

**Skin:** viral skin infections, urticaria, skin flakiness, disorders of sweat and sebum, sweating.

**Other:** viral infections, pain, bacterial infections, allergies, allergic reactions.

## Overdose and treatment

Chronic overdose of fluticasone may cause signs and symptoms of hypercorticism. Salmeterol overdose may cause seizures, angina, hypertension, hypotension, tachycardia, arrhythmias, nervousness, headache, tremor, muscle cramps, dry mouth, palpitations, nausea, prolonged QTc interval, ventricular arrhythmia, hypokalemia, hyperglycemia, cardiac arrest, and death.

Treatment consists of discontinuing drug and possibly using a cardioselective beta blocker. Cardiac monitoring is needed.

## Clinical considerations

■ Patients shouldn't be transferred from systemic corticosteroids to Advair Diskus because of HPA axis suppression. Death can occur from adrenal insufficiency.

■ Advair Diskus therapy shouldn't be started during rapidly deteriorating or potentially life-threatening episodes of asthma. Serious acute respiratory events, including death, can occur.

■ Drug shouldn't be used to treat status asthmaticus. When drug is prescribed, recommend making sure the patient has an inhaled, short-acting beta$_2$-agonist (such as albuterol) for acute symptoms.

■ A long-acting beta$_2$ agonist (such as Serevent, which is a form of salmeterol xinafoate) shouldn't be used with Advair Diskus.

■ Drug may produce paradoxical bronchospasm. If it does, recommend treating immediately with a short-acting inhaled broncho-

dilator (such as albuterol), and stopping Advair Diskus therapy.
- If patient is exposed to chickenpox, prophylaxis with varicella zoster immune globulin should be considered. If chickenpox develops, antiviral treatment should be considered.
- If patient is exposed to measles, prophylaxis with pooled I.M. immunoglobulin should be considered.
- Drug should be stored at controlled room temperature 68° to 77° F (20° to 25° C) in a dry place away from direct heat or sunlight. The device should be discarded 1 month after removal from the moisture-protective overwrap pouch or after every blister has been used, whichever comes first. One should not attempt to take the device apart.

### Therapeutic monitoring
- Advise clinician to monitor patient for urticaria, angioedema, rash, bronchospasm, or other signs of hypersensitivity, which may occur immediately after a dose of Advair Diskus.
- Advise clinician to monitor patient for increased use of inhaled short-acting beta$_2$-agonist. The dose of Advair Diskus may need to be increased.
- Advise clinician to monitor patient for hypercorticism and adrenal suppression. If these occur, dosage should be reduced slowly.
- Advise clinician to monitor patient for eosinophilia, vasculitic rash, worsening pulmonary symptoms, cardiac complications, or neuropathy, which may be signs of a serious eosinophilic condition.

### Special populations
**Breast-feeding patients.** It isn't known if the components of Advair Diskus appear in breast milk.
**Pediatric patients.** Recommend closely monitoring growth in children because growth suppression may occur. Child should be maintained on lowest effective dose to minimize potential for growth suppression. Safety and efficacy in children under age 12 have not been established.
**Geriatric patients.** No dosage adjustments are needed.

### Patient counseling
- Instruct patient on proper use of Diskus device to provide effective treatment.
- Tell patient to avoid exhaling into the Diskus and to activate and use the Diskus in a level, horizontal position.
- Instruct patient to keep the Diskus in a dry place, to avoid washing the mouthpiece or other parts of the device, and to avoid taking the Diskus apart.
- Tell patient to stop taking an oral or inhaled short-acting beta$_2$ agonist regularly when beginning treatment with Advair Diskus, and to

use the short-acting beta$_2$ agonist for relief from acute symptoms.
- Instruct patient to rinse mouth after inhalation to prevent oral candidiasis.
- Inform patient that improvement may be seen within 30 minutes after an Advair dose; however, the full benefit may not occur for 1 week or longer.
- Instruct patient not to exceed recommended prescribing dosage under any circumstances.
- Instruct patient not to relieve acute symptoms with Advair Diskus. Acute symptoms should be treated with an inhaled short-acting beta$_2$ agonist (such as albuterol).
- Instruct patient to report decreasing effects or use of increasing doses of his short-acting inhaled beta$_2$ agonist.
- Instruct patient not to use drug with a spacer device.
- Tell patient to report palpitations, chest pain, rapid heart rate, tremor, or nervousness.
- Instruct patient to contact prescriber before using drug if she is pregnant or breast-feeding.
- Instruct patient to contact prescriber immediately if exposed to chickenpox or measles.

# fluvastatin sodium
Lescol, Lescol-XL

*Pharmacologic classification:* HMG-CoA reductase inhibitor
*Therapeutic classification:* cholesterol-lowering antilipemic
*Pregnancy risk category X*

## Available forms
Available by prescription only
*Capsules:* 20 mg, 40 mg
*Extended-release tablets:* 80 mg

## Indications and dosages
*To reduce low-density lipoprotein cholesterol (LDL-C), total cholesterol, triglycerides, and apolipoprotein B levels and to increase high-density lipoprotein cholesterol in patients with primary hypercholesterolemia (types IIa and IIb) when response to diet and other nonpharmacologic measures has been inadequate; to slow progression of coronary atherosclerosis in patients with coronary artery disease*
*Adults:* 20 mg to 40 mg P.O. h.s. Increase dosage p.r.n. to a maximum of 80 mg daily (in divided doses).

For patients requiring LDL-C reduction to a goal of greater than or equal to 25%, the recommended starting dose is 40 mg as one capsule and 80 mg as one Lescol XL tablet P.O. as a single dose in the evening. Alternatively, 80 mg in divided doses of the 40 mg capsule given b.i.d. For patients requiring LDL-C reduction to a goal of < 25%, the recommended

starting dose is 20 mg P.O. in the evening. The recommended dosing range is 20 to 80 mg/day.
≡*Dosage adjustment.* With a persistent increase in ALT or AST level of at least three times the upper limit of normal, withdrawal of fluvastatin is recommended. Because fluvastatin is cleared hepatically, with less than 5% of the dose excreted into urine, dosage adjustments for mild to moderate renal impairment aren't needed. Exercise caution with severe impairment.

## Mechanism of action

*Antilipemic action:* Fluvastatin is a competitive inhibitor of HMG-CoA reductase, which is responsible for the conversion of HMG-CoA to mevalonate, a precursor of sterols, including cholesterol. This enzyme is an early (and rate-limiting) step in the synthetic pathway of cholesterol. Fluvastatin increases high-density lipoproteins and decreases low-density lipoproteins, very-low-density lipoproteins, and plasma triglycerides.

## Pharmacokinetics

*Absorption:* Absorbed rapidly and virtually completely (98%) after oral administration on an empty stomach.
*Distribution:* Over 98% of circulating drug is plasma protein–bound.
*Metabolism:* Completely metabolized in the liver. It has no active metabolites.
*Excretion:* About 5% is excreted in urine and 90% in feces.

| Route | Onset | Peak | Duration |
|-------|-------|------|----------|
| P.O. | Unknown | 1 hr | Unknown |

## Contraindications and precautions

Contraindicated in patients hypersensitive to drug; in those with active liver disease or conditions with unexplained persistent elevations of serum transaminase levels; in pregnant and breast-feeding women; and in women of childbearing age unless there's no risk of pregnancy.

Use cautiously in patients with impaired renal function and history of hepatic disease or heavy alcohol consumption.

## Interactions

**Drug-drug.** *Cholestyramine or colestipol:* May bind fluvastatin in the GI tract and decrease absorption. Fluvastatin should be given h.s., at least 2 hours after the resin, to avoid significant interaction from the drug binding to the resin.
*Cimetidine, omeprazole, and ranitidine:* Decreased fluvastatin metabolism. Advise clinician to monitor patient closely for adverse reactions.
*Cyclosporine and other immunosuppressants, erythromycin, gemfibrozil, and niacin:* Increased risk of polymyositis and rhabdomyol-

ysis when given with fluvastatin. Avoid use together.
*Digoxin:* Altered pharmacokinetics of digoxin. Advise clinician to monitor patient's serum digoxin levels carefully.
*Rifampin:* Enhanced fluvastatin metabolism and decreased plasma levels. Advise clinician to monitor lipid levels periodically.
*Warfarin:* Increased anticoagulant effect with bleeding. Recommend watching patient closely and monitoring INR and PT.
**Drug-herb.** *Red yeast rice:* Contains similar components to those of statin drugs, increasing the risk of adverse events or toxicity. Discourage use together.
**Drug-lifestyle.** *Alcohol use:* Increased risk of hepatotoxicity. Advise clinician to monitor patient carefully.

## Adverse reactions

**CNS:** headache, fatigue, dizziness, insomnia.
**EENT:** sinusitis, rhinitis, pharyngitis.
**GI:** dyspepsia, diarrhea, nausea, vomiting, abdominal pain, constipation, flatulence.
**Hepatic:** increased liver enzyme levels, increased bilirubin levels.
**Hematologic:** *thrombocytopenia, leukopenia, hemolytic anemia.*
**Metabolic:** abnormal thyroid function test results.
**Musculoskeletal:** arthropathy, muscle pain.
**Respiratory:** *upper respiratory tract infection,* cough, bronchitis.
**Skin:** hypersensitivity reactions (rash, pruritus).
**Other:** tooth disorder.

## Overdose and treatment

No specific information on overdose is available. If an accidental overdose occurs, patient should be treated symptomatically and supportive measures instituted as required. The dialyzability of fluvastatin and its metabolites in humans is unknown.

## Clinical considerations

■ Fluvastatin therapy should be started only after diet and other nonpharmacologic therapies have proven ineffective.
■ Drug may be taken without regard to meals; however, efficacy is enhanced if drug is taken in the evening.

### Therapeutic monitoring

■ Advise clinician to monitor patient closely for signs of myositis.
■ Liver function tests should be performed at the start of therapy, every 4 to 6 weeks during the first 3 months of therapy, every 6 to 12 weeks during the next 12 months, and at 6-month intervals thereafter.

### Special populations
**Pregnant patients.** Drug shouldn't be used during pregnancy.
**Breast-feeding patients.** Preclinical data suggest that drug appears in breast milk in a 2:1 ratio (milk:plasma). The potential for serious adverse reactions in nursing infants indicates that breast-feeding women shouldn't take fluvastatin.
**Pediatric patients.** Safety and efficacy in patients under age 18 haven't been established. Use in pediatric patients isn't recommended.

### Patient counseling
■ Instruct patient to take fluvastatin at bedtime to enhance effectiveness.
■ Warn patient to restrict alcohol intake because of potentially serious adverse effects.
■ Tell patient to report to prescriber adverse reactions, particularly muscle aches and pains.

## fluvoxamine maleate
Luvox

*Pharmacologic classification:* selective serotonin reuptake inhibitor (SSRI)
*Therapeutic classification:* anticompulsive
*Pregnancy risk category C*

### Available forms
Available by prescription only
*Tablets:* 25 mg, 50 mg, 100 mg

### Indications and dosages
*Obsessive-compulsive disorder*
*Adults:* Initially, 50 mg P.O. daily h.s. Increase in 50-mg increments q 4 to 7 days until maximum benefit is achieved. Maximum daily dose is 300 mg. Give total daily doses exceeding 100 mg in two divided doses.
≡*Dosage adjustment.* Because geriatric patients and patients with hepatic impairment have been observed to have decreased clearance of fluvoxamine maleate, dosage adjustment may be appropriate.

### Mechanism of action
*Anticompulsive action:* The exact mechanism of action is unknown. Fluvoxamine is a potent selective inhibitor of the neuronal uptake of serotonin, which is thought to improve obsessive-compulsive behavior.

### Pharmacokinetics
*Absorption:* Absolute bioavailability of drug is 53%.
*Distribution:* Mean apparent volume of distribution is about 25 L/kg. About 80% of drug is bound to plasma protein (mostly albumin).
*Metabolism:* Extensively metabolized in the liver, mostly by oxidative demethylation and deamination.

*Excretion:* Metabolites are primarily excreted in urine.

| Route | Onset | Peak | Duration |
|-------|-------|------|----------|
| P.O. | Unknown | 3-8 hr | Unknown |

### Contraindications and precautions
Contraindicated in patients hypersensitive to drug or to other phenylpiperazine antidepressants and within 14 days of MAO inhibitor therapy.
    Use cautiously in patients with hepatic dysfunction, concomitant conditions that may affect hemodynamic responses or metabolism, or history of mania or seizures.

### Interactions
**Drug-drug.** *Benzodiazepines, theophylline, and warfarin:* Reduced clearance of these drugs. Use together cautiously. However, diazepam shouldn't be coadministered with fluvoxamine. An adjustment in diazepam dosage may be needed.
*Carbamazepine, clozapine, methadone, metoprolol, propranolol, and tricyclic antidepressants:* Elevated serum levels of fluvoxamine. Use together with caution; recommend monitoring patient closely for adverse reactions. Dosage adjustments may be needed.
*Diltiazem:* May cause bradycardia. Advise clinician to monitor patient's heart rate.
*Lithium and tryptophan:* May enhance effects of fluvoxamine; use together cautiously.
*MAO inhibitors:* May cause severe excitation, hyperpyrexia, myoclonus, delirium, and coma. Avoid use together.
**Drug-herb.** *St. John's wort:* Serotonin levels may rise too high, causing serotonin syndrome. Discourage use together.
**Drug-lifestyle.** *Smoking:* May decrease effectiveness of drug. Advise patient to avoid smoking.

### Adverse reactions
**CNS:** headache, asthenia, somnolence, insomnia, nervousness, dizziness, tremor, anxiety, hypertonia, agitation, depression, CNS stimulation.
**CV:** palpitations, vasodilation.
**EENT:** amblyopia.
**GI:** *nausea, diarrhea, constipation, dyspepsia,* anorexia, *vomiting,* flatulence, dysphagia, *dry mouth,* taste perversion.
**GU:** abnormal ejaculation, urinary frequency, impotence, anorgasmia, urine retention.
**Respiratory:** upper respiratory tract infection, dyspnea, yawning.
**Skin:** sweating.
**Other:** flu syndrome, chills, decreased libido, tooth disorder.

### Overdose and treatment
Common signs and symptoms of fluvoxamine overdose include drowsiness, vomiting, diar-

---

rhea, and dizziness; coma, tachycardia, brady-cardia, hypotension, ECG abnormalities, liver function abnormalities, and seizures may also occur. Symptoms such as aspiration pneumonitis, respiratory difficulties, or hypokalemia may occur because of loss of consciousness or vomiting.

Treatment is supportive. Besides maintaining an open airway and monitoring vital signs and ECG, administration of activated charcoal may be as effective as emesis or lavage. Because absorption with overdose may be delayed, measures to minimize absorption may be needed for up to 24 hours after ingestion. Dialysis isn't believed to be beneficial.

### Clinical considerations
■ Advise prescriber to allow at least 14 days after stopping fluvoxamine before starting patient on an MAO inhibitor.
■ Advise prescriber to allow at least 14 days after MAO inhibitor therapy has been discontinued before starting patient on fluvoxamine. Fluvoxamine has been used in the treatment of bulimia nervosa (unlabeled use).

#### Therapeutic monitoring
■ Advise clinician to monitor patient for suicidal tendencies and allow a minimum supply of drug.

#### Special populations
**Pregnant patients.** Drug shouldn't be used during pregnancy.
**Breast-feeding patients.** Drug appears in breast milk and shouldn't be given to breast-feeding women.
**Pediatric patients.** Safety and efficacy in children under age 18 haven't been established.
**Geriatric patients.** Drug clearance is decreased by about 50% in geriatric patients compared with younger patients. Drug should be given cautiously in this age group and dosage is adjusted slowly when therapy starts.

### Patient counseling
■ Warn patient not to engage in hazardous activity until CNS effects are known and to avoid alcoholic beverages.
■ Alert patient that smoking may decrease the effectiveness of drug.
■ Inform patient that several weeks of therapy may be required to obtain the full antidepressant effect. Once improvement is seen, advise patient not to discontinue the drug until directed by prescriber.
■ Advise patient to contact prescriber before taking OTC drugs because of possible drug interactions.
**H ALERT** If the patient wishes to switch from an SSRI to St. John's wort, recommend waiting a few weeks for the SSRI to wash out of his system before the patient takes the herb.

The exact time required depends on which SSRI the patient is taking.

# folic acid
Folvite

*Pharmacologic classification:* folic acid derivative
*Therapeutic classification:* vitamin supplement
*Pregnancy risk category A*

### Available forms
Available by prescription only
*Tablets:* 1 mg
*Injection:* 10-ml vials (folic acid 5 mg/ml contains 1.5% benzyl alcohol and EDTA; Folvite 5 mg/ml contains 1.5% benzyl alcohol)
Available without a prescription
*Tablets:* 0.4 mg, 0.8 mg

### Indications and dosages
***Megaloblastic or macrocytic anemia secondary to folic acid deficiency, hepatic disease, alcoholism, intestinal obstruction, excessive hemolysis***
*Pregnant and breast-feeding patients:* 0.8 mg P.O., S.C., or I.M. daily.
*Adults and children ages 4 and older:* 0.4 mg P.O., S.C., or I.M. daily for 4 to 5 days. After anemia secondary to folic acid deficiency is corrected, proper diet and RDA supplements are needed to prevent recurrence.
*Children under age 4:* Up to 0.3 mg P.O., S.C., or I.M. daily.
***Prevention of megaloblastic anemia of pregnancy and fetal damage***
*Adults:* 1 mg P.O., S.C., or I.M. daily during pregnancy.
***Nutritional supplement***
*Adults:* Give 0.15 to 0.2 mg P.O., S.C., or I.M. daily for men; give 0.15 to 0.18 mg P.O., S.C., or I.M. daily for women.
*Children:* 0.05 mg P.O. daily.
***Tropical sprue***
*Adults:* 3 to 15 mg P.O. daily.

### I.V. administration
■ Protect folic acid injections from light.
■ Dilute 1 ml of folic acid injection containing 5 mg of folic acid per ml with 49 ml of sterile water for injection to provide a solution containing 0.1 mg folic acid per ml.

#### Incompatibilities
Incompatible with calcium gluconate, dextrose 40% in water, dextrose 50% in water, doxapram, oxidizing and reducing drugs, and heavy metal ions.

### Mechanism of action
*Nutritional action:* Exogenous folate is required to maintain normal erythropoiesis and to per-

form nucleoprotein synthesis. Folic acid stimulates production of RBCs, WBCs, and platelets in certain megaloblastic anemias.

Dietary folic acid is present in foods, primarily as reduced folate polyglutamate. This vitamin may be absorbed only after hydrolysis, reduction, and methylation occur in the GI tract. Conversion to active tetrahydrofolate may require vitamin $B_{12}$.

Oral synthetic form of folic acid is a monoglutamate and is absorbed completely after administration, even in malabsorption syndromes.

## Pharmacokinetics
*Absorption:* Absorbed rapidly from the GI tract, mainly from the proximal part of the small intestine. Normal serum folate levels range from 0.005 to 0.015 mcg/ml. Usually, serum levels less than 0.005 mcg/ml indicate folate deficiency; those less than 0.002 mcg/ml usually result in megaloblastic anemia.
*Distribution:* The active tetrahydrofolic acid and its derivatives are distributed into all body tissues; the liver contains about half of the total body folate stores. Folate is actively concentrated in the CSF. Folic acid appears in breast milk.
*Metabolism:* Metabolized in the liver to *N*-methyltetrahydrofolic acid, the main form of folate storage and transport.
*Excretion:* A single 0.1-mg to 0.2-mg dose usually results in only a trace amount of drug in urine. After large doses are given, excessive folate is excreted unchanged in urine. Small amounts of folic acid have been recovered in feces. About 0.05 mg/day of normal body folate stores is lost through a combination of urinary and fecal excretion and oxidative cleavage of the molecule.

| Route | Onset | Peak | Duration |
|-------|-------|------|----------|
| P.O. | 20-30 min | 2-3 hr | 3-6 hr |
| I.V. | 5 min | 10 min | 3-6 min |
| I.M. | 10-20 min | < 1 hr | 3-6 hr |

## Contraindications and precautions
Contraindicated in patients with undiagnosed anemia because it may mask pernicious anemia, and in those with pernicious anemia and other megaloblastic anemias in which vitamin $B_{12}$ is deficient.

## Interactions
**Drug-drug.** *Aminosalicylic acid, chloramphenicol, methotrexate, oral contraceptives, pyrimethamine, triamterene, trimethoprim, sulfasalazine:* May act as antagonists to folic acid. Advise clinician to monitor patient for decreased drug effect.
*Anticonvulsants such as phenobarbital and phenytoin:* Increased anticonvulsant metabolism and decreased blood levels of the anti-

convulsants. Advise clinician to monitor serum blood levels.
*Phenytoin and primidone:* Decreased serum folate levels; symptoms of folic acid deficiency in long-term therapy. Advise clinician to monitor patient closely.
*Pyrimethamine:* Interference with antimicrobial actions of pyrimethamine against toxoplasmosis. Avoid use together.

## Adverse reactions
**CNS:** general malaise.
**Respiratory:** *bronchospasm.*
**Skin:** allergic reactions (rash, pruritus, erythema).

## Overdose and treatment
Folic acid is relatively nontoxic. Adverse GI and CNS effects have been reported rarely in patients receiving 15 mg of folic acid daily for 1 month.

## Clinical considerations
■ The RDA for folic acid is 25 to 200 mcg in children and 180 to 200 mcg in adults; 100 mcg per day is considered an adequate oral supplement. Pregnant women require 400 mcg daily. During the first 6 months of breast-feeding, women require 280 mcg daily; during the second 6 months, this requirement decreases to 260 mcg daily.
■ The preferred route of administration for folic acid is P.O. The manufacturer recommends deep I.M., S.C., or I.V. only when P.O. treatment isn't feasible or when malabsorption is suspected.
■ Patients undergoing renal dialysis are at risk for folate deficiency.
■ Falsely low serum and erythrocyte folate levels may occur with the *Lactobacillus casei* assay in patients receiving anti-infectives, such as tetracycline, which suppress the growth of this organism.

### Therapeutic monitoring
■ Advise clinician to monitor CBC to measure effectiveness of drug treatment.

### Special populations
**Pregnant patients.** Prepregnancy initiation of drug therapy may reduce risk of fetal neural tube defects.
**Breast-feeding patients.** Folic acid appears in breast milk. Daily doses of 0.8 mg are sufficient to maintain a normoblastic bone marrow after clinical symptoms have subsided and blood components have returned to normal.

## Patient counseling
■ Advise patient of potential adverse reactions.

# fomivirsen sodium

Vitravene

*Pharmacologic classification:* phosphorothioate oligonucleotide
*Therapeutic classification:* antiviral
*Pregnancy risk category C*

## Available forms

Available by prescription only
*Intravitreal injection:* Preservative-free, single-use vials containing 0.25 ml, 6.6 mg/ml

## Indications and dosages

*Local treatment of CMV retinitis in patients with AIDS, who are intolerant of or have a contraindication to other treatments or who were insufficiently responsive to previous treatments*
*Adults:* Induction dose is 330 mcg (0.05 ml) by intravitreal injection every other week for two doses. Subsequent maintenance dose is 330 mcg (0.05 ml) by intravitreal injection once every 4 weeks after induction.

## Mechanism of action

*Antiviral action:* Drug inhibits human CMV replication by binding to the target mRNA and subsequently inhibiting virus replication.

## Pharmacokinetics

No information available.

| Route | Onset | Peak | Duration |
|---|---|---|---|
| Intravitreal | Unknown | Unknown | Unknown |

## Contraindications and precautions

Contraindicated in patients hypersensitive to drug or its components or in those who have been treated within 2 to 4 weeks with either I.V. or intravitreal cidofovir because of an increased risk of exaggerated ocular inflammation.

## Interactions

None reported.

## Adverse reactions

**CNS:** asthenia, headache, abnormal thinking, depression, dizziness, neuropathy, pain.
**CV:** chest pain.
**EENT:** abnormal or blurred vision, anterior chamber inflammation, cataract, conjunctival hemorrhage, decreased visual acuity, desaturation of color vision, eye pain, floaters, increased intraocular pressure, *ocular inflammation, iritis,* photophobia, retinal detachment, retinal edema, retinal hemorrhage, retinal pigment changes, *uveitis, vitritis,* application site reaction, conjunctival hyperemia, conjunctivitis, corneal edema, decreased peripheral vision, eye irritation, hypotony, keratic precipitates, optic neuritis, photopsia, retinal vascular disease, visual field defect, vitreous hemorrhage, vitreous opacity, sinusitis.
**GI:** abdominal pain, anorexia, diarrhea, nausea, vomiting, oral candidiasis, *pancreatitis.*
**GU:** catheter infection, *renal failure.*
**Hematologic:** anemia, lymphoma-like reaction, *neutropenia, thrombocytopenia.*
**Hepatic:** abnormal liver function test results, increased GGT.
**Metabolic:** decreased weight, dehydration.
**Musculoskeletal:** back pain.
**Respiratory:** bronchitis, dyspnea, increased cough, pneumonia.
**Skin:** rash, sweating.
**Other:** allergic reactions, cachexia, fever, flu syndrome, infection, *sepsis,* systemic CMV.

## Overdose and treatment

None reported.

## Clinical considerations

**H ALERT** Drug is for ophthalmic use by intravitreal injection only.
■ Drug provides localized therapy limited to the treated eye and doesn't provide treatment for systemic CMV disease.
■ Ocular inflammation (uveitis) is most common during induction dosing.

### Therapeutic monitoring

■ Advise clinician to monitor light perception and optic nerve head perfusion postinjection.
■ Advise clinician to monitor patient for increased intraocular pressure. This is usually transient and returns to normal without treatment or with temporary use of topical drugs.
■ Advise clinician to monitor patient for extraocular CMV disease or disease in the contralateral eye.

### Special populations

**Pregnant patients.** Safety and efficacy in pregnant women haven't been reported.
**Breast-feeding patients.** It's unknown if drug appears in breast milk. Recommend discontinuing drug or nursing.
**Pediatric patients.** Safety and efficacy in children haven't been established.
**Geriatric patients.** Safety and efficacy in patients over age 65 haven't been established.

## Patient counseling

■ Inform patient that drug isn't a cure for CMV retinitis and that some patients continue to experience progression of retinitis during and after treatment.
■ Tell patient that drug treats only the eye in which it has been injected and that CMV may also exist in the body. Stress importance of follow-up visits to monitor progress and to check for additional infections.
■ Advise HIV-infected patient to continue taking antiretroviral therapy as indicated.

---

* Canada only    ◇ Unlabeled clinical use

# formoterol fumarate inhalation powder

Foradil Aerolizer

*Pharmacologic classification:* long-acting selective beta$_2$ receptor agonist
*Therapeutic classification:* bronchodilator
*Pregnancy risk category C*

## Available forms

Available by prescription only.
*Capsules for inhalation:* 12 mcg

## Indications and dosages

**Maintenance treatment and prevention of bronchospasm in patients with reversible obstructive airway disease or nocturnal asthma, who usually require treatment with short-acting inhaled beta$_2$ agonists**
*Adults and children ages 5 and older:* One 12-mcg capsule by inhalation via Aerolizer inhaler every 12 hours. Total daily dose shouldn't exceed one capsule b.i.d. (24 mcg/day). If symptoms are present between doses, use a short-acting beta$_2$ agonist for immediate relief.
**Prevention of exercise-induced bronchospasm**
*Adults and children ages 12 and older:* One 12-mcg capsule by inhalation via Aerolizer inhaler at least 15 minutes before exercise given occasionally on a p.r.n. basis. Don't give additional doses within 12 hours of first dose.
**Maintenance treatment of COPD**
*Adults:* One 12-mcg capsule every 12 hours using the Aerolizer inhaler.
Total daily dose of greater than 24 mcg is not recommended.

## Mechanism of action

Formoterol fumarate acts locally in the lung to cause bronchodilation via long-acting selective beta$_2$ adrenergic receptor agonist activity. At a cellular level, formoterol stimulates intracellular adenyl cyclase, the enzyme responsible for catalyzing the conversion of adenosine triphosphate (ATP) to cyclic-3', 5'-adenosine monophosphate (cAMP). This increase in cAMP leads to relaxation of bronchial smooth muscle and inhibition of mediator release from mast cells. Because some beta$_2$ receptors are also present in the heart, adrenergic stimulation may occur in the CV system with use of formoterol.

## Pharmacokinetics

*Absorption:* Rapidly absorbed into plasma. Drug levels peak within 5 minutes after a 120-mcg dose. Similar to other products for oral inhalation, a majority of the inhaled dose is likely swallowed and subsequently absorbed from the GI tract.

*Distribution:* 61% to 64% bound to human plasma proteins.
*Metabolism:* Occurs primarily via direct glucuronidation and O-demethylation (involving cytochrome P-450 isoenzymes 2D6, 2C19, 2C9, and 2A6). Doesn't appear to inhibit CYP-450 enzymes at therapeutic levels.
*Excretion:* 59% to 62% eliminated in urine and 32% to 34% eliminated in feces over 104 hours. When 12 to 24 mcg formoterol was given to asthma patients, about 10% of total dose was excreted in urine as unchanged drug and about 15% to 18% was eliminated in urine as direct glucuronide conjugates of formoterol.

| Route | Onset | Peak | Duration |
|-------|-------|------|----------|
| Oral, inhalation | ≤ 15 min | 1-3 hr | 12 hr |

## Contraindications and precautions

Contraindicated in patients hypersensitive to drug or its components.

Use cautiously in patients with CV disease, particularly coronary insufficiency, cardiac arrhythmias, and hypertension, and in those who are unusually responsive to sympathomimetic amines. Also use cautiously in patients with preexisting diabetes mellitus because instances of hyperglycemia and ketoacidosis have occurred rarely with the use of beta agonists. Also use cautiously in patients with seizure disorders or thyrotoxicosis.

## Interactions

**Drug-drug.** *Adrenergics:* Possible potentiation of sympathetic effects of formoterol. Use with caution.
*Beta blockers:* Possible antagonized effects of beta agonists, causing bronchospasm in asthmatic patients. Avoid use except when benefit outweighs risks. Cardioselective beta blockers should be used with caution to minimize risk of bronchospasm.
*Diuretics, steroids, xanthine derivatives:* Possible potentiation of hypokalemic effect of formoterol and possible worsening of ECG changes. Use with caution.
*MAO inhibitors, tricyclic antidepressants, other drugs that prolong QT interval:* Possible increased risk of ventricular arrhythmias. Use with caution.

## Adverse reactions

**CNS:** tremor, dizziness, insomnia, nervousness, headache, fatigue, malaise.
**CV:** chest pain, angina, hypertension, hypotension, tachycardia, ***arrhythmias,*** palpitations.
**EENT:** dry mouth, tonsillitis, dysphonia.
**GI:** nausea.
**Metabolic:** hypokalemia, hyperglycemia, metabolic acidosis.
**Musculoskeletal:** muscle cramps.

---

**Respiratory:** bronchitis, chest infection, dyspnea.
**Skin:** rash.
**Other:** viral infection.

## Overdose and treatment

Signs and symptoms of overdose include excessive beta-adrenergic stimulation and exaggeration of adverse effects. Cardiac arrest and death may result.

Treatment of overdose should include discontinuation of drug, cardiac monitoring, appropriate symptomatic relief or supportive therapy, and possibly judicious use of cardioselective beta blockers. It's unknown if dialysis is beneficial.

## Clinical considerations

■ Drug isn't indicated for patients who are able to control asthma symptoms with just occasional use of inhaled, short-acting beta$_2$ agonists or for treatment of acute bronchospasm requiring immediate reversal with short-acting beta$_2$ agonists.
■ Drug may be used with short-acting beta$_2$ agonists, inhaled corticosteroids, and theophylline therapy for management of asthma.
■ Patients using drug twice daily shouldn't use additional doses for prevention of exercise-induced bronchospasm.
■ Drug isn't a substitute for short-acting beta$_2$ agonists for immediate relief of bronchospasm or a substitute for inhaled or oral corticosteroids.
■ Advise prescriber not to begin use in patients with rapidly deteriorating or significantly worsening asthma.
■ If usual dose doesn't control symptoms of bronchoconstriction and patient's short-acting beta$_2$ agonist becomes less effective, recommend reevaluating patient and treatment regimen.
■ For patients formerly using regularly scheduled short-acting beta$_2$ agonists, use of the short-acting drug should be decreased to an as-needed basis when long-acting formoterol is started.
■ As with all beta$_2$ agonists, formoterol may produce life-threatening paradoxical bronchospasm. If bronchospasm occurs, recommend stopping formoterol immediately and using an alternative drug.
■ Foradil capsules should be given only via oral inhalation and only used with the Aerolizer inhaler. They aren't for oral ingestion. Patient shouldn't exhale into the device. Capsules should remain in the unopened blister until administration time and should only be removed immediately before use.
■ Don't use Foradil Aerolizer with a spacer device.
■ Capsules should be pierced only once. In rare instances, the gelatin capsule may break into small pieces and get delivered to the mouth or throat upon inhalation. However, the Aerolizer contains a screen that should catch any broken pieces before they leave the device. To minimize the possibility of shattering the capsule, strictly follow storage and use instructions.
■ Before dispensing, store drug in refrigerator. Once dispensed to patient, drug may be stored at room temperature.

### Therapeutic monitoring

■ Advise clinician to monitor patient for tachycardia, hypertension, and other CV adverse effects. If these occur, drug may need to be discontinued.
■ Recommend watching for immediate hypersensitivity reactions, such as anaphylaxis, urticaria, angioedema, rash, and bronchospasm.

### Special populations

**Breast-feeding patients.** It's unknown if drug appears in breast milk. Use cautiously in breast-feeding women.
**Pediatric patients.** Safety and efficacy in children under age 5 haven't been established.
**Geriatric patients.** No overall differences in safety or efficacy have been observed in geriatric patients. However, increased sensitivity of some geriatric patients is possible.

## Patient counseling

■ Tell patient not to increase the dosage or frequency of use without medical advice.
■ Warn patient not to stop or reduce other drugs taken for asthma.
■ Advise patient that drug isn't to be used for acute asthmatic episodes.
■ Advise patient to report worsening symptoms or if treatment becomes less effective or if use of short-acting beta$_2$ agonists increases.
■ Tell patient to report nausea, vomiting, shakiness, headache, fast or irregular heartbeat, or sleeplessness.
■ Warn patient not to exceed the recommended daily dose.
■ Tell patient being treated for exercise-induced bronchospasm to take drug at least 15 minutes before exercise and that additional doses can't be taken for 12 hours.
■ Tell patient that adverse effects, such as palpitations, chest pain, rapid heart rate, tremor, and nervousness, may occur.
■ Tell patient not to use the Foradil Aerolizer with a spacer device or to exhale or blow into the Aerolizer inhaler.
■ Advise patient to avoid washing the Aerolizer and to always keep it dry. A new device comes with each refill. The new device should replace the old one.
■ Tell patient to avoid exposing capsules to moisture and to handle them only with dry hands.
■ Advise women to notify their prescriber if they become pregnant or are breast-feeding.

---

## foscarnet sodium (phosphonoformic acid)

Foscavir

*Pharmacologic classification:* pyrophosphate analogue
*Therapeutic classification:* antiviral
*Pregnancy risk category C*

### Available forms
Available by prescription only
*Injection:* 24 mg/ml in 250-ml and 500-ml vials

### Indications and dosages
*Cytomegalovirus (CMV) retinitis in patients with AIDS*
*Adults:* Initially, 60 mg/kg I.V. as an induction treatment in patients with normal renal function. Give as an I.V. infusion over 1 hour q 8 hours for 2 or 3 weeks, depending on response. Follow with a maintenance infusion of 90 mg/kg daily given over 2 hours; increase as needed and tolerated to 120 mg/kg daily if disease shows signs of progression.
*Mucocutaneous acyclovir-resistant herpes simplex virus (HSV) infection*
*Adults:* 40 mg/kg I.V. Give as an I.V. infusion over 1 hour q 8 to 12 hours for 2 or 3 weeks, depending on response.
◇ *Varicella zoster infection*
*Adults:* 40 mg/kg I.V. q 8 hours for 10 to 21 days.
≡ *Dosage adjustment.* For adult patients with renal failure, calculate weight-adjusted creatinine clearance (ml/minute/kg).
*For men:*

$$\frac{\text{creatinine}}{\text{clearance}} = \frac{(140 - \text{age})}{(\text{serum creatinine} \times 72)};$$
(per kg)

*For women:* Multiply the above value by 0.85.
Give the drug according to the tables on page 557.

### I.V. administration
■ Drug is given by slow I.V. infusion. It should not be given by rapid I.V. infusion or direct I.V. injection.
■ No dilution of drug is needed if it is given via a central vein. For infusion via a peripheral vein, dilute to concentration of 12 mg/ml using normal saline solution or $D_5W$.
■ Manufacturer recommends injection of 750 to 1,000 ml of $D_5W$ or normal saline solution before first dose to establish diuresis. With subsequent doses, 750 to 1,000 ml of fluid should be given with dose of 90 to 120 mg/kg and 500 ml with each dose of 40 to 60 mg/kg.

### Incompatibilities
Incompatible with dextrose 30%, lactated Ringer's, or solution containing calcium, such as total parenteral nutrition. Use only $D_5W$ or normal saline for dilution. Immediate precipitation occurs with acyclovir, amphotericin B, cotrimoxazole, ganciclovir, pentamidine, trimetrexate, and vancomycin. Delayed precipitation occurs with dobutamine, droperidol, haloperidol, and phenytoin. Gas production occurs with diazepam, digoxin, lorazepam, midazolam, and promethazine. Cloudiness or color change may occur when drug is mixed with diphenhydramine, leucovorin, or prochlorperazine.

### Mechanism of action
*Antiviral action:* An analogue of pyrophosphate (important in enzymatic reactions), drug inhibits known herpes viruses in vitro by blocking the pyrophosphate binding site on DNA polymerases and reverse transcriptases.

### Pharmacokinetics
*Absorption:* Administered I.V.
*Distribution:* About 14% to 17% bound to plasma proteins; drug is deposited in bone.
*Metabolism:* Unknown.
*Excretion:* About 80% to 90% appears in urine unchanged. Drug clearance is dependent on renal function. Plasma half-life is about 3 hours.

| Route | Onset | Peak | Duration |
|-------|-------|------|----------|
| I.V. | Unknown | Immediate | Unknown |

### Contraindications and precautions
Contraindicated in patients hypersensitive to drug.
Use with extreme caution in patients with impaired renal function.

### Interactions
**Drug-drug.** *Nephrotoxic drugs, such as amphotericin B and aminoglycosides:* Increased risk of nephrotoxicity. Avoid use together.
*Pentamidine:* Increased risk of nephrotoxicity; severe hypocalcemia has also been reported. Avoid use together.
*Zidovudine:* Increased risk or severity of anemia. Advise clinician to monitor blood counts.

### Adverse reactions
**CNS:** *headache, seizures,* fatigue, malaise, asthenia, paresthesia, dizziness, hypoesthesia, neuropathy, tremor, ataxia, generalized spasms, dementia, stupor, sensory disturbances, meningitis, aphasia, abnormal coordination, EEG abnormalities, depression, confusion, anxiety, insomnia, somnolence, nervousness, amnesia, agitation, aggressive reaction, hallucinations.
**CV:** *hypertension, palpitations, ECG abnormalities, sinus tachycardia,* cerebrovascular disorder, first-degree AV block, *hypotension,* edema.

## HSV INFECTION

**Induction dose**

| Creatinine clearance (ml/min/kg) | Equivalent to 80 mg/kg/day (40 mg/kg q 12 hr) | Equivalent to 120 mg/kg/day (40 mg/kg q 8 hr) |
| --- | --- | --- |
| > 1.4 | 40  q 12 hr | 40 q 8 hr |
| > 1.0 – 1.4 | 30 q 12 hr | 30 q 8 hr |
| > 0.8 – 1.0 | 20 q 12 hr | 35 q 12 hr |
| > 0.6 – 0.8 | 35 q 24 hr | 25 q 12 hr |
| > 0.5 – 0.6 | 25 q 24 hr | 40 q 24 hr |
| ≥ 0.4 – 0.5 | 20 q 24 hr | 35 q 24 hr |
| < 0.4 | Not recommended | Not recommended |

## CMV INFECTION

**Induction dose**

| Creatinine clearance (ml/min/kg) | Equivalent to 180 mg/kg/day (60 mg/kg q 8 hr) | Equivalent to 180 mg/kg/day (90 mg/kg q 12 hr) |
| --- | --- | --- |
| > 1.4 | 60 q 8 hr | 90 q 12 hr |
| > 1.0 – 1.4 | 45 q 8 hr | 70 q 12 hr |
| > 0.8 – 1.0 | 50 q 12 hr | 50 q 12 hr |
| > 0.6 – 0.8 | 40 q 12 hr | 80 q 24 hr |
| > 0.5 – 0.6 | 60 q 24 hr | 60 q 24 hr |
| ≥ 0.4 – 0.5 | 50 q 24 hr | 50 q 24 hr |
| < 0.4 | Not recommended | Not recommended |

**Maintenance dose**

| Creatinine clearance (ml/min/kg) | Equivalent to 90 mg/kg/day (Once daily) | Equivalent to 120 mg/kg/day (Once daily) |
| --- | --- | --- |
| > 1.4 | 90 q 24 hr | 120 q 24 hr |
| > 1.0 – 1.4 | 70 q 24 hr | 90 q 24 hr |
| > 0.8 – 1.0 | 50 q 24 hr | 65 q 24 hr |
| > 0.6 – 0.8 | 80 q 48 hr | 105 q 48 hr |
| > 0.5 – 0.6 | 60 q 48 hr | 80 q 48 hr |
| ≥ 0.4 – 0.5 | 50 q 48 hr | 65 q 48 hr |
| < 0.4 | Not recommended | Not recommended |

**EENT:** visual disturbances, eye pain, conjunctivitis, sinusitis, pharyngitis, rhinitis.
**GI:** *nausea, diarrhea, vomiting, abdominal pain, anorexia,* constipation, dysphagia, rectal *hemorrhage,* dry mouth, dyspepsia, melena, flatulence, ulcerative stomatitis, *pancreatitis,* taste perversion.
**GU:** *abnormal renal function, decreased creatinine clearance and increased serum creatinine levels, albuminuria, dysuria, polyuria, urethral disorder, urine retention, urinary tract infections, acute renal failure,* candidiasis.
**Hematologic:** *anemia, granulocytopenia, leukopenia, bone marrow suppression, throm-*
*bocytopenia,* platelet abnormalities, thrombocytosis, WBC count abnormalities.
**Hepatic:** abnormal hepatic function, increased liver enzyme levels.
**Metabolic:** hypokalemia, hypomagnesemia, hypophosphatemia or hyperphosphatemia, hypocalcemia.
**Musculoskeletal:** leg cramps, back or chest pain, arthralgia, myalgia.
**Respiratory:** *cough, dyspnea,* pneumonitis, respiratory insufficiency, pulmonary infiltration, stridor, pneumothorax, *bronchospasm,* hemoptysis.

**Skin:** *rash, increased sweating,* pruritus, skin ulceration, erythematous rash, seborrhea, skin discoloration, facial edema, *flushing,* inflammation and pain at infusion site.
**Other:** *fever,* lymphadenopathy, pain, infection, **sepsis,** rigors, lymphoma-like disorder, sarcoma, bacterial or fungal infections, abscess, flulike symptoms.

## Clinical considerations

■ Anemia is common (up to 33% of patients treated with drug) and may be severe enough to require transfusions.
■ Don't exceed the recommended dosage, infusion rate, or frequency of administration. All doses must be individualized according to patient's renal function.
■ An infusion pump must be used to give foscarnet.
■ Foscarnet may be active against certain CMV strains resistant to ganciclovir.

### Therapeutic monitoring
■ Advise clinician to monitor renal function and patient for anemia.

### Special populations
**Breast-feeding patients.** It's unknown if drug appears in breast milk. Use with caution.
**Pediatric patients.** Safety and efficacy in children haven't been established.
**Geriatric patients.** It's unknown if age alters drug response. However, geriatric patients are likely to have preexisting renal function impairment, which requires alterations in dosage.

## Patient counseling
■ Warn patient of the high frequency of adverse reactions and the need for ongoing laboratory studies.
■ Advise patient to report to prescriber perioral tingling, numbness in the limbs, and paresthesia.

# fosinopril sodium
Monopril

*Pharmacologic classification:* ACE inhibitor
*Therapeutic classification:* antihypertensive
*Pregnancy risk category C (D, second and third trimesters)*

## Available forms
Available by prescription only
*Tablets:* 10 mg, 20 mg, 40 mg

## Indications and dosages
*Hypertension*
*Adults:* Initially, 10 mg P.O. daily; adjust dosage based on blood pressure response at peak and trough levels. *Usual dose:* 20 to 40 mg daily;

maximum up to 80 mg daily. Dose may be divided.
*Heart failure*
*Adults:* Initially, 10 mg P.O. daily; maximum dose up to 40 mg daily. Doses may be divided.

## Mechanism of action
*Antihypertensive action:* Fosinopril is believed to lower blood pressure primarily by suppressing the renin-angiotensin-aldosterone system, although it's also been effective in patients with low-renin hypertension.

## Pharmacokinetics
*Absorption:* Absorbed slowly through GI tract, primarily via proximal small intestine.
*Distribution:* More than 95% is protein-bound.
*Metabolism:* Hydrolyzed primarily in the liver and gut wall by esterases.
*Excretion:* Part of drug (50%) is excreted in urine, the remainder in feces.

| Route | Onset | Peak | Duration |
|-------|-------|------|----------|
| P.O. | 1 hr | 3 hr | 24 hr |

## Contraindications and precautions
Contraindicated in patients hypersensitive to drug or other ACE inhibitors and in breast-feeding women.
Use cautiously in patients with impaired renal or hepatic function.

## Interactions
**Drug-drug.** *Antacids:* May impair absorption of fosinopril; recommend separating administration by at least 2 hours.
*Diuretics and other antihypertensives:* Excessive hypotension may occur. Effect may be minimized by stopping diuretic.
*Lithium:* Increased serum lithium levels and lithium toxicity may occur. Advise clinician to monitor lithium levels frequently.
*Potassium supplements or potassium-sparing diuretics:* Concurrent use may result in hyperkalemia. Advise clinician to monitor potassium levels.
**Drug-herb.** *Capsaicin:* Increased risk of cough. Discourage use together.
*Licorice:* May cause sodium retention and increase blood pressure, interfering with the therapeutic effects of ACE inhibitors. Discourage use together.
**Drug-food.** *Salt substitutes containing potassium:* Risk of hyperkalemia. Advise patient to avoid use of potassium salt substitutes.

## Adverse reactions
**CNS:** headache, dizziness, fatigue, syncope, paresthesia, sleep disturbance, *CVA.*
**CV:** chest pain, angina, *MI, hypertensive crisis,* rhythm disturbances, palpitations, hypotension, orthostatic hypotension.
**EENT:** tinnitus, sinusitis.

**GI:** nausea, vomiting, diarrhea, *pancreatitis,* dry mouth, abdominal distention, abdominal pain, constipation.
**GU:** sexual dysfunction, elevations of BUN and serum creatinine, renal insufficiency.
**Hematologic:** decreased hematocrit or hemoglobin levels.
**Hepatic:** elevated liver function test results, *hepatitis.*
**Metabolic:** hyperkalemia.
**Musculoskeletal:** arthralgia, musculoskeletal pain, myalgia, gout.
**Respiratory:** *dry, persistent, tickling, nonproductive cough; bronchospasm.*
**Skin:** urticaria, rash, photosensitivity, pruritus.
**Other:** decreased libido, *angioedema.*

## Overdose and treatment
Overdose has never been reported; however, the most common sign of overdose is likely to be hypotension.
Recommend treating with infusion of normal saline. Hemodialysis and peritoneal dialysis aren't effective in removing the drug.

## Clinical considerations
■ Diuretic therapy is usually discontinued 2 to 3 days before the start of ACE inhibitor therapy to reduce risk of hypotension. If fosinopril doesn't adequately control blood pressure, diuretic may be reinstituted with care.
■ Risk of orthostatic hypotension is low.
■ Blood pressure is lowered within 1 hour of a single dose of 10 to 40 mg.
■ False low measurements of digoxin levels may result with the digi-tab radioimmunoassay kit for digoxin; other kits may be used.

### *Therapeutic monitoring*
■ Advise clinician to monitor potassium levels.
■ Recommend performing CBC with differential counts before therapy, then every 2 weeks for 3 months, and periodically thereafter.

### *Special populations*
**Pregnant patients.** Drug is Category D in second and third trimesters of pregnancy.
**Breast-feeding patients.** Avoid use of drug; significant levels appear in breast milk.
**Pediatric patients.** Safety and efficacy in children haven't been established.
**Geriatric patients.** No age-related differences have been observed.

## Patient counseling
■ Tell patient to take dose 1 hour before or 2 hours after food or antacids.
■ Advise patient to report to prescriber light-headedness in the first few days of therapy and signs of infection, such as fever or sore throat. He should also contact his prescriber and discontinue drug immediately if the following occur: swelling of tongue, lips, face, mucous membranes, eyes, lips, or limbs; difficulty swallowing or breathing; or hoarseness.
■ Advise patient to maintain the same salt intake as before therapy because salt restriction can lead to precipitous decrease in blood pressure with initial doses of this drug. Large reductions in blood pressure may also occur with excessive perspiration and dehydration.
■ Warn patient to avoid sudden position changes until effect of drug is known; however, orthostatic hypotension is infrequent.

# fosphenytoin sodium
Cerebyx

*Pharmacologic classification:* hydantoin derivative
*Therapeutic classification:* anticonvulsant
*Pregnancy risk category D*

## Available forms
Available by prescription only
*Injection:* 2 ml (150 mg fosphenytoin sodium equivalent to 100 mg phenytoin sodium), 10 ml (750 mg fosphenytoin sodium equivalent to 500 mg phenytoin sodium)

## Indications and dosages
**Status epilepticus**
*Adults:* Give 15 to 20 mg phenytoin sodium equivalent (PE)/kg I.V. at 100 to 150 PE/minute as a loading dose and then, 4 to 6 mg PE/kg/day I.V. as a maintenance dose. (Phenytoin may be used instead of fosphenytoin as maintenance using the appropriate dose.)
**Prevention and treatment of seizures during neurosurgery**
*Adults:* Give 10 to 20 mg PE/kg I.M. or I.V. at an I.V. infusion rate not exceeding 150 mg PE/minute as a loading dose. Maintenance dose is 4 to 6 mg PE/kg/day I.V.
**Short-term substitution for oral phenytoin therapy**
*Adults:* Same total daily dose as oral phenytoin sodium therapy given as a single daily dose I.M. or I.V. at an I.V. infusion rate not exceeding 150 mg PE/minute. (Some patients may require more frequent dosing.)

## I.V. administration
■ Give dose of I.V. fosphenytoin used to treat status epilepticus at a maximum rate of 150 mg PE/minute.
■ The typical infusion of drug given to a 50-kg (110-lb) patient takes 5 to 7 minutes, whereas that of an identical molar dose of phenytoin can't be accomplished in less than 15 to 20 minutes because of the untoward CV effects that accompany the direct I.V. administration of phenytoin at rates of more than 50 mg/minute.

### Incompatibilities
Don't infuse with other drugs.

## Mechanism of action
*Anticonvulsant action:* Because fosphenytoin is a prodrug of phenytoin, its anticonvulsant action is that of phenytoin. Phenytoin stabilizes neuronal membranes and limits seizure activity by modulating voltage-dependent sodium channels of neurons, inhibiting calcium flux across neuronal membranes, modulating voltage-dependent calcium channels of neurons, and enhancing sodium-potassium adenosine triphosphatase activity of neurons and glial cells.

## Pharmacokinetics
*Absorption:* No information available.
*Distribution:* About 95% to 99% is bound to plasma proteins, primarily albumin. Volume of distribution increases with dose and rate and ranges from 4.3 to 10.8 L.
*Metabolism:* Conversion half-life of fosphenytoin to phenytoin is about 15 minutes. Phosphatases are believed to play a major role in the conversion.
*Excretion:* Unknown, although it isn't excreted in urine.

| Route | Onset | Peak | Duration |
|-------|-------|------|----------|
| I.V. | Unknown | End of infusion | Unknown |
| I.M. | Unknown | 30 min | Unknown |

## Contraindications and precautions
Contraindicated in patients hypersensitive to the drug or its components, phenytoin, or other hydantoins. Also contraindicated in patients with sinus bradycardia, SA block, second- and third-degree AV block, and Adams-Stokes syndrome because of the effect of parenteral phenytoin on ventricular automaticity.

Use cautiously in patients with hypotension, severe myocardial insufficiency, impaired renal or hepatic function, hypoalbuminemia, porphyria, diabetes mellitus, and history of hypersensitivity to similarly structured drugs, such as barbiturates and succinimides.

## Interactions
**Drug-drug.** *Drugs that may increase plasma phenytoin levels (and thus its therapeutic effects), such as amiodarone, chloramphenicol, chlordiazepoxide, cimetidine, diazepam, dicumarol, disulfiram, estrogens, ethosuximide, fluoxetine, H$_2$-antagonists, halothane, isoniazid, methylphenidate, phenothiazines, phenylbutazone, salicylates, succinimides, sulfonamides, tolbutamide, and trazodone:* Increased plasma phenytoin levels. Advise clinician to monitor patient carefully.
*Carbamazepine or reserpine:* Plasma phenytoin levels may be decreased. Use together cautiously.

*Coumarin, digitoxin, doxycycline, estrogens, furosemide, oral contraceptives, rifampin, quinidine, theophylline, and vitamin D:* Efficacy may be decreased by phenytoin because of increased hepatic metabolism.
*Phenobarbital, sodium valproate, valproic acid:* May increase or decrease plasma phenytoin levels. Advise clinician to monitor patient closely.
*Tricyclic antidepressants:* Lower seizure threshold and may require adjustments in phenytoin dosage.
**Drug-lifestyle.** *Acute alcohol use:* Increased plasma phenytoin level.
*Long-term alcohol use:* Decreased plasma phenytoin levels. Advise patient to avoid alcohol.

## Adverse reactions
**CNS:** increased or decreased reflexes, speech disorders, dysarthria, asthenia, *intracranial hypertension, cerebral hemorrhage,* thinking abnormalities, nervousness, hypesthesia, extrapyramidal syndrome, brain edema, headache, *nystagmus, dizziness, somnolence, ataxia,* stupor, incoordination, paresthesia, agitation, tremor, vertigo.
**CV:** hypertension, *cardiac arrest,* palpitation, *bradycardia,* atrial flutter, *bundle branch block,* cardiomegaly, orthostatic hypotension, QT interval prolongation, thrombophlebitis, ventricular extrasystoles, *HF,* vasodilation, tachycardia, hypotension.
**EENT:** deafness, visual field defect, eye pain, conjunctivitis, photophobia, hyperacusis, mydriasis, parosmia, ear pain, tinnitus, diplopia, amblyopia, pharyngitis, sinusitis, rhinitis, epistaxis.
**GI:** constipation, dyspepsia, diarrhea, anorexia, GI hemorrhage, increased salivation, tenesmus, tongue edema, dysphagia, flatulence, gastritis, ileus, nausea, dry mouth, vomiting, taste perversion, taste loss.
**GU:** urine retention, oliguria, dysuria, vaginitis, albuminuria, genital edema, kidney failure, polyuria, urethral pain, urinary incontinence, vaginal candidiasis.
**Hematologic:** *thrombocytopenia,* anemia, leukocytosis, hypochromic anemia, *leukopenia, agranulocytosis, granulocytopenia, pancytopenia,* ecchymosis.
**Hepatic:** elevated liver enzyme levels.
**Metabolic:** diabetes insipidus, hypokalemia, hyperglycemia, hypophosphatemia, alkalosis, acidosis, dehydration, hyperkalemia, ketosis, decreased serum levels of T$_4$.
**Musculoskeletal:** myasthenia, myopathy, leg cramps, arthralgia, myalgia, pelvic pain, back pain.
**Respiratory:** cyanosis, pneumonia, hyperventilation, *apnea,* aspiration pneumonia, asthma, dyspnea, atelectasis, increased cough, increased sputum, hypoxia, pneumothorax, hemoptysis, bronchitis, *pulmonary embolus.*

---

**Skin:** petechia, rash, maculopapular rash, urticaria, sweating, skin discoloration, contact dermatitis, pustular rash, skin nodule, *pruritus.*
**Other:** lymphadenopathy.

## Overdose and treatment

There have been no reports of fosphenytoin overdose. However, because it's a prodrug of phenytoin, overdose may be similar. Early signs of phenytoin overdose may include drowsiness, nausea, vomiting, nystagmus, ataxia, dysarthria, tremor, and slurred speech; hypotension, respiratory depression, and coma may follow. Death is caused by respiratory and circulatory depression. Estimated lethal dose of phenytoin in adults is 2 to 5 g.

Formate and phosphate are metabolites of fosphenytoin and, therefore, may contribute to signs of toxicity after overdose. Signs of formate toxicity are similar to those of methanol toxicity and are associated with severe anion-gap metabolic acidosis. Large amounts of phosphate, delivered rapidly, could potentially cause hypocalcemia with paresthesia, muscle spasms, and seizures. Ionized free calcium levels can be measured and, if low, used to guide treatment.

Treatment is with gastric lavage or emesis followed by supportive treatment. Advise clinician to monitor vital signs and fluid and electrolyte balance. Forced diuresis is of little or no value. Hemodialysis or peritoneal dialysis may be helpful.

## Clinical considerations

■ Always prescribe and dispense fosphenytoin in phenytoin sodium equivalent units (PE). Adjustments in the recommended dosages shouldn't be made when fosphenytoin is substituted for phenytoin and vice versa.
■ Patients receiving fosphenytoin at doses of 20 mg PE/kg at 150 mg PE/minute are expected to experience some sensory discomfort, with the groin being the most common location. The occurrence and intensity of the discomfort can be lessened by slowing or temporarily stopping the infusion.
■ The phosphate load provided by fosphenytoin (0.0037 mmol phosphate/mg PE fosphenytoin) must be taken into consideration when treating patients who require phosphate restriction, such as those with severe renal impairment.
■ Drug should be stopped in patients with acute hepatotoxicity; advise prescriber not to readminister to these patients.
■ I.M. drug administration generates systemic phenytoin levels similar enough to oral phenytoin sodium to allow essentially interchangeable use.
■ A dose of 15 to 20 mg PE/kg of fosphenytoin infused I.V. at 100 to 150 mg PE/minute yields plasma-free phenytoin levels over time that approximate those achieved when an equivalent dose of phenytoin sodium (such as parenteral dilantin) is given at 50 mg/minute I.V.
■ Interpretation of total phenytoin plasma levels should be made cautiously in patients with renal or hepatic disease or hypoalbuminemia caused by an increased fraction in unbound phenytoin. Unbound phenytoin levels may be more useful in these patients. Also, these patients are at increased risk for both the frequency and severity of adverse reactions when fosphenytoin is administered I.V.
■ I.M. fosphenytoin shouldn't be used because therapeutic phenytoin levels may not be reached as rapidly as with I.V. administration.
■ Fosphenytoin may produce artificially low results in dexamethasone or metyrapone tests.

### Therapeutic monitoring

■ Advise clinician to monitor patient's ECG, blood pressure, and respiration continuously throughout the period when maximal serum phenytoin levels occur, about 10 to 20 minutes after the end of fosphenytoin infusions. Severe CV complications are most commonly encountered in geriatric or gravely ill patients. Reduction in rate of administration or discontinuation of dosing may be needed.
■ Drug should be stopped if rash appears. If rash is exfoliative, purpuric, or bullous or if lupus erythematosus, Stevens-Johnson syndrome, or toxic epidermal necrolysis is suspected, use of drug shouldn't be resumed; alternative therapy should be used. If rash is mild (measles-like or scarlatiniform), therapy may be resumed after it has completely disappeared. If rash recurs on reinstitution of therapy, further fosphenytoin or phenytoin administration is contraindicated.
■ After drug administration, it's recommended that phenytoin levels not be monitored until conversion to phenytoin is essentially complete; about 2 hours after the end of an I.V. infusion or 4 hours after I.M. administration.

### Special populations

**Breast-feeding patients.** Because it's unknown if fosphenytoin appears in breast milk, breast-feeding isn't recommended.
**Pediatric patients.** Safety and efficacy in children haven't been established.
**Geriatric patients.** Geriatric patients metabolize and excrete phenytoin slowly; therefore, fosphenytoin should be given cautiously to older adults.

## Patient counseling

■ Warn patient that sensory disturbances may occur with I.V. drug administration.
■ Tell patient to report adverse reactions, especially rash, immediately.

# furosemide
Apo-Furosemide*, Lasix, Lasix
Special*, Novosemide*, Uritol*

*Pharmacologic classification:* loop
diuretic
*Therapeutic classification:* diuretic,
antihypertensive
*Pregnancy risk category C*

## Available forms
Available by prescription only
*Tablets:* 20 mg, 40 mg, 80 mg
*Solution:* 10 mg/ml, 40 mg/5 ml
*Injection:* 10 mg/ml

## Indications and dosages
*Acute pulmonary edema*
*Adults:* 40 mg I.V. injected slowly; then 80 mg
I.V. within 1 hour, p.r.n.
*Infants and children:* 1 mg/kg I.M. or I.V. q 2
hours until response is achieved; maximum
dose is 6 mg/kg/day. If needed, the initial dose
may be increased by 1 mg/kg no more often
than every 2 hours.
*Edema*
*Adults:* 20 to 80 mg P.O. daily in morning, with
second dose given in 6 to 8 hours, carefully adjusted up to 600 mg daily, p.r.n.; or 20 to 40 mg
I.M. or I.V. Increase by 20 mg q 2 hours until
desired response is achieved. I.V. dosage should
be given slowly over 1 to 2 minutes.
*Infants and children:* 2 mg/kg/day P.O., increased by 1 to 2 mg/kg in 6 to 8 hours, p.r.n.,
carefully adjusted not to exceed 6 mg/kg/day.
*Hypertension*
*Adults:* 40 mg P.O. b.i.d. Adjust dosage according to response.
◇ *Hypercalcemia*
*Adults:* 80 to 100 mg I.V. q 1 to 2 hours; or
120 mg P.O. daily.

## I.V. administration
■ Give I.V. furosemide slowly, over 1 to 2 minutes.
■ For I.V. infusion, dilute furosemide in $D_5W$,
normal saline solution, or lactated Ringer's solution, and use within 24 hours.
■ If high-dose furosemide therapy is needed,
give as a controlled infusion not exceeding
4 mg/minute.

### Incompatibilities
Incompatible with acidic solutions, aminoglycosides, amiodarone, amsacrine, bleomycin,
buprenorphine, chlorpromazine, diazepam,
dobutamine, doxapram, doxorubicin, droperidol, erythromycin, esmolol, fluconazole, fructose 10% in water, gentamicin, hydralazine,
idarubicin, invert sugar 10% in electrolyte #2,
isoproterenol, meperidine, metoclopramide,
milrinone, morphine, netilmicin, ondansetron,
prochlorperazine, promethazine, quinidine,
vinblastine, and vincristine.

## Mechanism of action
*Antihypertensive action:* This drug effect may
be the result of renal and peripheral vasodilatation and a temporary increase in glomerular filtration rate and a decrease in peripheral
vascular resistance.
*Diuretic action:* Loop diuretics inhibit sodium
and chloride reabsorption in the proximal part
of the ascending loop of Henle, promoting the
excretion of sodium, water, chloride, and potassium.

## Pharmacokinetics
*Absorption:* About 60% is absorbed from the
GI tract after oral administration. Food delays
absorption but doesn't alter diuretic response.
Diuresis begins in 30 to 60 minutes; peak diuresis occurs 1 to 2 hours after oral administration. Diuresis follows I.V. administration
within 5 minutes and peaks in 20 to 60 minutes.
*Distribution:* About 95% plasma protein–
bound. It crosses the placenta and appears in
breast milk.
*Metabolism:* Metabolized minimally by the
liver.
*Excretion:* About 50% to 80% of a dose is excreted in urine; plasma half-life is about 30
minutes. Duration of action is 6 to 8 hours after oral administration and about 2 hours after
I.V. administration.

| Route | Onset | Peak | Duration |
|---|---|---|---|
| P.O. | 20-30 min | 1-2 hr | 6-8 hr |
| I.V. | 5 min | ½ hr | 2 hr |

## Contraindications and precautions
Contraindicated in patients with anuria or those
hypersensitive to drug.
   Use cautiously in hepatic cirrhosis and during pregnancy.

## Interactions
**Drug-drug.** *Aminoglycoside antibiotics, cisplatin, and ethacrynic acid:* Can potentiate ototoxicity. Shouldn't be used together.
*Amphotericin B, corticosteroids, corticotropin,
metolazone:* Increased risk of hypokalemia.
Advise clinician to monitor potassium levels.
*Antidiabetics:* Decreased hypoglycemic effects. Advise clinician to monitor glucose
levels.
*Other antihypertensives:* Increased risk of hypotension. Recommend checking blood pressure frequently.
*Cardiac glycosides, lithium, and neuromuscu-
lar blockers:* Increased risk of toxicity. Advise
clinician to monitor potassium levels.
*NSAIDs:* May inhibit diuretic response. Use
together cautiously.

---

*Salicylates:* May cause salicylate toxicity. Use together cautiously.

*Sucralfate:* May reduce diuretic and antihypertensive effect. Recommend separating administration by 2 hours.

**Drug-herb.** *Aloe:* May increase drug effects. Advise using caution.

*Dandelion:* Possible interference with diuretic activity. Discourage use together.

*Ginseng:* Decreased diuretic effect. Discourage use together.

**Drug-lifestyle.** *Sun exposure:* Potentiates photosensitivity reactions. Advise patient to use sunblock.

## Adverse reactions

**CNS:** vertigo, headache, dizziness, paresthesia, restlessness.

**CV:** volume depletion and dehydration, orthostatic hypotension.

**EENT:** transient deafness with too rapid I.V. injection, blurred vision.

**GI:** abdominal discomfort and pain, diarrhea, anorexia, nausea, vomiting, constipation, *pancreatitis.*

**GU:** nocturia, polyuria, frequent urination, altered renal function test results, oliguria.

**Hematologic:** *agranulocytosis, leukopenia, thrombocytopenia,* azotemia, anemia, *aplastic anemia.*

**Hepatic:** altered liver function test results.

**Metabolic:** hypokalemia; hypochloremic alkalosis; asymptomatic hyperuricemia; fluid and electrolyte imbalances, including dilutional hyponatremia, hypocalcemia, hypomagnesemia; hyperglycemia and impaired glucose tolerance.

**Musculoskeletal:** muscle spasm, weakness.

**Skin:** dermatitis, purpura.

**Other:** fever, transient pain (at I.M. injection site), thrombophlebitis (with I.V. administration).

## Overdose and treatment

Signs and symptoms of overdose include profound electrolyte and volume depletion, which may precipitate circulatory collapse. Treatment is chiefly supportive; recommend replacing fluids and electrolytes.

## Clinical considerations

■ To prevent nocturia, give P.O. and I.M. preparations in the morning. Give second dose in early afternoon.

■ If oliguria or azotemia develops or increases, drug may need to be discontinued.

■ Watch for signs of hypokalemia, such as muscle weakness and cramps.

■ Furosemide may not be well absorbed orally in patient with severe HF. Drug may need to be given I.V. even if patient is taking other oral drugs.

■ Store tablets in light-resistant container to prevent discoloration (doesn't affect potency).

Don't use discolored (yellow) injectable preparation. Refrigerate oral furosemide solution to ensure drug stability.

### Therapeutic monitoring

■ Advise clinician to monitor weight, blood pressure, and pulse rate routinely with long-term use and during rapid diuresis.

■ Furosemide may lead to profound water and electrolyte depletion. Advise clinician to monitor fluid intake and output and electrolyte, BUN, and carbon dioxide levels frequently.

### Special populations

**Pregnant patients.** Use cautiously.

**Breast-feeding patients.** Drug shouldn't be used by breast-feeding women.

**Pediatric patients.** Drug should be used with caution in neonates. The usual pediatric dosage can be used, but recommend extending dosing intervals. Sorbitol content of oral preparations may cause diarrhea, especially at high doses.

**Geriatric patients.** Geriatric and debilitated patients require close observation because they're more susceptible to drug-induced diuresis.

## Patient counseling

■ Advise patient to take drug with food to prevent GI upset, and to take drug in morning to prevent nocturia. If second dose is needed, tell patient to take it in early afternoon, 6 to 8 hours after morning dose.

■ Advise patient to immediately report ringing in ears, severe abdominal pain, or sore throat and fever; these may indicate toxicity.

**H** *ALERT* Discourage patient from storing different types of drugs in the same container, increasing the risk of drug errors. The most popular strengths of furosemide and digoxin are white tablets about equal in size.

■ Teach patient to use protective clothing and a sunblock because of risk of photosensitivity reactions.

# gabapentin
Neurontin

*Pharmacologic classification:* 1-amino-
methyl cyclohexoneacetic acid
*Therapeutic classification:* anticonvulsant
*Pregnancy risk category C*

## Available forms
Available by prescription only
*Capsules:* 100 mg, 300 mg, 400 mg
*Film-coated tablets:* 600 mg, 800 mg
*Solution*: 250 mg/5 ml

## Indications and dosages
***Adjunctive treatment of partial seizures
with and without secondary generalization***
*Adults and adolescents over 12 years:* 900 mg
to 1.8 g P.O. daily in three divided doses. Initial dosage is 300 mg P.O. t.i.d. Doses up to
3,600 mg/day have been well tolerated.
*Starting dosage, children ages 3 to 12:* 10 to
15 mg/kg/day P.O. in three divided doses, adjusting over 3 days to reach effective dosages.
*Effective dosage, children ages 5 to 12:* 25 to
35 mg/kg/day P.O. in three divided doses.
*Effective dosage, children ages 3 to 4:*
40 mg/kg/day P.O. in three divided doses.
**≣ *Dosage adjustment.*** In adult patients with
renal impairment, if creatinine clearance is
more than 60 ml/minute, give 400 mg P.O. t.i.d.;
if creatinine clearance is between 30 and 60 ml/
minute, give 300 mg P.O. b.i.d.; if creatinine
clearance is between 15 and 30 ml/minute, give
300 mg P.O. daily; and if creatinine clearance
is less than 15 ml/minute, give 300 mg P.O.
every other day. Patients on hemodialysis
should receive a loading dose of 300 to 400 mg
P.O.; then 200 mg to 300 mg P.O. after each 4-
hour session of hemodialysis. The use of
gabapentin in children 3 to 12 years of age with
impaired renal function has not been established.

## Mechanism of action
*Anticonvulsant action:* The mechanism of action of gabapentin is unknown. Although it's
structurally related to gamma-aminobutyric
acid (GABA), it doesn't interact with GABA
receptors, isn't converted metabolically into
GABA or a GABA agonist, and doesn't inhibit
GABA uptake or degradation. Gabapentin
doesn't exhibit affinity for other common receptor sites.

## Pharmacokinetics
*Absorption:* Drug bioavailability isn't dose
proportional. A 400-mg dose, for example, is
about 25% less bioavailable than a 100-mg
dose. Over the recommended dose range of
300 to 600 mg t.i.d., however, differences in
bioavailability aren't large, and bioavailability is about 60%. Food has no effect on the rate
or extent of absorption.
*Distribution:* Circulates largely unbound (less
than 3%) to plasma protein. Drug crosses the
blood-brain barrier with about 20% of the corresponding plasma levels found in CSF.
*Metabolism:* Not appreciably metabolized in
humans. Clearance is more rapid in children
younger than age 5 compared with those older than age 5. Children 3 to 4 years old may
need higher dosage. Variable clearance in children under age 1.
*Excretion:* Eliminated from the systemic circulation by renal excretion as unchanged drug.
Its elimination half-life is 5 to 7 hours. Drug
can be removed from plasma by hemodialysis.

| Route | Onset | Peak | Duration |
|-------|-------|------|----------|
| P.O. | Unknown | Unknown | Unknown |

## Contraindications and precautions
Contraindicated in patients hypersensitive to
drug.

## Interactions
**Drug-drug.** *Antacids:* Decrease absorption of
gabapentin. Recommend separating administration of the two drugs by at least 2 hours.

## Adverse reactions
**CNS:** *fatigue, somnolence, dizziness, ataxia,
nystagmus, tremor,* nervousness, dysarthria,
amnesia, depression, abnormal thinking,
twitching, incoordination; in children 3 to 12
years of age: emotional lability, hostility including aggressive behavior, hyperkinesia,
dizziness, fatigue, headache, **seizures,** thought
disorders.
**CV:** peripheral edema, vasodilation.
**EENT:** *diplopia, rhinitis,* pharyngitis, dry
throat, *amblyopia.*

---

**GI:** nausea, vomiting, dyspepsia, dry mouth, constipation; in children ages 3 to 12: diarrhea, anorexia.
**GU:** impotence.
**Hematologic:** *leukopenia,* decreased WBC count.
**Metabolic:** increased appetite, weight gain.
**Musculoskeletal:** back pain, myalgia, fractures.
**Respiratory:** cough.
**Skin:** pruritus, abrasion.
**Other:** dental abnormalities.

## Overdose and treatment

Acute overdose of gabapentin may cause double vision, slurred speech, drowsiness, lethargy, and diarrhea. Supportive care is recommended. Gabapentin can be removed by hemodialysis and may be indicated by the patient's clinical state or in patients with significant renal impairment.

## Clinical considerations

■ Other anticonvulsant drugs shouldn't be suddenly withdrawn in patients starting gabapentin therapy. Recommend stopping drug therapy or substituting alternative drug gradually over at least 1 week to minimize risk of precipitating seizures.
■ Drug can be taken without regard to meals.
■ With t.i.d. dosing, interval between doses should not exceed 12 hours.
■ Gabapentin, when added to other antiepileptics, causes false-positive results with the Ames N-Multistix SG dipstick test for urinary protein. The more specific sulfosalicylic acid precipitation procedure is recommended to determine the presence of urine protein.

### Therapeutic monitoring

■ Routine monitoring of plasma drug levels isn't needed. Drug doesn't appear to alter plasma levels of other anticonvulsants.
■ Sulfosalicylic acid precipitation procedure is recommended to determine the presence of urine protein. Ames N-Multistix SG dipstick shouldn't be used to test for urine protein; false-positive results can occur.

### Special populations

**Pregnant patients.** Data concerning use during pregnancy are inadequate.
**Breast-feeding patients.** It's unknown if drug appears in breast milk. Recommend stopping breast-feeding if gabapentin therapy is initiated because of potential for serious adverse reactions.
**Pediatric patients.** Safety and efficacy in children under age 12 haven't been established.

## Patient counseling

■ Instruct patient to take first dose at bedtime to minimize drowsiness, dizziness, fatigue, and ataxia.

■ Warn patient to avoid driving or operating heavy machinery until adverse CNS effects of drug are known.
■ Inform patient that drug can be taken without regard to meals.

# galantamine hydrobromide
Reminyl

*Pharmacologic classification:* reversible, competitive acetylcholinesterase inhibitor
*Therapeutic classification:* cholinomimetic
*Pregnancy risk category B*

## Available forms

Available by prescription only
*Tablets:* 4 mg, 8 mg, 12 mg
*Oral solution:* 4 mg/ml

## Indications and dosages

*Mild to moderate dementia of Alzheimer's type*
*Adults:* Initially, 4 mg b.i.d., preferably with morning and evening meals. If dose is well tolerated after minimum of 4 weeks of therapy, increase dose to 8 mg b.i.d. A further increase to 12 mg b.i.d. may be attempted, but only after at least 4 weeks of therapy at the previous dose. Recommended dosage range is 16 to 24 mg daily in two divided doses.
≡*Dosage adjustment.* For patients with moderately impaired hepatic function (Child-Pugh score of 7 to 9), dose usually should not exceed 16 mg daily. For patients with severe hepatic impairment (Child-Pugh score of 10 to 15), drug isn't recommended. For patients with moderate renal impairment, dose usually should not exceed 16 mg daily. For patients with severe renal impairment (creatinine clearance < 9 ml/min), drug isn't recommended.

## Mechanism of action

*Anticholinesterase action:* Exact mechanism of action is unknown. Drug is a competitive and reversible inhibitor of acetylcholinesterase, which is believed to enhance cholinergic function by increasing the level of acetylcholine in the brain.

## Pharmacokinetics

*Absorption:* Rapidly and well absorbed, with an oral bioavailability of about 90%. Levels peak in about 1 hour. In geriatric patients, drug levels are 30% to 40% higher than in young healthy people.
*Distribution:* Primarily distributed to blood cells. Protein-binding isn't significant.
*Metabolism:* Metabolized in the liver by cytochrome P-450 enzymes (CYP 2D6 and CYP 3A4) and glucuronidated. Concurrent therapy with inhibitors of these enzyme systems may

result in modest increases in bioavailability of galantamine.

*Excretion:* Excreted in urine unchanged as the glucuronide, and as metabolites. Terminal half-life is about 7 hours.

| Route | Onset | Peak | Duration |
|-------|-------|------|----------|
| P.O. | Unknown | 1 hr | Unknown |

## Contraindications and precautions

Contraindicated in patients hypersensitive to drug or its components.

Use drug cautiously in patients with supraventricular cardiac conduction disorders and in those taking other drugs that significantly slow heart rate. Use cautiously during or before procedures involving anesthesia using succinylcholine-type or similar neuromuscular blockers. Use cautiously in patients with history of peptic ulcer disease and in those taking NSAIDs. Because of the potential for cholinomimetic effects, use drug cautiously in patients with bladder outflow obstruction, seizures, asthma, or COPD.

## Interactions

**Drug-drug.** *Amitriptyline, fluoxetine, fluvoxamine, quinidine:* Decreased galantamine clearance. Advise clinician to monitor patient closely.
*Anticholinergics:* Possible antagonized anticholinergic activity. Advise clinician to monitor patient.
*Cholinergics (such as bethanechol, succinylcholine):* Synergistic effect. Advise clinician to monitor patient closely. May need to avoid use before procedures using general anesthesia with succinylcholine-type neuromuscular blockers.
*Cimetidine, erythromycin, ketoconazole, paroxetine:* Increased galantamine bioavailability. Advise clinician to monitor patient closely.

## Adverse reactions

**CNS:** dizziness, headache, tremor, depression, insomnia, somnolence, fatigue, syncope.
**CV:** *bradycardia.*
**EENT:** rhinitis.
**GI:** *nausea, vomiting,* anorexia, *diarrhea,* abdominal pain, dyspepsia, anorexia.
**GU:** urinary tract infection, hematuria.
**Hematologic:** anemia.
**Metabolic:** weight loss.

## Overdose and treatment

Signs and symptoms of overdose are similar to those of other cholinergics and generally involve the CNS, parasympathetic nervous system, and neuromuscular junctions. In addition to muscle weakness or fasciculations, some or all of the following signs of cholinergic crisis may be present: severe nausea, vomiting, GI cramping, salivation, lacrimation, urination, defecation, sweating, bradycardia, hypoten-

sion, respiratory depression, collapse, and seizures. Increasing muscle weakness is possible and may result in death if respiratory muscles are involved.

Contact a poison control center for the latest recommendations for the management of a drug overdose. Treatment is supportive and symptomatic. Atropine I.V. may be used as an antidote for galantamine overdose. An initial dose of 0.5 to 1 mg is recommended, with subsequent doses based on clinical response. It's unknown if drug is removed by dialysis.

## Clinical considerations

■ Bradycardia and heart block have been reported in patients with and without underlying cardiac conduction abnormalities. Consider all patients at risk for adverse effects on cardiac conduction.
■ Drug should be given with food and antiemetics and adequate fluid intake to decrease the risk of nausea and vomiting.
■ If drug is stopped for several days or longer, it should be restarted at the lowest dose and increased, at 4-week intervals or longer, to the previous dosage level.
■ Oral solution and tablets are bioequivalent.
■ Use proper technique while dispensing the oral solution with the pipette. The measured amount should be dispensed in a nonalcoholic beverage and given right away.

### Therapeutic monitoring

■ Because of the risk of increased gastric acid secretion, advise clinician to monitor patients closely for symptoms of active or occult GI bleeding, especially those with an increased risk of developing ulcers.

### Special populations

**Breast-feeding patients.** It isn't known if drug appears in breast milk. There is no indication for use in breast-feeding mothers.
**Pediatric patients.** Safety and efficacy in children haven't been established.
**Geriatric patients.** No specific dosage adjustments are needed.

## Patient counseling

■ Advise patient to take drug with morning and evening meals.
■ Inform patient that nausea and vomiting are common adverse effects.
■ Advise patient and caregiver that the most common adverse effects can be minimized by following the recommended dosing and administration schedule.
■ Urge patient to report bradycardia immediately.
■ Advise patient that drug is believed to enhance cognitive function, but there is no evidence that it alters the underlying disease process.

- Teach proper technique for measuring the oral solution with the pipette.
- The measured amount of oral solution should be dispensed in a nonalcoholic beverage and consumed immediately.

# ganciclovir (DHPG)
Cytovene

*Pharmacologic classification:* synthetic nucleoside
*Therapeutic classification:* antiviral
*Pregnancy risk category C*

## Available forms
Available by prescription only
*Injection:* 500-mg vial
*Capsules:* 250 mg, 500 mg

## Indications and dosages
*Treatment of cytomegalovirus (CMV) retinitis*
*Adults:* Initially, 5 mg/kg I.V. (given at a constant rate over 1 hour) q 12 hours for 14 to 21 days; followed by a maintenance dose of 5 mg/kg I.V. every day; or 6 mg/kg I.V. once daily for 5 days per week. These I.V. infusions should be given at a constant rate over 1 hour. Alternatively, a maintenance dose of 1,000 mg P.O. t.i.d. or 500 mg P.O. q 3 hours while awake (6 times daily) may be used.

*Prevention of CMV in transplant recipients*
*Adults:* 5 mg/kg I.V. over 1 hour q 12 hours for 7 to 14 days, followed by a maintenance dose of 5 mg/kg every day or 6 mg/kg once daily 5 days per week.

*Other CMV infections*
*◊ 5 mg/kg I.V. over 1 hour q 12 hours for 14 to 21 days; or 2.5 mg/kg I.V. over 1 hour q 8 hours for 14 to 21 days.*

*Dosage adjustment.* Adjust dosage in patients with renal impairment. Consider dosage reduction for patients with neutropenia, anemia, or thrombocytopenia.

## Administration
- Reconstitute with sterile water for injection. Don't constitute with bacteriostatic water for injection because this may lead to the formation of a precipitate. Reconstituted solutions are stable for 12 hours. Don't refrigerate.
- For intermittent I.V. infusion, add 10 ml sterile water for injection to vial of 500 mg of ganciclovir to provide solution of 50 mg/ml. Shake vial to ensure complete dissolution. The appropriate dose should then be withdrawn and further diluted in 50 to 250 ml of compatible I.V. solution.
- For use in fluid-restricted patients, drug may be diluted to no more than 10 mg/ml.
- Recommend giving drug over 1 hour because of high potential for toxicity.

## Incompatibilities
Incompatible with parabens, a bacteriostatic drug. Also incompatible with amsacrine, cytarabine, doxorubicin, fludarabine, foscarnet, ondansetron, piperacillin sodium, sargramostim, tazobactam, and vinorelbine. Don't mix with other drugs.

## Mechanism of action
*Antiviral action:* Ganciclovir is a synthetic nucleoside analogue of 2´-deoxyguanosine. It competitively inhibits viral DNA polymerase, and may be incorporated within viral DNA to cause early termination of DNA replication. It has shown activity against CMV, herpes simplex virus type 1 and type 2 (HSV-1 and HSV-2), varicella zoster virus, Epstein-Barr virus, and hepatitis B virus.

## Pharmacokinetics
*Absorption:* Less than 7% is absorbed after oral administration.
*Distribution:* Only 2% to 3% protein-bound. It preferentially concentrates within CMV-infected cells because of action of cellular kinases that convert it to ganciclovir triphosphate.
*Metabolism:* Most (over 90%) is excreted unchanged.
*Excretion:* Elimination half-life is about 3 hours in patients with normal renal function; it can be as long as 30 hours in patients with severe renal failure. The primary route of excretion is through the kidneys by glomerular filtration and some renal tubular secretion.

| Route | Onset | Peak | Duration |
|-------|-------|------|----------|
| P.O. | Unknown | 1¼-3 hr | Unknown |
| I.V. | Unknown | Immediate | Unknown |

## Contraindications and precautions
Contraindicated in patients hypersensitive to drug and those with an absolute neutrophil count less than 500/mm³ or a platelet count less than 25,000/mm³.

Use cautiously in patients with impaired renal function.

## Interactions
**Drug-drug.** *Cytotoxic drugs:* Additive toxicity (bone marrow depression, stomatitis, alopecia). Advise clinician to monitor patient closely.
*Didanosine:* Increased plasma levels of didanosine. Advise clinician to monitor patient closely for didanosine toxicity.
*Imipenem-cilastatin:* Increased risk of seizures. Advise clinician to monitor patient closely.
*Immunosuppressants, such as azathioprine, corticosteroids, cyclosporine:* Enhanced immune and bone marrow suppression. Use together cautiously.

---

*Probenecid:* Decreased renal clearance of ganciclovir. Advise clinician to monitor patient closely for adverse reactions.
*Zidovudine:* Higher risk of neutropenia. Advise clinician to monitor patient closely for signs of neutropenia (fever, chills, and other flulike symptoms).

## Adverse reactions
**CNS:** altered dreams, confusion, ataxia, headache, *seizures, coma,* dizziness, somnolence, tremor, abnormal thinking, agitation, amnesia, anxiety, neuropathy, paresthesia, asthenia.
**EENT:** retinal detachment (in CMV retinitis patients).
**GI:** *nausea, vomiting, diarrhea, anorexia, abdominal pain,* flatulence, dyspepsia, dry mouth.
**GU:** increased serum creatinine levels.
**Hematologic:** *granulocytopenia, thrombocytopenia, leukopenia,* anemia.
**Hepatic:** abnormal liver function test results.
**Respiratory:** pneumonia.
**Skin:** *rash; sweating;* pruritus, inflammation, pain (at injection site).
**Other:** phlebitis, chills, *sepsis, fever,* infection.

## Overdose and treatment
Overdose may result in emesis, neutropenia, or GI disturbances.
   Treatment should be symptomatic and supportive. Hemodialysis may be useful. Recommend hydrating the patient to reduce plasma levels.

## Clinical considerations
■ Drug has a high potential for toxicity; use only when the potential for benefit outweighs risk.
■ **ALERT** Don't give S.C., I.M., or as a rapid I.V. bolus.

### Therapeutic monitoring
■ Advise clinician to monitor CBC to detect neutropenia, which may occur in as many as 40% of patients. It usually appears after about 10 days of therapy, and may be caused by a high dosage (15 mg/kg/day). Neutropenia is reversible, but may necessitate discontinuation of therapy. Patient may resume drug therapy when blood counts return to normal.
■ Adverse reactions occur frequently, can be reduced with reduction of dose, and generally resolve when drug therapy is discontinued.

### Special populations
**Breast-feeding patients.** Don't use drug in breast-feeding women. Instruct women to discontinue breast-feeding until at least 72 hours after last treatment.
**Pediatric patients.** Few data are available on drug use in children under age 12. Drug should be used with extreme caution, keeping in mind the potential for carcinogenic and reproductive toxicity.

**Geriatric patients.** Use drug cautiously in geriatric patients with compromised renal function.

## Patient counseling
■ Inform patient that maintenance infusions are needed to prevent recurrence of disease.
■ Instruct patient to have regular eye examinations to monitor retinitis.
■ Advise patient to immediately report signs or symptoms of infection (fever, sore throat) or easy bruising or bleeding.
■ Instruct patient to take oral dose with food

---

# ganirelix acetate
Antagon

*Pharmacologic classification:*
gonadotropin-releasing hormone
(GnRH) antagonist
*Therapeutic classification:* fertility
drug
*Pregnancy risk category X*

## Available forms
Available by prescription only
*Injection:* 250 mcg/0.5 ml in prefilled syring

## Indications and dosages
*Inhibition of premature luteinizing hormone (LH) surges in women undergoing medically supervised, controlled ovarian hyperstimulation*
*Adults:* 250 mcg S.C. once daily during ea
to midfollicular phase of menstrual cycle. Co
tinue daily until enough follicles of sufficio
size are confirmed by ultrasound; human cho
onic gonadotropin is then given to induce
nal maturation of follicles.

## Mechanism of action
*LH suppression action:* GnRH, secreted by t
pituitary gland, stimulates the synthesis a
secretion of gonadotropins, LH, and follicl
stimulating hormone (FSH). In midcycle,
large increase in GnRH leads to a large surg
in LH secretion, causing ovulation, an increa
in progesterone levels, and a decrease in estr
diol levels. Ganirelix blocks pituitary GnR
receptors and suppresses LH and, to a smal
er degree, FSH secretions. By suppressing L
and FSH secretions in the early to mid men
strual cycle, ganirelix stops premature go
nadotropin surges that could interfere with
trial of medically supervised, controlled ovar
ian hyperstimulation.

## Pharmacokinetics
*Absorption:* Rapidly absorbed after S.C. in
jection with an average of 91.1% absorbed.
*Distribution:* Most (81.9%) is plasma protein-
bound.

---

*Metabolism:* Unmetabolized drug is found in urine up to 24 hours after dose. Two metabolites have been detected in feces.
*Excretion:* Primary excretion route is fecal; metabolites can be detected nearly 8 days after a dose.

| Route | Onset | Peak | Duration |
|-------|-------|------|----------|
| S.C. | Unknown | Unknown | Unknown |

## Contraindications and precautions
Contraindicated in patients hypersensitive to ganirelix or its components or to GnRH or GnRH analogue. Also contraindicated in pregnant women.

Use drug with caution in patients with potential hypersensitivity to GnRH and in those with latex allergies because the product packaging contains natural rubber latex.

## Interactions
None reported.

## Adverse reactions
**CNS:** headache.
**GI:** abdominal pain, nausea.
**GU:** vaginal bleeding, gynecologic abdominal pain, ovarian hyperstimulation syndrome.
**Skin:** injection site reaction.
**Other:** *fetal death.*

## Overdose and treatment
No information available.

## Clinical considerations
■ Only prescribers experienced in infertility treatments should prescribe this drug.
■ Before starting treatment, prescriber should ensure that patient isn't pregnant.
■ The natural rubber latex packaging of this product may cause allergic reaction in hypersensitive patients.

### Therapeutic monitoring
■ After first injection, patients who report previous or potential hypersensitivity to GnRH must be monitored closely.
■ Increased WBC count and decreased bilirubin levels and hematocrit have occurred in patients receiving ganirelix injections.

### Special populations
**Pregnant patients.** Drug may cause fetal death; don't use in pregnancy.
**Breast-feeding patients.** The amount of drug that appears in breast milk is unknown; drug shouldn't be used by breast-feeding women.
**Pediatric patients.** Ganirelix use hasn't been studied in pediatric patients.
**Geriatric patients.** Ganirelix use hasn't been sufficiently studied in patients ages 65 and older.

## Patient counseling
■ Tell patient that the correct use of ganirelix injection is extremely important to the success of the infertility treatments.
■ Provide patient with information on proper technique for S.C. administration of drug.
■ Advise patient to store drug at room temperature, away from heat and light, and out of children's reach.
■ Instruct patient to discontinue drug and contact prescriber as soon as pregnancy is suspected.

# gatifloxacin
Tequin

*Pharmacologic classification:* fluoroquinolone antibiotic
*Therapeutic classification:* antibiotic
*Pregnancy risk category C*

## Available forms
Available by prescription only
*Injection:* 200 mg/20-ml vial, 400 mg/40-ml vial, 200 mg in 100 ml $D_5W$, 400 mg in 200 ml $D_5W$
*Tablets:* 200 mg, 400 mg

## Indications and dosages
*Acute bacterial exacerbation of chronic bronchitis caused by Streptococcus pneumoniae, Haemophilus influenzae, H. parainfluenzae, Moraxella catarrhalis, or Staphylococcus aureus*
*Adults:* 400 mg I.V. or P.O. daily for 5 days.
*Complicated urinary tract infection caused by Escherichia coli, Klebsiella pneumoniae, or Proteus mirabilis; acute pyelonephritis caused by E. coli*
*Adults:* 400 mg I.V. or P.O. daily for 7 to 10 days.
*Acute sinusitis caused by S. pneumoniae or H. influenzae*
*Adults:* 400 mg I.V. or P.O. daily for 10 days.
*Community-acquired pneumonia caused by S. pneumoniae, H. influenzae, H. parainfluenzae, M. catarrhalis, S. aureus, Mycoplasma pneumoniae, Chlamydia pneumoniae, or Legionella pneumophila*
*Adults:* 400 mg I.V. or P.O. daily for 7 to 14 days.
*Uncomplicated urethral gonorrhea in men and cervical gonorrhea or acute uncomplicated rectal infections in women caused by Neisseria gonorrhoeae*
*Adults:* 400 mg P.O. or I.V. as single dose.
*Uncomplicated urinary tract infection caused by E. coli, K. pneumoniae, or P. mirabilis*
*Adults:* 400 mg I.V. or P.O. as single dose, or 200 mg I.V. or P.O. daily for 3 days.
≡*Dosage adjustment.* For patients with creatinine clearance less than 40 ml/min, those on

hemodialysis, and those on continuous peritoneal dialysis, initial dose is 400 mg I.V. or P.O. daily, and subsequent doses are 200 mg I.V. or P.O. daily. For patients on hemodialysis, administer after hemodialysis session is complete.

## I.V. administration
- Dilute drug in single-use vials with $D_5W$ or normal saline solution to a final concentration of 2 mg/ml before administration. Diluted solutions are stable for 14 days at room temperature or refrigerated. Frozen solutions are stable up to 6 months, except for 5% sodium bicarbonate solutions. Thaw at room temperature. After thawing, solutions are stable for 14 days when stored at room temperature or under refrigeration.
- Don't mix with other drugs.
- Infuse over 60 minutes.
- Discard any unused portion of the single-dose vials.

### Incompatibilities
Additives and other drugs should not be added to gatifloxacin injection in single-use vials or gatifloxacin I.V. solutions.

## Mechanism of action
*Antibiotic action:* Gatifloxacin inhibits DNA gyrase and topoisomerase, preventing cell replication and division. It is active against gram-positive and gram-negative organisms, including *S. aureus, S. pneumoniae, E. coli, H. influenzae, H. parainfluenzae, K. pneumoniae, M. catarrhalis, N. gonorrhoeae, P. mirabilis, C. pneumoniae, L. pneumophilia,* and *M. pneumoniae.*

## Pharmacokinetics
*Absorption:* 96% is absorbed after oral administration; levels peak in 1 to 2 hours.
*Distribution:* 20% protein-bound. It is widely distributed into many tissues and fluids.
*Metabolism:* Limited biotransformation.
*Excretion:* More than 70% is excreted unchanged by the kidneys. Serum half-life is 7 to 14 hours.

| Route | Onset | Peak | Duration |
|-------|-------|------|----------|
| P.O. | Unknown | 1-2 hr | Unknown |
| I.V. | Unknown | Unknown | Unknown |

## Contraindications and precautions
Contraindicated in patients hypersensitive to fluoroquinolones. Drug shouldn't be used in patients with prolongation of QTc interval or in patients with uncorrected hypokalemia.

Use drug cautiously in patients with clinically significant bradycardia, acute myocardial ischemia, known or suspected CNS disorders, or renal insufficiency.

## Interactions
**Drug-drug.** *Antacids that contain aluminum or magnesium, ferrous sulfate; didanosine buffered tablets, buffered powder, or buffered solution; products that contain zinc, magnesium, or iron:* Decreased gatifloxacin absorption. Recommend giving gatifloxacin 4 hours before these products.
*Antidiabetics (glyburide, insulin):* Possible symptomatic hypoglycemia or hyperglycemia. Advise clinician to monitor blood glucose level.
*Antipsychotics, erythromycin, tricyclic antidepressants:* Possible prolonged QTc interval. Use drug cautiously.
*Class IA antiarrhythmics (procainamide, quinidine), class III antiarrhythmics (amiodarone, sotalol):* Potential for prolonged QTc interval. Avoid use together.
*Digoxin:* Possible increase in digoxin levels. Recommend watching for signs of digoxin toxicity.
*NSAIDs:* Increased risk of CNS stimulation and seizures. Use together cautiously.
*Probenecid:* Increased gatifloxacin levels and prolonged half-life. Advise clinician to monitor patient closely for adverse reactions.
*Warfarin:* Possible enhanced effects of warfarin. Advise clinician to monitor PT and INR.
**Drug-lifestyle.** *Sun exposure:* Photosensitivity reactions may occur. Urge patient to take precautions.

## Adverse reactions
**CNS:** headache, dizziness, abnormal dreams, insomnia, paresthesia, tremor, vertigo.
**CV:** palpitations, chest pain.
**EENT:** tinnitus, abnormal vision, pharyngitis.
**GI:** nausea, diarrhea, abdominal pain, constipation, dyspepsia, oral candidiasis, glossitis, stomatitis, mouth ulcer, vomiting, taste perversion.
**GU:** dysuria, hematuria, vaginitis.
**Musculoskeletal:** back pain.
**Respiratory:** dyspnea.
**Skin:** rash, sweating.
**Other:** allergic reaction, redness at injection site, chills, fever, peripheral edema.

## Overdose and treatment
Signs of overdose include decreased respiratory rate, vomiting, tremors, and convulsions.

To treat an overdose of oral gatifloxacin, recommend emptying the stomach by inducing vomiting or performing gastric lavage. Recommend providing symptomatic and supportive treatment, monitoring ECG, and maintaining hydration. Gatifloxacin is not removed by hemodialysis or peritoneal dialysis.

## Clinical considerations

■ In patients being treated for gonorrhea, recommend testing for syphilis at time of diagnosis.
■ Pseudomembranous colitis may occur in patients taking antibiotics.
■ Recommend stopping drug if patient experiences seizures, increased intracranial pressure, psychosis, or CNS stimulation leading to tremors, restlessness, light-headedness, confusion, hallucinations, paranoia, depression, nightmares, and insomnia.
■ Recommend stopping drug if patient experiences pain, inflammation, or rupture of a tendon.
■ Recommend stopping drug for skin rash or other sign of hypersensitivity.

### Therapeutic monitoring

■ Advise clinician to monitor glucose levels in patients with diabetes.
■ Advise clinician to monitor patients receiving digoxin for signs and symptoms of digoxin toxicity.
■ Advise clinician to monitor kidney function in patients with renal insufficiency.

### Special populations

**Breast-feeding patients.** It isn't known if gatifloxacin appears in breast milk. Use cautiously when giving gatifloxacin to a breast-feeding woman.
**Pediatric patients.** Safety and effectiveness of gatifloxacin have not been established in patients under age 18.
**Geriatric patients.** No dosage adjustment is needed based on age.

## Patient counseling

■ Tell patient to take drug as prescribed and to finish all of it even if symptoms disappear.
■ Advise patient to take drug 4 hours before intake of products that contain aluminum, magnesium, zinc, or iron.
■ Urge patient to use sunblock and to wear protective clothing when exposed to excessive sunlight.
■ Warn patient to avoid hazardous tasks until adverse CNS effects of drugs are known.
■ Advise diabetic patient to monitor glucose levels and notify prescriber if hypoglycemia occurs.
■ Urge patient to immediately report symptoms of allergic reaction, such as palpitations, fainting spells, rash, hives, difficulty swallowing or breathing, tightness in throat, hoarseness, and swelling of the lips, tongue, or face.
■ Advise patient to stop drug, refrain from exercise, and notify prescriber if pain, inflammation, or rupture of a tendon occurs.

# gemcitabine hydrochloride
Gemzar

*Pharmacologic classification:* nucleoside analogue
*Therapeutic classification:* antitumor
*Pregnancy risk category D*

## Available forms

Available by prescription only
*Powder for injection:* 200-mg/10 ml, 1-g/50 ml vials

## Indications and dosages

*Locally advanced (nonresectable stage II or stage III) or metastatic pancreatic adenocarcinoma (stage IV) and in patients previously treated with fluorouracil*
*Adults:* 1,000 mg/m² I.V. over 30 minutes once weekly for up to 7 weeks or until toxicity necessitates reducing or holding a dose. Treatment course of 7 weeks is followed by 1 week rest. Subsequent dosage cycles consist of one infusion weekly for 3 out of 4 consecutive weeks.
≡*Dosage adjustment.* Adjust dosage if bone marrow suppression is detected. Give full dose if absolute granulocyte count (AGC) is 1,000/mm³ or more and platelet count is 100,000/mm³ or more. If AGC is 500/mm³ to 999/mm³, or if platelet count is 50,000/mm³ to 99,000/mm³, give 75% of dose. Hold dose if AGC is less than 500/mm³ or platelet count is less than 50,000/mm³. Adjust dosage for subsequent cycles based on AGC and platelet count nadirs and degree of nonhematologic toxicity.
*Advanced non–small-cell lung cancer*
*Adults:* 1,000 mg/m² I.V. over 30 minutes once weekly for up to 7 weeks or until toxicity necessitates reducing or holding a dose. Treatment course of 7 weeks is followed by 1 week rest. Subsequent dosage cycles consist of one infusion weekly for 3 out of 4 consecutive weeks.
*Inoperable, locally advanced (stage IIIA or IIIB) or metastatic (stage IV) non–small-cell lung carcinoma as initial treatment with cisplatin*
**4-week schedule**
*Adults:* 1,000 mg/m² I.V. over 30 minutes on days 1, 8, and 15 of each 28-day cycle. Cisplatin is given on day 1 after gemcitabine administration is completed.
**3-week schedule**
*Adults:* 1,250 mg/m² I.V. over 30 minutes on days 1 and 8 of each 21-day cycle. Cisplatin is given on day 1 after gemcitabine administration is completed.
≡*Dosage adjustment.* When used with cisplatin, reduce dosage by 50% in the occurrence of severe nonhematologic toxicity.

◇*Advanced or metastatic bladder cancer*
*Adults:* 1,200 mg/m² to 1,250 mg/m² I.V. over 30 minutes, once a week for 3 weeks of a 4-week cycle.

## I.V. administration
**⊞ ALERT** Preparation and administration of parenteral form of drug may cause mutagenic, teratogenic, and carcinogenic risks for personnel.
▪ Vials containing 200 mg or 1 g of drug should be reconstituted with 5 or 25 ml, respectively, of normal saline solution and shaken to dissolve.
▪ The reconstituted solutions can be infused without further dilution, or as solutions that have been further diluted with normal saline solution to concentrations as low as 0.1 mg/ml.
▪ Infuse drug over 30 minutes.
▪ Reconstituted drug is stable for 24 hours at controlled room temperatures of 68° to 77° F (20° to 25° C).

### Incompatibilities
None reported.

## Mechanism of action
*Cytotoxic action:* Drug is cell-phase specific; it inhibits DNA synthesis and blocks progression of cells through G1/S-phase boundary.

## Pharmacokinetics
*Absorption:* Administered I.V.
*Distribution:* Volume of distribution ($V_d$) increases with increased infusion time. After an infusion lasting under 70 minutes, $V_d$ was 50 L/m², suggesting that drug isn't extensively distributed. The $V_d$ increased to 370 L/m² for longer infusions, reflecting slow equilibration of gemcitabine with the tissue compartment. Plasma protein–binding is negligible. Longer infusion time results in longer drug half-life.
*Metabolism:* Metabolized to an inactive uracil metabolite.
*Excretion:* Drug clearance decreases with increasing age; it's also less efficient in women than men. This results in an increased half-life with increased age and in women. A total of 92% to 98% of drug has been recovered almost entirely in urine.

| Route | Onset | Peak | Duration |
|-------|-------|------|----------|
| I.V. | Unknown | Unknown | Unknown |

## Contraindications and precautions
Contraindicated in patients hypersensitive to drug.

## Interactions
None reported.

## Adverse reactions
**CNS:** *paresthesia, somnolence.*
**CV:** *edema, peripheral edema.*
**GI:** *constipation, diarrhea, nausea, stomatitis, vomiting.*
**GU:** *elevated BUN* and creatinine, *hematuria, proteinuria.*
**Hematologic:** *anemia,* LEUKOPENIA, NEUTROPENIA, THROMBOCYTOPENIA, HEMORRHAGE.
**Hepatic:** *elevated liver enzyme levels.*
**Respiratory:** *bronchospasm, dyspnea.*
**Skin:** *alopecia, rash.*
**Other:** *fever, flulike symptoms,* INFECTION, *pain.*

## Overdose and treatment
There's no known antidote for drug overdose. If overdose is suspected, advise clinician to monitor patient with appropriate blood counts and provide supportive therapy.

## Clinical considerations
▪ Prolongation of infusion time beyond 60 minutes and dosing more frequent than weekly have been shown to increase drug toxicity.
▪ Age, gender, and renal impairment may predispose patient to toxicity.
▪ Exercise caution when drug is used for patients with renal and hepatic impairment.
▪ Drug is currently being investigated for treatment of advanced epithelial ovarian cancer.

### Therapeutic monitoring
▪ Advise clinician to monitor renal and hepatic function test results before treatment and periodically thereafter.
▪ Advise clinician to monitor CBC, differential, and platelet count before giving each dose. Drug can suppress bone marrow function as manifested by leukopenia, thrombocytopenia, and anemia.
▪ When drug is used with cisplatin, advise clinician to monitor levels of creatinine, potassium, calcium, and magnesium.

### Special populations
**Breast-feeding patients.** It's unknown if drug appears in breast milk. Avoid use in breast-feeding women.
**Pediatric patients.** Drug hasn't been studied in pediatric patients.
**Geriatric patients.** Drug clearance is affected by age; however, dosage adjustment isn't indicated.

## Patient counseling
▪ Advise patient to take temperature daily and to watch for signs of infection (fever, sore throat, fatigue) and bleeding (easy bruising, nosebleeds, bleeding gums, melena).

---

# gemfibrozil
Lopid

*Pharmacologic classification:* fibric acid derivative
*Therapeutic classification:* antilipemic
*Pregnancy risk category C*

## Available forms
Available by prescription only
*Tablets:* 600 mg

## Indications and dosages
**Type IV hyperlipidemia (hypertriglyceridemia) and severe hypercholesterolemia unresponsive to diet and other drugs; reduction of risk for cardiac disease, only in type IIb patients without history of disease**
*Adults:* 1,200 mg P.O. given in two divided doses 30 minutes before morning and evening meals.

## Mechanism of action
*Antilipemic action:* Gemfibrozil decreases serum triglyceride levels and very-low-density lipoprotein (VLDL) cholesterol while increasing serum high-density lipoprotein cholesterol, inhibits lipolysis in adipose tissue, and reduces hepatic triglyceride synthesis. Drug is closely related to clofibrate pharmacologically.

## Pharmacokinetics
*Absorption:* Well absorbed from GI tract. Plasma levels of VLDL decrease in 2 to 5 days with decreases in plasma VLDL levels occurring over several months.
*Distribution:* 95% protein-bound.
*Metabolism:* Metabolized by the liver.
*Excretion:* Eliminated mostly in urine but some is excreted in feces. After a single dose, half-life is 1½ hours; after multiple doses, half-life decreases to about 1⅓-1½ hours.

| Route | Onset | Peak | Duration |
|-------|-------|------|----------|
| P.O. | 2-5 days | 4 wk | Unknown |

## Contraindications and precautions
Contraindicated in patients hypersensitive to drug and those with hepatic or severe renal dysfunction (including primary biliary cirrhosis) and preexisting gallbladder disease.

## Interactions
**Drug-drug.** *Oral anticoagulants:* Enhanced effect of oral anticoagulants, increasing risk of hemorrhage. Recommend adjusting anticoagulant dose to maintain the desired PT and INR, and monitoring patient frequently.
*Atorvastatin, fluvastatin, lovastatin, pravastatin, simvastatin:* Myopathy with rhabdomyolysis can occur. Avoid use together.

## Adverse reactions
**CNS:** headache, fatigue, vertigo.
**CV:** atrial fibrillation.
**GI:** abdominal and epigastric pain, diarrhea, nausea, vomiting, *dyspepsia,* constipation, acute appendicitis.
**Hematologic:** anemia, *leukopenia,* eosinophilia, *thrombocytopenia.*
**Hepatic:** bile duct obstruction, elevated liver enzyme levels.
**Metabolic:** hypokalemia.
**Skin:** rash, dermatitis, pruritus, eczema.

## Overdose and treatment
In overdose, recommend immediately inducing emesis or starting gastric lavage.

## Clinical considerations
■ Because drug is pharmacologically related to clofibrate, adverse reactions from clofibrate may also occur with gemfibrozil. Some studies suggest clofibrate increases risk of death from cancer, postcholecystectomy complications, and pancreatitis. These hazards haven't been studied in gemfibrozil, however.
■ Before gemifibrozil therapy starts, treatment through behavioral changes (diet and exercise), as well as identification and treatment of possible underlying causes of hyperlipoproteinemia, should be aggressively attempted.
■ American College of Cardiology and American Heart Association recommend initiation of antilipemic therapy (with other drugs) for the treatment of chronic stable angina in patients with suspected or documented HF and LDL-C greater than 130 mg/dl. This is an unlabeled use.

### Therapeutic monitoring
■ Advise clinician to monitor lipoprotein levels regularly; recommend stopping drug if a substantial lipid response isn't obtained.

### Special populations
**Breast-feeding patients.** Safety in breast-feeding women hasn't been established.
**Pediatric patients.** Safety and efficacy in children under age 18 haven't been established.

## Patient counseling
■ Instruct patient to report adverse reactions promptly and to comply with prescribed regimen, diet, and exercise.
■ Warn patient not to exceed prescribed dose.

# gemtuzumab ozogamicin
Mylotarg

*Pharmacologic classification:* antibody–cytotoxic antitumor antibiotic conjugate
*Therapeutic classification:* chemotherapeutic
*Pregnancy risk category D*

## Available forms
Available by prescription only
*Powder for injection:* 5 mg

## Indications and dosages
**Treatment of patients with CD33-positive acute myeloid leukemia in first relapse and who are not considered candidates for cytotoxic chemotherapy**
Adults ages 60 and older: 9 mg/m$^2$ I.V. infusion over 2 hours every 14 days for a total of two doses. Premedicate with diphenhydramine 50 mg P.O. and acetaminophen 650 to 1,000 mg P.O. 1 hour before infusion.

## I.V. administration
**✋ALERT** Drug is light sensitive and must be protected from direct and indirect sunlight and unshielded fluorescent light during preparation and administration of the infusion.
■ Give in 100 ml of saline solution injection. Place the 100-ml I.V. bag into an ultraviolet-protectant bag. The resulting drug solution in the I.V. bag should be used immediately.
■ A separate I.V. line equipped with a low–protein-binding 1.2-micron terminal filter must be used to administer drug. May be infused by central or peripheral line.
**✋ALERT** Don't give as an I.V. push or bolus.

### Incompatibilities
None reported.

## Mechanism of action
*CD33-binding action:* Thought to bind to the CD33 antigen expressed on the surface of leukemic blasts in more than 80% of patients with acute myeloid leukemia. This results in formation of a complex that is internalized by the cell. The calicheamicin derivative is then released inside the cell, causing DNA double-strand breaks and cell death.

## Pharmacokinetics
*Absorption:* Administered I.V.
*Distribution:* Unknown.
*Metabolism:* Unknown. Studies suggest that liver microsomal enzymes are involved.
*Excretion:* The elimination half-lives of total and unconjugated calicheamicin are about 45 and 100 hours, respectively, after the first dose. After the second dose, the elimination half-life of total calicheamicin is increased to 60 hours.

| Route | Onset | Peak | Duration |
|-------|-------|------|----------|
| I.V. | Unknown | Unknown | Unknown |

## Contraindications and precautions
Contraindicated in patients hypersensitive to gemtuzumab ozogamicin or any of its components.
    Use drug cautiously in patients with hepatic impairment.

## Interactions
None known.

## Adverse reactions
**CNS:** *asthenia, depression, dizziness, headache, insomnia.*
**CV:** *hypertension, hypotension, tachycardia, peripheral edema.*
**EENT:** *epistaxis, pharyngitis, rhinitis.*
**GI:** *enlarged abdomen, abdominal pain, anorexia, constipation, diarrhea, dyspepsia, nausea, stomatitis, vomiting.*
**GU:** *hematuria, vaginal hemorrhage.*
**Hematologic:** *ecchymoses, anemia,* HEMORRHAGE, LEUKOPENIA, NEUTROPENIA, THROMBOCYTOPENIA.
**Hepatic:** *hepatotoxicity, increased liver enzyme levels.*
**Metabolic:** *hyperglycemia, hypokalemia, hypomagnesemia, increased LDH level.*
**Musculoskeletal:** *arthralgia, back pain.*
**Respiratory:** *increased cough, dyspnea,* **hypoxia,** *pneumonia.*
**Skin:** *local reaction, petechiae, rash.*
**Other:** *herpes simplex, chills, fever, pain,* NEUTROPENIC FEVER, SEPSIS.

## Overdose and treatment
Signs and symptoms of overdose are unknown. Provide general supportive measures in case of overdose. Blood pressure and blood counts should be carefully monitored. Gemtuzumab isn't dialyzable.

## Clinical considerations
■ Drug should be used only under the supervision of a clinician experienced in the use of chemotherapy drugs.
■ Gemtuzumab can produce a postinfusion symptom complex of chills, fever, hypotension, hypertension, hyperglycemia, hypoxia, and dyspnea that may occur during the first 24 hours after administration.
■ Recommend premedicating with diphenhydramine and acetaminophen. Additional doses of acetaminophen 650 to 1,000 mg P.O. can be given every 4 hours p.r.n.
■ Tumor lysis syndrome may occur. Recommend providing adequate hydration and treating with allopurinol to prevent hyperuricemia.

## Therapeutic monitoring

■ Advise clinician to monitor vital signs during infusion and for 4 hours after infusion.
■ Severe myelosuppression will occur in all patients given the recommended dose of this drug. Careful hematologic monitoring is required.
■ Advise clinician to monitor electrolytes, hepatic function, CBC, and platelets during therapy.

## Special populations

**Breast-feeding patients.** It isn't known if gemtuzumab ozogamicin appears in breast milk. Because of the potential for serious adverse reactions in nursing infants, a decision should be made whether to discontinue nursing or to discontinue drug, taking into account the importance of the drug to the mother.
**Pediatric patients.** Safety and effectiveness haven't been established.

## Patient counseling

■ Advise patient about postinfusion symptoms. Tell patient to continue taking acetaminophen 650 to 1,000 mg every 4 hours p.r.n.
■ Advise patient to watch for signs of infection, including fever, sore throat, fatigue, and bleeding (easy bruising, nosebleeds, bleeding gums, and melena). Tell patient to take temperature daily.

# gentamicin sulfate

Cidomycin*, Garamycin, Genoptic, Genoptic S.O.P., Gentacidin, Gentafair, Gentak, Gentasol, Jenamicin

*Pharmacologic classification:* aminoglycoside
*Therapeutic classification:* antibiotic
*Pregnancy risk category NR*

## Available forms

Available by prescription only
*Injection:* 40 mg/ml (adult), 10 mg/ml (pediatric), 2 mg/ml (intrathecal)
*Ophthalmic ointment:* 3 mg/g
*Ophthalmic solution:* 3 mg/ml
*Topical cream or ointment:* 0.1%

## Indications and dosages

*Serious infections caused by susceptible organisms*
*Adults with normal renal function:* 3 mg/kg/day I.M. or I.V. infusion (in 50 to 100 ml of normal saline solution or D₅W infused over 30 minutes to 2 hours) daily in divided doses q 8 hours. May be given by direct I.V. push if needed. For life-threatening infections, patient may receive up to 5 mg/kg/day in three to four divided doses.
*Children with normal renal function:* 2 to 2.5 mg/kg I.M. or I.V. infusion q 8 hours.

*Infants and neonates over age 1 week with normal renal function:* 2.5 mg/kg I.M. or I.V. infusion q 8 hours.
*Neonates under age 1 week:* 2.5 mg/kg I.M. or I.V. infusion q 12 hours. For I.V. infusion, dilute in normal saline solution or D₅W and infuse over 30 minutes to 2 hours.
*Meningitis*
*Adults:* Systemic therapy as previously noted for serious infections; may also use 4 to 8 mg intrathecally daily.
*Children:* Systemic therapy as previously noted for serious infections; may also use 1 to 2 mg intrathecally daily.
*Endocarditis prophylaxis for GI or GU procedure or surgery*
*Adults:* 1.5 mg/kg I.M. or I.V. 30 to 60 minutes before procedure or surgery and q 8 hours after, for two doses. Give separately with aqueous penicillin G or ampicillin.
*Children:* 2 mg/kg I.M. or I.V. 30 to 60 minutes before procedure or surgery and q 8 hours after, for two doses. Give separately with aqueous penicillin G or ampicillin.
*External ocular infections caused by susceptible organisms*
*Adults and children:* Instill 1 to 2 drops in eye q 4 hours. In severe infections, may use up to 2 drops q hour. Apply ointment to lower conjunctival sac b.i.d. or t.i.d.
*Primary and secondary bacterial infections; superficial burns; skin ulcers; and infected lacerations, abrasions, insect bites, or minor surgical wounds*
*Adults and children over age 1:* Rub in small amount gently t.i.d. or q.i.d., with or without gauze dressing.
*Pelvic inflammatory disease*
*Adults:* Initially, 2 mg/kg I.M. or I.V.; then 1.5 mg/kg q 8 hours.
≡*Dosage adjustment.* In patients with renal failure, initial dose is same as for those with normal renal function. Subsequent doses and frequency determined by renal function studies and blood levels; keep peak serum levels at between 4 and 10 mcg/ml and trough serum levels at between 1 and 2 mcg/ml. One method is to give 1-mg/kg doses and adjust the dosing interval based on steady-state serum creatinine, using the following formula:

$$\frac{\text{Creatinine}}{\text{(mg/100 ml)}} \times 8 = \frac{\text{dosing interval}}{\text{(hours)}}$$

*Posthemodialysis to maintain therapeutic blood levels*
*Adults:* 1 to 1.7 mg/kg I.M. or I.V. infusion after each dialysis.
*Children:* 2 to 2.5 mg/kg I.M. or I.V. infusion after each dialysis.

## I.V. administration

■ For adults, the dosage should be diluted in 50 to 200 ml of normal saline solution or D₅W and should be infused over 30 minutes to 2 hours.

■ For pediatric patients, the volume for dilution depends on the needs of the patient, but it should allow for an infusion period of 30 minutes to 2 hours.

## Incompatibilities

Incompatible with ampicillin, cefazolin, cefuroxime, cephapirin, cytarabine, dopamine, fat emulsions, furosemide, heparin, hetastarch, idarubicin, nafcillin, certain parenteral nutrition formulations, and ticarcillin. Manufacturer recommends not mixing gentamicin with other drugs.

## Mechanism of action

*Antibiotic action:* Gentamicin is bactericidal; it binds directly to the 30S ribosomal subunit, thus inhibiting bacterial protein synthesis. Its spectrum of activity includes many aerobic gram-negative organisms (including most strains of *Pseudomonas aeruginosa*) and some aerobic gram-positive organisms. Gentamicin may act against some bacterial strains resistant to other aminoglycosides; bacterial strains resistant to gentamicin may be susceptible to tobramycin, netilmicin, or amikacin.

## Pharmacokinetics

*Absorption:* Absorbed poorly after oral administration.

*Distribution:* Distributed widely after parenteral administration; intraocular penetration is poor. CSF penetration is low even in patients with inflamed meninges. Intraventricular administration produces high levels throughout the CNS. Protein-binding is minimal. Gentamicin crosses the placenta.

*Metabolism:* Not metabolized.

*Excretion:* Excreted primarily in urine by glomerular filtration; small amounts may be excreted in bile and appear in breast milk. Drug's elimination half-life in adults is 2 to 3 hours. In patients with severe renal damage, half-life may extend to 24 to 60 hours.

| Route | Onset | Peak | Duration |
|---|---|---|---|
| I.V. | Immediate | 30-90 min | Unknown |
| I.M. | Unknown | 30-90 min | Unknown |
| Intrathecal | Unknown | Unknown | Unknown |
| Topical | Unknown | Unknown | Unknown |
| Ophthalmic | Unknown | Unknown | Unknown |

## Contraindications and precautions

Contraindicated in patients hypersensitive to drug or in those who may exhibit cross-sensitivity with other aminoglycosides such as neomycin.

Systemic treatment should be used cautiously in neonates, infants, geriatric patients, or patients with renal or neuromuscular disorders.

## Interactions

*Drug-drug. Acyclovir, amphotericin B, capreomycin, cephalosporins, cisplatin, methoxyflurane, other aminoglycosides, polymyxin B, vancomycin:* May increase the hazard of nephrotoxicity, ototoxicity, or neurotoxicity. Use together cautiously.

*Bumetanide, ethacrynic acid, furosemide, mannitol, urea:* Increased hazard of ototoxicity. Use cautiously.

*Dimenhydrinate, other antiemetic and antivertigo drugs:* May mask gentamicin-induced ototoxicity. Use with caution.

*General anesthetics or neuromuscular blockers (such as succinylcholine and tubocurarine):* Increased neuromuscular blockade. Advise clinician to monitor patient closely.

*Indomethacin:* Increased serum peak and trough levels of gentamicin. Advise clinician to monitor gentamicin levels closely.

*Penicillin:* Results in synergistic bactericidal effect against *P. aeruginosa, Escherichia coli, Klebsiella, Citrobacter, Enterobacter, Serratia,* and *Proteus mirabilis;* however, the drugs are physically and chemically incompatible and are inactivated when mixed or given together. Don't mix drugs together.

## Adverse reactions

**CNS:** headache, lethargy, encephalopathy, confusion, dizziness, *seizures,* numbness, peripheral neuropathy (with injected form).
**CV:** hypotension (with injected form).
**EENT:** *ototoxicity,* blurred vision (with injected form); burning, stinging, blurred vision (with ophthalmic ointment), transient irritation (with ophthalmic solution), conjunctival hyperemia (with ophthalmic form).
**GI:** vomiting, nausea (with injected form).
**GU:** *nephrotoxicity* (with injected form).
**Hematologic:** anemia, eosinophilia, *leukopenia, thrombocytopenia, granulocytopenia* (with injected form).
**Musculoskeletal:** muscle twitching, myasthenia gravis-like syndrome.
**Respiratory:** *apnea* (with injected form).
**Skin:** rash, urticaria, pruritus, tingling (with injected form); minor skin irritation, possible photosensitivity, allergic contact dermatitis (with topical administration).
**Other:** fever, *anaphylaxis,* pain at injection site (with injected form); hypersensitivity reactions, overgrowth of nonsusceptible organisms (with ophthalmic form and long-term use).

Note: Systemic absorption from excessive use may cause systemic toxicities.

## Overdose and treatment

Signs of overdose include ototoxicity, nephrotoxicity, and neuromuscular toxicity. Drug can be removed by hemodialysis or peritoneal dialysis. Treatment with calcium salts or anticholinesterases reverses neuromuscular blockade.

## Clinical considerations

**⛔ ALERT** Use preservative-free formulations when intrathecal route is ordered.

■ Because drug is dializable, patients undergoing hemodialysis may need dosage adjustments.

### Therapeutic monitoring

■ Increased risk of toxicity may occur with prolonged peak serum level of more than 10 mcg/ml and trough serum level of more than 2 mcg/ml.

### Patient counseling

■ Inform patient of the proper administration technique.

■ Instruct patient to promptly report to prescriber if lesions worsen or skin irritation occurs.

---

# glimepiride

Amaryl

*Pharmacologic classification:* sulfonylurea
*Therapeutic classification:* antidiabetic
*Pregnancy risk category C*

## Available forms

Available by prescription only
*Tablets:* 1 mg, 2 mg, 4 mg

## Indications and dosages

*Adjunct to diet and exercise to lower blood glucose level in patients with type 2 (non–insulin-dependent) diabetes mellitus whose hyperglycemia can't be managed by diet and exercise alone*

*Adults:* Initially, 1 to 2 mg P.O. once daily with first main meal of the day; usual maintenance dose is 1 to 4 mg P.O. once daily. Maximum recommended dose is 8 mg once daily. After dose of 2 mg is reached, increase dosage in increments not exceeding 2 mg at 1- to 2-week intervals based on patient's blood glucose response.

*Adjunct to insulin therapy in patients with type 2 (non–insulin-dependent) diabetes mellitus whose hyperglycemia can't be managed by diet and exercise in conjunction with an oral hypoglycemic drug*

*Adults:* 8 mg P.O. once daily with first main meal of the day with low-dose insulin. Upward adjustments of insulin should be made weekly p.r.n. and guided by patient's blood glucose response.

*Adjunct to metformin therapy in patients with type 2 (non–insulin-dependent) diabetes mellitus whose hyperglycemia can't be managed by diet, exercise, and glimepiride or metformin alone*

*Adults:* 8 mg P.O. once daily with first main meal of the day, with metformin if patient doesn't respond adequately to glimepiride monotherapy. Adjust dosages based on patient's blood glucose response to determine minimum effective dosage of each drug.

**≡ Dosage adjustment.** Patients with renal impairment require cautious dosing. Give 1 mg P.O. once daily with first main meal of the day, followed by appropriate dosage adjustment p.r.n.

## Mechanism of action

*Antidiabetic action:* Exact mechanism of glimepiride to lower blood glucose level appears to depend on stimulating the release of insulin from functioning pancreatic beta cells. Also, drug can lead to increased sensitivity of peripheral tissues to insulin.

## Pharmacokinetics

*Absorption:* Completely absorbed from the GI tract.
*Distribution:* Protein-binding is greater than 99.5%.
*Metabolism:* Completely metabolized by oxidative biotransformation.
*Excretion:* Metabolites are excreted in urine (about 60%) and feces (about 40%).

| Route | Onset | Peak | Duration |
|-------|-------|------|----------|
| P.O. | Unknown | 2-3 hr | > 24 hr |

## Contraindications and precautions

Contraindicated in patients hypersensitive to drug and in those with diabetic ketoacidosis (with or without coma) because this condition should be treated with insulin. Recommend that prescriber use cautiously in debilitated or malnourished patients and in those with adrenal, pituitary, hepatic, or renal insufficiency because these patients are more susceptible to the hypoglycemic action of glucose-lowering drugs.

## Interactions

**Drug-drug.** *Beta blockers:* May mask symptoms of hypoglycemia. Advise clinician to monitor patient carefully.

*Corticosteroids, estrogens, isoniazid, nicotinic acid, oral contraceptives, phenothiazines, phenytoin, sympathomimetics, thiazides and other diuretics, and thyroid hormones:* Tend to produce hyperglycemia. May require dosage adjustment.

*Insulin:* Increased potential for hypoglycemia. May require dosage adjustment.

*NSAIDs and other drugs that are highly protein-bound, such as beta blockers, chloramphenicol, coumarins, MAO inhibitors, probenecid, salicylates, and sulfonamides:* May potentiate the hypoglycemic action of sulfonylureas such as glimepiride. May require dosage adjustment.

**Drug-herb.** *Aloe, bilberry leaf, bitter melon, burdock, dandelion, fenugreek, garlic, and ginseng:* Use together may improve blood sugar control, requiring a reduction of antidiabetics.

---

Advise patient to discuss the use of herbal medicines with his prescriber before use.

**Drug-lifestyle.** *Alcohol use:* Alters glycemic control, most commonly hypoglycemia. May also cause disulfiram-like reaction. Advise patient to avoid alcohol.

## Adverse reactions

**CNS:** dizziness, asthenia, headache.
**EENT:** changes in accommodation, blurred vision.
**GI:** vomiting, abdominal pain, nausea, diarrhea.
**Hematologic:** *leukopenia,* hemolytic anemia, *agranulocytosis, thrombocytopenia, aplastic anemia, pancytopenia.*
**Hepatic:** cholestatic jaundice, elevated transaminase levels.
**Metabolic:** hypoglycemia.
**Skin:** allergic skin reactions (pruritus, erythema, urticaria, morbilliform or maculopapular eruptions).

## Overdose and treatment

Overdose of sulfonylureas may produce hypoglycemia. Mild hypoglycemic symptoms without loss of consciousness or neurologic findings should be treated aggressively with oral glucose and adjustments in drug dosage and meal patterns. Advise clinician to monitor patient closely until he's out of danger.

Severe hypoglycemic reactions with coma, seizure, or other neurologic impairment occur infrequently but constitute medical emergencies requiring immediate hospitalization. If hypoglycemic coma occurs or is suspected, recommend giving a rapid I.V. injection of concentrated (50%) glucose solution followed by continuous infusion of a more dilute (10%) glucose solution at a rate that will maintain the blood glucose at a level of more than 100 mg/dl. Advise clinician to monitor patient closely for at least 24 to 48 hours because hypoglycemia may recur after apparent clinical recovery.

## Clinical considerations

■ In geriatric, debilitated, or malnourished patients or in patients with renal or hepatic insufficiency, the initial dosing, dose increments, and maintenance dose should be conservative to avoid hypoglycemic reactions.
■ Oral hypoglycemic drugs have been linked to an increased risk of CV mortality compared with diet or diet and insulin therapy.

### Therapeutic monitoring

■ Advise clinician to monitor fasting blood glucose level periodically to determine therapeutic response. Also advise clinician to monitor glycosylated hemoglobin, usually every 3 to 6 months, to more precisely assess long-term glycemic control.
■ During maintenance therapy, discontinue glimepiride if satisfactory lowering of blood glucose level is no longer achieved. Secondary failures to glimepiride monotherapy can be treated with glimepiride-insulin combination therapy.

### Special populations

**Breast-feeding patients.** It's unknown if drug appears in breast milk. Because of the potential for hypoglycemia in nursing infants, drug shouldn't be given to breast-feeding women.
**Pediatric patients.** Safety and efficacy in children haven't been established.
**Geriatric patients.** Geriatric patients may be more sensitive to the effects of drug because of reduced metabolism and elimination.

## Patient counseling

■ Instruct patient to take drug with first meal of the day.
■ Make sure patient understands that therapy relieves symptoms but doesn't cure disease.
■ Stress importance of adhering to specific diet, weight-reduction, exercise, and personal hygiene programs. Explain how and when to perform self-monitoring of glucose level.
■ Teach patient how to recognize and manage signs and symptoms of hyperglycemia and hypoglycemia.
■ Advise patient to carry medical identification regarding diabetic status.

# glipizide

Glucotrol, Glucotrol XL

*Pharmacologic classification:* sulfonylurea
*Therapeutic classification:* antidiabetic
*Pregnancy risk category C*

## Available forms

Available by prescription only
*Tablets:* 5 mg, 10 mg
*Tablets (extended-release):* 2.5 mg, 5 mg, 10 mg

## Indications and dosages

*Adjunct to diet to lower blood glucose levels in patients with type 2 (non–insulin-dependent) diabetes mellitus*
*Adults:* Initially, 5 mg P.O. daily 30 minutes before breakfast; adjust dosage in increments of 2.5 to 5 mg. Usual maintenance dose is 10 to 15 mg daily. Maximum recommended daily dose is 40 mg. Divide total daily doses of more than 15 mg except when using extended-release tablets.
≡ *Dosage adjustment.* Initial dose in geriatric patients or those with hepatic disease may be 2.5 mg.
**Extended-release tablets**
*Adults:* Initially, 5 mg P.O. daily. May increase to 10 mg after 3 months based on glycosylated hemoglobin measurement. Subsequent

dosage adjustments should be based on glycosylated hemoglobin measurements at 3-month intervals. If no response after 3 months on higher dose, previous dose should be resumed. Maximum daily dose is 20 mg.

*To replace insulin therapy*

*Adults:* If insulin dose is more than 20 units daily, patient may be started at usual dose of glipizide plus 50% of insulin dosage. If insulin dose is less than 20 units, insulin may be stopped.

## Mechanism of action

*Antidiabetic action:* Glipizide decreases blood glucose levels by stimulating insulin release from functioning beta cells in the pancreas. After prolonged administration, the hypoglycemic effects of the drug appear to reflect extrapancreatic effects, possibly including reduction of basal hepatic glucose production and enhanced peripheral sensitivity to insulin.

## Pharmacokinetics

*Absorption:* Absorbed rapidly and completely from the GI tract.

*Distribution:* Probably distributed within the extracellular fluid. It's about 92% to 99% protein-bound.

*Metabolism:* Metabolized almost completely by the liver to inactive metabolites.

*Excretion:* Excreted primarily in urine; small amounts are excreted in feces. Renal clearance of unchanged glipizide increases with increasing urinary pH. Duration of action is 10 to 24 hours; half-life is 2 to 4 hours.

| Route | Onset | Peak | Duration |
|-------|-------|------|----------|
| P.O. | 15-30 min | 1-3 hr | 4 hr |
| P.O. (extended-release) | 2-3 hr | 6-12 hr | 24 hr |

## Contraindications and precautions

Contraindicated in patients hypersensitive to drug or with diabetic ketoacidosis with or without coma, and during pregnancy or breast-feeding.

Use drug cautiously in patients with impaired renal or hepatic function and in geriatric, malnourished, or debilitated patients.

## Interactions

**Drug-drug.** *Adrenocorticoids, amphetamines, baclofen, corticotropin, epinephrine, estrogens, ethacrynic acid, furosemide, glucocorticoids, oral contraceptives, phenytoin, thiazide diuretics, thyroid hormones, triamterene:* May increase glucose levels. Dosage adjustments may be needed.

*Anabolic steroids, chloramphenicol, clofibrate, guanethidine, insulin, MAO inhibitors, probenecid, salicylates, sulfonamides:* Enhanced hypoglycemic effect by displacing glipizide from protein-binding sites. Advise clinician to monitor patient.

*Anticoagulants:* Increased plasma levels of both drugs and, after continued therapy, may reduce plasma levels and effectiveness of the anticoagulant. Advise clinician to monitor patient carefully.

*Antifungal antibiotics, such as fluconazole, miconazole:* Increased plasma levels of glipizide and hypoglycemia. Advise clinician to monitor patient.

*Beta blockers, including ophthalmics:* May mask symptoms of hypoglycemia. Advise clinician to monitor and observe patient closely.

*Cimetidine:* Potentiates hypoglycemic effects by preventing hepatic metabolism. Advise clinician to monitor patient closely.

*Corticosteroids, glucagon, rifampin, thiazide diuretics:* May decrease hypoglycemic response. Advise clinician to monitor patient closely.

*Hydantoins:* Increased blood levels of hydantoins. Advise clinician to monitor levels.

**Drug-herb.** *Aloe, bilberry leaf, bitter melon, burdock, dandelion, fenugreek, garlic, and ginseng:* Use together may improve blood sugar control, requiring a reduction of antidiabetic drugs. Advise patient to discuss the use of herbal medicines with his prescriber before use.

**Drug-lifestyle.** *Alcohol use:* Altered glycemic control. May also cause a disulfiram-like reaction. Advise patient to avoid alcohol.

*Smoking:* Increased corticosteroid release, requiring higher dosages. Discourage smoking.

## Adverse reactions

**CNS:** *asthenia,* dizziness, drowsiness, headache, pain, tremor, nervousness, insomnia, anxiety, depression, hypesthesia, paresthesia.

**GI:** nausea, constipation, diarrhea, flatulence, dyspepsia, vomiting.

**GU:** altered BUN level.

**Hematologic:** *leukopenia,* hemolytic anemia, *agranulocytosis, thrombocytopenia, aplastic anemia.*

**Hepatic:** cholestatic jaundice, altered liver enzyme levels.

**Metabolic:** altered cholesterol, *hypoglycemia,* weight gain.

**Skin:** rash, pruritus.

## Overdose and treatment

Signs and symptoms include low blood glucose levels, tingling of lips and tongue, hunger, nausea, decreased cerebral function, increased sympathetic activity, and, ultimately, seizures, stupor, and coma.

Mild hypoglycemia responds to treatment with oral glucose and dosage adjustments. If patient loses consciousness or experiences other neurologic changes, he should receive a rapid injection of dextrose 50%, followed by continuous infusion of dextrose 10% at a rate to maintain glucose levels at more than 100 mg/dl.

Advise clinician to monitor patient for 24 to 48 hours.

## Clinical considerations

■ To improve glucose control in patients who receive 15 mg/day or more, doses can be divided and given 30 minutes before the morning and evening meals.

■ Some patients taking glipizide can be controlled on a once-daily regimen; others show better response with divided dosing.

■ Drug has a mild diuretic effect that may be useful in patients with HF or cirrhosis.

■ Patients who may be more sensitive to drug, such as geriatric, debilitated, or malnourished patients, should begin therapy with lower doses (2.5 mg once daily).

■ Oral antidiabetics may cause an increased risk of CV mortality as compared with diet or diet and insulin therapy.

### Therapeutic monitoring

■ When substituting glipizide for chlorpropamide, advise clinician to monitor patient carefully during the first week because of the prolonged retention of chlorpropamide.

■ Advise clinician to monitor blood glucose, urine glucose, ketone levels, and glycosylated hemoglobin.

### Special populations

**Pregnant patients.** Use in pregnancy is usually not recommended. If glipizide must be used, manufacturer recommends that drug be discontinued at least 1 month before expected delivery to prevent neonatal hypoglycemia.

**Pediatric patients.** Safety and efficacy in children haven't been established. However, the American Diabetes Association states that most pediatric diabetologists use oral antidiabetics with type 2 diabetes mellitus because of greater patient compliance and convenience for patient's family.

**Geriatric patients.** Geriatric patients may be more sensitive to the effects of drug. Hypoglycemia causes a greater number of neurologic symptoms in geriatric patients.

## Patient counseling

■ Emphasize importance of following prescribed diet, exercise, and medical regimen.

■ Tell patient that, if a dose is missed, it should be taken immediately, unless it's almost time to take the next dose. Patient shouldn't double the dose.

■ Advise patient to avoid alcohol and products containing alcohol when taking glipizide.

■ Suggest that drug be taken with food if glipizide causes GI upset.

■ Provide patient with instruction on how to monitor blood glucose, urine glucose, and ketone levels, as prescribed.

■ Teach patient how to recognize and manage the signs and symptoms of hyperglycemia and hypoglycemia.

# glucagon

*Pharmacologic classification:* antihypoglycemic
*Therapeutic classification:* antihypoglycemic, diagnostic
*Pregnancy risk category B*

## Available forms

Available by prescription only
*Powder for injection:* 1 mg (1 unit)/vial, 10 mg (10 units)/vial

## Indications and dosages

### Severe hypoglycemia

*Adults and children weighing over 20 kg (44 lb):* 1 mg S.C., I.M., or I.V. May repeat dose after 15 minutes if patient fails to respond. When patient responds, give supplemental carbohydrates.
*Children weighing under 20 kg:* 0.5 mg S.C., I.M., or I.V. Alternatively, 20 to 30 mcg/kg. May repeat dose after 15 minutes if patient fails to respond. When patient responds, give supplemental carbohydrates.

### Diagnostic aid for radiographic examination of stomach, duodenum, and small intestine

*Adults:* 1 or 2 mg I.M. or 0.25 to 2 mg I.V. For relaxation of the stomach, use 0.5 mg I.V. or 2 mg I.M.

## I.V. administration

■ For I.V. drip infusion, glucagon is compatible with dextrose solution but forms a precipitate in chloride solutions.

■ After reconstitution, solutions must be used immediately. Discard unused portion.

### Incompatibilities

Incompatible with sodium chloride solution and other solutions with a pH of 3 to 9.5 because drug may cause precipitation.

## Mechanism of action

*Antihypoglycemic action:* Glucagon increases plasma glucose levels and causes smooth muscle relaxation and an inotropic myocardial effect because of the stimulation of adenylate cyclase to produce cAMP, which initiates a series of reactions that leads to the degradation of glycogen to glucose. Hepatic stores of glycogen are needed for glucagon to exert an antihypoglycemic effect.
*Diagnostic action:* The mechanism by which glucagon relaxes the smooth muscles of the GI tract hasn't been fully defined.

---

## Pharmacokinetics

*Absorption:* Glucagon is destroyed in the GI tract; therefore, it must be given parenterally. Administration to comatose hypoglycemic patients (with normal liver glycogen stores) usually produces a return to consciousness within 20 minutes.

*Distribution:* Not fully understood.

*Metabolism:* Degraded extensively by the liver, in the kidneys and plasma, and at its tissue receptor sites in plasma membranes.

*Excretion:* Metabolic products are excreted by the kidneys. Half-life is about 3 to 10 minutes.

| Route | Onset | Peak | Duration |
|-------|-------|------|----------|
| I.V. | Immediate | ½ hr | 60-90 min |
| I.M., S.C. | Unknown | Unknown | Unknown |

## Contraindications and precautions

Contraindicated in patients with pheochromocytoma or those hypersensitive to drug.

Use drug cautiously in patients with insulinoma.

## Interactions

**Drug-drug.** *Epinephrine:* Increases and prolongs hyperglycemic effects. Advise clinician to monitor glucose levels.

*Phenytoin:* Appears to inhibit glucagon-induced insulin release. Use with caution as a diagnostic drug in patients with diabetes mellitus.

## Adverse reactions

**CV:** hypotension.
**GI:** nausea, vomiting.
**Metabolic:** hypokalemia.
**Respiratory:** respiratory distress.
**Other:** hypersensitivity reactions (*bronchospasm*, rash, dizziness, light-headedness).

## Overdose and treatment

Signs and symptoms of overdose include nausea, vomiting, and hypokalemia. Patient should be treated symptomatically.

## Clinical considerations

■ Glucagon should be used only under direct medical supervision.
■ Glucagon has positive inotropic and chronotropic actions on the heart and may be used to treat overdose of beta blockers.

### Therapeutic monitoring

■ If patient experiences nausea and vomiting from glucagon administration and can't retain some form of sugar for 1 hour, consider administration of I.V. dextrose.

### Special populations

**Breast-feeding patients.** It's unknown if drug appears in breast milk. Exercise caution when administering drug.

**Pediatric patients.** Glucagon has been used safely and effectively for the treatment of hypoglycemia in children. Safety and efficacy in diagnostic procedures haven't been established.

## Patient counseling

■ Provide patient with instructions on how to mix and inject drug properly.
■ Tell patient to expect response usually within 20 minutes after injection.

# glyburide

DiaBeta, Glynase PresTab, Micronase

*Pharmacologic classification:* sulfonylurea
*Therapeutic classification:* antidiabetic
*Pregnancy risk category C*

## Available forms

Available by prescription only
*Tablets:* 1.25 mg, 2.5 mg, 5 mg
*Tablets (micronized):* 1.5 mg, 3 mg, 4.5 mg, 6 mg

## Indications and dosages

*Adjunct to diet to lower blood glucose levels in patients with type 2 (non–insulin-dependent) diabetes mellitus*
*Adults:* Initially, 2.5 to 5 mg P.O. daily with breakfast. Start patients who are more sensitive to hypoglycemic drugs at 1.25 mg daily. Usual maintenance dose is 1.25 to 20 mg daily, either as a single dose or in divided doses.

For micronized tablets, initially give 1.5 to 3 mg P.O. with breakfast. Usual maintenance dose is 0.75 to 12 mg P.O. daily.

≡*Dosage adjustment.* In geriatric, debilitated, or malnourished patients or those with renal or liver dysfunction, start therapy with 1.25 mg once daily.

*To replace insulin therapy*
*Adults:* If insulin dose is more than 40 units/day, patient may be started on 5 mg of glyburide daily plus 50% of the insulin dose. Patients maintained on less than 20 units/day should receive 2.5 to 5 mg/day; those maintained on 20 to 40 units/day should receive 5 mg/day. In all patients, glyburide is substituted and insulin discontinued abruptly.

For micronized tablets, if insulin dose is more than 40 units/day, give 3 mg P.O. with a 50% reduction in insulin. Patients maintained on 20 to 40 units/day should receive 3 mg P.O. as a single daily dose; those maintained on less than 20 units/day should receive 1.5 to 3 mg/day as a single dose.

## Mechanism of action

*Antidiabetic action:* Glyburide decreases blood glucose levels by stimulating insulin release from functioning beta cells in the pancreas. After prolonged administration, the hypoglycemic effects of the drug appear to be related to extrapancreatic effects, possibly including reduction of basal hepatic glucose production and enhanced peripheral sensitivity to insulin. The latter may result either from an increase in the number of insulin receptors or from changes in events subsequent to insulin binding.

## Pharmacokinetics

*Absorption:* Almost completely absorbed from the GI tract. A micronized tablet results in significant absorption; a 3-mg micronized tablet provides blood levels similar to a 5-mg conventional tablet.

*Distribution:* 99% protein-bound. Its distribution isn't fully understood.

*Metabolism:* Metabolized completely by the liver to inactive metabolites.

*Excretion:* Excreted as metabolites in urine and feces in equal proportions. Its duration of action is 24 hours; its half-life is 10 hours.

| Route | Onset | Peak | Duration |
|-------|-------|------|----------|
| P.O. | 1-4 hr | 4 hr | 24 hr |

## Contraindications and precautions

Contraindicated in patients hypersensitive to drug or those with diabetic ketoacidosis with or without coma, and during pregnancy or breast-feeding. Use drug cautiously in patients with impaired renal or hepatic function and in geriatric, malnourished, or debilitated patients.

## Interactions

**Drug-drug.** *Adrenocorticoids, amphetamines, baclofen, corticotropin, diazoxide, epinephrine, ethacrynic acid, furosemide, glucagon, glucocorticoids, phenytoin, rifampin, thiazide diuretics, thyroid hormones, triamterene:* Increased glucose levels. Dosage adjustments may be needed.

*Anabolic steroids, chloramphenicol, clofibrate, guanethidine, insulin, MAO inhibitors, probenecid, salicylates, sulfonamides:* Enhanced hypoglycemic effect by displacing glyburide from its protein-binding sites. Advise clinician to monitor glucose levels; advise clinician to monitor patient carefully.

*Anticoagulants:* May increase plasma levels of both drugs and, after continued therapy, may reduce plasma levels and anticoagulant effect. Advise clinician to monitor glucose levels and PT and INR.

*Beta blockers, including ophthalmics:* Increased risk of hypoglycemia. Use together cautiously.

*Hydantoins:* May increase levels of hydantoins. Advise clinician to monitor levels.

**Drug-herb.** *Aloe, bilberry leaf, bitter melon, burdock, dandelion, fenugreek, garlic, and ginseng:* Use together may improve blood sugar control, requiring a reduction in antidiabetics.

Advise patient to discuss the use of herbal medicines with his prescriber before use.

**Drug-lifestyle.** *Alcohol use:* Altered glycemic control, most commonly hypoglycemia. May also cause a disulfiram-like reaction consisting of nausea, vomiting, abdominal cramps, and headaches. Discourage use together.

*Smoking:* May increase corticosteroid release; patients who smoke may require higher dosages of glyburide. Advise patient to stop smoking.

## Adverse reactions

**EENT:** changes in accommodation or blurred vision.

**GI:** nausea, epigastric fullness, heartburn.

**GU:** altered BUN levels.

**Hematologic:** *leukopenia,* hemolytic anemia, *agranulocytosis, thrombocytopenia, aplastic anemia.*

**Hepatic:** cholestatic jaundice, *hepatitis,* abnormal liver function.

**Metabolic:** altered cholesterol level, *hypoglycemia,* weight gain, hyponatremia, SIADH.

**Musculoskeletal:** arthralgia, myalgia.

**Skin:** rash, pruritus, other allergic reactions.

**Other:** *angioedema.*

## Overdose and treatment

Signs and symptoms of overdose include low glucose levels, tingling of lips and tongue, hunger, nausea, decreased cerebral function (lethargy, yawning, confusion, agitation, and nervousness), increased sympathetic activity (tachycardia, sweating, and tremor) and, ultimately, seizures, stupor, and coma.

Mild hypoglycemia, without loss of consciousness or neurologic findings, responds to treatment with oral glucose and dosage adjustments. Patient with severe hypoglycemia should be hospitalized immediately. If hypoglycemic coma is suspected, the patient should receive rapid injection of dextrose 50%, followed by a continuous infusion of dextrose 10% at a rate to maintain glucose levels greater than 100 mg/dl. Advise clinician to monitor patient for 24 to 48 hours.

## Clinical considerations

■ To improve control in patients receiving 10 mg/day or more, divided doses, usually given before the morning and evening meals, are recommended.

■ Some patients taking glyburide may be controlled effectively on a once-daily regimen, whereas others show better response with divided dosing.

■ Glyburide is a second-generation sulfonylurea oral antidiabetic. It appears to cause fewer adverse reactions than first-generation drugs.

■ Drug has a mild diuretic effect that may be useful in patients with HF or cirrhosis.

- Oral antidiabetics may cause an increased risk of CV mortality compared with diet or diet and insulin therapy.
- Combined therapy with insulin may be useful in some patients with type 2 diabetes mellitus whose glucose is not controlled with oral antidiabetics and as a means of providing more flexibility with respect to timing of meals and amount of food ingested. It also may delay progression either to intensive insulin monotherapy or to a second daytime injection of insulin. There may be an increased risk of hypoglycemic reactions, and further study is required to more fully investigate the potential long-term benefits and risks.
- Glyburide therapy alters cholesterol, alkaline phosphatase, and BUN levels.

### Therapeutic monitoring
- When substituting glyburide for chlorpropamide, advise clinician to monitor patient closely during the first week because of the prolonged retention of chlorpropamide in the body.
- Advise clinician to monitor blood glucose, urine glucose, and ketone levels.

### Special populations
**Pediatric patients.** Glyburide is ineffective in type 1 (insulin-dependent, juvenile-onset) diabetes. Safety and efficacy in children haven't been established. However, the American Diabetes Association states that most pediatric diabetologists use oral antidiabetics with type 2 diabetes mellitus because of greater patient compliance and convenience for patient's family.
**Geriatric patients.** Geriatric patients may be more sensitive to effects of drug because of reduced metabolism and elimination. Hypoglycemia causes a greater number of neurologic symptoms in geriatric patients.

### Patient counseling
- Emphasize importance of following prescribed diet, exercise, and medical regimen.
- Advise patient to avoid alcohol and alcohol-containing products while taking glyburide.
- Suggest drug be taken with food if GI upset occurs.
- Provide patient with instruction on how to monitor blood glucose, urine glucose, and ketone levels.
- Inform patient of the signs and symptoms of hyperglycemia and hypoglycemia and what to do if these occur.

# glyburide and metformin hydrochloride
Glucovance

*Pharmacologic classification:* combination sulfonylurea and biguanide
*Therapeutic classification:* antidiabetic
*Pregnancy risk category B*

## Available forms
*Tablets:* 1.25 mg glyburide and 250 mg metformin, 2.5 mg glyburide and 500 mg metformin, 5 mg glyburide and 500 mg metformin

## Indications and dosages
*Adjunct to diet and exercise to improve glycemic control in patients with type 2 diabetes whose hyperglycemia cannot be controlled with diet and exercise alone*
*Adults:* Initially, 1.25 mg/250 mg P.O. once daily or b.i.d. with meals. In patients whose hyperglycemia cannot be managed with diet and exercise alone, start with 1.25 mg/250 mg once daily with meals. In patients with glycosylated hemoglobin above 9% or a fasting plasma glucose above 200 mg/dl, start with 1.25 mg/250 mg b.i.d. with morning and evening meals. Daily dose may be increased in increments of 1.25 mg/250 mg per day every 2 weeks up to the minimum dose needed to adequately control glucose. Maximum 20 mg glyburide and 2,000 mg metformin daily.
*Second-line therapy in patients with type 2 diabetes when diet, exercise, and initial treatment with a sulfonlyurea or metformin do not provide adequate glycemic control*
*Adults:* Initially 2.5 mg/500 mg or 5 mg/500 mg b.i.d. with meals. Increase in increments of no more than 5 mg/500 mg up to the minimum effective dose needed to adequately control glucose. Maximum, 20 mg glyburide and 2,000 mg metformin daily.
≡*Dosage adjustment.* Initial and maintenance dosing should be conservative in geriatric patients because of the likelihood of decreased renal function. Any dosage adjustment requires careful assessment of renal function. Geriatric, debilitated, and malnourished patients should not be given the maximum dose to avoid the risk of hypoglycemia.

## Mechanism of action
*Hypoglycemic action:* Glyburide appears to lower glucose levels by stimulating the release of insulin from the pancreas. The mechanism by which glyburide lowers glucose levels during long-term administration is not clearly established. Metformin decreases hepatic glucose production and intestinal absorption of glucose and improves insulin sensitivity.

## Pharmacokinetics
### glyburide
*Absorption:* Absorbed almost completely from the GI tract.
*Distribution:* Extensively protein-bound.
*Metabolism:* Metabolized completely by the liver to weakly active metabolites.
*Excretion:* Excreted as metabolites in urine and bile in equal proportions. Half-life is 10 hours.
### metformin hydrochloride
*Absorption:* Absorbed from GI tract, with food decreasing extent and slightly delaying rate of absorption.
*Distribution:* Negligibly plasma protein–bound.
*Metabolism:* Not metabolized.
*Excretion:* Excreted unchanged in urine. Half-life is 6.2 hours.

| Route | Onset | Peak | Duration |
|---|---|---|---|
| P.O. (glyburide) | 1 hr | 4 hr | 24 hr |
| P.O. (metformin) | Unknown | Unknown | Unknown |

## Contraindications and precautions
Contraindicated in patients hypersensitive to glyburide or metformin and patients with renal disease, renal dysfunction, or metabolic acidosis (including diabetic ketoacidosis). Contraindicated in HF that needs pharmacologic treatment.

Use drug cautiously in geriatric, hepatically impaired, debilitated, or malnourished patients and those with adrenal or pituitary insufficiency because of increased risk of hypoglycemia.

Renal or hepatic insufficiency in patients receiving fixed combination with metformin hydrochloride may increase blood levels of both drugs. Hepatic insufficiency may diminish glucogenetic capacity, both of which increase the risk of hypoglycemic reactions.

## Interactions
**Drug-drug.** *Beta blockers, chloramphenicol, ciprofloxacin, coumarins, highly protein-bound drugs, MAO inhibitors, miconazole, NSAIDs, probenecid, salicylates, sulfonamides:* Increased hypoglycemic activity of glyburide. Advise clinician to monitor glucose level.
*Calcium channel blockers, corticosteroids, estrogens, isoniazid, nicotinic acid, oral contraceptives, phenothiazines, phenytoin, sympathomimetics, thiazides and other diuretics, thyroid hormones:* Increased risk of hyperglycemia. Advise clinician to monitor patient's glucose level.
*Cationic drugs (such as amiloride, cimetidine, digoxin, morphine, procainamide, quinidine, quinine, ranitidine, triamterene, trimethoprim, vancomycin):* May increase metformin levels. Advise clinician to monitor patient.

*Furosemide:* Increased metformin levels and decreased furosemide levels. Advise clinician to monitor patient closely.
*Nifedipine:* Increased metformin levels. Metformin dosage may need to be decreased.
**Drug-herb.** *Aloe, bilberry leaf, bitter melon, burdock, dandelion, fenugreek, garlic, and ginseng:* Use together may improve blood sugar control, requiring a reduction in antidiabetics. Advise patient to discuss the use of herbal medicines with his prescriber before use.
**Drug-lifestyle.** *Alcohol use:* Altered glycemic control, most commonly hypoglycemia. May also cause disulfiram-like reaction with glyburide component. Avoid concomitant use.

## Adverse reactions
**CNS:** headache, dizziness.
**GI:** *diarrhea,* nausea, vomiting, abdominal pain.
**Metabolic:** *hypoglycemia.*
**Respiratory:** *upper respiratory tract infection.*

## Overdose and treatment
Glyburide overdose can produce hypoglycemia. Mild hypoglycemic symptoms, without loss of consciousness or neurological findings, should be treated aggressively with oral glucose and adjustments in drug, dosage, or meal patterns. Severe hypoglycemic reactions with coma, seizure, or other neurological impairment occur infrequently but demand immediate hospitalization. If hypoglycemic coma is diagnosed or suspected, the patient should be given a rapid I.V. injection of concentrated (50%) glucose solution followed by continuous infusion of a more dilute (10%) glucose solution at a rate that will maintain the glucose at a level above 100 mg/dl. Any patient with hypoglycemia should be monitored closely until out of danger and, if the reaction is severe, for a minimum of 24 to 48 hours, because hypoglycemia may recur after apparent clinical recovery.

Metformin overdose has not been linked to hypoglycemia, but lactic acidosis may occur. Hemodialysis may remove metformin, but not glyburide.

## Clinical considerations
■ For patients previously treated with glyburide or metformin, the starting dose of Glucovance should not exceed the daily dose of the glyburide (or equivalent dose of another sulfonylurea) and metformin already being taken.
■ Lactic acidosis is a rare, but serious (50% fatal), metabolic complication that can result from metformin accumulation. Reported cases have occurred primarily in diabetic patients with significant renal insufficiency; with multiple medical or surgical problems; and with multiple drug regimens. The risk of lactic acidosis increases with the degree of renal impairment and patient's age.

---

- Early symptoms of lactic acidosis may include malaise, myalgias, respiratory distress, increasing somnolence, and nonspecific abdominal distress.
- GI symptoms that occur after a patient is stabilized on any dose level of Glucovance are unlikely to be drug-related and could result from lactic acidosis or other serious disease.
- Lactic acidosis should be suspected in any diabetic patient with metabolic acidosis lacking evidence of ketoacidosis.
- Recommend stopping drug if CV collapse, acute HF, acute MI, or other conditions characterized by hypoxemia occur, because these conditions may be related to lactic acidosis and may cause prerenal azotemia.
- Acute alteration in renal function is noted in patients undergoing radiologic studies involving intravascular administration of iodinated contrast materials.

### Therapeutic monitoring
- Recommend assessing glucose level before therapy and regularly thereafter. Advise clinician to monitor glycosylated hemoglobin to assess long-term therapy.
- Recommend obtaining baseline renal function test results; drug shouldn't be started if serum creatinine levels are greater than or equal to 1.5 mg/dl for men or 1.4 mg/dl for women. Advise clinician to monitor renal function at least once yearly while the patient takes drug, and more often in those with increased risk of renal dysfunction. If renal impairment is detected, drug should be discontinued.
- Advise clinician to monitor patient closely during times of increased stress, such as infection, fever, surgery, or trauma; insulin therapy may be needed. Drug therapy should be temporarily suspended for any surgical procedure that requires restricted intake of food and fluids and should not be restarted until oral intake has resumed.
- Advise clinician to monitor patient's hematologic status for megaloblastic anemia. Patients with inadequate vitamin $B_{12}$ or calcium intake or absorption seem predisposed to developing subnormal vitamin $B_{12}$ levels when taking metformin. They should have serum vitamin $B_{12}$ level determinations every 2 to 3 years.
- Recommend evaluating patient who develops laboratory abnormalities or clinical illness for evidence of ketoacidosis or lactic acidosis, including serum electrolytes, ketones, blood glucose, blood pH, and lactate, pyruvate, and metformin levels. Drug should be stopped if evidence of acidosis occurs.

### Special populations
**Breast-feeding patients.** Drug is not recommended for breast-feeding women.
**Pediatric patients.** Safety and efficacy have not been established in children.

**Geriatric patients.** All patients should have a baseline serum creatinine that indicates normal renal function before starting therapy. Treatment shouldn't begin in patients ages 80 or older unless creatinine clearance measurement shows that renal function is not reduced. In geriatric patients, renal function should be monitored regularly and, generally, Glucovance should not be adjusted to the maximum dose.

### Patient counseling
- Tell patient to take once-daily dose with breakfast and twice-daily dose with breakfast and dinner.
- Teach the patient about diabetes and the importance of following therapeutic regimen; adhering to diet, weight-reduction, regular exercise and hygiene programs; and avoiding infection.
- Explain how and when to monitor glucose level and how to differentiate between hypoglycemia and hyperglycemia.
- Instruct patient to stop drug and report unexplained hyperventilation, myalgia, malaise, unusual somnolence, or other symptoms of early lactic acidosis.
- Tell patient that GI symptoms are common early in drug therapy. GI symptoms that occur after prolonged therapy may be related to lactic acidosis or other serious disease and should be reported promptly.
- Counsel patient against excessive alcohol intake, either acute or chronic.
- Advise patient not to take any other drugs, including OTC drugs, without checking with prescriber.
- Instruct patient to wear or carry medical identification.

## glycopyrrolate
Robinul, Robinul Forte

*Pharmacologic classification:* anticholinergic
*Therapeutic classification:* antimuscarinic, GI antispasmodic
*Pregnancy risk category B*

### Available forms
Available by prescription only
*Tablets:* 1 mg, 2 mg
*Injection:* 0.2 mg/ml in 1-ml, 2-ml, 5-ml, 20-ml vials

### Indications and dosages
*Blockade of cholinergic effects of anticholinesterase drugs used to reverse neuromuscular blockade*
*Adults and children:* 0.2 mg I.V. for each 1 mg of neostigmine or 5 mg of pyridostigmine. May be given I.V. without dilution or may be added to dextrose injection and infused.

*Preoperatively to diminish secretions and block cardiac vagal reflexes*
Adults and children over age 2: 0.0044 mg/kg of body weight given I.M. 30 to 60 minutes before anesthesia.
*Adjunctive therapy in peptic ulcers and other GI disorders*
Adults: 1 to 2 mg P.O. t.i.d. or 0.1 mg I.M. t.i.d. or q.i.d. Dosage should be individualized.

## I.V. administration

■ Drug may be given via the tubing of a running I.V. infusion of a compatible solution.
■ When used together with neostigmine or physostigmine, drug may be given in the same syringe.

### Incompatibilities

Incompatible with drugs having an alkaline pH and with chloramphenicol sodium succinate, dexamethasone sodium phosphate, diazepam, dimenhydrinate, methohexital, methylprednisolone sodium succinate, pentazocine lactate, pentobarbital sodium, secobarbital sodium, sodium bicarbonate, and thiopental.

## Mechanism of action

*Anticholinergic action:* Glycopyrrolate inhibits muscarinic actions of acetylcholine on autonomic effectors innervated by postganglionic cholinergic nerves. That action blocks adverse muscarinic effects from anticholinesterase drugs used to reverse curariform-induced neuromuscular blockade. Glycopyrrolate decreases secretions and GI motility by the same mechanism. Glycopyrrolate blocks cardiac vagal reflexes by blocking vagal inhibition of the SA node.

## Pharmacokinetics

*Absorption:* Poorly absorbed from GI tract (10% to 25%) after oral administration.
*Distribution:* Rapidly distributed. Because it's a quaternary amine, it doesn't cross the blood-brain barrier or enter the CNS.
*Metabolism:* Exact metabolic fate is unknown.
*Excretion:* Small amount of drug is eliminated in the urine as unchanged drug and metabolites. Drug is mostly excreted unchanged in feces or bile.

| Route | Onset | Peak | Duration |
|---|---|---|---|
| P.O. | Unknown | Unknown | 8-12 hr |
| I.V. | 1 min | Unknown | 3-7 hr |
| I.M., S.C. | 15-30 min | 30-45 min | 3-7 hr |

## Contraindications and precautions

Contraindicated in patients hypersensitive to drug and in those with glaucoma, obstructive uropathy, obstructive disease of the GI tract, myasthenia gravis, paralytic ileus, intestinal atony, unstable CV status in acute hemorrhage, severe ulcerative colitis, or toxic megacolon.

Use drug cautiously in patients with autonomic neuropathy, hyperthyroidism, coronary artery disease, arrhythmias, HF, hypertension, hiatal hernia, hepatic or renal disease, and ulcerative colitis. Also use with caution in hot or humid conditions where drug-induced heatstroke may occur.

## Interactions

**Drug-drug.** *Amantadine, antihistamines, antiparkinsonians, disopyramide, glutethimide, meperidine, phenothiazines, procainamide, quinidine, tricyclic antidepressants:* Additive adverse effects. Avoid use together.
*Antacids:* Decrease oral absorption of anticholinergics. Glycopyrrolate should be given at least 1 hour before antacids.
*Digoxin tablets (slowly dissolving):* May yield higher serum digoxin levels when given with anticholinergics. Use cautiously; dosage adjustment may be needed.
*Ketoconazole, levodopa:* Decreased GI absorption. Separate administration times by 2 to 3 hours.
*Oral potassium supplements, especially wax-matrix formulations:* Increased risk of potassium-induced GI ulcerations. Use cautiously.

## Adverse reactions

**CNS:** weakness, nervousness, insomnia, drowsiness, dizziness, headache, confusion or excitement (in geriatric patients).
**CV:** palpitations, tachycardia.
**EENT:** *dilated pupils, blurred vision,* photophobia, increased intraocular pressure.
**GI:** *constipation, dry mouth,* nausea, loss of taste, abdominal distention, vomiting, epigastric distress.
**GU:** *urinary hesitancy, urine retention,* impotence.
**Skin:** urticaria, decreased sweating or anhidrosis, other dermal manifestations.
**Other:** allergic reactions *(anaphylaxis),* fever.

## Overdose and treatment

Clinical effects of overdose include such peripheral effects as dilated, nonreactive pupils; blurred vision; flushed, hot, dry skin; dryness of mucous membranes; dysphagia; decreased or absent bowel sounds; urine retention; hyperthermia; tachycardia; hypertension; and increased respiration.

Treatment is primarily symptomatic and supportive p.r.n. If patient is alert, recommend inducing emesis (or using gastric lavage) and following with a saline cathartic and activated charcoal to prevent further drug absorption. In severe life-threatening cases, physostigmine may be given to block antimuscarinic effects of glycopyrrolate. Fluids may be given p.r.n.

---

Reactions may be *common*, uncommon, *life-threatening*, or COMMON AND LIFE-THREATENING.

to treat shock. If urine retention occurs, catheterization may be needed.

## Clinical considerations
■ Even slight overdose may lead to toxicity.
■ For immediate treatment of bradycardia, some prescribers prefer atropine over glycopyrrolate.

### Therapeutic monitoring
■ Advise clinician to monitor patient closely for toxicity.
■ Advise clinician to monitor patient for CNS effects and for urinary hesitancy or urine retention.

### Special populations
**Breast-feeding patients.** Drug may appear in breast milk, possibly causing infant toxicity. Breast-feeding women should avoid this drug, which may decrease milk production.
**Pediatric patients.** Drug not recommended for peptic ulcer in children under age 12. Manufacturer recommends that drug not be used in neonates under age 1 month because glycopyrrolate injection contains benzyl alcohol.
**Geriatric patients.** Give glycopyrrolate cautiously to geriatric patients. However, glycopyrrolate may be the preferred anticholinergic in geriatric patients.

## Patient counseling
■ Instruct patient to take oral drug 30 to 60 minutes before meals.
■ Warn patient to avoid activities that require alertness until CNS effects of drug are known.
■ Advise patient to contact prescriber to report signs of urinary hesitancy or urine retention.

# gold sodium thiomalate
Aurolate

*Pharmacologic classification:* gold salt
*Therapeutic classification:* antiarthritic
*Pregnancy risk category C*

## Available forms
Available by prescription only
*Injection:* 50 mg/ml with benzyl alcohol

## Indications and dosages
**Rheumatoid arthritis in patients whose symptoms progress despite an adequate regimen of NSAIDs; those with ◇psoriatic arthritis, or ◇Felty's syndrome**
*Adults:* Initially, 10 mg I.M.; then 25 mg in second week and continue for a third dose the following week. Continue until 1 g (cumulative) has been given, unless toxicity occurs. If improvement occurs without toxicity before initial 1-g dose, a maintenance dose of 25 to 50 mg every other week for 2 to 20 weeks may be started. Then continue to every third then

every fourth week indefinitely. Weekly injections may be restarted anytime, if needed. If patient doesn't respond after reaching initial 1-g dose, discontinue therapy, or give 25 to 50 mg I.M. for an additional 10 weeks, or increase dose by 10 mg q 1 to 4 weeks (maximum dose per injection is 100 mg).
*Children:* Initiate therapy with 10-mg test dose, then give 1 mg/kg weekly. Continue dosage and administration as listed for adults. Maximum single dose for children under age 12 is 50 mg.
◇ **Palindromic rheumatism**
*Adults:* Initially, 10 to 15 mg I.M. weekly until dose of 1 g is reached.
◇ **Pemphigus**
*Adults:* Initially, 10 mg I.M.; then 25 mg I.M. for second week, then 50 mg I.M. weekly. When patient is off corticosteroid therapy, maintenance dose of 25 to 50 mg I.M. q 2 weeks may be given.

## Mechanism of action
*Antiarthritic action:* Gold sodium thiomalate is thought to be effective against rheumatoid arthritis by altering the immune system to reduce inflammation. Although the exact mechanism of action remains unknown, these compounds have reduced serum levels of immunoglobulins and rheumatoid factors in patients with arthritis.

## Pharmacokinetics
*Absorption:* Absorption is rapid.
*Distribution:* Higher tissue levels occur with parenteral gold salts, with a mean steady-state plasma level of 1 to 5 mcg/ml. Drug is distributed widely throughout the body in lymph nodes, bone marrow, kidneys, liver, spleen, and tissues. About 85% to 90% is protein-bound.
*Metabolism:* Not broken down into its elemental form. The half-life with cumulative dosing is 14 to 40 days.
*Excretion:* About 70% is excreted in the urine, 30% in feces.

| Route | Onset | Peak | Duration |
|---|---|---|---|
| I.M. | Unknown | 3-6 hr | Unknown |

## Contraindications and precautions
Contraindicated in patients hypersensitive to drug; in those with history of severe toxicity from previous exposure to gold or heavy metals, hepatitis, or exfoliative dermatitis; and in patients with severe uncontrollable diabetes, renal disease, hepatic dysfunction, uncontrolled HF, systemic lupus erythematosus, colitis, or Sjögren's syndrome. Also contraindicated in patients with urticaria, eczema, hemorrhagic conditions, or severe hematologic disorders and in those who have recently received radiation therapy.

Use drug with extreme caution in patients with rash, marked hypertension, compromised cerebral or CV function, or history of renal or hepatic disease, drug allergies, or blood dyscrasias.

## Interactions
**Drug-drug.** *Other drugs known to cause blood dyscrasias:* Additive risk of hematologic toxicity. Avoid use together.
**Drug-lifestyle.** *Sun or ultraviolet light exposure:* May cause photosensitivity reactions. Advise patient to use precautions.

## Adverse reactions
**CNS:** confusion, hallucinations, *seizures.*
**CV:** *bradycardia,* hypotension.
**EENT:** corneal gold deposition, corneal ulcers.
**GI:** *metallic taste, stomatitis, diarrhea,* anorexia, abdominal cramps, nausea, vomiting, ulcerative enterocolitis.
**GU:** albuminuria, proteinuria, *nephrotic syndrome,* nephritis, acute tubular necrosis, hematuria, *acute renal failure.*
**Hematologic:** *thrombocytopenia* (with or without purpura), *aplastic anemia, agranulocytosis, leukopenia,* eosinophilia, anemia.
**Hepatic:** *hepatitis,* jaundice, elevated liver function test results.
**Skin:** diaphoresis, photosensitivity, *rash, dermatitis,* erythema, exfoliative dermatitis.
**Other:** *anaphylaxis, angioedema.*

## Overdose and treatment
When severe reactions to gold occur, corticosteroids, dimercaprol (a chelating drug), or penicillamine may be given to aid in the recovery. Prednisone 40 to 100 mg/day in divided doses is recommended to manage severe renal, hematologic, pulmonary, or enterocolitic reactions to gold. Dimercaprol may be used with corticosteroids to facilitate removal of the gold when the corticosteroid treatment alone is ineffective.

## Clinical considerations
■ Recommend giving all gold salts I.M., preferably intragluteally. Normal color of drug is pale yellow; don't use it if it darkens.
■ Patient should remain recumbent for 10 to 20 minutes and remain under medical observation for 30 minutes after administration because of possible anaphylactic reaction.
■ Vasomotor adverse effects are more common with gold sodium thiomalate than with other gold salts.
■ Serum protein–bound iodine test, especially when performed by the chloric acid digestion method, gives false readings during and for several weeks after gold therapy.
■ Adverse reactions to gold are severe and potentially life-threatening.

## Therapeutic monitoring
■ Recommend obtaining patient's urine for analysis for protein and sediment changes before each injection.
■ Advise clinician to monitor patient's CBC and platelet count monthly or before every other injection. Drug should be stopped if platelet count decreases to less than 100,000/mm³.
■ Most adverse reactions are readily reversible if drug is discontinued immediately.
■ If adverse reactions are mild, some rheumatologists order resumption of gold therapy after 2 to 3 weeks' rest.

## Special populations
**Breast-feeding patients.** Drug isn't recommended for use in breast-feeding women.
**Pediatric patients.** Use in children under age 6 isn't recommended.
**Geriatric patients.** Usual adult dose should be given. Use cautiously in patients with decreased renal function.

## Patient counseling
■ Inform patient that beneficial drug effect may be delayed for 3 months.
■ Explain that vasomotor adverse reactions—faintness, weakness, dizziness, flushing, nausea, vomiting, diaphoresis—may occur immediately after injection. Advise patient to lie down until symptoms subside.
■ Tell patient that stomatitis is often preceded by a metallic taste; this symptom must be reported to prescriber immediately.
■ Advise patient to report rash or other skin problems to prescriber immediately.

# gonadorelin acetate
Lutrepulse

*Pharmacologic classification:* gonadotropin-releasing hormone (GnRH)
*Therapeutic classification:* fertility
*Pregnancy risk category B*

## Available forms
Available by prescription only
*Injection:* 0.8 mg/10 ml, 3.2 mg/10 ml, in 10-ml vials
Supplied as a kit with I.V. supplies and portable infusion pump

## Indications and dosages
*To induce ovulation in women with primary hypothalamic amenorrhea*
*Adults:* 5 mcg I.V. q 90 minutes (using a Lutrepulse pump, 0.8 mg solution at 50 microliters/pulse) for 21 days. If no response after three treatment intervals, dosage may be increased. Usual dose is 1 to 20 mcg.

## I.V. administration

- The pulse period is set at 1 minute (drug is infused over 1 minute); pulse interval is set at 90 minutes.

### Incompatibilities

None reported.

## Mechanism of action

*Ovulation-stimulating action:* Mimics the action of GnRH, which results in the synthesis and release of luteinizing hormone (LH) from the anterior pituitary. LH subsequently acts on the reproductive organs to regulate hormone synthesis.

## Pharmacokinetics

*Absorption:* Administered I.V. using a portable pump.
*Distribution:* Low plasma volume of distribution (10 to 15 L) and high rate of clearance from plasma.
*Metabolism:* Rapidly metabolized. Several biologically inactive peptide fragments have been identified.
*Excretion:* Excreted primarily in urine. The high initial clearance rate (half-life of 2 to 10 minutes) is followed by a somewhat slower terminal half-life of 10 to 40 minutes.

| Route | Onset | Peak | Duration |
|-------|-------|------|----------|
| I.V. | Unknown | Unknown | 10-40 min |

## Contraindications and precautions

Contraindicated in patients hypersensitive to drug, in women with conditions that could be complicated by pregnancy (such as prolactinoma), in those who are anovulatory from any cause other than a hypothalamic disorder, and in those with ovarian cysts.

## Interactions

**Drug-drug.** *Ovary-stimulating drugs:* Risk of ovarian hyperstimulation. Avoid use together.

## Adverse reactions

**GU:** multiple pregnancy, ovarian hyperstimulation.
**Skin:** hematoma, local infection, inflammation, mild phlebitis.

## Overdose and treatment

No harmful effects are expected if the pump were to malfunction and deliver the entire contents of the highest-concentration vial (3.2 mg). Bolus doses of up to 3,000 mcg haven't proved harmful in clinical trials; however, continuous exposure (nonpulsatile administration) to gonadorelin may temporarily reduce pituitary responsiveness.

## Clinical considerations

- To mimic the action of the naturally occurring hormone, gonadorelin requires a pulsatile administration with a special portable infusion pump.

### Therapeutic monitoring

- Close monitoring of dosage and ultrasonography of the ovaries are needed to monitor drug response. Patients usually require pelvic ultrasound on days 7 and 14 after establishment of a baseline scan, although the interval between scans may be shortened.
- Regular pelvic examinations and midluteal phase serum progesterone determinations are needed.
- Similar drugs have caused anaphylaxis; advise clinician to monitor patients for signs and symptoms of anaphylaxis.

### Special populations

**Breast-feeding patients.** It's unknown if drug appears in breast milk; however, there's no reason to give drug to a breast-feeding woman.
**Pediatric patients.** Safety and efficacy in patients under age 18 haven't been established.

## Patient counseling

- Inform patient of the signs and symptoms of hypersensitivity reactions (hives, wheezing, difficulty breathing) and instruct her to report them immediately.
- Stress that a multiple pregnancy is possible (incidence about 12%).

# goserelin acetate
Zoladex, Zoladex 3-month

*Pharmacologic classification:* synthetic decapeptide
*Therapeutic classification:* luteinizing hormone-releasing hormone (LHRH; GnRH) analogue
*Pregnancy risk category X (10.8-mg implant); D (3.6-mg implant)*

## Available forms

Available by prescription only
*Implant:* 3.6 mg, 10.8 mg

## Indications and dosages

*Palliative treatment of advanced carcinoma of the prostate, endometriosis, advanced breast carcinoma*
*Adults:* One (3.6 mg) implant S.C. q 28 days into the upper abdominal wall for 6 months. Treatment of endometriosis shouldn't exceed 6 months.
*Palliative treatment of advanced carcinoma of the prostate*
*Men:* One (10.8 mg) implant S.C. q 12 weeks into the upper abdominal wall.

## Mechanism of action
*Hormonal action:* Chronic administration of goserelin, an LHRH, acts on the pituitary to decrease the release of follicle-stimulating hormone (FSH) and luteinizing hormone. In men, the result is dramatically decreased serum levels of testosterone.

## Pharmacokinetics
*Absorption:* Slowly absorbed from implant site.
*Distribution:* Administration of the implant results in measurable levels of drug in serum throughout the dosing period.
*Metabolism:* Clearance of goserelin after S.C. administration of the drug is rapid and occurs via a combination of hepatic metabolism and urinary excretion.
*Excretion:* Elimination half-life is about 4½ hours in patients with normal renal function. Substantial renal impairment prolongs half-life, but this doesn't appear to increase the risk of adverse effects.

| Route | Onset | Peak | Duration |
|-------|-------|------|----------|
| S.C. | Unknown | 12-15 days | Unknown |

## Contraindications and precautions
Contraindicated in patients hypersensitive to LHRH, LHRH agonist analogues, or goserelin acetate. Also contraindicated during pregnancy and in breast-feeding women. The 10.8-mg implant is contraindicated for use in women.

Use drug cautiously in patients at risk for osteoporosis, chronic alcohol or tobacco abuse, or use of anticonvulsants or corticosteroids.

## Interactions
None reported.

## Adverse reactions
**CNS:** *CVA,* lethargy, pain (worsened in the first 30 days), dizziness, *insomnia, asthenia,* anxiety, *depression, headache,* chills, *emotional lability.*
**CV:** edema, *HF, arrhythmias, peripheral edema,* hypertension, *MI,* peripheral vascular disorder, chest pain.
**GI:** nausea, vomiting, diarrhea, constipation, ulcer, anorexia, abdominal pain.
**GU:** *impotence, sexual dysfunction, lower urinary tract symptoms,* renal insufficiency, urinary obstruction, *vaginitis,* urinary tract infection, amenorrhea, increased serum testosterone levels during the first week of therapy.
**Hematologic:** anemia.
**Metabolic:** increased serum acid phosphatase initially (will decrease by week 4), hyperglycemia, weight increase.
**Musculoskeletal:** gout, back pain.
**Respiratory:** COPD, upper respiratory tract infection.

**Skin:** rash, *diaphoresis, acne, seborrhea,* hirsutism.
**Other:** *changes in libido, hot flashes, infection,* breast swelling and tenderness, *changes in breast size,* breast pain.

## Overdose and treatment
No information is available regarding accidental or intentional overdose.

## Clinical considerations
■ Drug should be given every 28 days for the 3.6-mg implant and every 12 weeks for the 10.8-mg implant, always under direct medical supervision. Local anesthesia may be used before injection.
■ In the unlikely event of the need to surgically remove goserelin, it may be localized by ultrasound.

### Therapeutic monitoring
■ Advise clinician to monitor patient for adverse reactions.
■ Advise clinician to monitor drug serum levels.

### Special populations
**Breast-feeding patients.** It's unknown if drug appears in breast milk.
**Pediatric patients.** Safety and efficacy in children under age 18 haven't been established.

## Patient counseling
■ Advise patient to report on time for each new implant.
■ Advise patient to immediately report to prescriber any implant-site reactions or other adverse reactions.

# granisetron hydrochloride
Kytril

*Pharmacologic classification:* selective 5-hydroxytryptamine (5-HT$_3$) receptor antagonist
*Therapeutic classification:* antiemetic, antinauseant
*Pregnancy risk category B*

## Available forms
Available by prescription only
*Tablets:* 1 mg
*Injection:* 1 mg/ml

## Indications and dosages
*Prevention of nausea and vomiting from emetogenic cancer chemotherapy*
*Adults and children ages 2 to 16:* 10 mcg/kg I.V. infused over 5 minutes or given by direct I.V. injection. Give within 30 minutes before administration of chemotherapy. Give only on days when chemotherapy is given. Continued

treatment while patient is not on chemotherapy hasn't been found to be useful.

*Adults:* 1 mg P.O. b.i.d. Give the first 1-mg tablet 1 hour before chemotherapy administration and the second tablet 12 hours after the first. Alternatively, 2 mg P.O. daily given up to 1 hour before chemotherapy. Give only on days when chemotherapy is given. Continued treatment while patient is not on chemotherapy hasn't been found to be useful.

*Prevention of radiation-induced nausea and vomiting in adults undergoing total body irradiation or daily fractionated radiation to the abdomen*
*Adults:* 2 mg P.O. once daily within 1 hour of radiation.

### I.V. administration

■ For I.V. infusion, dilute drug in D$_5$W or normal saline solution injection to a total volume of 20 to 50 ml and infuse over 5 minutes. For direct I.V. injection, give drug undiluted over 30 seconds.
■ Diluted solutions are stable for 24 hours at room temperature.

*Incompatibilities*
Don't mix in solution with other drugs.

### Mechanism of action

*Antiemetic action:* Granisetron as a selective 5-hydroxytryptamine (5-HT$_3$) receptor antagonist is thought to bind to serotonin receptors of the 5-HT$_3$ type located peripherally on vagal nerve terminals and centrally in the chemoreceptor trigger zone of the area postrema. This binding blocks serotonin stimulation and subsequent vomiting after emetogenic stimuli, such as cisplatin.

### Pharmacokinetics

*Absorption:* Not determined.
*Distribution:* Distributed freely between plasma and RBCs. Plasma protein–binding is about 65%.
*Metabolism:* Metabolized by the liver, possibly mediated by the cytochrome P-450 3A subfamily.
*Excretion:* About 12% is eliminated unchanged in the urine in 48 hours; the remainder is excreted as metabolites: 48% in the urine and 38% in the feces.

| Route | Onset | Peak | Duration |
|-------|-------|------|----------|
| P.O., I.V. | Unknown | Unknown | Unknown |

### Contraindications and precautions

Contraindicated in patients hypersensitive to drug.

### Interactions

**Drug-herb.** *Horehound:* Enhanced serotonergic effects. Discourage use together.

### Adverse reactions

**CNS:** *headache, asthenia,* somnolence, dizziness, anxiety.
**CV:** hypertension.
**GI:** diarrhea, *constipation,* abdominal pain, *nausea,* vomiting, decreased appetite.
**Hematologic:** *leukopenia,* anemia, **thrombocytopenia.**
**Hepatic:** elevated liver function test results.
**Skin:** alopecia.
**Other:** fever.

### Overdose and treatment

No antidote for overdose exists. Recommend giving symptomatic treatment. Overdose of up to 38.5 mg of granisetron has been reported without symptoms or only the occurrence of a slight headache.

### Clinical considerations

■ No dosage adjustment is recommended for patients with renal impairment or hepatic disease.

*Therapeutic monitoring*
■ Advise clinician to monitor patient for decreased symptoms and for any increase in nausea or abdominal pain.

*Special populations*
**Breast-feeding patients.** It's unknown if drug appears in breast milk.
**Pediatric patients.** Safety and efficacy in children under age 2 haven't been established. Safety and efficacy in children haven't been established for the oral form.

### Patient counseling

■ Tell patient to watch for signs of an anaphylactoid reaction—local or generalized hives, chest tightness, wheezing, and dizziness or weakness—and to report them immediately.

## griseofulvin microsize
Fulvicin-U/F, Grifulvin V, Grisactin

## griseofulvin ultramicrosize
Fulvicin P/G, Grisactin Ultra, Gris-PEG

*Pharmacologic classification:* penicillium antibiotic
*Therapeutic classification:* antifungal
*Pregnancy risk category C*

### Available forms

Available by prescription only
**Microsize**
*Capsules:* 250 mg
*Tablets:* 250 mg, 500 mg
*Oral suspension:* 125 mg/5 ml

**Ultramicrosize**
*Tablets:* 125 mg, 165 mg, 250 mg, 330 mg
*Tablets (film-coated):* 125 mg, 250 mg

## Indications and dosages
*Tinea corporis, tinea capitis, tinea barbae, or tinea cruris infections*
*Adults:* 330 mg ultramicrosize P.O. daily, or 500 mg microsize P.O. daily.
*Children weighing 14 to 23 kg (30 to 50 lb):* 82.5 to 165 mg ultramicrosize P.O. daily, or 125 to 250 mg microsize P.O. daily.
*Children weighing over 23 kg:* 165 to 330 mg ultramicrosize P.O. daily, or 250 to 500 mg microsize P.O. daily.
*Tinea pedis or tinea unguium infections*
*Adults:* 660 mg ultramicrosize P.O. daily or 1 g microsize P.O. daily.
*Children weighing 14 to 23 kg (30 to 50 lb):* 82.5 to 165 mg ultramicrosize P.O. daily, or 125 to 250 mg microsize P.O. daily.
*Children weighing over 23 kg:* 165 to 330 mg ultramicrosize P.O. daily, or 250 to 500 mg microsize P.O. daily.

## Mechanism of action
*Antifungal action:* Griseofulvin disrupts fungal cell's mitotic spindle, interfering with cell division; it also may inhibit DNA replication. Drug also enters keratin precursor cells, slowing fungal growth. Active against *Trichophyton, Microsporum,* and *Epidermophyton.*

## Pharmacokinetics
*Absorption:* Absorbed primarily in the duodenum, and rate of absorption varies among individuals. Ultramicrosize preparations are absorbed almost completely; microsize absorption ranges from 25% to 70% and may be increased by giving with a high-fat meal.
*Distribution:* Concentrates in skin, hair, nails, fat, liver, and skeletal muscle; it's tightly bound to new keratin.
*Metabolism:* Oxidatively demethylated and conjugated with glucuronic acid to inactive metabolites in the liver.
*Excretion:* About 50% of drug and its metabolites is excreted in urine and 33% in feces within 5 days. Less than 1% of a dose appears unchanged in urine. Drug is also excreted in perspiration. Elimination half-life is 9 to 24 hours.

| Route | Onset | Peak | Duration |
|-------|-------|------|----------|
| P.O. | Unknown | 4-8 hr | Unknown |

## Contraindications and precautions
Contraindicated in those hypersensitive to drug and in those with porphyria or hepatocellular failure. Also contraindicated in pregnant women and women who intend to become pregnant during therapy.

Use drug cautiously in penicillin-sensitive patients.

## Interactions
**Drug-drug.** *Barbiturates:* Impaired absorption of griseofulvin. Dosage may need to be increased.
*Oral contraceptives:* Decreased efficacy of contraceptives. Alternative method of contraception should be suggested.
*Phenobarbital:* Decreased griseofulvin blood levels as a result of decreased absorption or increased metabolism. Avoid use together.
*Warfarin:* Decreased PT and INR. Dosage adjustment may be needed.
**Drug-food.** *High-fat meals:* Increased absorption. May be given together.
**Drug-lifestyle.** *Alcohol use:* Increased alcohol effect, producing tachycardia, diaphoresis, and flushing. Advise patient to avoid alcohol.

## Adverse reactions
**CNS:** headache (in early stages of treatment), transient decrease in hearing, fatigue with large doses, occasional mental confusion, impaired performance of routine activities, psychotic symptoms, dizziness, insomnia, paresthesia of the hands and feet after extended therapy.
**EENT:** oral thrush.
**GI:** nausea, vomiting, flatulence, diarrhea, epigastric distress, *bleeding.*
**GU:** proteinuria, menstrual irregularities.
**Hematologic:** *leukopenia, **granulocytopenia*** (requires discontinuation of drug), porphyria.
**Hepatic:** *hepatotoxicity.*
**Skin:** *rash, urticaria,* photosensitivity, angioneurotic edema.
**Other:** lupus erythematosus.

## Overdose and treatment
Symptoms of overdose include headache, lethargy, confusion, vertigo, blurred vision, nausea, vomiting, and diarrhea. Treatment is supportive. After recent ingestion (within 4 hours), recommend emptying stomach by induced emesis or gastric lavage. Follow with activated charcoal to decrease absorption. A cathartic may also be helpful.

## Clinical considerations
■ Confirm identification of organism before therapy begins.
■ Recommend giving drug with or after meals consisting of a high fat content (if allowed), to minimize GI distress.
■ Treatment of tinea pedis may require combined oral and topical therapy.
**ᴴ ALERT** Because griseofulvin ultramicrosize is dispersed in polyethylene glycol, it's absorbed more rapidly and completely than microsize and is effective at one-half to two-thirds the usual griselfulvin dose. Don't interchange preparations.

---

Reactions may be *common,* uncommon, *life-threatening,* or COMMON AND LIFE-THREATENING.

### Therapeutic monitoring
■ Assess nutrition and monitor food intake; drug may alter taste sensation, suppressing appetite.
■ Check CBC regularly for possible adverse effects; advise clinician to monitor renal and liver function test results periodically.

### Special populations
**Pregnant patients.** Contraindicated in pregnant women and women who intend to become pregnant during therapy.
**Breast-feeding patients.** Safety hasn't been established in breast-feeding women.
**Pediatric patients.** Microsize griseofulvin has been used in children as young as 3 months. Manufacturer states that dosage of ultramicrosize griseofulvin has not been established in children ages 2 years and younger.

### Patient counseling
■ Encourage patient to maintain adequate nutritional intake.
■ Stress importance of completing prescribed regimen to prevent relapse even though symptoms may abate quickly.
■ Tell patient to report adverse reactions to prescriber immediately.
■ Advise patient to avoid exposure to intense indoor light and sunlight to reduce the risk of photosensitivity reactions.
■ Explain that drug may potentiate alcohol effects, and advise patient to avoid alcohol during therapy.

# guaifenesin
Amonidrin, Anti-Tuss, Balminil Expectorant*, Breonesin, Duratuss-G, Fenesin, Gee-Gee, Genatuss, GG-Cen, Glyate, Glycotuss, Glytuss, Guaifenex L.A., Guiatuss, Humibid L.A., Humibid Pediatric, Humibid Sprinkle, Hytuss, Hytuss 2X, Malotuss, Mytussin, Naldecon Senior EX, Organidin NR, Respa-GF, Resyl*, Robitussin, Scot-Tussin

*Pharmacologic classification:* propanediol derivative
*Therapeutic classification:* expectorant
*Pregnancy risk category C*

## Available forms
**Available by prescription only**
*Capsules (sustained-release):* 300 mg, 600 mg
*Tablets:* 200 mg
*Tablets (extended-release):* 600 mg, 800 mg, 1,200 mg
*Tablets (sustained-release):* 600 mg, 1,200 mg
*Liquid:* 100 mg/5 ml
**Available without a prescription**
*Tablets:* 100 mg, 200 mg

*Capsules:* 200 mg
*Syrup:* 100 mg/5 ml, 200 mg/5 ml

## Indications and dosages
**Expectorant**
*Adults and children ages 12 and older:* 200 to 400 mg P.O. q 4 hours; maximum dose is 2.4 g/day.
*Children ages 6 to 11:* 100 to 200 mg P.O. q 4 hours; maximum dose is 1.2 g/day.
*Children ages 2 to 5:* 50 to 100 mg P.O. q 4 hours; maximum dose is 600 mg/day.
*Children under age 2:* Individualize dosage.
**Extended-release and sustained-release**
*Adults and children over age 12:* 600 to 1,200 mg P.O. q 12 hours, not to exceed 2,400 mg in 24 hours.
*Children ages 6 to 11:* 600 mg P.O. q 12 hours, not to exceed 1,200 mg in 24 hours.
*Children ages 2 to 5:* 300 mg P.O. q 12 hours, not to exceed 600 mg in 24 hours.

## Mechanism of action
*Expectorant action:* Guaifenesin increases respiratory tract fluid by reducing adhesiveness and surface tension, decreasing viscosity of the secretions and thereby facilitating their removal.

## Pharmacokinetics
Unknown.

| Route | Onset | Peak | Duration |
|-------|-------|------|----------|
| P.O. | Unknown | Unknown | Unknown |

## Contraindications and precautions
Contraindicated in patients hypersensitive to drug.

## Interactions
None significant.

## Adverse reactions
**CNS:** dizziness, headache.
**GI:** vomiting and nausea (with large doses).
**Skin:** rash.

## Overdose and treatment
No information available.

## Clinical considerations
■ Efficacy of guaifenesin as an expectorant hasn't been clearly established because of conflicting results of clinical studies.
■ Drug may cause color interference with tests for 5-hydroxyindoleacetic acid and vanillylmandelic acid.

### Therapeutic monitoring
■ Patient should be reevaluated if symptoms persist for longer than 1 week, if cough recurs, or if cough is accompanied by fever, rash, or persistent headache.

### Special populations
**Breast-feeding patients.** It's unknown if drug appears in breast milk. Safety in breast-feeding women hasn't been established.
**Pediatric patients.** Individualize dosage for children under age 2.
**Geriatric patients.** No specific recommendations are available. Most liquid preparations contain alcohol (3.5% to 10%).

### Patient counseling
■ Advise patient to take drug with a full glass of water to help loosen mucus in lungs.
■ Advise patient to use sugarless throat lozenges to decrease throat irritation and associated cough and to report cough that persists longer than 7 days.

---

# guanabenz acetate
Wytensin

*Pharmacologic classification:* centrally acting antiadrenergic
*Therapeutic classification:* antihypertensive
*Pregnancy risk category C*

### Available forms
Available by prescription only
*Tablets:* 4 mg, 8 mg

### Indications and dosages
*Hypertension (generally considered a step 2 drug)*
*Adults:* Initially, 2 to 4 mg P.O. b.i.d. Dosage may be increased in increments of 4 to 8 mg/day q 1 to 2 weeks. The usual maintenance dose ranges from 8 to 16 mg daily. Maximum dose is 32 mg b.i.d.
*Children ages 12 and older:* Initially, 0.5 to 4 mg P.O. daily; maintenance dose ranges from 4 to 24 mg daily, given in two divided doses.
◇ *Management of opiate withdrawal*
*Adults:* 4 mg P.O. b.i.d. to q.i.d.

### Mechanism of action
*Antihypertensive action:* Guanabenz decreases blood pressure by stimulating central alpha₂-adrenergic receptors, decreasing cerebral sympathetic outflow and thus decreasing peripheral vascular resistance. Guanabenz may also antagonize antidiuretic hormone (ADH) secretion and ADH activity in the kidney.

### Pharmacokinetics
*Absorption:* After oral administration, 70% to 80% is absorbed from the GI tract.
*Distribution:* Appears to be distributed widely into the body, and is about 90% protein-bound.
*Metabolism:* Metabolized extensively in the liver; several metabolites are formed.

*Excretion:* Guanabenz and its metabolites are excreted primarily in urine; remaining drug is excreted in feces.

| Route | Onset | Peak | Duration |
|-------|-------|------|----------|
| P.O. | 1 hr | 2-5 hr | 6-12 hr |

### Contraindications and precautions
Contraindicated in patients hypersensitive to drug.
    Use drug cautiously in geriatric patients and in patients with impaired renal or hepatic function, severe coronary insufficiency, recent MI, or cerebrovascular disease.

### Interactions
**Drug-drug.** *Barbiturates, benzodiazepines, phenothiazines, other sedatives:* Increased CNS depressant effects. Use together cautiously.
*Diuretics and other antihypertensives:* Increased risk of excessive hypotension. Advise clinician to monitor blood pressure frequently.
*MAO inhibitors, tricyclic antidepressants:* Inhibit antihypertensive effects of guanabenz. Advise clinician to monitor blood pressure frequently.
**Drug-lifestyle.** *Alcohol use:* Increased CNS depressant effects. Advise patient to avoid alcohol.

### Adverse reactions
**CNS:** *drowsiness, sedation, dizziness, weakness,* headache.
**CV:** *rebound hypertension.*
**GI:** *dry mouth.*
**Hepatic:** elevations in liver enzyme levels.
**Metabolic:** may reduce serum cholesterol and total triglyceride levels slightly.

### Overdose and treatment
Clinical signs of overdose include bradycardia, CNS depression, respiratory depression, hypothermia, apnea, seizures, lethargy, agitation, irritability, diarrhea, and hypotension.
    Emesis shouldn't be induced; CNS depression occurs rapidly. After adequate respiration is assured, recommend emptying stomach by gastric lavage, then giving activated charcoal and a saline cathartic to decrease absorption. Symptomatic and supportive care should follow.

### Clinical considerations
■ Abrupt discontinuation of guanabenz causes severe rebound hypertension; dosage should be reduced gradually over 2 to 4 days.
■ Reduced dosages may be needed in patients with hepatic impairment.

### Therapeutic monitoring
■ Advise clinician to monitor patient for adverse reactions, including CNS effects.
■ Advise clinician to monitor liver enzyme level and serum triglyceride levels.

---

Reactions may be *common,* uncommon, *life-threatening,* or COMMON AND LIFE-THREATENING.

### Special populations
**Breast-feeding patients.** It's unknown if guanabenz appears in breast milk; an alternative feeding method is recommended during therapy.
**Pediatric patients.** Drug has been used to treat hypertension in a limited number of children over age 12; safety and efficacy in younger children haven't been established.
**Geriatric patients.** Geriatric patients may be more sensitive to antihypertensive and sedative effects of guanabenz.

### Patient counseling
■ Explain signs and symptoms of adverse effects and importance of reporting them.
■ Warn patient to avoid hazardous activities that require mental alertness and to avoid alcohol and other CNS depressants.
■ Suggest taking drug at bedtime until tolerance develops to sedation, drowsiness, and other CNS effects.
■ Warn patient to seek medical approval before taking OTC cold preparations.
■ Advise patient not to discontinue drug suddenly; severe rebound hypertension may occur.

# guanethidine monosulfate
Ismelin

*Pharmacologic classification:* adrenergic neuron blocker
*Therapeutic classification:* antihypertensive
*Pregnancy risk category C*

### Available forms
Available by prescription only
*Tablets:* 10 mg, 25 mg

### Indications and dosages
*Moderate to severe hypertension, ◇ signs and symptoms of thyrotoxicosis*
*Adults:* Initially, 10 mg P.O. once daily; increase by 10 mg at weekly to monthly intervals, p.r.n. Usual dose is 25 to 50 mg once daily; some patients may require up to 300 mg.

### Mechanism of action
*Antihypertensive action:* Guanethidine acts peripherally; it decreases arteriolar vasoconstriction and reduces blood pressure by inhibiting norepinephrine release and depleting norepinephrine stores in adrenergic nerve endings.

### Pharmacokinetics
*Absorption:* Absorbed incompletely from the GI tract. Maximal antihypertensive effects usually aren't evident for 1 to 3 weeks.

*Distribution:* Distributed throughout the body; it's not protein-bound but shows extensive tissue binding.
*Metabolism:* Undergoes partial hepatic metabolism to pharmacologically less active metabolites.
*Excretion:* Drug and metabolites are excreted primarily in urine; small amounts are excreted in feces. Elimination half-life after long-term administration is biphasic.

| Route | Onset | Peak | Duration |
|-------|-------|------|----------|
| P.O. | Unknown | 8 hr | 3-4 days |

### Contraindications and precautions
Contraindicated in patients with pheochromocytoma or frank HF, and in those hypersensitive to drug or receiving MAO inhibitors.
Use drug cautiously in patients with severe cardiac disease, recent MI, cerebrovascular disease, peptic ulcer, impaired renal function, or bronchial asthma, and in those taking other antihypertensives.

### Interactions
**Drug-drug.** *Amphetamines, ephedrine, MAO inhibitors, methylphenidate, norepinephrine, oral contraceptives, phenothiazines, or tricyclic antidepressants:* May antagonize the antihypertensive effect of guanethidine. MAO inhibitor therapy should be discontinued 1 week before guanethidine is started. Dosage may need adjustment.
*Cardiac glycosides:* May result in additive bradycardia. Monitor patient closely.
*Diuretics, other antihypertensives, levodopa:* May potentiate antihypertensive effect of guanethidine. Use together cautiously.
*Metaraminol, norepinephrine, oral sympathomimetic nasal decongestants:* Guanethidine potentiates pressor effects of such drugs. Advise clinician to monitor blood pressure closely.
*Rauwolfia alkaloids (reserpine):* May cause excessive orthostatic hypotension, bradycardia, and mental depression. Monitor patient for these effects.
**Drug-lifestyle.** *Alcohol use:* Increased hypotensive effect of guanethidine. Advise patient to avoid alcohol.

### Adverse reactions
**CNS:** *syncope, fatigue, headache, drowsiness, paresthesia, confusion.*
**CV:** *palpitations, chest pain, orthostatic hypotension, peripheral edema,* **bradycardia, HF.**
**EENT:** *visual disturbances,* glossitis.
**GI:** *diarrhea, indigestion, constipation, anorexia,* nausea, vomiting.
**GU:** *nocturia, urination frequency, ejaculation disturbances,* impotence.
**Metabolic:** *weight gain.*
**Musculoskeletal:** *aching limbs, leg cramps.*
**Respiratory:** shortness of breath, cough.

## Overdose and treatment
Signs of overdose include hypotension, blurred vision, syncope, bradycardia, and severe diarrhea.

After acute ingestion, recommend emptying stomach by induced emesis or gastric lavage and giving activated charcoal to reduce absorption. Further treatment is usually symptomatic and supportive.

## Clinical considerations
■ When drug is replacing MAO inhibitors, recommend waiting at least 1 week before starting guanethidine; if replacing ganglionic blockers, they should be withdrawn slowly to prevent a spiking blood pressure response during the transfer period.
■ Dosage requirements may be reduced in the presence of fever.
■ Recommend stopping drug 2 to 3 weeks before elective surgery to reduce risk of CV collapse during anesthesia.
■ The goal of hypertensive management is to achieve and maintain a systolic blood pressure less than 130 mm Hg and a diastolic blood pressure less than 85 mm Hg.

### Therapeutic monitoring
■ If diarrhea develops, atropine or paregoric may be prescribed.
■ Advise clinician to monitor patient for adverse reactions.
■ Systolic blood pressure is considered the therapeutic endpoint, especially in middle-aged and geriatric patients.

### Special populations
**Breast-feeding patients.** Small amounts of drug appear in breast milk; recommend alternative feeding method during therapy.
**Pediatric patients.** Safety and efficacy in children haven't been established.
**Geriatric patients.** Geriatric patients may be more sensitive to drug's antihypertensive effects.

## Patient counseling
■ Tell patient to report persistent diarrhea and excessive weight gain (2.25 kg [5 lb] weekly). Advise patient not to discontinue the drug but to call prescriber for further instructions.
■ Warn patient to avoid hazardous activities that require mental alertness and to take drug at bedtime until tolerance develops to sedation, drowsiness, and other CNS effects.
■ Advise patient to avoid sudden position changes, strenuous exercise, heat, and hot showers, to minimize orthostatic hypotension; and to relieve dry mouth with ice chips, hard candy, or gum.
■ Tell patient if a dose is missed not to double the next scheduled dose but to take only the next scheduled dose.

■ Advise patient to seek medical approval before taking OTC cold preparations.

# Haemophilus b vaccines

## Haemophilus b conjugate vaccine, diphtheria CRM protein conjugate (HbOC)
HibTITER

## Haemophilus b conjugate vaccine, meningococcal protein conjugate (PRP-OMP)
PedvaxHIB

## Haemophilus b polysaccharide conjugate vaccine, tetanus toxoid (PRP-T)
ActHIB

*Pharmacologic classification:* vaccine
*Therapeutic classification:* bacterial vaccine
*Pregnancy risk category C*

## Available forms
Available by prescription only
**Conjugate vaccine, diphtheria CRM$_{197}$**
*Injection:* 10 mcg of purified *Haemophilus* b saccharide and about 25 mcg CRM$_{197}$ protein per 0.5 ml
**Conjugate vaccine, meningococcal protein conjugate**
*Injection:* 7.5 mcg *Haemophilus* b capsular polysaccharide, 125 mcg *Neisseria meningitidis* OMPC per 0.5 ml
**Conjugate vaccine, tetanus toxoid**
*Powder for injection:* 10 mcg *Haemophilus* b purified capsular polysaccharide, 24 mcg of tetanus toxoid, and 8.5% sucrose

## Indications and dosages
### Routine immunization
**Haemophilus b conjugate vaccine, diphtheria CRM$_{197}$ protein conjugate**
*Children ages 2 to 6 months:* 0.5 ml I.M.; repeat in 2 months and again in 4 months (for total of three doses). A booster dose is required at age 15 months.
*Previously unvaccinated children ages 7 to 11 months:* 0.5 ml I.M.; repeat in 2 months (for total of two doses before age 15 months). A booster dose is required at age 15 months (but no sooner than 2 months after last vaccination).
*Previously unvaccinated children ages 12 to 14 months:* 0.5 ml I.M. A booster dose is required at age 15 months (but no sooner than 2 months after last vaccination).
*Previously unvaccinated children ages 15 to 60 months:* 0.5 ml I.M.
**Haemophilus b conjugate vaccine, meningococcal protein conjugate**
*Previously unvaccinated infants ages 2 to 10 months:* 0.5 ml I.M. ideally at 2 months. Repeat 2 months later (or as soon as possible thereafter). Give a booster dose of 0.5 ml I.M. at 12 to 15 months (but no sooner than 2 months after last vaccination).
*Previously unvaccinated children ages 11 to 14 months:* 0.5 ml I.M.; repeat in 2 months.
*Previously unvaccinated children ages 15 to 71 months:* 0.5 ml I.M.
**Haemophilus b polysaccharide conjugate vaccine, tetanus toxoid**
*Previously unvaccinated children ages 2 to 6 months:* Three 0.5-ml I.M. doses, at 8-week intervals followed by a booster dose at age 15 to 18 months.
*Previously unvaccinated children ages 7 to 11 months:* Two 0.5-ml I.M. doses at 8-week intervals, followed by a booster dose at ages 15 to 18 months.
*Previously unvaccinated children ages 12 to 14 months:* 0.5 ml I.M., followed by a booster dose at ages 15 to 18 months. Give no earlier than 2 months after previous dose.
*Previously unvaccinated children ages 15 to 60 months:* 0.5 ml I.M.

## Mechanism of action
*Prophylactic action:* Vaccine promotes active immunity to *H. influenzae* type b.

## Pharmacokinetics
*Absorption:* After I.M. or S.C. administration, increases in *H. influenzae* type b capsular antibody levels in serum are detectable in about 2 weeks and peak within 3 weeks.
*Distribution:* Limited data indicate that antibodies to *H. influenzae* type b can be detected in fetal blood and in breast milk after administration of the vaccine to pregnant and breastfeeding patients.

---

*Metabolism:* No information available.
*Excretion:* The vaccine polysaccharide has been detected in urine for up to 11 days after administration to children.

| Route | Onset | Peak | Duration |
|-------|-------|------|----------|
| I.M. | 2 wk after last dose | Unknown | Several yr |

## Contraindications and precautions

Contraindicated in patients with acute illness or hypersensitivity to any component of vaccine, including thimerosal. Drug shouldn't be given to patients less than 10 days before or during treatment with immunosuppressive drugs or irradiation.

Because of the natural latex proteins found in some of the packaging components, recommend taking precautions when drug is administered to patients with latex sensitivity.

## Interactions

**Drug-drug.** *Corticosteroids or immunosuppressants:* May impair immune response to the vaccine. Avoid vaccination under these circumstances.

## Adverse reactions

**CNS:** irritability.
**GI:** diarrhea, vomiting.
**Skin:** *erythema, pain at injection site.*
**Other:** *anaphylaxis,* fever.

## Overdose and treatment

No information available.

## Clinical considerations

■ Advise clinician that epinephrine solution 1:1,000 should be available to treat allergic reactions.
**ℍ ALERT** Vaccine types are age specific. Check labeling as well as current U.S. Health Service Advisory Committee on Immunization Practices (ACIP) and American Academy of Pediatrics (AAP) recommendations.
■ Vaccine may be given simultaneously with diphtheria, tetanus, and pertussis (DTP) vaccine; measles, mumps, and rubella (MMR) vaccine; poliovirus vaccine, inactivated (IPV); meningococcal vaccine; or pneumococcal vaccine, but should be given at different sites using different syringes.
■ Recommend administering same vaccine throughout the vaccination series; no data are available to support the interchangeability of the vaccines.
■ Children under age 24 months in whom invasive *H. influenzae* type b disease develops should be vaccinated because natural immunity may not develop.
■ Vaccination shouldn't be used to prevent invasive *H. influenzae* type b disease because

of the time required for the patient to develop immunity. Chemoprophylaxis (with drugs such as rifampin) should instead be used in both vaccinated and unvaccinated individuals because children with immunity may carry and transmit the organism. However, if every child in a household or day-care group has been fully vaccinated, chemoprophylaxis isn't needed.
■ A conjugate vaccine containing meningococcal proteins won't prevent meningococcal disease; one containing diphtheria proteins won't produce immunity against diphtheria; and one containing the tetanus toxoid conjugate won't produce immunity against tetanus toxoid. Recommend giving DTP vaccine according to the recommended schedule.
■ Some vaccine products may contain thimerosal.
■ For days or weeks after administration, *Haemophilus* b (Hib) may interfere with antigen detection tests.

### Therapeutic monitoring
■ Adverse reactions generally occur within the first 24 hours.
■ Advise clinician to monitor patient for anaphylaxis, injection site reactions, and fever.

### Special populations
**Pregnant patients.** Generally not recommended for use in pregnant women.
**Pediatric patients.** Safety and efficacy of PRP-OMP haven't been established for patients under age 2 months. Safety and efficacy of PRP-T haven't been established for patients under age 6 weeks.

## Patient counseling
■ *H. influenzae* type b is a cause of meningitis in infants and preschool children. Explain to parents that this vaccine will protect children only against meningitis caused by this organism.
■ Tell parents that child may experience swelling and inflammation at injection site and fever. Recommend acetaminophen liquid for fever.
■ Tell parents to report worrisome or persistent adverse reactions promptly.

# haloperidol

Apo-Haloperidol*, Haldol, Novo-
Peridol*, Peridol*

# haloperidol decanoate

Haldol Decanoate, Haldol Decanoate
100, Haldol LA*

# haloperidol lactate

Haldol, Haldol Concentrate,
Haloperidol Intensol

*Pharmacologic classification:* butyrophenone
*Therapeutic classification:* antipsychotic
*Pregnancy risk category C*

## Available forms

Available by prescription only
**haloperidol**
*Tablets:* 0.5 mg, 1 mg, 2 mg, 5 mg, 10 mg,
20 mg
**haloperidol decanoate**
*Injection:* 50 mg/ml, 100 mg/ml
**haloperidol lactate**
*Oral concentrate:* 2 mg/ml
*Injection:* 5 mg/ml

## Indications and dosages

*Psychotic disorders,* ◇ *alcohol dependence*
*Adults:* Dosage varies for each patient and variable symptoms. Initial dosage range is 0.5 to
5 mg P.O. b.i.d. or t.i.d.; or 2 to 5 mg I.M. q 4
to 8 hours, increased rapidly if needed for
prompt control. Maximum dose is 100 mg P.O.
daily. Doses of more than 100 mg have been
used to treat patients who have severely resistant conditions.
*Psychotic patients who require prolonged
therapy*
*Adults:* 100 mg I.M. of haloperidol decanoate
q 4 weeks. Experience with doses of more than
450 mg monthly is limited.
*Control of tics, vocal utterances in
Tourette syndrome*
*Adults:* 0.5 to 5 mg P.O. b.i.d. or t.i.d., increased,
p.r.n.
*Children ages 3 to 12:* 0.05 to 0.075 mg/kg/day
given b.i.d. or t.i.d.
◇ *Delirium*
*Adults:* 1 to 2 mg I.V. every 2 to 4 hours.

## I.V. administration

■ Haloperidol lactate has been given by direct
I.V. injection or infusion for delirium (unlabeled use).
**ᴴ ALERT** Don't administer haloperidol de-
conoate I.V.
■ Advise clinician to monitor QT interval and
stop drug or reduce dosage if prolongation occurs.

## Incompatibilities

None reported.

## Mechanism of action

*Antipsychotic action:* Haloperidol is thought
to exert its antipsychotic effects by strong postsynaptic blockade of CNS dopamine receptors, thereby inhibiting dopamine-mediated effects; its pharmacologic effects are most similar
to those of piperazine antipsychotics. Its mechanism of action in Tourette syndrome is unknown.
    Haloperidol has many other central and pe-
ripheral effects; it has weak peripheral anticholinergic effects and antiemetic effects, produces both alpha and ganglionic blockade, and
counteracts histamine- and serotonin-mediated
activity. Its most prominent adverse reactions
are extrapyramidal.

## Pharmacokinetics

*Absorption:* Rate and extent of absorption vary
with route of administration.
*Distribution:* Distributed widely into the body,
with high levels in adipose tissue. Drug is 90%
to 92% protein-bound.
*Metabolism:* Metabolized extensively by the
liver; there may be only one active metabolite
that's less active than parent drug.
*Excretion:* About 40% of a given dose is excreted in urine within 5 days; about 15% is excreted in feces via the biliary tract.

| Route | Onset | Peak | Duration |
|-------|-------|------|----------|
| P.O. | Unknown | 3-6 hr | Unknown |
| I.M. (decanoate) | Unknown | 3-9 days | Unknown |
| I.M. (lactate) | Unknown | 10-20 min | Unknown |

## Contraindications and precautions

Contraindicated in patients hypersensitive to
drug and in those experiencing parkinsonism,
coma, or CNS depression.
    Haloperidol should be used cautiously in
geriatric or debilitated patients; in patients with
history of seizures, EEG abnormalities, CV
disorders, allergies, angle-closure glaucoma,
or urine retention; and in those receiving anticoagulants, anticonvulsants, antiparkinsonians, or lithium drugs.

## Interactions

**Drug-drug.** *Aluminum- and magnesium-
containing antacids and antidiarrheals:* Separate administration times of oral haloperidol
and these drugs by 2 hours.
*Antiarrhythmics, disopyramide, procainamide,
quinidine:* Increased risk of arrhythmias and
conduction defects. Avoid use together.
*Atropine or other anticholinergics, including
antidepressants, antihistamines, MAO inhibitors, meperidine, phenothiazines, and antiparkinsonians:* Oversedation, paralytic ileus,

visual changes, and severe constipation. Use with caution.

*Beta blockers:* May inhibit haloperidol metabolism, increasing plasma levels and toxicity. Use with caution.

*Bromocriptine:* Haloperidol antagonizes the therapeutic effect of bromocriptine on prolactin secretion. Avoid concurrent use.

*Centrally acting antihypertensives (such as clonidine, guanabenz, guanadrel, guanethidine, methyldopa, reserpine):* Inhibited blood pressure response. Advise clinician to monitor blood pressure carefully.

*CNS depressants (including analgesics, barbiturates, narcotics, tranquilizers), general, spinal, or epidural anesthetics, or parenteral magnesium sulfate:* Increased CNS depression. Avoid use together.

*Dopamine:* Decreased vasoconstricting effects. Avoid use together

*Levodopa:* Decreased effectiveness of levodopa. Avoid use together.

*Lithium:* May result in severe neurologic toxicity with an encephalitis-like syndrome, and a decreased therapeutic response to haloperidol. Use with caution; recommend monitoring patient.

*Metrizamide:* Increased risk of seizures. Avoid use together.

*Nitrates:* Hypotension. Advise clinician to monitor blood pressure frequently.

*Phenobarbital:* Enhanced renal excretion. Advise clinician to monitor patient closely.

*Phenytoin:* Inhibited metabolism and increased toxicity of phenytoin. Avoid use together.

*Propylthiouracil:* Increased risk of agranulocytosis. Avoid use together.

*Rifampin:* Decreased haloperidol levels; decreased efficacy. Advise clinician to monitor patient carefully.

*Sympathomimetics, including epinephrine, phenylephrine, and ephedrine (often found in nasal sprays), and appetite suppressants:* May decrease stimulatory and pressor effects of these drugs. Advise clinician to monitor patient carefully.

**Drug-herb.** *Nutmeg:* Loss of symptom control; interference with existing therapy for psychiatric illnesses. Discourage use together.

**Drug-lifestyle.** *Heavy smoking:* Increased metabolism of haloperidol. Discourage smoking.

## Adverse reactions

**CNS:** *severe extrapyramidal reactions, tardive dyskinesia,* sedation, drowsiness, lethargy, headache, insomnia, confusion, vertigo, *seizures, neuroleptic malignant syndrome.*

**CV:** tachycardia, hypotension, hypertension, ECG changes.

**EENT:** *blurred vision.*

**GI:** dry mouth, anorexia, constipation, diarrhea, nausea, vomiting, dyspepsia.

**GU:** urine retention, menstrual irregularities, priapism.

**Hematologic:** *leukopenia,* leukocytosis.

**Hepatic:** altered liver function test results, jaundice.

**Skin:** rash, other skin reactions, diaphoresis.

**Other:** gynecomastia.

## Overdose and treatment

Overdose is manifested as greater acuity of adverse reactions, which can include deep, unarousable sleep, coma, hypotension, hypertension, extrapyramidal symptoms, dystonia, abnormal involuntary muscle movements, agitation, seizures, arrhythmias, ECG changes (may show QT interval prolongation and torsades de pointes), hypothermia, hyperthermia, and autonomic nervous system dysfunction. Overdose with long-acting decanoate requires prolonged recovery time.

Treatment is symptomatic and supportive, including maintaining vital signs, airway, stable body temperature, and fluid and electrolyte balance. Ipecac may be used to induce vomiting, with due regard for antiemetic properties of haloperidol and hazard of aspiration. Gastric lavage also may be used, followed by activated charcoal and saline cathartics; dialysis doesn't help.

Recommend regulating body temperature p.r.n. Recommend treating hypotension with I.V. fluids; epinephrine shouldn't be given. Recommend treating seizures with parenteral diazepam or barbiturates; arrhythmias, with parenteral phenytoin (1 mg/kg I.V. with rate titrated to blood pressure not to exceed 50 mg/minute with ECG monitoring; may repeat every 5 minutes up to 10 mg/kg); extrapyramidal reactions with benztropine at 1 to 2 mg or parenteral diphenhydramine at 10 to 50 mg.

## Clinical considerations

■ Drug has few CV adverse effects and may be preferred in patients with cardiac disease.

■ Dose of 2 mg is therapeutic equivalent of 100 mg chlorpromazine.

■ When changing from tablets to decanoate injection, patient should initially receive 10 to 20 times the oral dose once monthly (not more than 100 mg).

### Therapeutic monitoring

■ Recommend assessing patient periodically for extrapyramidal reactions and tardive dyskinesia.

■ Drug shouldn't be withdrawn abruptly except when required because abrupt withdrawal may cause severe adverse reaction.

### Special populations

**Pediatric patients.** Safety and efficacy of drug injection in children haven't been established and oral drug isn't recommended for children under age 3.

**Geriatric patients.** Drug is especially useful for agitation from senile dementia. Tardive dyskinesia may occur more often, especially in elderly women. Geriatric patients usually require lower initial doses and a more gradual dosage titration.

### Patient counseling
■ Warn patient against activities that require alertness and good psychomotor coordination until CNS response to drug is determined. Drowsiness and dizziness usually subside after a few weeks.
■ Tell patient to report adverse effects to prescriber.
■ Instruct patient to avoid combining with alcohol or other depressants.

# heparin sodium
Heparin Lock Flush, Hep-Lock, Hep-Lock U/P, Liquaemin

*Pharmacologic classification:* anticoagulant
*Therapeutic classification:* anticoagulant
*Pregnancy risk category C*

### Available forms
Available products are derived from bovine lung or porcine intestinal mucosa. All are injectable and available by prescription only.
**heparin sodium**
*Vials:* 1,000 units/ml, 5,000 units/ml, 10,000 units/ml, 20,000 units/ml, 40,000 units/ml
*Unit-dose ampules:* 1,000 units/ml, 5,000 units/ml, 10,000 units/ml
*Disposable syringes:* 1,000 units/ml, 2,500 units/ml, 5,000 units/ml, 7,500 units/ml, 10,000 units/ml, 20,000 units/ml
*Carpuject:* 5,000 units/ml
*Premixed I.V. solutions:* 1,000 units in 500 ml normal saline solution; 2,000 units in 1,000 ml normal saline solution; 12,500 units in 250 ml 0.45% saline solution; 25,000 units in 250 ml 0.45% saline solution; 25,000 units in 500 ml 0.45% saline solution; 10,000 units in 100 ml $D_5W$; 12,500 units in 250 ml $D_5W$; 25,000 units in 250 ml $D_5W$; 25,000 units in 500 ml $D_5W$
**heparin sodium flush**
*Vials:* 10 units/ml, 100 units/ml
*Disposable syringes:* 10 units/ml, 25 units/ 2.5 ml, 2,500 units/2.5 ml

### Indications and dosages
*Deep vein thrombosis, pulmonary embolism*
*Adults (based on weight of 68 kg): Full dose continuous I.V. infusion:* 5,000 units I.V. injection followed by infusion of 20,000 to 40,000 units in 1 L of normal saline or other compatible solution. For most patients, give over 24 hours. *Full dose intermittent I.V. therapy:* 10,000 units I.V. followed by 5,000 to 10,000

units every 4 to 6 hours. *Full dose S.C. therapy:* 5,000 units I.V. and 10,000 to 20,000 units S.C. followed by 8,000 to 10,000 units S.C. every 8 hours or 15,000 to 20,000 units every 12 hours.
*Children: Full dose continuous I.V. therapy:* 50 units/kg I.V. followed by 20,000 units/m² per 24 hours. *Full dose intermittent therapy:* 100 units/kg I.V. followed by 50 to 100 units/kg I.V. every 4 hours.
*Embolism prophylaxis*
*Adults:* 5,000 units S.C. 1 to 2 hours before surgery and every 8 to 12 hours after surgery for 5 to 7 days or until patient is ambulatory, whichever is longer.
*Open-heart surgery*
*Adults:* (total body perfusion) 150 to 400 units/kg continuous I.V. infusion.
*Disseminated intravascular coagulation*
*Adults:* 50 to 100 units/kg I.V. every 4 hours as a single injection or constant infusion. Discontinue if no improvement in 4 to 8 hours.
*Children:* 25 to 50 units/kg I.V. every 4 hours, as a single injection or constant infusion. Discontinue if no improvement in 4 to 8 hours.
*To maintain patency of I.V. indwelling catheters*
*Adults and children:* 10 to 100 units as an I.V. flush (not intended for therapeutic use).
◊ *Unstable angina*
*Adults:* 70 to 80 units/kg loading dose, followed by infusion maintaining PTT at 1.5 to 2 times control during first week of anginal pain.
*Anticoagulation in blood transfusion and samples*
*Transfusions and samples:* Mix 7,500 units and 100 ml of normal saline and add 6 to 8 ml of mixture to each 100 ml of whole blood or 70 to 150 units to each 10 to 20 ml of blood sample.
◊ *Post MI,* ◊ *cerebral thrombosis in evolving CVA,* ◊ *left ventricular thrombi,* ◊ *HF,* ◊ *history of embolism,* ◊ *atrial fibrillation*
*Adults:* 5,000 units S.C. every 12 hours empirically. Alternatively, 75 units/kg continuous infusion to maintain PTT at 1.5 to 2 times control value, followed by warfarin sodium.
Note: Heparin dosing is highly individualized, depending on disease state, age, weight, and renal and hepatic status.

### I.V. administration
■ When drug is added to I.V. solution, invert bag at least 6 times to ensure adequate mixing.
■ Intermittent injections can be given diluted in 50 to 100 ml of normal saline solution or undiluted.

### Incompatibilities
Incompatible with alteplase, amikacin, amacrine, amiodarone, ampicillin sodium, atracurium, cephalothin, chlorpromazine, ciprofloxacin, codeine phosphate, cytarabine, dacarbazine,

daunorubicin, dextrose 4.3% in 0.18% sodium chloride, diazepam, diltiazem, dobutamine, doxorubicin, droperidol, ergotamine, erythromycin glucepate or lactobionate, fentanyl sulfate and droperidol, filgrastim, gentamicin, haloperidol lactate, hyaluronidase, hydrocortisone sodium succinate, hydroxyzine hydrochloride, idarubicin, kanamycin, levorphanol, meperidine, methadone, methicillin, methotrimeprazine, methylprednisone sodium succinate, morphine sulfate, netilmicin, penicillin G potassium, penicillin G sodium, pentazocine lactate, phenytoin sodium, polymyxin B sulfate, prochlorperazine edisylate, promethazine hydrochloride, quinidine gluconate, 1/6 M sodium lactate, streptomycin, tobramycin sulfate, trifluoperazine, triflupromazine, vancomycin, and vinblastine.

Drug may also be incompatible with solutions containing a phosphate buffer, sodium carbonate, or sodium oxalate.

## Mechanism of action

*Anticoagulant action:* Heparin accelerates formation of antithrombin III-thrombin complex; it inactivates thrombin and prevents conversion of fibrinogen to fibrin.

## Pharmacokinetics

*Absorption:* Not absorbed from GI tract and must be given parenterally.
*Distribution:* Extensively bound to lipoprotein, globulins, and fibrinogen; it doesn't cross the placenta.
*Metabolism:* Although metabolism isn't completely described, drug is thought to be removed by the reticuloendothelial system, with some metabolism occurring in the liver.
*Excretion:* Little is known; a small fraction is excreted in urine as unchanged drug. Drug doesn't appear in breast milk. Plasma half-life is 1 to 2 hours.

| Route | Onset | Peak | Duration |
|-------|-------|------|----------|
| I.V. | Immediate | Unknown | Variable |
| S.C. | 20-60 min | 2-4 hr | Variable |

## Contraindications and precautions

Contraindicated in patients hypersensitive to drug. Conditionally contraindicated in patients with active bleeding; blood dyscrasia; or bleeding tendencies, such as hemophilia, thrombocytopenia, or hepatic disease with hypoprothrombinemia; suspected intracranial hemorrhage; suppurative thrombophlebitis; inaccessible ulcerative lesions (especially of GI tract) and open ulcerative wounds; extensive denudation of skin; ascorbic acid deficiency and other conditions that cause increased capillary permeability; during or after brain, eye, or spinal cord surgery; during spinal tap or spinal anesthesia; during continuous tube drainage of stomach or small intestine; subacute bacterial endocarditis; shock; advanced

renal disease; threatened abortion; or severe hypertension. Although heparin use is clearly hazardous in these conditions, its risks and benefits must be evaluated.

Use cautiously in postpartum women or women during menses; in patients with mild hepatic or renal disease, alcoholism, or history of asthma, allergies, or GI ulcer; or in those with occupations that have a high risk of accidents.

## Interactions

**Drug-drug.** *Antihistamines, cardiac glycosides, nicotine, tetracyclines:* May partially counteract the anticoagulant action of heparin. Dosage adjustment may be needed.
*Antithrombin III:* Enhanced anticoagulant effect. Reduce heparin dose during concurrent treatment.
*Oral anticoagulants, hydroxychloroquine, and platelet inhibitors:* Increased anticoagulant effect. Advise clinician to monitor INR, PT, and PTT.
**Drug-herb.** *Motherwort or red clover:* May risk increased bleeding. Discourage use together.

## Adverse reactions

**Hematologic:** *hemorrhage* (with excessive dosage), *overly prolonged clotting time, thrombocytopenia.*
**Hepatic:** increased ALT, increased AST, cholestatic reaction.
**Skin:** erythema, local irritation, hematoma, mild pain, ulceration, cutaneous or S.C. necrosis.
**Other:** *white clot syndrome;* hypersensitivity reactions (including chills, fever, pruritus, rhinitis, urticaria, *anaphylactoid reactions*).

## Overdose and treatment

The major sign of overdose is hemorrhage. Immediate withdrawal of drug usually allows the hemorrhage to resolve; however, severe hemorrhage may require treatment with protamine sulfate. Usually, 1 mg protamine sulfate neutralizes 90 units of bovine heparin or 115 units of porcine heparin.

Heparin administered by I.V. route disappears rapidly from the blood, so the protamine dose depends on when heparin was given. Give protamine slowly by I.V. injection (over 3 minutes); no more than 50 mg should be given in any 10-minute period.

Heparin administered by S.C. route is slowly absorbed. Give protamine as a 25- to 50-mg loading dose, followed by constant infusion of the remainder of the calculated dose over 8 to 16 hours.

For severe bleeding, transfusions may be required.

## Clinical considerations
- Many I.V. drugs are incompatible with heparin, and may form precipitates if they come in contact with heparin.
- Avoid I.M. administration of other drugs, if possible, to prevent or minimize hematoma.
- Abrupt withdrawal may increase coagulability; heparin is usually followed by prophylactic oral anticoagulant therapy.
- Hep-lock solution is not for systemic anticoagulation and should not be injected by any parenteral route of administration.
- Valid PT results in the presence of concurrent coumarin or indanedione therapy can be obtained only when blood samples are drawn 4 to 6 hours after I.V. heparin dose or 12 to 24 hours after S.C. heparin dose. Continuous I.V. heparin dose doesn't affect reliability of PT result. Heparin interferes with sulfobromophthalein test, causing an upward shift in the absorption peak; heparin also causes falsely elevated thyroxine level results when competitive protein-binding methods of testing are used. Heparinized blood shouldn't be used for erythrocyte sedimentation rates, platelet counts, fragility tests, or tests involving complement or isoagglutinins.
- Drug may cause false elevations in plasma AST.

### Therapeutic monitoring
- Recommend obtaining pretherapy baseline INR, PT, and PTT; PTT should be measured regularly. Anticoagulation is present when PTT values are 1½ to 2 times control values.
- Advise clinician to monitor platelet count and assess patient regularly for signs and symptoms of abnormal bleeding.

### Special populations
**Pregnant patients.** Heparin doesn't cross the placental barrier. Heparin should be used with caution during pregnancy, especially during the third trimester and postpartum period because of the increased risks of uteroplacental junction bleeding and maternal hemorrhage. Heparin therapy lasting longer than 1 month during pregnancy may cause maternal osteopenia and osteoporosis.
**Breast-feeding patients.** Heparin doesn't appear in breast milk.
**Pediatric patients.** Because of the risk of overdose, recommend avoiding heparin lock flush solutions containing heparin sodium 100 mg/ml for use in neonates, especially those with a low birth weight. When required, a preservative-free solution should be used. Heparin should be used with caution in infants with concomitant conditions causing an increased risk of hemorrhage.
**Geriatric patients.** At least one manufacturer reports a greater risk of hemorrhage in women over age 60. These patients may have increased heparin plasma levels and prolonged PTT. Use cautiously.

## Patient counseling
- Teach injection technique and methods of record keeping if patient or family will be giving drug.
- Encourage compliance with drug schedule and follow-up appointments, and need for routine monitoring of blood studies; teach patient and family signs of bleeding, and stress importance of immediately reporting first sign of excess bleeding.
- Caution patient against trying to make up missed doses.
- Instruct patient to inform dentist or other prescribers of his heparin therapy.
- Advise consulting prescriber before taking any other drugs, including OTC products or herbal medicines.

# hepatitis A vaccine, inactivated
Havrix, Vaqta

*Pharmacologic classification:* vaccine
*Therapeutic classification:* viral vaccine
*Pregnancy risk category C*

## Available forms
Available by prescription only
*Injection:* 720 ELISA units (EL.U.)/0.5 ml, 1,440 EL.U./1 ml (Havrix); 25 units/0.5 ml, 50 units/0.5 ml (Vaqta)

## Indications and dosages
*Immunization against disease caused by hepatitis A virus*
*Adults:* 1,440 EL.U./1 ml (Havrix) I.M. as a single dose. Give booster dose of 1,440 EL.U./1 ml I.M. 6 to 12 months after initial dose. Or 50 units (Vaqta) I.M. and booster dose 6 months after initial dose.
*Children ages 2 to 18:* 720 EL.U./1 ml (Havrix) I.M. as a single dose and booster dose 6 to 12 months after initial dose.
*Children ages 2 to 17:* Single dose of 25 units (Vaqta) I.M. and booster dose 6 to 18 months after initial dose.

## Mechanism of action
*Immunostimulant action:* Hepatitis A vaccine, inactivated, promotes active immunity to hepatitis A virus. Immunity isn't permanent or completely predictable.

## Pharmacokinetics
No information available.

| Route | Onset | Peak | Duration |
|-------|-------|------|----------|
| I.M. | 1-15 days | Unknown | 6 mo |

## Contraindications and precautions

Contraindicated in patients hypersensitive to any component of vaccine.

Use cautiously in patients with thrombocytopenia or bleeding disorders or in those taking anticoagulants; bleeding may occur after I.M. injection in these individuals.

## Interactions

None significant.

## Adverse reactions

**CNS:** *malaise, fatigue,* headache, insomnia, photophobia, vertigo.
**EENT:** pharyngitis.
**GI:** *anorexia, nausea,* abdominal pain, diarrhea, dysgeusia, vomiting.
**Hepatic:** jaundice, *hepatitis.*
**Musculoskeletal:** arthralgia, myalgia.
**Respiratory:** upper respiratory tract infection.
**Skin:** pruritus, *rash,* urticaria, *induration, redness, swelling,* hematoma.
**Other:** *fever,* lymphadenopathy, hypertonic episode, elevation of CK.

## Overdose and treatment

No information available.

## Clinical considerations

■ As with any vaccine, administration of hepatitis A vaccine should be delayed, if possible, in patients with febrile illness.
■ Although anaphylaxis is rare, epinephrine should be available to treat this reaction.
■ If vaccine is given to immunosuppressed persons or those receiving immunosuppressive therapy, the expected immune response may not be obtained.
■ There are no data to support routine vaccination of individuals with chronic hepatitis B or C who lack evidence of chronic liver disease.
■ Persons who should receive the vaccine include people traveling to or living in areas of high endemicity for hepatitis A (Africa, Asia [except Japan], the Mediterranean basin, Eastern Europe, the Middle East, Central and South America, Mexico, and parts of the Caribbean), military personnel, natives of Alaska and the Americas, persons engaging in high-risk sexual activity, and users of illicit injectable drugs. Also, certain institutional workers, child daycare workers, laboratory workers who handle live hepatitis A virus, and handlers of primate animals may benefit from immunization.
■ A positive result in the absence of infection may occur in individuals who have received hepatitis A vaccine and who are being evaluated by serology to detect IgM anti-HAV.

## Therapeutic monitoring

■ Serologic confirmation of immunity isn't needed.

## Special populations

**Breast-feeding patients.** It's unknown if vaccine appears in breast milk. Advise giving cautiously in breast-feeding women.
**Pediatric patients.** Vaccine is well tolerated, highly immunogenic, and effective in children ages 2 and older.

## Patient counseling

■ Inform patient that vaccine won't prevent hepatitis caused by other drugs such as hepatitis B virus, hepatitis C virus, hepatitis E virus, or other pathogens known to infect the liver.

# hepatitis B immune globulin, human (HBIG)

H-BIG, Hep-B-Gammagee, HyperHep

*Pharmacologic classification:* immune serum
*Therapeutic classification:* hepatitis B prophylaxis
*Pregnancy risk category C*

## Available forms

Available by prescription only
*Injection:* 1-ml, 4-ml, and 5-ml vials
*Prefilled syringe:* 0.5 ml

## Indications and dosages

*Hepatitis B exposure*
*Adults and children:* 0.06 ml/kg I.M. within 7 days after exposure. Repeat 28 days after exposure.
*Neonates born to HBsAg-positive women:* 0.5 ml I.M. within 12 hours of birth. Initiation of HB vaccination is also indicated.

The American College of Obstetricians and Gynecologists recommends use of HBIG in pregnancy for postexposure prophylaxis. Hepatitis B immune globulin should be given only if clearly needed.

## Mechanism of action

*Prophylactic action:* HBIG provides passive immunity to hepatitis B.

## Pharmacokinetics

*Absorption:* Absorbed slowly after I.M. injection. Antibodies to hepatitis B surface antigen (HBsAg) appear in serum within 1 to 6 days, peak within 3 to 11 days, and persist for about 2 to 6 months.
*Distribution:* Although specific information isn't available, HBIG probably crosses the placenta, as do other immunoglobulins.
*Metabolism:* No information available.

*Excretion:* Serum half-life for antibodies to HBsAg is reportedly 21 days.

| Route | Onset | Peak | Duration |
|-------|-------|------|----------|
| I.M. | 1-6 days | 3-11 days | 2 mo |

## Contraindications and precautions
Contraindicated in patients with history of anaphylactic reactions to immune serum or thimerosal allergy.

## Interactions
**Drug-drug.** *Vaccination with live-virus vaccines, such as measles, mumps, and rubella:* HBIG may interfere with immune response to vaccination. Give live virus vaccine 2 weeks before or 3 months after HBIG whenever possible.

## Adverse reactions
**Skin:** urticaria, pain, tenderness (at injection site).
**Other:** *anaphylaxis, angioedema.*

## Overdose and treatment
Manufacturers report the only anticipated manifestation would be injection site pain and tenderness. No treatment has been identified.

## Clinical considerations
■ Store at between 36° and 46° F (2° and 8° C). Don't freeze.
■ Epinephrine solution 1:1,000 should be available to treat allergic reactions.
■ Administer drug I.M. only. Severe, even fatal, reactions may occur if administered I.V.
■ HBIG may be given simultaneously, but at different sites, with hepatitis B vaccine.
■ HBIG hasn't been linked to a higher incidence of AIDS. The immune globulin is devoid of HIV. Immune globulin recipients don't develop antibodies to HIV.

### Therapeutic monitoring
■ Advise clinician to monitor patient for adverse reactions.

### Special populations
**Pregnant patients.** It's unknown if drug can cause harm to fetus; it should be used only when potential risk from exposure to hepatitis B infection outweighs potential risk of adverse drug event.
**Breast-feeding patients.** It's unknown if HBIG appears in breast milk.

## Patient counseling
■ Explain that patient's chances of getting AIDS after receiving HBIG are very small.
■ Inform patient that HBIG provides temporary protection against hepatitis B only.
■ Tell patient what to expect after vaccination: local pain, swelling, and tenderness at the in-

jection site. Recommend acetaminophen to relieve minor discomfort.
■ Encourage patient to promptly report headache, skin changes, or difficulty breathing.

# hepatitis B vaccine, recombinant
Engerix-B, Recombivax HB, Recombivax HB Dialysis Formulation, Recombivax HB Pediatric/Adolescent Formulation

*Pharmacologic classification:* vaccine
*Therapeutic classification:* viral vaccine
*Pregnancy risk category C*

## Available forms
Available by prescription only
*Injection:* 5 mcg HBsAg/0.5 ml (Recombivax HB pediatric/adolescent formulation); 10 mcg HBsAg/0.5 ml (Engerix-B, pediatric/adolescent injection); 10 mcg HBsAg/ml (Recombivax HB); 20 mcg HBsAg/ml (Engerix-B); 40 mcg HBsAg/ml (Recombivax HB Dialysis Formulation)

## Indications and dosages
*Immunization against infection from all known subtypes of hepatitis B; primary preexposure prophylaxis against hepatitis B; postexposure prophylaxis (when given with hepatitis B immune globulin)*
**Engerix-B**
*Adults ages 20 and older:* Initially, give 20 mcg (1-ml adult formulation) I.M., followed by a second dose of 20 mcg I.M. 30 days later. Give a third dose of 20 mcg I.M. 6 months after the initial dose.
*Neonates and children up to age 19:* Initially, give 10 mcg (0.5-ml pediatric/adolescent formulation) I.M., followed by a second dose of 10 mcg I.M. 30 days later. Give a third dose of 10 mcg I.M. 6 months after the initial dose.
*Adults undergoing dialysis or receiving immunosuppressant therapy:* Initially, give 40 mcg I.M. (divided into two 20-mcg doses and given at different sites). Follow with a second dose of 40 mcg I.M. in 30 days, a third dose after 2 months, and a final dose of 40 mcg I.M. 6 months after the initial dose.
Note: Alternative dosing schedule in certain populations (neonates born to infected mothers, persons recently exposed to the virus, and travelers to high-risk areas) who may receive the initial vaccine dose (20 mcg for adults and children over age 10, and 10 mcg for neonates and children up to age 10 for this dosing schedule) followed by a second dose in 1 month and the third dose after 2 months. For prolonged maintenance of protective antibody

titers, a booster dose is recommended 12 months after the initial dose.

**Recombivax HB**

*Adults ages 20 and older:* Initially, give 10 mcg (1-ml adult formulation) I.M., followed by a second dose of 10 mcg I.M. 30 days later. Give a third dose of 10 mcg I.M. 6 months after the initial dose.

*Neonates and children up to age 19:* Initially, give 5 mcg (0.5-ml pediatric/adolescent formulation) I.M., followed by a second dose of 5 mcg I.M. 30 days later. Give a third dose of 5 mcg I.M. 6 months after inital dose. Alternatively, adolescents ages 11 to 15 years can be given two doses of the Recombivax HB Adult formulation (10 mcg/dose), with the second dose given 4 to 6 months after the first.

*Neonates born to HBsAg-positive mothers:* Initially, give 5 mcg (0.5-ml pediatric/adolescent formulation) I.M. with 0.5 ml hepatitis B immune globulin. Follow with a second dose of 5 mcg I.M. 30 days later. Give a third dose of 5 mcg I.M. 6 months after the initial dose.

*Adults undergoing dialysis or receiving immunosuppressant therapy:* Initially, give 40 mcg I.M. (1-ml dialysis formulation). Follow with a second dose of 40 mcg I.M. in 30 days, and give a final dose of 40 mcg I.M. 6 months after the initial dose.

## Mechanism of action

*Prophylactic action:* Hepatitis B vaccine promotes active immunity to hepatitis B.

## Pharmacokinetics

No information available.

| Route | Onset | Peak | Duration |
|-------|-------|------|----------|
| I.M. | 2 weeks after last dose | > 6 mo | > 3 yr |

## Contraindications and precautions

Contraindicated in patients hypersensitive to yeast; recombinant vaccines are derived from yeast cultures.

Use cautiously in patients with active infection or compromised cardiac and pulmonary status or in those to whom a febrile or systemic reaction could pose a risk.

Immunization of individuals with moderate or severe febrile illness should be deferred until they have recovered.

## Interactions

**Drug-drug.** *Corticosteroids:* May impair the immune response to hepatitis B vaccine. Larger-than-usual doses of vaccine may be needed to develop adequate circulating antibody levels.

*Immunosuppressants:* Reduced response to vaccine. Recommend giving vaccine 2 weeks before initiation of immunosuppressive therapy or 3 months after discontinuation. Increased doses of vaccine may be needed.

## Adverse reactions

**CNS:** headache, dizziness, insomnia, paresthesia, neuropathy, transient malaise.
**EENT:** pharyngitis.
**GI:** nausea, anorexia, diarrhea, vomiting.
**Musculoskeletal:** arthralgia, myalgia.
**Skin:** local inflammation, *soreness* (at injection site).
**Other:** slight fever, flulike symptoms.

## Overdose and treatment

No information available.

## Clinical considerations

- Recommend having epinephrine solution 1:1,000 available.
- The Centers for Disease Control and Prevention reports that response to hepatitis B vaccine is significantly better after injection into the deltoid rather than the gluteal muscle.
- Hepatitis B vaccine may be administered S.C., but only to persons, such as hemophiliacs and patients with thrombocytopenia, who are at risk of hemorrhage from I.M. injection. Advise prescriber not to administer I.V.
- Hepatitis B vaccine may be given simultaneously, but at different sites, with hepatitis B immune globulin, influenza virus vaccine, *Haemophilus influenzae* type B conjugate vaccine, polyvalent pneumococcal vaccine, or DTP.
- Recombivax HB pediatric/adolescent formulation without preservative should be used promptly after being withdrawn from the single-dose vial and the vial should be discarded.
- Two-dose regimen appears to be as effective as the three-dose regimen, but long-term protection (greater than 2 years) is unknown.
- Immunologic memory may persist 10 to 15 years, and it has been suggested that booster doses in immunocompetent individuals should be given even if antibody titers decline after vaccination.

### Therapeutic monitoring

- Although not needed for most patients, serologic testing (to confirm immunity to hepatitis B after the three-dose regimen) is recommended for patients over age 50, those at high risk of needlestick injury (who might require postexposure prophylaxis), hemodialysis patients, immunocompromised patients, and those who inadvertently received one or more injections into the gluteal muscle. Some experts also recommend testing for health care workers.

### Special populations

**Pregnant patients.** Use drug in pregnant women only when benefits outweigh risks.
**Breast-feeding patients.** Use drug with caution in breast-feeding women.
**Pediatric patients.** Routine immunization is recommended for all neonates, regardless of whether the mother tests positive or negative

for HBsAg. It's usually well tolerated and highly immunogenic in children and infants of all ages. However, it's most effective in neonates weighing 2 kg (4.4 lb) or more. To minimize cumulative exposure to mercury in infants under age 6 months, especially neonates and those born prematurely, the use of thimerosal-free hepatitis B vaccine is recommended.

## Patient counseling
■ Tell patient that there's no risk of contracting HIV infection or AIDS from hepatitis B vaccine because it's synthetically derived.
■ Explain that hepatitis B vaccine provides protection against hepatitis B only, not against hepatitis A or hepatitis C.
■ Tell patient to expect some discomfort at injection site and possible fever, headache, or upset stomach. Recommend acetaminophen to relieve such effects. Encourage patient to report distressing adverse reactions.

# hetastarch (HES, hydroxyethyl starch)
Hespan

*Pharmacologic classification:* amylopectin derivative
*Therapeutic classification:* plasma volume expander
*Pregnancy risk category C*

## Available forms
Available by prescription only
*Injection:* 500 ml (6 g/100 ml in normal saline solution)

## Indications and dosages
*Plasma expander in shock and cardiopulmonary bypass surgery*
*Adults:* 500 to 1,000 ml I.V. dependent on amount of blood lost and resultant hemoconcentration. Total dose usually shouldn't exceed 20 ml/kg, up to 1,500 ml/day. Up to 20 ml/kg (1.2 g/kg)/hour may be used in hemorrhagic shock; in burns or septic shock, rate should be reduced.
*Leukapheresis adjunct*
Hetastarch is an adjunct in leukapheresis to improve harvesting and increase the yield of granulocytes.
*Adults:* Hetastarch 250 to 700 ml is infused at a constant fixed ratio, usually 1:8, to venous whole blood during continuous flow centrifugation (CFC) procedures. Up to 2 CFC procedures weekly, with total number of 7 to 10 procedures using hetastarch, have been found safe and effective. Safety of larger numbers of procedures is unknown.
  Note: Hetastarch can be used as a priming fluid in pump oxygenators for perfusion during extracorporeal circulation or as a cryopro-

tective drug for long-term storage of whole blood.

## I.V. administration
■ Up to 20 ml/kg hourly may be used in hemorrhagic shock. Slower rates of administration are typically used in patients with burns or septic shock.
■ Advise clinician to monitor I.V. site for signs of infiltration and phlebitis.
■ Discard partially used bottle because it doesn't contain a preservative.
■ Store drug at room temperature 77° F (25° C); avoid freezing.

### Incompatibilities
Incompatible with amikacin, ampicillin sodium, cefamandole, cefoperazone, cefotaxime, cefoxitin, cephalothin, cefonicid, gentamicin, ranitidine hydrochloride, theophylline, and tobramycin sulfate.

## Mechanism of action
*Leukapheresis adjunctive action:* Hetastarch enhances yield of granulocytes obtained by centrifugal means.
*Plasma volume expanding action:* Hetastarch has an average molecular weight of 450,000 and exhibits colloidal properties similar to human albumin. After an I.V. infusion of hetastarch 6%, the plasma volume expands slightly in excess of the volume infused because of the colloidal osmotic effect. Maximum plasma volume expansion occurs in a few minutes and decreases over 24 to 36 hours. Hemodynamic status may improve for 24 hours or longer.

## Pharmacokinetics
*Absorption:* Administered I.V.
*Distribution:* Distributed in blood plasma.
*Metabolism:* Hetastarch molecules larger than 50,000 molecular weight are slowly enzymatically degraded to molecules that can be excreted.
*Excretion:* Forty percent of hetastarch molecules smaller than 50,000 molecular weight are excreted in urine within 24 hours. Hetastarch molecules that aren't hydroxyethylated are slowly degraded to glucose. About 90% of dose is eliminated from the body with an average half-life of 17 days; remainder has a half-life of 48 days.

| Route | Onset | Peak | Duration |
|-------|-------|------|----------|
| I.V. | Immediate | Immediate | Unknown |

## Contraindications and precautions
Contraindicated in patients with severe bleeding disorders, severe HF, or renal failure with oliguria and anuria.

## Interactions
None reported.

## Adverse reactions
**CNS:** headache.
**CV:** peripheral edema of legs.
**EENT:** periorbital edema.
**GI:** nausea, vomiting.
**Musculoskeletal:** muscle pain.
**Respiratory:** wheezing.
**Skin:** urticaria.
**Other:** mild fever, chills.

## Overdose and treatment
Signs and symptoms of overdose include the adverse reactions listed previously. Infusion should be stopped if an overdose occurs, and treatment should be supportive.

## Clinical considerations
■ When added to whole blood, hetastarch increases the erythrocyte sedimentation rate.
■ Shouldn't be given as a substitute for blood or plasma.

### Therapeutic monitoring
■ To avoid circulatory overload, advise clinician to carefully monitor patients with impaired renal function and those at high risk of pulmonary edema or HF. Hetastarch 6% in normal saline contains 77 mEq sodium and chloride per 500 ml.
■ Advise clinician to monitor CBC, total leukocyte and platelet counts, leukocyte differential count, hemoglobin, hematocrit, PT, PTT, electrolyte, BUN, and creatinine levels.
■ Advise clinician to assess vital signs and cardiopulmonary status to obtain baseline at start of infusion to prevent fluid overload.
■ Advise clinician to observe patient for edema.

### Special populations
**Pregnant patients.** Hetastarch shouldn't be used in pregnant women, especially during early pregnancy. Drug should be used only when benefit to mother outweighs risk to fetus.
**Breast-feeding patients.** Advise prescriber to discontinue breast-feeding temporarily in women receiving hetastarch.
**Pediatric patients.** Safety and efficacy in children haven't been established.
**Geriatric patients.** Hetastarch should be used with caution in geriatric patients because of the potential for fluid overload; a lower dosage may be sufficient to produce desired plasma volume expansion.

## Patient counseling
■ Explain use and administration of drug to patient and family.
■ Instruct patient to report adverse reactions promptly.

# homatropine hydrobromide
AK-Homatropine, I-Homatrine, Isopto Homatropine, Minims Homatropine*

*Pharmacologic classification:* anticholinergic
*Therapeutic classification:* cycloplegic, mydriatic
*Pregnancy risk category C*

## Available forms
Available by prescription only
*Ophthalmic solution:* 2%, 5%

## Indications and dosages
### Cycloplegic refraction
*Adults:* Instill 1 to 2 drops of 2% or 1 drop of 5% solution in eye; repeat in 5 to 10 minutes, p.r.n.
*Children:* Instill 1 drop of 2% solution in eye; repeat at 10-minute intervals, p.r.n.
### Uveitis
*Adults:* Instill 1 to 2 drops of 2% or 5% solution in eye up to q 3 or 4 hours.
*Children:* Instill 1 drop of 2% solution in eye b.i.d. or t.i.d.

## Mechanism of action
*Cycloplegic and mydriatic actions:* Anticholinergic action prevents the sphincter muscle of the iris and the muscle of the ciliary body from responding to cholinergic stimulation, resulting in unopposed adrenergic influence and producing pupillary dilation (mydriasis) and paralysis of accommodation (cycloplegia).

## Pharmacokinetics
**Absorption:** Unknown.
**Distribution:** Unknown.
**Metabolism:** Unknown.
**Excretion:** Recovery from cycloplegic and mydriatic effects usually occurs within 1 to 3 days.

| Route | Onset | Peak | Duration |
|-------|-------|------|----------|
| Ophthalmic | Rapid | 40-60 min | 1-3 days |

## Contraindications and precautions
Contraindicated in patients hypersensitive to drug or other belladonna alkaloids such as atropine, and in those with glaucoma or who have adhesions between the iris and lens.
    Use cautiously in geriatric patients and in those with increased ocular pressure.

## Interactions
**Drug-drug.** *Carbachol, cholinesterase inhibitors, pilocarpine:* Interference with the antiglaucoma effects of these drugs. Avoid use together.

## Adverse reactions
**CNS:** confusion, somnolence, headache.
**CV:** tachycardia.

**EENT:** eye irritation, *blurred vision, photophobia,* increased intraocular pressure, transient stinging and burning, conjunctivitis, vascular congestion, edema.
**GI:** dry mouth.
**Skin:** dryness, rash.

## Overdose and treatment
Signs and symptoms of overdose include flushed dry skin, dry mouth, blurred vision, ataxia, dysarthria, hallucinations, tachycardia, and decreased bowel sounds.

Accidental ingestion should be treated by emesis or activated charcoal. Recommend using physostigmine to antagonize anticholinergic activity of homatropine in severe toxicity; propranolol may be used to treat symptomatic tachyarrhythmias unresponsive to physostigmine.

## Clinical considerations
■ Drug may produce symptoms of atropine sulfate poisoning, such as severe mouth dryness and tachycardia.
■ Patient may be photophobic and may benefit from wearing dark glasses to minimize discomfort.

### Therapeutic monitoring
■ Patient should be monitored for adverse reactions and to ascertain therapeutic result.

### Special populations
**Pediatric patients.** Use drug cautiously in young children and infants. There's an increased chance of sensitivity in children with Down syndrome, spastic paralysis, or brain damage. Feeding intolerance may result.
**Geriatric patients.** Use cautiously in geriatric patients because of the potential risk of undiagnosed glaucoma and increased sensitivity to effects of drug.

## Patient counseling
■ Provide patient with information on correct method of administration.
■ Inform patient that vision will be temporarily blurred after instillation, and advise caution when driving or operating machinery.
■ Inform patient that drug may produce drowsiness.

# hyaluronidase
Wydase

*Pharmacologic classification:* protein enzyme
*Therapeutic classification:* adjunctive drug
*Pregnancy risk category C*

## Available forms
Available by prescription only

*Injection (lyophilized powder):* 150 USP units/vial, 1,500 USP units/vial
*Injection (solution):* 150 USP units/ml in 1-ml and 10-ml vials

## Indications and dosages
*Adjunct to increase absorption and dispersion of other injected drugs*
*Adults and children:* Add 150 USP units to solution containing other drug.
*Adjunct to increase absorption rate of fluids given by hypodermoclysis*
*Adults and children:* Inject 150 USP units into the rubber tubing close to the needle of the running clysis solution. Generally, 150 USP units will facilitate absorption of 1 L or more of solution; individualize dosage administration and type of solution.
*Adjunct in excretory urography*
*Adults and children:* Give 75 USP units S.C. over each scapula before administration of the contrast medium.

## Mechanism of action
*Diffusing action:* Hyaluronidase is a spreading or diffusing substance that modifies the permeability of connective tissue through the hydrolysis of hyaluronic acid. Drug enhances the diffusion of substances injected S.C. as long as local interstitial pressure is adequate.

## Pharmacokinetics
No information available.

| Route | Onset | Peak | Duration |
|-------|-------|------|----------|
| S.C. | Immediate | Unknown | 1-2 days |

## Contraindications and precautions
Contraindicated in patients hypersensitive to drug.

## Interactions
**Drug-drug.** *Local anesthetics:* May increase analgesia, hasten onset, and reduce local swelling, but may also increase systemic absorption, increase toxicity, and shorten duration of action. Use caution.

## Adverse reactions
**Skin:** allergic reactions.

## Overdose and treatment
Up to 75,000 units have been given without ill effect; local adverse effects would be anticipated. Recommend treating symptomatically.

## Clinical considerations
■ Recommend giving skin test for sensitivity before use with an intradermal injection, using about 0.02 ml of hyaluronidase solution; a wheal with pseudopods appearing within 5 minutes after injection and lasting for 20 to 30 minutes along with urticaria indicates a positive reaction.

- Because of the potential for allergic reaction, although rare, epinephrine, corticosteroids, and antihistamines should be available for emergency treatment.
- Avoid contact with eyes; if it occurs, recommend flooding with water immediately.
- Drug also may be used to diffuse local anesthetics at injection site, especially in nerve block anesthesia. It also has been used to enhance the diffusion of drugs in management of I.V. extravasation.

### Therapeutic monitoring
- Advise clinician to monitor patient for adverse drug events.

### Special populations
**Pregnant patients.** Use drug during pregnancy only when clearly indicated.
**Breast-feeding patients.** It's unknown if drug appears in breast milk. Use with caution in breast-feeding women.
**Pediatric patients.** If drug is given for hypodermoclysis, care should be taken to avoid overhydration. In children under age 3, clysis should not exceed 200 ml; in premature neonates, clysis shouldn't exceed 25 ml/kg and the rate shouldn't exceed 2 ml/minute.

### Patient counseling
- Instruct patient to report unusual and significant adverse effects after injection.

---

# hydralazine hydrochloride
Apresoline, Novo-Hylazin

*Pharmacologic classification:* peripheral vasodilator
*Therapeutic classification:* antihypertensive
*Pregnancy risk category C*

### Available forms
Available by prescription only
*Tablets:* 10 mg, 25 mg, 50 mg, 100 mg
*Injection:* 20 mg/ml

### Indications and dosages
*Moderate to severe hypertension*
*Adults:* Initially, 10 mg P.O. q.i.d. for 2 to 4 days, then increased to 25 mg q.i.d. for remainder of week. If needed, increase dosage to 50 mg q.i.d. Maximum recommended dose is 200 mg daily, but some patients may require 300 to 400 mg daily.
For severe hypertension, 10 to 50 mg I.M. or 10 to 20 mg I.V. repeated, p.r.n. Switch to oral antihypertensives as soon as possible.
For hypertensive crisis associated with pregnancy, initially 5 mg I.V., followed by 5 to 10 mg I.V. q 20 to 30 minutes until adequate reduction in blood pressure is achieved. Usual range is 5 to 20 mg.

*Children:* Initially, 0.75 mg/kg P.O. daily in four divided doses (25 mg/m$^2$ daily); may increase gradually to 7.5 mg/kg daily.
I.M. or I.V. drug dosage is 0.4 to 1.2 mg/kg daily or 50 to 100 mg/m$^2$ daily in four to six divided doses. Initial parenteral dose should not exceed 20 mg.
◊ *Management of severe heart failure*
*Adults:* Initially, 50 to 75 mg P.O., then adjusted according to patient response. Most patients respond to 200 to 600 mg daily, divided q 6 to 12 hours, but doses as high as 3 g daily have been used.

### I.V. administration
- Drug should be injected as soon as possible after draining through needle into syringe; drug changes color after contact with metal.
- A color change develops when drug is diluted with most I.V. solutions. Generally, a color change over 8 to 12 hours doesn't indicate a loss of potency when the solution is stored at 30° C (86° F) or lower.
- Freezing should be avoided.
- Advise clinician to monitor blood pressure every 5 minutes until stable, then every 15 minutes.

### Incompatibilities
Avoid mixing with other drugs in same container. Incompatible with aminophylline, ampicillin sodium, chlorothiazide, dextrose 10% in lactated Ringer's solution, dextrose 10% in normal saline, D$_5$W, diazoxide, edetate calcium disodium, ethacrynate, fructose 10% in normal saline, fructose 10% in water, furosemide, hydrocortisone sodium succinate, mephentermine, methohexital, nitroglycerin, phenobarbital sodium, and verapamil.

### Mechanism of action
*Antihypertensive action:* Hydralazine has a direct vasodilating effect on vascular smooth muscle, thus lowering blood pressure. The effect of hydralazine on resistance vessels (arterioles and arteries) is greater than that on capacitance vessels (venules and veins).

### Pharmacokinetics
*Absorption:* Absorbed rapidly from GI tract after oral administration; peak plasma levels occur in 1 hour; bioavailability is 30% to 50%. Antihypertensive effect occurs 20 to 30 minutes after oral dose, 5 to 20 minutes after I.V. administration, and 10 to 30 minutes after I.M. administration. Food enhances absorption.
*Distribution:* Distributed widely throughout the body; drug is about 88% to 90% protein-bound.
*Metabolism:* Metabolized extensively in the GI mucosa and the liver. Hydralazine is subject to polymorphic acetylation. Slow acetyla-

---

tors have higher plasma levels, generally requiring lower doses.

*Excretion:* Mostly excreted in urine, primarily as metabolites; about 10% of an oral dose is excreted in feces. Antihypertensive effect persists 2 to 4 hours after an oral dose and 2 to 6 hours after I.V. or I.M. administration.

| Route | Onset | Peak | Duration |
|-------|-------|------|----------|
| P.O. | 20-30 min | 1-2 hr | 2-4 hr |
| I.V. | 5-20 min | 10-80 min | 2-6 hr |
| I.M. | 10-30 min | 1 hr | 2-6 hr |

## Contraindications and precautions

Contraindicated in patients hypersensitive to drug, and in those with coronary artery disease or mitral valvular rheumatic heart disease. Use cautiously in patients with suspected cardiac disease, CVA, or severe renal impairment, and in those receiving other antihypertensives.

## Interactions

**Drug-drug.** *Diazoxide, MAO inhibitors:* May cause severe hypotension. Use together cautiously.

*Diuretics and other antihypertensives:* Increased effects of these drugs. Use with caution.

*Epinephrine:* Decreased pressor response. Advise clinician to monitor patient closely.

## Adverse reactions

**CNS:** peripheral neuritis, *headache,* dizziness.
**CV:** orthostatic hypotension, *tachycardia,* edema, angina, *palpitations.*
**GI:** *nausea, vomiting, diarrhea, anorexia,* constipation.
**Hematologic:** *neutropenia, leukopenia, agranulocytosis.*
**Skin:** rash.
**Other:** *lupuslike syndrome* (especially with high doses).

## Overdose and treatment

Signs and symptoms of overdose include hypotension, tachycardia, headache, and skin flushing; arrhythmias and shock may occur.

After acute ingestion, recommend emptying stomach by emesis or gastric lavage and giving activated charcoal to reduce absorption. Symptomatic and supportive care should follow.

## Clinical considerations

■ The goal of hypertension management and prevention is to achieve and maintain a systolic blood pressure less than 140 mm Hg and a diastolic blood pressure less than 90 mm Hg, if tolerated.

■ Risk of drug-induced systemic lupus erythematosus (SLE) syndrome is greatest in patients receiving more than 200 mg/day for prolonged periods.

■ Food enhances oral absorption and helps minimize gastric irritation.

■ Some preparations contain tartrazine, which may precipitate allergic reactions, especially in aspirin-sensitive patients.

■ Patients with renal impairment may respond to lower maintenance doses of hydralazine.

### *Therapeutic monitoring*

■ Recommend performing CBC, lupus erythematosus (LE) cell preparation, and ANA titer determinations before therapy and at regular intervals during long-term therapy.

■ Headache and palpitations may occur 2 to 4 hours after first oral dose but should subside spontaneously.

■ Sodium retention may occur with long-term use.

Systolic blood pressure is considered the primary clinical endpoint, especially in middle-age and geriatric patients.

### *Special populations*

**Breast-feeding patients.** It's unknown if drug appears in breast milk. An alternative feeding method is recommended during therapy.
**Pediatric patients.** Drug has had limited use in children. Safety and efficacy in children haven't been established; use only if potential benefit outweighs risk.
**Geriatric patients.** Geriatric patients may be more sensitive to antihypertensive effects. Use with special caution in patients with history of CVA or impaired renal function; patients with renal impairment may respond to lower maintenance doses.

## Patient counseling

■ Instruct patient that drug should be taken exactly as prescribed, even when he is feeling well; warn against stopping drug suddenly because severe rebound hypertension may occur.

■ Explain adverse reactions and advise patient to report unusual effects, especially symptoms of SLE (sore throat, fever, rash, and muscle and joint pain).

■ Reassure patient that headaches and palpitations occurring 2 to 4 hours after initial dose usually subside spontaneously.

■ Instruct patient to report weight gain that exceeds 5 lb weekly.

■ Warn patient to seek medical approval before taking OTC cold preparations.

# hydrochlorothiazide
Apo-Hydro*, Aquazide-H, Diuchlor H*,
Esidrix, Hydro-chlor, Hydro-D,
HydroDIURIL, Microzide, Mictrin,
Neo-Codema*, Novo-Hydrazide*,
Oretic, Urozide*

*Pharmacologic classification:* thiazide
diuretic
*Therapeutic classification:* diuretic,
antihypertensive
*Pregnancy risk category B*

## Available forms
Available by prescription only
*Capsules:* 12.5 mg
*Tablets:* 25 mg, 50 mg
*Solution:* 50 mg/5 ml, 100 mg/ml

## Indications and dosages
### Edema
*Adults:* Initially, 25 to 200 mg P.O. daily for
several days or until dry weight is attained.
Maintenance dose is 25 to 100 mg P.O. daily
or intermittently. A few refractory cases may
require up to 200 mg daily.
### Hypertension
*Adults:* 12.5 to 50 mg P.O. once daily. Daily
dose increased or decreased based on blood
pressure.
*Children ages 2 to 12:* 2.2 mg/kg or 60 mg/m$^2$
daily in two divided doses. Usual dosage range
is 37.5 to 100 mg/day.
*Children ages 6 months to 2 years:* 2.2 mg/kg
or 60 mg/m$^2$ daily in two divided doses.
Usual dosage range is 12.5 to 37.5 mg/day.
*Children under 6 months:* Up to 3.3 mg/kg
daily in two divided doses.

## Mechanism of action
*Diuretic action:* Hydrochlorothiazide increases urinary excretion of sodium and water by
inhibiting sodium reabsorption in the cortical
diluting tubule of the nephron, thus relieving
edema.
*Antihypertensive action:* Exact mechanism of
antihypertensive effect of drug is unknown. It
may result partially from direct arteriolar vasodilation and a decrease in total peripheral resistance.

## Pharmacokinetics
*Absorption:* Absorbed from the GI tract; rate
and extent of absorption vary with different
formulations.
*Distribution:* Unknown.
*Metabolism:* None.
*Excretion:* Excreted unchanged in urine, usually
within 24 hours; half-life is 5½ to 14½ hours.

| Route | Onset | Peak | Duration |
|-------|-------|------|----------|
| P.O. | 2 hr | 4-5 hr | 6-12 hr |

## Contraindications and precautions
Contraindicated in patients with anuria and in
those hypersensitive to other thiazides or other sulfonamide derivatives.
    Use cautiously in patients with severely im-
paired renal or hepatic function or progressive
hepatic disease.

## Interactions
**Drug-drug.** *Amphetamine, quinidine, methenamine compounds (such as methenamine mandelate):* Alkaline urine, decreased urinary excretion of some amines, decreased therapeutic
efficacy. Advise clinician to monitor patient
for drug effect.
*Antihypertensives:* Increased hypotensive effect; this may be used to therapeutic advantage. Recommend checking blood pressure frequently.
*Cholestyramine, colestipol:* May bind hydrochlorothiazide, preventing its absorption.
Recommend giving drugs 1 hour apart.
*Diazoxide:* Increased hyperglycemic, hypotensive, and hyperuricemic effects. Insulin
dosage may require adjustment.
*Lithium:* Reduced renal clearance, elevating
serum lithium levels. Reduction in lithium
dosage by 50% may be needed.
**Drug-herb.** *Dandelion:* Possible interference
with diuretic activity. Discourage use together.
*Licorice root:* May contribute to the potassium depletion caused by thiazides. Discourage
patient from using this herb.

## Adverse reactions
**CNS:** dizziness, vertigo, headache, paresthesia, weakness, restlessness.
**CV:** volume depletion and dehydration, orthostatic hypotension, allergic myocarditis, vasculitis.
**GI:** anorexia, nausea, *pancreatitis,* epigastric
distress, vomiting, abdominal pain, diarrhea,
constipation.
**GU:** polyuria, frequent urination, *renal failure,* interstitial nephritis.
**Hematologic:** *aplastic anemia, agranulocytosis, leukopenia, thrombocytopenia,* hemolytic anemia.
**Hepatic:** jaundice.
**Metabolism:** hypokalemia; asymptomatic hyperuricemia; hyperglycemia and impaired glucose tolerance; fluid and electrolyte imbalances, including dilutional hyponatremia,
hypochloremia, metabolic alkalosis, and hypercalcemia.
**Musculoskeletal:** muscle cramps.
**Respiratory:** respiratory distress, pneumonitis.
**Skin:** dermatitis, photosensitivity, rash, purpura, alopecia.
**Other:** hypersensitivity reactions; gout; *anaphylactic reactions.*

## Overdose and treatment

Clinical signs of overdose include GI irritation and hypermotility, diuresis, and lethargy, which may progress to coma.

Treatment is mainly supportive; recommend monitoring and assisting respiratory, CV, and renal function as indicated. Advise clinician to monitor fluid and electrolyte balance. Recommend inducing vomiting with ipecac in conscious patient; otherwise, recommend using gastric lavage to avoid aspiration. Cathartics shouldn't be given; these promote additional loss of fluids and electrolytes.

## Clinical considerations

■ Recommendations for preparation and use of hydrochlorothiazide are the same as those for all thiazide diuretics.

■ Hydrochlorothiazide may interfere with tests for parathyroid function and should be discontinued before such tests.

### Therapeutic monitoring

■ Drug may cause glucose intolerance in some people. Advise clinician to monitor blood glucose in diabetic patients. Dosage adjustment of insulin or oral antidiabetic may be required.

### Special populations

**Breast-feeding patients.** Drug appears in breast milk; safety and efficacy in breast-feeding women haven't been established.

**Pediatric patients.** Drug can be used in pediatric patients; single daily dose of 1 mg/kg is recommended.

**Geriatric patients.** Geriatric and debilitated patients require close observation and may require reduced dosages. They're more sensitive to excess diuresis because of age-related changes in CV and renal function. Excess diuresis promotes orthostatic hypotension, dehydration, hypovolemia, hyponatremia, hypomagnesemia, and hypokalemia.

## Patient counseling

■ Instruct patient to take drug with food to avoid GI upset, to take drug in morning or early afternoon to avoid nocturia, and to avoid sudden postural changes.

■ Advise patient to use sunblock to avoid photosensitivity reactions.

■ Tell patient to consult prescriber before taking OTC drugs.

# hydrocortisone (systemic)

Cortef, Cortenema, Hycort*, Hydrocortone

# hydrocortisone acetate

Cortifoam

# hydrocortisone cypionate

Cortef

# hydrocortisone sodium phosphate

Hydrocortone Phosphate

# hydrocortisone sodium succinate

A-hydroCort, Solu-Cortef

*Pharmacologic classification:* glucocorticoid, mineralocorticoid
*Therapeutic classification:* adrenocorticoid replacement
*Pregnancy risk category C*

## Available forms

Available by prescription only
**hydrocortisone**
*Tablets:* 5 mg, 10 mg, 20 mg
*Injection:* 25-mg/ml, 50-mg/ml suspension
*Enema:* 100 mg/60 ml
**hydrocortisone acetate**
*Injection:* 25-mg/ml, 50-mg/ml suspension
*Enema:* 10% aerosol foam (provides 90 mg/application)
**hydrocortisone cypionate**
*Oral suspension:* 10 mg/5 ml
**hydrocortisone sodium phosphate**
*Injection:* 50-mg/ml solution
**hydrocortisone sodium succinate**
*Injection:* 100 mg/vial, 250 mg/vial, 500 mg/vial, 1,000 mg/vial

## Indications and dosages

*Severe inflammation, adrenal insufficiency*
**hydrocortisone**
*Adults:* 5 to 30 mg P.O. b.i.d., t.i.d., or q.i.d. (as much as 80 mg P.O. q.i.d. may be given in acute situations).
*Children:* 2 to 8 mg/kg or 60 to 240 mg/m$^2$ P.O. daily.
**hydrocortisone acetate**
*Adults:* 10 to 75 mg into joints or soft tissue at 2- or 3-week intervals. Dose varies with size of joint. In many cases, local anesthetics are injected with dose.
**hydrocortisone sodium phosphate**
*Adults:* 15 to 240 mg S.C., I.M., or I.V. daily in divided doses q 12 hours.

**hydrocortisone sodium succinate**
*Adults:* Initially, 100 to 500 mg I.M. or I.V., then 50 to 100 mg I.M. as indicated.
*Shock (other than adrenal crisis)*
**hydrocortisone sodium phosphate**
*Children:* 0.16 to 1 mg/kg I.M. daily or b.i.d.
**hydrocortisone sodium succinate**
*Adults:* 100 to 500 mg I.M. or I.V. q 2 to 6 hours.
*Children:* 0.16 to 1 mg/kg or 6 to 30 mg/m$^2$ I.M. or I.V. daily to b.i.d.
*Life-threatening shock*
**hydrocortisone sodium succinate**
*Adults:* 0.5 to 2 g I.V. initially, repeated at 2- to 6-hour intervals, p.r.n. High-dose therapy should be continued only until patient's condition has stabilized. Therapy shouldn't be continued beyond 48 to 72 hours.
*Adjunctive treatment of ulcerative colitis and proctitis*
**hydrocortisone**
*Adults:* One enema (100 mg) nightly for 21 days.
**hydrocortisone acetate (rectal foam)**
*Adults:* 90 mg (1 applicatorful) once or twice daily for 2 or 3 weeks; decrease frequency to every other day thereafter.

## I.V administration
■ I.V. therapy is generally reserved for those patients unable to take the drug orally or for emergency situations.
■ Parenteral injections must be given at 4- to 6-hour intervals to keep the blood level of drug elevated.

### Incompatibilities
Incompatible with amobarbital, ampicillin sodium, bleomycin, cephalothin sodium with aminophylline, ciprofloxacin, colistimethate, cytarabine, diazepam, dimenhydrinate, diphenhydramine, doxapram, doxorubicin, ephedrine, ergotamine, furosemide, heparin sodium, hydralazine, idarubicin, kanamycin, metaraminol, methicillin, methylprednisolone sodium succinate, mitoxantrone, nafcillin, pentobarbital sodium, phenobarbital sodium, phenytoin, prochlorperazine edisylate, promethazine hydrochloride, sargramostim, secobarbital, and vitamin B complex with C.

## Mechanism of action
*Adrenocorticoid replacement action:* Hydrocortisone is an adrenocorticoid with both glucocorticoid and mineralocorticoid properties. It's a weak anti-inflammatory but a potent mineralocorticoid, having potency similar to that of cortisone and twice that of prednisone. Hydrocortisone (or cortisone) is usually the drug of choice for replacement therapy in patients with adrenal insufficiency. It's usually not used for immunosuppressant activity because of the extremely large doses needed and the unwanted mineralocorticoid effects.

Hydrocortisone and hydrocortisone cypionate may be given orally. Hydrocortisone sodium phosphate may be given by I.M., S.C., or I.V. injection or by I.V. infusion, usually at 12-hour intervals. Hydrocortisone sodium succinate may be given by I.M. or I.V. injection or I.V. infusion every 2 to 10 hours, depending on the clinical situation. Hydrocortisone acetate is a suspension that may be given by intra-articular, intrasynovial, intrabursal, intralesional, or soft-tissue injection. It has a slow onset but a long duration of action. Injectable forms are usually used only when the oral dosage forms can't be used.

## Pharmacokinetics
*Absorption:* Absorbed readily after oral administration. After oral and I.V. administration, peak effects occur in about 1 to 2 hours. The acetate suspension for injection has a variable absorption over 24 to 48 hours, depending on whether it's injected into an intra-articular space or a muscle, and the nature of the blood supply to that muscle.
*Distribution:* Removed rapidly from the blood and distributed to muscle, liver, skin, intestines, and kidneys. Hydrocortisone is bound extensively to plasma proteins (transcortin and albumin). Only the unbound portion is active. Adrenocorticoids appear in breast milk and pass through the placenta.
*Metabolism:* Metabolized in the liver to inactive glucuronide and sulfate metabolites.
*Excretion:* Inactive metabolites and small amounts of unmetabolized drug are excreted by the kidneys. Insignificant quantities of drug are excreted in feces. Biologic half-life of hydrocortisone is 8 to 12 hours.

| Route | Onset | Peak | Duration |
|---|---|---|---|
| P.O., I.V., I.M., P.R. | Variable | Variable | Variable |

## Contraindications and precautions
Contraindicated in patients allergic to any component of the formulation, in those with systemic fungal infection, and in premature infants (with hydrocortisone sodium succinate).

Use hydrocortisone sodium phosphate or succinate cautiously in patients with recent MI, GI ulcer, renal disease, hypertension, osteoporosis, diabetes mellitus, hypothyroidism, cirrhosis, diverticulitis, ulcerative colitis, recent intestinal anastomosis, thromboembolic disorders, seizures, myasthenia gravis, HF, tuberculosis, ocular herpes simplex, emotional instability, and psychotic tendencies.

## Interactions
**Drug-drug.** *Antacids, cholestyramine, colestipol:* Decrease corticosteroid effect by adsorbing the oral corticosteroid, thereby decreasing the amount absorbed. May require dosage adjustment.

---

Reactions may be *common*, uncommon, *life-threatening*, or COMMON AND LIFE-THREATENING.

*Barbiturates, phenytoin, rifampin:* May decrease corticosteroid effects because of increased hepatic metabolism. May require increased corticosteroid dosage.

*Cardiac glycosides:* Increased risk of toxicity. Advise clinician to monitor patient closely.

*Diuretic or amphotericin B:* May result in hypokalemia. Advise clinician to monitor serum potassium levels.

*Estrogens:* Reduced metabolism of corticosteroids. Advise clinician to monitor patient for drug effect.

*Isoniazid and salicylates:* Increased metabolism of these drugs. Advise clinician to monitor patient carefully.

*Oral anticoagulants:* Decreased effects of oral anticoagulants by unknown mechanisms. Advise clinician to monitor PT and INR.

*Ulcerogenic drugs (such as NSAIDs):* Increased risk of GI ulceration. Avoid use together.

### Adverse reactions

**CNS:** *euphoria, insomnia,* psychotic behavior, pseudotumor cerebri, vertigo, headache, paresthesia, *seizures.*

**CV:** *HF,* hypertension, edema, *arrhythmias,* thrombophlebitis, *thromboembolism.*

**EENT:** cataracts, glaucoma.

**GI:** *peptic ulceration,* GI irritation, increased appetite, *pancreatitis,* nausea, vomiting.

**GU:** menstrual irregularities.

**Metabolic:** possible hypokalemia, hyperglycemia (requiring dosage adjustment in diabetics).

**Musculoskeletal:** muscle weakness, osteoporosis, growth suppression in children, carbohydrate intolerance.

**Skin:** delayed wound healing, acne, various skin eruptions, easy bruising, hirsutism.

**Other:** susceptibility to infections; cushingoid state (moonface, buffalo hump, central obesity), *acute adrenal insufficiency with increased stress (infection, surgery, trauma) or abrupt withdrawal (after long-term therapy).*

**After abrupt withdrawal:** rebound inflammation, fatigue, weakness, arthralgia, fever, dizziness, lethargy, depression, fainting, orthostatic hypotension, dyspnea, anorexia, hypoglycemia. *After prolonged use, sudden withdrawal may be fatal.*

### Overdose and treatment

Acute ingestion, even in massive doses, is rarely a clinical problem. Toxic signs and symptoms rarely occur if drug is used for less than 3 weeks, even at large doses. However, chronic use causes adverse physiologic effects, including suppression of the hypothalamic-pituitary-adrenal axis, cushingoid appearance, muscle weakness, and osteoporosis.

### Clinical considerations

■ Most adverse reactions to corticosteroids are dose- or duration-dependent.

■ Hydrocortisone suppresses reactions to skin tests, causes false-negative results in nitroblue tetrazolium tests for systemic bacterial infections, and decreases $^{131}I$ uptake and protein-bound iodine levels in thyroid function test results.

*Therapeutic monitoring*

■ Advise clinician to monitor patient for adverse reactions.

*Special populations*

**Pediatric patients.** Long-term use of hydrocortisone in children and adolescents may delay growth and maturation.

### Patient counseling

■ Caution patient to take drug as directed.

■ Inform patient of potential adverse effects and instruct him to contact prescriber immediately to report serious adverse events.

## hydrocortisone (topical)

Acticort 100, Aeroseb-HC, Ala-Cort, Ala-Scalp, Anusol-HC, Bactine, Barriere-HC*, CaldeCORT, Cetacort, CortaGel, Cortaid, Cortate*, Cort-Dome, Cortizone, Dermacort, DermiCort, Dermolate, Dermtex HC, Emo-Cort*, Hi-Cor, Hydro-Tex, Hytone, LactiCare-HC, Nutracort, Penecort, Rectocort*, S-T Cort, Synacort, Texacort, Unicort*

## hydrocortisone acetate

Anusol-HC, CaldeCORT, Cortaid, Cort-Dome, Cortef, Corticaine, Corticreme*, Cortoderm*, Gynecort, Hyderm*, Lanacort, Novohydrocort*, Orabase-HCA, Pharma-Cort, Rhulicort

## hydrocortisone buteprate

Pandel

## hydrocortisone butyrate

Locoid

## hydrocortisone valerate

Westcort

*Pharmacologic classification:* glucocorticoid
*Therapeutic classification:* anti-inflammatory
*Pregnancy risk category C*

### Available forms

Available by prescription only
**hydrocortisone**
*Cream:* 2.5%
*Ointment:* 0.5%, 1%, 2.5%
*Lotion:* 0.25%, 0.5%, 1%, 2%, 2.5%

*Gel:* 0.5%, 1%
*Solution:* 0.5%, 1%, 2.5%
*Aerosol:* 0.5%, 1%
*Pledgets (saturated with solution):* 0.5%, 1%
**hydrocortisone acetate**
*Cream:* 1%
*Ointment:* 0.5%, 1%
*Lotion:* 0.5%
*Suppositories:* 25 mg
*Rectal foam:* 10%
*Paste:* 0.5%
*Solution:* 1%
**hydrocortisone buteprate**
*Cream:* 0.1%
**hydrocortisone butyrate**
*Cream, ointment, solution:* 0.1%
**hydrocortisone valerate**
*Cream, ointment:* 0.2%
Available without a prescription
**hydrocortisone**
*Cream:* 0.5%, 1%
**hydrocortisone acetate**
*Cream:* 0.5%

## Indications and dosages
*Inflammation of corticosteroid-responsive dermatoses, including those on face, groin, armpits, and under breasts; seborrheic dermatitis of scalp*
*Adults and children:* Apply cream, lotion, ointment, foam, or aerosol sparingly once daily to q.i.d.
**Aerosol administration**
Shake can well. Direct spray onto affected area from a distance of 15 cm (6 inches). Apply for only 3 seconds (to avoid freezing tissues). Apply to dry scalp after shampooing; no need to massage or rub drug into scalp after spraying. Apply daily until acute phase is controlled, then reduce dosage to once to three times weekly, p.r.n., to maintain control.
**Rectal administration**
Shake can well. Apply once daily or b.i.d. for 2 to 3 weeks, then every other day, p.r.n.
*Dental lesions*
*Adults and children:* Apply paste b.i.d. to t.i.d. and at h.s.

## Mechanism of action
*Anti-inflammatory action:* Hydrocortisone stimulates the synthesis of enzymes needed to decrease the inflammatory response. Hydrocortisone, a corticosteroid secreted by the adrenal cortex, is about 1.25 times more potent an anti-inflammatory than equivalent doses of cortisone, but both have twice the mineralocorticoid activity of the other glucocorticoids.

Hydrocortisone 0.5% and 1%, and hydrocortisone acetate 0.5% are available without a prescription for the temporary relief of minor skin irritation, itching, and rashes caused by eczema, insect bites, soaps, and detergents.

Hydrocortisone is also given rectally as a retention enema for the temporary treatment of acute ulcerative colitis. Hydrocortisone acetate suspension is also available as a rectal suppository or aerosol foam suspension for the temporary treatment of inflammatory conditions of the rectum, such as hemorrhoids, cryptitis, proctitis, and pruritus ani.

## Pharmacokinetics
*Absorption:* Absorption depends on potency of preparation, amount applied, and nature of skin at application site. It ranges from about 1% in areas with a thick stratum corneum (such as the palms, soles, elbows, and knees) to as high as 36% in areas where the stratum corneum is thinnest (face, eyelids, and genitals). Absorption increases in areas of skin damage, inflammation, or occlusion. Some systemic absorption occurs, especially through the oral mucosa.
*Distribution:* After topical application, drug is distributed throughout the local skin layers. Any drug absorbed into circulation is removed rapidly from the blood and distributed into muscle, liver, skin, intestines, and kidneys.
*Metabolism:* After topical administration, hydrocortisone is metabolized primarily in the skin. The small amount absorbed into systemic circulation is metabolized primarily in the liver to inactive compounds.
*Excretion:* Inactive metabolites are excreted by the kidneys, primarily as glucuronides and sulfates, but also as unconjugated products. Small amounts of metabolites are also excreted in feces.

| Route | Onset | Peak | Duration |
|---|---|---|---|
| P.R., topical | Unknown | Unknown | Unknown |

## Contraindications and precautions
Contraindicated in patients hypersensitive to drug.

## Interactions
None significant.

## Adverse reactions
**GU:** glucosuria.
**Metabolic:** hyperglycemia.
**Skin:** burning, pruritus, irritation, dryness, erythema, folliculitis, hypertrichosis, hypopigmentation, acneiform eruptions, allergic contact dermatitis; *maceration, secondary infection, atrophy, striae, miliaria* (with occlusive dressings).
**Other:** *hypothalamic-pituitary-adrenal axis suppression,* Cushing's syndrome.

## Overdose and treatment
No information available.

## Clinical considerations
■ Recommendations for use of hydrocortisone are the same as those for all topical adrenocorticoids.

### Therapeutic monitoring
■ Recommendations for therapeutic monitoring of hydrocortisone are the same as those for all topical adrenocorticoids.

### Special populations
■ Recommendations are the same as those for all topical adrenocorticoids.

### Patient counseling
■ Recommendations are the same as those for all topical adrenocorticoids.

# hydromorphone hydrochloride
Dilaudid, Dilaudid-HP, Hydrostat IR

*Pharmacologic classification:* opioid
*Therapeutic classification:* analgesic, antitussive
*Pregnancy risk category C*
*Controlled substance schedule II*

### Available forms
Available by prescription only
*Tablets:* 1 mg, 2 mg, 3 mg, 4 mg, 8 mg
*Oral liquid:* 5 mg/5 ml
*Injection:* 1 mg/ml, 2 mg/ml, 3 mg/ml, 4 mg/ml, 10 mg/ml
*Suppository:* 3 mg

### Indications and dosages
*Moderate to severe pain*
*Adults:* 2 to 10 mg P.O. q 3 to 6 hours, p.r.n., or around-the-clock; or 2 to 4 mg I.M., S.C., or I.V. q 4 to 6 hours, p.r.n., or around-the-clock (give I.V. dose over 3 to 5 minutes); or 3-mg rectal suppository q 6 to 8 hours, p.r.n., or around-the-clock. (Give 1- to 14-mg Dilaudid-HP S.C. or I.M. q 4 to 6 hours.)
Note: Give hydromorphone hydrochloride in the smallest effective dosage to minimize the development of tolerance and physical dependence. Dosage must be individually adjusted based on patient's severity of pain, age, and size.
*Cough*
*Adults:* 1 mg P.O. q 3 to 4 hours, p.r.n.
*Children ages 6 to 12:* 0.5 mg P.O. q 3 to 4 hours, p.r.n.

### I.V. administration
■ Drug should be given by slow I.V. injection over at least 2 to 3 minutes.
■ Attention should be paid to the possibility of respiratory depression and hypotension.
■ Injection should be protected from light and stored at 59° to 86° F (15° to 30° C). Avoid freezing.

### Incompatibilities
Incompatible with alkalies, ampicillin sodium, bromides, cefazolin, cloxacillin, dexamethasone, diazepam, gallium, iodides, minocycline, phenobarbital sodium, phenytoin sodium, prochlorperazine edisylate, sargramostim, sodium bicarbonate, sodium phosphate, and thiopental.

### Mechanism of action
*Analgesic action:* Hydromorphone has analgesic properties related to opiate receptor affinity and is recommended for moderate to severe pain. There's no intrinsic limit to the analgesic effect of hydromorphone, unlike other opioids.
*Antitussive action:* Hydromorphone acts directly on the cough center in the medulla, producing an antitussive effect.

### Pharmacokinetics
*Absorption:* Well absorbed after oral, rectal, or parenteral administration.
*Distribution:* Unknown.
*Metabolism:* Metabolized primarily in the liver, where it undergoes conjugation with glucuronic acid.
*Excretion:* Excreted primarily in urine as the glucuronide conjugate. Duration of action is 4 to 5 hours.

| Route | Onset | Peak | Duration |
|---|---|---|---|
| P.O. | 30 min | 1½-2 hr | 4 hr |
| I.V. | 10-15 min | 15-30 min | 2-3 hours |
| I.M. | 15 min | ½-1 hr | 4-5 hr |
| S.C. | 15 min | ½-1½ hr | 4 hr |
| P.R. | Unknown | Unknown | 4 hr |

### Contraindications and precautions
Contraindicated in patients hypersensitive to drug, in those with intracranial lesions with increased intracranial pressure, and whenever ventilator function is depressed, such as in status asthmaticus, COPD, cor pulmonale, emphysema, and kyphoscoliosis.
Use cautiously in geriatric or debilitated patients and in those with hepatic or renal disease, Addison's disease, hypothyroidism, prostatic hyperplasia, or urethral strictures.

### Interactions
**Drug-drug.** *Anticholinergics:* Use of drug with anticholinergics may cause paralytic ileus. Avoid use together.
*Cimetidine:* Increases respiratory and CNS depression, causing confusion, disorientation, apnea, or seizures; reduced dosage of hydromorphone is usually required.
*Digitoxin, phenytoin, rifampin:* Drug accumulation and enhanced effects may result. Advise clinician to monitor patient closely.
*Other CNS depressants (narcotic analgesics, general anesthetics, antihistamines, barbiturates, benzodiazepines, muscle relaxants,*

*phenothiazines, sedative-hypnotics, tricyclic antidepressants):* Increase respiratory and CNS depression, sedation, and hypotensive effects of drug. Use together with extreme caution.

*General anesthetics:* Severe CV depression may result. Avoid use together.

*Narcotic antagonist:* Patients who become physically dependent on drug may experience acute withdrawal syndrome. Avoid use together.

**Drug-lifestyle.** *Alcohol use:* Increases CNS effects of drug. Advise patient to avoid alcohol.

## Adverse reactions
**CNS:** *sedation, somnolence, clouded sensorium,* dizziness, *euphoria.*
**CV:** *hypotension, **bradycardia.***
**EENT:** blurred vision, diplopia, nystagmus.
**GI:** *nausea, vomiting, constipation,* ileus.
**GU:** *urine retention.*
**Respiratory:** RESPIRATORY DEPRESSION, **bronchospasm.**
**Other:** induration (with repeated S.C. injections), physical dependence.

## Overdose and treatment
The most common signs and symptoms of hydromorphone overdose are CNS depression, respiratory depression, and miosis (pinpoint pupils). Other acute toxic effects include hypotension, bradycardia, hypothermia, shock, apnea, cardiopulmonary arrest, circulatory collapse, pulmonary edema, and seizures.

To treat an acute overdose, recommend first establishing adequate respiratory exchange via a patent airway and ventilation p.r.n.; recommend giving a narcotic antagonist (naloxone) to reverse respiratory depression. (Because the duration of action of hydromorphone is longer than that of naloxone, repeated dosing is needed.) Naloxone shouldn't be given unless patient has clinically significant respiratory or CV depression. Advise clinician to monitor vital signs closely.

If patient is seen within 2 hours of ingestion of an oral overdose, recommend emptying the stomach immediately by inducing emesis (ipecac syrup) or using gastric lavage. Advise prescriber to use caution to avoid risk of aspiration. Recommend giving activated charcoal via nasogastric tube for further removal of an oral overdose.

Symptomatic and supportive treatment (continued respiratory support, correction of fluid or electrolyte imbalance) should be provided. Advise clinician to monitor laboratory values, vital signs, and neurologic status closely.

Contact the local or regional poison control center for further information.

## Clinical considerations
■ Oral dosage form is particularly convenient for patients with chronic pain because tablets are available in several strengths, enabling patient to adjust his own dosage precisely.
■ Dilaudid-HP, a highly concentrated form (10 mg/ml), may be given in smaller volumes, preventing discomfort from large-volume injections.
■ Increased biliary tract pressure resulting from contraction of the sphincter of Oddi may interfere with hepatobiliary imaging studies.

### Therapeutic monitoring
■ Advise clinician to monitor patient for adverse reactions and response to dosage adjustments.

### Special populations
**Breast-feeding patients.** It's unknown if drug appears in breast milk; use with caution in breast-feeding women.
**Geriatric patients.** Lower doses are usually indicated for geriatric patients because they may be more sensitive to the therapeutic and adverse effects of drug.

## Patient counseling
■ Instruct patient to take or ask for drug before pain becomes intense.
■ Warn patient to avoid hazardous activities that require mental alertness.
■ Advise patient to avoid alcohol.

# hydroxychloroquine sulfate
Plaquenil Sulfate

*Pharmacologic classification:* 4-aminoquinoline
*Therapeutic classification:* antimalarial, anti-inflammatory
*Pregnancy risk category C*

## Available forms
Available by prescription only
*Tablets:* 200 mg (155-mg base)

## Indications and dosages
***Suppressive prophylaxis of malarial attacks***
*Adults:* 400 mg of sulfate (310-mg base) P.O. weekly on exactly the same day each week. (Begin 2 weeks before entering the endemic area and continue for 8 weeks after leaving.)
*Infants and children:* 5 mg, calculated as base per kilogram of body weight (shouldn't exceed the adult dosage regardless of weight) on exactly the same day each week. Start 2 weeks before exposure. If unable to do so, give 10-mg base/kg in two divided doses 6 hours apart.
***Treatment of acute attack of malaria***
*Adults:* 800 mg (620-mg base) followed by 400 mg (310-mg base) in 6 to 8 hours and

400 mg (310-mg base) on each of 2 consecutive days.

*Infants and children:* Initial dose, 10-mg base/kg (but not exceeding a single dose of 620-mg base). Second dose, 5-mg base/kg (but not exceeding a single dose of 310-mg base), is given 6 hours after first dose. Third dose, 5-mg base/kg, is given 18 hours after second dose. Fourth dose, 5-mg base/kg, is given 24 hours after third dose.

*Lupus erythematosus (chronic discoid and systemic)*
*Adults:* 400 mg P.O. daily or b.i.d., continued for several weeks or months, based on response. Prolonged maintenance dose is 200 to 400 mg P.O. daily.

◇*Rheumatoid arthritis*
*Adults:* Initially, 400 to 600 mg P.O. daily. When good response occurs (usually in 4 to 12 weeks), reduce dosage by half.

## Mechanism of action
*Amebicidal action:* Mechanism of action is unknown.

*Anti-inflammatory action:* Mechanism of action is unknown. Drug may antagonize histamine and serotonin and inhibit prostaglandin effects by blocking conversion of arachidonic acid to prostaglandin $F_2$; it may also inhibit chemotaxis of polymorphonuclear leukocytes, macrophages, and eosinophils.

*Antimalarial action:* Hydroxychloroquine binds to DNA, interfering with protein synthesis. It also inhibits DNA and RNA polymerases. It's active against asexual erythrocytic forms of *Plasmodium malariae, P. ovale, P. vivax,* and many strains of *P. falciparum.*

## Pharmacokinetics
*Absorption:* Absorbed readily and almost completely.

*Distribution:* Plasma protein–bound. It concentrates in the liver, spleen, kidneys, heart, and brain and is strongly bound to melanin-containing cells.

*Metabolism:* Metabolized by the liver to desethylchloroquine and desethyl hydroxychloroquine.

*Excretion:* Most of a given dose is excreted unchanged in urine. Drug and its metabolites are excreted slowly in urine; unabsorbed drug is excreted in feces. Small amounts of drug may be present in urine for months after it's discontinued. Drug appears in breast milk.

| Route | Onset | Peak | Duration |
|-------|-------|------|----------|
| P.O. | Unknown | 2-4½ hr | Unknown |

## Contraindications and precautions
Contraindicated in patients hypersensitive to drug, in long-term therapy for children, and in patients with retinal or visual field changes or porphyria.

Use cautiously in patients with severe GI, neurologic, or blood disorders.

## Interactions
**Drug-drug.** *Digoxin:* May increase serum digoxin levels. Advise clinician to monitor digoxin levels; patient requires close monitoring for signs of digoxin toxicity.

*Kaolin or magnesium trisilicate:* Decreased absorption of hydroxychloroquine. Drugs should be given at separate times.

**Drug-lifestyle.** *Prolonged, unprotected sun exposure:* May cause drug-induced dermatoses. Advise patient to use sunblock.

## Adverse reactions
**CNS:** irritability, nightmares, ataxia, *seizures,* psychosis, vertigo, nystagmus, dizziness, hypoactive deep tendon reflexes, ataxia, lassitude, headache.

**EENT:** visual disturbances (blurred vision; difficulty in focusing; reversible corneal changes; typically irreversible, sometimes progressive or delayed retinal changes, such as narrowing of arterioles; macular lesions; pallor of optic disk; optic atrophy; visual field defects; patchy retinal pigmentation, commonly leading to blindness), ototoxicity (irreversible nerve deafness, tinnitus, labyrinthitis).

**GI:** anorexia, abdominal cramps, diarrhea, nausea, vomiting.

**Hematologic:** *agranulocytosis, leukopenia, thrombocytopenia, hemolysis (in patients with G6PD deficiency), aplastic anemia.*

**Metabolic:** weight loss.

**Musculoskeletal:** skeletal muscle weakness.

**Skin:** alopecia, bleaching of hair, pruritus, lichen planus eruptions, skin and mucosal pigmentary changes, pleomorphic skin eruptions.

## Overdose and treatment
Symptoms of drug overdose may appear within 30 minutes after ingestion and may include headache, drowsiness, visual changes, CV collapse, and seizures followed by respiratory and cardiac arrest.

Treatment is symptomatic. Recommend emptying stomach by emesis or lavage. After lavage, activated charcoal in an amount at least five times the estimated amount of drug ingested may be helpful if given within 30 minutes of ingestion.

Ultra-short–acting barbiturates may help control seizures. Intubation may become necessary. Peritoneal dialysis and exchange transfusions may also be useful. Forced fluids and acidification of the urine are helpful after the acute phase.

## Clinical considerations
**⋈ ALERT** Dosage may be discussed in mg or mg-base; be aware of the difference.

■ Recommend giving drug immediately before or after meals on the same day each week to minimize gastric distress.
■ Drug isn't effective for chloroquine-resistant strains of *P. falciparum*.
■ Drug may cause inversion or depression of the T wave or widening of the QRS complex on ECG.

### Therapeutic monitoring
■ Advise clinician to monitor patient for blurred vision, increased sensitivity to light, hearing loss, pronounced GI disturbances, or muscle weakness.
■ Baseline and periodic ophthalmologic examinations are needed in prolonged or high-dosage therapy.

### Special populations
**Pregnant patients.** Avoid use of drug in patients with rheumatoid arthritis; disease can be managed with corticosteroids. In patients taking drug for systemic lupus erythematosus, some clinicians state that the benefits outweigh the risks to the fetus.
**Breast-feeding patients.** Safety hasn't been established. Use with caution in breast-feeding women.
**Pediatric patients.** Children are extremely susceptible to toxicity; recommend monitoring patient closely for adverse effects. Don't use drug for long-term therapy in children and don't exceed recommended dosage.

### Patient counseling
■ To prevent drug-induced dermatoses, warn patient to avoid excessive sun exposure.

# hydroxyurea
Droxia, Hydrea, Mylocel

*Pharmacologic classification:* antimetabolite (cell cycle–phase specific, S phase)
*Therapeutic classification:* antineoplastic
*Pregnancy risk category NR*

### Available forms
Available by prescription only
*Capsules:* 200 mg, 300 mg, 400 mg, 500 mg
*Tablets:* 1,000 mg

### Indications and dosages
Dosage and indications for hydroxyurea may vary. Check current literature for recommended protocol.
*Solid tumors*
*Adults:* 80 mg/kg P.O. as a single dose q 3 days; or 20 to 30 mg/kg P.O. as a single daily dose.
*Head and neck cancers, excluding the lip*
*Adults:* 80 mg/kg P.O. as a single dose q 3 days.

*Resistant chronic myelocytic leukemia*
*Adults:* 20 to 30 mg/kg P.O. as a single daily dose.

### Mechanism of action
*Antineoplastic action:* The exact mechanism of the cytotoxic action of hydroxyurea is unclear. Hydroxyurea inhibits DNA synthesis without, however, interfering with RNA or protein synthesis. Drug may act as an antimetabolite, inhibiting the incorporation of thymidine into DNA, and it may also damage DNA directly.

### Pharmacokinetics
*Absorption:* Well absorbed after oral administration. Higher serum levels are achieved if drug is given as a large, single dose rather than in divided doses.
*Distribution:* Hydroxyurea crosses the blood-brain barrier.
*Metabolism:* About 50% of an oral dose is degraded in the liver.
*Excretion:* The remaining 50% is excreted in urine as unchanged drug. The metabolites are excreted through the lungs as carbon dioxide and in urine as urea.

| Route | Onset | Peak | Duration |
|-------|-------|------|----------|
| P.O. | Unknown | 2 hr | 24 hr |

### Contraindications and precautions
Contraindicated in patients hypersensitive to drug and in those with marked bone marrow depression (leukopenia [less than 2,500 WBCs/mm$^3$], thrombocytopenia [less than 100,000 platelets/mm$^3$], or severe anemia).

Use cautiously in patients with impaired renal function. Advise prescriber not to give to pregnant women or women of childbearing age who may become pregnant unless potential benefit to patient outweighs possible risk to fetus.

### Interactions
**Drug-drug.** *Didanosine, indinavir, stavudine:* Fatal pancreatitis has occurred with concomitant use of these drugs. Avoid use together.
*Fluorouracil:* Neurotoxicity may occur when these two drugs are given together. Avoid concomitant use.
*Hydroxyurea and other myelosuppressive drugs or radiation therapy:* May increase likelihood of bone marrow depression or other adverse effects. Dosage adjustments may be needed.

### Adverse reactions
**CNS:** hallucinations, headache, dizziness, disorientation, *seizures,* malaise.
**GI:** *anorexia, nausea, vomiting, diarrhea,* stomatitis, constipation, *fatal pancreatitis.*
**GU:** increased BUN and serum creatinine levels.

**Hematologic:** *leukopenia, thrombocytopenia,* anemia, *megaloblastosis, bone marrow suppression,* with rapid recovery (dose-limiting and dose-related).
**Skin:** rash, alopecia, erythema.
**Other:** fever, chills.
Note: Drug may potentiate some adverse reactions typically observed with radiation therapy alone, such as gastric distress and mucositis.

## Overdose and treatment
Signs and symptoms of overdose include myelosuppression, ulceration of buccal and GI mucosa, facial erythema, maculopapular rash, disorientation, hallucinations, and impairment of renal tubular function.
Treatment is usually supportive and includes transfusion of blood components.

## Clinical considerations
■ Dosage modification may be required after other chemotherapy or radiation therapy.
■ Auditory and visual hallucinations and blood toxicity increase when decreased renal function exists.
■ Avoid all I.M. injections when platelet counts are below 100,000/mm³.
■ Store capsules in tight container at room temperature. Avoid exposure to excessive heat.
■ Drug is currently under investigation for the treatment of sickle cell anemia. Widespread use of drug for this disease isn't recommended because of the potential for toxicity.
■ Although drug is labeled for the treatment of melanoma and recurrent, metastatic, or inoperable ovarian cancer, other drugs are preferred.
■ Unlabeled use is for the treatment of cervical cancer, although other drugs are preferred.

### Therapeutic monitoring
■ Advise clinician to monitor intake and output levels; patient must remain hydrated.
■ Recommend obtaining BUN, uric acid, and serum creatinine levels routinely.
■ Drug may exacerbate postirradiation erythema.

### Special populations
**Pregnant patients.** Drug isn't to be given to pregnant women or women of childbearing age who may become pregnant unless potential benefit to patient outweighs possible risk to fetus.
**Breast-feeding patients.** It's unknown if drug appears in breast milk. However, because of risk of serious adverse reactions, mutagenicity, and carcinogenicity in the infant, breast-feeding isn't recommended.
**Pediatric patients.** Safety and efficacy have not been established in children.

**Geriatric patients.** Geriatric patients may be more sensitive to effects of drug, requiring a lower dosage.

## Patient counseling
■ Emphasize importance of continuing drug therapy despite nausea and vomiting.
■ Encourage daily fluid intake of ten to twelve 8-ounce glasses to increase urine output and facilitate excretion of uric acid.
■ Advise patient of potential for adverse reactions and instruct to immediately report postdose vomiting, and unusual bruising or bleeding.
■ Advise patient to avoid exposure to people with infection and to report signs of infection immediately.
■ Instruct patient to keep drug out of reach of children.
■ Tell patient that if the contents of the capsule are spilled, the powder should be wiped up immediately with a damp disposable towel and discarded in a closed container.

# hydroxyzine hydrochloride
Anxanil, Apo-Hydroxyzine*, Atarax, Hydroxacen, Hyzine-50, Multipax*, Novo-Hydroxyzin*, Quiess, Vistacon, Vistazine-50

# hydroxyzine pamoate
Vistaril

*Pharmacologic classification:* antihistamine (piperazine derivative)
*Therapeutic classification:* antianxiety, sedative, antipruritic, antiemetic, antispasmodic
*Pregnancy risk category C*

## Available forms
Available by prescription only
**hydroxyzine hydrochloride**
*Capsules:* 10 mg, 25 mg, 50 mg
*Tablets:* 10 mg, 25 mg, 50 mg, 100 mg
*Syrup:* 10 mg/5 ml
*Injection:* 25 mg/ml, 50 mg/ml
**hydroxyzine pamoate**
*Capsules:* 25 mg, 50 mg, 100 mg
*Oral suspension:* 25 mg/5 ml

## Indications and dosages
*Anxiety, tension, hyperkinesia*
*Adults:* 50 to 100 mg P.O. q.i.d.
*Children ages 6 and older:* 50 to 100 mg P.O. daily in divided doses.
*Children under age 6:* 50 mg P.O. daily in divided doses.
*Preoperative and postoperative adjunctive sedation*
*Adults:* 50 to 100 mg P.O. or 25 to 100 mg I.M.
*Children:* 0.6 mg/kg P.O. or 1.1 mg/kg I.M.

*Control of acutely disturbed and hysterical patients and for the management of agitation caused by alcohol withdrawal*
*Adults:* 50 to 100 mg I.M. p.r.n. every 4 to 6 hours.
*Management of pruritus caused by allergic conditions*
*Adults:* 25 mg P.O. t.i.d. or q.i.d.
*Children ages 6 and older:* 50 to 100 mg P.O. daily in divided doses.
*Children under age 6:* 50 mg P.O. daily in divided doses.
*Control of nausea and vomiting (except from pregnancy)*
*Adults:* 25 to 100 mg I.M. Subsequent dosing can be based on patient's response.
*Children:* 1.1 mg/kg I.M. Subsequent dosing can be based on patient's response.
*Control of emesis, to permit decreased opiate dosage, or to allay anxiety in prepartum and postpartum states*
*Adults:* 25 to 100 mg I.M. Subsequent dosing can be based on patient's response.

## Mechanism of action

*Antipruritic action:* Drug is a direct competitor of histamine for binding at cellular receptor sites.
*Anxiolytic and sedative actions:* Hydroxyzine produces its sedative and antianxiety effects through suppression of activity at subcortical levels; analgesia occurs at high doses.
*Other actions:* Hydroxyzine is used as a preoperative and postoperative adjunct for its sedative, antihistaminic, and anticholinergic activity.

## Pharmacokinetics

*Absorption:* Absorbed rapidly and completely after oral administration. Peak serum levels occur within 2 to 4 hours. Sedation and other clinical effects are usually noticed in 15 to 30 minutes.
*Distribution:* Not well understood.
*Metabolism:* Metabolized almost completely in the liver.
*Excretion:* Metabolites are excreted primarily in urine; small amounts of drug and metabolites are found in feces. Half-life of drug is 3 hours. Sedative effects can last for 4 to 6 hours, and antihistaminic effects can persist for up to 4 days.

| Route | Onset | Peak | Duration |
|-------|-------|------|----------|
| P.O. | 15-30 min | 2 hr | 4-6 hr |
| I.M. | Unknown | Unknown | 4-6 hr |

## Contraindications and precautions

Contraindicated in patients hypersensitive to drug and during early pregnancy.
Use cautiously with adjustments in dosage in geriatric or debilitated patients.

## Interactions

**Drug-drug.** *Barbiturates, opioids, tranquilizers, other CNS depressants:* Increased CNS effects. Recommend reducing dosage of CNS depressants by 50%.
*Epinephrine:* Concurrent use blocks vasopressor action. If a vasoconstrictor is needed, use norepinephrine or phenylephrine.
*Other anticholinergics:* Cause additive anticholinergic effects. Advise clinician to monitor patient closely.
**Drug-lifestyle.** *Alcohol use:* Additive effects. Advise patient to avoid alcohol.

## Adverse reactions

**CNS:** *drowsiness,* involuntary motor activity.
**GI:** *dry mouth.*
**Other:** marked discomfort at I.M. injection site, hypersensitivity reactions (wheezing, dyspnea, chest tightness).

## Overdose and treatment

Signs and symptoms of overdose include excessive sedation and hypotension; seizures may occur.
Treatment is supportive only. For recent oral ingestion, recommend emptying gastric contents through emesis or lavage. Recommend correcting hypotension with fluids and vasopressors (phenylephrine or metaraminol). Epinephrine shouldn't be given because hydroxyzine may counteract its effect.

## Clinical considerations

■ Carefully review patient's drug sensitivities and the use of CNS depressants for potential dosage adjustments.
■ Drug therapy causes falsely elevated urinary 17-hydroxycorticosteroid levels. It also may cause false-negative skin allergen test results by attenuating or inhibiting the cutaneous response to histamine.

### Therapeutic monitoring

■ Recommend observing patient for excessive sedation, especially if he's receiving other CNS depressants.

### Special populations

**Pregnant patients.** Drug isn't to be used during early pregnancy because of potential risk to the fetus. Safety and efficacy in pregnant women haven't been determined.
**Breast-feeding patients.** It's unknown if drug appears in breast milk. Safety hasn't been established in breast-feeding women.
**Geriatric patients.** Geriatric patients may experience greater CNS depression and anticholinergic effects. Lower doses are indicated.

## Patient counseling

■ Advise patient to avoid tasks that require mental alertness or physical coordination until CNS effects of drug are known.

■ Advise patient against use of other CNS depressants with hydroxyzine unless prescribed. Advise him to avoid alcohol and alcohol-containing products.

■ Instruct patient to seek medical approval before taking OTC cold or allergy preparations that contain antihistamine, which may potentiate the effects of hydroxyzine.

# hyoscyamine
Cystospaz

# hyoscyamine sulfate
Anaspaz, Cystospaz-M, Levsin, Levsin Drops, Levsinex Timecaps, Neoquess

*Pharmacologic classification:* belladonna alkaloid
*Therapeutic classification:* anticholinergic
*Pregnancy risk category C*

## Available forms
Available by prescription only
**hyoscyamine**
*Tablets:* 0.15 mg
**hyoscyamine sulfate**
*Tablets:* 0.125 mg
*Capsules (extended-release):* 0.375 mg
*Tablets (extended-release):* 0.375 mg
*Oral solution:* 0.125 mg/ml
*Elixir:* 0.125 mg/5 ml
*Injection:* 0.5 mg/ml

## Indications and dosages
**GI tract disorders caused by spasm; adjunctive therapy for peptic ulcers**
*Adults:* 0.125 to 0.25 mg P.O. or S.L. q.i.d. before meals and h.s.; 0.375 to 0.75 mg P.O. (extended-release form) q 12 hours; or 0.25 to 0.5 mg I.M., I.V., or S.C. q 4 hours b.i.d. to q.i.d. (Substitute oral medication when symptoms are controlled.)
*Children ages 2 to 12:* 0.033 mg at about 10 kg (22 lb); at about 20 kg (44 lb), 0.0625 mg; at about 40 kg (88 lb), 0.0938 mg; at about 50 kg (110 lb), 0.125 mg. May repeat q 4 hours, p.r.n. Maximum dose 0.75 mg/day.
*Children under age 2:* 0.0125 mg at about 2.3 kg (5 lb); at about 3.4 kg (7.5 lb), 0.0167 mg; at about 5 kg (11 lb), 0.02 mg; at about 6.8 kg (15 lb), 0.025 mg; at about 10 kg (22 lb), 0.033 mg; at about 15 kg (33 lb), 0.05 mg. May repeat q 4 hours, p.r.n. Maximum daily doses 0.075 mg, 0.1 mg, 0.125 mg, 0.15 mg, 0.2 mg, and 0.275 mg, respectively.
**Endoscopy or hypotonic duodenography**
*Adults:* 0.25 to 0.5 mg I.V., I.M., or S.C., 5 to 10 minutes before procedure.

*Preoperative medication*
*Adults and children over age 2:* 5 mcg/kg I.V., I.M., or S.C. 30 to 60 minutes before induction of anesthesia.

## I.V. administration
■ Parenteral solutions should be visually inspected for particulate matter and discoloration.

### Incompatibilities
None reported.

## Mechanism of action
*Antispasmodic and antiulcer action:* Hyoscyamine competitively blocks acetylcholine at cholinergic neuroeffector sites, decreasing GI motility and inhibiting gastric acid secretion.

## Pharmacokinetics
*Absorption:* Well absorbed when taken orally.
*Distribution:* Well distributed throughout the body and crosses the blood-brain barrier. About 50% of dose is plasma protein–bound.
*Metabolism:* Metabolized in the liver. Usual duration of effect is up to 4 hours with standard oral and parenteral administration and up to 12 hours for the extended-release preparation.
*Excretion:* Excreted in the urine.

| Route | Onset | Peak | Duration |
|---|---|---|---|
| P.O. | 20-30 min | ½-1 hr | 4-12 hr |
| P.O. (extended) | 20-30 min | 40-90 min | 12 hr |
| I.V. | 2 min | 15-30 min | 4 hr |
| I.M., S.C. | Unknown | 15-30 min | 4-12 hr |
| S.L. | 5-20 min | ½-1 hr | 4 hr |

## Contraindications and precautions
Contraindicated in patients with glaucoma, obstructive uropathy, obstructive disease of the GI tract, severe ulcerative colitis, myasthenia gravis, hypersensitivity to anticholinergics, paralytic ileus, intestinal atony, unstable CV status in acute hemorrhage, or toxic megacolon.

Use cautiously in patients with autonomic neuropathy, hyperthyroidism, coronary artery disease, arrhythmias, HF, hypertension, hiatal hernia with reflux esophagitis, hepatic or renal disease, and ulcerative colitis. Also use cautiously in hot or humid environments where drug-induced heatstroke can occur.

## Interactions
**Drug-drug.** *Amantadine:* Increased anticholinergic effects. Avoid use together.
*Antacids, antidiarrheals:* Decrease absorption of oral hyoscyamine. Oral hyoscyamine should be taken 1 hour before these drugs.

*Haloperidol or phenothiazines:* Reduced antipsychotic effectiveness. Advise clinician to monitor patient carefully.

*Phenothiazines:* Increase adverse anticholinergic effects of hyoscyamine. Avoid use together.

**Drug-herb.** *Jimsonweed:* May adversely effect CV function. Discourage use together.

## Adverse reactions

**CNS:** headache, insomnia, drowsiness, dizziness, nervousness, weakness; *confusion, excitement* (in geriatric patients).

**CV:** *palpitations,* tachycardia.

**EENT:** *blurred vision,* mydriasis, increased intraocular pressure, cycloplegia, photophobia.

**GI:** *dry mouth,* dysphagia, *constipation,* heartburn, loss of taste, nausea, vomiting, *paralytic ileus.*

**GU:** *urinary hesitancy, urine retention,* impotence.

**Skin:** urticaria, decreased sweating or possible anhidrosis, other dermal manifestations.

**Other:** fever, allergic reactions.

## Overdose and treatment

Signs and symptoms of overdose include curare-like symptoms, such as respiratory paralysis; central stimulation followed by depression; and such psychotic symptoms as disorientation, confusion, hallucinations, delusions, anxiety, agitation, and restlessness. Peripheral effects may include dilated, nonreactive pupils; blurred vision; flushed, hot, dry skin; dryness of mucous membranes; dysphagia; decreased or absent bowel sounds; urine retention; hyperthermia; headache; tachycardia; hypertension; and increased respiration.

Treatment is primarily symptomatic and supportive. Recommend maintaining patent airway. If patient is alert, recommend inducing emesis (or using gastric lavage) and following with a saline cathartic and activated charcoal to prevent further drug absorption. In severe cases, physostigmine may be given to block antimuscarinic effects. Fluids should be given, p.r.n., to treat shock; diazepam to control psychotic symptoms; and pilocarpine (instilled into the eyes) to relieve mydriasis. If urine retention occurs, catheterization may be needed.

## Clinical considerations

■ Consider the recommendations relevant to all anticholinergics.

■ Hyoscyamine is given P.O. Hyoscyamine sulfate usually is given P.O. or S.L., but may be given I.V., I.M., or S.C. when therapeutic effect is needed or if oral administration isn't possible.

### Therapeutic monitoring

■ Drug regimen is adjusted based on patient's response and tolerance.

### Special populations

**Breast-feeding patients.** Drug may appear in breast milk, possibly resulting in infant toxicity. Avoid use in breast-feeding women. Drug may also decrease milk production.

**Pediatric patients.** Safety and efficacy for use in children haven't been reported.

**Geriatric patients.** Use drug cautiously in geriatric patients; lower doses are indicated.

## Patient counseling

■ Advise patient to avoid driving or performing other hazardous activities if drowsiness, dizziness, or blurred vision occurs.

■ Advise patient to avoid using jimsonweed with hyoscyamine.

■ Tell patient to drink fluids to avoid constipation.

■ Instruct patient to report rash or other skin eruptions.

■ Advise patient that extended-release tablets may not completely disintegrate and tablet fragments may be excreted in stools in some patients.

■ Tell patient not to crush or chew extended-release tablets.

# ibuprofen

Advil, Children's Advil, Medipren, Motrin, Motrin IB, Nuprin, Pediacare Fever, PediaProfen, Rufen, Trendar

*Pharmacologic classification:* NSAID
*Therapeutic classification:* nonnarcotic analgesic, antipyretic, anti-inflammatory
*Pregnancy risk category B (D, in third trimester)*

## Available forms

Available without a prescription
*Tablets:* 100 mg, 200 mg
*Tablets (chewable):* 50 mg, 100 mg
*Oral suspension:* 100 mg/5 ml
Available by prescription only
*Tablets:* 100 mg, 300 mg, 400 mg, 600 mg, 800 mg
*Oral suspension:* 100 mg/5 ml
*Oral drops:* 40 mg/ml

## Indications and dosages

*Arthritis, gout, and postextraction dental pain*
*Adults:* 300 to 800 mg P.O. t.i.d. or q.i.d. Don't exceed 3,200 mg as total daily dose.
*Primary dysmenorrhea*
*Adults:* 400 mg P.O. q 4 to 6 hours.
*Mild to moderate pain*
*Adults:* 400 mg P.O. q 4 to 6 hours.
*Children:* 10 mg/kg P.O. q 6 to 8 hours; maximum dose, 40 mg/kg.
*Juvenile arthritis*
*Children:* 20 to 40 mg/kg/day P.O., divided into three or four doses. For mild disease, 20 mg/kg/day in divided doses.
*Fever reduction*
*Adults:* 200 to 400 mg P.O. q 4 to 6 hours, p.r.n. Don't exceed 1,200 mg/day or take longer than 3 days.
*Children ages 6 months to 12 years:* 5 mg/kg P.O. q 6 to 8 hours, p.r.n., if baseline temperature is 102.5° F (39.2° C) or below; 10 mg/kg P.O. q 6 to 8 hours, p.r.n., if baseline temperature is more than 102.5° F. Recommended daily maximum dose, 40 mg/kg.

## Mechanism of action

*Analgesic, antipyretic, and anti-inflammatory actions:* Mechanisms of action are unknown; ibuprofen is thought to inhibit prostaglandin synthesis.

## Pharmacokinetics

*Absorption:* Part of oral dose (80%) is absorbed from GI tract.
*Distribution:* Highly protein-bound.
*Metabolism:* Undergoes biotransformation in the liver.
*Excretion:* Excreted mainly in urine, with some biliary excretion. Plasma half-life ranges from 2 to 4 hours.

| Route | Onset | Peak | Duration |
|-------|-------|------|----------|
| P.O. | Variable | Variable | Variable |

## Contraindications and precautions

Contraindicated in patients hypersensitive to drug or in those who have the syndrome of nasal polyps, angioedema, and bronchospastic reaction to aspirin or other NSAIDs.

Use cautiously in patients with impaired renal or hepatic function, GI disorders, peptic ulcer disease, cardiac decompensation, hypertension, or known coagulation defects. Because chewable tablets contain aspartame, use cautiously in patients with phenylketonuria. Ibuprofen is contraindicated during the last trimester of pregnancy because it may cause problems with the fetus or complications during delivery.

## Interactions

**Drug-drug.** *ACE inhibitors:* Reduced response when used together; may result in acute reduction in renal function. Advise clinician to monitor patient closely.
*Antacids:* May decrease the absorption of ibuprofen. Patient should take drugs at separate times.
*Anticoagulants, thrombolytics (coumarin derivatives, heparin, streptokinase, urokinase):* Increased anticoagulant effects. Dosage adjustment may be needed. Advise clinician to monitor coagulation studies.
*Aspirin:* May decrease the bioavailability of ibuprofen. Advise clinician to monitor patient for drug effect.
*Aspirin, carbenicillin, cefamandole, cefoperazone, dextran, dipyridamole, mezlocillin, piperacillin, plicamycin, salicylates, sulfinpyrazone, ticarcillin, valproic acid, corticosteroids, or other anti-inflammatory drugs:* Increased risk of bleeding or adverse GI reactions. Avoid use together.

---

*\* Canada only     ◇ Unlabeled clinical use*

*Coumarin derivatives, nifedipine, phenytoin, verapamil:* Toxicity may occur with concurrent use; avoid use together.

*Diuretics, antihypertensives:* Concurrent use may decrease effectiveness of these drugs; diuretics may increase nephrotoxicity. Advise clinician to monitor patient closely.

*Gold compounds, other anti-inflammatory drugs, or acetaminophen:* Increased nephrotoxicity may occur. Use with caution.

*Insulin or oral antidiabetics:* May potentiate hypoglycemic effects. Dosage adjustment may be needed.

*Lithium, methotrexate:* Decreased renal clearance of these drugs. Use together cautiously. Advise clinician to monitor patient for adverse reactions; if needed, lithium blood levels should be drawn.

**Drug-herb.** *Dong quai, feverfew, garlic, ginger, ginkgo biloba, horse chestnut, red clover:* Possible increased risk of bleeding. Discourage use together.

*Feverfew:* Decreased effectiveness of NSAID. Discourage use together.

*St. John's wort, dong quai:* Increased risk of photosensitivity. Advise patient to avoid unprotected exposure to sunlight.

## Adverse reactions

**CNS:** *headache, dizziness,* nervousness, aseptic meningitis.
**CV:** *peripheral edema,* fluid retention, edema.
**EENT:** *tinnitus.*
**GI:** *epigastric distress, nausea, occult blood loss, peptic ulceration,* diarrhea, constipation, dyspepsia, flatulence, heartburn, decreased appetite.
**GU:** *acute renal failure,* azotemia, cystitis, hematuria.
**Hematologic:** prolonged bleeding time, anemia, *neutropenia, pancytopenia, thrombocytopenia, aplastic anemia, leukopenia, agranulocytosis.*
**Hepatic:** elevated liver enzyme levels.
**Respiratory:** *bronchospasm.*
**Skin:** pruritus, *rash,* urticaria, *Stevens-Johnson syndrome.*

## Overdose and treatment

Signs and symptoms of overdose include dizziness, drowsiness, paresthesia, vomiting, nausea, abdominal pain, headache, sweating, nystagmus, apnea, and cyanosis.

To treat drug overdose, recommend emptying stomach immediately by inducing emesis with ipecac syrup or by gastric lavage. Recommend giving activated charcoal via nasogastric tube. Recommend providing symptomatic and supportive measures (respiratory support and correction of fluid and electrolyte imbalances). Advise clinician to monitor laboratory effects and vital signs closely. Alkaline diuresis may enhance renal excretion. Dialysis is of minimal value because ibuprofen is strongly protein-bound.

## Clinical considerations

■ Maximum results in arthritis may require 1 to 2 weeks of continuous therapy with ibuprofen. Improvement may be seen, however, within 7 days.

■ Recommend giving drug on an empty stomach, 1 hour before or 2 hours after meals for maximum absorption. However, it may be given with meals to lessen GI upset.

■ For patients at high risk for complications from NSAID-induced ulceration, misoprostol, a proton pump inhibitor, or an $H_2$ blocker may be considered for preventative therapy.

■ For patients with rheumatoid arthritis, a disease-modifying antirheumatic drug may be considered for patients without adequate response to NSAIDs.

### *Therapeutic monitoring*

■ Advise clinician to monitor auditory and ophthalmic functions periodically during ibuprofen therapy.

■ Advise clinician to monitor cardiopulmonary status closely, and monitor vital signs, especially heart rate and blood pressure.

■ Advise clinician to observe patient for possible fluid retention and GI bleed.

### *Special populations*

**Pregnant patients.** Drug shouldn't be used in third trimester unless specifically directed by a prescriber.

**Breast-feeding patients.** Drug doesn't appear in breast milk in significant quantities. However, manufacturer recommends alternative feeding methods during ibuprofen therapy.

**Pediatric patients.** Safety and efficacy in children under age 6 months haven't been established.

**Geriatric patients.** Patients over age 60 may be more susceptible to the toxic effects of ibuprofen, especially adverse GI reactions. Use lowest possible effective dose. The effect of drug on renal prostaglandins may cause fluid retention and edema, a significant drawback for geriatric patients, especially those with HF.

## Patient counseling

■ Instruct patient to seek medical approval before taking OTC drugs.

■ Advise patient not to self-medicate with ibuprofen for longer than 10 days for analgesic use and not to exceed maximum dose of six tablets (1.2 g) daily for self-medication. Caution patient not to take drug if fever lasts longer than 3 days, unless prescribed.

■ Tell patient to report adverse reactions; they're usually dose-related.

■ Instruct patient in safety measures to prevent injury. Caution him to avoid hazardous activities that require mental alertness until CNS effects of drug are known.

■ Encourage patient to adhere to prescribed drug regimen and stress importance of medical follow-up.

# ibutilide fumarate
Corvert

*Pharmacologic classification:* ibutilide derivative
*Therapeutic classification:* supraventricular antiarrhythmic
*Pregnancy risk category C*

## Available forms
Available by prescription only
*Injection:* 0.1 mg/ml

## Indications and dosages
*Rapid conversion of atrial fibrillation or atrial flutter of recent onset to sinus rhythm*
*Adults weighing 60 kg (132 lb) or more:* 1 mg I.V. over 10 minutes.
*Adults weighing under 60 kg:* 0.01 mg/kg I.V. over 10 minutes.

## I.V. administration
■ Admixtures of the product, with approved diluents, are chemically and physically stable for 24 hours at room temperature and for 48 hours at refrigerated temperatures.

■ Drug may be given undiluted or diluted over 10 minutes.

■ Infusion should be stopped if arrhythmia is terminated or if sustained or nonsustained ventricular tachycardia or marked prolongation of QT or QTc interval occurs. If arrhythmia doesn't terminate within 10 minutes after infusion ends, a second 10-minute infusion of equal strength may be given.

### Incompatibilities
None reported.

## Mechanism of action
*Antiarrhythmic action:* An antiarrhythmic with predominantly class III properties, ibutilide prolongs action potential duration in isolated cardiac myocytes and increases both atrial and ventricular refractoriness.

## Pharmacokinetics
*Absorption:* Administered I.V.
*Distribution:* Highly distributed and about 40% protein-bound.
*Metabolism:* Not clearly defined.

*Excretion:* Excreted mainly in urine with the rest in feces; half-life of drug is about 6 hours.

| Route | Onset | Peak | Duration |
|---|---|---|---|
| I.V. | Unknown | Unknown | Unknown |

## Contraindications and precautions
Contraindicated in patients hypersensitive to drug or its components and in those with history of polymorphic ventricular tachycardia, such as torsades de pointes.

Use cautiously in patients with hepatic or renal dysfunction.

## Interactions
**Drug-drug.** *Class Ia antiarrhythmics (disopyramide, procainamide, quinidine) and other class III drugs (amiodarone, sotalol):* Increase the potential for prolonged refractoriness. Avoid concurrent administration and dosing for at least five half-lives before administration of ibutilide and for 4 hours after ibutilide dosing. Supraventricular arrhythmias may mask the cardiotoxicity from excessive digoxin levels. Use cautiously.

*$H_1$-receptor antagonist antihistamines, phenothiazines, tetracyclic antidepressants, tricyclic antidepressants, and other drugs that prolong QT interval:* Increase the risk for proarrhythmia. Patient requires ECG monitoring.

## Adverse reactions
**CNS:** headache.
**CV:** ventricular extrasystoles, nonsustained ventricular tachycardia, hypotension, bundle branch block, *sustained ventricular tachycardia, AV block,* hypertension, QT-segment prolongation, *bradycardia,* palpitations, tachycardia.
**GI:** nausea.

## Overdose and treatment
Overdose could exaggerate the expected prolongation of repolarization seen at usual clinical doses. Treatment should be supportive and appropriate for the condition.

## Clinical considerations
■ Proper equipment and facilities, including cardiac monitoring, intracardiac pacing facilities, cardioverter-defibrillator, and drug for treatment of sustained ventricular tachycardia, should be available during and after drug administration.

■ Hypokalemia and hypomagnesemia should be corrected before therapy begins to reduce the potential for proarrhythmia.

### Therapeutic monitoring
■ Patients with atrial fibrillation of longer than 2 to 3 days' duration must be given adequate anticoagulants, generally for at least 2 weeks.

■ Advise clinician to monitor patient's ECG continuously throughout drug administration and for at least 4 hours afterward or until QTc interval has returned to baseline because drug can induce or worsen ventricular arrhythmias in some patients. Longer monitoring is required if arrhythmic activity is noted.

### Special populations
**Breast-feeding patients.** It's unknown if drug appears in breast milk; discourage breast-feeding during drug therapy.
**Pediatric patients.** Safety and efficacy in children under age 18 haven't been established.

### Patient counseling
■ Tell patient to report adverse reactions at once.
■ Instruct patient to report discomfort at I.V. injection site.

# idarubicin
Idamycin

*Pharmacologic classification:* antibiotic antineoplastic
*Therapeutic classification:* antineoplastic
*Pregnancy risk category D*

### Available forms
Available by prescription only
*Injection:* 5 mg, 10 mg, 20 mg (lyophilized powder) in single-dose vials with 50-, 100-, or 200-mg lactose

### Indications and dosages
***Treatment of acute myelocytic leukemia in adults, including French-American-British classifications M1 through M7, with other approved antileukemic drugs***
*Adults:* 12 mg/m$^2$ daily by slow I.V. injection (over 10 to 15 minutes) for 3 days. Give with cytarabine 100 mg/m$^2$ daily by continuous infusion for 7 days, or give cytarabine as a 25-mg/m$^2$ bolus followed by 200 mg/m$^2$ daily by continuous I.V. infusion for 5 days. A second course may be given if needed.
≣ *Dosage adjustment.* If patient experiences severe mucositis, delay administration until recovery is complete and reduce dosage by 25%. Also, reduce dosage in patients with hepatic or renal impairment. Idarubicin shouldn't be given if bilirubin level is greater than 5 mg/dl.
Dosage and indications may vary. Check current literature for recommended protocol.

### I.V. administration
■ Follow usual chemotherapy mixing precautions. Vial is under negative pressure.
■ Reconstituted solutions are stable for 3 days (72 hours) at controlled room temperature (59°

to 86° F [15° to 30° C]); 7 days, if refrigerated. Discard unused solutions appropriately.
■ If extravasation or signs of extravasation occur, recommend stopping the infusion immediately and restarting in another vein. Recommend treating the site with intermittent ice packs for 30 minutes q.i.d. for 4 days.

### Incompatibilities
Don't mix with other drugs unless specific compatibility data are available. Precipitation occurs with heparin. Drug will degrade with prolonged contact with alkaline solutions.
Incompatible with acyclovir sodium, allopurinol, ampicillin sodium, cefazolin, cefepime, ceftazidime, clindamycin phosphate, dexamethasone sodium phosphate, etoposide, furosemide, gentamicin, hydrocortisone sodium succinate, lorazepam, meperidine, methotrexate sodium, mezlocillin, piperacillin sodium, sodium carbonate, sulbactam, tazobactam, vancomycin, and vincristine.

### Mechanism of action
*Antineoplastic action:* Idarubicin inhibits nucleic acid synthesis by intercalation and interacts with the enzyme topoisomerase II. It's highly lipophilic, which results in an increased rate of cellular uptake.

### Pharmacokinetics
*Absorption:* Administered I.V.
*Distribution:* Highly lipophilic and excessively tissue-bound (97%), with highest levels in nucleated blood and bone marrow cells. Its metabolite, idarubicinol, is detected in CSF; clinical significance of this is under evaluation.
*Metabolism:* Extensive extrahepatic metabolism is indicated. Metabolite has cytotoxic activity.
*Excretion:* Excreted predominantly by biliary excretion as its metabolite and, to a lesser extent, by renal elimination. Mean terminal half-life is 22 hours (range, 4 to 46 hours) when used as a single drug and 20 hours (range, 7 to 38 hours) when combined with cytarabine. Plasma levels of metabolite are sustained for longer than 8 days.

| Route | Onset | Peak | Duration |
|-------|-------|------|----------|
| I.V. | Unknown | Unknown | Unknown |

### Contraindications and precautions
No known contraindications. Use cautiously in patients with impaired renal or hepatic function and in those with bone marrow suppression induced by previous drug therapy or radiation therapy.

### Interactions
None reported.

---

## Adverse reactions

**CNS:** *headache, changed mental status,* peripheral neuropathy, *seizures.*
**CV:** *HF,* atrial fibrillation, chest pain, *MI,* asymptomatic decline in left ventricular ejection fraction, *myocardial insufficiency, arrhythmias, hemorrhage, myocardial toxicity.*
**GI:** *nausea, vomiting, cramps, diarrhea, mucositis, severe enterocolitis with perforation.*
**GU:** decreased renal function.
**Hematologic:** *myelosuppression.*
**Hepatic:** changes in hepatic function.
**Metabolic:** hyperuricemia.
**Skin:** *alopecia, rash, urticaria, bullous erythrodermatous rash on palms and soles,* hives (at injection site), erythema (at previously irradiated sites), tissue necrosis at injection site (if extravasation occurs).
**Other:** INFECTION, *fever,* hypersensitivity reactions.

## Overdose and treatment

Severe and prolonged myelosuppression and possibly increased severity of GI toxicity are anticipated. Supportive treatment, including platelet transfusions, antibiotics, and treatment of mucositis, is required. Acute cardiac toxicity with severe arrhythmias and delayed cardiac failure may also occur. Peritoneal dialysis or hemodialysis isn't effective.

## Clinical considerations

■ Hyperuricemia may result from rapid lysis of leukemic cells; appropriate preventive measures should be taken (including adequate hydration) before treatment is started.
■ Systemic infections should be controlled before therapy begins.

### Therapeutic monitoring

■ Recommend frequently monitoring CBC and hepatic and renal function.

### Special populations

**Breast-feeding patients.** It's unknown if idarubicin appears in breast milk. To avoid risk of serious adverse reactions in the infant, breastfeeding should be discontinued before therapy with idarubicin is started.
**Pediatric patients.** Safety and efficacy in children haven't been established.

## Patient counseling

■ Instruct patient to recognize signs and symptoms of extravasation and to report them immediately if they occur.
■ Tell patient to report signs and symptoms of infection, including persistent fever or sore throat.
■ Advise patient to minimize dangerous behavior that can cause bleeding and to report bleeding or abnormal bruising.

■ Instruct patients to report adverse symptoms, especially nausea, vomiting, diahrrea, and mucositis.

# ifosfamide
Ifex

*Pharmacologic classification:* alkylating drug (cell cycle–phase nonspecific)
*Therapeutic classification:* antineoplastic
*Pregnancy risk category D*

## Available forms

Available by prescription only
*Injection:* 1-g, 3-g vials

## Indications and dosages

**Germ cell testicular cancer**
*Adults:* 1.2 g/m²/day I.V. for 5 days with other chemotherapy drugs. Regimen is usually repeated q 3 weeks. Drug may be given by slow I.V. push, by intermittent infusion over at least 30 minutes, or by continuous infusion. Dosage and indications may vary. Check current literature for recommended protocol.
◊*lung cancer,* ◊*Hodgkin's and* ◊*malignant lymphoma,* ◊*breast cancer,* ◊*acute lymphocytic leukemia,* ◊*ovarian cancer,* ◊*gastric cancer,* ◊*pancreatic cancer,* ◊*sarcomas,* ◊*cervical cancer,* ◊ *uterine cancer*
*Adults:* 1.2 to 2.5 g/m²/day I.V. for 3 to 5 days, with cycles of therapy repeated p.r.n.

## I.V. administration

■ Drug can be further diluted with D₅W or normal saline solution for I.V. infusion. This solution is stable for 7 days at room temperature and 6 weeks at 41° F (5° C).
■ Drug may be given by I.V. push injection in a minimum of 75 ml normal saline solution over 30 minutes.
■ Infusing each dose over 2 hours or longer decreases the possibility of cystitis.

### Incompatibilities

Incompatible with cefepime.

## Mechanism of action

*Antineoplastic action:* Ifosfamide requires activation by hepatic microsomal enzymes to exert its cytotoxic activity. The active compound cross-links strands of DNA and also breaks the DNA chain.

## Pharmacokinetics

*Absorption:* Administered I.V.
*Distribution:* Crosses the blood-brain barrier with its metabolites.
*Metabolism:* About 50% of dose is metabolized in the liver.

---

***Excretion:*** Excreted primarily in the urine. The terminal half-life is reported to be about 7 hours at doses of 1.6 to 2.4 g/m²/day and about 15 hours at a single dose of 3.8 to 5 g/m².

| Route | Onset | Peak | Duration |
|-------|-------|------|----------|
| I.V. | Unknown | Unknown | Unknown |

## Contraindications and precautions

Contraindicated in patients with severe bone marrow suppression or those hypersensitive to drug.

Use cautiously in patients with renal or hepatic impairment, compromised bone marrow reserve as indicated by granulocytopenia, bone marrow metastases, prior radiation therapy, or therapy with cytotoxic drugs. Contraindicated in pregnancy because of possible embryotoxic and teratogenic effects on the fetus.

## Interactions

**Drug-drug.** *Chloral hydrate, phenobarbital, phenytoin:* May increase the activity of ifosfamide by induction of hepatic microsomal enzymes, increasing the conversion of ifosfamide to its active form. Advise prescriber to be alert for possible combined drug actions, desirable or undesirable, involving ifosfamide, even though it has been used successfully together with other drugs, including other cytotoxic drugs.

## Adverse reactions

**CNS:** *somnolence, confusion,* **coma, seizures,** ataxia, hallucinations, depressive psychosis, dizziness, disorientation, cranial nerve dysfunction.
**GI:** *nausea, vomiting.*
**GU:** *hemorrhagic cystitis, hematuria,* **nephrotoxicity.**
**Hematologic:** *leukopenia, thrombocytopenia, myelosuppression.*
**Hepatic:** elevated liver enzyme levels, liver dysfunction.
**Metabolic:** *metabolic acidosis.*
**Skin:** *alopecia,* phlebitis.
**Other:** infection.

## Overdose and treatment

Signs and symptoms of overdose include myelosuppression, nausea, vomiting, alopecia, and hemorrhagic cystitis.

Treatment is usually supportive and includes transfusion of blood components, antiemetics, and bladder irrigation.

## Clinical considerations

■ Follow all established procedures for the safe handling, administration, and disposal of chemotherapeutic drugs.
■ Recommend pushing fluids (3 L daily) and giving with mesna (Mesnex) to prevent hemorrhagic cystitis. Advise prescriber to avoid giving drug at bedtime, because infrequent voiding during the night may increase the pos-sibility of cystitis. Bladder irrigation with normal saline solution may decrease the possibility of cystitis.

### Therapeutic monitoring

■ Recommend assessing patient for changes in mental status and cerebellar dysfunction. Dosage may have to be decreased.
■ Advise clinician to monitor CBC and renal and liver function test results.
■ Sterile phlebitis may occur at the injection site; warm compresses should be applied.

### Special populations

**Pregnant patients.** If the patient becomes pregnant while taking drug, she should be informed of the potential hazard to the fetus.
**Breast-feeding patients.** Drug appears in breast milk. Because of the potential for serious adverse reactions, mutagenicity, and carcinogenicity in the infant, breast-feeding isn't recommended.
**Pediatric patients.** Safety and efficacy in children haven't been established.

## Patient counseling

■ Tell patient to ensure adequate fluid intake to prevent bladder toxicity and to facilitate excretion of uric acid.
■ Warn patient to avoid exposure to infection and to report signs of infection or unusual bleeding immediately.
■ Reassure patient that hair should grow back after treatment has ended.
■ Tell patient to contact prescriber immediately if blood appears in the urine.
■ Advise both men and women to use contraceptive measures during therapy.

# imatinib mesylate

Gleevec

*Pharmacologic classification:* protein-tyrosine kinase inhibitor
*Therapeutic classification:* antineoplastic
*Pregnancy risk category D*

## Available forms

*Capsules:* 100 mg

## Indications and dosages

***Chronic myeloid leukemia (CML) in blast crisis, in accelerated phase, or in chronic phase after failure of interferon-alpha therapy***
*Adults: Chronic-phase CML:* 400 mg P.O. daily as single dose with a meal and large glass of water. *Accelerated-phase CML or blast crisis:* 600 mg P.O. daily as single dose with a meal and large glass of water. Continue treatment as long as patient continues to benefit. May increase daily dose to 600 mg P.O. in

## DOSAGE ADJUSTMENTS FOR NEUTROPENIA AND THROMBOCYTOPENIA

| Type of chronic myeloid leukemia (CML) | Laboratory values | Treatment guidelines |
|---|---|---|
| Chronic-phase CML or gastrointestinal stromal tumor (GIST) (starting dose 400 mg) | Absolute neutrophil count (ANC) < 1 × 10⁹/L or platelets < 50 × 10⁹/L | 1. Stop Gleevec until ANC ≥ 1.5 × 10⁹/L and platelets ≥ 75 × 10⁹/L.<br>2. Resume treatment at 400 mg.<br>3. If recurrence of ANC < 1 × 10⁹/L, or platelets < 50 × 10⁹/L, repeat step 1 and resume Gleevec at reduced dose of 300 mg. |
| Accelerated phase CML and blast crisis or GIST (starting dose 600 mg) | ANC < 0.5 × 10⁹/L occurring after at least 1 month of treatment or platelets < 10 × 10⁹/L | 1. Check if cytopenia is related to leukemia via marrow aspirate or biopsy.<br>2. If cytopenia is unrelated to leukemia, reduce dose of Gleevec to 400 mg.<br>3. If cytopenia persists 2 weeks, reduce further to 300 mg.<br>4. If cytopenia persists 4 weeks and is still unrelated to leukemia, stop Gleevec until ANC ≥ 1 × 10⁹/L and platelets ≥ 20 × 10⁹/L and then resume treatment at 300 mg. |

chronic phase or to 800 mg P.O. (400 mg P.O. b.i.d.) in accelerated phase or blast crisis.

Consider dosage increases only if there is an absence of severe adverse reactions and absence of severe non–leukemia-related neutropenia or thrombocytopenia in the following circumstances: disease progression (at any time), failure to achieve a satisfactory hematologic response after at least 3 months of treatment, or loss of a previously achieved hematologic response.

***Treatment of patients with Kit (CD117)-positive unresectable or metastatic malignant gastrointestinal stromal tumors (GIST)***

*Adults:* 400 or 600 mg P.O. daily.

≡ *Dosage adjustment.* For severe nonhematologic adverse reactions (severe hepatotoxicity or severe fluid retention), withhold drug until event has resolved; resume treatment as appropriate based on initial severity of event. For elevations in bilirubin level more than three times the institutional upper limit of normal (IULN), or liver transaminase levels more than five times IULN, withhold drug until bilirubin level returns to less than 1.5 IULN and transaminase levels to less than 2.5 IULN. May then resume drug at reduced daily dose (400 mg to 300 mg or 600 mg to 400 mg).

For dosage adjustments for neutropenia and thrombocytopenia, see the table above.

## Mechanism of action

*Antineoplastic action:* Drug inhibits Bcr-Abl tyrosine kinase, which is the abnormal tyrosine kinase created by the Philadelphia chromosome abnormality in CML; in vivo, it inhibits tumor growth of Bcr-Abl–transfected murine myeloid cells as well as Bcr-Abl–positive leukemia lines derived from CML patients in blast crisis.

## Pharmacokinetics

Inhibits proliferation and induces apoptosis in Bcr-Abl–positive cell lines as well as fresh leukemic cells from Philadelphia chromosome–positive CML.

*Absorption:* Well absorbed orally.

*Distribution:* 98% protein-bound.

*Metabolism:* Metabolized via cytochrome P-450 system, primarily CYP 3A4.

*Excretion:* Excreted primarily in feces as metabolites.

| Route | Onset | Peak | Duration |
|---|---|---|---|
| P.O. | Unknown | 2-4 hr | Unknown |

## Contraindications and precautions

Contraindicated in patients hypersensitive to drug or its components.

Use cautiously in patients with hepatic impairment.

## Interactions

**Drug-drug.** *CYP 3A4 inhibitors (clarithromycin, erythromycin, itraconazole, ketoconazole):* Decreased metabolism and increased imatinib levels. Advise clinician to monitor patient for toxicity.

*CYP 3A4 inducers (carbamazepine, dexamethasone, phenobarbital, phenytoin, rifampin):* Increased metabolism and decreased imatinib levels. Use cautiously.

*Dihydropyridine–calcium channel blockers, certain HMG-CoA reductase inhibitors, cyclosporine, pimozide, triazolo-benzodiazepines:* Increased levels of these drugs. Advise clinician to monitor patient for toxicity and obtaining drug levels, if appropriate.

*Warfarin:* Altered metabolism of warfarin. Avoid use together; use standard heparin or a low-molecular-weight heparin.

---

* Canada only    ◇ Unlabeled clinical use

**Drug-herb.** *St. John's wort:* May decrease imatinib effects. Warn patient not to use together.

## Adverse reactions
**CNS:** *headache,* CEREBRAL HEMORRHAGE, *fatigue, weakness.*
**CV:** *edema.*
**EENT:** nasopharyngitis, *epistaxis.*
**GI:** *anorexia, nausea, diarrhea, abdominal pain, constipation, vomiting, dyspepsia,* GI HE-MORRHAGE.
**GU:** Increased creatinine.
**Hematologic:** HEMORRHAGE, NEUTROPENIA, THROMBOCYTOPENIA, *anemia.*
**Hepatic:** increased bilirubin, alkaline phosphatase, AST, and ALT levels.
**Metabolic:** *hypokalemia,* weight increase.
**Musculoskeletal:** *myalgia, muscle cramps, musculoskeletal pain, arthralgia.*
**Respiratory:** *cough, dyspnea, pneumonia.*
**Skin:** *rash,* pruritus, *petechiae.*
**Other:** *pyrexia, night sweats.*

## Overdose and treatment
Experience with doses greater than 800 mg is limited.
    Advise clinician to observe patient and give supportive treatment, p.r.n.

## Clinical considerations
■ Because GI irritation is common, patients should take drug with food.

### *Therapeutic monitoring*
■ Advise clinician to monitor CBC weekly for first month, then decrease to biweekly for second month, and periodically thereafter.
■ Advise clinician to monitor patient's weight daily and to evaluate and treat unexpected rapid weight gain.
■ Advise clinician to monitor patients closely for fluid retention, which can be severe.
■ Advise clinician to monitor liver function test results carefully because hepatotoxicity (occasionally severe) may occur, and to decrease dosage p.r.n.
■ Although there are no data on long-term safety of this drug, advise clinician to monitor renal and liver toxicity and immunosuppression carefully.

### *Special populations*
**Breast-feeding patients.** It's unknown if drug appears in breast milk. Because of possible adverse reactions, women shouldn't breast-feed while taking this drug.
**Pediatric patients.** Safety and efficacy in children haven't been established.
**Geriatric patients.** Geriatric patients may have an increased risk of edema when taking this drug. Advise clinician to monitor patient's fluid status.

## Patient counseling
■ Tell patient to take drug with food and a large glass of water.
■ Advise patient to report adverse effects such as fluid retention to prescriber.
■ Advise patient to obtain periodic liver and kidney function tests and blood work to determine blood counts.

# imipenem and cilastatin sodium
Primaxin I.M., Primaxin I.V.

*Pharmacologic classification:* carbapenem (thienamycin class), beta-lactam antibiotic
*Therapeutic classification:* antibiotic
*Pregnancy risk category C*

## Available forms
Available by prescription only
*Powder (for I.M. injection):* 500-mg, 750-mg vial
*Injection:* 250-mg, 500-mg vials, ADD-Vantage, and infusion bottles

## Indications and dosages
*Mild to moderate lower respiratory tract, skin and skin-structure, or gynecologic infection*
*Adults weighing at least 70 kg (154 lb):* 500 to 750 mg I.M. q 12 hours.
*Mild to moderate intra-abdominal infections*
*Adults weighing at least 70 kg:* 750 mg I.M. q 12 hours.
*Serious respiratory and urinary tract infections; intra-abdominal, gynecologic, bone, joint, or skin infections; bacterial septicemia; endocarditis*
*Adults weighing at least 70 kg:* 250 mg to 1 g by I.V. infusion q 6 to 8 hours. Maximum daily dose is 50 mg/kg/day or 4 g/day, whichever is less.
*Children:* 15 to 25 mg/kg q 6 hours.
≡*Dosage adjustment.* In patients with renal failure and creatinine clearance of 6 to 20 ml/minute/1.73 m², 125 to 250 mg I.V. q 12 hours for most pathogens. There may be an increased risk of seizures when doses of 500 mg q 12 hours are given to these patients. When creatinine clearance is 5 ml/minute/1.73 m² or less, imipenem shouldn't be given unless hemodialysis is instituted within 48 hours.
    Note: In patients weighing less than 70 kg or those with impaired renal function, dosages vary. Check current literature for recommended protocol.

## I.V. administration
■ Drug isn't to be given by direct I.V. bolus injection.

■ Infuse 250- or 500-mg dose over 20 to 30 minutes; infuse 1-g dose over 40 to 60 minutes.
■ If nausea occurs, recommend slowing infusion.

### Incompatibilities
Drug shouldn't be mixed with other antibiotics. Incompatible with $D_5W$ in lactated Ringer's injection. Manufacturer doesn't recommend mixing drug in same solution or tubing as other drugs.

Drug may be physically incompatible with aminoglycosides; don't mix together.

## Mechanism of action
*Antibacterial action:* A bactericidal drug, imipenem inhibits bacterial cell wall synthesis. Its spectrum of antimicrobial activity includes many gram-positive, gram-negative, and anaerobic bacteria, including *Staphylococcus* and *Streptococcus* species, *Escherichia coli, Klebsiella, Proteus, Enterobacter* species, *Pseudomonas aeruginosa,* and *Bacteroides* species, including *B. fragilis.* Resistant bacteria include methicillin-resistant staphylococci, *Clostridium difficile,* and other *Pseudomonas* species.

Cilastatin inhibits the enzymatic breakdown of imipenem in the kidneys, making it effective in treating urinary tract infections.

## Pharmacokinetics
*Absorption:* After I.M. administration, imipenem blood levels peak within 2 hours; cilastatin levels reach their peak within 1 hour. After I.V. administration, peak levels of both drugs appear in about 20 minutes. Imipenem is about 75% bioavailable and cilastatin is about 95% bioavailable after I.M. administration compared with I.V. administration.
*Distribution:* Distributed rapidly and widely. About 20% of imipenem is protein-bound; 40% of cilastatin is protein-bound.
*Metabolism:* Imipenem is metabolized by kidney dehydropeptidase I, resulting in low urine levels. Cilastatin inhibits this enzyme, thereby reducing metabolism of imipenem.
*Excretion:* About 70% of imipenem and cilastatin dose is excreted unchanged by the kidneys (when imipenem is combined with cilastatin) through tubular secretion and glomerular filtration. Imipenem is cleared by hemodialysis; therefore, a supplemental dose is required after this procedure. Half-life of drug is about 1 hour after I.V. administration. The prolonged absorption that occurs after I.M. administration results in a longer half-life (2 to 3 hours).

| Route | Onset | Peak | Duration |
|-------|-------|------|----------|
| I.M. | Unknown | 1-2 hr | Unknown |
| I.V. | Unknown | Unknown | Unknown |

## Contraindications and precautions
Contraindicated in patients hypersensitive to drug. Imipenem and cilastatin sodium reconstituted with lidocaine hydrochloride for I.M. injection is contraindicated in patients hypersensitive to local anesthetics of the amide type and in patients with severe shock or heart block.

Drug should be cautiously in patients with impaired renal function, seizure disorders, or allergy to penicillins or cephalosporins.

## Interactions
**Drug-drug.** *Chloramphenicol:* May impede the bactericidal effects of imipenem. Recommend giving chloramphenicol a few hours after imipenem and cilastatin.
*Ganciclovir:* Generalized seizures have occurred in several patients during combined imipenem and cilastatin and ganciclovir therapy. Advise clinician to monitor patient closely.
*Probenecid:* May prevent tubular secretion of cilastatin (but not imipenem) and prolong plasma cilastatin half-life.

## Adverse reactions
**CNS:** *seizures,* dizziness, somnolence.
**CV:** hypotension.
**GI:** nausea, vomiting, diarrhea, *pseudomembranous colitis.*
**Hematologic:** *agranulocytosis,* thrombocytosis.
**Hepatic:** transient increases in liver enzyme levels.
**Skin:** rash, urticaria, pruritus, pain at injection site.
**Other:** hypersensitivity reactions *(anaphylaxis),* thrombophlebitis, fever.

## Overdose and treatment
If overdose occurs, recommend stopping drug, treating symptomatically, and instituting supportive measures p.r.n. Although imipenem and cilastatin sodium are hemodialyzable, use of hemodialysis in treating drug overdose is questionable.

## Clinical considerations
■ Culture and sensitivity tests should be performed before therapy starts.
■ Drug has broadest antibacterial spectrum of any available antibiotic. It's most valuable for empiric treatment of unidentified infections and for mixed infections that would otherwise require combination of antibiotics, possibly including an aminoglycoside.

### Therapeutic monitoring
■ Recommend continuing use of anticonvulsants in patients with known seizure disorders. Patients who exhibit CNS toxicity should receive phenytoin or benzodiazepines. Recommend reducing dosage or stopping drug if CNS toxicity continues.
■ Prolonged use may result in overgrowth of nonsusceptible organisms. In addition, use of

imipenem and cilastatin as a sole course of therapy has resulted in resistance during therapy.

### Special populations
**Breast-feeding patients.** It's unknown if drug appears in breast milk. Give cautiously to breast-feeding women.
**Pediatric patients.** Safety and efficacy in children under age 12 haven't been established; however, drug has been used in children ages 3 months to 13 years. Dosage range is 15 to 25 mg/kg every 6 hours.
**Geriatric patients.** Give cautiously to geriatric patients because they may also have renal dysfunction.

### Patient counseling
■ Advise patient of potential adverse reactions.
■ Instruct patient to report to prescriber immediately any serious adverse drug events.

---

# imipramine hydrochloride
Apo-Imipramine*, Impril*, Novopramine*, Tofranil

# imipramine pamoate
Tofranil-PM

*Pharmacologic classification:* dibenzazepine tricyclic antidepressant
*Therapeutic classification:* antidepressant
*Pregnancy risk category B*

### Available forms
Available by prescription only
**imipramine hydrochloride**
*Tablets:* 10 mg, 25 mg, 50 mg
**imipramine pamoate**
*Capsules:* 75 mg, 100 mg, 125 mg, 150 mg

### Indications and dosages
*Depression*
*Adults:* Initially, 75 to 100 mg P.O. daily in divided doses, with 25- to 50-mg increments, up to 200 mg. Alternatively, some patients can start with lower doses (25 mg P.O.) and dosage is adjusted slowly in 25-mg increments every other day. Maximum dose, 300 mg daily. Alternatively, entire dosage may be given h.s. Maximum dose is 200 mg/day for outpatients, 300 mg/day for inpatients, 100 mg/day for geriatric patients.
◊ *Childhood enuresis*
*Children ages 6 and older:* 25 to 75 mg P.O. daily, 1 hour before bedtime. Usual dose 1.5 mg/kg/day in three divided doses. Maximum dose, 5 mg/kg/day.

### Mechanism of action
*Antidepressant action:* Imipramine is thought to exert its antidepressant effects by inhibiting reuptake of norepinephrine and serotonin in CNS nerve terminals (presynaptic neurons), which results in increased levels and enhanced activity of these neurotransmitters in the synaptic cleft. Drug also has anticholinergic activity and is used to treat nocturnal enuresis in children over age 6.

### Pharmacokinetics
*Absorption:* Absorbed rapidly from GI tract and muscle tissue after oral and I.M. administration.
*Distribution:* Distributed widely into the body, including the CNS; drug appears in breast milk. Drug is 90% protein-bound. Steady state is achieved within 2 to 5 days. Therapeutic plasma levels (parent drug and metabolite) are thought to range from 150 to 300 ng/ml.
*Metabolism:* Metabolized by the liver to the active metabolite desipramine. A significant first-pass effect may explain variability of serum levels in different patients taking the same dosage.
*Excretion:* Mostly excreted in urine.

| Route | Onset | Peak | Duration |
|-------|-------|------|----------|
| P.O. | Unknown | ½-2 hr | Unknown |

### Contraindications and precautions
Contraindicated during acute recovery phase of MI, in patients hypersensitive to drug, and in those receiving MAO inhibitors.

Use with caution in patients at risk for suicide; in those with impaired renal or hepatic function, history of urine retention, angle-closure glaucoma, increased intraocular pressure, CV disease, or hyperthyroidism; and in patients receiving thyroid hormones.

### Interactions
**Drug-drug.** *Barbiturates:* Induce imipramine metabolism and decrease therapeutic efficacy. Avoid use together.
*Beta blockers, cimetidine, methylphenidate, oral contraceptives, propoxyphene:* Inhibit imipramine metabolism, increasing plasma levels and toxicity. Use together cautiously.
*Centrally acting antihypertensives, such as clonidine, guanabenz, guanadrel, guanethidine, methyldopa, and reserpine:* Decreased hypotensive effects of antihypertensives. Use cautiously.
*CNS depressants, including analgesics, barbiturates, narcotics, tranquilizers, and anesthetics (oversedation); atropine or other anticholinergics, including antihistamines, antiparkinsonians, meperidine, and phenothiazines:* Oversedation, paralytic ileus, visual changes, and severe constipation. Avoid use together.
*Disulfiram or ethchlorvynol:* May cause delirium and tachycardia. Recommend observing patient closely.
*Haloperidol and phenothiazines:* Decrease metabolism of imipramine, decreasing therapeu-

tic efficacy. Advise clinician to monitor patient closely.

*Metrizamide:* Increased risk of seizures. Advise clinician to monitor patient closely.

*Pimozide, thyroid hormones, and antiarrhythmics (disopyramide, procainamide, quinidine):* May increase risk of arrhythmias and conduction defects. Avoid use together.

*Sympathomimetics, including ephedrine, epinephrine, and phenylephrine (often found in nasal sprays):* May increase blood pressure. Patient needs frequent blood pressure checks.

*Warfarin:* May prolong PT and cause bleeding. Advise clinician to monitor PT and INR.

**Drug-herb.** *Evening primrose oil:* Possible additive or synergistic effect resulting in lower seizure threshold, increasing the risk of seizure. Discourage use together.

*St. John's wort, SAMe, yohimbe:* Use with some tricyclic antidepressants may cause elevation of serotonin levels. Discourage use together.

**Drug-lifestyle.** *Alcohol use:* Additive CNS depressive effects. Advise patient to avoid alcohol use.

*Heavy smoking:* Induces imipramine metabolism and decreases therapeutic efficacy. Advise clinician to monitor patient for therapeutic effect.

## Adverse reactions
**CNS:** *CVA, drowsiness, dizziness,* excitation, tremor, confusion, hallucinations, anxiety, ataxia, paresthesia, nervousness, EEG changes, *seizures,* extrapyramidal reactions.
**CV:** *orthostatic hypotension, tachycardia, ECG changes,* hypertension, *MI, arrhythmias, heart block,* precipitation of HF.
**EENT:** blurred vision, tinnitus, mydriasis.
**GI:** *dry mouth, constipation,* nausea, vomiting, anorexia, paralytic ileus, abdominal cramps.
**GU:** *urine retention,* testicular swelling, impotence.
**Metabolic:** increased or decreased serum glucose levels, inappropriate antidiuretic hormone secretion syndrome.
**Skin:** rash, urticaria, photosensitivity, pruritus, *diaphoresis.*
**Other:** galactorrhea and breast enlargement (in females), altered libido, hypersensitivity reaction, gynecomastia (in males).
**After abrupt withdrawal of long-term therapy:** nausea, headache, malaise (does not indicate addiction).

## Overdose and treatment
Drug overdose is frequently life-threatening, particularly when combined with alcohol. The first 12 hours after acute ingestion is a stimulatory phase characterized by excessive anticholinergic activity, including agitation, irritation, confusion, hallucinations, hyperthermia, parkinsonian symptoms, seizure, urine retention, dry mucous membranes, pupillary dilatation, constipation, and ileus. This is followed

by CNS depressant effects, including hypothermia, decreased or absent reflexes, sedation, hypotension, cyanosis, and cardiac irregularities, including tachycardia, conduction disturbances, and quinidine-like effects on the ECG.

Severity of overdose is best indicated by widening of the QRS complex, which usually represents a serum level in excess of 1,000 ng/ml; serum levels are usually not helpful. Metabolic acidosis may follow hypotension, hypoventilation, and seizures.

Treatment is symptomatic and supportive, including maintaining airway, stable body temperature, and fluid or electrolyte balance. Recommend inducing emesis if patient is conscious; follow with gastric lavage and activated charcoal to prevent further absorption. Dialysis is of little use.

Recommend treating seizures with parenteral diazepam or phenytoin and arrhythmias with parenteral phenytoin or lidocaine. Quinidine, procainamide, and atropine aren't to be used during an overdose. Recommend treating acidosis with sodium bicarbonate. Advise prescriber not to give barbiturates; these may enhance CNS and respiratory depressant effects.

## Clinical considerations
■ Drug causes a high risk of orthostatic hypotension.
■ Recommend stopping drug at least 48 hours before surgical procedures.
■ Drug shouldn't be withdrawn abruptly, but tapered gradually over time.

### Therapeutic monitoring
■ Advise clinician to monitor sitting and standing blood pressures after initial dose.
■ Tolerance to sedative effects of drug usually develops over several weeks.

### Special populations
**Breast-feeding patients.** Drug appears in breast milk in low levels. The potential benefit to the woman should outweigh possible risks to the infant.
**Pediatric patients.** Drug isn't recommended for treating depression in patients under age 12. Pamoate salt shouldn't be used for enuresis in children.
**Geriatric patients.** Recommended dose is 30 to 40 mg P.O. daily, not to exceed 100 mg daily. Therapy should be started at low doses (10 mg) and adjusted slowly. Geriatric patients may be at greater risk for adverse cardiac reactions.

## Patient counseling
■ Tell patient to take drug exactly as prescribed.
■ Explain that full effects of drug may not become apparent for up to 4 to 6 weeks after initiation of therapy.
■ Warn patient not to discontinue drug abruptly, not to share drug with others, and not to drink alcoholic beverages while taking drug.

- Advise patient to take drug with food or milk if it causes stomach upset.
- Suggest relieving dry mouth with sugarless chewing gum or hard candy. Encourage good dental prophylaxis because persistent dry mouth may lead to increased risk of dental caries.
- Encourage patient to report unusual or troublesome effects immediately, including confusion, movement disorders, rapid heartbeat, dizziness, fainting, or difficulty urinating.

# immune globulin (gamma globulin [IG] immune serum globulin [ISG])

## immune globulin for I.M. use (IGIM)
BayGam, Gammar

## immune globulin for I.V. use (IGIV)
Gamimune N (5%, 10%), Gammagard S/D, Gammar-P IV, Iveegam, Panglobulin, Polygam S/D, Sandoglobulin, Venoglobulin-I, Venoglobulin-S

*Pharmacologic classification:* immune serum
*Therapeutic classification:* antibody production stimulator
*Pregnancy risk category C*

## Available forms
Available by prescription only
**IGIM**
*Injection:* 2-ml, 10-ml vials
**IGIV**
*I.V.:* Gamimune N—5% and 10% solution in 10-ml, 50-ml, 100-ml, and 250-ml single-use vials; Gammagard S/D—2.5-g, 5-g, and 10-g single-use vials for reconstitution; Gammar-P IV—1-g, 2.5-g, and 5-g vials with diluent and 10-g vials with administration set and diluent; Iveegam—1-g, 2.5-g, and 5-g vials with diluent; Polygam S/D—2.5-g, 5-g, and 10-g single-use vials with diluent; Sandoglobulin—1-g, 3-g, 6-g, and 12-g vials or kits with diluent or bulk packs without diluent; Venoglobulin-I—2.5-g and 5-g vials with or without reconstitution kits with sterile water, 10-g vials with reconstitution kit and administration set, and 0.5-g vials with reconstitution kit; Venoglobulin-S—5% and 10% in 50-ml, 100-ml, and 200-ml vials.

## Indications and dosages
*Agammaglobulinemia, hypogammaglobulinemia, immune deficiency (IGIV)*
*Adults and children:* For Gamimune N only, 100 to 200 mg/kg or 2 to 4 ml/kg I.V. infusion

monthly. Infusion rate is 0.01 to 0.02 ml/kg/minute for 30 minutes. Rate can then be increased to maximum of 0.08 ml/kg/minute for remainder of infusion.
For Gammagard S/D only, initially 200 to 400 mg/kg I.V., followed by 100 mg/kg monthly. Initiate infusion at 0.5 ml/kg/hour, gradually increasing to maximum of 4 ml/kg/hour.
For Gammar-P IV only, 200 to 400 mg/kg q 3 to 4 weeks. Infusion rate is 0.01 ml/kg/minute, increasing to 0.02 ml/kg/minute after 15 to 30 minutes, with gradual increase to 0.06 ml/kg/minute.
For Iveegam only, 200 mg/kg I.V. monthly. If response is inadequate, doses may be increased up to 800 mg/kg or the drug may be given more frequently. Infuse at 1 to 2 ml/minute.
For Polygam S/D only, 100 mg/kg I.V. monthly. An initial dose of 200 to 400 mg/kg may be given. Initiate infusion at 0.5 ml/kg/hour, gradually increasing to maximum of 4 ml/kg/hour.
For Sandoglobulin and Panglobulin, 200 mg/kg I.V. monthly. Start with 0.5 to 1 ml/minute of a 3% solution; increase up to 2.5 ml/minute gradually after 15 to 30 minutes.
For Venoglobulin-I only, 200 mg/kg I.V. monthly; may be increased to 300 to 400 mg/kg and may be repeated more frequently than once monthly. Infuse at 0.01 to 0.02 ml/kg/minute for 30 minutes, then increase to 0.04 ml/kg/minute or higher, if tolerated.
For Venoglobulin-S only, 200 mg/kg I.V. monthly. Increase dose to 300 to 400 mg/kg monthly or give more frequently if adequate IgI levels aren't achieved. Initiate infusion at 0.01 to 0.02 ml/kg/minute for 30 minutes, then increase 5% solutions to 0.04 ml/kg/minute and 10% solutions to 0.05 ml/kg/minute, if tolerated.
*Hepatitis A exposure (IGIM)*
*Adults and children:* 0.02 to 0.04 ml/kg I.M. as soon as possible after exposure. Up to 0.1 ml/kg may be given after prolonged or intense exposure.
*Measles exposure (IGIM)*
*Adults and children:* 0.2 to 0.25 ml/kg within 6 days after exposure.
*Postexposure prophylaxis of measles (IGIM) for immunosuppressed patients*
*Adults and children:* 0.5 ml/kg I.M. within 6 days after exposure.
*Chickenpox exposure (IGIM)*
*Adults and children:* 0.6 to 1.2 ml/kg I.M. as soon as exposed.
*Rubella exposure in first trimester of pregnancy (IGIM)*
*Women:* 0.55 ml/kg I.M. as soon as exposed.
*Idiopathic thrombocytopenic purpura (IGIV)*
*Adults and children:* Initially, 400 mg/kg daily of Sandoglobulin, Panglobulin, or Gamimune N (5% or 10%) I.V. for 2 to 5 consecutive days

depending on platelet count and clinical response. Maintenance dose is 400 to 1,000 mg/kg I.V. of Gamimune N 5%, 10%, or Sandoglobulin as a single infusion to maintain a platelet count greater than 30,000/mm³.

*Bone marrow transplantation (IGIV)*
*Adults over age 20:* Gamimune N 10%, 500 mg/kg on day 7 and day 2 before transplantation; then weekly through 90 days after transplantation.

## I.V. administration
■ Reconstitute Gammagard S/D with diluent (sterile water for injection) and transfer device provided by manufacturer. Administration set (provided) contains a 15-micron in-line filter that must be used during administration.
■ Reconstitute Sandoglobulin with diluent supplied (normal saline solution).
■ Gamimune N can be diluted with D₅W.
■ Store Sandoglobulin and Gammagard S/D at room temperature not exceeding 77° F (25° C); Gamimune-N and Iveegam, at 36° to 46° F (2° to 8° C) but don't freeze; Gammar-P IV, at room temperature below 86° F (30° C) but don't freeze; Venoglobulin-I at room temperature below 86° F (30° C).

### Incompatibilities
Don't mix with other drugs or fluids. Give in separate infusion line.

## Mechanism of action
*Immune action:* Immune globulin provides passive immunity by increasing antibody titer. The mechanism by which IGIV increases platelet counts in idiopathic thrombocytopenic purpura isn't fully known.

## Pharmacokinetics
*Absorption:* Slow I.M. absorption.
*Distribution:* Distributes evenly between intravascular and extravascular spaces.
*Metabolism:* Unknown.
*Excretion:* Serum half-life is reportedly 21 to 24 days in immunocompetent patients.

| Route | Onset | Peak | Duration |
|---|---|---|---|
| I.V. | Immediate | Immediate | Unknown |
| I.M. | Unknown | 2-5 hr | Unknown |

## Contraindications and precautions
Contraindicated in patients hypersensitive to drug.

## Interactions
**Drug-drug.** *Live-virus vaccines:* Immune globulin may interfere with the immune response to live-virus vaccines (such as measles, mumps, rubella). Live-virus vaccines must not be given within 3 months after administration of immune globulin.

## Adverse reactions
**CNS:** faintness, headache, malaise, aseptic meningitis syndrome.
**CV:** chest pain, chest tightness.
**GI:** nausea, vomiting.
**GU:** increased serum creatinine and BUN, oliguria, anuria, acute renal failure, acute tubular necrosis, proximal tubular nephropathy, osmotic nephrosis.
**Musculoskeletal:** hip pain, joint pain, muscle stiffness (at injection site).
**Respiratory:** dyspnea, shortness of breath.
**Skin:** erythema, urticaria.
**Other:** fever, *anaphylaxis,* chills, infusion reactions.

## Overdose and treatment
Excessively rapid I.V. infusion rate can precipitate an anaphylactoid reaction.

## Clinical considerations
■ Recommend obtaining a thorough history of allergies and reactions to immunizations.
■ Epinephrine solution 1:1,000 should be available to treat allergic reactions.
■ Advise prescriber to inject I.M. formulation into different sites, preferably into buttocks. It isn't advisable to inject more than 3 ml per injection site.
■ Shouldn't be given for hepatitis A exposure if 2 weeks or more have elapsed since exposure or after onset of clinical illness.
■ Although pregnancy isn't a contraindication to use, it's unknown if immune globulin can cause fetal harm.
■ Immune globulin has been studied in the treatment of various conditions, including Kawasaki disease, asthma, allergic disorders, autoimmune neutropenia, myasthenia gravis, and platelet transfusion rejection. It also has been used in the prophylaxis of infection in immunocompromised patients.

### Therapeutic monitoring
■ Advise clinician to closely monitor blood pressure in patient receiving IGIV, especially if it's patient's first infusion of immune globulin.

### Special populations
**Breast-feeding patients.** It's unknown if immune globulin appears in breast milk. Use with caution in breast-feeding women.

## Patient counseling
■ Explain that the patient's chances of getting AIDS or hepatitis after receiving immune globulin are minute because of stringent government standards that require testing for these viruses.
■ Instruct patient to promptly report headache, skin changes, or difficulty breathing; decreased urine output; sudden weight gain; swelling; and shortness of breath.

# inamrinone lactate

Inocor

*Pharmacologic classification:* bipyridine derivative
*Therapeutic classification:* inotropic, vasodilator
*Pregnancy risk category C*

## Available forms

Available by prescription only
*Injection:* 5 mg/ml

## Indications and dosages

***Short-term management of heart failure***
*Adults:* Initially, 0.75 mg/kg I.V. bolus over 2 to 3 minutes; then begin maintenance infusion of 5 to 10 mcg/kg/minute. Additional bolus of 0.75 mg/kg may be given 30 minutes after therapy is initiated. Maximum daily dose is 10 mg/kg.
***Cardiac life support in patients for whom other preferred drugs cannot be used for pump failure and acute pulmonary edema***
*Adults:* 0.75 mg/kg I.V. bolus over 2 to 3 minutes, then 5 to 15 mcg/kg/minute.

## I.V. administration

■ Dispense drug as supplied or dilute in normal or half-normal saline solution to concentration of 1 to 3 mg/ml.
■ Don't administer furosemide in I.V. lines containing inamrinone because a chemical reaction occurs immediately.
■ Store at room temperature and protect from light.

### Incompatibilities

Don't dilute drug with solutions containing dextrose because a slow chemical reaction occurs over 24 hours. However, inamrinone can be injected into running dextrose infusions through a Y-connector or directly into tubing. Use diluted solution within 24 hours.

## Mechanism of action

*Inotropic action:* The mechanism of action responsible for the apparent inotropic effect isn't fully understood; however, it may be linked to inhibition of phosphodiesterase activity, resulting in increased cellular levels of adenosine 3',5'-cyclic phosphate; this, in turn, may alter intracellular and extracellular calcium levels. The role of calcium homeostasis hasn't been determined. Clinical effects include increased cardiac output mediated by reduced afterload and, possibly, inotropism.
*Vasodilating action:* The primary vasodilating effect of inamrinone seems to stem from a direct effect on peripheral vessels.

## Pharmacokinetics

*Absorption:* Administered I.V.

*Distribution:* Distribution volume is 1.2 L/kg. Distribution sites are unknown. Protein-binding ranges from 10% to 49%. Therapeutic steady state serum levels range from 0.5 to 7 mcg/ml (ideal level: 3 mcg/ml).
*Metabolism:* Metabolized in the liver to several metabolites of unknown activity.
*Excretion:* In normal patients, inamrinone is excreted in the urine, with a terminal elimination half-life of about 4 hours. Half-life may be prolonged slightly in patients with HF.

| Route | Onset | Peak | Duration |
|-------|-------|------|----------|
| I.V. | 2-5 min | 10 min | ½-2 hr |

## Contraindications and precautions

Contraindicated in patients hypersensitive to inamrinone or bisulfites. It shouldn't be used in patients with severe aortic or pulmonic valvular disease in place of surgical intervention or during an acute phase of MI.

## Interactions

**Drug-drug.** *Cardiac glycosides:* Increased inotropic effect. This is a benefit in certain conditions.
*Disopyramide:* May cause severe hypotension. Avoid use together.

## Adverse reactions

**CV:** *arrhythmias,* hypotension, chest pain.
**GI:** nausea, vomiting, anorexia, abdominal pain.
**Hematologic:** *thrombocytopenia.*
**Hepatic:** elevated liver enzyme levels.
**Metabolic:** decreased serum potassium.
**Skin:** burning at injection site.
**Other:** hypersensitivity reactions (pericarditis, ascites, myositis vasculitis, pleuritis), fever.

## Overdose and treatment

Sign of overdose is severe hypotension. Treatment may include administration of a potent vasopressor, such as norepinephrine, as well as other general supportive measures, including cautious fluid volume replacement.

## Clinical considerations

■ Inamrinone is prescribed primarily for patients who haven't responded to therapy with cardiac glycosides, diuretics, and vasodilators.

### Therapeutic monitoring

■ Advise clinician to monitor blood pressure and heart rate throughout infusion. Prescriber should slow or stop infusion if patient's blood pressure decreases or if arrhythmias (ventricular or supraventricular) occur. Dosage may need to be reduced.
■ Advise clinician to monitor platelet counts. A count below 150,000/mm$^3$ usually necessitates dosage reduction. Thrombocytopenia usually occurs after prolonged treatment.

---

- Advise clinician to monitor electrolyte levels (especially potassium) because drug increases cardiac output, which may cause diuresis.
- Hemodynamic monitoring may be useful in guiding therapy.
- Advise clinician to monitor liver function test results to detect hepatic damage.
- Advise clinician to observe patient for adverse GI effects (such as nausea, vomiting, and diarrhea); recommend reducing dosage or stopping drug.

### Special populations
**Breast-feeding patients.** Drug may appear in breast milk. Safety in breast-feeding women hasn't been established.
**Pediatric patients.** Safety and efficacy in children under age 18 haven't been established.

### Patient counseling
- Warn patient that burning may occur at the injection site.
- Tell patient to report adverse reactions promptly.

# indapamide
Lozol

*Pharmacologic classification:* thiazide-like diuretic
*Therapeutic classification:* diuretic, antihypertensive
*Pregnancy risk category B*

### Available forms
Available by prescription only
*Tablets:* 1.25 mg, 2.5 mg

### Indications and dosages
#### Edema of heart failure
*Adults:* 2.5 mg P.O. as a single daily dose taken in the morning; increase dose to 5 mg daily after 1 week if response is poor.
#### Hypertension
*Adults:* 1.25 mg P.O. as a single daily dose taken in the morning; increase dose to 2.5 mg daily after 4 weeks if response is poor. Maximum daily dose, 5 mg.

### Mechanism of action
*Antihypertensive action:* Exact mechanism of antihypertensive effect of indapamide is unknown. This effect may result from direct arteriolar vasodilatation through calcium channel blockade. Drug also reduces total body sodium.
*Diuretic action:* Indapamide increases urinary excretion of sodium and water by inhibiting sodium reabsorption in the cortical diluting tubule of the nephron, thus relieving edema.

### Pharmacokinetics
*Absorption:* Absorbed completely from the GI tract.
*Distribution:* Distributes widely into body tissues because of its lipophilicity; drug is 71% to 79% plasma protein–bound.
*Metabolism:* Indapamide undergoes significant hepatic metabolism.
*Excretion:* About 60% of drug dose is excreted in urine within 48 hours; about 16% to 23% is excreted in feces.

| Route | Onset | Peak | Duration |
|---|---|---|---|
| P.O. | Unknown | 2-5 hr | 18 hr |

### Contraindications and precautions
Contraindicated in patients with anuria and in those hypersensitive to other sulfonamide-derived drugs.

Drug should be cautiously in patients with severely impaired renal or hepatic function and progressive hepatic disease.

### Interactions
**Drug-drug.** *Amphetamine, quinidine:* Indapamide turns urine slightly more alkaline and may decrease urinary excretion of some amines, such as alkaline urine. Advise clinician to monitor patient.
*Other antihypertensives:* Indapamide potentiates hypotensive effects. This may be used to therapeutic advantage.
*Cholestyramine and colestipol:* May bind indapamide, preventing its absorption. Drugs should be given 1 hour apart.
*Diazoxide:* Increased hyperglycemic, hypotensive, and hyperuricemic effects of diazoxide. Advise clinician to monitor patient closely; insulin dosage may need adjustment.
*Lithium:* Reduced renal clearance, elevating serum lithium levels. May necessitate reduction in lithium dosage by 50%.
*Methenamine compounds (such as methenamine mandelate):* Decreased therapeutic efficacy of these drugs. Advise clinician to monitor patient closely.
**Drug-herb.** *Licorice root:* May contribute to the potassium depletion caused by thiazides. Discourage patient from using this herb.

### Adverse reactions
**CNS:** headache, nervousness, dizziness, lightheadedness, weakness, vertigo, restlessness, drowsiness, fatigue, anxiety, depression, numbness of limbs, irritability, agitation.
**CV:** volume depletion and dehydration, orthostatic hypotension, palpitations, PVCs, irregular heartbeat, vasculitis.
**EENT:** rhinorrhea.
**GI:** anorexia, nausea, epigastric distress, vomiting, abdominal pain, diarrhea, constipation.
**GU:** nocturia, polyuria, frequent urination, impotence.

**Metabolic:** asymptomatic hyperuricemia; fluid and electrolyte imbalances, including dilutional hyponatremia and hypochloremia, metabolic alkalosis, and hypokalemia; gout; weight loss.
**Musculoskeletal:** muscle cramps and spasms.
**Skin:** rash, pruritus, flushing.

## Overdose and treatment
Clinical signs of overdose include GI irritation and hypermotility, diuresis, and lethargy, which may progress to coma.

Treatment is mainly supportive; recommend monitoring and assisting respiratory, CV, and renal function as indicated. Advise clinician to monitor fluid and electrolyte balance. Vomiting should be induced with ipecac in conscious patient; otherwise, recommend using gastric lavage to avoid aspiration. Cathartics shouldn't be given; these promote additional loss of fluids and electrolytes.

## Clinical considerations
■ Clinical considerations for use of indapamide are the same as those for all thiazide and thiazide-like diuretics.
■ Indapamide therapy may interfere with tests for parathyroid function and should be discontinued before such tests are done.

### *Therapeutic monitoring*
■ Therapeutic monitoring considerations for use of indapamide are the same as those for all thiazide and thiazide-like diuretics.

### *Special populations*
**Breast-feeding patients.** Drug appears in breast milk; its safety and effectiveness in breast-feeding women haven't been established.
**Pediatric patients.** Safety and efficacy in children haven't been established.
**Geriatric patients.** Geriatric and debilitated patients require close observation and may require reduced dosages. They're more sensitive to excess diuresis because of age-related changes in CV and renal function. Excess diuresis promotes orthostatic hypotension, dehydration, hypovolemia, hyponatremia, hypomagnesemia, and hypokalemia.

## Patient counseling
■ Patient counseling considerations for use of indapamide are the same as those for all thiazide and thiazide-like diuretics.

# indinavir sulfate
Crixivan

*Pharmacologic classification:* HIV protease inhibitor
*Therapeutic classification:* antiviral
*Pregnancy risk category C*

## Available forms
Available by prescription only
*Capsules:* 100 mg, 200 mg, 333 mg, 400 mg

## Indications and dosages
*Treatment of patients with HIV infection when antiretroviral therapy is warranted*
*Adults:* 800 mg P.O. q 8 hours with other antiretroviral drugs. Indinavir shouldn't be used as monotherapy.
≡*Dosage adjustment.* Reduce dosage to 600 mg P.O. q 8 hours in patients with mild to moderate hepatic insufficiency resulting from cirrhosis.

## Mechanism of action
*Antiviral action:* Indinavir sulfate inhibits HIV protease, an enzyme required for the proteolytic cleavage of viral polyprotein precursors into individual functional proteins found in infectious HIV. By binding to the protease active site, indinavir prevents cleavage of the viral polyproteins, resulting in formation of immature noninfectious viral particles.

## Pharmacokinetics
*Absorption:* Rapidly absorbed in GI tract when it is given on an empty stomach. A meal high in calories, fat, and protein significantly interferes with drug absorption, whereas lighter meals don't.
*Distribution:* About 60% is plasma protein–bound.
*Metabolism:* Metabolized to at least seven metabolites. Cytochrome P-450 3A4 (CYP 3A4) is the major enzyme responsible for formation of the oxidative metabolites.
*Excretion:* Less than 20% is excreted unchanged in urine.

| Route | Onset | Peak | Duration |
|-------|-------|------|----------|
| P.O. | Unknown | Unknown | Unknown |

## Contraindications and precautions
Contraindicated in patients hypersensitive to any component of drug. Contraindicated if the patient is also given rifampin.

Use cautiously in patients with hepatic insufficiency resulting from cirrhosis.

## Interactions
**Drug-drug.** *Amprenavir, saquinavir:* Increased plasma levels of these drugs. Dosage adjustments are probably not needed when used together.

*Carbamazepine:* Decreased indinavir AUC. Advise prescriber to consider an alternative drug.

*Clarithromycin:* Altered plasma levels of clarithromycin. Dosage adjustments are probably not needed when used together.

*Delavirdine, itraconazole, ketoconazole:* Causes an increase in the plasma levels of indinavir. Advise prescriber to consider a dosage reduction of indinavir to 600 mg every 8 hours.

*Didanosine:* A normal gastric pH may be needed for optimal absorption of indinavir. Recommend giving these drugs at least 1 hour apart on an empty stomach.

*Efavirenz, nevirapine:* Decreased plasma levels of indinavir. Advise prescriber to increase indinavir to 1,000 mg every 8 hours.

*HMG-CoA reductase inhibitors, such as atorvastatin, lovastatin, and simvastatin:* Increased levels of these drugs; therefore, increased risk of myopathy, including rhabdomyolysis. Avoid use together.

*Lopinavir/ritonavir fixed combination:* May increase plasma levels of indinavir. Advise prescriber to consider adjusting the dose of indinavir to 600 mg b.i.d.

*Midazolam, triazolam:* Competition for CYP 3A4 by indinavir could result in inhibition of the metabolism of these drugs and could create the potential for serious or life-threatening events, such as arrhythmias or prolonged sedation. These drugs shouldn't be given with indinavir.

*Nelfinavir:* Increased levels of indinavir by 50%, and nelfinavir by 80%. There are limited data regarding adjusting the dose to indinavir 1,200 mg b.i.d. and nelfinavir 1,250 mg b.i.d.

*Rifabutin:* Increased plasma levels of rifabutin and decreased levels of indinavir. Recommend giving indinavir 1,000 mg q 8 hours and decreasing the rifabutin dose to either 150 mg daily or 300 mg 2 to 3 times a week.

*Rifampin:* Potent inducer of CYP 3A4, which could markedly diminish plasma levels of indinavir; coadministration of indinavir and rifampin isn't recommended.

*Ritonavir:* Increased levels of indinavir by 2 to 5 times. Advise prescriber to adjust dose to indinavir 400 mg b.i.d. and ritonavir 400 mg b.i.d.; or indinavir 800 mg b.i.d. and ritonavir 100 to 200 mg b.i.d.

*Sildenafil:* Increased sildenafil plasma levels; may result in an increase in sildenafil-associated adverse events, including hypotension, visual changes, and priapism. Advise patient not to exceed 25 mg in a 48-hour period.

**Drug-herb.** *St. John's wort:* Decreased plasma level of indinavir. Discourage use together.

**Drug-food.** *Grapefruit juice:* Plasma levels and therapeutic effect of indinavir may be decreased. Patient should take with liquid other than grapefruit juice.

## Adverse reactions

**CNS:** malaise; headache, insomnia, dizziness, somnolence, asthenia, fatigue.

**GI:** abdominal pain, *nausea,* diarrhea, vomiting, acid regurgitation, anorexia, dry mouth, taste perversion.

**GU:** nephrolithiasis.

**Hematologic:** decreased hemoglobin, platelet count, or neutrophil count.

**Hepatic:** elevations in ALT, AST, and serum amylase; *hyperbilirubinemia,* jaundice.

**Musculoskeletal:** flank pain, back pain.

## Overdose and treatment

Symptoms of acute or chronic overdose have been reported as renal and GI effects.

Treatment is supportive, and the patient is observed closely. It's not known if indinavir is removed by hemodialysis or peritoneal dialysis.

## Clinical considerations

■ Dosage of indinavir is the same if drug is used alone or with other antiretroviral drugs. However, antiretroviral activity of indinavir may be increased when used with approved reverse transcriptase inhibitors. Synergistic effects are noted when combined with zidovudine and lamivudine.

■ An antiretroviral pregnancy registry has been established at: 1-800-258-4263 to monitor maternal-fetal outcomes of pregnant women who become exposed to the drug.

### Therapeutic monitoring

■ Recommend periodic measuring of HIV-RNA, CD4+.

■ Drug may cause nephrolithiasis. If signs and symptoms of nephrolithiasis occur, advise prescriber to consider stopping drug for 1 to 3 days during the acute phase. To prevent nephrolithiasis, patient should maintain adequate hydration.

### Special populations

**Pregnant patients.** There are no adequate studies to date for use during pregnancy.

**Breast-feeding patients.** Drug may appear in breast milk. Because of the potential for indinavir to cause adverse effects in nursing infants and to prevent transmitting infection to the infant, breast-feeding isn't recommended.

**Pediatric patients.** Safety and efficacy in children haven't been established. High risk of mild to severe renal effects with pediatric patients.

## Patient counseling

■ Inform patient that indinavir isn't a cure for HIV infection. Opportunistic infections and other complications with HIV disease may continue to develop. Drug has also not been shown to reduce risk of transmitting HIV to others

through sexual contact or blood contamination.
■ Caution patient not to adjust dosage or discontinue indinavir therapy without medical approval.
■ Tell patient to store capsules in the original container and to keep the desiccant in the bottle because the capsules are sensitive to moisture.
■ Instruct patient to take drug on an empty stomach with water 1 hour before or 2 hours after a meal. Alternatively, he may take it with other liquids (such as skim milk, juice, coffee, or tea) or with a light meal. Inform patient that a meal high in calories, fat, and protein reduces the absorption of indinavir.
■ Advise patient that, if a dose of indinavir is missed, therapy should be resumed with the next dose, and a double dose shouldn't be taken.
■ Instruct patient to drink at least 1.5 L of fluid daily.
■ Patients receiving sildenafil should be advised that they may be at an increased risk of sildenafil-associated adverse events, including hypotension, visual changes, and priapism; they should promptly report any symptoms to their prescribers.

---

## indomethacin, indomethacin sodium trihydrate

Apo-Indomethacin*, Indameth, Indochron E-R, Indocid*, Indocin, Indocin SR, Novomethacin*

*Pharmacologic classification:* NSAID
*Therapeutic classification:* nonnarcotic analgesic, antipyretic, anti-inflammatory
*Pregnancy risk category NR*

### Available forms
Available by prescription only
*Capsules:* 25 mg, 50 mg
*Capsules (sustained-release):* 75 mg
*Suspension:* 25 mg/5 ml
*Injection:* 1-mg vials
*Suppositories:* 50 mg

### Indications and dosages
**Moderate to severe arthritis, ankylosing spondylitis**
*Adults:* 25 mg P.O. b.i.d. or t.i.d. with food or antacids; dose may be increased by 25 to 50 mg daily q 7 days up to 200 mg daily; or 50 mg P.R. q.i.d. Alternatively, sustained-release capsules may be given: 75 mg to start, in the morning or h.s., followed, if needed, by 75 mg b.i.d.
**Acute gouty arthritis**
*Adults:* 50 mg t.i.d. Reduce dosage as soon as possible, then stop it. Don't use sustained-release capsules for this condition.

**Juvenile arthritis**
*Children ages 2 to 14:* 2 mg/kg P.O. daily in divided doses. Up to 4 mg/kg daily, but not exceeding 150 to 200 mg daily, in divided doses.
**To close a hemodynamically significant patent ductus arteriosus in premature infants (I.V. form only)**
*Neonate under age 48 hours:* 0.2 mg/kg I.V. followed by 2 doses of 0.1 mg/kg at 12- to 24-hour intervals.
*Neonate ages 2 to 7 days:* 0.2 mg/kg I.V. followed by 2 doses of 0.2 mg/kg at 12- to 24-hour intervals.
*Neonate over age 7 days:* 0.2 mg/kg I.V. followed by 2 doses of 0.25 mg/kg at 12- to 24-hour intervals.
**Acute shoulder pain**
*Adults:* 75 to 150 mg P.O. b.i.d. or t.i.d. with food or antacids; usual treatment is 7 to 14 days.
◇**Pericarditis**
*Adults:* 75 to 200 mg P.O. daily in three or four divided doses.
◇**Dysmenorrhea**
*Adults:* 25 mg P.O. t.i.d. with food or antacids.
◇**Bartter's syndrome**
*Adults:* 150 mg/day P.O. with food or antacids.
*Children:* 0.5 to 2 mg/kg in divided doses.

### I.V. administration
■ Reconstitute 1-mg vial of I.V. dose with 1 to 2 ml of sterile water for injection or normal saline injection. Prepare solution immediately before use to prevent deterioration. Don't use solution if it's discolored or contains a precipitate.
■ Use I.V. administration only for premature neonates with patent ductus arteriosus. Don't give a second or third I.V. dose if anuria or marked oliguria exists.
■ If ductus arteriosus reopens, a second course of one to three doses may be given. If ineffective, surgery may be needed.

### Incompatibilities
Incompatible with solutions with pH less than 6. Also incompatible with amino acid injection, calcium gluconate, cimetidine, dextrose injection, dobutamine, dopamine, gentamicin, tobramycin sulfate, and tolazoline.

### Mechanism of action
*Analgesic, antipyretic, and anti-inflammatory actions:* Exact mechanisms of action are unknown; indomethacin is thought to produce its analgesic, antipyretic, and anti-inflammatory effects by inhibiting prostaglandin synthesis and possibly by inhibiting phosphodiesterase.
*Closure of patent ductus arteriosus:* Mechanism of action is unknown, but it is believed to be through inhibition of prostaglandin synthesis.

---

## Pharmacokinetics
**Absorption:** Absorbed rapidly and completely from the GI tract.
**Distribution:** Highly protein-bound.
**Metabolism:** Metabolized in the liver.
**Excretion:** Excreted mainly in urine, with some biliary excretion.

| Route | Onset | Peak | Duration |
|---|---|---|---|
| P.O., I.V., P.R. | Unknown | Unknown | Unknown |

## Contraindications and precautions
Contraindicated in patients hypersensitive to drug and in those with a history of aspirin- or NSAID-induced asthma, rhinitis, or urticaria; in pregnancy, or in breast-feeding women. Also contraindicated in infants with untreated infection, active bleeding, coagulation defects or thrombocytopenia, congenital heart disease in those for whom patency of the ductus arteriosus is needed for satisfactory pulmonary or systemic blood flow, necrotizing enterocolitis, or impaired renal function. Suppositories are contraindicated in patients with a history of proctitis or recent rectal bleeding.

Use cautiously in geriatric patients and in patients with history of GI disease, impaired renal or hepatic function, epilepsy, parkinsonism, CV disease, infection, mental illness, or depression.

## Interactions
**Drug-drug.** *Anticoagulants and thrombolytics (such as coumarin derivatives, heparin, streptokinase, urokinase):* May potentiate anticoagulant effects. Advise clinician to monitor PT, PTT, and INR.
*Antihypertensives and diuretics:* Concurrent use may decrease their effectiveness.
*Aspirin:* May decrease the bioavailability of indomethacin. Avoid use together.
*Aspirin, cefamandole, cefoperazone, dextran, dipyridamole, mezlocillin, parenteral carbenicillin, piperacillin, plicamycin, salicylates, sulfinpyrazone, ticarcillin, valproic acid, or other anti-inflammatory drugs, corticotropin, or corticosteroids:* Bleeding problems may occur. Advise clinician to monitor patient closely.
*Coumarin derivatives, nifedipine, phenytoin, verapamil:* Toxicity may occur. Advise clinician to monitor patient carefully.
*Gold compounds, other anti-inflammatory drugs, acetaminophen:* Increased nephrotoxicity may occur. Don't use together.
*Insulin or oral antidiabetics:* Concurrent use may potentiate hypoglycemic effects. Avoid use together.
*Lithium, methotrexate:* Indomethacin may decrease the renal clearance of these drugs. Advise clinician to monitor patient closely.
*Triamterene and other diuretics:* Potential nephrotoxicity. Avoid use together.
**Drug-herb.** *Dong quai, feverfew, garlic, ginger, horse chestnut, red clover:* Possible increased risk of bleeding. Discourage use together.
*Senna:* May block diarrheal effects. Discourage use together.
*St. John's wort, dong quai:* Increased risk of photosensitivity. Advise patient to avoid unprotected exposure to sunlight.
**Drug-lifestyle.** *Alcohol use:* May increase GI adverse effects. Advise patient to avoid alcohol.

## Adverse reactions
**Oral and rectal forms**
**CNS:** *headache, dizziness,* depression, drowsiness, confusion, somnolence, fatigue, peripheral neuropathy, *seizures,* psychic disturbances, syncope, *vertigo.*
**CV:** hypertension, *edema, HF.*
**EENT:** blurred vision, corneal and retinal damage, hearing loss, tinnitus.
**GI:** nausea, anorexia, *diarrhea, peptic ulceration, GI bleeding,* constipation, dyspepsia, *pancreatitis.*
**GU:** hematuria, *acute renal failure,* proteinuria, interstitial nephritis; proteinuria and interstitial nephritis (I.V. form).
**Hematologic:** *hemolytic anemia, aplastic anemia, agranulocytosis, leukopenia, thrombocytopenic purpura,* iron-deficiency anemia.
**Metabolic:** hyperkalemia.
**Skin:** pruritus, urticaria, *Stevens-Johnson syndrome.*
**Other:** hypersensitivity (rash, respiratory distress, *anaphylaxis, angioedema*).

## Overdose and treatment
Signs and symptoms of overdose include dizziness, nausea, vomiting, intense headache, mental confusion, drowsiness, tinnitus, sweating, blurred vision, paresthesias, and seizures.

To treat overdose, recommend emptying stomach immediately by inducing emesis with ipecac syrup or by gastric lavage. Recommend giving activated charcoal via nasogastric tube. Recommend providing symptomatic and supportive measures (respiratory support and correction of fluid and electrolyte imbalances). Advise clinician to monitor laboratory parameters and vital signs closely. Dialysis may be of little value because indomethacin is strongly protein-bound.

## Clinical considerations
■ Oral suspension shouldn't be mixed with liquids or antacids before administering.
■ Patient should retain suppository in the rectum for at least 1 hour after insertion to ensure maximum absorption.
■ For patients at high risk for complications from NSAID-induced gastric ulceration, misoprostol, a proton-pump inhibitor, or $H_2$-blocker, may be considered for preventative therapy.

---

■ In arthritic patients without adequate response, a disease-modifying antirheumatic drug should be considered.

■ Drug therapy may interfere with dexamethasone suppression test results. It may also interfere with urinary 5-hydroxyindoleacetic acid determinations.

### Therapeutic monitoring

■ Advise clinician to monitor patient carefully for bleeding and for reduced urine output.

■ Advise clinician to monitor cardiopulmonary status for significant changes. Recommend watching for signs and symptoms of fluid overload, and checking weight and intake and output daily.

■ Advise clinician to monitor renal function test results before start of therapy and frequently during therapy to prevent adverse effects.

■ Severe headache may occur. If headache persists, advise prescriber to decrease dose.

### Special populations

**Breast-feeding patients.** Drug appears in breast milk in levels similar to those in maternal plasma; use in breast-feeding women should be avoided.

**Pediatric patients.** Safety of long-term drug use in children under age 14 hasn't been established. Use of I.V. indomethacin in premature infants for patent ductus arteriosus is considered an alternative to surgery.

**Geriatric patients.** Patients over age 60 may be more susceptible to the toxic effects of indomethacin. The effect of drug on renal prostaglandins may cause fluid retention and edema, a significant drawback for geriatric patients and those with HF.

### Patient counseling

■ Instruct patient in proper administration of dosage form prescribed, such as suppository, sustained-release capsule, or suspension.

■ Advise patient to seek medical approval before taking OTC drugs.

■ Caution patient to avoid hazardous activities that require alertness or concentration.

■ Tell patient to report signs and symptoms of adverse reactions and to adhere to prescribed drug regimen.

# infliximab

Remicade

*Pharmacologic classification:* monoclonal antibody $IgG_{1k}$
*Therapeutic classification:* antiinflammatory
*Pregnancy risk category C*

### Available forms

Available by prescription only
*Injection:* 100 mg/20-ml vial

### Indications and dosages

*Reduction of signs and symptoms in patients with moderately to severely active Crohn's disease with inadequate response to conventional therapy*
Adults: 5 mg/kg single I.V. infusion over a period of not less than 2 hours.
*Reduction in the number of draining enterocutaneous fistulas in patients with fistulizing Crohn's disease*
Adults: 5 mg/kg I.V. infused over a period of not less than 2 hours. Give additional doses of 5 mg/kg at 2 and 6 weeks after initial infusion.
*Reduction of signs and symptoms of rheumatoid arthritis and reduction of progress of structural damage in patients who respond inadequately to methotrexate*
Adults: 3 mg/kg I.V. over 2 hours. Additional doses given at 2 and 6 weeks after the first infusion and then every 8 weeks. If response is inadequate, dose may be increased to maximum of 10 mg/kg or infusions may be given every 4 weeks.

### I.V. administration

■ Vials don't contain antibacterial preservatives.

■ Dilute total volume of reconstituted dose to 250 ml with normal saline injection. Infusion concentration range is 0.4 to 4 mg/ml. Infusion should begin within 3 hours of preparation and must be given over a period of not less than 2 hours.

### Incompatibilities

Incompatible with PVC equipment and devices; should be prepared only in glass infusion bottles or polypropylene or polyolefin infusion bags and given through polyethylene-lined administration sets. Drug shouldn't be infused in the same I.V. line with other drugs.

### Mechanism of action

*Anti-inflammatory action:* Drug is a monoclonal antibody that binds to human tumor necrosis factor (TNF)-alpha to neutralize its activity and inhibit its binding with receptors, reducing the infiltration of inflammatory cells and TNF-alpha production in inflamed areas of the intestine.

### Pharmacokinetics

*Absorption:* Administered I.V.
*Distribution:* Not reported.
*Metabolism:* Not reported.
*Excretion:* Terminal half-life is 9½ days.

| Route | Onset | Peak | Duration |
|-------|-------|------|----------|
| I.V. | Unknown | Unknown | Unknown |

### Contraindications and precautions

Contraindicated in patients hypersensitive to murine proteins or other components of the drug. Use with caution in geriatric patients. Patients with congestive HF should not begin using this drug, because of clinical trials showing that heart patients on Remicade got much sicker than those patients who were not using the drug. Tuberculosis (frequently disseminated or extrapulmonary at clinical presentation), invasive fungal infections, and other opportunistic infections have been observed in patients receiving infliximab. Some of these infections have been fatal.

## Interactions
None reported.

## Adverse reactions
**CNS:** *headache, fatigue,* dizziness, malaise, insomnia.
**CV:** hypertension, hypotension, tachycardia, chest pain, peripheral edema.
**EENT:** pharyngitis, rhinitis, sinusitis, conjunctivitis.
**GI:** *nausea, abdominal pain,* vomiting, constipation, dyspepsia, flatulence, intestinal obstruction, oral pain, ulcerative stomatitis, toothache.
**GU:** dysuria, increased micturition frequency.
**Hematologic:** anemia, hematoma, ecchymosis.
**Hepatic:** elevated liver enzyme levels.
**Musculoskeletal:** myalgia, arthralgia, arthritis, back pain.
**Respiratory:** *upper respiratory tract infections,* bronchitis, cough, dyspnea, flu syndrome, respiratory tract allergic reaction.
**Skin:** rash, pruritus, acne, alopecia, eczema, erythema, erythematous rash, maculopapular rash, papular rash, dry skin, increased sweating, urticaria, flushing.
**Other:** *fever,* chills, pain, hot flashes, abscess, fungal infection.

## Overdose and treatment
Single doses up to 20 mg/kg have been given without direct toxic effects. If overdose should occur, recommend monitoring patient for signs and symptoms of adverse events and giving symptomatic treatment.

## Clinical considerations
■ Advise clinician to monitor patient for adverse effects.
■ Advise prescriber to reevaluate Remicade therapy for patients with HF, a heart weakened by age, damage from an MI, or some other condition.
■ Patients should be evaluated for latent tuberculosis infection with a tuberculin skin test. Treatment of latent tuberculosis infection should be started before therapy with infliximab is begun.
■ Cases of histoplasmosis, listeriosis, pneumocystosis, and tuberculosis have been observed in patients receiving infliximab. For patients who have lived in regions where histoplasmosis is endemic, the benefits and risks of infliximab therapy should be carefully considered before the therapy starts.

### Therapeutic monitoring
■ Infusion-related reactions, such as fever, chills, pruritus, urticaria, dyspnea, hypotension, hypertension, and chest pain may occur. If an infusion reaction occurs, recommend stopping drug, notifying prescriber, and being prepared to give acetaminophen, antihistamines, corticosteroids, and epinephrine p.r.n.
■ Advise clinician to monitor patient for development of lymphoma and infection. Patients with long duration of Crohn's disease and chronic exposure to immunosuppressant therapies are more susceptible to development of lymphoma and infection.
■ Drug may affect normal immune responses. Autoimmune antibodies and lupuslike syndrome may develop; recommend stopping drug therapy. Symptoms can be expected to resolve.
■ Remicade treatment should stop if a patient's heart condition gets worse.

### Special populations
**Breast-feeding patients.** It's unknown if infliximab appears in breast milk. Patient should discontinue either drug or breast-feeding.
**Pediatric patients.** Safety and efficacy of drug use in children haven't been established.
**Geriatric patients.** Use with caution in patients over age 65.

## Patient counseling
■ Tell patient about infusion-reaction symptoms and instruct to report adverse events.
■ Inform patient of postinfusion side effects and instruct him to report them promptly.

# influenza virus vaccine, 2001-2002 trivalent types A & B (purified surface antigen)
Fluvirin

# influenza virus vaccine, 2001-2002 trivalent types A & B (subvirion)
Fluogen, FluShield, Fluzone

*Pharmacologic classification:* vaccine
*Therapeutic classification:* viral vaccine
*Pregnancy risk category C*

## Available forms
Available by prescription only
*Injection:* 0.5-ml prefilled syringe; 5-ml vials

## Indications and dosages

*Annual influenza prophylaxis in high-risk patients*
*Adults and children ages 9 and older:* 0.5 ml I.M. (subvirion or purified surface antigen).
*Children ages 3 to 8:* 0.5 ml I.M. (subvirion or purified surface antigen).
*Infants and children ages 6 to 36 months:* 0.25 ml I.M. (subvirion or purified surface antigen).

Check package insert for annual changes and additional dosing recommendations.

Two-dose regimen is recommended for children ages 6 months to 8 years who are receiving the vaccine for the first time. A second dose should be given at least 4 weeks after the first. However, a single dose is sufficient in children who have previously received at least one dose of any influenza vaccine.

## Mechanism of action

*Influenza prophylaxis:* Vaccine promotes active immunity to influenza by inducing antibody production. Protection is provided only against those strains of virus from which the vaccine is prepared (or closely related strains).

## Pharmacokinetics

*Absorption:* Duration of immunity varies widely.
*Distribution:* No information available.
*Metabolism:* No information available.
*Excretion:* No information available.

| Route | Onset | Peak | Duration |
|-------|-------|------|----------|
| I.M. | Unknown | Unknown | About 1 yr |

## Contraindications and precautions

Contraindicated in patients hypersensitive to chicken eggs or any component of the vaccine such as thimerosal. Vaccination should be deferred in patients with acute respiratory or other active infection and immunization delayed in those with an active neurologic disorder.

## Interactions

**Drug-drug.** *Corticosteroids or immunosuppressants:* Concurrent use may impair the immune response to the vaccine. Avoid use together.
*Phenytoin and aminopyrine:* Decreased serum phenytoin and aminopyrine levels. Advise clinician to monitor patient and drug levels.
*Theophylline:* Increased serum theophylline levels. Advise clinician to monitor theophylline levels.
*Warfarin:* Rare prolonged PT, GI bleeding, transient gross hematuria, and epistaxis. Advise clinician to monitor patient closely.

## Adverse reactions

**CNS:** malaise.
**Musculoskeletal:** myalgia.

**Skin:** erythema, induration, and *soreness at injection site.*
**Other:** *anaphylaxis,* fever.

Note: Fever and malaise reactions occur most often in children and in others not exposed to influenza viruses. Severe reactions in adults are rare.

## Overdose and treatment

No information available.

## Clinical considerations

■ Patients hypersensitive to egg protein should have a skin test to assess sensitivity to vaccine. A scratch test should be given with 0.05 to 0.1 ml of a 1:100 dilution in normal saline solution for injection. Patients with positive skin test reactions shouldn't receive the influenza virus vaccine.
■ Epinephrine solution 1:1,000 should be available to treat allergic reactions.
■ Influenza vaccine shouldn't be given to patients with active influenza infection. Such infection should be treated with amantadine.
■ To reduce the frequency of adverse reactions, only the split-virus or purified surface antigen vaccine should be used in children.
■ Pneumococcal vaccine, DTP, or live attenuated measles virus vaccine may be given simultaneously but at a different injection site.
■ Store vaccine between 36° and 46° F (2° and 8° C). Don't freeze.
■ Advisory Committee on Immunization Practices states that short-term prophylaxis with antiviral drugs may be indicated as an adjunct to influenza virus vaccine for high-risk individuals and health care personnel who receive vaccine after influenza activity begins.

### Therapeutic monitoring

■ Advise clinician to monitor patient for adverse drug reactions.

### Special populations

**Pregnant patients.** If given during pregnancy, the influenza vaccine should be given during the second trimester to avoid a coincidental association with spontaneous abortion, which is common in the first trimester.
**Breast-feeding patients.** Breast-feeding isn't a contraindication for receiving vaccine.
**Pediatric patients.** Influenza vaccine is contraindicated in children under age 6 months.
**Geriatric patients.** Annual vaccination is highly recommended for patients over age 65.

## Patient counseling

■ Advise patient of potential injection site discomfort, fever, malaise, and muscle aches.
■ Encourage patient to report distressing adverse reactions promptly.
■ Warn patient that many cases of Guillain-Barré syndrome were reported after vaccination for the swine flu of 1976. This condi-

---

*Reactions may be* common, uncommon, *life-threatening,* or COMMON AND LIFE-THREATENING.

tion usually causes reversible paralysis and muscle weakness, but it can be fatal in some individuals. Influenza vaccines made after 1976 don't have as high a risk of Guillain-Barré syndrome, but the condition still occurs, albeit rarely. Patients with history of Guillain-Barré syndrome have a greater risk for repeat episodes.

# insulin (regular)
Humulin-R, Novolin R, Novolin R PenFill, Pork Regular Iletin II, Regular (Concentrated) Iletin II, Regular Insulin, Regular Purified Pork Insulin, Velosulin Human*, Velosulin BR

# insulin (lispro)
Humalog, Humalog Mix 75/25

# isophane insulin suspension (NPH)
Humulin N, Novolin N, Novolin N PenFill, NPH-N, Pork NPH Iletin II

# insulin zinc suspension (lente)
Humulin L, Lente Iletin II, Lente L, Novolin L

# extended zinc insulin suspension (ultralente)
Humulin U Ultralente, Ultralente*

# isophane insulin suspension and insulin injection (70% isophane insulin and 30% insulin injection)
Humulin 70/30, Novolin 70/30, Novolin 70/30 PenFill

# isophane insulin suspension and insulin injection (50% isophane insulin and 50% insulin injection)
Humulin 50/50

*Pharmacologic classification:* pancreatic hormone
*Therapeutic classification:* antidiabetic
*Pregnancy risk category NR*

## Available forms
Available without a prescription
**insulin (regular)**
*Injection (pork):* 100 units/ml
*Injection (human):* 100 units/ml
**isophane insulin suspension (NPH)**
*Injection (pork):* 100 units/ml
*Injection (human):* 100 units/ml

**insulin zinc suspension (lente)**
*Injection (pork):* 100 units/ml
*Injection (human):* 100 units/ml
**extended zinc insulin suspension (ultralente)**
*Injection (human):* 100 units/ml
Available by prescription only
**insulin (lispro)**
*Injection (human):* 100 units/ml, 25 units/ml with insulin lispro protamine 75 units/ml
*Cartridge (human):* 1.5 ml
**regular (concentrated) Iletin II insulin**
*Injection (pork):* 500 units/ml

## Indications and dosages
*Diabetic ketoacidosis (regular insulin)*
*Adults:* Administer loading dose of 0.15 unit/kg I.V. followed by 0.1 unit/kg/hour as a continuous infusion. Decrease rate of insulin infusion when plasma glucose level reaches 300 mg/dl. Start infusion of $D_5W$ separately from the insulin infusion when plasma glucose reaches 250 mg/dl. Thirty minutes before discontinuing insulin infusion, administer a dose of insulin S.C.; intermediate-acting insulin is recommended.

Alternative dosage schedule is 50 to 100 units I.V. and 50 to 100 units S.C. immediately; base subsequent doses on therapeutic response and glucose, acetone, or ketone levels monitored at 1- to 2-hour intervals, or 2.4 to 7.2 units I.V. loading dose followed by 2.4 to 7.2 units/hour.
*Children:* 0.5 to 1 unit/kg in two divided doses, one given I.V. and the other S.C., followed by 0.5 to 1 unit/kg I.V. q 1 to 2 hours; or 0.1 unit/kg I.V. bolus, then 0.1 unit/kg/hour continuous I.V. infusion until serum glucose decreases to 250 mg/dl; then start S.C. insulin.
*Ketosis-prone and juvenile-onset diabetes mellitus, diabetes mellitus inadequately controlled by diet and oral antidiabetics*
*Adults and children:* Individualized dosage adjusted based on patient's serum and urine glucose levels.
*Hyperkalemia*
*Adults:* 5 to 10 units of regular insulin with 50 ml of $D_5W$ over 5 minutes. Alternatively, 25 units of regular insulin given S.C. and an infusion of 1,000 ml dextrose 10% in water with 90 mEq sodium bicarbonate; infuse 330 ml over 30 minutes and the balance over 3 hours.
*Provocative test for growth hormone secretion*
*Adults:* Rapid I.V. injection of regular insulin 0.05 to 0.15 unit/kg.
*Control of hyperglycemia with longer-acting insulin in patients with type 1 diabetes mellitus and with sulfonylureas in patients with type 2 diabetes mellitus*
*Adults and children over age 3:* Dosage varies among patients and must be determined by a health care professional familiar with patient's metabolic needs, eating habits, and other

## COMPARING INSULIN PREPARATIONS

The table below lists the various forms of insulin and their times of onset, peak, and duration.
Individual responses can vary.

| Preparation | Purified† | Onset (hr) | Peak (hr) | Duration (hr) |
|---|---|---|---|---|
| **Rapid-acting insulins** | | | | |
| **insulin injection (regular, crystalline zinc)** | | | | |
| Regular Insulin | No | ½ | 2½-5 | 8 hr |
| Pork Regular Iletin II | Yes | ½ | 2-4 | 6-8 |
| Velosulin BR Human | Yes | ½ | 1-3 | 8 |
| Regular Purified Pork Insulin | Yes | ½ | 2½-5 | 8 |
| Humulin R | N.A. | ½ | 2-4 | 6-8 |
| Novolin R/Novolin R PenFill | N.A. | ½ | 2½-5 | 8 |
| **insulin injection (lispro)** | | | | |
| Humalog | Yes | < ½ | ½-1½ | < 6 |
| **Intermediate-acting insulins** | | | | |
| **isophane insulin suspension (NPH)** | | | | |
| NPH | No | 1½ | 4-12 | 24 |
| Pork NPH Iletin II | Yes | 1-2 | 6-12 | 18-24 |
| Humulin N | N.A. | 1-2 | 6-12 | 18-24 |
| Novolin N/Novolin N PenFill | N.A. | 1½ | 4-12 | 24 |
| **insulin zinc suspension (lente)** | | | | |
| Lente Iletin II | Yes | 1-3 | 6-12 | 18-24 |
| Lente L | Yes | 2½ | 7-15 | 22 |
| Humulin L | N.A. | 1-3 | 6-12 | 18-24 |
| Novolin L | N.A. | 2½ | 7-15 | 22 |
| **isophane (NPH) 70%, regular insulin 30%** | | | | |
| Humulin 70/30 | N.A. | ½ | 4-8 | 24 |
| Novolin 70/30/Novolin 70/30 PenFill | N.A. | ½ | 2-12 | 24 |
| **isophane (NPH) 50%, regular insulin 50%** | | | | |
| Humulin 50/50 | N.A. | ½ | 4-8 | 24 |
| **Long-acting insulins** | | | | |
| **extended insulin zinc suspension (ultralente)** | | | | |
| Ultralente | No | 4 | 10-30 | 36 |
| Humulin U Ultralente | Yes | 4-6 | 8-20 | 24-28 |

N.A. indicates not applicable.
† Purified insulins contain < 10 parts per million proinsulin.

lifestyle variables. Inject S.C. within 15 minutes before or immediately after a meal.

### I.V. administration
▪ Insulin (regular) is the only type of insulin that can be given I.V.
▪ I.V. route should be used only for patients with circulatory collapse, diabetic ketoacidosis, or hyperkalemia, or to evaluate growth hormone reserve.

▪ Insulin (regular) should be diluted with normal saline solution for I.V. infusion.

### Incompatibilities
Incompatible with aminophylline, amobarbital, chlorothiazide, cytarabine, dobutamine, methylprednisolone sodium succinate, pentobarbital sodium, phenobarbital sodium, phenytoin sodium, secobarbital, sodium bicarbonate, and thiopental.

## Mechanism of action

*Antidiabetic action:* Insulin is used as a replacement for the physiologic production of endogenous insulin in patients with type 2 (insulin-dependent) diabetes mellitus (IDDM) and diabetes mellitus inadequately controlled by diet and oral hypoglycemic drugs. Insulin increases glucose transport across muscle and fat-cell membranes to reduce blood glucose levels. It also promotes conversion of glucose to its storage form, glycogen; triggers amino acid uptake and conversion to protein in muscle cells and inhibits protein degradation; stimulates triglyceride formation and inhibits release of free fatty acids from adipose tissue; and stimulates lipoprotein lipase activity, which converts circulating lipoproteins to fatty acids. Insulin is available in various forms and these differ mainly in onset, peak, and duration of action. Characteristics of the various insulin preparations are compared in the following chart.

## Pharmacokinetics

*Absorption:* Insulin must be given parenterally because it's destroyed in the GI tract. Commercially available preparations are formulated to differ in onset, peak, and duration after subcutaneous administration. They're classified as rapid-acting (½- to 1-hour onset), intermediate-acting (1- to 2-hour onset), and long-acting (4- to 8-hour onset). The accompanying chart summarizes major pharmacokinetic differences.
*Distribution:* Distributed widely throughout the body.
*Metabolism:* Some insulin is bound and inactivated by peripheral tissues, but the majority appears to be degraded in the liver and kidneys.
*Excretion:* Filtered by renal glomeruli and undergoes some tubular reabsorption. Plasma half-life is about 9 minutes after I.V. administration.

| Route | Onset | Peak | Duration |
|---|---|---|---|
| I.V. | Immediate | Unknown | Unknown |
| S.C. (rapid) | 0.5-1.5 hr | 2-3 hr | 5-7 hr |
| S.C. (intermediate) | 1-2.5 hr | 4-15 hr | 12-24 hr |
| S.C. (long-acting) | 4-8 hr | 10-30 hr | 36 hr |

## Contraindications and precautions

No known contraindications.

## Interactions

**Drug-drug.** *Anabolic steroids, beta blockers, clofibrate, fenfluramine, MAO inhibitors, salicylates, tetracycline:* Prolonged hypoglycemic effect. Advise clinician to monitor blood glucose carefully.

*Corticosteroids, dextrothyroxine sodium, epinephrine, and thiazide diuretics:* Diminish insulin response. Advise clinician to monitor patient for hyperglycemia.
*Rosiglitazone:* May increase the risk of HF and other CV effects in patients. Advise clinician to monitor patient closely and check liver function tests periodically.
**Drug-herb.** *Aloe, bilberry leaf, bitter melon, burdock, dandelion, fenugreek, garlic, and ginseng:* Use together may improve blood glucose control, requiring a reduction of antidiabetic drugs. Advise patient to discuss the use of herbal products with his prescriber.
*Basil, bay, bee pollen, burdock, ginseng, glucomannian, horehound, marshmallow, myrrh, sage:* May affect glycemic control. Advise clinician to monitor blood glucose carefully and discourage patient from using together.
**Drug-lifestyle.** *Alcohol use:* May cause a prolonged hypoglycemic effect. Advise patient to avoid alcohol.
*Marijuana use:* May increase insulin requirements. Advise patient to avoid marijuana use.
*Smoking:* Decreases absorption of insulin administered S.C. Advise patient to avoid smoking within 30 minutes of insulin injection.

## Adverse reactions

**Metabolic:** *hypoglycemia,* hyperglycemia (rebound, or Somogyi, effect).
**Skin:** urticaria, pruritus, swelling, redness, stinging, warmth at injection site, *lipoatrophy, lipohypertrophy.*
**Other:** hypersensitivity reactions (*anaphylaxis,* rash).

## Overdose and treatment

Insulin overdose may produce signs and symptoms of hypoglycemia (tachycardia, palpitations, anxiety, hunger, nausea, diaphoresis, tremors, pallor, restlessness, headache, and speech and motor dysfunction).

Treatment is directed toward treating hypoglycemia and is based on patient's symptoms. If patient is responsive, recommend giving 10 to 15 g of a fast-acting oral carbohydrate. If patient's signs and symptoms persist after 15 minutes, recommend giving an additional 10 g carbohydrate. If patient is unresponsive, an I.V. bolus of dextrose 50% solution should immediately increase glucose levels. Some prefer to use dextrose 25% in water because it's less irritating should extravasation occur. A common infusion rate is based on glucose content: 10 to 20 mg/kg/minute. Parenteral glucagon or epinephrine S.C. may also be given; both drugs elevate blood glucose levels in a few minutes by stimulating glycogenolysis. Fluid and electrolyte imbalance may require I.V. fluids and electrolyte (such as potassium) replacement.

## Clinical considerations

■ Human insulin may be advantageous for non-insulin-dependent patients requiring intermittent or short-term therapy (such as pregnancy, surgery, infection, or total parenteral nutrition therapy), for patients with insulin resistance, or for those with lipoatrophy.

■ Lente, semilente, and ultralente insulins may be mixed in any proportion.

■ Regular insulin may be mixed with NPH or lente insulins in any proportion. However, in vitro binding occurs over time until an equilibrium is reached. Give these mixtures either immediately after preparation or after stability occurs (5 to 15 minutes for NPH regular, 24 hours for lente regular) to minimize variability in patient response. Note that switching from separate injections to a prepared mixture also may alter the patient's response. When mixing two insulins, one should always draw regular insulin into the syringe first.

■ Lispro insulin may be mixed with Humulin N or Humulin U and given within 15 minutes before a meal to prevent a hypoglycemic reaction. The effects of mixing lispro insulin with insulins of animal source or insulin preparations produced by other manufacturers haven't been studied and may require a change in dosage.

■ Insulin should be stored in a cool area. Refrigeration is desirable but not essential, except with regular glucose concentrated.

■ Administration route is S.C. because it allows slower absorption and causes less pain than I.M. injections. Ketosis-prone, juvenile-onset, severely ill, and newly diagnosed diabetics with very high blood glucose levels may require hospitalization and I.V. treatment with regular fast-acting insulin. Ketosis-resistant diabetics may be treated as outpatients with intermediate-acting insulin after they have received instructions on how to alter dosage according to self-performed urine or blood glucose determinations. Some patients, primarily pregnant or brittle diabetics, may use a dextrometer to perform fingerstick blood glucose tests at home.

■ Injection sites should be rotated; however, unstable diabetics may achieve better control if injection site is rotated within same anatomic region.

■ In pregnant diabetic women, insulin requirements increase, sometimes drastically, then decline immediately postpartum.

### Therapeutic monitoring

■ With regular insulin concentrated, a secondary hypoglycemic reaction may occur 18 to 24 hours after injection. This may be caused by a repository effect of drug and the high level of insulin in the preparation (500 units/ml).

■ Some patients may develop insulin resistance and require large insulin doses to control symptoms of diabetes. Iletin, II, Regular Purified Pork, 500 units/ml may be used for these patients.

■ Patient should notify pharmacist several days before prescription refill is needed in case U-500 is not in stock. Hospital pharmacy should be given sufficient notice before refill of in-house prescription.

■ U-500 insulin should never be stored in same area with other insulin preparations because of danger of severe overdose if given accidentally to other patients. U-500 insulin must be administered with a U-100 syringe because no syringes are made for this drug.

■ Pregnant women may require specialized laboratory testing and diagnostic tests and frequent monitoring.

### Special populations

**Pregnant patients.** Advise clinician to monitor insulin use during pregnancy. The target preprandial glucose level is 70 to 100 mg/dl, or preprandial glucose levels of 80 to 110 mg/dl. The goals for 1- and 2-hour postprandial glucose levels are less than 140 mg/dl and less than 120 mg/dl, respectively, or 1- and 2-hour postprandial glucose levels of less than 155 mg/dl or less than 135 mg/dl, respectively.

**Breast-feeding patients.** Advise clinician to monitor drug use closely in breast-feeding women.

**Geriatric patients.** There may be an increased risk of hypoglycemia from insulin therapy and an increased potential for CVA and heart attack in older patients.

## Patient counseling

■ Instruct patient to strictly adhere to manufacturer's instructions regarding assembly, administration, and care of specialized delivery systems, such as insulin pumps.

■ Emphasize importance of regular meal times and that meals must not be omitted.

■ Teach patient that glucose monitoring is an essential guide to correct dosage and to therapeutic success.

■ Emphasize importance of recognizing hypoglycemic symptoms because insulin-induced hypoglycemia is hazardous and may cause brain damage if prolonged.

■ Advise patient to always wear a medical identification bracelet or pendant, to carry ample insulin supply and syringes on trips, to have carbohydrates (sugar or candy) on hand for emergency, and to note time-zone changes for dose schedule when traveling.

■ Instruct patient not to change the order of mixing insulins or change the model or brand of syringe or needle. Make sure he knows when mixing two insulins, always to draw regular insulin into the syringe first.

■ Inform patient that use of marijuana may increase insulin requirements.

■ Inform patient that cigarette smoking decreases absorption of insulin administered S.C.

Advise him not to smoke within 30 minutes after insulin injection.
■ Instruct patient on the appropriate measures for safe disposal of needles.

# insulin aspart (rDNA origin) injection
NovoLog

*Pharmacologic classification:* human insulin analogue
*Therapeutic classification:* antidiabetic
*Pregnancy risk category C*

## Available forms
Available by prescription only
*Injection:* 100 units of insulin aspart per ml (U-100) in 3-ml PenFill cartridges or 10-ml vial

## Indications and dosages
*Control of hyperglycemia in patients with diabetes mellitus*
*Adults:* Dosage is individualized based on the patient's needs. Typical daily insulin requirements are 0.5 to 1 unit/kg daily divided in a meal-related treatment regimen. About 50% to 70% of this dose may be provided with Novo-Log and the remainder by an intermediate-acting or long-acting insulin. Give within 5 to 10 minutes of start of meal by S.C. injection in the abdominal wall, thigh, or upper arm.

## Mechanism of action
*Antidiabetic action:* Thought to bind to insulin receptors on muscle and fat cells to lower glucose levels and to facilitate the cellular uptake of glucose and inhibit the output of glucose from the liver.

## Pharmacokinetics
*Absorption:* NovoLog is as bioavailable as regular human insulin. It has a faster absorption and onset and shorter duration of action compared with regular human insulin.
*Distribution:* Low plasma protein–binding (0% to 9%), similar to regular insulin.
*Metabolism:* No information available.
*Excretion:* Half-life is shorter than that of regular human insulin (81 minutes compared with 141 minutes, respectively).

| Route | Onset | Peak | Duration |
|-------|-------|------|----------|
| S.C. | Rapid | 1-3 hr | 3-5 hr |

## Contraindications and precautions
Contraindicated during hypoglycemia and in patients hypersensitive to NovoLog or one of its excipients.

Use drug cautiously in patients prone to hypoglycemia and hypokalemia, such as those who are fasting, have autonomic neuropathy, or are using potassium-lowering drugs or drugs sensitive to serum potassium levels.

## Interactions
**Drug-drug.** *ACE inhibitors, disopyramide, fibrates, fluoxetine, MAO inhibitors, oral antidiabetics, propoxyphene, salicylates, somatostatin analogue (octreotide), sulfonamide antibiotics:* May enhance glucose-lowering effects of insulin and may potentiate hypoglycemia. Advise clinician to monitor glucose levels and patient for signs of hypoglycemia. May require insulin dosage adjustment.
*Beta blockers, clonidine:* May potentiate or weaken glucose-lowering effect of insulin, causing hypoglycemia or hyperglycemia. May mask signs and symptoms of hypoglycemia (may be reduced or absent). Advise clinician to monitor glucose level.
*Corticosteroids; danazol; diuretics; estrogens and progestogens such as in oral contraceptives; isoniazid; niacin; phenothiazine derivatives; somatropin; sympathomimetics such as epinephrine, salbutamol, and terbutaline; thyroid hormones:* May reduce the glucose-lowering effect of insulin and may cause hyperglycemia. Advise clinician to monitor glucose level. May require insulin dosage adjustment.
*Guanethidine, reserpine:* May mask signs and symptoms of hypoglycemia (may be reduced or absent). Advise clinician to monitor glucose level.
*Lithium salts, pentamidine:* May potentiate or weaken glucose-lowering effect of insulin, causing hypoglycemia or hyperglycemia. Pentamidine may cause hypoglycemia, which may sometimes be followed by hyperglycemia. Advise clinician to monitor glucose level.
**Drug-herb.** *Aloe, bilberry leaf, bitter melon, burdock, dandelion, fenugreek, garlic, and ginseng:* Use together may improve blood glucose control, requiring a reduction of antidiabetics. Advise patient to discuss the use of herbal medicines with his prescriber before use.
**Drug-lifestyle.** *Alcohol use:* May potentiate or weaken blood glucose-lowering effect of insulin, resulting in hypoglycemia or hyperglycemia. Advise clinician to monitor glucose level.

## Adverse reactions
**Metabolic:** hypoglycemia.
**Skin:** injection site reactions, lipodystrophy, pruritus, rash.
**Other:** allergic reactions.

## Overdose and treatment
Hypoglycemia may occur from an excess of insulin relative to food intake, energy expenditure, or both. Warning signs and symptoms of hypoglycemia include shaking, sweating, dizziness, fatigue, hunger, irritability, confu-

sion, blurred vision, headaches, or nausea and vomiting.

Mild hypoglycemia can be treated with oral glucose. Adjustments in drug dosage, meal patterns, or exercise may be needed. More severe episodes involving coma, seizure, or neurologic impairment may be treated with I.M. or S.C. glucagon or concentrated I.V. glucose. Sustained carbohydrate intake and observation may be needed because hypoglycemia may recur after apparent recovery.

## Clinical considerations
■ Store drug at between 36° and 46° F (2° to 8° C); don't freeze. Vials shouldn't be exposed to excessive heat or sunlight. Open vials of NovoLog are stable at room temperature for 28 days.
■ Insulin vials should be inspected visually before use. NovoLog should be clear and colorless. It should never contain particulate matter, appear cloudy or viscous, or be discolored. Drug shouldn't be used after its expiration date.
■ NovoLog should be given 5 to 10 minutes before the start of a meal. Because of rapid onset and short duration of action, patients may need the addition of longer-acting insulins to prevent premeal hyperglycemia. Drug should be given by S.C. injection into the abdominal wall, thigh, or upper arm. It's important to rotate sites to minimize lipodystrophies.

### Therapeutic monitoring
■ Advise clinician to monitor warning signs of hypoglycemia and the patient's glucose levels while patient is receiving NovoLog.

### Special populations
**Breast-feeding patients.** It isn't known if insulin aspart appears in breast milk. Caution should be used when drug is given to nursing mother.
**Pediatric patients.** Safety and effectiveness haven't been studied.
**Geriatric patients.** The effect of age on the pharmacokinetics and mechanism of action of NovoLog hasn't been studied.

## Patient counseling
■ Inform patient of the possible risks and benefits of NovoLog.
■ Teach patient to recognize hypoglycemia and hyperglycemia and how to treat them.
■ Instruct patient on injection techniques, timing of dose to meals, adherence to meal planning, importance of regular glucose monitoring and periodic glycosylated hemoglobin testing, proper storage of insulin, and safe disposal of used needles.
■ Tell women to notify prescriber about planned, suspected, or known pregnancy because information about drug use during pregnancy and breast-feeding isn't available.

# insulin glargine (rDNA) injection
Lantus

*Pharmacologic classification:* pancreatic hormone
*Therapeutic classification:* antidiabetic
*Pregnancy risk category C*

## Available forms
Available by prescription only
*Injection:* 100 units/ml

## Indications and dosages
*Management of type 1 diabetes mellitus in patients who need basal (long-acting) insulin for the control of hyperglycemia*
*Adults and children over age 6:* Individualize dosage and administer S.C. once daily h.s.
*Management of type 2 diabetes mellitus in patients who need basal (long-acting) insulin for control of hyperglycemia*
*Adults:* Individualize dosage and administer S.C. once daily h.s.

## Mechanism of action
*Antidiabetic action:* Regulates glucose metabolism by stimulating peripheral glucose uptake, especially by skeletal muscle and fat, and by inhibiting hepatic glucose production.

## Pharmacokinetics
*Absorption:* After S.C. injection of insulin glargine in healthy patients and in patients with diabetes, the insulin serum levels indicate a slower, more prolonged absorption and a relatively constant level and time profile over 24 hours with no pronounced peak compared with NPH insulin.
*Distribution:* No information available.
*Metabolism:* Partly metabolized to form two active metabolites with in vitro activity similar to that of insulin.
*Excretion:* No information available.

| Route | Onset | Peak | Duration |
|-------|-------|------|----------|
| S.C. | Slow | None | 11-24 hr |

## Contraindications and precautions
Lantus is contraindicated in patients who are hypersensitive to insulin glargine or its excipients. Avoid use during episodes of hypoglycemia.

Use drug cautiously in patients with renal or hepatic impairment.

## Interactions
**Drug-drug.** *ACE inhibitors, disopyramide, fibrates, fluoxetine, MAO inhibitors, octreotide, oral antidiabetics, propoxyphene, salicylates, somatostatin analogue, sulfonamide antibi-*

*otics:* May cause hypoglycemia and increased insulin effect. Advise clinician to monitor glucose level. Dosage adjustments of insulin may be required.

*Beta blockers, clonidine, guanethidine, reserpine:* May mask signs of hypoglycemia. Use cautiously. Advise clinician to monitor glucose level.

*Beta blockers, clonidine, lithium:* May potentiate or weaken glucose-lowering effect of insulin. Advise clinician to monitor glucose level. Insulin dosage may need adjustment.

*Corticosteroids, danazol, diuretics, estrogens and progestins (including oral contraceptives), isoniazid, phenothiazine derivatives, somatropin, sympathomimetics (such as albuterol, epinephrine, and terbulaline), thyroid hormones:* May reduce glucose-lowering effect of insulin. Advise clinician to monitor glucose level. Insulin dosage may need adjustment.

*Pentamidine:* May cause hypoglycemia, which may be followed by hyperglycemia. Use cautiously. Advise clinician to monitor glucose level.

**Drug-herb.** *Aloe, bilberry leaf, bitter melon, burdock, dandelion, fenugreek, garlic, and ginseng.* Use together may improve blood glucose control, requiring a reduction of antidiabetic drugs. Advise patient to discuss the use of herbal products with his prescriber before use.

**Drug-lifestyle.** *Alcohol, emotional stress:* May potentiate or weaken the blood glucose–lowering effect of insulin. Advise clinician to monitor glucose level. Dosage adjustments of insulin may be needed.

## Adverse reactions
**Metabolic:** hypoglycemia.
**Skin:** lipodystrophy, pruritus, rash, injection site reaction (pain).
**Other:** allergic reactions.

## Overdose and treatment
Hypoglycemia may result from excessive insulin dose or from lower insulin requirements caused by increased work or exercise without eating, food not being absorbed in the usual manner because of postponement or omission of a meal, or illness with vomiting, fever, or diarrhea. Symptoms may include fatigue, weakness, confusion, headache, convulsions, dizziness, hunger, nausea, numbness, and pale skin.

Mild episodes of hypoglycemia can be treated with oral glucose or other carbohydrates. Adjustments in drug dosage, meal patterns, or exercise may be needed. More severe episodes with coma, seizure, or neurologic impairment may be treated with I.M./S.C. glucagon or concentrated I.V. glucose. Sustained carbohydrate intake and observation may be needed because hypoglycemia may recur after apparent clinical recovery.

## Clinical considerations
■ Insulin glargine isn't intended for I.V. administration. It is only meant for S.C. administration.

■ Because of the prolonged duration of insulin glargine, it's not the insulin of choice for diabetic ketoacidosis.

■ Note that the prolonged duration of activity of insulin glargine is dependent on injection into S.C. space.

■ The absorption, onset, and duration of action may be affected by exercise and other variables such as illness and emotional stress.

■ Insulin glargine must not be diluted or mixed with any other insulin or solution.

■ As with any insulin therapy, lipodystrophy may occur at the site of injection and delay insulin absorption. Recommend continuously rotating the injection site within a given area to reduce lipodystrophy.

■ Hypoglycemia is the most common adverse effect of insulin. Early symptoms may be different or less pronounced in patients with long duration of diabetes, diabetic nerve disease, or intensified diabetes control. Advise clinician to monitor glucose level closely in these patients because severe hypoglycemia may result before the patient develops symptoms.

### Therapeutic monitoring
■ As with any insulin, the desired blood glucose levels as well as the doses and timing of antidiabetics must be determined individually. Glucose monitoring is recommended for all patients with diabetes.

### Special populations
**Breast-feeding patients.** It isn't known if insulin glargine appears in significant amounts in breast milk. Because many drugs do, including human insulin, caution should be used when Lantus is given to a nursing woman. Breast-feeding women may need adjustments in insulin dosage and diet.
**Pediatric patients.** Safety and effectiveness have been established in 6- to 15-year-olds with type 1 diabetes. Administration to children under age 6 hasn't been studied. Based on the results of clinical trials, the dosage recommendation for children is the same as for adults.
**Geriatric patients.** Because hypoglycemia may be difficult to recognize in geriatric patients with diabetes, the initial dosing, dose increments, and maintenance dose should be conservative to avoid hypoglycemic reactions.

## Patient counseling
■ Educate patient on proper blood glucose monitoring techniques, proper diabetes management, and safe disposal of used needles.

**◢ ALERT** Educate diabetic patients on the signs and symptoms of hypoglycemia, such as fatigue, weakness, confusion, headache, and pale skin.
■ Advise patient to treat mild episodes of hypoglycemia with oral glucose tablets. Encourage patient to always carry glucose tablets in case of a hypoglycemic episode.
■ Teach patient the importance of maintaining a diabetic diet and that adjustments in drug dosage, meal patterns, and exercise may be needed to regulate glucose levels.
**◢ ALERT** Any change of insulin should be made cautiously and only under medical supervision. Changes in insulin, strength, manufacturer, type (such as regular, NPH, or insulin analogs), species (animal, human), or method of manufacturer (rDNA versus animal source insulin) may result in the need for a change in dosage. Oral antidiabetic treatment also being taken may need to be adjusted.
■ Tell patient to consult prescriber before using OTC drugs.
**◢ ALERT** Warn patient not to dilute or mix any other insulin or solution with insulin glargine. If the solution is cloudy, advise the patient to discard the vial.
■ Tell patient to store unopened vials and cartridges in the refrigerator.

---

# interferon alfa-2a, recombinant
Roferon-A

# interferon alfa-2b, recombinant
Intron A

*Pharmacologic classification:* biological response modifier
*Therapeutic classification:* antineoplastic, antiviral
*Pregnancy risk category C*

## Available forms
Available by prescription only
**alfa-2a**
*Solution for injection:* 3 million IU/vial, 9 million IU/vial, 9 million IU/multidose vial, 18 million IU/multidose vial, 36 million IU/multidose vial
*Powder for injection with diluent:* 18 million IU/multidose vial
**alfa-2b**
*Powder for injection with diluent:* 3 million IU/vial; 5 million IU/vial; 10 million IU/vial; 18 million IU/multidose vial; 25 million IU/vial; 50 million IU/vial
*Solution for injection:* 10 million IU/vial, 18 million IU/multidose vial, 25 million IU/vial

## Indications and dosages
*Hairy cell leukemia*
**alfa-2a**
*Adults:* For induction, 3 million IU S.C. or I.M. daily for 16 to 24 weeks. For maintenance, 3 million IU S.C. or I.M. three times weekly.
**alfa-2b**
*Adults:* For induction and maintenance, 2 million IU/m² I.M. or S.C. three times weekly.
*Condylomata acuminata*
**alfa-2b**
*Adults:* 1 million IU per lesion, intralesionally, three times weekly for 3 weeks.
*Kaposi's sarcoma*
**alfa-2a**
*Adults:* For induction, 36 million IU S.C. or I.M. daily for 10 to 12 weeks; for maintenance, 36 million IU three times weekly. Doses may begin at 3 million IU and be escalated upward every 3 days until patient is given 36 million IU daily, to decrease toxicity.
**alfa-2b**
*Adults:* 30 million IU/m² S.C. or I.M. three times weekly. Maintain dose unless disease progresses rapidly or intolerance occurs.
*Chronic hepatitis C*
**alfa-2a**
*Adults:* 3 million IU 3 times a week S.C. or I.M. for 12 months (48 to 52 weeks). Alternatively, induction dose of 6 million IU 3 times weekly for the first 3 months (12 weeks) followed by 3 million IU 3 times weekly for 9 months (36 weeks). If no response after 3 months, therapy should be stopped. Retreatment with either 3 or 6 million IU 3 times weekly for 6 to 12 months may be considered.
**alfa-2b**
*Adults:* 3 million IU S.C. or I.M. three times weekly. If response occurs, recommend continuing therapy for 6 months. If no response by 12 to 16 weeks, recommend stopping therapy.
*Chronic hepatitis B*
**alfa-2b**
*Adults:* 30 to 35 million IU (alfa-2b) S.C. or I.M. weekly as either 5 million IU daily or 10 million IU three times weekly for 16 weeks.
*Children ages 1 to 17 years old:* 3 million IU/m² S.C. 3 times weekly for 1 week, then escalate dose to 6 million IU/m² S.C. 3 times weekly (up to 10 million IU/m² S.C. 3 times weekly) for 16 to 24 weeks.
*Chronic myelogenous leukemia*
**alfa-2a**
*Adults:* 9 million IU daily I.M or S.C. An escalating dosing regimen in which daily doses of 3 million and 6 million IU are given over 3 days, followed by 9 million IU daily for remainder of therapy, may produce increased short-term tolerance.
*Children:* 2.5 to 5 million IU /m² daily.

---

*Malignant melanoma*
**alfa-2b**
*Adults:* 20 million IU/m² daily given as I.V. infusion 5 days in a row for 4 weeks. For maintenance therapy, 10 million IU/m² S.C. three times weekly for 48 weeks. If adverse effects occur, recommend stopping therapy until they abate and then resuming therapy at 50% of the previous dose. If intolerance persists, therapy should be stopped.
*Initial treatment of clinically aggressive follicular non-Hodgkin's lymphoma with anthracycline-containing combination chemotherapy*
**alfa-2b**
*Adults:* 5 million IU S.C. 3 times weekly for up to 18 months.
◊ *Renal cell carcinoma*
*Adults:* 5 to 20 million IU daily or three times weekly.

## Mechanism of action

*Antineoplastic action:* Interferon alfa is a sterile protein product produced by recombinant DNA techniques applied to genetically engineered *Escherichia coli* bacteria. The interferons are naturally occurring small protein molecules produced and secreted by cells in response to viral infections or synthetic and biological inducers. Their exact mechanism of action is unknown but appears to involve direct antiproliferative action against tumor cells or viral cells to inhibit replication and modulation of host immune response by enhancing the phagocytic activity of macrophages and augmenting specific cytotoxicity of lymphocytes for target cells. To date, three major classes of interferons have been identified: alfa, beta, and gamma.

## Pharmacokinetics

*Absorption:* More than 80% of dose is absorbed after I.M. or S.C. injection.
*Distribution:* Not applicable.
*Metabolism:* Appears to be metabolized in the liver and kidney.
*Excretion:* Reabsorbed from glomerular filtrate with minor biliary elimination.

| Route | Onset | Peak | Duration |
|---|---|---|---|
| I.M., S.C. | Unknown | Unknown | Unknown |

## Contraindications and precautions

Contraindicated in patients hypersensitive to drug or to murine (mouse) immunoglobulin. Use drug cautiously in patients with CV or pulmonary disease, diabetes mellitus, coagulation disorders, or myelosuppression. Contraindicated in pregnant women and in male partners of pregnant women.

Use cautiously in breast-feeding women; it isn't known if drug appears in breast milk.

## Interactions

**Drug-drug.** *Blood dyscrasia–causing drugs, bone marrow depressant therapy, radiation therapy:* Increased bone marrow depressant effects. Dosage reduction may be required.
*CNS depressants:* Enhanced CNS depression. Advise clinician to monitor patient closely.
*Live-virus vaccine:* May potentiate replication of vaccine virus, increase adverse effects, and decrease patient's antibody response. Avoid use together.
*Methylxanthines, such as aminophylline and theophylline:* Increased half-life of these drugs, perhaps by interfering with cytochrome P-450 drug-metabolizing enzymes. Advise clinician to monitor patient closely.

## Adverse reactions

**CNS:** *dizziness, confusion,* paresthesia, numbness, lethargy, *depression, decreased mental status,* forgetfulness, ***coma,*** nervousness, insomnia, sedation, apathy, anxiety, irritability, fatigue, vertigo, gait disturbances, incoordination.
**CV:** hypotension, chest pain, ***arrhythmias,*** palpitations, syncope, ***HF,*** hypertension, edema, ***MI.***
**EENT:** *dryness or inflammation of the oropharynx,* rhinorrhea, sinusitis, conjunctivitis, earache, eye irritation.
**GI:** *anorexia, nausea, diarrhea, vomiting,* abdominal fullness, *abdominal pain,* flatulence, constipation, hypermotility, gastric distress, *change in taste,* excessive salivation.
**GU:** transient impotence.
**Hematologic:** *leukopenia, mild thrombocytopenia.*
**Hepatic:** *hepatitis.*
**Metabolic:** *weight loss,* cyanosis.
**Respiratory:** *cough,* dyspnea.
**Skin:** diaphoresis, *rash, dryness, pruritus, partial alopecia,* urticaria, flushing, inflammation at injection site.
**Other:** *flulike syndrome (fever, fatigue, myalgia, headache, chills, arthralgia),* night sweats, hot flashes.

## Overdose and treatment

No information available.

## Clinical considerations

■ When preparing antineoplastics for injection, special precautions should be taken because of their potential for carcinogenicity and mutagenicity. Use of a biological containment cabinet is recommended. Vials shouldn't be shaken.
**H** *ALERT* S.C. administration route should be used in patients whose platelet count is less than 50,000/mm³.
■ Different brands of interferons may not be therapeutically interchangeable.
■ Administration of drug at bedtime minimizes inconvenience of fatigue.

■ When using interferon alfa-2b for condylomata acuminata by intralesional injection, one should use only the 10 million-IU vial reconstituted with 1 ml of diluent. Using other strengths or more diluent would produce a hypertonic solution. For administration, a 25G to 30G needle and a tuberculin syringe should be used. Up to five lesions may be treated simultaneously.

■ The following indications aren't included in U.S. labeling, but drug may be used for these applications: chronic myelocytic leukemia; treatment of superficial bladder carcinoma; treatment of malignant lymphomas, especially nodular, poorly differentiated types; multiple myeloma; mycosis fungoides; papillomas; minimal residual epithelial ovarian cancer (intraperitoneal administration); and laryngeal papillomatosis (interferon alfa-2b).

### Therapeutic monitoring

■ Almost all patients experience flulike symptoms at the beginning of therapy; these effects tend to diminish with continued therapy.

■ Dosage reduction may be needed if headaches persist. Hypotension may result from fluid depletion; supportive treatment may be required.

■ Advise clinician to monitor blood pressure, BUN, hematocrit, platelet count, ALT, AST, LD, alkaline phosphatase, serum bilirubin, creatinine, uric acid, total and differential leukocyte count, and ECG.

■ Advise clinician to monitor patient for CNS adverse reactions, such as decreased mental status and dizziness. Periodic neuropsychiatric monitoring is recommended.

### Special populations

**Pregnant patients.** Contraindicated in pregnancy. Women of childbearing age should use an effective method of contraception during therapy with interferon-alpha preparations.
**Breast-feeding patients.** Drug has potential for serious adverse effects on breast-fed infants; a decision should be made to discontinue breast-feeding or discontinue drug.
**Pediatric patients.** Safety and efficacy in children under age 18 haven't been established.
**Geriatric patients.** Neurotoxicity and cardiotoxicity are more common in geriatric patients, especially those with underlying CNS or cardiac impairment.

### Patient counseling

■ Instruct patient that the bone marrow–depressant effects of interferon may cause an increased risk of microbial infection, delayed healing, and gingival bleeding. A decrease in salivary flow may also occur.

■ Advise patient not to take a missed dose or to double the next dose, but to call for further instructions.

■ Inform patient to store drug in refrigerator and to keep it from freezing.

■ Caution patient against driving or performing tasks requiring alertness until response to drug is known.

■ Advise patient to seek medical approval before taking OTC drugs for colds, coughs, allergies, and similar disorders; explain that interferons commonly cause flulike symptoms and patient may need to take acetaminophen before each dose.

■ Tell patient that drug may cause temporary loss of some hair. Normal hair growth should return when drug is discontinued.

■ Inform patient to avoid use of aspirin and chronic alcohol intake because these may increase risk of GI bleeding.

# interferon beta-1a

Avonex

*Pharmacologic classification:* biological response modifier
*Therapeutic classification:* antiviral, immunoregulator
*Pregnancy risk category C*

## Available forms

Available by prescription only
*Lyophilized powder for injection:* 33 mcg (6.6 million IU) of interferon beta-1a

## Indications and dosages

*To slow progression of physical disability and decrease the frequency of clinical exacerbations in relapsing multiple sclerosis*
*Adults:* 30 mcg I.M. once weekly.

## Mechanism of action

*Antiviral and immunoregulator actions:* The mechanisms by which interferon beta-1a exerts its actions in multiple sclerosis aren't clearly understood. However, it's known that the biological response-modifying properties of interferon beta-1a are mediated through its interactions with specific cell receptors found on the surface of human cells. The binding to these receptors induces the expression of a number of interferon-induced gene products that are believed to be the mediators of the biological actions of interferon beta-1a.

## Pharmacokinetics

None known.

| Route | Onset | Peak | Duration |
|-------|-------|------|----------|
| I.M. | Unknown | Unknown | Unknown |

## Contraindications and precautions

Contraindicated in pregnancy and in patients hypersensitive to natural or recombinant interferon-beta, human albumin, or any other component of the formulation.

---

Reactions may be *common*, uncommon, *life-threatening*, or COMMON AND LIFE-THREATENING.

Use drug cautiously in patients with depression, seizure disorders, or severe cardiac conditions.

## Interactions
None reported.

## Adverse reactions
**CNS:** malaise, *asthenia, headache, sleep difficulty, dizziness,* syncope, suicidal tendency, *seizure,* speech disorder, ataxia.
**CV:** chest pain, vasodilation.
**EENT:** otitis media, decreased hearing, sinusitis.
**GI:** *nausea, diarrhea, dyspepsia,* anorexia, abdominal pain.
**GU:** ovarian cyst, vaginitis.
**Hematologic:** anemia, elevated eosinophil levels, decreased hematocrit.
**Hepatic:** elevated AST levels.
**Musculoskeletal:** *muscle ache,* muscle spasm, arthralgia.
**Respiratory:** *upper respiratory tract infection,* dyspnea.
**Skin:** ecchymosis (at injection site), injection site reaction, urticaria, alopecia, nevus, herpes zoster, herpes simplex.
**Other:** *flulike symptoms, pain, fever, chills, infection,* hypersensitivity reaction.

## Overdose and treatment
No information available.

## Clinical considerations
■ Recommend exercising caution when giving drug to patients with preexisting seizure disorders.
■ Vials of drug should be stored in the refrigerator. If refrigeration is unavailable, drug can be stored at 77° F (25° C) for up to 30 days. Drug shouldn't be exposed to high temperatures or freezing.

### Therapeutic monitoring
■ Recommend the following laboratory tests before therapy starts and at periodic intervals thereafter: complete and differential WBC counts, platelet counts, and blood chemistries, including liver function test results.
■ Use of interferon beta-1a may cause depression and suicidal ideation. It isn't known if these symptoms may be related to the underlying neurologic basis of multiple sclerosis, to interferon beta-1a treatment, or to a combination of both. Advise clinician to closely monitor patient for these symptoms and consider cessation of therapy if they occur.
■ Advise clinician to monitor patient with cardiac disease, such as angina, HF, or arrhythmia, for worsening of clinical condition during initiation of therapy. Although drug doesn't have any known direct-acting cardiac toxicity, it does cause flulike symptoms, which may be

stressful to patients with severe cardiac conditions.

### Special populations
**Pregnant patients.** Therapy should be stopped if pregnancy occurs.
**Breast-feeding patients.** It's unknown if drug appears in breast milk. Consider risks and benefits before continuing either breast-feeding or drug therapy.
**Pediatric patients.** Safety and effectiveness in children under age 18 haven't been established.

## Patient counseling
■ Caution patient not to change dosage or administration schedule. If a dose is missed, tell him to take it as soon as he remembers. The regular schedule may then be resumed, but two injections shouldn't be given within 2 days of each other.
■ Instruct patient how to store drug properly.
■ Inform patient that flulike symptoms are common after therapy starts. Recommend use of acetaminophen to lessen the impact of these symptoms.
■ Advise patient to report depression, suicidal ideation, or other adverse reactions.
■ Advise women of childbearing age not to become pregnant while taking interferon beta-1a because of the abortifacient potential of drug. If pregnancy does occur, instruct patient to discontinue treatment and call prescriber immediately.

# interferon beta-1b
Betaseron

*Pharmacologic classification:* biological response modifier
*Therapeutic classification:* antiviral, immunoregulator
*Pregnancy risk category C*

## Available forms
Available by prescription only
*Powder for injection, lyophilized:* 9.6 million IU (0.3 mg)

## Indications and dosages
*Reduction of the frequency of exacerbations in relapsing-remitting multiple sclerosis*
*Adults:* 8 million IU (0.25 mg) S.C. every other day.

## Mechanism of action
*Antiviral and immunoregulator actions:* The mechanisms by which interferon beta-1b exerts its actions in multiple sclerosis aren't clearly understood. However, it's known that the biological response-modifying properties of interferon beta-1b are mediated through its in-

teractions with specific cell receptors found on the surface of human cells. The binding to these receptors induces the expression of a number of interferon-induced gene products that are believed to be the mediators of the biological actions of interferon beta-1b.

## Pharmacokinetics
*Absorption:* Serum levels are undetectable after the recommended dose.
*Distribution:* No information available.
*Metabolism:* No information available.
*Excretion:* No information available on patients with multiple sclerosis; however, in clinical studies involving healthy patients, elimination half-life ranged from 8 minutes to 4 hours.

| Route | Onset | Peak | Duration |
|-------|-------|------|----------|
| S.C. | Unknown | 1-8 hr | Unknown |

## Contraindications and precautions
Contraindicated in patients hypersensitive to interferon beta or human albumin.

Use drug cautiously in women of childbearing age; drug is contraindicated in pregnancy.

## Interactions
None significant.

## Adverse reactions
**CNS:** *malaise,* depression, anxiety, emotional lability, depersonalization, *suicidal tendencies,* confusion, somnolence, *hypertonia, asthenia, migraine, seizures,* headache, dizziness.
**CV:** palpitations, hypertension, tachycardia, peripheral vascular disorder, hemorrhage.
**EENT:** laryngitis, *sinusitis, conjunctivitis,* abnormal vision.
**GI:** *diarrhea, constipation, abdominal pain, vomiting.*
**GU:** *menstrual disorders (bleeding or spotting, early or delayed menses, fewer days of menstrual flow, menorrhagia).*
**Hematologic:** *decreased WBC and absolute neutrophil count.*
**Hepatic:** *elevated ALT level; elevated bilirubin level.*
**Metabolic:** hypothyroidism, SIADH secretion.
**Respiratory:** dyspnea.
**Skin:** *inflammation, pain, and necrosis at injection site; alopecia; diaphoresis.*
**Other:** *flulike symptoms (fever, chills, myalgia, diaphoresis);* breast pain, *pelvic pain; lymphadenopathy,* generalized edema, *myasthenia,* Cushing's syndrome, diabetes insipidus, diabetes mellitus.

## Overdose and treatment
No information available.

## Clinical considerations
■ Drug is being investigated in the treatment of AIDS, AIDS-related Kaposi's sarcoma, metastatic renal cell carcinoma, malignant melanoma, cutaneous T-cell lymphoma, and acute hepatitis C as unlabeled uses.
■ Drug should be injected immediately after preparation.
■ Refrigerate drug or reconstituted product (up to 3 hours) at 36° to 46° F (2° to 8° C); don't freeze.

### Therapeutic monitoring
■ Recommend performing the following laboratory tests before therapy starts and at periodic intervals thereafter: hemoglobin, complete and differential WBC counts, platelet counts, and blood chemistries, including liver function tests.
■ Drug use may cause depression and suicidal ideation. Other mental disorders have been observed and can include anxiety, emotional lability, depersonalization, and confusion. It's not known if these symptoms may be related to the underlying neurologic basis of multiple sclerosis, to interferon beta-1b treatment, or to a combination of both. Advise clinician to closely monitor patient with these symptoms and consider stopping therapy.

### Special populations
**Pregnant patients.** Therapy should be stopped if pregnancy occurs.
**Breast-feeding patients.** It's unknown if drug appears in breast milk. Consider risks and benefits before continuing either breast-feeding or drug therapy.
**Pediatric patients.** Safety and efficacy in children under age 18 haven't been established.

## Patient counseling
■ Caution patient to take protective measures (such as sunscreens, protective clothing) against exposure to ultraviolet light or sunlight until tolerance is determined.
■ Teach patient how to self-administer S.C. injections, including solution preparation, use of aseptic technique, rotation of injection sites, and equipment disposal. Periodically reevaluate patient's technique.
■ Instruct patient to rotate injection sites to minimize local reactions.
■ Inform patient that flulike symptoms are common after therapy starts. Recommend taking drug at bedtime to help minimize the symptoms.
■ Caution patient not to change dosage or schedule of administration without medical consultation.
■ Advise patient to report depression or suicidal ideation.
■ Inform women of childbearing age about abortifacient potential of drug.

# interferon gamma-1b

Actimmune

*Pharmacologic classification:* biological response modifier
*Therapeutic classification:* antineoplastic
*Pregnancy risk category C*

## Available forms

Available by prescription only
*Injection:* 100 mcg (3 million IU)/0.5 ml in single-dose vials

## Indications and dosages

**To decrease the frequency and severity of serious infection of chronic granulomatous disease**
*Adults with body surface area over 0.5 m²:* 50 mcg/m² (1.5 million IU /m²) S.C. three times weekly (such as Monday, Wednesday, and Friday).
*Adults with body surface area of 0.5 m² or less:* 1.5 mcg/kg S.C. three times weekly (such as Monday, Wednesday, and Friday).
**To delay disease progression in patients with severe, malignant osteopetrosis**
*Adults with body surface area over 0.5 m²:* 50 mcg/m² (1 million IU/m²) S.C. three times weekly in the deltoid or anterior thigh.
*Adults with body surface area of 0.5 m² or less:* 1.5 mcg/kg/dose S.C. three times weekly in the deltoid or anterior thigh.

## Mechanism of action

*Antineoplastic action:* Interferon gamma-1b is a single-chain polypeptide containing 140 amino acids, produced by fermentation of genetically engineered *Escherichia coli.* It has potent phagocytic activity not seen with other interferons. Exact mechanism of action is unknown, but growing evidence suggests it interacts functionally with other interleukin molecules, and all form part of a complex lymphokine network. A broad range of biological activities has been noted, including enhancement of oxidative metabolism of tissue macrophages, antibody-dependent cellular cytotoxicity, natural killer cell activity, and effects on Fc receptor expression on monocytes and major histocompatibility antigen expression. In chronic granulomatous disease, interferon gamma-1b provides enhancement of phagocyte function, including elevation of superoxide levels and improved killing of *Staphylococcus aureus.*

## Pharmacokinetics

*Absorption:* About 90% is absorbed after S.C. injection.
*Distribution:* Unknown.
*Metabolism:* Unknown.
*Excretion:* Unknown. Mean elimination half-life after S.C. dosing is about 6 hours.

| Route | Onset | Peak | Duration |
|-------|-------|------|----------|
| P.O. | Unknown | 7 hr | Unknown |

## Contraindications and precautions

Contraindicated in patients hypersensitive to drug or to genetically engineered products derived from *Escherichia coli.*

Use drug cautiously in patients with CV disease (arrhythmias, HF, or ischemia), compromised CNS function, or seizure disorders and in those receiving myelosuppressive drugs.

## Interactions

**Drug-drug.** *Drugs that use this metabolic degradation pathway:* Interferon gamma-1b can decrease hepatic microsomal cytochrome P-450 levels, which could lead to decreased metabolism of drug. Use with caution.
*Myelosuppressive drugs:* Additive effects. Use together cautiously.

## Adverse reactions

**CNS:** *fatigue,* decreased mental status, gait disturbance, dizziness.
**GI:** *nausea, vomiting, diarrhea,* abdominal pain.
**GU:** proteinuria.
**Hematologic: *neutropenia, thrombocytopenia.***
**Hepatic:** elevated liver enzyme levels (at high doses).
**Metabolic:** weight loss.
**Musculoskeletal:** back pain.
**Skin:** *rash; erythema, tenderness* (at injection site).
**Other:** flulike syndrome (headache, fever, chills, myalgia, arthralgia).

## Overdose and treatment

No information available.

## Clinical considerations

■ Store drug in refrigerator immediately; don't freeze. Excessive or vigorous agitation should be avoided. Drug shouldn't be shaken. Unopened or unentered vials shouldn't be left at room temperature longer than 12 hours before use. Vials that exceed these limits shouldn't be returned to refrigerator; they should be discarded.
■ Each vial is designed for single use only.

### *Therapeutic monitoring*

■ If acute hypersensitivity reaction occurs, recommend stopping drug immediately and instituting symptomatic and supportive treatment.
■ Transient cutaneous rash hasn't required discontinuation of therapy.

■ If severe adverse reactions occur, recommend reducing dose by 50% or stopping therapy until reaction subsides.

### Special populations
**Breast-feeding patients.** It's unknown if drug appears in breast milk. Risks and benefits should be considered before either breast-feeding or drug therapy is continued.
**Pediatric patients.** Safety and efficacy haven't been established in children under age 1.

### Patient counseling
■ Thoroughly review the patient information package insert with patient.

---

# ipecac syrup
*Pharmacologic classification:* alkaloid emetic
*Therapeutic classification:* emetic
*Pregnancy risk category C*

---

### Available forms
Available with and without a prescription
*Syrup:* 70 mg powdered ipecac/ml

### Indications and dosages
*To induce vomiting in poisoning*
*Adults:* 15 to 30 ml P.O., followed by 200 to 300 ml of water.
*Children ages 1 to 11:* 15 ml P.O., followed by about 200 ml of water or other clear liquid.
*Children under age 1:* 5 to 10 ml P.O., followed by 100 to 200 ml of water or other clear liquid.
    May repeat dose once after 20 minutes, if needed.

### Mechanism of action
*Emetic action:* Ipecac syrup directly irritates the GI mucosa and directly stimulates the chemoreceptor trigger zone through the effects of emetine and cephalin, its two alkaloids.

### Pharmacokinetics
*Absorption:* Absorbed in significant amounts mainly when it doesn't produce emesis.
*Distribution:* Unknown.
*Metabolism:* Unknown.
*Excretion:* Emetine is excreted in urine slowly, over a period lasting up to 60 days.

| Route | Onset | Peak | Duration |
|---|---|---|---|
| P.O. | 20 min | Unknown | 20-25 min |

### Contraindications and precautions
Contraindicated in semicomatose or unconscious patients or those with severe inebriation, seizures, shock, or loss of gag reflex. Drug shouldn't be given after ingestion of gasoline, kerosene, volatile oils, or caustic substances (lye).

### Interactions
**Drug-drug.** *Activated charcoal:* May inactivate ipecac syrup and shouldn't be taken together. Activated charcoal may be given after patient vomits.
*Antiemetics:* Decreased effectiveness of ipecac. Avoid use together.
**Drug-food.** *Carbonated beverages:* May cause abdominal distention. Avoid use together.
*Milk (or milk products):* May decrease therapeutic effectiveness of ipecac syrup. Avoid use together.
*Vegetable oil:* Delays absorption. Shouldn't be taken together.

### Adverse reactions
**CNS:** depression, *drowsiness*.
**CV:** *arrhythmias,* bradycardia, hypotension; atrial fibrillation, *fatal myocarditis* (with excessive doses).
**GI:** diarrhea.

### Overdose and treatment
Clinical effects of overdose include diarrhea, persistent nausea or vomiting (longer than 30 minutes), stomach cramps or pain, arrhythmias, hypotension, myocarditis, difficulty breathing, and unusual fatigue or weakness.
    Toxicity from chronic ipecac overdose usually involves use of the concentrated fluid extract in dosage appropriate for the syrup. Clinical effects of cardiotoxicity include tachycardia, T-wave depression, atrial fibrillation, depressed myocardial contractility, HF, and myocarditis. Other toxic effects include bloody stools and vomitus, hypotension, shock, seizures, and coma. The usual cause of death is HF.
    Treatment requires discontinuation of drug followed by symptomatic and supportive care, which may include digitalis and pacemaker therapy to treat cardiotoxic effects. However, no antidote exists for the cardiotoxic effects of ipecac, which may be fatal despite intensive treatment.

### Clinical considerations
■ Ipecac syrup usually empties the stomach completely within 30 minutes (in over 90% of patients); average emptying time is 20 minutes.
■ In antiemetic toxicity, ipecac syrup is usually effective if less than 1 hour has passed since ingestion of antiemetic.
■ Ipecac syrup may be used in small amounts as an expectorant in cough preparations; however, this use has doubtful therapeutic benefit.
**H ALERT** Don't confuse ipecac syrup with ipecac fluidextract, which is rarely used but is 14 times more potent. Never store these two drugs together—the wrong drug could cause death.

---

### Therapeutic monitoring
■ Little if any systemic toxicity occurs with doses of 30 ml or less.
■ Drug may be abused by patients with eating disorders (such as bulimia or anorexia nervosa).

### Special populations
**Breast-feeding patients.** Safety in breast-feeding women hasn't been established; possible risks must be weighed against benefits of drug.
**Pediatric patients.** Advise parents to keep ipecac syrup at home at all times but to keep it out of children's reach.

### Patient counseling
■ Instruct patient to take syrup with 1 or 2 glasses of water.
■ Advise patient to take activated charcoal only after vomiting has stopped.

# ipratropium bromide
Atrovent

*Pharmacologic classification:* anticholinergic
*Therapeutic classification:* bronchodilator
*Pregnancy risk category B*

### Available forms
Available by prescription only
*Inhaler:* each metered dose supplies 18 mcg
*Inhalation solution:* 0.02%
*Nasal spray:* 0.03%, 0.06%

### Indications and dosages
**Bronchospasm in chronic bronchitis and emphysema**
*Adults:* Usually, 2 inhalations (36 mcg) q.i.d.; patient may take additional inhalations, p.r.n., but shouldn't exceed 12 inhalations in 24 hours or 500 mcg q 6 to 8 hours via oral nebulizer.
**Rhinorrhea from allergic and nonallergic perennial rhinitis**
**0.03% nasal spray**
*Adults and children ages 6 and older:* 2 sprays (42 mcg) per nostril b.i.d. or t.i.d.
**Rhinorrhea associated with the common cold**
**0.06% nasal spray**
*Adults and children ages 12 and older:* 2 sprays (84 mcg) per nostril t.i.d. or q.i.d.
*Children ages 5 to 11:* 2 sprays (84 mcg) per nostril t.i.d.

### Mechanism of action
*Anticholinergic action:* Ipratropium appears to inhibit vagally mediated reflexes by antagonizing the action of acetylcholine. Anticholinergics prevent the increases in intracellular level of cyclic guanosine monophosphate (cyclic GMP) that result from interaction of acetyl-choline with the muscarinic receptor on bronchial smooth muscle.
The bronchodilation after inhalation is primarily a local, site-specific effect, not a systemic one.

### Pharmacokinetics
*Absorption:* Not readily absorbed into the systemic circulation either from the surface of the lung or from the GI tract as confirmed by blood levels and renal excretion studies. Much of an inhaled dose is swallowed.
*Distribution:* Not applicable.
*Metabolism:* Metabolism is hepatic; elimination half-life is about 2 hours.
*Excretion:* Most of an administered dose is excreted unchanged in feces. Absorbed drug is excreted in urine and bile.

| Route | Onset | Peak | Duration |
|---|---|---|---|
| Inhalation | Unknown | Unknown | Unknown |
| Intranasal | Unknown | Unknown | Unknown |

### Contraindications and precautions
Contraindicated in patients hypersensitive to drug or atropine or its derivatives and in those hypersensitive to soya lecithin or related food products, such as soybeans and peanuts.
Use drug cautiously in patients with angle-closure glaucoma, prostatic hyperplasia, and bladder-neck obstruction.

### Interactions
**Drug-drug.** *Antimuscarinics, including ophthalmic preparations:* Concurrent use may produce additive effects. Avoid use together.
*Fluorocarbon propellant–containing oral inhalants, such as adrenocorticoids, cromolyn, glucocorticoids, and sympathomimetics:* Increased risk of fluorocarbon toxicity may result from too-closely timed administration of ipratropium and other fluorocarbon propellant–containing oral inhalants. A 5-minute interval between administration of such drugs is recommended.
**Drug-herb.** *Jaborandi tree, pill-bearing spurge:* Products may decrease therapeutic effect of drug. Advise clinician to monitor patient closely.

### Adverse reactions
**CNS:** dizziness, headache, nervousness.
**CV:** palpitations, chest pain.
**EENT:** cough, blurred vision, rhinitis, sinusitis, pharyngitis.
**GI:** nausea, GI distress, dry mouth.
**Musculoskeletal:** back pain.
**Respiratory:** *upper respiratory tract infection, bronchitis,* cough, dyspnea, ***bronchospasm,*** increased sputum.
**Skin:** rash.
**Other:** pain, flulike symptoms.

## Overdose and treatment

Acute overdose by inhalation is unlikely because ipratropium isn't well absorbed systemically after aerosol or oral administration.

## Clinical considerations

- Because of delayed onset of bronchodilation, drug isn't recommended to treat acute respiratory distress.
- Initial nasal spray pump requires priming with seven actuations of the pump. If used regularly as recommended, no further priming is needed. If not used for longer than 24 hours, the pump will require two actuations. If not used for longer than 7 days, the pump will require seven actuations to reprime.

### Therapeutic monitoring

- Advise clinician to monitor patient for adverse drug events and therapeutic effect.

### Special populations

**Breast-feeding patients.** It's unknown if drug appears in breast milk. Although lipid-insoluble quaternary bases pass into breast milk, ipratropium is unlikely to reach the infant, especially when taken by aerosol. Use caution when giving to breast-feeding women.
**Pediatric patients.** Safety and efficacy in children under age 5 haven't been established.

## Patient counseling

- Instruct patient on correct method of administration.
- Advise patient to allow 1 minute between inhalations.
- Instruct patient to take a missed dose as soon as possible, unless it is almost time for the next scheduled dose, in which case he should skip the missed dose. Warn him to never double the dose.
- Suggest sugarless hard candy, gum, ice, or saliva substitute to relieve dry mouth. Tell patient to report dry mouth to prescriber if it persists longer than 2 weeks.
- Instruct patient to call prescriber if he experiences no benefits within 30 minutes after administration, or if condition worsens.

---

# irbesartan

Avapro

*Pharmacologic classification:* angiotensin II receptor antagonist
*Therapeutic classification:* antihypertensive
*Pregnancy risk category C (D, in second and third trimesters)*

## Available forms

Available by prescription only
*Tablets:* 75 mg, 150 mg, 300 mg

## Indications and dosages

*Treatment of hypertension—alone, or with other antihypertensives*
*Adults:* Initially 150 mg P.O. once daily, increased to maximum of 300 mg once daily if needed, without regard to food.
≣ *Dosage adjustment.* In volume- and salt-depleted patients, give 75 mg P.O. initially.

## Mechanism of action

*Antihypertensive action:* Irbesartan blocks the vasoconstrictor and aldosterone-secreting effects of angiotensin II by selectively blocking the binding of angiotensin II to its receptor sites.

## Pharmacokinetics

*Absorption:* Absorbed rapidly and completely. The average absolute bioavailability is 60% to 80%, and it isn't affected by food.
*Distribution:* Drug is 90% plasma protein–bound. It may cross the blood-brain barrier and placenta. Steady state is achieved within 3 days. Drug is widely distributed.
*Metabolism:* Metabolized by conjugation and oxidation. Cytochrome P-450 2C9 is the major enzyme responsible for formation of the oxidative metabolites. Metabolites don't appear to add appreciably to the pharmacologic activity.
*Excretion:* Excreted in the bile and urine. 20% is excreted in the urine and the rest in the feces. Drug may also appear in breast milk. Elimination half-life is 11 to 15 hours.

| Route | Onset | Peak | Duration |
|-------|-------|------|----------|
| P.O. | Unknown | 1¼-2 hr | 24 hr |

## Contraindications and precautions

Contraindicated in patients who are hypersensitive to drug or its components and in pregnant or breast-feeding women.

Use cautiously in volume- or salt-depleted patients, in patients whose renal function may depend on the activity of the renin-angiotensin-aldosterone system (such as patients with severe HF), and in those with unilateral or bilateral renal artery stenosis.

## Interactions

None reported.

## Adverse reactions

**CNS:** fatigue, anxiety, dizziness, headache.
**CV:** chest pain, edema, tachycardia.
**EENT:** pharyngitis, rhinitis, sinus abnormality.
**GI:** diarrhea, dyspepsia, abdominal pain, nausea, vomiting.
**GU:** urinary tract infection.
**Musculoskeletal:** musculoskeletal trauma or pain.
**Respiratory:** upper respiratory tract infection.
**Skin:** rash.

---

## Overdose and treatment
No information available. The most likely signs and symptoms of an overdose are expected to be hypotension and tachycardia, and possibly bradycardia. Drug isn't removed by hemodialysis. If hypotension occurs, patient should be placed in supine position and, if needed, given an I.V. infusion of normal saline.

## Clinical considerations
■ Pharmacokinetics of drug aren't altered in patients with renal impairment or in patients on hemodialysis. Irbesartan isn't removed by hemodialysis. Dosage adjustment isn't needed in patients with mild to severe renal impairment unless patient with renal impairment is also volume depleted.
■ Dosage adjustment isn't needed in patients with hepatic insufficiency.
■ Patients not adequately treated by the maximum 300-mg once-daily dose are unlikely to derive additional benefit from a higher dose or twice-daily dosing.

### Therapeutic monitoring
■ Advise clinician to monitor blood pressure regularly. A transient hypotensive response isn't a contraindication to further treatment. Therapy with irbesartan can usually be continued once blood pressure has stabilized. Systolic blood pressure is now principal endpoint.

### Special populations
**Pregnant patients.** Contraindicated during pregnancy because of potential danger to the fetus. The patient should immediately call prescriber if pregnancy is suspected.
**Breast-feeding patients.** Because of the potential for serious adverse reactions in breast-fed infants, alternative feeding method should be used during drug therapy.
**Pediatric patients.** Safety and efficacy in children under age 18 have not been established.

## Patient counseling
■ Instruct patient on proper administration of the drug and potential adverse reactions.
■ Advise patient that if a dose is missed, he should take it as soon as possible, but not double the dose.
■ Warn patient about symptoms of hypotension and what to do if these develop.
■ Caution patient not to discontinue drug without medical approval.

# irinotecan hydrochloride
Camptosar

*Pharmacologic classification:* topoisomerase inhibitor
*Therapeutic classification:* antineoplastic
*Pregnancy risk category D*

## Available forms
Available by prescription only
*Injection:* 20 mg/ml

## Indications and dosages
***Treatment of metastatic carcinoma of the colon or rectum in which the disease has recurred or progressed following fluorouracil (5-FU)-based therapy***
*Adults:* Initially, 125 mg/m$^2$ I.V. infusion over 90 minutes. Recommended treatment regimen is 125 mg/m$^2$ I.V. given once weekly for 4 weeks, followed by a 2-week rest period. Thereafter, additional courses of treatment may be repeated q 6 weeks (4 weeks on therapy, followed by 2 weeks off therapy). Subsequent doses may be adjusted to as high as 150 mg/m$^2$ or to as low as 50 mg/m$^2$ in 25- to 50-mg/m$^2$ increments depending on patient's tolerance. Treatment with additional courses may continue indefinitely in patients who attain a response or in those whose disease remains stable provided intolerable toxicity does not occur.
***First-line treatment of carcinoma of the colon or rectum with 5-FU and leucovorin***
*Adults:* 125 mg/m$^2$ I.V. infusion over 90 minutes on days 1, 8, 15 and 22, with leucovorin 20 mg/m$^2$ I.V. bolus immediately after Camptosar and 5-FU 500 mg/m$^2$ I.V. bolus immediately after leucovorin; or, 180 mg/m$^2$ I.V. infusion over 90 minutes on days 1, 15, and 29, with leucovorin 200 mg/m$^2$ I.V. infusion over 2 hours on days 1, 2, 15, 16, 29, and 30; 5-FU 400 mg/m$^2$ I.V. bolus on days 1, 2, 15, 16, 29, and 30; and 600 mg/m$^2$ 5-FU I.V. over 22 hours on days 1, 2, 15, 16, 29, and 30.

## I.V. administration
■ Drug solution is stable for up to 24 hours at controlled room temperature of 77° F (25° C) and in ambient fluorescent lighting. Store solutions diluted in D$_5$W in refrigerator (35° to 46° F [2° to 8° C]) and protect from light; these are stable for 48 hours. However, because of possible microbial contamination during dilution, use admixture within 24 hours if refrigerated or within 6 hours if kept at room temperature. Refrigeration of admixtures using normal saline isn't recommended because of a low and sporadic incidence of visible particulates.
■ Freezing of drug and admixtures should be avoided because drug may precipitate.

■ Irinotecan must be diluted before infusion with D$_5$W injection (preferred) or normal saline injection to a final concentration range of 0.12 to 1.1 mg/ml.

### Incompatibilities
Other drugs shouldn't be added to an irinotecan infusion.

## Mechanism of action
*Antineoplastic action:* Irinotecan is a derivative of camptothecin. Camptothecins interact specifically with the enzyme topoisomerase I, which relieves torsional strain in DNA by inducing reversible single-strand breaks. Irinotecan and its active metabolite bind to the topoisomerase I–DNA complex and prevent religation of these single-strand breaks.

## Pharmacokinetics
*Absorption:* Administered I.V.
*Distribution:* About 30% to 68% plasma protein–bound, whereas its active metabolite, SN-38, is about 95% bound.
*Metabolism:* Undergoes metabolic conversion in the liver to its active metabolite SN-38.
*Excretion:* Small amounts of drug and SN-38 are excreted in urine. Terminal half-life of irinotecan is 6 hours in patients ages 65 and older and 5½ hours in patients under age 65; mean terminal elimination half-life of SN-38 is about 10 hours.

| Route | Onset | Peak | Duration |
|-------|-------|------|----------|
| I.V. | Unknown | Unknown | Unknown |

## Contraindications and precautions
Contraindicated in patients hypersensitive to drug.

Use cautiously in geriatric patients and in those who have previously received pelvic or abdominal irradiation because of increased risk of severe myelosuppression. Because of possible fetal risk, drug shouldn't be used during pregnancy.

## Interactions
**Drug-drug.** *Other antineoplastics:* May cause additive adverse effects such as myelosuppression and diarrhea. Advise clinician to monitor patient closely.

## Adverse reactions
**CNS:** *insomnia, dizziness, asthenia, headache.*
**CV:** *vasodilation, edema.*
**EENT:** *rhinitis.*
**GI:** DIARRHEA, *nausea, vomiting, anorexia, constipation, flatulence, stomatitis, dyspepsia, abdominal cramping and pain, abdominal enlargement.*
**Hematologic:** LEUKOPENIA, *anemia,* NEUTROPENIA.
**Hepatic:** *increased alkaline phosphatase, increased AST levels.*

**Metabolic:** *weight loss, dehydration.*
**Musculoskeletal:** *back pain.*
**Respiratory:** *dyspnea, increased coughing.*
**Skin:** *alopecia, sweating, rash.*
**Other:** *fever, pain, chills, minor infection.*

## Overdose and treatment
The adverse effects of overdose are similar to those reported with the recommended dosage and regimen. There's no known antidote for drug overdose. Maximum supportive care should be instituted to prevent dehydration because of diarrhea and to treat any infectious complications.

## Clinical considerations
■ Irinotecan can induce severe forms of diarrhea.
■ Routine administration of a colony-stimulating factor isn't needed but may be helpful in patients experiencing significant neutropenia.

### Therapeutic monitoring
■ Careful monitoring of the WBC count with differential, hemoglobin, and platelet count is recommended before each dose of irinotecan.
■ Recommend temporarily stopping therapy if neutropenic fever occurs or if the absolute neutrophil count drops below 500/mm$^3$. Recommend reducing drug dosage if there's a clinically significant decrease in the total WBC count (less than 2,000/mm$^3$), neutrophil count (less than 1,000/mm$^3$), hemoglobin (less than 8 g/dl), or platelet count (less than 100,000/mm$^3$). Recommend consulting manufacturer for dosage guidelines in these situations.

### Special populations
**Pregnant patients.** Drug may be harmful to fetus.
**Breast-feeding patients.** It's unknown if drug appears in breast milk. Because of the potential for serious adverse reactions in breast-fed infants, breast-feeding should be stopped during irinotecan therapy.
**Pediatric patients.** Safety and efficacy in children haven't been established.
**Geriatric patients.** Caution should be used when drug is given to geriatric patients, especially those with history of HF and hypotension.

## Patient counseling
■ Advise women of childbearing age to avoid pregnancy because drug may cause fetal harm.
■ Inform patient about risk of diarrhea and when and how to treat it if it occurs.
■ Tell patient to call prescriber if vomiting occurs, fever or evidence of infection develops, or symptoms of dehydration (fainting, lightheadedness, or dizziness) occur after drug administration.
■ Warn patient that alopecia may occur.

---

# iron dextran

DexFerrum, InFeD

*Pharmacologic classification:* parenteral iron supplement
*Therapeutic classification:* hematinic
*Pregnancy risk category C*

## Available forms

Available by prescription only
*Injection:* 50 mg elemental iron/ml in 2-ml single-dose vials

## Indications and dosages

*Iron-deficiency anemia*
*Adults and children:* Dosage is highly individualized and is based on patient's weight and hemoglobin level. Drug is usually given I.M.; preservative-free solution can be given I.V. Check current literature for recommended protocol.

## I.V. administration

■ I.V. use is controversial, and some health care facilities don't allow it. I.V. is route of choice if patient has insufficient muscle mass for deep injection, impaired absorption from muscle because of stasis or edema, risk of uncontrolled I.M. bleeding from trauma (as in hemophilia), or need for massive and prolonged parenteral therapy (as in chronic substantial blood loss).
■ Give no more than 50 mg of iron per minute (1 ml per minute) if using drug undiluted.
■ Vein must be flushed with 10 ml normal saline injection to minimize local irritation.

### Incompatibilities

Don't mix with other drugs or add to parenteral nutrition solutions for I.V. infusion.

## Mechanism of action

*Hematinic action:* Iron dextran is a complex of ferric hydroxide and dextran in a colloidal solution. After I.M. injection, 10% to 50% remains in the muscle for several months; remainder enters bloodstream, increasing plasma iron level for up to 2 weeks. Iron is an essential component of hemoglobin.

## Pharmacokinetics

*Absorption:* I.M. doses are absorbed in two stages: 60% after 3 days, and up to 90% by 3 weeks. Remainder is absorbed over several months or longer.
*Distribution:* During first 3 days, local inflammation facilitates passage of drug into the lymphatic system; drug is then ingested by macrophages, which enter lymph and blood.
*Metabolism:* After I.M. or I.V. administration, iron dextran is cleared from plasma by reticuloendothelial cells of the liver, spleen, and bone marrow.

*Excretion:* In doses of 500 mg or less, half-life is 6 hours. Traces appear in breast milk and are excreted in urine, bile, and feces. Drug can't be removed by hemodialysis.

| Route | Onset | Peak | Duration |
|-------|-------|------|----------|
| I.M., I.V. | Unknown | Unknown | Unknown |

## Contraindications and precautions

Contraindicated in patients hypersensitive to drug, in those with all types of anemia except iron-deficiency anemia, and in those with acute infectious renal disease.

Use cautiously in patients with impaired hepatic function, rheumatoid arthritis, and other inflammatory diseases.

## Interactions

**Drug-herb.** *Black cohosh, chamomile, feverfew, gossypol, hawthorn, nettle, plantain, St. John's wort:* Decreased iron absorption. Discourage use together.
*Oregano:* Reduced iron absorption. Separate administration by at least 2 hours when giving with iron supplements or iron-containing foods.

## Adverse reactions

**CNS:** headache, transitory paresthesia, dizziness, malaise.
**CV:** *hypotensive reaction, peripheral vascular flushing (with overly rapid I.V. administration),* bradycardia.
**GI:** nausea, anorexia.
**Musculoskeletal:** arthralgia, myalgia.
**Respiratory:** *bronchospasm,* dyspnea.
**Skin:** rash, urticaria, purpura, *brown skin discoloration (at I.M. injection site); local phlebitis (at I.V. injection site),* sterile abscess, necrosis, atrophy, fibrosis.
**Other:** *soreness, inflammation, anaphylaxis,* delayed sensitivity reactions, fever, chills.

## Overdose and treatment

Injected iron has much greater bioavailability than oral iron, but data on acute overdose are limited.

## Clinical considerations

■ Oral iron should be discarded before iron dextran is given.
■ Recommend giving a test dose of 0.5 ml iron dextrose I.M. or I.V. and monitoring patient for drug reactions, including anaphylaxis. Recommend keeping epinephrine (0.5 ml of a 1:1,000 solution) readily available for such an emergency.
■ I.V. use is controversial, and some health care facilities don't allow it. I.V. is route of choice if patient has insufficient muscle mass for deep injection, impaired absorption from muscle because of stasis or edema, risk of uncontrolled I.M. bleeding from trauma (as in hemophilia), or need for massive and prolonged parenteral therapy (as in chronic substantial blood loss).

Give no more than 50 mg of iron per minute (1 ml per minute) if using drug undiluted. Vein must be flushed with 10 ml normal saline injection to minimize local irritation.

■ Large doses (more than 250 mg iron) may color the serum brown. Iron dextran may cause false elevations of serum bilirubin level and false reductions in serum calcium level. Iron dextran prevents meaningful measurement of serum iron level and total iron binding capacity for up to 3 weeks; I.M. injection may cause dense areas of activity on bone scans using technetium 99m diphosphonate, for 1 to 6 days.

### Therapeutic monitoring
■ Advise clinician to monitor hemoglobin, hematocrit, and reticulocyte count during therapy. An increase of about 1 g/dl weekly in hemoglobin is usual.
■ Advise clinician to monitor patient for tissue damage and adverse events.

### Special populations
**Breast-feeding patients.** Traces of unmetabolized iron dextran appear in breast milk; impact on infant is unknown.
**Pediatric patients.** Drug isn't recommended for use in children under age 4 months.

## Patient counseling
■ Warn patient of possibility of skin staining with I.M. injections.

---

# iron sucrose injection
Venofer

*Pharmacologic classification:* polynuclear iron (III)-hydroxide in sucrose
*Therapeutic classification:* hematinic
*Pregnancy risk category B*

## Available forms
Available by prescription only
*Injection:* 20 mg/ml of elemental iron

## Indications and dosages
*Iron-deficiency anemia in patients undergoing long-term hemodialysis who are receiving supplemental erythropoietin therapy*
*Adults:* 100 mg (5 ml) of elemental iron I.V. directly into the dialysis line either by slow injection (1 ml per minute) or by infusion over 15 minutes during the dialysis session one to three times weekly to a total of 1,000 mg in 10 doses. Repeat if needed.

## I.V. administration
■ Inspect for particulate matter and discoloration before administration.
■ For administration by slow injection, give 1 ml (20 mg elemental iron) undiluted solution per minute, not exceeding one vial (100 mg elemental iron) per injection.
■ For administration by infusion, dilute to a maximum of 100 ml in normal saline solution immediately before infusion, and infuse 100 mg elemental iron over at least 15 minutes.

### Incompatibilities
Don't mix with other drugs or add to parenteral nutrition solutions of I.V. infusion.

## Mechanism of action
*Iron replacement action:* Iron is essential to the synthesis of hemoglobin to maintain oxygen transport and to the function and formation of other physiologically important heme and non-heme compounds. After administration, drug is dissociated by the reticuloendothelial system into iron and sucrose. The released iron component eventually replenishes depleted body iron stores, resulting in significant increases in serum iron and serum ferritin and significant decreases in total iron binding capacity.

## Pharmacokinetics
*Absorption:* Administered I.V.
*Distribution:* Distributed mainly in blood and somewhat in extravascular fluid. A significant amount of iron is also distributed in the liver, spleen, and bone marrow.
*Metabolism:* Dissociated by the reticuloendothelial system into iron and sucrose.
*Excretion:* About 75% of sucrose and 5% of the iron component are eliminated by urinary excretion in 24 hours. In healthy adults, elimination half-life is 6 hours.

| Route | Onset | Peak | Duration |
|-------|-------|------|----------|
| I.V. | Unknown | Unknown | Variable |

## Contraindications and precautions
Contraindicated in patients with evidence of iron overload, patients hypersensitive to drug or any of its inactive components, and patients with anemia not caused by iron deficiency.

## Interactions
**Drug-drug.** *Oral iron preparations:* Reduced absorption of these compounds. Avoid use together.
**Drug-herb.** *Black cohosh, chamomile, feverfew, gossypol, hawthorn, nettle, plantain, St. John's wort:* Decreased iron absorption. Use together should be discouraged.

## Adverse reactions
**CNS:** headache, asthenia, malaise, dizziness.
**CV:** *hypotension,* chest pain, hypertension, fluid retention.
**GI:** nausea, vomiting, diarrhea, abdominal pain.
**Hepatic:** elevated liver enzyme levels.
**Musculoskeletal:** *leg cramps,* bone and muscle pain.

---

**Respiratory:** dyspnea, pneumonia, cough.
**Skin:** pruritus, application site reaction.
**Other:** fever, accidental injury, pain.

## Overdose and treatment

Symptoms of overdose or too-rapid infusion include hypotension, headache, nausea, dizziness, joint aches, paresthesia, abdominal and muscle pain, edema, and CV collapse.

Administering the solution more slowly and treating with I.V. fluids, hydrocortisone, or antihistamines may alleviate most symptoms.

## Clinical considerations

■ Rare but fatal hypersensitivity reactions characterized by anaphylaxis, loss of consciousness, collapse, hypotension, dyspnea, or convulsion have been reported.
■ Administering by infusion may reduce the risk of hypotension.
■ Dose should be withheld in patients with evidence of iron overload.

### Therapeutic monitoring

■ Transferrin saturation values increase rapidly after I.V. administration of iron sucrose. Advise clinician to obtain serum iron values 48 hours after I.V. dosing.
■ Advise clinician to monitor hemoglobin, hematocrit, serum ferritin, and transferrin saturation.

### Special populations

**Breast-feeding patients.** It's not known if drug appears in breast milk. Use cautiously when giving to breast-feeding women.
**Pediatric patients.** Safety and efficacy haven't been established.
**Geriatric patients.** Dose selection in geriatric patients should be conservative because of the possibility that they have decreased hepatic, renal, and cardiac function; concomitant disease; and other drug therapy.

## Patient counseling

■ Instruct patient to notify prescriber if symptoms of overdose occur, such as headache, nausea, dizziness, joint aches, paresthesia, or abdominal and muscle pain.

# isoniazid (INH)

Isotamine*, Laniazid, Laniazid C.T., Nydrazid, PMS Isoniazid*

*Pharmacologic classification:* isonicotinic acid hydrazine
*Therapeutic classification:* antitubercular
*Pregnancy risk category C*

## Available forms

Available by prescription only
*Tablets:* 50 mg, 100 mg, 300 mg
*Oral solution:* 50 mg/5 ml
*Injection:* 100 mg/ml

## Indications and dosages

*Primary treatment against actively growing tubercle bacilli*
*Adults:* 5 to 10 mg/kg P.O. or I.M. daily in a single dose, up to 300 mg/day.
*Infants and children:* 10 to 20 mg/kg P.O. or I.M. daily in a single dose, up to 300 to 500 mg/day.

Note: Concomitant administration of at least one other effective antitubercular drug is recommended, and therapy should be continued long enough to prevent relapse.
*Treatment of latent tuberculosis infection*
*Adults:* 300 mg P.O. daily single dose, or 15 mg/kg (not to exceed 900 mg/day) twice weekly continued for 9 months.
*Infants and children:* 10 to 15 mg/kg P.O. daily single dose, up to 300 mg/day, continued for 6 months to 1 year, or 20 to 30 mg/kg (up to 900 mg) twice weekly for 9 months. In HIV-infected infants and children, therapy should continue for a minimum of 9 to 12 months.

## Mechanism of action

*Antitubercular action:* INH interferes with lipid and DNA synthesis, thus inhibiting bacterial cell wall synthesis. Its action is bacteriostatic or bactericidal, depending on organism susceptibility and drug level at infection site. INH is active against *Mycobacterium tuberculosis, M. bovis,* and some strains of *M. kansasii.*

Resistance by *M. tuberculosis* develops rapidly when INH is used to treat tuberculosis, and it's usually combined with another antitubercular drug to prevent or delay resistance. During prophylaxis, however, resistance isn't a problem and isoniazid can be used alone.

## Pharmacokinetics

*Absorption:* Rapidly and completely absorbed from the GI tract after oral administration. INH also is absorbed readily after I.M. injection.
*Distribution:* Distributed widely into body tissues and fluids, including ascitic, synovial, pleural, and cerebrospinal fluids; lungs and other organs; and sputum and saliva. Drug crosses the placenta and appears in breast milk in levels similar to plasma.
*Metabolism:* Inactivated primarily in the liver by genetically controlled acetylation. Rate of metabolism varies individually; fast acetylators metabolize drug five times as rapidly as others. About 50% of blacks and whites are slow acetylators of INH, whereas more than 80% of Chinese, Japanese, and Eskimos are fast acetylators.
*Excretion:* About 75% of a dose is excreted in urine in 24 hours as unchanged drug and metabolites; some drug is excreted in saliva, sputum, and feces, and appears in breast milk. Plasma half-life in adults is 1 to 4 hours, de-

pending on metabolic rate. Drug is removed by peritoneal dialysis or hemodialysis.

| Route | Onset | Peak | Duration |
|-------|-------|------|----------|
| P.O. | Unknown | 1-2 hr | Unknown |
| I.M. | Unknown | Unknown | Unknown |

## Contraindications and precautions

Contraindicated in patients with acute hepatic disease or drug-associated hepatic damage.

Use cautiously in geriatric patients and in patients with severe, non-INH-associated hepatic disease, seizure disorders (especially those taking phenytoin), severe renal impairment, or chronic alcoholism.

## Interactions

**Drug-drug.** *Antacids:* Decreased oral absorption of INH. Antacid should be given at least 1 hour before INH.

*Anticoagulants:* May increase anticoagulant activity. Dosage adjustment may be needed.

*Benzodiazepines (such as diazepam), carbamazepine, phenytoin:* INH-induced inhibition of metabolism and elevation of serum levels, causing toxicity. Advise clinician to monitor patient closely.

*Corticosteroids:* May decrease INH efficacy. Advise clinician to monitor patient for drug effects.

*Cycloserine:* Increased hazard of CNS toxicity, drowsiness, and dizziness. Advise clinician to monitor patient for safety.

*Disulfiram:* May cause coordination difficulties and psychotic episodes. Patient requires close observation.

*Rifampin:* May accelerate INH metabolism to hepatotoxic metabolites. Use with caution.

**Drug-lifestyle.** *Alcohol use:* Increased risk of INH-induced hepatitis and seizures. Advise patient to avoid alcohol.

## Adverse reactions

**CNS:** *peripheral neuropathy* (dose-related and especially in patients who are malnourished, alcoholic, diabetic, or slow acetylators), usually preceded by paresthesia of hands and feet, *seizures,* toxic encephalopathy, memory impairment, toxic psychosis.

**EENT:** optic neuritis, atrophy.

**GI:** nausea, vomiting, epigastric distress.

**Hematologic:** *agranulocytosis,* hemolytic anemia, *aplastic anemia,* eosinophilia, *thrombocytopenia,* sideroblastic anemia.

**Hepatic:** *hepatitis* (occasionally severe and sometimes fatal, especially in geriatric patients), jaundice, *elevated serum transaminase levels,* bilirubinemia.

**Metabolic:** hyperglycemia, metabolic acidosis, pyridoxine deficiency, hypocalcemia, hypophosphatemia.

**Skin:** irritation at I.M. injection site.

**Other:** rheumatic and lupuslike syndromes, hypersensitivity reactions (fever, rash, lymphadenopathy, vasculitis), gynecomastia.

## Overdose and treatment

Early signs of overdose include nausea, vomiting, slurred speech, dizziness, blurred vision, and visual hallucinations, occurring 30 minutes to 3 hours after ingestion; gross overdose causes CNS depression progressing from stupor to coma, with respiratory distress, intractable seizures, and death.

To treat, recommend establishing ventilation and controlling seizures with diazepam. Pyridoxine is given to equal dose of INH. Initial dose is 1 to 4 g pyridoxine I.V., followed by 1 g every 30 minutes thereafter, until the entire dose is given. Recommend clearing drug with gastric lavage after seizure control and correcting acidosis with parenteral sodium bicarbonate; recommend forcing diuresis with I.V. fluids and osmotic diuretics, and, if needed, enhancing clearance of the drug with hemodialysis or peritoneal dialysis.

## Clinical considerations

- At least 12 months of preventive therapy is recommended for patients with past tuberculosis and HIV-infected patients.
- If compliance is a problem, twice-weekly supervised drug administration may be used.
- Oral doses should be taken on empty stomach for maximum absorption, or with food if gastric irritation occurs.
- Aluminum-containing antacids or laxatives should be taken 1 hour after oral dose of INH.
- Drug may hinder stabilization of glucose level in patients with diabetes mellitus.
- Pyridoxine 50 mg P.O. daily is sometimes recommended to prevent peripheral neuropathy from large doses of INH. It may also be useful in patients at risk of developing peripheral neuropathy (malnourished patients, diabetics, and alcohol abusers). Pyridoxine (50 to 200 mg daily) has been used to treat drug-induced neuropathy.
- Because drug is dialyzable, patients undergoing hemodialysis or peritoneal dialysis may need dosage adjustments.
- INH alters results of urine glucose tests that use cupric sulfate method (Benedict's reagent, Diastix, or Chemstrip uG). Elevated liver function test results occur in about 15% of cases; most abnormalities are mild and transient, but some persist throughout treatment.

### Therapeutic monitoring

- Advise clinician to monitor patient for adverse effects, especially hepatic dysfunction, CNS toxicity, and optic neuritis.
- Advise clinician to monitor blood, renal, and hepatic function test results before and periodically during therapy to minimize toxicity; recommend assessing visual function periodically.

- Hepatotoxicity appears to be age-related and may limit use for prophylaxis. Alcohol consumption and history of alcohol-related liver disease also increases risk of hepatotoxicity.
- Improvement is usually evident after 2 to 3 weeks of therapy.

### Special populations
**Pregnant patients.** Safe use of drug during pregnancy hasn't been established. Potential benefits to the woman should be weighed against the risks to the fetus.
**Breast-feeding patients.** Drug appears in breast milk; use with caution in breast-feeding women and recommend monitoring infants for possible INH-induced toxicity.
**Pediatric patients.** Infants and children tolerate larger doses of drug.
**Geriatric patients.** Use with caution in geriatric patients; risk of hepatic effects is increased after age 35. Drug prophylaxis in patients with a positive purified protein derivative test may not be indicated in older patients because of risk of hepatotoxicity.

### Patient counseling
- Instruct patient on proper administration of the drug and the potential for adverse reactions.
- Advise patient to avoid alcohol.
- Urge patient to comply with and complete prescribed regimen.
- Advise patient not to discontinue drug without medical approval.
- Explain importance of follow-up appointments.

# isoproterenol
Isuprel

# isoproterenol hydrochloride
Isuprel, Isuprel Mistometer

# isoproterenol sulfate
Medihaler-Iso

*Pharmacologic classification:* adrenergic
*Therapeutic classification:* bronchodilator, cardiac stimulant
*Pregnancy risk category C*

### Available forms
Available by prescription only
**isoproterenol**
*Nebulizer inhaler:* 0.25%, 0.5%, 1%
**isoproterenol hydrochloride**
*Aerosol inhaler:* 120 mcg/metered spray, 131 mcg/metered spray
*Injection:* 20 mcg/ml, 200 mcg/ml
**isoproterenol sulfate**
*Aerosol inhaler:* 80 mcg/metered spray

## Indications and dosages
*Complete heart block after closure of ventricular septal defect*
*Adults:* I.V. bolus, 0.04 to 0.06 mg (2 to 3 ml of a 1:50,000 dilution).
*Children:* I.V. bolus, 0.01 to 0.03 mg (0.5 to 1.5 ml of a 1:50,000 dilution).
*Bronchospasm during mild acute asthma attacks*
**isoproterenol hydrochloride**
*Adults and children:* Via aerosol inhalation, 1 inhalation initially, repeated, p.r.n. after 1 to 5 minutes, to maximum 6 inhalations daily. Maintenance dosage is 1 to 2 inhalations four to six times daily at 3- to 4-hour intervals. Via hand-bulb nebulizer, 5 to 15 deep inhalations of a 0.5% solution; if needed, may be repeated in 5 to 10 minutes. May be repeated up to five times daily.

Alternatively, 3 to 7 deep inhalations of a 1% solution, repeated once in 5 to 10 minutes if needed. May be repeated up to five times daily.
**isoproterenol sulfate**
*Adults and children:* For acute dyspneic episodes, 1 inhalation initially; repeated if needed after 2 to 5 minutes. Maximum 6 inhalations daily. Maintenance dosage is 1 to 2 inhalations up to six times daily.
*Bronchospasm in COPD*
**isoproterenol hydrochloride**
*Adults and children: Via hand-bulb nebulizer:* 5 to 15 deep inhalations of a 0.5% solution, or 3 to 7 deep inhalations of a 1% solution no more frequently than q 3 to 4 hours.
*Bronchospasm during mild acute asthma attacks or in COPD*
**isoproterenol hydrochloride**
*Adults and children:* Oral inhalation of 2 ml of 0.125% solution or 2.5 ml of 0.1% solution up to five times daily.
*Acute asthma attacks unresponsive to inhalation therapy or control of bronchospasm during anesthesia*
**isoproterenol hydrochloride**
*Adults:* 0.01 to 0.02 mg (0.5 to 1 ml of a 1:50,000 dilution) I.V. Repeat, if needed.
*Emergency treatment of arrhythmias*
**isoproterenol hydrochloride**
*Adults:* Initially, 0.02 to 0.06 mg I.V. bolus. Subsequent doses 0.01 to 0.2 mg I.V. Alternatively, 5 mcg/minute titrated to patient's response. Range, 2 to 20 mcg/minute. Alternatively, 0.2 mg I.M. or S.C.; subsequent doses 0.02 to 1 mg I.M. or 0.15 to 0.2 mg S.C. In extreme cases, 0.02 mg (0.1 of 1:5,000) intracardiac injection.
*Immediate temporary control of atropine-resistant hemodynamically significant bradycardia*
**isoproterenol hydrochloride**
*Adults:* 2 to 10 mcg/minute I.V. infusion, titrated to patient's response.

---

*Children:* 0.1 mcg/kg/minute, titrated to patient's response. Maximum rate, 1 mcg/kg/minute.

**Heart block, Stokes-Adams attacks, and shock**

**isoproterenol hydrochloride**

*Adults and children:* 0.5 to 5 mcg/minute by continuous I.V. infusion titrated to patient's response; or 0.02 to 0.06 mg I.V. boluses with 0.01 to 0.2 mg additional doses; or 0.2 mg I.M. or S.C. with 0.02 to 1 mg I.M. or 0.15 to 0.2 mg additional doses.

**Postoperative cardiac patients with bradycardia**

**isoproterenol**

*Children:* I.V. infusion of 0.029 mcg/kg/minute.

**As an aid in diagnosing the etiology of mitral regurgitation**

*Adults:* 4 mcg/min I.V. infusion.

**As an aid in diagnosing coronary artery disease or lesions**

*Adults:* 1 to 3 mcg/min I.V. infusion.

**Status asthmaticus**

*Children:* 0.08 to 1.7 mcg/kg/minute I.V. infusion. Advise clinician to monitor cardiac function.

## I.V. administration

■ Drug must be diluted and given via slow I.V. infusion. Discard remaining contents.

■ Prescribed I.V. infusion rate should include specific guidelines for regulating flow or terminating infusion in relation to heart rate, premature beats, ECG changes, precordial distress, blood pressure, and urine flow. Because of danger of precipitating arrhythmias, rate of infusion is usually decreased or infusion may be temporarily discontinued if heart rate exceeds 110 beats per minute.

■ Continuously monitor ECG during I.V. administration.

### Incompatibilities

Incompatible with alkalies, aminophylline, furosemide, metals, and sodium bicarbonate.

## Mechanism of action

*Bronchodilator action:* Isoproterenol relaxes bronchial smooth muscle by direct action on beta$_2$-adrenergic receptors, relieving bronchospasm, increasing vital capacity, decreasing residual volume in lungs, and facilitating passage of pulmonary secretions. It also produces relaxation of GI and uterine smooth muscle via stimulation of beta$_2$ receptors. Peripheral vasodilation, cardiac stimulation, and relaxation of bronchial smooth muscle are the main therapeutic effects.

*Cardiac stimulant action:* Isoproterenol acts on beta$_1$-adrenergic receptors in the heart, producing a positive chronotropic and inotropic effect; it usually increases cardiac output. In patients with AV block, isoproterenol shortens conduction time and the refractory period of the AV node and increases the rate and strength of ventricular contraction.

## Pharmacokinetics

*Absorption:* After injection or oral inhalation, absorption is rapid; after S.L. or rectal administration, absorption is variable and often unreliable.

*Distribution:* Distributed widely.

*Metabolism:* Metabolized by conjugation in the GI tract and by enzymatic reduction in liver, lungs, and other tissues.

*Excretion:* Excreted primarily in urine as unchanged drug and its metabolites.

| Route | Onset | Peak | Duration |
|---|---|---|---|
| I.V. | Immediate | Unknown | Few minutes |
| S.C. | Immediate | Unknown | 2 hr |
| Oral inhalation | Immediate | Unknown | Unknown |

## Contraindications and precautions

Contraindicated in patients with tachycardia caused by digitalis intoxication, in patients with preexisting arrhythmias (other than those that may respond to treatment with isoproterenol), and in those with angina pectoris.

Use cautiously in geriatric patients and in patients with impaired renal function, CV disease, coronary insufficiency, diabetes, hyperthyroidism, or sensitivity to sympathomimetic amines.

## Interactions

**Drug-drug.** *Beta blockers:* Antagonize cardiac-stimulating, bronchodilating, and vasodilating effects of isoproterenol. Advise clinician to monitor patient closely.

*Cardiac glycoside, potassium-depleting drugs, or other drugs that affect cardiac rhythm:* Arrhythmias may occur. Advise clinician to monitor patient's ECG.

*Cyclopropane or halogenated hydrocarbon general anesthetics:* Increased risk of arrhythmias. Use together should be avoided.

*Epinephrine and other sympathomimetics:* May cause additive CV reactions. Drugs may be used together if at least 4 hours elapse between administration of the two drugs. Use together cautiously.

*Ergot alkaloids:* May increase blood pressure. Use with caution.

*Xanthine derivatives, I.V. corticosteroids:* May have additive cardiotoxic effects. Advise clinician to monitor patient closely.

## Adverse reactions

**CNS:** *headache, mild tremor,* weakness, dizziness, *nervousness,* insomnia, **Stokes-Adams attacks.**

**CV:** palpitations, *tachycardia, anginal pain,* **arrhythmias, cardiac arrest,** *rapid increase and decrease in blood pressure.*

---

**GI:** *nausea, vomiting, heartburn.*
**Metabolic:** hyperglycemia.
**Respiratory:** *bronchospasm,* bronchitis, sputum increase, pulmonary edema.
**Skin:** diaphoresis.
**Other:** swelling of parotid glands (with prolonged use).

## Overdose and treatment
Signs and symptoms of overdose include exaggeration of common adverse reactions, particularly arrhythmias, extreme tremors, nausea, vomiting, and profound hypotension.

Treatment includes symptomatic and supportive measures. Advise clinician to monitor vital signs closely. Sedatives (barbiturates) may be used to treat CNS stimulation. Recommend using cardioselective beta blockers to treat tachycardia and arrhythmias. These drugs should be used with caution; they may induce asthmatic attack.

## Clinical considerations
- Drug doesn't replace administration of blood, plasma, fluids, or electrolytes in patients with blood volume depletion.
- Severe paradoxical airway resistance may follow oral inhalations.
- Hypotension must be corrected before isoproterenol is given.
- Isoproterenol has also been used to aid diagnosis of coronary artery disease and of mitral regurgitation.
- Risk factors for cardiotoxicity with I.V. infusions for the treatment of severe asthma include hypercapnia and concomitant use of a theophylline derivative or corticosteroids.
- Use for temporary immediate control of hemodynamically significant bradycardia is limited to when atropine and dobutamine have failed and when transcutaneous and transvenous pacing are not available.
- Isoproterenol may reduce the sensitivity of spirometry in the diagnosis of asthma.

### Therapeutic monitoring
- Advise clinician to carefully monitor response to therapy by frequent determinations of heart rate, ECG pattern, blood pressure, and central venous pressure, as well as (for patients in shock) urine volume, blood pH, and $Pco_2$ levels.
- Advise clinician to monitor patient for rebound bronchospasm when effects of drug end.
- If three to five treatments within 6 to 12 hours provide minimal or no relief, reevaluate therapy.

### Special populations
**Pregnant patients.** Drug should be given during pregnancy only when clearly indicated.
**Breast-feeding patients.** It's unknown if drug appears in breast milk; therefore, it should be used cautiously in breast-feeding women.

**Pediatric patients.** Safety and efficacy have not been established. Use with caution in children.
**Geriatric patients.** Geriatric patients may be more sensitive to therapeutic and adverse effects of drug.

## Patient counseling
- Urge patient to call prescriber if no relief is gained or condition worsens.
- Advise patient to store oral forms away from heat and light (not in bathroom medicine cabinet where heat and moisture will cause deterioration of the drug) and to keep drug out of the reach of children.
**Inhalation**
- Give patient instructions on proper use of inhaler.
- Tell patient that saliva and sputum may appear red or pink after oral inhalation, because isoproterenol turns red on exposure to air.
- Advise patient to rinse mouth with water after drug is absorbed completely and between doses.
**Sublingual**
- Tell patient to allow S.L. tablet to dissolve under tongue, without sucking, and not to swallow saliva (may cause epigastric pain) until drug has been absorbed completely.
- Warn patient that frequent use of S.L. tablets may damage teeth because of acidity of drug.

# isosorbide dinitrate
Apo-ISDN\*, Coronex\*, Dilatrate-SR,
Iso-Bid, Isonate, Isordil, Isordil
Titradose, Isotrate, Novosorbide\*,
Sorbitrate, Sorbitrate SA

*Pharmacologic classification:* nitrate
*Therapeutic classification:* antianginal, vasodilator
*Pregnancy risk category C*

## Available forms
Available by prescription only
*Tablets:* 5 mg, 10 mg, 20 mg, 30 mg, 40 mg
*Tablets (S.L.):* 2.5 mg, 5 mg, 10 mg
*Tablets (extended-release):* 40 mg
*Tablets (chewable):* 5 mg, 10 mg
*Capsules (extended-release):* 40 mg

## Indications and dosages
*Acute relief of angina pectoris or prophylaxis in situations likely to provoke angina attacks in patients who don't respond to nitroglycerin lingual or S.L. preparations*
Adults: 2.5 to 5 mg S.L., intrabuccally, or as a chewable tablet. Additional doses may be given at 5- to 10-minute intervals (up to 3 doses in a 15- to 30-minute period). For prophylaxis, 2.5 to 5 mg should be placed under the tongue about 15 minutes before activity.

***Long-term prophylaxis of angina pectoris***
*Adults:* 5 to 40 mg b.i.d. or t.i.d. P.O. of conventional tablets.

◇ ***Adjunctive treatment of heart failure***
*Adults:* 80 mg daily P.O with hydralazine. Maximum 160 mg isosorbide dinitrate and 300 mg hydralazine.

◇ ***Diffuse esophageal spasm without gastroesophageal reflux***
*Adults:* 10 to 30 mg P.O. q.i.d.

## Mechanism of action
*Antianginal action:* Drug reduces myocardial oxygen demand through peripheral vasodilation, resulting in decreased venous filling pressure (preload) and, to a lesser extent, decreased arterial impedance (afterload). These combined effects result in decreased cardiac work and, consequently, reduced myocardial oxygen demands. Drug also redistributes coronary blood flow from epicardial to subendocardial regions.
*Vasodilating action:* Drug dilates peripheral vessels (primarily venous), helping to manage pulmonary edema and HF caused by decreased venous return to the heart (preload). Arterial vasodilatory effects also decrease arterial impedance (afterload) and thus left ventricular work, benefiting the failing heart. These combined effects may help some patients with acute MI. (Use of isosorbide dinitrate in patients with HF and acute MI is currently unapproved.)

## Pharmacokinetics
*Absorption:* Oral form is well absorbed from the GI tract but undergoes first-pass metabolism, resulting in bioavailability of about 50% (depending on dosage form used).
*Distribution:* Limited information is available on plasma protein–binding and distribution of drug. Like nitroglycerin, it's distributed widely throughout the body.
*Metabolism:* Metabolized in the liver to active metabolites.
*Excretion:* Metabolites are excreted in the urine; elimination half-life is about 5 to 6 hours with oral administration; 2 hours with S.L. administration. About 80% to 100% of absorbed dose is excreted in urine within 24 hours. Duration of effect is longer than that of S.L. preparations.

| Route | Onset | Peak | Duration |
|---|---|---|---|
| P.O. | 30 min | Unknown | 5-6 hr |
| S.L., P.O. (chewable) | 3 min | Unknown | ½-2 hr |
| P.O. (extended) | 1 hr | Unknown | 5-6 hr |

## Contraindications and precautions
Contraindicated in patients with hypersensitivity or idiosyncrasy to nitrates, severe hypotension, shock, or acute MI with low left ventricular filling pressure.

Use cautiously in patients with hypotension or blood volume depletion (such as from diuretic therapy).

## Interactions
**Drug-drug.** *Antihypertensives, calcium channel blockers, phenothiazines, vasodilators:* Additive hypotensive effects. Recommend using with caution and checking blood pressure frequently.
**Drug-lifestyle.** *Alcohol use:* Additive hypotensive effects. Advise patient to avoid alcohol.

## Adverse reactions
**CNS:** *headache* (sometimes with throbbing), dizziness, weakness.
**CV:** *flushing, orthostatic hypotension, tachycardia, palpitations, ankle edema,* fainting.
**GI:** nausea, vomiting, S.L. burning.
**Skin:** cutaneous vasodilation, rash.
**Other:** hypersensitivity reactions.

## Overdose and treatment
Clinical effects of overdose result primarily from vasodilation and methemoglobinemia and include hypotension, persistent throbbing headache, palpitations, visual disturbance, flushing of the skin and sweating (with skin later becoming cold and cyanotic), nausea and vomiting, colic and bloody diarrhea, orthostatism, initial hyperpnea, dyspnea, slow respiratory rate, bradycardia, heart block, increased intracranial pressure with confusion, fever, paralysis, and tissue hypoxia, which can lead to cyanosis, metabolic acidosis, coma, clonic seizures, and circulatory collapse. Death may result from circulatory collapse or asphyxia.

Treatment includes gastric lavage followed by administration of activated charcoal to remove remaining gastric contents. Advise clinician to monitor blood gas measurements and methemoglobin levels, as indicated. Supportive care includes respiratory support and oxygen administration, passive movement of limbs to aid venous return, recumbent positioning (Trendelenburg position, if needed), maintenance of adequate body temperature, and administration of I.V. fluids.

An I.V. adrenergic agonist (such as phenylephrine) may be considered if further treatment is required. For methemoglobinemia, methylene blue (1 to 2 mg/kg I.V.) may be given. (Epinephrine and related compounds are contraindicated in isosorbide dinitrate overdose.)

## Clinical considerations
■ Drug should be stored in a cool place, in a tightly closed container away from light.
■ Maintenance of continuous 24-hour plasma levels may result in refractory tolerance. Dosing regimens should include dose-free intervals, which vary based on form of drug used.

- Drug may cause orthostatic hypotension. To minimize this, patient should change to upright position slowly, walk up and down stairs carefully, and lie down at first sign of dizziness.
- Drug shouldn't be stopped abruptly because this may cause coronary vasospasm.
- Additional dose may be given before anticipated stress or at bedtime if angina is nocturnal.
- Isosorbide dinitrate may interfere with serum cholesterol determination tests using the Zlatkis-Zak color reaction, causing a falsely decreased value.

### Therapeutic monitoring
- Advise clinician to monitor blood pressure and intensity and duration of patient's response to drug.
- Drug may cause headache, especially at first. Dosage may need to be reduced temporarily, but tolerance to this effect usually develops. In the interim, patient may relieve headache with aspirin or acetaminophen.

### Special populations
**Breast-feeding patients.** It's unknown if drug appears in breast milk. It should be used cautiously in breast-feeding women.
**Pediatric patients.** Methemoglobinemia may occur in infants receiving large doses of isosorbide dinitrate.

## Patient counseling
- Instruct patient to take drug regularly, as prescribed, and to keep it easily accessible at all times. Drug is physiologically needed but not addictive.
- Warn patient that headache may occur initially, but may respond to usual headache remedies or dosage reduction. Assure patient that headache usually subsides gradually with continued treatment.
- Tell patient to take oral tablets on an empty stomach, either 30 minutes before or 1 to 2 hours after meals; to swallow oral tablets whole; and to chew chewable tablets thoroughly before swallowing.
- Advise patient to sit when self-administering S.L. tablets. He should lubricate tablet with saliva or place a few milliliters of fluid under tongue with tablet. If patient experiences tingling sensation with drug placed S.L., he may try to hold tablet in buccal pouch. If no relief occurs, he should call or go to hospital emergency department.
- Warn patient to make positional changes gradually to avoid excessive dizziness.
- Instruct patient to avoid alcohol while taking drug because severe hypotension and CV collapse may occur.
- Advise patient to report blurred vision, dry mouth, or persistent headache.
- Caution patient not to stop long-term therapy abruptly.

# isosorbide mononitrate
Imdur, ISMO, Monoket

*Pharmacologic classification:* nitrate
*Therapeutic classification:* antianginal
*Pregnancy risk category C*

## Available forms
Available by prescription only
*Tablets:* 10 mg, 20 mg
*Tablets (extended-release):* 30 mg, 60 mg, 120 mg

## Indications and dosages
*Prevention of angina pectoris from coronary artery disease (but not to abort acute anginal attacks)*
Adults: 20 mg P.O. b.i.d., with doses 7 hours apart and first dose on awakening. For extended-release tablets, 30 to 60 mg P.O. once daily, on arising; after several days, dosage may be increased to 120 mg once daily; rarely, 240 mg may be required; extended-release tablets shouldn't be crushed or chewed.

## Mechanism of action
*Antianginal action:* Drug is the major active metabolite of isosorbide dinitrate. It relaxes vascular smooth muscle and consequently dilates peripheral arteries and veins. Dilation of the veins promotes peripheral pooling of blood and decreases venous return to the heart, thereby reducing left ventricular end-diastolic pressure and pulmonary capillary wedge pressure (preload). Arteriolar relaxation reduces systemic vascular resistance, systolic arterial pressure, and mean arterial pressure (afterload). Dilation of the coronary arteries also occurs.

## Pharmacokinetics
*Absorption:* Absolute bioavailability is almost 100%.
*Distribution:* Volume of distribution is about 0.6 L/kg. Less than 4% is bound to plasma proteins.
*Metabolism:* Drug isn't subject to first-pass metabolism in the liver.
*Excretion:* Less than 1% of isosorbide mononitrate is eliminated in urine. Overall elimination half-life of drug is about 5 hours.

| Route | Onset | Peak | Duration |
|---|---|---|---|
| P.O. | Unknown | 30-60 min | Unknown |

## Contraindications and precautions
Contraindicated in patients with hypersensitivity or idiosyncrasy to nitrates, severe hypotension, shock, or acute MI with low left ventricular filling pressure.

Use cautiously in patients with hypotension or blood volume depletion (such as from diuretic therapy).

## Interactions
**Drug-drug.** *Calcium channel blockers and organic nitrates:* Marked symptomatic orthostatic hypotension. Dosage adjustments of either class of drugs may be needed.
**Drug-lifestyle.** *Alcohol use:* Increased vasodilation. Advise patient to avoid alcohol.

## Adverse reactions
**CNS:** *headache* (sometimes with throbbing), dizziness, weakness.
**CV:** *orthostatic hypotension, tachycardia, palpitations, ankle edema,* fainting.
**GI:** nausea, vomiting.
**Musculoskeletal:** arthralgia.
**Respiratory:** bronchitis, pneumonia, upper respiratory tract infection.
**Skin:** cutaneous vasodilation, rash, *flushing.*
**Other:** hypersensitivity reactions, S.L. burning.

## Overdose and treatment
Symptoms of overdose may include increased intracranial pressure; persistent, throbbing headache; confusion; moderate fever; vertigo; palpitations; visual disturbances; nausea and vomiting (possibly with colic and even bloody diarrhea); syncope (especially with upright position); air hunger; dyspnea, later followed by reduced ventilatory effort; diaphoresis, with skin either flushed or cold and clammy; heart block and bradycardia; paralysis; coma; seizures; and death.

No specific antagonist to vasodilator effects of drug is known. However, drug is significantly removed from the blood during hemodialysis.

If drug is ingested, recommend inducing emesis or performing gastric lavage followed by activated charcoal administration. Because drug is rapidly and completely absorbed, however, gastric lavage may be effective only with recent ingestion. Recommend treating severe hypotension and reflex tachycardia by elevating legs and administering I.V. fluids. Epinephrine is ineffective in reversing severe hypotension from overdose, and epinephrine and related compounds are contraindicated. Recommend giving oxygen and artificial ventilation if needed. Advise clinician to monitor methemoglobin levels as indicated.

## Clinical considerations
■ Drug-free interval sufficient to avoid tolerance to drug isn't completely defined. The recommended regimen involves two daily doses given 7 hours apart, with a gap of 17 hours between the second dose of 1 day and the first dose of the next day. Considering the relatively long half-life of drug, this result is consistent with those obtained for other organic nitrates.
■ The asymmetric twice-daily regimen successfully avoids significant rebound or withdrawal effects. In studies of other nitrates, the risk and magnitude of such phenomena appear to be highly dependent on the schedule of nitrate administration.
■ Onset of action of oral drug isn't sufficiently rapid to be useful in aborting an acute anginal episode.

### Therapeutic monitoring
■ Benefits of drug in patients with acute MI or HF have not been established. Because effects of drug are difficult to terminate rapidly, its use isn't recommended in such patients. If it's used, however, careful clinical or hemodynamic monitoring must be performed to avoid the hazards of hypotension and tachycardia.
■ Advise clinician to monitor blood pressure, especially in those susceptible to hypotension.
■ Methemoglobinemia has occurred in patients receiving other organic nitrates and probably could occur as an adverse reaction. Significant methemoglobinemia has occurred in association with moderate overdoses of organic nitrates. Methemoglobinemia should be suspected in patients who exhibit signs of impaired oxygen delivery despite adequate cardiac output and adequate $Pao_2$. Classically, methemoglobinemic blood is chocolate brown, without color change on exposure to air. Treatment of choice for methemoglobinemia is methylene blue, 1 to 2 mg/kg I.V.

### Special populations
**Breast-feeding patients.** It's unknown if drug appears in breast milk. Caution should be used when drug is given to breast-feeding women.
**Pediatric patients.** Safety and efficacy in children haven't been established.

## Patient counseling
■ Tell patient to follow prescribed dosing schedule carefully (two doses taken 7 hours apart) to maintain antianginal effect and to prevent tolerance.
■ Warn patient that daily headaches sometimes accompany treatment with nitrates, including isosorbide mononitrate, and are a marker of drug activity. Patient shouldn't alter treatment schedule, because loss of headache may occur with simultaneous loss of antianginal efficacy. Tell patient to treat headaches with aspirin or acetaminophen.
■ Warn patient to avoid alcohol while taking drug because of increased risk of lightheadedness.
■ Tell patient to rise slowly from recumbent or seated position to avoid light-headedness caused by sudden decrease in blood pressure.

# isotretinoin
Accutane

*Pharmacologic classification:* retinoic
acid derivative
*Therapeutic classification:* antiacne,
keratinization stabilizer
*Pregnancy risk category X*

## Available forms
Available by prescription only
*Capsules:* 10 mg, 20 mg, 40 mg

## Indications and dosages
**Severe recalcitrant nodular acne**
*Adults and adolescents:* 0.5 to 2 mg/kg P.O.
daily given in two divided doses and continued for 15 to 20 weeks.
◇**Keratinization disorders resistant to conventional therapy,** ◇**prevention of skin
cancer**
*Adults:* Dosage varies with specific disease and
severity of the disorder; dosages up to 2 to
4 mg/kg P.O. daily have been used. Consult
current literature for specific recommendations.
◇**Squamous cell cancer of the head and
neck**
*Adults:* 50 to 100 mg/m².

## Mechanism of action
*Antiacne action:* Exact mechanism of action
is unknown; isotretinoin decreases the size and
activity of sebaceous glands, which decreases
secretion and probably explains the rapid clinical improvement. A reduction in *Propioni-
bacterium acnes* in the hair follicles occurs as
a secondary result of decreased nutrients.
*Keratinizing action:* Isotretinoin has anti-
inflammatory and keratinizing effects. The
mechanism is unknown.

## Pharmacokinetics
*Absorption:* When given orally, drug is absorbed rapidly from the GI tract. Therapeutic
range for isotretinoin hasn't been established.
*Distribution:* Distributed widely. In animals,
it's found in most organs and is known to cross
the placenta. In humans, degree of placental
transfer and the degree of secretion in breast
milk are unknown. Isotretinoin is 99.9%
protein-bound, primarily to albumin.
*Metabolism:* Metabolized in the liver and possibly in the gut wall. The major metabolite is
4-oxo-isotretinoin, with tretinoin and 4-oxo-
tretinoin also found in the blood and urine.
*Excretion:* Elimination process is not fully
known, although renal and biliary pathways
are known to be used.

| Route | Onset | Peak | Duration |
|-------|-------|------|----------|
| P.O. | Unknown | 3 hr | Unknown |

## Contraindications and precautions
Contraindicated in women of childbearing age
unless patient has had a negative serum pregnancy test within 2 weeks before beginning
therapy, will begin drug therapy on day 2 or 3
of next menstrual period, and will comply with
stringent contraceptive measures for 1 month
before therapy, during therapy, and for at least
1 month after therapy. Severe fetal abnormalities may occur if used during pregnancy. Also
contraindicated in patients hypersensitive to
parabens, which are used as preservatives.
    Drug should not be used in patients with
hypertriglyceridemia and should be used cautiously in patients with preexisting elevated
fasting serum triglyceride levels and those patients with an increased tendency to develop
hypertriglyceridemia. Use should be discontinued if pancreatitis, tinnitus, or impaired hearing occurs.

## Interactions
**Drug-drug.** *Carbamazepine:* Decreased carbamazepine levels. Advise clinician to monitor patient carefully.
*Medicated soaps and cleansers, medicated
cover-ups, topical resorcinol peeling drugs
(benzoyl peroxide), and alcohol-containing
preparations:* Cumulative drying effect. Use
cautiously.
*Tetracyclines:* May increase the potential for
the development of pseudotumor cerebri. Avoid
use together.
*Vitamin A products:* Additive toxic effect. Avoid
use together.
**Drug-lifestyle.** *Alcohol use:* Increased plasma
triglyceride levels.

## Adverse reactions
**CNS:** headache, fatigue, *pseudotumor cerebri*
(benign intracranial hypertension).
**EENT:** *conjunctivitis, drying of mucous mem-
branes,* corneal deposits, dry eyes, visual dis-
turbances, *epistaxis, dry nose,* color vision dis-
turbances, hearing impairment.
**GI:** nonspecific GI symptoms, gum bleeding
and inflammation, *nausea, vomiting,* anorex-
ia, *dry mouth, abdominal pain.*
**GU:** glomerulonephritis.
**Hematologic:** anemia, elevated platelet count.
**Hepatic:** *hypertriglyceridemia,* elevated AST,
ALT, and alkaline phosphatase levels.
**Metabolic:** hyperglycemia.
**Musculoskeletal:** *musculoskeletal pain (skeletal hyperostosis).*
**Respiratory:** bronchospasm.
**Skin:** *cheilosis, rash, dry skin, facial skin
desquamation,* peeling of palms and toes, skin
infection, photosensitivity, *cheilitis, pruritus,
fragility, petechiae, brittle nails,* thinning of
hair.

## Overdose and treatment
Signs and symptoms of overdose are rare and would be extensions of adverse reactions.

## Clinical considerations
■ For women of childbearing age, a negative blood test for pregnancy must be obtained before therapy.
■ Drug should be given with or shortly after meals.
■ Therapy usually lasts 15 to 20 weeks, followed by at least 8 weeks off drug before a second course is begun.
■ Contact lenses may be uncomfortable during treatment; recommend use of artificial tears.
■ Drug has been used in a limited number of patients to treat psoriasis (combined with psoralen and ultraviolet light); it has also been used to treat cutaneous neoplasms.

### Therapeutic monitoring
■ Advise clinician to monitor patient for visual problems.
■ Pregnancy tests must be repeated monthly to avoid administration during pregnancy.

### Special populations
**Pregnant patients.** Drug is a potent teratogen and shouldn't be taken during pregnancy. Clinician should report any cases of pregnancy with specific information on contraception used during drug therapy. Pregnancy registry: 1-800-526-6367; Medwatch: 1-800-FDA-1088.
**Breast-feeding patients.** It's unknown if drug appears in breast milk; breast-feeding isn't recommended during drug therapy.

## Patient counseling
■ Recommend taking drug with or shortly after meals to ease GI discomfort.
■ To reduce risk of hypertriglyceridemia, advise patient to avoid alcohol.
■ Warn patient to be cautious when driving, particularly at night because drug causes decreased night vision.
■ Advise patient not to take vitamin supplements containing vitamin A while taking drug.
■ Instruct patient to avoid prolonged exposure to sunlight or sun lamps to prevent photosensitivity.

# isradipine
DynaCirc

*Pharmacologic classification:* calcium channel blocker
*Therapeutic classification:* antihypertensive
*Pregnancy risk category C*

## Available forms
Available by prescription only
*Capsules:* 2.5 mg, 5 mg

## Indications and dosages
*Management of hypertension*
*Adults:* Individualize dosage. Initially, 2.5 mg P.O. b.i.d. alone or with thiazide diuretic. Maximal response may require 2 to 4 weeks; therefore, dosage adjustments of 5 mg daily should be made at 2- to 4-week intervals up to maximum of 20 mg daily. Doses of 10 mg or more per day haven't been shown to be more effective but rather to lead to increased risk of adverse reactions. Same starting dose is used in geriatric, hepatically impaired, and renally impaired patients.

## Mechanism of action
*Antihypertensive action:* A dihydropyridine calcium channel blocker, isradipine binds to calcium channels and inhibits calcium flux into cardiac and smooth muscle, which results in dilation of arterioles. This dilation reduces systemic resistance and lowers blood pressure while producing small increases in resting heart rate.

## Pharmacokinetics
*Absorption:* About 90% to 95% is absorbed after oral administration.
*Distribution:* 95% plasma protein–bound.
*Metabolism:* Completely metabolized before elimination, with extensive first-pass metabolism.
*Excretion:* About 60% to 65% is excreted in urine; 25% to 30%, in feces.

| Route | Onset | Peak | Duration |
|-------|-------|------|----------|
| P.O. | Unknown | 1½ hr | Unknown |

## Contraindications and precautions
Contraindicated in patients hypersensitive to drug.
   Use cautiously in patients with HF, especially if combined with a beta blocker.

## Interactions
**Drug-drug.** *Fentanyl anesthesia:* Severe hypotension has been reported with concomitant use of a beta blocker and a calcium channel blocker. Use together should be avoided.

## Adverse reactions
**CNS:** dizziness, *headache,* fatigue.
**CV:** edema, flushing, syncope, angina, tachycardia.
**GI:** nausea, diarrhea, abdominal discomfort, vomiting.
**Respiratory:** dyspnea.
**Skin:** rash.

## Overdose and treatment
No well-documented cases of overdose have been reported; however, presumably excessive peripheral vasodilation with marked and prolonged systemic hypotension may occur. Provide symptomatic and supportive treatment,

including active CV support, monitoring of input and output and cardiac and respiratory function, elevation of legs, and fluid replacement p.r.n. Use vasoconstrictors only when not specifically contraindicated.

## Clinical considerations
■ Drug has no significant effect on heart rate and no adverse effects on cardiac contractility, conduction or digitalis clearance, or lipid or renal function.
■ Administration with food significantly increases the time to reach peak levels by about 1 hour. However, food has no effect on total bioavailability of drug.

### Therapeutic monitoring
■ Elevated liver function test results have been reported in some patients.
■ Dosage should be individualized. Advise clinician to allow 2 to 4 weeks between dosage adjustments.

### Special populations
**Breast-feeding patients.** It's unknown if isradipine appears in breast milk. The potential risk of serious adverse reactions in the infant should be considered.
**Pediatric patients.** Safety and efficacy haven't been established in children under age 18.
**Geriatric patients.** No age-related problems have been reported.

## Patient counseling
■ Instruct patient to report irregular heartbeat, shortness of breath, swelling of hands or feet, pronounced dizziness, constipation, nausea, or hypotension.

# itraconazole
Sporanox

*Pharmacologic classification:* synthetic triazole
*Therapeutic classification:* antifungal
*Pregnancy risk category C*

## Available forms
Available by prescription only
*Capsules:* 100 mg
*Injection:* 10 mg/ml
*Oral solution:* 10 mg/ml

## Indications and dosages
*Treatment of blastomycosis (pulmonary and extrapulmonary), histoplasmosis (including chronic cavitary pulmonary disease and disseminated nonmeningeal histoplasmosis)*
*Adults:* 200 mg P.O. once daily. If condition doesn't improve or shows evidence of progressive fungal disease, increase dosage in 100-mg increments to maximum of 400 mg

daily. Give doses of more than 200 mg/day in two divided doses. Alternatively, 200 mg I.V. b.i.d. for 4 doses, then decrease to 200 mg I.V. once daily for up to 14 days.
*Aspergillosis (pulmonary and extrapulmonary) in patients who are intolerant of or refractory to amphotericin B therapy*
*Adults:* 200 to 400 mg P.O. daily, or 200 mg I.V. b.i.d. for 4 doses, then decrease to 200 mg I.V. daily for up to 14 days.
*Oropharyngeal candidiasis*
*Adults:* 200 mg (20 ml) oral solution P.O. daily for 1 to 2 weeks.
*Esophageal candidiasis*
*Adults:* 100 mg (10 ml) oral solution P.O. daily for at least 3 weeks.
◊ *Treatment of superficial mycoses (dermatophytoses, pityriasis versicolor, sebopsoriasis, candidiasis [vaginal, oral, or chronic mucocutaneous], onychomycosis),* ◊ *systemic mycoses (candidiasis, cryptococcal infections [meningitis, disseminated],* ◊ *dimorphic infections [paracoccidioidomycosis, coccidioidomycosis]),* ◊ *S.C. mycoses (sporotrichosis, chromomycosis),* ◊ *cutaneous leishmaniasis,* ◊ *fungal keratitis,* ◊ *alternariatoxicosis, and* ◊ *zygomycosis*
*Adults:* 50 to 400 mg P.O. daily. Duration of therapy varies from 1 day to more than 6 months, depending on the condition and mycologic response.
   Note: Drug should be stopped if clinical signs and symptoms develop that are consistent with liver disease and may be attributable to itraconazole.
   Before treatment starts, appropriate nail specimens for laboratory testing (KOH preparation, fungal culture, or nail biopsy) should be obtained to confirm the diagnosis of onychomycosis.

## I.V. administration
■ Drug must be diluted before I.V. infusion, using the normal saline solution diluent provided by the manufacturer.
■ The infusion should be given over 60 minutes.
■ After infusion, the infusion set should be flushed and the entire I.V. line should be discarded.

### Incompatibilities
Drug should not be given with or admixed with other drugs.

## Mechanism of action
*Antifungal action:* Itraconazole is a synthetic triazole antifungal drug. In vitro, itraconazole inhibits the cytochrome P-450–dependent synthesis of ergosterol, a vital component of fungal cell membranes.

## Pharmacokinetics

*Absorption:* Oral bioavailability of drug is maximal when taken with food; absolute oral bioavailability is 55%.

*Distribution:* Plasma protein–binding of drug is 99.8%; 99.5% for its metabolite, hydroxyitraconazole.

*Metabolism:* Extensively metabolized by the liver into a large number of metabolites, including hydroxyitraconazole, the major metabolite.

*Excretion:* Fecal excretion of parent drug varies between 3% and 18% of the dose. Renal excretion of parent drug is less than 0.03% of dose. About 40% of dose is excreted as inactive metabolites in the urine. Drug isn't removed by hemodialysis.

| Route | Onset | Peak | Duration |
|-------|-------|------|----------|
| P.O. | Unknown | Unknown | Unknown |

## Contraindications and precautions

Contraindicated in patients hypersensitive to drug, in patients receiving terfenadine, and in breast-feeding women because drug appears in breast milk. Contraindicated in patients with ventricular dysfunction (CHF) or history of CHF. If signs and symptoms of CHF occur, itraconazole should be discontinued.

Use cautiously in patients with hypochlorhydria or HIV infection and in those receiving drugs that are highly protein-bound.

## Interactions

**Drug-drug.** *Cyclosporine:* Itraconazole may increase cyclosporine plasma levels. Cyclosporine dosage should be reduced by 50% when itraconazole doses greater than 100 mg/day are used. Advise clinician to monitor cyclosporine levels.

*Digoxin:* Increased digoxin levels. Advise clinician to monitor digoxin levels.

*Dofetilide, pimozide, or quinidine:* Contraindicated because of increased plasma level of these drugs by CYP 3A4 metabolism, causing serious CV events, including torsades de pointes, QT prolongation, ventricular tachycardia, cardiac arrest, or sudden death.

*$H_2$ antagonists, isoniazid, phenytoin, rifampin:* May reduce plasma itraconazole levels. Advise clinician to monitor patient for drug effect.

*HMG-CoA reductase inhibitors:* Contraindicated during treatment with itraconazole. Shouldn't be used together.

*Nonsedating antihistamines:* Rare instances of life-threatening arrhythmias and death. Shouldn't be used together.

*Phenytoin:* Altered phenytoin metabolism. Advise clinician to monitor phenytoin levels.

*Sulfonylureas:* Concurrent use may cause hypoglycemia. Advise clinician to monitor serum glucose.

*Warfarin:* Enhanced anticoagulant effect. Advise clinician to monitor PT.

**Drug-food.** *Grapefruit juice:* Plasma levels and therapeutic effect of itraconazole may be decreased. Recommend taking with liquid other than grapefruit juice.

## Adverse reactions

**CNS:** malaise, fatigue, headache, dizziness, somnolence.

**CV:** edema, hypertension.

**GI:** *nausea,* vomiting, diarrhea, abdominal pain, anorexia.

**GU:** albuminuria, impotence.

**Hepatic:** impaired hepatic function.

**Metabolic:** hypokalemia.

**Skin:** rash, pruritus.

**Other:** fever, decreased libido.

## Overdose and treatment

In the event of accidental overdose, supportive measures should be used, including gastric lavage with sodium bicarbonate. Itraconazole isn't removed by dialysis.

## Clinical considerations

■ In life-threatening situations, the recommended loading dose is 200 mg three times daily (600 mg/day) for first 3 days. Treatment should be continued for minimum of 3 months and until clinical parameters and laboratory tests indicate that the active fungal infection has subsided. An inadequate period of treatment may lead to recurrence of active infection.

■ Instruct prescriber to obtain specimens for fungal cultures and other relevant laboratory studies (wet mount, histopathology, serology) before therapy to isolate and identify causative organisms. Therapy may be instituted before results of cultures and other laboratory studies are known; once results become available, anti-infective therapy should be adjusted accordingly.

■ The clinical course of histoplasmosis in HIV-infected patients is more severe and usually requires maintenance therapy to prevent relapse. Because hypochlorhydria has occurred in HIV-infected patients, absorption of itraconazole may be decreased.

■ Itraconazole shouldn't be given to a patient with creatinine clearance under 30 ml per minute.

### Therapeutic monitoring

■ Advise clinician to monitor hepatic enzyme test values in patients with preexisting hepatic function abnormalities.

### Special populations

**Pregnant patients.** Drug shouldn't be given during pregnancy because of potential risk to fetus.

---

**Breast-feeding patients.** Because drug appears in breast milk, its use is contraindicated in breast-feeding women.

**Pediatric patients.** Safety and efficacy in children haven't been established.

## Patient counseling

■ Instruct patient to take drug with food to enhance absorption.

■ Tell patient to swish oral solution vigorously before swallowing.

■ Tell patient to report signs and symptoms that may suggest liver dysfunction (jaundice, unusual fatigue, anorexia, nausea, vomiting, dark urine, pale stool) so appropriate laboratory testing can be performed.

## ketamine hydrochloride
Ketalar

*Pharmacologic classification:* dissociative anesthetic
*Therapeutic classification:* anesthetic
*Pregnancy risk category NR*

### Available forms
Available by prescription only
*Injection:* 10 mg/ml, 50 mg/ml, 100 mg/ml

### Indications and dosages
***Induction of general anesthesia, especially for short diagnostic or surgical procedures not requiring skeletal muscle relaxation; adjunct to other general anesthetics or low-potency drugs, such as nitrous oxide***
*Adults and children:* 1 to 4.5 mg/kg I.V. administered over 60 seconds; or 6.5 to 13 mg/kg I.M. To maintain anesthesia, repeat in increments of half to full initial dose.

### I.V. administration
■ For direct injection, dilute 100 mg/ml concentration with an equal volume of sterile water for injection, normal saline, or $D_5W$. For continuous infusion, prepare a 1-mg/ml solution by adding 5 ml from the 100 mg/ml vial to 500 ml of $D_5W$ or normal saline.
■ If patient must restrict fluids, prepare a 2-mg/ml solution by adding 10 ml of 50 mg/ml or 5 ml of 100 mg/ml of drug to 250 ml of diluent.
■ Store at room temperature, and protect from light and heat.

### Incompatibilities
Incompatible with barbiturates and diazepam. Barbiturates are incompatible in the same syringe.

### Mechanism of action
*Anesthetic action:* Ketamine induces a profound sense of dissociation from the environment by direct action on the cortex and limbic system.

### Pharmacokinetics
*Absorption:* Absorbed rapidly and well after I.M. injection.
*Distribution:* Rapidly enters the CNS.
*Metabolism:* Metabolized by the liver to an active metabolite with one-third the potency of parent drug.
*Excretion:* Excreted in urine.

| Route | Onset | Peak | Duration |
|-------|-------|------|----------|
| I.V. | 30 sec | Unknown | 5-10 min |
| I.M. | 3-4 min | Unknown | 12-25 min |

### Contraindications and precautions
Contraindicated in patients with schizophrenia or other acute psychosis because it may exacerbate the condition; in those with CV disease for whom a sudden increase in blood pressure would be harmful; and in patients allergic to drug.

### Interactions
**Drug-drug.** *Barbiturates or narcotics:* Concurrent use may cause prolonged recovery time. Advise clinician to monitor patient closely.
*Halothane and enflurane:* Myocardial depression and hypotension. Avoid use together.
*Thyroid hormones:* May cause hypertension and tachycardia. Advise clinician to monitor patient closely.
*Tubocurarine and other nondepolarizing muscle relaxants:* Increased neuromuscular effects; prolonged respiratory depression. Advise clinician to monitor patient closely.

### Adverse reactions
**CNS:** tonic-clonic movements, hallucinations, confusion, excitement, dreamlike states, irrational behavior, psychic abnormalities.
**CV:** *hypertension; tachycardia;* hypotension, **bradycardia** (if used with halothane); ***arrhythmias.***
**EENT:** diplopia, nystagmus, **laryngospasm.**
**GI:** mild anorexia, nausea, vomiting, excessive salivation.
**Respiratory:** *respiratory depression* in high doses, *apnea* (if given too rapidly).
**Skin:** transient erythema, measleslike rash.

### Overdose and treatment
Clinical signs include respiratory depression. Advise prescriber to support respiration, using mechanical ventilation if needed.

### Clinical considerations
■ Recommend keeping verbal, tactile, and visual stimulation to a minimum during induction and recovery.

- The effect of ketamine on blood pressure makes it particularly useful in hypovolemic patients as an induction drug that supports blood pressure.
- Emergency reactions may be reduced by using lower dosage of ketamine with I.V. diazepam and can be treated with short- or ultrashort-acting barbiturates.
- Risk of emergency reactions is lower in patients under age 15 or over age 65 and when drug is given I.M.
- Dissociative and hallucinatory adverse effects have led to drug abuse.

### Therapeutic monitoring
- Patients require physical support because of rapid induction; advise clinician to monitor vital signs perioperatively. Blood pressure begins to increase shortly after injection, peaks at 10% to 50% above preanesthetic levels, and returns to baseline within 15 minutes. Clinical signs of overdose include respiratory depression.
- Emergency reactions occur in 12% of patients, including dreams, visual imagery, hallucinations, and delirium, and may occur for up to 24 hours postoperatively.

### Special populations
**Pediatric patients.** Drug is safe and especially useful in managing minor surgical or diagnostic procedures or in repeated procedures that require large amounts of analgesia, such as the changing of burn dressings.
**Geriatric patients.** Use with caution, especially in patients with suspected CVA, hypertension, or cardiac disease.

### Patient counseling
- Warn patient to avoid tasks requiring motor coordination and mental alertness for 24 hours after anesthesia.

# ketoconazole
Nizoral, Nizoral A-D

*Pharmacologic classification:* imidazole derivative
*Therapeutic classification:* antifungal
*Pregnancy risk category C*

### Available forms
Available by prescription only
*Tablets:* 200 mg
*Cream:* 2%
*Shampoo:* 2%
Available without prescription
*Shampoo:* 1%

### Indications and dosages
***Severe fungal infections caused by susceptible organisms***
*Adults:* Initially, 200 mg P.O. daily as a single dose. Dose may be increased to 400 mg once daily in patients who don't respond to lower dosage.
*Children over age 2:* 3.3 to 6.6 mg/kg P.O. daily as a single dose.
***Topical treatment of tinea corporis, tinea cruris, tinea versicolor, and tinea pedis***
*Adults and children:* Apply daily or b.i.d. for about 2 weeks; for tinea pedis, apply for 6 weeks.
***Seborrheic dermatitis***
*Adults and children:* Apply b.i.d. for about 4 weeks.
***Dandruff***
*Adults:* Apply for 1 minute, rinse, then reapply for 3 minutes. Shampoo twice weekly for 4 weeks with at least 3 days between shampoos.
***Prostatic carcinoma; disseminated intravascular coagulation (DIC) associated with prostatic cancer***
*Adults:* 400 mg P.O. q 8 hours.

## Mechanism of action
*Antifungal action:* Drug is fungicidal and fungistatic, depending on levels. It inhibits demethylation of lanosterol, thereby altering membrane permeability and inhibiting purine transport. The in vitro spectrum of activity includes most pathogenic fungi. However, CSF levels after oral administration aren't predictable. It shouldn't be used to treat fungal meningitis, and specimens should be obtained for susceptibility testing before therapy. Currently available tests may not accurately reflect in vivo activity, so results should be interpreted with caution.

Drug is used orally to treat disseminated or pulmonary coccidioidomycosis, paracoccidioidomycosis, or histoplasmosis; oral candidiasis; and candiduria (but low renal clearance may limit its usefulness).

It's also useful in some dermatophytoses, including tinea capitis, tinea cruris, tinea pedis, tinea manus, and tinea unguium (onychomycosis) caused by *Epidermophyton, Microsporum,* or *Trichophyton.*

## Pharmacokinetics
*Absorption:* Converted to the hydrochloride salt before absorption. Absorption is erratic; it's decreased by raised gastric pH and may be increased in extent and consistency by food.
*Distribution:* Distributed into bile, saliva, cerumen, synovial fluid, and sebum; CSF penetration is erratic and considered minimal. It is 84% to 99% plasma protein–bound.
*Metabolism:* Converted into several inactive metabolites in the liver.
*Excretion:* More than 50% of a dose is excreted in feces within 4 days; drug and metabolites are secreted in bile. About 13% is excreted unchanged in urine. It probably appears in

---

breast milk. Half-life is biphasic, initially 2 hours, with a terminal half-life of 8 hours.

| Route | Onset | Peak | Duration |
|-------|-------|------|----------|
| P.O. | Unknown | 1-4 hr | Unknown |
| Topical | Unknown | Unknown | Unknown |

## Contraindications and precautions
Contraindicated in patients hypersensitive to drug.

Oral form should be used cautiously in patients with hepatic disease. Because CSF levels of ketoconazole are unpredictable after oral administration, drug shouldn't be used alone to treat fungal meningitis.

## Interactions
**Drug-drug.** *Corticosteroids:* May increase corticosteroid levels. Advise clinician to monitor patient carefully.
*Cyclosporine:* Drug may raise serum levels as a result of interference with metabolism. Advise clinician to monitor patient closely.
*Drugs that raise gastric pH (antacids, antimuscarinics, cimetidine, famotidine, ranitidine):* Decreased absorption of ketoconazole. Should be given 2 hours after ketoconazole.
*Oral sulfonylureas:* Effects of sulfonylureas may be intensified. Advise clinician to monitor patient closely.
*Other hepatotoxic drugs:* Drug may enhance toxicity. Advise clinician to monitor patient closely.
*Phenytoin:* Serum levels of both drugs may be altered. Advise clinician to monitor patient response to drug, and drug levels.
*Rifampin:* May decrease serum level of ketoconazole to ineffective levels. Advise clinician to monitor patient for drug effect.
*Tacrolimus:* Increased plasma levels of tacrolimus. Use with caution. Advise clinician to monitor renal function and tacrolimus level.
*Warfarin:* May enhance anticoagulant effect. Advise clinician to monitor PT and INR.
**Drug-herb.** *Yew preparations:* Inhibit ketoconazole metabolism. Discourage use together.
**Drug-lifestyle.** *Alcohol use:* May cause a disulfiram-like reaction. Advise patient to avoid alcohol.

## Adverse reactions
**CNS:** headache, nervousness, dizziness, somnolence, photophobia, *suicidal tendencies,* severe depression (with oral administration).
**GI:** *nausea, vomiting,* abdominal pain, diarrhea (with oral administration).
**GU:** impotence (with oral administration).
**Hematologic:** *thrombocytopenia,* hemolytic anemia, *leukopenia* (with oral administration).
**Hepatic:** elevated liver enzyme levels, *fatal hepatotoxicity* (with oral administration).
**Skin:** pruritus; severe irritation, stinging (with topical administration).

**Other:** fever, chills; gynecomastia with tenderness (with oral administration).

## Overdose and treatment
Overdose may cause dizziness, tinnitus, headache, nausea, vomiting, or diarrhea; patients with adrenal hypofunction or patients on long-term corticosteroid therapy may show signs of adrenal crisis.

Treatment includes induced emesis and sodium bicarbonate lavage, followed by activated charcoal and a cathartic; supportive measures should be provided p.r.n.

## Clinical considerations
■ Recommend identifying organism, but not delaying therapy for laboratory test results.
■ P.O. drug should be given with citrus juice.
■ P.O. drug requires acidity for absorption; administration adjustments needed for patients with achlorhydria.

### Therapeutic monitoring
■ Advise prescriber to monitor for signs of hepatotoxicity: persistent nausea, unusual fatigue, jaundice, dark urine, and pale stools.

### Special populations
**Pregnant patients.** Ketoconazole shouldn't be given to pregnant women.
**Breast-feeding patients.** Drug may appear in breast milk. Alternative feeding methods are recommended.
**Pediatric patients.** Safe use in children under age 2 hasn't been established. Use should be considered in pediatric patients only when the benefits outweigh the risks.

## Patient counseling
■ Instruct achlorhydric patients how to dissolve each tablet in 4 ml of 0.2N hydrochloric acid solution or take with 200 ml of 0.1N hydrochloric acid. A glass or plastic straw should be used to avoid damaging tooth enamel. Each dose should be followed with a glass of water.
■ Tell patient to avoid driving or performing other hazardous activities if dizziness or drowsiness occur; these often occur early in treatment but abate as treatment continues.
■ Caution patient not to alter dose or dosage interval or to discontinue drug without medical approval; therapy must continue until active fungal infection is completely eradicated, to prevent recurrence.
■ Reassure patient that nausea will subside; to minimize reaction, patient may take drug with food or may divide dosage into two doses.
■ Advise patient to avoid self-prescribed preparations for GI distress (such as antacids); some may alter gastric pH levels and interfere with drug action.
■ Caution patient concerning drug-drug and drug-herb interactions.

# ketoprofen
Actron, Orudis, Orudis KT, Oruvail

*Pharmacologic classification:* NSAID
*Therapeutic classification:* nonnarcotic
analgesic, anti-inflammatory, antipyretic
*Pregnancy risk category B*

## Available forms
Available by prescription only
*Capsules:* 25 mg, 50 mg, 75 mg
*Capsules (extended-release):* 100 mg, 150 mg,
200 mg
Available without a prescription
*Tablets:* 12.5 mg

## Indications and dosages
**Rheumatoid arthritis and osteoarthritis**
*Adults:* Usual dose is 75 mg t.i.d. or 50 mg q.i.d.
P.O. Maximum dose is 300 mg/day; or 200 mg
(extended-release capsules) P.O. daily.
**Mild to moderate pain; dysmenorrhea**
*Adults:* 25 to 50 mg P.O. q 6 to 8 hours, p.r.n.
**Temporary relief of mild aches and pain,
fever (self-medication)**
*Adults:* 12.5 mg q 4 to 6 hours. Don't exceed
75 mg in a 24-hour period.

## Mechanism of action
*Analgesic, antipyretic, and anti-inflammatory
actions:* Mechanisms of action are unknown;
ketoprofen is thought to inhibit prostaglandin
synthesis.

## Pharmacokinetics
*Absorption:* Absorbed rapidly and completely from the GI tract.
*Distribution:* Highly protein-bound. Extent of
body tissue fluid distribution isn't known, but
therapeutic levels range from 0.4 to 6 mcg/ml.
*Metabolism:* Metabolized in the liver.
*Excretion:* Excreted in urine as parent drug
and its metabolites.

| Route | Onset | Peak | Duration |
|---|---|---|---|
| P.O., P.R. | 1-2 hr | ½-2 hr | 3-4 hr |

## Contraindications and precautions
Contraindicated in patients hypersensitive to
drug or with history of aspirin-induced or
NSAID-induced asthma, urticaria, or other
allergic-type reactions.
  Use cautiously in patients with impaired re-
nal or hepatic function, peptic ulcer disease,
HF, hypertension, or fluid retention.

## Interactions
**Drug-drug.** *Antihypertensives and diuretics:*
Decreased effectiveness of these drugs; in-
creased nephrotoxic potential from diuretics.
Use together should be avoided.

*Aspirin:* Decreases the bioavailability of ketoprofen. Use together should be avoided.
*Coumarin derivatives, heparin, streptokinase,
urokinase, nifedipine, phenytoin, or verapamil:*
Toxicity may occur, along with increased risk
of bleeding. Advise patient to closely monitor
patient PT and INR.
*Gold compounds, other anti-inflammatory
drugs, or acetaminophen:* Increased nephrotoxicity.
*Insulin or oral antidiabetics:* Because of the
influence of prostaglandins on glucose metabolism, concurrent use may potentiate hypoglycemic effects. Advise clinician to monitor blood glucose levels.
*Lithium and methotrexate:* Decreased renal
clearance of lithium and methotrexate. Advise
clinician to monitor patient closely
*Other drugs that inhibit platelet aggregation,
such as aspirin, parenteral carbenicillin,
cefamandole, cefoperazone, dextran, dipyridamole, mezlocillin, piperacillin, plicamycin,
salicylates, sulfinpyrazone, ticarcillin, valproic
acid, or other anti-inflammatory drugs:* Bleeding problems may occur. Advise clinician to
monitor patient for signs of bleeding.
*Salicylates, anti-inflammatory drugs, corti-
cotropin, or corticosteroids:* May cause GI ulceration and hemorrhage. Use together should
be avoided.
**Drug-herb.** *Dong quai, feverfew, garlic, ginger, horse chestnut, red clover:* Possible increased risk of bleeding. Use together should
be discouraged.
*St. John's wort, dong quai:* Increased risk of
photosensitivity. Advise patient to avoid unprotected exposure to sunlight.
**Drug-lifestyle.** *Alcohol use:* Increased GI adverse effects, including ulceration and hemorrhage. Advise patient to avoid alcohol.
*Prolonged sun exposure:* Increased risk of photosensitivity reaction. Advise patient to take
precautions.

## Adverse reactions
**CNS:** *headache, dizziness, CNS excitation* or
depression.
**EENT:** tinnitus, visual disturbances, *laryngeal
edema.*
**GI:** *nausea, abdominal pain, diarrhea, con-
stipation, flatulence, peptic ulceration,* dys-
pepsia, anorexia, vomiting, stomatitis, *peptic
ulceration.*
**GU:** *nephrotoxicity,* elevated BUN.
**Hematologic:** prolonged bleeding time, *throm-
bocytopenia, agranulocytosis.*
**Hepatic:** elevated liver enzyme levels.
**Respiratory:** dyspnea, *bronchospasm.*
**Skin:** rash, photosensitivity, *exfoliative der-
matitis.*
**Other:** peripheral edema.

## Overdose and treatment

Signs and symptoms of overdose include nausea and drowsiness.

Recommend inducing emesis with ipecac syrup or emptying stomach via gastric lavage; recommend giving activated charcoal via nasogastric tube. Symptomatic and supportive measures (respiratory support and correction of fluid and electrolyte imbalances) should be provided. Advise clinician to monitor laboratory parameters and vital signs closely. Hemodialysis may be useful in removing ketoprofen and assisting in care of renal failure.

## Clinical considerations

■ Tablets should be given on an empty stomach either 30 minutes before or 2 hours after meals to ensure adequate absorption. However, capsules may be taken with foods or antacids to minimize GI distress.
■ Disease-modifying antirheumatic drugs may be considered in arthritic patients who do not respond adequately to NSAIDs.
■ For patients at high risk for complications from NSAID-induced GI ulceration, misoprostol, a proton-pump inhibitor, or an $H_2$ blocker may be considered.
■ In vitro interactions with glucose determinations have been reported with glucose oxidase and peroxidase methods, resulting in falsely elevated glucose levels.
■ Ketoprofen may interfere with serum iron determination (false increases or decreases depending on method used) and may cause falsely elevated serum bilirubin levels.

### Therapeutic monitoring

■ Advise prescriber to monitor patient for CNS effects and possible photosensitivity reactions.
■ Advise clinician to monitor laboratory test results for abnormalities.

### Special populations

**Breast-feeding patients.** Most NSAIDs appear in breast milk; however, distribution of ketoprofen is unknown. Use of ketoprofen should be avoided in breast-feeding women.
**Pediatric patients.** Safe use in children under age 12 hasn't been established.
**Geriatric patients.** Patients over age 60 may be more susceptible to the toxic effects of ketoprofen. It should be used with caution. The effects of drug on renal prostaglandins may cause fluid retention and edema, a significant drawback for geriatric patients and those with HF. The manufacturer recommends that initial dose be reduced by 33% to 50% in geriatric patients.

## Patient counseling

■ Instruct patient about prescribed drug regimen and proper drug administration, to avoid alcoholic beverages during therapy, and to report adverse reactions.

■ Tell patient to seek medical approval before taking OTC drugs (especially aspirin and aspirin-containing products).
■ Caution patient to avoid activities that require alertness or concentration; stress need for safety measures to prevent injury.
■ Advise patient of potential photosensitivity reactions. Advise patient to use sunblock.

# ketorolac tromethamine
Toradol

*Pharmacologic classification:* NSAID
*Therapeutic classification:* analgesic
*Pregnancy risk category C*

## Available forms

Available by prescription only
*Tablets:* 10 mg
*Injection:* 15 mg/ml (1-ml cartridge), 30 mg/ml (1-ml and 2-ml cartridges)

## Indications and dosages

*Short-term management of pain*
*Adults under age 65:* Dosage should be based on patient response; initially, 60 mg I.M. or 30 mg I.V. as a single dose, or multiple doses of 30 mg I.M. or I.V. q 6 hours. Maximum daily dose shouldn't exceed 120 mg.
≡*Dosage adjustment.* In patients ages 65 or older, renally impaired patients, and those weighing less than 50 kg (110 lb), 30 mg I.M. or 15 mg I.V. initially as a single dose, or multiple doses of 15 mg I.M. or I.V. q 6 hours. Maximum daily dose shouldn't exceed 60 mg.
*Short-term management of moderately severe, acute pain when switching from parenteral to oral administration*
*Adults under age 65:* 20 mg P.O. as a single dose followed by 10 mg P.O. q 4 to 6 hours, not to exceed 40 mg/day.
≡*Dosage adjustment.* In patients ages 65 or older, renally impaired patients, and those weighing under 50 kg (110 lb), 10 mg P.O. as a single dose, followed by 10 mg P.O. q 4 to 6 hours, not to exceed 40 mg/day.

## I.V. administration

■ Solutions should be inspected for particulate matter and discoloration before administration whenever solution and container permit.
■ I.V. adminstration must be given over no less than 15 seconds.

### Incompatibilities

Incompatible with solutions of opiate agonists that cause a relatively low pH, such as meperidine and morphine sulfate, because precipitation can occur.

---

## Mechanism of action
*Analgesic action:* Ketorolac is an NSAID that acts by inhibiting the synthesis of prostaglandins.

## Pharmacokinetics
*Absorption:* Completely absorbed after I.M. administration. After oral administration, food delays absorption but doesn't decrease total amount of drug absorbed.
*Distribution:* Mean peak plasma levels occur about 30 minutes after a 50-mg dose and range from 2.2 to 3 mcg/ml. Drug is highly protein-bound.
*Metabolism:* Metabolism is primarily hepatic; a para-hydroxy metabolite and conjugates have been identified; less than 50% of a dose is metabolized. Liver impairment doesn't substantially alter drug clearance.
*Excretion:* Primary excretion is in urine (more than 90%); the rest in feces. Terminal plasma half-life is 3¾ to 6⅓ hours (average 4½ hours) in young adults; it's substantially prolonged in patients with renal failure.

| Route | Onset | Peak | Duration |
|-------|-------|------|----------|
| P.O. | ½ -1 hr | ½ -1 hr | 6-8 hr |
| I.V. | Immediate | Immediate | 6-8 hr |
| I.M. | 10 min | ½ -1 hr | 6-8 hr |

## Contraindications and precautions
Contraindicated in patients hypersensitive to drug, or those with active peptic ulcer disease, recent GI bleeding or perforation, advanced renal impairment, risk for renal impairment from volume depletion, suspected or confirmed cerebrovascular bleeding, hemorrhagic diathesis, incomplete hemostasis, or high risk of bleeding.

Also contraindicated in patients with history of peptic ulcer disease or GI bleeding, past allergic manifestations to aspirin or other NSAIDs, and during labor and delivery or breast-feeding. In addition, drug is contraindicated as prophylactic analgesic before major surgery or intraoperatively when hemostasis is critical; in patients receiving aspirin, an NSAID, or probenecid; and in those requiring analgesics to be administered epidurally or intrathecally.

Use cautiously in patients with impaired renal or hepatic function.

## Interactions
**Drug-drug.** *Diuretics:* Decreased efficacy of diuretic; increased risk of nephrotoxicity. Advise clinician to monitor patient closely.
*Free (unbound) salicylates or warfarin:* Increased blood levels of salicylates or warfarin. Use with extreme caution; advise clinician to monitor patient closely.

*Lithium:* Increased lithium levels and decreased methotrexate clearance, increasing its toxicity. Advise clinician to monitor patient closely.
**Drug-herb.** *Dong quai, feverfew, garlic, ginger, horse chestnut, red clover:* Possible increased risk of bleeding. Use together should be discouraged.
*St. John's wort, dong quai:* Increased risk of photosensitivity. Advise patient to avoid unprotected exposure to sunlight.
**Drug-lifestyle.** *Alcohol use:* Increased GI effects, including ulceration and hemorrhage. Advise patient to avoid alcohol.

## Adverse reactions
**CNS:** *drowsiness, sedation,* dizziness, *headache.*
**CV:** edema, hypertension, palpitations, *arrhythmias.*
**GI:** *nausea, dyspepsia, GI pain,* diarrhea, peptic ulceration, vomiting, constipation, flatulence, stomatitis.
**GU:** *renal failure.*
**Hematologic:** decreased platelet adhesion, purpura, *thrombocytopenia.*
**Skin:** pain (at injection site), pruritus, rash, diaphoresis.

## Overdose and treatment
There is no experience with overdose in humans. Recommend withholding drug and providing supportive treatment.

## Clinical considerations
■ Hypovolemia should be corrected before therapy with ketorolac is initiated.
■ The combined duration of ketorolac I.M., I.V., or P.O. shouldn't exceed 5 days. Oral use is only for continuation of I.V. or I.M. therapy.

### Therapeutic monitoring
■ I.M. injections in patients with coagulopathies or those receiving anticoagulants may cause bleeding and hematoma at the site of injection.

### Special populations
**Breast-feeding patients.** Because drug appears in breast milk, its use is contraindicated in breast-feeding women.
**Pediatric patients.** Drug isn't recommended for use in children because safety and efficacy haven't been established.
**Geriatric patients.** Use lower initial doses (30 mg I.M.) in patients over age 65 or weighing under 110 lb. In clinical trials, geriatric subjects have exhibited a longer terminal half-life of drug (average 7 hours in geriatric patients compared with 4½ hours in healthy young adults).

## Patient counseling
■ Instruct patient to avoid aspirin, aspirin-containing products, and alcoholic beverages during therapy.

■ Warn patient that GI ulceration, bleeding, and perforation can occur at any time, with or without warning, in anyone taking NSAIDs on a long-term basis. Inform patient of signs and symptoms of GI bleeding.

# ketorolac tromethamine (ophthalmic)

Acular, Acular PF

*Pharmacologic classification:* NSAID
*Therapeutic classification:* ophthalmic anti-inflammatory
*Pregnancy risk category C*

## Available forms

Available by prescription only
*Ophthalmic solution:* 0.5%

## Indications and dosages

*Relief of ocular itching caused by seasonal allergic conjunctivitis*
*Adults:* Instill 1 drop (250 mcg) in conjunctival sac q.i.d. Efficacy hasn't been established beyond 1 week of continued use.
*Prevention and relief of postoperative ocular inflammation in patients undergoing cataract extaction*
*Adults:* 1 drop of a 0.5% solution (250 mcg) in the eye undergoing surgery q.i.d. beginning 24 hours after surgery and continuing for 2 weeks.
◊*Prevention and relief of postoperative cystoid macular edema from cataract extraction*
*Adults:* 1 or 2 drops of a 0.5% solution (250 or 500 mcg) every 6 to 8 hours beginning 24 hours before surgery and continuing for 3 to 4 weeks after surgery.
◊*Active treatment of chronic aphakic or pseudophakic cystoid macular edema*
*Adults:* 1 or 2 drops of a 0.5% solution (250 or 500 mcg) to the affected eye q.i.d. for 2 to 3 months.
*Reduction of ocular pain and photophobia in patients undergoing ocular incisional refractive surgery*
*Adults:* 1 drop of a 0.5% solution (250 mcg) q.i.d. in the operated eye for up to 3 days after surgery.

## Mechanism of action

*Anti-inflammatory action:* Anti-inflammatory action of ketorolac tromethamine is thought to be a result, in part, of its ability to inhibit prostaglandin biosynthesis. Drug reduces prostaglandin $E_2$ levels in aqueous humor with ocular administration. It has also shown analgesic and antipyretic activity because of the same mechanism of action.

## Pharmacokinetics

No information available.

| Route | Onset | Peak | Duration |
|---|---|---|---|
| Ophthalmic | Unknown | Unknown | Unknown |

## Contraindications and precautions

Contraindicated in patients hypersensitive to any component of the formulation and in those wearing soft contact lenses.
Use cautiously in patients hypersensitive to other NSAIDs or aspirin and in those with bleeding disorders.

## Interactions

None reported.

## Adverse reactions

**EENT:** *transient stinging and burning on instillation,* superficial keratitis, superficial ocular infections, ocular irritation.
**Other:** hypersensitivity reactions.

## Overdose and treatment

Overdose will not ordinarily cause acute problems. If accidentally ingested, have the patient drink fluids to dilute.

## Clinical considerations

■ Ophthalmic solution has been safely given with other ophthalmic drugs, such as antibiotics, beta blockers, carbonic anhydrase inhibitors, cycloplegics, and mydriatics.
■ Drug should be stored at room temperature and protected from light.

### Therapeutic monitoring

■ Advise clinician to monitor patient for adverse reactions, including superficial ocular infections and hypersensitivity reactions.

### Special populations

**Breast-feeding patients.** Use cautiously in breast-feeding women.
**Pediatric patients.** Safety and efficacy in children haven't been established.

## Patient counseling

■ Teach patient how to administer eyedrops and stress importance of not touching dropper to eye or surrounding area.
■ Advise patient not to use more drops than prescribed and to use only as prescribed.

# ketotifen fumarate
Zaditor

*Pharmacologic classification:* histamine ($H_1$-receptor) antagonist and mast cell stabilizer
*Therapeutic classification:* ophthalmic antihistamine
*Pregnancy risk category C*

## Available forms
Available by prescription only
*Ophthalmic solution:* 0.025%; supplied as 5-ml solution in 7.5-ml bottles

## Indications and dosages
*Temporary prevention of ocular itching caused by allergic conjunctivitis*
*Adults and children ages 3 and older:* Instill one drop in affected eye q 8 to 12 hours.

## Mechanism of action
*Antihistamine action:* Selective, noncompetitive histamine antagonist ($H_1$-receptor) and mast cell stabilizer that inhibits release of mediators from cells involved in hypersensitivity reactions, thus providing temporary prevention of eye itching.

## Pharmacokinetics
*Absorption:* Effect occurs within minutes after administration.
*Distribution:* No information available.
*Metabolism:* No information available.
*Excretion:* No information available.

| Route | Onset | Peak | Duration |
|---|---|---|---|
| Ophthalmic | Rapid | Unknown | Unknown |

## Contraindications and precautions
Contraindicated in patients hypersensitive to drug or its components.

## Interactions
None reported.

## Adverse reactions
**CNS:** *headache.*
**EENT:** *conjunctival infection, rhinitis,* ocular allergic reactions, burning or stinging of eyes, conjunctivitis, eye discharge, dry eyes, eye pain, eyelid disorder, itching of eyes, keratitis, lacrimation disorder, mydriasis, photophobia, ocular rash, pharyngitis.
**Other:** flu syndrome.

## Clinical considerations
■ Drug is for ophthalmic use only, and not for injection or oral use.
■ Drug isn't indicated for irritation caused by contact lenses.

■ Preservative in drug may be absorbed by soft contact lenses. Contact lenses shouldn't be inserted until 10 minutes after drug is instilled.

### Therapeutic monitoring
■ Advise clinician to monitor patient for sensitivity reactions.
■ Advise clinician to monitor patient for signs of infection.

### Special populations
**Breast-feeding patients.** It's unknown if topical ocular drug appears in breast milk. It should be used cautiously in breast-feeding women.
**Pediatric patients.** Safety and effectiveness in children under age 3 haven't been established.

## Patient counseling
■ Teach patient proper instillation technique. Tell him to avoid contaminating dropper tip and solution and not to touch eyelids or surrounding areas with dropper tip of bottle.
■ Tell patient not to wear contact lenses if eyes are red. Warn patient not to use drug to treat irritation related to contact lenses.
■ Instruct patient who wears soft contact lenses and whose eyes aren't red to wait at least 10 minutes after instilling drug before inserting contact lenses.
■ Advise patient to report adverse reactions to drug.
■ Advise patient to keep bottle tightly closed when not in use.

# labetalol hydrochloride
Normodyne, Trandate

*Pharmacologic classification:* alpha
and beta blocker
*Therapeutic classification:* antihypertensive
*Pregnancy risk category C*

## Available forms
Available by prescription only
*Tablets:* 100 mg, 200 mg, 300 mg
*Injection:* 5 mg/ml in 20-, 40-, and 60-ml vials
and 4- and 8-ml disposable syringes

## Indications and dosages
*Hypertension, ◇ pheochromocytoma*
*Adults:* 100 mg P.O. b.i.d. with or without a
diuretic. Dosage may be increased by 100 mg
b.i.d. q 2 or 3 days until optimum response
is reached. Usual maintenance dose is 200
to 600 mg b.i.d.; maximum daily dose is
2,400 mg.
*Severe hypertension and hypertensive*
*emergencies; ◇ clonidine withdrawal*
*hypertension*
*Adults:* Initially, 20 to 80 mg I.V. bolus slowly over 2 minutes; may repeat injections of 40
to 80 mg q 10 minutes to maximum dose of
300 mg.
  Alternatively, drug may be given as continuous I.V. infusion at an initial rate of 0.5 to
2 mg/minute until satisfactory response is
obtained. Usual effective, cumulative dose is
50 to 200 mg although up to 300 mg may be
needed.
  *Oral dose following I.V. therapy:* 200 mg
P.O. followed by 200 to 400 mg in 6 to 12 hours
(depending on blood pressure response); then
increase in usual increments at 1-day intervals
while patient is hospitalized to achieve desired
effects.
*◇ Controlled hypotension during anesthesia*
*Adults:* Initially, 10 to 30 mg I.V. bolus slowly; may repeat injections of 5 to 10 mg I.V.,
p.r.n.
*Elderly:* Use a lower maintenance dose of 100
to 200 mg P.O. b.i.d.

## I.V. administration
■ For I.V. infusion, dilute labetalol injection to
an appropriate concentration (such as 200 mg

of drug added to 160 ml of $D_5W$ or normal
saline solution to provide a concentration of
1 mg/ml). Administer using a controlled infusion device.
■ Patients receiving I.V. labetalol infusion must
be kept in the supine position during the infusion and for 3 hours after the infusion.
■ Drug may be given by slow, direct I.V. injection over 2 minutes at 10-minute intervals.
■ During direct I.V. injection, advise clinician
to monitor blood pressure before and at 5-minute intervals after each injection; maximum
hypotensive effect usually occurs in 5 to 15
minutes after each injection.

### Incompatibilities
Incompatible with cefoperazone, nafcillin, and
sodium bicarbonate. Avoid giving drug in same
infusion line with other alkaline solutions (such
as furosemide).

## Mechanism of action
*Antihypertensive action:* Labetalol inhibits catecholamine access to both beta- and postsynaptic alpha-adrenergic receptor sites. Drug may
also have a vasodilating effect.

## Pharmacokinetics
*Absorption:* Oral absorption is high (90% to
100%); however, drug undergoes extensive
first-pass metabolism in the liver, and only
about 25% of an oral dose reaches systemic
circulation unchanged.
*Distribution:* Distributed widely throughout
the body; about 50% protein-bound.
*Metabolism:* Orally administered drug is metabolized extensively in the liver and possibly
in GI mucosa.
*Excretion:* About 5% of a dose is excreted unchanged in urine; remainder is excreted as
metabolites in urine and feces (biliary elimination). Plasma half-life is about 5½ hours after I.V. administration or 6 to 8 hours after oral
administration.

| Route | Onset | Peak | Duration |
|-------|-------|------|----------|
| P.O. | 20 min | 2-4 hr | 8-12 hr |
| I.V. | 2-5 min | 5 min | 2-4 hr |

## Contraindications and precautions
Contraindicated in patients with a history of
obstructive airway disease such as bronchial
asthma, overt cardiac failure, greater than first-degree heart block, cardiogenic shock, severe

bradycardia, other conditions caused by severe and prolonged hypotension, and those hypersensitive to drug.

Use cautiously in patients with HF, hepatic failure, chronic bronchitis, emphysema, preexisting peripheral vascular disease, and pheochromocytoma.

Ejaculation failure and impotence in males and decreased libido have been reported.

## Interactions

**Drug-drug.** *Beta agonists:* Labetalol may antagonize bronchodilation produced by these drugs. Avoid use together.

*Cimetidine:* May increase bioavailability of oral labetalol. If used together, labetalol dosage may require adjustment.

*Diuretics, other antihypertensives:* Labetalol may potentiate antihypertensive effects of these drugs. Advise clinician to monitor patient closely.

*Glutethimide:* May decrease bioavailability of oral labetalol. Adjustment in labetalol dosage may be needed.

*Halothane:* Synergistic antihypertensive effect and significant myocardial depression. Advise clinician to monitor patient closely.

*Nitroglycerin:* Labetalol blunts the reflex tachycardia produced by nitroglycerin without preventing its hypotensive effect. In patients with angina, additional antihypertensive effects may occur. Use with caution.

*Tricyclic antidepressants:* May increase risk of labetalol-induced tremor. Avoid use together.

## Adverse reactions

**CNS:** vivid dreams, fatigue, headache, paresthesia, syncope, transient scalp tingling.
**CV:** *orthostatic hypotension, dizziness,* **ventricular arrhythmias.**
**EENT:** nasal stuffiness.
**GI:** nausea, vomiting, diarrhea.
**GU:** sexual dysfunction, urine retention.
**Metabolic:** blocks signs and symptoms hypoglycemia.
**Musculoskeletal:** muscle spasm, toxic myopathy.
**Respiratory:** dyspnea, *bronchospasm.*
**Skin:** rash.

## Overdose and treatment

Signs and symptoms of overdose include severe hypotension, bradycardia, HF, and bronchospasm.

After acute ingestion, advise clinician to empty stomach by induced emesis or gastric lavage and give activated charcoal to reduce absorption. Subsequent treatment is usually symptomatic and supportive.

## Clinical considerations

■ Unlike other beta blockers, labetalol doesn't decrease resting heart rate or cardiac output.

■ Dosage may need to be reduced in patients with hepatic insufficiency and severe renal impairment.

■ Dizziness tends to occur in early stages of treatment and in patients taking diuretics or receiving higher doses.

■ Beta blockers can increase the risk of developing diabetes mellitus.

■ Investigational uses include managing chronic stable angina pectoris, excessive sympathetic activity associated with tetanus, and uncontrolled hypertension before and during anesthesia.

■ It may be more cost-effective for patient to take drug b.i.d. rather than once daily.

■ Store tablets and injection at 36° to 86° F (2° to 30° C) and protect from light, moisture, and freezing.

■ Drug may cause a false-positive increase of urine free and total catecholamine levels when measured by a nonspecific trihydroxindole fluorometric method.

### Therapeutic monitoring

■ Advise clinician to use specific radioenzyme or high-performance liquid chromatography assay techniques to reduce risk of false-positive urine free and total catecholamine levels.

■ Advise clinician to monitor blood pressure closely during and after I.V. infusion; after infusion, recommend monitoring blood pressure every 5 minutes for 30 minutes, then at 30-minute intervals for 2 hours, then hourly for 6 hours.

### Special populations

**Pregnant patients.** Labetalol has been effective for management of hypertension from pregnancy and with reduced proteinuria and prevention of eclampsia. Rarely, transient hypotension, bradycardia, respiratory depression, and hypoglycemia have occurred in neonates.

**Breast-feeding patients.** Small amounts of drug appear in breast milk; use cautiously in breast-feeding women.

**Pediatric patients.** Safety and efficacy in children haven't been established; use drug only if potential benefit outweighs risk.

**Geriatric patients.** Geriatric patients may require lower maintenance dosages of labetalol because of increased bioavailability or delayed metabolism; they also may experience enhanced adverse effects. Use drug with caution in geriatric patients.

### Patient counseling

■ Advise patient that transient scalp tingling may occur when therapy starts but that it usually subsides quickly.

■ Tell patient to take drug as prescribed to maintain adequate blood pressure control.

# lactulose
Calulose, Catulac, Cephulac, Cholac,
Chronulac, Constilac, Constulose,
Duphalac, Enulose, Generlac,
Kristalose

*Pharmacologic classification:* disaccharide
*Therapeutic classification:* laxative
*Pregnancy risk category B*

## Available forms
Available by prescription only
*Powder:* 10 g/packet, 20 g/packet
*Syrup:* 10 g/15 ml
*Rectal solution:* 3.33 g/5 ml

## Indications and dosages
*Constipation*
*Adults:* 10 to 20 g P.O. daily (may increase to 40 g if needed).
◇ *Children:* 5 g P.O. daily as single dose after breakfast.
*To prevent and treat portal-systemic encephalopathy, including hepatic precoma and coma in patients with severe hepatic disease*
*Adults:* Initially, 20 to 30 g (30 to 45 ml) P.O. t.i.d. or q.i.d., until two or three soft stools are produced daily. Usual dosage is 60 to 100 g daily in divided doses; can also be given by retention enema. Mix 200 g of lactulose with 700 ml of water or normal saline solution for retention for 60 minutes. May repeat q 4 to 6 hours. May repeat immediately if retention is less than 30 minutes.
*Infants:* Initially, 1.67 to 6.67 g P.O. daily in divided doses. Adjust doses q 1 to 2 days to produce two to three loose stools daily.
*Older children and adolescents:* Initially, 27 to 60 g P.O. daily in divided doses. Adjust doses q 1 to 2 days to produce two to three loose stools daily.
◇ *After barium meal examination*
*Adults:* 3.3 to 6.7 g, P.O. b.i.d. for 1 to 4 weeks.
◇ *To restore bowel movements after hemorrhoidectomy*
*Adults:* 10 g P.O. twice during day before surgery and for 5 days postoperatively.

## Mechanism of action
*Laxative action:* Because lactulose is indigestible, it passes through the GI tract to the colon unchanged, where it's digested by normally occurring bacteria. The weak acids produced in this manner increase the fluid content of the stool and cause distention, thus promoting peristalsis and bowel evacuation.

Lactulose also is used to reduce serum ammonia levels in patients with hepatic disease. Lactulose breakdown acidifies the colon, which, in turn, converts ammonia ($NH_3$) to ammonium ($NH_4^+$), which isn't absorbed and is excreted in the stool. Furthermore, this "ion trapping" effect causes ammonia to diffuse from the blood into the colon, where it's excreted as well.

## Pharmacokinetics
*Absorption:* Absorbed minimally.
*Distribution:* Distributed locally, primarily in the colon.
*Metabolism:* Metabolized by colonic bacteria (absorbed portion isn't metabolized).
*Excretion:* Mostly excreted in feces; absorbed portion is excreted in urine.

| Route | Onset | Peak | Duration |
|-------|-------|------|----------|
| P.O. | 24-48 hr | Variable | Variable |
| P.R. | Unknown | Unknown | Unknown |

## Contraindications and precautions
Contraindicated in patients on a low-galactose diet. Use cautiously in patients with diabetes mellitus. Use cautiously in patients who may require electrocautery procedures during proctoscopy or colonoscopy.

## Interactions
*Drug-drug. Neomycin, other antibiotics:* May theoretically decrease lactulose effectiveness by eliminating bacteria needed to digest it into the active form. Advise clinician to monitor patient for effect.
*Nonabsorbable antacids:* May decrease lactulose effectiveness by preventing a decrease in the pH of the colon. Avoid use together.

## Adverse reactions
GI: *abdominal cramps, belching, gaseous distention, flatulence,* nausea, vomiting, *diarrhea* (with excessive dosage).

## Overdose and treatment
No cases of overdose have been reported. Clinical effects include diarrhea and abdominal cramps.

## Clinical considerations
■ After drug is given through nasogastric tube, tube should be flushed with water to clear it and ensure passage of drug to stomach.
■ Recommend diluting drug with water or fruit juice to minimize its sweet taste.
■ For oral administration, reconstitute powder by dissolving 10- to 20-g packet in 120 ml of water.
■ For administration by retention enema, patient should retain drug for 30 to 60 minutes. If retained less than 30 minutes, dose should be repeated immediately. Recommend beginning oral therapy before stopping retention enemas.
■ Drug shouldn't be given with other laxatives because resulting loose stools may falsely indicate adequate dosage of lactulose.

---

■ Store at 59° to 86° F (15° to 30° C); avoid freezing.

### Therapeutic monitoring
■ Advise clinician to monitor frequency and consistency of stools.
■ Advise clinician to monitor serum potassium, chloride, and carbon dioxide in long-term treatment.

### Special populations
**Breast-feeding patients.** It's unknown if drug appears in breast milk. Use with caution in breast-feeding women.
**Geriatric patients.** Advise clinician to monitor patient's serum electrolyte levels; geriatric patients are more sensitive to possible hypernatremia.

### Patient counseling
■ Advise patient that taking drug with juice may improve the taste.
■ Instruct patient to contact prescriber if unusual diarrhea condition occurs.

# lamivudine (3TC)
Epivir, Epivir-HBV

*Pharmacologic classification:* synthetic nucleoside analogue
*Therapeutic classification:* antiviral
*Pregnancy risk category C*

### Available forms
Available by prescription only
**Epivir**
*Tablets:* 150 mg
*Oral solution:* 10 mg/ml
**Epivir-HBV**
*Tablets:* 100 mg
*Oral solution:* 5 mg/ml

### Indications and dosages
*Treatment of patients with HIV infection (should be used with other antiretrovirals)*
*Adults weighing 50 kg (110 lb) or more and children ages 16 and older:* 150 mg P.O. b.i.d.
*Adults weighing less than 50 kg:* 2 mg/kg P.O., b.i.d.
*Children ages 3 months to 16 years:* 4 mg/kg P.O. b.i.d. Maximum dose is 150 mg b.i.d.
◇ *Neonates 30 days and younger:* 2 mg/kg P.O. b.i.d.
≡ *Dosage adjustment.* For children with renal impairment, consider decreasing the dose or increasing the dosage interval. For adults and adolescents with renal impairment, refer to the following table.

| Creatinine clearance (ml/min) | Recommended dosage |
|---|---|
| 30-49 | 150 mg once daily |
| 15-29 | 150 mg first dose; then 100 mg once daily |
| 5-14 | 150 mg first dose; then 50 mg once daily |
| < 5 | 50 mg first; then 25 mg once daily |

*Treatment of chronic hepatitis B with evidence of hepatitis B viral replication and active liver inflammation*
*Adults:* 100 mg P.O. once daily. Safety and efficacy of treatment beyond 1 year haven't been established; optimum duration of treatment isn't known. Formulation and dosage of lamivudine in Epivir-HBV aren't appropriate for those dually infected with hepatitis B virus (HBV) and HIV; test patients for HIV before treatment is initiated. If lamivudine is given to patients with HBV and HIV, use the higher dosage indicated for HIV therapy as part of an appropriate combination regimen.
*Children ages 2 to 17:* 3 mg/kg once daily, up to a maximum dose of 100 mg. Safety and efficacy of treatment beyond 1 year haven't been established; optimum duration of treatment isn't known.
≡ *Dosage adjustment.* For patients with renal impairment (ages 16 and older), if creatinine clearance is 30 to 49 ml/minute, 100 mg P.O. on the first day, then 50 mg P.O. once daily thereafter. If clearance is 15 to 29 ml/minute, 100 mg on the first day, then 25 mg P.O. once daily thereafter. If clearance is 5 to 14 ml/ minute, 35 mg on the first day, then 15 mg once daily thereafter. If creatinine clearance is less than 5 ml/minute, 35 mg on the first day, then 10 mg P.O. once daily thereafter.
◇ *Postexposure prophylaxis following occupational exposure to HIV*
*Adults:* 150 mg P.O. b.i.d. with oral zidovudine (600 mg daily); oral indinavir (800 mg q 8 hours) or oral nelfinavir (750 mg P.O. t.i.d.) is added if risk of transmission is likely. Initiate within a few hours and continue for 28 days.

### Mechanism of action
*Antiviral action:* Lamivudine inhibits HIV reverse transcription via viral DNA chain termination. RNA- and DNA-dependent DNA polymerase activities are also inhibited.

### Pharmacokinetics
*Absorption:* Rapidly absorbed after oral administration in HIV-infected patients.
*Distribution:* Believed to be distributed into extravascular spaces. Volume of distribution is independent of dose and doesn't correlate with

body weight. Less than 36% is bound to plasma proteins.

*Metabolism:* Metabolism is minor route of elimination. The only known metabolite is the trans-sulfoxide metabolite.

*Excretion:* Primarily eliminated unchanged in urine. Mean elimination half-life is 5 to 7 hours.

| Route | Onset | Peak | Duration |
|-------|-------|------|----------|
| P.O. | Unknown | 1-3 hr | Unknown |

## Contraindications and precautions

Contraindicated in patients hypersensitive to drug. Use drug with extreme caution and only if there's no satisfactory alternative therapy in children with history of pancreatitis or other significant risk factors for development of pancreatitis. Treatment with lamivudine should be stopped immediately if signs, symptoms, or laboratory abnormalities suggest pancreatitis.

Use cautiously in children with a history of prior therapy with nucleoside reverse transcriptase inhibitors, and in patients with impaired renal function; use dosage reduction.

Lactic acidosis and severe hepatomegaly with steatosis have been reported in patients receiving lamivudine. Treatment should be stopped if signs of lactic acidosis or hepatotoxicity develop.

## Interactions

**Drug-drug.** *Co-trimoxazole:* Decreased clearance of lamivudine may cause increased blood levels of lamivudine. Advise clinician to monitor patient closely.

## Adverse reactions

Adverse reactions are related to the combination therapy of lamivudine and zidovudine.
**CNS:** *malaise, headache, fatigue, neuropathy, dizziness, insomnia and other sleep disorders,* depressive disorders.
**EENT:** *nasal symptoms, sore throat.*
**GI:** *nausea, diarrhea, vomiting, anorexia,* abdominal pain, abdominal cramps, dyspepsia, *pancreatitis* (in children ages 3 months to 12 years).
**Hematologic:** *neutropenia,* anemia, *thrombocytopenia.*
**Hepatic:** elevated liver enzymes and bilirubin levels.
**Musculoskeletal:** *musculoskeletal pain,* myalgia, arthralgia.
**Respiratory:** *cough.*
**Skin:** rash.
**Other:** *fever, chills.*

## Overdose and treatment

No information available.

## Clinical considerations

■ When used in treatment of HIV infection, drug must be given with zidovudine. It isn't intended for use as monotherapy.
■ Safety and efficacy of treatment of HBV for periods longer than 1 year or in patients with decompensated liver disease or organ transplant haven't been established.
**⚠ ALERT** Monotherapy with lamivudine in patients with HIV-HBV co-infection in HBV dosage is inadequate and may lead to rapid emergence of HIV resistance. Counseling and testing for HIV infection before and periodically during treatment are recommended. Use higher dosage with other appropriate antiretrovirals.
■ Lamivudine has been used in combination therapy for the preventive treatment of maternal-fetal transmission of HIV.

### Therapeutic monitoring

■ Advise clinician to monitor CBC, platelet count, and liver function test results throughout therapy.

### Special populations

**Pregnant patients.** An antiretroviral pregnancy registry has been established to monitor maternal-fetal outcomes of pregnant women exposed to lamivudine. Pregnant patients can be registered by calling 1-800-258-4263.
**Breast-feeding patients.** To avoid transmitting HIV to the infant, HIV-positive women shouldn't breast-feed.
**Pediatric patients.** Safety and efficacy in treatment of HIV infection haven't been established in children under age 3 months.

## Patient counseling

■ Inform patient that long-term effects of drug are unknown.
■ Stress importance of taking drug exactly as prescribed.
■ Instruct parents of children receiving drug about signs and symptoms of pancreatitis and tell them to report these immediately.
■ Inform patients receiving dosage of less than therapeutic levels for HIV treatment that HIV testing is recommended.

# lamivudine/zidovudine
Combivir

*Pharmacologic classification:* reverse transcriptase inhibitor
*Therapeutic classification:* antiretroviral
*Pregnancy risk category C*

## Available forms

Available by prescription only
*Tablets:* Each tablet contains 150 mg lamivudine and 300 mg zidovudine

---

Reactions may be *common,* uncommon, *life-threatening,* or COMMON AND LIFE-THREATENING.

## Indications and dosages
### Treatment of HIV infection
*Adults and children over age 12 and weighing 50 kg (110 lb) or more:* One tablet P.O. b.i.d.

## Mechanism of action
*Antiretroviral action:* Lamivudine and zidovudine are phosphorylated intracellularly to active metabolites that inhibit reverse transcriptase by way of DNA chain termination. Both drugs are also weak inhibitors of mammalian DNA polymerase. Together, they have synergistic antiretroviral activity. Combination therapy with lamivudine and zidovudine aims to suppress or delay emergence of phenotypic and genotypic resistant strains that can occur with retroviral monotherapy, because more mutations are needed to develop dual resistance.

## Pharmacokinetics
*Absorption:* Both lamivudine and zidovudine are rapidly absorbed following oral administration with respective oral bioavailability of 86% and 64%.
*Distribution:* Both drugs are extensively distributed and exhibit low protein binding.
*Metabolism:* Only about 5% of lamivudine is metabolized whereas zidovudine is primarily (74%) metabolized in the liver.
*Excretion:* Lamivudine is primarily eliminated unchanged in the urine. Zidovudine and its major metabolite are primarily eliminated in the urine. Elimination half-lives of lamivudine and zidovudine are 5 to 7 hours and ½ to 3 hours, respectively. Because renal excretion is a principal route of elimination, dosage adjustments are needed in patients with compromised renal function, making this fixed ratio combination unsuitable. Hemodialysis and peritoneal dialysis have negligible effect on the removal of zidovudine, but removal of its metabolite, GZDV, is enhanced. The effect of dialysis on lamivudine is unknown.

| Route | Onset | Peak | Duration |
|-------|-------|------|----------|
| P.O. | Unknown | Unknown | Unknown |

## Contraindications and precautions
Contraindicated in patients hypersensitive to components of drug and in those weighing under 50 kg (110 lb), those with creatinine clearance less than 50 ml/minute, and those experiencing dose-limiting adverse effects.

Use combination with caution in patients with bone marrow suppression or renal insufficiency. Lactic acidosis and severe hepatomegaly with steatosis have been reported in patients receiving lamivudine and zidovudine alone and in combination. Stop treatment if signs of lactic acidosis or hepatotoxicity develop. Hepatotoxic events may be more severe in patients with decompensated liver function from hepatitis B. Myopathy and myositis from prolonged use of zidovudine may occur.

## Interactions
*Drug-drug. Atovaquone, fluconazole, methadone, probenecid, valproic acid coadministered with zidovudine:* Increased bioavailability of zidovudine. Dosage modification isn't needed.
*Ganciclovir, interferon-alpha, other bone marrow suppressive or cytotoxic drugs:* May increase hematologic toxicity of zidovudine. Most drug interaction studies haven't been completed. Use cautiously as with other reverse transcriptase inhibitors.
*Nelfinavir, ritonavir:* Decreased bioavailability of zidovudine may occur with concurrent administration. Dosage modification isn't needed.
*Nelfinavir, co-trimoxazole coadministered with lamivudine:* Increased bioavailability of lamivudine. Dosage modification isn't needed.

## Adverse reactions
**CNS:** *headache,* malaise, *fatigue, insomnia, dizziness, neuropathy,* depression.
**GI:** *nausea, diarrhea, vomiting, anorexia,* abdominal pain, abdominal cramps, dyspepsia, *pancreatitis.*
**EENT:** *nasal signs and symptoms.*
**Hematologic:** *neutropenia,* anemia.
**Musculoskeletal:** *musculoskeletal pain,* myalgia, arthralgia, myopathy, myositis.
**Respiratory:** *cough.*
**Skin:** rash.
**Other:** *fever, chills.*

## Overdose and treatment
Overdose (6 g) with lamivudine results in normal hematologic tests and no adverse signs or symptoms. Overdoses of zidovudine, with exposure up to 50 g, result in only nausea and vomiting. No antidote is known for lamivudine/zidovudine overdose.

## Clinical considerations
■ Don't use combination drug therapy in children or in patients requiring dosage adjustments, such as those with renal dysfunction.
■ Combination may be given with or without food.

### Therapeutic monitoring
■ Advise clinician to monitor patient for bone marrow toxicity with frequent blood counts, particularly patients with advanced HIV infection.
■ Advise clinician to monitor patient for signs of lactic acidosis and hepatotoxicity.
■ Advise clinician to monitor patient's fine motor skills and peripheral sensation for evidence of peripheral neuropathies.

### Special populations
**Pregnant patients.** Contact 1-800-722-9292, extension 39437, for patients exposed to drug during pregnancy.
**Breast-feeding patients.** Although zidovudine appears in breast milk at levels similar to those in serum, it's unknown if lamivudine/zidovudine appears in breast milk.
**Pediatric patients.** Don't use in patients under age 12 because the fixed-dose combination treatment can't be adjusted for this patient group.
**Geriatric patients.** Safety and efficacy in patients over age 65 haven't been established.

### Patient counseling
■ Advise patient that combination drug therapy isn't a cure for HIV infection, and that he may continue to experience illness, including opportunistic infections.
■ Warn patient that transmission of HIV virus can still occur with drug therapy.
■ Teach patient signs and symptoms of neutropenia and anemia, and instruct him to report such occurrences.
■ Advise patient to consult prescriber before taking other drugs.
■ Warn patient to report abdominal pain immediately.
■ Stress importance of taking combination drug therapy exactly as prescribed to reduce the development of resistance.

---

# lamotrigine
Lamictal

*Pharmacologic classification:* phenyltriazine
*Therapeutic classification:* anticonvulsant
*Pregnancy risk category C*

### Available forms
Available by prescription only
*Tablets:* 25 mg, 100 mg, 150 mg, 200 mg
*Chewable tablets:* 2 mg, 5 mg, 25 mg

### Indications and dosages
*Adjunct therapy in treatment of partial seizures caused by epilepsy and Lennox-Gastout syndrome*
*Adults and children ages 16 and older (12 and older for Lennox-Gastaut syndrome):* 50 mg P.O. daily for 2 weeks, followed by 100 mg daily in two divided doses for 2 weeks. Thereafter, usual maintenance dose is 300 to 500 mg P.O. daily given in two divided doses. For patients also taking valproic acid, give 25 mg P.O. every other day for 2 weeks, followed by 25 mg P.O. daily for 2 weeks. Thereafter, increase 25 to 50 mg q 1 to 2 weeks. Effective maintenance dose is 100 to 400 mg daily in 1 or 2 divided doses.
*Adjunct treatment of Lennox-Gastaut syndrome in patients receiving hepatic-enzyme–inducing anticonvulsants without concomitant valproic acid therapy*
*Children ages 2 to 12:* 0.6 mg/kg P.O. daily (rounded down to the nearest 5 mg) in two divided doses for 2 weeks. During subsequent 2 weeks, 1.2 mg/kg (rounded down to the nearest 5 mg) daily in two divided doses. Then, increase q 1 to 2 weeks by 1.2 mg/kg (rounded down to the nearest 5 mg) until effective daily dose of about 5 to 15 mg/kg (maximum of 400 mg/day in two divided doses) is reached.
*Adjunct treatment of Lennox-Gastaut syndrome in patients receiving hepatic-enzyme–inducing anticonvulsants with concomitant valproic acid therapy*
*Children ages 2 to 12:* 0.15 mg/kg P.O. daily (rounded down to the nearest 5 mg) in one or two divided doses for 2 weeks. If the initial calculated daily dose of lamotrigine is 2.5 to 5 mg, a 5-mg dose should be given on alternate days for the first 2 weeks. During subsequent 2 weeks, 0.3 mg/kg (rounded down to the nearest 5 mg) daily in one dose or two divided doses. Then, increase q 1 to 2 weeks by 0.3 mg/kg (rounded down to the nearest 5 mg) until effective daily dose of about 1 to 5 mg/kg (maximum of 200 mg/day in one or two divided doses) is reached.

### Mechanism of action
*Anticonvulsant action:* Mechanism unknown. Possibly related to inhibition of release of glutamate and aspartate in the brain. This may occur by acting on voltage-sensitive sodium channels.

### Pharmacokinetics
*Absorption:* Rapidly and completely absorbed from the GI tract with negligible first-pass metabolism. Absolute bioavailability is 98%.
*Distribution:* About 55% plasma protein–bound.
*Metabolism:* Metabolized predominantly by glucuronic acid conjugation; the major metabolite is an inactive 2-N-glucuronide conjugate.
*Excretion:* Excreted primarily in urine with only a small portion being excreted in feces.

| Route | Onset | Peak | Duration |
|-------|-------|------|----------|
| P.O. | Unknown | 1½-4¾ hr | Unknown |

### Contraindications and precautions
Contraindicated in patients hypersensitive to drug. Use cautiously in patients with impaired renal, hepatic, or cardiac function.

---

Reactions may be *common,* uncommon, *life-threatening,* or COMMON AND LIFE-THREATENING.

## Interactions

**Drug-drug.** *Carbamazepine, phenobarbital, phenytoin, primidone:* Decreased lamotrigine steady-state levels. Advise clinician to monitor patient carefully.

*Folate inhibitors such as co-trimoxazole, methotrexate:* May be affected by lamotrigine because it inhibits dihydrofolate reductase, an enzyme involved in the synthesis of folic acid. Advise clinician to monitor patient closely because drug may have an additive effect.

*Valproic acid:* Decreased lamotrigine clearance, which increases steady-state levels of drug. Advise clinician to monitor patient closely for toxicity.

**Drug-lifestyle.** *Sun exposure:* Possible photosensitivity reactions. Advise patient to take precautions.

## Adverse reactions

**CNS:** *dizziness, headache, ataxia, somnolence,* malaise, incoordination, insomnia, tremor, depression, anxiety, *seizures,* irritability, speech disorder, decreased memory, concentration disturbance, sleep disorder, emotional lability, vertigo, mind racing, *suicide attempts.*
**CV:** palpitations.
**EENT:** *diplopia, blurred vision,* epistaxis, vision abnormality, rhinitis, pharyngitis, nystagmus.
**GI:** *nausea, vomiting,* diarrhea, dyspepsia, abdominal pain, constipation, anorexia, dry mouth, rectal hemorrhage, peptic ulcer.
**GU:** dysmenorrhea, vaginitis, amenorrhea, bronchitis.
**Metabolic:** weight loss
**Musculoskeletal:** dysarthria, muscle spasm, neck pain.
**Respiratory:** cough, dyspnea.
**Skin:** *Stevens-Johnson syndrome, rash,* pruritus, hot flashes, alopecia, acne, epidermal neurolyisis, photosensitivity, contact dermatitis, dry skin, sweating.
**Other:** flulike syndrome, fever, infection, chills, peripheral edema, lupus-like syndrome, tooth disorder, vasculitis.

## Overdose and treatment

Limited information available. Following a suspected overdose, treatment should be supportive. Recommend inducing emesis or performing gastric lavage, if needed. It isn't known if hemodialysis is effective.

## Clinical considerations

■ Drug may be given without regard to meals. Chewable tablets may be swallowed whole, chewed and swallowed with a small amount of water or diluted fruit juice, or dispersed in about 5 ml of liquid for about 1 minute and consumed immediately.

■ Drug shouldn't be stopped abruptly because of risk of increasing seizure frequency. Instead, drug should be tapered over at least 2 weeks.
■ Drug should be stopped immediately if drug-induced rash occurs.
■ If lamotrigine is added to a multidrug regimen that includes valproate, recommend reducing dose of lamotrigine and using a lower maintenance dose in patients with severe renal impairment.
■ Exacerbation of parkinsonian signs and symptoms in patients with preexisting parkinsonian syndrome is possible.
**H ALERT** Don't confuse Lamictal with Lamisil.

## Therapeutic monitoring

■ Evaluate patient for reduction in the frequency and duration of seizures.
■ Check adjunct serum levels of anticonvulsant.

## Special populations

**Pregnant patients.** Safety for use during pregnancy hasn't been established. To monitor fetal outcomes in pregnant patients exposed to drug, pregnancy registries have been established. Clinicians may call to register: Lamotrigine Pregnancy Registry, 1-800-336-2176, or patients may call the North American Antiepileptic Drug Pregnancy Registry, 1-888-233-2334.
**Breast-feeding patients.** Drug use in breast-feeding women isn't recommended.
**Pediatric patients.** Recommended use in children ages 2 to 12 is very limited. Drug must be carefully given following the detailed guidelines provided with the drug. The risk of severe, potentially life-threatening rash in children is much higher than that reported in adults.
**Geriatric patients.** Safety and efficacy in patients over age 65 haven't been established.

## Patient counseling

■ Inform patient that rash may occur, especially during first 6 weeks of therapy and in children. Combination therapy of valproic acid and lamotrigine is likely to precipitate a serious rash. Although it may resolve with continued therapy, tell patient to report rash immediately in case drug needs to be discontinued.
■ Warn patient not to perform hazardous activities until CNS effects are known.
■ Advise patient to take protective measures against photosensitivity reactions until tolerance is known.

# lansoprazole
Prevacid

*Pharmacologic classification:* acid (proton) pump inhibitor
*Therapeutic classification:* antiulcerative
*Pregnancy risk category B*

## Available forms
Available by prescription only
*Capsules (delayed-release):* 15 mg, 30 mg

## Indications and dosages
*Short-term treatment of active duodenal ulcer*
*Adults:* 15 mg P.O. daily before meals for 4 weeks.
*Short-term treatment of erosive esophagitis*
*Adults:* 30 mg P.O. daily before meals for up to 8 weeks. If healing doesn't occur, an additional 8 weeks of therapy may be needed.
*Long-term treatment of pathologic hypersecretory conditions, including Zollinger-Ellison syndrome*
*Adults:* Initially, 60 mg P.O. once daily. Increase dosage, p.r.n. Give daily doses exceeding 120 mg in divided doses.
*Maintenance of healed duodenal ulcer*
*Adults:* 15 mg P.O. once daily.
*Short-term treatment of gastric ulcer*
*Adults:* 30 mg P.O. daily for up to 8 weeks.
*Short-term treatment of symptomatic gastroesophageal reflux disease (GERD)*
*Adults:* 15 mg P.O. daily for up to 8 weeks.
**Helicobacter pylori** *eradication to reduce risk of duodenal ulcer recurrence*
*Adults:* For patients receiving dual therapy, 30 mg P.O. lansoprazole with 1 g P.O. amoxicillin, each given q 8 hours for 14 days. For patients receiving triple therapy, 30 mg P.O. lansoprazole with 1 g P.O. amoxicillin and 500 mg P.O. clarithromycin, all given q 12 hours for 10 to 14 days.
*Treatment of NSAID-related ulcer in patients who continue to take NSAIDs*
*Adults:* 30 mg P.O. daily for 8 weeks.
*Reduction in risk of NSAID-related ulcer in patients who have a history of gastric ulcer but who need NSAIDs*
*Adults:* 15 mg P.O. daily for up to 12 weeks.

## Mechanism of action
*Antiulcer action:* Lansoprazole inhibits activity of the acid (proton) pump and binds to hydrogen-potassium ATPase, located at the secretory surface of the gastric parietal cells, to block the formation of gastric acid.

## Pharmacokinetics
*Absorption:* Rapidly absorbed with absolute bioavailability of more than 80%.

*Distribution:* 97% plasma protein–bound.
*Metabolism:* Extensively metabolized in the liver.
*Excretion:* About two-thirds of dose is excreted in feces; one-third in urine.

| Route | Onset | Peak | Duration |
|-------|-------|------|----------|
| P.O. | Unknown | 1¾ hr | Unknown |

## Contraindications and precautions
Contraindicated in patients hypersensitive to drug.

## Interactions
**Drug-drug.** *Ampicillin esters, iron salts, ketoconazole:* Lansoprazole may interfere with the absorption of these drugs. Advise clinician to monitor patient closely.
*Sucralfate:* Delays lansoprazole absorption. Give lansoprazole at least 30 minutes before sucralfate.
*Theophylline:* May cause mild increase in theophylline excretion. Use together cautiously. Dosage adjustment of theophylline may be needed.
**Drug-herb.** *Male fern:* Inactivated in alkaline stomach environment. Discourage use together.

## Adverse reactions
**CNS:** headache.
**GI:** diarrhea, nausea, abdominal pain.

## Overdose and treatment
No adverse effects have been reported with drug overdose. Drug isn't removed from the circulation by hemodialysis. If required, treatment should be supportive.

## Clinical considerations
■ Dosage adjustment may be required for patients with severe liver disease.
■ Drug shouldn't be used as maintenance therapy for patients with duodenal ulcer disease or erosive esophagitis.
■ Contents of capsule can be mixed with 40 ml of apple juice in a syringe and given within 3 to 5 minutes via a nasogastric tube. Recommend flushing with additional apple juice to give entire dose and maintain patency of the tube.
■ Contents of capsule can also be sprinkled on a tablespoon of applesauce, liquid dietary supplement, pudding, etc., and ingested immediately.
■ Contents of capsule can be emptied into a small volume (60 ml) of orange or tomato juice, mixed briefly, and swallowed immediately.

### Therapeutic monitoring
■ Advise clinician to monitor liver function test results in long-term therapy.

## Special populations

**Breast-feeding patients.** Because it isn't known if lansoprazole appears in breast milk, a decision to discontinue either breast-feeding or drug should be made.

**Pediatric patients.** Safety and efficacy in children haven't been established.

**Geriatric patients.** Although initial dosage regimen need not be altered for geriatric patients, subsequent doses over 30 mg/day shouldn't be given unless additional gastric acid suppression is needed.

## Patient counseling

- Instruct patient to take drug before meals.
- Caution patient not to open, chew, or crush capsules; capsules should be swallowed whole.
- Instruct patient who mixes drug in orange or tomato juice to rinse glass after consumption with 120 ml or more of juice and then to swallow the contents. This will ensure that entire dose is consumed.

# latanoprost
Xalatan

*Pharmacologic classification:* prostaglandin analogue
*Therapeutic classification:* antiglaucoma drug; ocular antihypertensive
*Pregnancy risk category C*

## Available forms
Available by prescription only
*Ophthalmic solution:* 0.005%

## Indications and dosages
*Increased intraocular pressure (IOP) in patients with ocular hypertension or open-angle glaucoma who are intolerant of other IOP-lowering drugs or insufficiently responsive to another IOP-lowering drug*
Adults: 1 drop in conjunctival sac of affected eyes once daily in the evening.

## Mechanism of action
*Antiglaucoma and ocular antihypertensive actions:* Exact mechanism of action unknown. Drug may lower IOP by increasing the outflow of aqueous humor.

## Pharmacokinetics
*Absorption:* Absorbed through the cornea.
*Distribution:* Distribution volume is about 0.16 L/kg. The acid of latanoprost could be measured in aqueous humor during first 4 hours and in plasma only during first hour after local administration.
*Metabolism:* Hydrolyzed by esterases in the cornea to the biologically active acid. The active acid of drug reaching the systemic circulation is primarily metabolized by the liver.

*Excretion:* Metabolites are mainly eliminated in urine.

| Route | Onset | Peak | Duration |
|---|---|---|---|
| Ophthalmic | 2-4 hr | 8-12 hr | Unknown |

## Contraindications and precautions
Contraindicated in patients hypersensitive to drug, benzalkonium chloride, or other ingredients in the product.

Use cautiously when giving to patients with impaired renal or hepatic function. Use with caution in patients with active ocular inflammation (iritis, uveitis), patients at risk for macular edema, aphakic patients, and pseudophakic patients.

## Interactions
**Drug-drug.** *Thimerosal:* Precipitation occurs when eyedrops containing thimerosal are mixed with latanoprost. If such drugs are used together, advise clinician to give them at least 5 minutes apart.

*Topical beta blockers (betaxolol, carteolol, levobunolol, metipranolol, timolol), topical dipivefrin, topical epinephrine, oral carbonic anhydrase inhibitor (acetazolamide), topical carbonic anhydrase inhibitor (dorzolamide):* IOP-lowering effects of theses drugs may be additive. This may be a therapeutic advantage, but if using other topical drugs, recommend separating administration times by 5 minutes.

## Adverse reactions
**CNS:** migraine headache
**CV:** chest pain; angina pectoris.
**EENT:** *blurred vision; burning; stinging;* itching; conjunctival hyperemia; foreign body sensation; increased pigmentation of iris; punctate epithelial keratopathy; dry eye; excessive tearing; photophobia; conjunctivitis; diplopia; eye pain or discharge; retinal detachment; lid crusting, edema, erythema, discomfort, or pain; herpes simplex keratitis, corneal edema and erosions.
**Musculoskeletal:** muscle, joint, or back pain.
**Respiratory:** upper respiratory tract infection, asthma.
**Skin:** rash; allergic skin reaction.
**Other:** cold, flu.

## Overdose and treatment
Apart from ocular irritation and conjunctival or episcleral hyperemia, ocular effects of latanoprost at high doses aren't known. Treatment should be symptomatic if overdose occurs.

## Clinical considerations
- Latanoprost may gradually change eye color, increasing the amount of brown pigment in the iris. The change in iris color occurs slowly and may not be noticeable for several months

to years. The increased pigmentation may be permanent.
■ Protect drug from light; refrigerate unopened bottle.

### Therapeutic monitoring
■ Advise clinician to monitor IOP-lowering effects of drug.

### Special populations
**Breast-feeding patients.** It isn't known if drug appears in breast milk. Use caution when giving drug to breast-feeding women.
**Pediatric patients.** Safety and efficacy in children haven't been established.

### Patient counseling
■ Tell patient receiving treatment in only one eye about the potential for increased brown pigmentation in the treated eye as well as heterochromia between the eyes.
■ Teach patient to instill drops. Advise him to wash hands before and after instilling solution, and warn him not to touch dropper or tip to eye or surrounding tissue.
■ Advise patient to apply light finger pressure on lacrimal sac for 1 minute after instillation to minimize systemic absorption of drug.
■ Instruct patient to report ocular reactions, especially conjunctivitis and lid reactions.
■ Tell patient using contact lenses to remove them before administration of the solution and not to reinsert the contact lenses for 15 minutes after administration.
■ Advise patient that if more than one topical ophthalmic is being used, to give the drugs at least 5 minutes apart.
■ Stress importance of compliance with recommended therapy.

# leflunomide
Arava

*Pharmacologic classification:* pyrimidine synthesis inhibitor
*Therapeutic classification:* antirheumatic
*Pregnancy risk category X*

### Available forms
Available by prescription only
*Tablets:* 10 mg, 20 mg, 100 mg

### Indications and dosages
*To reduce signs and symptoms of active rheumatoid arthritis and to slow structural damage as evidenced by erosions and joint space narrowing seen on X-ray*
*Adults:* 100 mg P.O. q 24 hours for 3 days, followed by 20 mg (maximum daily dose) P.O. q 24 hours. Dosage may be decreased to 10 mg daily if higher dose isn't well tolerated (for example, because of hepatic enzyme elevations).

### Mechanism of action
*Immunomodulatory action:* Drug inhibits dihydroorotate dehydrogenase, an enzyme involved in de novo pyrimidine synthesis, and has antiproliferative activity and anti-inflammatory effects.

### Pharmacokinetics
*Absorption:* Bioavailability is 80%. Without loading dose, plasma levels peak in about 2 months.
*Distribution:* Extensively plasma protein–bound.
*Metabolism:* Metabolized to an active metabolite (M1), responsible for most of its activity.
*Excretion:* Eliminated by renal and direct biliary excretion. About 43% is excreted in the urine and 48% in the feces. Half-life of the active metabolite is about 2 weeks.

| Route | Onset | Peak | Duration |
|-------|-------|------|----------|
| P.O. | Unknown | 6-12 hr | Unknown |

### Contraindications and precautions
Contraindicated in patients hypersensitive to drug or its components and in women who are or may become pregnant or who are breastfeeding. Drug isn't recommended for patients with hepatic insufficiency, hepatitis B or C, severe immunodeficiency, bone marrow dysplasia, or severe uncontrolled infections. Drug isn't recommended for use by men attempting to father a child.

Vaccination with live vaccines isn't recommended. Consider the long half-life of drug when contemplating administration of a live vaccine after stopping drug treatment.

The risk of malignancy, particularly lymphoproliferative disorders, increases with use of some immunosuppressants, including leflunomide. Use cautiously in patients with renal insufficiency.

### Interactions
**Drug-drug.** *Activated charcoal, cholestyramine:* Decreased plasma levels of leflunomide. They are sometimes used for this effect in treating overdose.
*Methotrexate, other hepatotoxic drugs:* Increased risk of hepatotoxicity. Advise clinician to monitor liver enzyme levels as appropriate.
*Rifampin:* Increased level of active leflunomide metabolite. Use together cautiously.

### Adverse reactions
**CNS:** asthenia, dizziness, headache, paresthesia, malaise, migraine, sleep disorder, vertigo, neuritis, anxiety, depression, insomnia, neuralgia.
**CV:** angina pectoris, *hypertension,* chest pain, palpitation, tachycardia, vasculitis, vasodilation, varicose veins, peripheral edema.

**EENT:** pharyngitis, rhinitis, sinusitis, epistaxis, enlarged salivary glands, blurred vision, cataract, conjunctivitis, eye disorder.

**GI:** stomatitis, taste perversion, dry mouth, mouth ulcer, oral candidiasis, anorexia, *diarrhea,* dyspepsia, gastroenteritis, nausea, abdominal pain, vomiting, cholelithiasis, colitis, constipation, esophagitis, flatulence, gastritis, melena.

**GU:** urinary tract infection, albuminuria, cystitis, dysuria, hematuria, menstrual disorder, pelvic pain, vaginal candidiasis, prostate disorder, urinary frequency.

**Hematologic:** anemia, ecchymoses, hyperlipidemia.

**Hepatic:** elevated liver enzyme levels.

**Metabolic:** increased CK, diabetes mellitus, hyperglycemia, hyperthyroidism, hypokalemia, weight loss.

**Musculoskeletal:** arthrosis, back pain, bursitis, muscle cramps, myalgia, bone necrosis, bone pain, arthralgia, leg cramps, joint disorder, neck pain, synovitis, tendon rupture, tenosynovitis.

**Respiratory:** bronchitis, increased cough, pneumonia, *respiratory infection,* asthma, dyspnea, lung disorder.

**Skin:** *alopecia,* eczema, pruritus, *rash,* dry skin, acne, contact dermatitis, fungal dermatitis, hair discoloration, nail disorder, skin nodule, subcutaneous nodule, maculopapular rash, skin disorder, skin discoloration, skin ulcer, increased sweating.

**Other:** hematoma, herpes simplex, herpes zoster, tooth disorder, gingivitis, ***allergic reaction,*** fever, flu syndrome, injury or accident, pain, abscess, cyst, hernia.

## Overdose and treatment

No overdose has been reported in humans. If overdose occurs, activated charcoal (50 g every 6 hours for 24 hours) reduces plasma levels. Cholestyramine may also be given as 8 g P.O. t.i.d. for 11 days.

## Clinical considerations

■ Leflunomide can cause fetal harm when given to pregnant women; it's recommended that women planning to become pregnant discontinue leflunomide therapy and consult their prescriber.

■ Men planning to father a child should discontinue drug therapy and follow recommended leflunomide removal protocol (cholestyramine 8 g, P.O. t.i.d. for 11 days).

■ Aspirin, other NSAIDs, and low-dose corticosteroids may be continued during treatment; however, combined use of drug with antimalarials, intramuscular or oral gold, penicillamine, azathioprine, or methotrexate hasn't been adequately studied.

### Therapeutic monitoring

■ Advise clinician to monitor liver enzyme (ALT and AST) levels before starting therapy and monthly thereafter until stable. Frequency can then be decreased based on clinical situation.

### Special populations

**Breast-feeding patients.** Drug shouldn't be used by breast-feeding women.

**Pediatric patients.** Safety in children and adolescents hasn't been established. Not recommended for patients under age 18.

## Patient counseling

■ Explain the need and frequency of required blood tests and monitoring.

■ Instruct patient to use birth control during course of treatment and until it has been determined that drug is no longer active.

■ Warn female patient to immediately notify prescriber if signs or symptoms of pregnancy occur (such as late menses or breast tenderness).

# letrozole
Femara

*Pharmacologic classification:* aromatase inhibitor
*Therapeutic classification:* hormone
*Pregnancy risk category D*

## Available forms

Available by prescription only
*Tablets:* 2.5 mg

## Indications and dosages

***Metastatic breast cancer in postmenopausal women with disease progression following antiestrogen therapy***
*Adults:* 2.5 mg P.O. as a single daily dose, without regard to meals.

***First-line treatment of hormone receptor–positive or hormone receptor–unknown, locally advanced or metastatic breast cancer in postmenopausal women***
*Adults:* 2.5 mg P.O. once daily until tumor progression is evident.

## Mechanism of action

*Hormone action:* Letrozole inhibits conversion of androgens to estrogens by competitive inhibition of the aromatase enzyme system. Decreased estrogens are likely to lead to decreased tumor mass or delayed progression of tumor growth in some women.

## Pharmacokinetics

***Absorption:*** Rapidly and completely absorbed. Food doesn't affect bioavailability. Steady-state plasma levels are reached in 2 to 6 weeks after daily dosing.

*Distribution:* Large volume of distribution (1.9 L/kg). It's weakly protein-bound.
*Metabolism:* Slowly metabolized to an inactive form. In human liver microsomes, letrozole strongly inhibits cytochrome P-450 isozyme 2A6 and moderately inhibits isozyme 2C19.
*Excretion:* The inactive glucuronide metabolite is eliminated in the urine.

| Route | Onset | Peak | Duration |
|-------|-------|------|----------|
| P.O. | Unknown | 2 days | Unknown |

## Contraindications and precautions
Contraindicated in patients hypersensitive to drug or its components. Avoid use in pregnant patients because drug may cause fetal harm.

Use cautiously in patients with severe liver impairment.

## Interactions
None reported.

## Adverse reactions
**CNS:** headache, somnolence, dizziness, fatigue, asthenia.
**CV:** edema, hypertension, *thromboembolism*, chest pain.
**GI:** *nausea,* vomiting, constipation, diarrhea, abdominal pain, anorexia, dyspepsia.
**Hematologic:** hypercholesterolemia.
**Metabolic:** weight gain.
**Musculoskeletal:** *bone, limb, and back pain;* arthralgias.
**Respiratory:** dyspnea, coughing.
**Skin:** hot flashes, rash, pruritus.
**Other:** viral infections.

## Overdose and treatment
There have been no reports of overdose during clinical trials with letrozole. If overdose occurs, recommend considering inducing emesis if patient is alert; recommend providing supportive care and monitoring vital signs frequently.

## Clinical considerations
■ No dosage adjustment is needed in patients with mild to moderate liver dysfunction or in renally impaired patients with creatinine clearance of 10 ml/minute or more.
■ Patients treated with letrozole don't need glucocorticoid or mineralocorticoid replacement therapy. Letrozole significantly lowers serum estrone, estradiol, and estrone sulfate, but hasn't been shown to significantly affect adrenal corticosteroid synthesis, aldosterone synthesis, or synthesis of thyroid hormones.

### Therapeutic monitoring
■ Advise clinician to monitor patient for decreased tumor progression.

### Special populations
**Breast-feeding patients.** It's unknown if letrozole appears in breast milk. Use caution when giving letrozole to breast-feeding women.

## Patient counseling
■ Instruct patient to take drug exactly as prescribed.
■ Tell patient that drug can be taken with or without food.
■ Advise patient that drug treatment is long-term, and stress importance of follow-up appointments.
■ Tell patient to inform prescriber if pregnancy is suspected or is being planned.

# leucovorin calcium (citrovorum factor or folinic acid)
Wellcovorin

*Pharmacologic classification:* formyl derivative (active reduced form of folic acid)
*Therapeutic classification:* vitamin, antidote
*Pregnancy risk category C*

## Available forms
Available by prescription only
*Tablets:* 5 mg, 10 mg, 15 mg, 25 mg
*Injection:* 1-ml ampule (3 mg/ml with 0.9% benzyl alcohol, 5 mg/ml with methyl and propyl parabens); 50-mg, 100-mg, 200-mg (preservative free), 350-mg, and 500-mg (preservative free) vials for reconstitution (contain no preservatives)
*Injection:* 10 mg/ml (preservative free)

## Indications and dosages
*Overdose of folic acid antagonist*
*Adults and children:* I.M., or I.V. dose equivalent to weight of antagonist given as soon as possible after the overdose.
*Leucovorin rescue after large methotrexate dose in treatment of cancer*
*Adults and children:* Begin 24 hours after last dose of methotrexate according to protocol. Initially, 10 mg/m² I.M. or I.V.; then give 10 mg/m² orally q 6 hours until serum methotrexate level is less than $5 \times 10^{-8}$ M (0.05 micromolar). Adjust subsequent doses based upon serum creatinine and methotrexate levels.
*Toxic effects of methotrexate used to treat severe psoriasis*
*Adults and children:* 4 to 8 mg I.M. 2 hours after methotrexate dose.
*Hematologic toxicity from pyrimethamine therapy*
*Adults and children:* Dosage highly individualized depending on dosage of folic acid antagonist and patient's clinical status.

---

Reactions may be *common*, uncommon, *life-threatening*, or COMMON AND LIFE-THREATENING.

*Prevention of toxicities in* **Pneumocystis carinii** *patients receiving trimetrexate glucuronate*
*Adults:* 20 mg/m$^2$ P.O. or I.V. over 5 to 10 minutes q 6 hours (total daily dose of 80 mg/m$^2$). If given orally, round up to the next 25-mg dose. Leucovorin should be continued at least 72 hours after last trimetrexate dose. Adjust dosages of both drugs based on hematologic response of patient.
*Advanced colorectal cancer*
*Adults:* 200 mg /m$^2$ by slow I.V. injection over 3 minutes followed by 5-fluorouracil (5-FU) or 20 mg/m$^2$ by slow I.V. injection over 3 minutes followed by 5-FU. Repeat treatment for 5 days. May repeat course at 4-week intervals for two courses and then at 4- to 5-week intervals as long as the patient has recovered from toxic effects of previous treatment. Dosage of 5-FU should be individualized.
*Megaloblastic anemia from congenital enzyme deficiency*
*Adults and children:* 3 to 6 mg I.M. daily.
*Folate-deficient megaloblastic anemias*
*Adults and children:* Up to 1 mg of leucovorin I.M. daily. Duration of treatment depends on hematologic response.

## I.V. administration

■ Reconstitute drug by adding 5 to 10 ml of sterile water for injection or bacteriostatic water for injection (which contains benzyl alcohol) to vial containing 50 or 100 mg of leucovorin, respectively. Solution will contain 10 mg/ml. Add 17 ml of sterile water for injection or bacteriostatic water for injection to vial containing 350 mg of leucovorin for a resulting concentration of 20 mg/ml. When parenteral doses greater than 10 mg/m$^2$ are needed, only reconstitute with sterile water for injection. If reconstituted with sterile water for injection, use immediately. If reconstituted with bacteriostatic water for injection, use within 7 days.
■ Leucovorin admixed with D$_{10}$W dextrose injection, normal saline injection, Ringer's or lactated Ringer's injection is stable for 24 hours when stored at room temperature and protected from light.
■ Maximum rate of leucovorin infusion shouldn't exceed 160 mg/minute because of calcium level of solution.

### Incompatibilities
Incompatible with droperidol and foscarnet.

## Mechanism of action

*Reversal of folic acid antagonism:* Leucovorin is a derivative of tetrahydrofolic acid, the reduced form of folic acid. Leucovorin performs as a cofactor in 1-carbon transfer reactions in the biosynthesis of purines and pyrimidines of nucleic acids. Impairment of thymidylate synthesis in patients with folic acid deficiency may account for defective DNA synthesis, mega-

loblast formation, and megaloblastic and macrocytic anemias. Leucovorin is a potent antidote for the hematopoietic and reticuloendothelial toxic effects of folic acid antagonists (trimethoprim, pyrimethamine, and methotrexate). "Leucovorin rescue" is used to prevent or decrease toxicity of massive methotrexate doses. Folinic acid rescues normal cells without reversing the oncolytic effect of methotrexate.

## Pharmacokinetics

*Absorption:* After oral administration, leucovorin is absorbed rapidly. The increase in plasma and serum folate activity after oral administration is mainly from 5-methyltetrahydrofolate (the major transport and storage form of folate in the body).
*Distribution:* Tetrahydrofolic acid and its derivatives are distributed throughout the body; the liver contains about half of the total body folate stores.
*Metabolism:* Metabolized in the liver.
*Excretion:* Excreted by the kidneys as 10-formyl tetrahydrofolate and 5,10-methenyl tetrahydrofolate.

| Route | Onset | Peak | Duration |
|-------|-------|------|----------|
| P.O. | 20-30 min | 2-3 hr | 3-6 hr |
| I.V. | 5 min | 10 min | 3-6 hr |
| I.M. | 10-20 min | < 1 hr | 3-6 hr |

## Contraindications and precautions
Contraindicated in patients with pernicious anemia and other megaloblastic anemias that result from the lack of vitamin B$_{12}$.

## Interactions
**Drug-drug.** *Fluorouracil:* When given together, leucovorin increases toxicity of fluorouracil. Use lower doses of fluorouracil.
*Phenytoin:* Decreased serum phenytoin levels and increased frequency of seizures. Although this interaction has occurred solely in patients receiving folic acid, it should be considered when leucovorin is given. Phenytoin dosage should be adjusted.
*Phenytoin, primidone:* May decrease serum folate levels, producing symptoms of folate deficiency. Advise clinician to monitor patient carefully.

## Adverse reactions
**Skin:** hypersensitivity reactions, urticaria, *anaphylactic reactions.*

## Overdose and treatment
Leucovorin is relatively nontoxic; no specific recommendations for overdose have been reported. However, an excessive amount of leucovorin may nullify the chemotherapeutic effect of folic acid antagonists such as methotrexate.

## Clinical considerations

- Drug administration continues until plasma methotrexate levels are less than $5 \times 10^{-8}$ M.
- Shouldn't be used as sole treatment of pernicious anemia or vitamin $B_{12}$ deficiency.
- To treat overdose of folic acid antagonists, the drug should be used within 1 hour; it isn't effective after a 4-hour delay.
- When giving more than 25 mg, drug should be administered parenterally.
- Store at room temperature in a light-resistant container, not in high-moisture areas.

### Therapeutic monitoring

- Advise clinician to monitor patient for signs of drug allergy, such as rash, wheezing, pruritus, and urticaria.
- Advise clinician to monitor serum creatinine level daily to detect possible renal function impairment.
- When used with fluorouracil, advise clinician to monitor CBC and platelet count before each course of therapy and repeat weekly during first two courses of therapy. Also, advise clinician to monitor serum electrolyte levels and liver function test results before each course of therapy for three courses and then before every other course.

### Special populations

**Breast-feeding patients.** It's unknown if leucovorin appears in breast milk; use with caution in breast-feeding women.
**Pediatric patients.** Drug may increase frequency of seizures in susceptible children. Don't use diluents containing benzyl alcohol when reconstituting drug for neonates.

## Patient counseling

- Emphasize importance of taking leucovorin only under medical supervision.

## leuprolide acetate

Lupron, Lupron Depot, Lupron Depot-Ped, Lupron Depot-3 Month, Lupron Depot-4 month

*Pharmacologic classification:* gonadotropin-releasing hormone
*Therapeutic classification:* antineoplastic; luteinizing hormone-releasing hormone (LHRH) analogue
*Pregnancy risk category X*

### Available forms

Available by prescription only
*Injection:* 5 mg/ml in 2.8-ml multiple-dose vials
*Suspension for depot injection:* 3.75 mg, 7.5 mg, 11.25 mg, 15 mg, 22.5 mg, 30 mg

## Indications and dosages

Dosage and indications may vary. Check current literature for recommended protocol. The four different depot preparations aren't interchangeable.
*Management of advanced prostate cancer*
*Adults:* 7.5 mg I.M. (depot injection) once monthly or 1 mg S.C. daily; or 22.5 mg I.M. (depot injection) q 3 months or 30 mg I.M. q 4 months (depot injection).
*Treatment of endometriosis*
*Adults:* 3.75 mg I.M. (depot injection) once monthly for a maximum of 6 months.
*Correction of anemia associated with uterine fibroids before surgery*
*Adults:* 3.75 mg I.M. q 1 month for up to 3 consecutive months with iron therapy
◊ *Central precocious puberty*
*Children (girls under age 8 and boys under age 9):* Starting dose 0.3 mg/kg (minimum 7.5 mg), given as a single I.M. or S.C. dose (depot injection) q 4 weeks. An initial dose of 7.5 mg if weight is 25 kg (55 lb) or less; 11.25 mg if weight is 25 to 37.5 kg (55 to 82½ lb); and 15 mg if weight is more than 37.5 kg (82½ lb). Titrate upward in increments of 3.75 mg q 4 weeks until clinical or laboratory tests indicate no progression of the disease. If leuprolide acetate injection is used, initial dose is 50 mcg/kg S.C. daily. Titrate upward by 10 mcg/kg daily.

## Mechanism of action

*Antineoplastic action:* Leuprolide is a synthetic analogue of LHRH. It inhibits gonadotropin secretion and androgen or estrogen synthesis. Because of this effect, leuprolide may inhibit the growth of hormone-dependent tumors.
*Hormonal action:* Because leuprolide lowers levels of sex hormones, it reduces the size of endometrial implants, resulting in decreased dysmenorrhea and pelvic pain in women with endometriosis.

## Pharmacokinetics

*Absorption:* Leuprolide is a polypeptide molecule that's destroyed in the GI tract. After S.C. administration, drug is rapidly and essentially completely absorbed.
*Distribution:* Distribution hasn't been determined, but high levels may distribute into kidney, liver, pineal, and pituitary tissue. About 7% to 15% of dose is plasma protein–bound.
*Metabolism:* Metabolism is unclear, but drug may be metabolized in the anterior pituitary and hypothalamus, similar to endogenous gonadotropin-releasing hormone.
*Excretion:* Plasma elimination half-life is 3 hours.

| Route | Onset | Peak | Duration |
|---|---|---|---|
| I.M., S.C. | < 2-4 wk | 1-2 mo | 60-90 days |

## Contraindications and precautions

Contraindicated in patients hypersensitive to drug or other gonadotropin-releasing hormone analogues, during pregnancy or lactation, and in women with undiagnosed vaginal bleeding.

Use cautiously in patients hypersensitive to benzyl alcohol.

## Interactions

None reported.

## Adverse reactions

**CNS:** *dizziness, depression, headache, pain,* insomnia, *asthenia.*
**CV:** *arrhythmias,* angina, *MI, peripheral edema, ECG changes,* hypertension, murmur.
**EENT:** sinus congestion.
**GI:** *nausea, vomiting,* anorexia, constipation.
**GU:** *impotence, vaginitis,* urinary frequency, hematuria, urinary tract infection.
**Hematologic:** anemia.
**Hepatic:** elevated liver enzyme levels.
**Metabolic:** *weight gain or loss,* initially increased then decreased with continued therapy serum acid phosphatase and testosterone levels.
**Musculoskeletal:** transient bone pain during first week of treatment, joint disorder, myalgia, neuromuscular disorder.
**Respiratory:** dyspnea, pulmonary fibrosis.
**Skin:** skin reactions at injection site, dermatitis.
**Other:** gynecomastia, *hot flashes, androgen-like effects.*

## Clinical considerations

■ Experimental uses include male contraception, treatment of endocrine disorders, hypogonadism, delayed puberty, oligospermia, anovulation, and amenorrhea.
■ When treating endometriosis, advise clinician to give for a maximum of 6 months. Safety and efficacy of retreatment are unknown.
■ To reconstitute suspension containing 3.75, 7.5, 11.25, or 15 mg of drug/dose, add 1 ml of provided diluent to leuprolide acetate powder for injection using a 22G needle; 1.5 ml of provided diluent is added to the 22.5 or 30 mg drug/dose vial using a 23G needle. Shake well. Resulting suspension is milky. Use 22.5 and 30 mg concentration immediately.
■ Advise clinician to use a 22G needle for monthly injection and a 23G needle for 3-month injection.
■ A 0.5-ml, low dose, U-100 insulin syringe may be used if needed to replace manufacturer-provided syringes to inject leuprolide acetate injection; fill syringe to the 20-unit mark.
■ Discard solution if particulate matter is visible or if the solution is discolored.
■ Erythema or induration may develop at injection site.
■ When treating prostate cancer, leuprolide may aggravate signs and symptoms of disease during first 1 to 2 weeks of therapy. Temporary paresthesia and weakness may occur during first week of therapy.
■ No unusual adverse effects were observed in patients who had received 20 mg daily for 2 years.
■ Refrigerate leuprolide vials for injection until used. Don't freeze. Vial in use may be stored at room temperature. Leuprolide powder for injection suspension may be stored at room temperature. Reconstituted suspension is stable for 24 hours.

### Therapeutic monitoring

■ Recommend measuring serum testosterone and acid phosphatase levels before and during therapy.
■ Recommend measuring serum testosterone, prostate specific antigen, and prostatic acid phosphatase levels before and during therapy in patients with prostate cancer.
■ Advise clinician to monitor liver function test results.

### Special populations

**Pregnant patients.** Reversible suppression of fertility in men and women has occurred.

## Patient counseling

■ Reassure patient that bone pain is transient and will disappear after about 1 week.
■ Inform patient that a temporary reaction of burning, itching, and swelling at injection site may occur. Tell him to report persistent reactions.
■ Advise patient to continue taking drug even if he experiences a sense of well-being.
■ Instruct women of childbearing age to use an effective nonhormonal method of contraception during therapy, and to discontinue drug and notify prescriber if pregnancy occurs.

---

# levalbuterol hydrochloride
Xopenex

*Pharmacologic classification:* beta$_2$ agonist
*Therapeutic classification:* bronchodilator
*Pregnancy risk category C*

## Available forms

Available by prescription only
*Solution for inhalation:* 0.63 mg or 1.25 mg in 3-ml vials

## Indications and dosages

*To prevent or treat bronchospasm in patients with reversible obstructive airway disease*
*Adults and adolescents ages 12 and older:* 0.63 mg given t.i.d. q 6 to 8 hours, by oral inhalation via a nebulizer. Patients with more severe asthma who don't respond adequately to

a dose of 0.63 mg may benefit from a dosage of 1.25 mg t.i.d.

## Mechanism of action
*Bronchodilator action:* Levalbuterol activates beta$_2$ receptors on airway smooth muscle, which leads the smooth muscle in all airways—from the trachea to the terminal bronchioles—to relax, thereby relieving bronchospasm and reducing airway resistance. Drug also inhibits the release of mediators from mast cells in the airway.

## Pharmacokinetics
No information available.

| Route | Onset | Peak | Duration |
|---|---|---|---|
| Inhalation | Unknown | Unknown | Unknown |

## Contraindications and precautions
Contraindicated in patients hypersensitive to levalbuterol or racemic albuterol.

Use cautiously in patients with CV disorders, especially coronary insufficiency, hypertension, and arrhythmias. Also use cautiously in patients with seizure disorders, hyperthyroidism, or diabetes mellitus and in patients who are unusually responsive to sympathomimetic amines.

## Interactions
**Drug-drug.** *Beta blockers:* May cause reduced pulmonary effect of the drug and, possibly, severe bronchospasm. Don't use together, if possible. If use together is needed, a cardioselective beta blocker may be considered, but advise clinician to give with caution.
*Digoxin:* Decreased digoxin levels (up to 22%). Advise clinician to monitor digoxin levels.
*Loop or thiazide diuretics:* May cause ECG changes and hypokalemia from concurrent administration of these non–potassium-sparing diuretics. Use together cautiously.
*MAO inhibitors, tricyclic antidepressants:* Potentiate the action of levalbuterol on the vascular system. Advise clinician to give with extreme caution in patients being given MAO inhibitors or tricyclic antidepressants, or within 2 weeks of discontinuation of these drugs.
*Other short-acting sympathomimetic aerosol bronchodilators, epinephrine:* May cause increased adrenergic adverse effects. To avoid serious CV effects, advise clinician to use additional adrenergics with caution.

## Adverse reactions
**CNS:** dizziness, migraine, nervousness, tremor, anxiety, pain.
**CV:** tachycardia.
**EENT:** *rhinitis,* sinusitis, turbinate edema.
**GI:** dyspepsia.
**Musculoskeletal:** leg cramps.
**Respiratory:** increased cough, *viral infection.*
**Other:** flu syndrome, accidental injury.

## Overdose and treatment
Signs and symptoms of overdose are those of excessive beta-receptor stimulation, including seizures, angina, hypertension or hypotension, tachycardia with rates up to 200 beats per minute, arrhythmias, nervousness, headache, tremor, dry mouth, palpitation, nausea, dizziness, fatigue, malaise, and sleeplessness. Hypokalemia may also occur. As with other sympathomimetics, abuse of levalbuterol may result in cardiac arrest and death.

Treatment consists of stopping the drug and giving symptomatic therapy. A cardioselective beta-receptor blocker may be used, but keep in mind that beta-receptor blockers can cause bronchospasm. It's unknown if dialysis is beneficial in managing levalbuterol overdose.

## Clinical considerations
**◪ ALERT** Like other inhaled beta agonists, levalbuterol may produce paradoxical bronchospasm, which may be life-threatening. If this occurs, drug should be stopped immediately and alternative therapy should be instituted.
▪ Small, transient increases in blood glucose levels may occur after oral inhalation.
▪ Serum potassium levels may decrease slightly, but potassium supplementation is usually unnecessary.
▪ Keep unopened vials in foil pouch. Once the foil pouch is opened, use the vials within 2 weeks. If vials are removed from pouch but not used immediately, protect from light and excessive heat and use within 1 week.

### Therapeutic monitoring
▪ Advise clinician to monitor patient for clinical effect of drug and for worsening of symptoms.

### Special populations
**Pregnant patients.** Use drug only if benefits outweigh risk to the fetus.
**Breast-feeding patients.** Plasma levels of levalbuterol are very low following inhalation of therapeutic dosages. It's unknown if drug appears in breast milk. Give cautiously to breast-feeding women.
**Pediatric patients.** Safety and efficacy of levalbuterol in children under age 12 are unknown.
**Geriatric patients.** Safety and efficacy of levalbuterol are unknown in patients ages 65 and older. In general, patients in this age group should be started at a dose of 0.63 mg.

## Patient counseling
▪ Warn patient that he may experience paradoxical bronchospasm (difficulty breathing). Tell him to discontinue drug and contact his prescriber immediately if this occurs.

---

- Inform patient that common adverse effects include palpitations, rapid heart rate, headache, dizziness, tremor, and nervousness.
- Inform patient that the effects of levalbuterol may last up to 8 hours.
- Warn patient not to increase dose or frequency without consulting his prescriber.
- Advise patient to seek medical attention immediately if levalbuterol becomes less effective for treating signs and symptoms, signs and symptoms become worse, or he's using levalbuterol more frequently than usual.
- Caution patient to use other inhalants and antasthmatics only as directed while taking levalbuterol.
- Advise female patient to inform prescriber about the use of levalbuterol if she becomes pregnant or is breast-feeding.
- Instruct patient not to use levalbuterol after the expiration date stamped on the container.
- Inform patient that once the foil pouch is opened, the vials should be used within 2 weeks. If opened pouch isn't used immediately, vials should be protected from light and excessive heat, and used within 1 week.
- Tell patient to discard any vials containing discolored solution.

# levetiracetam
Keppra

*Pharmacologic classification:* anticonvulsant
*Therapeutic classification:* anticonvulsant
*Pregnancy risk category C*

## Available forms
Available by prescription only
*Tablets:* 250 mg, 500 mg, 750 mg

## Indications and dosages
### Adjunctive therapy for partial seizures
*Adults:* Initially, 500 mg b.i.d. Dosage can be increased by 500 mg b.i.d., p.r.n., for seizure control at 2-week intervals to maximum dosage of 1,500 mg b.i.d.
≡*Dosage adjustment.* For patients with renal insufficiency, if creatinine clearance is 50 to 80 ml/minute, give 500 to 1,000 mg q 12 hours; if 30 to 50 ml/minute, give 250 to 750 mg q 12 hours; if less than 30 ml/minute, give 250 to 500 mg q 12 hours. For end-stage renal disease dialysis patients, give 500 to 1,000 mg q 24 hours. A 250- to 500-mg dose should be given after dialysis.

## Mechanism of action
*Anticonvulsant action:* Mechanism of action is unknown. Levetiracetam is thought to inhibit kindling activity in hippocampus, thus preventing simultaneous neuronal firing that leads to seizure activity.

## Pharmacokinetics
*Absorption:* Rapidly absorbed in GI tract; serum levels peak in about 1 hour. Can be taken with food, but time to reach peak levels is delayed by about 1½ hours with slightly lower serum levels. Steady-state serum levels reached in about 2 days.
*Distribution:* Minimal protein-binding.
*Metabolism:* No active metabolites; isn't metabolized through cytochrome P-450 system.
*Excretion:* 66% of drug eliminated unchanged by glomerular filtration and tubular reabsorption. Elimination half-life is about 7 hours in patients with normal renal function.

| Route | Onset | Peak | Duration |
|-------|-------|------|----------|
| P.O. | Rapid | 1 hr | Unknown |

## Contraindications and precautions
Contraindicated in patients hypersensitive to drug. Use cautiously in immunocompromised patients and in those with poor renal function.

## Interactions
**Drug-drug.** *Antihistamines, benzodiazepines, narcotics, tricyclic antidepressants, other drugs that cause drowsiness:* Possible severe sedation. Avoid concomitant use.
**Drug-lifestyle.** *Alcohol use:* Possible severe sedation. Discourage use together.

## Adverse reactions
**CNS:** *asthenia, headache, somnolence,* dizziness, depression, vertigo, paresthesia, nervousness, hostility, emotional lability, ataxia, amnesia, anxiety.
**EENT:** diplopia, sinusitis, pharyngitis, rhinitis.
**GI:** anorexia.
**Hematologic:** *leukopenia, neutropenia.*
**Musculoskeletal:** pain.
**Respiratory:** cough, infection.

## Overdose and treatment
For overdose, emesis or gastric lavage may be helpful in early stages of treatment. Hemodialysis removes about 50% of drug if performed within 4 hours of overdose.

## Clinical considerations
- For patients with renal insufficiency, dosage reduction is based on creatinine clearance.
- Seizures may occur if drug is stopped abruptly. Tapering is recommended.
- Drug is approved only as an adjunctive drug for partial seizures.
- Drug can be taken with or without food.

### Therapeutic monitoring
- Baseline CBC with periodic follow-up may be advisable in immunocompromised patients because of reports of leukopenia and neutropenia.

- Advise clinician to monitor patient closely for such adverse reactions as dizziness, which may lead to falls.

### Special populations

**Breast-feeding patients.** It's unknown if drug appears in breast milk. Determine risks and benefits before giving to breast-feeding women.
**Pediatric patients.** Drug isn't recommended for children under age 16.
**Geriatric patients.** Advise patient to use extra care when sitting up or standing to avoid falling.

### Patient counseling

- Tell patient to call prescriber and not to stop drug suddenly if adverse reactions occur.
- Warn patient to use extra care when sitting or standing to avoid falling.
- Advise patient to take this drug in addition to other prescribed seizure drugs.

---

# levobunolol hydrochloride

AKBeta, Betagan

*Pharmacologic classification:* beta blocker
*Therapeutic classification:* antiglaucoma
*Pregnancy risk category C*

### Available forms

Available by prescription only
*Ophthalmic solution:* 0.25%, 0.5%

### Indications and dosages

*Chronic open-angle glaucoma and ocular hypertension*
*Adults:* Instill 1 to 2 drops (0.5% solution) daily or 1 to 2 drops (0.25% solution) b.i.d. in eye.

### Mechanism of action

*Antiglaucoma action:* Levobunolol is a nonselective beta-blocker that reduces intraocular pressure. Exact mechanism is unknown, but drug appears to reduce formation of aqueous humor.

### Pharmacokinetics

*Absorption:* Systemic absorption is undetermined, but may occur.
*Distribution:* Unknown.
*Metabolism:* Unknown.
*Excretion:* Unknown.

| Route | Onset | Peak | Duration |
|-------|-------|------|----------|
| Ophthalmic | 1 hr | 2-6 hr | 24 hr |

### Contraindications and precautions

Contraindicated in patients hypersensitive to drug, and those with bronchial asthma, history of bronchial asthma or severe COPD, sinus bradycardia, second- or third-degree AV block, cardiac failure, or cardiogenic shock. Use cautiously in patients with chronic bronchitis, emphysema, diabetes mellitus, hyperthyroidism, and myasthenia gravis.

### Interactions

**Drug-drug.** *Carbonic anhydrase inhibitors, epinephrine, pilocarpine:* Increased reductions in intraocular pressure. Use together cautiously.
*Catecholamine-depleting drugs, reserpine:* Enhance the hypotensive and bradycardiac effects of these drugs. Advise clinician to monitor patient carefully.
*Oral beta blockers:* Increased systemic effects. Advise clinician to monitor patient carefully.

### Adverse reactions

**CNS:** headache, depression, insomnia.
**CV:** slight reduction in resting heart rate.
**EENT:** *transient eye stinging and burning,* tearing, erythema, itching, keratitis, corneal punctate staining, photophobia; decreased corneal sensitivity (with long-term use).
**GI:** nausea.
**Skin:** urticaria.
**Other:** evidence of beta blockade and systemic absorption *(hypotension, **bradycardia**, syncope, **asthmatic attacks in patients with history of asthma**, HF).*

### Overdose and treatment

Overdose is extremely rare with ophthalmic use. However, usual symptoms include bradycardia, hypotension, bronchospasm, heart block, and cardiac failure.

After accidental ingestion, emesis is most effective if initiated within 30 minutes, providing patient isn't obtunded, comatose, or having seizures. Recommend following with activated charcoal. Recommend treating bradycardia, conduction defects, and hypotension with I.V. fluids, glucagon, atropine, or isoproterenol. Recommend treating bronchoconstriction with I.V. aminophylline, and seizures with I.V. diazepam.

### Clinical considerations

**◼ ALERT** Drug contains sodium metabisulfite, which may precipitate an allergic reaction in susceptible individuals.
- Levobunolol is faster acting than timolol.
- Because levobunolol has little or no effect on pupil size, drug shouldn't be used alone in patients with angle-closure glaucoma; use with a miotic.
- Store at 59° to 86° F (15° to 30° C) in light-resistant container.

### Therapeutic monitoring

- Cardiac output is reduced in both healthy patients and those with heart disease. Drug may decrease heart rate and blood pressure and produces beta blockade in bronchi and bronchioles. No effect on pupil size or accommodation has been noted. Advise clinician to monitor patient for these effects.

■ In some patients, a few weeks' treatment may be required to stabilize pressure-lowering response; intraocular pressure should be determined after 4 weeks of treatment.

### Special populations
**Geriatric patients.** Use drug with caution in geriatric patients with cardiac or pulmonary disease who may experience exacerbation of symptoms, depending on extent of systemic absorption.

### Patient counseling
■ Warn patient not to touch dropper to eye or surrounding tissue.

■ Show patient how to instill drug. Teach him to press lacrimal sac lightly for 1 minute after drug administration, to decrease chance of systemic absorption.

■ Remind patient not to blink more than usual or to close eyes tightly during treatment.

■ Tell patient to report severe reaction, although transient stinging and discomfort are common.

# levobupivacaine
Chirocaine

*Pharmacologic classification:* amino amide local anesthetic
*Therapeutic classification:* local anesthetic
*Pregnancy risk category B*

### Available forms
Available by prescription only
*Injection:* 2.5 mg/ml (0.25%), 5 mg/ml (0.5%), 7.5 mg/ml (0.75%)

### Indications and dosages
*Epidural for surgery*
*Adults:* 50 to 150 mg (10 to 20 ml) 0.5% to 0.75% solution.
*Epidural for cesarean section*
*Adults:* 100 to 150 mg (20 to 30 ml) 0.5% solution.
*Peripheral nerve block*
*Adults:* 75 to 150 mg (30 ml) or 1 to 2 mg/kg (0.4 ml/kg) 0.25% to 0.5% solution.
*Ophthalmic block*
*Adults:* 37.5 to 112.5 mg (5 to 15 ml) 0.75% solution.
*Local infiltration*
*Adults:* 150 mg (60 ml) 0.25% solution.
*Labor analgesia*
*Adults:* 25 to 50 mg (10 to 20 ml) 0.25% solution as epidural bolus.
*Postoperative pain*
*Adults:* 5 to 25 mg/hr (4 to 10 ml/hr) 0.125% to 0.25% solution as epidural infusion.

Note: Dosage will differ depending on anesthetic procedure, area to be anesthetized, vascularity of area, number of neuronal segments to be blocked, degree of block, duration of anesthesia desired, and individual patient conditions and tolerance. Always use incremental doses.

### Mechanism of action
*Anesthetic action:* Levobupivacaine blocks the generation and conduction of nerve impulses by increasing the threshold for electrical excitation in the nerve, slowing propagation of the nerve impulse, and reducing the rate of the action potential.

### Pharmacokinetics
*Absorption:* Depends on dose and route of administration because absorption from the site of administration is affected by vascularity of tissue. Blood levels peak 30 minutes after epidural administration.
*Distribution:* Plasma protein–binding is greater than 97%. Drug is widely distributed to all tissues after parenteral administration.
*Metabolism:* Widely metabolized by hepatic enzyme systems with no unchanged drug excreted in the urine or feces. In vitro studies show that CYP3A4 isoform and CYP1A2 isoform mediate the metabolism of levobupivacaine.
*Excretion:* After I.V. administration 71% is recovered from urine and 24% from feces. Elimination half-life is 3.3 hours after I.V. administration with a terminal half-life of 1.3 hours.

| Route | Onset | Peak | Duration |
|---|---|---|---|
| Epidural, local injection | Variable | 30 min | 1.3 hr |

### Contraindications and precautions
Contraindicated in patients hypersensitive to levobupivacaine or to any local anesthetic of the amide type. Drug shouldn't be used in emergency situations in which a fast onset of surgical anesthesia is needed. 0.75% levobupivacaine should be avoided in obstetric patients and solutions of levobupivacaine shouldn't be used for the production of obstetric paracervical block anesthesia. Drug shouldn't be used for I.V. regional anesthesia (Bier block).

Advise clinician to use caution when giving large volumes of higher concentrations because cardiac toxicity can occur. Use with caution in patients with hepatic disease, hypotension, hypovolemia, or impaired CV function, especially heart block.

### Interactions
**Drug-drug.** *Calcium channel blockers, clarithromycin, erythromycin, ketoconazole, ritonavir:* Possible decreased hepatic metabolism and increased effect of levobupivacaine. Dosage adjustment of levobupivacaine should be considered.

---

* Canada only   ◇ Unlabeled clinical use

*Drugs related to amide-type local anesthetics, other local anesthetics:* Increased toxic effects of these drugs. Use cautiously.

*Omeprazole, phenobarbital, phenytoin, rifampin:* Possible increased hepatic metabolism with decreased levobupivacaine effect. Advise clinician to monitor patient closely.

## Adverse reactions

**CNS:** dizziness, *headache,* paresthesia, somnolence, anxiety, hypesthesia.
**CV:** hypotension, abnormal ECG, ***bradycardia,*** tachycardia, hypertension.
**EENT:** diplopia.
**GI:** nausea, vomiting, enlarged abdomen, constipation, flatulence, abdominal pain, dyspepsia, diarrhea.
**GU:** albuminuria, urinary incontinence, decreased urine flow, urinary tract infection, hematuria, abnormal urine.
**Hematologic:** anemia, leukocytosis.
**Musculoskeletal:** back pain.
**Respiratory:** coughing.
**Skin:** pruritus, purpura.
**Other:** postoperative pain, fever, fetal distress, delayed delivery, pain, rigors, hypothermia, hemorrhage in pregnancy, breast pain, increased wound drainage, local anesthesia.

## Overdose and treatment

Acute emergencies are generally related to high plasma levels or high dermatomal level. Toxic reactions may include CNS stimulation, seizures, circulatory depression, apnea, and respiratory depression.

To treat toxic reactions, recommend immediately establishing and maintaining a patent airway or give controlled ventilation with 100% oxygen. If needed, advise clinician to use I.V. barbiturates, anticonvulsants, or muscle relaxants to control seizures. Supportive treatment of circulatory depression may require the administration of I.V. fluids or appropriate vasopressors. If maintaining a patent airway is difficult or prolonged ventilatory support is necessary, endotracheal intubation may be indicated.

If maternal hypotension or fetal bradycardia occurs in the pregnant patient, recommend maintaining patient in the left lateral decubitus position, if possible, or manually displacing the uterus off the great vessels to prevent aortocaval compression of the uterus. Resuscitation in pregnant patients may take longer than in nonpregnant patients. Rapid delivery of the fetus may improve the response to resuscitation efforts.

## Clinical considerations

**H ALERT** Local anesthetics should only be given by prescribers experienced in the diagnosis and management of drug-related toxicity and other acute emergencies that may occur.

■ Resuscitative equipment, drugs, and oxygen should be immediately available.
■ Disinfectants containing heavy metals, which cause the release of ions, shouldn't be used for skin or mucous membrane disinfection because they may cause swelling and edema.
**H ALERT** Unintended I.V. injection is possible and may cause cardiac arrest.
**H ALERT** Pregnant patients have a high risk of cardiac arrhythmias, cardiac and circulatory arrest, and death if drug is inadvertently administered I.V.
■ Advise clinician to give a test dose of a local anesthetic with a fast onset, preferably a solution containing epinephrine, before epidural anesthesia with levobupivacaine. Advise clinician to monitor patient for CNS and CV toxicity.
■ Recommend aspirating for blood or CSF before injecting any dose of levobupivacaine to avoid intravascular or intrathecal injection.
**H ALERT** An intravascular injection is still possible even if aspirations for blood are negative.
■ Advise clinician to give smallest dose and concentration required to produce desired result.
■ During epidural administration, advise clinician to give in incremental volumes of 3 to 5 ml with sufficient time between doses to detect toxicity.
■ Small doses of local anesthetics injected into the head and neck area may produce adverse reactions similar to those seen with systemic toxicity that occurs with unintentional intravascular injections of larger doses.
■ Local anesthetics rapidly cross the placental barrier and can cause maternal, fetal, and neonatal toxicity. Adverse reactions may involve alterations in the CNS, peripheral vascular tone, and cardiac function, including maternal hypotension, fetal bradycardia, and fetal decelerations. Advise clinician to monitor fetal heart rate continuously.
■ The 0.75% concentration is indicated for nonobstetric surgery patients requiring long duration of profound muscle relaxation.
■ The 0.125% solution is used only as adjunct therapy with fentanyl or clonidine.
■ Levobupivacaine diluted in normal saline solution is stable when stored in polyvinyl chloride bags at room temperature for up to 24 hours.

### *Therapeutic monitoring*

■ Advise clinician to monitor patient for ECG changes, hypotension, and bradycardia.
■ Recommend continuously monitoring CV and respiratory status and patient's state of consciousness after each injection. Restlessness, anxiety, incoherent speech, light-headedness, numbness and tingling of mouth and lips, metallic taste, tinnitus, dizziness, blurred vision, tremors, twitching, depression, or drowsiness may be early signs of CNS toxicity.

---

### Special populations
**Breast-feeding patients.** Some local anesthetics appear in breast milk. Use with caution in breast-feeding women.
**Pediatric patients.** Safety and effectiveness haven't been established.
**Geriatric patients.** No differences in safety and effectiveness have been observed in geriatric patients.

### Patient counseling
■ Advise patient that temporary loss of sensation and motor activity in anesthetized part of body may occur.

# levodopa
Larodopa

*Pharmacologic classification:* dopamine precursor
*Therapeutic classification:* antiparkinsonian
*Pregnancy risk category C*

### Available forms
Available by prescription only
*Tablets:* 100 mg, 250 mg, 500 mg
*Capsules:* 100 mg, 250 mg, 500 mg

### Indications and dosages
*Parkinsonism*
Levodopa is indicated in treating idiopathic, postencephalitic, arteriosclerotic parkinsonism, and symptomatic parkinsonism that may follow injury to the nervous system by carbon monoxide intoxication and manganese intoxication.
*Adults:* Initially, 0.5 to 1 g P.O. daily, given b.i.d., t.i.d., or q.i.d. with food; increase 100 to 750 mg daily q 3 to 7 days, as tolerated. Usual optimal dose is 3 to 6 g daily divided into three or more doses. Maximum recommended dose is 8 g daily; some patients may need more. A significant therapeutic response may not be obtained for 6 months. Larger dose requires close supervision.

### Mechanism of action
*Antiparkinsonian action:* Precise mechanism hasn't been established. A small percentage of each dose crossing the blood-brain barrier is decarboxylated. The dopamine then stimulates dopaminergic receptors in the basal ganglia to enhance the balance between cholinergic and dopaminergic activity, resulting in improved modulation of voluntary nerve impulses transmitted to the motor cortex.

### Pharmacokinetics
*Absorption:* Absorbed rapidly from the small intestine by an active amino acid transport system, with 30% to 50% reaching general circulation.

*Distribution:* Distributed widely to most body tissues, but not to the CNS, which receives less than 1% of dose because of extensive metabolism in the periphery.
*Metabolism:* Most (95%) is converted to dopamine by l-aromatic amino acid decarboxylase enzyme in the lumen of the stomach and intestines and on the first pass through the liver.
*Excretion:* Excreted primarily in urine; 80% of dose is excreted within 24 hours as dopamine metabolites. Half-life is 1 to 3 hours.

| Route | Onset | Peak | Duration |
|-------|-------|------|----------|
| P.O. | Unknown | 1-3 hr | 5 hr |

### Contraindications and precautions
Contraindicated in concurrent therapy with MAO inhibitors within 14 days, in patients hypersensitive to drug, and those with acute angle-closure glaucoma, melanoma, or undiagnosed skin lesions.
Use cautiously in patients with severe renal, CV, hepatic, and pulmonary disorders; peptic ulcer; psychiatric illness; MI with residual arrhythmias; bronchial asthma; emphysema; and endocrine disorders.

### Interactions
**Drug-drug.** *Anesthetics, hydrocarbon inhalation:* Possible arrhythmias because of increased endogenous dopamine level. Levodopa should be stopped 6 to 8 hours before administration of anesthetics such as halothane.
*Antacids containing calcium, magnesium, or sodium bicarbonate:* Possible increased absorption of levodopa. Antacids should be given 1 hour after levodopa.
*Anticholinergics:* Use with levodopa may produce a mild synergy and increased efficacy. Gradual reduction in anticholinergic dosage is needed.
*Anticonvulsants (such as hydantoins, phenytoin), benzodiazepines, haloperidol, papaverine, phenothiazines, rauwolfia alkaloids, thioxanthenes:* Possible decreased therapeutic effects of levodopa. Advise clinician to monitor patient for decreased effectiveness.
*Antihypertensives:* Increased hypotensive effect. Advise clinician to monitor blood pressure.
*Bromocriptine:* Possible additive effects. Reduced levodopa dosage may be needed.
*Methyldopa:* Possible alteration of antiparkinsonian effects of levodopa and production of additive toxic CNS effects. Avoid use together.
*MAO inhibitors:* Possible hypertensive crisis. MAO inhibitors should be stopped for 2 to 4 weeks before starting levodopa.
*Pyridoxine:* A small dose (10 mg) reverses antiparkinsonian effects of levodopa. Don't give together.

---

*Sympathomimetics:* Possible increased risk of arrhythmias. Dosage reduction of the sympathomimetic is recommended; administration of carbidopa with levodopa reduces the tendency of sympathomimetics to cause dopamine-induced arrhythmias. Recommend reducing levodopa dosage.

*Tricyclic antidepressants:* Possible increased sympathetic activity, with sinus tachycardia and hypertension. Avoid use together, if possible.

**Drug-herb.** *Jimsonweed:* Possible adverse effect on CV function. Discourage use together.

*Kava:* Possible increased parkinsonian symptoms. Discourage use together.

*Rauwolfia:* Possible decreased effectiveness of levodopa. Discourage use together.

## Adverse reactions

**CNS:** *aggressive behavior; choreiform, dystonic, and dyskinetic movements; involuntary grimacing, head movements, myoclonic body jerks, seizures,* ataxia, tremor, muscle twitching; bradykinetic episodes; psychiatric disturbances; mood changes, nervousness, anxiety, disturbing dreams, euphoria, malaise, fatigue; severe depression, *suicidal tendencies,* dementia, delirium, hallucinations.

**CV:** *orthostatic hypotension,* cardiac irregularities, phlebitis.

**EENT:** blepharospasm, blurred vision, diplopia, mydriasis or miosis, activation of latent Horner's syndrome, oculogyric crises, excessive salivation.

**GI:** dry mouth, bitter taste, *nausea, vomiting, anorexia,* constipation, flatulence, diarrhea, abdominal pain.

**GU:** urinary frequency, urine retention, incontinence, darkened urine, priapism.

**Hematologic:** *hemolytic anemia, leukopenia, agranulocytosis.*

**Hepatic:** elevated liver enzyme levels, *hepatotoxicity.*

**Metabolic:** weight loss (at start of therapy).

**Respiratory:** hyperventilation, hiccups.

**Other:** dark perspiration.

## Overdose and treatment

Signs and symptoms of overdose include spasm or closing of eyelids, irregular heartbeat, or palpitations. Treatment includes immediate gastric lavage, maintenance of an adequate airway, and judicious administration of I.V. fluids and may include antiarrhythmics, if needed. Pyridoxine 10 to 25 mg P.O. has been reported to reverse toxic and therapeutic effects of levodopa. (Its usefulness hasn't been established in acute overdose.)

## Clinical considerations

■ Advise clinician to give drug between meals and with low-protein snack to maximize drug absorption and minimize GI upset. Foods high in protein appear to interfere with transport of drug.

■ Tablets and capsules may be crushed and mixed with applesauce or baby-food fruits for patients who have difficulty swallowing pills.

■ Maximum effectiveness of drug may not occur for several weeks or months after therapy begins.

■ Because of risk of precipitating a symptom complex resembling neuroleptic malignant syndrome, recommend observing patient closely if levodopa dosage is reduced abruptly or discontinued.

■ If restarting therapy after a long period of interruption, recommend adjusting drug dosage gradually to previous level.

■ Patients undergoing surgery should continue levodopa as long as oral intake is permitted, usually 6 to 24 hours before surgery. Drug should be resumed as soon as patient is able to take oral drug.

■ Although controversial, a medically supervised period of drug discontinuance (drug holiday) may reestablish the effectiveness of a lower dose regimen.

■ Combination of levodopa-carbidopa usually reduces amount of levodopa needed, thus reducing risk of adverse reactions.

■ Levodopa has also been used to relieve pain of herpes zoster, management of bone pain in metastatic disease, and management of hepatic coma.

■ Protect drug from heat, light, and moisture. If preparation darkens, it has lost potency and should be discarded.

■ Coombs' test occasionally becomes positive during extended therapy. Colorimetric test for uric acid has shown false elevations. False-positive results have been noted on tests for urine glucose using the copper-reduction method; false-negative results have occurred with the glucose oxidase method. Levodopa also may interfere with tests for urine ketones, urine norepinephrine, and urine protein determinations.

### Therapeutic monitoring

■ Advise clinician to monitor patient also receiving antihypertensive for possible drug interactions. Recommend stopping MAO inhibitors at least 2 weeks before levodopa therapy begins.

■ Advise clinician to monitor vital signs, especially while adjusting dose.

■ Advise clinician to monitor patient for muscle twitching and blepharospasm (twitching of eyelids), which may be an early sign of drug overdose.

■ Patients on long-term therapy should be tested regularly for diabetes and acromegaly; check blood tests and liver and kidney function test results periodically for adverse effects. Leukopenia may require cessation of therapy.

---

Reactions may be *common*, uncommon, *life-threatening*, or COMMON AND LIFE-THREATENING.

■ Advise clinician to monitor serum laboratory test results periodically. Coombs' test occasionally becomes positive during extended use. Expect uric acid elevation with colorimetric method but not with uricase method.

■ Alkaline phosphatase, AST, ALT, LDH, bilirubin, BUN, and protein-bound iodine levels show transient elevations in patients receiving levodopa; WBC, hemoglobin level, and hematocrit show occasional reduction.

### Special populations
**Breast-feeding patients.** Drug may inhibit lactation and shouldn't be used by breast-feeding women.
**Pediatric patients.** Safety of levodopa in children under age 12 hasn't been established.
**Geriatric patients.** Smaller doses may be required because of reduced tolerance to effects of drug. Geriatric patients, especially those with osteoporosis, should resume normal activity gradually, because increased mobility may increase risk of fractures. Geriatric patients are more likely to develop adverse effects, such as anxiety, confusion, or nervousness; those with preexisting heart disease are more susceptible to cardiac effects of levodopa.

### Patient counseling
■ Warn patient and family not to increase drug dose without specific instruction. (They may be tempted to do this as parkinsonian symptoms progress.)

■ Explain that therapeutic response may not occur for up to 6 months.

■ Advise patient and family that multivitamin preparations, fortified cereals, and certain OTC products may contain pyridoxine (vitamin $B_6$), which can reverse the effects of levodopa.

■ Warn patient of possible dizziness and orthostatic hypotension, especially at start of therapy. Tell patient to change position slowly and dangle legs before getting out of bed. Instruct patient in use of elastic stockings to control this adverse reaction if appropriate.

■ Inform patient of signs and symptoms of adverse reactions and therapeutic effects and need to report changes.

■ Tell patient to take a missed dose as soon as possible, to skip dose if next scheduled dose is within 2 hours, but not to double the dose.

■ Advise patient not to take drug with food, and that eating something about 15 minutes after administration may help reduce GI upset.

■ Warn patient of possible darkening of urine, sweat, and other body fluids.

# levodopa-carbidopa
Atamet, Sinemet 10-100, Sinemet 25-100, Sinemet 25-250, Sinemet CR 25-100, Sinemet CR 50-200

*Pharmacologic classification:* decarboxylase inhibitor/dopamine precursor combination
*Therapeutic classification:* antiparkinsonian
*Pregnancy risk category C*

### Available forms
Available by prescription only
*Tablets:* 10 mg carbidopa with 100 mg levodopa (Sinemet 10-100), 25 mg carbidopa with 100 mg levodopa (Sinemet 25-100), 25 mg carbidopa with 250 mg levodopa (Sinemet 25-250)
*Tablets (sustained-release):* 50 mg carbidopa with 200 mg levodopa (Sinemet CR 50-200), 25 mg carbidopa with 100 mg levodopa (Sinemet CR 25-100)

### Indications and dosages
*Parkinsonism*
*Adults:* Most patients respond to a 25 mg/100 mg combination (1 tablet P.O. t.i.d.). Dose may be increased q 1 or 2 days to maximum of 8 tablets or 1 tablet of 10 mg/100 mg t.i.d. or q.i.d. up to 2 tablets q.i.d.; or 1 sustained-release tablet b.i.d. at intervals at least 6 hours apart. Intervals may be adjusted based on patient response. Usual dose is 2 to 8 tablets daily in divided doses every 4 to 8 hours while awake.

Maintenance therapy must be carefully adjusted based on patient tolerance and desired therapeutic response. Usual maintenance dose is 3 to 6 tablets of 25 mg carbidopa/250 mg levodopa P.O. daily in divided doses. Don't exceed 8 tablets of 25 mg carbidopa/250 mg levodopa daily. Optimum daily dose must be determined by careful adjustment for each patient.

Daily dose of carbidopa should be 70 to 100 mg or more to suppress the peripheral metabolism of levodopa.

### Mechanism of action
*Decarboxylase-inhibiting action:* Carbidopa inhibits the peripheral decarboxylation of levodopa, thus slowing its conversion to dopamine in extracerebral tissues. This results in an increased availability of levodopa for transport to the brain, where it undergoes decarboxylation to dopamine.

### Pharmacokinetics
*Absorption:* A total of 40% to 70% of dose is absorbed after oral administration. Plasma levodopa levels are increased when carbidopa and

levodopa are given together because carbidopa inhibits the peripheral metabolism of levodopa.
*Distribution:* Carbidopa is distributed widely in body tissues except the CNS. Levodopa also appears in breast milk.
*Metabolism:* Carbidopa isn't metabolized extensively. It inhibits metabolism of levodopa in the GI tract, thus increasing its absorption from the GI tract and its level in plasma.
*Excretion:* Some (30%) of the dose is excreted unchanged in urine within 24 hours. When given with carbidopa, the amount of levodopa excreted unchanged in urine is increased by about 6%. Half-life is 1 to 2 hours.

| Route | Onset | Peak | Duration |
|-------|-------|------|----------|
| P.O. | Unknown | 40-150 min | Unknown |

## Contraindications and precautions
Contraindicated in patients hypersensitive to drug, those with acute angle-closure glaucoma, melanoma, or undiagnosed skin lesions, and within 14 days of MAO inhibitor therapy.

Use cautiously in patients with severe CV, endocrine, pulmonary, renal, or hepatic disorders; peptic ulcer; psychiatric illness; MI with residual arrhythmias; bronchial asthma; emphysema; and well-controlled chronic open-angle glaucoma.

## Interactions
**Drug-drug.** *Anesthetics, hydrocarbon inhalation:* May cause arrhythmias because of increased endogenous dopamine level. Levodopa should be stopped 6 to 8 hours before administration of anesthetics such as halothane.
*Antacids containing calcium, magnesium, or sodium bicarbonate:* May increase absorption of levodopa. Advise clinician to give antacids 1 hour after levodopa.
*Anticonvulsants (such as hydantoins, phenytoin), benzodiazepines, haloperidol, papaverine, phenothiazines, rauwolfia alkaloids, thioxanthenes:* May decrease therapeutic effects of levodopa. Advise clinician to monitor patient for decreased effectiveness.
*Antihypertensives:* Increased hypotensive effect. Advise clinician to monitor blood pressure.
*Bromocriptine:* May produce additive effects. Reduced levodopa dosage may be needed.
*Methyldopa:* May alter the antiparkinsonian effects of levodopa and may produce additive toxic CNS effects. Avoid use together.
*MAO inhibitors:* May cause a hypertensive crisis. Recommend stopping MAO inhibitors for 2 to 4 weeks before starting levodopa.
*Molindone:* May inhibit antiparkinsonian effects of levodopa by blocking dopamine receptors in the brain. Avoid use together.
*Sympathomimetics:* May increase the risk of arrhythmias. Dosage reduction of the sympathomimetic is recommended; the administration of carbidopa with levodopa reduces the tendency of sympathomimetics to cause

dopamine-induced arrhythmias. Recommend reducing levodopa dose.

## Adverse reactions
**CNS:** *choreiform, dystonic, dyskinetic movements; involuntary grimacing, head movements, myoclonic body jerks, ataxia,* tremor, muscle twitching; bradykinetic episodes; psychiatric disturbances, anxiety, disturbing dreams, euphoria, malaise, fatigue; severe depression, *suicidal tendencies,* dementia, delirium, hallucinations (may necessitate reduction or withdrawal of drug), confusion, insomnia, agitation.
**CV:** *orthostatic hypotension, cardiac irregularities,* phlebitis.
**EENT:** blepharospasm, blurred vision, diplopia, mydriasis or miosis, oculogyric crises, excessive salivation.
**GI:** *dry mouth,* bitter taste, *nausea, vomiting, anorexia,* constipation; flatulence; diarrhea; abdominal pain.
**GU:** urinary frequency, elevated BUN, urine retention, urinary incontinence, darkened urine, priapism.
**Hematologic:** *hemolytic anemia, thrombocytopenia, leukopenia, agranulocytosis.*
**Hepatic:** elevated levels of ALT, AST, alkaline phosphatase, serum bilirubin, LDH; *hepatotoxicity.*
**Metabolic:** weight loss (at start of therapy); elevated levels of serum protein-bound iodine; elevated serum gonadotropin levels.
**Respiratory:** hyperventilation, hiccups.
**Other:** dark perspiration.

## Overdose and treatment
There have been no reports of overdose with carbidopa. Signs and symptoms of levodopa overdose are irregular heartbeat and palpitations, severe continuous nausea and vomiting, and spasm or closing of eyelids.

Treatment of overdose includes immediate gastric lavage and antiarrhythmic, if needed. Pyridoxine isn't effective in reversing the actions of carbidopa and levodopa combinations.

## Clinical considerations
■ Muscle twitching and blepharospasm (twitching of eyelids) may be an early sign of overdose.
■ If patient is being treated with levodopa, recommend stopping it at least 8 hours before starting levodopa-carbidopa. Initial combination therapy should provide no more than 20% to 25% of previous levodopa dosage.
■ The combination drug usually reduces the amount of levodopa needed by 75%, thereby reducing the risk of adverse reactions.
■ Sustained-release tablets may be split, but never crushed or chewed.
■ For patients being transferred from conventional levodopa-carbidopa preparation to an

extended-release preparation, the extended-release tablet should provide 10% to 30% more levodopa daily.

- Pyridoxine (vitamin B₆) doesn't reverse beneficial effects of levodopa-carbidopa. Multivitamins can be taken without fear of losing control of symptoms.
- If therapy is interrupted temporarily, usual daily dosage may be given as soon as patient resumes oral drugs.
- Maximum effectiveness of drug may not occur for several weeks or months after therapy begins.
- Antiglobulin determinations (Coombs' test) are occasionally positive after long-term use. Thyroid function determinations may inhibit thyroid-stimulating hormone response to protirelin.
- Serum and urine uric acid determinations may show false elevations. Urine glucose determinations using copper reduction method may show false-positive results; with the glucose oxidase method, false-negative results. Urine ketone determination using dip-stick method, urine norepinephrine determinations, and urine protein determinations using Lowery test may show false-positive results.

### Therapeutic monitoring
- Recommend carefully monitoring patients who also receive antihypertensive or hypoglycemic drugs. MAO inhibitors should be stopped at least 2 weeks before therapy begins.
- Dosage adjustment is based on patient's response and tolerance to drug. Therapeutic and adverse reactions occur more rapidly with levodopa-carbidopa combination than with levodopa alone.
- Recommend observing and monitoring vital signs, especially while dosage is being adjusted.
- Test patients on long-term therapy regularly for diabetes and acromegaly; periodically repeat blood test and liver and kidney function test results.

### Special populations
**Breast-feeding patients.** Because levodopa may inhibit lactation, don't use drug in breast-feeding women.
**Pediatric patients.** Safety of drug in children under age 18 hasn't been established.
**Geriatric patients.** Smaller doses may be required in geriatric patients because of their reduced tolerance to the effects of levodopa-carbidopa. Geriatric patients, especially those with osteoporosis, should resume normal activity gradually because increased mobility may increase the risk of fractures. Geriatric patients are especially vulnerable to CNS adverse effects, such as anxiety, confusion, or nervousness; those with preexisting heart disease are more susceptible to cardiac effects.

### Patient counseling
- Instruct patient to report adverse reactions and therapeutic effects.
- Warn patient of possible dizziness or orthostatic hypotension, especially when therapy starts. Tell patient to change position slowly and dangle legs before getting out of bed. Elastic stockings may be helpful in some patients.
- Tell patient to take food shortly after taking drug to relieve gastric irritation.
- Inform patient that drug may cause urine or sweat to darken.
- Tell patient to take a missed dose as soon as possible, to skip a missed dose if next scheduled dose is within 2 hours, and never to double the dose.

# levofloxacin
Levaquin

*Pharmacologic classification:* fluorinated carboxyquinolone
*Therapeutic classification:* broad-spectrum antibacterial
*Pregnancy risk category C*

### Available forms
Available by prescription only
*Tablets:* 250 mg, 500 mg
*Single-use vials:* 500 mg
*Infusion (premixed):* 250 mg in 50 ml D₅W, 500 mg in 100 ml D₅W

### Indications and dosages
*Acute maxillary sinusitis caused by susceptible strains of* **Streptococcus pneumoniae, Moraxella catarrhalis,** *or* **Haemophilus influenzae**
*Adults:* 500 mg P.O. or I.V. daily for 10 to 14 days.
*Acute bacterial exacerbation of chronic bronchitis caused by* **Staphylococcus aureus, S. pneumoniae, M. catarrhalis, H. influenzae,** *or* **H. parainfluenzae**
*Adults:* 500 mg P.O. or I.V. daily for 7 days.
*Community-acquired pneumonia caused by* **S. aureus, S. pneumoniae, M. catarrhalis, H. influenzae, H. parainfluenzae, Klebsiella pneumoniae, Chlamydia pneumoniae, Legionella pneumoniae,** *or* **Mycoplasma pneumoniae**
*Adults:* 500 mg P.O. or I.V. daily for 7 to 14 days.
*Uncomplicated skin and skin-structure infections (mild to moderate) caused by* **S. aureus** *or* **Streptococcus pyogenes**
*Adults:* 500 mg P.O. or I.V. daily for 7 to 10 days.
≣*Dosage adjustment.* If creatinine clearance is 20 to 49 ml/minute, initial dose is 500 mg,

and subsequent doses are half the initial dose.
If creatinine clearance is 10 to 19 ml/minute,
subsequent doses are half the initial dose, and
the interval is prolonged to q 48 hours.
**Complicated skin and skin-structure
infections**
*Adults:* 750 mg P.O. or I.V. daily for 7 to 14
days.
**Acute mild to moderate pyelonephritis
caused by Escherichia coli; complicated
mild to moderate urinary tract infections
(UTIs) caused by Enterococcus faecalis,
Enterobacter cloacae, E. coli, K. pneumoniae, Proteus mirabilis, or Pseudomonas aeruginosa; uncomplicated UTIs**
*Adults:* 250 mg P.O. or I.V. daily for 10 days
(only 3 days for uncomplicated UTIs).
≡ **Dosage adjustment.** If creatinine clearance
is 10 to 19 ml/minute, dosage interval is increased to q 48 hours.
◇ **Traveler's diarrhea**
*Adults:* 500 mg P.O. single dose with loperamide hydrochloride.
◇ **Prophylaxis of traveler's diarrhea**
*Adults:* 500 mg P.O. once daily during period
of risk, for up to 3 weeks.

## I.V. administration
■ Single-dose vial must be diluted with $D_5W$
or normal saline solution to concentration of
5 mg/ml.
■ Reconstituted solution should be clear, slightly yellow, and free of particulate matter.
■ Because a rapid or bolus administration may
result in hypotension, I.V. levofloxacin should
only be administered by slow infusion.
■ Administer 250- to 500-mg doses over 60
minutes. Administer 750-mg doses over 90
minutes.
■ Don't mix with other drugs.

### Incompatibilities
Don't give through same I.V. line with solutions containing multivalent cations such as
magnesium.

## Mechanism of action
*Antibacterial action:* Levofloxacin inhibits bacterial DNA gyrase, an enzyme required for
DNA replication, transcription, repair, and recombination in susceptible bacteria.

## Pharmacokinetics
*Absorption:* The plasma level after I.V. administration is comparable to that observed for
equivalent oral doses (on a mg/mg basis).
Therefore, oral and I.V. routes can be considered interchangeable.
*Distribution:* Mean volume of distribution
ranges from 89 to 112 L after single and multiple 500-mg doses, indicating widespread distribution into body tissues. Drug also penetrates well into lung tissues, generally twofold
to fivefold higher than plasma levels.

*Metabolism:* Undergoes limited metabolism
in humans. The only identified metabolites
are the desmethyl and N-oxide metabolites,
which have little relevant pharmacologic activity.
*Excretion:* Primarily excreted unchanged in
the urine. Mean terminal half-life is about 6
to 8 hours.

| Route | Onset | Peak | Duration |
|---|---|---|---|
| P.O., I.V. | Unknown | 1-2 hr | Unknown |

## Contraindications and precautions
Contraindicated in patients hypersensitive to
drug, its components, or quinolone antimicrobials. Safety and efficacy of levofloxacin in
children, adolescents (under age 18), and pregnant and breast-feeding women haven't been
established.
    Use cautiously in patients with history of
seizure disorders or other CNS diseases, such
as cerebral arteriosclerosis, because quinolones
can cause CNS stimulation and increased intracranial pressure. This may lead to seizures
(lowered seizure threshold), toxic psychoses,
tremors, restlessness, anxiety, light-headedness,
confusion, hallucinations, paranoia, depression, nightmares, insomnia and, rarely, suicidal thoughts or acts. These can occur after the
first dose.

## Interactions
**Drug-drug.** *Antacids containing aluminum or
magnesium, iron salts, products containing
zinc, sucralfate:* May interfere with GI absorption of levofloxacin. Give these drugs at
least 2 hours apart.
*Antidiabetics:* May alter blood glucose levels.
Advise clinician to monitor glucose levels
closely.
*NSAIDs:* May increase CNS stimulation.
Advise clinician to monitor patient for seizure
activity.
*Theophylline:* Coadministration may result in
decreased clearance of theophylline. Advise
clinician to monitor theophylline levels.
*Warfarin and derivatives:* May cause increased
effect of oral anticoagulant with some fluoroquinolones. Advise clinician to monitor PT and
INR.
**Drug-lifestyle.** *Sun exposure:* Increased photosensitivity. Advise patient to take precautions.

## Adverse reactions
**CNS:** headache, insomnia, dizziness, encephalopathy, paresthesia, abnormal EEG,
*seizures.*
**CV:** chest pain, palpitations, vasodilation.
**GI:** nausea, diarrhea, constipation, vomiting,
abdominal pain, dyspepsia, flatulence, *pseudomembranous colitis.*
**GU:** vaginitis.
**Hematologic:** eosinophilia, hemolytic anemia,
decreased lymphocyte count.

---

Reactions may be *common*, uncommon, *life-threatening*, or COMMON AND LIFE-THREATENING.

**Metabolic:** decreased glucose level.
**Musculoskeletal:** back pain, tendon rupture.
**Respiratory:** allergic pneumonitis.
**Skin:** rash, photosensitivity, pruritus, erythema multiforme, *Stevens-Johnson syndrome.*
**Other:** pain, hypersensitivity reactions, injection site reaction, *anaphylaxis, multisystem organ failure.*

## Overdose and treatment
No information available. If acute overdose occurs, advise clinician to empty the stomach, maintain hydration, and observe patient. Drug isn't effectively removed by hemodialysis or peritoneal dialysis.

## Clinical considerations
■ If patient experiences symptoms of excessive CNS stimulation (restlessness, tremor, confusion, hallucinations), recommend stopping drug and instituting seizure precautions.
■ Ruptures of tendons and tendonitis have occurred with quinolone therapy. Drug should be stopped if pain, inflammation, or rupture of a tendon occurs. These ruptures can occur after therapy has been stopped.

### Therapeutic monitoring
■ Advise clinician to monitor blood glucose and renal, hepatic, and hematopoietic test results as indicated.
■ Advise clinician to monitor renal function closely, especially in geriatric patient.

### Special populations
**Breast-feeding patients.** Based on data from ofloxacin, it can be presumed that levofloxacin does appear in breast milk. Because of potential for serious adverse reactions in breast-fed infants, a decision should be made to discontinue either breast-feeding or drug.
**Pediatric patients.** Safety and efficacy in children under age 18 haven't been established.
**Geriatric patients.** Because of decreased renal function in these patients, dosage adjustment may be needed.

## Patient counseling
■ Tell patient to take drug as prescribed, even if symptoms disappear.
■ Advise patient to take drug with plenty of fluids and to avoid antacids, sucralfate, and products containing iron or zinc for at least 2 hours before and after each dose.
■ Warn patient to avoid hazardous tasks until adverse CNS effects of drug are known.
■ Advise patient to use sunblock and wear protective clothing when exposed to excessive sunlight.
■ Tell patient to stop drug and report if rash or other signs of hypersensitivity develop.
■ Tell patient to report pain or inflammation.

■ Tell diabetic patient to monitor glucose levels and report if a hypoglycemic reaction occurs.

# levonorgestrel implants
Norplant System

*Pharmacologic classification:* progestin
*Therapeutic classification:* contraceptive
*Pregnancy risk category X*

## Available forms
Available by prescription only
*Implants:* 36 mg in each of six Silastic capsules; kits also include trocar, scalpel, forceps, syringe, two needles, package of skin closures, three packages of gauze sponges, stretch bandages, and surgical drape

## Indications and dosages
*Long-term (up to 5 years), reversible prevention of pregnancy*
*Adults:* Six Silastic capsules containing 36 mg each for a total of 216 mg are surgically implanted in the superficial plane beneath the skin of a woman's upper arm during first 7 days of onset of menses.

## Mechanism of action
*Contraceptive action:* Levonorgestrel is a synthetic, biologically active progestin, exhibiting no significant estrogenic activity. A continuous low dose of levonorgestrel is diffused through the wall of each capsule. Pregnancy is prevented by at least two mechanisms: inhibition of ovulation and thickening of cervical mucus.

## Pharmacokinetics
*Absorption:* 100% bioavailable. Plasma levels average 0.3 ng/ml over 5 years but are highly variable as a function of individual metabolism and body weight.
*Distribution:* Bound by the circulating protein sex hormone-binding globulin (SHBG).
*Metabolism:* Metabolized by the liver.
*Excretion:* Metabolites are excreted in the urine.

| Route | Onset | Peak | Duration |
|-------|-------|------|----------|
| Subdermal | 24 hr | 24 hr | Unknown |

## Contraindications and precautions
Contraindicated in patients with active thrombophlebitis or thromboembolic disorders, undiagnosed abnormal genital bleeding, acute liver disease, malignant or benign liver tumors, known or suspected breast cancer, known or suspected pregnancy, history of idiopathic intracranial hypertension, and hypersensitivity

to levonorgestrel or components of the Norplant System.

Use cautiously in diabetic and prediabetic patients and in those with history of depression or hyperlipidemia.

### Interactions
**Drug-drug.** *Carbamazepine, phenytoin:* Reduced efficacy of levonorgestrel. Patient should take additional precautions to avoid pregnancy.

### Adverse reactions
**CNS:** headache, nervousness, dizziness, depression, tingling, numbness.
**GI:** nausea, *abdominal discomfort,* appetite change.
**GU:** *amenorrhea, many days of bleeding or prolonged bleeding, spotting, irregular onset of bleeding, frequent onset of bleeding, scanty bleeding, cervicitis, vaginitis, leukorrha.*
**Metabolic:** decreased thyroxine levels, increased $T_3$ uptake, weight gain.
**Musculoskeletal:** mastalgia, *musculoskeletal pain.*
**Skin:** dermatitis, acne, hirsutism, hypertrichosis, alopecia; infection, transient pain, itching (at implant site).
**Other:** adnexal enlargement, *removal difficulty, breast discharge.*

### Overdose and treatment
Overdose may occur if more than six Silastic capsules are in situ, resulting in fluid retention with its associated effects and uterine bleeding irregularities. All previously implanted capsules should be removed before insertion of a new set.

### Clinical considerations
■ The total implanted dose is 216 mg. Implantation of all six capsules should be performed during the first 7 days of menstrual cycle. Insertion is subdermal in the midportion of the inside of the upper arm, 8 to 10 cm above the elbow crease.
■ Each capsule is 2.4 mm in diameter and 34 mm in length.
■ Determine whether patient has allergies to the antiseptic or anesthetic to be used, or contraindications to progestin-only contraception.
■ During insertion, special attention must be given to asepsis and correct placement of capsules; careful technique minimizes tissue trauma.
■ Patients should receive a copy of patient information booklet and should be made aware of potential adverse reactions and of risks and benefits of the system and of other forms of contraception.
■ Store at room temperature away from excess heat and moisture.

### Therapeutic monitoring
■ Patients should be reexamined at least yearly; examinations should focus on implant site, blood pressure, breasts, abdominal and pelvic organs, including cervical cytology, and related laboratory tests.
■ Patient should be monitored for recurrent or abnormal vaginal bleeding.
■ Patients with strong family history of breast cancer should be monitored for breast nodules.

### Patient counseling
■ Tell patient that altered bleeding patterns tend to become more regular after 9 to 12 months.
■ Warn patient to report heavy bleeding.
■ Advise patient to avoid bumping or wetting the insertion site for at least 3 days after insertion.
■ Explain that some tenderness in the implant area may occur for 1 to 2 days.
■ Tell patient that insertion usually takes 10 to 15 minutes and causes little or no discomfort because of the local anesthetic.
■ Advise patient that, when laboratory studies are ordered, she should inform all prescribers that levonorgestrel implants are being used.
■ Tell patient who takes phenytoin or carbamazepine that she may need to use additional contraceptive measures.
■ Advise patient to thoroughly review patient information booklet.

# levothyroxine sodium ($T_4$ or L-thyroxine sodium)
Eltroxin, Levo-T, Levothroid, Levoxine, Levoxyl, Synthroid

*Pharmacologic classification:* thyroid hormone
*Therapeutic classification:* thyroid hormone replacement
*Pregnancy risk category A*

### Available forms
Available by prescription only
*Tablets:* 25 mcg, 50 mcg, 75 mcg, 88 mcg, 100 mcg, 112 mcg, 125 mcg, 137 mcg, 150 mcg, 175 mcg, 200 mcg, 300 mcg
*Injection:* 200 mcg/vial, 500 mcg/vial

### Indications and dosages
*Congenital hypothyroidism*
*Neonates:* 37.5 mcg (25 to 50 mcg) P.O. daily. *Premature neonates under 2 kg (4.4 lb) and those at risk for cardiac failure:* 25 mcg P.O. daily initially; dosage may be increased to 50 mcg daily in 4 to 6 weeks.
*Children under age 1:* Initially, 25 to 50 mcg P.O. daily.
*Children ages 1 and older:* 3 to 5 mcg/kg P.O. daily until adult dose (150 mcg) is reached in early or mid-adolescence.

Alternatively, the following dosing guidelines may be used:

*Children over age 12:* Over 150 mcg or 2 to 3 mcg/kg/day.

*Children ages 6 to 12:* 100 to 150 mcg or 4 to 5 mcg/kg/day.

*Children ages 1 to 5:* 75 to 100 mcg or 5 to 6 mcg/kg/day.

*Children ages 6 to 12 months:* 50 to 75 mcg or 6 to 8 mcg/kg/day.

*Children under age 6 months:* 25 to 50 mcg or 8 to 10 mcg/kg/day.

*Myxedema coma*
*Adults:* 300 to 500 mcg I.V. If no response in 24 hours, give an additional 100 to 300 mcg I.V. in 48 hours. maintenance dose of 50 to 200 mcg may be given until condition stabilizes and drug can be given orally.

*Thyroid hormone replacement for atrophy of gland, surgical removal, excessive radiation or antithyroid drugs, or congenital defect*
*Adults:* For mild hypothyroidism—initially, 50 mcg P.O. daily, increased by 25 to 50 mcg P.O. daily q 2 to 4 weeks until desired response is achieved; may be administered I.V. or I.M. when P.O. ingestion is precluded for long periods. Usual dose is 100 to 200 mcg daily.

For severe hypothyroidism—12.5 to 25 mcg P.O. daily, increased by 25 to 50 mcg daily q 2 to 4 weeks until desired response is achieved.

*Elderly:* Initially, 12.5 to 50 mcg P.O. daily and increase in 12.5- to 25-mcg increments q 3 to 8 weeks.

≡ *Dosage adjustment.* For patients with CV disease, start at 50 mcg daily and increase in 50-mcg increments at 2- to 4-week intervals.

### I.V administration

■ Levothyroid powder for injection or levothyroxine sodium powder is reconstituted by adding 2 ml or 5 ml of normal saline solution to vial containing 200 or 500 mcg, respectively. Shake until a clear solution is obtained. Concentration is about 100 mcg/ml.

■ Synthroid powder for injection is reconstituted by adding 5 ml of normal saline solution or bacteriostatic sodium chloride injection with benzyl alcohol to 200 or 500 mcg vial. Shake until a clear solution is obtained. Concentration is 40 or 100 mcg/ml, respectively. Use reconstituted solutions immediately and don't coadminister with other I.V. infusion solutions.

### Incompatibilities

Don't mix with other solutions for I.V. infusion.

### Mechanism of action

*Thyroid hormone replacement:* Levothyroxine affects protein and carbohydrate metabolism, promotes gluconeogenesis, increases the use and mobilization of glycogen stores, stimulates protein synthesis, and regulates cell growth and differentiation.

## Pharmacokinetics

*Absorption:* Between 50% and 80% is absorbed from the GI tract. Full effects don't occur for 1 to 3 weeks after oral therapy begins. After I.M. administration, absorption is variable and poor. After an I.V. dose in patients with myxedema coma, increased responsiveness may occur within 6 to 8 hours, but maximum therapeutic effect may not occur for up to 24 hours.

*Distribution:* Distribution isn't fully described; however, drug is distributed into most body tissues and fluids. The highest levels are found in the liver and kidneys; 99% is protein-bound.

*Metabolism:* Metabolized in peripheral tissues, primarily in the liver, kidneys, and intestines. About 85% of metabolized levothyroxine is deiodinated.

*Excretion:* Fecal excretion eliminates 20% to 40% of levothyroxine. Half-life is 6 to 7 days.

| Route | Onset | Peak | Duration |
|-------|-------|------|----------|
| P.O. | 24 hr | Unknown | Unknown |
| I.V. | Unknown | Unknown | Unknown |
| I.M. | Unknown | Unknown | Unknown |

## Contraindications and precautions

Contraindicated in patients hypersensitive to drug, acute MI and thyrotoxicosis uncomplicated by hypothyroidism, or uncorrected adrenal insufficiency.

Use cautiously in the elderly and in patients with renal impairment, angina pectoris, hypertension, ischemia, or other CV disorders.

## Interactions

**Drug-drug.** *Aluminum hydroxide, calcium carbonate, ferrous sulfate, infant soybean formula, sodium polystyrene sulfonate, sucralfate:* When used concomitanlty, decreased absorption of levothyroxine may occur. Avoid concomitant use if possible.

*Anticoagulants:* May alter anticoagulant effect. An increase in levothyroxine dosage may necessitate a decrease in anticoagulant dosage.

*Beta blockers:* May decrease conversion of levothyroxine to liothyronine. Advise clinician to monitor patient.

*Cholestyramine:* May delay absorption of levothyroxine. Don't give together.

*Corticotropin:* Concurrent use causes changes in thyroid status. Advise clinician to monitor patient; dosage adjustment of both drugs may be needed.

*Estrogens:* Increase levothyroxine requirements. Advise clinician to monitor patient for decreased levothyroxine effect.

*Hepatic enzyme inducers such as phenytoin:* May increase hepatic degradation of levothyroxine and increase dosage requirements of levothyroxine. Recommend adjusting dosages p.r.n.

*Insulin, oral antidiabetics:* Altered serum glucose levels. Recommend adjusting doses of these drugs p.r.n.

*Somatrem:* May accelerate epiphyseal maturation. Avoid concurrent use in children if possible.

*Sympathomimetics, tricyclic antidepressants:* May increase the effects of any or all of these drugs and may lead to coronary insufficiency or arrhythmias. Recommend close monitoring if concurrent use is needed.

*Theophylline:* Decreased theophylline clearance can be expected in hypothyroid patients. Clearance returns to normal when euthyroid state is achieved.

## Adverse reactions

**CNS:** *nervousness, insomnia, tremor,* headache.

**CV:** *tachycardia, palpitations, **arrhythmias**, angina pectoris, **cardiac arrest**.*

**GI:** diarrhea, vomiting.

**GU:** menstrual irregularities.

**Metabolic:** weight loss.

**Skin:** diaphoresis, allergic skin reactions.

**Other:** heat intolerance, fever.

## Overdose and treatment

Evidence of overdose includes signs and symptoms of hyperthyroidism, including weight loss, increased appetite, palpitations, nervousness, diarrhea, abdominal cramps, sweating, tachycardia, increased blood pressure, widened pulse pressure, angina, arrhythmias, tremor, headache, insomnia, heat intolerance, fever, and menstrual irregularities.

Treatment of overdose requires reduction of GI absorption and efforts to counteract central and peripheral effects, primarily sympathetic activity. Advise clinician to use gastric lavage or induce emesis (followed by activated charcoal up to 4 hours after ingestion). If the patient is comatose or is having seizures, inflate cuff on endotracheal tube to prevent aspiration. Treatment may include oxygen and artificial ventilation p.r.n. to support respiration. It also should include appropriate measures to treat heart failure and to control fever, hypoglycemia, and fluid loss. Propranolol (or another beta blocker) may be used to combat many of the effects of increased sympathetic activity. Levothyroxine should be gradually withdrawn over 2 to 6 days, then resumed at a lower dose.

## Clinical considerations

■ Levothyroxine has predictable effects because of standard hormonal content; therefore, it's the usual drug of choice for thyroid hormone replacement.

■ Give as a single dose before breakfast.

■ Patient with history of lactose intolerance may be sensitive to Levothroid, which contains lactose.

■ Synthroid 100- and 300-mcg tablets contain tartrazine, a dye that causes allergic reactions in susceptible individuals.

■ When switching from levothyroxine to liothyronine, levothyroxine dosage should be stopped when liothyronine treatment begins. After residual effects of levothyroxine have disappeared, liothyronine dosage can be increased in small increments. When switching from liothyronine to levothyroxine, levothyroxine therapy can begin several days before withdrawing liothyronine to avoid relapse.

■ Protect drug from moisture and light.

■ Levothyroxine therapy alters radioactive iodine ($^{131}$I) thyroid uptake, protein-bound iodine levels, and liothyronine uptake.

## Therapeutic monitoring

■ Carefully observe patient for adverse effects during initial dose adjustment phase.

■ Advise clinician to monitor patient for aggravation of concurrent diseases, such as Addison's disease or diabetes mellitus.

■ Patient taking levothyroxine who requires $^{131}$I uptake tests must stop drug 4 weeks before test.

## Special populations

**Breast-feeding patients.** Minimal amounts of drug appear in breast milk. Use with caution in breast-feeding women.

**Pediatric patients.** Partial and temporary hair loss may occur during the first few months of therapy.

**Geriatric patients.** Geriatric patients are more sensitive to effects of drug. In patients over age 60, initial dosage should be 25% lower than usual recommended dosage.

## Patient counseling

■ Advise taking drug at same time each day; encourage morning dosing to avoid insomnia.

■ Tell patient to report headache, diarrhea, nervousness, excessive sweating, heat intolerance, chest pain, increased pulse rate, or palpitations.

■ Encourage patient to use the same product consistently because all brands don't have equal bioavailability.

■ Advise patient to store drug in cool, dry place to prevent deterioration of product.

■ Tell patient that replacement therapy is to be taken essentially for life, except in cases of transient hypothyroidism.

# lidocaine (lignocaine)
Xylocaine

# lidocaine hydrochloride
Anestacon, Dilocaine, L-Caine,
Lidoderm Patch, Lidoject, LidoPen
Auto-Injector, Nervocaine, Xylocaine,
Xylocaine Viscous, Zilactin-L

*Pharmacologic classification:* amide
derivative
*Therapeutic classification:* ventricular
antiarrhythmic, local anesthetic
*Pregnancy risk category B*

## Available forms
Available by prescription only
*Injection:* 5 mg/ml, 10 mg/ml, 15 mg/ml,
20 mg/ml, 40 mg/ml, 100 mg/ml, 200 mg/ml
*Premixed solutions:* 2 mg/ml, 4 mg/ml, 8 mg/ml
in $D_5W$
*Parenteral injection:* 0.5%, 1%, 1.5%, 2%, 4%
(lidocaine with epinephrine combinations also
available)
*Ointment:* 5%
*Topical solution:* 2%, 4%
*Jelly:* 2%
*Spray:* 10%
Available without a prescription
*Ointment:* 2.5%
*Liquid:* 2.5%
*Cream:* 0.5%
*Spray:* 0.5%
*Gel:* 0.5%, 2.5%
*Transdermal patch:* 5%

## Indications and dosages
*Ventricular arrhythmias from MI, cardiac
manipulation, or cardiac glycosides*
*Adults:* 50 to 100 mg (0.7 to 1.4 mg/kg) I.V.
bolus at 25 to 50 mg/minute. If the desire
effect isn't obtained, give a second dose of
25 to 50 mg 5 minutes after completion of
the first injection. Don't exceed 300-mg total
bolus during a 1-hour period. Simultaneously, begin constant infusion of 1 to 4 mg/minute.
If single bolus has been given, repeat smaller bolus (usually one-half initial bolus) 5
to 10 minutes after start of infusion to maintain therapeutic serum level. After 24 hours
of continuous infusion, decrease rate by one-
half.
　　For I.M. administration in all adults, 300 mg
(4.3 mg/kg) in deltoid muscle has been used
in early stages of acute MI. If necessary, may
be repeated in 60 to 90 minutes.
*Children:* 0.5 to 1 mg/kg by I.V. bolus; may
repeat bolus if needed, not to exceed 3 to
5 mg/kg, followed by infusion of 10 to 50 mcg/
kg/minute. In advanced cardiac life support,
1 mg/kg I.V. bolus, followed by an infusion of

20 to 50 mcg/kg/minute if needed after defibrillation or cardioversion.
*Elderly:* Give half the bolus amount and use
slower infusion rate.
≡ *Dosage adjustment.* Give half the bolus
amount to lightweight patients and to those
with HF or hepatic disease. Use slower infusion rate in those with HF or hepatic disease
and in patients weighing under 50 kg (110 lb).
◇ *Status epilepticus*
*Adults:* 1 mg/kg I.V. bolus; then, if seizure
continues, give 0.5 mg/kg 2 minutes after first
dose; infusion at 30 mcg/kg/minute may be
used.
*Local anesthesia of skin or mucous mem-
branes, pain from dental extractions,
stomatitis*
*Adults and children:* Apply 2% to 5% solution
or ointment or 15 ml of Xylocaine Viscous q
3 to 4 hours to oral or nasal mucosa.
*Local anesthesia in procedures involving
the male or female urethra*
*Adults:* Instill about 15 ml (male) or 3 to 5 ml
(female) into urethra.
*Pain, burning, or itching caused by burns,
sunburn, or skin irritation*
*Adults and children:* Apply topical agent liberally.
*Relief of pain from postherpetic neuralgia*
*Adults:* Apply 1 to 3 patches to intact skin, covering most painful area, once daily for up to
12 hours each day. Smaller areas of treatment
are recommended in patients who are debilitated or have poor elimination. Excessive dosing by applying patch to larger areas or for
longer than recommended wearing time could
cause increased absorption of lidocaine and
high lidocaine levels, leading to serious adverse effects.
*Lidocaine hydrochloride injection used as
procedural anesthetic*
*Adults:* Lidocaine with epinephrine, 7 mg/kg
(no more than 500 mg total); lidocaine without epinephrine, 4.4 mg/kg (no more than
300 mg total). For continuous epidural or caudal anesthesia, maximum doses shouldn't be
given at intervals less than 90 minutes. Maximum recommended dose in paracervical block
is 200 mg total. For I.V. regional anesthesia,
dose shouldn't exceed 4 mg/kg. See table below.
*Children:* Based on age and weight. For I.V.
regional anesthesia, use dilute solutions (0.25%
to 0.5%) not to exceed 3 mg/kg.
　　The suggested concentrations and volumes
in the table on page 720 serve only as a guide.
Other volumes and concentrations may be
used as long as the total maximum recommended dose isn't exceeded.

## RECOMMENDED DOSAGES

### Injection (without epinephrine)

| Procedure | Concen- tration (%) | Volume (ml) | Total dose (mg) |
|---|---|---|---|
| *Infiltration* | | | |
| Percutaneous | 0.5 or 1 | 1-60 | 5-300 |
| I.V. regional | 0.5 | 10-60 | 50-300 |
| *Peripheral nerve blocks* | | | |
| Brachial | 1.5 | 15-20 | 225-300 |
| Dental | 2 | 1-5 | 20-100 |
| Intercostal | 1 | 3 | 30 |
| Paravertebral | 1 | 3-5 | 30-50 |
| Pudendal (each side) | 1 | 10 | 100 |
| *Paracervical* | | | |
| Obstetrical analgesia (each side) | 1 | 10 | 100 |
| *Sympathetic nerve blocks* | | | |
| Cervical (stellate ganglion) | 1 | 5 | 50 |
| Lumbar | 1 | 5-10 | 50-100 |
| *Central neural blocks* | | | |
| Epidural* | | | |
| Thoracic | 1 | 20-30 | 200-300 |
| Lumbar | | | |
| Analgesia | 1 | 25-30 | 250-300 |
| Anesthesia | 1.5 | 15-20 | 225-300 |
| | 2 | 10-15 | 200-300 |
| Caudal | | | |
| Obstetrical analgesia | 1 | 20-30 | 200-300 |
| Surgical anesthesia | 1.5 | 15-20 | 225-300 |

*Dose determined by number of dermatomes to be anesthetized (2-3 ml/dermatome)

≡ *Dosage adjustment.* Dosages are reduced for children, geriatric patients, debilitated patients, and patients with cardiac or liver disease.

## I.V. administration

■ For I.V. regional anesthesia, advise clinician to use 50 ml Xylocaine 0.5% injection.
■ I.V. infusions are prepared by adding 1 g of lidocaine (using 25 ml of a commercially available 4% or 5 ml of a 20% injection) to 1 L of $D_5W$ to provide a level of 1 mg/ml. Alternatively, 0.2% or 0.4% is available. In fluid-restricted patients, an 8 mg/ml concentration may be used. Don't add to blood transfusion assemblies.

**H** *ALERT* Lidocaine injections, additive syringes, and single-use vials containing 40, 100, or 200 mg/ml are for I.V. infusion preparation and must be diluted before use.

### Incompatibilities

Incompatible with amphotericin B, ampicillin sodium, cefazolin, hydromorphone, methohexital, and phenytoin.

## Mechanism of action

*Local anesthetic action:* As a local anesthetic, lidocaine acts to block initiation and conduction of nerve impulses by decreasing the permeability of the nerve cell membrane to sodium ions.

*Ventricular antiarrhythmic action:* One of the oldest antiarrhythmics, lidocaine remains among the most widely used drugs for treating acute ventricular arrhythmias. As a class IB antiarrhythmic, it suppresses automaticity and shortens the effective refractory period and action potential duration of His-Purkinje fibers and suppresses spontaneous ventricular depolarization during diastole. Therapeutic levels don't significantly affect conductive atrial tissue and AV conduction.

Unlike quinidine and procainamide, lidocaine doesn't significantly alter hemodynamics when given in usual doses. Drug seems to act preferentially on diseased or ischemic myocardial tissue; exerting its effects on the conduction system, it inhibits reentry mechanisms and halts ventricular arrhythmias.

## Pharmacokinetics

*Absorption:* Absorbed after oral administration; however, a significant first-pass effect occurs in the liver and only about 35% of drug reaches the systemic circulation. Oral doses high enough to achieve therapeutic blood levels result in an unacceptable toxicity, probably from high levels of lidocaine.

*Distribution:* Distributed widely throughout the body; it has a high affinity for adipose tissue. After I.V. bolus administration, an early, rapid decline in plasma levels occurs, mainly because of distribution into highly perfused tissues, such as the kidneys, lungs, liver, and heart, followed by a slower elimination phase in which metabolism and redistribution into skeletal muscle and adipose tissue occur. The first (early) distribution phase occurs rapidly, calling for initiation of a constant infusion after an initial bolus dose. Distribution volume declines in patients with liver or hepatic disease, resulting in toxic levels with usual doses. About 60% to 80% of circulating drug is plasma protein-bound. Usual therapeutic drug level is 1.5 to 5 mcg/ml. Although toxicity may occur within this range, levels greater than 5 mcg/ml are considered toxic and warrant dosage reduction.

***Metabolism:*** Metabolized in the liver to two active metabolites. Less than 10% of a parenteral dose escapes metabolism and reaches the kidneys unchanged. Metabolism is affected by hepatic blood flow, which may decrease after MI and with heart failure. Liver disease also may limit metabolism.

***Excretion:*** Half-life undergoes a biphasic process, with an initial phase of 7 to 30 minutes followed by a terminal half-life of 1½ to 2 hours. Elimination half-life may be prolonged in patients with heart failure or liver disease. Continuous infusions longer than 24 hours also may cause an apparent half-life increase.

| Route | Onset | Peak | Duration |
|---|---|---|---|
| I.V. | Immediate | Immediate | 10-20 min |
| I.M. | 5-15 min | 10 min | 2 hr |
| Peripheral injection | Variable | Variable | Variable |
| Topical | 30-60 sec | Unknown | Variable |

## Contraindications and precautions

Contraindicated in patients hypersensitive to amide-type local anesthetics, and those with Stokes-Adams syndrome, Wolff-Parkinson-White syndrome, and severe degrees of SA, AV, or intraventricular block in absence of artificial pacemaker. Also contraindicated in patients with inflammation or infection in puncture region, septicemia, severe hypertension, spinal deformities, and neurologic disorders.

Use cautiously in geriatric patients; in patients with renal or hepatic disease, complete or second-degree heart block, sinus bradycardia, or heart failure; and in those weighing less than 50 kg (110 lb).

## Interactions

**Drug-drug.** *Beta blockers:* Enhanced sympathomimetic effects. Drug shouldn't be used with lidocaine and epinephrine.

*Beta blockers, cimetidine:* May cause lidocaine toxicity from reduced hepatic clearance. Avoid use together.

*Butyrophenones, phenothiazines:* May reduce or reverse the pressor effects of epinephrine. Advise clinician to monitor patient for drug effect.

*Cyclic antidepressants, MAO inhibitors:* Prolonged and severe hypertension when lidocaine with epinephrine is used. Avoid use together.

*Ergot-type oxytocics, vasopressors:* Severe, persistent hypertension or CVA. Avoid using lidocaine with epinephrine.

*High-dose lidocaine, succinylcholine:* May increase neuromuscular effects of succinylcholine. Use together cautiously.

*Other antiarrhythmics, including phenytoin, procainamide, propranolol, quinidine:* May cause additive or antagonist effects as well as additive toxicity. Avoid use together.

**Drug-herb.** *Pareira:* May add to or potentiate the effects of neuromuscular blockade. Discourage use together.

## Adverse reactions

**CNS:** anxiety, nervousness, lethargy, somnolence, paresthesia, muscle twitching; *confusion, tremor, stupor, restlessness, light-headedness,* hallucinations, apprehension, unconsciousness, confusion, tremors, stupor, restlessness, slurred speech, euphoria, depression, *seizures.*

**CV:** CARDIAC ARREST; *hypotension, new or worsened arrhythmias* (with systemic form); hypotension, myocardial depression, *arrhythmias* (with topical use), edema, *bradycardia, asystole.*

**EENT:** *tinnitus, blurred or double vision* (with systemic form); tinnitus, blurred or double vision (with topical use).

**GI:** nausea, vomiting (with topical use).

**Respiratory:** *respiratory arrest, status asthmaticus.*

**Skin:** dermatologic reactions, sensitization, diaphoresis (with topical use), rash (with topical use).

**Other:** *anaphylaxis;* soreness at injection site, sensation of cold (with systemic form).

## Overdose and treatment

Effects of overdose include signs and symptoms of CNS toxicity, such as seizures or respiratory depression, and CV toxicity (as indicated by hypotension).

Treatment includes general supportive measures and drug discontinuation. A patent airway should be maintained and other respiratory support measures carried out immediately. Diazepam or thiopental may be given to treat any seizures. To treat significant hypotension, vasopressors (including dopamine and norepinephrine) may be given.

## Clinical considerations

◼ *ALERT* Lidocaine isn't used to treat supraventricular arrhythmias.

◼ Lidocaine with epinephrine (for local anesthesia) shouldn't be given to treat arrhythmias. Solutions with epinephrine should be used cautiously in CV disorders and in body areas with limited blood supply (ears, nose, fingers, toes).

◼ Patient receiving lidocaine I.M. will show a sevenfold increase in CK level. Such CK originates in skeletal muscle, not the heart. Recommend testing isoenzyme levels to confirm MI, if using I.M. route.

◼ When larger volumes are required for local anesthesia, advise clinician to use a solution containing epinephrine.

◼ Preparations used for epidural, spinal, or caudal anesthesia should contain no bacteriostatic drugs.

- In many severely ill patients, seizures may
be the first sign of toxicity. However, severe
reactions are usually preceded by somnolence,
confusion, and paresthesia. All signs and symptoms of toxicity should be regarded as serious;
recommend promptly reducing dosage or stopping therapy. Continued infusion could lead to
seizures and coma. Advise clinician to give
oxygen through nasal cannula, if not contraindicated. Oxygen and resuscitation equipment should be kept nearby.
- Doses of up to 400 mg I.M. have been ad-
vocated in prehospital phase of acute MI.
**H ALERT** Advise against the use of solutions
containing preservatives for spinal, epidural,
or caudal block or I.V. injection.
- With epidural use, recommend injecting a 2-
to 5-ml test dose at least 5 minutes before giving total dose to check for intravascular or
subarachnoid injection. Motor paralysis and
extensive sensory anesthesia indicate subarachnoid injection.
- Partially used vials containing no preservatives should be discarded.
- Because I.M. lidocaine therapy may increase
CK levels, isoenzyme tests should be performed
for differential diagnosis of acute MI.

### Therapeutic monitoring
- Patient requires constant cardiac monitoring
when receiving I.V. lidocaine. Advise clinician
to use infusion pump or microdrip system and
timer to monitor infusion precisely. Never exceed infusion rate of 4 mg/minute, if possible.
A faster rate greatly increases risk of toxicity.
- Advise clinician to monitor vital signs and
serum electrolyte, BUN, and creatinine levels.
- Advise clinician to monitor ECG constantly if administering drug I.V., especially in patients with liver disease, HF, hypoxia, respiratory depression, hypovolemia, or shock,
because these conditions may affect drug metabolism, excretion, or distribution volume,
predisposing patient to drug toxicity.
- Advise clinician to monitor patient for signs
of excessive depression of cardiac conductivity (such as sinus node dysfunction, PR interval prolongation, QRS complex widening, and
appearance or exacerbation of arrhythmias). If
they occur, recommend reducing dosage or
stopping drug.
- Therapeutic serum levels range from 2 to
5 mcg/ml.

### Special populations
**Pediatric patients.** Safety and efficacy in children haven't been established. Use of an I.M.
autoinjector device isn't recommended.
**Geriatric patients.** Because of prevalence of
concurrent disease states and declining organ
system function in geriatric patients, conservative lidocaine doses should be used.

### Patient counseling
- Advise patient to report adverse effects
promptly.

## lindane (gamma benzene hexachloride)
G-well, Kwell, Scabene

*Pharmacologic classification:* chlori-
nated hydrocarbon insecticide
*Therapeutic classification:* scabicide,
pediculicide
*Pregnancy risk category B*

### Available forms
Available by prescription only
*Lotion:* 1%
*Shampoo:* 1%

### Indications and dosages
*Scabies*
*Adults and children:* Apply a thin layer of cream
or lotion and gently massage it on all skin surfaces, moving from the neck to the toes. For
adults and children ages 6 and older, 30 to
60 ml; for children under age 6, 30 ml. After
8 to 12 hours, remove drug by bathing and
scrubbing well. Treatment may be repeated after 1 week if needed.
*Pediculosis*
*Adults and children:* Apply shampoo to clean,
dry, affected area and wait 4 minutes. Then add
a small amount of water and lather for 4 to 5
minutes; rinse thoroughly. Comb hair to remove nits. Treatment may be repeated after 1
week if needed.

### Mechanism of action
*Scabicide and pediculicide actions:* Lindane
is toxic to the parasitic mite *Sarcoptes scabiei*
and its eggs, and to lice *(Pediculus capitis,
Pediculus corporis,* and *Phthirus pubis).* Drug
is absorbed through the organism's exoskele-
ton, causing its death.

### Pharmacokinetics
*Absorption:* About 10% of topical dose may
be absorbed in 24 hours.
*Distribution:* Stored in body fat.
*Metabolism:* Metabolism occurs in the liver.
*Excretion:* Excreted in urine and feces.

| Route | Onset | Peak | Duration |
|---|---|---|---|
| Topical | 190 min | Unknown | Unknown |

### Contraindications and precautions
Contraindicated in patients hypersensitive to
drug, in those with raw or inflamed skin or
seizure disorders, and in premature infants. Use
cautiously in young patients (including infants).

## Interactions
None reported. However, avoid using with other oils or ointments.

## Adverse reactions
**CNS:** *dizziness, seizures.*
**Skin:** *irritation* (with repeated use).

## Overdose and treatment
Accidental ingestion may cause extreme CNS toxicity; symptoms include CNS stimulation, dizziness, and seizures. To treat lindane ingestion, advise clinician to empty stomach by appropriate measures (emesis or lavage), followed with saline catharsis (do not use oil laxative). Seizures should be treated with pentobarbital, phenobarbital, or diazepam, p.r.n.

## Clinical considerations
■ Make sure patient's body is clean and dry before application.
■ Avoid applying drug to acutely inflamed skin or raw, weeping surfaces.
■ Avoid contact with face, eyes, mucous membranes, and urethral meatus.
**⚠ ALERT** No one should use more than 2 ounces in one application.
■ Place hospitalized patient in isolation with linen-handling precautions.

### Therapeutic monitoring
■ Advise clinician to monitor patient for need of retreatment.
■ Advise clinician to monitor patient for signs of systemic toxicity.

### Special populations
**Pregnant patients.** The Centers for Disease Control and Prevention (CDC) states that lindane isn't for use in pregnant women.
**Breast-feeding patients.** Because drug appears in breast milk in low levels, an alternative method of feeding may be used for 4 days if there's any concern.
**Pediatric patients.** Use cautiously, especially in infants and small children, who are much more susceptible to CNS toxicity. Discourage thumb-sucking in children using lindane, to prevent ingestion of drug. The CDC recommends other scabicide therapies for children under age 10.
**Geriatric patients.** Use reduced dose in geriatric patients because of their increased susceptibility to percutaneous absorption.

## Patient counseling
■ Explain correct use of drug.
■ The CDC recommends that bathing before application be avoided because toxicity (such as seizures) has been caused by such application. If the patient does bathe, the skin should be allowed to dry and cool completely before application of lotion. Before application of

shampoo, the hair should be washed with plain shampoo and dried.
■ Warn patient that itching may continue for several weeks, even if treatment is effective, especially in scabies infestation.
■ If drug contacts eyes, tell patient to flush with water and call prescriber for further instructions. He should avoid inhaling vapor.
■ Explain that reapplication usually isn't needed unless live mites are found; advise reapplication if drug is accidentally washed off, but caution against overuse.
■ Tell patient he may use drug to clean combs and brushes, and to wash them thoroughly afterward; advise patient that all clothing and bed linen that may have been contaminated by him within the past 2 days should be machine-washed in hot water and dried in hot dryer or dry cleaned to avoid reinfestation or transmission of organism.
■ Discourage repeated use of drug, which may irritate skin and cause systemic toxicity.
■ Caution patient to avoid using with other oils or ointments.
■ Advise patient that family and close contacts, including sexual contacts, should be treated at the same time.
■ Warn patient not to use if open wounds, cuts, or sores are present on scalp or groin, unless directed by his prescriber.

# linezolid
Zyvox

*Pharmacologic classification:* oxazolidinone
*Therapeutic classification:* antibiotic
*Pregnancy risk category C*

## Available forms
Available by prescription only
*Tablets:* 400 mg, 600 mg
*Powder for oral suspension:* 100 mg/5 ml when constituted
*Injection:* 2 mg/ml

## Indications and dosages
**Vancomycin-resistant Enterococcus faecium *infections, including those with concurrent bacteremia***
*Adults:* 600 mg I.V. or P.O. q 12 hours for 14 to 28 days.
**Nosocomial pneumonia caused by Staphylococcus aureus *(methicillin-susceptible [MSSA] and methicillin-resistant [MRSA] strains) or* Streptococcus pneumoniae *(penicillin-susceptible strains only); complicated skin and skin-structure infections caused by* S. aureus *(MSSA and MRSA),* Streptococcus pyogenes, *or* Streptococcus agalactiae; *community-acquired pneumonia caused by* S. pneumoniae *(penicillin-susceptible strains only), including those***

*with concurrent bacteremia, or* **S. aureus**
*(MSSA only)*
*Adults:* 600 mg I.V. or P.O. q 12 hours for 10
to 14 days.
*Uncomplicated skin and skin-structure
infections caused by* **S. aureus** *(MSSA
only) or* **Streptococcus pyogenes**
*Adults:* 400 mg P.O. q 12 hours for 10 to 14
days.

## I.V. administration
■ Linezolid is compatible with D$_5$W, normal
saline solution for injection, and lactated
Ringer's injection. Flush I.V. line before and
after infusion.
■ Infuse drug over 30 to 120 minutes and don't
infuse in a series connection.
■ Inspect for particulate matter and leaks.

### Incompatibilities
Incompatible with amphotericin B, ceftriaxone sodium, chlorpromazine hydrochloride,
diazepam, erythromycin lactobionate, pentamidine isothionate, phenytoin sodium, and
trimethoprim-sulfamethoxazole.

## Mechanism of action
*Antibacterial action:* Linezolid is bacteriostatic against enterococci and staphylococci,
and bactericidal against most strains of streptococci. It exerts its antimicrobial effects by
interfering with bacterial protein synthesis.
Linezolid binds to the 23S ribosomal DNA on
the bacterial 50S ribosomal subunit. This action prevents the formation of a functional 70S
ribosomal subunit, thereby blocking the trans-
lation step of bacterial protein synthesis.

## Pharmacokinetics
*Absorption:* Rapidly and completely absorbed
after oral dosing. Levels peak in 1 to 2 hours.
Bioavailability is about 100%.
*Distribution:* Distributed readily into well-
perfused tissues. Protein-binding is about 31%.
*Metabolism:* Undergoes oxidative metabolism
to two inactive metabolites. Drug doesn't appear to be metabolized by the cytochrome P-450
oxidative system.
*Excretion:* At steady state, about 30% of dose
appears in urine as linezolid and about 50% as
metabolites. Linezolid undergoes significant
renal tubular reabsorption, such that renal clearance is low. Nonrenal clearance accounts for
about 65% of the total clearance.

| Route | Onset | Peak | Duration |
|-------|-------|------|----------|
| P.O. | Unknown | 1-2 hr | Unknown |
| I.V. | Unknown | ½ hr | Unknown |

## Contraindications and precautions
Contraindicated in patients hypersensitive to
linezolid or its components.
    Use cautiously in patients with uncontrolled
hypertension, pheochromocytoma, carcinoid

syndrome, or untreated hyperthyroidism because effects of linezolid in these patients is
unknown.

## Interactions
**Drug-drug.** *Adrenergics (such as dopamine,
epinephrine, pseudoephedrine):* Possible hypertension. Advise clinician to monitor blood
pressure and heart rate. Recommend starting
continuous infusion of dopamine and epinephrine at lower doses and adjusting to response.
*Serotoninergics:* Increased risk of serotonin
syndrome (confusion, delirium, restlessness,
tremors, blushing, diaphoresis, hyperpyrexia).
If symptoms develop, stop serotoninergic drug.
**Drug-food.** *Foods and beverages high in tyramine, such as aged cheeses, air-dried meats,
red wines, sauerkraut, soy sauce, tap beers:*
Increased blood pressure. Tyramine content of
meals shouldn't exceed 100 mg.

## Adverse reactions
**CNS:** headache, insomnia, dizziness.
**GI:** diarrhea, nausea, vomiting, constipation,
elevated amylase and lipase levels, altered taste,
tongue discoloration, oral candidiasis.
**GU:** elevated BUN level, vaginal candidiasis.
**Hematologic:** anemia, *leukopenia, neutrope-
nia, thrombocytopenia.*
**Hepatic:** elevated liver enzyme levels.
**Skin:** rash.
**Other:** fever, fungal infection.

## Overdose and treatment
Limited information is available. Signs and
symptoms of overdose include vomiting,
tremors, decreased activity, and ataxia. Treatment is supportive, with maintenance of
glomerular filtration. Hemodialysis may be
useful in increasing the elimination of linezolid. Effectiveness of peritoneal dialysis and
hemoperfusion in eliminating drug is unknown.

## Clinical considerations
■ Advise clinician to obtain samples for culture and sensitivity testing before linezolid therapy starts.
■ To reconstitute powder for oral suspension,
gently tap bottle to loosen powder. Using a total of 123 ml distilled water, pour half the volume of distilled water into container and shake
vigorously to wet powder. Add second portion
of distilled water and shake vigorously to obtain uniform suspension. Each 5 ml contains
100 mg of drug.
■ Before administering dose, invert container
three to five times (don't shake) to gently mix.
■ Store reconstituted suspension at room temperature and use within 21 days.
■ No dosage adjustment is needed when
switching from I.V. to P.O. forms.
■ Safety and efficacy of linezolid therapy lasting longer than 28 days are unknown.

---

Reactions may be *common,* uncommon, *life-threatening,* or COMMON AND LIFE-THREATENING.

- Pseudomembranous colitis and superinfection may occur. Consider these possibilities in patients who have persistent diarrhea or secondary infections.
- Because inappropriate use of antibiotics may encourage development of resistant organisms, recommend carefully considering alternative drugs before starting linezolid therapy, especially in the outpatient setting.
- Store drug at room temperature in its protective overwrap. Solution may develop a yellow coloration, but this doesn't affect drug's potency.

### Therapeutic monitoring
- Linezolid may cause thrombocytopenia; advise clinician to monitor platelet count in patients at increased risk for bleeding, in those with thrombocytopenia or receiving other drugs that may cause thrombocytopenia, and in patients receiving linezolid for longer than 14 days.

### Special populations
**Pediatric patients.** Safety and efficacy in children haven't been determined.

### Patient counseling
- Inform patient that tablets and oral suspension may be taken without regard to meals.
- Stress importance of completing entire course of therapy, even if patient feels better.
- Advise patient to alert prescriber about hypertension, use of cough or cold preparations, or treatment with selective serotonin reuptake inhibitors or other antidepressants.
- If patient has phenylketonuria, explain that each 5 ml of linezolid oral suspension contains 20 mg of phenylalanine. Linezolid tablets and injection don't contain phenylalanine.
- Tell patient to limit foods and beverages containing tyramine so that his intake is less than 100 mg of tyramine per meal. Foods high in tyramine include those that may have undergone protein changes by aging, fermentation, pickling, or smoking to improve flavor (such as aged cheeses, sauerkraut, soy sauce, beer, and red wine).

---

# liothyronine sodium (T₃)
Cytomel, Triostat

*Pharmacologic classification:* thyroid hormone
*Therapeutic classification:* thyroid hormone replacement
*Pregnancy risk category A*

### Available forms
Available by prescription only
*Tablets:* 5 mcg, 25 mcg, 50 mcg
*Injection:* 10 mcg/ml

## Indications and dosages
*Congenital hypothyroidism*
*Children:* 5 mcg P.O. daily, increased by 5 mcg q 3 to 4 days until desired response occurs.
*Myxedema*
*Adults:* Initially, 5 mcg daily, increased by 5 to 10 mcg q 1 to 2 weeks. maintenance dose is 50 to 100 mcg daily.
*Myxedema coma, precoma*
*Adults:* Initially, 25 to 50 mcg I.V.; reassess after 4 to 12 hours, then switch to P.O. as soon as possible. Patients with known or suspected cardiac disease should receive 10 to 20 mcg I.V.
*Nontoxic goiter*
*Adults:* Initially, 5 mcg P.O. daily; may be increased by 5 to 10 mcg daily at intervals of 1 to 2 weeks until dosage of 25 mcg daily is reached. Thereafter, dosage may be increased by 12.5 to 25 mcg daily at intervals of 1 to 2 weeks until desired response is noted. Usual maintenance dose is 75 mcg daily.
*Adults over age 65:* Initially, 5 mcg P.O. daily, increased by 5-mcg increments q 1 to 2 weeks until desired response is obtained.
*Children:* Initially, 5 mcg P.O. daily, increased by 5-mcg increments at weekly intervals until desired response is achieved.
*Thyroid hormone replacement*
*Adults:* Initially, 25 mcg P.O. daily, increased by 12.5 to 25 mcg q 1 to 2 weeks until satisfactory response is achieved. Usual maintenance dose is 25 to 75 mcg daily.
*Liothyronine suppression test to differentiate hyperthyroidism from euthyroidism*
*Adults:* 75 to 100 mcg daily for 7 days.

## I.V. administration
- Dose is based on initial and continuous monitoring of patient's status.
- Subsequent dose should be given at least 4 hours after initial dose to allow for adequate assessment of therapeutic response, but no longer than 12 hours after initial dose.

### Incompatibilities
None reported.

## Mechanism of action
*Thyroid hormone replacement:* Liothyronine is usually a second-line drug in the treatment of hypothyroidism, myxedema, and cretinism. This component of thyroid hormone affects protein and carbohydrate metabolism, promotes gluconeogenesis, increases the use and mobilization of glycogen stores, stimulates protein synthesis, and regulates cell growth and differentiation. The major effect of liothyronine is to increase the metabolic rate of tissue. It may be most useful in syndromes of thyroid hormone resistance.

## Pharmacokinetics
*Absorption:* 95% absorbed from the GI tract.

---

*Distribution:* Highly protein-bound. Its distribution hasn't been fully described.
*Metabolism:* Not fully understood.
*Excretion:* Half-life is 1 to 2 days.

| Route | Onset | Peak | Duration |
|-------|-------|------|----------|
| P.O. | Unknown | 2-3 days | 3 days |
| I.V. | Unknown | Unknown | Unknown |

## Contraindications and precautions
Contraindicated in patients hypersensitive to drug, and those with acute MI uncomplicated by hypothyroidism, untreated thyrotoxicosis, or uncorrected adrenal insufficiency.

Use cautiously in geriatric patients and in patients with angina pectoris, hypertension, ischemia, other CV disorders, renal insufficiency, diabetes, or myxedema.

## Interactions
**Drug-drug.** *Adrenocorticoids, corticotropin:* Altered thyroid status. Changes in liothyronine dosages may require dosage changes in the adrenocorticoid or corticotropin as well.
*Anticoagulants:* Altered PT and INR. Advise clinician to monitor patient for potential dosage adjustment.
*Estrogens:* Increased serum thyroxine-binding globulin levels. May increase liothyronine requirements.
*Insulin, oral antidiabetics:* May affect dosage requirements of these drugs. Advise clinician to monitor patient for potential dosage adjustment.
*Sympathomimetics, tricyclic antidepressants:* May increase the effects of any or all of these drugs, causing coronary insufficiency or arrhythmias. Use together cautiously.

## Adverse reactions
**CNS:** *nervousness, insomnia, tremor,* headache.
**CV:** *tachycardia, arrhythmias,* angina pectoris, **cardiac decompensation and collapse.**
**GI:** diarrhea, vomiting.
**GU:** menstrual irregularities.
**Metabolic:** weight loss.
**Musculoskeletal:** accelerated bone maturation in infants and children.
**Skin:** diaphoresis, skin reactions.
**Other:** heat intolerance.

## Overdose and treatment
Signs and symptoms of overdose include signs and symptoms of hyperthyroidism, including weight loss, increased appetite, palpitations, diarrhea, nervousness, abdominal cramps, sweating, headache, tachycardia, increased blood pressure, widened pulse pressure, angina, arrhythmias, tremor, insomnia, heat intolerance, fever, and menstrual irregularities.

Treatment of overdose reduces GI absorption and counteracts central and peripheral effects, primarily sympathetic activity. Advise

clinician to use gastric lavage or induce emesis (followed by activated charcoal up to 4 hours after ingestion). If patient is comatose or having seizures, inflate the cuff on an endotracheal tube to prevent aspiration. Treatment may include oxygen and ventilation to maintain respiration. It also should include appropriate measures to treat HF and to control fever, hypoglycemia, and fluid loss. Propranolol (or another beta blocker) may be used to counteract many of the effects of increased sympathetic activity. Liothyronine should be withdrawn gradually over 2 to 6 days, then resumed at a lower dose.

## Clinical considerations
■ Liothyronine may be preferred when rapid effect is desired or when GI absorption or peripheral conversion of levothyroxine to liothyronine is impaired.
■ Oral absorption may be reduced in patients with heart failure.
■ When switching from levothyroxine to liothyronine, recommend stopping levothyroxine and starting liothyronine at low dosage, increasing in small increments after residual effects of levothyroxine have disappeared. When switching from liothyronine to levothyroxine, recommend starting levothyroxine several days before withdrawing liothyronine to avoid relapse.
■ Recommend stopping drug 7 to 10 days before patient undergoes radioactive iodine uptake tests.
■ Liothyronine therapy alters radioactive iodine ($^{131}$I) uptake, protein-bound iodine levels, and liothyronine uptake.

### *Therapeutic monitoring*
■ Advise clinician to monitor thyroid test results to assess response to drug therapy.

### *Special populations*
**Breast-feeding patients.** Minimal amounts of drug appear in breast milk. Use with caution in breast-feeding women.
**Pediatric patients.** Partial hair loss may occur during first few months of therapy. Reassure child and parents that this is temporary. Infants and children may experience an accelerated rate of bone maturation.
**Geriatric patients.** Geriatric patients are more sensitive to effects of the drug. In patients over age 60, initial dosage should be 25% lower than usual recommended dosage.

## Patient counseling
■ Tell patient to report headache, diarrhea, nervousness, excessive sweating, heat intolerance, chest pain, increased pulse rate, or palpitations.
■ Advise patient not to store drug in warm, humid areas, such as the bathroom, to prevent deterioration of drug.

---

■ Encourage patient to take drug at the same time each day, preferably in the morning, to avoid insomnia.

# liotrix
Thyrolar

*Pharmacologic classification:* thyroid hormone
*Therapeutic classification:* thyroid hormone replacement
*Pregnancy risk category A*

## Available forms
Available by prescription only
*Tablets:*
Thyrolar-¼—levothyroxine sodium 12.5 mcg and liothyronine sodium 3.1 mcg
Thyrolar-½—levothyroxine sodium 25 mcg and liothyronine sodium 6.25 mcg
Thyrolar-1—levothyroxine sodium 50 mcg and liothyronine sodium 12.5 mcg
Thyrolar-2—levothyroxine sodium 100 mcg and liothyronine sodium 25 mcg
Thyrolar-3—levothyroxine sodium 150 mcg and liothyronine sodium 37.5 mcg

## Indications and dosages
*Hypothyroidism*
Dosages must be individualized to approximate deficit in patient's thyroid secretion.
*Adults:* Initially, 12.5 to 30 mg thyroid equivalent (usually, Thyrolar-¼ or Thyrolar-½ ) P.O. daily; increased q 1 to 2 weeks until desired response is achieved.
*Children over age 12:* 2 to 3 mcg/kg/day.
*Children ages 6 to 12:* 4 to 5 mcg/kg/day.
*Children ages 1 to 5:* 5 to 6 mcg/kg/day.
*Children ages 6 to 12 months:* 6 to 8 mcg/kg/day.
*Children under age 6 months:* 8 to 10 mcg/kg/day.

## Mechanism of action
*Thyroid stimulant and replacement:* Liotrix affects protein and carbohydrate metabolism, promotes gluconeogenesis, increases the use and mobilization of glycogen stores, stimulates protein synthesis, and regulates cell growth and differentiation. The major effect of liotrix is to increase the metabolic rate of tissue. It's used to treat hypothyroidism (myxedema, cretinism, and thyroid hormone deficiency).

Liotrix is a synthetic preparation combining levothyroxine sodium and liothyronine sodium in a 4 to 1 ratio by weight. Such combination products were developed because circulating $T_3$ was assumed to result from direct release from the thyroid gland. About 80% of $T_3$ is known to be derived from deiodination of $T_4$ in peripheral tissues, and patients receiving only $T_4$ have normal serum $T_3$ and $T_4$ levels. Therefore, there's no clinical advantage

to combining thyroid hormones; such combination could result in excessive $T_3$ level.

## Pharmacokinetics
*Absorption:* About 50% to 95% is absorbed from the GI tract.
*Distribution:* Distribution isn't fully understood.
*Metabolism:* Metabolized partially in peripheral tissues (liver, kidneys, and intestines).
*Excretion:* Excreted partially in feces.

| Route | Onset | Peak | Duration |
|-------|-------|------|----------|
| P.O. | Unknown | Unknown | Unknown |

## Contraindications and precautions
Contraindicated in patients hypersensitive to drug, and those with acute MI uncomplicated by hypothyroidism, untreated thyrotoxicosis, or uncorrected adrenal insufficiency.

Use cautiously in the elderly and in patients with impaired renal function, ischemia, angina pectoris, hypertension, other CV disorders, myxedema, and diabetes mellitus or insipidus.

## Interactions
**Drug-drug.** *Adrenocorticoids, corticotropin:* Altered thyroid status. Changes in liothyronine dosages may require dosage changes in the adrenocorticoid or corticotropin as well.
*Anticoagulants:* Altered PT and INR. Advise clinician to monitor patient for potential dosage adjustment.
*Beta blockers:* May decrease the conversion of $T_4$ to $T_3$. Advise clinician to monitor patient for effect.
*Cholestyramine:* May delay absorption of $T_4$. Separate doses by 4 to 5 hours.
*Estrogens:* Increased serum thyroxine-binding globulin levels. May increase liothyronine requirements.
*Hepatic enzyme inducers such as phenytoin:* May increase hepatic degradation of $T_4$, resulting in increased requirements of $T_4$. Advise clinician to monitor patient for drug effect.
*Insulin, oral antidiabetics:* May affect dosage requirements of these drugs. Advise clinician to monitor patient for potential dosage adjustment.
*Somatrem:* May accelerate epiphyseal maturation. Advise clinician to monitor patient for effect.
*Sympathomimetics, tricyclic antidepressants:* Drug may increase the effects of any or all of these drugs, causing coronary insufficiency or arrhythmias. Use together cautiously.

## Adverse reactions
**CNS:** nervousness, insomnia, tremor, headache, heat intolerance.
**CV:** *tachycardia, arrhythmias,* angina pectoris, *cardiac decompensation and collapse.*
**GI:** diarrhea, vomiting.
**GU:** menstrual irregularities.

---

* Canada only   ◇ Unlabeled clinical use

**Metabolic:** weight loss.
**Musculoskeletal:** accelerated rate of bone maturation in infants and children.
**Skin:** diaphoresis, allergic skin reactions.

## Overdose and treatment
Evidence of overdose includes signs and symptoms of hyperthyroidism, including weight loss, increased appetite, palpitations, nervousness, diarrhea, abdominal cramps, sweating, tachycardia, increased pulse rate and blood pressure, angina, arrhythmias, tremor, headache, insomnia, heat intolerance, fever, and menstrual irregularities.

Treatment requires reduction of GI absorption and efforts to counteract central and peripheral effects, primarily sympathetic activity. Advise clinician to use gastric lavage or induce emesis, then follow with activated charcoal, if less than 4 hours since ingestion. If patient is comatose or having seizures, recommend inflating the cuff on an endotracheal tube to prevent aspiration. Treatment may include oxygen and artificial ventilation p.r.n. to maintain respiration. It should also include appropriate measures to treat heart failure and to control fever, hypoglycemia, and fluid loss. Propranolol (or atenolol, metoprolol, acebutolol, nadolol, or timolol) may be used to combat many of the effects of increased sympathetic activity. Thyroid therapy should be withdrawn gradually over 2 to 6 days, then resumed at a lower dosage.

## Clinical considerations
■ Note that $T_4$ is drug of choice for hypothyroidism. Hepatic conversion of $T_4$ to $T_3$ is usually adequate. Excessive exogenous supplementation of $T_3$ usually causes toxicity.
■ The two commercially prepared liotrix brands contain different amounts of each ingredient; don't change from one brand to the other without considering the differences in potency.
■ Recommend starting dosages at lower limits in geriatric patients, in patients with long-standing disease, other endocrinopathies, or CV disease, and in patients with severe hypothyroidism.
■ Protect drug from heat and moisture.
■ Liotrix therapy alters radioactive iodine ($^{131}$I) thyroid uptake, protein-bound iodine levels, and $T_3$ uptake.

### Therapeutic monitoring
■ Advise clinician to monitor patient's pulse rate and blood pressure.
■ Advise clinician to monitor thyroid test results for clinical response to doses given and for dose adjustment.

### Special populations
**Breast-feeding patients.** Minimal amounts of drug appear in breast milk. Use with caution in breast-feeding women.

**Pediatric patients.** Partial hair loss may occur during first few months of therapy. Reassure child and parents that this is temporary. Infants and children may experience accelerated rate of bone maturation.
**Geriatric patients.** Geriatric patients are more sensitive to effects of drug and may require a lower dosage.

## Patient counseling
■ Tell patient to report headache, diarrhea, nervousness, excessive sweating, heat intolerance, chest pain, increased pulse rate, or palpitations.
■ Advise patient not to store liotrix in warm and humid areas, such as the bathroom.
■ Encourage patient to take a single daily dose in the morning to avoid insomnia.

# lisinopril
Prinivil, Zestril

*Pharmacologic classification:* ACE inhibitor
*Therapeutic classification:* antihypertensive
*Pregnancy risk category C (D, second and third trimesters)*

## Available forms
Available by prescription only
*Tablets:* 5 mg, 10 mg, 20 mg, 40 mg

## Indications and dosages
*Mild to severe hypertension*
*Adults:* Initially, 5 to 10 mg P.O. daily. Most patients are well controlled on 20 to 40 mg daily as a single dose. Doses up to 80 mg have been used.
*Heart failure*
*Adults:* Initially, 2.5 to 5 mg P.O. daily. Most patients are well controlled on 5 to 20 mg daily as a single dose.
*Acute MI*
*Adults:* Initially, 5 mg P.O.; then give 5 mg after 24 hours, 10 mg after 48 hours, and 10 mg daily for 6 weeks.

For patients with acute MI with low systolic blood pressure (less than 120 mm Hg), give 2.5 mg P.O. when treatment is started or during the first 3 days after an infarct. If hypotension occurs, a daily maintenance dose of 5 mg may be given with temporary reductions to 2.5 mg, if needed.
≡*Dosage adjustment.* For adults with renal impairment, initially, 5 mg P.O. if creatinine clearance is between 10 and 30 ml/minute, and 2.5 mg/day P.O. if it's less than 10 ml/minute. Dosage may be adjusted upward until blood pressure is controlled or to maximum of 40 mg daily. Dosage for patients with HF who have a creatinine clearance of less than 30 ml/minute is 2.5 mg/day P.O. Adults with HF, hyponatremia (serum sodium less than

130 mEq/L), or moderate to severe renal impairment (creatinine clearance less than 30 ml/min) should receive an initial dose of 2.5 mg.

## Mechanism of action

*Antihypertensive action:* Lisinopril inhibits ACE, preventing the conversion of angiotensin I to angiotensin II, a potent vasoconstrictor. Reduced formation of angiotensin II decreases peripheral arterial resistance and aldosterone secretion, thereby reducing sodium and water retention and blood pressure.

## Pharmacokinetics

*Absorption:* Variable absorption occurs after oral administration; an average of about 25% of an oral dose has been absorbed by test subjects.
*Distribution:* Distributed widely in tissues. Plasma protein–binding appears insignificant. Minimal amounts enter the brain. Preclinical studies indicate that it crosses the placenta.
*Metabolism:* Not metabolized.
*Excretion:* Excreted unchanged in the urine.

| Route | Onset | Peak | Duration |
|-------|-------|------|----------|
| P.O. | 1 hr | 7 hr | 24 hr |

## Contraindications and precautions

ACE inhibitor therapy shouldn't be initiated in hypotensive patients who are at immediate risk for cardiogenic shock and require I.V. administration of a vasopressor.

Contraindicated in patients hypersensitive to ACE inhibitors or history of angioedema related to previous treatment with ACE inhibitor, and in patients during the second and third trimesters of pregnancy.

Use cautiously in patients at risk for hyperkalemia and in those with impaired renal function.

## Interactions

**Drug-drug.** *Diuretics:* May cause excessive hypotension. Advise clinician to monitor blood pressure closely.
*Indomethacin:* May attenuate the hypotensive effect of lisinopril. Advise clinician to monitor patient closely.
*Lithium:* May increase plasma lithium levels. Advise clinician to monitor lithium levels.
*Potassium-sparing diuretics, potassium supplements:* May lead to hyperkalemia. Advise clinician to monitor serum potassium levels.
**Drug-food.** *Salt substitutes containing potassium:* May lead to hyperkalemia. Advise clinician to monitor serum potassium levels.

## Adverse reactions

**CNS:** *dizziness, headache, fatigue, paresthesia.*
**CV:** hypotension, *orthostatic hypotension,* chest pain.

**EENT:** *nasal congestion.*
**GI:** *diarrhea,* nausea, dyspepsia.
**GU:** impotence.
**Hematologic:** *neutropenia, agranulocytopenia.*
**Metabolic:** hyperkalemia.
**Respiratory:** *dry, persistent, tickling, nonproductive cough;* dyspnea.
**Skin:** rash.
**Other:** *angioedema, anaphylaxis.*

## Overdose and treatment

The most likely sign of overdose would be hypotension. Recommended treatment is I.V. infusion of normal saline solution.

## Clinical considerations

- Drug absorption is unaffected by food.
- Diuretics should be stopped 2 to 3 days before lisinopril therapy to reduce the risk of hypotension.
- If drug doesn't adequately control blood pressure, diuretics may be added.
- Lower dosage is needed in patients with impaired renal function.
- Recommend starting drug therapy in the hospital for HF patients because of the risk of severe hypotension.
- Drug shouldn't be used after acute MI in patients at risk for severe hemodynamic deterioration or cardiogenic shock.
- Beneficial effects of lisinopril may require several weeks of therapy.

### Therapeutic monitoring

- Recommend reviewing WBC and differential counts before treatment, every 2 weeks for 3 months, and periodically thereafter.
- Advise clinician to monitor patient's peak and trough blood pressures to assess clinical response.

### Special populations

**Breast-feeding patients.** Drug may appear in breast milk, but effect on infant is unknown; use with caution in breast-feeding women.
**Pediatric patients.** Safety and efficacy in children haven't been established; use only if potential benefits outweigh risks.
**Geriatric patients.** Geriatric patients may require lower doses because of impaired drug clearance. They may also be more sensitive to hypotensive effects of drug.

## Patient counseling

- Tell patient to report light-headedness, especially in first few days of treatment, so dosage can be adjusted; signs of infection, such as sore throat or fever, because drug may decrease WBC count; facial swelling or difficulty breathing, because drug may cause angioedema; and loss of taste, which may necessitate discontinuation of drug.

- To minimize orthostatic hypotension, advise patient to avoid sudden postural changes.
- Warn patient to seek medical approval before taking OTC cold preparations.
- Instruct patient to avoid potassium-containing salt substitutes.
- Warn women of childbearing age of the need to avoid pregnancy during therapy.
- Instruct patient to report any adverse events, including persistent dry cough.

# lithium carbonate
Carbolith*, Duralith*, Eskalith, Eskalith CR, Lithane, Lithizine*, Lithobid, Lithonate

# lithium citrate
Cibalith-S

*Pharmacologic classification:* alkali metal
*Therapeutic classification:* antimanic drug, antipsychotic drug
*Pregnancy risk category D*

## Available forms
Available by prescription only
**lithium carbonate**
*Capsules:* 150 mg, 300 mg, 600 mg
*Tablets:* 300 mg
*Tablets (sustained-release):* 300 mg, 450 mg
*Tablets (film-coated):* 300 mg
*Tablets (extended-release, film-coated):* 300 mg
**lithium citrate**
*Syrup (sugarless):* 300 mg/5 ml (with 0.3% alcohol)

## Indications and dosages
*Prevention or control of mania; prevention of depression in patients with bipolar illness*
*Adults:* For acute episodes: 1.8 g or 30 ml of lithium citrate P.O. daily in two or three divided doses or 20 to 30 mg/kg/day in two or three divided doses to maintain lithium levels at 1 to 1.5 mEq/L. For maintenance dose: 900 mg to 1.2 g or 15 to 20 ml of oral solution P.O. daily in two to four divided doses to maintain serum lithium level of 0.6 to 1.2 mEq/L. Usual maintenance dose doesn't exceed 2.4 g daily.
*Elderly:* 600 to 900 mg daily.
◇ *Major depression,* ◇ *schizoaffective disorder,* ◇ *schizophrenic disorder,* ◇ *alcohol dependence*
*Adults:* 300 mg lithium carbonate P.O. t.i.d. or q.i.d.
◇ *Apparent mixed bipolar disorder in children*
*Children:* Initially, 15 to 60 mg/kg or 0.5 to 1.5 g/m² lithium carbonate P.O. daily in three divided doses. Don't exceed usual adult dosage. Adjust dosage based on patient response and

serum lithium levels; usual dosage range is 150 to 300 mg daily in divided doses to maintain lithium levels of 0.5 to 1.2 mEq/L.
◇ *Chemotherapy-induced neutropenia in children and patients with AIDS receiving zidovudine*
*Adults and children:* 300 to 1,000 mg P.O. daily.

## Mechanism of action
*Antimanic and antipsychotic actions:* Lithium is thought to exert its antipsychotic and antimanic effects by competing with other cations for exchange at the sodium-potassium ion pump, thus altering cation exchange at the tissue level. It also inhibits adenyl cyclase, reducing intracellular levels of cAMP and, to a lesser extent, cyclic guanosine monophosphate (cGMP).

## Pharmacokinetics
*Absorption:* Rate and extent of absorption vary with dosage form; absorption is complete within 6 hours of oral administration from conventional tablets and capsules.
*Distribution:* Distributed widely into the body; appears in breast milk; levels in thyroid gland, bone, and brain tissue exceed serum levels. Steady-state serum level achieved in 12 hours: therapeutic effect begins in 5 to 10 days and is maximal within 3 weeks. Therapeutic and toxic serum levels and therapeutic effects show good correlation. Therapeutic range is 0.6 to 1.2 mEq/L; adverse reactions increase as level reaches 1.5 to 2 mEq/L; such levels may be needed in acute mania. Toxicity usually occurs at levels above 2 mEq/L.
*Metabolism:* Not metabolized.
*Excretion:* Excreted 95% unchanged in urine; about 50% to 80% of a given dose is excreted within 24 hours. Level of renal function determines elimination rate.

| Route | Onset | Peak | Duration |
|-------|-------|------|----------|
| P.O. | Unknown | ½-3 hr | Unknown |

## Contraindications and precautions
Contraindicated if therapy can't be closely monitored and during pregnancy. Use cautiously in the elderly; in patients with thyroid disease, seizure disorders, renal or CV disease, severe dehydration or debilitation, or sodium depletion; and in those receiving neuroleptics, neuromuscular blockers, and diuretics.

## Interactions
**Drug-drug.** *Antacids, other drugs containing aminophylline, caffeine, calcium, sodium, theophylline:* May increase lithium excretion by renal competition for elimination, thus decreasing therapeutic effect of lithium. Advise clinician to monitor patient closely.
*Carbamazepine, mazindol, methyldopa, phenytoin, tetracyclines:* May increase lithium toxicity. Advise clinician to monitor patient closely.

*Chlorpromazine:* Decreased effects of chlorpromazine. Avoid giving together.

*Electroconvulsive therapy (ECT):* Acute neurotoxicity with delirium has occurred in patients receiving lithium and ECT. Recommend reducing lithium dosage or withdrawing drug before ECT.

*Fluoxetine:* Increases lithium serum levels. Advise clinician to monitor patient closely.

*Haloperidol:* May result in severe encephalopathy characterized by confusion, tremors, extrapyramidal effects, and weakness. Use this combination with caution.

*Indomethacin, phenylbutazone, piroxicam, other NSAIDs:* Decreased renal excretion of lithium. May require a 30% reduction in lithium dosage.

*Neuromuscular blockers, such as atracurium, pancuronium, and succinylcholine:* May potentiate the effects of these drugs. Advise clinician to monitor patient closely.

*Selected serotonin-reuptake inhibitors:* Adverse effects possibly from increased serum lithium concentrations, lithium toxicity, and serotonin syndrome can occur with concomitant use with lithium. Use with caution when giving concurrently.

*Sympathomimetics, especially norepinephrine:* Lithium may interfere with pressor effects of these drugs. Advise clinician to monitor patient closely.

*Thiazide diuretics:* May decrease renal excretion and enhance lithium toxicity. Diuretic dosage may need to be reduced by 30%.

**Drug-herb.** *Parsley:* May promote or produce serotonin syndrome. Discourage use together.

*Psyllium seed:* Inhibited GI absorption. Discourage use together.

**Drug-food.** *Dietary sodium:* May alter renal elimination of lithium. Increased sodium intake may increase elimination of drug; decreased intake may decrease elimination. Advise clinician to monitor serum lithium levels.

**Drug-lifestyle.** *Caffeine:* Interferes with effectiveness of drug. Advise patient to avoid caffeine use.

## Adverse reactions

**CNS:** tremors, drowsiness, headache, confusion, restlessness, dizziness, psychomotor retardation, lethargy, *coma,* blackouts, *epileptiform seizures,* EEG changes, worsened organic mental syndrome, impaired speech, ataxia, muscle weakness, incoordination.

**CV:** *reversible ECG changes, arrhythmias,* hypotension, *bradycardia, peripheral vascular collapse.*

**EENT:** tinnitus, blurred vision.

**GI:** dry mouth, metallic taste, nausea, vomiting, anorexia, diarrhea, *thirst,* abdominal pain, flatulence, indigestion.

**GU:** *polyuria,* glycosuria, renal toxicity with long-term use, decreased creatinine clearance, albuminuria.

**Hematologic:** *leukocytosis with WBC count of 14,000 to 18,000/mm³* (reversible); elevated neutrophil count.

**Metabolic:** goiter, transient hyperglycemia, hypothyroidism (lowered $T_3$, $T_4$, and protein-bound iodine, but elevated radioactive iodine uptake [$^{131}I$]), hyponatremia.

**Skin:** pruritus, rash, diminished or absent sensation, drying and thinning of hair, psoriasis, acne, alopecia.

**Other:** ankle and wrist edema.

## Overdose and treatment

Vomiting and diarrhea occur within 1 hour of acute ingestion (induce vomiting in noncomatose patients if it is not spontaneous). Death has occurred in patients ingesting 10 to 60 g of lithium; patients have ingested 6 g with minimal toxic effects. Serum lithium levels above 3.4 mEq/L are potentially fatal.

Overdose with long-term lithium ingestion may follow altered pharmacokinetics, drug interactions, or volume or sodium depletion; sedation, confusion, hand tremors, joint pain, ataxia, muscle stiffness, increased deep tendon reflexes, visual changes, and nystagmus may occur. Symptoms may progress to coma, movement abnormalities, tremors, seizures, and CV collapse.

Treatment is symptomatic and supportive; recommend closely monitoring vital signs. If emesis isn't feasible, recommend treating with gastric lavage. Advise clinician to monitor fluid and electrolyte balance and correct sodium depletion with normal saline solution. Recommend starting hemodialysis if serum level is above 3 mEq/L, and in severely symptomatic patients unresponsive to fluid and electrolyte correction, or if urine output decreases significantly. Serum rebound of tissue lithium stores (from high volume distribution) commonly occurs after dialysis and may necessitate prolonged or repeated hemodialysis. Peritoneal dialysis may help but is less effective.

## Clinical considerations

■ Lithium is used investigationally to increase WBC count in patients undergoing cancer chemotherapy. It has also been used investigationally to treat cluster headaches, aggression, organic brain syndrome, aggressive outbursts in children with ADHD from broken homes, and tardive dyskinesia. Drug has been used to treat SIADH.

■ EEG changes include diffuse slowing, widening of frequency spectrum, potentiation, and disorganization of background rhythm.

■ Recommend shaking syrup formulation before administration.

■ Drug should be stopped before ECT therapy.

■ Advise clinician to give drug with food or milk to reduce GI upset.

■ Expect lag of 1 to 3 weeks before beneficial effects of drug are noticed. Other psychotropic drugs (such as chlorpromazine) may be needed during interim period.

■ Recommend adjusting fluid and salt ingestion to compensate if excessive loss occurs through protracted sweating or diarrhea. Patient should have fluid intake of 2½ to 3 L daily and a balanced diet with adequate salt intake.

■ Lithane tablets contain tartrazine, a dye that may precipitate an allergic reaction in certain individuals, particularly asthmatics sensitive to aspirin.

■ Drug causes false-positive test results on thyroid function tests.

### Therapeutic monitoring

■ Advise clinician to monitor baseline ECG, thyroid and renal studies, and electrolyte levels. Advise clinician to monitor lithium blood levels 8 to 12 hours after first dose, usually before morning dose, two or three times weekly the first month, then weekly to monthly on maintenance therapy.

■ Determination of serum drug levels is crucial to safe use of drug. Don't use drug in patients who can't have regular serum drug level checks. Be sure patient or responsible family member can comply with instructions.

■ When lithium blood levels are below 1.5 mEq/L, adverse reactions usually remain mild.

■ Advise clinician to monitor fluid intake and output, especially when surgery is scheduled.

■ Recommend observing patient for signs of edema or sudden weight gain.

■ Outpatient follow-up of thyroid and renal functions should occur every 6 to 12 months. Thyroid should be palpated to check for enlargement.

■ Recommend checking urine for specific gravity below 1.015, which may indicate diabetes insipidus.

■ Drug may alter glucose tolerance in diabetic patients. Advise clinician to monitor blood glucose levels closely.

■ Advise clinician to monitor serum levels and signs of impending toxicity.

■ Advise clinician to monitor drug dosing carefully when patient's initial manic symptoms begin to subside because the ability to tolerate high serum lithium levels decreases as symptoms resolve. Dosage must be adjusted based on lithium level, patient tolerance, and clinical response.

### Special populations

**Pregnant patients.** Lithium has been used during pregnancy in life-threatening situations and severe disease when other therapies couldn't be used or were ineffective. Fetal toxicity includes increased risk of CV abnormalities, Down syndrome, clubfoot, meningomyelocele, transient hypothyroidism with goiter, transient nephrogenic diabetes insipidus, muscular hypotonia, and apnea.

**Breast-feeding patients.** Lithium level in breast milk is 33% to 50% that of maternal serum level. Women should avoid breast-feeding during treatment with lithium.

**Pediatric patients.** Drug isn't recommended for use in children under age 12.

**Geriatric patients.** Geriatric patients are more susceptible to chronic overdose and toxic effects, especially dyskinesias. These patients usually respond to a lower dosage.

### Patient counseling

■ Explain that lithium has a narrow therapeutic margin of safety. A serum drug level that's even slightly high may be dangerous.

■ Warn patient and family to watch for signs of toxicity (diarrhea, vomiting, dehydration, drowsiness, muscle weakness, tremor, fever, and ataxia) and to expect transient nausea, polyuria, thirst, and discomfort during first few days. If toxic symptoms occur, tell patient to withhold one dose and report symptoms promptly.

■ Warn ambulatory patient to avoid activities that require alertness and good psychomotor coordination until CNS response to drug is determined.

■ Advise patient to maintain adequate water intake and adequate—but not excessive—salt in diet.

■ Explain importance of regular follow-up visits to measure lithium serum levels.

■ Tell patient to avoid large amounts of caffeine, which will interfere with effectiveness of drug.

■ Advise patient to seek medical approval before starting weight-loss program.

■ Tell patient not to switch brands of lithium or take other prescription or OTC drugs without medical approval. Different brands may not provide equivalent effect.

■ Tell patient to take drug with food or milk.

■ Warn patient against stopping this drug abruptly.

■ Tell patient to explain to close friend or family members the signs of lithium overdose, in case emergency aid is needed.

■ Instruct patient to carry identification and instruction card with toxicity and emergency information.

# lomefloxacin hydrochloride
Maxaquin

*Pharmacologic classification:* fluoro-quinolone
*Therapeutic classification:* broad-spectrum antibiotic
*Pregnancy risk category C*

# Available forms

Available by prescription only
*Tablets:* 400 mg

# Indications and dosages

*Acute bacterial exacerbations of chronic bronchitis caused by* **Haemophilus influenzae** *or* **Moraxella catarrhalis**
*Adults:* 400 mg P.O. daily for 10 days.
*Uncomplicated urinary tract infections (cystitis) caused by* **Escherichia coli, Klebsiella pneumoniae, Proteus mirabilis,** *or* **Staphylococcus saprophyticus**
*Adults:* 400 mg P.O. daily for 10 days.
*Complicated urinary tract infections caused by* **E. coli, K. pneumoniae, P. mirabilis,** *or* **Pseudomonas aeruginosa;** *possibly effective against infections caused by* **Citrobacter diversus** *or* **Enterobacter cloacae**
*Adults:* 400 mg P.O. daily for 14 days.
*Prophylaxis of infections after transurethral surgical procedures*
*Adults:* 400 mg P.O. 2 to 6 hours before surgery as a single dose.
*Prophylaxis for patient undergoing transrectal prostate biopsy procedure*
*Adults:* 400 mg P.O. 1 to 6 hours before procedure, as a single dose.
◊ *Uncomplicated gonorrhea*
*Adults:* 400 mg P.O. as a single dose.
≡ *Dosage adjustment.* For adults with renal impairment and creatinine clearance of 10 to 40 ml/minute, give loading dose of 400 mg P.O. on first day, followed by 200 mg P.O. daily for duration of therapy. Periodic determination of blood drug levels is recommended. Hemodialysis removes negligible amounts of drug.

# Mechanism of action

*Antibiotic action:* Lomefloxacin inhibits bacterial DNA gyrase, an enzyme needed for bacterial replication. Drug is bactericidal.

# Pharmacokinetics

*Absorption:* Rapidly absorbed from the GI tract; absolute bioavailability is 95% to 98%. Food impairs absorption by reducing total amount absorbed and slowing absorption rate.
*Distribution:* Only 10% plasma protein–bound.
*Metabolism:* About 10% is metabolized in the liver.
*Excretion:* Mostly excreted unchanged in urine; about 10% is excreted as metabolites. Solubility in urine is pH dependent. About 10% of a dose appears unchanged in the feces. Half-life is 8 hours. Steady state is reached after 2 days of once-daily therapy.

| Route | Onset | Peak | Duration |
|-------|-------|------|----------|
| P.O. | Unknown | 1½ hr | Unknown |

# Contraindications and precautions

Contraindicated in patients hypersensitive to drug or other fluoroquinolones. Use cautiously in patients with known or suspected CNS disorders, such as seizures or cerebral arteriosclerosis.

# Interactions

*Drug-drug. Antacids, minerals, sucralfate:* Bind with lomefloxacin in the GI tract and impair its absorption. Give antacids and sucralfate no less than 4 hours before or 2 hours after lomefloxacin.
*Cimetidine:* Other quinolones show substantially increased plasma half-lives. Advise clinician to monitor patient for toxicity.
*Cyclosporine, warfarin:* Other quinolones also increase the effects or serum levels of these drugs. Lomefloxacin hasn't been tested for these effects. Advise clinician to monitor patient for toxicity.
*Probenecid:* Decreases excretion of lomefloxacin. Don't give together.
*Drug-lifestyle. Sun exposure:* Photosensitivity reactions may occur. Advise patient to use sunblock.

# Adverse reactions

**CNS:** cerebrovascular disorder, *dizziness, headache,* abnormal dreams, fatigue, malaise, asthenia, agitation, anorexia, anxiety, confusion, depersonalization, depression, increased appetite, insomnia, nervousness, somnolence, *seizures, coma,* hyperkinesia, tremor, vertigo, paresthesia, twitching, paranoid reactions, impaired concentration.
**CV:** flushing, hypotension, hypertension, edema, syncope, *arrhythmias,* tachycardia, *bradycardia,* extrasystoles, cyanosis, angina pectoris, *MI, cardiac failure, pulmonary embolism,* cardiomyopathy, phlebitis.
**EENT:** epistaxis, abnormal vision, conjunctivitis, eye pain, earache, tinnitus, tongue discoloration, photophobia, abnormal lacrimation.
**GI:** taste perversion, *diarrhea, nausea,* thirst, dry mouth, pseudomembranous colitis, abdominal pain, dyspepsia, vomiting, flatulence, constipation, inflammation, dysphagia, bleeding, stomatitis.
**GU:** dysuria, hematuria, anuria, leukorrhea, epididymitis, orchitis, vaginitis, vaginal candidiasis, intermenstrual bleeding, perineal pain, albuminuria.
**Hematologic:** thrombocythemia, *thrombocytopenia,* lymphadenopathy, increased fibrinolysis, anemia, *hemolytic anemia,* leukocytosis.
**Hepatic:** elevated liver enzyme levels.
**Metabolic:** hypoglycemia.
**Musculoskeletal:** Achilles, shoulder and hand tendon ruptures, leg cramps, arthralgia, myalgia.

---

* Canada only    ◊ Unlabeled clinical use

**Respiratory:** dyspnea, *bronchospasm,* respiratory disorder or infection, increased sputum, stridor.
**Skin:** pruritus, skin disorder, skin exfoliation, eczema, increased diaphoresis, rash, urticaria, *photosensitivity.*
**Other:** *anaphylaxis,* chest or back pain, chills, allergic reaction, facial edema, flulike symptoms, decreased heat tolerance, gout.

## Overdose and treatment
Treatment of overdose includes emptying the stomach by induced vomiting or gastric lavage, observing patient closely, and providing supportive care. Drug isn't significantly removed by hemodialysis or peritoneal dialysis.

## Clinical considerations
■ Drug shouldn't be used for empiric treatment of acute exacerbations of chronic bronchitis when suspected pathogen is *Streptococcus pneumoniae* because this organism shows resistance to drug. Because blood drug levels don't readily exceed the minimum inhibitory concentration against *Pseudomonas aeruginosa,* drug shouldn't be used to treat bacteremia caused by this organism, but it has been used successfully to treat complicated urinary tract *Pseudomonas* infections.
**◪ ALERT** Drug may cause false-positive opiate results in urinary assays.
■ Achilles and other tendon ruptures have been reported. Discontinue drug if pain, inflammation, or tendon rupture occurs.

*Therapeutic monitoring*
■ Advise clinician to monitor renal and hepatic function test results and CBC in patients with impairments.

*Special populations*
**Breast-feeding patients.** It's unknown if drug appears in breast milk. Because of risk of serious adverse effects in the infant, a decision should be made to either discontinue drug or breast-feeding.
**Pediatric patients.** Because studies have shown that quinolones can cause arthropathy in immature animals, avoid using these drugs in children.

## Patient counseling
■ Remind patient to take all of drug prescribed, even after he feels better.
■ Advise patient to take drug on an empty stomach.
■ Tell patient to avoid hazardous tasks that require alertness, such as driving, until adverse CNS effects of drug are known.
■ Instruct patient to avoid sunlight or artificial ultraviolet light, and to call prescriber immediately if signs of photosensitivity occur.
■ Tell patient that sucralfate or antacids containing magnesium or aluminum shouldn't be

taken within 4 hours before or 2 hours after taking drug.
■ Instruct patient to drink fluids liberally.

# lomustine (CCNU)
CeeNU, CeeNU Dose Pack

*Pharmacologic classification:* alkylating drug, nitrosourea (cell cycle–phase nonspecific)
*Therapeutic classification:* antineoplastic
*Pregnancy risk category D*

## Available forms
Available by prescription only
*Capsules:* 10 mg, 40 mg, 100 mg
*Dose pack:* 2 capsules lomustine 10 mg, 2 capsules lomustine 40 mg, 2 capsules lomustine 100 mg

## Indications and dosages
Dosage and indications may vary. Check current literature for recommended protocol. Wait at least 6 weeks between repeat courses.
*Brain tumors, Hodgkin's disease, lymphomas*
*Adults and children:* Initially, 130 mg/m² P.O. given as a single dose. Drug is given q 6 weeks.
**≣ *Dosage adjustment.*** For patients with compromised bone marrow function, initial dose is usually 100 mg/m². Subsequent doses should be reduced according to bone marrow depression using the following guidelines.

| Nadir after prior dose | | Percentage of prior dose to be given |
|---|---|---|
| WBCs/mm³ | Platelets/mm³ | |
| > 4,000 | > 100,000 | 100% |
| 3,000-3,999 | 75,000-99,999 | 100% |
| 2,000-2,999 | 25,000-74,999 | 70% |
| < 2,000 | < 25,000 | 50% |

Repeat doses shouldn't be given until WBC count is more than 4,000/mm³ and platelet count is more than 100,000/mm³. Hematologic toxicity is delayed and cumulative; don't give repeat courses before 6 weeks.

## Mechanism of action
*Antineoplastic action:* Lomustine exerts its cytotoxic activity through alkylation, resulting in the inhibition of DNA and RNA synthesis. As with other nitrosourea compounds, lomustine is known to modify cellular proteins and alkylate proteins, resulting in an inhibition of pro-

---

tein synthesis. Cross-resistance exists between lomustine and carmustine.

## Pharmacokinetics
*Absorption:* Rapidly and well absorbed across the GI tract after oral administration.
*Distribution:* Distributed widely into body tissues. Because of its high lipid solubility, drug and its metabolites cross the blood-brain barrier to a significant extent.
*Metabolism:* Metabolized rapidly and extensively in the liver. Some of the metabolites have cytotoxic activity.
*Excretion:* Metabolites are excreted primarily in urine, with smaller amounts excreted in feces and through the lungs. Plasma elimination of drug is biphasic, with an initial phase half-life of 6 hours and a terminal phase of 1 to 2 days. Extended half-life of the terminal phase is thought to be caused by enterohepatic circulation and protein-binding.

| Route | Onset | Peak | Duration |
|-------|-------|------|----------|
| P.O. | Unknown | Unknown | Unknown |

## Contraindications and precautions
Contraindicated in patients hypersensitive to drug. Use cautiously in patients with decreased platelet, WBC, or RBC counts and in those receiving other myelosuppressants.

## Interactions
None reported.

## Adverse reactions
**CNS:** disorientation, lethargy, ataxia.
**GI:** *nausea, vomiting,* stomatitis.
**GU:** *nephrotoxicity,* progressive azotemia, *renal failure.*
**Hematologic:** *anemia, leukopenia,* delayed up to 6 weeks, lasting 1 to 2 weeks; *thrombocytopenia,* delayed up to 4 weeks, lasting 1 to 2 weeks; *bone marrow suppression,* delayed up to 6 weeks.
**Hepatic:** *hepatotoxicity.*
**Respiratory:** pulmonary fibrosis.
**Skin:** alopecia.
**Other:** *secondary malignant disease.*

## Overdose and treatment
Signs and symptoms of overdose include myelosuppression, nausea, and vomiting. Treatment is usually supportive, including antiemetics and transfusion of blood components.

## Clinical considerations
■ Drug has been used investigationally to treat bronchiogenic carcinoma, non-Hodgkin's lymphoma, malignant melanoma, breast cancer, renal cell carcinoma, and GI carcinoma.
■ Give drug 2 to 4 hours after meals. Drug is more completely absorbed if taken when the stomach is empty. To avoid nausea, give antiemetic before administering.

■ Anorexia may persist for 2 to 3 days after a given dose.
■ Dosage adjustment may be required in event of decreased platelet, WBC, or RBC count.
■ Avoid all I.M. injections when platelet count is below 100,000/mm³.
■ Use anticoagulants cautiously. Recommend watching patient closely for signs of bleeding.
■ Because drug crosses the blood-brain barrier, it may be used to treat primary brain tumors.

### Therapeutic monitoring
■ Advise clinician to monitor CBC weekly. Drug is usually not given more than every 6 weeks; bone marrow toxicity is cumulative and delayed.
■ Recommend frequent assessment of renal and hepatic status.

### Special populations
**Breast-feeding patients.** Metabolites of lomustine appear in breast milk. Breast-feeding should be stopped because of increased risk of serious adverse reactions, mutagenicity, and carcinogenicity in the infant.

## Patient counseling
■ Emphasize importance of continuing drug despite nausea and vomiting.
■ Stress importance of taking the exact dose.
■ Tell patient to immediately report if vomiting occurs shortly after a dose is taken.
■ Advise patient to avoid exposure to people with infections.
■ Caution patient to avoid alcohol for a short period after taking drug.
■ Warn patient to avoid products containing aspirin.
■ Tell patient to promptly report a sore throat, fever, or unusual bruising or bleeding.
■ Advise patient to use effective contraceptive measures during drug therapy.

# loperamide hydrochloride
Imodium, Imodium A-D, Kaopectate II

*Pharmacologic classification:* piperidine derivative
*Therapeutic classification:* antidiarrheal
*Pregnancy risk category B*

## Available forms
Available by prescription only
*Capsules:* 2 mg
Available without a prescription
*Tablets:* 2 mg
*Solution:* 1 mg/5 ml

## Indications and dosages
*Acute, nonspecific diarrhea*
**Adults and children over age 12:** Initially, 4 mg P.O., then 2 mg after each unformed stool. Maximum dose, 16 mg daily.

*Children ages 9 to 11:* 2 mg P.O. t.i.d. on first day.

*Children ages 6 to 8:* 2 mg P.O. b.i.d. on first day.

*Children ages 2 to 5:* 1 mg P.O. t.i.d. on first day.

Maintenance dose is one-third to one-half the initial dose (0.1 mg/kg only after each unformed stool) not to exceed dose recommended on the first day. Discontinue if no improvement after 48 hours.

*Chronic diarrhea*

*Adults:* Initially, 4 mg P.O., then 2 mg after each unformed stool until diarrhea subsides. Adjust dose to individual response. Discontinue if 16 mg is used for at least 10 days.

◊ *Children:* 0.08 to 0.24 mg/kg daily in 2 to 3 divided doses.

**Directions for patient self-medication**

*Adults:* 4 teaspoons or 2 tablets P.O. after the first loose bowel movement, followed by 2 teaspoons or 1 tablet after each subsequent loose bowel movement. Don't exceed 8 mg daily.

*Children ages 9 to 11 (27 to 43 kg [60 to 95 lb]):* 2 teaspoons or 1 tablet P.O. after first loose bowel movement, followed by 1 teaspoon or ½ tablet after each subsequent loose bowel movement. Don't exceed 6 mg daily.

*Children ages 6 to 8 (22 to 27 kg [48 to 59 lb]):* 2 teaspoons or 1 tablet P.O. after first loose bowel movement, followed by 1 teaspoon or ½ tablet after each subsequent loose bowel movement. Don't exceed 4 mg daily.

## Mechanism of action

*Antidiarrheal action:* Loperamide reduces intestinal motility by acting directly on intestinal mucosal nerve endings; tolerance to antiperistaltic effect doesn't develop. Drug also may inhibit fluid and electrolyte secretion by an unknown mechanism. Although it's chemically related to opiates, it hasn't shown any physical dependence characteristics in humans, and it possesses no analgesic activity.

## Pharmacokinetics

*Absorption:* Absorbed poorly from the GI tract.
*Distribution:* Distribution isn't well characterized.
*Metabolism:* Absorbed loperamide is metabolized in the liver.
*Excretion:* Excreted primarily in feces; less than 2% is excreted in urine.

| Route | Onset | Peak | Duration |
|-------|-------|------|----------|
| P.O. | Unknown | 2½-5 hr | 24 hr |

## Contraindications and precautions

Contraindicated in children under age 2, in patients hypersensitive to drug, or when constipation must be avoided. Also, OTC use is contraindicated in patients with a fever exceeding 101° F (38.3° C) or if blood is present in the stool. Use cautiously in patients with hepatic impairment.

## Interactions

*Opioid analgesics:* May cause severe constipation. Avoid use together.

## Adverse reactions

**CNS:** drowsiness, fatigue, dizziness.
**GI:** dry mouth; abdominal pain, distention, or discomfort; *constipation;* nausea; vomiting.
**Skin:** rash, hypersensitivity reactions.

## Overdose and treatment

Effects of overdose include constipation, GI irritation, and CNS depression. Treatment is with activated charcoal if ingestion was recent. If patient is vomiting, activated charcoal may be given in a slurry when patient can retain fluids. Alternatively, gastric lavage may be performed, followed by administration of activated charcoal slurry. Advise clinician to monitor patient for CNS depression and treat respiratory depression with naloxone.

## Clinical considerations

■ After administration via nasogastric tube, tube should be flushed to clear it and ensure passage of drug to stomach.

*Therapeutic monitoring*

■ Advise clinician to monitor patient for reduced stools or lack of improvement.
■ Advise clinician to monitor fluid and electrolytes if severe diarrhea occurs.

*Special populations*

**Breast-feeding patients.** It's unknown if drug appears in breast milk. Use with caution in breast-feeding women.
**Pediatric patients.** Drug is approved for use in children ages 2 and older; however, children may be more susceptible to untoward CNS effects.

## Patient counseling

■ Warn patient to take drug only as directed and not to exceed recommended dose.
■ Caution patient to avoid driving and other tasks requiring alertness because drug may cause drowsiness and dizziness.
■ Instruct patient to call if no improvement occurs in 48 hours or if fever develops.

# lopinavir/ritonavir

Kaletra

*Pharmacologic classification:* protease inhibitor
*Therapeutic classification:* antiviral
*Pregnancy risk category C*

## Available forms

*Capsules:* lopinavir 133.3 mg/ritonavir 33.3 mg
*Solution:* lopinavir 400 mg/ritonavir 100 mg per 5 ml (80 mg/20 mg per ml)

## Indications and dosages

***Treatment of HIV infection in combination therapy with other antiretroviral agents***

*Adults and children over age 12:* 400 mg lopinavir/100 mg ritonavir (3 capsules or 5 ml) P.O. b.i.d. with food. In treatment-experienced patient also taking efavirenz or nevirapine, where reduced susceptibility to lopinavir might be suspected, consider a dose of 533/133 mg (4 capsules or 6.5 ml) P.O. b.i.d. with food.

*Children ages 6 months to 12 years weighing 15 to 40 kg (33 to 88 lb):* 10 mg/kg (lopinavir content) P.O. b.i.d. with food, up to a maximum of 400/100 mg in children weighing over 40 kg. In treatment-experienced patient also taking efavirenz or nevirapine who weighs 15 to 50 kg, where reduced susceptibility to lopinavir might be suspected, consider a dose of 11 mg/kg (lopinavir content) P.O. b.i.d. Treatment-experienced children who weigh over 50 kg can receive the adult dose.

*Children ages 6 months to 12 years weighing 7 to < 15 kg (15 to < 33 lb):* 12 mg/kg (lopinavir content) P.O. b.i.d. with food. In treatment-experienced patient also taking efavirenz or nevirapine, where reduced susceptibility to lopinavir might be suspected, consider a dose of 13 mg/kg (lopinavir content) P.O. b.i.d. with food.

## Mechanism of action

*Antiviral action:* Lopinavir inhibits the HIV protease, thus preventing cleavage of the Gag-Pol polyprotein, resulting in the production of immature, noninfectious viral particles. Ritonavir inhibits metabolism of lopinavir, thereby increasing plasma levels of lopinavir.

## Pharmacokinetics

*Absorption:* Levels peak in 4 hours. Drug is better absorbed when taken with food.
*Distribution:* 98% to 99% plasma protein-bound.
*Metabolism:* Extensively metabolized by the CYP3A isoenzyme, which is part of the P-450 pathway. Ritonavir is a potent inhibitor of the CYP3A, which inhibits the metabolism of lopinavir, and therefore increases plasma levels of lopinavir.

*Excretion:* Excreted in urine and feces. Less than 3% excreted unchanged. Half-life is 5 to 6 hours.

| Route | Onset | Peak | Duration |
|-------|-------|------|----------|
| P.O. | Unknown | 4 hr | 5-6 hr |

## Contraindications and precautions

Contraindicated in patients hypersensitive to drug or its components. Use cautiously in patients with a history of pancreatitis or with hepatic impairment, hepatitis B or C, marked elevations in liver enzyme levels, or hemophilia. Also use cautiously in elderly patients.

## Interactions

**Drug-drug.** *Amiodarone, bepridil, lidocaine, quinidine:* Increased antiarrhythmic levels. Use cautiously; Advise clinician to monitor drug levels if possible.

*Amprenavir, indinavir, saquinavir:* Increased levels of these drugs. Avoid use together.

*Antiarrhythmics (flecainide, propafenone), pimozide:* Increased risk of cardiac arrhythmias. Don't use together.

*Atorvastatin:* Increased levels of these drugs. Advise clinician to use lowest possible dose and monitor patient carefully.

*Atovaquone, methadone:* Decreased levels of these drugs. Recommend considering increased doses of these drugs.

*Carbamazepine, dexamethasone, phenobarbital, phenytoin:* Decreased lopinavir level. Use cautiously.

*Clarithromycin:* Increased clarithromycin level in patients with renal impairment. Clarithromycin dose should be adjusted.

*Cyclosporine, rapamycin, tacrolimus:* Increased levels of these drugs. Advise clinician to monitor therapeutic levels.

*Delavirdine, ritonavir:* Increased lopinavir level. Avoid use together.

*Didanosine:* Decreased absorption of didanosine because lopinavir/ritonavir is taken with food. Advise clinician to give didanosine 1 hour before or 2 hours after lopinavir/ritonavir.

*Dihydroergotamine, ergonovine, ergotamine, methylergonovine:* Increased risk of ergot toxicity characterized by peripheral vasospasm and ischemia. Don't use together.

*Disulfiram, metronidazole:* Risk of disulfiram-like reaction. Avoid concomitant use.

*Efavirenz, nevirapine:* Decreased lopinavir levels. Consider increased lopinavir/ritonavir dosage.

*Felodipine, nicardipine, nifedipine:* Increased levels of these drugs. Use cautiously. Advise clinician to monitor patient.

*Itraconazole, ketoconazole:* Increased levels of these drugs. Don't give more than 200 mg daily of these drugs.

*Lovastatin, simvastatin:* Increased risk of adverse reactions, such as myopathy and rhabdomyolysis. Avoid concomitant use.

---

* Canada only    ◇ Unlabeled clinical use

*Midazolam, triazolam:* Increased risk of prolonged or increased sedation or respiratory depression. Don't use together.

*Oral contraceptives (ethinyl estradiol):* Decreased effectiveness of contraceptives. Recommend alternative contraception measures.

*Rifabutin:* Increased rifabutin level. Decrease rifabutin dose by 75%, and monitor patient for adverse reactions.

*Rifampin:* Decreased effectiveness of lopinavir/ritonavir. Avoid concomitant use.

*Sildenafil:* Increased sildenafil level. Reduce sildenafil dose. Use cautiously, and monitor patient for adverse reactions.

*Warfarin:* Possible effect on warfarin level. Advise clinician to monitor PT and INR.

**Drug-herb.** *St. John's wort:* Loss of virologic response and possible resistance to lopinavir/ritonavir. Discourage concomitant use.

**Drug-food.** *Any food:* Increased absorption of drug. Advise clinician to give drug with food.

## Adverse reactions

**CNS:** asthenia, headache, insomnia, malaise, abnormal dreams, agitation, amnesia, anxiety, ataxia, confusion, depression, dizziness, dyskinesia, emotional lability, encephalopathy, hypertonia, nervousness, neuropathy, paresthesia, peripheral neuritis, somnolence, abnormal thinking, tremors.

**CV:** chest pain, *deep vein thrombosis,* hypertension, palpitations, thrombophlebitis, vasculitis, edema.

**EENT:** sinusitis, abnormal vision, eye disorder, otitis media, tinnitus.

**GI:** abdominal pain, abnormal stools, *diarrhea, nausea,* vomiting, anorexia, cholecystitis, constipation, dry mouth, dyspepsia, dysphagia, enterocolitis, eructation, esophagitis, fecal incontinence, flatulence, gastritis, gastroenteritis, GI disorder, hemorrhagic colitis, increased appetite, *pancreatitis,* sialadenitis, stomatitis, ulcerative stomatitis, elevated amylase level.

**GU:** abnormal ejaculation, taste perversion, hypogonadism, renal calculus, urine abnormality.

**Hematologic:** anemia, *leukopenia, neutropenia; thrombocytopenia in children.*

**Hepatic:** elevated liver enzyme levels, hyperbilirubinemia in children.

**Metabolic:** Cushing's syndrome, hypothyroidism, dehydration, decreased glucose tolerance, lactic acidosis, weight loss, hyperglycemia, hyperuricemia, *hypercholesterolemia, elevated triglycerides;* hyponatremia in children.

**Musculoskeletal:** back pain, athralgia, arthrosis, myalgia.

**Respiratory:** bronchitis, dyspnea, lung edema.

**Skin:** rash, acne, alopecia, dry skin, exfoliative dermatitis, furunculosis, nail disorder, pruritus, benign skin neoplasm, skin discoloration, sweating.

**Other:** pain, chills, facial edema, fever, flu syndrome, viral infection, lymphadenopathy, peripheral edema, decreased libido, gynecomastia.

## Overdose and treatment

Experience of acute overdose with lopinavir/ritonavir is limited. There's no known antidote.

Treatment of overdose is supportive and symptomatic. Recommend inducing emesis or performing gastric lavage. Activated charcoal may be used to remove unabsorbed drug. Dialysis is unlikely to help with drug removal. Oral solution contains 42% alcohol. Ingestion of the product by young child may cause alcohol-related toxicity.

## Clinical considerations

■ To monitor maternal-fetal outcomes of pregnant women exposed to lopinavir/ritonavir, an antiretroviral registry has been established. Prescribers are encouraged to enroll patients by calling 1-800-258-4263.

**H** *ALERT* Many drug interactions are possible. Review drugs that patient is taking.

■ Advise clinician to give drug with food.

■ Refrigerated drug remains stable until expiration date on package. If stored at room temperature, drug should be used within 2 months.

### Therapeutic monitoring

■ Advise clinician to monitor patient for signs of fat redistribution, including central obesity, buffalo hump, peripheral wasting, breast enlargement, and cushingoid appearance.

■ Advise clinician to monitor total cholesterol and triglyceride levels before starting therapy and periodically thereafter.

■ Advise clinician to monitor patient for signs of pancreatitis: nausea, vomiting, abdominal pain, and increased lipase and amylase values.

■ Advise clinician to monitor patient for signs of bleeding.

### Special populations

**Breast-feeding patients.** It's not known if drug appears in breast milk. To avoid HIV transmission, the CDC recommends that HIV-infected mothers not breast-feed their infants.

**Pediatric patients.** Safety and efficacy in children under age 6 months haven't been established.

## Patient counseling

■ Tell patient to take drug with food.

■ Tell patient also taking didanosine to take it 1 hour before or 2 hours after lopinavir/ritonavir.

■ Advise patient to report adverse reactions to prescriber.

■ Tell patient to immediately report severe nausea, vomiting, or abdominal pain.

■ Warn patient to tell prescriber about any other prescription or nonprescription medicine that he's taking, including herbal supplements.

---

Reactions may be *common,* uncommon, *life-threatening,* or COMMON AND LIFE-THREATENING.

- Tell patient that drug isn't a cure for HIV.

# loracarbef
Lorabid

*Pharmacologic classification:* synthetic beta-lactam antibiotic of carbacephem class
*Therapeutic classification:* antibiotic
*Pregnancy risk category B*

## Available forms
Available by prescription only
*Pulvules:* 200 mg, 400 mg
*Powder for oral suspension:* 100 mg/5 ml, 200 mg/5 ml

## Indications and dosages
**Secondary bacterial infections of acute bronchitis**
*Adults and adolescents ages 13 and older:* 200 to 400 mg P.O. q 12 hours for 7 days.
**Acute bacterial exacerbations of chronic bronchitis**
*Adults and adolescents ages 13 and older:* 400 mg P.O. q 12 hours for 7 days.
**Pneumonia**
*Adults and adolescents ages 13 and older:* 400 mg P.O. q 12 hours for 14 days.
**Pharyngitis or tonsillitis**
*Adults and adolescents ages 13 and older:* 200 mg P.O. q 12 hours for 10 days.
*Children ages 6 months to 12 years:* 15 mg/kg P.O. daily in divided doses q 12 hours for 10 days.
**Sinusitis**
*Adults and adolescents ages 13 and older:* 400 mg P.O. q 12 hours for 10 days.
*Children ages 6 months to 12 years:* 15 mg/kg P.O. q 12 hours for 10 days.
**Acute otitis media**
*Children ages 6 months to 12 years:* 30 mg/kg (oral suspension) P.O. daily in divided doses q 12 hours for 10 days.
**Uncomplicated skin and skin-structure infections**
*Adults and adolescents ages 13 and older:* 200 mg P.O. q 12 hours for 7 days.
**Impetigo**
*Children:* 15 mg/kg P.O. daily in divided doses q 12 hours for 7 days.
**Uncomplicated cystitis**
*Adults and adolescents ages 13 and older:* 200 mg P.O. daily for 7 days.
**Uncomplicated pyelonephritis**
*Adults and adolescents ages 13 and older:* 400 mg P.O. q 12 hours for 14 days.
≡*Dosage adjustment.* Adults and children with creatinine clearance of 10 to 49 ml/minute should receive half the usual dose at same interval or normal recommended dose at twice the usual dosage interval; for those with creatinine clearance below 10 ml/minute, usual

dose q 3 to 5 days. Hemodialysis patients should be given another dose after dialysis.

## Mechanism of action
*Antibiotic action:* Loracarbef exerts its bactericidal action by binding to essential target proteins of the bacterial cell wall, leading to inhibition of cell-wall synthesis. Loracarbef is active against gram-positive aerobes, such as *Staphylococcus aureus, S. saprophyticus, Streptococcus pneumoniae,* and *S. pyogenes;* and gramnegative aerobes, such as *Escherichia coli, Haemophilus influenzae,* and *Moraxella catarrhalis.*

## Pharmacokinetics
*Absorption:* After oral administration, drug is about 90% absorbed from the GI tract. When pulvules are taken with food, peak plasma levels are 50% to 60% of those achieved on an empty stomach. (Effect of food on rate and extent of absorption of suspension form has not been studied to date.) Absorption of suspension form is greater than that of pulvule.
*Distribution:* About 25% of circulating drug is plasma protein–bound.
*Metabolism:* Doesn't appear to be metabolized.
*Excretion:* Eliminated primarily in urine. Elimination half-life in patients with normal renal function averages 1 hour.

| Route | Onset | Peak | Duration |
|-------|-------|------|----------|
| P.O. | Unknown | ½-1 hr | Unknown |

## Contraindications and precautions
Contraindicated in patients hypersensitive to drug or other cephalosporins and in patients with diarrhea caused by pseudomembranous colitis. Use cautiously in pregnant and breast-feeding women.

## Interactions
*Probenecid:* Decreased excretion of loracarbef, causing increased plasma levels. Advise clinician to monitor patient for toxicity.

## Adverse reactions
**CNS:** headache, somnolence, nervousness, insomnia, dizziness.
**CV:** vasodilation.
**GI:** diarrhea, nausea, vomiting, abdominal pain, anorexia, *pseudomembranous colitis.*
**GU:** vaginal candidiasis, transient increases in BUN and creatinine levels.
**Hematologic:** *transient thrombocytopenia, leukopenia,* eosinophilia.
**Hepatic:** transient elevations in AST, ALT, and alkaline phosphatase levels.
**Skin:** rash, urticaria, pruritus, *erythema multiforme.*
**Other:** hypersensitivity reactions, including *anaphylaxis.*

## Overdose and treatment
Toxic symptoms after overdose of beta-lactams, such as loracarbef, may include nausea, vomiting, epigastric distress, and diarrhea. Forced diuresis, peritoneal dialysis, hemodialysis, or hemoperfusion haven't been established as beneficial for an overdose of loracarbef. Hemodialysis is effective in hastening the elimination of loracarbef from plasma in patients with chronic renal failure.

## Clinical considerations
■ Consider the increased rate of absorption if oral suspension is to be substituted for pulvule. Pulvules shouldn't be substituted for oral suspension when treating otitis media.
■ Pseudomembranous colitis has been reported with nearly all antibacterial drugs and may range from mild to life-threatening. Therefore, diagnosis must be considered in patients with diarrhea subsequent to drug administration.
■ To reconstitute powder for oral suspension, add 30 ml of water in two portions to the 50-ml bottle or 60 ml of water in two portions to the 100-ml bottle; shake after each addition.
■ After reconstitution, oral suspension is stable for 14 days at controlled room temperature (59° to 86° F [15° to 30° C]).

### Therapeutic monitoring
■ Culture and sensitivity tests should be performed before giving first dose. Therapy may begin pending test results.
■ Drug may cause overgrowth of nonsusceptible bacteria or fungi. Advise clinician to monitor patient for signs and symptoms of superinfection.

### Special populations
**Breast-feeding patients.** It isn't known if drug appears in breast milk. Use caution when giving drug to breast-feeding women.
**Pediatric patients.** Safety and efficacy in infants under age 6 months haven't been established.

## Patient counseling
■ Instruct patient to take drug at least 1 hour before or at least 2 hours after eating.
■ Tell patient to take drug exactly as prescribed, even after he feels better.
■ Inform patient that oral suspension can be stored at room temperature for 14 days. Instruct patient to discard unused portion after 14 days.

# loratadine
Claritin

*Pharmacologic classification:* tricyclic antihistamine
*Therapeutic classification:* antihistamine
*Pregnancy risk category B*

## Available forms
Available by prescription only
*Tablets:* 10 mg
*Tablets (rapidly distintegrating):* 10 mg
*Syrup:* 1 mg/ml

## Indications and dosages
**Symptomatic treatment of seasonal allergic rhinitis and indicated for treatment of idiopathic chronic urticaria**
*Adults and children ages 6 and older:* 10 mg P.O. daily.
*Children ages 2 to 5:* 5 mg (1 teaspoon) of syrup P.O. once daily.
≣*Dosage adjustment.* For patients with liver failure or glomerular filtration rate below 30 ml/minute, adjust dosage to 10 mg every other day.
◇*Perennial allergic rhinitis*
*Adults:* 10 mg P.O. daily.

## Mechanism of action
*Antihistaminic action:* Loratadine is a long-acting tricyclic antihistamine with selective peripheral $H_1$-receptor antagonistic activity.

## Pharmacokinetics
*Absorption:* Readily absorbed. Because loratadine's peak plasma level may be delayed by 1 hour with a meal, give drug on an empty stomach.
*Distribution:* About 97% plasma protein–bound. Drug doesn't readily cross the blood-brain barrier.
*Metabolism:* Extensively metabolized to an active metabolite (descarboethoxyloratadine). The specific enzyme systems responsible for metabolism haven't been identified.
*Excretion:* About 80% of total dose given can be found equally distributed between urine and feces. Mean elimination half-life is 8½ hours for loratadine. Drug isn't eliminated by hemodialysis; it's unknown if drug is eliminated by peritoneal dialysis.

| Route | Onset | Peak | Duration |
|-------|-------|------|----------|
| P.O. | 1-3 hr | 8-10 hr | 24 hr |

## Contraindications and precautions
Contraindicated in patients hypersensitive to drug. Use cautiously in patients with hepatic impairment and in breast-feeding women.

## Interactions

**Drug-drug.** *Drugs known to inhibit hepatic metabolism:* Should be coadministered with caution until definitive interaction studies can be completed.
**Drug-herb.** *Licorice:* May prolong the QT interval and be potentially additive. Discourage use together.

## Adverse reactions

**CNS:** headache, somnolence, fatigue.
**GI:** dry mouth.

## Overdose and treatment

Somnolence, tachycardia, and headache have been reported with overdoses greater than 10 ml (40 to 180 mg). If overdose occurs, symptomatic and supportive measures should be instituted promptly and maintained for as long as needed.

Treatment consists of emesis (ipecac syrup), except in patients with impaired consciousness, followed by administration of activated charcoal to adsorb any remaining drug. If vomiting is unsuccessful or contraindicated, gastric lavage should be performed with normal saline. Saline cathartics also may be of value for rapid dilution of bowel contents.

## Clinical considerations

■ No information exists to indicate that drug abuse or dependency occurs.
■ Store drug in a cool, dry place away from heat and direct sunlight.

### Therapeutic monitoring

■ Advise clinician to monitor renal and hepatic function in patients with preexisting conditions.

### Special populations

**Breast-feeding patients.** Loratadine passes easily into breast milk. Antihistamine therapy is contraindicated in breast-feeding women.
**Pediatric patients.** Safety and efficacy in children under age 6 haven't been established.

## Patient counseling

■ Instruct patient to take drug on an empty stomach at least 2 hours after a meal and to avoid eating for at least 1 hour after taking drug.
■ Tell patient to take drug only once daily. Tell him to call if symptoms persist or worsen.
■ Warn patient to stop taking drug 4 days before allergy skin tests to preserve accuracy of tests.

# lorazepam

Apo-Lorazepam*, Ativan, Novo-Lorazem*

*Pharmacologic classification:* benzodiazepine
*Therapeutic classification:* anxiolytic, sedative-hypnotic
*Pregnancy risk category D*
*Controlled substance schedule IV*

## Available forms

Available by prescription only
*Tablets:* 0.5 mg, 1 mg, 2 mg
*Tablets (S.L.)*:* 1 mg, 2 mg
*Injection:* 2 mg/ml, 4 mg/ml
*Solution:* 2 mg/ml

## Indications and dosages

*Anxiety, tension, agitation, irritability, especially in anxiety neuroses or organic (especially GI or CV) disorders*
*Adults:* Initially, 2 to 3 mg P.O. daily in two to three divided doses. Usual range is 2 to 6 mg P.O. daily in divided doses; maximum dose, 10 mg/day.
*Insomnia*
*Adults:* 2 to 4 mg P.O. h.s.
*Preoperatively*
*Adults:* 0.05 mg/kg I.M. 2 hours before surgery (maximum, 4 mg). Alternatively, 0.044 mg/kg (maximum total dose, 2 mg) I.V. 15 to 20 minutes before surgery; for adults under age 50, dosage may be increased to 0.05 mg/kg (maximum, 4 mg) I.V. when increased lack of recall of preoperative events is desired.
◇ *Management of nausea and vomiting associated with emetogenic cancer chemotherapy*
*Adults:* 2.5 mg P.O. the evening before chemotherapy and repeat just after the initiation of chemotherapy. Alternatively, 1.5 mg/m² (maximum 3 mg) I.V. over 5 minutes 45 minutes before chemotherapy.
*Elderly:* Initially, 1 to 2 mg P.O. daily in divided doses. Then dosage is divided, p.r.n.
◇ *Status epilepticus*
*Adults and children:* 0.05 to 0.1 mg/kg I.V. Doses may be repeated at 10- to 15-minute intervals p.r.n. for seizure control. Alternatively, adults may be given 4 to 8 mg I.V.

## I.V. administration

■ Dilute lorazepam with an equal volume of a compatible diluent, such as $D_5W$, sterile water for injection, or normal saline solution.
■ Drug may be injected directly into a vein or into the tubing of a compatible I.V. infusion, such as normal saline solution or $D_5W$ solution. The rate of lorazepam I.V. injection shouldn't exceed 2 mg/minute. Emergency resuscitative equipment should be available when administering I.V.

■ Diluted lorazepam solutions must be given immediately.

### Incompatibilities
Incompatible with idarubicin.

## Mechanism of action
*Anxiolytic and sedative actions:* Lorazepam depresses the CNS at the limbic and subcortical levels of the brain. It produces an antianxiety effect by influencing the effect of the neurotransmitter gamma-aminobutyric acid (GABA) on its receptor in the ascending reticular activating system, which increases inhibition and blocks both cortical and limbic arousal after stimulation of the reticular formation.

## Pharmacokinetics
*Absorption:* When given orally, is well absorbed through the GI tract.
*Distribution:* Distributed widely throughout the body. Drug is about 85% protein-bound.
*Metabolism:* Metabolized in the liver to inactive metabolites.
*Excretion:* Metabolites are excreted in urine as glucuronide conjugates.

| Route | Onset | Peak | Duration |
|-------|-------|------|----------|
| P.O. | 1 hr | 2 hr | 12-24 hr |
| I.V. | 5 min | 1-1½ hr | 6-8 hr |
| I.M. | 15-30 min | 1-1½ hr | 6-8 hr |

## Contraindications and precautions
Contraindicated in patients with acute angle-closure glaucoma and those hypersensitive to drug, other benzodiazepines, or its vehicle (used in parenteral dosage form).

Use cautiously in patients with pulmonary, renal, or hepatic impairment and in geriatric, acutely ill, or debilitated patients. Don't use in pregnant women, especially during the first trimester of pregnancy.

## Interactions
**Drug-drug.** *Antidepressants, antihistamines, barbiturates, general anesthetics, MAO inhibitors, narcotics, phenothiazines:* Lorazepam potentiates the CNS depressant effects of these drugs. Use together cautiously.
*Cimetidine, possibly disulfiram:* Diminished hepatic metabolism of lorazepam, which increases its plasma level. Avoid use together.
*Scopolamine:* Combined use of parenteral lorazepam and scopalamine may be associated with an increased risk of hallucinations, irrational behavior, and increased sedation. Use together cautiously.
**Drug-lifestyle.** *Alcohol use:* Lorazepam potentiates the CNS depressant effects of alcohol. Advise patient to avoid alcohol.
*Heavy smoking:* Accelerated lorazepam metabolism, thus lowering clinical effectiveness. Encourage patient to quit smoking.

## Adverse reactions
**CNS:** *drowsiness,* amnesia, insomnia, agitation, *sedation,* dizziness, weakness, unsteadiness, disorientation, depression, headache.
**EENT:** visual disturbances.
**GI:** abdominal discomfort, nausea, change in appetite.
**Other:** *acute withdrawal syndrome* (after sudden discontinuation in physically dependent persons).

## Overdose and treatment
Signs and symptoms of overdose include somnolence, confusion, coma, hypoactive reflexes, dyspnea, labored breathing, hypotension, bradycardia, slurred speech, and unsteady gait or impaired coordination.

Treatment requires support of blood pressure and respiration until drug effects subside; Advise clinician to monitor vital signs. Mechanical ventilatory assistance via endotracheal tube may be required to maintain a patent airway and support adequate oxygenation. Flumazenil, a specific benzodiazepine antagonist, may be useful. Advise clinician to use I.V. fluids and vasopressors, such as dopamine and phenylephrine to treat hypotension, if needed. If patient is conscious, recommend inducing emesis. Advise clinician to use gastric lavage if ingestion was recent, but only if an endotracheal tube is present to prevent aspiration. After emesis or lavage, activated charcoal should be given with a cathartic as a single dose. Dialysis is of limited value.

## Clinical considerations
■ Lorazepam is one of the preferred benzodiazepines for patients with hepatic disease.
■ Advise clinician to use lowest possible effective dose to avoid oversedation.
■ Parenteral lorazepam appears to possess potent amnestic effects.
■ For the oral concentrated solution, recommend adding dose to 30 ml or more of water, juice, or soda, or to semisolid foods.
■ Oral drug is given in divided doses, with the largest dose given before bedtime.
**⚠ ALERT** Arteriospasm may result from intra-arterial injection of lorazepam. Advise against administering by this route.
■ Don't use drug solutions if they're discolored or contain a precipitate.
■ I.M. doses of lorazepam are given undiluted, deep into a large muscle mass.

### Therapeutic monitoring
■ Advise clinician to monitor hepatic function test results to prevent cumulative effects and to ensure adequate drug metabolism.
■ Advise clinician to monitor renal function test results.

---

Reactions may be *common*, uncommon, *life-threatening*, or COMMON AND LIFE-THREATENING.

### Special populations
**Breast-feeding patients.** Drug may appear in breast milk. Don't give to breast-feeding women.
**Pediatric patients.** Safety of oral lorazepam in children under age 12 hasn't been established. Safety of S.L. or parenteral lorazepam in children under age 18 hasn't been established. Neonates haven't been closely observed for withdrawal symptoms when mother took lorazepam for a prolonged period during pregnancy.
**Geriatric patients.** Geriatric patients are more sensitive to CNS-depressant effects of lorazepam. They may require supervision with ambulation and activities of daily living when therapy starts or changes. Lower doses usually are effective in geriatric patients because of decreased elimination. Parenteral administration of drug is more likely to cause apnea, hypotension, bradycardia, and cardiac arrest in geriatric patients.

### Patient counseling
■ Caution patient not to make changes in drug regimen without specific instructions.
■ Teach safety measures, as appropriate, to protect from injury, such as gradual position changes and supervised walking.
■ Advise patient of possible retrograde amnesia after I.V. or I.M. use.
■ Tell patient to avoid large amounts of caffeine-containing products, which may interfere with effectiveness of drug.
■ Advise patient of potential for physical and psychological dependence with long-term use.
■ Tell patient to discontinue drug slowly (over 8 to 12 weeks) after long-term therapy.

# losartan potassium
Cozaar

*Pharmacologic classification:* angiotensin II receptor antagonist
*Therapeutic classification:* antihypertensive
*Pregnancy risk category C (D second and third trimesters)*

### Available forms
Available by prescription only
*Tablets:* 25 mg, 50 mg, 100 mg

### Indications and dosages
*Hypertension*
*Adults:* Initially, 25 to 50 mg P.O. daily. Maintenance dose is 25 to 100 mg P.O. once daily or b.i.d.

### Mechanism of action
*Antihypertensive action:* Losartan is an angiotensin II receptor antagonist; it blocks the vasoconstrictor and aldosterone-secreting effects of angiotensin II by selectively blocking the binding of angiotensin II to its receptor sites found in many tissues, including vascular smooth muscle.

### Pharmacokinetics
*Absorption:* Well absorbed and undergoes substantial first-pass metabolism; systemic bioavailability is about 33%.
*Distribution:* Both losartan and its active metabolite are highly bound to plasma proteins, primarily albumin.
*Metabolism:* Cytochrome P-450 2C9 and 3A4 are involved in the biotransformation of drug to its metabolites.
*Excretion:* Drug and its metabolites are primarily excreted in feces with a small amount excreted in urine.

| Route | Onset | Peak | Duration |
|-------|-------|------|----------|
| P.O. | Unknown | 1 hr | Unknown |

### Contraindications and precautions
Contraindicated in patients hypersensitive to drug. Use cautiously in patients with impaired renal or hepatic function.

### Interactions
None significant.

### Adverse reactions
**CNS:** dizziness, insomnia.
**EENT:** nasal congestion, sinus disorder, sinusitis.
**GI:** diarrhea, dyspepsia.
**Musculoskeletal:** muscle cramps, myalgia, back or leg pain.
**Respiratory:** cough, upper respiratory tract infection.
**Other:** *angioedema.*

### Overdose and treatment
The most likely signs are hypotension and tachycardia; bradycardia may occur from parasympathetic stimulation. If symptomatic hypotension occurs, supportive treatment should be started. Neither losartan nor its active metabolite can be removed by hemodialysis.

### Clinical considerations
■ Advise clinician to use the lowest dose (25 mg) initially in patients with impaired hepatic function and in those who are intravascularly volume-depleted (receiving diuretic therapy).
■ Drug can be used alone or with other antihypertensives.
■ If antihypertensive effect measured at trough (using once-daily dosing) is inadequate, a twice-daily regimen at the same total daily dose or an increased dose may give a more satisfactory response.
■ Patients with severe heart failure whose renal function depends on the angiotensin-aldosterone system have experienced acute renal failure during therapy with ACE inhibitors.

Manufacturer of losartan states that drug would be expected to do the same. Recommend closely monitoring patient, especially during first few weeks of therapy.

### Therapeutic monitoring
■ Advise clinician to monitor blood pressure at regular intervals during therapy. Goal of therapy is to maintain systolic blood pressure < 140 mm Hg and diastolic blood pressure < 90 mm Hg.
■ Advise clinician to monitor patient taking diuretics concurrently in treatment of hypertension for symptomatic hypotension.
■ Advise clinician to monitor patient's renal function (serum creatinine and BUN levels).

### Special populations
**Pregnant patients.** Drugs such as losartan that act directly on the renin-angiotensin system can cause fetal and neonatal morbidity and death when given to pregnant women; these problems haven't been detected when exposure has been limited to the first trimester. If pregnancy is suspected, drug should be stopped.
**Breast-feeding patients.** It isn't known if drug appears in breast milk. Because of the potential for adverse effects in the breast-fed infant, a decision should be made whether to discontinue the drug or breast-feeding, taking into account the importance of drug to the woman.
**Pediatric patients.** Safety and efficacy in children haven't been established.

### Patient counseling
■ Instruct patient not to stop drug abruptly.
■ Tell patient to avoid sodium substitutes; these products may contain potassium, which can cause hyperkalemia in patients taking losartan.
■ Inform woman of childbearing age about the consequences of second- and third-trimester exposure to losartan; instruct her to call prescriber immediately if pregnancy is suspected.

# lovastatin
Mevacor

*Pharmacologic classification:* lactone, HMG-CoA reductase inhibitor
*Therapeutic classification:* cholesterol-lowering drug
*Pregnancy risk category X*

### Available forms
Available by prescription only
*Tablets:* 10 mg, 20 mg, 40 mg

### Indications and dosages
***Reduction of low-density lipoprotein and total cholesterol levels in patients with primary hypercholesterolemia (types IIa and IIb), atherosclerosis***
*Adults:* Initially, 20 mg P.O. once daily with evening meal. For patients with severely ele-

vated cholesterol levels (> 300 mg/dl), initial dose should be 40 mg. Recommended range is 20 to 80 mg in single or divided doses.
≡ *Dosage adjustment.* For patients also taking immunosuppressants, 10 mg P.O. daily, not to exceed 20 mg daily.

### Mechanism of action
*Antilipemic action:* Lovastatin, an inactive lactone, is hydrolyzed to the beta-hydroxy acid, which specifically inhibits HMG-CoA reductase. This enzyme is an early (and rate-limiting) step in the synthetic pathway of cholesterol. At therapeutic doses, the enzyme isn't blocked, and biologically necessary amounts of cholesterol can still be synthesized.

### Pharmacokinetics
*Absorption:* About 30% of an oral dose is absorbed in animals. Administration of drug with food improves plasma levels of total inhibitors by about 30%. Onset of action is about 3 days, with maximal therapeutic effects seen in 4 to 6 weeks.
*Distribution:* Less than 5% of an oral dose reaches the systemic circulation because of extensive first-pass hepatic extraction; the liver is the principal site of action for the drug. Both the parent compound and its principal metabolite are highly plasma protein–bound (more than 95%). Lovastatin can cross the placenta and the blood-brain barrier.
*Metabolism:* Converted to the active B hydroxy acid form in the liver. Other metabolites include the 6 hydroxy derivative and two unidentified compounds.
*Excretion:* About 80% is excreted primarily in feces, about 10% in urine.

| Route | Onset | Peak | Duration |
|-------|-------|------|----------|
| P.O.  | Unknown | 2 hr | Unknown |

### Contraindications and precautions
Contraindicated in patients hypersensitive to drug, in those with active liver disease or conditions associated with unexplained persistent elevations of serum transaminase levels, in pregnant and breast-feeding women, and in women of childbearing age unless there's no risk of pregnancy.

Use cautiously in patients who consume excessive amounts of alcohol or have history of liver disease.

### Interactions
**Drug-drug.** *Cholestyramine, colestipol:* May enhance lipid-reducing effects but may decrease bioavailability of lovastatin. Advise clinician to monitor patient closely.
*Cyclosporine, erythromycin, gemfibrozil, niacin:* May increase risk of severe myopathy or rhabdomyolysis. Use together cautiously.

---

*Isradipine:* May increase clearance of lovastatin and its metabolites. Advise clinician to monitor patient carefully.

*Itraconazole:* Administration with lovastatin increases HMG-CoA reductase inhibitor levels. Therapy with lovastatin should be temporarily interrupted if systemic azole antifungal treatment is required.

*Warfarin:* Increased anticoagulant effect. Advise clinician to monitor PT and INR.

**Drug-food.** *Grapefruit juice:* Concomitant use may cause increased plasma levels of drug. Instruct patient to avoid ingestion of large quantities (> 1 quart/day) of grapefruit juice.

**Drug-lifestyle.** *Alcohol use:* May increase hepatic effects. Advise patient to avoid alcohol. *Sun exposure:* Photosensitivity reaction. Advise patient to use sunblock.

## Adverse reactions
**CNS:** headache, dizziness, peripheral neuropathy, insomnia.
**CV:** chest pain.
**EENT:** blurred vision.
**GI:** constipation, diarrhea, dyspepsia, flatulence, abdominal pain or cramps, heartburn, nausea, vomiting.
**Hepatic:** elevated serum transaminase levels, abnormal liver test results.
**Musculoskeletal:** muscle cramps, myalgia, myositis, *rhabdomyolysis.*
**Skin:** rash, pruritus, alopecia.
**Other:** photosensitivity.

## Overdose and treatment
No information available.

## Clinical considerations
■ Drug therapy should start only after diet and other nonpharmacologic therapies have proved ineffective. Patient should be on a standard cholesterol-lowering diet and continue on this diet during therapy.
■ Recommend giving drug with evening meal; absorption is enhanced and cholesterol biosynthesis is greater in the evening.
■ Therapeutic response occurs in about 2 weeks, with maximum effects in 4 to 6 weeks.
■ Store tablets at room temperature in a light-resistant container.
■ Drug shouldn't exceed 20 mg/day if patient is receiving immunosuppressive drugs.

### Therapeutic monitoring
■ Advise clinician to monitor patient for signs of myositis; have patient report muscle aches and pains.
■ Liver function tests are needed frequently when therapy starts and periodically thereafter.
■ Advise clinician to monitor serum lipoprotein, triglycerides, and serum cholesterol levels periodically during therapy.

### Special populations
**Breast-feeding patients.** Drug is contraindicated for use in breast-feeding women.
**Pediatric patients.** Safety and efficacy in children haven't been established.

## Patient counseling
■ Stress importance of lowering cholesterol.
■ Advise patient to restrict alcohol intake.
■ Instruct patient to take drug with evening meal.
■ Tell patient to report adverse reactions, particularly muscle aches and pains, and to take precautions with exposure to sun and other ultraviolet light until tolerance is determined.

# loxapine hydrochloride
Loxitane C, Loxitane IM

# loxapine succinate
Loxapac*, Loxitane

*Pharmacologic classification:* dibenzoxazepine
*Therapeutic classification:* antipsychotic drug
*Pregnancy risk category NR*

## Available forms
Available by prescription only
*Capsules:* 5 mg, 10 mg, 25 mg, 50 mg
*Oral concentrate:* 25 mg/ml
*Injection:* 50 mg/ml

## Indications and dosages
*Psychotic disorders*
*Adults:* Initially, 10 mg P.O. b.i.d. (in severe schizophrenia, 50 mg P.O. daily); usual therapeutic and maintenance dose is 60 to 100 mg P.O. daily b.i.d. to q.i.d. for most patients (dose varies from patient to patient) or 12.5 to 50 mg I.M. q 4 to 6 hours or longer. Maximum daily dose, 250 mg. After desired symptom control, change to oral therapy. Don't administer drug I.V.

## Mechanism of action
*Antipsychotic action:* Loxapine is the only tricyclic antipsychotic; it's structurally similar to amoxapine. Loxapine is thought to exert its antipsychotic effects by postsynaptic blockade of CNS dopamine receptors, thus inhibiting dopamine-mediated effects. Loxapine has many other central and peripheral effects; its most prominent adverse reactions are extrapyramidal.

## Pharmacokinetics
*Absorption:* Absorbed rapidly and completely from the GI tract. First-pass metabolism results in lower systemic availability.

*Distribution:* Distributed widely into the body; appears in breast milk. Steady-state serum level is achieved within 3 to 4 days. Drug is 91% to 99% protein-bound.

*Metabolism:* Metabolized extensively by the liver, forming a few active metabolites; duration of action is 12 hours.

*Excretion:* Mostly excreted as metabolites in urine; some is excreted in feces by way of the biliary tract. About 50% is excreted in urine and feces within 24 hours.

| Route | Onset | Peak | Duration |
|-------|-------|------|----------|
| P.O., I.M. | ½ hr | 1½-3 hr | 12 hr |

## Contraindications and precautions

Contraindicated in patients hypersensitive to dibenzoxazepines and in patients experiencing coma, severe CNS depression, or drug-induced depressed states. Use cautiously in patients with seizure or CV disorders, glaucoma, or history of urine retention.

## Interactions

**Drug-drug.** *Aluminum- and magnesium-containing antacids and antidiarrheals:* Decrease loxapine absorption and its therapeutic effects. Separate administration times.

*Antiarrhythmics, disopyramide, procainamide, quinidine:* Increased risk of arrhythmias and conduction defects. Use together cautiously.

*Atropine and other anticholinergics, including antidepressants, antihistamines, MAO inhibitors, meperidine, phenothiazines, and antiparkinsonians:* Oversedation, paralytic ileus, visual changes, and severe constipation. Avoid use together.

*Beta blockers:* May inhibit loxapine metabolism, increasing plasma levels and toxicity. Use together cautiously.

*Bromocriptine:* Loxapine may antagonize therapeutic effect of bromocriptine on prolactin secretion. Advise clinician to monitor patient for effect.

*CNS depressants, including analgesics, barbiturates, narcotics, tranquilizers, anesthetics (general, spinal, and epidural), and parenteral magnesium sulfate (oversedation, respiratory depression, and hypotension):* Additive effects are likely after use of loxapine with these drugs. Use together cautiously.

*Centrally acting antihypertensives, such as clonidine, guanabenz, guanadrel, guanethidine, methyldopa, and reserpine:* Loxapine may inhibit blood pressure response. Use together cautiously.

*Dopamine:* Decreased vasoconstricting effects of high-dose dopamine. Avoid use together.

*Levodopa:* Decreased effectiveness and increased toxicity of levodopa (by dopamine blockade). Avoid use together.

*Lithium:* May result in severe neurologic toxicity with an encephalitis-like syndrome and a decreased therapeutic response to loxapine. Avoid use together.

*Nitrates:* May cause hypotension. Use together cautiously.

*Sympathomimetics, including epinephrine, phenylephrine, and ephedrine (often found in nasal sprays), and appetite suppressants:* Decreased stimulatory and pressor effects. Loxapine may cause epinephrine reversal, an inhibition of the vasopressor effect of epinephrine. Use together cautiously.

**Drug-lifestyle.** *Alcohol use:* Additive effects are likely. Advise patient to avoid alcohol.

## Adverse reactions

**CNS:** *neuroleptic malignant syndrome, extrapyramidal reactions, sedation, drowsiness, seizures,* numbness, confusion, syncope, *tardive dyskinesia,* pseudoparkinsonism, EEG changes, dizziness.

**CV:** *orthostatic hypotension, tachycardia,* ECG changes, hypertension.

**EENT:** *blurred vision,* nasal congestion.

**GI:** *dry mouth, constipation,* nausea, vomiting, paralytic ileus.

**GU:** *urine retention,* menstrual irregularities.

**Hematologic:** *leukopenia, agranulocytosis, thrombocytopenia.*

**Hepatic:** jaundice.

**Metabolic:** weight gain.

**Skin:** *mild photosensitivity,* allergic reactions, rash, pruritus.

**Other:** gynecomastia.

## Overdose and treatment

CNS depression is characterized by deep, unarousable sleep and possible coma, hypotension or hypertension, extrapyramidal symptoms, abnormal involuntary muscle movements, agitation, seizures, arrhythmias, ECG changes, hypothermia or hyperthermia, and autonomic nervous system dysfunction. Treatment is symptomatic and supportive, including maintaining vital signs, airway, stable body temperature, and fluid and electrolyte balance.

Vomiting shouldn't be induced: drug inhibits cough reflex, and aspiration may occur. Advise clinician to use gastric lavage, then activated charcoal and saline cathartics; hemodialysis may be helpful. Body temperature should be regulated p.r.n. Recommend treating hypotension with I.V. fluids; epinephrine shouldn't be given. Recommend treating seizures with parenteral diazepam or barbiturates; arrhythmias with parenteral phenytoin (1 mg/kg with rate adjusted to blood pressure); and extrapyramidal reactions with benztropine at 1 to 2 mg or parenteral diphenhydramine at 10 to 50 mg.

## Clinical considerations

■ Tardive dyskinesia may occur, usually after prolonged use. It may not appear until months or years after treatment and may disappear spontaneously or persist for life.

- Drug shouldn't be combined with alcohol or other depressants.
- Recommend diluting liquid concentrate with orange or grapefruit juice just before giving.
- Dose of 10 mg is therapeutic equivalent of 100 mg chlorpromazine.
- Photosensitivity warnings may apply with loxapine.
- Drug causes false-positive test results for urinary porphyrins, urobilinogen, amylase, and 5-hydroxyindoleacetic acid (5-HIAA) because of darkening of urine by metabolites; it also causes false-positive urine pregnancy test results using human chorionic gonadotropin.

### Therapeutic monitoring
- Recommend assessing patient periodically for abnormal body movement.
- Baseline blood pressure measurements should be obtained before therapy starts and monitored regularly.
- Periodic ophthalmic testing should be performed.

### Special populations
**Pediatric patients.** Drug isn't recommended for children under age 16.
**Geriatric patients.** Geriatric patients are highly sensitive to antimuscarinic, hypotensive, and sedative effects of drug and have a higher risk of extrapyramidal adverse reactions, such as parkinsonism and tardive dyskinesia. Higher plasma levels develop in these patients and, therefore, they require lower initial dosage and more gradual dosage adjustment.

### Patient counseling
- Warn patient against activities that require alertness and good psychomotor coordination until CNS response to drug is determined. Drowsiness and dizziness usually subside after first few weeks.
- Recommend sugarless gum or candy, mouthwash, ice chips, or artificial saliva to help alleviate dry mouth.
- Advise patient to get up slowly to avoid orthostatic hypotension.

# Lyme disease vaccine (recombinant OspA)
LYMErix

*Pharmacologic classification:* vaccine, bacterial-recombinant
*Therapeutic classification:* biological
*Pregnancy risk category C*

### Available forms
Available by prescription only
*Single-dose vials and prefilled syringes:* 30 mcg/0.5 ml

### Indications and dosages
*Active immunization against Lyme disease*
*Children and adults ages 15 to 70:* 30 mcg I.M. in deltoid region; repeat dose at 1 and 12 months after first dose. Safety and efficacy of this vaccine are based on administration of second and third doses several weeks before the onset of the disease transmission season.

### Mechanism of action
*Lyme disease prophylaxis:* The vaccine stimulates specific antibodies directed against *Borrelia burgdorferi* (a bacterial spirochete that causes Lyme disease). The vaccine contains lipoprotein OspA, an outer surface protein of *B. burgdorferi.*

### Pharmacokinetics
No information available.

| Route | Onset | Peak | Duration |
|-------|-------|------|----------|
| I.M. | Unknown | Unknown | Unknown |

### Contraindications and precautions
Contraindicated in patients hypersensitive to vaccine or its components. Don't give vaccine to patients with treatment-resistant Lyme arthritis (antibiotic refractory) or moderate or severe febrile illness. Lyme disease vaccine shouldn't be given to patients receiving anticoagulants unless potential benefit outweighs risk of administration.

Use cautiously in immunosuppressed patients and in those receiving immunosuppressive therapy because the expected immune response may not occur. For patients receiving immunosuppressive therapy, consider deferring vaccination for 3 months after therapy.

Also use cautiously in persons who may have allergic reactions to packaging for the LYMErix syringe, which contains dry natural rubber. Note that the vial packaging doesn't contain rubber.

### Interactions
None reported.

### Adverse reactions
**CNS:** *headache, fatigue,* dizziness, depression, hypoesthesia, paresthesia.
**EENT:** pharyngitis, rhinitis, sinusitis.
**GI:** diarrhea, nausea.
**Musculoskeletal:** *arthralgia,* back pain, achiness, myalgia, arthritis, arthrosis, stiffness, tendinitis.
**Respiratory:** bronchitis, coughing, upper respiratory tract infection.
**Skin:** *rash, injection site pain, redness, soreness, swelling,* injection site reaction, contact dermatitis.
**Other:** chills or rigors, fever, viral infection, flulike symptoms.

## Overdose and treatment
No information available.

## Clinical considerations
- Before immunization, recommend reviewing the patient's history for possible vaccine sensitivity, allergies, previous vaccination-related adverse reactions, and occurrence of any adverse-event related symptoms or signs. Epinephrine injection (1:1,000) and other appropriate drugs used for control of immediate allergic reactions must be immediately available.
- Recommend shaking well before withdrawal and use. Recommend inspecting visually for particulate matter or discoloration before administration. With thorough agitation, LYMErix is a turbid white suspension. It should be discarded if it appears otherwise. Vaccine should be used as supplied; no dilution or reconstitution is needed. Any vaccine remaining in a single-dose vial should be discarded.
- Packaging for vaccine prefilled syringe contains dry natural rubber, which may cause allergic reactions; packaging for the vial doesn't contain natural rubber.
- A separate sterile syringe and needle or a sterile disposable unit must be used for each patient to prevent transmission of infectious drugs. Needles should be disposed properly; don't recap.
- Administer vaccine by I.M. injection in the deltoid region. Vaccine shouldn't be injected I.V., intradermally, or subcutaneously.
- No data are available on the immune response to vaccine when given concurrently with other vaccines. When concomitant administration of other vaccines is required, they should be given with different syringes and at different injection sites.
- It's recommended that vaccine not be given to antibiotic-resistant Lyme arthritis patients.
- As with other I.M. injections, vaccine shouldn't be given to individuals on anticoagulant therapy or with clotting disorders, unless the potential benefit clearly outweighs the risk of administration.
- Store between 36° and 46° F (2° and 8° C). Don't freeze; discard if product has been frozen.
- LYMErix vaccination may result in a positive IgG enzyme-linked immunosorbent assay in the absence of infection.

### Therapeutic monitoring
- Advise clinician to monitor patient for adverse reactions and report any such reactions to 1-800-822-7967.

### Special populations
**Pregnant patients.** Prescribers are encouraged to register pregnant women who received the vaccine by calling 1-800-366-8900.

**Breast-feeding patients.** It isn't known if vaccine appears in breast milk; use cautiously in breast-feeding women.
**Pediatric patients.** Safety and efficacy in children under age 15 haven't been evaluated. Avoid giving to this age group.
**Geriatric patients.** Vaccine isn't indicated for patients over age 70.

## Patient counseling
- Inform patient that this vaccine is specific for preventing, not treating, Lyme disease.
- Inform patients, parents, or guardians of the benefits and risks of immunization with the vaccine, and of the importance of completing the immunization series.
- Ask patient regarding the occurrence of any symptoms or signs after a previous dose of the same vaccine and advise him to report any adverse events.
- Instruct patient to tell prescriber giving vaccine if he's taking anticoagulants (warfarin, heparin) or other blood-thinning drugs such as aspirin.
- Advise patient of ways to prevent other tick-borne diseases (wearing long-sleeved shirts, long pants, tucking pants into socks, and treating clothing with tick repellents). In addition, tell patient to carefully check himself when returning from endemic areas for the presence of ticks.
- Instruct patient on the appropriate way to remove ticks (use fine-pointed tweezers to avoid squashing the tick during removal from skin).

# lymphocyte immune globulin (antithymocyte globulin [equine], ATG)
Atgam

*Pharmacologic classification:* immunoglobulin
*Therapeutic classification:* immunosuppressant
*Pregnancy risk category C*

## Available forms
Available by prescription only
*Injection:* 50 mg of equine IgG per ml, in 5-ml ampules

## Indications and dosages
***Prevention of acute renal allograft rejection***
*Adults and children:* 15 mg/kg/day I.V. for 14 days, then same dosage every other day for next 14 days (to a total of 21 doses in 28 days). Give the first dose of ATG within 24 hours before or after transplantation.

*Treatment of acute renal allograft rejection*
*Adults and children:* 10 to 15 mg/kg/day I.V. for 14 days; if needed, same dosage may be given every other day for another 14 days (to a total of 21 doses in 28 days). Begin ATG therapy at the first sign of acute rejection.
*Aplastic anemia*
*Adults and children:* 10 to 20 mg/kg I.V. daily for 8 to 14 days, followed by alternate-day therapy for an additional 14 days (total of 21 doses in 28 days).
◇ *Skin allotransplantation*
*Adults:* 10 mg/kg I.V. 24 hours before allograft; then 10 to 15 mg/kg every other day. Maintenance dose is variable and can range from 5 to 40 mg/kg/day, based on clinical response and clinical indicators of immunosuppressive activity. Therapy usually continues until allografts cover less than 20% of total body surface area; often, this requires 40 to 60 days of treatment.
*Bone marrow allotransplantation; ◇ graft-versus-host disease after bone marrow transplantation*
*Adults:* 7 to 10 mg/kg I.V. every other day for six doses.

## I.V. administration
■ Dilute drug concentrate for injection before I.V. infusion. Dilute required dose of ATG in normal saline or half-normal saline injection (usually 250 to 1,000 ml); final level preferably shouldn't exceed 1 mg of equine IgG per ml. Recommend infusing over at least 4 hours.
■ Infusion in dextrose or highly acidic solutions isn't recommended.
■ Invert I.V. infusion solution container into which ATG concentrate is added to prevent contact of undiluted ATG with air inside the container. Refrigerate diluted solutions of ATG at 36° to 46° F (2° to 8° C) if administration is delayed. Reconstituted solutions shouldn't be used after 12 hours (including actual infusion time), even if stored at 36° to 46° F.

### Incompatibilities
None reported.

## Mechanism of action
*Immunosuppressive action:* The exact mechanism hasn't been fully defined but may involve elimination of antigen-reactive T cells (T lymphocytes) in peripheral blood or alteration of T-cell function. The effects of antilymphocyte preparations, including ATG, on T cells are variable and complex. Whether the effects of ATG are mediated through a specific subset of T cells hasn't been determined.

## Pharmacokinetics
*Absorption:* Administered I.V.

*Distribution:* Distribution of ATG into body fluids and tissues hasn't been fully described. Because antilymphocyte serum reportedly is poorly distributed into lymphoid tissues (such as spleen, lymph nodes), it's likely that ATG is also poorly distributed into these tissues.
No information is available on transplacental distribution of ATG. However, such distribution is likely because other immunoglobulins cross the placenta. Virtually all transplacental passage of immunoglobulins occurs during the last 4 weeks of pregnancy.
*Metabolism:* Not known.
*Excretion:* Plasma half-life of equine IgG reportedly averages about 6 days (range 1.5 to 13 days). About 1% of a dose of ATG is excreted in urine, principally as unchanged equine IgG. In one report, mean urinary level of equine IgG was about 4 mcg/ml after about 21 doses of ATG over 28 days.

| Route | Onset | Peak | Duration |
|-------|-------|------|----------|
| I.V. | Varies | Unknown | 6 days |

## Contraindications and precautions
Contraindicated in patients hypersensitive to drug. An intradermal skin test is recommended at least 1 hour before first dose. Marked local swelling or erythema larger than 10 mm indicates an increased potential for severe systemic reaction, such as anaphylaxis. Severe reactions to skin test, such as hypotension, tachycardia, dyspnea, generalized rash, or anaphylaxis, usually preclude further administration of drug.
Use cautiously in patients receiving other immunosuppressive drugs, such as corticosteroids or azathioprine.

## Interactions
**Drug-drug.** *Other immunosuppressive therapy (azathioprine, corticosteroids, graft irradiation):* May intensify immunosuppression, an effect that can be used to therapeutic advantage; however, such therapy may increase vulnerability to infection and possibly the risk of lymphoma or lymphoproliferative disorders. Advise clinician to monitor patient closely.

## Adverse reactions
**CNS:** malaise, *seizures,* headache.
**CV:** *hypotension,* chest pain, thrombophlebitis, tachycardia, edema, iliac vein obstruction, renal artery stenosis.
**EENT:** *laryngospasm.*
**GI:** *nausea, vomiting, diarrhea,* epigastric pain, abdominal distention, stomatitis.
**Hematologic:** LEUKOPENIA, THROMBOCYTOPENIA, *hemolysis, aplastic anemia.*
**Hepatic:** elevated liver enzyme levels.
**Metabolic:** hyperglycemia.
**Musculoskeletal:** *myalgia, arthralgia.*

**Respiratory:** hiccups, *dyspnea,* ***pulmonary edema.***
**Skin:** *rash, pruritus, urticaria.*
**Other:** *febrile reactions,* serum sickness, ***anaphylaxis,*** *infections,* night sweats, lymphadenopathy, *chills.*

## Overdose and treatment
No information available.

## Clinical considerations
■ Drug has been used to treat aplastic anemia, lymphoma, agranulocytosis, and as an adjunct in bone marrow, cardiac allotransplantation, and skin allotransplantation.
■ To minimize risks of leukopenia and infection, some prescribers recommend that azathioprine and corticosteroid dosages be reduced by 50% when ATG is used with these drugs for the prevention or treatment of renal allograft rejection.
■ Some prescribers elect to give prophylactic platelet transfusion in patients receiving drug for aplastic anemia because of high risk of thrombocytopenia.
■ Because of risk of severe systemic reaction (anaphylaxis), manufacturer recommends an intradermal skin test before administration of initial dose of ATG. The skin test procedure consists of intradermal injection of 0.1 ml of a 1:1,000 dilution of ATG concentrate for injection in normal saline injection (5 mcg of equine IgG). Advise clinician to give a control test using normal saline injection in the other arm to facilitate interpretation of the results. If a wheal or area of erythema exceeding 10 mm in diameter (with or without pseudopod formation) and itching or marked local swelling develops, infusion of ATG requires extreme caution; severe and potentially fatal systemic reactions may occur in patients with a positive skin test. A systemic reaction to the skin test, such as generalized rash, tachycardia, dyspnea, hypotension, or anaphylaxis rules out further administration of ATG. The predictive value of the ATG skin test hasn't been clearly established, and an allergic reaction may occur despite a negative skin test.
■ The manufacturer hasn't yet determined the total number of ATG doses (10 to 20 mg/kg per dose) that can be given safely to a patient. Some renal allograft recipients have received up to 50 doses in 4 months; others, up to four 28-day courses of 21 doses each without an increased risk of adverse effects.

### Therapeutic monitoring
■ Anaphylaxis may occur at any time during drug therapy and may be indicated by hypotension, respiratory distress, or pain in the chest, flank, or back. Advise clinician to monitor patient closely.

■ Recommend observing patient receiving drug for signs of leukopenia, thrombocytopenia, and concurrent infection.
■ Advise clinician to monitor peripheral blood levels of rosette-forming cells (RFCs) in order to guide therapy in allograft recipient (maintain RFCs at 10% of treatment level).
■ Advise clinician to monitor patient for signs of infection during ATG therapy.

### Special populations
**Breast-feeding patients.** Although it's unknown if drug appears in breast milk, other immunoglobulins appear in breast milk. Breast-feeding women should consider an alternative feeding method.
**Pediatric patients.** Safety and efficacy in children haven't been established. Drug has had limited use in children ages 3 months to 19 years.

## Patient counseling
■ Warn patient that a febrile reaction is likely.

# magaldrate (aluminum magnesium hydroxide sulfate)

Lowsium, Riopan Plus

*Pharmacologic classification:*
aluminum-magnesium salt
*Therapeutic classification:* antacid
*Pregnancy risk category C*

## Available forms
Available without a prescription
*Suspension:* 540 mg/5 ml

## Indications and dosages
***Indigestion or hyperacidity from peptic ulcer, gastritis, peptic esophagitis, hiatal hernia***
Adults: 5 to 10 ml (suspension) P.O. between meals and h.s. with water.

## Mechanism of action
*Antacid action:* Magaldrate neutralizes gastric acid, reducing the direct acid irritant effect. This increases gastric pH, which inactivates pepsin. Magaldrate also enhances mucosal barrier integrity and improves gastroesophageal sphincter tone.

## Pharmacokinetics
*Absorption:* Aluminum may be absorbed systemically. Magnesium also may be absorbed, posing a risk to patients with renal failure. Absorption is unrelated to mechanism of action.
*Distribution:* Distribution is primarily local.
*Metabolism:* None.
*Excretion:* Excreted in feces; some aluminum and magnesium may appear in breast milk. Duration of action is prolonged.

| Route | Onset | Peak | Duration |
|-------|-------|------|----------|
| P.O. | 20 min | Unknown | 20-180 min |

## Contraindications and precautions
Contraindicated in patients with severe renal disease. Use cautiously in patients with mild renal impairment.

## Interactions
**Drug-drug.** *Anticoagulants, antimuscarinics, chenodiol, chlordiazepoxide, diazepam, digoxin, isoniazid, phenothiazines (especially chlor-*

*promazine), phosphates, quinolones, tetracycline, vitamin A, warfarin:* Decreased absorption, thus lessening their effectiveness. Separate administration times.
*Enterically coated drugs:* Magaldrate may cause premature release of these drugs. Separate doses of magaldrate and all oral drugs by 1 to 2 hours.
*Levodopa:* Concurrent administration may increase levodopa absorption, increasing risk of toxicity. Separate administration times.
**Drug-herb.** *Melatonin:* Additive inhibitory effects on the *N*-methyl-*D*-aspartate receptor. Discourage use together.

## Adverse reactions
**GI:** mild constipation, diarrhea.
**GU:** increased urine pH levels.
**Metabolic:** decreased serum potassium levels, increased serum gastrin levels.

## Overdose and treatment
No information available.

## Clinical considerations
■ Recommend shaking suspension well and giving with small amounts of water or fruit juice.
■ After administration through nasogastric tube, recommend flushing tube with water to clear it and ensure passage of drug to stomach.
■ Advise clinician to give drug at least 1 hour apart from enterically coated drugs.
■ Suspension contains saccharin and sorbitol.
■ Most formulations contain less than 0.5 mg of sodium per tablet (or 5 ml of liquid).
■ Magaldrate may antagonize effect of pentagastrin during gastric acid secretion tests.

### Therapeutic monitoring
■ Advise clinician to monitor renal function and serum phosphate, potassium, and magnesium levels in patients with renal disease.

### Special populations
**Breast-feeding patients.** Some aluminum and magnesium may appear in breast milk. However, no problems have been linked to use in breast-feeding women.
**Pediatric patients.** Use of drug as an antacid in children under age 6 requires a well-established diagnosis because children typically give vague descriptions of symptoms.

### Patient counseling
- Caution patient to take drug only as directed and 1 or 2 hours apart from other oral drugs.
- Remind patient to shake suspension well or to chew tablets thoroughly.
- Warn patient not to take more than 18 teaspoonfuls in a 24-hour period.

---

# magnesium hydroxide (milk of magnesia)

Milk of Magnesia, Phillips' Milk of Magnesia, Concentrated Phillips' Milk of Magnesia

*Pharmacologic classification:* magnesium salt
*Therapeutic classification:* antiulcerative, antacid, laxative
*Pregnancy risk category NR*

### Available forms
Available without a prescription
*Tablets:* 300 mg, 600 mg
*Tablets (chewable):* 311 mg
*Liquid:* 400 mg/5 ml, 800 mg/5 ml
*Suspension (concentrated):* 10 ml (equivalent to 30 ml of milk of magnesia)
*Suspension:* 77.5 mg/g

### Indications and dosages
*Constipation, bowel evacuation before surgery*
*Adults and children over age 6:* 10 to 20 ml concentrated milk of magnesia P.O.; 15 to 60 ml milk of magnesia P.O.
*Laxative*
*Adults:* 30 to 60 ml P.O., usually h.s.
*Children ages 6 to 12:* 15 to 30 ml P.O.
*Children ages 2 to 6:* 5 to 15 ml P.O.
*Antacid*
*Adults:* 5 to 15 ml (liquid) P.O., p.r.n., up to q.i.d.; 2.5 to 7.5 ml (liquid concentrate) P.O., p.r.n., up to q.i.d.; 2 to 4 tablets P.O., p.r.n., up to q.i.d.
*Children:* 2.5 to 5 ml P.O., p.r.n.

### Mechanism of action
*Antiulcer action:* Magnesium hydroxide neutralizes gastric acid, decreasing the direct acid irritant effect. This increases pH, which, in turn, leads to pepsin inactivation. Magnesium hydroxide also enhances mucosal barrier integrity and improves gastric and esophageal sphincter tone.

*Antacid action:* Drug reacts rapidly with hydrochloric acid in the stomach to form magnesium chloride and water.

*Laxative action:* Magnesium hydroxide produces its laxative effect by increasing the osmotic gradient in the gut and drawing in water, causing distention that stimulates peristalsis and bowel evacuation.

### Pharmacokinetics
*Absorption:* About 15% to 30% may be absorbed systemically (posing a potential risk to patients with renal failure).
*Distribution:* None.
*Metabolism:* None.
*Excretion:* Unabsorbed drug is excreted in feces; absorbed drug is excreted rapidly in urine.

| Route | Onset | Peak | Duration |
|-------|-------|------|----------|
| P.O. | ½-3 hr | Variable | Variable |

### Contraindications and precautions
Contraindicated in patients with abdominal pain, nausea, vomiting, or other symptoms of appendicitis or acute surgical abdomen and in those with myocardial damage, heart block, fecal impaction, rectal fissures, intestinal obstruction or perforation, renal disease. Also contraindicated in patients about to deliver.

Use cautiously in patients with rectal bleeding.

### Interactions
**Drug-drug.** *Chlordiazepoxide, chlorpromazine, dicumarol, digoxin, iron salts, isoniazid:* Use of magnesium hydroxide with aluminum hydroxide may decrease the absorption rate of these drugs. Separate administration times.
*Enteric-coated tablets:* Premature release of enterically coated drugs. Recommend separating administration times.
*Quinolones, tetracyclines:* Decreased absorption. Recommend separating administration times.

### Adverse reactions
**GI:** *abdominal cramping, nausea, diarrhea,* laxative dependence (with long-term or excessive use).
**Metabolic:** fluid and electrolyte disturbances (with daily use).

### Overdose and treatment
No information available.

### Clinical considerations
- Advise clinician to give drug at least 1 hour apart from enterically coated drugs and shake suspension well.
- After administration of the drug through nasogastric tube, recommend flushing tube with water to clear it.

### *Therapeutic monitoring*
- Advise clinician to monitor patient for signs and symptoms of hypermagnesemia, especially if patient has impaired renal function.

### *Special populations*
**Breast-feeding patients.** Some magnesium may appear in breast milk, but no problems have been reported with use by breast-feeding women.

---

Reactions may be *common*, uncommon, *life-threatening*, or COMMON AND LIFE-THREATENING.

**Pediatric patients.** Use as an antacid in children under age 6 requires a well-established diagnosis because children tend to give vague descriptions of symptoms.

## Patient counseling
■ Caution patient to avoid overuse to prevent laxative dependence.
■ Instruct patient to shake suspension well or to chew tablets well.
■ Encourage patient using drug as a laxative to maintain adequate fluid intake, diet, and exercise.

# magnesium sulfate

*Pharmacologic classification:* mineral, electrolyte
*Therapeutic classification:* anticonvulsant
*Pregnancy risk category A*

## Available forms
Available by prescription only
*Parenteral injection:* 10%, 12.5%, 50%
*Injection for I.V. use:* 4% (4, 20, and 40 g); 8% (4 g)
*Parenteral injection for I.V. use:* 1% (1 and 10 g) in $D_5W$; 2% (10 and 20 g) in $D_5W$

## Indications and dosages
*Hypomagnesemic seizures*
*Adults:* 1 g I.V. or I.M. Alternatively, 1 to 2 g (as 10% solution) I.V. over 15 minutes, then 1 g I.M. q 4 to 6 hours, based on patient's response and magnesium blood levels.
*Seizures secondary to hypomagnesemia in acute nephritis*
*Children:* 0.2 ml/kg of 50% solution I.M. q 4 to 6 hours, p.r.n., or 100 to 200 mg/kg as a 1% to 3% solution I.V. given slowly over 1 hour with the first half of dose in the first 15 to 20 minutes. Also, 0.1 to 0.2 ml/kg of 20% solution (20 to 40 mg/kg) I.M. Titrate dosage according to magnesium blood levels and seizure response.
*Life-threatening arrhythmias*
*Adults:* For patients with sustained ventricular tachycardia or torsades de pointes, give 1 to 6 g I.V. over several minutes followed by 3 to 20 mg/minute I.V. infusion for 5 to 48 hours depending on patient response and serum magnesium levels. For patients with paroxysmal atrial tachycardia, give 3 to 4 g I.V. over 30 seconds.
*Prevention or control of seizures in preeclampsia or eclampsia*
*Adults:* Initially, 4 g I.V. in 250 ml $D_5W$ and 4 to 5 g deep I.M. into each buttock (using undiluted 50% magnesium sulfate injection); then 4 to 5 g deep I.M. into alternate buttock q 4 hours, p.r.n. Alternatively, 4 g I.V. as a loading dose followed by 1 to 3 g hourly as an I.V.

infusion. Maximum daily dose, 30 to 40 g. Alternatively, 8 to 15 g (depending on weight of patient—8 g for 45-kg [100-lb] patient and 15 g for 90-kg [198-lb] patient); 4 g of magnesium sulfate (as magnesium sulfate injection or magnesium sulfate in $D_5W$) is given I.V. and the remaining dose is given I.M. using undiluted 50% magnesium sulfate injection. Dosage over next 24 hours based on serum level and urinary excretion of magnesium following the initial dose. Subsequent doses should be sufficient to replace magnesium excreted in urine, about 65% of the initial dose administered I.M. q 6 hours.
≡*Dosage adjustment.* For patients with severe renal insufficiency, maximum dose is 20 g in 48 hours.
*Barium poisoning,* ◇*asthma*
*Adults:* 1 to 2 g I.V.
◇*Management of preterm labor*
*Adults:* 4 to 6 g I.V. over 20 minutes as a loading dose, followed by maintenance infusions of 2 to 4 g/hour for 12 to 24 hours as tolerated after contractions subside.
*Mild hypomagnesemia*
*Adults:* 1 to 3 g I.M. q 6 hours for 4 doses; or 5 g in 1 L of $D_5W$, or dextrose 5% in normal saline solution I.V. over 3 hours.
*Reduction of CV morbidity and mortality associated with acute MI*
*Adults:* 2 g I.V. over 5 to 15 minutes, followed by infusion of 18 g over 24 hours (12.5 mg/min). Initiate therapy as soon as possible, but no longer than 6 hours after MI.

## I.V. administration
■ I.V. bolus must be injected slowly to avoid respiratory or cardiac arrest.
■ If possible, recommend administering by constant infusion pump; maximum infusion rate is 150 mg/minute. Rapid drip causes feeling of heat.
■ Level of magnesium sulfate shouldn't exceed 20% at a rate no greater than 150 mg/minute (1.5 ml of a 10% concentration or equivalent).

## Incompatibilities
Incompatible with alcohol, alkali carbonates and bicarbonates, calcium gluceptate, calcium gluconate, cefepime, ciprofloxacin, dobutamine, hydrocortisone sodium succinate, I.V. fat emulsion 10%, polymyxin B, procaine, sodium bicarbonate, and soluble phosphates.

## Mechanism of action
*Anticonvulsant action:* Magnesium sulfate has CNS and respiratory depressant effects. It acts peripherally, causing vasodilation; moderate doses cause flushing and sweating, whereas high doses cause hypotension. It prevents or controls seizures by blocking neuromuscular transmission.

Drug is sometimes used in pregnant women to prevent or control preeclamptic or eclamptic seizures; it also is used to treat hypomagnesemic seizures in adults, and in children with acute nephritis.

## Pharmacokinetics
*Absorption:* Effective anticonvulsant serum levels are 2.5 to 7.5 mEq/L.
*Distribution:* Magnesium sulfate is distributed widely throughout the body.
*Metabolism:* None.
*Excretion:* Excreted unchanged in urine; some appears in breast milk.

| Route | Onset | Peak | Duration |
|-------|-------|------|----------|
| I.V. | 1-2 min | Rapid | ½ hr |
| I.M. | 1 hr | Unknown | 3-4 hr |

## Contraindications and precautions
Parenteral administration of drug contraindicated in patients with heart block or myocardial damage. Use cautiously in patients with impaired renal function and in women in labor. Don't give in toxemia of pregnancy during the 2 hours preceding delivery.

## Interactions
**Drug-drug.** *Antidepressants, antipsychotics, anxiolytics, barbiturates, general anesthetics, hypnotics, narcotics:* May increase CNS depressant effects. Reduced dosages may be required.
*Cardiac glycosides:* Changes in cardiac conduction in digitalized patients may lead to heart block if I.V. calcium is given. Avoid use together, if possible.
*Succinylcholine, tubocurarine:* Potentiated and prolonged neuromuscular blocking action of these drugs. Use with caution.
**Drug-lifestyle.** *Alcohol use:* Increased CNS depressant effects. Avoid use together.

## Adverse reactions
**CNS:** drowsiness, *depressed reflexes,* flaccid paralysis.
**CV:** *hypotension, flushing, **circulatory collapse,*** depressed cardiac function.
**Metabolic:** hypocalcemia.
**Respiratory:** *respiratory paralysis.*
**Skin:** diaphoresis.
**Other:** hypothermia.

## Overdose and treatment
Signs and symptoms of overdose with magnesium sulfate include a sharp decrease in blood pressure and respiratory paralysis, ECG changes (increased PR, QRS, and QT intervals), heart block, and asystole.

Treatment requires artificial ventilation and I.V. calcium salt to reverse respiratory depression and heart block. Usual dose is 5 to 10 mEq of calcium (10 to 20 ml of a 10% calcium gluconate solution).

## Clinical considerations
**◨ ALERT** Read label closely to ensure proper dosage and concentration is given.
■ Drug should be stopped as soon as needed effect is achieved.
■ For I.M. administration in adults, levels of 25% or 50% are generally used; in infants and children, levels shouldn't exceed 20% (200 mg/ml).
■ To calculate grams of magnesium in a percentage of solution: X% = X g/100 ml (for example, 25% = 25 g/100 ml = 250 mg/ml).

### Therapeutic monitoring
■ Respiratory rate must be 16 breaths/minute or more before each dose. Recommend keeping I.V. calcium gluconate 20% on hand.
■ Advise clinician to monitor serum magnesium level and clinical status to avoid overdose.
■ When giving repeated doses, recommend testing knee jerk reflex before each dose; if absent, magnesium should be stopped. Use of drug beyond this point risks respiratory center failure.
■ When used as a tocolytic drug, patient requires monitoring for magnesium toxicity and of I.V. fluids infused to avoid circulatory overload.
■ After use in toxemic women within 24 hours before delivery, newborn requires observation for signs of magnesium toxicity, including neuromuscular and respiratory depression.

### Special populations
**Breast-feeding patients.** Drug appears in breast milk; in patients with normal renal function, all magnesium sulfate is excreted within 24 hours of discontinuing drug. Alternative feeding method is recommended during therapy.
**Pediatric patients.** Drug isn't indicated for pediatric use.

## Patient counseling
■ Advise patient to report adverse effects promptly.

# mannitol
Osmitrol, Resectisol

*Pharmacologic classification:* osmotic diuretic
*Therapeutic classification:* diuretic
*Pregnancy risk category C*

## Available forms
Available by prescription only
*Injection:* 5%, 10%, 15%, 20%, 25%
*Urogenital solution:* 5 g/100 ml distilled water

---

## Indications and dosages

**Test dose for marked oliguria or suspected inadequate renal function**

*Adults and children over age 12:* 200 mg/kg or 12.5 g as a 15% or 20% solution I.V. over 3 to 5 minutes. Response is adequate if 30 to 50 ml urine/hour is excreted over 2 to 3 hours. May repeat test dose one time if response is inadequate the first time.

◇ *Children under age 12:* 0.2 g/kg or 6 g/m² I.V. over 3 to 5 minutes.

**Treatment of oliguria**

*Adults and children over age 12:* 50 to 100 g as a 15% to 20% solution I.V. over 90 minutes to several hours.

*Children under age 12:* 2 g/kg or 60 g/m² I.V.

**Prevention of oliguria or acute renal failure**

*Adults and children over age 12:* 50 to 100 g followed by a 5% to 10% solution I.V. Exact level is determined by fluid requirements.

**Treatment of edema and ascites**

*Adults and children over age 12:* 100 g as a 10% to 20% solution I.V. over 2 to 6 hours.

◇ *Children under age 12:* 2 g/kg or 60 g/m² I.V. as a 15% to 20% solution over 2 to 6 hours.

**To reduce intraocular pressure or intracranial pressure**

*Adults and children over age 12:* 1.5 to 2 g/kg as a 15% to 25% solution I.V. over 30 to 60 minutes (give 60 to 90 minutes before surgery if used preoperatively).

◇ *Children under age 12:* 2 g/kg or 60 g/m² I.V. as a 15% to 20% solution over 30 to 60 minutes.

**To promote diuresis in drug intoxication**

*Adults and children over age 12:* 25 g loading dose followed by an infusion maintaining 100 to 500 ml urine output/hour and positive fluid balance (of 1 to 2 L). For patients with barbiturate poisoning, give 0.5 g/kg followed by a 5% to 10% solution. Alternatively, 1 L of 10% solution during first hour. Subsequent dosing based on urine output, urine pH, and fluid balance.

◇ *Children under age 12:* 2 g/kg or 60 g/m² of 5% to 10% solution p.r.n.

**Urologic irrigation**

*Adults:* 2.5% to 5 % irrigating solution via indwelling urethral catheter.

## I.V. administration

■ Give drug by intermittent or continuous infusion via an in-line filter at prescribed rate.
■ Direct injection isn't recommended.

### Incompatibilities

Incompatible with imipenem-cilastatin and blood products. If blood must be given with mannitol, recommend adding 20 mEq of sodium chloride to each liter of mannitol.

## Mechanism of action

*Diuretic action:* Mannitol increases the osmotic pressure of glomerular filtrate, inhibiting tubular reabsorption of water and electrolytes, thus promoting diuresis. This action also promotes urinary elimination of certain drugs. This effect is useful for prevention and management of acute renal failure or oliguria. This action is also useful for reduction of intracranial or intraocular pressure because mannitol elevates plasma osmolality, enhancing flow of water into extracellular fluid.

## Pharmacokinetics

*Absorption:* Administered I.V.; it lowers intracranial pressure in 15 minutes and intraocular pressure in 30 to 60 minutes; it produces diuresis in 1 to 3 hours.

*Distribution:* Remains in the extracellular compartment. It doesn't cross the blood-brain barrier.

*Metabolism:* Metabolized minimally to glycogen in the liver.

*Excretion:* Filtered by the glomeruli; half-life in adults with normal renal function is about 100 minutes.

| Route | Onset | Peak | Duration |
|-------|-------|------|----------|
| I.V. | ¼-1 hr | 1-3 hr | 3-8 hr |

## Contraindications and precautions

Contraindicated in patients hypersensitive to drug and in those with anuria, severe pulmonary congestion, frank pulmonary edema, severe heart failure, severe dehydration, metabolic edema, progressive renal disease or dysfunction, or active intracranial bleeding except during craniotomy. Use cautiously in pregnant patients.

## Interactions

**Drug-drug.** *Cardiac glycosides:* May enhance the possibility of digitalis toxicity. Advise clinician to monitor serum digoxin levels.

*Diuretics, including carbonic anhydrase inhibitors:* Increased effects of these drugs. Advise clinician to monitor patient closely.

*Lithium:* Enhanced renal excretion of lithium and lower serum lithium levels. Advise clinician to monitor lithium levels.

## Adverse reactions

**CNS:** *seizures,* dizziness, headache.
**CV:** edema, thrombophlebitis, hypotension, hypertension, *HF,* tachycardia, angina-like chest pain.
**EENT:** blurred vision, rhinitis, dry mouth.
**GI:** thirst, nausea, vomiting, *diarrhea.*
**GU:** urine retention.
**Metabolic:** fluid and electrolyte imbalance, dehydration.
**Skin:** urticaria.
**Other:** local pain, fever, chills.

## Overdose and treatment

Signs and symptoms of overdose include polyuria, cellular dehydration, hypotension, and CV collapse.

Recommend stopping infusion and instituting supportive measures. Hemodialysis removes mannitol and decreases serum osmolality.

## Clinical considerations

■ For maximum pressure reduction during surgery, advise clinician to give drug 1 to 1½ hours preoperatively.

■ Advise against giving with whole blood; agglutination will occur.

■ Mannitol solutions commonly crystallize at low temperatures; recommend placing crystallized solutions in a hot water bath, shaking vigorously to dissolve crystals, and cooling to body temperature before use. Solutions with undissolved crystals shouldn't be used.

■ Fluid administration shouldn't exceed 1 L per day in excess of urine output.

■ Store drug at 59° to 86° F (15° to 30° C) and protect from freezing.

■ Drug therapy may interfere with tests for inorganic phosphorus level or blood ethylene glycol.

### Therapeutic monitoring

■ Use with extreme caution in patients with compromised renal function; monitoring should include vital signs (including CVP) hourly and input and output, weight, renal function, fluid balance, and serum and urinary sodium and potassium levels daily.

### Special populations

**Breast-feeding patients.** Safety of drug in breast-feeding women hasn't been established.
**Pediatric patients.** Dosage for children under age 12 hasn't been established.
**Geriatric patients.** Geriatric or debilitated patients require close observation and may require lower dosage. Excessive diuresis promotes rapid dehydration, leading to hypovolemia, hypokalemia, and hyponatremia.

## Patient counseling

■ Tell patient he may feel thirsty or experience mouth dryness, and emphasize importance of drinking only the amount of fluids provided.

■ With initial doses, warn patient to change position slowly, especially when rising from lying or sitting position, to prevent dizziness from orthostatic hypotension.

■ Instruct patient to immediately report pain in the chest, back, or legs; shortness of breath; or apnea.

# measles, mumps, and rubella virus vaccine, live
M-M-R II

*Pharmacologic classification:* vaccine
*Therapeutic classification:* viral vaccine
*Pregnancy risk category C*

## Available forms

Available by prescription only
*Injection:* Single-dose vial containing not less than 1,000 $TCID_{50}$ (tissue culture infective doses) of attenuated measles virus derived from Enders' attenuated Edmonston strain (grown in chick embryo culture); 20,000 $TCID_{50}$ of the Jeryl Lynn (B level) mumps strain (grown in chick embryo culture); and 1,000 $TCID_{50}$ of the Wistar RA 27/3 strain of rubella virus (propagated in human diploid cell culture)

## Indications and dosages

*Measles, mumps, and rubella immunization*
*Adults (born after 1957):* Two doses of 0.5 ml S.C. in outer aspect of upper arm, given at least 1 month apart.
*Children:* Initially, 0.5 ml S.C. in outer aspect of upper arm at age 12 to 15 months; second dose at age 4 to 6 years. Second dose may be given earlier if at least 4 weeks have elapsed since first dose and both doses are given beginning at or after age 12 months.

## Mechanism of action

*Measles, mumps, and rubella prophylaxis:* This vaccine promotes active immunity to measles (rubeola), mumps, and German measles (rubella) by inducing production of antibodies.

## Pharmacokinetics

*Absorption:* Antibodies are usually evident 2 to 3 weeks after injection. Duration of vaccine-induced immunity is expected to be lifelong.
*Distribution:* No information available.
*Metabolism:* No information available.
*Excretion:* No information available.

| Route | Onset | Peak | Duration |
|-------|-------|------|----------|
| S.C. | Unknown | Unknown | < 11 yr |

## Contraindications and precautions

Contraindicated in immunosuppressed patients; in those with cancer, blood dyscrasias, gamma globulin disorders, fever, active untreated tuberculosis, or anaphylactic or anaphylactoid reactions to neomycin or eggs; in those receiving corticosteroid or radiation therapy; and in pregnant women. Use cautiously in patients with history of cerebral injury, individual or family history of seizures, or any other condition in which stress from fever should be avoided.

## Interactions
**Drug-drug.** *Immune serum globulin, transfusions of blood or blood products:* May interfere with the immune response to the vaccine. Whenever possible, defer vaccination for 3 months in these situations.
*Immunosuppressants:* May interfere with the response to vaccine. Avoid use together if possible.

## Adverse reactions
**CNS:** syncope, malaise, headache.
**EENT:** otitis media, conjunctivitis, sore throat.
**GI:** diarrhea, vomiting.
**Respiratory:** cough.
**Skin:** urticaria, rash.
**Other:** fever, regional lymphadenopathy, *anaphylaxis,* vasculitis, erythema at injection site.

## Overdose and treatment
No information available.

## Clinical considerations
**⛔ ALERT** Vaccine shouldn't be administered I.V. Recommend using a 25G, ⅝-inch needle and inject S.C., preferably into the outer aspect of the upper arm. Use a sterile syringe free of preservatives, antiseptics, and detergents for each injection because these substances may inactivate the live virus vaccine.
■ Recommend using only the diluent supplied. Reconstituted solution should be discarded after 8 hours.
■ Solution may be used if red, pink, or yellow, but it must be clear.
■ Drug can be given to patient with HIV infection who doesn't have severe immunosuppression.
■ Recommend obtaining a thorough history of allergies, especially to antibiotics, eggs, chicken, or chicken feathers, and of reactions to immunizations.
■ Recommend performing a skin test to assess vaccine sensitivity (against a control of normal saline solution in the opposing extremity) in patients with history of anaphylactoid reactions to egg ingestion. Advise clinician to give a prick (intracutaneous) or scratch test with a 1:10 dilution. Read results after 5 to 30 minutes. A positive reaction is a wheal with or without pseudopodia and surrounding erythema.
■ Epinephrine solution 1:1,000 should be available to treat allergic reactions.
■ Most adults born before 1957 are believed to have been infected with naturally occurring disease, and vaccination isn't needed; however, vaccination should be offered if they are considered susceptible.
■ Vaccine shouldn't be given less than 1 month before or after immunization with other live virus vaccines—except for monovalent or triva-

lent live oral poliovirus vaccine or poliovirus vaccine, inactivated, which may be given simultaneously at separate sites using separate syringes.
■ Vaccine may not offer any protection when given within a few days after exposure to natural measles, mumps, or rubella.
■ Advise clinician to give passive immunization with immune serum globulin, if needed, when immediate protection against measles is required in patients who cannot receive the measles vaccine component. Advise against giving any live virus vaccine component simultaneously with immune serum globulin.
■ Revaccination is unnecessary if the child received two doses of vaccine at least 1 month apart, beginning after the first birthday.
■ Store vaccine at 36° to 46° F (2° to 8° C) and protect from light.
■ Measles, mumps, and rubella vaccine may temporarily decrease the response to tuberculin skin testing. If a tuberculin skin test is needed, advise clinician to give it either before or simultaneously with this vaccine.

### *Therapeutic monitoring*
■ Advise clinician to monitor patient for allergic reactions.

### *Special populations*
**Breast-feeding patients.** No data are available regarding distribution of measles or mumps virus components in breast milk. Some reports have shown transfer of rubella virus or virus antigen into breast milk in about 68% of women. Few adverse effects have been linked to breast-feeding after immunization with rubella-containing vaccines. The risk-benefit ratio suggests that breast-feeding women may be immunized with the rubella component, if needed.
**Pediatric patients.** Children under age 15 months may not respond to one, two, or all three of vaccine components because retained maternal antibodies may interfere with immune response. However, vaccination at age 12 months is recommended if child lives in a high-risk area because the benefits outweigh the risk of a slightly lower efficacy of vaccine.

## Patient counseling
■ Tell patient what to expect after vaccination: tingling sensations in the limbs or joint aches and pains that may resemble arthritis, beginning several days to several weeks after vaccination. These symptoms usually resolve within 1 week. Other effects include pain and inflammation at the injection site and a low-grade fever, rash, or difficulty breathing. Recommend acetaminophen to alleviate adverse reactions, such as fever.
■ Tell patient to report distressing adverse reactions.

■ Advise women of childbearing age not to become pregnant for 3 months after receiving vaccine.

# measles and rubella virus vaccine, live, attenuated

M-R-Vax II

*Pharmacologic classification:* vaccine
*Therapeutic classification:* viral vaccine
*Pregnancy risk category C*

## Available forms

Available by prescription only
*Injection:* Single-dose vial containing not less than 1,000 $TCID_{50}$ (tissue culture infective doses) each of attenuated measles virus derived from Enders' attenuated Edmonston strain (grown in chick embryo culture) and the Wistar RA 27/3 strain of rubella virus (propagated in human diploid cell culture)
    Note: 10-dose and 50-dose vials are available to government agencies and institutions only.

## Indications and dosages

**Measles and rubella immunization**
*Adults and children ages 15 months and older:* 0.5 ml in outer aspect of the upper arm. For adequate protection against measles, a two-dose schedule is recommended (at least 1 month between doses).

## Mechanism of action

*Measles and rubella prophylaxis:* Vaccine promotes active immunity to measles (rubeola) and German measles (rubella) virus by inducing production of antibodies.

## Pharmacokinetics

*Absorption:* Antibodies are usually detectable 2 to 3 weeks after injection. Duration of vaccine-induced immunity is expected to be lifelong.
*Distribution:* No information available.
*Metabolism:* No information available.
*Excretion:* No information available.

| Route | Onset | Peak | Duration |
|-------|-------|------|----------|
| S.C. | Unknown | Unknown | < 11 yr |

## Contraindications and precautions

Contraindicated in immunosuppressed patients; in those with cancer, blood dyscrasias, gamma globulin disorders, fever, active untreated tuberculosis, or anaphylactic or anaphylactoid reactions to eggs or neomycin; in those receiving corticosteroid or radiation therapy; and in pregnant women. Use cautiously in patients with history of cerebral injury, individual or family history of seizures, or any other condi-

tion in which stress resulting from fever should be avoided.

## Interactions

**Drug-drug.** *Immune serum globulin, transfusions of blood or blood products:* May interfere with the immune response to the vaccine. Whenever possible, defer vaccination for 3 months in these situations.
*Immunosuppressants:* May interfere with response to vaccine. Avoid use together if possible.

## Adverse reactions

**CNS:** syncope, malaise, headache.
**EENT:** sore throat.
**GI:** vomiting, diarrhea.
**Respiratory:** cough.
**Skin:** rash.
**Other:** fever, lymphadenopathy, erythema, burning, or stinging (at injection site); vasculitis, *anaphylaxis.*

## Overdose and treatment

No information available.

## Clinical considerations

**H ALERT** Advise against administering I.V. Recommend using a 25G, ⅝-inch needle and inject S.C., preferably into the outer aspect of the upper arm.
■ Recommend using a sterile syringe free of preservatives, antiseptics, and detergents for each injection because these substances may inactivate the live virus vaccine.
■ Recommend using only diluent supplied. Reconstituted solution should be discarded after 8 hours.
■ Solution may be used if red, pink, or yellow, but it must be clear.
■ Drug can be given to patient with HIV infection who doesn't have severe immunosuppression.
■ Recommend obtaining a thorough history of allergies, especially to antibiotics, eggs, chicken, or chicken feathers, and of reactions to immunizations.
■ Skin testing is needed to assess vaccine sensitivity (against a control of normal saline solution in the opposing extremity) in patients with history of anaphylactoid reactions to eggs. Advise clinician to give a prick (intracutaneous) or scratch test with a 1:10 dilution. Results may be read after 5 to 30 minutes. A positive reaction is a wheal with or without pseudopodia and surrounding erythema.
■ Epinephrine solution 1:1,000 should be available to treat allergic reactions.
■ Vaccine shouldn't be given less than 1 month before or after immunization with other live virus vaccines, except for mumps virus vaccine and monovalent or trivalent live oral poliovirus vaccine, and poliovirus vaccine, inactivated, which may be given simultaneously.

---

■ Vaccine may not offer protection when given within a few days' exposure to natural measles or rubella.

■ According to Centers for Disease Control and Prevention recommendations, measles, mumps and rubella (MMR) is the preferred vaccine.

■ Passive immunization is given with immune serum globulin when immediate protection against measles is required in patients who can't receive the measles vaccine component. Don't give either vaccine component simultaneously with immune serum globulin.

■ Store vaccine at 36° to 46° F (2° to 8° C) and protect from light.

■ Revaccination is usually given between 4 to 6 years of age. Measles virus vaccine, live, MMR II, or MR-VAX II may be used.

■ Measles and rubella vaccine may temporarily decrease response to tuberculin skin testing. If a tuberculin skin test is needed, give it either before or simultaneously with measles and rubella vaccine.

## Therapeutic monitoring

■ Advise clinician to monitor patient for adverse allergic reaction.

## Special populations

**Breast-feeding patients.** No data are available regarding distribution of measles and rubella virus components in breast milk. Some reports have shown transfer of rubella virus or virus antigen into breast milk in about 68% of patients. Few adverse effects have been linked to breast-feeding after immunization with rubella-containing vaccines. The risk-benefit ratio suggests that breast-feeding women may be immunized with the rubella component, if needed. **Pediatric patients.** Children under age 15 months may not respond to one or both of the vaccine components because retained maternal antibodies may interfere with the immune response; revaccination is recommended after age 15 months.

## Patient counseling

■ Tell patient to expect tingling sensations in the limbs or joint aches and pains that may resemble arthritis, beginning several days to several weeks after vaccination. These symptoms usually resolve within 1 week. Other effects include pain and inflammation at the injection site and a low-grade fever, rash, or difficulty breathing. Recommend acetaminophen for relief of fever.

■ Encourage patient to report distressing adverse reactions.

■ Advise women of childbearing age not to become pregnant for 3 months after receiving the vaccine.

# measles virus vaccine, live, attenuated

Attenuvax

*Pharmacologic classification:* vaccine
*Therapeutic classification:* viral vaccine
*Pregnancy risk category C*

## Available forms

Available by prescription only
*Injection:* Single-dose vial containing not less than $1,000$ $TCID_{50}$ (tissue culture infective doses) per 0.5 ml of attenuated measles virus derived from Enders' attenuated Edmonston strain grown in chick embryo culture.

Note: 10-dose and 50-dose vials are available to government agencies and institutions only.

## Indications and dosages

*Immunization*
*Adults and children ages 15 months and older:* 0.5 ml (1,000 units) S.C. in outer aspect of the upper arm. Give two doses at least 1 month apart. For children, usual schedule is the first dose at age 15 months and a second dose at the entry of school (ages 4 to 6 years).

## Mechanism of action

*Measles prophylaxis:* Measles virus vaccine promotes active immunity to measles virus by inducing production of antibodies.

## Pharmacokinetics

*Absorption:* Antibodies are usually evident 2 to 3 weeks after injection. Duration of vaccine-induced immunity is at least 13 to 16 years and probably lifelong in most immunized persons.
*Distribution:* No information available.
*Metabolism:* No information available.
*Excretion:* No information available.

| Route | Onset | Peak | Duration |
|-------|-------|------|----------|
| S.C. | Few days | Unknown | $\geq 13$ yr |

## Contraindications and precautions

Contraindicated in immunosuppressed patients; in those with HIV, cancer, blood dyscrasias, gamma globulin disorders, fever, active untreated tuberculosis, or anaphylactic or anaphylactoid reactions to neomycin or eggs; in those receiving corticosteroid or radiation therapy; and in pregnant patients. Use cautiously in patients with history of cerebral injury, individual or family history of seizures, or any other condition where stress resulting from fever should be avoided.

## Interactions

**Drug-drug.** *Immune serum globulin, transfusions of blood or blood products:* May interfere with the immune response to the vaccine. Whenever possible, defer vaccination for 3 months in these situations.

*Immunosuppressants:* May interfere with the response to vaccine. Avoid use together.

*Meningococcal vaccine:* If given together, can result in reduced seroconversion rate to meningococci. Avoid administration together.

## Adverse reactions

**CNS:** *febrile seizures* (in susceptible children).
**GI:** anorexia.
**Hematologic:** *leukopenia.*
**Skin:** rash, erythema, swelling, tenderness (at injection site).
**Other:** fever, lymphadenopathy, *anaphylaxis.*

## Overdose and treatment

No information available.

## Clinical considerations

■ Recommend obtaining a thorough history of allergies, especially to antibiotics, eggs, chicken, or chicken feathers, and of reactions to immunizations.

■ Measles vaccine shouldn't be given less than 1 month before or after immunization with other live virus vaccines, except for mumps virus vaccine, rubella virus vaccine, or monovalent or trivalent live oral poliovirus vaccine or poliovirus vaccine, inactivated, which may be given simultaneously.

■ Measles, mumps, and rubella (MMR) vaccine may be given concurrently with pneumococcal conjugate-7-valent vaccine at a different site using a separate syringe.

■ Vaccine may offer some protection when given within a few days after exposure to natural measles and substantial protection when given a few days before exposure.

■ According to Centers for Disease Control and Prevention recommendations, MMR is the preferred vaccine.

■ Passive immunization is given with immune serum globulin if immediate protection against measles is required in patients who can't receive the measles vaccine.

■ Patients who received measles vaccine live when under age 1 year should be considered susceptible to measles, and therefore should be revaccinated.

■ Epinephrine solution 1:1,000 should be available to treat allergic reactions.

■ Drug shouldn't be administered I.V. Use a 25G, ⅝-inch needle and inject S.C., preferably into the outer aspect of the upper arm. Use a sterile syringe free of preservatives, antiseptics, and detergents for each injection, because these substances may inactivate the live virus vaccine.

■ Recommend using diluent supplied. Reconstituted solution shouldn't be discarded after 8 hours.

■ Store vaccine at 35° to 46° F (2° to 8° C), and protect from light. Solution may be used if red, pink, or yellow, but it must be clear.

■ Measles vaccine may temporarily decrease the response to tuberculin skin testing. If a tuberculin skin test is needed, advise clinician to give it either before or simultaneously with the measles vaccine.

### Therapeutic monitoring

■ Patients with a history of anaphylactoid reactions to eggs should first have a skin test to assess vaccine sensitivity (against a control of normal saline solution in the other arm). Advise clinician to give a prick (intracutaneous) or scratch test with a 1:10 dilution. Results may be read after 5 to 30 minutes. A positive reaction is a wheal with or without pseudopodia and surrounding erythema.

### Special populations

**Breast-feeding patients.** It's unknown if vaccine appears in breast milk. Use with caution in breast-feeding women.

**Pediatric patients.** Children under age 15 months may not respond to the vaccine, because retained maternal antibodies may interfere with the immune response, revaccination is recommended after age 15 months.

## Patient counseling

■ Tell patient to expect pain and inflammation at the injection site, fever, rash, general malaise, or difficulty breathing. Recommend acetaminophen for relief of fever.

■ Encourage patient to report distressing adverse reactions.

■ Advise women of childbearing age not to become pregnant for 3 months after receiving the vaccine.

---

# mebendazole

Vermox

*Pharmacologic classification:* benzimidazole
*Therapeutic classification:* anthelmintic
*Pregnancy risk category C*

## Available forms

Available by prescription only
*Tablets (chewable):* 100 mg

## Indications and dosages

*Pinworm infestations*
*Adults and children over age 2:* 100 mg P.O. as a single dose. If infection persists 3 weeks later, repeat treatment.

*Roundworm,* ◇ *whipworm, and hookworm infestations,* ◇ *trichostrongylosis,*

◇ *eosinophilic enterocolitis caused by dog hookworm*
*Adults and children over age 2:* 100 mg P.O. b.i.d. for 3 days. If infection persists 3 weeks later, repeat treatment. Alternatively, for treatment of hookworm, whipworm, or roundworm, 500 mg P.O. as a single dose.

◇ *Trichinosis*
*Adults and children over age 2:* 200 to 400 mg P.O. t.i.d. for 3 days, then 400 to 500 mg t.i.d. for 10 days.

◇ *Capillariasis*
*Adults and children over age 2:* 200 mg P.O. b.i.d. for 20 days.

◇ *Toxocariasis*
*Adults and children:* 100 to 200 mg P.O. b.i.d. for 5 days.

◇ *Dracunculiasis*
*Adults and children over age 2:* 400 to 800 mg P.O. daily for 6 days.

◇ **Mansonella perstans** *infestations*
*Adults and children over age 2:* 100 mg P.O. b.i.d. for 30 days.

◇ **Angiostrongylus cantonensis** *infestations*
*Adults and children:* 100 mg P.O. b.i.d. for 5 days.

◇ **Angiostrongylus costaricensis**
*Adults and children over age 2:* 200 to 400 mg P.O. t.i.d. for 10 days.

◇ *Onchocerciasis*
*Adults:* 1 g P.O. b.i.d. for 28 days.

◇ *Treatment of hydatid disease (echinococcosis)*
*Adults:* 40 mg/kg P.O. for 1 to 6 months. Alternatively, sequential 2-week courses of 50 mg/kg daily; 200 mg/kg daily; and 50 mg/kg daily for 21 to 30 days.

## Mechanism of action
*Anthelmintic action:* Mebendazole inhibits uptake of glucose and other low–molecular-weight nutrients in susceptible helminths, depleting the glycogen stores they need for survival and reproduction. It has a broad spectrum and may be useful in mixed infections. It's considered a drug of choice in the treatment of ascariasis, capillariasis, enterobiasis, trichuriasis, and uncinariasis; it has been used investigationally to treat echinococciasis, onchocerciasis, and trichinosis.

## Pharmacokinetics
*Absorption:* About 5% to 10% of a given dose is absorbed. Absorption varies widely among patients.
*Distribution:* Highly plasma protein–bound; crosses the placenta.
*Metabolism:* Metabolized to inactive 2-amino-5(6)-benzimidazolyl phenylketone.
*Excretion:* Most of a dose is excreted in feces; 2% to 10% is excreted in urine in 48 hours as either unchanged drug or the 2-amine metabolite. Half-life is 3 to 9 hours. It's unknown if drug appears in breast milk.

| Route | Onset | Peak | Duration |
|---|---|---|---|
| P.O. | Unknown | 2-4 hr | Variable |

## Contraindications and precautions
Contraindicated in patients hypersensitive to drug.

## Interactions
**Drug-drug.** *Anticonvulsants, including carbamazepine and phenytoin:* May enhance the metabolism of mebendazole and decrease its efficacy. Advise clinician to monitor patient for clinical effect.
*Cimetidine:* Inhibits mebendazole metabolism and may result in increased plasma levels of drug. Use together cautiously.

## Adverse reactions
**GI:** occasional, transient abdominal pain and diarrhea in massive infection and expulsion of worms.
**Other:** fever.

## Overdose and treatment
Signs and symptoms of overdose may include GI disturbances and altered mental status. No specific recommendations exist; treatment is supportive. After recent ingestion (within 4 hours), recommend emptying stomach by induced emesis or gastric lavage. Recommend following with activated charcoal to decrease absorption.

## Clinical considerations
■ Tablets may be chewed, swallowed whole, or crushed and mixed with food.
■ Laxatives, enemas, or dietary restrictions are unnecessary.
■ Stool specimens should be collected in a clean, dry container and transferred to a properly labeled container to send to laboratory; ova may be destroyed by toilet bowl water, urine, and some drugs.
■ Store drug at 59° to 77° F (15° to 25° C) in well-closed container; product expires 3 years from date of manufacture.

### Therapeutic monitoring
■ High-dose treatment of hydatid disease and trichinosis is investigational. Advise clinician to monitor WBC counts to detect drug toxicity, especially during initial therapy.

### Special populations
**Breast-feeding patients.** Safety in breast-feeding women hasn't been established.
**Pediatric patients.** Drug may be given to children under age 2 only when potential benefits justify risks.

## Patient counseling

■ Teach patient and family members personal hygiene measures to prevent reinfection: washing perianal area and changing undergarments and bedclothes daily; washing hands and cleaning fingernails before meals and after defecation; and sanitary disposal of feces.
■ Advise patient to bathe often, by showering, if possible.
■ Advise patient to keep hands away from mouth, to keep fingernails short, and to wear shoes to avoid hookworm; explain that ova are easily transmitted directly and indirectly by hands, food, or contaminated articles. Washing clothes in household washing machine will destroy ova.
■ Instruct patient to handle bedding carefully because shaking will send ova into the air, and to disinfect toilet facilities and vacuum or damp-mop floors daily to reduce number of ova.
■ Encourage patient's family and contacts to be checked for infestation and treated, if needed.

---

## mechlorethamine hydrochloride (nitrogen mustard)
Mustargen

*Pharmacologic classification:* alkylating drug (cell cycle–phase nonspecific)
*Therapeutic classification:* antineoplastic
*Pregnancy risk category D*

## Available forms

Available by prescription only
*Injection:* 10-mg vials

## Indications and dosages

Dosage and indications may vary. Check current literature for recommended protocols.
*Hodgkin's disease, bronchogenic carcinoma, chronic lymphocytic leukemia, chronic myelocytic leukemia, lymphosarcoma, polycythemia vera*
*Adults:* 0.4 mg/kg I.V. per course of therapy as a single dose or 0.1 to 0.2 mg/kg on 2 to 4 successive days q 3 to 6 weeks. Give through running I.V. infusion. Dose reduced in prior radiation therapy or chemotherapy to 0.2 to 0.4 mg/kg. Dose based on ideal or actual body weight, whichever is less.
*Intracavitary doses for neoplastic effusions*
*Adults:* 0.2 to 0.4 mg/kg.
*Treatment of advanced Hodgkin's disease (MOPP regimen)*
*Adults:* 6 mg/m$^2$ given I.V. on days 1 and 8 of 28-day cycle. In subsequent cycles, dose is based on leukocyte count.

## I.V. administration

■ To reconstitute powder, use 10 ml of sterile water for injection or normal saline solution to give a concentration of 1 mg/ml.
■ When reconstituted, drug is a clear colorless solution. Don't use if solution is discolored or if droplets of water are visible within vial before reconstitution.
■ Solution is very unstable. Prepare immediately before infusion and use within 15 minutes. Discard unused solution.
■ Dilution of drug into a large volume of I.V. solution isn't recommended because it may react with the diluent and isn't stable for a prolonged period.
■ Drug may be administered I.V. push over a few minutes into the tubing of a freely flowing I.V. infusion. Following administration, recommend flushing vein for 2.5 minutes with running I.V. solution or injecting 5 to 10 ml of solution into sidearm.

### *Incompatibilities*
Incompatible with methohexital.

## Mechanism of action

*Antineoplastic action:* Mechlorethamine exerts its cytotoxic activity through the basic processes of alkylation. Drug causes crosslinking of DNA strands, single-strand breakage of DNA, abnormal base pairing, and interruption of other intracellular processes, resulting in cell death.

## Pharmacokinetics

*Absorption:* Administered I.V. After intracavitary administration, mechlorethamine is absorbed incompletely, probably from deactivation by body fluids in the cavity.
*Distribution:* Doesn't cross the blood-brain barrier.
*Metabolism:* Undergoes rapid chemical transformation and reacts quickly with various cellular components before being deactivated.
*Excretion:* Metabolites are excreted in urine. Less than 0.01% of an I.V. dose is excreted unchanged in urine.

| Route | Onset | Peak | Duration |
|---|---|---|---|
| I.V., intracavitary | Few sec-few min | Unknown | Unknown |

## Contraindications and precautions

Contraindicated in patients hypersensitive to drug and those with known infectious diseases. Use cautiously in patients with severe anemia or depressed neutrophil or platelet count and in those who have recently undergone chemotherapy or radiation therapy.

## Interactions

None reported.

## Adverse reactions

**CNS:** weakness, vertigo.
**EENT:** tinnitus; deafness (with high doses).
**GI:** *nausea, vomiting, anorexia* (beginning within minutes, lasting 8 to 24 hours).
**GU:** menstrual irregularities, impaired spermatogenesis.
**Hematologic:** *thrombocytopenia, lymphocytopenia, agranulocytosis,* nadir of myelosuppression occurring by days 4 to 10 and lasting 10 to 21 days; mild anemia begins in 2 to 3 weeks.
**Hepatic:** jaundice.
**Metabolic:** hyperuricemia.
**Skin:** *alopecia,* rash, sloughing, severe irritation (if drug extravasates or touches skin).
**Other:** herpes zoster, *anaphylaxis,* thrombophlebitis, amyloidosis.

### Overdose and treatment

Signs and symptoms of overdose include severe leukopenia, anemia, thrombocytopenia, and a hemorrhagic diathesis with subsequent delayed bleeding. Death may follow.

Treatment is usually supportive and includes transfusion of blood components and antibiotic treatment of complicating infections.

### Clinical considerations

■ Avoid contact with skin or mucous membranes. Wear gloves when preparing solution and during administration to prevent accidental skin contact. If contact occurs, wash with copious amounts of water.
■ To prevent hyperuricemia with resulting uric acid nephropathy, allopurinol may be given; recommend keeping patient well hydrated.
■ Drug has been used topically to treat mycosis fungoides.
■ Treatment of extravasation includes local injections of a 1/6 M sodium thiosulfate solution. Prepare solution by mixing 4 ml of sodium thiosulfate 10% with 6 ml of sterile water for injection. Also, recommend applying ice packs for 6 to 12 hours to minimize local reactions.
■ During intracavitary administration, patient should be turned from side to side every 15 minutes for 1 hour to distribute drug.
■ All I.M. injections should be avoided when platelet count is low.

#### Therapeutic monitoring

■ Advise clinician to monitor uric acid levels, CBC, and liver function test results.
■ Recommend using anticoagulants cautiously. Recommend watching patient closely for signs of bleeding.
■ Advise clinician to monitor site closely for extravasation of drug.

#### Special populations

**Breast-feeding patients.** It isn't known if drug appears in breast milk. However, because of the potential for serious adverse reactions, mutagenicity, and carcinogenicity in the infant, breast-feeding isn't recommended.

### Patient counseling

■ Tell patient to avoid exposure to people with infections.
■ Advise patient that adequate fluid intake is very important to facilitate excretion of uric acid.
■ Reassure patient that hair should grow back after treatment has ended.
■ Tell patient to promptly report signs or symptoms of bleeding or infection.
■ Advise patient to use contraception while using drug.

## meclizine hydrochloride

Antivert, Antivert/25, Antrizine, Bonine, Dizmiss, Meclizine, Meni-D, Ru-Vert-M

*Pharmacologic classification:* piperazine-derivative antihistamine
*Therapeutic classification:* antiemetic, antivertigo drug
*Pregnancy risk category B*

### Available forms

Available with or without a prescription
*Tablets:* 12.5 mg, 25 mg, 50 mg
*Tablets (chewable):* 25 mg
*Capsules:* 25 mg

### Indications and dosages

*Dizziness*
*Adults and children ages 12 and older:* 25 to 100 mg P.O. daily in divided doses. Dosage varies with patient response.
*Motion sickness*
*Adults and children ages 12 and older:* 25 to 50 mg P.O. 1 hour before travel; may repeat dose daily for duration of journey.

### Mechanism of action

*Antiemetic action:* Meclizine probably inhibits nausea and vomiting by centrally decreasing sensitivity of labyrinth apparatus that relays stimuli to the chemoreceptor trigger zone and stimulates the vomiting center in the brain.

*Antivertigo action:* Drug decreases labyrinth excitability and conduction in vestibular-cerebellar pathways.

### Pharmacokinetics

*Absorption:* Well absorbed.
*Distribution:* Well distributed throughout the body and crosses the placenta.
*Metabolism:* Probably metabolized in the liver.

*Excretion:* Half-life is about 6 hours. Drug is excreted unchanged in feces; metabolites are found in urine.

| Route | Onset | Peak | Duration |
|-------|-------|------|----------|
| P.O. | 1 hr | Unknown | 8-24 hr |

## Contraindications and precautions
Contraindicated in patients hypersensitive to drug. Use cautiously in patients with asthma, glaucoma, or prostatic hyperplasia.

## Interactions
**Drug-drug.** *CNS depressants, such as anxiolytics, barbiturates, sleeping aids, and tranquilizers:* Additive sedative. Use together cautiously.
*Other ototoxic drugs, such as aminoglycosides, cisplatin, loop diuretics, salicylates, and vancomycin:* Meclizine may mask signs of ototoxicity. Avoid use together.
**Drug-lifestyle.** *Alcohol use:* Additive sedative and CNS depressant effects. Advise patient to avoid alcohol.

## Adverse reactions
**CNS:** *drowsiness,* restlessness, excitation, nervousness, auditory and visual hallucinations.
**CV:** hypotension, palpitations, tachycardia.
**EENT:** blurred vision, diplopia, tinnitus, dry nose and throat.
**GI:** dry mouth, constipation, anorexia, nausea, vomiting, diarrhea.
**GU:** urine retention, urinary frequency.
**Skin:** urticaria, rash.

## Overdose and treatment
Signs and symptoms of moderate overdose may include hyperexcitability alternating with drowsiness. Seizures, hallucinations, and respiratory paralysis may occur in profound overdose. Anticholinergic symptoms, such as dry mouth, flushed skin, fixed and dilated pupils, and GI symptoms, are common, especially in children.

Recommend treating overdose by administering gastric lavage to empty stomach contents; emesis with ipecac syrup may be ineffective. Recommend treating hypotension with vasopressors, and controlling seizures with diazepam or phenytoin. Stimulants shouldn't be given.

## Clinical considerations
- Tablets may be placed in mouth and allowed to dissolve without water, or they may be chewed or swallowed whole.
- Abrupt withdrawal of drug after long-term use may cause paradoxical reactions or sudden reversal of improved state.
- Meclizine should be stopped 4 days before diagnostic skin tests to avoid preventing, reducing, or masking test response.

## Therapeutic monitoring
- Advise clinician to monitor patient for excessive CNS effects.

## Special populations
**Breast-feeding patients.** Safety in breast-feeding women hasn't been established.
**Pediatric patients.** Safety and efficacy for use in children haven't been established. Don't use in children under age 12; infants and children under age 6 may experience paradoxical hyperexcitability.
**Geriatric patients.** Geriatric patients are usually more sensitive to adverse effects of antihistamines and are especially likely to experience a greater degree of dizziness, sedation, hyperexcitability, dry mouth, and urine retention than younger patients.

## Patient counseling
- Instruct patient to avoid activities that require mental alertness and physical coordination, such as driving and operating dangerous machinery.

# medroxyprogesterone acetate
Amen, Cycrin, Depo-Provera, Provera

*Pharmacologic classification:* progestin
*Therapeutic classification:* progestin, antineoplastic
*Pregnancy risk category X*

## Available forms
Available by prescription only
*Tablets:* 2.5 mg, 5 mg, 10 mg
*Injection:* 150 mg/ml, 400 mg/ml

## Indications and dosages
*Abnormal uterine bleeding from hormonal imbalance*
*Adults:* 5 to 10 mg P.O. daily for 5 to 10 days beginning on day 16 to 21 of menstrual cycle. If patient has received estrogen, then 10 mg P.O. daily for 10 days beginning on day 16 of cycle. If bleeding is controlled satisfactorily, give two subsequent cycles of combination therapy.
*Secondary amenorrhea*
*Adults:* 5 to 10 mg P.O. daily for 5 to 10 days, preferably beginning on day 16 to 21 of menstrual cycle. If patient has received estrogen, then 10 mg P.O. daily for 10 days.
*Endometrial or renal carcinoma (adjunct)*
*Adults:* 400 to 1,000 mg I.M. weekly. If disease improves or stabilizes in a few weeks or months, 400 mg/month.

◇ *Paraphilia in males*
*Adults:* Initially, 200 mg I.M. b.i.d. or t.i.d. or 500 mg I.M. weekly. Adjust dosage based on response.
*Contraception in females*
*Adults:* 150 mg I.M. q 3 months; give first injection on first 5 days of menstrual cycle.

## Mechanism of action
*Progestational action:* Parenteral medroxyprogesterone suppresses ovulation, causes thickening of cervical mucus, and induces sloughing of the endometrium.
*Antineoplastic action:* Drug may inhibit growth progression of progestin-sensitive endometrial or renal cancer tissue by an unknown mechanism.

## Pharmacokinetics
*Absorption:* Absorption is slow after I.M. administration.
*Distribution:* Not well characterized.
*Metabolism:* Primarily hepatic; not well characterized.
*Excretion:* Primarily renal; not well characterized.

| Route | Onset | Peak | Duration |
|-------|-------|------|----------|
| P.O., I.M. | Unknown | Unknown | Unknown |

## Contraindications and precautions
Contraindicated in patients hypersensitive to drug, those with active thromboembolic disorders, history of thromboembolic disorders or of cerebral vascular disease or apoplexy, breast cancer, undiagnosed abnormal vaginal bleeding, missed abortion, hepatic dysfunction, and during pregnancy. Tablets are also contraindicated in patients with liver dysfunction or known or suspected malignant disease of the genital organs.

Use cautiously in patients with diabetes mellitus, seizures, migraines, cardiac or renal disease, asthma, or mental depression.

## Interactions
**Drug-drug.** *Aminoglutethimide:* May increase the hepatic metabolism of medroxyprogesterone, possibly decreasing its therapeutic effect. Avoid use together.
*Bromocriptine:* Progestins may cause amenorrhea or galactorrhea, thus interfering with the action of bromocriptine. Avoid use together.

## Adverse reactions
**CNS:** depression, *CVA.*
**CV:** thrombophlebitis, *pulmonary embolism,* edema, *thromboembolism.*
**EENT:** exophthalmos, diplopia.
**GU:** breakthrough bleeding, dysmenorrhea, amenorrhea, cervical erosion, abnormal secretions,
**Hepatic:** cholestatic jaundice.
**Metabolic:** changes in weight.

**Skin:** rash, pain, induration, sterile abscesses, acne, pruritus, melasma, alopecia, hirsutism.
**Other:** breast tenderness, enlargement, or secretion.

## Overdose and treatment
No information available.

## Clinical considerations
■ Parenteral form is for I.M. administration only. Recommend injecting deep into large muscle mass, preferably the gluteal muscle. Advise clinician to monitor patient for development of sterile abscesses. Suspension must be shaken vigorously immediately before each use to ensure complete suspension of drug.
■ Drug has been used to treat obstructive sleep apnea and to manage paraphilia.
■ When used as a long-acting contraceptive in females, pregnancy should be ruled out before therapy starts.
■ Store drug between 59° and 86° F (15° and 30° C); avoid freezing.

### Therapeutic monitoring
■ Advise clinician to monitor glucose level in diabetic patient.

### Special populations
**Breast-feeding patients.** Detectable amounts of drug appear in breast milk. Infants exposed to drug via breast milk have been studied for developmental and behavioral effects through puberty; no adverse effects have been noted.

## Patient counseling
■ Tell patient not to take drug if she becomes pregnant.
■ Advise patient to report chest pain, difficulty breathing, or leg pain.
■ Inform patient about signs of CVA.

# megestrol acetate
Megace

*Pharmacologic classification:* progestin
*Therapeutic classification:* antineoplastic
*Pregnancy risk category X*

## Available forms
Available by prescription only
*Tablets:* 20 mg, 40 mg
*Suspension:* 200 mg/5 ml

## Indications and dosages
Dosage and indications may vary. Check current literature for recommended protocol.
*Palliative treatment of breast carcinoma*
*Adults:* 40 mg (tablets) P.O. q.i.d.

---

*Palliative treatment of endometrial carcinoma*
Adults: 40 to 320 mg (tablets) P.O. daily in divided doses.
*Anorexia, cachexia, or weight loss in patients with AIDS*
Adults: 800 mg (suspension) P.O. daily; 100 to 400 mg for AIDS-related cachexia.
◇ *Anorexia or cachexia in patients with neoplastic disease*
Adults: 480 to 600 mg P.O. daily.

## Mechanism of action
*Antineoplastic action:* Megestrol inhibits growth and causes regression of progestin-sensitive breast and endometrial cancer tissue by an unknown mechanism.
*Treatment of anorexia, cachexia, or weight loss:* Mechanism for weight gain is unknown. Megestrol may stimulate appetite by interfering with the production of mediators such as cachectin.

## Pharmacokinetics
*Absorption:* Well absorbed across the GI tract after oral administration.
*Distribution:* Appears to be stored in fatty tissue and is highly plasma protein–bound.
*Metabolism:* Completely metabolized in the liver.
*Excretion:* Metabolites are eliminated primarily through the kidneys.

| Route | Onset | Peak | Duration |
|-------|-------|------|----------|
| P.O. | Unknown | Unknown | Unknown |

## Contraindications and precautions
Contraindicated in patients hypersensitive to drug and during pregnancy (especially first 4 months). Use cautiously in patients with history of thrombophlebitis.

## Interactions
**Drug-drug.** *Bromocriptine:* May cause amenorrhea or galactorrhea, interfering with the action of bromocriptine. Use of these drugs together isn't recommended.

## Adverse reactions
**CV:** thrombophlebitis, hypertension, edema, chest pain.
**EENT:** pharyngitis.
**GI:** increased appetite, nausea, vomiting, diarrhea, flatulence.
**GU:** breakthrough menstrual bleeding, impotence.
**Hepatic:** hepatomegaly.
**Metabolic:** weight gain, hyperglycemia.
**Musculoskeletal:** carpal tunnel syndrome.
**Respiratory:** *pulmonary embolism,* dyspnea, pneumonia, cough.
**Skin:** alopecia, rash, pruritus, candidiasis.
**Other:** decreased libido.

## Overdose and treatment
No information available.

## Clinical considerations
■ Investigational uses include prevention of contraception, treatment of prostatic hypertrophy, endometriosis, and endometrial hyperplasias.
■ Store tablets between 59° and 86° F (15° and 30° C) and oral suspension at 77° F (25° C) or less.

### Therapeutic monitoring
■ Advise clinician to monitor hemapoietic function and liver function.

## Patient counseling
■ Recommendations for care and teaching of the patient during therapy are the same as those for all progestins.

# meloxicam
Mobic

*Pharmacologic classification:* enolic acid NSAID
*Therapeutic classification:* anti-inflammatory, analgesic
*Pregnancy risk category C*

## Available forms
Available by prescription only
*Tablets:* 7.5 mg

## Indications and dosages
*Relief of signs and symptoms of osteoarthritis*
Adults: 7.5 mg P.O. once daily. May increase p.r.n. to maximum dose of 15 mg daily.

## Mechanism of action
*Anti-inflammatory and analgesic actions:* Mechanism of action may be related to prostaglandin (cyclooxygenase) synthetase inhibition.

## Pharmacokinetics
*Absorption:* Bioavailability after oral administration is 89% and doesn't appear to be affected by either food or antacids. Steady-state conditions are reached after 5 days of daily administration.
*Distribution:* 99.4% bound to human plasma proteins (primarily albumin).
*Metabolism:* Almost completely metabolized to pharmacologically inactive metabolites.
*Excretion:* Excreted in both urine and feces primarily as metabolites. Elimination half-life ranges from 15 to 20 hours.

| Route | Onset | Peak | Duration |
|-------|-------|------|----------|
| P.O. | Unknown | Unknown | Unknown |

## Contraindications and precautions

Contraindicated in patients hypersensitive to meloxicam and in patients who have experienced asthma, urticaria, or allergic-type reactions after taking aspirin or other NSAIDs. Avoid use in late pregnancy.

Use with extreme caution in patients with a history of ulcers or GI bleeding. Use cautiously in patients with dehydration, anemia, hepatic disease, renal disease, hypertension, fluid retention, HF, or preexisting asthma. Also use cautiously in geriatric and debilitated patients because of increased risk of fatal GI bleeding.

## Interactions

**Drug-drug.** *ACE inhibitors:* Diminished antihypertensive effects. Advise clinician to monitor blood pressure.
*Aspirin:* Increased risk of adverse effects. Avoid concurrent use.
*Furosemide, thiazide diuretics:* Reduced sodium excretion, leading to sodium retention. Advise clinician to monitor patient for edema and increased blood pressure.
*Lithium:* Increased lithium levels. Advise clinician to monitor plasma lithium levels closely during treatment.
*Warfarin:* May increase PT or INR and increase risk of bleeding complications. Advise clinician to monitor PT and INR, and patient for bleeding.
**Drug-herb.** *Dong quai, feverfew, garlic, ginger, horse chestnut, red clover:* Possible increased risk of bleeding. Discourage use together.
**Drug-lifestyle.** *Alcohol use, smoking:* Increased risk of GI irritation and bleeding. Discourage use while on drug therapy, and monitor patient for bleeding if used concomitantly.

## Adverse reactions

**CNS:** dizziness, headache, insomnia, fatigue, *seizures,* paresthesia, tremor, vertigo, anxiety, confusion, depression, nervousness, somnolence, malaise, syncope.
**CV:** *arrhythmias,* palpitations, tachycardia, angina, *HF,* hypertension, hypotension, *MI,* edema.
**EENT:** pharyngitis, abnormal vision, conjunctivitis, tinnitus.
**GI:** abdominal pain, diarrhea, dyspepsia, flatulence, nausea, constipation, colitis, dry mouth, duodenal ulcer, esophagitis, gastric ulcer, gastritis, gastroesophageal reflux, *hemorrhage, pancreatitis,* vomiting, increased appetite, taste perversion.
**GU:** albuminuria, elevated BUN and creatinine levels, hematuria, urinary frequency, *renal failure,* urinary tract infection.
**Hematologic:** anemia, *leukopenia,* purpura, *thrombocytopenia.*
**Hepatic:** elevated liver function test results, bilirubinemia, *hepatitis.*

**Metabolic:** dehydration, weight increase or decrease.
**Musculoskeletal:** arthralgia, back pain.
**Respiratory:** upper respiratory tract infection, asthma, *bronchospasm,* dyspnea, coughing.
**Skin:** rash, pruritus, alopecia, bullous eruption, photosensitivity, sweating, urticaria.
**Other:** accidental injury, allergic reaction, fever, *angioedema,* flulike symptoms.

## Overdose and treatment

Symptoms following acute overdose of NSAIDs include lethargy, drowsiness, nausea, vomiting, epigastric pain, and GI bleeding. Severe poisoning may result in acute renal failure, hepatic dysfunction, respiratory depression, coma, seizures, CV collapse, and cardiac arrest. Anaphylactoid reactions may also occur.

There is no antidote, and patients should be managed with symptomatic and supportive care. Within 1 hour of the overdose, recommend inducing vomiting or performing gastric lavage. Activated charcoal is recommended for patients seen 1 to 2 hours after overdose. Activated charcoal may be given repeatedly for substantial overdose or severely symptomatic patient. Cholestyramine may be useful following an overdose. Forced diuresis, alkalinization of urine, hemodialysis, or hemoperfusion may not be useful because of high protein-binding.

## Clinical considerations

**⊞ ALERT** Drug may produce allergy-type reactions in patients hypersensitive to aspirin and other NSAIDs.
■ Patients with a history of ulcers or GI bleeding have a higher risk of GI bleeding while taking NSAIDs such as meloxicam. Other risk factors for GI bleeding include treatment with corticosteroids or anticoagulants, longer duration of NSAID treatment, smoking, alcoholism, older age, and poor overall health.
■ Recommend rehydrating patients who are dehydrated before starting treatment with meloxicam.
■ Recommend periodic monitoring of CBC and chemistry profile for patients on long-term treatment.

### Therapeutic monitoring

■ Advise clinician to monitor patient for signs and symptoms of overt and occult bleeding.
■ NSAIDs such as meloxicam can cause fluid retention; recommend closely monitoring patients who have hypertension, edema, or HF.
■ Meloxicam may be hepatotoxic and elevation of ALT or AST levels has been reported and should be monitored if it occurs. If signs and symptoms consistent with liver disease develop, or if systemic manifestations such as

eosinophilia rash occur, drug should be discontinued.

## Special populations

**Breast-feeding patients.** It's unknown if drug appears in breast milk. However, because it may enter breast milk and has the potential for serious adverse reactions in breast-fed infants, a decision should be made to discontinue either breast-feeding or drug, taking into account the importance of drug to the mother.

**Pediatric patients.** Safety and efficacy in children under age 18 haven't been established.

**Geriatric patients.** As with any NSAID, use cautiously when treating this age-group.

## Patient counseling

- Tell patient to report any history of allergic reactions to aspirin or other NSAIDs before starting therapy.
- Teach patient signs and symptoms of GI ulcerations and bleeding (vomiting blood, blood in stool, and black, tarry stools) and instruct him to contact prescriber if these occur.
- Instruct patient to report skin rash, weight gain, or edema.
- Advise patient to report warning signs of hepatotoxicity (nausea, fatigue, lethargy, pruritus, jaundice, right upper quadrant tenderness and flulike symptoms).
- Warn patient with prior history of asthma to stop taking drug and notify prescriber if asthma recurs while he's taking meloxicam.
- Tell woman to notify prescriber if she becomes pregnant or is planning to become pregnant while taking this drug.
- Inform patient that it may take several days before consistent pain relief is achieved.

---

# melphalan (phenylalanine mustard)

Alkeran

*Pharmacologic classification:* alkylating drug (cell cycle–phase nonspecific)
*Therapeutic classification:* antineoplastic
*Pregnancy risk category D*

## Available forms

Available by prescription only
*Tablets (scored):* 2 mg
*Powder for injection:* 50 mg

## Indications and dosages

Dosage and indications may vary. Check current literature for recommended protocol.
*Multiple myeloma*
*Adults:* 6 mg P.O. daily for 2 to 3 weeks; then stop therapy for 4 weeks. When WBC and platelet count begin to increase, start mainte-

nance dose of 2 mg P.O. daily. Alternatively, give 0.15 mg/kg/day P.O. for 7 days or 0.25 mg/kg/day P.O. for 4 days at 4- to 6-week intervals, usually with prednisone. Advise clinician to monitor patient's blood counts. Other dosing methods: 10 mg P.O. for 7 to 10 days. When platelet and leukocyte counts exceed 100,000/mm$^3$ and 4,000/mm$^3$, respectively, initiate maintenance therapy at 2 mg P.O. daily. Dosage adjusted by 1 to 3 mg based on hematologic response.

For I.V. administration, give 16 mg/m$^2$ over 15 to 20 minutes once at 2-week intervals for four doses. Advise clinician to monitor patient's blood counts and reduce dosage p.r.n. After satisfactory recovery, repeat dose at 4-week intervals.
*Epithelial ovarian cancer*
*Adults:* 200 mcg/kg/day P.O. for 5 days, repeated q 4 to 5 weeks if blood counts return to normal.

≋ *Dosage adjustment.* For patients with renal impairment, reduce I.V. melphalan dosage by 50% to reduce risk of severe leukopenia and drug-related death.

## I.V. administration

- Follow facility policy to reduce risks. Preparation and administration of parenteral form are linked to carcinogenic, mutagenic, and teratogenic risks for staff.
- Because drug isn't stable in solution, reconstitute immediately before administering with 10 ml of sterile diluent supplied by manufacturer. Shake vigorously until solution is clear. The resulting solution will contain 5 mg/ml of melphalan. Immediately dilute required dose in normal saline solution for injection. Final concentration shouldn't exceed 0.45 mg/ml. Give infusion over 15 to 20 minutes.
- Promptly dilute and administer; reconstituted product begins to degrade within 30 minutes. After final dilution, nearly 1% of drug degrades every 10 minutes. Don't refrigerate reconstituted product because a precipitate will form. Administration must be completed within 60 minutes of reconstitution.

## Incompatibilities

Incompatible with amphotericin B, chlorpromazine D$_5$W, and lactated Ringer's injection. Compatibility with normal saline injection depends on the level; don't prepare solutions with a concentration exceeding 0.45 mg/ml.

## Mechanism of action

*Antineoplastic action:* Melphalan exerts its cytotoxic activity by forming cross-links of strands of DNA and RNA and inhibiting protein synthesis.

---

## Pharmacokinetics

*Absorption:* Absorption from GI tract is incomplete and variable. One study found that absorption ranged from 25% to 89% after an oral dose of 0.6 mg/kg.

*Distribution:* Distributed rapidly and widely into total body water. Drug is initially 50% to 60% plasma protein–bound and eventually increases to 80% to 90% over time.

*Metabolism:* Extensively deactivated by the process of hydrolysis.

*Excretion:* Elimination has been described as biphasic, with an initial half-life of 8 minutes and a terminal half-life of 2 hours. Melphalan and its metabolites are excreted primarily in urine, with 10% of an oral dose excreted as unchanged drug.

| Route | Onset | Peak | Duration |
|-------|-------|------|----------|
| P.O., I.V. | Unknown | Unknown | Unknown |

## Contraindications and precautions

Contraindicated in patients hypersensitive to drug and in those whose disease is known to be resistant to drug. Patients hypersensitive to chlorambucil may have cross-sensitivity to melphalan.

Use cautiously in patients with impaired renal function, severe leukopenia, thrombocytopenia, anemia, or chronic lymphocytic leukemia.

## Interactions

**Drug-drug.** *Cimetidine:* Inhibits GI absorption. Avoid administration together.

*Cisplatin, cyclosporine:* May increase nephrotoxicity. Advise clinician to monitor renal function closely in patients receiving melphalan and cyclosporine together or melphalan and cisplatin together.

*Interferon alpha:* May cause a decrease in melphalan serum levels. Advise clinician to monitor patient carefully.

**Drug-food.** *Any food:* Reduces bioavailability of melphalan. Advise patient to take drug on an empty stomach.

## Adverse reactions

**CNS:** transient paralysis, peripheral neuritis.

**CV:** hypotension, tachycardia, edema, thrombosis, phlebitis, *pulmonary embolism.*

**GI:** nausea, vomiting, diarrhea, oral ulceration.

**Hematologic:** *thrombocytopenia, leukopenia, bone marrow suppression, hemolytic anemia.*

**Hepatic:** *hepatotoxicity.*

**Respiratory:** *pneumonitis, pulmonary fibrosis,* dyspnea, *bronchospasm.*

**Skin:** pruritus, alopecia, urticaria.

**Other:** *anaphylaxis,* hypersensitivity, *secondary malignancy,* vesiculation and tissue necrosis.

## Overdose and treatment

Signs and symptoms of overdose include myelosuppression, hypocalcemia, severe nausea, vomiting, ulceration of the mouth, decreased consciousness, seizures, muscular paralysis, and cholinomimetic effects.

Treatment is usually supportive and includes transfusion of blood components.

## Clinical considerations

- Fever may enhance elimination of the drug.
- Recommend using anticoagulants, aspirin, and aspirin-containing products cautiously.
- Oral dose may be taken all at one time.
- Advise clinician to give drug on an empty stomach because absorption is decreased by food.
- Recommend stopping therapy temporarily or reducing dosage if WBC count goes below 3,000/mm$^3$ or platelet count goes below 100,000/mm$^3$.
- Avoid I.M. injections when platelet count is less than 100,000/mm$^3$.
- Increased bone marrow suppression was observed in patients with BUN levels of 30 mg/dl or more.
- Recommend following procedure for proper handling and disposal of antineoplastics.

### Therapeutic monitoring

- Frequent hematologic monitoring, including CBC, is needed for accurate dosage adjustments and prevention of toxicity.
- Advise clinician to monitor renal function, especially if BUN level is greater than 30 mg/dl.

### Special populations

**Breast-feeding patients.** It isn't known if melphalan appears in breast milk. However, because of risk of serious adverse reactions, mutagenicity, and carcinogenicity in the infant, breast-feeding isn't recommended.

## Patient counseling

- Instruct patient to continue taking drug despite nausea and vomiting.
- Tell patient to call prescriber immediately if vomiting occurs shortly after taking a dose.
- Explain that adequate fluid intake is important to facilitate excretion of uric acid.
- Instruct patient to avoid exposure to people with infections.
- Reassure patient that hair should grow back after treatment has ended.
- Tell patient to promptly report signs and symptoms of infection or bleeding.
- Advise women of childbearing age to avoid becoming pregnant while receiving drug therapy.

# meningococcal polysaccharide vaccine
Menomune-A/C/Y/W-135

*Pharmacologic classification:* vaccine
*Therapeutic classification:* bacterial vaccine
*Pregnancy risk category C*

## Available forms
Available by prescription only
*Injection:* A killed bacterial vaccine in single-dose, 10-dose, and 50-dose vials with vial of diluent

## Indications and dosages
**Meningococcal meningitis prophylaxis**
*Adults and children over age 2:* 0.5 ml S.C.
◇ *Children ages 3 to 18 months:* 0.5 ml S.C. for two doses 3 months apart.

## Mechanism of action
*Meningitis prophylaxis:* Vaccine promotes active immunity to meningitis caused by *Neisseria meningitidis.*

## Pharmacokinetics
No information available.

| Route | Onset | Peak | Duration |
|-------|-------|------|----------|
| S.C. | Unknown | Unknown | 3 yr |

## Contraindications and precautions
Contraindicated in immunosuppressed patients hypersensitive to thimerosal. Defer vaccination in patients with acute illness. Avoid use during pregnancy unless clearly needed.

## Interactions
**Drug-drug.** *Vaccines containing whole-cell pertussis or whole-cell typhoid antigens:* Combined endotoxin effect. Don't use together.

## Adverse reactions
**CNS:** headache, malaise.
**GU:** nephropathy.
**Musculoskeletal:** muscle cramps.
**Other:** *pain, tenderness, erythema, induration* (at injection site); *anaphylaxis,* chills, fever.

## Overdose and treatment
No information available.

## Clinical considerations
■ Recommend obtaining a thorough history of patient's allergies and reactions to immunizations.
■ Meningitis vaccine shouldn't be given intradermally, I.M., or I.V.; safety and efficacy haven't been established.
■ Epinephrine solution 1:1,000 should be available to treat allergic reactions.

■ Booster responses to second doses of vaccine are poor and unpredictable.
■ In a child age 3 to 6 months, vaccine may provide short-term protection against serotype A meningococcal disease.
■ In a child as young as 6 months, vaccine may provide short-term protection against serotype C meningococcal disease.
■ Older children and adults in high-risk exposure areas should consider revaccination every 3 to 5 years.
■ Children under age 4 vaccinated in high-risk exposure areas should be revaccinated 2 to 3 years after primary immunization.
■ Meningococcal polysaccharide vaccine groups A, C, Y, and W-135 is recommended for outbreak control to prevent additional cases among specific populations when meningococcal outbreaks occur and serogroup C is involved.
■ The 50-dose vial of vaccine is intended for jet injector administration only and generally shouldn't be given using syringes and needles. Discard any unused vaccine.
■ Reconstitute vaccine with diluent provided. Shake until dissolved. Discard reconstituted solution after 5 days.
■ Store vaccine between 36° and 46° F (2° and 8° C).
■ Protective antibody levels may be achieved within 10 to 14 days after vaccination.

### Therapeutic monitoring
■ Advise clinician to monitor patient for adverse allergic reactions.

### Special populations
**Breast-feeding patients.** It isn't known if vaccine appears in breast milk. Use with caution in breast-feeding women.
**Pediatric patients.** Vaccine isn't recommended for children under age 2, but has been used investigationally in children ages 3 to 24 months.

## Patient counseling
■ Tell patient that pain and inflammation may occur at injection site. Recommend acetaminophen to alleviate adverse reactions, such as fever.
■ Encourage patient to report distressing adverse reactions.
■ Advise patient on use of contraceptives, if needed.
■ Explain that vaccine will provide immunity only to meningitis caused by one type of bacteria.

## menotropins
Humegon, Pergonal

*Pharmacologic classification:* gonado-tropin
*Therapeutic classification:* ovulation stimulant, spermatogenesis stimulant
*Pregnancy risk category X*

### Available forms
Available by prescription only
*Injection:* 75 IU of luteinizing hormone (LH) and 75 IU of follicle-stimulating hormone (FSH) activity per ampule; 150 IU of LH and 150 IU of FSH activity per ampule

### Indications and dosages
*Production of follicular maturation*
*Adults:* 75 IU each of FSH and LH I.M. daily for 9 to 12 days, followed by 10,000 United States Pharmacopeia (USP) units chorionic go-nadotropin (CG) I.M. 1 day after last dose of menotropins; may repeat for two more menstrual cycles if evidence of ovulation, but pregnancy doesn't occur. Then, if ovulation or follicular development doesn't occur, increase to 150 IU each of FSH and LH I.M. daily for 9 to 12 days, followed by 10,000 USP units CG I.M. 1 day after last dose of menotropins; may repeat for two menstrual cycles if evidence of ovulation, but pregnancy doesn't occur.
Note: If the ovaries are abnormally enlarged or if total urinary estrogen excretion is > 100 mcg daily, or if urinary estriol excretion is > 50 mcg daily, hold CG dose because hy-perstimulation syndrome is more likely to oc-cur.
*Stimulation of spermatogenesis*
*Adults:* After 5,000 USP units of CG I.M. 3 times weekly for 4 to 6 months of treatment; 1 ampule (75 IU FSH/LH) I.M. three times weekly (given with 2,000 USP units CG twice weekly) for at least 4 months. If no improve-ment occurs after 4 months, treatment may con-tinue with 75 IU FSH/LH three times weekly or 150 IU FSH/LH three times weekly. Dosage of CG doesn't change.

### Mechanism of action
*Ovulation stimulant action:* Menotropins causes growth and maturation of the ovarian follicle in women who don't have primary ovarian fail-ure by mimicking the action of endogenous LH and FSH. Additional treatment with CG is usually required to achieve ovulation.
*Spermatogenesis stimulant action:* Meno-tropins causes spermatogenesis when given with CG in men with primary or secondary pi-tuitary hypofunction.

### Pharmacokinetics
*Absorption:* Must be administered parenteral-ly for effectiveness.

*Distribution:* Unknown.
*Metabolism:* Not fully known.
*Excretion:* Excreted in urine.

| Route | Onset | Peak | Duration |
|-------|-------|------|----------|
| I.M. | 9-12 days | Unknown | Unknown |

### Contraindications and precautions
Contraindicated in patients hypersensitive to drug; in women with primary ovarian failure, uncontrolled thyroid or adrenal dysfunction, pituitary tumor, abnormal uterine bleeding, uterine fibromas, or ovarian cysts or enlarge-ment; in pregnant women; and in men with normal pituitary function, primary testicular failure, or infertility disorders other than hypo-gonadotropic hypogonadism.

### Interactions
None reported.

### Adverse reactions
**CNS:** headache, malaise, dizziness.
**CV:** *CVA,* tachycardia.
**GI:** nausea, vomiting, diarrhea, abdominal cramps, bloating.
**GU:** *ovarian enlargement with pain and ab-dominal distention, ovarian hyperstimulation syndrome* (sudden severe abdominal pain, dis-tention, nausea, vomiting, weight gain, and dyspnea followed by hypovolemia, hemocon-centration, electrolyte imbalance, pleural ef-fusion, ascites, and hemoperitoneum), gyneco-mastia, ovarian cysts, ectopic pregnancy.
**Musculoskeletal:** musculoskeletal aches, joint pains.
**Respiratory:** *atelectasis, acute respiratory distress syndrome, pulmonary embolism, pul-monary infarction, arterial occlusion,* dys-pnea, tachypnea.
**Skin:** rash.
**Other:** fever, multiple births, hypersensitivi-ty, *anaphylactic reactions,* chills.

### Overdose and treatment
The most common dose-related adverse effect appears to be ovarian hyperstimulation syn-drome. Drug should be discontinued. Symp-tomatic and supportive care includes bed rest, fluid and electrolyte replacement, and anal-gesics.

### Clinical considerations
**⊩ ALERT** Drug is administered by I.M. route only.
■ Reconstitute drug with 1 to 2 ml of sterile saline injection. Use immediately and discard any unused portion.
■ Pregnancies that follow ovulation induced with menotropins show a relatively high fre-quency of multiple births.
■ Store drug at 37° to 86° F (3° to 30° C).

### Therapeutic monitoring
■ Advise clinician to monitor patient at least every other day for enlarged ovaries or hyperstimulation syndrome during and for 2 weeks after therapy.

### Special populations
**Breast-feeding patients.** Drug isn't indicated for use in breast-feeding women.

### Patient counseling
■ Teach patient signs and tests that indicate time of ovulation, such as increase in basal body temperature and increase in the appearance and volume of cervical mucus.
■ Warn patient to immediately report symptoms of ovarian hyperstimulation syndrome, such as abdominal distention and pain, dyspnea, and vaginal bleeding.
■ Warn patient that multiple births are possible. Ectopic pregnancy and congenital malformations have been reported in pregnancies following treatment.
■ Encourage daily intercourse from day before CG is given until ovulation occurs.
■ Advise patient that she should be examined at least every other day for signs of excessive ovarian stimulation during therapy and for 2 weeks after treatment is discontinued.

---

# meperidine hydrochloride (pethidine hydrochloride)
Demerol

*Pharmacologic classification:* opioid
*Therapeutic classification:* analgesic, adjunct to anesthesia
*Pregnancy risk category C*
*Controlled substance schedule II*

### Available forms
Available by prescription only
*Tablets:* 50 mg, 100 mg
*Oral solution:* 50 mg/5 ml
*Injection:* 10 mg/ml, 25 mg/ml, 50 mg/ml, 75 mg/ml, 100 mg/ml

### Indications and dosages
*Moderate to severe pain*
*Adults:* 50 to 150 mg P.O., I.M., or S.C. q 3 to 4 hours; or continuous infusion of 15 to 35 mg/hour.
*Children:* 1.1 to 1.8 mg/kg P.O., I.M., or S.C. q 3 to 4 hours or 175 mg/m² daily in six divided doses. Maximum single dose for children shouldn't exceed 100 mg.
*Preoperatively*
*Adults:* 50 to 100 mg I.M. or S.C. 30 to 90 minutes before surgery.
*Children:* 1 to 2 mg/kg I.M. or S.C. 30 to 90 minutes before surgery. Don't exceed adult dose.

### Support of anesthesia
*Adults:* Repeated slow I.V. injections of fractional doses (10 mg/ml) or continuous I.V. infusion of 1 mg/ml. Titrate dose to meet patient's needs.
### Obstetric analgesia
*Adults:* 50 to 100 mg I.M. or S.C. when pain becomes regular; may repeat at 1- to 3-hour intervals.

### I.V. administration
■ Concentration of 10 mg/ml should only be used with compatible infusion device and doesn't require further dilution.
■ Meperidine may be given slowly through an I.V., preferably as a diluted solution.
■ During I.V. administration, tachycardia may occur, possibly as a result of atropine-like effects of the drug.

### Incompatibilities
Incompatible with aminophylline, amobarbital, ephedrine, heparin, methicillin, morphine, phenobarbital sodium, phenytoin, sodium bicarbonate, sodium iodide, sulfadiazine, thiamylal, and thiopental.

### Mechanism of action
*Analgesic action:* Meperidine is a narcotic agonist with actions and potency similar to those of morphine, with principal actions at the opiate receptors. It's recommended for the relief of moderate to severe pain.

### Pharmacokinetics
*Absorption:* Given orally, drug is only half as effective as it is parenterally.
*Distribution:* Distributed widely throughout the body and is 60% to 80% plasma protein–bound.
*Metabolism:* Metabolized primarily by hydrolysis in the liver to an active metabolite, normeperidine.
*Excretion:* About 30% is excreted in urine as the *N*-demethylated derivative; about 5% is excreted unchanged. Excretion is enhanced by acidifying the urine. Half-life of parent compound is 3 to 5 hours and the half-life of metabolite is 8 to 21 hours.

| Route | Onset | Peak | Duration |
|-------|-------|------|----------|
| P.O. | 15 min | 1-1½ hr | 2-4 hr |
| I.V. | 1 min | 5-7 min | 2-4 hr |
| I.M. | 10-15 min | 30-50 min | 2-4 hr |
| S.C. | 10-15 min | 40-60 min | 2-4 hr |

### Contraindications and precautions
Contraindicated in patients hypersensitive to drug and in those who have received MAO inhibitors within the past 14 days.

Use cautiously in geriatric or debilitated patients and in those with increased intracranial pressure, head injury, asthma, other respiratory conditions, supraventricular tachycardia, seizures, acute abdominal conditions, renal or hepatic disease, hypothyroidism, Addison's disease, urethral stricture, and prostatic hyperplasia.

## Interactions

**Drug-drug.** *Anticholinergics:* May cause paralytic ileus. Advise clinician to monitor patient closely.

*Cimetidine:* May increase respiratory and CNS depression, causing confusion, disorientation, apnea, or seizures. Dosage of meperidine should be reduced.

*General anesthetics:* Severe CV depression may result from use together. Use together cautiously.

*Isoniazid:* Meperidine can potentiate adverse effects of isoniazid. Avoid use together.

*MAO inhibitors:* May precipitate unpredictable and occasionally fatal reactions, even in patients who may receive MAO inhibitors within 14 days of receiving meperidine. Avoid use together.

*Narcotic antagonist:* Patients who become physically dependent on drug may experience acute withdrawal syndrome if given a narcotic antagonist. Avoid use together.

*Other CNS depressants, such as antihistamines, barbiturates, benzodiazepines, general anesthetics, muscle relaxants, narcotic analgesics, phenothiazines, sedative-hypnotics, and tricyclic antidepressants:* Potentiate respiratory and CNS depression, sedation, and hypotensive effects of drugs. Use together cautiously.

**Drug-herb.** *Parsley:* May promote or produce serotonin syndrome. Discourage use together.

**Drug-lifestyle.** *Alcohol use:* Potentiates respiratory and CNS depression, sedation, and hypotensive effects of drug. Discourage use together.

## Adverse reactions

**CNS:** *sedation, somnolence, clouded sensorium, euphoria, dizziness,* paradoxical excitement, tremor, *seizures* (with large doses), headache, hallucinations, syncope, *light-headedness.*
**CV:** *hypotension, bradycardia,* tachycardia, *cardiac arrest, shock.*
**GI:** *constipation,* ileus, dry mouth, *nausea, vomiting,* biliary tract spasms.
**GU:** *urine retention.*
**Respiratory:** *respiratory depression, respiratory arrest.*
**Skin:** pruritus, urticaria, *diaphoresis.*
**Other:** physical dependence, muscle twitching; phlebitis (after I.V. delivery); pain (at injection site); local tissue irritation, induration (after S.C. injection).

## Overdose and treatment

The most common signs and symptoms of meperidine overdose are CNS depression, respiratory depression, skeletal muscle flaccidity, cold and clammy skin, mydriasis, bradycardia, and hypotension. Other acute toxic effects include hypothermia, shock, apnea, cardiopulmonary arrest, circulatory collapse, pulmonary edema, and seizures.

To treat acute overdose, recommend first establishing adequate respiratory exchange via a patent airway and ventilation p.r.n.; a narcotic antagonist (naloxone) should be given to reverse respiratory depression. (Because the duration of action of meperidine is longer than that of naloxone, repeated dosing is needed.) Naloxone shouldn't be given unless the patient has clinically significant respiratory or CV depression. Advise clinician to monitor vital signs.

If patient presents within 2 hours of ingestion of an oral overdose, recommend emptying the stomach immediately by inducing emesis (ipecac syrup) or using gastric lavage. Caution should be taken to avoid risk of aspiration. Advise clinician to give activated charcoal via nasogastric tube for further removal of meperidine, and acidify urine to help remove drug.

Recommend providing symptomatic and supportive treatment (continued respiratory support, correction of fluid or electrolyte imbalance). Advise clinician to monitor laboratory values, vital signs, and neurologic status closely.

## Clinical considerations

■ Drug may be given to patients allergic to morphine.

■ Commercial preparations contain sodium metabisulfite, which may cause allergic reactions in susceptible individuals.

■ Question patient carefully regarding possible use of MAO inhibitors within the past 14 days.

■ Because drug toxicity commonly appears after several days of treatment, this drug isn't recommended for treatment of chronic pain.

■ S.C. injection is very painful.

■ Oral dose is less than half as effective as parenteral dose. Advise clinician to give I.M. if possible. When changing from parenteral to oral route, dosage should be increased.

■ Syrup has local anesthetic effect. Advise clinician to give with water.

■ Alternating meperidine with a peripherally active nonopioid analgesic, such as aspirin, acetaminophen or NSAIDs, may improve pain control while allowing lower opioid dosages.

■ Injectable meperidine is compatible with sodium chloride and $D_5W$ solutions and their combinations, and with lactated Ringer's and sodium lactate solution.

■ Drug increases plasma amylase or lipase levels through increased biliary tract pressure; levels may be unreliable for 24 hours after meperidine administration.

### Therapeutic monitoring
- Meperidine and its active metabolite normeperidine accumulate. Advise clinician to monitor patient for neurotoxic effects, especially in burn patients and those with poor renal function, sickle cell anemia, or cancer.
- When administered I.V., recommend closely monitoring heart rate and respiratory rate.

### Special populations
**Breast-feeding patients.** Drug appears in breast milk; use with caution in breast-feeding women.
**Pediatric patients.** Drug shouldn't be given to infants under age 6 months.
**Geriatric patients.** Lower doses are usually indicated for geriatric patients because they may be more sensitive to the therapeutic and adverse effects of drug.

### Patient counseling
- Caution patient about CNS drug effects. Warn patient to avoid driving and other potentially hazardous activities that require mental alertness until CNS effects of drug are known.
- Advise patient to avoid alcohol.
- Tell patient to take drug before pain becomes intense.

# mephenytoin
Mesantoin

*Pharmacologic classification:* hydantoin derivative
*Therapeutic classification:* anticonvulsant
*Pregnancy risk category NR*

### Available forms
Available by prescription only
*Tablets:* 100 mg

### Indications and dosages
**Generalized tonic-clonic or complex-partial seizures**
*Adults:* 50 to 100 mg P.O. daily; may increase by 50 to 100 mg at weekly intervals; usual maintenance dose is 200 to 600 mg daily given in three equally divided doses. Doses up to 800 mg/day may be required.
*Children:* Initially, 50 to 100 mg P.O. daily. May increase slowly by 50 to 100 mg at weekly intervals. Dosage must be adjusted individually. Usual maintenance dose is 100 to 400 mg/day (or 3 to 15 mg/kg/day or 100 to 450 mg/m$^2$/day) given in three equally divided doses.

### Mechanism of action
*Anticonvulsant action:* Like other hydantoin derivatives, mephenytoin stabilizes the neuronal membranes and limits seizure activity either by increasing efflux or by decreasing influx of sodium ions across cell membranes in the motor cortex during generation of nerve impulses. Like phenytoin, mephenytoin appears to have antiarrhythmic effects.

Mephenytoin is used for prophylaxis of tonic-clonic (grand mal), psychomotor, focal, and jacksonian-type partial seizures in patients refractory to less toxic drugs. It's usually combined with phenytoin, phenobarbital, or primidone; phenytoin is preferred because it causes less sedation than barbiturates. Mephenytoin also is used with succinimides to control combined absence and tonic-clonic disorders; combined use with oxazolidinediones, paramethadione or trimethadione isn't recommended because of the increased hazard of blood dyscrasias.

### Pharmacokinetics
*Absorption:* Absorbed from the GI tract.
*Distribution:* Distributed widely throughout the body; good seizure control without toxicity occurs when serum levels of drug and major metabolite reach 25 to 40 mcg/ml.
*Metabolism:* Metabolized by the liver.
*Excretion:* Excreted in urine.

| Route | Onset | Peak | Duration |
|-------|-------|------|----------|
| P.O. | 30 min | Unknown | 24-48 hr |

### Contraindications and precautions
Contraindicated in patients with hydantoin hypersensitivity.

### Interactions
**Drug-drug.** *Antihistamines, chloramphenicol, cimetidine, diazepam, diazoxide, disulfiram, isoniazid, oral anticoagulants, phenylbutazone, salicylates, sulfamethizole, valproate:* Therapeutic effects and toxicity of mephenytoin may be increased by use with these drugs. Advise clinician to monitor patient closely.
*Folic acid:* Therapeutic effects of mephenytoin may be decreased. Use together cautiously.
*Oral contraceptives:* Decreased effects of oral contraceptives. Recommend alternative means of contraception.
**Drug-lifestyle.** *Alcohol use:* May reduce therapeutic effects of drug. Avoid use together.

### Adverse reactions
**CNS:** ataxia, *drowsiness,* fatigue, irritability, choreiform movements, depression, tremor, insomnia, dizziness (usually transient).
**EENT:** conjunctivitis, diplopia, nystagmus, gingival hyperplasia (with prolonged use).
**GI:** nausea and vomiting (with prolonged use).
**Hematologic:** *leukopenia, neutropenia, agranulocytosis, thrombocytopenia,* eosinophilia, leukocytosis.
**Hepatic:** elevated liver function test results.
**Musculoskeletal:** polyarthropathy.
**Respiratory:** *pulmonary fibrosis.*
**Skin:** rash, *exfoliative dermatitis, Stevens-Johnson syndrome, fatal dermatitides.*

---

Reactions may be *common,* uncommon, *life-threatening,* or COMMON AND LIFE-THREATENING.

**Other:** edema, lymphadenopathy.

## Overdose and treatment

Signs of acute mephenytoin toxicity may include restlessness, dizziness, drowsiness, nausea, vomiting, nystagmus, ataxia, dysarthria, tremor, and slurred speech; hypotension, respiratory depression, and coma may follow. Death may result from respiratory and circulatory depression.

Recommend treating overdose with gastric lavage or emesis and following up with supportive treatment. Recommend carefully monitoring vital signs and fluid and electrolyte balance. Forced diuresis is of little or no value. Hemodialysis or peritoneal dialysis may be helpful.

## Clinical considerations

■ Decreased alertness and coordination are most pronounced at start of treatment. Patient may need help with walking and other activities for first few days.
■ Drug shouldn't be discontinued abruptly. Transition from mephenytoin to other anticonvulsant drug should progress over 6 weeks.
■ When patient is receiving phenobarbital, recommend continuing phenobarbital until the transition to the other anticonvulsant is completed. Then, a gradual withdrawal of phenobarbital should be attempted.
■ Safe use of mephenytoin during pregnancy hasn't been established. Use drug during pregnancy only when clearly needed.

### Therapeutic monitoring

■ CBC and platelet counts should be performed before therapy, after 2 weeks of initial therapy, and after 2 weeks on maintenance dose; they should be repeated every month for 1 year and, subsequently, at 3-month intervals. If neutrophil count declines to 1,600 to 2,500/mm³, recommend obtaining CBC every 2 weeks.
■ Drug should be stopped if neutrophil count is less than 1,600/mm³.

### Special populations

**Breast-feeding patients.** Safe use during breast-feeding hasn't been established. Alternative feeding method is recommended.

## Patient counseling

■ Tell patient never to discontinue drug or change dosage except as prescribed and to avoid alcohol, which decreases effectiveness of drug and increases sedative effects.
■ Explain that follow-up laboratory tests are essential for safe use.
■ Instruct patient to report unusual changes immediately (cutaneous reaction, sore throat, glandular swelling, fever, mucous membrane swelling).

# meprobamate

Apo-Meprobamate*, Equanil, MB-Tab, Meprospan, Miltown, Neuramate

*Pharmacologic classification:* carbamate
*Therapeutic classification:* anxiolytic
*Pregnancy risk category D*
*Controlled substance schedule IV*

## Available forms

Available by prescription only
*Tablets:* 200 mg, 400 mg, 600 mg
*Capsules (sustained-release):* 200 mg, 400 mg

## Indications and dosages

### Anxiety and tension

*Adults:* 1.2 to 1.6 g P.O. daily in three or four equally divided doses. Maximum dose, 2.4 g daily (sustained-release capsules, 400 to 800 mg b.i.d.).
*Children ages 6 to 12:* 100 to 200 mg P.O. b.i.d. or t.i.d. Alternatively, 25 mg/kg/day or 700 mg/m²/day in two or three divided doses. Sustained-release capsules, 200 mg b.i.d. Not recommended for children under age 6.

### Preoperative sedation and relief of anxiety

*Adults:* 400 mg P.O.
*Children:* 200 mg P.O.

## Mechanism of action

*Anxiolytic action:* While the cellular mechanism is unknown, drug causes nonselective CNS depression similar to that seen with use of barbiturates. Meprobamate acts at multiple sites in the CNS, including the thalamus, hypothalamus, limbic system, and spinal cord, but not the medulla or reticular activating system.

## Pharmacokinetics

*Absorption:* Well absorbed after oral administration. Sedation usually occurs within 1 hour.
*Distribution:* Distributed throughout the body; 20% is protein-bound. Drug appears in breast milk at two to four times the serum level; meprobamate crosses the placenta.
*Metabolism:* Metabolized rapidly in the liver to inactive glucuronide conjugates. Half-life of drug is 6 to 17 hours.
*Excretion:* Metabolites of drug and 10% to 20% of a single dose as unchanged drug are excreted in urine.

| Route | Onset | Peak | Duration |
|-------|-------|------|----------|
| P.O. | Unknown | Unknown | Unknown |

## Contraindications and precautions

Contraindicated in patients hypersensitive to meprobamate or related compounds, such as carisoprodol, mebutamate, tybamate, and carbromal, and in those with porphyria. Avoid use of drug during first trimester of pregnancy and in breast-feeding women.

Use cautiously in geriatric or debilitated patients and in those with impaired renal or hepatic function, seizure disorders, or suicidal tendencies.

### Interactions
**Drug-drug.** *Antihistamines, barbiturates, narcotics, tranquilizers, other CNS depressants:* Potentiated effects. Use together cautiously.
**Drug-lifestyle.** *Alcohol use:* Potentiated effects. Use together cautiously.

### Adverse reactions
**CNS:** *drowsiness,* ataxia, dizziness, slurred speech, headache, syncope, vertigo, *seizures.*
**CV:** palpitations, tachycardia, hypotension, *arrhythmias.*
**GI:** nausea, vomiting, diarrhea.
**Hematologic:** *aplastic anemia, thrombocytopenia, agranulocytosis.*
**Skin:** pruritus, urticaria, erythematous maculopapular rash, *hypersensitivity reactions.*
**After abrupt withdrawal of long-term therapy:** severe generalized tonic-clonic seizures may occur.

### Overdose and treatment
Signs and symptoms of overdose include drowsiness, lethargy, ataxia, coma, hypotension, shock, and respiratory depression.

Treatment of overdose is supportive and symptomatic, including maintaining adequate ventilation and a patent airway, with mechanical ventilation, if needed.

Recommend treating hypotension with fluids and vasopressors p.r.n. Recommend emptying gastric contents by emesis or lavage if ingestion was recent, followed by activated charcoal and a cathartic. Treat seizures with parenteral diazepam. Peritoneal dialysis and hemodialysis may effectively remove drug. Serum levels of more than 100 mcg/ml may be fatal.

### Clinical considerations
■ Safety precautions are needed; such as raised bed rails, especially for geriatric patients, when treatment starts or changes. Patient may need assistance when walking.
■ Drug abuse and addiction may occur.
■ Drug should be withdrawn gradually; otherwise, withdrawal symptoms may occur if patient has been taking drug for a long time.
■ Store drug at 59° to 86° F (15° to 30° C); expires 2 to 5 years from date of manufacture.
■ Drug therapy may falsely elevate urinary 17-ketosteroids, 17-ketogenic steroids (as determined by the Zimmerman reaction), and 17-hydroxycorticosteroid levels (as determined by the Glenn-Nelson technique).

### Therapeutic monitoring
■ Frequent assessment of level of consciousness and vital signs is needed.
■ Periodic evaluation of CBC is recommended during long-term therapy.
■ Advise clinician to monitor hepatic and renal function.

### Special populations
**Breast-feeding patients.** Drug appears in breast milk at two to four times the serum level. Don't use in breast-feeding women.
**Pediatric patients.** Safety hasn't been established in children under age 6.
**Geriatric patients.** Geriatric patients may have more pronounced CNS effects. Use lowest dose possible.

### Patient counseling
■ Tell patient to avoid alcohol and other CNS depressants, such as antihistamines, narcotics, and tranquilizers, while taking drug, unless prescribed.
■ Advise patient not to increase dose or frequency and not to abruptly discontinue or decrease dose unless prescribed.
■ Tell patient to avoid tasks that require mental alertness or physical coordination until CNS effects of drug are known.
■ Recommend sugarless candy or gum or ice chips to relieve dry mouth.
■ Advise patient to report sore throat, fever, or unusual bleeding or bruising.
■ Inform patient of potential for physical or psychological dependence with long-term use.

# mercaptopurine (6-MP)
Purinethol

*Pharmacologic classification:* antimetabolite (cell cycle–phase specific, S phase)
*Therapeutic classification:* antineoplastic
*Pregnancy risk category D*

### Available forms
Available by prescription only
*Tablets (scored):* 50 mg

### Indications and dosages
Dosage and indications may vary. Check current literature for recommended protocols.
*Acute lymphoblastic leukemia (in children), chronic myelocytic leukemia*
*Adults:* 2.5 mg/kg P.O. daily as a single dose; increase to 5 mg/kg daily (only if, after 4 weeks, there's no clinical improvement or signs of toxicity). Alternatively, 80 to 100 mg/m²/day. Maintenance dose is 1.5 to 2.5 mg/kg daily.
*Children:* 2.5 mg/kg P.O. daily. Alternatively, 70 mg/m²/day. Maintenance dose is 1.5 to 2.5 mg/kg/day.

---

◇ *Acute myeloblastic leukemia*
*Adults:* 500 mg/m$^2$/day P.O. with other therapies.

## Mechanism of action

*Antineoplastic action:* Mercaptopurine is converted intracellularly to its active form, which exerts its cytotoxic antimetabolic effects by competing for an enzyme required for purine synthesis. This results in inhibition of DNA and RNA synthesis. Cross-resistance exists between mercaptopurine and thioguanine.

## Pharmacokinetics

*Absorption:* Absorption after an oral dose is incomplete and variable; about 50% of a dose is absorbed. Peak serum levels occur in 2 hours.
*Distribution:* Distributed widely into total body water. Drug crosses the blood-brain barrier, but the CSF level is too low for treatment of meningeal leukemias.
*Metabolism:* Extensively metabolized in the liver. It appears to undergo extensive first-pass metabolism, contributing to its low bioavailability.
*Excretion:* Excreted in urine.

| Route | Onset | Peak | Duration |
|-------|-------|------|----------|
| P.O. | Unknown | Unknown | Unknown |

## Contraindications and precautions

Contraindicated in patients whose disease has shown resistance to drug. Use cautiously in pregnancy or after chemotherapy or radiation therapy in patients with depressed neutrophil or platelet counts and in those with impaired renal or hepatic function.

## Interactions

**Drug-drug.** *Allopurinol at doses of 300 to 600 mg/day:* Increased toxic effects of mercaptopurine, especially myelosuppression. Reduce dosage by 25% to 30% when giving with allopurinol.
*Co-trimoxazole:* Enhanced marrow suppression. Use together cautiously.
*Other hepatotoxic drugs:* Increased potential for hepatotoxicity. Use together cautiously.
*Warfarin:* Decreased anticoagulant activity of warfarin with use together. Advise clinician to monitor PT and INR.

## Adverse reactions

**GI:** *nausea, vomiting, anorexia, painful oral ulcers, diarrhea, **pancreatitis**, GI ulceration.*
**Hematologic:** *leukopenia, thrombocytopenia,* anemia (all may persist several days after drug is stopped).
**Hepatic:** *jaundice, **hepatotoxicity.***
**Metabolic:** hyperuricemia.
**Skin:** rash, hyperpigmentation.

## Overdose and treatment

Signs and symptoms of overdose include myelosuppression, nausea, vomiting, and hepatic necrosis.

Treatment is usually supportive and includes transfusion of blood components and antiemetics. Hemodialysis is thought to be of marginal use because of the rapid intracellular incorporation of mercaptopurine into active metabolites with long persistence.

## Clinical considerations

■ Investigational uses include prevention of rejection of homografts, treatment of various autoimmune diseases, treatment of Crohn's disease, and treatment of chronic active hepatitis.
■ Drug is sometimes called 6-mercaptopurine or 6-MP.
■ Dosage modifications may be required following chemotherapy or radiation therapy, in depressed neutrophil or platelet count, and in impaired hepatic or renal function.
■ Hepatic dysfunction is reversible when drug is stopped. Recommend watching for jaundice, clay-colored stools, and frothy dark urine. Drug should be stopped if hepatic tenderness occurs. Advise clinician to monitor hepatic function during initiation of therapy.
■ All I.M. injections should be avoided when platelet count is less than 100,000/mm$^3$.
■ Store tablets at room temperature and protect from light.

### Therapeutic monitoring

■ Monitor weekly blood counts; watch for precipitous decline.
■ Monitor intake and output. Push fluids (3 L/day).
■ Evaluate hepatic function and hematologic values weekly during therapy.
■ Monitor serum uric acid levels. If allopurinol is needed, use very cautiously.
■ Observe patient for signs of bleeding and infection.

### Special populations

**Breast-feeding patients.** It isn't known if drug appears in breast milk. However, because of the potential for serious adverse reactions, mutagenicity, and carcinogenicity in the infant, breast-feeding isn't recommended.
**Pediatric patients.** Adverse GI reactions are less common in children than in adults.

## Patient counseling

■ Warn patient that improvement may take 2 to 4 weeks or longer.
■ Tell patient to continue drug despite nausea and vomiting.
■ Instruct patient to immediately report vomiting that occurs shortly after taking a dose.
■ Warn patient to avoid alcoholic beverages while taking drug.

- Urge patient to ensure adequate fluid intake to increase urine output and facilitate the excretion of uric acid.
- Advise patient to avoid exposure to people with infections. Tell patient to immediately report signs of unusual bleeding or infection.
- Advise women of childbearing age not to become pregnant while taking drug.

# meropenem
Merrem I.V.

*Pharmacologic classification:* carbapenem derivative
*Therapeutic classification:* antibiotic
*Pregnancy risk category B*

## Available forms
Available by prescription only
*Powder for injection:* 500 mg/15 ml, 500 mg/20 ml, 500 mg/100 ml, 1 g/15 ml, 1 g/30 ml, 1 g/100 ml

## Indications and dosages
*Complicated appendicitis and peritonitis caused by viridans group streptococci,* Escherichia coli, Klebsiella pneumoniae, Pseudomonas aeruginosa, Bacteroides fragilis, B. thetaiotaomicron, *and* Peptostreptococcus *species; bacterial meningitis caused by* Streptococcus pneumoniae, Haemophilus influenzae, *and* Neisseria meningitidis
**Recommended level not to exceed 50 mg/ml**
*Adults:* Administer 1 g I.V. q 8 hours over 15 to 30 minutes as I.V. infusion or over about 3 to 5 minutes as I.V. bolus injection (5 to 20 ml).
*Children ages 3 months and older weighing 50 kg (110 lb) or less:* Give 20 mg/kg (intraabdominal infection) or 40 mg/kg (bacterial meningitis) q 8 hours over 15 to 30 minutes as I.V. infusion or over about 3 to 5 minutes as I.V. bolus injection (5 to 20 ml).
　　Note: For children weighing over 50 kg, give 1 g q 8 hours for treating intra-abdominal infections and 2 g q 8 hours for treating meningitis.
≡*Dosage adjustment.* For adults with renal impairment, give 1 g q 12 hours if creatinine clearance is 26 to 50 ml/minute, 500 mg q 12 hours if it's 10 to 25 ml/minute, and 500 mg q 24 hours if it's less than 10 ml/minute. There's no clinical experience in children with renal impairment.

## I.V. administration
- For I.V. bolus administration, add 10 ml of sterile water for injection to 500 mg/20-ml vial size or 20 ml to 1 g/30-ml vial size to provide concentration of 50 mg/ml. Shake to dissolve and let stand until clear.
- For I.V. infusion, infusion vials (500 mg/100 ml and 1 g/100 ml) may be directly reconstituted with a compatible infusion fluid to provide a concentration of 2.5 to 50 mg/ml. Alternatively, an injection vial may be reconstituted, then the resulting solution added to an I.V. container and further diluted with an appropriate infusion fluid.
- For ADD-Vantage vials, reconstitute only with half-normal saline injection, normal saline injection, or $D_5W$ injection in 50-, 100-, or 250-ml Abbott ADD-Vantage flexible diluent containers. Follow manufacturer guidelines closely when using ADD-Vantage vials.
- Drug should be infused over 15 to 30 minutes.

## Incompatibilities
Don't mix with or physically add meropenem to solutions containing other drugs.

## Mechanism of action
*Antibiotic action:* Meropenem inhibits cell-wall synthesis in bacteria. It readily penetrates the cell wall of most gram-positive and gram-negative bacteria to reach penicillin-binding protein targets.

## Pharmacokinetics
*Absorption:* Administered I.V.
*Distribution:* Distributed into most body fluids and tissues, including CSF. It's only about 2% plasma protein–bound.
*Metabolism:* Thought to undergo minimal metabolism. One inactive metabolite has been identified.
*Excretion:* Excreted unchanged primarily in urine. Elimination half-life of drug in adults with normal renal function and children ages 2 and older is about 1 hour and 1½ hours in children ages 3 months to 2 years.

| Route | Onset | Peak | Duration |
|-------|-------|------|----------|
| I.V. | Unknown | 1 hr | Unknown |

## Contraindications and precautions
Contraindicated in patients hypersensitive to any component of drug or other drugs in the same class and in those who have shown anaphylactic reactions to beta-lactams. Use cautiously in patients with history of seizure disorders or impaired renal function.

## Interactions
**Drug-drug.** *Probenecid:* Competes with meropenem for active tubular secretion and thus inhibits the renal excretion of meropenem. Sometimes used together for this effect.

## Adverse reactions
**CNS:** headache, syncope, insomnia, agitation, delirium, confusion, dizziness, *seizures,* nervousness, paresthesia, hallucinations, somnolence, anxiety, depression.

**CV:** *HF, cardiac arrest, MI, pulmonary embolism,* tachycardia, chest pain, hypertension, *bradycardia,* hypotension.

**GI:** diarrhea, nausea, vomiting, constipation, abdominal pain or enlargement, oral candidiasis, anorexia.

**GU:** dysuria, *renal failure,* increased creatinine clearance or BUN levels, presence of RBCs in urine.

**Hematologic:** anemia, increased or decreased platelet count, increased eosinophil count, prolonged or shortened PT and INR or PTT, positive direct or indirect Coombs' test, decreased hemoglobin or hematocrit, decreased WBC count.

**Hepatic:** *hepatic failure,* cholestatic jaundice, jaundice, flatulence, ileus; increased levels of ALT, AST, alkaline phosphatase, LDH, and bilirubin.

**Musculoskeletal:** back pain.

**Respiratory:** *apnea, hypoxia,* respiratory disorder, dyspnea.

**Skin:** rash, pruritus, urticaria, sweating.

**Other:** hypersensitivity, *anaphylactic reactions;* inflammation, pain, edema, phlebitis, or thrombophlebitis at injection site; bleeding events, pain, *sepsis, shock,* fever, peripheral edema.

## Overdose and treatment

Signs and symptoms and treatment of overdose are unknown. If overdose occurs, discontinue drug and give general supportive treatment until renal elimination occurs. Meropenem and its metabolite are readily dialyzable and effectively removed by hemodialysis.

## Clinical considerations

■ Don't use to treat methicillin-resistant staphylococci.

■ Obtain specimen for culture and sensitivity tests before giving first dose. Therapy may begin pending test results.

**H** *ALERT* Serious and occasionally fatal hypersensitivity (anaphylactic) reactions have been reported in patients receiving therapy with beta-lactams. Before therapy starts, it should be known if previous hypersensitivity reactions to penicillins, cephalosporins, other beta-lactams, and other allergens have occurred.

■ Drug should be stopped immediately if an allergic reaction occurs. Serious anaphylactic reactions require immediate emergency treatment with epinephrine, oxygen, I.V. steroids, and airway management. Other therapy may also be required as indicated by the patient's condition.

■ Seizures and other CNS adverse reactions from meropenem therapy commonly occur in patients with CNS disorders, bacterial meningitis, and compromised renal function.

■ If seizures occur during meropenem therapy, dosage should be decreased or meropenem stopped.

■ Use freshly prepared solutions of meropenem immediately whenever possible. Stability of drug varies with type of drug used (injection vial, infusion vial, or ADD-Vantage container). Consult manufacturer's literature for details.

### Therapeutic monitoring

■ Drug may cause overgrowth of nonsusceptible bacteria or fungi. Advise clinician to monitor patient for signs and symptoms of superinfection.

■ Periodic assessment of organ system functions, including renal, hepatic, and hematopoietic, is recommended during prolonged therapy.

### Special populations

**Breast-feeding patients.** It isn't known if drug appears in breast milk; use cautiously in breast-feeding women.

**Pediatric patients.** Safety and efficacy haven't been established in children under age 3 months.

**Geriatric patients.** Use cautiously in geriatric patients because of decreased renal function. Dosage adjustment is recommended in patients with advanced age whose creatinine clearance levels are less than 50 ml/minute.

### Patient counseling

■ Tell patient to report pain, inflammation or swelling at I.V. site to prescriber.

■ Advise breast-feeding patient of risk of transmitting drug to infant through breast milk.

■ Instruct patient to report adverse reactions or symptoms of superinfection to prescriber.

# mesalamine (5-aminosalicylic acid)

Asacol, Pentasa, Rowasa

*Pharmacologic classification:* salicylate
*Therapeutic classification:* anti-inflammatory
*Pregnancy risk category B*

## Available forms

Available by prescription only
*Capsules (controlled-release):* 250 mg
*Tablets (delayed-release):* 400 mg
*Suppositories:* 500 mg
*Rectal suspension:* 4 g/60 ml, in units of seven disposable bottles

## Indications and dosages

***Active mild to moderate distal ulcerative colitis, proctosigmoiditis, proctitis***
*Adults:* 800 mg (delayed-release tablets) P.O. t.i.d. for 6 weeks or 1 g (controlled-release capsules) q.i.d. for up to 8 weeks.

Alternatively, 1 rectal suppository b.i.d. for 3 to 6 weeks. For maximum benefit, the suppository should be retained for 1 to 3 hours or longer. Usual dosage of mesalamine suspension enema in 60-ml units is one rectal instillation (4 g) once daily, preferably h.s., retained for about 8 hours.

◇ Lower doses of suspension enemas of 4 g q 2 to 3 nights or 1 g daily have been effective.
◇ *Maintenance of remission of ulcerative colitis*
*Adults:* 1.6 g P.O. daily in divided doses for 6 months. Alternatively, 60 ml (4 g) rectal suspension q 2 to 3 nights or 1 to 3 g rectal suspension daily.

## Mechanism of action

*Anti-inflammatory action:* Mechanism of action of mesalamine (and sulfasalazine) is unknown, but appears to be topical rather than systemic. Mucosal production of arachidonic acid (AA) metabolites, both through cyclooxygenase pathways (such as prostaglandins [PGs]) and lipoxygenase pathways (such as leukotrienes [LTs] and hydroxyeicosatetraenoic acids [HETEs]) is increased in patients with chronic inflammatory bowel disease; possibly, mesalamine may diminish inflammation by blocking cyclooxygenase and inhibiting PG production in the colon.

Sulfasalazine is split by bacterial action in the colon into sulfapyridine (SP) and mesalamine (5-ASA). The mesalamine component is considered therapeutically active in ulcerative colitis.

## Pharmacokinetics

*Absorption:* Drug administered rectally as a suppository or suspension enema is poorly absorbed from the colon. Extent of absorption depends on retention time, with considerable individual variation. Oral tablets are coated with an acrylic resin that delays the release of drug until tablet is beyond the terminal ileum. About 72% of a dose reaches the colon; 28% of a dose is absorbed. Absorption isn't affected by food. Capsules are formulated to release therapeutic levels throughout the GI tract. About 20% to 30% is absorbed.
*Distribution:* Maximum plasma levels of oral mesalamine and *N*-acetyl 5-ASA are about twice as high as those seen with sulfasalazine therapy. At steady state, about 10% to 30% of daily 4-g rectal dose can be recovered in cumulative 24-hour urine collections.
*Metabolism:* Undergoes acetylation, but site is unknown. Most absorbed drug is excreted in urine as the *N*-acetyl-5-ASA metabolite. Elimination half-life of drug is ½ to 1½ hours; half-life of acetylated metabolite is 5 to 10 hours. Steady-state plasma levels show no accumulation of either free or metabolized drug during repeated daily administrations.

*Excretion:* After rectal administration, drug is mostly excreted in the feces as parent drug and metabolite. After oral administration, drug is mostly excreted in the urine as metabolite.

| Route | Onset | Peak | Duration |
| --- | --- | --- | --- |
| P.O., P.R. | Unknown | 3-12 hr | Unknown |

## Contraindications and precautions

Contraindicated in patients allergic to mesalamine, salicylates, or components of the preparation; also contraindicated in children. Use cautiously in geriatric, pregnant, and breast-feeding patients, and in those with renal dysfunction.

## Interactions

None reported.

## Adverse reactions

**CNS:** headache, dizziness, fatigue, malaise, asthenia, chills, anxiety, depression, hyperesthesia, paresthesia, tremor.
**CV:** chest pain.
**GI:** abdominal pain, cramps, discomfort, flatulence, diarrhea, rectal pain, bloating, nausea, *pancolitis,* **pancreatitis,** vomiting, constipation, eructation.
**GU:** dysuria, hematuria, urinary urgency.
**Musculoskeletal:** arthralgia, myalgia, back pain.
**Respiratory:** wheezing.
**Skin:** itching, rash, urticaria, hair loss.
**Other:** *anaphylaxis,* fever, hypertonia.

## Overdose and treatment

No information available.

## Clinical considerations

■ Drug has been used to treat Crohn's disease.
■ Rectal suspension contains potassium metabisulfite, which may produce an allergic reaction in susceptible individuals.
■ While effects of drug may be evident in 3 to 21 days, usual course of therapy is 3 to 6 weeks depending on symptoms and sigmoidoscopic findings. Clinical studies haven't determined if suspension enema will modify relapse rates after the 6-week, short-term treatment.

### Therapeutic monitoring

■ Advise clinician to monitor renal function test results during therapy.

### Special populations

**Breast-feeding patients.** It isn't known if drug or its metabolites appear in breast milk. Avoid breast-feeding during therapy.
**Pediatric patients.** Safety and efficacy for use in children haven't been established.

## Patient counseling

■ Tell patient to swallow tablets whole and not to crush or chew them.

■ Tell patient to retain suppository as long as possible (at least 1 to 3 hours) for maximum effectiveness.

■ Instruct patient in correct use of rectal suspension:

– Shake bottle well to make sure the suspension is homogeneous.

– Remove the protective sheath from the applicator tip. Holding the bottle at the neck will not cause drug to be discharged.

– To administer, lie on the left side (to facilitate migration into the sigmoid colon) with the lower leg extended and the upper right leg flexed forward for balance; or may use the knee-chest position.

– Gently insert the applicator tip in the rectum, pointing toward the umbilicus.

– Steadily squeeze the bottle to discharge the preparation into the colon.

■ Patient instructions are included with every seven units.

---

## mesna
Mesnex

*Pharmacologic classification:* thiol derivative
*Therapeutic classification:* uroprotectant
*Pregnancy risk category B*

---

### Available forms
Available by prescription only
*Injection:* 100 mg/ml in 2- and 10-ml ampules

### Indications and dosages
**Prevention of ifosfamide-induced hemorrhagic cystitis**
*Adults:* Calculate daily dose as 60% of the ifosfamide dose. Give in three equally divided bolus doses: Give first dose at time of ifosfamide injection. Subsequent doses are given at 4 and 8 hours following ifosfamide. Alternatively, give dose in four divided doses just before ifosfamide dose, then at 4, 8, and 12 hours after ifosfamide; or, at time of ifosfamide dose and then at 3, 6, and 9 hours after ifosfamide dose.

Protocols that use 1.2 g/m² ifosfamide would employ 240 mg/m² mesna at 0, 4, and 8 hours after ifosfamide.

◇ Continuous mesna I.V. infusion is given at 100% ifosfamide dosage and may be mixed in the same I.V. solution. Continue regimen as long as ifosfamide is given; it may have to continue for additional 8 to 24 hours as a result of shorter mesna half-life.

◇ *Prophylaxis in bone marrow recipients receiving cyclophosphamides*
*Adults:* 60% to 160% of the cyclophosphamide daily dose given in three to five divided doses or by continuous infusion. Alternatively, in patients receiving cyclophosphamide, 50 to 60 mg/kg I.V. daily for 2 to 4 days; give

10 mg/kg I.V. loading dose of mesna followed by 60 mg/kg by way of continuous I.V. infusion over 24 hours. Give mesna regimen with each cyclophosphamide dose and continue for an additional 24 hours.

### I.V. administration
■ Dilute appropriate dose in D₅W injection, normal saline solution injection, or lactated Ringer's injection to a level of 20 mg/ml. Once diluted, solution is stable for 24 hours at room temperature. However, the manufacturer recommends refrigerating the solution and using within 6 hours (contains no preservatives).

■ Infuse I.V. solution over 15 to 30 minutes.

*Incompatibilities*
Incompatible with cisplatin.

### Mechanism of action
*Uroprotectant action:* Mesna disulfide is reduced to mesna in the kidney and reacts with the urotoxic metabolites of ifosfamide to detoxify the drug and protect the urinary system.

### Pharmacokinetics
*Absorption:* Administered I.V.
*Distribution:* Remains in the vascular compartment; doesn't distribute through tissues.
*Metabolism:* Rapidly metabolized to mesna disulfide, its only metabolite.
*Excretion:* In the kidneys, 33% of the dose is eliminated in the urine in 24 hours; half-life of mesna and mesna disulfide are ½ and 1¼ hours, respectively.

| Route | Onset | Peak | Duration |
|-------|-------|------|----------|
| I.V. | Unknown | Unknown | Unknown |

### Contraindications and precautions
Contraindicated in patients hypersensitive to mesna or thiol-containing compounds.

### Interactions
None reported.

### Adverse reactions
**CNS:** headache, fatigue.
**CV:** hypotension.
**GI:** soft stools, nausea, vomiting, diarrhea, dysgeusia.
**Musculoskeletal:** limb pain.
**Other:** *allergy.*

### Overdose and treatment
No information available. There's no known antidote.

### Clinical considerations
■ Because mesna is used with ifosfamide and other chemotherapeutic drugs, it's difficult to determine adverse reactions attributable solely to mesna.

---

■ The parenteral form of the drug has been administered orally by preparing extemporaneous oral solutions by mixing injection with flavored syrup to produce a concentration of 20 to 50 mg/ml. Solutions are stable for 7 days at 75° F (24° C). If carbonated beverages, apple juice, or orange juice is used, solution is stable for at least 24 hours at 41° F (5° C).

■ Patients receiving mesna for ifosfamide-induced hemorrhagic cystitis should be adequately hydrated (2 L of oral or I.V. fluid before and during ifosfamide therapy).

■ Mesnex multidose vials may be stored and used for up to 8 days.

■ Discard unused mesna from open ampules. It will form an inactive oxidation product (dimesna) upon exposure to oxygen.

■ Mesna is physically incompatible with cisplatin or carboplatin. Don't add mesna to cisplatin infusions.

■ Store drug at 59° to 86° F (15° to 30° C); expires 5 years from date of manufacture.

■ Mesna may produce a false-positive test for urinary ketones. A red-violet color will return to violet with the addition of glacial acetic acid.

### Therapeutic monitoring
■ Advise clinician to monitor morning urine specimen for erythrocytes, which may precede hemorrhagic cystitis.

### Special populations
**Breast-feeding patients.** It isn't known if mesna appears in breast milk.

**Pediatric patients.** Safety in children hasn't been established. However, drug has been used for prophylaxis of ifosfamide-induced hemorrhagic cystitis in infants and children ages 4 to 16 and for prophylaxis of cyclophosphamide-induced hemorrhagic cystitis in children ages 5 months and older.

Note: Multidose vials contain benzyl alcohol.

### Patient counseling
■ Instruct patient to report hematuria or allergy immediately.

## mesoridazine besylate
Serentil

*Pharmacologic classification:* phenothiazine (piperidine derivative)
*Therapeutic classification:* antipsychotic drug
*Pregnancy risk category NR*

### Available forms
Available by prescription only
*Tablets:* 10 mg, 25 mg, 50 mg, 100 mg
*Oral concentrate:* 25 mg/ml (0.6% alcohol)
*Injection:* 25 mg/ml

## Indications and dosages
*Psychotic disorders*
**Adults:** Initially, 50 mg P.O. t.i.d. to maximum of 400 mg/day; or 25 mg I.M. repeated in 30 to 60 minutes, p.r.n., not to exceed 200 mg I.M. daily.

## Mechanism of action
*Antipsychotic action:* Mesoridazine, a metabolite of thioridazine, is thought to exert its antipsychotic effects by postsynaptic blockade of CNS dopamine receptors, thereby inhibiting dopamine-mediated effects.

Drug has many other central and peripheral effects; it produces both alpha and ganglionic blockade and counteracts histamine- and serotonin-mediated activity. Its most prominent adverse reactions are antimuscarinic and sedative; it causes fewer extrapyramidal effects than other antipsychotics.

## Pharmacokinetics
*Absorption:* Appears to be well absorbed from the GI tract following oral administration. I.M. dosage form is absorbed rapidly.
*Distribution:* Distributed widely into the body; appears in breast milk. Steady-state serum level is achieved within 4 to 7 days. Drug is 91% to 99% protein-bound.
*Metabolism:* Metabolized extensively by the liver; no active metabolites are formed.
*Excretion:* Mostly excreted as metabolites in urine; some excreted in feces via biliary tract.

| Route | Onset | Peak | Duration |
|-------|-------|------|----------|
| P.O., I.M. | Unknown | 2-4 hr | 4-6 hr |

## Contraindications and precautions
Contraindicated in patients hypersensitive to drug or in those experiencing severe CNS depression or comatose states.

## Interactions
**Drug-drug.** *Aluminum- and magnesium-containing antacids and antidiarrheals:* Decreased absorption. Separate administration times.
*Antiarrhythmics, disopyramide, procainamide, quinidine:* Increased risk of arrhythmias and conduction defects. Avoid use together.
*Atropine and other anticholinergics, including antidepressants, antihistamines, MAO inhibitors, meperidine, phenothiazines, and antiparkinsonians:* Oversedation, paralytic ileus, visual changes, and severe constipation. Use together cautiously.
*Beta blockers:* May inhibit mesoridazine metabolism, increasing plasma levels and toxicity. Advise clinician to monitor patient for signs of toxicity.
*Bromocriptine:* Mesoridazine may antagonize therapeutic effect of bromocriptine on prolactin secretion. Use together cautiously.

*Centrally acting antihypertensives, such as clonidine, guanabenz, guanadrel, guanethidine, methyldopa, and reserpine:* Mesoridazine may inhibit blood pressure response to these drugs. Advise clinician to monitor blood pressure frequently.

*CNS depressants, including analgesics, barbiturates, opioids, tranquilizers, and general, spinal, or epidural anesthetics, or parenteral magnesium sulfate:* Oversedation, respiratory depression, and hypotension. Avoid use together.

*High-dose dopamine:* Decreased vasoconstricting effects. Advise clinician to monitor patient for clinical effects.

*Levodopa:* Decreased effectiveness and increased toxicity of levodopa. Use together cautiously.

*Lithium:* May result in severe neurologic toxicity with an encephalitis-like syndrome and a decreased therapeutic response to mesoridazine. Avoid use together.

*Metrizamide:* Increased risk of seizures. Use together cautiously.

*Nitrates:* Hypotension. Advise clinician to monitor blood pressure.

*Phenobarbital:* Enhanced renal excretion of mesoridazine. Advise clinician to monitor patient for clinical effects.

*Phenytoin:* Mesoridazine may inhibit metabolism and increase toxicity of phenytoin. Decreased phenytoin dosage may be needed.

*Propylthiouracil:* Increased risk of agranulocytosis. Advise clinician to monitor hematopoietic studies.

*Sympathomimetics, including epinephrine, phenylephrine, phenylpropanolamine, and ephedrine (often found in nasal sprays), or appetite suppressants:* May decrease their stimulatory and pressor effects. Use together cautiously.

**Drug-food.** *Caffeine:* Increased metabolism of drug. Advise patient to limit caffeine use.

**Drug-lifestyle.** *Alcohol use:* Additive effects. Advise patient to avoid alcohol.

*Heavy smoking:* Increased metabolism. Advise patient to avoid smoking.

*Sun exposure:* Increased risk of photosensitivity reactions. Recommend patient use sun screen or limit exposure.

## Adverse reactions

**CNS:** *neuroleptic malignant syndrome,* extrapyramidal reactions, *tardive dyskinesia, sedation, drowsiness, tremor, rigidity, weakness, EEG changes, dizziness.*

**CV:** *hypotension, tachycardia, ECG changes.*

**EENT:** *ocular changes, blurred vision, retinitis pigmentosa, nasal congestion.*

**GI:** *dry mouth, constipation, nausea, vomiting.*

**GU:** *urine retention, menstrual irregularities, inhibited ejaculation.*

**Hematologic:** *leukopenia, agranulocytosis, aplastic anemia,* eosinophilia, *thrombocytopenia.*

**Hepatic:** jaundice, abnormal liver function test results.

**Metabolic:** weight gain, elevated tests for protein-bound iodine.

**Skin:** *mild photosensitivity, allergic reactions, pain at I.M. injection site, sterile abscess, rash.*

**Other:** *gynecomastia.*

**After abrupt withdrawal of long-term therapy:** gastritis, nausea, vomiting, dizziness, tremor, feeling of warmth or cold, diaphoresis, tachycardia, headache, insomnia.

## Overdose and treatment

CNS depression is characterized by deep, unarousable sleep and possible coma, hypotension or hypertension, extrapyramidal symptoms, abnormal involuntary muscle movements, agitation, seizures, arrhythmias, ECG changes, hypothermia or hyperthermia, and autonomic nervous system dysfunction.

Treatment is symptomatic and supportive, including maintaining vital signs, airway, stable body temperature, and fluid and electrolyte balance.

Vomiting shouldn't be induced; drug inhibits cough reflex, and aspiration may occur. Recommend using gastric lavage, then activated charcoal and saline cathartics; dialysis doesn't help. Body temperature should be regulated p.r.n. Recommend treating hypotension with I.V. fluids; epinephrine shouldn't be given. Recommend treating seizures with parenteral diazepam or barbiturates; arrhythmias, with parenteral phenytoin (15 mg to 18 mg/kg not exceeding 50 mg/min, with rate titrated to blood pressure); recommend treating extrapyramidal reactions with benztropine at 1 to 2 mg or parenteral diphenhydramine at 10 to 50 mg.

## Clinical considerations

**⚠ ALERT** Dose-related serious cardiac adverse effects, including torsades de pointes, and sudden death have been reported with drug therapy.

■ I.M. form is irritating.

■ Mesoridazine causes false-positive test results for urinary porphyrins, urobilinogen, amylase, and 5-hydroxyindoleacetic acid because of darkening of urine by metabolites; it also causes false-positive urine pregnancy test results using human chorionic gonadotropin.

### Therapeutic monitoring

■ Recommend obtaining baseline ECG and serum potassium and periodically thereafter, especially during dosage adjustment.

■ Advise clinician to monitor vital signs, especially during parenteral therapy.

■ Advise clinician to monitor hematopoietic and liver function test results.

## Patient counseling
- Warn patient to avoid activities that require alertness and good psychomotor coordination until CNS effects of drug are known. Tell patient that drowsiness and dizziness usually subside after a few weeks.
- Advise patient to change position slowly.
- Warn patient to avoid alcohol while taking this drug.
- Instruct patient to relieve dry mouth with sugarless gum or hard candy.
- Advise patient to use sunblock and to wear protective clothing to avoid photosensitivity reactions.

# metaproterenol sulfate
Alupent

*Pharmacologic classification:* adrenergic
*Therapeutic classification:* bronchodilator
*Pregnancy risk category C*

## Available forms
Available by prescription only
*Tablets:* 10 mg, 20 mg
*Syrup:* 10 mg/5 ml
*Aerosol inhaler:* 0.65 mg/metered spray
*Nebulizer inhaler:* 0.4%, 0.6%, 5% solution

## Indications and dosages
**Bronchial asthma and reversible bronchospasm**
**Oral**
*Adults and children over age 9 or weighing over 27 kg (60 lb):* 20 mg P.O. t.i.d. or q.i.d.
*Children ages 6 to 9 or weighing under 27 kg:* 10 mg P.O. t.i.d. or q.i.d.
◊ *Children under age 6:* 1.3 to 2.6 mg/kg P.O. daily in divided doses.
**Inhalation**
*Adults and children ages 12 and older:* Administered by metered aerosol, 2 or 3 inhalations q 3 to 4 hours with at least 2 minutes between inhalations; no more than 12 inhalations in 24 hours. Administered by hand-bulb nebulizer, 10 inhalations of an undiluted 5% solution or, alternatively, administered by intermittent positive pressure breathing, 0.3 ml (range, 0.2 to 0.3 ml of a 5% solution diluted in about 2.5 ml of a normal saline solution or 2.5 ml of a commercially available 0.4% or 0.6% solution for nebulization).
*Children ages 6 to 11:* 0.1 ml (range 0.1 to 0.2 ml) of 5% solution diluted with normal saline solution to final volume of 3 ml. Administer by nebulizer.
Note: To relieve acute bronchospasm, usually don't need to repeat more than q 4 hours. If part of bronchospastic pulmonary disease treatment regimen, give three to four times daily.

## Mechanism of action
*Bronchodilator action:* Metaproterenol relaxes bronchial smooth muscle and peripheral vasculature by stimulating beta$_2$-adrenergic receptors, thus decreasing airway resistance by way of bronchodilation. It has lesser effect on beta$_1$ receptors and has little or no effect on alpha-adrenergic receptors. In high doses, it may cause CNS and cardiac stimulation, resulting in tachycardia, hypertension, or tremors.

## Pharmacokinetics
*Absorption:* Well-absorbed from the GI tract.
*Distribution:* Widely distributed throughout the body.
*Metabolism:* Extensively metabolized on first pass through the liver.
*Excretion:* Excreted in urine, mainly as glucuronic acid conjugates.

| Route | Onset | Peak | Duration |
|---|---|---|---|
| P.O. | 15 min | 1 hr | 1-4 hr |
| Inhalation | 1 min | 1 hr | 1-2½ hr |
| Nebulizer | 5-30 min | 1 hr | 1-2½ hr |

## Contraindications and precautions
Contraindicated in patients hypersensitive to drug or its ingredients, in use during anesthesia with cyclopropane or halogenated hydrocarbon general anesthetics, and in those with tachycardia and arrhythmias caused by tachycardia, peripheral or mesenteric vascular thrombosis, profound hypoxia, or hypercapnia.
Use cautiously in patients with hypertension, hyperthyroidism, heart disease, diabetes, or cirrhosis and in those receiving cardiac glycosides.

## Interactions
**Drug-drug.** *Beta blockers, especially propranolol:* Antagonize bronchodilating effects of metaproterenol. Avoid use together.
*General anesthetics (especially chloroform, cyclopropane, halothane, trichloroethylene), cardiac glycosides, levodopa, theophylline derivatives, thyroid hormones:* May increase the potential for cardiac effects, including severe ventricular tachycardia, arrhythmias, and coronary insufficiency. Use together cautiously.
*MAO inhibitors, tricyclic antidepressants:* May potentiate their CV actions. Use together cautiously.
*Other sympathomimetics:* May produce additive effects and toxicity. Use together cautiously.
*Xanthines, other sympathomimetics, other CNS-stimulating drugs:* Increased CNS stimulation. Advise clinician to monitor patient closely.

---

## Adverse reactions

**CNS:** *nervousness, weakness, drowsiness, tremor, vertigo, headache.*
**CV:** *tachycardia, hypertension, palpitations, **cardiac arrest** (with excessive use).*
**GI:** *vomiting, nausea, heartburn, dry mouth.*
**Respiratory: *paradoxical bronchiolar constriction with excessive use,* cough, dry and irritated throat.
**Skin:** rash, hypersensitivity reactions.

## Overdose and treatment

Signs and symptoms of overdose include exaggeration of common adverse reactions, particularly nausea and vomiting, arrhythmias, angina, hypertension, and seizures.

Treatment includes supportive and symptomatic measures. Advise clinician to monitor vital signs closely. Recommend supporting CV status. Recommend using cardioselective beta blockers (acebutolol, atenolol, metoprolol) with extreme caution to treat symptoms; they may induce severe bronchospasm or asthmatic attack.

## Clinical considerations

- Adverse reactions are dose-related and characteristic of sympathomimetics, and may persist a long time because of the long duration of action of metaproterenol.
- Excessive or prolonged use may lead to decreased effectiveness.
- Avoid simultaneous administration of adrenocorticoid inhalation aerosol. Allow at least 5 minutes to lapse between using the two aerosols.
- Aerosol treatments may be used with oral tablet dosing.
- Store tablets and oral solution at 59° to 86° F (15° to 30° C) in tight, light-resistant containers. Store oral inhalation and nebulizer solution at 50° to 86° F (15° to 30° C).
- Drug may reduce sensitivity of spirometry in diagnosis of asthma.

### Therapeutic monitoring

- Advise clinician to monitor patient for signs and symptoms of toxic effects, such as nausea and vomiting, tremors, and arrhythmias.

### Special populations

**Pediatric patients.** Oral inhalation in children under age 12 isn't recommended because safety and efficacy haven't been established. Safety and efficacy of oral preparations in children under age 6 haven't been established.
**Geriatric patients.** Geriatric patients may be more sensitive to the therapeutic and adverse effects of drug.

## Patient counseling

- Instruct patient to use only as directed and to take no more than two inhalations at one time with 1- to 2-minute intervals between. Remind patient to save applicator; refills may be available.
- Tell patient to take missed dose if remembered within 1 hour. If beyond 1 hour, patient should skip dose and resume regular schedule. Patient shouldn't double the dose.
- Tell patient to store drug away from heat and light, and safely out of reach of children.
- Inform patient to immediately report if no relief occurs or condition worsens.
- Warn patient to avoid simultaneous use of adrenocorticoid aerosol and to allow at least 5 minutes to lapse between using the two aerosols.
- Tell patient that he may experience bad taste in mouth after using oral inhaler.
- Instruct patient to shake container, exhale through nose as completely as possible, then give aerosol while inhaling deeply through mouth, and hold breath for 10 seconds before exhaling slowly. Patient should wait 1 to 2 minutes before repeating inhalations.
- Tell patient that drug may have shorter duration of action after prolonged use. Advise patient to report failure to respond to usual dose.
- Warn patient not to increase dose or frequency unless prescribed; serious adverse reactions are possible.

# metaraminol bitartrate
Aramine

*Pharmacologic classification:* adrenergic
*Therapeutic classification:* vasopressor
*Pregnancy risk category C*

## Available forms

Available by prescription only
*Injection:* 10 mg/ml parenteral

## Indications and dosages

*Prevention of hypotension*
*Adults:* 2 to 10 mg I.M. or S.C. At least 10 minutes should elapse before repeat dosing.
*Children:* 0.1 mg/kg or 3 mg/m² S.C. or I.M.
*Hypotension in severe shock*
*Adults:* 0.5 to 5 mg direct I.V. followed by I.V. infusion. If needed, mix 15 to 100 mg (up to 500 mg has been used) in 500 ml normal saline solution or $D_5W$; titrate infusion based on blood pressure response.
*Children:* 0.01 mg/kg or 0.3 mg/m² direct I.V. followed by I.V. infusion (dilution of 1 mg in 25 ml of diluent) if needed, of 0.4 mg/kg or 12 mg/m² diluted and titrated to maintain desired blood pressure.
◊ *Priapism*
*Adults:* 1 to 2 mg injected into corpus cavernosum of the penis.

## I.V. administration

- Dilute drug before I.V. use. Preferred solutions for dilution are normal saline solution or D₅W injection.
- Injection site should be selected carefully. I.V. route is preferred, using large veins. Extravasation should be avoided.
- Advise clinician to monitor infusion rate; use of infusion-controlling device preferred.
- Drug should be withdrawn gradually; recurrent hypotension may follow abrupt withdrawal.

### Incompatibilities

Incompatible with amphotericin B, barbiturates, dexamethasone sodium phosphate, erythromycin lactobionate, fibrinogen, hydrocortisone sodium succinate, methicillin, methylprednisolone sodium succinate, penicillin G potassium, phenytoin sodium, prednisolone sodium phosphate, ranitidine, and thiopental.

## Mechanism of action

*Vasopressor action:* Drug acts predominantly by direct stimulation of alpha-adrenergic receptors, which constrict both capacitance and resistance blood vessels, resulting in increased total peripheral resistance; increased systolic and diastolic blood pressure; decreased blood flow to vital organs, skin, and skeletal muscle; and constriction of renal blood vessels, which reduces renal blood flow. It also has a direct stimulating effect on beta₁ receptors of the heart, producing a positive inotropic response, and an indirect effect, releasing norepinephrine from its storage sites, which, with repeated use, may result in tachyphylaxis. Metaraminol also acts as a weak or false neurotransmitter by replacing norepinephrine in sympathetic nerve endings. Its main effects are vasoconstriction and cardiac stimulation. It doesn't usually cause CNS stimulation but may cause contraction of pregnant uterus and uterine blood vessels because of its alpha-adrenergic effects.

## Pharmacokinetics

*Absorption:* Pressor effects may persist 20 to 90 minutes, depending on route of administration and patient variability.
*Distribution:* Not completely known.
*Metabolism:* In vitro tests suggest that metaraminol is not metabolized. Effects appear to be terminated by uptake of drug into tissues and by urinary excretion.
*Excretion:* Excreted in urine; may be accelerated by acidifying urine.

| Route | Onset | Peak | Duration |
|-------|-------|------|----------|
| I.V. | 1-2 min | Unknown | 20 min |
| I.M. | 10 min | Unknown | < 90 min |
| S.C. | 5-20 min | Unknown | < 90 min |

## Contraindications and precautions

Contraindicated in patients hypersensitive to drug and in those receiving anesthesia with cyclopropane and halogenated hydrocarbon anesthetics.

Use cautiously in patients with cardiac or thyroid disease, hypertension, peripheral vascular disease, cirrhosis, history of malaria, or sulfite sensitivity; in those receiving cardiac glycosides; and during pregnancy.

## Interactions

**Drug-drug.** *Alpha adrenergic blockers:* Pressor effects may be decreased, but not completely blocked. Use together cautiously.
*Atropine:* Blocks the reflex bradycardia caused by metaraminol and enhances its pressor response. Use together cautiously.
*Beta blockers:* Mutual inhibition of therapeutic effects with increased potential for hypertension, and excessive bradycardia with possible heart block. Avoid use together.
*Cardiac glycosides, general anesthetics, levodopa, maprotiline, other sympathomimetics, thyroid hormones:* Increased cardiac effects may result. Use together cautiously.
*Doxapram, ergot alkaloids, mazindol, methylphenidate, trimethaphan:* Possible increased pressor effects. Use together cautiously.
*Guanadrel, guanethidine, rauwolfia alkaloids, diuretics used as antihypertensives:* Decreased hypotensive effects. Advise clinician to monitor blood pressure frequently.
*MAO inhibitors:* Possible prolonged and intensified cardiac stimulant and vasopressor effects. Don't give metaraminol until 14 days after MAO inhibitors have been discontinued.

## Adverse reactions

**CNS:** apprehension, dizziness, headache, tremor.
**CV:** hypertension; hypotension; palpitations; ***arrhythmias,*** including sinus or ***ventricular tachycardia; cardiac arrest.***
**GI:** nausea.
**Skin:** flushing, diaphoresis.
**Other:** abscess, necrosis, sloughing upon extravasation.

## Overdose and treatment

Signs and symptoms of overdose include severe hypertension, arrhythmias, seizures, cerebral hemorrhage, acute pulmonary edema, and cardiac arrest.

Treatment requires discontinuation of drug followed by supportive and symptomatic measures. Advise clinician to monitor vital signs closely. Recommend using atropine for reflex bradycardia and propranolol for tachyarrhythmias. Recommend using a sympatholytic drug to relieve hypertension.

---

## Clinical considerations

■ Commercial preparations contain sodium bisulfite, which may cause allergic reactions in susceptible individuals.

■ Recommend correcting blood volume depletion before administration. Metaraminol isn't a substitute for blood, plasma, fluids, or electrolyte replacement.

■ When administering I.M. or S.C., at least 10 minutes should elapse before additional doses are given because maximum effect isn't immediately apparent.

■ To treat extravasation, recommend infiltrating site promptly with 10 to 15 ml normal saline solution containing 5 to 10 mg phentolamine, using fine needle.

■ Cumulative effect possible after prolonged use. Excessive vasopressor response may persist after drug is withdrawn.

■ Recommend keeping emergency drugs on hand to reverse effect of metaraminol: atropine for reflex bradycardia, phentolamine for extravasation, and propranolol for tachyarrhythmias.

■ Don't mix in bag or syringe with other drugs.

### Therapeutic monitoring

■ Blood pressure, heart rate and rhythm should be checked during and after metaraminol administration until patient is stable.

■ Advise clinician to monitor diabetic patients closely. Insulin adjustments may be needed.

■ Advise clinician to monitor fluid and electrolyte status carefully.

### Special populations

**Breast-feeding patients.** It isn't known if drug appears in breast milk. Use cautiously in breast-feeding women.

**Pediatric patients.** Because safety hasn't been fully established, use cautiously.

**Geriatric patients.** Geriatric patients may be more sensitive to effects of drug.

### Patient counseling

■ Ask patient about sulfite allergy before giving drug; vials contain sodium bisulfite.

■ Inform patient that he'll need frequent assessment of vital signs.

■ Advise patient to report adverse reactions.

---

# metformin hydrochloride

Glucophage, Glucophage XR

*Pharmacologic classification:*
biguanide
*Therapeutic classification:* antidiabetic
*Pregnancy risk category B*

### Available forms

Available by prescription only
*Tablets:* 500 mg, 850 mg, 1,000 mg
*Tablets (extended-release):* 500 mg

## Indications and dosages

*Adjunct to diet and exercise to lower blood glucose in patients with type 2 diabetes*

*Adults:* Initially, 500 mg P.O. b.i.d. with morning and evening meals or 850 mg P.O. once daily with morning meal. When 500-mg dose is used, increase dose by 500 mg weekly to maximum dose of 2,500 mg daily, p.r.n. Alternatively, 500 mg P.O. b.i.d. May be increased to 850 mg P.O. b.i.d. after 2 weeks. When 850-mg dose is used, increase dose 850 mg every other week to maximum daily dose of 2,550 mg, p.r.n.

Note: If patient requires more than 2 g daily, give in three divided doses.

For extended-release tablets: *Adults:* 500 mg P.O. daily with evening meal. May increase by 500 mg intervals to a maximum dose of 2 g daily.

Note: If 2 g daily dose not sufficient for glycemic control, may switch to 1 g b.i.d. If greater than 2 g daily dose is needed, patient should be switched to conventional form of metformin. (Maximum daily dose of conventional form is 2.5 g, given in divided doses.)

## Mechanism of action

*Antidiabetic action:* Drug decreases hepatic glucose production and intestinal absorption of glucose and improves insulin sensitivity (increases peripheral glucose uptake and utilization).

## Pharmacokinetics

*Absorption:* Absorbed from GI tract with absolute bioavailability being about 50% to 60%. Food decreases the extent and slightly delays absorption.

*Distribution:* Negligibly plasma protein–bound. It partitions into erythrocytes, most likely as a function of time.

*Metabolism:* Not metabolized.

*Excretion:* 90% is excreted in urine. Elimination half-life is about 6¼ hours in plasma and 17½ hours in blood.

| Route | Onset | Peak | Duration |
|-------|-------|------|----------|
| P.O. | Unknown | Unknown | Unknown |

## Contraindications and precautions

Contraindicated in patients with HF, renal disease, metabolic acidosis, and those with hypersensitivity to drug. Drug should be temporarily withheld in patients undergoing radiologic studies involving parenteral administration of iodinated contrast materials because use of such products may cause acute renal dysfunction. Drug should be stopped if a hypoxic state develops. Avoid use in patients with hepatic disease.

Use cautiously in geriatric, debilitated, or malnourished patients and in those with adrenal or pituitary insufficiency because of increased susceptibility to developing hypoglycemia.

---

## Interactions

**Drug-drug.** *Calcium channel blockers, corticosteroids, estrogens, isoniazid, nicotinic acid, oral contraceptives, phenothiazines, phenytoin, sympathomimetics, thiazides or other diuretics, thyroid hormones:* May produce hyperglycemia. Advise clinician to monitor patient's glycemic control. Metformin dosage may need to be increased.

*Cationic drugs such as amiloride, cimetidine, digoxin, morphine, procainamide, quinidine, quinine, ranitidine, triamterene, trimethoprim, vancomycin:* Potential to compete for common renal tubular transport systems, which may increase metformin plasma levels. Advise clinician to monitor patient's blood glucose level.

*Nifedipine:* Increased metformin plasma levels. Advise clinician to monitor patient closely. Metformin dosage may need to be decreased.

## Adverse reactions

**GI:** unpleasant or metallic taste, diarrhea, nausea, vomiting, abdominal bloating, flatulence, anorexia.
**Hematologic:** *megaloblastic anemia.*
**Metabolic:** *lactic acidosis.*
**Skin:** rash, dermatitis.

## Overdose and treatment

Hypoglycemia hasn't been observed with ingestion of up to 85 g of metformin, although lactic acidosis has occurred. Hemodialysis may be useful for removing accumulated drug from patients in whom metformin overdose is suspected.

## Clinical considerations

■ Advise clinician to give drug with meals; recommend giving conventional form once-daily dose with breakfast, twice-daily dose with breakfast and dinner. Advise clinician to give extended-release form once daily dose with dinner.

■ When transferring patients from standard oral hypoglycemic drugs other than chlorpropamide to metformin, no transition period is needed. When transferring patients from chlorpropamide, recommend using caution during the first 2 weeks because of prolonged retention of chlorpropamide in the body, increasing risk of hypoglycemia during this time.

■ If patient doesn't respond to 4 weeks of maximum dose of metformin, recommend adding an oral sulfonylurea while continuing metformin at the maximum dose. If patient still doesn't respond after several months of concomitant therapy at maximum doses, recommend stopping both drugs and starting insulin therapy.

■ Risk of drug-induced lactic acidosis is very low. Reported cases have occurred primarily in diabetic patients with significant renal insufficiency, multiple concomitant medical or surgical problems, and multiple concomitant drugs. Risk of lactic acidosis increases with advanced age and degree of renal impairment.

■ Recommend stopping drug immediately if patient develops conditions related to hypoxemia or dehydration because of risk of lactic acidosis caused by these conditions.

■ Recommend suspending therapy temporarily for surgical procedures (except minor procedures not needing restricted intake of food and fluids) or radiologic procedures involving parenteral administration of iodinated contrast; therapy shouldn't be resumed until patient's oral intake has resumed and renal function is normal.

## Therapeutic monitoring

■ Patient's renal function is assessed before beginning therapy and then annually thereafter. If renal impairment is detected, another antidiabetic should be prescribed.

■ Advise clinician to monitor patient's blood glucose level regularly to evaluate effectiveness.

■ Patient requires close monitoring during times of increased stress, such as infection, fever, surgery, or trauma. Insulin therapy may be required in these situations.

■ Advise clinician to monitor patient's hematologic status for megaloblastic anemia. Patients with inadequate vitamin $B_{12}$ or calcium intake or absorption appear to be predisposed to developing subnormal vitamin $B_{12}$ levels. These patients should have serum vitamin $B_{12}$ levels checked routinely at 2- to 3-year intervals.

■ Advise clinician to monitor glycosylated hemoglobin q 3 months to monitor continued response.

## Special populations

**Breast-feeding patients.** It isn't known if metformin appears in breast milk. Because of the potential for serious adverse effects in breast-feeding infants, drug shouldn't be given to breast-feeding women.
**Pediatric patients.** Safety and efficacy in children haven't been established. Studies in maturity-onset diabetes of the young haven't been conducted.
**Geriatric patients.** Because aging causes decreased renal function, give cautiously to geriatric patients.

## Patient counseling

■ Instruct patient to discontinue drug immediately and report unexplained hyperventilation, myalgia, malaise, unusual somnolence, or other nonspecific symptoms of early lactic acidosis.

■ Warn patient not to consume excessive amounts of alcohol while taking metformin.

---

Reactions may be *common,* uncommon, *life-threatening,* or COMMON AND LIFE-THREATENING.

- Instruct patient about nature of diabetes, importance of following therapeutic regimen, adhering to specific diet, weight reduction, exercise and personal hygiene programs; and avoiding infection. Explain how and when to perform self-monitoring of blood glucose level, and teach recognition of hypoglycemia and hyperglycemia.
- Tell patient not to change drug dosage without medical approval. Encourage him to report abnormal blood glucose levels.
- Advise patient not to take other drugs, including OTC drugs, without medical approval.
- Instruct patient to carry medical identification regarding diabetic status.

# methadone hydrochloride
Dolophine, Methadose, Physeptone*

*Pharmacologic classification:* opioid
*Therapeutic classification:* analgesic, narcotic detoxification adjunct
*Pregnancy risk category C*
*Controlled substance schedule II*

## Available forms
Available by prescription only
*Tablets:* 5 mg, 10 mg, 40 mg for oral solution (for narcotic abstinence syndrome)
*Oral solution:* 5 mg/5 ml, 10 mg/5 ml, 10 mg/ml (concentrate)
*Injection:* 10 mg/ml

## Indications and dosages
**Severe pain**
*Adults:* 2.5 to 10 mg P.O., I.M., or S.C. q 3 to 4 hours, p.r.n., or around-the-clock.
◊ *Children:* 0.7 mg/kg P.O. q 4 to 6 hours.
**Relief of severe, chronic pain**
*Adults:* 5 to 20 mg P.O. q 6 to 8 hours.
**Narcotic abstinence syndrome**
*Adults:* 15 to 20 mg P.O. daily (highly individualized). Maintenance dosage is 20 to 120 mg P.O. daily. Adjust dosage, p.r.n. Daily doses above 120 mg require special state and federal approval. If patient feels nauseated, give one-fourth of total P.O. dose in two injections, S.C. or I.M. Treatment is 30 (short-term) to 180 (long-term) days.

## Mechanism of action
*Analgesic action:* Methadone is an opiate agonist that has analgesic activity via an affinity for the opiate receptors similar to that of morphine. It's recommended for severe, chronic pain and is also used in detoxification and maintenance of patients with opiate abstinence syndrome.

## Pharmacokinetics
*Absorption:* Well absorbed from the GI tract. Oral administration delays onset and prolongs

duration of action as compared to parenteral administration.
*Distribution:* Highly tissue protein–bound, which may explain its cumulative effects and slow elimination.
*Metabolism:* Metabolized primarily in the liver by N-demethylation.
*Excretion:* Half-life is prolonged (7 to 11 hours) in patients with hepatic dysfunction. Urinary excretion, the major route, is dose-dependent. Methadone metabolites are also excreted in the feces via the bile.

| Route | Onset | Peak | Duration |
|-------|-------|------|----------|
| P.O. | ½-1 hr | ½-2 hr | 4-6 hr |
| I.M. | 10-20 min | 1-2 hr | 4-5 hr |

## Contraindications and precautions
Contraindicated in patients hypersensitive to drug. Use cautiously in geriatric or debilitated patients and in those with severe renal or hepatic impairment, acute abdominal conditions, hypothyroidism, Addison's disease, prostatic hyperplasia, urethral stricture, head injury, increased intracranial pressure, asthma, or other respiratory disorders.

## Interactions
**Drug-drug.** *Cimetidine:* Increased respiratory and CNS depression, causing confusion, disorientation, apnea, or seizures. Such use usually requires reduced dosage of methadone.
*Opioid antagonist:* Patients who become physically dependent on drug may experience acute withdrawal syndrome if given with methadone. Use with caution; advise clinician to monitor patient closely.
*Other CNS depressants, such as antidepressants, antihistamines, barbiturates, benzodiazepines, general anesthetics, muscle relaxants, narcotic analgesics, phenothiazines, and sedative-hypnotics:* Potentiated respiratory and CNS depression, sedation, and hypotensive effects. Use together cautiously.
*Rifampin:* May reduce blood level of methadone. Advise clinician to monitor patient.
**Drug-lifestyle.** *Alcohol use:* Potentiated respiratory and CNS depression, sedation, and hypotensive effects. Advise patient to avoid alcohol.

## Adverse reactions
**CNS:** *sedation, somnolence, clouded sensorium, euphoria, dizziness, choreic movements, seizures* (with large doses), headache, insomnia, agitation, *light-headedness,* syncope.
**CV:** *hypotension, bradycardia, shock, cardiac arrest,* palpitations, edema.
**EENT:** visual disturbances.
**GI:** *nausea, vomiting, constipation, ileus, dry mouth, anorexia, biliary tract spasm,* increased plasma amylase levels.
**GU:** *urine retention.*

---

**Respiratory:** *respiratory depression, respiratory arrest.*
**Skin:** *diaphoresis,* pruritus, urticaria.
**Other:** physical dependence; pain at injection site; tissue irritation, induration (after S.C. injection), *decreased libido.*

## Overdose and treatment
The most common signs and symptoms of drug overdose are CNS depression, respiratory depression, and miosis (pinpoint pupils). Others include hypotension, bradycardia, hypothermia, shock, apnea, cardiopulmonary arrest, circulatory collapse, pulmonary edema, and seizures. Toxicity may result from accumulation of drug over several weeks.

To treat acute overdose, recommend first establishing adequate respiratory exchange by way of a patent airway and ventilation p.r.n.; advise clinician to give an opioid antagonist (naloxone) to reverse respiratory depression. Because the duration of action of methadone is longer than that of naloxone, repeated naloxone dosing is needed. The antagonist naloxone shouldn't be given unless the patient has clinically significant respiratory or CV depression. Advise clinician to monitor vital signs closely.

If patient is seen within 2 hours of ingestion of an oral overdose, recommend emptying the stomach immediately by inducing emesis (ipecac syrup) or using gastric lavage. Recommend using caution to avoid risk of aspiration. Advise clinician to give activated charcoal through nasogastric tube for further removal of drug in an oral overdose.

Symptomatic and supportive treatment (continued respiratory support, correction of fluid or electrolyte imbalance) should be provided. Advise clinician to monitor laboratory values, vital signs, and neurologic status closely.

## Clinical considerations
■ Recommend verifying that patient is in a methadone maintenance program for management of narcotic addiction and, if so, at what dosage, and continuing that program appropriately.
■ Dispersible tablets may be dissolved in 4 ounces (120 ml) of water or fruit juice; oral concentrate must be diluted to at least 30 ml, but when used for detoxification, must be diluted with at least 3 ounces (90 ml) of water before administration.
**H ALERT** Diluents used for diluting methadone and levomethadyl acetate should differ in color and taste in any specific clinic setting to avoid confusion.
■ Oral liquid form (not tablets) is legally required and is the only form available in drug maintenance programs.
■ Regimented scheduling (around-the-clock) is beneficial in severe, chronic pain. When used for severe, chronic pain, tolerance may develop with long-term use, requiring a higher dose to achieve the same degree of analgesia.
■ Patient treated for narcotic abstinence syndrome usually requires an additional analgesic if pain control is needed.
■ Physical and psychological tolerance or dependence may occur. Be aware of potential for abuse.

### Therapeutic monitoring
■ Recommend observing patient for increased sedation, respiratory depression, stabilization of symptoms of withdrawal, or for pain relief.

### Special populations
**Breast-feeding patients.** Methadone appears in breast milk; it may cause physical dependence in breast-feeding infants of women on methadone maintenance therapy.
**Pediatric patients.** Drug isn't recommended for use in children. Safe use as maintenance drug in adolescent addicts hasn't been established.
**Geriatric patients.** Lower doses are usually indicated for geriatric patients because they may be more sensitive to the therapeutic and adverse effects of drug.

## Patient counseling
■ If appropriate, tell patient that constipation is often severe during maintenance with methadone. Instruct him to take a stool softener or other laxative.
■ Caution patient to avoid activities that require full alertness, such as driving and operating machinery, because of potential for drowsiness.

# methamphetamine hydrochloride
Desoxyn

*Pharmacologic classification:* amphetamine
*Therapeutic classification:* CNS stimulant, short-term adjunctive anorexigenic, sympathomimetic amine
*Pregnancy risk category C*
*Controlled substance schedule II*

## Available forms
Available by prescription only
*Tablets:* 5 mg

## Indications and dosages
*Attention deficit hyperactivity disorder*
*Children ages 6 and older:* Initially, 5 mg P.O. once daily or b.i.d., with 5-mg increments weekly, p.r.n. Usual effective dose is 20 to 25 mg daily.

---

Reactions may be *common,* uncommon, *life-threatening,* or COMMON AND LIFE-THREATENING.

*Short-term adjunct in exogenous obesity*
Adults: 2.5 to 5 mg P.O. b.i.d. to t.i.d. 30 minutes before meals. Don't use for longer than a few weeks.

## Mechanism of action

*CNS stimulant action:* Amphetamines are sympathomimetic amines with CNS stimulant activity; in hyperactive children, they have a paradoxical calming effect.

*Anorexigenic action:* Anorexigenic effects are thought to occur in the hypothalamus, where decreased smell and taste acuity decreases appetite; they may involve other systemic and metabolic effects. They may be tried for short-term control of refractory obesity, with caloric restriction and behavior modification.

The cerebral cortex and reticular activating system appear to be the primary sites of activity; amphetamines release nerve terminal stores of norepinephrine, promoting nerve impulse transmission. At high dosages, effects are mediated by dopamine.

Amphetamines are used to treat narcolepsy and as adjuncts to psychosocial measures in attention deficit disorder in children. The precise mechanisms of action in these conditions are unknown.

## Pharmacokinetics

*Absorption:* Rapidly absorbed from the GI tract after oral administration.

*Distribution:* Widely distributed throughout the body. Drug crosses the placenta and appears in breast milk.

*Metabolism:* Metabolized in the liver to at least seven metabolites.

*Excretion:* Excreted in urine.

| Route | Onset | Peak | Duration |
|-------|-------|------|----------|
| P.O. | Unknown | Unknown | 24 hr |

## Contraindications and precautions

Contraindicated in patients with moderate to severe hypertension, hyperthyroidism, symptomatic CV disease, advanced arteriosclerosis, glaucoma, hypersensitivity or idiosyncrasy to sympathomimetic amines, or history of drug abuse; within 14 days of MAO inhibitor therapy; and in agitated patients.

Use cautiously in geriatric, debilitated, asthenic, or psychopathic patients and in those with history of suicidal or homicidal tendencies.

## Interactions

**Drug-drug.** *Acetazolamide, antacids, sodium bicarbonate.* Enhances reabsorption of methamphetamine and prolongs duration of action. Advise clinician to monitor patient closely.

*Antihypertensives:* May antagonize their effects. Advise clinician to monitor patient closely.

*Ascorbic acid:* Enhances methamphetamine excretion and shortens duration of action. May need to increase methamphetamine dose.

*Barbiturates:* Antagonize methamphetamine by CNS depression. Avoid use together.

*General anesthesia:* Increased risk of arrhythmias. Advise clinician to monitor patient closely.

*Haloperidol, phenothiazines:* Decreased methamphetamine effects. Advise clinician to monitor patient closely.

*Insulin:* Drug may alter insulin requirements. Advise clinician to monitor serum glucose level.

*MAO inhibitors (or drugs with MAO-inhibiting activity, such as furazolidone) or within 14 days of such therapy:* May cause hypertensive crisis. Avoid use together.

*Other CNS stimulants:* Additive effects. Avoid use together.

**Drug-herb.** *Melatonin:* Enhances monoaminergic effects of methamphetamine and may exacerbate insomnia. Discourage use together.

**Drug-food.** *Caffeine:* Additive effects. Discourage use together.

## Adverse reactions

**CNS:** *nervousness, insomnia, irritability,* talkativeness, dizziness, headache, hyperexcitability, tremor, euphoria.

**CV:** hypertension, *tachycardia, palpitations, arrhythmias.*

**EENT:** blurred vision, mydriasis.

**GI:** dry mouth, metallic taste, diarrhea, constipation, anorexia.

**GU:** impotence.

**Metabolic:** elevated plasma corticosteroid levels.

**Skin:** urticaria.

**Other:** altered libido.

## Overdose and treatment

Symptoms of overdose include increasing restlessness, tremor, hyperreflexia, tachypnea, confusion, aggressiveness, hallucinations, and panic; fatigue and depression usually follow the excitement stage. Other symptoms may include arrhythmias, shock, alterations in blood pressure, nausea, vomiting, diarrhea, and abdominal cramps; death is usually preceded by seizures and coma.

Recommend treating overdose symptomatically and supportively. If ingestion is recent (within 4 hours), recommend using gastric lavage or emesis and sedating with barbiturate; advise clinician to monitor vital signs and fluid and electrolyte balance. I.V. phentolamine is suggested for treatment of severe acute hypertension. Chlorpromazine is useful in decreasing CNS stimulation and sympathomimetic effects. Urinary acidification may enhance excretion. Saline catharsis (magnesium citrate) may hasten GI evacuation of unabsorbed long-acting forms. Hemodialysis or peritoneal dialysis may be effective in severe cases.

## Clinical considerations
■ Drug isn't recommended for first-line treatment of obesity.
■ Rapid withdrawal after prolonged use may lead to depression, somnolence, and increased appetite.
■ Drug may interfere with urinary steroid determinations.

### *Therapeutic monitoring*
■ When treating behavioral disorders in children, a periodic discontinuation of the drug should be considered to evaluate effectiveness and the need for continued therapy.

### *Special populations*
**Breast-feeding patients.** Amphetamines appear in breast milk. An alternative to breast-feeding should be used.
**Pediatric patients.** Drug isn't recommended for weight reduction in children under age 12.
**Geriatric patients.** Geriatric or debilitated patients may be especially sensitive to effects of methamphetamine. Use drug with caution.

## Patient counseling
■ Warn patient that potential for abuse is high. Discourage use to combat fatigue.
■ Advise patient to avoid caffeine- and alcohol-containing drinks, to take drug 1 hour before next meal, and to take last daily dose at least 6 hours before bedtime to prevent insomnia.
■ Warn patient not to increase dosage unless prescribed.
■ Inform patient that methamphetamine may impair ability to engage in potentially hazardous activities, such as operating machinery or driving a motor vehicle.

---

# methimazole
Tapazole

*Pharmacologic classification:* thyroid hormone antagonist
*Therapeutic classification:* antihyperthyroid drug
*Pregnancy risk category D*

## Available forms
Available by prescription only
*Tablets:* 5 mg, 10 mg

## Indications and dosages
### *Hyperthyroidism, preparation for thyroidectomy, thyrotoxic crisis*
*Adults:* 15 mg P.O. daily if mild; 30 to 40 mg P.O. daily if moderately severe; 60 mg P.O. daily if severe; all are given in three equally divided doses q 8 hours. Continue until patient is euthyroid, then start maintenance dose of

5 to 15 mg daily. Continue initial dosage for 2 months.
*Children:* 0.4 mg/kg/day P.O. divided q 8 hours. Continue until patient is euthyroid, then start maintenance dose of 0.2 mg/kg/day divided q 8 hours.

## Mechanism of action
*Antithyroid action:* In treating hyperthyroidism, methimazole inhibits synthesis of thyroid hormone by interfering with the incorporation of iodide into tyrosyl. Methimazole also inhibits the formation of iodothyronine. As preparation for thyroidectomy, methimazole inhibits synthesis of the thyroid hormone and causes a euthyroid state, reducing surgical problems during thyroidectomy; as a result, the mortality for a single-stage thyroidectomy is low. Iodide reduces the vascularity of the gland, making it less friable. For treating thyrotoxic crisis (thyrotoxicosis), propylthiouracil (PTU) theoretically is preferred over methimazole because it inhibits peripheral deiodination of thyroxine to triiodothyronine.

## Pharmacokinetics
*Absorption:* Absorbed rapidly from the GI tract (80% to 95% bioavailable).
*Distribution:* Readily crosses the placenta and appears in breast milk. Drug is concentrated in the thyroid, and isn't protein-bound.
*Metabolism:* Undergoes hepatic metabolism.
*Excretion:* About 80% of drug and its metabolites are excreted renally; 7% is excreted unchanged. Half-life is between 5 and 13 hours.

| Route | Onset | Peak | Duration |
|---|---|---|---|
| P.O. | < 5 days | ½-1 hr | Unknown |

## Contraindications and precautions
Contraindicated in patients hypersensitive to drug and in breast-feeding women. Use cautiously in pregnant women.

## Interactions
**Drug-drug.** *Anticoagulants:* Antivitamin K action of methimazole potentiates the action of anticoagulants. Advise clinician to monitor PT and INR.
*Iodinated glycerol, lithium, potassium iodide:* May potentiate hypothyroid and goitrogenic effects. Use together cautiously.
*Other bone marrow depressants:* Increased risk of agranulocytosis. Advise clinician to monitor CBC.
*Other hepatotoxic drugs:* Increases the risk of hepatotoxicity. Advise clinician to monitor liver function test results and use together cautiously.
*PTU and adrenocorticoids or corticotropin:* May require a dosage adjustment of the steroid when thyroid status changes. Advise clinician to monitor patient closely.

---

Reactions may be *common*, uncommon, *life-threatening*, or COMMON AND LIFE-THREATENING.

## Adverse reactions

**CNS:** headache, drowsiness, vertigo, paresthesia, neuritis, neuropathies, CNS stimulation, depression.
**GI:** diarrhea, nausea, vomiting (may be dose-related), salivary gland enlargement, loss of taste, epigastric distress.
**GU:** nephritis.
**Hematologic:** *agranulocytosis, leukopenia, thrombocytopenia, aplastic anemia.*
**Hepatic:** jaundice, hepatic dysfunction, *hepatitis.*
**Metabolic:** hypothyroidism (mental depression; cold intolerance; hard, nonpitting edema; hypoprothrombinemia and bleeding).
**Musculoskeletal:** arthralgia, myalgia.
**Skin:** rash, urticaria, discoloration, pruritus, erythema nodosum, exfoliative dermatitis, lupus-like syndrome.
**Other:** fever, lymphadenopathy.

## Overdose and treatment

Signs and symptoms of overdose include nausea, vomiting, epigastric distress, fever, headache, arthralgia, pruritus, edema, and pancytopenia. Treatment is supportive; recommend performing gastric lavage or inducing emesis, if possible. If bone marrow depression develops, fresh whole blood, corticosteroids, and anti-infectives may be required.

## Clinical considerations

■ Best response occurs if dosage is given around-the-clock and given at the same time each day with respect to meals.
■ Doses of more than 40 mg per day increase the risk of agranulocytosis.
■ A beta blocker, usually propranolol, is given to manage the peripheral signs of hyperthyroidism, primarily tachycardia.
■ Euthyroid state may take several months to develop.
■ Sulfonamide-type adverse reactions can occur.

### *Therapeutic monitoring*

■ Advise clinician to monitor CBC in patients with signs and symptoms of illness.
■ Advise clinician to monitor liver function test results, especially if hepatic dysfunction is suspected.

### *Special populations*

**Pregnant patients.** Drug may induce goiter and hypothyroidism in developing fetus. The manufacturer states that the drug may be used judiciously to treat hyperthyroidism complicated by pregnancy.
**Breast-feeding patients.** Patient should discontinue breast-feeding before beginning therapy because drug appears in breast milk. However, if breast-feeding is needed, PTU is the preferred antithyroid hormone.

## Patient counseling

■ Tell patient to take drug at regular intervals around-the-clock and to take it at the same time each day in relation to meals.
■ If GI upset occurs, advise patient to take drug with meals.
■ Tell patient to promptly report fever, sore throat, malaise, unusual bleeding, yellowing of eyes, nausea, or vomiting.
■ Advise patient not to store drug in bathroom; heat and humidity cause it to deteriorate.
■ Tell patient to inform other prescribers and dentists of drug use.
■ Teach patient how to recognize the signs of hyperthyroidism and hypothyroidism and what to do if they occur.

---

# methocarbamol
Robaxin

*Pharmacologic classification:* carbamate derivative of guaifenesin
*Therapeutic classification:* skeletal muscle relaxant
*Pregnancy risk category C*

## Available forms

Available by prescription only
*Tablets:* 500 mg, 750 mg
*Tablets (film-coated):* 500 mg, 750 mg
*Injection:* 100 mg/ml parenteral in 10 ml vial

## Indications and dosages

*Adjunct in acute, painful musculoskeletal conditions*
*Adults:* 1.5 g P.O. q.i.d. for 2 to 3 days. Maintenance dose, 4 to 4.5 g P.O. daily in three to six divided doses. Alternatively, 1 g I.M. or I.V. For severe conditions, I.M. or I.V. doses may be given at 8-hour intervals. Maximum dosage, 3 g daily I.M. or I.V. for 3 consecutive days. Patient may resume I.M. or I.V. use after drug-free interval of 2 days.
*Supportive therapy in tetanus management*
*Adults:* 1 to 2 g I.V. push (300 mg/minute) and an additional 1 to 2 g may be added to I.V. solution. Total initial I.V. dosage, 3 g. Repeat I.V. infusion of 1 to 2 g q 6 hours until nasogastric tube can be inserted. Maximum P.O. dose is 24 g daily to manage tetanus.
*Children:* 15 mg/kg or 500 mg/m$^2$ I.V. Don't inject faster than 180 mg/m$^2$/minute. May be repeated q 6 hours, if needed, to total dosage of 1.8 g/m$^2$ daily for 3 consecutive days.

## Mechanism of action

*Skeletal muscle relaxant action:* Drug doesn't relax skeletal muscle directly. Its effects appear to be related to its sedative action; however, the exact mechanism of action is unknown.

---

## I.V. administration

■ Advise clinician to give I.V. undiluted at a rate not exceeding 300 mg/minute. May also be given by I.V. infusion after diluting in $D_5W$ or normal saline solution.

■ For I.V. administration, dilute 1 g of drug with up to 250 ml of $D_5W$ or normal saline injection. Don't refrigerate I.V. solution because precipitate and haze may occur.

■ Patient should be supine during and for at least 10 to 15 minutes after I.V. injection.

### Incompatibilities

None reported.

### Pharmacokinetics

*Absorption:* Rapidly and completely absorbed from the GI tract.

*Distribution:* Widely distributed throughout the body.

*Metabolism:* Extensively metabolized in liver by way of dealkylation and hydroxylation. Half-life of drug is between 1 and 2 hours.

*Excretion:* Rapidly and almost completely excreted in urine, mainly as its glucuronide and sulfate metabolites (40% to 50%), as unchanged drug (10% to 15%), and the rest as unidentified metabolites.

| Route | Onset | Peak | Duration |
|-------|-------|------|----------|
| P.O. | 30 min | 2 hr | Unknown |
| I.V. | Immediate | Immediate | Unknown |
| I.M. | Unknown | Unknown | Unknown |

### Contraindications and precautions

Contraindicated in patients hypersensitive to drug, and those with impaired renal function (injectable form), or seizure disorder (injectable form). Safe use of methocarbamol in regard to fetal development hasn't been established. Therefore, drug shouldn't be used in women who are or may become pregnant, especially during early pregnancy, unless the benefits outweigh the possible hazards.

### Interactions

**Drug-drug.** *Anticholinesterase drugs:* In patients with myasthenia gravis, severe weakness may result if given methocarbamol. Avoid use together.

*Other CNS depressants, including anxiolytics, narcotics, psychotics, and tricyclic antidepressants:* May cause additive CNS depression. Use together cautiously.

**Drug-lifestyle.** *Alcohol use:* May cause additive CNS depression. Advise patient to avoid alcohol.

### Adverse reactions

**CNS:** drowsiness, dizziness, light-headedness, headache, syncope, mild muscular incoordination (with I.M. or I.V. use), *seizures* (with I.V. use only), vertigo.

**CV:** flushing, hypotension, *bradycardia* (with I.M. or I.V. use).

**EENT:** blurred vision, conjunctivitis, nystagmus, diplopia.

**GI:** nausea, GI upset, metallic taste.

**GU:** hematuria (with I.V. use only), discoloration of urine.

**Skin:** urticaria, pruritus, rash.

**Other:** thrombophlebitis, extravasation (with I.V. use only), fever, *anaphylactic reactions* (with I.M. or I.V. use).

### Overdose and treatment

Signs and symptoms of overdose include extreme drowsiness, nausea and vomiting, and arrhythmias.

Treatment includes symptomatic and supportive measures. If ingestion is recent, recommend emptying stomach by emesis or gastric lavage (may reduce absorption). Recommend maintaining adequate airway, monitoring urine output and vital signs, and giving I.V. fluids, if needed.

### Clinical considerations

■ Drug shouldn't be administered S.C.

■ Methocarbamol solutions containing 4 mg/ml in sterile water for injection, $D_5W$, or normal saline injection are stable for 6 days at room temperature.

■ Inspect all solutions before administration for particles and haze.

■ To give via nasogastric tube, recommend crushing tablets and suspending in water or normal saline solution.

■ When used in tetanus, follow manufacturer's instructions.

■ Patient's urine may turn black, blue, brown, or green if left standing.

■ Patient needs assistance in walking after parenteral administration.

■ Extravasation of I.V. solution may cause thrombophlebitis and sloughing from hypertonic solution.

■ Oral administration should replace parenteral use as soon as feasible.

■ Adverse reactions after oral administration are usually mild and transient and subside with dosage reduction.

■ For I.M. administration, advise against giving more than 500 mg in each gluteal region.

■ Store at 59° to 86° F (15° to 30° C). Avoid freezing injection.

■ Methocarbamol therapy alters results of laboratory tests for urine 5-hydroxyindoleacetic acid (5-HIAA) using quantitative method of Udenfriend (false-positive) and for urine vanillylmandelic acid (false-positive when Gitlow screening test used; no problem when quantitative method of Sunderman used).

### Therapeutic monitoring

■ Advise clinician to monitor vital signs during I.V. or I.M. administration.

### Special populations
**Breast-feeding patients.** Drug appears in breast milk in small amounts. Patient shouldn't breast-feed during treatment with methocarbamol.
**Pediatric patients.** For children under age 12, use only as recommended for tetanus.
**Geriatric patients.** Lower doses are indicated because geriatric patients are more sensitive to effects of drug.

## Patient counseling
■ Tell patient that urine may turn black, blue, green, or brown.
■ Warn patient that drug may cause drowsiness. Patient should avoid hazardous activities that require alertness until degree of CNS depression can be determined.
■ Advise patient to make position changes slowly, particularly from recumbent to upright position, and to dangle legs before standing.
■ Advise patient to avoid alcoholic beverages and use OTC cold or cough preparations carefully because some contain alcohol.
■ Tell patient to store drug away from heat and light (not in bathroom medicine cabinet) and safely out of reach of children.
■ Tell patient to take missed dose if remembered within 1 hour. Beyond 1 hour, patient should skip that dose and resume regular schedule. He shouldn't double the dose.
■ Inform athletes that skeletal muscle relaxants are banned in competition and tested for by the U.S. Olympic Committee and the National Collegiate Athletic Association.

---

## methotrexate, methotrexate sodium
Folex, Mexate, Mexate-AQ, Rheumatrex Dose Pack

*Pharmacologic classification:* antimetabolite (cell cycle–phase specific, S phase)
*Therapeutic classification:* antineoplastic
*Pregnancy risk category X*

## Available forms
Available by prescription only
*Tablets (scored):* 2.5 mg
*Injection:* 20-mg, 25-mg, 50-mg, 100-mg, 250-mg, 1-g vials, lyophilized powder, preservative-free; 25-mg/ml vials, preservative-free solution; 2.5-mg/ml, 25-mg/ml vials, lyophilized powder, preserved

## Indications and dosages
Dosage and indications may vary. Check current literature for recommended protocols.

*Trophoblastic tumors (choriocarcinoma, hydatidiform mole)*
*Adults:* 15 to 30 mg P.O. or I.M. daily for 5 days. Repeat after 1 or more weeks, according to response or toxicity.
◊ *Adults:* 10 to 15 mg via the hypogastric artery until toxicity or therapeutic response occurs; three to five courses are usually needed.
*Acute lymphoblastic leukemia*
*Adults and children:* 3.3 mg/m$^2$ P.O. daily for 4 to 6 weeks or until remission occurs; then 20 to 30 mg/m$^2$ P.O. or I.M. twice weekly or 2.5 mg/kg I.V. q 14 days. (Used with prednisone.)
*Prophylaxis against meningeal leukemia*
12 mg/m$^2$ or 15 mg intrathecally. Consult specific references for intervals and dosing.
*Meningeal leukemia*
*Adults and children:* 12 mg/m$^2$ intrathecally to a maximum dose of 15 mg q 2 to 5 days until CSF is normal. Alternatively, 12 mg/m$^2$ once weekly for 2 weeks, then once monthly. Use only vials of powder with no preservatives; dilute using normal saline solution injection without preservatives. Use only new vials of drug and diluent. Use immediately after reconstitution.
*Burkitt's lymphoma (stage I or II)*
*Adults:* 10 to 25 mg P.O. daily for 4 to 8 days with 7- to 10-day rest intervals.
*Lymphosarcoma (stage III; malignant lymphoma)*
*Adults:* 0.625 to 2.5 mg/kg daily P.O., I.M., or I.V.
*Mycosis fungoides (advanced)*
*Adults:* 2.5 to 10 mg P.O. daily or 50 mg I.M. weekly; or 25 mg I.M. twice weekly for several weeks to months.
*Psoriasis (severe)*
*Adults:* Initially, a 5- to 10-mg test dose should be given 1 week before therapy. Then, 2.5 to 5 mg P.O. at 12-hour intervals for three doses each week or at 8-hour intervals for four doses each week. May increase by 2.5 mg/week, not to exceed 25 or 30 mg/week. Alternatively, 10 to 25 mg P.O., I.M., or I.V. as single weekly dose. May increase by 2.5 to 5 mg/week, not to exceed 50 mg/week. Alternatively, 2.5 mg P.O. daily for 5 days followed by a 2-day rest period. Dosage shouldn't exceed 6.25 mg/day. Improvement within 4 weeks should be noted with optimum results in 2 to 3 months.
*Rheumatoid arthritis (severe, refractory)*
*Adults:* 7.5 to 20 mg weekly P.O. in single or divided doses.
◊ *Adults:* 7.5 to 15 mg I.M. once weekly.
*Adjunct treatment in osteosarcoma*
*Adults:* Give 12 g/m$^2$ as a 4-hour I.V. infusion.
◊ *Head and neck carcinoma*
*Adults:* 40 to 60 mg/m$^2$ I.V. once weekly. Response limited to 4 months.

---

## I.V. administration

■ Methotrexate may be given undiluted by I.V. push injection.
■ Drug can be diluted to a higher volume with normal saline solution for I.V. infusion.

### Incompatibilities

Incompatible with bleomycin, chlorpromazine, droperidol, fluorouracil, metoclopramide, prednisolone, promethazine, and sodium phosphate.

## Mechanism of action

*Antineoplastic action:* Methotrexate exerts its cytotoxic activity by tightly binding with dihydrofolic acid reductase, an enzyme crucial to purine metabolism, resulting in an inhibition of DNA, RNA, and protein synthesis.

## Pharmacokinetics

*Absorption:* Absorption across the GI tract appears to be dose related. Lower doses are essentially completely absorbed, while absorption of larger doses is incomplete and variable. I.M. doses are absorbed completely.
*Distribution:* Distributed widely throughout the body, with the highest levels found in the kidneys, gallbladder, spleen, liver, and skin. Drug crosses the blood-brain barrier but doesn't achieve therapeutic levels in the CSF. About 50% of the drug is plasma protein–bound.
*Metabolism:* Metabolized only slightly in the liver.
*Excretion:* Excreted primarily into urine as unchanged drug. Elimination has been described as biphasic, with a first phase half-life averaging 1.5 to 3.5 hours and a terminal phase half-life of 8 to 15 hours.

| Route | Onset | Peak | Duration |
|-------|-------|------|----------|
| P.O. | Unknown | 1-2 hr | Unknown |
| I.V. | Unknown | Immediate | Unknown |
| I.M. | Unknown | ½-1 hr | Unknown |
| Intrathecal | Unknown | Unknown | Unknown |

## Contraindications and precautions

Contraindicated in patients hypersensitive to drug and during pregnancy or breast-feeding. Also contraindicated in patients with psoriasis or rheumatoid arthritis who also are alcoholics and in those with alcoholic liver, chronic liver disease, immunodeficiency syndromes, or pre-existing blood dyscrasias.

Use cautiously in very young or geriatric or debilitated patients and in those with impaired renal or hepatic function, bone marrow suppression, aplasia, leukopenia, thrombocytopenia, anemia, folate deficiency, infection, peptic ulcer, or ulcerative colitis. Drug exits slowly from third space compartments resulting in a prolonged terminal plasma half-life and risk of toxicity.

## Interactions

**Drug-drug.** *Folic acid:* May decrease the effectiveness of methotrexate. Use together cautiously.
*Immunizations:* May not be effective when given during methotrexate therapy. Vaccines shouldn't be given during methotrexate therapy.
*MTX; other potentially hepatotoxic drugs, such as azathiopine, retinoids, and sulfasalazine:* Increased risk of hepatoxicity. Advise clinician to monitor patient closely.
*NSAIDs, salicylates, sulfonamides, sulfonylureas:* May increase the therapeutic and toxic effects of methotrexate by displacing methotrexate from plasma proteins, increasing the levels of free methotrexate. Avoid use together if possible.
*Oral antibiotics, such as chloramphenicol, nonabsorbable broad-spectrum antibiotics, and tetracycline:* May decrease absorption of the drug. Use together cautiously.
*Phenytoin:* Increased risk of seizures. Advise clinician to monitor patient closely.
*Probenecid:* Increases the therapeutic and toxic effects of methotrexate. Combined use of these drugs requires a lower dosage of methotrexate.
*Pyrimethamine:* Similar pharmacologic action. Avoid use together.
**Drug-food.** *Any food:* Delayed absorption and reduced peak levels of methotrexate. Advise clinician to give on empty stomach.
**Drug-lifestyle.** *Sun exposure:* Increased risk of photosensitivity reactions. Advise patient to use sunblock.

## Adverse reactions

**CNS:** *arachnoiditis* (within hours of intrathecal use), subacute *neurotoxicity* (may begin a few weeks later), *necrotizing demyelinating leukoencephalopathy* (may occur a few years later), malaise, fatigue, dizziness, headache, drowsiness, *seizures.*
**EENT:** pharyngitis, gingivitis, blurred vision.
**GI:** stomatitis, diarrhea, abdominal distress, anorexia, GI ulceration and bleeding, enteritis, *nausea, vomiting.*
**GU:** nephropathy, *tubular necrosis, renal failure,* hyperuricemia, hematuria, menstrual dysfunction, defective spermatogenesis, cystitis.
**Hematologic:** WBC and platelet count nadirs occurring on day 7; anemia, *leukopenia, thrombocytopenia* (all dose-related).
**Hepatic:** acute toxicity (elevated transaminase level), *chronic toxicity (cirrhosis, hepatic fibrosis).*
**Metabolic:** diabetes.
**Musculoskeletal:** arthralgia, myalgia, osteoporosis (in children, with long-term use).
**Respiratory:** *pulmonary fibrosis, pulmonary interstitial infiltrates, pneumonitis;* dry, nonproductive cough.

---

Reactions may be *common*, uncommon, *life-threatening*, or COMMON AND LIFE-THREATENING.

**Skin:** alopecia, *urticaria, pruritus, hyperpig-mentation, erythematous rash, ecchymoses, psoriatic lesions (aggravated by exposure to sun), rash, photosensitivity.*
**Other:** fever, chills, reduced resistance to infection, soft tissue necrosis, osteonecrosis, *septicemia, sudden death.*

## Overdose and treatment
Signs and symptoms of overdose include myelosuppression, anemia, nausea, vomiting, dermatitis, alopecia, and melena.

The antidote for hematopoietic toxicity of methotrexate (diagnosed or anticipated) is calcium leucovorin, started as soon as possible and within 1 hour after the administration of methotrexate. The dosage of leucovorin should produce plasma levels higher than those of methotrexate. Because leucovorin blunts therapeutic response of methotrexate, consult specific disease protocol for details.

## Clinical considerations
■ Methotrexate has been used to treat breast cancer, bladder carcinoma, and various solid tumors. In addition, it has been used investigationally for its immunosuppressive and anti-inflammatory effects in various conditions.
■ Methotrexate is also used as second-line defense therapy for recurrent small cell lung cancer.
■ For patients with rheumatoid arthritis, methotrexate is used as the initial or anchor disease-modifying antirheumatic drug.
■ Use reconstituted solutions of preservative-free drug within 24 hours after mixing.
■ For intrathecal administration, use preservative-free formulations only. Dilute with unpreserved normal saline.
■ Dose modification may be required in impaired hepatic or renal function, bone marrow depression, aplasia, leukopenia, thrombocytopenia, or anemia. Use cautiously in infection, peptic ulcer, ulcerative colitis, and in very young, old, or debilitated patients.
■ GI adverse reactions may require drug discontinuation.
■ Rash, redness, or ulcerations in mouth or pulmonary adverse reactions may signal serious complications.
■ Recommend alkalinizing urine by giving sodium bicarbonate tablets to prevent precipitation of drug, especially with high doses. Urine pH should be maintained at more than 6.5. Recommend reducing dose if BUN level is 20 to 30 mg/dl or serum creatinine level is 1.2 to 2 mg/dl. Recommend stopping drug if BUN level is more than 30 mg/dl or serum creatinine level is more than 2 mg/dl.
■ All I.M. injections should be avoided in patients with thrombocytopenia.
■ Leucovorin rescue is needed with high-dose protocols (doses greater than 100 mg).

■ Methotrexate may alter results of the laboratory assay for folate by inhibiting the organism used in the assay, thus interfering with the detection of folic acid deficiency.

### Therapeutic monitoring
■ Advise clinician to monitor uric acid levels and BUN.
■ Advise clinician to monitor intake and output daily. Recommend forcing fluids (2 to 3 L daily).
■ Recommend watching for increases in AST, ALT, and alkaline phosphatase levels, which may signal hepatic dysfunction. Methotrexate shouldn't be used when the potential for "third spacing" exists.
■ Advise clinician to monitor patient for bleeding (especially GI) and infection.
■ Advise clinician to monitor temperature daily, and watch for cough, dyspnea, and cyanosis.

### Special populations
**Breast-feeding patients.** Drug appears in breast milk. To avoid risk of serious adverse reactions, mutagenicity, and carcinogenicity in the infant, patient should discontinue breast-feeding during therapy.

## Patient counseling
■ Emphasize importance of continuing drug despite nausea and vomiting. Advise patient to call immediately if vomiting occurs shortly after taking a dose.
■ Encourage patient to maintain adequate fluid intake to increase urine output, to prevent nephrotoxicity, and to facilitate excretion of uric acid.
■ Instruct patients also taking leucovorin to take exactly as prescribed to avoid potentially serious adverse effects.
■ Warn patient to avoid alcoholic beverages during therapy.
■ Caution patient to avoid conception during and immediately after therapy because of possible abortion or congenital anomalies.
■ Tell patient to avoid prolonged exposure to sunlight and to use a highly protective sunblock when exposed to sunlight.
■ Teach patient good mouth care to prevent superinfection of oral cavity.
■ Tell patient to take methotrexate tablets on an empty stomach for best results.
■ Advise patient that hair should grow back after treatment has ended.
■ Recommend salicylate-free analgesics for pain relief or fever reduction.
■ Tell patient to avoid exposure to people with infections and to report signs of infection immediately.
■ Advise patient to report unusual bruising or bleeding promptly.

# methylcellulose
Citrucel

*Pharmacologic classification:* adsorbent
*Therapeutic classification:* bulk-forming laxative
*Pregnancy risk category C*

## Available forms
Available without a prescription
*Powder:* 105 mg/g, 196 mg/g

## Indications and dosages
*Chronic constipation*
*Adults:* Maximum dose is 6 g P.O. daily, divided into 0.45 to 3 g/dose.
*Children ages 6 to 12:* Maximum dose is 3 g P.O. daily, divided into 0.45 to 1.5 g/dose.

## Mechanism of action
*Laxative action:* Methylcellulose adsorbs intestinal fluid and serves as a source of indigestible fiber, stimulating peristaltic activity.

## Pharmacokinetics
*Absorption:* Not absorbed.
*Distribution:* Distributed locally, in the intestine.
*Metabolism:* None.
*Excretion:* Excreted in feces.

| Route | Onset | Peak | Duration |
|---|---|---|---|
| P.O. | 12-24 hr | < 3 days | Variable |

## Contraindications and precautions
Contraindicated in patients with abdominal pain, nausea, vomiting, or other symptoms of appendicitis or acute surgical abdomen and in those with intestinal obstruction or ulceration, disabling adhesions, or difficulty swallowing.

## Interactions
**Drug-drug.** *Oral medications:* When used together, methylcellulose may absorb other drugs. Separate administration times by at least 1 hour.

## Adverse reactions
**GI:** *nausea, vomiting, diarrhea* (with excessive use); *esophageal, gastric, small intestinal, or colonic strictures* (when drug is chewed or taken in dry form); abdominal cramps, especially in severe constipation; laxative dependence (with long-term or excessive use).

## Overdose and treatment
No information available.

## Clinical considerations
■ Give drug with water or juice (at least 8 ounces).
■ Drug may absorb oral medications; schedule at least 1 hour apart from all other drugs.

■ Bulk laxatives most closely mimic natural bowel function and don't promote laxative dependence.
■ Drug is especially useful in patients with postpartum constipation, long-term laxative abuse, irritable bowel syndrome, diverticular disease, or colostomies; in debilitated patients; and to empty colon before barium enema examinations.

### Therapeutic monitoring
■ Advise clinician to monitor patient for clinical response.

### Special populations
**Breast-feeding patients.** Because drug isn't absorbed, use probably poses no risk to breast-feeding infants.

## Patient counseling
■ Instruct patient to take other oral medications 1 hour before or after methylcellulose.
■ Explain that full effect of drug may not occur for 2 to 3 days.

# methyldopa
Apo-Methyldopa*, Dopamet*, Novomedopa*

*Pharmacologic classification:* centrally acting antiadrenergic
*Therapeutic classification:* antihypertensive
*Pregnancy risk category B (oral); C (I.V.)*

## Available forms
Available by prescription only
*Tablets:* 125 mg, 250 mg, 500 mg
*Injection (as methyldopate hydrochloride):* 250 mg/5 ml in 5-ml vials

## Indications and dosages
*Moderate to severe hypertension*
*Adults:* Initially, 250 mg P.O. b.i.d. or t.i.d. in first 48 hours, then increased or decreased, p.r.n., q 2 days. Alternatively, 250 to 500 mg I.V. q 6 hours (maximum dose, 1 g q 6 hours). Adjust dosage if other antihypertensives are added to or deleted from therapy.

Maintenance dose is 500 mg to 2 g P.O. daily in two to four divided doses. Maximum recommended daily dose is 3 g. I.V. infusion dose is 250 to 500 mg given over 30 to 60 minutes q 6 hours. Maximum I.V. dose, 1 g q 6 hours.
*Children:* Initially, 10 mg/kg P.O. daily or 300 mg/m$^2$ P.O. daily in two to four divided doses; or 20 to 40 mg/kg I.V. daily or 0.6 to 1.2 g/m$^2$ I.V. daily in four divided doses. Increase dosage at least q 2 days until desired response occurs. Maximum daily dose is 65 mg/kg, 2 g/m$^2$, or 3 g, whichever is least.

## I.V. administration

■ Add required dose of drug to 100 ml of D₅W injection. Alternatively, a concentration of 100 mg/ml may be used.
■ ADD-Vantage vials contain 50 mg/ml and should be reconstituted per manufacturer direction.
■ Recommend administering I.V. infusion over 30 to 60 minutes.

### Incompatibilities
Incompatible with amphotericin B, methohexital, and some total parenteral nutrition solutions. Mix cautiously with drugs that have poor solubility in acidic media, such as barbiturates and sulfonamides.

## Mechanism of action
*Antihypertensive action:* Exact mechanism unknown. Antihypertensive action thought to be caused by a metabolite of methyldopa, alpha-methylnorepinephrine, which stimulates central inhibitory alpha-adrenergic receptors, decreasing total peripheral resistance; drug may act as a false neurotransmitter. Drug may also reduce plasma renin activity.

## Pharmacokinetics
*Absorption:* Absorbed partially from the GI tract. Absorption varies, but usually about 50% of an oral dose is absorbed. No correlation exists between plasma level and antihypertensive effect. After I.V. administration, blood pressure usually begins to decrease in 4 to 6 hours.
*Distribution:* Distributed throughout the body and is bound weakly to plasma proteins.
*Metabolism:* Metabolized extensively in the liver and intestinal cells.
*Excretion:* Drug and its metabolites are excreted in urine; unabsorbed drug is excreted unchanged in feces. Elimination half-life is about 2 hours.

| Route | Onset | Peak | Duration |
|-------|---------|--------|----------|
| P.O. | Unknown | 4-6 hr | 12-48 hr |
| I.V. | Unknown | 4-6 hr | 10-16 hr |

## Contraindications and precautions
Contraindicated in patients hypersensitive to drug or those with active hepatic disease (such as acute hepatitis) and active cirrhosis. Also contraindicated if previous methyldopa therapy has been related to liver disorders. Use cautiously in patients with impaired hepatic function, in those receiving MAO inhibitors, and in breast-feeding women.

## Interactions
**Drug-drug.** *Anesthetics:* Increased effects. Patients undergoing surgery may require reduced dosages of anesthetics.
*Diuretics:* May increase hypotensive effect of methyldopa. Use together cautiously.

*Haloperidol:* May produce dementia and sedation. Use together cautiously.
*Lithium:* May increase risk of lithium toxicity. Advise clinician to monitor lithium levels.
*Oral iron therapy:* May decrease hypotensive effects and increase serum levels of levodopa. Use together cautiously.
*Other antihypertensives:* Potentiated antihypertensive effects. Use together cautiously.
*Phenothiazines, tricyclic antidepressants:* May cause a reduction in antihypertensive effects. Advise clinician to monitor blood pressure.
*Phenoxybenzamine:* May cause reversible urinary incontinence. Avoid use together.
*Sympathomimetic amines such as phenylpropanolamine:* Potentiated pressor effects. Use together cautiously.
*Tolbutamide:* Methyldopa may impair tolbutamide metabolism. Advise clinician to monitor serum glucose levels.
**Drug-herb.** *Capsicum:* May reduce antihypertensive effectiveness of drug. Discourage use together.

## Adverse reactions
**CNS:** *sedation, headache, weakness, dizziness,* decreased mental acuity, paresthesia, parkinsonism, involuntary choreoathetoid movements, psychic disturbances, depression, nightmares.
**CV:** ***bradycardia,*** *orthostatic hypotension, aggravated angina, myocarditis,* edema.
**EENT:** *nasal congestion.*
**GI:** nausea, vomiting, diarrhea, *pancreatitis, dry mouth,* constipation.
**GU:** amenorrhea, impotence, altered serum creatinine, altered urine uric acid.
**Hematologic:** *hemolytic anemia, thrombocytopenia, leukopenia, bone marrow depression.*
**Hepatic:** *hepatic necrosis,* abnormal liver function test results, *hepatitis.*
**Skin:** rash.
**Other:** decreased libido, galactorrhea, gynecomastia, drug-induced fever.

## Overdose and treatment
Signs and symptoms of overdose include sedation, hypotension, impaired atrioventricular conduction, and coma.

After recent (within 4 hours) ingestion, recommend emptying stomach by induced emesis or gastric lavage. Advise clinician to give activated charcoal to reduce absorption, then treat symptomatically and supportively. In severe cases, hemodialysis may be considered.

## Clinical considerations
■ Patients with impaired renal function may require smaller maintenance dosages of drug.
■ Multiple dosing may decrease patient compliance, but b.i.d. dosing may provide adequate control with decreased cost.

■ Methyldopate hydrochloride is administered I.V.; I.M. or S.C. administration isn't recommended because of unpredictable absorption.
■ Patients receiving methyldopa may become hypertensive after dialysis because drug is dialyzable.
■ Sedation and drowsiness usually disappear with continued therapy; bedtime dosage will minimize this effect. Orthostatic hypotension may indicate a need for dosage reduction. Some patients tolerate receiving the entire daily dose in the evening or h.s.
■ Tolerance may develop after 2 to 3 weeks.
■ Signs of hepatotoxicity may occur 2 to 4 weeks after therapy begins.
■ Methyldopa may cause falsely high levels of urine catecholamines, interfering with the diagnosis of pheochromocytoma. A positive direct antiglobulin (Coombs') test may also occur.

### Therapeutic monitoring

■ At the start of, and periodically throughout therapy, advise clinician to monitor hemoglobin level, hematocrit, and RBC count for hemolytic anemia, and liver function test results.
■ Recommend taking blood pressure in supine, sitting, and standing positions during dosage adjustment; recommend taking blood pressure at least every 30 minutes during I.V. infusion until patient is stable.
■ Advise clinician to monitor intake and output and daily weights to detect sodium and water retention; voided urine exposed to air may darken because of the breakdown of methyldopa or its metabolites.
■ Advise clinician to monitor patient for signs and symptoms of drug-induced depression.

### Special populations

**Pregnant patients.** Methyldopa is the most extensively used hypotensive in pregnant women.
**Breast-feeding patients.** Drug appears in breast milk; the American Academy of Pediatrics considers methyldopa to be compatible with breast-feeding.
**Pediatric patients.** Safety and efficacy in children haven't been established; use only if potential benefits outweigh risks.
**Geriatric patients.** Dosage reductions may be needed in geriatric patients because they're more sensitive to sedation and hypotension.

### Patient counseling

■ Teach patient signs and symptoms of adverse effects, such as "jerky" movements, and about the need to report them; he should also report excessive weight gain (5 lb [2.25 kg ] weekly), signs of infection, or fever.
■ Teach patient to minimize adverse effects by taking drug at bedtime until tolerance develops to sedation, drowsiness, and other CNS effects; by avoiding sudden position changes to minimize orthostatic hypotension; and by using ice chips, hard candy, or gum to relieve dry mouth.
■ Warn patient to avoid hazardous activities that require mental alertness until sedative effects subside.
■ Instruct patient to call prescriber for instructions before taking OTC cold preparations.

---

# methylergonovine maleate
Methergine

*Pharmacologic classification:* ergot alkaloid
*Therapeutic classification:* oxytocic
*Pregnancy risk category C*

## Available forms
Available by prescription only
*Tablets:* 0.2 mg
*Injection:* 0.2 mg/ml ampule

## Indications and dosages
***Prevention and treatment of postpartum hemorrhage caused by uterine atony or subinvolution***
*Adults:* 0.2 mg I.M. or I.V. q 2 to 4 hours, p.r.n. for maximum five doses. Following initial I.M. or I.V. dose, may give 0.2 to 0.4 mg P.O. q 6 to 12 hours for maximum 7 days. Decrease dose if severe cramping occurs.
◊ ***Diagnosis of coronary artery spasm***
*Adults:* 0.1 to 0.4 mg I.V.

## I.V. administration
■ Drug shouldn't be administered I.V. routinely because of the possibility of inducing sudden hypertensive and CV accidents.
■ If I.V. administration is considered essential as a life-saving measure, dilute desired dose with normal saline injection to a volume of 5 ml and give slowly over no less than 60 seconds.
■ Store I.V. solutions below 77° F (25° C). Give only if solution is clear and colorless.

## Incompatibilities
None reported.

## Mechanism of action
*Oxytocic action:* Drug stimulates contractions of uterine and vascular smooth muscle. The intense uterine contractions are followed by periods of relaxation. Drug produces vasoconstriction primarily of capacitance blood vessels, causing increased central venous pressure and elevated blood pressure. Drug increases the amplitude and frequency of uterine contractions and tone, which therefore impedes uterine blood flow.

## Pharmacokinetics
*Absorption:* Absorption is rapid, with 60% of an oral dose appearing in the bloodstream.

---

*Distribution:* Distribution appears to be rapidly distributed into tissues.
*Metabolism:* Extensive first-pass metabolism precedes hepatic metabolism.
*Excretion:* Excreted primarily in the feces, with a small amount in urine.

| Route | Onset | Peak | Duration |
|-------|-------|------|----------|
| P.O. | 5-10 min | 30 min | 3 hr |
| I.V. | Immediate | Unknown | 45 min |
| I.M. | 2-5 min | Unknown | 3 hr |

## Contraindications and precautions
Contraindicated in patients with hypertension, toxemia, or sensitivity to ergot preparations and in pregnant women. Use cautiously in patients with renal or hepatic disease, sepsis, or obliterative vascular disease and during the first stage of labor.

## Interactions
**Drug-drug.** *Local anesthetics with vasoconstrictors (lidocaine with epinephrine):* Enhanced vasoconstriction. Use together cautiously.
*Other ergot alkaloids, sympathomimetic amines:* Enhanced vasoconstrictor potential. Use together cautiously.
**Drug-lifestyle.** *Smoking (nicotine):* Enhanced vasoconstriction caused by drug. Avoid use together.

## Adverse reactions
**CNS:** dizziness, headache, *seizures, CVA* (with I.V. use), hallucinations.
**CV:** hypertension, transient chest pain, palpitations, hypotension.
**EENT:** tinnitus, nasal congestion, foul taste.
**GI:** *nausea, vomiting, diarrhea.*
**GU:** hematuria.
**Musculoskeletal:** leg cramps.
**Respiratory:** dyspnea.
**Skin:** diaphoresis.
**Other:** thrombophlebitis.

## Overdose and treatment
Signs and symptoms of overdose include seizures and gangrene with nausea, vomiting, diarrhea, dizziness, fluctuations in blood pressure, weak pulse, chest pain, tingling, and numbness and coldness in limbs.

Treatment of oral overdose requires that the patient drink tap water, milk, or vegetable oil to delay absorption, then follow with gastric lavage or emesis, then activated charcoal and cathartics. Recommend treating seizures with anticonvulsants and hypercoagulability with heparin; vasodilators should be used to improve blood flow as required. Gangrene may require surgical amputation.

## Clinical considerations
■ Contractions begin 5 to 15 minutes after P.O. administration, 2 to 5 minutes after I.M. injection, and immediately following I.V. injection; continue 3 hours or more after P.O. or I.M. administration, 45 minutes after I.V.
■ Store tablets in tightly closed, light-resistant containers. Discard if discolored.

### Therapeutic monitoring
■ Advise clinician to monitor blood pressure, pulse rate, and uterine response. Recommend observing patient for sudden change in vital signs, frequent periods of uterine relaxation, and character and amount of vaginal bleeding.

### Special populations
**Breast-feeding patients.** Ergot alkaloids inhibit lactation. Drug appears in breast milk, and ergotism has been reported in breast-fed infants.

### Patient counseling
■ Advise smoking cessation during therapy.
■ Warn patient of adverse reactions.

# methylphenidate hydrochloride
Concerta, Metadate, Metadate CD, Metadate ER, Methylin, Methylin ER, Ritalin, Ritalin-SR

*Pharmacologic classification:* piperidine CNS stimulant
*Therapeutic classification:* CNS stimulant (analeptic)
*Pregnancy risk category NR (C for Concerta and Metadate CD)*
*Controlled substance schedule II*

## Available forms
Available by prescription only
*Tablets:* 5 mg, 10 mg, 20 mg
*Tablets (sustained-release):* 20 mg
*Tablets (extended-release):* 10 mg, 18 mg, 20 mg, 36 mg, 54 mg
*Capsules (extended-release):* 20 mg

## Indications and dosages
*Attention deficit hyperactivity disorder (ADHD; Metadate, Methylin, Ritalin)*
*Children ages 6 and older:* Initially 5 mg P.O. daily before breakfast and lunch, increased in 5- to 10-mg increments weekly, p.r.n., until an optimum daily dose of 2 mg/kg is reached, not to exceed 60 mg daily.
*ADHD (Concerta)*
*Children ages 6 and older not currently taking methylphenidate or who are taking stimulants other than methylphenidate:* 18 mg P.O. (extended-release) once daily in the morning. Adjust dosage by 18 mg at weekly intervals to

a maximum of 54 mg daily taken once daily in the morning.

*Children ages 6 and older currently on methylphenidate:* If previous methylphenidate daily dose is 5 mg b.i.d. or t.i.d. or 20 mg sustained-release, recommended dose is 18 mg P.O. every morning. If previous methylphenidate daily dose is 10 mg b.i.d. or t.i.d. or 40 mg sustained-release, recommended dose is 36 mg P.O. every morning. If previous methylphenidate daily dose is 15 mg b.i.d. or t.i.d. or 60 mg sustained-release, recommended dose 54 mg P.O. every morning. Maximum daily dose is 54 mg.

*ADHD (Metadate CD)*
*Children ages 6 and older:* Initially, 20 mg P.O. daily before breakfast; increased in 20-mg increments weekly to maximum of 60 mg daily.

*Narcolepsy (Ritalin, Methylin)*
*Adults:* 10 mg P.O. b.i.d. or t.i.d. 30 to 45 minutes before meals. Dosage varies with patient needs; average dose is 40 to 60 mg daily.

When using sustained-release tablets, calculate regular dose in q-8-hour intervals and give as such.

## Mechanism of action
*Analeptic action:* The cerebral cortex and reticular activating system appear to be the primary sites of activity; methylphenidate releases nerve terminal stores of norepinephrine, promoting nerve impulse transmission. At high doses, effects are mediated by dopamine.

Drug is used to treat narcolepsy and as an adjunct to psychosocial measures in ADHD. Like amphetamines, it has a paradoxical calming effect in hyperactive children.

## Pharmacokinetics
*Absorption:* Absorbed rapidly and completely after oral administration.
*Distribution:* Unknown.
*Metabolism:* Metabolized by the liver.
*Excretion:* Excreted in urine.

| Route | Onset | Peak | Duration |
|-------|-------|------|----------|
| P.O. | Unknown | 2-5 hr | Unknown |

## Contraindications and precautions
Contraindicated in patients hypersensitive to drug, glaucoma, motor tics, family history of or diagnosis of Tourette syndrome, or history of marked anxiety, tension, or agitation.

Use cautiously in patients with history of seizures, drug abuse, hypertension, or EEG abnormalities.

## Interactions
**Drug-drug.** *Anticonvulsants (phenobarbital, phenytoin, primidone), coumarin anticoagulants, phenylbutazone, tricyclic antidepressants:* Methylphenidate may inhibit metabolism and increase the serum levels of these drugs. Dosage adjustment may be needed if concomitant therapy is needed.

*Bretylium, guanethidine:* Decreased hypotensive effects. Advise clinician to monitor patient for clinical effect.

*MAO inhibitors (or drugs with MAO-inhibiting activity) or within 14 days of such therapy:* May cause severe hypertension. Avoid use together.

**Drug-lifestyle.** *Caffeine:* May enhance CNS stimulant effects of methylphenidate and decrease effectiveness of drug in ADHD. Discourage caffeine use.

## Adverse reactions
**CNS:** *nervousness, insomnia, Tourette syndrome, dizziness, headache, akathisia, dyskinesia, seizures,* drowsiness.
**CV:** *palpitations, angina, tachycardia, changes in blood pressure and pulse rate, arrhythmias.*
**GI:** nausea, abdominal pain, anorexia.
**Hematologic:** *thrombocytopenia, thrombocytopenic purpura, leukopenia,* anemia.
**Metabolic:** weight loss.
**Skin:** rash, urticaria, *exfoliative dermatitis, erythema multiforme.*

## Overdose and treatment
Symptoms of overdose may include euphoria, confusion, delirium, coma, toxic psychosis, agitation, headache, vomiting, dry mouth, mydriasis, self-injury, fever, diaphoresis, tremors, hyperreflexia, hyperpyrexia, muscle twitching, seizures, flushing, hypertension, tachycardia, palpitations, and arrhythmias.

Treat overdose symptomatically and supportively: Recommend using gastric lavage or emesis in patients with intact gag reflex. Airway and circulation should be maintained. Recommend closely monitoring vital signs and fluid and electrolyte balance. Recommend maintaining patient in cool room, monitoring temperature, minimizing external stimulation, and protecting him against self-injury. External cooling blankets may be needed.

## Clinical considerations
- Methylphenidate is the drug of choice for ADHD. Therapy is usually stopped after puberty.
- If paradoxical aggravation of symptoms occurs during therapy, recommend reducing dosage or stopping drug.
- Drug may decrease seizure threshold in seizure disorders.
- Intermittent drug-free periods when stress is least evident (weekends, school holidays) may help prevent development of tolerance and permit decreased dosage when drug is resumed. Sustained-release form allows convenience of single, at-home dosing for school children.
- Drug has abuse potential; discourage use to combat fatigue. Some abusers dissolve tablets and inject drug.

**H** *ALERT* After high-dose and long-term use, abrupt withdrawal may unmask severe depression. Dosage should be lowered gradually to prevent acute rebound depression.
■ Drug impairs ability to perform tasks requiring mental alertness.
■ Be sure patient obtains adequate rest; fatigue may result as drug wears off.
■ Discourage methylphenidate use for analeptic effect; CNS stimulation superimposed on CNS depression may cause neuronal instability and seizures.
■ Don't give drug to women of childbearing age unless potential benefits outweigh possible risks.
■ Store drug in tight, light-resistant containers.

### Therapeutic monitoring
■ Advise clinician to monitor patient closely when therapy starts; drug may precipitate Tourette syndrome.
■ Recommend checking vital signs regularly for increased blood pressure or other signs of excessive stimulation; avoid late-day or evening dosing, especially of long-acting dosage forms, to minimize insomnia.
■ Advise clinician to monitor CBC, differential, and platelet counts when patient is taking drug long-term.
■ Advise clinician to monitor height and weight; drug has caused growth suppression.

### Special populations
**Pediatric patients.** Drug isn't recommended for ADHD in children under age 6. It has caused growth suppression; all patients should be monitored.

### Patient counseling
■ Explain reason for therapy and the risks and benefits that may be anticipated.
■ Tell patient to avoid drinks containing caffeine to prevent added CNS stimulation and not to alter dosage unless prescribed.
■ Advise narcoleptic patient to take first dose on awakening; advise ADHD patient to take last dose several hours before bedtime to avoid insomnia.
■ Tell patient not to chew or crush sustained-release dosage forms.
■ Warn patient not to use drug to mask fatigue, to be sure to obtain adequate rest, and to call prescriber if excessive CNS stimulation occurs.
■ Advise patient to avoid potentially hazardous activities that require mental alertness until degree of sedative effect is determined.

# methylprednisolone (systemic)
Medrol, Meprolene

# methylprednisolone acetate
Depo-Medrol

# methylprednisolone sodium succinate
A-methaPred, Solu-Medrol

*Pharmacologic classification:* glucocorticoid
*Therapeutic classification:* anti-inflammatory, immunosuppressant
*Pregnancy risk category C*

## Available forms
Available by prescription only
**methylprednisolone**
*Tablets:* 2 mg, 4 mg, 8 mg, 16 mg, 24 mg, 32 mg
**methylprednisolone acetate**
*Injection:* 20 mg/ml, 40 mg/ml, 80 mg/ml suspension
**methylprednisolone sodium succinate**
*Injection:* 40 mg, 125 mg, 500 mg, 1,000 mg, 2,000 mg/vial

## Indications and dosages
*Multiple sclerosis*
**methylprednisolone**
*Adults:* 200 mg P.O. daily for 1 week, followed by 80 mg every other day for 1 month.
*Inflammation*
**methylprednisolone**
*Adults:* 2 to 60 mg P.O. daily in four divided doses, depending on disease being treated.
*Children:* 0.117 to 1.66 mg/kg daily or 3.3 to 50 mg/m$^2$ P.O. daily in three to four divided doses.
**methylprednisolone acetate**
*Adults:* 10 to 80 mg I.M. daily; or 4 to 80 mg into joints and soft tissue, p.r.n., q 1 to 5 weeks; or 20 to 60 mg intralesionally.
**methylprednisolone sodium succinate**
*Adults:* 10 to 250 mg I.M. or I.V. q 4 hours.
*Children:* 0.03 to 0.2 mg/kg or 1 to 6.25 mg/m$^2$ I.M. or I.V. daily in one or two divided doses.
*Shock*
**methylprednisolone sodium succinate**
*Adults:* 100 to 250 mg I.V. at 2- to 6-hour intervals or 30 mg/kg I.V. initially and repeat q 4 to 6 hours, p.r.n. Alternatively, after original I.V. push dose, 30 mg/kg I.V. infusion q 12 hours for 24 to 48 hours.
◊ *Severe lupus nephritis*
**methylprednisolone sodium succinate**
*Adults:* 1 g I.V. over 1 hour for 3 days. Therapy is then continued orally at 0.5 mg/kg/day.
*Children:* 30 mg/kg I.V. every other day for six doses.

◊ *Treatment or minimization of motor and sensory defects caused by acute spinal cord injury*
*Adults:* Initially, 30 mg/kg I.V. over 15 minutes followed in 45 minutes by I.V. infusion of 5.4 mg/kg/hour for 23 hours.

◊ *Adjunct to moderate-severe* **Pneumocystis carinii** *pneumonia*
*Adults and children over age 13:* 30 mg I.V. b.i.d. for 5 days; 30 mg I.V. daily for 5 days; 15 mg I.V. daily for 11 days (or until completion of anti-infective regimen).

## I.V. administration

■ Methylprednisolone sodium succinate is reconstituted for I.V. use with bacteriostatic water for injection containing 0.9% benzyl alcohol. Reconstitute per manufacturer instruction.
■ I.V. bolus administration is over at least 1 minute.
■ For I.V. infusion, further dilute with compatible I.V. solution (such as normal saline solution or $D_5W$). Reconstituted drug should be clear. Discard after 48 hours.

### Incompatibilities

Incompatible with calcium gluconate, cephalothin, cytarabine, filgrastim, glycopyrrolate, metaraminol, nafcillin, and penicillin G sodium.

## Mechanism of action

*Anti-inflammatory action:* Methylprednisolone stimulates the synthesis of enzymes needed to decrease the inflammatory response. It suppresses the immune system by reducing activity and volume of the lymphatic system, thus producing lymphocytopenia (primarily of T lymphocytes), decreasing immunoglobulin and complement levels, decreasing passage of immune complexes through basement membranes, and possibly by depressing reactivity of tissue to antigen-antibody interactions.

Drug is an intermediate-acting glucocorticoid. It has essentially no mineralocorticoid activity but is a potent glucocorticoid, with five times the potency of an equal weight of hydrocortisone. It's used primarily as an anti-inflammatory and immunosuppressant.

Methylprednisolone may be administered orally. Methylprednisolone sodium succinate may be administered by I.M. or I.V. injection or by I.V. infusion, usually at 4- to 6-hour intervals.

Methylprednisolone acetate suspension may be administered by intra-articular, intrasynovial, intrabursal, intralesional, or soft-tissue injection. It has a slow onset but a long duration of action. Injectable forms are usually used only when the oral dosage forms can't be used.

## Pharmacokinetics

*Absorption:* Absorbed readily after oral administration.

*Distribution:* Distributed rapidly to muscle, liver, skin, intestines, and kidneys. Adrenocorticoids appear in breast milk and through the placenta.
*Metabolism:* Metabolized in the liver to inactive glucuronide and sulfate metabolites.
*Excretion:* Inactive metabolites and small amounts of unmetabolized drug are excreted by the kidneys. Insignificant quantities of drug are excreted in feces. Biological half-life of methylprednisolone is 18 to 36 hours.

| Route | Onset | Peak | Duration |
|---|---|---|---|
| P.O. | Rapid | 2-3 hr | 30-36 hr |
| I.V. | Rapid | Immediate | 7 days |
| I.M. | 6-48 hr | 4-8 days | 1-4 wk |
| Intra-articular | Rapid | 7 days | 1-5 wk |

## Contraindications and precautions

Contraindicated in patients allergic to any component of the formulation, in those with systemic fungal infections, and in premature infants (acetate and succinate).

Use cautiously in patients with renal disease, GI ulceration, hypertension, osteoporosis, diabetes mellitus, hypothyroidism, cirrhosis, diverticulitis, nonspecific ulcerative colitis, recent intestinal anastomoses, thromboembolic disorders, seizures, myasthenia gravis, HF, tuberculosis, emotional instability, ocular herpes simplex, and psychotic tendencies.

## Interactions

**Drug-drug.** *Amphotericin B, diuretic therapy:* May enhance hypokalemia. Advise clinician to monitor serum potassium.
*Antacids, cholestyramine, colestipol:* Decreased corticosteroid effect. Separate administration times.
*Anticholinesterase:* Profound weakness. Use together cautiously.
*Barbiturates, phenytoin, rifampin:* May cause decreased corticosteroid effects because of increased hepatic metabolism. Advise clinician to monitor patient for potential dosage adjustment.
*Cyclosporine:* Levels of cyclosporine may increase. Use together cautiously.
*Estrogens:* Reduced metabolism of corticosteroids. Dosage adjustment may be needed.
*Insulin, oral antidiabetics:* Hyperglycemia. Dosage adjustment may be needed.
*Isoniazid, salicylates:* Increased metabolism. May require dosage adjustment of isoniazid or salicylates.
*Oral anticoagulants:* Decreased effectiveness. Advise clinician to monitor PT and INR.
*Ulcerogenic drugs such as NSAIDs:* Increased risk of GI ulceration. Use together cautiously.
*Vaccines:* Decreased effectiveness of vaccines. Don't give vaccine during steroid therapy.

---

## Adverse reactions
Most adverse reactions to corticosteroids are dose-dependent or duration-dependent.

**CNS:** *euphoria, insomnia,* psychotic behavior, pseudotumor cerebri, vertigo, headache, paresthesia, *seizures.*

**CV:** *HF,* hypertension, edema, *arrhythmias,* thrombophlebitis, *thromboembolism, fatal arrest or circulatory collapse* (following rapid administration of large I.V. doses).

**EENT:** cataracts, glaucoma.

**GI:** *peptic ulceration,* GI irritation, increased appetite, *pancreatitis,* nausea, vomiting.

**GU:** menstrual irregularities, increased urine glucose levels.

**Metabolic:** hypokalemia, hyperglycemia, hypocalcemia, decreased $T_4$ and $T_3$ levels, carbohydrate intolerance, growth suppression in children, cushingoid state (moonface, buffalo hump, central obesity).

**Musculoskeletal:** muscle weakness, osteoporosis.

**Skin:** hirsutism, delayed wound healing, acne, various skin eruptions.

**Other:** susceptibility to infections, *acute adrenal insufficiency that may occur with increased stress (infection, surgery, or trauma) or abrupt withdrawal after long-term therapy.*

**After abrupt withdrawal:** rebound inflammation, fatigue, weakness, arthralgia, fever, dizziness, lethargy, depression, fainting, orthostatic hypotension, dyspnea, anorexia, hypoglycemia. *After prolonged use, sudden withdrawal may be fatal.*

## Overdose and treatment
Acute ingestion, even in massive doses, is rarely a clinical problem. Toxic signs and symptoms rarely occur if drug is used for less than 3 weeks, even at large doses. However, long-term use causes adverse physiologic effects, including suppression of the hypothalamus-pituitary-adrenal axis, cushingoid appearance, muscle weakness, and osteoporosis.

## Clinical considerations
■ Methylprednisolone sodium succinate is reconstituted for I.M. use with bacteriostatic water for injection containing 0.9% benzyl alcohol.

■ Store drug at 68° to 77° F (20° to 25° C); avoid freezing methylprednisolone acetate.

■ Drug suppresses reactions to skin tests; causes false-negative results in the nitroblue tetrazolium test for systemic bacterial infections, and decreases radioactive iodine ($^{131}$I) uptake and protein-bound iodine levels in thyroid function tests.

### Therapeutic monitoring
■ Advise clinician to monitor patient for adverse effects.

### Special populations
**Pediatric patients.** Long-term use of adrenocorticoids in children and adolescents may delay growth and maturation.

**Geriatric patients.** In geriatric patients, compare risks and benefits of steroid use; lower doses are recommended. Advise clinician to monitor blood pressure and blood glucose and electrolyte levels at least every 6 months.

## Patient counseling
■ Tell patient not to stop drug abruptly or without prescriber's consent.

■ Instruct patient to take oral form of drug with food.

■ Teach patient early signs of adrenal insufficiency: fatigue, muscular weakness, joint pain, fever, anorexia, nausea, dyspnea, dizziness and fainting.

■ Tell patient to carry a card identifying need for supplemental systemic steroids during stress. Drug, dose, and name of prescriber should be on card.

■ Teach patient on long-term therapy to notify prescriber of sudden weight gain or swelling.

■ Tell patient on long-term therapy to consult with prescriber about the need for vitamin D or calcium supplement, or a physical exercise program.

■ Warn patient to avoid exposure to infections (such as chicken pox or measles) and to contact prescriber if such exposure occurs.

# metoclopramide hydrochloride
Apo-Metoclop*, Clopra, Maxeran*, Maxolon, Octamide PFS, Reclomide, Reglan

*Pharmacologic classification:* para-aminobenzoic acid (PABA) derivative
*Therapeutic classification:* antiemetic, GI stimulant
*Pregnancy risk category B*

## Available forms
Available by prescription only
*Tablets:* 5 mg, 10 mg
*Syrup:* 5 mg/5 ml
*Injection:* 5 mg/ml
*Solution:* 10 mg/ml

## Indications and dosages
*Prevention or reduction of nausea and vomiting induced by highly emetogenic chemotherapy*
*Adults:* 1 to 2 mg/kg I.V. q 2 hours for two doses, beginning 30 minutes before emetogenic chemotherapy drug administration, then q 3 hours for three doses. ◇ Some clinicians have used up to 2.75 mg/kg I.V. infusion to control nausea and vomiting. Diphenhydramine 50 mg

I.M. may be needed to control extrapyramidal symptoms at this dose.

*Facilitation of small-bowel intubation and to aid in radiologic examinations*
*Adults and adolescents ages 14 and older:* 10 mg I.V. as a single dose over 1 to 2 minutes.
*Children ages 6 to 14:* 2.5 to 5 mg I.V.
*Children under age 6:* 0.1 mg/kg I.V.

*Delayed gastric emptying secondary to diabetic gastroparesis*
*Adults:* 10 mg P.O. 30 minutes before meals and h.s. for 2 to 8 weeks, depending on response; or 10 mg I.M. or I.V. over 2 minutes.

*Gastroesophageal reflux*
*Adults:* 10 to 15 mg P.O. q.i.d., p.r.n., taken 30 minutes before meals and h.s. for up to 12 weeks.

Geriatric patients may only require 5 mg per dose.

*Postoperative nausea and vomiting*
*Adults:* 10 to 20 mg I.M. near end of surgical procedure, repeated q 4 to 6 hours, p.r.n.
≡ *Dosage adjustment.* If creatinine clearance is less than 40 ml/minute, initial doses should be 50% of usual recommended doses and adjusted as tolerated.

## I.V. administration

■ For I.V. push administration, recommend using undiluted and injecting over a 1- to 2-minute period. For I.V. infusion, dilute with 50 ml of D₅W, dextrose 5% in half-normal saline injection, Ringer's injection, or lactated Ringer's injection, and infuse over at least 15 minutes. Solution is stable for 48 hours when stored at 39° to 86° F (4° to 30° C) and protected from light or for 24 hours when exposed to normal light.
■ Recommend administering by I.V. infusion 30 minutes before chemotherapy.

### Incompatibilities

Incompatible with allopurinol, ampicillin, calcium gluconate, cefepime, cephalosporins, cephalothin, chloramphenicol, chloramphenicol sodium succinate, cisplatin, erythromycin lactobionate, furosemide, methotrexate, penicillin G potassium, and sodium bicarbonate.

## Mechanism of action

*Antiemetic action:* Metoclopramide inhibits dopamine receptors in the chemoreceptor trigger zone of the brain to inhibit or reduce nausea and vomiting.
*GI stimulant action:* Drug relieves esophageal reflux by increasing lower esophageal sphincter tone and reduces gastric stasis by stimulating motility of the upper GI tract, thus reducing gastric emptying time.

## Pharmacokinetics

*Absorption:* After oral administration, drug is absorbed rapidly and thoroughly from the GI

tract. After I.M. administration, about 74% to 96% of drug is bioavailable.
*Distribution:* Distributed to most body tissues and fluids, including the brain. Drug crosses the placenta and appears in breast milk.
*Metabolism:* Not metabolized extensively; a small amount is metabolized in the liver.
*Excretion:* Mostly excreted in urine and feces. Hemodialysis and renal dialysis remove minimal amounts.

| Route | Onset | Peak | Duration |
|-------|-------|------|----------|
| P.O. | ½-1 hr | 1-2 hr | 1-2 hr |
| I.V. | 1-3 min | Unknown | 1-2 hr |
| I.M. | 10-15 min | Unknown | 1-2 hr |

## Contraindications and precautions

Contraindicated in patients in whom stimulation of GI motility might be dangerous (such as those with hemorrhage, obstruction, or perforation), in those hypersensitive to drug, and those with pheochromocytoma, or seizure disorders. Use cautiously in patients with history of depression, Parkinson's disease, and hypertension.

## Interactions

**Drug-drug.** *Acetaminophen, aspirin, cyclosporine, diazepam, levodopa, lithium, tetracycline:* Increased absorption of these drugs. Advise clinician to monitor patient closely.
*Anticholinergics, opiates:* May antagonize effect of metoclopramide on GI motility. Avoid use together if possible.
*Antihypertensives, CNS depressants (such as sedatives and tricyclic antidepressants):* May lead to increased CNS depression. Advise clinician to monitor patient closely.
*Butyrophenone antipsychotics, phenothiazine:* May potentiate extrapyramidal reactions. Avoid use together if possible.
*Cyclosporine:* Increased absorption, possibly increasing its immunosuppressive and toxic effects. Advise clinician to monitor patient carefully.
*Digoxin:* Decreased absorption. Advise clinician to monitor serum digoxin levels.
*MAO inhibitors:* Increased blood pressure. Use together cautiously.
**Drug-lifestyle.** *Alcohol use:* May lead to increased CNS depression. Advise patient to avoid alcohol.

## Adverse reactions

**CNS:** *restlessness, anxiety, drowsiness, fatigue, lassitude, depression, akathisia, insomnia, confusion, **suicidal ideation, seizures,*** hallucinations, headache, dizziness, extrapyramidal symptoms, tardive dyskinesia, dystonic reactions.
**CV:** transient hypertension, hypotension, AV block, supraventricular tachycardia, *bradycardia.*

---

Reactions may be *common,* uncommon, *life-threatening,* or COMMON AND LIFE-THREATENING.

GI: nausea, bowel disturbances, diarrhea.
GU: urinary frequency, incontinence, prolactin secretion.
Hematologic: *neutropenia, agranulocytosis,* sulfhemoglobinemia.
Respiratory: *bronchospasm.*
Skin: rash, urticaria.
Other: fever, loss of libido, porphyria.

## Overdose and treatment
Clinical effects of overdose (which is rare) include drowsiness, dystonia, seizures, and extrapyramidal effects.

Treatment includes administration of antimuscarinics, antiparkinsonians, or antihistamines with antimuscarinic activity (such as 50 mg diphenhydramine, given I.M.).

## Clinical considerations
■ Drug has been used investigationally to treat anorexia nervosa, dizziness, migraine, intractable hiccups, and to promote postpartum lactation; oral dose form is being used investigationally to treat nausea and vomiting.
■ Don't use drug for longer than 12 weeks.
■ Metoclopramide is photosensitive and will degrade when exposed to light. Protect all forms from light. Store at 59° to 86° F (15° to 30° C).
■ Drug may be used to facilitate nasoduodenal tube placement.
■ When oral concentrate is used, recommend diluting with water, juice, carbonated beverages, or mixing with semisolid food.
■ Diphenhydramine may be used to counteract extrapyramidal effects of high-dose metoclopramide.

### *Therapeutic monitoring*
■ Advise clinician to monitor renal and hepatic test results.
■ Advise clinician to monitor ECG for changes.

### *Special populations*
Breast-feeding patients. Because drug appears in breast milk, use caution when giving to breast-feeding women.
Pediatric patients. Children have an increased risk of adverse CNS effects.
Geriatric patients. Use drug with caution, especially if patient has impaired renal function; dosage may need to be decreased. Geriatric patients are more likely to experience extrapyramidal symptoms and tardive dyskinesia.

## Patient counseling
■ Warn patient to avoid driving for 2 hours after each dose because drug may cause drowsiness. Until extent of CNS effect is known, advise patient not to consume alcohol.
■ Tell patient to report twitching or involuntary movement.
■ Instruct patient to take drug 30 minutes before each meal.

# metolazone
Mykrox, Zaroxolyn

*Pharmacologic classification:* quinazoline derivative (thiazide-like) diuretic
*Therapeutic classification:* diuretic, antihypertensive
*Pregnancy risk category B*

## Available forms
Available by prescription only
*Tablets:* 2.5 mg, 5 mg, 10 mg
*Tablets (rapid-acting):* 0.5 mg (Mykrox)

## Indications and dosages
Tablets
*Edema (heart failure)*
*Adults:* 5 to 10 mg P.O. daily.
*Edema (renal disease)*
*Adults:* 5 to 20 mg P.O. daily.
*Hypertension*
*Adults:* 2.5 to 10 mg P.O. daily; maintenance dose based on patient's blood pressure. If using stepped-care approach, initial dose is 1.25 to 2.5 mg.
Rapid-acting tablets
*Hypertension*
*Adults:* 0.5 mg P.O. once daily; may be increased to maximum of 1 mg daily.

## Mechanism of action
*Diuretic action:* Metolazone increases urinary excretion of sodium and water by inhibiting sodium reabsorption in the cortical diluting tubule of the nephron, thus relieving edema. Metolazone may be more effective in edema associated with impaired renal function than thiazide or thiazide-like diuretics.

*Antihypertensive action:* Exact mechanism is unknown; antihypertensive effect may result from direct arteriolar vasodilatation. Metolazone also reduces total body sodium levels and total peripheral resistance.

## Pharmacokinetics
*Absorption:* About 65% of a given dose of metolazone is absorbed after oral administration to healthy subjects; in cardiac patients, absorption falls to 40%. However, rate and extent of absorption vary among preparations.
*Distribution:* Metolazone is 50% to 70% erythrocyte-bound and about 33% protein-bound.
*Metabolism:* Insignificant.
*Excretion:* About 70% to 95% of metolazone is excreted unchanged in urine. Half-life is about 14 hours in healthy subjects; it may be prolonged in patients with decreased creatinine clearance.

| Route | Onset | Peak | Duration |
|-------|-------|------|----------|
| P.O. | 1 hr | 2-8 hr | 12-24 hr |

## Contraindications and precautions

Contraindicated in patients with anuria, hepatic coma or precoma, or hypersensitivity to thiazides or other sulfonamide-derived drugs. Use cautiously in patients with impaired renal or hepatic function.

## Interactions

**Drug-drug.** *Amphetamine, quinidine:* Decreased urinary excretion. Advise clinician to monitor patient closely.

*Cholestyramine, colestipol:* May bind metolazone, preventing its absorption. Give drugs 1 hour apart.

*Diazoxide:* Metolazone may potentiate hyperglycemic, hypotensive, and hyperuricemic effects of diazoxide. Use together cautiously.

*Digoxin:* Increased risk of digoxin toxicity. Advise clinician to monitor electrolytes.

*Furosemide:* Excessive volume and electrolyte depletion. Advise clinician to monitor fluid and electrolytes.

*Insulin, sulfonylurea:* Increased requirements in diabetic patients. Advise clinician to monitor patient closely.

*Lithium:* Elevated serum lithium levels. May necessitate a 50% reduction in lithium dosage.

*Methenamine mandelate:* Decreased therapeutic effect. Advise clinician to monitor patient closely.

*Other antihypertensives:* Potentiated effects. This may be used to therapeutic advantage.

**Drug-lifestyle.** *Sun exposure:* Increased risk of photosensitivity reactions. Recommend patient use adequate protection or avoid excessive sun exposure.

## Adverse reactions

**CNS:** *dizziness, headache, fatigue, vertigo, paresthesia, weakness, restlessness, drowsiness, anxiety, depression, nervousness, blurred vision.*

**CV:** volume depletion and dehydration, orthostatic hypotension, palpitations, vasculitis.

**GI:** anorexia, nausea, ***pancreatitis***, epigastric distress, vomiting, abdominal pain, diarrhea, constipation, dry mouth.

**GU:** nocturia, polyuria, frequent urination, impotence.

**Hematologic:** *aplastic anemia, agranulocytosis, leukopenia.*

**Hepatic:** jaundice, *hepatitis.*

**Metabolic:** hyperglycemia and glucose tolerance impairment; fluid and electrolyte imbalances, including hypokalemia, dilutional hyponatremia and hypochloremia, metabolic alkalosis, hypercalcemia.

**Musculoskeletal:** muscle cramps.

**Skin:** dermatitis, photosensitivity, rash, purpura, pruritus, urticaria.

## Overdose and treatment

Signs and symptoms of overdose include orthostatic hypotension, dizziness, electrolyte abnormalities, GI irritation and hypermotility, diuresis, and lethargy, which may progress to coma.

Treatment is mainly supportive; advise clinician to monitor and assist respiratory, CV, and renal function as indicated. Advise clinician to monitor fluid and electrolyte balance. Recommend inducing vomiting with ipecac in conscious patient, otherwise, using gastric lavage to avoid aspiration. Cathartics shouldn't be given; these promote additional loss of fluids and electrolytes.

## Clinical considerations

■ Drug is effective in patients with decreased renal function.

■ Metolazone is used as an adjunct in furosemide-resistant edema.

■ Drug has been used with furosemide to induce diuresis in patients who didn't respond to either diuretic alone.

■ Rapid-acting form (Mykrox) isn't interchangeable with other forms of metolazone. Dosage and uses vary.

■ Store at room temperature in tight, light-resistant containers.

■ Drug therapy may interfere with tests for parathyroid function and should be discontinued before such tests.

### Therapeutic monitoring

■ Advise clinician to monitor renal and hepatic function, electrolyte levels (potassium, sodium, chloride, calcium), and glucose level.

### Special populations

**Breast-feeding patients.** Drug may appear in breast milk. Safety and efficacy in breast-feeding women haven't been established.

**Pediatric patients.** Safety and efficacy in children haven't been established.

**Geriatric patients.** Geriatric and debilitated patients require close observation and may require reduced dosages. They are more sensitive to excess diuresis because of age-related changes in CV and renal function. Excess diuresis promotes orthostatic hypotension, dehydration, hypovolemia, hyponatremia, hypomagnesemia, and hypokalemia.

## Patient counseling

■ Tell patient to take drug in the morning to prevent nocturia.

■ Advise patient to avoid sudden posture changes and to rise slowly to avoid orthostatic hypotension.

■ Instruct patient to use a sunblock to prevent photosensitivity reactions.

---

Reactions may be *common,* uncommon, *life-threatening,* or COMMON AND LIFE-THREATENING.

# metoprolol succinate
Toprol XL

# metoprolol tartrate
Lopressor

*Pharmacologic classification:* beta blocker
*Therapeutic classification:* antihypertensive, adjunctive treatment of acute MI
*Pregnancy risk category C*

## Available forms
Available by prescription only
*Tablets:* 50 mg, 100 mg
*Tablets (extended-release):* 25 mg, 50 mg, 100 mg, 200 mg
*Injection:* 1 mg/ml in 5-ml ampules or prefilled syringes

## Indications and dosages
**Mild to severe hypertension**
*Adults:* Initially, 50 to 100 mg P.O. daily in single or divided doses; usual maintenance dose is 100 to 450 mg daily. Alternatively, 50 to 100 mg P.O. extended-release tablets daily (maximum dose, 400 mg daily). Dosages may be increased weekly or p.r.n. to desired effect.
**Early intervention in acute MI**
*Adults:* 2.5 to 5 mg rapid I.V. injections at 2- to 5-minute intervals up to a total of 15 mg over 10 to 15 minutes. Then give 50 mg P.O. 15 minutes after the last I.V. dose, and continue 50 mg P.O. every 6 hours for 48 hours. Maintenance dose, 100 mg P.O. b.i.d.
◇ *Atrial tachyarrythmias following acute MI*
*Adults:* 2.5 to 5 mg I.V. q 2 to 5 minutes to control rate up to 15 mg over a 10- to 15-minute period. Once heart rate is controlled or normal sinus rhythm restored, therapy may continue with 50 mg P.O. b.i.d. for 24 hours starting 15 minutes after the last I.V. dose. Increase dose to 100 mg P.O. b.i.d. as tolerated. Discontinue when therapeutic efficacy is achieved or if systolic blood pressure is less than 100 mm Hg or heart rate is less than 50 beats/minute.
**Angina**
*Adults:* 100 mg P.O. per day in two divided doses. Maintenance dose, 100 to 400 mg daily. Alternatively, 100 mg P.O. extended-release tablets daily (maximum dose, 400 mg daily). Dosages may be increased weekly or p.r.n.
**Treatment of stable, symptomatic heart failure (New York Heart Association class II) resulting from ischemia, hypertension, or cardiomyopathy**
*Adults:* 25 mg P.O. once daily for 2 weeks. Double the dose every 2 weeks as tolerated to a maximum of 200 mg daily.

≡ *Dosage adjustment.* For patients with more severe HF, start with 12.5 mg P.O. once daily for 2 weeks.

## I.V. administration
■ I.V. administration is used as initial treatment during early phase of definite or suspected acute MI.
■ I.V. treatment is halted when therapeutic effect is achieved (as evidenced by heart rate, ECG, and blood pressure), or if systolic blood pressure drops to 100 mm Hg or heart rate drops to 50 beats per minute.

## Incompatibilities
None reported.

## Mechanism of action
*Antihypertensive action:* Exact mechanism unknown. Metoprolol is classified as a cardioselective beta$_1$ antagonist. Drug may reduce blood pressure by blocking adrenergic receptors, thus decreasing cardiac output; by decreasing sympathetic outflow from the CNS; or by suppressing renin release.
*Action after acute MI:* Exact mechanism by which metoprolol decreases mortality after MI is unknown. In patients with MI, metoprolol reduces heart rate, systolic blood pressure, and cardiac output. Drug also appears to decrease the occurrence of ventricular fibrillation in these patients.

## Pharmacokinetics
*Absorption:* Orally administered metoprolol is absorbed rapidly and almost completely from GI tract; food enhances absorption.
*Distribution:* Distributed widely throughout the body; about 12% protein-bound.
*Metabolism:* Metabolized in the liver.
*Excretion:* About 95% of a given dose of metoprolol is excreted in urine within 72 hours, largely as metabolites.

| Route | Onset | Peak | Duration |
|---|---|---|---|
| P.O. | 15 min | 1 hr | 6-12 hr |
| P.O. (extended) | 15 min | 6-12 hr | 24 hr |
| I.V. | 5 min | 20 min | 5-8 hr |

## Contraindications and precautions
Contraindicated in patients hypersensitive to drug or other beta blockers. Also contraindicated in patients with sinus bradycardia, heart block greater than first-degree, cardiogenic shock, or overt cardiac failure when used to treat hypertension or angina. When used to treat MI, drug also is contraindicated in patients with heart rate less than 45 beats per minute, second- or third-degree heart block, PR interval of 0.24 second or longer with first-degree heart block, systolic blood pressure less than 100 mm Hg, or moderate to severe cardiac failure.

---

* Canada only     ◇ Unlabeled clinical use

Use cautiously in patients with diabetes mellitus, impaired hepatic or respiratory function, diabetes, or HF.

## Interactions
**Drug-drug.** *Cardiac glycosides:* Enhanced bradycardia. Advise clinician to monitor patient closely.
*Diuretics, other antihypertensives:* Potentiated antihypertensive effects. Advise clinician to monitor patient carefully.
*Sympathomimetics:* Antagonized beta-adrenergic effects of sympathomimetics. Advise clinician to monitor patient for drug effect.
*Verapamil:* May decrease bioavailability of metoprolol when given with antiarrhythmics. Advise clinician to monitor patient for drug effect.

## Adverse reactions
**CNS:** *fatigue, dizziness,* depression.
**CV:** *bradycardia, hypotension, HF.*
**GI:** nausea, diarrhea.
**Respiratory:** dyspnea, *bronchospasm.*
**Skin:** rash.

## Overdose and treatment
Signs and symptoms of overdose include severe hypotension, bradycardia, HF, and bronchospasm.

After acute ingestion, recommend emptying stomach by induced emesis or gastric lavage, and giving activated charcoal to reduce absorption. Subsequent treatment is usually symptomatic and supportive.

## Clinical considerations
■ Metoprolol may be given daily as a single dose or in divided doses. If a dose is missed, patient should take only the next scheduled dose.
■ Advise clinician to give drug with meals to enhance absorption.
■ Recommend reducing dosage in patients with impaired hepatic function.
■ Late-evening doses should be avoided to minimize insomnia.
■ Beta blockers may increase the risk of developing diabetes, or may mask signs and symptoms of hypoglycemia.
■ Store drug at 59° to 86° F (15° to 30° C).

## Therapeutic monitoring
■ Advise clinician to monitor heart rate, blood pressure, and ECG during I.V. administration.
■ Recommend checking blood pressure during dosage adjustment and every 3 to 6 months while patient is on maintenance therapy.
■ Recommend observing patient for signs of mental depression.

## Special populations
**Breast-feeding patients.** Metoprolol appears in breast milk. An alternative to breast-feeding is recommended during therapy.
**Pediatric patients.** Safety and efficacy in children haven't been established. No dosage recommendation exists for children.
**Geriatric patients.** Geriatric patients may require lower maintenance doses of metoprolol because of delayed metabolism; they may also experience enhanced adverse effects. Use with caution.

## Patient counseling
■ Instruct patient to take drug exactly as prescribed and to take it with meals.
■ Inform patient not to stop drug abruptly and to notify the prescriber for adverse reactions. Inform him that drug must be withdrawn gradually over 1 to 2 weeks.

# metronidazole
Apo-Metronidazole*, Flagyl, Flagyl ER, Metric-21, Novonidazol*, Protostat

# metronidazole hydrochloride
Flagyl I.V., Flagyl I.V. RTU, Metro I.V.

*Pharmacologic classification:* nitroimidazole
*Therapeutic classification:* antibacterial, antiprotozoal, amebicide
*Pregnancy risk category B*

## Available forms
Available by prescription only
*Tablets:* 250 mg, 500 mg
*Tablets (film-coated):* 250 mg, 500 mg
*Tablet (extended-release, film-coated):* 750 mg
*Capsules:* 375 mg
*Powder for injection:* 500-mg single-dose vials
*Injection:* 500 mg/dl ready to use

## Indications and dosages
*Amebic hepatic abscess*
*Adults:* 500 to 750 mg P.O. t.i.d. for 5 to 10 days. Alternatively, 2.4 g P.O. daily for 1 to 2 days or 500 mg I.V. q 6 hours for 10 days.
*Children:* 30 to 50 mg/kg P.O. daily (in three doses) for 5 to 10 days. Alternatively, 1.3 g/m$^2$ P.O. daily in three divided doses for 5 to 10 days.
*Intestinal amebiasis*
*Adults:* 750 mg P.O. t.i.d. for 5 to 10 days. Centers for Disease Control and Prevention recommends addition of iodoquinol 650 mg P.O. t.i.d. for 20 days. Alternatively, 2.4 g P.O. daily for 1 to 2 days or 500 mg I.V. q 6 hours for 10 days.
◇ *Children:* 30 to 50 mg/kg P.O. daily (in three divided doses) for 5 to 10 days. Follow this therapy with oral iodoquinol. Alternatively,

1.3 g/m² P.O. daily in three divided doses for 5 to 10 days.

**Trichomoniasis**
*Adults (both men and women concurrently):* 375-mg capsule P.O. b.i.d. for 7 days, or 500-mg tablet P.O. b.i.d. for 7 days or a single dose of 2 g P.O. or divided into two doses given on same day.

◇ *Children:* 15 mg/kg P.O. daily (in three doses) for 7 to 10 days. Alternatively, 40 mg/kg P.O. as a single dose. Dose shouldn't exceed 2 g.

**Refractory trichomoniasis**
*Adults (women):* 500 mg P.O. b.i.d. for 7 days. If repeated failure, 2 g P.O. daily for 3 to 5 days. Alternatively (for repeated failure), 2 to 3.5 g P.O. daily for 3 to 21 days depending on in vitro susceptibility testing.

**Bacterial infections caused by anaerobic microorganisms**
*Adults:* Loading dose is 15 mg/kg I.V. infused over 1 hour (about 1 g for a 154-lb [70-kg] adult). Maintenance dose is 7.5 mg/kg I.V. or P.O. q 6 hours (about 500 mg for a 154-lb adult). Give first maintenance dose 6 hours after the loading dose. Maximum dose shouldn't exceed 4 g daily. Continue therapy for 7 days to 3 weeks.

◇ **Giardiasis**
*Adults:* 250 mg P.O. t.i.d. for 5 days, or 2 g once daily for 3 days. If coexistent amebiasis, 750 mg P.O. t.i.d. for 5 to 10 days.
*Children:* 5 mg/kg P.O. t.i.d. for 5 to 7 days.

**Prevention of postoperative infection in contaminated or potentially contaminated colorectal surgery**
*Adults:* 15 mg/kg infused over 30 to 60 minutes and completed about 1 hour before surgery. Then 7.5 mg/kg infused over 30 to 60 minutes at 6 and 12 hours after initial dose. If used with oral neomycin or oral kanamycin, 750 mg P.O. b.i.d. to t.i.d. beginning 2 days before surgery. Alternatively, 500 mg to 1 g I.V. 1 hour before surgery followed by 500 mg I.V. at 8 and 16 hours postoperatively. Or, 500 mg I.V. metronidazole with 1 to 2 g I.V. cefazolin just before surgery. For prolonged procedures, additional intraoperative doses may be given every 4 to 8 hours, for the duration of the procedure.

◇ **Bacterial vaginosis**
*Adults:* 500 mg P.O. b.i.d. for 7 days; or 2 g P.O. as a single dose. Alternatively, 250 mg P.O. t.i.d. for 7 days. In pregnant women, 250 mg P.O. t.i.d. for 7 days or 2 g P.O. as a single dose. In nonpregnant women, 750 mg (extended-release) P.O. daily for 7 days.

**Pelvic inflammatory disease**
*Adults:* 500 mg I.V. q 12 hours with I.V. ofloxacin or I.V. ciprofloxacin and I.V. or oral doxycycline.

◇ **Pelvic inflammatory disease (ambulatory patients)**
*Adults:* 500 mg P.O. b.i.d. for 14 days (given with 400 mg b.i.d. of ofloxacin).

◇ **Infection with Clostridium difficile**
*Adults:* 750 mg to 2 g P.O. daily, in three to four divided doses for 7 to 14 days. Alternatively, 500 to 750 mg I.V. q 6 to 8 hours when oral dosing isn't feasible.

◇ **Helicobacter pylori *with peptic ulcer disease***
*Adults:* 250 to 500 mg P.O. t.i.d. to q.i.d. (with other drugs). Continue for 7 to 14 days depending on regimen used.
*Children:* 15 to 20 mg/kg P.O. daily, divided in two doses for 4 weeks (with other drugs).

◇ **Amebiasis caused by Dientamoeba fragilis**
*Children:* 250 mg P.O. t.i.d. for 7 days.

◇ **Entamoeba polecki *infection***
*Adults:* 750 mg P.O. t.i.d. for 10 days.
*Children:* 35 to 50 mg/kg P.O. daily in three divided doses for 10 days.

◇ **Dracunculiasis caused by Dracunculus medinensis *(guinea worm infection)***
*Adults:* 250 mg P.O. t.i.d. for 10 days.
*Children:* 25 mg/kg daily P.O. in three divided doses (up to 750 mg daily) for 10 days.

◇ **Balantidiasis caused by Balantidium coli**
*Adults:* 750 mg P.O. t.i.d. for 5 days.
*Children:* 35 to 50 mg/kg P.O. daily in three divided doses for 5 days.

◇ **Symptomatic Blastocystis hominis *infection***
*Adults:* 750 mg P.O. t.i.d. for 10 days.

◇ **Active Crohn's disease**
*Adults:* 400 mg P.O. b.i.d. For refractory perineal disease, 20 mg/kg (1 to 1.5 g) in three to five divided doses daily.

◇ **Prophylaxis in sexual assault victims**
*Adults:* 2 g P.O. (with other drugs).

## I.V. administration

■ When preparing powder for injection, follow manufacturer's instructions carefully; use solution prepared from powder within 24 hours. I.V. solutions must be prepared in three steps: reconstitution with 4.4 ml of normal saline solution injection (with or without bacteriostatic water); dilution with lactated Ringer's injection, D₅W, or normal saline solution; and neutralization with sodium bicarbonate, 5 mEq/500 mg metronidazole. Final concentration should be 8 mg/ml or less.

■ Advise clinician to give by slow infusion only; if used with a primary I.V. fluid system, recommend stopping the primary fluid during the infusion; drug shouldn't be given by I.V. push.

**⚠ ALERT** Recommend infusing drug over at least 1 hour. I.V. push shouldn't be given.

## Incompatibilities

Incompatible with aluminum, amino acid 10%, and dopamine. Manufacturer recommends not mixing other drugs with metronidazole.

## Mechanism of action

*Bactericidal, trichomonacidal, and amebicidal actions:* The nitro group of metronidazole is reduced inside the infecting organism; this reduction product disrupts DNA and inhibits nucleic acid synthesis. Drug is active in intestinal and extraintestinal sites. It's active against most anaerobic bacteria and protozoa, including *Bacteroides fragilis, B. melaninogenicus, Fusobacterium, Veillonella, Clostridium, Peptococcus, Peptostreptococcus, Entamoeba histolytica, Trichomonas vaginalis, Giardia lamblia,* and *Balantidium coli.*

## Pharmacokinetics

*Absorption:* About 80% of an oral dose is absorbed; food delays the rate but not the extent of absorption.

*Distribution:* Distributed into most body tissues and fluids, including CSF, bone, bile, saliva, pleural and peritoneal fluids, vaginal secretions, seminal fluids, middle ear fluid, and hepatic and cerebral abscesses. CSF levels approach serum levels in patients with inflamed meninges; they reach about 50% of serum levels in patients with uninflamed meninges. Less than 20% of metronidazole is plasma protein–bound. It readily crosses the placenta.

*Metabolism:* Metabolized to an active 2-hydroxymethyl metabolite and also to other metabolites.

*Excretion:* About 60% to 80% of dose is excreted as parent compound or its metabolites. About 20% of a metronidazole dose is excreted unchanged in urine; about 6% to 15% is excreted in feces. Half-life of drug is 6 to 8 hours in adults with normal renal function; its half-life may be prolonged in patients with impaired hepatic function.

| Route | Onset | Peak | Duration |
|-------|-------|------|----------|
| P.O. | Unknown | 2 hr | Unknown |
| I.V. | Immediate | 1 hr | Unknown |

## Contraindications and precautions

Contraindicated in patients hypersensitive to drug or other nitroimidazole derivatives. Use cautiously in patients with history of blood dyscrasia or alcoholism, hepatic disease, retinal or visual field changes, or CNS disorders and in those receiving hepatotoxic drugs.

## Interactions

**Drug-drug.** *Barbiturates, phenytoin:* Reduced antimicrobial effectiveness of metronidazole. Patient may need higher doses of metronidazole.

*Cimetidine:* Decreased clearance of metronidazole. Advise clinician to monitor patient for adverse effects.

*Disulfiram:* May precipitate psychosis and confusion. Avoid use together.

*Lithium:* May increase lithium levels. Advise clinician to monitor serum lithium levels.

*Oral anticoagulants:* Prolonged PT and INR. Advise clinician to monitor patient for this effect.

**Drug-lifestyle.** *Alcohol use:* May cause disulfiram-like reaction (nausea, vomiting, headache, abdominal cramps, and flushing) with drug. Advise patient to avoid alcohol.

## Adverse reactions

**CNS:** vertigo, headache, ataxia, dizziness, syncope, incoordination, confusion, irritability, depression, weakness, insomnia, *seizures,* peripheral neuropathy.

**CV:** ECG change (flattened T wave), edema (with I.V. RTU preparation).

**GI:** abdominal cramping, stomatitis, metallic taste, epigastric distress, nausea, vomiting, anorexia, diarrhea, constipation, proctitis, dry mouth.

**GU:** darkened urine, polyuria, dysuria, cystitis, dyspareunia, dryness of vagina and vulva, vaginal candidiasis.

**Hematologic:** *transient leukopenia, neutropenia.*

**Musculoskeletal:** fleeting joint pain.

**Skin:** flushing, rash.

**Other:** decreased libido, overgrowth of nonsusceptible organisms, especially *Candida* (glossitis, furry tongue); fever; thrombophlebitis (after I.V. infusion); sometimes resembling serum sickness.

## Overdose and treatment

Signs and symptoms of overdose include nausea, vomiting, ataxia, seizures, and peripheral neuropathy.

There's no known antidote for metronidazole; treatment is supportive. If patient doesn't vomit spontaneously, induced emesis or gastric lavage is indicated for an oral overdose; activated charcoal and a cathartic may be used. Diazepam or phenytoin may be used to control seizures.

## Clinical considerations

■ Injection contains 28 mEq of sodium per gram of metronidazole.

■ Trichomoniasis should be confirmed by wet smear and amebiasis by culture before giving metronidazole.

■ Drug may interfere with the chemical analyses of aminotransferases and triglyceride, leading to falsely decreased values.

### Therapeutic monitoring

■ Advise clinician to monitor patient on I.V. drug for candidiasis.

■ When treating amebiasis, advise clinician to monitor number and character of stools. Fecal specimens should be sent to the laboratory promptly; infestation is detectable only in warm specimens. Recommend repeated fecal studies at 3-month intervals to ensure elimination of organisms.

### Special populations
**Pregnant patients.** If drug is indicated during pregnancy for trichomoniasis, the 7-day regimen is preferred over the single-dose regimen. Avoid treatment with metronidazole during the first trimester.
**Breast-feeding patients.** Patient should discontinue breast-feeding while taking drug.
**Pediatric patients.** Neonates may eliminate drug more slowly than older infants and children.

### Patient counseling
■ Inform patient that drug may cause metallic taste and discolored (red-brown) urine.
■ Tell patient to take tablets with meals to minimize GI distress and that tablets may be crushed to facilitate swallowing.
■ Counsel patient on need for medical follow-up after discharge.
■ Advise patient to report adverse effects.
■ Tell patient to avoid alcohol and alcohol-containing drugs during therapy and for at least 48 hours after the last dose to prevent disulfiram-like reaction.
**Amebiasis patients**
■ Explain that follow-up examinations of stool specimens are needed for 3 months after treatment is discontinued to ensure elimination of amebae.
■ To help prevent reinfection, instruct patient and family members in proper hygiene, including disposal of feces and hand washing after defecation and before handling, preparing, or eating food, and about the risks of eating raw food and the control of contamination by flies.
■ Encourage other household members and suspected contacts to be tested and, if needed, treated.
**Trichomoniasis patients**
■ Teach correct personal hygiene, including perineal care.
■ Explain that asymptomatic sexual partners of patients being treated for trichomoniasis should be treated simultaneously to prevent reinfection; patient should refrain from intercourse during therapy or have partner use condom.

# metronidazole (topical)
MetroCream, MetroGel, MetroGel-Vaginal, Noritate

*Pharmacologic classification:* nitroimidazole
*Therapeutic classification:* antiprotozoal, antibacterial
*Pregnancy risk category B*

### Available forms
Available by prescription only
*Topical gel:* 0.75%, 1%
*Topical cream:* 0.75%
*Vaginal gel:* 0.75%

### Indications and dosages
*Topical treatment of acne rosacea,* ◇ *pressure ulcer, inflammatory papules or pustules*
*Adults:* Apply a thin film b.i.d. to affected area during the morning and evening (once daily for Noritate 1% topical gel). Significant results should be seen within 3 weeks and continue for first 9 weeks of therapy.
*Topical treatment of bacterial vaginosis*
*Adults:* One applicator b.i.d., vaginally, for 5 days or once h.s. (nonpregnant women).
◇ *Treatment of decubitus pressure ulcer*
*Adults:* Prepare a 1% aqueous solution or suspension from crushed metronidazole tablets (sterilized); apply t.i.d.

### Mechanism of action
*Anti-inflammatory action:* Although its exact mechanism of action is unknown, topical metronidazole probably exerts an anti-inflammatory effect through its antibacterial and antiprotozoal actions.

### Pharmacokinetics
*Absorption:* Under normal conditions, serum levels of metronidazole after topical administration are negligible.
*Distribution:* Less than 20% plasma protein–bound.
*Metabolism:* Unknown.
*Excretion:* Unknown after topical or intravaginal application.

| Route | Onset | Peak | Duration |
|-------|-------|------|----------|
| Topical | Unknown | Unknown | Unknown |
| Intravaginal | Unknown | 6-12 hr | Unknown |

### Contraindications and precautions
Contraindicated in patients hypersensitive to drug or its ingredients (such as parabens) and other nitroimidazole derivatives. Use cautiously in patients with history of blood dyscrasia. Use vaginal form cautiously in patients with history of CNS disease because risk of seizures or peripheral neuropathy exists.

### Interactions
**Drug-drug.** *Oral anticoagulants:* May potentiate anticoagulant effect. Advise clinician to monitor patient closely for adverse effects.
**Drug-lifestyle.** *Alcohol use:* May cause disulfiram-like reaction. Avoid use together.

### Adverse reactions
**CNS:** dizziness, light-headedness, headache (with vaginal form).
**EENT:** lacrimation (if topical gel is applied around the eyes).
**GI:** decreased appetite, cramps, pain, nausea, diarrhea, constipation, metallic or bad taste in mouth (with vaginal form).
**GU:** *cervicitis, vaginitis,* urinary frequency (with vaginal form).

**Skin:** rash, *transient redness, dryness, mild burning, stinging* (with vaginal form).
**Other:** overgrowth of nonsusceptible organisms (with vaginal form).

## Overdose and treatment
No information available. Overdose after topical application is unlikely.

## Clinical considerations
■ Topical metronidazole therapy hasn't caused the adverse reactions observed with parenteral or oral metronidazole therapy (including disulfiram-like reaction following alcohol ingestion). However, some of the drug can be absorbed following topical use. Limited clinical experience hasn't shown any of these adverse effects.

### Therapeutic monitoring
■ Advise clinician to monitor patient for clinical effect.

### Special populations
**Breast-feeding patients.** Drug appears in breast milk. A decision should be made to discontinue either drug or breast-feeding, after assessing the importance of drug to the woman.
**Pediatric patients.** Safety hasn't been established in children.

## Patient counseling
■ Advise patient to cleanse area thoroughly before applying the drug. Patient may use cosmetics after applying the drug.
■ Instruct patient to avoid use of drug on eyelids and to apply it cautiously if drug must be used around the eyes.
■ If local reactions occur, advise patient to apply drug less frequently or to discontinue use and call prescriber for specific instructions.

---

# mexiletine hydrochloride
Mexitil

*Pharmacologic classification:* lidocaine analogue, sodium channel antagonist
*Therapeutic classification:* ventricular antiarrhythmic
*Pregnancy risk category C*

## Available forms
Available by prescription only
*Capsules:* 150 mg, 200 mg, 250 mg

## Indications and dosages
*Life-threatening documented ventricular arrhythmias, including ventricular tachycardia*
*Adults:* 200 mg P.O. q 8 hours. May increase or decrease dosage in increments of 50 to 100 mg q 8 hours every 2 to 3 days if satisfactory control isn't obtained. Alternatively,

give a loading dose of 400 mg with maintenance dose of 200 mg P.O. q 8 hours. Some patients may respond well to 450 mg q 12 hours. Maximum daily dose shouldn't exceed 1,200 mg.
◇ *Diabetic neuropathy*
*Adults:* 150 mg P.O. daily for 3 days; then, 300 mg P.O. daily for 3 days followed by 10 mg/kg daily.

## Mechanism of action
*Antiarrhythmic action:* Mexiletine is structurally similar to lidocaine and exerts similar electrophysiologic and hemodynamic effects. A class IB antiarrhythmic, it suppresses automaticity and shortens the effective refractory period and action potential duration of His-Purkinje fibers and suppresses spontaneous ventricular depolarization during diastole. At therapeutic serum levels, the drug doesn't affect conductive atrial tissue or AV conduction.

Unlike quinidine and procainamide, mexiletine doesn't significantly alter hemodynamics when given in usual doses. Its effects on the conduction system inhibit reentry mechanisms and halt ventricular arrhythmias. Drug doesn't have a significant negative inotropic effect.

## Pharmacokinetics
*Absorption:* About 90% is absorbed from the GI tract. Absorption rate decreases with conditions that speed gastric emptying.
*Distribution:* Widely distributed throughout the body. About 50% to 60% of circulating drug is plasma protein–bound. Usual therapeutic drug level is 0.5 to 2 mcg/ml. Although toxicity may occur within this range, levels above 2 mcg/ml are considered toxic and are associated with an increased frequency of adverse CNS effects, warranting dosage reduction.
*Metabolism:* Metabolized in the liver to relatively inactive metabolites. Less than 10% of a parenteral dose escapes metabolism and reaches the kidneys unchanged. Metabolism is affected by hepatic blood flow, which may be reduced in patients who are recovering from MI and in those with HF. Liver disease also limits metabolism.
*Excretion:* In healthy patients, half-life of drug is 10 to 12 hours. Elimination half-life may be prolonged in patients with HF or liver disease. Urinary excretion increases with urine acidification and slows with urine alkalinization.

| Route | Onset | Peak | Duration |
|-------|-------|------|----------|
| P.O. | ½-2 hr | 2-3 hr | Unknown |

## Contraindications and precautions
Contraindicated in patients with cardiogenic shock or preexisting second- or third-degree AV block in the absence of an artificial pacemaker. Use cautiously in patients with hy-

---

potension, HF, first-degree heart block, ventricular pacemaker, preexisting sinus node dysfunction, or seizure disorders.

## Interactions

**Drug-drug.** *Ammonium chloride:* Enhances mexiletine excretion. Advise clinician to monitor patient closely.

*Antacids containing aluminum-magnesium hydroxide, atropine, narcotics:* May delay mexiletine absorption. Separate administration times.

*Cimetidine:* May decrease mexiletine metabolism, resulting in increased serum levels. Advise clinician to monitor patient closely.

*High-dose antacids, carbonic anhydrase inhibitors, sodium bicarbonate:* Decreases mexiletine excretion. Advise clinician to monitor patient closely.

*Metoclopramide:* May increase absorption. Advise clinician to monitor patient closely.

*Phenobarbital, phenytoin, rifampin:* May induce hepatic metabolism of mexiletine and thus reduce serum drug levels. Advise clinician to monitor patient closely.

*Theophylline:* Increased serum theophylline levels. Advise clinician to monitor serum theophylline levels.

## Adverse reactions

**CNS:** *tremor, dizziness, blurred vision, diplopia, confusion,* light-headedness, incoordination, changes in sleep habits, paresthesia, weakness, fatigue, speech difficulties, tinnitus, depression, *nervousness, headache.*
**CV:** *new or worsened arrhythmias,* palpitations, chest pain, nonspecific edema, angina.
**GI:** *nausea, vomiting, upper GI distress, heartburn, diarrhea, constipation, dry mouth,* changes in appetite, abdominal pain.
**Hepatic:** *altered liver function test results.*
**Skin:** rash.

## Overdose and treatment

Effects of overdose are primarily extensions of adverse CNS effects. Seizures are the most serious effect.

Treatment usually involves symptomatic and supportive measures. In acute overdose, emesis induction or gastric lavage should be performed. Urine acidification may accelerate drug elimination. If patient has bradycardia and hypotension, atropine may be given.

## Clinical considerations

■ Advise clinician to give dosage with meals, if possible.
■ Because of proarrhythmic effects, drug is generally not recommended for non–life-threatening arrhythmias.
■ Drug shouldn't be given within 1 hour of antacids containing aluminum-magnesium hydroxide.

■ When changing from lidocaine to mexiletine, recommend stopping infusion when first mexiletine dose is given. Infusion line should be kept open, however, until arrhythmia appears to be satisfactorily controlled.
■ When transferring patient from another Class I oral antiarrhythmic, initial dose of 200 mg should be initiated 6 to 12 hours after last dose of quinidine; 3 to 6 hours after last dose of procainamide; 6 to 12 hours after last dose of disopyramide; and 8 to 12 hours after last dose of tocainide.
■ Patient whose condition isn't controlled by dosing every 8 hours may respond to dosing every 6 hours.
■ Many patients who respond well to mexiletine (300 mg or less every 8 hours) can be maintained on an every 12-hour schedule. The same total daily dose is divided into twice-daily doses, which improves patient compliance.
■ Tremor (usually a fine hand tremor) is common in patients taking higher doses of mexiletine.

### Therapeutic monitoring

■ Advise clinician to monitor blood pressure and heart rate and rhythm for significant change.
■ Advise clinician to monitor hepatic function test results.

### Special populations

**Breast-feeding patients.** Drug appears in breast milk. An alternative to breast-feeding should be used during therapy.
**Geriatric patients.** Most geriatric patients require reduced dosages because of reduced hepatic blood flow and consequent decreased metabolism. Geriatric patients also may be more susceptible to CNS adverse effects.

## Patient counseling

■ Tell patient to take drug with food to reduce risk of nausea.
■ Instruct patient to report if the following occur: unusual bleeding or bruising; signs of infection, such as fever, sore throat, stomatitis, or chills; or fatigue.

# mezlocillin sodium
Mezlin

*Pharmacologic classification:* extended-spectrum penicillin, acyclaminopenicillin
*Therapeutic classification:* antibiotic
*Pregnancy risk category B*

## Available forms

Available by prescription only
*Injection:* 1 g, 2 g, 3 g, 4 g
*Infusion:* 2 g, 3 g, 4 g
*Pharmacy bulk package:* 20 g

---

## Indications and dosages

*Infections caused by susceptible organisms*

*Adults:* 200 to 300 mg/kg I.V. or I.M. daily given in four to six divided doses. Usual dosage is 3 g q 4 hours or 4 g q 6 hours. For serious infections, up to 24 g daily may be given. Therapy is usually 10 to 14 days.

*Children under age 12:* For mild to moderate infection, 50 to 100 mg/kg daily in four divided doses. For more severe infections, 200 to 300 mg/kg per day I.M. or I.V. in divided doses q 4 to 6 hours.

◇ *Neonates age 7 days and younger:* 75 mg/kg q 12 hours I.V. or I.M.

*Neonates age 8 days and older:* 75 mg/kg q 8 hours (if weight under 2 kg [4.4 lb]) or q 6 hours (if weight over 2 kg) I.V. or I.M.

*Uncomplicated urinary tract infections (UTIs)*

*Adults:* 100 to 125 mg/kg daily I.M. or I.V. in divided doses q 6 hours or 1.5 to 2 g q 6 hours.

*Complicated UTIs*

*Adults:* 150 to 200 mg/kg I.V. daily divided into q-6-hour doses or 3 g q 6 hours.

*Uncomplicated gonococcal urethritis caused by* Neisseria gonorrhoeae

*Adults:* 1 to 2 g I.M. or I.V. with 1 g of oral probenecid.

*Surgical prophylaxis*

*Adults:* 4 g I.V. 30 minutes to 1.5 hours before surgery and repeat I.V. 6 and 12 hours later.

≡ *Dosage adjustment.* For adult patients with renal impairment with creatinine clearance of 10 to 30 ml/minute, give 3 g q 6 to 8 hours for life-threatening or serious infection. For UTI, give 1.5 g q 6 to 8 hours. If creatinine clearance is less than 10 ml/minute, give 2 g q 6 to 8 hours for life-threatening or serious infection. For UTI, give 1.5 g q 8 hours.

Patients on hemodialysis should be given 3 to 4 g after each dialysis session, then q 12 hours. Patients on peritoneal dialysis may receive 3 g q 12 hours.

## I.V. administration

■ For direct I.V. injection, add 9 to 10 ml of sterile water for injection, D₅W injection, normal saline injection to each gram of mezlocillin. Shake vigorously and inject desired dose over 3 to 5 minutes. Don't exceed 100 mg/ml concentration.

■ For I.V. infusion, further dilute in 50 to 100 ml of a compatible I.V. solution (such as normal saline or D₅W) and infuse over 30 minutes. Reconstitute ADD-Vantage vial according to manufacturer instructions.

## Incompatibilities

Incompatible with amiodarone, aminoglycosides, filgrastim, and idarubicin and shouldn't be infused in the same I.V. line or solution as these drugs.

## Mechanism of action

*Antibiotic action:* Mezlocillin is bactericidal; it adheres to bacterial penicillin-binding proteins, thereby inhibiting bacterial cell-wall synthesis.

Extended-spectrum penicillins are more resistant to inactivation by certain beta-lactamases, especially those produced by gram-negative organisms, but are still liable to inactivation by certain others.

Spectrum of activity of drug includes many gram-negative aerobic and anaerobic bacilli, many gram-positive and gram-negative aerobic cocci, and some gram-positive aerobic and anaerobic bacilli, but a large number of these organisms are resistant to mezlocillin. Mezlocillin may be effective against some strains of carbenicillin-resistant and ticarcillin-resistant gram-negative bacilli. Mezlocillin shouldn't be used as sole therapy because of the rapid development of resistance. Some clinicians believe that there's no evidence that it has any advantages over ticarcillin or carbenicillin, at least with respect to cure rates. Drug is less active against *Pseudomonas aeruginosa* than other members of this class, such as piperacillin.

## Pharmacokinetics

*Absorption:* Well absorbed.

*Distribution:* Distributed widely. It penetrates minimally into CSF with uninflamed meninges, crosses the placenta, and is 16% to 42% protein-bound.

*Metabolism:* Partially metabolized; about 15% of a dose is metabolized to inactive metabolites.

*Excretion:* Excreted primarily (39% to 72%) in urine by glomerular filtration and renal tubular secretion; up to 30% of a dose is excreted in bile, and some appears in breast milk. Elimination half-life in adults is ¾ to 1½ hours; in extensive renal impairment, half-life is extended to 2 to 14 hours. Mezlocillin is removed by hemodialysis but not by peritoneal dialysis.

| Route | Onset | Peak | Duration |
|-------|-------|------|----------|
| I.V. | Immediate | Immediate | Unknown |
| I.M. | Unknown | 45-90 min | Unknown |

## Contraindications and precautions

Contraindicated in patients hypersensitive to drug or other penicillins. Use cautiously in patients with bleeding tendencies, uremia, hypokalemia, or allergy to cephalosporins.

## Interactions

**Drug-drug.** *Aminoglycoside antibiotics:* Synergistic bactericidal effect against *P. aeruginosa, Escherichia coli, Klebsiella, Citrobacter, Enterobacter, Serratia,* and *Proteus mirabilis.* This is a therapeutic advantage.

*Clavulanic acid:* Synergistic bactericidal effect against certain beta-lactamase-producing bacteria. This is a therapeutic advantage.

*Methotrexate:* Delayed elimination and elevated serum levels of methotrexate. Advise clinician to monitor patient closely.

*Probenecid:* Blocked tubular secretion of penicillins, raising their serum levels. Advise clinician to monitor patient carefully.

*Vecuronium bromide:* Prolonged neuromuscular blockade. Advise clinician to monitor patient closely.

## Adverse reactions

**CNS:** neuromuscular irritability, *seizures.*
**GI:** nausea, diarrhea, vomiting, abnormal taste, pseudomembranous colitis.
**GU:** interstitial nephritis.
**Hematologic:** *bleeding* (with high doses), *neutropenia, thrombocytopenia,* eosinophilia, *leukopenia, hemolytic anemia.*
**Metabolic:** *hypokalemia.*
**Other:** *hypersensitivity reactions (anaphylaxis,* edema, fever, chills, rash, pruritus, urticaria), overgrowth of nonsusceptible organisms, *pain at injection site, vein irritation, phlebitis.*

## Overdose and treatment

Signs of overdose include neuromuscular sensitivity or seizures; a 4- to 6-hour hemodialysis will remove 20% to 30% of mezlocillin.

## Clinical considerations

■ Mezlocillin may be more suitable than carbenicillin or ticarcillin for patients on salt-free diets; mezlocillin contains only 1.85 mEq of sodium per gram.
■ Drug is almost always used with another antibiotic, such as an aminoglycoside, in life-threatening infections.
■ For I.M. reconstitution, for each gram, add 3 to 4 ml of sterile water for injection or 1% lidocaine without epinephrine and dissolve.
■ Recommend injecting I.M. dose slowly over 12 to 15 seconds to minimize pain. Don't exceed 2 g per site.
■ Solutions are stable for 24 hours to 7 days depending on solution used and storage temperature.
■ If precipitate forms during refrigerated storage, warm to 98.6° F (37° C) in warm water bath and shake well. Solution should be clear.
■ Because drug is partially dialyzable, dosage may need adjustment in patients undergoing hemodialysis.
■ Drug alters tests for urinary or serum proteins; it interferes with turbidimetric methods that use sulfosalicylic acid, trichloroacetic acid, acetic acid, or nitric acid. Positive Coombs' tests have been reported in patients taking carbenicillin disodium.
**H ALERT** Beware of sound-alikes: methicillin and mezlocillin.

## Therapeutic monitoring

■ Advise clinician to monitor serum potassium level and liver function test results.
■ Advise clinician to monitor patient with high serum levels for seizures.

### Special populations

**Breast-feeding patients.** Drug appears in breast milk; safe use in breast-feeding women hasn't been established. An alternative to breast-feeding is recommended during therapy.
**Geriatric patients.** Half-life may be prolonged in geriatric patients because of impaired renal function.

## Patient counseling

■ Instruct patient to report adverse reactions promptly.
■ Tell patient to alert prescriber if discomfort occurs.
■ Caution patient to limit salt intake during mezlocillin therapy because of high sodium content of drug.

# miconazole nitrate

Desenex Prescription Strength Jock Itch Spray Powder, Desenex Prescription Strength Shake Powder, Femizol-M, Lotrimin AF, Micatin, Monistat 3, Monistat 7, Monistat-Derm, Monistat Dual Pack, Ting Spray Liquid, Zeasorb AF

*Pharmacologic classification:* imidazole derivative
*Therapeutic classification:* antifungal
*Pregnancy risk category B*

## Available forms

Available by prescription only
*Vaginal suppositories:* 200 mg
*Vaginal cream:* 2%, 4%
*Aerosol:* 1%
*Lotion:* 1%, 2%
*Solution:* 1%
*Cream:* 1%, 2%
Available without a prescription
*Cream:* 2%
*Powder:* 2%
*Spray:* 2%
*Vaginal cream:* 2%
*Vaginal suppositories:* 100 mg, 200 mg

## Indications and dosages

*Cutaneous or mucocutaneous fungal infections caused by susceptible organisms*
**Topical use**
*Adults and children:* Apply to affected areas b.i.d. for 2 to 4 weeks.
*Treatment of pityriasis (tinea vericolor)*
*Adults and children over age 2:* Apply cream to affected area once daily.

**Vaginal use**
*Adults:* Insert 200-mg suppository h.s. for 3 days, or 100-mg suppository or 1 applicatorful of vaginal cream h.s. for 7 days.

## Mechanism of action
*Antifungal action:* Miconazole is both fungistatic and fungicidal, depending on drug level, in *Coccidioides immitis, Candida albicans, Cryptococcus neoformans, Histoplasma capsulatum, Candida tropicalis, C. parapsilosis, Paracoccidioides brasiliensis, Sporothrix schenckii, Aspergillus flavus, Microsporum canis, Curvularia, Pseudallescheria boydii,* dermatophytes, and some gram-positive bacteria. Miconazole causes thickening of the fungal cell wall, altering membrane permeability; it also may kill the cell by interference with peroxisomal enzymes, causing accumulation of peroxide within the cell wall. It attacks virtually all pathogenic fungi.

## Pharmacokinetics
*Absorption:* About 50% of an oral dose is absorbed; however, no oral dosage form is currently available. A small amount of drug is systemically absorbed after vaginal administration.
*Distribution:* Penetrates well into inflamed joints, vitreous humor, and the peritoneal cavity. Distribution into sputum and saliva is poor, and CSF penetration is unpredictable. Over 90% plasma protein–bound.
*Metabolism:* Metabolized in the liver, predominantly to inactive metabolites.
*Excretion:* Elimination is triphasic; terminal half-life is about 24 hours. Between 10% and 14% of an oral dose is excreted in urine; 50% in feces. Up to 1% of a vaginal dose is excreted in urine; 14% to 22% of an I.V. dose is excreted in urine. It's unknown if it appears in breast milk.

| Route | Onset | Peak | Duration |
|-------|-------|------|----------|
| Topical, intravaginal | Unknown | Unknown | Unknown |

## Contraindications and precautions
Topical form contraindicated in patients hypersensitive to drug. Use cautiously in patients with hepatic insufficiency.

## Interactions
**Drug-drug.** *Amphotericin B:* Possible antagonized effects of amphotericin B. Advise clinician to monitor patient carefully.
*Phenytoin:* Increased phenytoin levels. Advise clinician to monitor phenytoin levels.
*Warfarin:* Increased anticoagulant effect. Advise clinician to monitor PT and INR.

## Adverse reactions
**CNS:** headache.
**GU:** vulvovaginal burning, pruritus, or irritation with vaginal cream; pelvic cramps.

**Skin:** irritation, burning, maceration, allergic contact dermatitis.

## Overdose and treatment
No information available.

## Clinical considerations
■ Recommend cleaning affected area before applying cream. After application, area should be gently massaged until cream disappears.
■ Topical therapy should continue for at least 1 month; improvement should begin in 1 to 2 weeks. If no improvement occurs by 4 weeks, diagnosis should be reevaluated.
■ Insert vaginal applicator high into vagina, except in pregnancy.

### Therapeutic monitoring
■ Advise clinician to monitor patient for clinical effects.

### Special populations
**Pregnant patients.** The 7-day vaginal treatment is preferred in pregnant women.
**Breast-feeding patients.** Safety hasn't been established in breast-feeding women.
**Pediatric patients.** Safety in children under age 1 hasn't been established.

## Patient counseling
■ Teach patient the symptoms of fungal infection, and explain treatment rationale.
■ Encourage patient to adhere to prescribed regimen and follow-up visits and to report adverse effects.
■ Teach patient correct procedure for intravaginal or topical applications.
■ To prevent vaginal reinfection, teach correct perineal hygiene and recommend that patient abstain from sexual intercourse during therapy.

# midazolam hydrochloride
Versed

*Pharmacologic classification:* benzodiazepine
*Therapeutic classification:* preoperative sedative, drug for conscious sedation, adjunct for induction of general anesthesia, amnestic
*Pregnancy risk category D*
*Controlled substance schedule IV*

## Available forms
Available by prescription only
*Injection:* 1 mg/ml in 2-ml, 5-ml, and 10-ml vials; 5 mg/ml in 1-ml, 2-ml, 5-ml, and 10-ml vials; 5 mg/ml in 2-ml disposable syringe
*Syrup:* 2 mg/ml in 118-ml bottle

---

## Indications and dosages

*Preoperative sedation (to induce sleepiness or drowsiness and relieve apprehension)*
*Adults under age 60:* 0.07 to 0.08 mg/kg I.M. about ½ to 1 hour before surgery. May be given with atropine or scopolamine and reduced doses of narcotics.

≡ *Dosage adjustment.* Reduce dosage in patients over age 60, those with COPD, those considered to be high-risk surgical patients, and those who have received concomitant narcotics or other depressants.

*Conscious sedation*
*Adults ages 60 and older:* 1.5 mg or less over at least 2 minutes. If additional titration is needed, give at a rate not exceeding 1 mg over 2 minutes. Total doses exceeding 3.5 mg aren't usually needed.
*Adults under age 60:* Initially, 1 to 2.5 mg I.V. administered over at least 2 minutes; repeat in 2 minutes, if needed, in small increments of initial dose over at least 2 minutes to achieve desired effect. Total dose up to 5 mg may be used. Additional doses to maintain desired level of sedation may be given by slow titration in increments of 25% of dose used to reach the sedation endpoint.

*Induction of general anesthesia*
*Unpremedicated adults ages 55 and older:* Initially, 0.3 mg/kg. For debilitated patients, initial dose is 0.2 to 0.25 mg/kg. For premedicated patients, 0.15 mg/kg may be sufficient.
*Unpremedicated adults under age 55:* 0.3 to 0.35 mg/kg I.V. over 20 to 30 seconds if patient hasn't received preanesthesia drug, or 0.15 to 0.35 mg/kg (usually 0.25 mg/kg) I.V. over 20 to 30 seconds if patient has received preanesthesia drug. Additional increments of 25% of the initial dose may be needed to complete induction.

*Continuous infusion for sedation of intubated and mechanically ventilated patients as a component of anesthesia or during treatment in a critical-care setting*
*Adults:* If a loading dose is needed to rapidly initiate sedation, give 0.01 to 0.05 mg/kg slowly or infused over several minutes, with dose repeated at 10- to 15-minute intervals until adequate sedation is achieved. For maintenance of sedation, usual infusion rate is 0.02 to 0.10 mg/kg/hour (1 to 7 mg/hour). Titrate infusion rate to the desired amount of sedation. Drug can be titrated up or down by 25% to 50% of the initial infusion rate to achieve optimal sedation without oversedation.
*Children:* After a loading dose of 0.05 to 0.2 mg/kg over 2 to 3 minutes in intubated patients only, an infusion may be initiated at 0.06 to 0.12 mg/kg/hour (1 to 2 mcg/kg/minute). Dose may be titrated up or down by 25% of the initial or subsequent infusion rate to obtain optimal sedation.
*Neonates:* Use only on intubated neonates. No loading dose is used in neonates. Neonates under age 32 weeks' gestation receive infusion rates of 0.03 mg/kg/hour (0.5 mcg/kg/minute). In neonates over age 32 weeks' gestation, infusion rates are 0.06 mg/kg/hour (1 mcg/kg/minute). Infusion may be run more rapidly in the first few hours to obtain a therapeutic blood level. Rate of infusion should be frequently and carefully reassessed to give the lowest possible amount of drug.

*Sedation, anxiolysis, and amnesia before diagnostic, therapeutic, or endoscopic procedures or before induction of anesthesia in children*
*Children ages 13 to 16:* 0.07 to 0.08 mg/kg I.M. ½ to 1 hour before surgery; for conscious sedation, 1 to 2.5 mg I.V. over at least 2 minutes.
*Children ages 6 to 12:* 25 to 50 mcg/kg I.V. up to 400 mcg/kg (usual dose doesn't exceed 10 mg).
*Children ages 6 months to 5 years:* Initially 50 to 100 mcg/kg I.V. up to 600 mcg/kg (usual dose doesn't exceed 6 mg).
*Children ages 6 months to 16 years:* 250 to 500 mcg/kg P.O. up to 20 mg or up to 1 mg/kg. Lower doses may provide adequate therapeutic effect for children age 6 months to 16 years or cooperative patients. Alternatively, 100 to 150 mcg/kg I.M. (up to 500 mcg/kg may be needed) not to exceed 10 mg.

## I.V. administration

■ When mixing infusion, use 5-mg/ml vial, and dilute to 0.5 mg/ml with $D_5W$ or normal saline solution.
■ Administer slowly over at least 2 minutes to prevent respiratory depression, and wait at least 2 minutes when titrating doses to effect.
■ Before administration, ensure the immediate availability of oxygen and resuscitative equipment. Apnea and death have been reported with rapid I.V. administration. Avoid intra-arterial injection because the hazards of this route are unknown. Avoid extravasation.

### Incompatibilities

Incompatible with dimenhydrinate, pentobarbital sodium, perphenazine, prochlorperazine edisylate, and rantidine hydrochloride.

## Mechanism of action

*Sedative and anesthetic actions:* Although exact mechanism is unknown, midazolam, like other benzodiazepines, is thought to facilitate the action of gamma-aminobutyric acid (GABA) to provide a short-acting CNS depressant action.
*Amnestic action:* Mechanism of action is unknown.

## Pharmacokinetics

*Absorption:* Absorption after I.M. administration appears to be 80% to 100%.
*Distribution:* Drug has a large volume of distribution and is about 97% protein-bound. Drug

crosses the placenta and enters fetal circulation.

*Metabolism:* Metabolized in the liver.
*Excretion:* Metabolites are excreted in urine. Half-life of drug is 1¼ to 12⅓ hours.

| Route | Onset | Peak | Duration |
|-------|-------|------|----------|
| P.O. | 10-20 min | 1-2 hr | 2-6 hr |
| I.V. | 1½-5 min | Rapid | 2-6 hr |
| I.M. | 15 min | 15-60 min | 2-6 hr |

## Contraindications and precautions

Contraindicated in patients hypersensitive to drug, those with acute angle-closure glaucoma, and in those experiencing shock, coma, or acute alcohol intoxication. Use cautiously in patients with uncompensated acute illnesses and in geriatric or debilitated patients.

## Interactions

**Drug-drug.** *Antidepressants, antihistamines, barbiturates, narcotics, tranquilizers, other CNS and respiratory depressants:* Potentiated effects. Use together cautiously.
*CYP3A4 inhibitors (azole antifungals, calcium channel blockers, HIV protease inhibitors, macrolides, quinupristin and dalfopristin):* Concomitant use may increase plasma level of midazolam and can increase and prolong sedative effect. Advise clinician to give concomitantly with caution and monitor patient closely.
*Droperidol, fentanyl, narcotics:* Potentiate the hypnotic effect of midazolam. Advise clinician to monitor patient closely.
*Erythromycin:* May decrease plasma clearance of midazolam. Advise clinician to monitor patient closely.
*Inhaled anesthetics:* Midazolam may decrease the needed dose of inhaled anesthetics by depressing respiratory drive. Anesthesia dosage may require adjustment.
*Isoniazid:* May decrease the metabolism of midazolam. Advise clinician to monitor patient closely.
**Drug-food.** *Grapefruit juice:* Increased bioavailability of oral syrup form of drug. Patient shouldn't use together.
**Drug-lifestyle.** *Alcohol use:* Potentiated effects of alcohol. Advise patient to avoid alcohol.

## Adverse reactions

**CNS:** headache, oversedation, drowsiness, amnesia.
**CV:** variations in blood pressure (hypotension) and pulse rate, *cardiac arrest.*
**GI:** *nausea,* vomiting.
**Respiratory:** *hiccups, decreased respiratory rate, apnea, respiratory arrest.*
**Other:** *pain, tenderness* (at injection site).

## Overdose and treatment

Signs and symptoms of overdose include confusion, stupor, coma, respiratory depression, and hypotension.

Treatment is supportive. Recommend maintaining patent airway and ensuring adequate ventilation with mechanical support, if needed. Advise clinician to monitor vital signs. Recommend using I.V. fluids or ephedrine to treat hypotension. Flumazenil, a specific benzodiazepine-receptor antagonist, is indicated for complete or partial reversal of the sedative effects.

## Clinical considerations

■ Individualized dosages are advised, using the smallest effective dose possible. Use with extreme caution and reduced dosage in geriatric and debilitated patients.

■ Medical personnel who administer midazolam should be familiar with airway management. Close monitoring of cardiopulmonary function is required. Recommend continuously monitoring patients who have received midazolam to detect potentially life-threatening respiratory depression.

**⚠ ALERT** Laryngospasm and bronchospasm may occur; countermeasures should be available.

■ Midazolam can be mixed in the same syringe with morphine, meperidine, atropine, and scopolamine.

■ Syrup form must be given only to patients visually monitored by health care professionals.

■ There is a potential for adverse effects, such as hypotension, metabolic acidosis, and kernicterus, related to neonate metabolism of benzyl alcohol. The amount of benzyl alcohol should be taken into account when giving high doses of drugs, including midazolam, containing the preservative.

■ I.M. dose should be administered deep into a large muscle mass to prevent tissue injury.

■ Solution that's discolored or contains a precipitate shouldn't be used.

### Therapeutic monitoring

■ Hypotension occurs more frequently in patients premedicated with narcotics. Advise clinician to monitor vital signs closely.

### Special populations

**Breast-feeding patients.** It isn't known if drug appears in breast milk; use with caution in breast-feeding women.
**Pediatric patients.** The safety and efficacy of oral solution in children under age 6 months haven't been established. Advise clinician to monitor the amount of benzyl alcohol when used in neonates.
**Geriatric patients.** Geriatric or debilitated patients, especially those with COPD, are at significantly increased risk for respiratory de-

---

pression and hypotension. Lower doses are indicated. Use with caution. Oral dosage forms aren't recommended for geriatric use.

### Patient counseling
■ Advise patient to postpone tasks that require mental alertness or physical coordination until the effects of the drug have worn off.
■ Instruct patient as needed in safety measures, such as supervised walking and gradual position changes, to prevent injury.
■ Advise patient to contact prescriber before taking OTC drugs.

# mifepristone
Mifeprex

*Pharmacologic classification:* synthetic steroid
*Therapeutic classification:* antiprogestational drug
*Pregnancy risk category NR*

### Available forms
*Tablets:* 200 mg

### Indications and dosages
*Termination of intrauterine pregnancy through 49th day of pregnancy*
*Adults:* On day 1,600 mg (three 200-mg tablets) P.O. as a single dose. On day 3, unless abortion is confirmed by clinical examination or ultrasonographic scan, give 400 mcg (two 200-mcg tablets) misoprostol P.O.

### Mechanism of action
*Antiprogestational action:* Mifeprex is a synthetic steroid with antiprogestational effects. It competitively interacts with progesterone at progesterone-receptor sites. Drug inhibits activity of endogenous and exogenous progesterone, resulting in termination of pregnancy.

### Pharmacokinetics
*Absorption:* Rapidly absorbed; levels peak in about 90 minutes.
*Distribution:* 98% bound to plasma proteins, albumin, and alpha$_1$-acid glycoprotein.
*Metabolism:* Metabolized by *N*-demethylation and terminal hydroxylation to three major metabolites. CYP-450 3A4 is primarily responsible for the metabolism.
*Excretion:* Excreted in feces and urine.

| Route | Onset | Peak | Duration |
|-------|-------|------|----------|
| P.O. | Rapid | 90 min | 11 days |

### Contraindications and precautions
Contraindicated in patients with confirmed or suspected ectopic pregnancy or undiagnosed adnexal mass and in patients with an intrauterine device in place. Also contraindicated in patients with chronic adrenal failure, those on concurrent long-term corticosteroid therapy, and those with history of allergy to mifepristone, misoprostol, or other prostaglandins. Contraindicated in patients with inherited porphyrias or hemorrhagic disorders and in those on concurrent anticoagulant therapy.

The treatment procedure is contraindicated in patients without access to a medical facility equipped to provide emergency treatment of incomplete abortion, blood transfusions, and emergency resuscitation during the period from the first visit until discharged by prescriber.

Don't give to any patient who may be unable to understand effects of the treatment procedure or to comply with its regimen.

Use cautiously in patients who are heavy smokers and in those with CV disease; hypertension; respiratory, renal, or hepatic disease; type 1 diabetes, or severe anemia. Also use cautiously in women who are over age 35 and who smoke 10 or more cigarettes per day because such patients were excluded from clinical trials of mifepristone.

### Interactions
**Drug-drug.** *Carbamazepine, dexamethasone, phenobarbital, phenytoin, rifampin:* Possible induced metabolism and reduced serum mifepristone level. Use together cautiously.
*Drugs that are CYP3A4 substrates and have narrow therapeutic ranges (general anesthetics):* Increased serum levels and prolonged elimination of these drugs. Use together cautiously.
*Erythromycin, itraconazole, ketoconazole:* Possible inhibited metabolism and increased serum mifepristone level. Use together cautiously.
**Drug-herb.** *St. John's wort:* Possible induced metabolism and decreased mifepristone level. Tell patient not to use together.
**Drug-food.** *Grapefruit juice:* Possible inhibited metabolism and increased mifepristone level. Tell patient to take drug with a different beverage.

### Adverse reactions
**CNS:** *headache, dizziness, fatigue,* insomnia, asthenia, anxiety, syncope, fainting.
**EENT:** sinusitis.
**GI:** *abdominal cramping, nausea, vomiting, diarrhea,* dyspepsia.
**GU:** vaginitis, *uterine cramping,* pelvic pain, uterine hemorrhage.
**Hematologic:** anemia, leukorrhea, decrease in hemoglobin of more than 2 g/dl.
**Musculoskeletal:** back pain, leg pain.
**Other:** fever, rigors, viral infections.

### Overdose and treatment
No serious adverse reactions occurred with three times the recommended dose of mifepristone. If patient ingests a massive overdose,

she should be observed closely for signs of adrenal failure.

## Clinical considerations
■ Drug is supplied only to licensed prescribers who sign and return a Prescriber's Agreement. It isn't available through pharmacies.

■ For purposes of this treatment, pregnancy is dated from the first day of the last menstrual period in a presumed 28-day cycle with ovulation occurring at midcycle. Duration of pregnancy may be determined from menstrual history and clinical examination. Ultrasonography should be used if duration of pregnancy is uncertain or if ectopic pregnancy is suspected.

■ Patient must read the drug guide and sign the patient agreement before drug is given.

■ Any intrauterine device must be removed before treatment with mifepristone begins.

■ Mifepristone and misoprostol treatment for termination of pregnancy requires three office visits by patient to prescriber for proper administration. Treatment may only be given in a clinic, medical office, or hospital, by or under the supervision of a prescriber able to assess the gestational age of an embryo and to diagnose ectopic pregnancies. Prescribers must also be able to provide surgical intervention in cases of incomplete abortion or severe bleeding, or have made plans to provide such care through others, and be able to assure patient access to medical facilities equipped to provide blood transfusions and resuscitation, if needed.

■ During the period following administration of misoprostol, the patient may need drug for cramps or GI symptoms.

■ Store mifepristone at controlled room temperature.

### Therapeutic monitoring
■ Patient must return for follow-up visit about 14 days after administration of mifepristone to determine by clinical examination or ultrasound that a complete termination of pregnancy has occurred and to assess the degree of bleeding. Patients who have an ongoing pregnancy at this visit have a risk of fetal malformation resulting from the treatment. Surgical termination is recommended.

■ Vaginal bleeding and uterine or abdominal cramping are expected effects of the drug. Vaginal bleeding or spotting occurs for an average of 9 to 16 days. Excessive bleeding may require treatment with vasoconstrictors, curettage, saline infusions, or blood transfusions. Persistence of moderate or heavy bleeding at the 14-day follow-up visit may indicate incomplete abortion.

### Special populations
**Breast-feeding patients.** It isn't known if drug appears in breast milk. Breast-feeding women should consult prescriber to decide if they should discard their breast milk for a few days following administration.

## Patient counseling
■ Give patient a copy of the drug guide and the patient agreement. Review them with patient and discuss any questions the patient has.

■ Inform patient of importance of completing treatment schedule, and stress need for follow-up visit about 14 days after taking mifepristone.

■ Tell patient to expect uterine cramping and vaginal bleeding that may be heavy at times.

■ Inform patient that vaginal bleeding isn't proof of a complete abortion and that she must return for follow-up visit to confirm the abortion.

■ Inform patient that, if treatment fails, surgical intervention may be needed.

■ Supply patient with a name and telephone number to contact in case of emergency.

■ Inform patient that she may become pregnant again as soon as termination of pregnancy is complete and before normal menses has returned.

■ Teach patient about forms of contraception.

# miglitol
Glyset

*Pharmacologic classification:* alpha-glucosidase inhibitor
*Therapeutic classification:* antidiabetic
*Pregnancy risk category B*

## Available forms
Available by prescription only
*Tablets:* 25 mg, 50 mg, 100 mg

## Indications and dosages
*Monotherapy adjunct to diet to improve glycemic control in patients with type 2 diabetes mellitus whose hyperglycemia can't be managed with diet alone, or with a sulfonylurea when diet plus either miglitol or sulfonylurea alone don't result in adequate glycemic control*
Adults: 25 mg P.O. t.i.d. at the start (with the first bite) of each main meal; dose may be increased after 4 to 8 weeks to 50 mg P.O. t.i.d. The dose may then be further increased after 3 months, based on the glycosylated hemoglobin level, to a maximum of 100 mg P.O. t.i.d.

## Mechanism of action
*Antidiabetic action:* Miglitol lowers blood glucose through reversible inhibition of the enzymes alpha-glucosidases in the brush border of the small intestine. Alpha-glucosidases are responsible for the conversion of oligosaccharides and disaccharides to glucose. Inhibition of these enzymes results in delayed glucose

absorption and a lowering of postprandial blood glucose. In contrast to sulfonylureas, miglitol has no effect on insulin secretion.

## Pharmacokinetics
*Absorption:* Shows saturable absorption at high doses. A 25-mg dose is completely absorbed, whereas a dose of 100 mg is only 50% to 70% absorbed.
*Distribution:* Distributes primarily into the extracellular fluid. Protein binding is negligible (less than 4%).
*Metabolism:* Not metabolized.
*Excretion:* Eliminated primarily by renal excretion. More than 95% of a given dose is recovered in the urine as unchanged drug. Elimination half-life is about 2 hours.

| Route | Onset | Peak | Duration |
|-------|-------|------|----------|
| P.O. | Unknown | 2-3 hr | Unknown |

## Contraindications and precautions
Miglitol is contraindicated in patients hypersensitive to the drug or its components. Also contraindicated in patients with diabetic ketoacidosis, inflammatory bowel disease, colonic ulceration, or partial intestinal obstruction, and in patients predisposed to intestinal obstruction or those with chronic intestinal diseases associated with marked disorders of digestion or absorption, or with conditions that may deteriorate as a result of increased gas formation in the intestine.

Drug isn't recommended in patients with significant renal dysfunction (serum creatinine more than 2 mg/dl). Use cautiously in patients also receiving insulin or oral sulfonylureas.

## Interactions
**Drug-drug.** *Digoxin, propranolol, ranitidine:* May decrease the bioavailability of these drugs. Advise clinician to monitor patient for loss of drug efficacy; dosage adjustment may be needed. *Intestinal absorbents such as charcoal; digestive enzyme preparations, such as amylase and pancreatin:* May reduce the effectiveness of miglitol. Avoid use together.
**Drug-herb.** *Aloe, bilberry leaf, bitter melon, burdock, fenugreek, garlic, ginseng:* May improve blood glucose control, requiring dosage reduction of antidiabetic. Advise patient to consult prescriber before taking any herbal preparations.

## Adverse reactions
**GI:** *abdominal pain, diarrhea, flatulence.*
**Metabolic:** decreased serum iron level.
**Skin:** rash.

## Overdose and treatment
Overdose may result in transient increases in GI adverse reactions. No serious systemic reactions are expected in the event of an overdose.

## Clinical considerations
■ An increased risk of hypoglycemia can occur when used with insulin or sulfonylureas; dosage adjustments of these drugs may be needed.
■ The management of type 2 diabetes should also include diet control, exercise program, and regular testing of urine and blood glucose.
■ Advise clinician to give miglitol with the first bite of each main meal.
■ Mild to moderate hypoglycemia may be treated with a form of dextrose such as glucose tablets or gel. Severe hypoglycemia may require I.V. glucose or glucagon administration.

### Therapeutic monitoring
■ When treatment starts or changes, 1-hour postprandial plasma glucose may be used to determine therapeutic response.
■ Advise clinician to monitor patients for an increased frequency of hypoglycemia.
■ Advise clinician to monitor blood glucose level regularly, especially during situations of increased stress, such as infection, fever, surgery, and trauma.
■ In addition to checking glucose levels regularly, advise clinician to monitor glycosylated hemoglobin every 3 months to evaluate long-term glycemic control.

### Special populations
**Breast-feeding patients.** Although the amount of miglitol appearing in breast milk is low, it's recommended that miglitol not be given to breast-feeding women.
**Pediatric patients.** Safety and efficacy of miglitol in children haven't been established.
**Geriatric patients.** No significant differences in the safety and effectiveness of miglitol have been observed in placebo-controlled clinical trials between older and younger patients.

## Patient counseling
■ Instruct patient about the importance of adhering to dietary, weight reduction, and exercise instructions and to have blood glucose and glycosylated hemoglobin tested regularly.
■ Inform patient that treatment with miglitol relieves symptoms but doesn't cure diabetes.
■ Teach patient to recognize signs and symptoms of hyperglycemia and hypoglycemia.
■ Instruct patient to treat hypoglycemia with glucose tablets and to have a source of glucose readily available to treat symptoms of hypoglycemia when miglitol is taken with a sulfonylurea or insulin.
■ Advise patient to seek medical advice promptly during periods of stress such as fever, trauma, infection, or surgery because drug requirements may change.
■ Instruct patient to take miglitol three times a day with the first bite of each main meal.
■ Show patient how and when to perform self-monitoring of glucose levels.

- Advise patient that adverse GI effects are most common during the first few weeks of therapy and should improve over time.
- Urge patient to carry medical identification at all times.

# milrinone lactate
Primacor

*Pharmacologic classification:* bipyridine phosphodiesterase inhibitor
*Therapeutic classification:* inotropic vasodilator
*Pregnancy risk category C*

## Available forms
Available by prescription only
*Solution:* 1 mg/ml in 10-ml and 20-ml vials
*Cartridge:* 5 ml
*Injection, premixed:* 200 mEq/ml in $D_5W$

## Indications and dosages
*Short-term I.V. therapy for heart failure*
*Adults:* Initial loading dose of 50 mcg/kg I.V. over 10 minutes, followed by continuous infusion/maintenance dose of 0.375 to 0.75 mcg/kg/minute. Adjust infusion dosage based on hemodynamic and clinical response.
≣ *Dosage adjustment.* For patients with renal impairment, refer to the table below.

| Creatinine clearance (ml/min) | Infusion rate (mcg/kg/min) |
|---|---|
| 50 | 0.43 |
| 40 | 0.38 |
| 30 | 0.33 |
| 20 | 0.28 |
| 10 | 0.23 |
| 5 | 0.20 |

Note: If hypotension occurs, administration of milrinone should be reduced or temporarily discontinued until patient's condition stabilizes.

## I.V. administration
- Milrinone must be further diluted before I.V. administration. Acceptable diluents include half normal saline or normal saline solution or $D_5W$.
- Prepare the 100 mcg/ml, 150 mcg/ml, or 200 mcg/ml solutions by adding 180 ml, 113 ml, or 80 ml to the 20-mg (20-ml) vial. Add one-half of the diluent amounts to the 10-ml vial to achieve same concentration.

## Incompatibilities
When furosemide is injected into an I.V. line containing milrinone, an immediate chemical interaction occurs, as evidenced by the formation of a precipitate. Therefore, furosemide shouldn't be given in an I.V. line that contains milrinone.

## Mechanism of action
*Inotropic and vasodilator actions:* Milrinone is a selective inhibitor of peak III cAMP phosphodiesterase isozyme in cardiac and vascular muscle. This inhibitory action is consistent with cAMP-mediated increases in intracellular ionized calcium and contractile force in cardiac muscle, as well as with cAMP-dependent contractile protein phosphorylation and relaxation in vascular muscle. In addition to increasing myocardial contractility, milrinone improves diastolic function, shown by improvements in left ventricular diastolic relaxation.

## Pharmacokinetics
*Absorption:* Administered I.V.
*Distribution:* About 70% is bound to human plasma protein.
*Metabolism:* About 12% is metabolized to a glucuronide metabolite.
*Excretion:* After I.V. administration, about 90% is excreted unchanged in urine within 8 hours.

| Route | Onset | Peak | Duration |
|---|---|---|---|
| I.V. | 5-15 min | 1-2 hr | 3-6 hr |

## Contraindications and precautions
Contraindicated in patients hypersensitive to drug, and those with severe aortic or pulmonic valvular disease in place of surgical correction, or during the acute phase of an MI.
    Use cautiously in patients with atrial fibrillation or flutter.

## Interactions
None reported.

## Adverse reactions
**CNS:** headache.
**CV:** *ventricular arrhythmias, ventricular ectopic activity, nonsustained ventricular tachycardia,* SUSTAINED VENTRICULAR TACHYCARDIA, VENTRICULAR FIBRILLATION, hypotension, angina.

## Overdose and treatment
Hypotension may occur with milrinone overdose because of its vasodilator effect. No specific antidote is known, but general measures for circulatory support should be taken.

## Clinical considerations
- Drug therapy isn't recommended for patients in acute phase of post-MI; clinical studies in this population are lacking.
- Duration of therapy depends on patient responsiveness. Patients have been maintained on infusions of milrinone for up to 5 days.

### Therapeutic monitoring
■ Advise clinician to monitor renal function and fluid and electrolyte changes during milrinone therapy. Hypokalemia should be corrected with potassium supplements before or during use of milrinone.

### Special populations
**Breast-feeding patients.** It isn't known if drug appears in breast milk. Use caution when giving drug to breast-feeding women.
**Pediatric patients.** Safety and efficacy in children haven't been established.

## Patient counseling
■ Instruct patient to report adverse effects, especially angina.
■ Instruct patient to report discomfort at I.V. site.

---

# minocycline hydrochloride
Dynacin, Minocin

*Pharmacologic classification:* tetracycline
*Therapeutic classification:* antibiotic
*Pregnancy risk category NR*

## Available forms
Available by prescription only
*Capsules:* 50 mg, 100 mg
*Tablets:* 50 mg, 100 mg
*Suspension:* 50 mg/5 ml
*Injection:* 100 mg/vial

## Indications and dosages
*Infections caused by sensitive organisms*
*Adults:* Initially, 200 mg P.O., I.V.; then 100 mg q 12 hours or 50 mg P.O. q 6 hours.
*Children over age 8:* Initially, 4 mg/kg P.O., I.V.; then 4 mg/kg P.O. daily, divided q 12 hours. Give I.V. in 500- to 1,000-ml solution without calcium over 6 hours.
*Gonorrhea in patients sensitive to penicillin*
*Adults:* Initially, 200 mg P.O.; then 100 mg q 12 hours for 4 days.
*Syphilis in patients sensitive to penicillin*
*Adults:* Initially, 200 mg P.O.; then 100 mg q 12 hours for 10 to 15 days.
*Meningococcal carrier state*
*Adults:* Initially, 200 mg P.O.; then 100 mg P.O. q 12 hours for 5 days.
*Uncomplicated urethral, endocervical, or rectal infection caused by* **Chlamydia trachomatis** *or* **Ureaplasma urealyticum**
*Adults:* 100 mg P.O. q 12 hours for at least 7 days.
*Uncomplicated gonococcal urethritis in men*
*Adults:* 100 mg P.O. q 12 hours for 5 days.
**Mycobacterium marinum**
*Adults:* 100 mg P.O. q 12 hours for 6 to 8 weeks.

*Cholera*
*Adults:* Initially, 200 mg P.O.; then 100 mg P.O. q 12 hours for 72 hours.
*Acne*
*Adults:* 50 mg P.O. daily to t.i.d.
◇ *Treatment of multibacillary leprosy*
*Adults:* 100 mg P.O. daily with clofazimine and ofloxacin for 6 months, followed by 100 mg P.O. daily for an additional 18 months in conjunction with clofazimine.
◇ *Nocardiosis*
*Adults:* Usual dose for 12 to 18 months.
◇ *Sclerosis drug for pleural effusions*
*Adults:* 300 mg mixed in 40 to 50 ml sodium chloride injection, instilled through a thoracostomy tube.
◇ *Nongonococcal urethritis caused by* **C. trachomatis** *or mycoplasma*
*Adults:* 100 mg P.O. daily in one or two divided doses for 1 to 3 weeks.

## I.V. administration
■ Reconstitute 100 mg powder with 5 ml sterile water for injection, with further dilution of 500 to 1,000 ml for I.V. infusion to a concentration of 100 to 200 mcg/ml. Recommend infusing over 6 hours.
■ Reconstituted solution is stable for 24 hours at room temperature. Use final diluted solution immediately.

## Incompatibilities
Avoid mixing with solutions containing calcium because precipitate may form. Drug is compatible with Ringer's injection and lactated Ringer's injection.

## Mechanism of action
*Antibacterial action:* Minocycline is bacteriostatic; it binds reversibly to ribosomal units, thus inhibiting bacterial protein synthesis.

Minocycline is active against many gram-negative and gram-positive organisms, *Mycoplasma, Rickettsia, Chlamydia,* and spirochetes; it may be more active against staphylococci than other tetracyclines.

The potential vestibular toxicity and cost of minocycline limit its usefulness. It may be more active than other tetracyclines against *Nocardia asteroides;* it's also effective against *Mycobacterium marinum* infections. It has been used for meningococcal meningitis prophylaxis because of its activity against *Neisseria meningitidis.*

## Pharmacokinetics
*Absorption:* About 90% to 100% is absorbed after oral administration.
*Distribution:* Widely distributed into body tissues and fluids, including synovial, pleural, prostatic, and seminal fluids, bronchial secretions, saliva, and aqueous humor; CSF penetration is poor. Drug crosses the placenta, and is 55% to 88% protein-bound.

---

* Canada only    ◇ Unlabeled clinical use

*Metabolism:* Metabolized partially.
*Excretion:* Excreted primarily unchanged in urine by glomerular filtration. Plasma half-life is 11 to 22 hours in adults with normal renal function. Some drug appears in breast milk.

| Route | Onset | Peak | Duration |
|-------|-------|------|----------|
| P.O. | Unknown | 1-4 hr | Unknown |
| I.V. | Immediate | Immediate | Unknown |

## Contraindications and precautions
Contraindicated in patients hypersensitive to drug or other tetracyclines. Use cautiously in patients with impaired renal or hepatic function, in children under age 8, and during the last half of pregnancy.

## Interactions
**Drug-drug.** *Antacids containing aluminum, calcium, or magnesium; laxatives containing magnesium; oral iron products; sodium bicarbonate:* Decreased oral absorption of minocycline because of chelation. Give drugs at separate times.
*Digoxin:* Increased bioavailability. Decreased digoxin dose may be needed.
*Oral anticoagulants:* Increased effects. Decreased anticoagulant dose may be needed.
*Oral contraceptives:* Possibly less effective when given with minocycline. Advise patient to use alternative method of birth control.
*Penicillins:* Tetracyclines may antagonize bactericidal effects of penicillin. Give penicillin 2 to 3 hours before minocycline.
**Drug-food.** *Any, food, milk, other dairy products:* Possible decreased absorption of minocycline. Avoid use together.
**Drug-lifestyle.** *Sun exposure:* Increased risk of photosensitivity reactions. Advise patient to use sunblock and limit sun exposure.

## Adverse reactions
**CNS:** headache, *intracranial hypertension (pseudotumor cerebri),* light-headedness, dizziness, vertigo.
**CV:** pericarditis.
**EENT:** dysphagia, glossitis.
**GI:** *anorexia, epigastric distress, oral candidiasis, nausea, vomiting, diarrhea,* enterocolitis, inflammatory lesions in anogenital region.
**GU:** increased BUN level.
**Hematologic:** *neutropenia,* eosinophilia, *thrombocytopenia,* hemolytic anemia.
**Hepatic:** elevated liver enzyme levels.
**Skin:** *maculopapular and erythematous rashes, photosensitivity, increased pigmentation,* urticaria.
**Other:** hypersensitivity reactions *(anaphylaxis);* permanent discoloration of teeth, enamel defects, and bone growth retardation if used in children under age 8; superinfection; *thrombophlebitis.*

## Overdose and treatment
Signs of overdose are usually limited to GI tract; advise clinician to give antacids or empty stomach by gastric lavage if ingestion occurred within the preceding 4 hours.

## Clinical considerations
**H** *ALERT* Check expiration date. Outdated or deteriorated tetracyclines have caused reversible nephrotoxicity (Fanconi's syndrome).
■ Drug causes false-negative results in urine glucose tests using glucose oxidase reagent (Clinistix or glucose enzymatic test strip). Minocycline causes false elevations in fluorometric test results for urinary catecholamines.
**H** *ALERT* Beware of sound-alikes: minocin, niacin, and mithracin.

### Therapeutic monitoring
■ Advise clinician to monitor renal and hepatic function in prolonged therapy.

### Special populations
**Breast-feeding patients.** Avoid use in breast-feeding women.
**Pediatric patients.** Drug isn't recommended for use in children under age 9.

## Patient counseling
■ Tell patient to take entire amount of drug prescribed, even after he feels better.
■ Instruct patient to take oral form of drug with a full glass of water. Drug may be taken with food. Tell patient not to take within 1 hour of bedtime to avoid esophageal irritation or ulceration.
■ Warn patient to avoid driving or other hazardous tasks because of possible adverse CNS effects.
■ Caution patient to avoid direct sunlight and ultraviolet light, wear protective clothing, and use sunblock. Photosensitivity reactions may occur within a few minutes to several hours after exposure. Photosensitivity persists for some time after discontinuation of therapy.

# minoxidil (systemic)
Loniten

*Pharmacologic classification:* peripheral vasodilator
*Therapeutic classification:* antihypertensive
*Pregnancy risk category C*

## Available forms
Available by prescription only
*Tablets:* 2.5 mg, 10 mg

## Indications and dosages
*Severe hypertension*
*Adults and children over age 12:* Initially, 2.5 to 5 mg P.O. as a single daily dose. Dose may

be increased at 3-day intervals (minimum) to 10 mg, 20 mg, and then 40 mg. If rapid control is needed, dosage may be adjusted q 6 hours. Effective dosage range is usually 10 to 40 mg daily in one to two divided doses. Maximum dose is 100 mg/day.

*Children under age 12:* 0.2 mg/kg (maximum 5 mg) as an initial single daily dose. Effective dosage range is usually 0.25 to 1 mg/kg daily in one or two doses. If needed, dose is increased after at least 3-day intervals in increments of 50% to 100% until optimal response is attained. If rapid control is needed, dosage may be adjusted q 6 hours. Maximum dose is 50 mg/day.

## Mechanism of action

*Antihypertensive action:* Drug produces its antihypertensive effect by a direct vasodilating effect on vascular smooth muscle; the effect on resistance vessels (arterioles and arteries) is greater than that on capacitance vessels (venules and veins).

## Pharmacokinetics

*Absorption:* Absorbed rapidly and almost completely from the GI tract.
*Distribution:* Distributed widely into body tissues; it isn't plasma protein–bound.
*Metabolism:* About 90% of a given dose is metabolized.
*Excretion:* Excreted primarily in urine. Average plasma half-life is 4¼ hours.

| Route | Onset | Peak | Duration |
|-------|-------|------|----------|
| P.O. | ½ hr | 2-3 hr | 2-5 days |

## Contraindications and precautions

Contraindicated in patients with pheochromocytoma or those hypersensitive to drug. Use cautiously in patients with impaired renal function or after acute MI.

## Interactions

**Drug-drug.** *Diuretics, guanethidine:* Possible profound orthostatic hypotension. Avoid use together.

## Adverse reactions

**CV:** *edema, tachycardia, pericardial effusion and tamponade, HF,* ECG changes, rebound hypertension.
**GI:** nausea, vomiting.
**Metabolic:** *weight gain.*
**Skin:** rash, *Stevens-Johnson syndrome.*
**Other:** *breast tenderness, hypertrichosis* (elongation, thickening, and enhanced pigmentation of fine body hair).

## Overdose and treatment

Signs of overdose include hypotension, tachycardia, headache, and skin flushing.

After acute ingestion, recommend emptying stomach by induced emesis or gastric lavage, and giving activated charcoal to reduce absorption. Further treatment is usually symptomatic and supportive. Advise clinician to give normal saline solution I.V. to maintain blood pressure. Sympathomimetic drugs, such as epinephrine and norepinephrine, should be avoided because of their excessive cardiac stimulating action.

## Clinical considerations

■ Drug therapy is usually given with other antihypertensives, such as diuretics, beta blockers, or sympathetic nervous system suppressants.
■ Patients with renal failure or on dialysis may require smaller maintenance doses of minoxidil. Because minoxidil is removed by dialysis, it's recommended that, on the day of dialysis, the drug be given immediately after dialysis if dialysis is at 9 a.m.; if dialysis is after 3 p.m., the daily dose is given at 7 a.m. (8 hours before dialysis).
■ After blood pressure is stabilized, patient should be reevaluated every 3 to 6 months.

### Therapeutic monitoring

■ Advise clinician to monitor blood pressure and pulse after administration; recommend assessing intake, output, and body weight for sodium and water retention.
■ Advise clinician to monitor patient for HF, pericardial effusion, and cardiac tamponade; have phenylephrine, dopamine, and vasopressin on hand to treat hypotension.

### Special populations

**Breast-feeding patients.** Drug appears in breast milk. An alternative to breast-feeding is recommended during therapy.
**Pediatric patients.** Because of limited experience in children, use with caution. Cautious drug adjustment is needed.
**Geriatric patients.** Geriatric patients may be sensitive to antihypertensive effects of drug. Dosage adjustment may be needed because of altered drug clearance. Advise clinician to monitor orthostatic blood pressure in geriatric patients.

## Patient counseling

■ Explain that drug is usually taken with other antihypertensives; emphasize importance of taking drug as prescribed.
■ Caution patient to report the following cardiac symptoms promptly: increased heart rate (over 20 beats per minute over normal), rapid weight gain, shortness of breath, chest pain, severe indigestion, dizziness, light-headedness, or fainting.
■ Tell patient to call prescriber for instructions before taking OTC cold preparations.
■ Advise patient that hypertrichosis will disappear 1 to 6 months after stopping drug.

---

## minoxidil (topical)
Hair Regrowth, Rogaine

*Pharmacologic classification:* direct-acting vasodilator
*Therapeutic classification:* hair-growth stimulant
*Pregnancy risk category C*

### Available forms
Available without a prescription
*Topical solution:* 2%, 5% in 60-ml bottle

### Indications and dosages
**Male-pattern baldness (alopecia androgenetica), diffuse hair loss or thinning in women,** ◇ **adjunct to hair transplantation**
*Adults:* Apply 1 ml to affected area b.i.d. for 4 months or longer.
◇ *Alopecia areata*
*Adults:* 1 ml of 1%, 3%, or 5% solution applied to scalp b.i.d.

### Mechanism of action
*Hair-growth stimulation:* Exact mechanism by which drug promotes hair growth is unknown. It may alter androgen metabolism in the scalp, or it may exert a local vasodilatation and enhance the microcirculation around the hair follicle. It may also directly stimulate the hair follicle.

### Pharmacokinetics
*Absorption:* Poorly absorbed through intact skin. About 0.3% to 4.5% of a topically applied dose reaches the systemic circulation.
*Distribution:* Serum levels are generally negligible.
*Metabolism:* Metabolism is not fully described.
*Excretion:* Eliminated primarily by the kidneys. About 95% of a topically applied dose is eliminated after 4 days.

| Route | Onset | Peak | Duration |
|-------|-------|------|----------|
| Topical | Unknown | Unknown | Unknown |

### Contraindications and precautions
Contraindicated in patients hypersensitive to drug or its components or during pregnancy. Use cautiously in patients with renal, cardiac, or hepatic disease; in those over age 50; and in breast-feeding women.

### Interactions
None reported.

### Adverse reactions
**CNS:** headache, dizziness, faintness, light-headedness.
**CV:** edema, chest pain, hypertension, hypotension, palpitations, increased or decreased pulse rate, *HF.*
**EENT:** sinusitis.

**GI:** diarrhea, nausea, vomiting.
**GU:** urinary tract infection, renal calculi, urethritis.
**Metabolic:** weight gain.
**Musculoskeletal:** back pain, tendinitis.
**Respiratory:** bronchitis, upper respiratory infection.
**Skin:** irritant dermatitis, allergic contact dermatitis, eczema, hypertrichosis, local erythema, pruritus, dry skin or scalp, flaking, alopecia, exacerbation of hair loss.

### Overdose and treatment
None reported. However, if topical use produces systemic adverse effects, recommend washing application site thoroughly with soap and water and treating symptoms, as appropriate. Treatment is symptomatic. Clinical signs of oral overdose include hypotension, tachycardia, headache, and skin flushing.

After acute ingestion, recommend emptying stomach by induced emesis or gastric lavage, and giving activated charcoal to reduce absorption. Further treatment is usually symptomatic and supportive.

### Clinical considerations
■ Before treatment with topical minoxidil, patient should provide a history and have a physical examination and should be advised of potential risks; a risk-benefit decision should be made. Patients with cardiac disease should realize that adverse effects may be especially serious. Alert patient to possibility of tachycardia and fluid retention, and advise clinician to monitor him for increased heart rate, weight gain, or other systemic effects.
■ Don't use with other topical agents such as corticosteroids, retinoids, and petroleum jelly, or drugs that enhance percutaneous absorption. Rogaine is for topical use only; each milliliter contains 20 or 50 mg minoxidil and accidental ingestion could cause adverse systemic effects.
■ The alcohol base will burn and irritate the eye and other sensitive surfaces (eye, abraded skin, and mucous membranes). If topical minoxidil contacts sensitive areas, recommend flushing copiously with cool water.
■ The 5% topical solution shouldn't be used in women.
■ Self-medication should cease and a clinician consulted if there is no hair growth in 8 months for women and 12 months for men using the 2% solution and in 4 months in men using the 5% solution.

### Therapeutic monitoring
■ Before treatment starts, recommend checking that patient has a normal, healthy scalp. Local abrasion or dermatitis may increase absorption and the risk of adverse effects.
■ Advise clinician to monitor patient 1 month after starting topical drug therapy and at least

every 6 months afterward. Topical minoxidil should be stopped if systemic effects occur.

### Special populations
**Breast-feeding patients.** Topical minoxidil shouldn't be given to breast-feeding women.
**Pediatric patients.** Safety and efficacy haven't been established for patients under age 18.

### Patient counseling
■ Tell patient to avoid inhaling the spray.
■ Teach patient to apply topical minoxidil as follows: Dry hair and scalp before application. Apply dose of 1 ml to the total affected areas twice daily. Total daily dose shouldn't exceed 2 ml. If the fingertips are used to apply the drug, wash the hands afterward.
■ Encourage patient to carefully review patient information leaflet, which is included with each package and in the full product information.
■ Inform patient that 4 months of use may be required before results become apparent.

## mirtazapine
Remeron

*Pharmacologic classification:* piperazinoazepine
*Therapeutic classification:* tetracyclic antidepressant
*Pregnancy risk category C*

### Available forms
Available by prescription only
*Tablets:* 15 mg, 30 mg, 45 mg

### Indications and dosages
*Depression*
*Adults:* Initially, 15 mg P.O. h.s. Maintenance dose ranges from 15 mg to 45 mg daily. Dosage adjustments should be made at intervals no less than 1 to 2 weeks apart.

### Mechanism of action
*Antidepressant action:* Mechanism of action unknown.

### Pharmacokinetics
*Absorption:* Rapidly and completely absorbed from the GI tract. Absolute bioavailability of drug is about 50%.
*Distribution:* About 85% plasma protein–bound.
*Metabolism:* Extensively metabolized in the liver.
*Excretion:* Predominantly eliminated in urine (75%) with 15% being excreted in feces. Half-life is between 20 and 40 hours.

| Route | Onset | Peak | Duration |
|-------|-------|------|----------|
| P.O. | Unknown | 2 hr | Unknown |

### Contraindications and precautions
Contraindicated in patients hypersensitive to drug. Administration with MAO inhibitors is contraindicated.

Use cautiously in patients with CV or cerebrovascular disease, seizure disorders, suicidal ideation, impaired hepatic and renal function, or history of mania or hypomania. Also use cautiously in patients with conditions that predispose them to hypotension, such as dehydration, hypovolemia, or treatment with antihypertensives, and in pregnancy.

### Interactions
**Drug-drug.** *Diazepam, other CNS depressants:* Possible additive CNS effects. Avoid use together.
*MAO inhibitors or within 14 days of initiating or discontinuing therapy with MAO inhibitors:* Potential for serious, sometimes fatal, reactions. Avoid use together.
**Drug-lifestyle.** *Alcohol use:* Additive CNS effects. Avoid use together.

### Adverse reactions
**CNS:** *somnolence,* dizziness, asthenia, abnormal dreams, abnormal thinking, tremor, confusion.
**CV:** edema.
**GI:** nausea, *increased appetite, dry mouth, constipation.*
**GU:** urinary frequency.
**Hematologic:** *agranulocytosis.*
**Metabolic:** *weight gain.*
**Musculoskeletal:** back pain, myalgia.
**Respiratory:** dyspnea.
**Other:** flu syndrome, peripheral edema.

### Overdose and treatment
Overdose may result in disorientation, drowsiness, impaired memory, and tachycardia. If overdose occurs, treat as for any antidepressant overdose. If patient is unconscious, recommend establishing an airway and providing adequate oxygenation. Recommend considering gastric lavage, induced emesis, or both, and also activated charcoal. Advise clinician to monitor cardiac and vital signs and provide general symptomatic and supportive measures.

### Clinical considerations
■ Use with caution in patients with increased intraocular pressure, history of urinary retention, or history of narrow-angle glaucoma because of anticholinergic properties.
■ There should be a drug-free interval of at least 2 weeks when switching from MAO inhibitor therapy to mirtazapine or from mirtazapine to an MAO inhibitor.

### Therapeutic monitoring
■ Although risk of agranulocytosis is rare, recommend stopping drug and monitoring patient

closely if he develops a sore throat, fever, stomatitis, or other signs of infection together with a low WBC count.
■ Patient requires close observation because it isn't known if mirtazapine causes physical or psychological dependence.

### Special populations
**Breast-feeding patients.** It isn't known if drug appears in breast milk; use cautiously in breast-feeding women.
**Pediatric patients.** Safety and efficacy in children haven't been established.
**Geriatric patients.** Give mirtazapine cautiously to geriatric patients because pharmacokinetic studies reveal a decreased clearance in geriatric patients.

### Patient counseling
■ Caution patient not to perform hazardous activities if somnolence occurs with drug use.
■ Instruct patient not to use alcohol or other CNS depressants while taking drug because of additive effect.
■ Tell patient to report signs and symptoms of infection, such as fever, chills, sore throat, mucous membrane ulceration, or other possible signs of infection, including any flulike complaints.
■ Stress importance of compliance with mirtazapine therapy.
■ Instruct patient not to take other drugs without medical approval.
■ Tell women of childbearing age to report suspected pregnancy immediately.

# misoprostol
Cytotec

*Pharmacologic classification:*
prostaglandin E$_1$ analogue
*Therapeutic classification:* antiulcerative, gastric mucosal protectant
*Pregnancy risk category X*

### Available forms
Available by prescription only
*Tablets:* 100 mcg, 200 mcg

### Indications and dosages
*Prevention of gastric ulcer induced by NSAIDs*
*Adults:* 200 mcg P.O. q.i.d with meals and h.s. Reduce dosage to 100 mcg P.O. q.i.d. in patients who can't tolerate this dosage.
◊ *Duodenal or gastric ulcer*
*Adults:* 100 to 200 mcg P.O. q.i.d. with meals and h.s. for 4 to 8 weeks.

### Mechanism of action
*Antiulcer action:* Misoprostol enhances the production of gastric mucous and bicarbonate, and decreases basal, nocturnal, and stimulated gastric acid secretion.

### Pharmacokinetics
*Absorption:* Rapidly absorbed after oral administration.
*Distribution:* Less than 90% plasma protein–bound.
*Metabolism:* Rapidly de-esterified to misoprostol acid, the biologically active metabolite. The de-esterified metabolite undergoes further oxidation in several body tissues.
*Excretion:* About 15% of an oral dose appears in the feces; the balance is excreted in urine. Terminal half-life is 20 to 40 minutes.

| Route | Onset | Peak | Duration |
|-------|-------|------|----------|
| P.O. | 30 min | 10-15 min | 3 hr |

### Contraindications and precautions
Contraindicated in pregnant and breast-feeding women and in those with a known allergy to prostaglandins.

### Interactions
None significant.

### Adverse reactions
**CNS:** headache.
**GI:** *diarrhea, abdominal pain, nausea, flatulence, dyspepsia, vomiting, constipation.*
**GU:** hypermenorrhea, dysmenorrhea, spotting, cramps, menstrual disorders.
**Other:** *anaphylaxis, uterine rupture and perforation in pregnant patient, fetal death,* maternal uterine tachysystole, abnormal fetal heart rate.

### Overdose and treatment
There is little clinical experience with overdose. Cumulative daily doses of 1,600 mcg have been given, with only minor GI discomfort noted. Treatment should be supportive.

### Clinical considerations
■ Drug has been used for treatment and prophylaxis of reflux esophagitis, alcohol-induced gastritis, hemorrhagic gastritis, fat malabsorption in cystic fibrosis, and NSAID-induced nephropathy.
■ Misoprostol shouldn't be prescribed for a woman of childbearing age unless she:
– needs NSAID therapy and is at high risk for development of gastric ulcers.
– is capable of complying with effective contraception practices.
– has received both oral and written warnings regarding the hazards of misoprostol therapy, the risk of possible contraception failure, and the hazards this drug would pose to other women of childbearing age who might take this drug by mistake.
– has had a negative serum pregnancy test within 2 weeks before beginning therapy and she'll

begin therapy on the second or third day of her next normal menstrual period.
- Diarrhea is usually dose-related and develops within the first 2 weeks of therapy. It can be minimized by giving the drug after meals and at bedtime, and by avoiding magnesium-containing antacids.
- Misoprostol produces a modest decrease in basal pepsin secretion.

### Therapeutic monitoring
- Advise clinician to monitor patient for GI distress, especially diarrhea.

### Special populations
**Pregnant patients.** Drug shouldn't be routinely used in women of childbearing age unless they're at high risk for development of ulcers or complications from NSAID-induced ulcers.
**Breast-feeding patients.** Breast-feeding isn't recommended because of potential for drug-induced diarrhea in infant.
**Pediatric patients.** Safety hasn't been established in children under age 18.

### Patient counseling
- Explain importance of not giving drug to anyone else.
- Make sure patient understands that a miscarriage could result if drug is taken by a pregnant woman.
- Advise patient to take drug as prescribed for duration of therapy.

---

## mitomycin (mitomycin-C; MTC)
Mutamycin

*Pharmacologic classification:* antineoplastic antibiotic (cell cycle–phase nonspecific)
*Therapeutic classification:* antineoplastic
*Pregnancy risk category NR*

---

### Available forms
Available by prescription only
*Injection:* 5-mg, 20-mg, 40-mg vials

### Indications and dosages
Dosage and indications may vary. Check current literature for recommended protocol. Not indicated as a single-agent primary therapy.
***Stomach and pancreatic adenocarcinoma (with other chemotherapeutic drugs); cancer of ◊ anus, ◊ breast, ◊ colon, ◊ rectum, ◊ head, ◊ neck, ◊ lung, ◊ cervix***
*Adults:* 20 mg/m² as a single dose. Repeat cycle q 6 to 8 weeks, adjusting dosage, if needed, according to the following table.

| Nadir after prior dose | | Percentage of prior dose to be given |
|---|---|---|
| WBCs/mm³ | Platelets/mm³ | |
| > 4,000 | > 100,000 | 100% |
| 3,000-3,999 | 75,000-99,999 | 100% |
| 2,000-2,999 | 25,000-74,999 | 70% |
| < 2,000 | < 25,000 | 50% |

**ALERT** Drug should be stopped if WBC count is less than 4,000/mm³ or platelet count is less than 150,000/mm³. No repeat dose should be given until blood counts go above these levels. If disease progresses after two courses of therapy, recommend stopping use.
◊ *Bladder cancer*
*Adults:* 20 to 60 mg intravesically once per week for 8 weeks.

### I.V. administration
- To reconstitute 5-mg vial, use 10 ml of sterile water for injection; to reconstitute 20-mg vial, use 40 ml of sterile water for injection; to reconstitute a 40-mg vial, use 80 ml sterile water for injection, to give a concentration of 0.5 mg/ml. Allow to stand at room temperature until complete dissolution occurs.
- Drug may be administered by I.V. push injection slowly over 5 to 10 minutes into the tubing of a freely flowing I.V. infusion.
- Drug can be further diluted to 100 to 150 ml with normal saline solution or D₅W for I.V. infusion (over 30 to 60 minutes or longer).

### Incompatibilities
Incompatible with bleomycin.

### Mechanism of action
*Antineoplastic action:* Mitomycin exerts its cytotoxic activity by a mechanism similar to that of the alkylating drugs. The drug is converted to an active compound which forms cross-links between strands of DNA, inhibiting DNA synthesis. Mitomycin also inhibits RNA and protein synthesis to a lesser extent.

### Pharmacokinetics
*Absorption:* Administered I.V.
*Distribution:* Distributes widely into body tissues; animal studies show that the highest levels are found in the kidneys followed by the muscle, eyes, lungs, intestines, and stomach. It doesn't cross the blood-brain barrier.
*Metabolism:* Metabolized by hepatic microsomal enzymes; deactivated in the kidneys, spleen, brain, and heart.

*Excretion:* Excreted in urine. A small portion is eliminated in bile and feces.

| Route | Onset | Peak | Duration |
|-------|-------|------|----------|
| I.V. | Unknown | Unknown | Unknown |

## Contraindications and precautions
Contraindicated in patients hypersensitive to drug, and those with thrombocytopenia, coagulation disorders, or an increase in bleeding tendency from other causes. Contraindicated as primary therapy as a single drug to replace surgery or radiotherapy.

## Interactions
**Drug-drug.** *Vinca alkaloids:* Acute shortness of breath and severe bronchospasm have occurred following use of vinca alkaloids in patients who had previously or simultaneously received mitomycin. Advise clinician to monitor patient closely.

## Adverse reactions
**CNS:** headache, neurologic abnormalities, confusion, drowsiness, asthenia, malaise, fatigue.
**EENT:** blurred vision.
**GI:** *nausea, vomiting, anorexia, diarrhea.*
**GU:** bladder fibrosis or contraction.
**Hematologic:** *thrombocytopenia, leukopenia* (may be delayed up to 8 weeks and may be cumulative with successive doses), *microangiopathic hemolytic anemia, characterized by thrombocytopenia, renal failure,* and hypertension.
**Respiratory:** *interstitial pneumonitis,* pulmonary edema, dyspnea, nonproductive cough, adult respiratory distress syndrome.
**Skin:** sloughing with extravasation, *reversible alopecia,* desquamation, induration, pruritus, pain at injection site.
**Other:** *septicemia,* cellulitis, ulceration, fever, pain.

## Overdose and treatment
Signs and symptoms of overdose include myelosuppression, nausea, vomiting, and alopecia.

Treatment is usually supportive and includes transfusion of blood components, antiemetics, and antibiotics for infections that may develop.

## Clinical considerations
■ Reconstituted solution remains stable for 1 week at room temperature and for 2 weeks if refrigerated.
■ Mitomycin has been used intra-arterially to treat certain tumors, for example, into hepatic artery for colon cancer. It has also been given as a continuous daily infusion.
■ Ulcers caused by extravasation develop late and dorsal to the extravasation site. Recommend applying cold compresses for at least 12 hours.

**H ALERT** Don't confuse this drug with mitoxantrone. Question any unfamiliar color of the drug.

### *Therapeutic monitoring*
■ Recommend observing patient for evidence of renal toxicity. Drug shouldn't be given to patient with a serum creatinine level over 1.7 mg/dl.
■ Continue CBC and blood studies at least 7 weeks after therapy is stopped. Advise clinician to monitor patient for signs of bleeding.

### *Special populations*
**Breast-feeding patients.** It isn't known if drug appears in breast milk. To avoid risk of serious adverse reactions, mutagenicity, and carcinogenicity in the infant, breast-feeding isn't recommended.
**Pediatric patients.** Safety and efficacy in children haven't been established.

## Patient counseling
■ Tell patient to avoid exposure to people with infections.
■ Warn patient not to receive immunizations during therapy and for several weeks afterward. Members of the same household shouldn't receive immunizations during the same period.
■ Reassure patient that hair should grow back after treatment has been discontinued.
■ Tell patient to call prescriber promptly if he develops a sore throat or fever or notices unusual bruising or bleeding.

# mitoxantrone hydrochloride
Novantrone

*Pharmacologic classification:* antibiotic antineoplastic
*Therapeutic classification:* antineoplastic
*Pregnancy risk category D*

## Available forms
Available by prescription only
*Injection:* 2 mg mitoxantrone base/ml in 10-ml, 12.5-ml, 15-ml vials

## Indications and dosages
*Initial treatment with other approved drugs for acute nonlymphocytic leukemia*
*Adults:* For induction (in combination chemotherapy), 12 mg/m$^2$ daily by I.V. infusion on days 1 to 3, and 100 mg/m$^2$ of cytosine arabinoside by continuous I.V. infusion (over 24 hours) on days 1 to 7 for 7 days.

Most complete remissions follow initial course of induction therapy. A second course may be given if antileukemic response is incomplete: Give mitoxantrone for 2 days and cytosine for 5 days using the same daily dosage levels. Withhold second course of therapy until toxicity clears if severe or life-threatening nonhematologic toxicity occurs.

***Combined initial therapy for pain from advanced hormone-refractory prostate cancer***
*Adults:* 12 to 14 mg/m$^2$ I.V. infusion over 15 to 30 minutes q 21 days.

## I.V. administration

■ To prepare, dilute solutions to at least 50 ml with either normal saline solution or D$_5$W. Inject slowly into tubing of a freely running I.V. solution of normal saline solution or D$_5$W over not less than 3 minutes. Discard unused infusion solutions appropriately. Don't mix for infusion with heparin; a precipitate may form. Specific compatibility data aren't available.
■ For I.V. infusion over 15 to 30 minutes, further dilute solution.

### Incompatibilities
Incompatible with heparin sodium. Manufacturer recommends not mixing with other drugs.

## Mechanism of action
*Antineoplastic action:* Mechanism of action isn't completely established. Drug is a DNA-reactive drug that has cytocidal effects on proliferating and nonproliferating cells, suggestive of lack of cell-phase specificity.

## Pharmacokinetics
*Absorption:* Administered I.V.
*Distribution:* 78% plasma protein–bound.
*Metabolism:* Metabolized by the liver.
*Excretion:* Excretion is via renal and hepatobiliary systems; 6% to 11% of dose is excreted in urine within 5 days: 65% is unchanged drug; 35% is two inactive metabolites. Within 5 days, 25% of dose is excreted in feces.

| Route | Onset | Peak | Duration |
|-------|-------|------|----------|
| I.V. | Unknown | Unknown | Unknown |

## Contraindications and precautions
Contraindicated in patients hypersensitive to mitoxantrone. Use cautiously in patients with prior exposure to anthracyclines or other cardiotoxic drugs. Contraindicated in pregnancy unless potential benefits outweigh potential hazards to fetus.

## Interactions
None reported.

## Adverse reactions
**CNS:** *seizures,* headache.
**EENT:** conjunctivitis, temporary blue color to sclera.
**CV:** *HF, arrhythmias,* tachycardia.
**GI:** *bleeding, abdominal pain, diarrhea, nausea, mucositis, vomiting,* stomatitis.
**GU:** *renal failure.*

**Hematologic:** *myelosuppression.*
**Hepatic:** jaundice.
**Metabolic:** hyperuricemia.
**Respiratory:** *dyspnea, cough.*
**Skin:** *alopecia, petechiae, ecchymoses.*
**Other:** *sepsis, fungal infections, fever.*

## Overdose and treatment
Accidental overdoses have occurred and have caused severe leukopenia with infection. Advise clinician to monitor hematologic effects and treat symptomatically. Antimicrobial therapy may be needed.

## Clinical considerations
■ Safety of administration by routes other than I.V. hasn't been established. Don't use intrathecally.
■ After penetration of container, undiluted mitoxantrone concentration may be stored no longer than 7 days at room temperature or 14 days if refrigerated.
■ If extravasation occurs, recommend stopping I.V. and restarting in another vein. Mitoxantrone is a nonvesicant and the possibility of severe local reactions is minimal.
■ Urine may appear blue-green for 24 hours after administration.
■ Bluish discoloration of sclera may occur; this may be a sign of myelosuppression.
**⚠ ALERT** Don't confuse this drug with mitomycin. Question any unfamiliar color of the drug.

### Therapeutic monitoring
■ Close and frequent monitoring of hematologic and chemical laboratory parameters, including serial CBC and liver function test results, with frequent patient observation is recommended.
■ Hyperuricemia may result from rapid lysis of tumor cells. Advise clinician to monitor serum uric acid levels. Hypouricemic therapy should be started before antileukemic therapy.
■ Transient elevations of AST and ALT levels have occurred 4 to 24 days after mitoxantrone therapy.

### Special populations
**Breast-feeding patients.** It isn't known if drug appears in breast milk. Because of potential for serious adverse reactions in infants, patient should discontinue breast-feeding before therapy.
**Pediatric patients.** Safety and efficacy in children haven't been established.

## Patient counseling
■ Tell patient urine may appear blue-green for 24 hours after administration, and sclera may appear bluish.
■ Advise patient to call prescriber promptly if signs and symptoms of myelosuppression de-

velop, such as fever, sore throat, easy bruising, or excessive bleeding.
■ Advise patient to use contraception; tell patient to report if pregnancy is suspected.
■ Tell patient to drink fluids to minimize uric acid nephropathy.

# mivacurium chloride
Mivacron

*Pharmacologic classification:* non-depolarizing neuromuscular blocker
*Therapeutic classification:* skeletal muscle relaxant
*Pregnancy risk category C*

## Available forms
Available by prescription only
*Injection:* 2 mg/ml in 5-ml and 10-ml vials
*Infusion:* 0.5 mg/ml, in 50 ml $D_5W$

## Indications and dosages
*Adjunct to general anesthesia, to facilitate endotracheal intubation, and to provide skeletal muscle relaxation during surgery or mechanical ventilation*
Dosage is highly individualized. All times of onset and duration of neuromuscular blockade are averages and considerable individual variation is normal.
*Adults:* Usually, 0.15 mg/kg I.V. push over 5 to 15 seconds provides adequate muscle relaxation within 2 to 3 minutes for endotracheal intubation. Clinically sufficient neuromuscular blockade usually lasts about 15 to 20 minutes. Alternatively, 0.2 mg/kg over 30 seconds or 0.25 mg/kg in doses of 0.15 mg/kg and 0.1 mg/kg 30 seconds later. Spontaneous recovery usually occurs in 25 to 35 minutes. Supplemental doses of 0.1 mg/kg I.V. q 15 to 25 minutes usually maintain muscle relaxation. Alternatively, maintain neuromuscular blockade with a continuous infusion of 4 mcg/kg/minute started simultaneously with initial dose, or 9 to 10 mcg/kg/minute started after evidence of spontaneous recovery of initial dose. When used with isoflurane or enflurane anesthesia, dosage is usually reduced about 35% to 40%.
≡ *Dosage adjustment.* Infusion rate needs to be reduced by 50% in end-stage renal and liver patients.
*Children ages 2 to 12:* 0.20 mg/kg I.V. push administered over 5 to 15 seconds.
    Neuromuscular blockade is usually evident in less than 2 minutes. Although supplemental doses of 0.1 mg/kg I.V. q 15 minutes usually maintain muscle relaxation in adults, maintenance doses are usually required more frequently in children. Alternatively, maintain neuromuscular blockade with a continuous infusion titrated to effect. Most children respond

to 5 to 31 mcg/kg/minute (average, 14 mcg/kg/minute).

## I.V. administration
■ Drug is compatible with $D_5W$, normal saline solution injection, dextrose 5% in normal saline solution injection, lactated Ringer's injection, and dextrose 5% in lactated Ringer's injection. Diluted solutions are stable for 24 hours at room temperature.
■ When diluted as directed, mivacurium is compatible with alfentanil, fentanyl, sufentanil, droperidol, and midazolam.
■ Drug is available as premixed infusion in $D_5W$. After removing the protective outer wrap, check container for minor leaks by squeezing the bag before administering. Don't add other drugs to the container, and don't use the container in series connections.

### *Incompatibilities*
Drug shouldn't be mixed with other drugs.

## Mechanism of action
*Neuromuscular blocking action:* Mivacurium competes with acetylcholine for receptor sites at the motor end-plate. Because this action may be antagonized by cholinesterase inhibitors, mivacurium is considered a competitive antagonist. Drug is a mixture of three stereoisomers, each possessing neuromuscular blocking activity: the cis-trans isomer (36% of the total) and the trans-trans isomer (57% of the total) are about 10 times as potent as the cis-cis isomer (only 6% of the total). The isomers don't interconvert in vivo.

## Pharmacokinetics
*Absorption:* Administered I.V.
*Distribution:* Volume of distribution is small, indicating that drug isn't extensively distributed to tissues.
*Metabolism:* Rapidly hydrolyzed by plasma pseudocholinesterase to inactive components.
*Excretion:* Metabolites are excreted in bile and urine. Of the highly active isomers, the cis-trans and trans-trans isomers each have an elimination half-life of less than 2.3 minutes. The less active cis-cis isomer, which is only a small portion of the total drug, has an elimination half-life of 55 minutes.

| Route | Onset | Peak | Duration |
|-------|-------|------|----------|
| I.V. | 1-2 min | 2-5 min | 20-35 min |

## Contraindications and precautions
Contraindicated in patients hypersensitive to drug. Use cautiously in patients with significant CV disease, metastatic cancer, severe electrolyte disturbances, or neuromuscular disease; in those who may be adversely affected by the release of histamine; and in those in whom neuromuscular blockade reversibility is difficult, such as patients with myasthenia gravis or

myasthenic syndrome. Use with extreme caution in patients with reduced plasma cholinesterase activity because drug may cause prolonged neuromuscular blockade.

## Interactions
**Drug-drug.** *Alkaline solutions such as barbiturate solutions:* Possible formation of precipitate. Don't administer drug through same I.V. line with any of these drugs.
*Aminoglycosides (gentamicin, kanamycin, neomycin, streptomycin), bacitracin, colistimethate, colistin, magnesium salts, polymyxin B, tetracyclines:* Possible increased muscle weakness. Advise clinician to monitor patient closely.
*Carbamazepine, phenytoin:* Possible prolonged time to maximal block or shortened duration of blockade with neuromuscular blockers. Advise clinician to monitor patient closely.
*Glucocorticosteroids, MAO inhibitors, oral contraceptives:* Possible diminished plasma cholinesterase activity with long-term use. Advise clinician to monitor patient closely.
*Inhalational anesthetics (especially enflurane, isoflurane), quinidine:* Possible enhanced activity or prolonged action. Advise clinician to monitor patient closely.

## Adverse reactions
**CNS:** dizziness.
**CV:** *flushing, tachycardia,* **bradycardia,** *arrhythmias, hypotension.*
**Musculoskeletal:** prolonged muscle weakness, muscle spasms.
**Respiratory:** *bronchospasm,* wheezing, *respiratory insufficiency or apnea.*
**Skin:** rash, urticaria, erythema.
**Other:** phlebitis.

## Overdose and treatment
Overdose may result in prolonged neuromuscular blockade. Recommend maintaining a patent airway and controlling respirations until patient recovers neuromuscular function. Antagonists shouldn't be given until there's some evidence of spontaneous recovery. In clinical trials, administration of 0.03 to 0.064 mg/kg neostigmine methylsulfate or 0.5 mg/kg edrophonium chloride to patients with spontaneous recovery of muscle function resulted in increased muscle strength of about 10% recovery to about 95% recovery within 10 minutes.

## Clinical considerations
■ When mivacurium is given I.V. push to adults receiving anesthetic combinations of nitrous oxide and opiates, neuromuscular blockade usually lasts 15 to 20 minutes; most patients recover 95% of muscle strength in 25 to 30 minutes.

■ Duration of drug effect is increased about 150% in patients with end-stage renal disease and 300% in patients with hepatic dysfunction.
■ Dosage should be adjusted to ideal body weight in obese patients (patients 30% or more above their ideal weight) because of reported prolonged neuromuscular blockade.
■ A nerve stimulator and train-of-four monitoring are recommended to document antagonism of neuromuscular blockade and recovery of muscle strength. Before attempting pharmacologic reversal with neostigmine methylsulfate or edrophonium chloride, some evidence of spontaneous recovery should be evident.
■ Experimental evidence suggests that acid-base and electrolyte balance may influence actions of and response to nondepolarizing neuromuscular blockers. Alkalosis may counteract paralysis; acidosis may enhance it.
■ Mivacurium, like other neuromuscular blockers, doesn't have an effect on consciousness or pain threshold. To avoid patient distress, this drug shouldn't be given until the patient's consciousness is obtunded by the general anesthetic.

### Therapeutic monitoring
■ Advise clinician to monitor vital signs and respirations until patient is fully recovered from neuromuscular blockade (as evidenced by hand grip, head lift, and ability to cough).

### Special populations
**Breast-feeding patients.** It isn't known if drug appears in breast milk. Use with caution in breast-feeding women.
**Pediatric patients.** As with other neuromuscular blockers, dosage requirements for children are higher on a mg/kg basis as compared with adults. Onset and recovery of neuromuscular blockade occur more rapidly in children.

## Patient counseling
■ Explain purpose of drug to patient and family.
■ Assure patient that he will be continuously monitored.

# modafinil
Provigil

*Pharmacologic classification:* nonamphetamine CNS stimulant
*Therapeutic classification:* analeptic
*Pregnancy risk category C*
*Controlled substance schedule IV*

## Available forms
Available by prescription only
*Tablets:* 100 mg, 200 mg

## Indications and dosages

*Improvement of wakefulness in patients with excessive daytime sleepiness from narcolepsy*
*Adults:* 200 mg P.O. daily, given as a single dose in the morning.
≡*Dosage adjustment.* For patients with severe hepatic impairment, 100 mg P.O. daily, given as a single dose in the morning.

## Mechanism of action

*CNS stimulant action:* The exact mechanism of action in which modafinil promotes wakefulness is unknown. Modafinil has wake-promoting actions like sympathomimetics including amphetamines, but modafinil is structurally distinct from amphetamines and doesn't appear to alter the release of either dopamine or norepinephrine to produce CNS stimulation.

## Pharmacokinetics

*Absorption:* Absorption is rapid.
*Distribution:* Well distributed in body tissue and is moderately bound to plasma protein (about 60%), primarily albumin.
*Metabolism:* Primarily metabolized (about 90%) in the liver, with subsequent renal elimination of the metabolites.
*Excretion:* Less than 10% is renally excreted as unchanged drug.

| Route | Onset | Peak | Duration |
|-------|-------|------|----------|
| P.O. | Unknown | 2-4 hr | Unknown |

## Contraindications and precautions

Contraindicated in patients hypersensitive to drug. Don't use in patients with history of left ventricular hypertrophy or ischemic ECG changes, chest pain, arrhythmias, or other clinically significant manifestations of mitral valve prolapse in association with CNS stimulant use.

Use with caution in patients with recent history of MI or unstable angina and in those with history of psychosis. Use cautiously, and in reduced dosages, in patients with severe hepatic impairment, with or without cirrhosis. Also use cautiously in patients concurrently treated with MAO inhibitors and those with a history of psychosis.

## Interactions

**Drug-drug.** *Carbamazepine; itraconazole, ketoconazole, or other inhibitors of CYP3A4; phenobarbital; rifampin; other inducers of CYP3A4:* Altered levels of modafinil. Advise clinician to monitor patient closely.
*Cyclosporine, theophylline:* Reduced serum levels. Use together cautiously.
*Diazepam, phenytoin, propranolol, other drugs metabolized by CYP2C19:* Increased serum levels of drugs metabolized by this enzyme. Use together cautiously. Dosage adjustment may be needed.

*Methylphenidate:* Possible delayed absorption of modafinil by about 1 hour when given together. Separate dosage administration times are recommended.
*Phenytoin, warfarin:* Increased serum levels of these drugs. Advise clinician to monitor patient closely for signs of toxicity.
*Steroidal contraceptives:* Reduced contraceptive effectiveness. Recommend alternative or concomitant method of contraception during modafinil therapy and for 1 month after drug is discontinued.
*Tricyclic antidepressants, such as clomipramine and desipramine:* Increased levels of these drugs. Dosage reduction of these drugs may be needed.

## Adverse reactions

**CNS:** *headache,* nervousness, dizziness, syncope, depression, anxiety, cataplexy, insomnia, paresthesia, dyskinesia, hypertonia, confusion, amnesia, emotional lability, ataxia, tremor.
**CV:** hypotension, hypertension, vasodilation, *arrhythmias,* chest pain.
**EENT:** *rhinitis,* pharyngitis, epistaxis, amblyopia, abnormal vision.
**GI:** gingivitis, mouth ulcer, *nausea,* diarrhea, dry mouth, anorexia, vomiting, thirst.
**GU:** abnormal urine, urine retention, abnormal ejaculation, albuminuria.
**Hematologic:** eosinophilia.
**Hepatic:** abnormal liver function.
**Metabolic:** hyperglycemia.
**Musculoskeletal:** joint disorder, neck pain, rigid neck.
**Respiratory:** lung disorder, dyspnea, asthma.
**Skin:** dry skin.
**Other:** herpes simplex, chills, fever.

## Overdose and treatment

No specific antidote to a modafinil overdose exists. In an overdose, supportive care should be initiated as appropriate, including CV monitoring. If there are no contraindications, induced emesis or gastric lavage should be considered. There are no data to suggest the utility of dialysis or urinary acidification or alkalinization in enhancing drug elimination.

## Clinical considerations

■ Safety and efficacy of dosage in patients with severe renal impairment haven't been determined.
■ Although dosages of 400 mg daily as a single dose have been well tolerated, there's no consistent evidence that this dosage confers additional benefit beyond the 200-mg dose.
■ Even though food has no effect on overall bioavailability, the absorption of modafinil may be delayed by about 1 hour if given with food.

### Therapeutic monitoring

■ Advise clinician to monitor patient for misuse or abuse.

---

■ Advise clinician to monitor liver function test results before and during drug therapy.

### Special populations

**Breast-feeding patients.** It isn't known if modafinil appears in breast milk. Because many drugs appear in breast milk, give modafinil cautiously to a breast-feeding woman.

**Pediatric patients.** Safety and efficacy in patients under age 16 haven't been established.

**Geriatric patients.** Safety and efficacy in patients over age 65 haven't been established. In geriatric patients, a lower dosage may be considered because elimination of drug and its metabolites may be reduced.

### Patient counseling

■ Advise female patient to notify prescriber if she becomes pregnant or intends to become pregnant during therapy.

■ Caution patient regarding the potential increased risk of pregnancy when using steroidal contraceptives (including depot or implantable contraceptives) with modafinil tablets. Recommend alternative or concomitant method of contraception during modafinil therapy and for 1 month after drug is discontinued.

■ Advise female patient to notify prescriber if she is breast-feeding.

■ Instruct patient to avoid taking any prescription or OTC drugs before consulting with prescriber because of the potential for interactions between modafinil and other drugs.

■ Advise patient to avoid alcohol while taking modafinil.

■ Tell patient to notify prescriber if he develops a rash, hives, or a related allergic reaction.

■ Modafinil may impair judgment. Advise patient to use caution while driving or during other activities requiring alertness until effects are known.

---

# molindone hydrochloride
Moban

*Pharmacologic classification:* dihydroindolone
*Therapeutic classification:* antipsychotic drug
*Pregnancy risk category NR*

### Available forms

Available by prescription only
*Tablets:* 5 mg, 10 mg, 25 mg, 50 mg, 100 mg
*Oral concentrate:* 20 mg/ml

### Indications and dosages

**Psychotic disorders**

*Adults:* 50 to 75 mg P.O. daily in three to four divided doses, increased 100 mg daily in 3 to 4 days to a maximum of 225 mg daily. Maintenance dose for mild disease is 5 to 15 mg t.i.d. or q.i.d., moderate disease is 10 to 25 mg t.i.d. or q.i.d., and severe disease is up to 225 mg daily.

◇ *Behavioral complications from mental retardation, mentally retarded schizophrenic child*

*Children ages 3 to 5:* 1 to 2.5 mg P.O. daily as a single dose.

### Mechanism of action

*Antipsychotic action:* Molindone is unrelated to all other antipsychotic drugs; it's thought to exert its antipsychotic effects by postsynaptic blockade of CNS dopamine receptors, thereby inhibiting dopamine-mediated effects.

Molindone has many other central and peripheral effects; it also produces alpha and ganglionic blockade. Its most prominent adverse reactions are extrapyramidal.

### Pharmacokinetics

*Absorption:* Data are limited, but absorption appears rapid.
*Distribution:* Distributed widely into the body.
*Metabolism:* Metabolized extensively. Half-life is approximately 2 hours.
*Excretion:* Most of drug is excreted as metabolites in urine; some is excreted in feces by way of the biliary tract. Overall, 90% of a given dose is excreted within 24 hours.

| Route | Onset | Peak | Duration |
| --- | --- | --- | --- |
| P.O. | Unknown | 1½ hr | 24-36 hr |

### Contraindications and precautions

Contraindicated in patients hypersensitive to drug and in those experiencing coma or severe CNS depression. Use cautiously in patients at risk for seizures or when high physical activity is harmful to patient.

### Interactions

**Drug-drug.** *Antiarrhythmics, disopyramide, procainamide, quinidine:* Increased risk of arrhythmias and conduction defects. Avoid use together.

*Atropine and other anticholinergics, including antidepressants, antihistamines, MAO inhibitors, meperidine, phenothiazines, and antiparkinsonians:* Oversedation, paralytic ileus, visual changes, and severe constipation. Use together cautiously.

*Beta blockers:* May inhibit molindone metabolism, increasing plasma levels and toxicity. Advise clinician to monitor patient for toxicity.

*Bromocriptine:* Molindone may antagonize therapeutic effect of bromocriptine on prolactin secretion. Use together cautiously.

*Centrally acting antihypertensives, such as clonidine, guanabenz, guanadrel, guanethidine, methyldopa, and reserpine:* Mesoridazine may inhibit blood pressure response to these drugs. Advise clinician to monitor blood pressure carefully.

---

*CNS depressants, including analgesics, barbiturates, opioids, tranquilizers, and general, spinal, or epidural anesthetics, or parenteral magnesium sulfate:* Oversedation, respiratory depression, and hypotension. Avoid use together.
*High-dose dopamine:* Decreased vasoconstricting effects. Advise clinician to monitor patient for clinical effects.
*Levodopa:* Decreased effectiveness and increased toxicity of levodopa. Use together cautiously.
*Metrizamide:* Increased risk of seizures. Use together cautiously.
*Nitrates:* Hypotension. Advise clinician to monitor blood pressure.
*Phenytoin, tetracycline:* Molindone may inhibit absorption. Advise clinician to monitor patient closely.
*Propylthiouracil:* Increased risk of agranulocytosis. Advise clinician to monitor hematopoietic studies.
*Sympathomimetics, including epinephrine, ephedrine (often found in nasal sprays), phenylephrine, or appetite suppressants:* May decrease their stimulatory and pressor effects. Use together cautiously.
**Drug-lifestyle.** *Alcohol use:* Additive effects. Advise patient to avoid alcohol.
*Sun exposure:* Increased risk of photosensitivity reactions. Recommend patient use sunblock and avoid excessive exposure to the sun.

## Adverse reactions

**CNS:** *neuroleptic malignant syndrome, extrapyramidal reactions, tardive dyskinesia, sedation, drowsiness, depression, euphoria, pseudoparkinsonism, EEG changes, dizziness,* insomnia, **suicidal tendencies.**
**CV:** *orthostatic hypotension, tachycardia, ECG changes.*
**EENT:** *blurred vision.*
**GI:** *dry mouth, constipation, nausea,* anorexia.
**GU:** *urine retention, menstrual irregularities, inhibited ejaculation.*
**Hematologic:** *leukopenia,* leukocytosis, eosinophilia.
**Hepatic:** jaundice, abnormal liver function test results.
**Skin:** *mild photosensitivity, **allergic reactions.***
**Other:** *gynecomastia,* increased libido.

## Overdose and treatment

CNS depression is characterized by deep, unarousable sleep and possible coma, hypotension or hypertension, extrapyramidal symptoms, abnormal involuntary muscle movements, agitation, seizures, arrhythmias, ECG changes, hypothermia or hyperthermia, and autonomic nervous system dysfunction.

Treatment is symptomatic and supportive, including maintaining vital signs, airway, stable body temperature, and fluid-electrolyte balance.

Vomiting shouldn't be induced; drug inhibits cough reflex, and aspiration may occur. Recommend using gastric lavage, then activated charcoal and saline cathartics; dialysis doesn't help. Recommend regulating body temperature p.r.n. Hypotension should be treated with I.V. fluids; epinephrine shouldn't be given. Recommend treating seizures with parenteral diazepam or barbiturates; arrhythmias, with parenteral phenytoin; extrapyramidal reactions, with benztropine at 1 to 2 mg or parenteral diphenhydramine at 10 to 50 mg.

## Clinical considerations

■ Some commercial preparations contain sodium metabisulfite, which may cause severe allergic reaction in susceptible individuals.
■ Drug may cause GI distress and should be given with food or fluids.
■ Concentrate should be diluted in 2 to 4 ounces of liquid, preferably soup, water, juice, carbonated drinks, milk, or puddings.
■ Drug may cause pink to brown discoloration of urine.
■ Protect liquid form from light and store at 59° to 86° F (15° to 30° C).
■ Drug causes false-positive results in urine pregnancy tests using human chorionic gonadotropin and has additive potential for causing seizures with metrizamide myelography.

### Therapeutic monitoring

■ Advise clinician to monitor patient for CNS adverse effects, especially drowsiness and extrapyramidal symptoms.
■ Advise clinician to monitor CBC and liver function test results in long-term therapy.

### Special populations

**Pediatric patients.** Drug isn't recommended for children under age 12.
**Geriatric patients.** Lower doses are recommended; 30% to 50% of usual dose may be effective. Geriatric patients are at greater risk for tardive dyskinesia and other extrapyramidal effects.

## Patient counseling

■ Explain risks of dystonic reaction and tardive dyskinesia to patient and advise him to report abnormal body movements.
■ Warn patient to avoid spilling liquid preparation on the skin; rash and irritation may result.
■ Advise patient to avoid temperature extremes (hot or cold baths, sunlamps, or tanning beds) because drug may cause thermoregulatory changes.
■ Suggest sugarless gum or candy, ice chips, or artificial saliva to relieve dry mouth.
■ Warn patient not to take drug with antacids or antidiarrheals; not to drink alcoholic beverages or take other drugs that cause sedation; not to stop taking drug or take any other drug

except as instructed; and to take drug exactly as prescribed, without doubling after missing a dose.

■ Warn patient about sedative effect. Tell him to report difficult urination, sore throat, dizziness, or fainting.

■ Advise patient to get up slowly from a recumbent or seated position to minimize effects of light-headedness.

■ Tell patient that drug may contain sodium metabisulfite, which can cause an allergic reaction to those with a sulfite allergy.

---

# montelukast sodium
Singulair

*Pharmacologic classification:*
leukotriene receptor antagonist
*Therapeutic classification:* antasthmatic
*Pregnancy risk category B*

## Available forms
Available by prescription only
*Tablets:* 10 mg
*Tablets (chewable):* 4 mg, 5 mg

## Indications and dosages
*Prophylaxis and chronic treatment of asthma*
*Adults and adolescents ages 15 and older:*
10 mg P.O. once daily in evening.
*Children ages 6 to 14:* 5 mg (chewable tablet) P.O. once daily in the evening.
*Children ages 2 to 5:* 4 mg (chewable tablet) P.O. once daily.
*Prevention of exercise-induced broncho-constriction*
*Adults and adolescents ages 15 and older:*
10 mg P.O. once daily.
◊ *Children ages 6 to 14:* 5 mg P.O. once daily.

## Mechanism of action
*Antasthmatic action:* Montelukast causes inhibition of airway cysteinyl leukotriene receptors. Drug binds with high affinity and selectivity to the $cysLT_1$ receptor, and inhibits the physiologic action of the cysteinyl leukotriene $LTD_4$. This receptor inhibition reduces early- and late-phase bronchoconstriction resulting from antigen challenge.

## Pharmacokinetics
*Absorption:* Rapidly absorbed after oral administration with mean oral bioavailability of 64%. Food doesn't affect absorption of drug. For chewable tablet, mean oral bioavailability is 73%.
*Distribution:* Minimally distributed to the tissues with a steady-state volume of distribution of 8 to 11 L. Highly plasma protein–bound.
*Metabolism:* Extensively metabolized, but plasma levels of metabolites at therapeutic doses are undetectable. In vitro studies with human liver microsomes show metabolism involvement by cytochromes P-450 3A4 and 2C9.
*Excretion:* About 86% of an oral dose is metabolized and excreted in the feces, indicating drug and its metabolites are excreted almost exclusively in the bile. Half-life is 2¾ to 5½ hours.

| Route | Onset | Peak | Duration |
|---|---|---|---|
| P.O. (film-coated) | Unknown | 3-4 hr | Unknown |
| P.O. (chewable) | Unknown | 2-2½ hr | Unknown |

## Contraindications and precautions
Contraindicated in patients hypersensitive to drug or its components. Also contraindicated in patients with acute asthmatic attacks or status asthmaticus. Although airway function is improved in patients with known aspirin hypersensitivity, these patients should avoid aspirin and NSAIDs.

## Interactions
**Drug-drug.** *Phenobarbital, rifampin:* Increased metabolism of drug. Advise clinician to monitor patient closely.

## Adverse reactions
**CNS:** *headache,* dizziness, fatigue, asthenia.
**EENT:** nasal congestion.
**GI:** dyspepsia, infectious gastroenteritis, abdominal pain.
**Respiratory:** cough, influenza.
**Skin:** rash.
**Other:** dental pain, fever, trauma.

## Overdose and treatment
No information is available on treatment of drug overdose. Recommend providing supportive measures for overdose, such as removal of unabsorbed material from the GI tract and clinical monitoring.

## Clinical considerations
■ Although dose of inhaled corticosteroids may be reduced gradually, montelukast shouldn't be abruptly substituted for inhaled or oral corticosteroids.
■ Drug shouldn't be used as monotherapy for management of exercise-induced bronchospasm.
■ No added benefit is achieved with doses above 10 mg daily.

### Therapeutic monitoring
■ Advise clinician to monitor patient for worsening asthmatic symptoms.

### Special populations
**Breast-feeding patients.** It isn't known if drug appears in breast milk. Use cautiously in breast-feeding women.

---

**Pediatric patients.** Safety and efficacy in children under age 6 haven't been established.

**Geriatric patients.** No difference in safety and effectiveness of drug has been reported between geriatric and younger patient populations.

## Patient counseling

- Advise patient to take drug daily, even if asymptomatic, and to contact prescriber if asthma isn't well controlled.
- Warn patient that drug isn't beneficial in acute asthma attacks, or in exercise-induced bronchospasm, and advise him to keep appropriate rescue drugs available.
- Advise patient sensitive to aspirin not to take aspirin and NSAIDs.
- Warn patient with phenylketonuria that chewable tablet contains phenylalanine, a component of aspartame.
- Advise patients to seek medical attention if short-acting bronchodilators are needed more often than usual or prescribed.

---

# moricizine hydrochloride
Ethmozine

*Pharmacologic classification:* sodium channel blocker
*Therapeutic classification:* antiarrhythmic
*Pregnancy risk category B*

## Available forms

Available by prescription only
*Tablets:* 200 mg, 250 mg, 300 mg

## Indications and dosages

***Treatment of documented, life-threatening ventricular arrhythmias when benefit of treatment outweighs risks***
*Adults:* Dosage must be individualized. Usual range is 600 to 900 mg P.O. daily, given q 8 hours in equally divided doses. Dosage may be adjusted within this range in increments of 150 mg daily at 3-day intervals until desired effect is obtained. Hospitalization is recommended for initiation of therapy because patient will be at high risk. Patients whose arrhythmias are well controlled during q-8-hour dosing may receive the same dose daily, divided q 12 hours to increase compliance.
≡ *Dosage adjustment.* For patients with hepatic impairment and significant renal dysfunction, give 600 mg or less daily. Advise clinician to monitor ECG before increasing dose.

## Mechanism of action

*Antiarrhythmic action:* Although moricizine is chemically related to the neuroleptic phenothiazines, it hasn't shown any dopaminergic activities. It does have potent local anesthetic activity and myocardial membrane-stabilizing effects. A Class I antiarrhythmic, it reduces the fast inward current carried by sodium ions. In patients with ventricular tachycardia, moricizine prolongs AV conduction but has no significant effect on ventricular repolarization. Intra-atrial conduction or atrial effective refractory periods aren't consistently affected and moricizine has minimal effect on sinus cycle length and sinus node recovery time. This may be significant in patients with sinus node dysfunction.

In patients with impaired left ventricular function, moricizine has minimal effects on measurements of cardiac performance: cardiac index, CVA volume, pulmonary artery wedge pressure, systemic or pulmonary vascular resistance, and ejection fraction either at rest or during exercise. A small but consistent increase in resting blood pressure and heart rate are seen. Moricizine has no effect on exercise tolerance in patients with ventricular arrhythmias, HF, or angina pectoris.

Moricizine has antiarrhythmic activity similar to that of disopyramide, propranolol, and quinidine. Arrhythmia "rebound" isn't noted after therapy stops.

## Pharmacokinetics

*Absorption:* Administration within 30 minutes of mealtime delays absorption and lowers peak plasma levels but has no effect on extent of absorption.
*Distribution:* 95% plasma protein–bound.
*Metabolism:* Undergoes significant first-pass metabolism resulting in an absolute bioavailability of about 38%. At least 26 metabolites have been identified with no single one representing at least 1% of the given dose. It has been shown to induce its own metabolism.
*Excretion:* About 56% is excreted in feces, 39% in urine; some is also recycled through enterohepatic circulation.

| Route | Onset | Peak | Duration |
|-------|-------|------|----------|
| P.O. | 2 hr | ½-2 hr | 10-24 hr |

## Contraindications and precautions

Contraindicated in patients with cardiogenic shock, those hypersensitive to drug, and those with preexisting second- or third-degree AV block or right bundle branch block when associated with left hemiblock (bifascicular block), unless an artificial pacemaker is present. Recommend stopping breast-feeding or drug because drug appears in breast milk.

Use cautiously in patients with impaired renal or hepatic function, sick sinus syndrome, coronary artery disease, or left ventricular function.

## Interactions

**Drug-drug.** *Cimetidine:* Decreased moricizine clearance by 49% when used together; no significant changes in efficacy or tolerance have

---

been observed. Patient should receive decreased doses of cimetidine (not more than 600 mg/day).
*Digoxin:* Prolongs the PR interval. Advise clinician to monitor patient closely.
*Propranolol:* May produce a small additive increase in the PR interval. Advise clinician to monitor patient carefully.
*Theophylline:* Theophylline clearance increases and plasma half-life decreases. Advise clinician to monitor theophylline levels.

## Adverse reactions
**CNS:** *dizziness, headache, fatigue,* hyperesthesia, anxiety, asthenia, nervousness, paresthesia, sleep disorders.
**CV:** *proarrhythmic events (ventricular tachycardia, PVCs, supraventricular arrhythmias),* ECG abnormalities (including *conduction defects, sinus pause, junctional rhythm,* or *AV block*), **HF,** palpitations, chest pain, *cardiac death,* hypotension, hypertension, vasodilation, cerebrovascular events.
**EENT:** blurred vision.
**GI:** *nausea, vomiting, abdominal pain, dyspepsia, diarrhea, dry mouth.*
**GU:** urine retention, urinary frequency, dysuria.
**Musculoskeletal:** musculoskeletal pain.
**Respiratory:** dyspnea.
**Skin:** diaphoresis, rash.
**Other:** drug-induced fever, thrombophlebitis.

## Overdose and treatment
Symptoms of overdose include emesis, lethargy, coma, syncope, hypotension, conduction disturbances, exacerbation of HF, MI, sinus arrest, arrhythmias, and respiratory failure. No specific antidote has been identified.

Treatment should be supportive and include careful monitoring of cardiac, respiratory, and CNS changes. Gastric evacuation to avoid aspiration may be used with care as well.

## Clinical considerations
■ When switching from another antiarrhythmic to moricizine, recommend withdrawing previous therapy one to two half-lives before starting moricizine. Moricizine should be started 6 to 12 hours after last dose of quinidine and disopyramide; 3 to 6 hours after last dose of procainamide; 8 to 12 after encainide, propafenone, tocainide, or mexiletine; and 12 to 24 hours after flecainide.
■ Initial dose for patients with renal or hepatic impairment is 600 mg daily or lower. Advise clinician to monitor patient (with ECG) before making dosage adjustments.

### *Therapeutic monitoring*
■ Electrolyte imbalances should be corrected before starting therapy; hypokalemia, hyperkalemia, or hypomagnesemia may alter effects of drug.

■ Advise clinician to monitor patient for increased dizziness and nausea with 12-hour dosing.

### *Special populations*
**Breast-feeding patients.** Drug appears in breast milk. Because of the potential for adverse reactions in the breast-fed infant, a decision whether to continue therapy must be made.
**Pediatric patients.** Safety and efficacy in children haven't been established.

## Patient counseling
■ Instruct patient to take drug as prescribed to maintain adequate arrhythmia control.

# morphine hydrochloride*
Morphitec*, M.O.S.*

# morphine sulfate
Astramorph PF, Duramorph, Epimorph*, Infumorph, MS Contin, MSIR, MS/L, MS/S, OMS Concentrate, Oramorph SR, RMS Uniserts, Roxanol, Statex*

*Pharmacologic classification:* opioid
*Therapeutic classification:* narcotic analgesic
*Pregnancy risk category C*
*Controlled substance schedule II*

## Available forms
Available by prescription only
**morphine hydrochloride***
*Tablets:* 10 mg, 20 mg, 40 mg, 60 mg
*Syrup:* 1 mg/ml, 5 mg/ml, 10 mg/ml, 20 mg/ml, 50 mg/ml
*Suppositories:* 20 mg, 30 mg
**morphine sulfate**
*Tablets:* 15 mg, 30 mg
*Tablets (extended-release):* 15 mg, 30 mg, 60 mg, 100 mg
*Tablets (soluble):* 10 mg, 15 mg, 30 mg
*Capsules:* 15 mg, 30 mg
*Oral solution:* 10 mg/5 ml, 20 mg/5 ml, 20 mg/ml, 100 mg/5 ml
*Injection (with preservative):* 1 mg/ml, 2 mg/ml, 3 mg/ml, 4 mg/ml, 5 mg/ml, 8 mg/ml, 10 mg/ml, 15 mg/ml, 25 mg/ml, 50 mg/ml
*Injection (without preservative):* 500 mcg/ml, 1 mg/ml, 10 mg/ml, 15 mg/ml, 25 mg/ml
*Suppositories:* 5 mg, 10 mg, 20 mg, 30 mg

## Indications and dosages
### *Severe pain*
*Adults:* 10 mg q 4 hours S.C. or I.M., or 10 to 30 mg P.O., or 10 to 20 mg P.R. q 4 hours, p.r.n., or around-the-clock. May be injected slow I.V. (over 4 to 5 minutes) 2.5 to 15 mg diluted in 4 to 5 ml water for injection. May also give controlled-release tablets 15 to 30 mg q 12

hours. As an intermittent epidural injection, 5 mg via an epidural catheter q 24 hours. For continuous epidural infusion (device not implanted surgically), initial dose is 2.4 mg per 24 hours. May increase 1 to 2 mg daily, p.r.n. For a surgically implanted device, 3.5 to 7.5 mg daily or 4.5 to 10 mg daily if opiate tolerant. Intrathecal dose is one-tenth epidural dose, 0.2 to 1 mg may provide adequate relief in patients not tolerant to opiates.

*Children:* 0.1 to 0.2 mg/kg S.C. or I.M. q 4 hours. Maximum dose is 15 mg. May also give 0.05 to 0.1 mg/kg I.V. very slowly. In some situations, morphine may be given by continuous I.V. infusion or by intraspinal and intrathecal injection.

***Severe chronic pain associated with cancer***

*Adults:* Initial loading dose of 15 mg followed by 0.8 to 10 mg/hour continuous I.V. or ◇ S.C. infusion. Titrate to effect.

*Children:* 0.025 to 2.6 mg/kg/hour by I.V. infusion or 0.025 to 1.79 mg/kg/hour by ◇ S.C. infusion.

***Preoperative sedation and adjunct to anesthesia***

*Adults:* 8 to 10 mg I.M., S.C., or I.V.

***Postoperative analgesia***

*Children:* 0.01 to 0.04 mg/kg/hour by continuous I.V. infusion.

◇ 0.015 to 0.02 mg/kg/hour by continuous I.V. infusion.

***Control of pain from acute MI***

*Adults:* Initially, 2 to 15 mg I.M., S.C., or I.V. Additional doses of 1 to 4 mg I.V. may be given q 5 minutes, p.r.n.

***Control of angina pain***

*Adults:* 2 to 5 mg I.V. q 5 to 30 minutes, p.r.n., for pain unrelieved by three doses of S.L. nitroglycerin.

***Adjunctive treatment of acute pulmonary edema***

*Adults:* 10 to 15 mg I.V. at a rate not exceeding 2 mg/minute.

***Analgesia during labor***

*Adults:* 10 mg I.M. or S.C.

## I.V. administration

■ Morphine sulfate 10 or 25 mg/ml injections are intended for use with continuous, controlled microinfusion devices.

■ Morphine 25 mg/ml is diluted to a concentration of 0.1 to 1 mg/ml in $D_5W$. A higher concentration may be used for patients with a fluid restriction.

### Incompatibilities

Incompatible with aminophylline, amobarbital, barbiturates that are soluble, cefepime, chlorothiazide, heparin sodium, meperidine, methicillin, phenobarbital sodium, phenytoin sodium, promethazine hydrochloride, sodium bicarbonate, sodium iodide, and thiopental.

## Mechanism of action

*Analgesic action:* Morphine is the principal opium alkaloid, the standard for opiate agonist analgesic activity. Mechanism of action is thought to be via the opiate receptors, altering patient's perception of pain. Morphine is particularly useful in severe, acute pain or severe, chronic pain. Morphine also has a central depressant effect on respiration and on the cough reflex center.

## Pharmacokinetics

*Absorption:* Variable absorption is from the GI tract.

*Distribution:* Distributed widely through the body.

*Metabolism:* Metabolized primarily in the liver. One metabolite, morphine 6-glucuromide, is active.

*Excretion:* Excreted in the urine and bile. Morphine 6-glucuromide may accumulate after continuous dosing in patients with renal failure, leading to enhanced and prolonged opiate activity.

| Route | Onset | Peak | Duration |
|---|---|---|---|
| P.O. | 1 hr | 1-2 hr | 4-12 hr |
| I.V. | 5 min | 20 min | 4-5 hr |
| I.M. | 10-30 min | 30-60 min | 4-5 hr |
| S.C. | 10-30 min | 50-90 min | 4-5 hr |
| P.R. | 20-30 min | 20-60 min | 4-5 hr |
| Epidural | 15-60 min | 15-60 min | 24 hr |
| Intrathecal | 15-60 min | 30-60 min | 24 hr |

## Contraindications and precautions

Contraindicated in patients hypersensitive to drug or those with conditions that would preclude administration of opioids by I.V. route (acute bronchial asthma or upper airway obstruction).

Use cautiously in geriatric or debilitated patients and in those with head injury, increased intracranial pressure, seizures, pulmonary disease, prostatic hyperplasia, hepatic or renal disease, acute abdominal conditions, hypothyroidism, Addison's disease, or urethral strictures.

## Interactions

**Drug-drug.** *Anticholinergics:* May cause paralytic ileus. Advise clinician to monitor patient carefully.

*Cimetidine:* Increased respiratory and CNS depression. Reduced dosage of morphine is usually needed.

*General anesthetics:* Severe CV depression may result. Use together cautiously.

*Narcotic antagonists:* Patients who become physically dependent on this drug may experience acute withdrawal syndrome if given a narcotic antagonist. Avoid use together.

*Other CNS depressants, such as antihistamines, barbiturates, benzodiazepines, general anes-*

---

*thetics, MAO inhibitors, muscle relaxants, narcotic analgesics, phenothiazines, sedative-hypnotics, and tricyclic antidepressants:* Potentiate respiratory and CNS depression, sedation, and hypotensive effects of drug. Use together cautiously.

**Drug-lifestyle.** *Alcohol use:* Potentiates effects of drug. Advise patient to avoid alcohol.

## Adverse reactions

**CNS:** *sedation, somnolence, clouded sensorium, euphoria, seizures* (with large doses), *dizziness,* nightmares (with long-acting oral forms), light-headedness, hallucinations, nervousness, depression, syncope.

**CV:** *hypotension, bradycardia, shock, cardiac arrest,* tachycardia, hypertension.

**GI:** *nausea, vomiting, constipation, ileus, dry mouth, biliary tract spasms, anorexia,* increased plasma amylase levels.

**GU:** *urine retention.*

**Hematologic:** *thrombocytopenia.*

**Respiratory:** *respiratory depression, apnea, respiratory arrest.*

**Skin:** pruritus, skin flushing (with epidural administration); *diaphoresis; edema.*

**Other:** *physical dependence, decreased libido.*

## Overdose and treatment

Rapid I.V. administration may result in overdose because of the delay in maximum CNS effect (30 minutes). The most common signs and symptoms of morphine overdose are respiratory depression with or without CNS depression, and miosis (pinpoint pupils). Other acute toxic effects include hypotension, bradycardia, hypothermia, shock, apnea, cardiopulmonary arrest, circulatory collapse, pulmonary edema, and seizures.

For treatment of acute overdose, recommend first establishing adequate respiratory exchange by way of a patent airway and ventilation, p.r.n., and giving a narcotic antagonist (naloxone) to reverse respiratory depression. (Because duration of action of morphine is longer than that of naloxone, repeated naloxone dosing is needed.) Naloxone shouldn't be given in the absence of clinically significant respiratory or CV depression. Advise clinician to monitor vital signs closely.

If patient is seen within 2 hours of ingestion of an oral overdose, recommend emptying the stomach immediately by inducing emesis (ipecac syrup) or using gastric lavage. Recommend using caution to avoid risk of aspiration. Activated charcoal should be given via nasogastric tube for further removal of drug in an oral overdose.

Recommend providing symptomatic and supportive treatment (continued respiratory support, correction of fluid or electrolyte imbalance). Advise clinician to monitor laboratory parameters, vital signs, and neurologic status closely.

## Clinical considerations

■ Morphine is the drug of choice in relieving pain of MI; it may cause transient decrease in blood pressure.

■ Regimented scheduling (around-the-clock) is beneficial in severe, chronic pain.

■ Oral solutions of various levels are available, as well as a new intensified oral solution.

■ There's a greater fluctuation in pain control with extended-release preparations.

■ Note the disparity between oral and parenteral doses.

**H *ALERT*** For continuous epidural or intrathecal infusion, morphine is administered via a controlled-infusion device. Take care when refilling the reservoir of such devices to ensure that drug is instilled into the proper port. A technical error could result in life-threatening respiratory depression.

■ Long-term therapy in patients with advanced renal disease may lead to toxicity as a result of accumulation of the active metabolite.

■ Some morphine injections contain sulfites that may cause allergic-type reactions.

■ For S.L. administration, measure oral solution with tuberculin syringe, and give dose a few drops at a time to allow maximal S.L. absorption and to minimize swallowing.

■ Refrigeration of rectal suppositories isn't needed. In some patients, rectal and oral absorption may not be equivalent.

■ Preservative-free preparations are available for epidural and intrathecal administration. The use of the epidural route is increasing.

■ Morphine may worsen or mask gallbladder pain.

**H *ALERT*** Don't confuse morphine with hydromorphone. Teach patient not to crush extended-release tablets.

### *Therapeutic monitoring*

■ Epidural morphine has proven to be an excellent analgesic for patients with postoperative pain. After epidural administration, advise clinician to monitor patient closely for respiratory depression up to 24 hours after the injection. Recommend checking respiratory rate and depth according to protocol (such as every 15 minutes for 2 hours, then hourly for 18 hours). Some clinicians advocate a dilute naloxone infusion of 5 to 10 mcg/kg/hour during the first 12 hours to minimize respiratory depression without altering pain relief.

■ Recommend carefully monitoring patient's vital signs during morphine administration.

### *Special populations*

**Breast-feeding patients.** Morphine appears in breast milk. Mother should wait 2 to 3 hours after last dose before breast-feeding to avoid sedating the infant.

**Pediatric patients.** Safety and efficacy of epidural and intrathecal dosing in children haven't been established. Safety and efficacy of morphine use in neonates haven't been established. Children may be more sensitive to opiates on a body-weight basis.

**Geriatric patients.** Lower doses are usually indicated for geriatric patients, who may be more sensitive to the therapeutic and adverse effects of drug.

## Patient counseling
■ Tell patient that oral liquid form of morphine may be mixed with a glass of fruit juice immediately before it's taken, if desired, to improve the taste.
■ Tell patient taking long-acting morphine tablets to swallow them whole. Tablets shouldn't be broken, crushed, or chewed before swallowing.

---

# moxifloxacin hydrochloride
Avelox, Avelox I.V.

*Pharmacologic classification:* fluoro-quinolone
*Therapeutic classification:* antibiotic
*Pregnancy risk category C*

## Available forms
Available by prescription only
*Tablets (film-coated):* 400 mg
*Injection:* 400 mg/250 ml

## Indications and dosages
*Acute bacterial sinusitis caused by* **Haemophilus influenzae, Moraxella catarrhalis,** *or* **Streptococcus pneumoniae**
*Adults:* 400 mg P.O. or I.V. once daily for 10 days.
*Acute bacterial exacerbation of chronic bronchitis caused by* **H. influenzae, Haemophilus parainfluenzae, Klebsiella pneumoniae, M. catarrhalis, Staphylococcus aureus,** *or* **S. pneumoniae**
*Adults:* 400 mg P.O. or I.V. once daily for 5 days.
*Mild to moderate community-acquired pneumonia caused by* **Chlamydia pneumoniae, H. influenzae, M. catarrhalis, Moraxella pneumoniae,** *or* **S. pneumoniae**
*Adults:* 400 mg P.O. or I.V. once daily for 7 to 14 days.
*Uncomplicated skin and skin-structure infections caused by* **S. aureus** *or* **Streptococcus pyogenes**
*Adults:* 400 mg P.O. or I.V. once daily for 7 days.

## I.V. administration
■ Give by direct infusion or via Y-type administration set over 60 minutes.
■ If I.V. line is used for other medications, flush before and after moxifloxacin administration with normal saline solution or $D_5W$.

■ Solution containing particulate matter should not be used.

## Incompatibilities
Data are limited. Don't mix with other drugs or infuse simultaneously via the same I.V. line.

## Mechanism of action
*Antibactericidal action:* Drug inhibits the activity of topoisomerase I (DNA gyrase) and topoisomerase IV in susceptible bacteria. These enzymes are needed for bacterial DNA replication, transcription, repair, and recombination.

## Pharmacokinetics
*Absorption:* Well absorbed after oral administration; absolute bioavailability of about 90%.
*Distribution:* Widely distributed. Plasma protein–binding about 50%. Penetrates well into nasal and bronchial secretions, sinus mucosa, and saliva.
*Metabolism:* Metabolized to inactive glucuronide and sulfate conjugates. About 14% of dose converted to glucuronide metabolite. Sulfate metabolite accounts for about 38% of dose.
*Excretion:* About 45% excreted unchanged, 20% in urine and 25% in feces. Mean elimination half-life is about 12 hours.

| Route | Onset | Peak | Duration |
|---|---|---|---|
| P.O., I.V. | Unknown | 1-3 hr | Unknown |

## Contraindications and precautions
Contraindicated in patients hypersensitive to drug or its components or fluoroquinolone antimicrobials.

Use cautiously in patients with prolonged QT interval and uncorrected hypokalemia. Also use cautiously in patients with CNS disorders and in the presence of other risk factors that may predispose patients to seizures or lower seizure threshold.

## Interactions
**Drug-drug.** *Antacids; didanosine; metal cations, such as aluminum, magnesium, iron, zinc; multivitamins; sucralfate:* Metal cations chelate with moxifloxacin, resulting in decreased absorption and lower serum levels. Give drug at least 8 hours before or 6 hours after drugs containing metal cations.
*Antipsychotic drugs, erythromycin, tricyclic antidepressants:* Possible additive effect when used with these drugs. Advise clinician to monitor patient and ECG closely; use drug cautiously.
*Class IA antiarrhythmics (such as procainamide, quinidine), Class III antiarrhythmics (such as amiodarone, sotalol):* Lack of clinical experience. Avoid concurrent use.
*NSAIDs:* Increased risk of CNS stimulation and seizures. Don't use together.
**Drug-lifestyle.** *Sun exposure:* Although photosensitivity hasn't occurred with moxifloxacin,

it has been reported with other fluoroquinolones. Tell patient to take precautions.

## Adverse reactions
**CNS:** dizziness, headache.
**CV:** *prolongation of QT interval.*
**GI:** taste perversion, abdominal pain, diarrhea,
dyspepsia, nausea, vomiting, hyperlipidemia,
increased amylase, GGT, and LDH levels.
**Hematologic:** thrombocythemia, *thrombocy-
topenia,* eosinophilia, *leukopenia,* increase or
decrease in PT.
**Hepatic:** abnormal liver function test results.
**Metabolic:** hyperglycemia.

## Overdose and treatment
In acute overdose, immediately empty the stomach. Advise clinician to monitor ECG closely
because of the risk of QT interval prolongation. Provide adequate hydration and supportive care. It isn't known if drug is dialyzable.

## Clinical considerations
■ Give at same time each day to provide consistent absorption. Provide liberal fluid intake.
■ Advise patient to complete entire course of
therapy.
■ NSAIDs may increase risk of CNS stimulation and seizures when used with fluoroquinolones such as moxifloxacin.
■ Rupture of Achilles and other tendons has
been linked to fluoroquinolones. If pain, inflammation, or rupture of a tendon occurs, drug
should be stopped.
**◾ ALERT** Drug may cause false-positive opiate results in urinary assays.
■ Drug hasn't been studied in patients with
moderate to severe hepatotoxicity (Child Pugh
Classes B and C) and isn't recommended in
this setting.
■ CNS reactions caused by fluoroquinolones
may occur after initial dose. Recommend stopping drug and starting appropriate therapy if
any of these reactions occurs.
■ Serious hypersensitivity reactions, including
anaphylaxis, have occurred in patients receiving fluoroquinolones. Recommend stopping
drug and starting supportive measures as indicated.
■ Pseudomembranous colitis may occur with
moxifloxacin as with other antimicrobials. This
diagnosis should be considered if diarrhea develops after start of therapy.

### Therapeutic monitoring
■ Recommend watching for hypersensitivity
reactions, CNS toxicities including seizures,
QT interval prolongation, pseudomembranous
colitis, phototoxicity, and tendon rupture.

### Special populations
**Breast-feeding patients.** Drug may appear in
breast milk. Benefits of drug must be weighed
against potential risks to breast-feeding infant.

**Geriatric patients.** Advise clinician to monitor patient for ECG changes, especially with
the I.V. form.

## Patient counseling
■ Tell patient to take drug at same time each
day.
■ Advise patient to finish entire course of therapy, even if condition has improved.
■ Tell patient to drink plenty of fluids.
■ Tell patient to avoid hazardous activities,
such as driving an automobile or operating machinery, until effects of drug are known.
■ Advise patient to call prescriber if he experiences allergic reaction, palpitations, fainting,
persistent diarrhea, sunburn, tendon injury, or
seizures.

# mumps virus vaccine, live
Mumpsvax

*Pharmacologic classification:* vaccine
*Therapeutic classification:* viral vac-
cine
*Pregnancy risk category C*

## Available forms
Available by prescription only
*Injection:* single-dose vial containing not less
than 20,000 TCID$_{50}$ (tissue culture infective
doses) of attenuated mumps virus derived from
Jeryl Lynn mumps strain (grown in chick embryo culture) and vial of diluent

## Indications and dosages
*Immunization*
*Adults and children over age 1:* 1 vial (0.5 ml)
S.C. in outer aspect of the upper arm.

## Mechanism of action
*Mumps prophylactic action:* Vaccine promotes
active immunity to mumps.

## Pharmacokinetics
*Absorption:* Antibodies usually are evident 2
to 3 weeks after injection. Duration of vaccine-
induced immunity is at least 20 years and prob-
ably lifelong.
*Distribution:* No information available.
*Metabolism:* No information available.
*Excretion:* No information available.

| Route | Onset | Peak | Duration |
|-------|-------|------|----------|
| S.C. | Unknown | Unknown | > 15 yr |

## Contraindications and precautions
Contraindicated in immunosuppressed patients;
in those with cancer, blood dyscrasias, gamma globulin disorders, fever, untreated active
tuberculosis, or anaphylactic or anaphylactoid
reactions to neomycin or eggs; in those receiving corticosteroid or radiation therapy; and
in pregnant women.

## Interactions

**Drug-drug.** *Immune serum globulin, transfusions of blood or blood products:* May interfere with immune response to vaccine. If possible, defer vaccination for 3 months in these situations.

*Immunosuppressants:* May interfere with response to vaccine. Avoid use together.

## Adverse reactions

**CNS:** *malaise*
**GI:** *diarrhea.*
**Skin:** *rash.*
**Other:** *slight fever, mild allergic reactions, mild lymphadenopathy, injection-site reaction.*

## Overdose and treatment

No information available.

## Clinical considerations

- Mumps vaccine shouldn't be used in delayed hypersensitivity (anergy) skin testing.
- Recommend obtaining a thorough history of patient's allergies, especially to antibiotics, eggs, chicken, or chicken feathers, and of reactions to immunizations.
- Skin testing is performed to assess vaccine sensitivity (against a control of normal saline solution in the opposite arm) in patients with history of anaphylactoid reactions to egg ingestion. Advise clinician to give an intradermal or scratch test with a 1:10 dilution and reading results after 5 to 30 minutes. A positive reaction is a wheal with or without pseudopodia and surrounding erythema. If sensitivity test is positive, desensitization should be considered.
- The FDA requires that the manufacturer, lot number, date of administration, and name, address, and title of person giving the vaccine be documented.
- Vaccine can be used in HIV-infected patients who don't have severe immunosuppression.
- Epinephrine solution 1:1,000 should be available to treat allergic reactions.
- Vaccine shouldn't be given I.V. Use a 25G, ⅝-inch needle and inject S.C., preferably into the outer aspect of the upper arm.
- Use only diluent supplied. Discard reconstituted solution after 8 hours.
- Store in refrigerator and protect from light. Solution may be used if red, pink, or yellow, but it must be clear.
- Don't give vaccine less than 1 month before or after immunization with other live virus vaccines—except for live, attenuated measles virus vaccine, live rubella virus vaccine, or monovalent or trivalent live oral poliovirus vaccine or poliovirus vaccine, inactivated, which may be given simultaneously.
- Vaccine doesn't offer protection when given after exposure to natural mumps.
- Revaccination is recommended at 4 to 6 years of age.
- The minimum interval between doses should be 4 weeks.
- Vaccine temporarily may decrease the response to tuberculin skin testing. If a tuberculin skin test is needed, it should be given either before or simultaneously with mumps vaccine.

### Therapeutic monitoring

- Advise clinician to monitor patient for allergic response.

### Special populations

**Breast-feeding patients.** It isn't known if vaccine appears in breast milk. No problems have been reported. Use vaccine cautiously in breast-feeding women.

**Pediatric patients.** Vaccine isn't recommended for children under age 1 because retained maternal mumps antibodies may interfere with immune response.

## Patient counseling

- Tell patient that he may experience pain and inflammation at the injection site and a low-grade fever, rash, or general malaise.
- Encourage patient to report distressing adverse reactions.
- Recommend acetaminophen to alleviate adverse reactions, such as fever.
- Tell women of childbearing age to avoid pregnancy for 3 months after vaccination. Provide contraceptive information, if needed.

# mupirocin (pseudomonic acid A)

Bactroban

# mupirocin calcium

Bactroban Nasal

*Pharmacologic classification:* antibiotic
*Therapeutic classification:* topical antibacterial
*Pregnancy risk category B*

## Available forms

Available by prescription only
*Ointment:* 2% (1-g single-use tubes, 15 g, 30 g)
*Cream:* 2%
*Ointment for intranasal use:* 2%

## Indications and dosages

*Topical treatment of impetigo caused by* **Staphylococcus aureus,** *beta-hemolytic* **streptococcus,** *and* **Streptococcus pyogenes**

*Adults and children:* Apply a small amount to affected area t.i.d. for 1 to 2 weeks. The area treated may be covered with a gauze dressing, if desired.

### Eradication of nasal colonization of methicillin-resistant S. aureus
*Adults:* Apply one-half of a single-use tube to each nostril b.i.d. for 5 days. Press and release the sides of the nose repeatedly for 1 minute to disperse the drug through the nares.

## Mechanism of action
*Antibacterial action:* Mupirocin is structurally unrelated to other drugs and is produced by fermentation of the organism *Pseudomonas fluorescens.* Mupirocin inhibits bacterial protein synthesis by reversibly and specifically binding to bacterial isoleucyl transfer-RNA synthetase. Mupirocin shows no cross-resistance with chloramphenical, erythromycin, gentamicin, lincomycin, methicillin, neomycin, novobiocin, penicillin, streptomycin, or tetracycline.

## Pharmacokinetics
*Absorption:* Normal subjects showed no absorption after 24-hour application under occlusive dressings.
*Distribution:* Highly protein-bound (about 95%). A substantial decrease in activity can be expected in the presence of serum (as in exudative wounds).
*Metabolism:* Slightly metabolized locally in the skin to monic acid.
*Excretion:* Eliminated locally by desquamation of the skin.

| Route | Onset | Peak | Duration |
|-------|-------|------|----------|
| Topical | Unknown | Unknown | Unknown |

## Contraindications and precautions
Contraindicated in patients hypersensitive to drug. Use cautiously in patients with burns or impaired renal function.

## Interactions
None reported.

## Adverse reactions
**CNS:** headache (with nasal use).
**EENT:** rhinitis, pharyngitis, burning (with nasal use).
**GI:** taste perversion.
**Respiratory:** upper respiratory congestions, cough (with nasal use).
**Skin:** burning, pruritus, stinging, rash, pain, erythema (with topical administration).

## Overdose and treatment
No information available.

## Clinical considerations
■ If sensitivity or chemical irritation occurs, recommend stopping treatment and starting appropriate alternative therapy.
■ When used on burns or to treat extensive open wounds, absorption of polyethylene glycol vehicle is possible and may result in serious renal toxicity.

## Therapeutic monitoring
■ Patients not showing a clinical response within 3 to 5 days should be reevaluated.
■ Recommend watching for superinfection. Use of antibiotics (prolonged or repeated) may result in bacterial or fungal overgrowth of nonsusceptible organisms.

## Special populations
**Breast-feeding patients.** It isn't known if drug appears in breast milk. Use with caution in breast-feeding women.

## Patient counseling
■ Advise patient to wash and dry affected areas thoroughly. Then apply thin film, rubbing in gently.
■ Tell patient to use single-use tube for nasal application for one application only, then discard tube. Apply one-half of the ointment from the tube into one nostril and the remaining into the other nostril, in the morning and evening.
■ Warn patient to avoid contact around eyes and mucous membranes.

# mycophenolate mofetil
CellCept

# mycophenolate mofetil hydochloride
CellCept Intravenous

*Pharmacologic classification:* mycophenolic acid derivative
*Therapeutic classification:* immunosuppressant
*Pregnancy risk category C*

## Available forms
Available by prescription only
*Capsules:* 250 mg
*Tablets:* 500 mg
*Powder for injection:* 500 mg

## Indications and dosages
*Prophylaxis of organ rejection in patients receiving allogeneic renal transplants*
*Adults:* 1 g P.O. or I.V. b.i.d. Use with corticosteroids and cyclosporine.
*Prophylaxis of organ rejection in patients receiving cardiac transplants*
*Adults:* 1.5 g P.O. or I.V. b.i.d. Use with corticosteroids and cyclosporine.
*Prophylaxis of organ rejection in patients receiving allogenic hepatic transplants*
*Adults:* 1 g I.V. b.i.d. over no less than 2 hours or 1.5 g P.O. b.i.d. Use with corticosteroids and cyclosporine.

## I.V. administration

■ I.V. solution shouldn't be administered by rapid or bolus method; it must be given over 2 hours or longer.

■ Reconstitute by injecting 14 ml $D_5W$ injection into a 500-mg vial; shake and inspect for particles or discoloration (solution is slightly yellow). Discard if particles or discoloration is present. To prepare a 1-g dose, further dilute two reconstituted vials in 140 ml of $D_5W$ injection. To prepare a 1.5-g dose, further dilute three reconstituted vials in 210 ml of $D_5W$ injection. The final concentration of both preparations is 6 mg/ml.

■ Use solution within 4 hours of reconstitution and dilution. Store at 77° F (25° C).

### Incompatibilities

Don't mix or give at the same time via the same infusion line with other I.V. drugs or I.V. admixtures.

### Mechanism of action

*Immunosuppressive action:* Mycophenolate inhibits proliferative responses of T and B lymphocytes, suppresses antibody formation by B lymphocytes, and may inhibit recruitment of leukocytes into sites of inflammation and graft rejection.

### Pharmacokinetics

*Absorption:* Absorbed from the GI tract. Absolute bioavailability of drug and active metabolite is 94%.
*Distribution:* About 97% plasma protein–bound.
*Metabolism:* Undergoes complete presystemic metabolism to mycophenolic acid.
*Excretion:* Primarily excreted in urine with a small amount excreted in feces. Half-life is about 18 hours.

| Route | Onset | Peak | Duration |
|-------|-------|------|----------|
| P.O. | Unknown | ½-1¼ hr | 7½-18 hr |
| I.V. | Unknown | Unknown | 10-17 hr |

### Contraindications and precautions

Contraindicated in patients hypersensitive to drug, mycophenolic acid, or components of product. Don't use during pregnancy unless the benefits outweigh the risks. Use cautiously in patients with GI disorders.

### Interactions

**Drug-drug.** *Acyclovir, ganciclovir:* Increased risk of toxicity for both drugs. Advise clinician to monitor patient closely.
*Antacids with magnesium and aluminum hydroxides:* Decreased absorption of mycophenolate mofetil. Give drugs separately.
*Cholestyramine:* May interfere with enterohepatic recirculation, causing a decrease in mycophenolate bioavailability. Don't give together.

*Oral contraceptives:* Mycophenolate may affect efficacy of oral contraceptives. Advise patient to use alternative contraceptive measures.

### Adverse reactions

**CNS:** *astenia, tremor,* insomnia, dizziness, *headache.*
**CV:** *chest pain, hypertension, edema.*
**EENT:** pharyngitis.
**GI:** *diarrhea, constipation, nausea, dyspepsia, vomiting, oral candidiasis, abdominal pain.*
**GU:** *urinary tract infection, hematuria,* renal tubular necrosis.
**Hematologic:** *anemia,* **leukopenia,** THROMBOCYTOPENIA, hypochromic anemia, leukocytosis.
**Metabolic:** *hypercholesterolemia, hypophosphatemia, hypokalemia,* hyperkalemia, hyperglycemia.
**Musculoskeletal:** *back pain.*
**Respiratory:** *dyspnea, cough,* bronchitis, pneumonia.
**Skin:** *acne,* rash.
**Other:** *pain, fever, sepsis, possible immunosuppression-induced infection or lymphoma.*

### Overdose and treatment

Although there's no reported experience of overdose in humans, doses of 4 to 5 g per day compared with 3 g per day caused an increase in nausea, vomiting, or diarrhea and occasional hematologic abnormalities in some patients. Treatment includes use of bile acid sequestrants to increase excretion of drug.

### Clinical considerations

■ Avoid doses exceeding 1 g b.i.d. in patients with severe chronic renal impairment (glomerular filtration rate below 25 ml per minute) outside the immediate posttransplant period.

**H ALERT** Because of potential teratogenic effects, don't open capsules and don't crush tablets. Also avoid inhalation or direct contact with skin or mucous membranes of the powder contained in the capsules. If such contact occurs, wash thoroughly with soap and water; rinse eyes with plain water.

■ Immunosuppression-induced infection or lymphoma may occur.

### Therapeutic monitoring

■ Advise clinician to monitor patient's CBC regularly. If neutropenia develops, recommend interrupting therapy, reducing dosage, performing appropriate diagnostic tests, or giving additional treatment.

### Special populations

**Breast-feeding patients.** It isn't known if drug appears in breast milk. Use in breast-feeding women isn't recommended.
**Pediatric patients.** Safety and efficacy in children haven't been established.

## Patient counseling

■ Warn patient not to open capsules or crush tablets; instruct him to swallow them whole on an empty stomach.

■ Instruct patient of need for repeated appropriate laboratory tests during drug therapy.

■ Give patient complete dosage instructions and inform him of increased risk of lymphoproliferative diseases and other malignancies.

■ Explain that drug is used with other drug therapies. Stress importance of not interrupting or stopping these drugs without medical approval.

■ Inform women that a pregnancy test should be taken within 1 week before therapy starts and that effective contraception must be used before, during, and for 6 weeks after therapy is completed, even when there's history of infertility (unless from hysterectomy). Also, two forms of contraception must be used simultaneously unless abstinence is chosen. If pregnancy occurs despite these measures, she must contact her prescriber immediately.

# nabumetone
Relafen

*Pharmacologic classification:* NSAID
*Therapeutic classification:* antarthritic
*Pregnancy risk category C*

## Available forms
Available by prescription only
*Tablets:* 500 mg, 750 mg

## Indications and dosages
***Acute and long-term treatment of rheumatoid arthritis or osteoarthritis***
*Adults:* Initially, 1,000 mg P.O. daily as a single dose or in divided doses b.i.d. Adjust dosage based on patient response. Maximum recommended daily dose, 2,000 mg.

## Mechanism of action
*Anti-inflammatory action:* Nabumetone probably acts by inhibiting the synthesis of prostaglandins. Drug also has analgesic and antipyretic action.

## Pharmacokinetics
*Absorption:* Well absorbed from the GI tract. After absorption, about 35% is rapidly transformed to 6-methoxy-2-naphthylacetic acid (6MNA), the principal active metabolite; the balance is transformed to unidentified metabolites. Administration with food increases the absorption rate and peak levels of 6MNA but doesn't change total drug absorbed.
*Distribution:* 6MNA is extensively plasma protein–bound.
*Metabolism:* 6MNA is metabolized to inactive metabolites in the liver.
*Excretion:* Metabolites are excreted primarily in urine. About 9% appears in the feces. Elimination half-life is about 24 hours. Half-life is increased in patients with renal failure.

| Route | Onset | Peak | Duration |
|-------|-------|------|----------|
| P.O. | Unknown | 2-4 hr | Unknown |

## Contraindications and precautions
Contraindicated in patients with hypersensitivity reactions, history of aspirin- or NSAID-induced asthma, urticaria, or other allergic-type reactions and during third trimester of pregnancy.

Use cautiously in patients with impaired renal or hepatic function, HF, hypertension, conditions that predispose to fluid retention, and history of peptic ulcer disease.

## Interactions
**Drug-drug.** *Drugs that are highly plasma protein–bound, such as warfarin:* Nabumetone may displace drug. Use together with caution.

## Adverse reactions
**CNS:** *dizziness, headache,* fatigue, insomnia, nervousness, somnolence.
**CV:** vasculitis, edema.
**EENT:** *tinnitus.*
**GI:** *diarrhea, dyspepsia, abdominal pain, constipation, flatulence, nausea,* dry mouth, gastritis, stomatitis, anorexia, vomiting, ***bleeding,*** ulceration.
**Respiratory:** dyspnea, pneumonitis.
**Skin:** *pruritus, rash,* increased diaphoresis.

## Overdose and treatment
After an accidental overdose, recommend emptying the stomach by induced emesis or lavage. Activated charcoal may limit the amount of drug absorbed.

## Clinical considerations
■ Because NSAIDs impair the synthesis of renal prostaglandins, they may decrease renal blood flow and lead to reversible renal function impairment, especially in patients with preexisting renal failure, liver dysfunction, and HF; in geriatric patients; and in those taking diuretics. Advise clinician to monitor these patients closely during therapy.

### Therapeutic monitoring
■ During long-term therapy, recommend periodic monitoring of renal and liver function, CBC, and hematocrit. Advise clinician to monitor patient carefully for signs and symptoms of GI bleeding.

### Special populations
**Breast-feeding patients.** The active metabolite of nabumetone, 6MNA, appears in the milk of laboratory rats. Because of risk of serious toxicity to the infant, use in breast-feeding women isn't recommended.
**Pediatric patients.** Safety and efficacy in children haven't been established.

Geriatric patients. No differences in safety or efficacy have been noted in geriatric patients.

## Patient counseling
■ Tell patient to take drug with food, milk, or antacids to enhance drug absorption.
■ Stress importance of follow-up examinations to detect adverse GI effects.
■ Teach patient signs and symptoms of GI bleeding, and tell him to report them to prescriber immediately.
■ Advise patient to limit alcohol intake because of risk of additive GI toxicity.

# nadolol
Corgard

*Pharmacologic classification:* beta blocker
*Therapeutic classification:* antihypertensive, antianginal
*Pregnancy risk category C*

## Available forms
Available by prescription only
*Tablets:* 20 mg, 40 mg, 80 mg, 120 mg, 160 mg

## Indications and dosages
*Hypertension*
*Adults:* Initially, 20 to 40 mg P.O. once daily. Dosage may be increased in 40- to 80-mg increments daily at 2- to 14-day intervals until optimum response occurs. Usual maintenance dose is 40 or 80 mg once daily. Doses of up to 240 or 320 mg daily may be needed. Rarely, up to 640 mg daily.
*Long-term prophylactic management of chronic stable angina pectoris*
*Adults:* Initially, 40 mg P.O. once daily. Dosage may be increased in 40- to 80-mg increments daily at 3- to 7-day intervals until optimum response occurs. Usual maintenance dose is 40 or 80 mg once daily. Doses of up to 160 or 240 mg daily may be needed.
◇ *Arrhythmias*
*Adults:* 60 to 160 mg P.O. daily.
◇ *Prophylaxis of vascular headache*
*Adults:* 20 to 40 mg P.O. once daily; may gradually increase to 120 mg daily, if needed.
≡ *Dosage adjustment.* For renally impaired patients, refer to the following table.

| Creatinine clearance (ml/min) | Dosing interval |
|---|---|
| 31-50 | q 24-36 hr |
| 10-30 | q 24-48 hr |
| < 10 | q 40-60 hr |

## Mechanism of action
*Antihypertensive action:* Mechanism of antihypertensive effect is unknown. Drug may reduce blood pressure by blocking adrenergic receptors, thus decreasing cardiac output; by decreasing sympathetic outflow from the CNS; or by suppressing renin release.
*Antianginal action:* Nadolol decreases myocardial oxygen consumption, thus relieving angina, by blocking catecholamine-induced increases in heart rate, myocardial contraction, and blood pressure.

## Pharmacokinetics
*Absorption:* 30% to 40% of a dose of nadolol is absorbed from the GI tract. Absorption isn't affected by food.
*Distribution:* Distributed throughout the body; drug is about 30% protein-bound.
*Metabolism:* Not metabolized.
*Excretion:* Most of a given dose is excreted unchanged in urine; the remainder is excreted in feces. Plasma half-life is about 20 hours. Antihypertensive and antianginal effects persist for about 24 hours.

| Route | Onset | Peak | Duration |
|---|---|---|---|
| P.O. | Unknown | 2-4 hr | Unknown |

## Contraindications and precautions
Contraindicated in patients with bronchial asthma, sinus bradycardia and greater than first-degree heart block, and cardiogenic shock. Use cautiously in patients with hyperthyroidism, HF, diabetes, chronic bronchitis, emphysema, and impaired renal or hepatic function and in those receiving general anesthesia before undergoing surgery.

## Interactions
**Drug-drug.** *Antimuscarinics such as atropine:* May antagonize nadolol-induced bradycardia. Use together cautiously.
*Diuretics, other antihypertensives and, at high doses, the neuromuscular blocking effect of tubocurarine and related drugs:* Potentiated antihypertensive effects. Use together cautiously.
*Other antiarrhythmics:* May have additive or antagonistic cardiac effects and additive toxic effects. Use together cautiously.
*Sympathomimetics, such as epinephrine and isoproterenol:* Antagonized effects of these drugs. Use together cautiously.
**Drug-lifestyle.** *Cocaine use:* Inhibited therapeutic effects of nadolol. Discourage use together.

## Adverse reactions
**CNS:** fatigue, dizziness.
**CV:** *bradycardia,* hypotension, *HF,* peripheral vascular disease, rhythm and conduction disturbances.

**GI:** nausea, vomiting, diarrhea, abdominal pain, constipation, anorexia.
**Respiratory:** *increased airway resistance.*
**Skin:** rash.
**Other:** fever.

## Overdose and treatment
Signs of overdose include severe hypotension, bradycardia, HF, and bronchospasm.

After acute ingestion, recommend emptying patient's stomach by induced emesis or gastric lavage, and giving activated charcoal to reduce absorption. Magnesium sulfate may be given orally as a cathartic. Subsequent treatment is usually symptomatic and supportive.

## Clinical considerations
- Dosage adjustments may be needed in patients with renal impairment.
- Nadolol has been used as an antiarrhythmic and as a prophylactic drug for migraine headaches.
- If long-term therapy is used, recommend gradually decreasing dosage over 1 to 2 weeks before discontinuing drug. Abrupt withdrawal may exacerbate angina and cause an MI.
- Beta blockers may mask the signs and symptoms of hypoglycemia.
- There may be an increased risk for patients to develop diabetes.

### Therapeutic monitoring
- Careful monitoring of blood pressure during initial dosing and adjustment is needed; once condition is stabilized, monitoring is done at 3- to 6-month intervals.
- Advise clinician to monitor patient for reflex bradycardia, which may be treated with atropine.
- Advise clinician to monitor patients with hyperthyroidism and diabetes carefully; symptoms may be masked by drug therapy.

### Special populations
**Breast-feeding patients.** Drug appears in breast milk; an alternative to breast-feeding is recommended during therapy.
**Pediatric patients.** Safety and efficacy in children haven't been established; use only if potential benefit outweighs risk.
**Geriatric patients.** Geriatric patients may require lower maintenance doses of nadolol because of increased bioavailability or delayed metabolism; they also may experience enhanced adverse effects.

## Patient counseling
- Tell patient not to discontinue nadolol abruptly. Drug should be tapered.

# nafcillin sodium
Nafcil, Nallpen, Unipen

*Pharmacologic classification:*
penicillinase-resistant penicillin
*Therapeutic classification:* antibiotic
*Pregnancy risk category B*

## Available forms
Available by prescription only
*Capsules:* 250 mg
*Tablets:* 500 mg
*Injection:* 500 mg, 1 g, 2 g
*Pharmacy bulk package:* 10 g
*I.V. infusion piggyback:* 1 g, 2 g

## Indications and dosages
***Systemic infections caused by susceptible organisms (methicillin-sensitive* Staphylococcus aureus)**
*Adults:* 250 to 500 mg P.O. q 4 to 6 hours for mild to moderate infections and 1 g q 4 to 6 hours for more severe infections. Alternatively, 500 mg I.M. q 4 hours or 500 to 1,000 mg I.V. q 4 hours depending on severity of the infection.
*Children over age 1 month:* 50 to 100 mg/kg P.O. daily, divided into doses given q 6 hours. Alternatively, 50 to 200 mg/kg/day I.M. or I.V. in divided doses q 4 to 6 hours depending on the severity of the infection.
*Neonates:* 30 to 40 mg/kg/day P.O. divided equally into three to four doses; or 20 mg/kg daily I.M. in two equally divided doses. Alternatively, 40 mg/kg/day I.M. in two equally divided doses q 12 hours if neonate is less than 7 days old and 60 to 200 mg/kg/day in equally divided doses q 8 hours if neonate is 7 to 28 days old. For mild to moderate infection, may give 50 to 100 mg/kg/day I.V. in divided doses q 6 hours. For more severe infections, 100 to 200 mg/kg/day I.V. divided q 4 to 6 hours. Alternatively, 25 mg/kg I.V. q 12 hours (if less than 7 days old and under 2 kg [4.4 lb]) or q 8 hours (if less than 7 days old and over 2 kg or over 7 days old and less than 2 kg) or q 6 hours (if over 7 days old and over 2 kg).
***Meningitis***
*Neonates over age 7 days and under 2 kg:* 50 mg/kg I.V. q 8 hours.
*Neonates over age 7 days and over 2 kg:* 50 mg/kg I.V. q 6 hours.
*Neonates under age 7 days and under 2 kg:* 50 mg/kg I.V. q 12 hours.
*Neonates under age 7 days and over 2 kg:* 50 mg/kg I.V. q 8 hours.
***Acute or chronic osteomyelitis caused by susceptible organisms***
*Adults:* 1 to 2 g I.V. q 4 hours for 4 to 8 weeks.
***Meningitis caused by susceptible organisms***
*Adults:* 100 to 200 mg/kg/day I.V. in divided doses q 4 to 6 hours.

*Native valve endocarditis caused by susceptible organisms*
Adults: 2 g I.V. q 4 hours for 4 to 6 weeks with gentamicin.

## I.V. administration
■ Recommend infusing I.V. nafcillin for short time periods (24 to 48 hours), if possible, to avoid risk of thrombophlebitis.

### Incompatibilities
Incompatible with aminoglycosides, aminophylline, ascorbic acid, aztreonam, bleomycin, cytarabine, droperidol, fentanyl, hydrocortisone sodium succinate, labetalol, metaraminol, meperidine, methylprednisolone sodium succinate, nalbuphine, pentazocine lactate, promazine, regular insulin, verapamil hydrochloride, and vitamin B complex with C.

## Mechanism of action
*Antibiotic action:* Nafcillin is bactericidal; it adheres to bacterial penicillin-binding proteins, thus inhibiting bacterial cell wall synthesis.

Nafcillin resists the effects of penicillinases—enzymes that inactivate penicillin—and is active against many strains of penicillinase-producing bacteria; this activity is most important against penicillinase-producing staphylococci; some strains may remain resistant. Nafcillin is also active against a few gram-positive aerobic and anaerobic bacilli but has no significant effect on gram-negative bacilli.

## Pharmacokinetics
*Absorption:* Absorbed erratically and poorly from the GI tract. Food decreases absorption.
*Distribution:* Distributed widely; CSF penetration is poor but enhanced by meningeal inflammation. Drug crosses the placenta and is 70% to 90% protein-bound.
*Metabolism:* Metabolized primarily in the liver; it undergoes enterohepatic circulation. Dosage adjustment isn't needed for patients in renal failure.
*Excretion:* Excreted primarily in bile; about 25% to 30% is excreted in urine unchanged. It may also appear in breast milk. Elimination half-life in adults is ½ to 1½ hours.

| Route | Onset | Peak | Duration |
|-------|-------|------|----------|
| P.O. | Unknown | ½-2 hr | Unknown |
| I.V. | Immediate | Immediate | Unknown |
| I.M. | Unknown | ½-1 hr | Unknown |

## Contraindications and precautions
Contraindicated in patients hypersensitive to drug or other penicillins. Use cautiously in patients with GI distress or sensitivity to cephalosporins.

## Interactions
**Drug-drug.** *Cyclosporines:* Subtherapeutic cyclosporine levels. Advise clinician to monitor cyclosporine levels.
*Hepatotoxic drugs:* May increase the risk of hepatotoxicity. Advise clinician to monitor patient closely.
**Drug-food.** *Carbonated beverages, fruit juice:* Acidity may inactivate drug. Don't give together.

## Adverse reactions
**GI:** *nausea,* vomiting, diarrhea.
**Hematologic:** *transient leukopenia, neutropenia, granulocytopenia, thrombocytopenia* with high doses.
**Other:** hypersensitivity reactions (chills, fever, rash, pruritus, urticaria, *anaphylaxis*), vein irritation, thrombophlebitis.

## Overdose and treatment
Signs and symptoms of overdose include neuromuscular irritability or seizures. There are no specific recommendations. Treatment is supportive. After recent ingestion (4 hours or less), recommend emptying stomach by induced emesis or gastric lavage, and following with activated charcoal to reduce absorption. Nafcillin isn't appreciably removed by hemodialysis.

## Clinical considerations
■ Advise clinician to give drug with water only; acid in fruit juice or carbonated beverage may inactivate drug.
■ Advise clinician to give dose on empty stomach; food decreases absorption.
■ If used to treat infections caused by group A beta-hemolytic streptococci, therapy should be continued for at least 10 days to decrease risk of rheumatic fever or glomerulonephritis.
■ Nafcillin alters tests for urinary and serum proteins; turbidimetric urine and serum proteins are often falsely positive or elevated in tests using sulfosalicylic acid or trichloroacetic acid.

### Therapeutic monitoring
■ Recommend evaluating renal, hepatic, and hematologic systems periodically during prolonged nafcillin therapy.

### Special populations
**Breast-feeding patients.** Nafcillin appears in breast milk; use drug with caution in breast-feeding women.
**Pediatric patients.** Nafcillin that's been reconstituted with bacteriostatic water for injection with benzyl alcohol shouldn't be used in neonates because of toxicity.
**Geriatric patients.** Half-life may be prolonged in geriatric patients because of impaired hepatic and renal function.

## Patient counseling
- Tell patient to report severe diarrhea or allergic reactions promptly.

# nalbuphine hydrochloride
Nubain

*Pharmacologic classification:* narcotic agonist-antagonist, opioid partial agonist
*Therapeutic classification:* analgesic, adjunct to anesthesia
*Pregnancy risk category NR*

## Available forms
Available by prescription only
*Injection:* 1.5 mg/ml, 10 mg/ml, 20 mg/ml

## Indications and dosages
*Moderate to severe pain*
*Adults:* 10 to 20 mg S.C., I.M., or I.V. q 3 to 6 hours, p.r.n., or around-the-clock. Maximum dose, 160 mg/day.
*Supplement to anesthesia*
*Adults:* 0.3 mg/kg to 3 mg/kg I.V. over 10 to 15 minutes; maintenance dose, 0.25 to 0.5 mg/kg I.V.

## I.V. administration
- Give doses by slow I.V. injection over 2 to 3 minutes into a vein or free-flowing I.V. solution of $D_5W$ or normal saline or Ringer's solution. Rapid I.V. injection increases the risk of adverse effects.

## Incompatibilities
Incompatible with allopurinol, cefepime, diazepam, detorolac, nafcillin, pentobarbital sodium, piperacillin and tazobactam sodium, promethazine, sargramostim, thiethylperazine, and tromethamine.

## Mechanism of action
*Analgesic action:* Analgesia is believed to result from action of drug at opiate receptor sites in the CNS, relieving moderate to severe pain. The narcotic antagonist effect may result from competitive inhibition at opiate receptors. Like other opioids, nalbuphine causes respiratory depression, sedation, and miosis. In patients with coronary artery disease or MI, it appears to produce no substantial changes in heart rate, pulmonary artery or wedge pressure, left ventricular end-diastolic pressure, pulmonary vascular resistance, or cardiac index.

## Pharmacokinetics
*Absorption:* When given orally, drug is about one-fifth as effective as an analgesic as it is when given I.M., apparently because of first-pass metabolism in the GI tract and liver.
*Distribution:* Not appreciably plasma protein–bound.

*Metabolism:* Metabolized in the liver.
*Excretion:* Excreted in urine and to some degree in bile.

| Route | Onset | Peak | Duration |
|-------|-------|------|----------|
| I.V. | 2-3 min | 30 min | 3-6 hr |
| I.M. | 15 min | 1 hr | 3-6 hr |
| S.C. | 15 min | Unknown | 3-6 hr |

## Contraindications and precautions
Contraindicated in patients hypersensitive to drug. Use cautiously in patients with history of drug abuse, emotional instability, head injury, increased intracranial pressure, impaired ventilation, MI accompanied by nausea and vomiting, upcoming biliary surgery, and hepatic or renal disease.

## Interactions
**Drug-drug.** *Barbiturate anesthetics such as thiopental:* Additive CNS and respiratory depressant effects and, possibly, apnea. Use together very cautiously.
*Cimetidine:* May increase narcotic nalbuphine toxicity. A narcotic antagonist may be needed if toxicity occurs.
*General anesthetics:* May cause severe CV depression. Avoid use together.
*Digitoxin, phenytoin, rifampin:* Drug accumulation and enhanced effects may result. Advise clinician to monitor patient carefully for toxicity.
*Narcotic antagonists:* Patients who become physically dependent on drug may experience acute withdrawal syndrome if given high doses of a narcotic antagonist. Use with caution; advise clinician to monitor patient closely.
*Other CNS depressants (antihistamines, barbiturates, benzodiazepines, muscle relaxants, narcotic analgesics, phenothiazines, sedativehypnotics, tricyclic antidepressants):* Potentiated respiratory and CNS depression, sedation, and hypotensive effects. Reduced doses of nalbuphine are usually needed.

## Adverse reactions
**CNS:** *headache, sedation, dizziness, vertigo,* nervousness, depression, restlessness, crying, euphoria, hostility, unusual dreams, confusion, hallucinations, speech difficulty, delusions.
**CV:** hypertension, hypotension, tachycardia, *bradycardia.*
**EENT:** blurred vision, *dry mouth.*
**GI:** cramps, dyspepsia, bitter taste, *nausea, vomiting,* constipation, biliary tract spasms.
**GU:** urinary urgency.
**Respiratory:** *respiratory depression,* dyspnea, asthma, *pulmonary edema.*
**Skin:** pruritus, burning, urticaria, *clamminess.*

---

Reactions may be *common,* uncommon, *life-threatening,* or COMMON AND LIFE-THREATENING.

## Overdose and treatment
The most common signs and symptoms of nalbuphine overdose are CNS depression, respiratory depression, and miosis (pinpoint pupils). Other acute toxic effects include hypotension, bradycardia, hypothermia, shock, apnea, cardiopulmonary arrest, circulatory collapse, pulmonary edema, and seizures.

To treat acute overdose, recommend first establishing adequate respiratory exchange via a patent airway and ventilation p.r.n., and giving a narcotic antagonist (naloxone) to reverse respiratory depression. Because the duration of action of nalbuphine is longer than that of naloxone, repeated naloxone dosing is needed. Naloxone shouldn't be given in the absence of clinically significant respiratory or CV depression. Advise clinician to monitor vital signs closely.

Recommend providing symptomatic and supportive treatment, such as continued respiratory support and correction of fluid or electrolyte imbalance. Advise clinician to monitor laboratory values, vital signs, and neurologic status closely.

## Clinical considerations
■ Some commercial preparations contain sodium metabisulfite which may cause allergic reactions in susceptible individuals.
■ Nalbuphine may obscure the signs and symptoms of an acute abdominal condition or worsen gallbladder pain.
■ Drug may cause orthostatic hypotension in ambulatory patients.
■ Before administration, visually inspect all parenteral products for particulate matter and discoloration.
■ Drug causes respiratory depression, which at 10 mg is equal to the respiratory depression produced by 10 mg of morphine.
■ Drug may interfere with enzymatic tests for detection of opioids.
■ Store at 59° to 86° F (15° to 30° C) and protect from light.

### Therapeutic monitoring
■ When drug is used during labor and delivery, recommend observing neonate for signs of respiratory depression.
■ Drug also acts as a narcotic antagonist; it may precipitate abstinence syndrome in narcotic-dependent patients. Advise clinician to give 25% of usual dose in these patients and monitor for signs and symptoms of withdrawal.

### Special populations
Breast-feeding patients. It isn't known if drug appears in breast milk. Use with caution in breast-feeding women.
Pediatric patients. Safety in children under age 18 hasn't been established.

Geriatric patients. Lower doses are usually indicated for geriatric patients, who may be more sensitive to therapeutic and adverse effects of drug.

## Patient counseling
■ Instruct patient to avoid driving or operating machinery because drug may cause dizziness and fatigue.

# naloxone hydrochloride
Narcan

*Pharmacologic classification:* narcotic (opioid) antagonist
*Therapeutic classification:* narcotic antagonist
*Pregnancy risk category B*

## Available forms
Available by prescription only
*Injection:* 0.4 mg/ml, 1 mg/ml with preservatives, and 0.02 mg/ml, 0.4 mg/ml paraben-free

## Indications and dosages
*Known or suspected narcotic-induced respiratory depression, including that caused by natural and synthetic narcotics, methadone, nalbuphine, pentazocine, and propoxyphene*
*Adults:* 0.4 to 2 mg I.V., S.C., or I.M., repeated q 2 to 3 minutes, p.r.n. If no response is observed after 10 mg have been given, question diagnosis of narcotic-induced toxicity. Also, 0.4 mg I.V. loading dose followed by 0.4 mg/hour infusion.
*Children:* 0.01 mg/kg I.V.; give a subsequent dose of 0.1 mg/kg if needed. Dosage for continuous infusion is 0.024 to 0.16 mg/kg/hour. If I.V. route not available, dose may be given I.M. or S.C. in divided doses. Alternatively, 0.1 mg/kg I.V. q. 2 to 3 minutes, p.r.n., in neonates and children up to age 5 and 2 mg I.V. q 2 to 3 minutes, p.r.n., in children ages 6 and older.
*Postoperative narcotic depression*
*Adults:* 0.1 to 0.2 mg I.V. q 2 to 3 minutes, p.r.n., until desired response is obtained. Alternatively, 0.005 mg/kg I.V. and repeat in 15 minutes, p.r.n., or administer 0.01 mg/kg I.M. for the second dose. May give continuous infusion at 0.0037 mg/kg/hour.
*Children:* 0.005 to 0.01 mg/kg dose I.M., I.V., or S.C., repeated q 2 to 3 minutes, p.r.n., until desired degree of reversal is obtained.
*Neonates (asphyxia neonatorum):* 0.01 mg/kg I.V. into umbilical vein repeated q 2 to 3 minutes, p.r.n.

Drug level for use in neonates and children is 0.02 mg/ml.

◊ *Naloxone challenge for diagnosing*
*opiate dependence*
*Adults:* 0.16 mg I.M. naloxone; if no signs of
withdrawal after 20 to 30 minutes, give second dose of 0.24 mg I.V.
◊ *Opiate addiction*
*Adults:* 200 mg to 3 g P.O. daily.

## I.V. administration
■ Naloxone can be diluted in $D_5W$ or normal
saline solution. Use within 24 hours after mixing.
■ Naloxone may be given by continuous I.V.
infusion, which is needed in many cases to control the adverse effects of epidurally administered morphine. Usual dose is 2 mg in 500 ml
of $D_5W$ or normal saline solution.
■ Injections are stable at pH of 2.5 to 5.

## Incompatibilities
Manufacturer recommends that naloxone not
be mixed with any drug, especially preparations containing bisulfite, sulfite, long-chain
or high-molecular-weight anions, or alkaline
solutions.

## Mechanism of action
*Narcotic (opioid) antagonism:* Naloxone is essentially a pure antagonist. In patients who
have received an opioid agonist or other analgesic with narcotic-like effects, naloxone
antagonizes most of the opioid effects, especially respiratory depression, sedation, and hypotension. Because the duration of action of
naloxone in most cases is shorter than that of
the opioid, opiate effects may return as those
of naloxone dissipate. Naloxone doesn't produce tolerance or physical or psychological dependence. The precise mechanism of action is
unknown, but is thought to involve competitive antagonism of more than one opiate receptor in the CNS.

## Pharmacokinetics
*Absorption:* Rapidly inactivated after oral administration; therefore, it's given parenterally.
The duration of action is longer after I.M. use
and higher doses, when compared with I.V. use
and lower doses.
*Distribution:* Rapidly distributed into body tissues and fluids.
*Metabolism:* Rapidly metabolized in the liver,
primarily by conjugation.
*Excretion:* Excreted in urine. Plasma half-life
has been reported to be from 60 to 90 minutes
in adults and 3 hours in neonates.

| Route | Onset | Peak | Duration |
|---|---|---|---|
| I.V. | 1-2 min | 5-15 min | Variable |
| I.M., S.C. | 2-5 min | 5-15 min | Variable |

## Contraindications and precautions
Contraindicated in patients hypersensitive to
drug. Use cautiously in patients with cardiac

irritability and opiate addiction. When giv-
en to a narcotic addict, naloxone may produce an acute abstinence syndrome. Use with
caution; advise clinician to monitor patient
closely.

## Interactions
**Drug-drug.** *Cardiotoxic drugs:* May have serious CV effects if also given naloxone. Use
together cautiously.

## Adverse reactions
**CNS:** tremors, *seizures.*
**CV:** tachycardia, hypertension (with higher-
than-recommended doses), hypotension, *ven-*
*tricular fibrillation, cardiac arrest.*
**GI:** nausea, vomiting (with higher-than-
recommended doses).
**Respiratory:** *pulmonary edema.*
**Skin:** diaphoresis.
**Other:** withdrawal symptoms (in narcotic-
dependent patients with higher-than-
recommended doses).

## Overdose and treatment
No serious adverse reactions to naloxone overdose are known except those of acute abstinence syndrome in narcotic-dependent persons.

## Clinical considerations
■ Before administration, visually inspect all
parenteral products for particulate matter and
discoloration.
■ Recommend taking a careful drug history to
rule out possible narcotic addiction, to avoid
inducing withdrawal symptoms (apply cau-
tions also to the baby of an addicted mother).
■ Because duration of activity of naloxone is
shorter than that of most narcotics, vigilance
and repeated doses are usually needed in the
management of an acute narcotic overdose in
a nonaddicted patient.
■ Naloxone isn't effective in treating respiratory depression caused by nonopioid drugs.
■ Naloxone is the safest drug to use when cause
of respiratory depression is uncertain.

### Therapeutic monitoring
■ Drug shouldn't be depended on too much;
recommend paying close attention to the airway, breathing, and circulation.
■ Recommend maintaining adequate respiratory and CV status at all times. Respiratory
"overshoot" may occur; advise clinician to
monitor patient for respiratory rate higher than
before respiratory depression. Respiratory rate
increases in 1 to 2 minutes, and effect lasts 1
to 4 hours.

### Special populations
**Breast-feeding patients.** It isn't known if drug
appears in breast milk.

---

Reactions may be *common,* uncommon, *life-threatening,* or COMMON AND LIFE-THREATENING.

**Geriatric patients.** Lower doses are usually indicated for geriatric patients because they may be more sensitive to therapeutic and adverse effects of drug.

## Patient counseling
■ Inform family about use and administration of drug.

# naltrexone hydrochloride
ReVia

*Pharmacologic classification:* narcotic (opioid) antagonist
*Therapeutic classification:* narcotic detoxification adjunct
*Pregnancy risk category C*

## Available forms
Available by prescription only
*Tablets:* 50 mg

## Indications and dosages
*Adjunct for maintenance of opioid-free state in detoxified individuals*
*Adults:* Don't attempt treatment until naloxone challenge is negative (0.2 mg I.V., if no signs of withdrawal after 30 seconds, give additional 0.6 mg I.V.; alternatively, administer 0.8 mg S.C. and observe for 20 minutes for signs of withdrawal). Don't attempt treatment until patient has remained opioid-free for 7 to 10 days, verified by analyzing urine for opioids. Initially, 25 mg P.O. If no withdrawal signs occur within 1 hour, give an additional 25 mg. Alternatively, 10- to 12.5-mg initial dose followed by 10- to 12.5-mg incremental increases daily to 50 mg, or 5 mg initially with incremental 10-mg increases hourly to 50 mg. Once patient has been started on 50 mg q 24 hours, flexible maintenance schedule may be used. From 50 to 150 mg may be given daily, depending on the schedule prescribed, but the average daily dose is 50 mg.
*Alcoholism (short-term therapy)*
*Adults:* 50 mg P.O. daily.

## Mechanism of action
*Opioid antagonism:* Naltrexone is essentially a pure opiate (narcotic) antagonist. Like naloxone, it has little or no agonist activity. Its precise mechanism of action is unknown, but it's thought to involve competitive antagonism of more than one opiate receptor in the CNS. When given to patients who haven't recently received opiates, it exhibits little or no pharmacologic effect. At oral doses of 30 to 50 mg daily, it produces minimal analgesia, only slight drowsiness, and no respiratory depression. However, pharmacologic effects, including psychotomimetic effects, increased systolic or diastolic blood pressure, respiratory depression, and decreased oral temperature, which are sug-

gestive of opiate agonist activity, have reportedly occurred in a few patients. In patients who have received single or repeated large doses of opiates, naltrexone attenuates or produces a complete but reversible block of the pharmacologic effects of the narcotic. Naltrexone doesn't produce physical or psychological dependence, and tolerance to its antagonist activity reportedly doesn't develop.

## Pharmacokinetics
*Absorption:* Well absorbed after oral administration. It undergoes extensive first-pass hepatic metabolism (only 5% to 20% of an oral dose reaches the systemic circulation unchanged).
*Distribution:* About 21% to 28% protein-bound. Extent and duration of antagonist activity of drug appear directly related to plasma and tissue levels of drug. It's widely distributed throughout the body, but considerable interindividual variation exists.
*Metabolism:* Oral naltrexone undergoes extensive first-pass hepatic metabolism. Its major metabolite is believed to be a pure antagonist also, and may contribute to its efficacy. Drug and hepatic metabolites may undergo enterohepatic recirculation.
*Excretion:* Excreted primarily by the kidneys. Elimination half-life is about 4 hours; that of its major active metabolite is about 13 hours.

| Route | Onset | Peak | Duration |
|-------|-------|------|----------|
| P.O. | 15-30 min | 12 hr | 24 hr |

## Contraindications and precautions
Contraindicated in patients receiving opioid analgesics, in opioid-dependent patients, in patients in acute opioid withdrawal, in those with positive urine screen for opioids, and in those with acute hepatitis or liver failure. Also contraindicated in patients hypersensitive to drug.

Use cautiously in patients with mild hepatic disease or history of hepatic impairment.

## Interactions
**Drug-drug.** *Drugs containing opioids, such as antidiarrheals, cough and cold preparations, and opioid analgesics:* Attenuated opioid activity. Avoid use together.
*Drugs that alter hepatic metabolism:* May increase or decrease serum naltrexone levels. Advise clinician to monitor patient for this effect.

## Adverse reactions
**CNS:** *insomnia, anxiety, nervousness, headache,* depression, dizziness, fatigue, somnolence, *suicidal ideation.*
**GI:** *nausea, vomiting,* anorexia, *abdominal pain,* constipation, increased thirst.
**GU:** delayed ejaculation, decreased potency.
**Hematologic:** lymphocytosis.
**Hepatic:** *hepatotoxicity.*

**Musculoskeletal:** *muscle and joint pain.*
**Skin:** rash.
**Other:** chills.

## Overdose and treatment
Overdose hasn't been documented. Test subjects have received 800 mg/day (16 tablets) for up to 1 week and showed no evidence of toxicity. In case of overdose, recommend providing symptomatic and supportive treatment in a closely supervised environment. Local or regional poison control center should be contacted for further information.

## Clinical considerations
■ Naltrexone has been used investigationally for the treatment of methadone dependence.
■ A naloxone (Narcan) challenge test may be given to the patient before naltrexone use. Naloxone (0.8 mg S.C. or I.V., incremental doses) is given and the patient closely monitored for signs and symptoms of opiate withdrawal. If acute abstinence signs and symptoms are present, naltrexone shouldn't be given. If results are inconclusive, may repeat challenge with 1.6 mg I.V.
■ Before administration, a careful drug history should be taken to rule out possible narcotic use. Treatment shouldn't be attempted until the patient has been opiate-free for 7 to 10 days. Verify self-reporting of abstinence from narcotics by urinalysis. No withdrawal signs or symptoms should be reported by patient or be evident.
■ Because naltrexone can precipitate potentially severe opiate withdrawal, it shouldn't be used in patients receiving opiates or in nondetoxified patients physically dependent on opiates.
■ Drug can cause hepatocellular injury if given at higher-than-recommended doses. Naltrexone can cause or exacerbate signs and symptoms of abstinence in anyone not completely opioid-free.

### Therapeutic monitoring
■ Recommend performing liver function tests before naltrexone use to establish a baseline and to evaluate possible drug-induced hepatotoxicity every 1 month for 6 months.
■ In an emergency requiring analgesia that can only be achieved by administering opiates, a patient who has been receiving naltrexone may need a higher dose than usual of narcotic, and the resulting respiratory depression may be deeper and more prolonged.

### Special populations
**Breast-feeding patients.** It isn't known if drug appears in breast milk. Use drug with caution in breast-feeding women, especially because of its known hepatotoxicity.
**Pediatric patients.** Safety in patients under age 18 hasn't been established.

**Geriatric patients.** Use in geriatric patients isn't documented, but reduced dosage would probably be needed.

## Patient counseling
■ Inform patient that opioid drugs, such as cough and cold preparations, antidiarrheal products, and narcotic analgesics may not be effective; recommend nonnarcotic alternative if available.
■ Warn patient not to self-administer narcotics while taking naltrexone because serious injury, coma, or death may result.
■ Explain that drug has no tolerance or dependence liability.
■ Tell patient to report withdrawal signs and symptoms (tremors, vomiting, bone or muscle pains, sweating, abdominal cramps).
■ Tell patient to carry an identification card that alerts medical personnel that naltrexone is taken, and to inform new prescriber that he's receiving drug.

# nandrolone decanoate
Androlone-D 200, Deca-Durabolin, Hybolin Decanoate-50, Hybolin Decanoate-100, Neo-Durabolic

*Pharmacologic classification:* anabolic steroid
*Therapeutic classification:* erythropoietic, anabolic
*Pregnancy risk category X*
*Controlled substance schedule III*

## Available forms
Available by prescription only
*Injection:* 50 mg/ml, 100 mg/ml, 200 mg/ml (in oil)

## Indications and dosages
*Anemia from renal insufficiency*
*Adults:* 100 to 200 mg I.M. weekly in men; 50 to 100 mg/week in women.
*Children ages 2 to 13:* 25 to 50 mg I.M. q 3 to 4 weeks.

## Mechanism of action
*Androgenic action:* Nandrolone exerts inhibitory effects on hormone-responsive breast tumors and metastases.
*Erythropoietic action:* Nandrolone stimulates kidney production of erythropoietin, leading to increases in RBC mass and volume.
*Anabolic action:* Nandrolone may reverse corticosteroid-induced catabolism and promote tissue development in severely debilitated patients.

## Pharmacokinetics
*Absorption:* Well absorbed.

*Distribution:* Slowly released from I.M. depot following injection and is hydrolyzed to free nandrolone by plasma esterase.

*Metabolism:* Metabolized in the liver.

*Excretion:* Both the unchanged drug and its metabolites are excreted in the urine. The elimination half-life of nandrolone is 6 to 8 days.

| Route | Onset | Peak | Duration |
|---|---|---|---|
| I.M. | Unknown | 3-6 days | Unknown |

## Contraindications and precautions

Contraindicated in patients hypersensitive to anabolic steroids, in men with breast cancer or prostate cancer, in patients with nephrosis, in those experiencing the nephrotic phase of nephritis, in women with breast cancer and hypercalcemia, during pregnancy, and in breast-feeding women.

Use cautiously in patients with renal, cardiac, or hepatic disease; diabetes; epilepsy; migraine; or other conditions that may be aggravated by fluid retention.

## Interactions

**Drug-drug.** *Adrenocorticosteroids, adrenocorticotropic hormone:* Increased potential for fluid and electrolyte retention. Advise clinician to monitor patient for this effect.

*Insulin, oral antidiabetics:* Decreased blood glucose levels; may require adjustment of antidiabetics or insulin.

*Warfarin-type anticoagulants:* Increases in PT and INR. Advise clinician to monitor PT and INR.

## Adverse reactions

**CNS:** excitation, insomnia, habituation, depression.

**CV:** edema.

**GI:** nausea, vomiting, diarrhea.

**GU:** bladder irritability.

**Hematologic:** elevated serum lipid levels, suppression of clotting factors.

**Hepatic:** reversible jaundice, *peliosis hepatis,* elevated liver enzyme levels, *liver cell tumors.*

**Metabolic:** increased serum sodium, potassium, calcium and phosphate; abnormal results of fasting plasma glucose, glucose tolerance, and metyrapone tests; decreased thyroid function test results and 17-ketosteroid levels.

**Skin:** pain and induration at injection site.

**Other:** *hypoestrogenic effects in women (flushing; diaphoresis; vaginitis, including itching, dryness, and burning; vaginal bleeding; nervousness; emotional lability; menstrual irregularities), excessive hormonal effects in men (prepubertal-premature epiphyseal closure,* acne, priapism, *growth of body and facial hair,* phallic enlargement; postpubertal-testicular atrophy, oligospermia, decreased ejaculatory volume, impotence, gynecomastia, epididymitis), androgenic effects in women (acne, edema, *weight gain, hirsutism,* hoarseness, clitoral enlargement, *decreased breast size,* changes in libido, male-pattern baldness, *oily skin or hair*).

## Overdose and treatment

No information available.

## Clinical considerations

■ Recommend administering nandrolone injections I.M. deeply into the gluteal muscle.

■ An adequate iron intake is needed for maximum response.

■ Therapy should be intermittent, if possible.

■ Duration is dependent on patient response and occurrence of adverse reactions.

■ Surgically induced anephric patients may be less responsive to effect on anemia.

### Therapeutic monitoring

■ Advise clinician to monitor liver function test results, serum lipid and cholesterol levels, and CBC periodically.

■ Prepubertal males and females should have X-ray studies every 6 months to evaluate bone age.

### Special populations

**Breast-feeding patients.** It isn't known if anabolic steroids appear in breast milk. Because of the potential for serious adverse reactions in breast-fed infants, a decision to discontinue breast-feeding or drug should be made.

**Pediatric patients.** The adverse effects of giving androgens to young children aren't fully understood, but the risk of serious disturbances (premature epiphyseal closure, masculinization of females, or precocious development in males) exists; recommend weighing the possible benefits before instituting therapy in young children.

**Geriatric patients.** Elderly men should be observed for the development of prostatic hyperplasia and prostatic carcinoma.

## Patient counseling

■ Instruct diabetic patient to monitor glucose closely because glucose tolerance may be altered.

■ Tell women to report menstrual irregularities, acne, deepening of voice, male-pattern baldness, or hirsutism.

■ Tell patient to notify prescriber if persistent GI upset, nausea, vomiting, changes in skin color, or ankle swelling occur.

# naphazoline hydrochloride

AK-Con, Albalon Liquifilm, Allerest,
Clear Eyes, Comfort Eye Drops,
Degest 2, Nafazair, Naphcon, Naphcon
Forte, VasoClear, Vasocon

*Pharmacologic classification:* sympathomimetic
*Therapeutic classification:* decongestant, vasoconstrictor
*Pregnancy risk category C*

## Available forms

Available by prescription only
*Ophthalmic solution:* 0.1%
Available without a prescription
*Ophthalmic solution:* 0.012%, 0.02%, 0.025%
(generic), 0.03%
*Nasal drops or sprays:* 0.05% (solution)

## Indications and dosages

*Ocular congestion, irritation, itching*
*Adults:* Instill 1 to 3 drops (0.1% solution) q 3
to 4 hours or 1 to 2 drops (0.012% to 0.03%
solution) in eye daily to q.i.d. for 3 to 4 days.
*Nasal congestion*
*Adults and children over age 12:* 1 or 2 drops
or sprays (0.05% solution), p.r.n. May repeat
doses q 3 to 6 hours. Treatment not to exceed
3 to 5 days.
*Children ages 6 to 12:* 1 to 2 drops or sprays
(0.025% solution), p.r.n.

## Mechanism of action

*Decongestant action:* Naphazoline produces
vasoconstriction by local and alpha-adrenergic
action on blood vessels of the conjunctiva or
nasal mucosa; therefore, it reduces blood flow
and nasal congestion.

## Pharmacokinetics

*Absorption:* Well absorbed intranasally.
*Distribution:* Unknown.
*Metabolism:* Unknown.
*Excretion:* Unknown.

| Route | Onset | Peak | Duration |
|---|---|---|---|
| Ophthalmic | 10 min | Unknown | 2-6 hr |
| Nasal | 10 min | Unknown | 2-6 hr |

## Contraindications and precautions

Contraindicated in patients hypersensitive to
ingredients of drug and in those with acute
angle-closure glaucoma. Use of 0.1% solution
is contraindicated in children. Use cautiously
in patients with hyperthyroidism, cardiac disease, hypertension, or diabetes mellitus.

## Interactions

**Drug-drug.** *MAO inhibitors:* May result in an
increased adrenergic response and hypertensive crisis. Avoid use together.

## Adverse reactions

**CNS:** headache, dizziness, nervousness, weakness (with ophthalmic form).
**CV:** hypertension, *cardiac irregularities.*
**EENT:** transient eye stinging, pupillary dilation, eye irritation, photophobia, blurred vision, increased intraocular pressure, keratitis,
lacrimation (with ophthalmic form); rebound
nasal congestion (with excessive or long-term
use), sneezing, stinging, dryness of mucosa
(with nasal administration).
**GI:** nausea (with ophthalmic form).
**Other:** diaphoresis (with ophthalmic form);
systemic effects in children after excessive or
long-term use, marked sedation (with nasal administration).

## Overdose and treatment

Signs and symptoms of overdose include CNS
depression, sweating, decreased body temperature, bradycardia, shocklike hypotension, decreased respiration, CV collapse, and coma.

Activated charcoal or gastric lavage may be
used initially to treat accidental ingestion; give
early before sedation occurs. Advise clinician
to monitor vital signs and ECG, p.r.n. Seizures
should be treated with I.V. diazepam.

## Clinical considerations

■ Naphazoline is the most widely used ocular
decongestant.
■ Don't shake container.

### Therapeutic monitoring

■ Advise clinician to monitor patient for blurred
vision, pain, or lid edema.

### Special populations

**Pediatric patients.** Use in infants and children
may result in CNS depression, leading to coma
and marked reduction in body temperature. Although drug is available without a prescription,
parents shouldn't use nasal solution containing 0.025% naphazoline hydrochloride in children under age 6, and 0.05% naphazoline hydrochloride in children under age 12.
**Geriatric patients.** Use drug with caution in
geriatric patients with severe cardiac disease
or poorly controlled hypertension and in diabetics prone to diabetic ketoacidosis.

## Patient counseling

■ Teach patient how to instill ophthalmic or
nasal drug; tell him not to share drug with
others.
■ Advise patient to report blurred vision, eye
pain, or lid swelling that occurs when using
ophthalmic product.
■ Inform patient using ophthalmic solution that
photophobia may follow pupil dilation; tell patient to report this effect promptly.
■ Warn patient not to exceed recommended
dosage; rebound nasal congestion and con-

---

junctivitis also may occur with frequent or prolonged use.

■ Tell patient to call prescriber if nasal congestion persists after 5 days of using nasal solution.

# naproxen
EC-Naprosyn, Naprosyn

# naproxen sodium
Aleve, Anaprox, Naprelan

*Pharmacologic classification:* NSAID
*Therapeutic classification:* nonnarcotic analgesic, antipyretic, anti-inflammatory
*Pregnancy risk category B*

## Available forms
Available by prescription only
**naproxen**
*Tablets:* 250 mg, 375 mg, 500 mg
*Tablets (delayed-release):* 375 mg, 500 mg
*Oral suspension:* 125 mg/5 ml
**naproxen sodium**
*Tablets (film-coated):* 275 mg, 550 mg
*Tablets (extended-release):* 375 mg, 500 mg
    Note: 220 mg, 275 mg, 550 mg of naproxen sodium = 200 mg, 250 mg, or 500 mg of naproxen, respectively.
Available without a prescription
**naproxen sodium**
*Tablets or capsules:* 220 mg

## Indications and dosages
*Mild to moderately severe musculoskeletal or soft-tissue irritation*
**naproxen**
*Adults:* 250 to 500 mg P.O. b.i.d. Alternatively, 250 mg in the morning and 500 mg in the evening; 375 to 500 mg P.O. b.i.d. (delayed-release), or 750 to 1,000 mg P.O. daily (controlled-release).
**naproxen sodium**
*Adults:* 275 to 550 mg P.O. b.i.d. Alternatively, 275 mg in the morning and 550 mg in the evening; 825 to 1,100 mg (extended-release) P.O. once daily.
*Mild to moderate pain; primary dysmenorrhea*
**naproxen**
*Adults:* 500 mg P.O. to start, followed by 250 mg P.O. q 6 to 8 hours, p.r.n. Maximum daily dose shouldn't exceed 1.25 g naproxen. Or, 1,000 mg P.O. daily (controlled-release); patients requiring greater analgesia, a 1,500-mg dose may be used for a limited period.
**naproxen sodium**
*Adults:* 550 mg P.O. to start, followed by 275 mg P.O. q 6 to 8 hours, p.r.n. Maximum daily dose is 1.375 g naproxen sodium.
*Self-medication:* 220 mg q 8 to 12 hours. Maximum daily dose is 440 mg for adults ages 65

and older, or three tablets for adults under age 65. Don't self-medicate for longer than 10 days.
*Acute gout*
**naproxen**
*Adults:* 750 mg P.O. initially, then 250 mg q 8 hours until episode subsides. Or, 1,000 mg to 1,500 mg (using naproxen sodium controlled-release tablets) P.O. daily on the first day, then 1,000 mg P.O. daily until attack subsides.
**naproxen sodium**
*Adults:* 825 mg P.O. initially, then 275 mg q 8 hours until attack has subsided.
*Juvenile rheumatoid arthritis*
**naproxen**
*Children:* 10 mg/kg/day P.O. in two divided doses.

## Mechanism of action
*Analgesic, antipyretic, and anti-inflammatory actions:* Mechanisms of action are unknown; naproxen is thought to inhibit prostaglandin synthesis.

## Pharmacokinetics
*Absorption:* Absorbed rapidly and completely from the GI tract.
*Distribution:* Highly protein-bound. It crosses the placenta and appears in breast milk.
*Metabolism:* Metabolized in the liver.
*Excretion:* Excreted in urine. Half-life is 10 to 20 hours.

| Route | Onset | Peak | Duration |
|-------|-------|------|----------|
| P.O. | 1 hr | 2-4 hr | 7 hr |

## Contraindications and precautions
Contraindicated in patients hypersensitive to drug and those with asthma, rhinitis, or nasal polyps. Use cautiously in geriatric patients and in patients with history of peptic ulcer disease or renal, CV, GI, or hepatic disease.

## Interactions
**Drug-drug.** *Acetaminophen, gold compounds, other anti-inflammatories:* Increased nephrotoxicity. Advise clinician to monitor renal function test results.
*Anticoagulants, thrombolytics, such as coumadin derivatives, heparin, streptokinase, and urokinase:* May potentiate anticoagulant effects. Advise clinician to monitor PT and INR.
*Antihypertensives, diuretics:* Decreased effects of these drugs. Using together may increase risk of nephrotoxicity. Avoid use together.
*Anti-inflammatories, corticosteroids, corticotropin, salicylates:* May cause increased GI adverse reactions, including ulceration and hemorrhage. Use together very cautiously.
*Aspirin:* May decrease the bioavailability of naproxen. Advise clinician to monitor patient for effect.
*Aspirin, parenteral carbenicillin, cefamandole, cefoperazone, dextran, dipyridamole, mezlocillin, piperacillin, plicamycin, salicylates,*

*sulfinpyrazone, ticarcillin, valproic acid, other anti-inflammatory drugs:* Bleeding problems. Use together very cautiously.

*Coumadin derivatives, nifedipine, phenytoin, verapamil:* Increased risk of toxicity. Advise clinician to monitor patient closely.

*Insulin, oral antidiabetics:* May potentiate hypoglycemic effects. Advise clinician to monitor serum glucose level.

*Lithium, methotrexate:* Increased nephrotoxicity may occur. Advise clinician to monitor renal function test results.

**Drug-herb.** *Dong quai, feverfew, garlic, ginger, horse chestnut, red clover:* Possible increased risk of bleeding. Discourage use together.

### Adverse reactions

**CNS:** *headache, drowsiness, dizziness,* vertigo.

**CV:** *edema,* palpitations.

**EENT:** visual disturbances, *tinnitus,* auditory disturbances.

**GI:** *epigastric distress, occult blood loss, nausea, peptic ulceration,* constipation, dyspepsia, heartburn, diarrhea, stomatitis, thirst.

**GU:** nephrotoxicity.

**Hematologic:** *thrombocytopenia,* eosinophilia, *agranulocytosis, neutropenia.*

**Hepatic:** elevated liver enzyme levels.

**Respiratory:** dyspnea.

**Skin:** *pruritus, rash,* urticaria, ecchymoses, diaphoresis, purpura.

### Overdose and treatment

Signs and symptoms of overdose include drowsiness, heartburn, indigestion, nausea, and vomiting.

To treat overdose of naproxen, recommend emptying stomach immediately by inducing emesis with ipecac syrup or by gastric lavage. Advise clinician to give activated charcoal via nasogastric tube. Symptomatic and supportive measures (respiratory support and correction of fluid and electrolyte imbalances) should be provided. Advise clinician to monitor laboratory parameters and vital signs closely. Hemodialysis is ineffective in naproxen removal.

### Clinical considerations

■ Recommend using lowest possible effective dose; 250 mg of naproxen is equivalent to 275 mg of naproxen sodium.

■ Relief usually begins within 2 weeks after beginning therapy with naproxen.

■ Recommend instituting safety measures to prevent injury resulting from possible CNS effects.

■ Naproxen and its metabolites may interfere with urinary 5-hydroxyindoleacetic acid and 17-hydroxy-corticosteroid determinations.

■ Use with misoprostol may be considered for patients at high risk of NSAID-induced GI ulceration.

### Therapeutic monitoring

■ Advise clinician to monitor fluid balance. Advise clinician to monitor patient for signs and symptoms of fluid retention, especially significant weight gain.

■ Advise clinician to monitor liver function test results, renal function test results, CBC, and bleeding times in long-term therapy.

### Special populations

**Breast-feeding patients.** Because naproxen and naproxen sodium appear in breast milk, these drugs should be avoided during breast-feeding.

**Pediatric patients.** Safety of naproxen in children under age 2 hasn't been established. Safety of naproxen sodium in children hasn't been established. No age-related problems have been reported.

**Geriatric patients.** Patients over age 60 are more sensitive to the adverse effects (especially GI toxicity) of drug. The effect of naproxen on renal prostaglandins may cause fluid retention and edema. This may be significant in geriatric patients, especially those with HF.

### Patient counseling

■ Caution patient to avoid taking naproxen with OTC drugs.

■ Teach patient signs and symptoms of possible adverse reactions and tell him to report them promptly.

■ Instruct patient to check his weight every 2 to 3 days and to report any gain of 3 lb (1.4 kg) or more within 1 week.

■ Instruct patient in safety measures; advise him to avoid activities that require alertness until CNS effects are known.

■ Warn patient against combining naproxen (Naprosyn) with naproxen sodium (Anaprox) because both drugs circulate in the blood as naproxen anion.

■ Teach patient not to break or crush controlled or delayed-release tablets.

# naratriptan hydrochloride
Amerge

*Pharmacologic classification:* selective 5-hydroxytryptamine$_1$ (5-HT$_1$) receptor subtype agonist
*Therapeutic classification:* antimigraine
*Pregnancy risk category C*

### Available forms

Available by prescription only
*Tablets:* 1 mg, 2.5 mg

### Indications and dosages

*Treatment of acute migraine headache attacks with or without aura*

*Adults:* 1 or 2.5 mg P.O. as a single dose. Dose should be individualized, depending on the possible benefit of the 2.5-mg dose and the greater risk of adverse events. If headache returns or if only partial response occurs, may repeat dose after 4 hours, for maximum dose of 5 mg within 24 hours.

≣ *Dosage adjustment.* For patients with mild to moderate renal or hepatic impairment, consider a lower initial dosage; don't exceed maximum dose of 2.5 mg over a 24-hour period. Don't use in patients with severe renal or hepatic impairment.

## Mechanism of action

*Antimigraine action:* Naratriptan binds with high affinity to 5-HT$_{1D}$ and 5-HT$_{1B}$ receptors. One theory suggests that activation of 5-HT$_{1D/1B}$ receptors located on intracranial blood vessels leads to vasoconstriction, which causes the migraine relief. Another hypothesis suggests that activation of 5-HT$_{1D/1B}$ receptors on sensory nerve endings in the trigeminal system results in the inhibition of proinflammatory neuropeptide release.

## Pharmacokinetics

*Absorption:* Well absorbed with about 70% oral bioavailability.
*Distribution:* Steady-state volume of distribution is 170 L; 28% to 31% plasma protein–bound.
*Metabolism:* In vitro, naratriptan is metabolized by many P-450 cytochrome isoenzymes to inactive metabolites.
*Excretion:* Predominantly eliminated in urine, with 50% of dose recovered unchanged and 30% as metabolites. Mean elimination half-life is 6 hours.

| Route | Onset | Peak | Duration |
|-------|-------|------|----------|
| P.O. | Unknown | 2-3 hr | Unknown |

## Contraindications and precautions

Contraindicated in patients hypersensitive to drug or its components and in those with history, symptoms, or signs of ischemic cardiac, cerebrovascular (such as CVA or transient ischemic attack), or peripheral vascular syndromes (such as ischemic bowel disease). Also contraindicated in patients with significant underlying CV diseases, including angina pectoris, MI, and silent myocardial ischemia. Drug shouldn't be given to patients with uncontrolled hypertension because of potential increase in blood pressure.

Contraindicated in patients with severe renal (creatinine clearance less than 15 ml/minute) or hepatic (Child-Pugh grade C) impairment and in those with hemiplegic or basilar migraine.

Drug or other 5-HT$_1$ agonists are also contraindicated in patients with potential risk factors for coronary artery disease, such as hypertension, hypercholesterolemia, obesity, diabetes, strong family history of coronary

artery disease, women with surgical or physiologic menopause, men over age 40, or smokers.

## Interactions

**Drug-drug.** *Ergot-containing or ergot-type drugs, other 5-HT$_1$ agonists:* Prolonged vasospastic reactions. Use of these drugs within 24 hours of naratriptan is contraindicated.
*Oral contraceptives:* Increased naratriptan levels. Advise clinician to monitor patient closely.
*Selective serotonin reuptake inhibitors (SSRIs), such as fluoxetine, fluvoxamine, paroxetine, and sertraline:* Weakness, hyperreflexia, and incoordination when coadministered with 5-HT$_1$ agonists. Use together cautiously.
**Drug-lifestyle.** *Smoking:* Increased clearance of naratriptan by 30%. Advise patient to avoid smoking.

## Adverse reactions

**CNS:** paresthesia, dizziness, drowsiness, malaise, fatigue, vertigo.
**CV:** palpitations, increased blood pressure, tachyarrhythmias, abnormal ECG changes (PR, QT prolongation, ST/T wave abnormalities, PVCs, atrial flutter or fibrillation), syncope.
**EENT:** ear, nose and throat infections, photophobia.
**GI:** nausea, hyposalivation, vomiting.
**Other:** warm or cold temperature sensations; pressure, tightness, heaviness sensations.

## Overdose and treatment

A significant increase in blood pressure has been observed with an overdose, occurring between 30 minutes and 6 hours after ingestion of drug. Blood pressure returned to normal within 8 hours without pharmacologic intervention in some patients, whereas in other antihypertensive patients, drug treatment was needed.

No specific antidote exists. Recommend performing ECG monitoring for evidence of ischemia. Advise clinician to monitor patient for at least 24 hours after an overdose or while symptoms persist. The effect of hemodialysis or peritoneal dialysis on drug is unknown.

## Clinical considerations

■ Recommend using drug only when a clear diagnosis of migraine has been established. It's not intended for prophylactic therapy of migraines or for use in the management of hemiplegic or basilar migraine.
■ Safety and effectiveness haven't been established for cluster headaches.

### Therapeutic monitoring

■ First dose should be given in a medically equipped facility for patients at risk for coronary artery disease but determined to have a satisfactory CV evaluation. ECG monitoring should be considered.

---

* Canada only     ◊ Unlabeled clinical use

■ Periodic cardiac reevaluation in patients who have or develop risk factors for coronary artery disease is needed.

### Special populations
**Pregnant patients.** To monitor fetal outcomes of patients exposed to naratriptan during pregnancy, call 1-800-722-9292, ext. 39441.
**Breast-feeding patients.** Use with caution in breast-feeding women.
**Pediatric patients.** Safety and efficacy in patients under age 18 haven't been established.
**Geriatric patients.** Don't use drug in geriatric patients.

### Patient counseling
■ Tell patient that drug is intended to relieve, and not prevent, migraine headaches.
■ Instruct patient not to use drug if pregnancy is suspected or during pregnancy itself.
■ Teach patient to alert prescriber of risk factors for coronary artery disease.
■ Instruct patient to take dose soon after headache starts. If there's no response to the first tablet, tell patient to seek medical approval before taking second tablet.
■ Tell patient that if more relief is needed after the first tablet, such as when a partial response occurs or if the headache returns, he may take a second tablet but not sooner than 4 hours after the first tablet. Inform him not to exceed two tablets within 24 hours.

## nateglinide
Starlix

*Pharmacologic classification:* amino acid derivative
*Therapeutic classification:* antidiabetic
*Pregnancy risk category C*

### Available forms
Available by prescription only
*Tablets:* 60 mg, 120 mg

### Indications and dosages
*Alone or with metformin, to lower blood glucose level in patients with type 2 diabetes whose hyperglycemia isn't adequately controlled by diet and exercise and who haven't received long-term treatment with other antidiabetics*
Adults: 120 mg P.O. t.i.d., taken 1 to 30 minutes before meals. If patient's glycosulated hemoglobin is near goal when treatment starts, may give 60 mg P.O. t.i.d.

### Mechanism of action
*Blood glucose–lowering action:* Nateglinide lowers blood glucose level by stimulating insulin secretion from the pancreas. This action is dependent on the presence of functioning beta cells in the pancreas. The extent of insulin release is relative to blood glucose level.

### Pharmacokinetics
*Absorption:* Rapidly absorbed when taken immediately before a meal. Levels peak within 1 hour. The rate of absorption is slower when nateglinide is taken with or after a meal, but extent of absorption is unaffected.
*Distribution:* 98% bound to plasma proteins, primarily albumin.
*Metabolism:* Metabolized in the liver by hydroxylation followed by glucuronide conjugation. Drug is mainly metabolized by the cytochrome P-450 isoenzymes CYP2C9 (70%) and CYP3A4 (30%).
*Excretion:* Nateglinide and its metabolites are rapidly and completely eliminated in urine and feces after oral use. Average elimination half-life in healthy people and those with type 2 diabetes is about 1.5 hours.

| Route | Onset | Peak | Duration |
|-------|-------|------|----------|
| P.O.  | 20 min | 1 hr | 4 hr |

### Contraindications and precautions
Contraindicated in patients hypersensitive to drug and in patients with type 1 diabetes or diabetic ketoacidosis.

Use cautiously in geriatric patients, malnourished patients, and patients with moderate to severe liver dysfunction or adrenal or pituitary insufficiency.

### Interactions
**Drug-drug.** *Corticosteroids, sympathomimetics, thiazides, thyroid products:* Possible reduced hypoglycemic action of nateglinide. Advise clinician to monitor patient for hyperglycemia and monitor blood glucose level closely.
*MAO inhibitors, nonselective beta blockers, NSAIDs, salicylates:* Possible potentiated hypoglycemic action of nateglinide. Advise clinician to monitor patient for hypoglycemia and monitor blood glucose level closely.

### Adverse reactions
**CNS:** dizziness.
**GI:** diarrhea.
**Metabolic:** hypoglycemia.
**Musculoskeletal:** back pain, arthropathy.
**Respiratory:** *upper respiratory tract infection,* bronchitis, coughing.
**Other:** flulike symptoms, accidental trauma.

### Overdose and treatment
No adverse events occurred at a dosage of 720 mg daily for 7 days. However, an overdose may result in hypoglycemia. Recommend treating hypoglycemic symptoms without loss of consciousness with oral glucose and adjustments in dosage, meal patterns, or both. Recommend treating severe hypoglycemic re-

actions, including coma, seizures, or other neurologic symptoms, with I.V. glucose. Dialysis isn't effective in removing nateglinide.

## Clinical considerations
■ Don't use with or instead of glyburide or other oral antidiabetics. Drug may be used with metformin.
■ Advise clinician to give drug 1 to 30 minutes before a meal. If patient misses a meal, the scheduled dose should be skipped.
■ Risk of hypoglycemia rises with strenuous exercise, alcohol ingestion, insufficient caloric intake, and use with other oral antidiabetics.
■ Symptoms of hypoglycemia may be masked in patients with autonomic neuropathy or in those who use beta blockers.
■ Insulin may be needed for glycemic control in patients with fever, infection, trauma, or impending surgery.
■ Effectiveness may decline over time.

### Therapeutic monitoring
■ Advise clinician to monitor blood glucose level regularly to evaluate drug effectiveness.
■ Recommend observing patient for evidence of hypoglycemia, including sweating, rapid pulse, trembling, confusion, headache, irritability, and nausea. To minimize the risk of hypoglycemia, the dose of nateglinide should be followed immediately by a meal. If hypoglycemia occurs and patient remains conscious, advise clinician to give an oral form of glucose. If unconscious, advise clinician to give I.V. glucose.
■ Advise clinician to monitor blood glucose level closely when other drugs are started or stopped to detect possible drug interactions.
■ Periodically monitor HbA1c level.

### Special populations
**Breast-feeding patients.** It isn't known if drug appears in breast milk. Avoid use in breast-feeding women.
**Pediatric patients.** The safety and efficacy of nateglinide in children hasn't been determined.

## Patient counseling
■ Tell patient to take drug 1 to 30 minutes before a meal.
■ To reduce the risk of hypoglycemia, advise patient to skip the scheduled dose if he skips a meal.
■ Educate patient about the risk of hypoglycemia and its signs and symptoms (sweating, rapid pulse, trembling, confusion, headache, irritability, and nausea). Advise patient to treat these symptoms by eating or drinking something containing sugar.
■ Teach patient how to monitor and record blood glucose levels to evaluate diabetes control.
■ Instruct patient to adhere to the prescribed diet and exercise regimen.

■ Explain possible long-term complications of diabetes and the importance of regular preventive therapy.
■ Encourage patient to wear or carry medical identification that shows he has diabetes.

# nefazodone hydrochloride
Serzone

*Pharmacologic classification:* phenylpiperazine
*Therapeutic classification:* antidepressant
*Pregnancy risk category C*

## Available forms
Available by prescription only
*Tablets:* 50 mg, 100 mg, 150 mg, 200 mg, 250 mg

## Indications and dosages
*Depression*
*Adults:* Initially, 200 mg/day P.O. divided into two doses. Dosage increased in 100- to 200-mg/day increments at intervals of no less than 1 week, p.r.n. Usual dosage range, 300 to 600 mg/day.
*Adults ages 65 and older:* Initially, 50 mg P.O. b.i.d. Increase slowly p.r.n. Usual dose is 200 to 400 mg/day.

## Mechanism of action
*Antidepressive action:* Action of drug isn't precisely defined. It inhibits neuronal uptake of serotonin and norepinephrine. It also occupies central 5-HT$_1$ (serotonin) and alpha receptors.

### Pharmacokinetics
*Absorption:* Rapidly and completely absorbed but, because of extensive metabolism, its absolute bioavailability is only about 20%.
*Distribution:* Extensively plasma protein–bound.
*Metabolism:* Extensively metabolized by n-dealkylation and aliphatic and aromatic hydroxylation.
*Excretion:* Excreted in urine. Half-life of drug is 2 to 4 hours.

| Route | Onset | Peak | Duration |
|-------|-------|------|----------|
| P.O. | Unknown | 1 hr | Unknown |

## Contraindications and precautions
Contraindicated in patients hypersensitive to drug or other phenylpiperazine antidepressants. Drug shouldn't be used within 14 days of MAO inhibitor therapy. Treatment shouldn't be initiated in patients with active liver disease. Use with carbamazepine or pimozide is contraindicated.

Use cautiously in patients with CV or cerebrovascular disease that could be exacerbated by hypotension (such as history of MI, angi-

na, or CVA) and conditions that would predispose patients to hypotension (such as, dehydration, hypovolemia, and antihypertensive
drug treatment). Use cautiously in patients with
history of mania.

## Interactions
**Drug-drug.** *Alprazolam, triazolam:* Potenti-
ated effects of these drugs. Don't give together. However, if needed, dosages of alprazolam
and triazolam may need to be reduced greatly.
*CNS active drugs:* May alter CNS activity. Use
together cautiously.
*Digoxin:* Increased serum digoxin levels. Use
together cautiously and monitor digoxin levels.
*MAO inhibitors:* May cause severe excitation,
hyperpyrexia, seizures, delirium, or coma.
Avoid use together.
*Other highly plasma protein–bound drugs:*
May increase risk and severity of adverse reactions. Advise clinician to monitor patient
closely.

## Adverse reactions
**CNS:** *headache, somnolence, dizziness, asthenia,* insomnia, *light-headedness, confusion,*
memory impairment, paresthesia, abnormal
dreams, decreased concentration, ataxia, incoordination, psychomotor retardation, tremor,
hypertonia.
**CV:** orthostatic hypotension, vasodilation, hypotension, peripheral edema.
**EENT:** *blurred vision, abnormal vision,*
pharyngitis, tinnitus, visual field defect.
**GI:** taste perversion, *dry mouth, nausea, constipation,* dyspepsia, diarrhea, increased appetite, vomiting, thirst.
**GU:** urinary frequency, urinary tract infection,
urine retention, vaginitis, breast pain.
**Musculoskeletal:** neck rigidity, arthralgia.
**Respiratory:** cough.
**Skin:** pruritus, rash.
**Other:** infection, flulike syndrome, chills, fever.

## Overdose and treatment
Common symptoms from overdose of nefazodone include nausea, vomiting, and somnolence. Other drug-associated adverse reactions
may occur. Recommend providing symptomatic and supportive treatment in the case of
hypotension or excessive sedation. Gastric
lavage should be used if needed.

## Clinical considerations
**H ALERT** Life-threatening hepatic failure has
occurred with administration of this drug.
■ Recommend allowing at least 1 week after
stopping drug before giving patient an MAO
inhibitor. Also, recommend allowing at least
14 days before patient is started on nefazodone
after MAO inhibitor therapy has been stopped.
■ Drug therapy may precipitate mania or hypomania in patients with bipolar or other affective disorders.

## Therapeutic monitoring
■ Advise clinician to monitor patient needs for
suicidal tendencies. Only a minimum supply
of drug should be allowed.
■ Advise clinician to monitor liver function test
results in patients with hepatic dysfunction.

## Special populations
**Breast-feeding patients.** It isn't known if nefazodone appears in breast milk; use caution
when giving drug to breast-feeding women.
**Pediatric patients.** Safety and efficacy in patients under age 18 haven't been established.
**Geriatric patients.** Because of increased systemic exposure to nefazodone, treatment should
begin at half the usual dose, but recommend
increasing dose over the same dosage range as
in younger patients. Usual precautions should
be taken in geriatric patients who have ongoing medical illnesses or are receiving other
drugs.

## Patient counseling
**H ALERT** Tell patient to immediately contact
prescriber if he experiences signs and symptoms of liver failure, including jaundice, anorexia, GI complaints, or malaise.
■ Warn patient not to engage in hazardous activities until CNS effects are known.
■ Instruct men that if prolonged or inappropriate erections occur, to stop drug immediately and seek medical attention.
■ Instruct women to report suspected pregnancy or if planning to become pregnant during therapy.
■ Instruct patient not to drink alcoholic during
therapy.
■ Tell patient to report rash, hives, or a related allergic reaction.
■ Inform patient that several weeks of therapy
may be required to obtain the full antidepressant effect. Once improvement is seen, advise
patient not to discontinue drug until directed.

# nelfinavir mesylate
Viracept

*Pharmacologic classification:* HIV
protease inhibitor
*Therapeutic classification:* antiviral
*Pregnancy risk category B*

## Available forms
Available by prescription only
*Tablets:* 250 mg
*Powder:* 50 mg/g of powder

## Indications and dosages
*Treatment of HIV infection when anti-
retroviral therapy is warranted*
*Adults and adolescents over age 13:* 750 mg
P.O. t.i.d or 1,250 mg b.i.d., with meal or light
snack.

*Children ages 2 to 13:* 20 to 30 mg/kg/dose P.O. t.i.d. with meal or light snack; don't exceed 750 mg t.i.d. Recommended pediatric dose given t.i.d. is shown in the table below.

| Body weight (kg) | No. of level 1-g scoops | No. of level tea-spoons | No. of tablets |
|---|---|---|---|
| 7 to < 8.5 | 4 | 1 | - |
| 8.5 to < 10.5 | 5 | 1.25 | - |
| 10.5 to < 12 | 6 | 1.5 | - |
| 12 to < 14 | 7 | 1.75 | - |
| 14 to < 16 | 8 | 2 | - |
| 16 to < 18 | 9 | 2.25 | - |
| 18 to < 23 | 10 | 2.5 | 2 |
| ≥ 23 | 15 | 3.75 | 3 |

◊ *Children ages 2 to 13 weighing 23 to 53 kg (50 to 116 lb):* 25 to 30 mg/kg P.O. t.i.d. up to 1,250 or 1,500 mg/dose.
◊ **Postexposure prophylaxis following occupational exposure to HIV**
*Adults:* 750 mg P.O. t.i.d. with oral zidovudine and lamivudine for 4 weeks.

## Mechanism of action
*Antiviral action:* Inhibition of the protease enzyme prevents cleavage of the viral polyprotein, resulting in the production of an immature, noninfectious virus.

## Pharmacokinetics
*Absorption:* Absolute bioavailability isn't determined. Food increases absorption of drug.
*Distribution:* Apparent volume of drug distribution is 2 to 7 L/kg. More than 98% of drug is bound to plasma protein.
*Metabolism:* Metabolized in the liver by multiple cytochrome P-450 isoforms, including CYP3A.
*Excretion:* Terminal half-life is 3½ to 5 hours. Drug is primarily excreted in the feces.

| Route | Onset | Peak | Duration |
|---|---|---|---|
| P.O. | Unknown | 2-4 hr | Unknown |

## Contraindications and precautions
Contraindicated in patients hypersensitive to drugs or its components. Use cautiously in patients with hepatic dysfunction or hemophilia types A and B.

## Interactions
**Drug-drug.** *Amiodarone, ergot derivatives, midazolam, quinidine, triazolam:* Increased plasma levels of these drugs, which may increase risk for serious or life-threatening adverse events. Avoid use together.

*Anti-HIV protease inhibitors, such as indinavir and saquinavir:* May increase plasma levels of both drugs. Use together cautiously.
*Carbamazepine, phenobarbital, phenytoin:* May reduce the effectiveness of nelfinavir by decreasing nelfinavir plasma levels. Use together cautiously.
*Drugs primarily metabolized by CYP3A, such as calcium channel blockers and dihydropyridine:* May result in increased levels of these drugs and decreased plasma level of nelfinavir. Use together cautiously.
*3-Hydroxy-3-methylglutaryl coenzyme A inhibitors such as lovastatin and simvastatin:* May increase plasma levels of antilipemic drugs. Avoid use together.
*Oral contraceptives:* Nelfinavir may decrease plasma levels of oral contraceptives. Advise patient to use appropriate contraceptive measures during therapy.
*Rifabutin:* Increased rifabutin plasma levels. Reduced dose of rifabutin to one-half the usual dose, or other change in regimen may be needed.
*Rifampin:* Decreased nelfinavir plasma levels. Don't use together.
*Ritonavir:* May increase level of nelfinavir. Use together cautiously.
*Sildenafil:* May increase adverse effects of sildenafil, including hypotension, visual changes, and priapism. Patient shouldn't exceed 25 mg of sildenafil in 48 hours.
**Drug-herb.** *St. John's wort:* may substantially reduce blood levels of the drug that could cause loss of therapeutic effects. Warn against concomitant use.

## Adverse reactions
**CNS:** anxiety, depression, dizziness, emotional lability, hyperkinesia, insomnia, malaise, migraine headache, paresthesia, *seizures,* sleep disorders, somnolence, *suicidal ideation.*
**EENT:** iritis, eye disorders, pharyngitis, rhinitis, sinusitis.
**GI:** abdominal pain, nausea, *diarrhea,* flatulence, anorexia, dyspepsia, epigastric pain, GI bleeding, *pancreatitis,* mouth ulceration, vomiting.
**GU:** sexual dysfunction, kidney calculus, urine abnormality.
**Hematologic:** anemia, *leukopenia, thrombocytopenia.*
**Hepatic:** *hepatitis.*
**Metabolic:** dehydration, diabetes mellitus, hyperlipidemia, hyperuricemia, hypoglycemia, fever.
**Musculoskeletal:** back pain, arthralgia, arthritis, cramps, myalgia, myasthenia, myopathy.
**Respiratory:** dyspnea, *bronchospasm.*
**Skin:** rash, dermatitis, folliculitis, fungal dermatitis, pruritus, sweating, urticaria.
**Other:** fever, redistribution or accumulation of body fat.

---

* Canada only   ◊ Unlabeled clinical use

## Overdose and treatment
Information is limited. Unabsorbed drug may be removed by emesis or gastric lavage; activated charcoal may also be used. Drug is removed by hemodialysis but not by peritoneal dialysis.

## Clinical considerations
- Decision to use drug is based on surrogate marker changes in patients who received drug with nucleoside analogues or alone for up to 24 weeks. There are no results from controlled trials evaluating the effect on survival or risk of opportunistic fungal infections.
- Drug dosage is same if used alone or with other antiretrovirals.
- Antiretroviral activity may be increased when used with approved reverse transcriptase inhibitors.
- Give oral powder in children unable to take tablets; may mix oral powder with water, milk, formula, soy formula, soy milk, or dietary supplements.
- Don't reconstitute with water in its original container.
- Use reconstituted powder within 6 hours.
- May mix crushed tablets in water. Mixture must be used within 6 hours.
- Acidic foods or juice aren't recommended because of their bitter taste.

### *Therapeutic monitoring*
- Advise clinician to monitor CBC with differential (especially neutrophils) and chemistries; low incidences of laboratory abnormalities were reported in clinical studies. Increases in alkaline phosphatase, amylase, CK, LDH, AST, ALT, and GGT levels may occur; advise clinician to monitor patient closely.
- Advise clinician to monitor patient for toxicity and disease progression.

### *Special populations*
**Pregnant patients.** Use only when clearly needed. To monitor maternal-fetal outcomes, register patient by calling 1-800-258-4263.
**Breast-feeding patients.** It isn't known if drug appears in breast milk. Although safety hasn't been established, advise HIV-infected women not to breast-feed to avoid HIV transmission to the infant.
**Pediatric patients.** Safety and efficacy haven't been established in children under age 2.
**Geriatric patients.** Safety and efficacy have not been established in patients 65 years of age and older.

## Patient counseling
- Advise patient to take drug with food.
- Inform patient that drug isn't a cure for HIV infection.
- Tell patient that long-term effects of drug are currently unknown and that there's evidence that drug reduces risk of HIV transmission to others.
- Advise patient to take drug daily as prescribed and not to alter dose or discontinue drug without medical approval.
- If patient misses a dose, tell him to take the dose as soon as possible and return to his normal schedule. If a dose is skipped, advise patient not to double the dose.
- Tell patient that diarrhea is the most common adverse effect and that it can be controlled with loperamide, if needed.
- Explain to patient that body fat may accumulate or redistribute during therapy.
- Instruct patient taking oral contraceptives to use alternate or additional contraceptive measures.
- Advise patient to report use of other prescribed or OTC drugs or herbal remedy use.

---

# neomycin sulfate
Mycifradin, Myciguent, Neo-Tabs

*Pharmacologic classification:* aminoglycoside
*Therapeutic classification:* antibiotic
*Pregnancy risk category C*

## Available forms
Available by prescription only
*Tablets:* 500 mg
*Oral solution:* 125 mg/5 ml
*Otic suspension:* 5 mg/ml (with polymyxin B sulfate 10,000 units/ml and hydrocortisone 1%)
Available without a prescription
*Cream:* 0.5%
*Ointment:* 0.5%

## Indications and dosages
*Infectious diarrhea caused by enteropathogenic* **Escherichia coli**
*Adults:* 50 mg/kg P.O. daily in four divided doses for 2 to 3 days.
*Children:* 50 to 100 mg/kg P.O. daily divided q 4 to 6 hours for 2 to 3 days.
*Suppression of intestinal bacteria preoperatively*
*Adults:* 1 g P.O. q 1 hour for four doses, then 1 g q 4 hours for rest of 24 hours. A saline cathartic should precede therapy.
*Children:* 40 to 100 mg/kg P.O. daily divided q 4 to 6 hours. First dose should be preceded by saline cathartic.
**For 2- to 3-day regimen**
*Adults and children:* 88 mg/kg P.O. in six equally divided doses at 4-hour intervals. Alternatively, for 8 a.m. surgery, 1 g of neomycin and 1 g of erythromycin base P.O. at 1 p.m., 2 p.m., and 11 p.m. on the day preceding surgery.

---

*Adjunctive treatment in hepatic coma*
*Adults:* 1 to 3 g P.O. q.i.d. for 5 to 6 days; 200 ml of 1% or 100 ml of 2% solution as enema retained for 20 to 60 minutes q 6 hours.
*Children:* 50 to 100 mg/kg P.O. daily in divided doses for 5 to 6 days.
◊ *Treatment of hypercholesterolemia*
*Adults:* 500 mg to 2 g P.O. daily in two or three divided doses.
**External ear canal infection**
*Adults and children:* 2 to 5 drops into ear canal t.i.d. or q.i.d. for 7 to 10 days.
**Topical bacterial infections, burns, wounds, skin grafts, following surgical procedure, lesions, pruritus, trophic ulcerations, and edema**
*Adults and children:* Rub in small amount gently b.i.d., t.i.d., or as directed.
≣ *Dosage adjustment.* Use reduced dosage in adults and children with renal impairment. Specific recommendations aren't available.

## Mechanism of action

*Antibiotic action:* Neomycin is bactericidal; it binds directly to the 30S ribosomal subunit, thus inhibiting bacterial protein synthesis. Its spectrum of action includes many aerobic gram-negative organisms and some aerobic gram-positive organisms. Drug is far less active against many gram-negative organisms than are amikacin, gentamicin, netilmicin, and tobramycin. Given orally or as retention enema, neomycin inhibits ammonia-forming bacteria in the GI tract, reducing ammonia and improving neurologic status of patients with hepatic encephalopathy. It's rarely given systemically because of its high potential for ototoxicity and nephrotoxicity. The FDA has revoked licensing of the parenteral preparation for this reason.

## Pharmacokinetics

*Absorption:* Absorbed poorly (about 3%) after oral administration, although oral administration is enhanced in patients with impaired GI motility or mucosal intestinal ulcerations. Neomycin isn't absorbed through intact skin; it may be absorbed from wounds, burns, or skin ulcers.
*Distribution:* Crosses the placenta. Oral administration restricts distribution to the GI tract.
*Metabolism:* Not metabolized.
*Excretion:* Excreted primarily in urine by glomerular filtration. Elimination half-life in adults is 2 to 3 hours; in severe renal damage, half-life may extend to 24 hours. After oral administration, neomycin is excreted primarily unchanged in feces.

| Route | Onset | Peak | Duration |
|---|---|---|---|
| P.O. | Unknown | 1-4 hr | 8 hr |
| Topical | Unknown | Unknown | Unknown |

## Contraindications and precautions

Contraindicated in patients hypersensitive to drug. Oral form contraindicated in patients sensitive to other aminoglycosides and in those with intestinal obstruction.

Use oral form cautiously in geriatric patients and in patients with impaired renal function, neuromuscular disorders, or ulcerative bowel lesions. Drug shouldn't be administered parenterally. Recommend using topical form cautiously in patients with extensive dermatologic conditions.

## Interactions

**Drug-drug.** *Oral anticoagulants:* Potentiated effects of anticoagulant. Dosage adjustment of anticoagulants may be needed.

## Adverse reactions

**EENT:** *ototoxicity* (with oral administration).
**GI:** nausea, vomiting, diarrhea, malabsorption syndrome, *Clostridium difficile*–associated colitis (with oral administration).
**GU:** *nephrotoxicity* (with oral administration).
**Musculoskeletal:** *neuromuscular blockade* (with topical administration).
**Skin:** *rash, contact dermatitis,* urticaria (with topical administration).

## Overdose and treatment

Signs of overdose include ototoxicity, nephrotoxicity, and neuromuscular toxicity. Recommend removing drug by hemodialysis or peritoneal dialysis; treatment with calcium salts or anticholinesterases reverses neuromuscular blockade. After recent ingestion (4 hours or less), recommend emptying the stomach by induced emesis or gastric lavage and following with activated charcoal to reduce absorption.

## Clinical considerations

■ In hepatic coma, recommend decreasing dietary protein and reassessing neurologic status frequently.
**Preoperative bowel contamination**
■ Recommend providing low-residue diet and cathartic immediately before administration of oral neomycin; follow-up enemas may be needed to completely empty bowel.
**Topical therapy**
■ Drug shouldn't be applied to more than 20% of body surface.
■ Drug shouldn't be applied to any body surface of patient with decreased renal function without considering risk-benefit ratio.
**Otic therapy**
■ Recommend reculturing persistent drainage.
■ Drug is best used with other antibiotics.
■ Ear shouldn't be touched with dropper.

### Therapeutic monitoring

■ Advise clinician to monitor patient for hypersensitivity or contact dermatitis.

- Advise clinician to monitor renal function during drug therapy.
- Recommend evaluating patient's hearing before and during prolonged drug therapy.
- Advise clinician to monitor patient for superinfection.

## Patient counseling
- Instruct patient to report adverse reactions promptly.
- Encourage adequate fluid intake.

# neostigmine bromide
# neostigmine methylsulfate
Prostigmin

*Pharmacologic classification:* cholinesterase inhibitor
*Therapeutic classification:* muscle stimulant
*Pregnancy risk category C*

## Available forms
Available by prescription only
*Tablets:* 15 mg
*Injection:* 0.5 mg/ml, 1 mg/ml

## Indications and dosages
*Antidote for nondepolarizing neuromuscular blockers*
*Adults:* 0.5 to 2 mg slow I.V. Repeat, p.r.n.; maximum total dose, 5 mg. Give 0.6 to 1.2 mg atropine sulfate I.V. before antidote dose if patient is bradycardic.
*Neonates, infants, and children:* 0.04 mg/kg/dose I.V. with atropine sulfate (0.02 mg/kg atropine) with each dose of neostigmine.
*Prevention of postoperative abdominal distention and bladder atony*
*Adults:* 0.25 mg I.M. or S.C. q 4 to 6 hours for 2 to 3 days.
*Treatment of postoperative abdominal distention and bladder atony*
*Adults:* 0.5 to 1 mg S.C. or I.M.; if for urine retention and there's no response in 1 hour, catheterize patient and repeat dose q 3 hours for five doses after bladder is emptied.
◊ *Diagnosis of myasthenia gravis*
*Adults:* 0.022 mg/kg I.M. Give atropine 0.011 mg/kg I.V. with dose or I.M. 30 minutes before dose. If cholinergic reaction occurs, discontinue test and give atropine sulfate 0.4 to 0.6 mg I.V. If results are inconclusive, retest on another day using 0.031 mg/kg I.M. of neostigmine preceded by atropine 0.01 g/kg.
*Children:* 0.025 to 0.04 mg/kg I.M. preceded by 0.011 mg/kg S.C. of atropine sulfate.
*Symptomatic control of myasthenia gravis*
*Adults:* 0.5 to 2.5 mg S.C., I.V., or I.M. Oral dose can range from 15 to 375 mg/day (average 150 mg in 24 hours). Subsequent dosages must be individualized, based on response and

tolerance of adverse effects. Therapy may be required day and night.
*Children:* 7.5 to 15 mg P.O. t.i.d. or q.i.d. Alternatively, 0.333 mg/kg or 10 mg/m$^2$ P.O. six times daily.
*Neonates:* 0.1 to 0.2 S.C. or 0.03 mg/kg I.M. q 2 to 4 hours or 1 to 4 mg P.O. q 2 to 3 hours. Gradual dosage reduction as symptoms improve.
◊ *Supraventricular tachycardia from tricyclic antidepressant overdose*
*Children:* 0.5 to 1 mg I.V. followed by 0.25 to 0.5 mg q 1 to 3 hours, p.r.n.
◊ *Decrease small bowel transit time during radiography*
*Adults:* 0.5 to 0.75 mg S.C.

## I.V. administration
- Give at a slow, controlled rate not exceeding 1 mg/minute in adults.

### Incompatibilities
None reported.

## Mechanism of action
*Muscle stimulant action:* Neostigmine blocks hydrolysis of acetylcholine by cholinesterase, resulting in acetylcholine accumulation at cholinergic synapses, which leads to increased cholinergic receptor stimulation at the myoneural junction.

## Pharmacokinetics
*Absorption:* Poorly absorbed (1% to 2%) from GI tract after oral administration.
*Distribution:* About 15% to 25% of dose is plasma protein–bound.
*Metabolism:* Hydrolyzed by cholinesterases and metabolized by microsomal liver enzymes. Duration of effect varies considerably, depending on patient's physical and emotional status and on disease severity.
*Excretion:* About 80% of dose is excreted in urine as unchanged drug and metabolites in the first 24 hours after administration.

| Route | Onset | Peak | Duration |
|---|---|---|---|
| P.O. | 45-75 min | 1-2 hr | 2-4 hr |
| I.V. | 4-8 min | 1-2 hr | 2-4 hr |
| I.M., S.C. | 20-30 min | 1-2 hr | 2-4 hr |

## Contraindications and precautions
Contraindicated in patients hypersensitive to cholinergics or to bromide and in those with peritonitis or mechanical obstruction of the intestine or urinary tract. Use cautiously in patients with bronchial asthma, bradycardia, seizure disorders, recent coronary occlusion, vagotonia, hyperthyroidism, arrhythmias, and peptic ulcer.

---

## Interactions
**Drug-drug.** *Atropine, corticosteroids, magnesium, procainamide, quinidine:* May reverse cholinergic effect of neostigmine on muscle. Advise clinician to monitor patient for drug effect.

*Other cholinergics:* May cause additive toxicity. Avoid use together.

*Succinylcholine:* May result in prolonged respiratory depression. Advise clinician to monitor patient closely.

## Adverse reactions
**CNS:** dizziness, *seizures,* headache, muscle weakness, loss of consciousness, drowsiness.

**CV:** *bradycardia,* hypotension, tachycardia, *AV block,* syncope, *cardiac arrest.*

**EENT:** blurred vision, lacrimation, miosis.

**GI:** *nausea, vomiting, diarrhea, abdominal cramps,* excessive salivation, flatulence, increased peristalsis.

**GU:** urinary frequency.

**Musculoskeletal:** *muscle cramps,* muscle fasciculations, arthralgia.

**Respiratory:** *bronchospasm,* dyspnea, *respiratory depression, respiratory arrest,* increased bronchial secretions.

**Skin:** rash, urticaria, diaphoresis, flushing.

**Other:** hypersensitivity reactions, *anaphylaxis.*

## Overdose and treatment
Signs and symptoms of overdose include headache, nausea, vomiting, diarrhea, blurred vision, miosis, excessive tearing, bronchospasm, increased bronchial secretions, hypotension, incoordination, excessive sweating, muscle weakness, cramps, fasciculations, paralysis, bradycardia or tachycardia, excessive salivation, and restlessness or agitation.

Recommend supporting respiration; bronchial suctioning may be performed. Drug should be stopped immediately. Atropine may be given to block muscarinic effects of neostigmine but won't counter paralytic effects of drug on skeletal muscle. Atropine overdose should be avoided, because it may lead to bronchial plug formation.

## Clinical considerations
■ If muscle weakness is severe, determine if this stems from drug toxicity or from exacerbation of myasthenia gravis. A test dose of edrophonium I.V. will aggravate drug-induced weakness but will temporarily relieve weakness resulting from the disease.

■ Hospitalized patients may be able to manage a bedside supply of tablets to take themselves.

■ Advise clinician to give drug with food or milk to reduce the chance for GI adverse effects.

■ In diagnosis of myasthenia gravis, all anticholinergics should be stopped for at least 8 hours before neostigmine administration.

■ When giving drug to patient with myasthenia gravis, recommend scheduling largest dose before anticipated periods of fatigue. If patient has dysphagia, this dose should be scheduled 30 minutes before each meal.

■ All other cholinergics should be stopped during neostigmine therapy because of risk of additive toxicity.

■ When administering neostigmine to prevent abdominal distention and GI distress, insertion of a rectal tube may be indicated to help passage of gas.

■ Administering atropine with neostigmine can relieve or eliminate adverse reactions; these symptoms may indicate neostigmine overdose and will be masked by atropine.

■ Patients may develop resistance to drug.

### *Therapeutic monitoring*
■ Advise clinician to monitor patient's vital signs, particularly pulse.

### *Special populations*
**Breast-feeding patients.** Neostigmine may appear in breast milk, possibly resulting in infant toxicity. Recommend evaluating patient's clinical status to see if breast-feeding or drug should be discontinued.

**Pediatric patients.** Safety and efficacy in children haven't been fully established.

**Geriatric patients.** Geriatric patients may be more sensitive to effects of neostigmine. Use with caution.

## Patient counseling
■ Instruct patient to observe and record changes in muscle strength.

# nevirapine
Viramune

*Pharmacologic classification:* nonnucleoside reverse transcriptase inhibitor
*Therapeutic classification:* antiviral
*Pregnancy risk category C*

## Available forms
Available by prescription only
*Tablets:* 200 mg
*Oral suspension:* 50 mg/5 ml

## Indications and dosages
*Treatment of patients with HIV-1 infection*
*Adults and adolescents:* 200 mg P.O. daily for first 14 days, followed by 200 mg P.O. q 12 hours with other antiretrovirals.

*Treatment in children infected with HIV-1 (with other antiretrovirals)*

*Children ages 2 months to 8 years:* 4 mg/kg P.O. once daily for first 14 days, followed by 7 mg/kg P.O. q 12 hours thereafter. Maximum daily dose shouldn't exceed 400 mg.

*Children ages 8 and older:* 4 mg/kg P.O. once daily for first 14 days, followed by 4 mg/kg P.O. q 12 hours thereafter. Maximum daily dose shouldn't exceed 400 mg. Alternatively, children may receive 120 mg/m$^2$ P.O. daily for first 14 days, followed by 120 to 200 mg/m$^2$ q 12 hours.

◊ *Neonates:* 5 mg/kg P.O. daily for first 14 days followed by 120 mg/m$^2$ q 12 hours for next 14 days, then 200 mg/m$^2$ q 12 hours.

## Mechanism of action

*Antiviral action:* Nevirapine binds directly to reverse transcriptase and blocks the RNA- and DNA-dependent DNA polymerase activities by causing a disruption of the catalytic site of the enzyme.

## Pharmacokinetics

*Absorption:* Readily absorbed.
*Distribution:* Widely distributed, crosses the placenta, and appears in breast milk. It's about 60% plasma protein–bound.
*Metabolism:* Extensively metabolized in the liver.
*Excretion:* Metabolites are primarily excreted in urine; a small amount of drug is excreted in feces.

| Route | Onset | Peak | Duration |
|-------|---------|------|----------|
| P.O. | Unknown | 4 hr | Unknown |

## Contraindications and precautions

Contraindicated in patients hypersensitive to drug. Use cautiously in patients with impaired renal or hepatic function because the pharmacokinetics of nevirapine haven't been evaluated in these patient groups.

## Interactions

**Drug-drug.** *Drugs extensively metabolized by P-450 CYP3A:* Nevirapine may lower the plasma levels of these drugs. Dosage adjustment of these drugs may be needed.
*Ketoconazole:* Decreased ketoconazole levels. Avoid use together.
*Methadone:* May decrease plasma levels of methadone and increase its metabolism. Advise clinician to monitor patient closely for opiate withdrawl; increased dose of methadone may be needed.
*Oral contraceptives, protease inhibitors:* Decreased plasma levels of these drugs. Don't give together.
**Drug-herb.** *St. John's wort:* Decreased nevirapine levels. Discourage use together.

## Adverse reactions

**CNS:** headache, peripheral neuropathy, paresthesia.
**GI:** nausea, diarrhea, abdominal pain, ulcerative stomatitis.
**Hematologic:** *neutropenia,* eosinophilia.
**Hepatic:** *hepatitis,* abnormal liver function test results, *hepatotoxicity.*
**Metabolic:** myalgia.
**Skin:** *rash, Stevens-Johnson syndrome,* facial edema, epidermic necrolysis.
**Other:** fever.

## Overdose and treatment

No information available.

## Clinical considerations

■ Nevirapine is generally used in three-drug combination regimens.
■ Use of a 200-mg dose as a lead-in period has been shown to decrease the evidence of a rash.
■ Resistant virus emerges rapidly when drug is given as monotherapy. Therefore, recommend always giving with at least one other antiretroviral drug.
■ Drug should be stopped if patient develops a severe rash or a rash accompanied by fever, blistering, oral lesions, conjunctivitis, swelling, muscle or joint aches, or general malaise. If rash occurs during the initial 14 days, dosage shouldn't be increased until it has resolved. Most rashes occur within the first 6 weeks of therapy.
■ Drug must be stopped temporarily in patients experiencing moderate or severe liver function test abnormalities (excluding GGT) until they've returned to baseline. May restart drug at half the previous dose level. If moderate or severe liver function test abnormalities recur, drug therapy should be stopped. Advise clinician to monitor liver function test results closely.
■ If therapy is interrupted for longer than 7 days, therapy should be resumed as if being given for the first time.
■ If disease progresses during therapy, alternative antiretroviral therapy must be considered.

### Therapeutic monitoring

■ Advise clinician to monitor clinical chemistry tests, including liver function test results, before therapy starts and regularly throughout therapy.
■ Advise clinician to monitor patient for development of rash.

### Special populations

**Breast-feeding patients.** Drug appears in breast milk. HIV-infected women shouldn't breast-feed.

**Pediatric patients.** Safety and efficacy in children haven't been established.

## Patient counseling

■ Inform patient that drug isn't a cure for HIV infection, and the illnesses caused by advanced HIV infection may still occur. Also tell patient that drug doesn't reduce risk of transmission of HIV to others through sexual contact or blood contamination.

■ Instruct patient to report rash immediately. Therapy may need to be stopped temporarily.

■ Stress importance of taking drug exactly as prescribed. If a dose is missed, tell patient to take the next dose as soon as possible. However, if a dose is skipped, he shouldn't double the next dose.

■ Tell patient not to use other drugs without medical approval.

■ Advise women of childbearing age to avoid oral contraceptives and other hormonal methods of birth control as a method of contraception during therapy.

# niacin (vitamin B₃, nicotinic acid)

Niaspan, Nico-400, Nicobid, Nicotinex, Slo-Niacin

*Pharmacologic classification:* B-complex vitamin
*Therapeutic classification:* vitamin B₃, antilipemic, peripheral vasodilator
*Pregnancy risk category A (C if greater than RDA)*

## Available forms

Available by prescription only
*Capsules:* 500 mg
*Tablets (extended-release):* 500 mg, 750 mg, and 1,000 mg; and 21-day starter pack (7 each) 375 mg, 500 mg, and 750 mg
Available without a prescription
*Tablets:* 25 mg, 50 mg, 100 mg, 125 mg, 250 mg, 400 mg, 500 mg
*Tablets (timed-release):* 250 mg, 500 mg, 750 mg
*Capsules (timed-release):* 125 mg, 250 mg, 300 mg, 400 mg, 500 mg, 750 mg
*Elixir:* 50 mg/5 ml

## Indications and dosages

*Pellagra*
*Adults:* 300 to 500 mg in divided doses P.O., depending on severity of niacin deficiency. Maximum recommended daily dose is 500 mg; should be divided into 10 doses, 50 mg each.
*Children:* 100 to 300 mg P.O. daily in divided doses, depending on severity of niacin deficiency.

To prevent recurrence after symptoms subside, advise adequate nutrition and adequate supplements to meet RDA.
*Peripheral vascular disease and circulatory disorders*
*Adults:* 100 to 150 mg P.O. three to five times daily.
*Adjunctive treatment of hyperlipidemias, especially those from hypercholesterolemia*
*Adults:* 1.5 to 6 g P.O. daily in two to four divided doses with or after meals; maximum dose is 9 g daily. Alternatively, initial dose is 100 mg P.O. t.i.d., increasing by 300 mg/day at 4- to 7-day intervals or 500 mg P.O. t.i.d. with gradual increase to desired effect.
*Hartnup disease*
*Adults:* 50 to 200 mg P.O. daily in divided doses.
*Dietary supplement*
*Adults:* 10 to 20 mg P.O. daily.

## Mechanism of action

*Vitamin replacement action:* As a vitamin, niacin functions as a coenzyme essential to tissue respiration, lipid metabolism, and glycogenolysis. Niacin deficiency causes pellagra, which manifests as dermatitis, diarrhea, and dementia; administration of niacin cures pellagra. Niacin lowers cholesterol and triglyceride levels by an unknown mechanism.
*Antilipemic action:* Mechanism of action is unknown. Nicotinic acid inhibits lipolysis in adipose tissues, decreases hepatic esterification of triglyceride, and increases lipoprotein lipase activity. It reduces serum cholesterol and triglyceride levels.
*Vasodilating action:* Niacin acts directly on peripheral vessels, dilating cutaneous vessels and increasing blood flow, predominantly in the face, neck, and chest.

## Pharmacokinetics

*Absorption:* Absorbed rapidly from the GI tract. Cholesterol and triglyceride levels decrease after several days.
*Distribution:* Coenzymes are distributed widely in body tissues; niacin appears in breast milk.
*Metabolism:* Metabolized by the liver to active metabolites.
*Excretion:* Excreted in urine.

| Route | Onset | Peak | Duration |
|-------|-------|------|----------|
| P.O. | Unknown | 45 min | Unknown |

## Contraindications and precautions

Contraindicated in patients with hepatic dysfunction, active peptic ulcer, severe hypotension, arterial hemorrhage, or hypersensitivity to drug. Use cautiously in patients with history of liver disease, peptic ulcer, allergy, gout, gallbladder disease, diabetes mellitus, or coronary artery disease.

## Interactions

**Drug-drug.** *Aspirin:* May decrease the metabolic clearance of nicotinic acid. Use together cautiously.

*Isoniazid:* If used long-term, drug may interfere with the conversion of dietary tryptophan to niacin. Niacin requirements may increase.

*Sympathetic blockers:* May cause added vasodilation and hypotension. Use together cautiously.

## Adverse reactions

Most reactions are dose-dependent.

**CV:** *excessive peripheral vasodilation,* hypotension, atrial fibrillation, ***arrhythmias.***

**EENT:** toxic amblyopia.

**GI:** *nausea, vomiting, diarrhea,* possible activation of peptic ulceration, epigastric or substernal pain.

**Hepatic:** *hepatic dysfunction.*

**Metabolic:** hyperglycemia, hyperuricemia.

**Skin:** *flushing,* pruritus, dryness, tingling.

## Overdose and treatment

Niacin is a water-soluble vitamin, which seldom causes toxicity in patients with normal renal function.

## Clinical considerations

■ RDA of niacin in men is 19 mg; in women, 15 mg; and in children, 5 to 20 mg.

■ Megadoses of niacin aren't usually recommended.

■ Advise clinician to monitor hepatic function and blood glucose levels during initial therapy.

■ Aspirin may reduce flushing response.

■ Niacin therapy alters fluorometric test results for urine catecholamines and results for urine glucose tests using cupric sulfate (Benedict's reagent).

### Therapeutic monitoring

■ Advise clinician to monitor hepatic function and blood glucose levels when therapy starts.

### Special populations

**Pregnant patients.** Normal supplementation of niacin hasn't caused problems. However, large doses should be avoided unless it is determined that the potential benefits outweigh the risks.

**Breast-feeding patients.** There have been no reports of problems in breast-feeding women taking normal daily doses as dietary requirement.

## Patient counseling

■ Explain disease process and reason for therapy; stress that use of niacin to treat hyperlipidemia or to dilate peripheral vessels is not simply "taking a vitamin," but is serious medicine. Emphasize importance of complying with therapy.

■ Instruct patient not to substitute sustained-release (timed) tablets for intermediate-release tablets in equivalent doses. Severe hepatic toxicity, including necrosis, has occurred.

■ Explain that cutaneous flushing and warmth commonly occur in the first 2 hours; this will cease on continued therapy.

■ Advise patient not to make sudden postural changes to minimize effects of orthostatic hypotension.

■ Instruct patient to avoid hot liquids when initially taking drug to reduce flushing response.

■ Advise patient to take drug with meals to minimize GI irritation.

# nicardipine hydrochloride
Cardene, Cardene SR

*Pharmacologic classification:* calcium channel blocker
*Therapeutic classification:* antianginal, antihypertensive
*Pregnancy risk category C*

## Available forms

Available by prescription only
*Capsules:* 20 mg, 30 mg
*Capsules (extended-release):* 30 mg, 45 mg, 60 mg
*Injection:* 2.5 mg/ml in 10-ml ampules

## Indications and dosages

**Hypertension; management of chronic stable angina**

*Adults:* Initially, 20 mg P.O. t.i.d. Adjust dosage based on patient response. Usual dosage range, 20 to 40 mg t.i.d. Extended-release capsules (for hypertension only) can be initiated at 30 mg b.i.d. Usual dose, 30 to 60 mg b.i.d.

**Short-term management of hypertension when oral therapy isn't feasible or possible**

*Adults:* Initially, 5 mg/hour I.V. infusion; titrate infusion upward by 2.5 mg/hour q 5 to 15 minutes up to a maximum of 15 mg/hour, p.r.n. Maintenance infusion is 3 mg/hour. When transferring to oral therapy, give P.O. of conventional capsule 1 hour before discontinuing infusion.

Note: If patient is already taking nicardipine and requires short-term I.V. management of hypertension, give 0.5 mg/hour if dose is 20 mg q 8 hours; 1.2 mg/hour if dose is 30 mg q 8 hours; and 2.2 mg/hour if dose is 40 mg q 8 hours.

## I.V. administration

■ Dilute with compatible I.V. solution before administration. Drug is compatible with $D_5W$, $D_5W$ in normal or half-normal saline solution, and normal or half-normal saline solution for 24 hours at room temperature.

■ Administer by slow I.V. infusion in a concentration of 0.1 mg/ml.
■ Closely monitor blood pressure during and after completion of infusion.
■ Titrate infusion rate, as ordered, if hypotension or tachycardia occurs.
■ Change peripheral infusion site every 12 hours to minimize risk of venous irritation.
■ When switching to oral therapy other than nicardipine, initiate therapy upon ending of infusion. If oral nicardipine is to be used, administer first dose of t.i.d. regimen 1 hour before stopping infusion.

### Incompatibilities
Incompatible with lactated Ringer's solution and sodium bicarbonate.

### Mechanism of action
*Antianginal and antihypertensive action:* Nicardipine inhibits the transmembrane flux of calcium ions into cardiac and smooth-muscle cells. Drug appears to act specifically on vascular muscle and may cause a smaller decrease in cardiac output than other calcium channel blockers because of its vasodilatory effect.

### Pharmacokinetics
*Absorption:* Completely absorbed after oral administration. Absorption may be decreased if drug is taken with food. Therapeutic serum levels are 28 to 50 ng/ml.
*Distribution:* Extensively (more than 95%) plasma protein–bound.
*Metabolism:* A substantial first-pass effect reduces absolute bioavailability to about 35%. Drug is extensively metabolized in the liver, and the process is saturable. Increasing dosage yields nonlinear increases in plasma levels.
*Excretion:* Elimination half-life of drug is about 8½ hours after steady-state levels are reached.

| Route | Onset | Peak | Duration |
|-------|-------|------|----------|
| P.O. (immediate) | ½-11½ min | Unknown | Unknown |
| P.O. (sustained) | 20 min | 1-4 hr | 12 hr |
| I.V. | Immediate | Immediate | Unknown |

### Contraindications and precautions
Contraindicated in patients hypersensitive to drug and in those with advanced aortic stenosis. Use cautiously in patients with impaired renal or hepatic function, cardiac conduction disturbances, hypotension, or HF.

### Interactions
**Drug-drug.** *Cimetidine:* Higher plasma levels of nicardipine. Advise clinician to monitor patient for increased effects.
*Cyclosporine:* Increased plasma levels of cyclosporine. Advise clinician to monitor patient closely.

*Digoxin:* Increased plasma levels of cardiac glycosides. Advise clinician to monitor serum digoxin level.
*Fentanyl anesthesia:* Severe hypotension. Advise clinician to monitor blood pressure frequently.
**Drug-food.** *Grapefruit juice:* Increased bioavailability of drug. Advise patient to avoid taking drug with grapefruit juice.

### Adverse reactions
**CNS:** dizziness, light-headedness, headache, paresthesia, asthenia.
**CV:** *peripheral edema, palpitations,* angina, tachycardia.
**GI:** nausea, abdominal discomfort, dry mouth.
**Skin:** rash, *flushing.*

### Overdose and treatment
Overdose may produce hypotension, bradycardia, drowsiness, confusion, and slurred speech. Treatment is supportive, with vasopressors given p.r.n. I.V. calcium gluconate may be useful to counteract the effects of drug.

### Clinical considerations
■ Allow at least 3 days between oral dosage changes to ensure achievement of steady-state plasma levels.
■ When treating patients with chronic stable angina, S.L. nitroglycerin, prophylactic nitrate therapy, and beta blockers may be continued.
■ In patients with hepatic dysfunction, therapy should begin at 20 mg P.O. b.i.d.; subsequent dosage should be carefully adjusted based on patient response.

### Therapeutic monitoring
■ When treating hypertension, recommend measuring blood pressure during times of plasma level trough (about 8 hours after dose, or immediately before subsequent doses). Because of prominent effects that may occur during plasma level peaks, recommend measuring blood pressure 1 to 2 hours after conventional dose and 2 to 4 hours after extended-release dose. Dosage adjustment should be based on blood pressure 2 to 4 hours after oral dose.
■ Advise clinician to monitor blood pressure during I.V. administration because nicardipine I.V. decreases peripheral resistance.

### Special populations
**Breast-feeding patients.** Substantial levels of drug appear in the breast milk of animals given nicardipine. Breast-feeding isn't recommended.
**Pediatric patients.** Safety in patients under age 18 hasn't been established.

### Patient counseling
■ Tell patient to take oral form of drug exactly as prescribed.

■ Advise patient to report chest pain to pre-scriber immediately. Some patients may ex-perience increased frequency, severity, or du-ration of chest pain at the beginning of therapy or during dosage adjustments.

# nicotine

Nicoderm, Nicoderm CQ, Nicotrol, Nicotrol NS

*Pharmacologic classification:* nicotinic cholinergic agonist
*Therapeutic classification:* smoking cessation aid
*Pregnancy risk category D*

## Available forms

Available by prescription only
**Nicotrol inhaler:** 10 mg cartridge, supplying 4 mg of nicotine
Available with and without a prescription
*Transdermal system:* Designed to release nico-tine at a fixed rate
**Nicoderm:** 21 mg/day, 14 mg/day, 7 mg/day
**Nicotrol:** 15 mg/day
*Nasal spray:* Metered spray pump
**Nicotrol NS:** 10 mg/ml

## Indications and dosages
*Relief of nicotine withdrawal symptoms in patients attempting smoking cessation*
*Adults:* One transdermal system applied to a nonhairy part of the upper trunk or upper out-er arm. Dosage varies slightly with product selected.
**Nicoderm**
Initially, apply one 21-mg/day system daily for 6 weeks. After 24 hours, remove system and apply a new system to a different site. Then, taper dosage to 14 mg/day for 2 to 4 weeks. Finally, taper dosage to 7 mg/day if needed. Nicotine substitution and gradual withdrawal should take 8 to 12 weeks.
≡ *Dosage adjustment.* Patients who weigh un-der 45 kg (100 lb), have CV disease, or who smoke less than half a pack of cigarettes dai-ly should start therapy with the 14-mg/day sys-tem.
**Nicotrol**
*Adults:* Apply one 15-mg/day system daily for 6 weeks. Apply system upon waking and re-move h.s. because patch provides systemic de-livery over 16 hours.
**Nicotrol NS**
*Adults:* Initially, one or two doses per hour (one dose = 2 sprays—one in each nostril). En-courage patient to use at least the recommended minimum of eight doses per day. Maximum recommended dose is 40 mg or 80 sprays/day. Duration of treatment shouldn't exceed 3 months with gradual dose reduction during those 3 months.

**Nicotrol inhaler**
*Adults:* Initial dose is 6 to 16 cartridges daily. Best effect is achieved with continuous puff-ing. Recommended treatment is up to 3 months and, if needed, gradual reduction over the next 6 to 12 weeks.

## Mechanism of action
*Nicotinic cholinergic action:* Nicotine trans-dermal system and nasal spray provide nico-tine, the chief stimulant alkaloid found in to-bacco products, which stimulates nicotinic acetylcholine receptors in the CNS, neuro-muscular junction, autonomic ganglia, and adrenal medulla.

## Pharmacokinetics
*Absorption:* Rapidly absorbed.
*Distribution:* Less than 5% bound to plasma protein.
*Metabolism:* Metabolized by the liver, kidney, and lungs. Over 20 metabolites have been iden-tified. Primary metabolites are cotinine (15%) and trans-3-hydroxycotinine (45%).
*Excretion:* Excreted primarily in urine as metabolites; about 10% is excreted unchanged. With high urine flow rates or acidified urine, up to 30% can be excreted unchanged.

| Route | Onset | Peak | Duration |
|---|---|---|---|
| Transdermal | Unknown | 3-9 hr | Unknown |
| Intranasal | Unknown | 4-15 min | Unknown |
| Inhalation | Unknown | 15 min | Unknown |

## Contraindications and precautions
Contraindicated in patients hypersensitive to nicotine or any components. Also contraindi-cated in nonsmokers and in patients with re-cent MI, life-threatening arrhythmias, and se-vere or worsening angina pectoris.
   Use cautiously in patients with hyperthy-roidism, pheochromocytoma, type 1 diabetes, or peptic ulcer disease.

## Interactions
**Drug-drug.** *Acetaminophen, caffeine, imipra-mine, oxazepam, pentazocine, propranolol, theophylline:* Cessation of smoking may de-crease induction of hepatic enzymes responsi-ble for metabolizing certain drugs. Dosage re-duction of such drugs may be needed.
*Adrenergic agonists, such as isoproterenol and phenylephrine; adrenergic antagonists, such as labetalol and prazosine:* Cessation of smok-ing may decrease levels of circulating cate-cholamines. Dosage adjustment of such drugs may be needed.
*Insulin:* Cessation of smoking may increase the amount of S.C. insulin absorbed. Insulin dosage should be adjusted.
**Drug-herb.** *Blue cohosh:* Increases effects of nicotine. Discourage use together.

---

Reactions may be *common*, uncommon, *life-threatening*, or COMMON AND LIFE-THREATENING.

## Adverse reactions

**CNS:** somnolence, dizziness, *headache, insomnia,* paresthesia, abnormal dreams, nervousness.
**CV:** hypertension.
**EENT:** pharyngitis, sinusitis.
**GI:** abdominal pain, constipation, dyspepsia, nausea, diarrhea, vomiting, dry mouth.
**GU:** dysmenorrhea.
**Musculoskeletal:** back pain, myalgia.
**Respiratory:** increased cough.
**Skin:** *local or systemic erythema, pruritus, burning at application site,* cutaneous hypersensitivity, rash, diaphoresis.

## Overdose and treatment

Overdose could produce the symptoms of acute nicotine poisoning, including nausea, vomiting, diarrhea, weakness, respiratory failure, hypotension, and seizures. Treatment is symptomatic. Barbiturates or benzodiazepines may be used to treat seizures, and atropine may attenuate excessive salivation or diarrhea. Advise clinician to give fluids to treat hypotension and increase urine flow to enhance elimination of drug.

## Clinical considerations

■ Transdermal nicotine has been used investigationally to manage ulcerative colitis.
■ Discourage use of transdermal system for more than 3 months. Long-term nicotine consumption by any route can be dangerous and habit-forming.
■ Transdermal system is usually applied as soon as patient wakes up.
■ If patients receiving 24-hour transdermal system experience sleep disruption, the system can be removed before bedtime or patient can be switched to 16-hour system.
■ Patients who can't stop cigarette smoking during the initial 4 weeks of therapy will probably not benefit from continued use of drug. Patients who were unsuccessful may benefit from counseling to identify factors that led to the unsuccessful attempt. Encourage patient to minimize or eliminate the factors that contributed to treatment failure and to try again, possibly after some interval, before the next attempt.
■ Health care workers' exposure to the nicotine within the transdermal systems should be minimal; however, avoid unnecessary contact with the system. After contact, wash hands with water alone because soap can enhance absorption.
■ Nicotrol NS isn't recommended in patients with chronic nasal disorders or severe reactive airway disease.
■ Increased cough is a common occurrence in patients using the inhaler.
■ Although use of nicotine replacement therapy isn't recommended in recent MI patients, it may be considered preferable to cigarette smoking in patients experiencing withdrawal.

### Therapeutic monitoring

■ Advise clinician to monitor patient for correct use of system to prevent overdose or failure of program.

### Special populations

**Breast-feeding patients.** Nicotine appears in breast milk and is readily absorbed after oral administration. Weigh the infant's risk of exposure to nicotine in drug against his risk of exposure from continued smoking by the mother.
**Pediatric patients.** Safety and efficacy in children haven't been established. According to the U.S. Public Health Services, adolescents may be considered for nicotine replacement therapy if there is evidence of nicotine dependence and a desire to quit tobacco use.

## Patient counseling

■ Tell patient to discontinue use of patch and to immediately report a generalized rash or persistent or severe local skin reactions, such as pruritus, edema, or erythema.
■ Make sure patient understands that nicotine can evaporate from the transdermal system once it's removed from its protective packaging. The patch shouldn't be altered in any way (folded or cut) before it's applied. It should be applied promptly after removal of the system's protective packaging. Tell patient not to store patch at temperatures above 86° F (30° C).
**◾ ALERT** The amount of nicotine contained in a patch could prove fatal to a child if ingested; even used patches contain a substantial amount of residual nicotine. Patients should ensure that both used and unused transdermal systems and metered spray bottles are kept out of the reach of children.
■ Teach patient how to dispose of transdermal system. After removal, fold the patch in half, bringing the adhesive sides together. If the system comes in a protective pouch, dispose of the used patch in the pouch that contained the new system. Careful disposal is needed to prevent accidental poisoning of children or pets.
■ Be sure that patient reads and understands the patient information that's dispensed with drug when the prescription is filled.
■ Inform patient to refrain from smoking while using the system; he may experience adverse effects from the increased nicotine levels.
■ Explain that patient is likely to experience nasal irritation with Nicotrol NS, which may become less bothersome with continued use.
■ Tell patient to store the inhaler and cartridge in an inside pocket or a warm area during cold weather.

# nicotine polacrilex (nicotine resin complex)

Nicorette

*Pharmacologic classification:* nicotinic agonist
*Therapeutic classification:* smoking cessation aid
*Pregnancy risk category X*

## Available forms

Available with and without a prescription
*Chewing gum:* 2 mg, 4 mg nicotine resin complex per square

## Indications and dosages

*Aid in managing nicotine dependence*
Serves as a temporary aid to smokers seeking to give up smoking while participating in a behavior modification program under medical supervision. Generally, a smoker with the "physical" type of nicotine dependence is most likely to benefit from use of nicotine chewing gum.
*Adults:* Chew one piece of gum slowly and intermittently for 30 minutes whenever the urge to smoke occurs. Most patients require about 9 to 12 pieces of gum daily during first month. Patients using the 2-mg strength shouldn't exceed 24 pieces of gum daily if unsupervised or 30 pieces if supervised; those using the 4-mg strength shouldn't exceed 24 pieces of gum daily.

## Mechanism of action

*Nicotine replacement action:* Nicotine is an agonist at the nicotinic receptors in the peripheral nervous system and CNS and produces both behavioral stimulation and depression. It acts on the adrenal medulla to aid in overcoming physical dependence on nicotine during withdrawal from habitual smoking.

CV effects of nicotine are usually dose-dependent. Nonsmokers have experienced CNS-mediated symptoms of hiccuping, nausea, and vomiting, even with a small dose. A smoker chewing a 2-mg piece of gum every hour usually doesn't experience CV adverse effects.

## Pharmacokinetics

*Absorption:* Bound to ion-exchange resin and is released only during chewing. The blood level depends upon the vigor with which the gum is chewed.
*Distribution:* Distribution into tissues hasn't been fully characterized. It crosses the placenta and appears in breast milk.
*Metabolism:* Metabolized mainly by the liver and less so by the kidneys and lungs. Main metabolites are cotinine and nicotine-19-*N*-oxide.

*Excretion:* Both nicotine and its metabolites are excreted in urine, with about 10% to 20% excreted unchanged. Excretion of nicotine is increased in acid urine and by high urine output.

| Route | Onset | Peak | Duration |
|-------|-------|------|----------|
| P.O. | Unknown | 15-30 min | Unknown |

## Contraindications and precautions

Contraindicated in nonsmokers; in patients with recent MI, life-threatening arrhythmias, severe or worsening angina pectoris, or active temporomandibular joint disease; and during pregnancy.

Use cautiously in patients with hyperthyroidism, pheochromocytoma, insulin-dependent diabetes, peptic ulcer disease, history of esophagitis, oral or pharyngeal inflammation, or dental conditions that might be exacerbated by chewing gum.

## Interactions

**Drug-drug.** *Adrenergic agonists, adrenergic blockers:* Nicorette gum and smoking can increase the circulating levels of cortisol and catecholamines. Dosage adjustments may be needed.
*Imipramine, pentazocine, theophylline:* Smoking cessation either with or without nicotine substitutes may reverse increased metabolism of smoking. Dosage adjustments may be needed.
*Propoxyphene:* Smoking cessation may reduce the first-pass metabolism of propoxyphene. Dosage adjustments may be needed.
**Drug-herb.** *Blue cohosh:* May increase effects of nicotine. Discourage use together.
**Drug-food.** *Beverages, any food:* Inhibited absorption. Advise patient to avoid eating and drinking 15 minutes before and during chewing of gum.
*Caffeine:* Smoking may increase the metabolism of caffeine. Advise clinician to monitor patient for effect.

## Adverse reactions

**CNS:** dizziness, light-headedness, irritability, insomnia, headache, paresthesia.
**CV:** atrial fibrillation.
**EENT:** throat soreness, jaw muscle ache (from chewing).
**GI:** nausea, vomiting, indigestion, eructation, anorexia, excessive salivation.
**Other:** hiccups, sweating.

## Overdose and treatment

The risk of overdose is minimized by early nausea and vomiting that result from excessive nicotine intake. Poisoning manifests as nausea, vomiting, salivation, abdominal pain, diarrhea, cold sweats, headache, dizziness, disturbed hearing and vision, mental confusion, and weakness.

Treatment includes emesis; advise clinician to give ipecac syrup if emesis hasn't occurred. A saline cathartic will speed the passage of the gum through the GI tract. Advise clinician to give gastric lavage followed by activated charcoal in unconscious patients. Recommend providing supportive treatment of respiratory paralysis and CV collapse, p.r.n.

## Clinical considerations
■ Patients most likely to benefit from Nicorette gum are smokers with a high physical dependence. Typically, they smoke over 15 cigarettes daily; prefer brands of cigarettes with high nicotine levels; usually inhale the smoke; smoke the first cigarette within 30 minutes of arising; and find the first morning cigarette the hardest to give up.
■ Patient may initiate reduction by reducing actual pieces of gum chewed or length of time gum is chewed.
■ Smoking cessation generally takes 2 to 3 months with gradual dose reduction.
■ Although nicotine replacement therapy isn't recommended in patients with recent MI, it may be considered preferable to cigarette smoking in patients experiencing nicotine withdrawal.

### Therapeutic monitoring
■ Recommend patient be reevaluated at least monthly to determine therapy response.

### Special populations
**Breast-feeding patients.** Nicotine appears in breast milk and is readily absorbed after oral administration. Weigh the infant's risk of exposure to nicotine from a transdermal patch against his risk of exposure from continued smoking by the mother.

## Patient counseling
■ Instruct patient to chew gum slowly and intermittently for about 30 minutes to promote slow and even buccal absorption of nicotine. Fast chewing allows faster absorption and produces more adverse reactions. After about 15 chews, advise the patient to "park" the gum between the cheek and gum for a few minutes.
■ Inform patient that he shouldn't eat or drink anything 15 minutes before or while chewing gum.
■ At the initial visit, instruct patient to chew one piece of gum whenever the urge to smoke occurs instead of having a cigarette. Most patients will require about ten pieces of gum daily during first month of treatment.
■ Tell patient who has successfully abstained to gradually withdraw gum use after 3 months; he shouldn't use gum for longer than 6 months.
■ Inform patient that gum is sugar-free and usually doesn't stick to dentures.

# nifedipine
Adalat, Adalat CC, Procardia, Procardia XL

*Pharmacologic classification:* calcium channel blocker
*Therapeutic classification:* antianginal
*Pregnancy risk category C*

## Available forms
Available by prescription only
*Capsules:* 10 mg, 20 mg
*Tablets (extended-release):* 30 mg, 60 mg, 90 mg

## Indications and dosages
*Management of Prinzmetal's or variant angina or chronic stable angina pectoris*
*Adults:* Starting dose is 10 mg P.O. t.i.d. Usual effective dosage range is 10 to 20 mg t.i.d. Some patients may require up to 30 mg q.i.d. Alternatively, 30 to 60 mg (extended-release preparation) P.O. daily. Doses are gradually increased at 7- to 14-day intervals or more frequently, if needed. Maximum daily dose for capsules is 180 mg; for extended-release tablets, 120 mg.
*Hypertension*
*Adults:* Initially, 30 to 60 mg P.O. once daily (extended-release tablets). Adjust dosage at 7- to 14-day intervals based on patient tolerance and response. Maximum daily dose is 120 mg.
◊ *Quick reduction of blood pressure*
*Adults:* 10 to 20 mg q 20 to 30 minutes; capsule should be bitten and then swallowed.

## Mechanism of action
*Antianginal action:* Nifedipine dilates systemic arteries, resulting in decreased total peripheral resistance and modestly decreased systemic blood pressure with a slightly increased heart rate, decreased afterload, and increased cardiac index. Reduced afterload and the subsequent decrease in myocardial oxygen consumption probably account for the value of nifedipine in treating chronic stable angina. In Prinzmetal's angina, nifedipine inhibits coronary artery spasm, increasing myocardial oxygen delivery.

## Pharmacokinetics
*Absorption:* About 90% of a dose is absorbed rapidly from the GI tract after oral administration; however, only about 65% to 70% of drug reaches the systemic circulation because of a significant first-pass effect in the liver. Therapeutic serum levels are 25 to 100 ng/ml.
*Distribution:* About 92% to 98% of circulating nifedipine is plasma protein–bound.
*Metabolism:* Metabolized in the liver.

*Excretion:* Excreted in urine and feces as inactive metabolites. Elimination half-life is 2 to 5 hours.

| Route | Onset | Peak | Duration |
|-------|-------|------|----------|
| P.O. | 20 min | ½-1 hr | 4-8 hr |
| P.O. | 20 min | 6 hr | 24 hr |

## Contraindications and precautions

Contraindicated in patients hypersensitive to drug. Use cautiously in geriatric patients and in patients with HF or hypotension. Use extended-release form cautiously in patients with GI narrowing.

Use with caution in patients with unstable angina who aren't currently taking a beta blocker because a higher incidence of MI has been reported.

## Interactions

**Drug-drug.** *Beta blockers:* May exacerbate angina, HF, and hypotension. Use together cautiously.

*Cimetidine:* May decrease metabolism of nifedipine. Use together cautiously.

*Digoxin:* May cause increased serum digoxin levels. Advise clinician to monitor serum digoxin level.

*Fentanyl:* May cause excessive hypotension. Use together cautiously.

*Hypotensive drugs:* May precipitate excessive hypotension. Use together cautiously.

*Phenytoin:* Drug may increase phenytoin levels. Advise clinician to monitor phenytoin levels.

*Quinupristin and dalfopristin:* May increase the plasma levels of nifedipine. Advise clinician to monitor patient closely.

**Drug-food.** *Grapefruit juice:* Increased bioavailability of drug. Advise patient to avoid taking drug with grapefruit juice.

## Adverse reactions

**CNS:** *dizziness, light-headedness, flushing, headache, weakness,* syncope, nervousness.
**CV:** *peripheral edema,* hypotension, palpitations, **HF, MI, pulmonary edema.**
**EENT:** nasal congestion.
**GI:** *nausea,* diarrhea, constipation, abdominal discomfort; increase in serum levels of alkaline phosphate, LDH, AST, and ALT.
**Metabolic:** hypokalemia.
**Musculoskeletal:** muscle cramps.
**Respiratory:** dyspnea, cough.
**Skin:** rash, pruritus.
**Other:** fever.

## Overdose and treatment

Effects of overdose are extensions of pharmacologic effects of the drug, primarily peripheral vasodilation and hypotension.

Treatment includes such basic support measures as hemodynamic and respiratory monitoring. If patient requires blood pressure support by a vasoconstrictor, norepinephrine may be given. Recommend elevating limbs and correcting any fluid deficit.

## Clinical considerations

■ Nifedipine has been used investigationally to treat Raynaud's phenomenon and preterm labor.

**H ALERT** Warn patient not to switch brands. Procardia XL and Adalat CC aren't therapeutically equivalent because of major differences in their pharmacokinetics.

■ Initial doses or dosage increase may exacerbate angina briefly. Reassure patient that this symptom is temporary.

■ Nifedipine isn't available in S.L. form. No advantage has been found in S.L. or intrabuccal use.

■ Although rebound effect hasn't been observed when drug is stopped, dosage should be reduced slowly.

### Therapeutic monitoring

■ Advise clinician to monitor blood pressure regularly, especially if patient is also taking beta blockers or antihypertensives.

### Special populations

**Geriatric patients.** Use drug with caution in geriatric patients because they may be more sensitive to effects of drug and duration of effect may be prolonged. Orthostatic blood pressures should be monitored.

## Patient counseling

■ Instruct patient to swallow capsules whole without breaking, crushing, or chewing them unless instructed otherwise.

■ Tell patient that he may experience annoying hypotensive effects during adjustment of dosage and urge compliance with therapy.

# nisoldipine
Sular

*Pharmacologic classification:* calcium channel blocker
*Therapeutic classification:* antihypertensive
*Pregnancy risk category C*

## Available forms

Available by prescription only
*Tablets (extended-release):* 10 mg, 20 mg, 30 mg, 40 mg

## Indications and dosages

### Hypertension

*Adults:* Initially, 20 mg P.O. once daily, then increased by 10 mg per week or at longer intervals, p.r.n. Usual maintenance dose, 20 to 40 mg once daily. Don't exceed 60 mg daily.

**≡ Dosage adjustment.** For patients over age 65 or those with hepatic dysfunction, give starting dose of 10 mg P.O. once daily. Advise clinician to monitor blood pressure closely during any dosage adjustment.

## Mechanism of action

*Antihypertensive action:* Nisoldipine prevents the entry of calcium ions into vascular smooth-muscle cells, causing dilation of the arterioles, which in turn decreases peripheral vascular resistance.

## Pharmacokinetics

*Absorption:* Relatively well absorbed from GI tract. High-fat foods significantly affect release of drug from the coat-core formulation.
*Distribution:* About 99% plasma protein–bound.
*Metabolism:* Extensively metabolized with five major metabolites identified.
*Excretion:* Excreted in urine; half-life ranges from 7 to 12 hours.

| Route | Onset | Peak | Duration |
|-------|-------|------|----------|
| P.O. | Unknown | 6-12 hr | 24 hr |

## Contraindications and precautions

Contraindicated in patients hypersensitive to dihydropyridine calcium channel blockers. Use cautiously in patients receiving beta blockers and in those who have compromised ventricular or hepatic function and HF.

## Interactions

**Drug-drug.** *Cimetidine:* Increased bioavailability of nisoldipine as well as increasing peak level. Use together cautiously.
*Quinidine:* Decreased bioavailability, but not peak level of nisoldipine. Advise clinician to monitor blood pressure.
**Drug-food.** *Grapefruit juice, high-fat meals:* May decrease absorption. Advise patient not to take drug with these foods.

## Adverse reactions

**CNS:** *headache,* dizziness.
**CV:** vasodilation, palpitations, chest pain, *peripheral edema.*
**EENT:** pharyngitis, sinusitis.
**GI:** nausea.
**Skin:** rash.

## Overdose and treatment

Overdose with similar drugs leads to pronounced hypotension. Treatment should focus on CV support, including monitoring of CV and respiratory function, elevation of limbs, and judicious use of calcium infusion, pressor agents, and fluids.

## Clinical considerations

■ Extended-release form of drug makes it unsuitable for use in hypertensive emergency.

### Therapeutic monitoring

■ Advise clinician to monitor patient carefully. Some patients, especially those with severe obstructive coronary artery disease, have increased frequency, duration, or severity of angina or even acute MI after initiation of calcium channel blocker therapy or at time of dosage increase.
■ Advise clinician to monitor blood pressure regularly, especially when treatment starts or changes.

### Special populations

**Breast-feeding patients.** It isn't known if drug appears in breast milk. Use of drug in breast-feeding women isn't recommended.
**Pediatric patients.** Safety and efficacy in children haven't been established.
**Geriatric patients.** Geriatric patients may have two- to threefold higher plasma levels than younger patients, requiring cautious dosing.

### Patient counseling

■ Tell patient to take drug exactly as prescribed, even if he feels better.
■ Advise patient to swallow tablet whole and not to chew, divide, or crush tablets, unless instructed otherwise.
■ Tell patient not to take drug with a high-fat meal or with grapefruit products.
■ Advise patient to rise slowly from supine position to avoid dizziness and hypotension, especially when therapy starts.

# nitrofurantoin macrocrystals
Macrobid, Macrodantin

# nitrofurantoin microcrystals
Furadantin

*Pharmacologic classification:* nitrofuran
*Therapeutic classification:* urinary tract anti-infective
*Pregnancy risk category B*

## Available forms

Available by prescription only
**macrocrystals**
*Capsules:* 25 mg, 50 mg, 100 mg
*Capsules (dual-release):* 100 mg
**microcrystals**
*Suspension:* 25 mg/5 ml

## Indications and dosages

*Initial or recurrent urinary tract infections caused by susceptible organisms*
*Adults and children over age 12:* 50 to 100 mg P.O. q.i.d. or 100 mg dual-release capsules q 12 hours for 7 days.

*Children ages 1 month to 12 years:* 5 to 7 mg/kg/24 hours P.O. daily, divided q.i.d.
**Long-term suppression therapy**
*Adults:* 50 to 100 mg P.O. daily h.s. as a single dose.
*Children:* As low as 1 mg/kg/day P.O. in a single dose or two divided doses.

## Mechanism of action
*Antibacterial action:* Nitrofurantoin has bacteriostatic action in low levels and possible bactericidal action in high levels. Although its exact mechanism of action is unknown, it may inhibit bacterial enzyme systems interfering with bacterial carbohydrate metabolism. Drug is most active at an acidic pH.
   Spectrum of activity includes many common gram-positive and gram-negative urinary pathogens, including *Escherichia coli, Staphylococcus aureus,* enterococci, and certain strains of *Klebsiella* and *Enterobacter.* Organisms that usually resist nitrofurantoin include *Acinetobacter, Proteus, Providencia, Pseudomonas,* and *Serratia.*

## Pharmacokinetics
*Absorption:* When given orally, drug is well absorbed (mainly by the small intestine) from GI tract. Presence of food aids dissolution of drug and speeds absorption. The macrocrystal form exhibits slower dissolution and absorption; it causes less GI distress.
*Distribution:* Crosses into bile and placenta. 60% plasma protein–bound. Plasma half-life is about 20 minutes. Peak urine levels occur in about 30 minutes when drug is given as microcrystals, somewhat later when given as macrocrystals.
*Metabolism:* Metabolized partially in the liver.
*Excretion:* About 30% to 50% of dose is eliminated by glomerular filtration and tubular secretion into urine as unchanged drug within 24 hours. Some drug may appear in breast milk.

| Route | Onset | Peak | Duration |
|-------|-------|------|----------|
| P.O.  | Unknown | Unknown | Unknown |

## Contraindications and precautions
Contraindicated in pregnant women at term (38 to 42 weeks' gestation), during labor and delivery, or when the onset of labor is imminent. Contraindicated in children ages 1 month and under and in patients with moderate to severe renal impairment, anuria, oliguria, or creatinine clearance under 60 ml per minute.
   Use cautiously in patients with impaired renal function, anemia, diabetes mellitus, electrolyte abnormalities, vitamin B deficiency, debilitating disease, or G6PD deficiency.

## Interactions
**Drug-drug.** *Anticholinergics:* Enhance bioavailability. Advise clinician to monitor patient carefully.

*Magnesium trisilicate antacids:* May decrease nitrofurantoin absorption. Separate administration times.
*Probenecid. sulfinpyrazone:* Reduced renal excretion of nitrofurantoin. Advise clinician to monitor patient for increased toxicity and decreased clinical effect.
*Quinolone derivatives, such as cinoxacin, ciprofloxacin, nalidixic acid, and norfloxacin:* May antagonize anti-infective effects. Advise clinician to monitor patient for decreased clinical effect
**Drug-food.** *Any food:* Enhances bioavailability of nitrofurantoin. Advise clinician to give drug with food.

## Adverse reactions
**CNS:** *peripheral neuropathy,* headache, dizziness, drowsiness, *ascending polyneuropathy* (with high doses or renal impairment).
**GI:** *anorexia, nausea, vomiting,* abdominal pain, *diarrhea.*
**GU:** overgrowth of nonsusceptible organisms in the urinary tract.
**Hematologic:** *hemolysis in patients with G6PD deficiency* (reversed after stopping drug), *agranulocytosis, thrombocytopenia.*
**Hepatic:** *hepatitis, hepatic necrosis,* elevated bilirubin and alkaline phosphatase.
**Metabolic:** decreased serum glucose level.
**Respiratory:** *pulmonary sensitivity reactions* (cough, chest pain, fever, chills, dyspnea, pulmonary infiltration with consolidation or pleural effusion), *asthmatic attacks in patients with history of asthma.*
**Skin:** maculopapular, erythematous, or eczematous eruption; transient alopecia; pruritus; urticaria; *exfoliative dermatitis; Stevens-Johnson syndrome.*
**Other:** hypersensitivity reactions *(anaphylaxis),* drug fever.

## Overdose and treatment
Acute overdose may result in nausea and vomiting. Treatment is symptomatic. No specific antidote is known. Recommend increasing fluid intake to promote urinary excretion of drug. Nitrofurantoin is dialyzable.

## Clinical considerations
■ Culture and sensitivity test results should be obtained before starting therapy, and repeated p.r.n.
■ Oral suspension may be mixed with water, milk, fruit juice, and formulas.
■ Drug may turn urine brown or rust-yellow.
■ Recommend continuing treatment for at least 3 days after sterile urine specimens have been obtained.
■ Long-term therapy may cause overgrowth of nonsusceptible organisms, especially *Pseudomonas.*
■ Nitrofurantoin may cause false-positive results in urine glucose tests using cupric sulfate

---

reagents (such as Benedict's test, Fehling's solution, or Clinitest) because it reacts with these reagents.

### Therapeutic monitoring
■ Advise clinician to monitor CBC regularly.
■ Advise clinician to monitor fluid intake and output and pulmonary status.

### Special populations
**Breast-feeding patients.** Safety hasn't been established. Although drug appears in low levels in breast milk, no adverse reactions have been reported, except in infants with G6PD deficiency, in whom hemolytic anemia may develop.
**Pediatric patients.** Contraindicated in infants under age 1 month because their immature enzyme systems increase risk of hemolytic anemia.

## Patient counseling
■ Instruct patient to take drug with food or milk to minimize GI distress. Have patient report any unpleasant side effects.
■ Caution patient that drug may cause false-positive results in urine glucose tests using cupric sulfate reduction method (Clinitest) but not in glucose oxidase test (glucose enzymatic test strip, Diastix, or Chemstrip uG).
■ Emphasize that bedtime dose is important because drug will remain in bladder longer.
■ Warn patient that drug may turn urine brown or rust-yellow.

---

## nitrofurazone
Furacin

*Pharmacologic classification:* synthetic antibacterial nitrofuran derivative
*Therapeutic classification:* topical antibacterial
*Pregnancy risk category C*

### Available forms
Available by prescription only
*Topical solution:* 0.2%
*Ointment:* 0.2% soluble dressing
*Cream:* 0.2%

### Indications and dosages
*Adjunct for major burns (especially when resistance to other anti-infectives occurs); prevention of skin-graft infection before or after surgery*
*Adults and children:* Apply directly to lesion or to dressings used to cover affected area daily or as indicated, depending on severity of burn. Apply once daily or q few days, depending on dressing technique.

## Mechanism of action
*Antibacterial action:* Exact mechanism of action is unknown. However, it appears that drug inhibits bacterial enzymes involved in carbohydrate metabolism. Nitrofurazone has a broad spectrum of activity against gram-positive and gram-negative organisms.

## Pharmacokinetics
*Absorption:* Limited drug absorption with topical use.
*Distribution:* None.
*Metabolism:* None.
*Excretion:* None.

| Route | Onset | Peak | Duration |
|-------|-------|------|----------|
| Topical | Unknown | Unknown | Unknown |

## Contraindications and precautions
Contraindicated in patients hypersensitive to drug. Use cautiously in patients with known or suspected renal impairment.

## Interactions
None reported.

## Adverse reactions
**Skin:** *erythema, pruritus,* burning, edema, severe reactions (vesiculation, denudation, ulceration), *allergic contact dermatitis.*

## Overdose and treatment
If overdose occurs, recommend stopping drug and cleansing area with mild soap and water.

## Clinical considerations
■ Investigationally, drug has been given orally for the treatment of refractory African trypanosomiasis, acute bacillary dysentry, and testicular tumors. Diluted nitrofurazone solution with 6 to 10 parts of sterile water has been used for bladder irrigation.
■ Avoid contact with eyes and mucous membranes.
■ If undiluted solution is cloudy, warm to 122° to 140° F (50° to 60° C).
■ Solutions for wet dressings are prepared by diluting nitrofurazone solution with distilled water (equal parts of each).
■ Use diluted solutions within 24 hours after preparation; discard diluted solution that becomes cloudy.

### Therapeutic monitoring
■ Advise clinician to monitor patient for overgrowth of nonsusceptible organisms, including fungi and *Pseudomonas.*

### Special populations
**Breast-feeding patients.** Safety in breast-feeding women hasn't been established. Potential benefits to mother must be weighed against risks to infant.

---

## Patient counseling
- Teach patient proper application of drug and to apply directly on lesion or place on gauze.
- Tell patient to avoid exposure of drug to direct sunlight, excessive heat, strong fluorescent lighting, and alkaline materials.

# nitroglycerin (glyceryl trinitrate)

*Oral, extended-release*
Niong, Nitro-Bid, Nitrocine, Nitroglyn

*Sublingual*
Nitroquick, Nitrostat

*Translingual*
Nitrolingual

*I.V.*
Nitro-Bid IV, Tridil

*Topical*
Nitro-Bid, Nitrol

*Transdermal*
Deponit, Minitran, Nitro-Derm, Nitrodisc, Nitro-Dur, Transderm-Nitro

*Transmucosal*
Nitrogard

*Pharmacologic classification:* nitrate
*Therapeutic classification:* antianginal, vasodilator
*Pregnancy risk category C*

## Available forms
Available by prescription only
*Tablets (S.L.):* 0.15 mg, 0.3 mg, 0.4 mg, 0.6 mg
*Tablets (buccal, controlled-release):* 1 mg, 2 mg, 3 mg
*Capsules (sustained-release):* 2.5 mg, 6.5 mg, 9 mg, 13 mg
*Aerosol (lingual):* 0.4 mg/metered spray
*I.V.:* 0.5 mg/ml, 0.8 mg/ml, 5 mg/ml
*I.V. premixed solutions in dextrose:* 100 mcg/ml, 200 mcg/ml, 400 mcg/ml
*Topical:* 2% ointment
*Transdermal:* 0.1-mg, 0.2-mg, 0.3-mg, 0.4-mg, 0.6-mg, 0.8-mg/hour systems

## Indications and dosages
**Prophylaxis against chronic anginal attacks**
*Adults:* 2.5 to 9 mg P.O. q 8 to 12 hours; or 2% ointment. Start with ½-inch ointment, increasing with ½-inch increments until headache occurs, then decreasing to previous dose. Range of dosage with ointment is 0.5 to 4 inches q 4 to 6 hours. Usual dose is 1 to 2 inches.

Alternatively, transdermal disc or pad may be applied to hairless site once daily. However, to prevent tolerance, topical forms shouldn't be worn overnight.
**Relief of acute angina pectoris, prophylaxis to prevent or minimize anginal attacks when taken immediately before stressful events**
*Adults:* One S.L. tablet dissolved under the tongue or in the buccal pouch immediately on indication of anginal attack. May repeat q 5 minutes for 15 to 30 minutes for a maximum of three doses. Or, using Nitrolingual spray, spray one or two doses into mouth, preferably onto or under the tongue. May repeat q 3 to 5 minutes to a maximum of three doses within a 15-minute period. Or, transmucosally, 1 to 3 mg q 3 to 5 hours during waking hours.
**Hypertension, heart failure, angina**
Nitroglycerin is indicated to control hypertension from surgery, to treat HF from MI, to relieve angina pectoris in acute situations, and to produce controlled hypotension during surgery (by I.V. infusion).
*Adults:* Initial infusion rate is 5 mcg/minute. May be increased by 5 mcg/minute q 3 to 5 minutes until a response is noted. If a 20-mcg/minute rate doesn't produce desired response, dosage may be increased by as much as 10 to 20 mcg/minute q 3 to 5 minutes.
**Acute myocardial infarction**
*Adults:* Initially, 12.5 to 25 mcg I.V. followed by an infusion at 10 to 20 mcg/minute; increase 5 to 10 mcg/minute q 5 to 10 minutes p.r.n. Maximum dose is 200 mcg/minute. Decrease or discontinue if mean arterial pressure is under 80 mm Hg or systolic blood pressure under 90 mm Hg.
◊ **Hypertensive crisis**
*Adults:* Infuse at 5 to 100 mcg/minute I.V.

## I.V. administration
- Administration as I.V. infusion requires special nonabsorbent tubing supplied by manufacturer because regular plastic tubing may absorb up to 80% of drug.
- Prepare infusion in a glass bottle or container.

### Incompatibilities
Incompatible with alteplase, hydralazine, and phenytoin sodium. Avoid mixing with other drugs.

## Mechanism of action
*Antianginal action:* Nitroglycerin relaxes vascular smooth muscle of both the venous and arterial beds, resulting in a net decrease in myocardial oxygen consumption. It also dilates coronary vessels, leading to redistribution of blood flow to ischemic tissue. Systemic and coronary vascular effects of drug, which may vary slightly with the various nitroglycerin forms, probably account for its value in treating angina.

*Vasodilating action:* Nitroglycerin dilates peripheral vessels, making it useful (in I.V. form) in producing controlled hypotension during surgical procedures and in controlling blood pressure in perioperative hypertension. Because peripheral vasodilation decreases venous return to the heart (preload), nitroglycerin also helps to treat pulmonary edema and HF. Arterial vasodilation decreases arterial impedance (afterload), thereby decreasing left ventricular work and aiding the failing heart. These combined effects may prove valuable in treating some patients with acute MI.

## Pharmacokinetics
*Absorption:* Well absorbed from the GI tract. However, because it undergoes first-pass metabolism in the liver, it's incompletely absorbed into the systemic circulation. Onset of action for oral preparations is slow (except for S.L. tablets). After S.L. administration, absorption from the oral mucosa is relatively complete. Nitroglycerin also is well absorbed after topical administration as an ointment or transdermal system.
*Distribution:* Distributed widely throughout the body. About 60% of circulating drug is plasma protein–bound.
*Metabolism:* Metabolized in the liver and serum to 1,3 glyceryl dinitrate; 1,2 glyceryl dinitrate; and glyceryl mononitrate. Dinitrate metabolites have a slight vasodilatory effect.
*Excretion:* Metabolites are excreted in urine; elimination half-life is about 1 to 4 minutes.

| Route | Onset | Peak | Duration |
|---|---|---|---|
| P.O. | 20-45 min | Unknown | 3-8 hr |
| Buccal | 3 min | Unknown | 3-5 hr |
| S.L. | 1-3 min | Unknown | ½-1 hr |
| I.V. | Immediate | Immediate | 3-5 min |
| Translingual | 2-4 min | Unknown | ½-1 hr |
| Topical | 30 min | Unknown | 2-12 hr |
| Transdermal | 30 min | Unknown | 24 hr |

## Contraindications and precautions
Contraindicated in patients hypersensitive to nitrates and in those with early MI (S.L. form), severe anemia, increased intracranial pressure, angle-closure glaucoma, orthostatic hypotension, and allergy to adhesives (transdermal form). I.V. form is contraindicated in patients hypersensitive to I.V. form, cardiac tamponade, restrictive cardiomyopathy, or constrictive pericarditis. Extended-release preparations shouldn't be used in patients with organic or functional GI hypermotility or malabsorption syndrome.

Use cautiously in patients with hypotension or volume depletion.

## Interactions
**Drug-drug.** *Antihypertensives, phenothiazines:* May cause additive hypotensive effects. Use together cautiously.
*Ergot alkaloids:* May precipitate angina. Avoid use together.
*Sildenafil:* Potentiates hypotensive effects of nitrates. Don't use together.
**Drug-lifestyle.** *Alcohol use:* May cause additive hypotensive effects. Discourage use together.

## Adverse reactions
**CNS:** *headache, sometimes with throbbing; dizziness;* weakness.
**CV:** *orthostatic hypotension, tachycardia, flushing, palpitations,* fainting.
**GI:** nausea, vomiting, S.L. burning.
**Skin:** cutaneous vasodilation, contact dermatitis (patch), rash.
**Other:** hypersensitivity reactions.

## Overdose and treatment
Effects of overdose result primarily from vasodilation and methemoglobinemia and include hypotension, persistent throbbing headache, palpitations, visual disturbances, flushing of the skin, sweating (with skin later becoming cold and cyanotic), nausea and vomiting, colic, bloody diarrhea, orthostasis, initial hyperpnea, dyspnea, slow respiratory rate, bradycardia, heart block, increased intracranial pressure with confusion, fever, paralysis, tissue hypoxia (from methemoglobinemia) leading to cyanosis, and metabolic acidosis, coma, clonic seizures, and circulatory collapse. Death may result from circulatory collapse or asphyxia.

Treatment includes gastric lavage followed by administration of activated charcoal to remove remaining gastric contents. Advise clinician to monitor blood gas measurements and methemoglobin levels, as indicated. Supportive care includes respiratory support and oxygen administration, passive movement of the limbs to aid venous return, and recumbent positioning.

## Clinical considerations
■ Ask patient about use of sildenafil before using nitrates.
■ Recommend using only S.L. and translingual forms to relieve acute angina attack.
■ S.L. dose may be given before anticipated stress or h.s. if angina is nocturnal.
■ To apply ointment, recommend spreading it in uniform thin layer to hairless part of skin except distal parts of arms or legs, because absorption won't be maximal at these sites. Don't rub in. Recommend covering with plastic film to aid absorption and to protect clothing. If using Tape-Surrounded Appli-Ruler (TSAR) system, recommend keeping TSAR on skin to protect patient's clothing and ensure that ointment remains in place. If serious adverse effects de-

velop in patients using ointment or transdermal system, product should be removed at once or ointment wiped from skin. Contact with ointment should be avoided.

■ Recommend removing transdermal patch before defibrillation. Because of patch's aluminum backing, electric current may cause patch to explode.

■ When terminating transdermal nitroglycerin treatment for angina, dosage and frequency of application should be gradually reduced over 4 to 6 weeks.

■ If drug causes headache, which is especially likely with initial doses, aspirin or acetaminophen may be indicated. Dosage may need to be reduced temporarily.

■ Drug may cause orthostatic hypotension. To minimize this, patient should change to upright position slowly, go up and down stairs carefully, and lie down at the first sign of dizziness.

■ To prevent withdrawal symptoms, dosage should be reduced gradually after long-term use of oral or topical preparations.

■ Nitrate tolerance may develop.

■ Nitroglycerin may interfere with serum cholesterol determination tests using the Zlatkis-Zak color reaction, resulting in falsely decreased values.

**⚠ ALERT** Don't confuse Nitro-Bid with Nicobid or nitroglycerin with nitroprusside.

### Therapeutic monitoring

■ When drug is given to patients during initial days after acute MI, advise clinician to monitor hemodynamic and clinical status carefully.

■ Advise clinician to monitor blood pressure and intensity and duration of patient's response to drug.

### Special populations
**Pediatric patients.** Methemoglobinemia may occur in infants receiving large doses of nitroglycerin.

## Patient counseling

■ Instruct patient to take drug regularly, as prescribed, and to keep S.L. form accessible at all times. Drug is physiologically needed but not addictive.

■ Teach to take oral tablet on empty stomach, either 30 minutes before or 1 to 2 hours after meals, to swallow oral tablets whole, and to chew chewable tablets thoroughly before swallowing.

■ Instruct patient to take S.L. tablet at first sign of angina attack. Tell him to wet tablet with saliva, place it under the tongue until completely absorbed, and sit down and rest. If no relief occurs after three tablets, he should call or go to hospital emergency room. If he complains of tingling sensation with drug placed S.L., he may try holding tablet in buccal pouch.

■ Advise patient to store S.L. tablets in original container or other container specifically approved for this use away from heat and light. Keep cap to bottle tightly closed.

■ Instruct patient not to use extended-release nitroglycerin for acute angina atttacks.

■ Instruct patient to place transmucosal tablet under upper lip or in buccal pouch, to let it dissolve slowly over a 3- to 5-hour period, and not to chew or swallow tablet. Advise him that dissolution rate may increase if he touches tablet with tongue or drinks hot liquids.

■ If patient is receiving nitroglycerin lingual aerosol (Nitrolingual), instruct him how to use this device correctly. Remind him not to inhale spray but to release it onto or under the tongue. Also tell him not to swallow immediately after administering the spray but to wait about 10 seconds before swallowing.

■ Caution patient to use care when wearing transdermal patch near a microwave oven because leaking radiation may heat metallic backing of patch and cause burns.

■ Warn patient that headache may follow initial doses but that this symptom may respond to usual headache remedies or dosage reduction (dosage should be reduced only with medical approval). Assure patient that headache usually subsides gradually with continued treatment.

■ Instruct patient to avoid alcohol while taking drug because severe hypotension and CV collapse may occur.

■ Warn patient that drug may cause dizziness or flushing and to move to an upright position slowly.

■ Tell patient to report blurred vision, dry mouth, or persistent headache.

## nitroprusside sodium
Nipride*, Nitropress

*Pharmacologic classification:* vasodilator
*Therapeutic classification:* antihypertensive
*Pregnancy risk category C*

## Available forms
Available by prescription only
*Injection:* 50 mg/2-ml, 50 mg/5-ml vials

## Indications and dosages
### Hypertensive emergencies
*Adults and children:* Initial dose is 0.25 to 3 mcg/kg/minute. I.V. infusion titrated to blood pressure, with a range of 0.3 to 10 mcg/kg/minute. Maximum infusion rate is 10 mcg/kg/minute for 10 minutes. If an adequate blood pressure response isn't achieved at this rate, discontinue infusion.
### Acute heart failure
*Adults and children:* I.V. infusion titrated to cardiac output and systemic blood pressure.

Same dosage range as for hypertensive emergencies.

## I.V. administration

■ Prepare solution using $D_5W$ solution; don't use bacteriostatic water for injection or sterile saline solution for reconstitution; because of light sensitivity, foil-wrap I.V. solution (but not tubing). Fresh solutions have faint brownish tint; discard after 24 hours.

■ The concentrated solution is further diluted in 250, 500, or 1,000 ml $D_5W$ to produce a concentration of 200, 100, or 50 mcg/ml, respectively.

■ Infuse drug with infusion pump.

■ Drug is best run piggyback through a peripheral line with no other drugs; rate of main I.V. line shouldn't be adjusted while drug is running because even small boluses can cause severe hypotension.

### Incompatibilities

Incompatible with bacteriostatic water for injection. Don't add any other drug or preservative to nitroprusside solution.

## Mechanism of action

*Antihypertensive action:* Nitroprusside acts directly on vascular smooth muscle, causing peripheral vasodilation.

## Pharmacokinetics

*Absorption:* Administered I.V.
*Distribution:* Unknown.
*Metabolism:* Metabolized rapidly in erythrocytes and tissues to a cyanide radical and then converted to thiocyanate in the liver.
*Excretion:* Excreted primarily as metabolites in urine. Blood pressure returns to pretreatment level 1 to 10 minutes after completion of infusion.

| Route | Onset | Peak | Duration |
|-------|-------|------|----------|
| I.V. | 1-2 min | Immediate | 10 min |

## Contraindications and precautions

Contraindicated in patients hypersensitive to drug and those with compensatory hypertension (such as in arteriovenous shunt or coarctation of the aorta), inadequate cerebral circulation, congenital optic atrophy, or tobacco-induced amblyopia.

Use cautiously in patients with renal or hepatic disease, increased intracranial pressure, hypothyroidism, hyponatremia, or low vitamin $B_{12}$ levels.

## Interactions

**Drug-drug.** *General anesthetics, particularly enflurane and halothane:* Potentiated hypotensive effects. Advise clinician to monitor blood pressure carefully.

*Nitroprusside:* May potentiate antihypertensive effects of other antihypertensives. Use together cautiously.

*Pressor drugs such as epinephrine:* May cause an increase in blood pressure during nitroprusside therapy. Advise clinician to monitor blood pressure carefully.

*Sildenafil:* Potentiates hypotensive effects of nitrates. Don't use together.

## Adverse reactions

**CNS:** *headache, dizziness, loss of consciousness, apprehension, **increased intracranial pressure**, restlessness.*
**CV:** ***bradycardia***, *hypotension, tachycardia, palpitations, ECG changes.*
**GI:** *nausea, abdominal pain, ileus.*
**GU:** *increased serum creatinine.*
**Metabolic:** *acidosis, methemoglobinemia, hypothyroidism.*
**Musculoskeletal:** *muscle twitching.*
**Skin:** pink color, flushing, rash, diaphoresis.
**Other:** *thiocyanate toxicity, cyanide toxicity, venous streaking, irritation at infusion site.*

## Overdose and treatment

Signs and symptoms of overdose include the adverse reactions listed above and increased tolerance to the antihypertensive effects of drug.

Recommend treating overdose by giving nitrites to induce methemoglobin formation. Recommend stopping drug and giving amyl nitrite inhalations for 15 to 30 seconds each minute until a 3% sodium nitrite solution can be prepared. Advise clinician to give amyl nitrite cautiously to minimize risk of additional hypotension secondary to vasodilation. Then the sodium nitrite solution should be administered by I.V. infusion at a rate not exceeding 2.5 to 5 ml/minute up to a total dose of 10 to 15 ml. Should be followed with I.V. sodium thiosulfate infusion (12.5 g in 50 ml of $D_5W$ solution) over 10 minutes. If needed, infusions of sodium nitrite and sodium thiosulfate may be repeated at half the initial doses. Further treatment involves symptomatic and supportive care.

## Clinical considerations

■ Ask patient about use of sildenafil before using nitrates.

■ Drug also may be used to produce controlled hypotension during anesthesia, to reduce bleeding from surgical procedure.

■ Hypertensive patients are more sensitive to nitroprusside than normotensive patients. Also, patients taking other antihypertensives are extremely sensitive to nitroprusside. Nitroprusside has been used in patients with acute MI, refractory HF, and severe mitral regurgitation.

■ The goal of therapy is to reduce the mean arterial pressure by 25% within minutes to 2 hours.

### Therapeutic monitoring
■ Advise clinician to monitor blood pressure at least every 5 minutes at start of infusion and every 15 minutes thereafter during infusion.
■ Nitroprusside can cause cyanide toxicity; therefore, check serum thiocyanate levels every 72 hours; levels above 100 mcg/ml indicate cyanide toxicity, which can produce profound hypotension, metabolic acidosis, dyspnea, ataxia, and vomiting. If such symptoms occur, recommend stopping infusion and reevaluating therapy.

### Special populations
**Breast-feeding patients.** It isn't known if drug appears in breast milk; give with caution to breast-feeding women.
**Geriatric patients.** Geriatric patients may be more sensitive to antihypertensive effects of drug.

## Patient counseling
■ Advise patient to report CNS symptoms, such as headache or dizziness, promptly.

---

# nizatidine
Axid, Axid AR

*Pharmacologic classification:* H$_2$-receptor antagonist
*Therapeutic classification:* antiulcerative
*Pregnancy risk category B*

## Available forms
Available by prescription only
*Capsules:* 150 mg, 300 mg
Available without a prescription
*Capsules:* 75 mg

## Indications and dosages
**Treatment of active duodenal ulcer, gastric ulcer**
*Adults:* 300 mg P.O. once daily h.s. Alternatively, may give 150 mg P.O. b.i.d. for up to 8 weeks.
**Maintenance therapy for duodenal ulcer patients**
*Adults:* 150 mg P.O. once daily h.s. for up to 1 year.
**Gastroesophageal reflux disease**
*Adults:* 150 mg P.O. b.i.d. up to 12 weeks.
**Heartburn (self-medication)**
*Adults and children ages 12 and older:* One 75-mg capsule P.O. 30 to 60 minutes before meals; use up to b.i.d. not to exceed continuous therapy for 2 weeks.
≡ *Dosage adjustment.* For adults with renal impairment, refer to the following table.

| Creatinine clearance (ml/min) | Active duodenal ulcer | Maintenance dose |
|---|---|---|
| 20-50 | 150 mg/day | 150 mg q other day |
| < 20 | 150 mg q other day | 150 mg q 3 days |

## Mechanism of action
*Antiulcer action:* Nizatidine is a competitive, reversible inhibitor of H$_2$ receptors, particularly those in the gastric parietal cells.

## Pharmacokinetics
*Absorption:* Well absorbed (more than 90%) after oral administration. Absorption may be slightly enhanced by food, and slightly impaired by antacids.
*Distribution:* About 35% plasma protein–bound.
*Metabolism:* Probably undergoes hepatic metabolism. About 40% of excreted drug is metabolized; the remainder is excreted unchanged.
*Excretion:* More than 90% of an oral dose is excreted in urine within 12 hours. Renal clearance is about 500 ml/minute, which indicates excretion by active tubular secretion. Less than 6% of a given dose is eliminated in the feces. Elimination half-life is 1 to 2 hours. Moderate to severe renal impairment significantly prolongs half-life and decreases clearance of nizatidine. In anephric persons, half-life is 3½ to 11 hours; plasma clearance is 7 to 14 L/hour.

| Route | Onset | Peak | Duration |
|---|---|---|---|
| P.O. | ½ hr | ½-3 hr | 12 hr |

## Contraindications and precautions
Contraindicated in patients hypersensitive to H$_2$-receptor antagonists. Use cautiously in patients with impaired renal function.

## Interactions
**Drug-drug.** *High doses of aspirin (3,900 mg/day) with nizatidine (150 mg twice-daily):* Increases serum salicylate levels. Advise clinician to monitor salicylate levels.
**Drug-food.** *Tomato-based mixed-vegetable juices:* May decrease potency of drug when used together. Advise patient not to use together.

## Adverse reactions
**CNS:** somnolence.
**CV:** *arrhythmias.*
**Hematologic:** eosinophilia.
**Hepatic:** hepatocellular injury, elevated liver function test results.
**Metabolic:** hyperuricemia.
**Skin:** *diaphoresis,* rash, urticaria.
**Other:** fever.

---

Reactions may be *common,* uncommon, **life-threatening,** or COMMON AND LIFE-THREATENING.

## Overdose and treatment
Expected effects of overdose are cholinergic, including lacrimation, salivation, emesis, miosis, and diarrhea. Treatment may include use of activated charcoal, emesis, or lavage, with clinical monitoring and supportive therapy.

## Clinical considerations
■ Because drug is excreted primarily by the kidneys, recommend reducing dosage in patients with moderate to severe renal insufficiency.
■ Nizatidine is partially metabolized in the liver. In patients with normal renal function and uncomplicated hepatic dysfunction, the disposition of nizatidine is similar to that in patients with normal hepatic function.
■ For patients on maintenance therapy, consider that effects of continuous drug therapy for over 1 year aren't known.
■ False-positive tests for urobilinogen may occur during nizatidine therapy.

### Therapeutic monitoring
■ Advise clinician to monitor liver function test results in prolonged therapy and BUN and creatinine levels in patients with renal impairment.

### Special populations
**Breast-feeding patients.** Use with caution in breast-feeding women.
**Pediatric patients.** Safety and efficacy in children haven't been established.
**Geriatric patients.** Safety and efficacy appear similar to those in younger patients. However, consider that geriatric patients have reduced renal function.

## Patient counseling
■ Advise patient not to smoke because this may increase gastric acid secretion and worsen the disease.
■ Tell patient not to mix drug with tomato-based mixed-vegetable juices.
■ Advise patient to report abdominal pain and blood in stools or emesis to prescriber immediately.

---

# norepinephrine bitartrate (formerly levarterenol bitartrate)
Levophed

*Pharmacologic classification:* adrenergic (direct-acting)
*Therapeutic classification:* vasopressor
*Pregnancy risk category C*

## Available forms
Available by prescription only
*Injection:* 1 mg/ml parenteral

## Indications and dosages
*Hypotension, shock, cardiopulmonary resuscitation*
*Adults:* Initially, 8 to 12 mcg/minute I.V. infusion; then titrated to maintain desired blood pressure; maintenance dose, 2 to 4 mcg/minute.
*Children:* Initially, 2 mcg/minute or 2 mcg/m²/minute I.V. infusion, then titrated to maintain desired blood pressure. For advanced cardiac life support, initial infusion rate is 0.1 mcg/kg/minute.
◇ *GI bleeding*
*Adults:* 8 mg in 250 ml normal saline solution given intraperitoneally, or 8 mg in 100 ml normal saline solution given via a nasogastric tube q hour for 6 to 8 hours then q 2 hours for 4 to 6 hours.

## I.V. administration
■ Prepare infusion solution by adding 4 mg norepinephrine to 1 L of $D_5W$. The resultant solution contains 4 mcg/ml.
■ Injection site should be selected carefully. Administration by I.V. infusion requires an infusion pump or other device to control flow rate. If possible, recommend infusing into antecubital vein of the arm or the femoral vein and changing injection sites for prolonged therapy. Must be diluted before use with $D_5W$ or saline (dilution with saline alone isn't recommended). Drug should be withdrawn gradually; recurrent hypotension may follow abrupt withdrawal.

### Incompatibilities
Incompatible with aminophylline, amobarbital, cephalothin, cephapirin, chlorothiazide, chlorpheniramine, lidocaine, pentobarbital sodium, phenobarbital sodium, phenytoin sodium, secobarbital, sodium bicarbonate, sodium iodide, streptomycin, thiopental, and whole blood. Don't mix drug with normal saline alone.

## Mechanism of action
*Vasopressor action:* Norepinephrine acts predominantly by direct stimulation of alpha-adrenergic receptors, constricting both capacitance and resistance blood vessels. This results in increased total peripheral resistance; increased systolic and diastolic blood pressure; decreased blood flow to vital organs, skin, and skeletal muscle; and constriction of renal blood vessels, which reduces renal blood flow. It also has a direct stimulating effect on beta₁ receptors of the heart, producing a positive inotropic response. Its main therapeutic effects are vasoconstriction and cardiac stimulation.

## Pharmacokinetics
*Absorption:* Administered I.V.
*Distribution:* Localizes in sympathetic nerve tissues. It crosses the placenta but not the blood-brain barrier.

---

*Metabolism:* Metabolized in the liver and other tissues to inactive compounds.

*Excretion:* Excreted in urine primarily as sulfate and glucuronide conjugates. Small amounts are excreted unchanged in urine.

| Route | Onset | Peak | Duration |
|-------|-------|------|----------|
| I.V. | Immediate | Immediate | 1-2 min after infusion ends |

## Contraindications and precautions

Contraindicated in patients with mesenteric or peripheral vascular thrombosis, profound hypoxia, hypercapnia, or hypotension resulting from blood volume deficit and during cyclopropane and halothane anesthesia.

Use cautiously in patients with sulfite allergies or in those receiving MAO inhibitors or triptyline- or imipramine-type antidepressants. Use with caution in patients with ischemic heart disease because the drug increases myoardial oxygen requirements.

## Interactions

**Drug-drug.** *Atropine:* Blocks the reflex bradycardia caused by norepinephrine and enhances its pressor effects. Use together cautiously.

*Beta blockers:* May result in an increased potential for hypertension; propranolol may be used to treat arrhythmias occurring during norepinephrine administration. Use together cautiously.

*Furosemide, other diuretics:* May decrease arterial responsiveness. Advise clinician to monitor blood pressure for effect.

*General anesthetics:* Norepinephrine may cause increased arrhythmias. Use together cautiously.

*Guanethidine, MAO inhibitors, methyldopa, parenteral ergot alkaloids, some antihistamines, tricyclic antidepressants:* Severe, prolonged hypertension. Avoid use together.

## Adverse reactions

**CNS:** anxiety, weakness, dizziness, tremor, restlessness, insomnia.

**CV:** *bradycardia, severe hypertension, arrhythmias.*

**Respiratory:** respiratory difficulties, *asthmatic episodes.*

**Other:** *anaphylaxis,* irritation or necrosis with extravasation.

## Overdose and treatment

Signs and symptoms of overdose include severe hypertension, photophobia, retrosternal or pharyngeal pain, intense sweating, vomiting, cerebral hemorrhage, seizures, and arrhythmias. Monitor vital signs closely.

Treatment includes supportive and symptomatic measures. Use atropine for reflex bradycardia, phentolamine for extravasation, and propranolol for tachyarrhythmias.

## Clinical considerations

■ Recommend correcting blood volume depletion before administration. Norepinephrine isn't a substitute for blood, plasma, fluid, or electrolyte replacement.

■ To treat extravasation, recommend infiltrating site promptly with 10 to 15 ml saline solution containing 5 to 10 mg phentolamine, using a fine needle.

■ Some clinicians add phentolamine (5 to 10 mg) to each liter of infusion solution as a preventive against sloughing, should extravasation occur.

■ In patients with previously normal blood pressure, recommend adjusting flow rate to maintain blood pressure at low normal (usually 80 to 100 mm Hg systolic); in hypertensive patients, recommend maintaining systolic no more than 40 mm Hg below preexisting pressure level.

■ Avoid contact of drug with iron salts, alkalies, or oxidizing drugs.

■ Protect solution from light. Discard solution that's discolored or contains a precipitate.

### Therapeutic monitoring

■ Advise clinician to monitor intake and output. Norepinephrine reduces renal blood flow, which may cause decreased urine output initially.

■ Recommend observing patient constantly during administration of norepinephrine. Recommend obtaining baseline blood pressure and pulse before therapy and repeating every 2 minutes until stabilization; should be repeated every 5 minutes during drug administration.

■ In addition to vital signs, advise clinician to monitor patient's mental state, skin temperature of limbs, and skin color (especially earlobes, lips, and nail beds).

### Special populations

**Pediatric patients.** Use with caution in children.

**Geriatric patients.** Drug hasn't been evaluated systematically in patients ages 65 and older. No specific dosage recommendations.

## Patient counseling

■ Inform patient of need for frequent monitoring of vital signs.

■ Advise patient to report adverse reactions.

# norethindrone
Micronor, Nor-Q.D.

# norethindrone acetate
Aygestin, Norlutate*

*Pharmacologic classification:* progestin
*Therapeutic classification:* contraceptive
*Pregnancy risk category X*

## Available forms
Available by prescription only
**norethindrone**
*Tablets:* 0.35 mg
**norethindrone acetate**
*Tablets:* 5 mg

## Indications and dosages
*Amenorrhea, abnormal uterine bleeding, endometriosis*
**norethindrone acetate**
*Adults:* 2.5 to 10 mg P.O. daily on days 5 to 10 of second half of menstrual cycle.
*Endometriosis*
**norethindrone acetate**
*Adults:* 5 mg P.O. daily for 14 days, then increase by 2.5 mg/day q 2 weeks up to 15 mg/day. Daily therapy may be continued consecutively for 6 to 9 months; if breakthrough bleeding occurs, temporarily discontinue therapy.
*Contraception*
**norethindrone**
*Adults:* 0.35 mg P.O. daily, beginning day 1 of menstrual cycle and continuing uninterrupted thereafter.

## Mechanism of action
*Contraceptive action:* Norethindrone suppresses ovulation, causes thickening of cervical mucus, and induces sloughing of the endometrium.

## Pharmacokinetics
*Absorption:* Well absorbed after oral administration.
*Distribution:* Distributed into bile, appears in breast milk, and is about 80% protein-bound.
*Metabolism:* Primarily metabolized in the liver, where it undergoes extensive first-pass metabolism.
*Excretion:* Excreted primarily in feces. Elimination half-life is 5 to 14 hours.

| Route | Onset | Peak | Duration |
|-------|-------|------|----------|
| P.O. | Unknown | Unknown | Unknown |

## Contraindications and precautions
Contraindicated in patients with thromboembolic disorders, cerebral apoplexy, or history of these conditions; breast cancer, undiagnosed abnormal vaginal bleeding; severe hepatic disease; missed abortion; during pregnancy; and in patients hypersensitive to drug.
Use cautiously in patients with diabetes mellitus, seizures, migraine, cardiac or renal disease, asthma, or mental depression.

## Interactions
**Drug-drug.** *Bromocriptine:* Amenorrhea or galactorrhea, thus interfering with the action of bromocriptine. Don't use together.

## Adverse reactions
**CNS:** depression, *CVA.*
**CV:** thrombophlebitis, *pulmonary embolism,* edema, *thromboembolism.*
**EENT:** exophthalmos, diplopia, retinal thrombosis.
**GU:** breakthrough bleeding, dysmenorrhea, amenorrhea, cervical erosion, abnormal secretions.
**Hepatic:** cholestatic jaundice.
**Metabolic:** changes in weight, decreased pregnanediol excretion, increased serum alkaline phosphatase and amino acid levels, glucose tolerance.
**Skin:** melasma, rash, acne, pruritus.
**Other:** breast tenderness, enlargement, or secretion.

## Overdose and treatment
No information available.

## Clinical considerations
**H ALERT** Norethindrone acetate is twice as potent as norethindrone. Norethindrone acetate shouldn't be used for contraception.
■ Use as a test for pregnancy isn't appropriate; drug may cause birth defects and masculinization of female fetus.
■ Preliminary estrogen treatment is usually needed in menstrual disorders.

### Therapeutic monitoring
■ Advise clinician to monitor liver function test results in patients with hepatic impairment.
■ Recommend observing patient for signs of edema; blood pressure should be monitored.

## Patient counseling
■ FDA regulations require that patient reads package insert explaining possible adverse reactions, before receiving first dose.
■ Tell patient to use drug at same time of day every day of the year when used as a contraceptive.
■ Tell patient with visual disturbances or migraine to stop drug and notify prescriber immediately.
■ Inform patient of procedure if drug dose is missed.

# norfloxacin (systemic)
Noroxin

*Pharmacologic classification:* fluoroquinolone
*Therapeutic classification:* broad-
spectrum antibiotic
*Pregnancy risk category C*

## Available forms
Available by prescription only
*Tablets:* 400 mg

## Indications and dosages
***Complicated and uncomplicated urinary
tract infections caused by various gram-
negative and gram-positive bacteria***
*Adults:* For complicated infection, 400 mg P.O.
b.i.d. for 10 to 21 days; for uncomplicated in-
fection, 400 mg P.O. b.i.d. for 3 to 10 days.
Don't exceed 800 mg/day. Patients with crea-
tinine clearance less than 30 ml/minute should
receive 400 mg/day for appropriate duration
of therapy.
***Uncomplicated gonorrhea***
*Adults:* 800 mg P.O. as a single dose.
***Prostatitis***
*Adults:* 400 mg P.O. q 12 hours for 28 days.
◇ ***Gastroenteritis***
*Adults:* 400 mg P.O. b.i.d. for 5 days.
◇ ***Treatment of traveler's diarrhea***
*Adults:* 400 mg P.O. b.i.d. for up to 3 days.

## Mechanism of action
*Antibacterial action:* Norfloxacin is generally
bactericidal. It inhibits DNA gyrase, blocking
DNA synthesis. Spectrum of activity includes
most aerobic gram-positive and gram-negative
urinary pathogens, including *Pseudomonas
aeruginosa.*

## Pharmacokinetics
*Absorption:* About 30% to 40% of dose is absorbed from the GI tract; as dose increases,
percentage of absorbed drug decreases. Food
may reduce absorption.
*Distribution:* Distributed into renal tissue, liver, gallbladder, prostatic fluid, testicles, seminal fluid, bile, and sputum. From 10% to 15%
plasma protein–bound.
*Metabolism:* Unknown.
*Excretion:* Most of systemically absorbed drug
is excreted by the kidneys, with about 30% appearing in feces. In patients with normal renal
function, plasma half-life is 3 to 4 hours; up to
8 hours in severe renal impairment.

| Route | Onset | Peak | Duration |
|-------|-------|------|----------|
| P.O. | Unknown | ½-2 hr | Unknown |

## Contraindications and precautions
Contraindicated in patients hypersensitive to
fluoroquinolones. Use cautiously in patients
with renal impairment or conditions predisposing them to seizure disorders, such as cerebral arteriosclerosis.

## Interactions
**Drug-drug.** *Antacids:* Decreased absorption.
Give drugs at separate times.
*Multivitamins containing divalent or trivalent
cations:* May interfere with absorption of norfloxacin. Give drugs at separate times.
*Nitrofurantoin:* Antagonizes antibacterial activity of norfloxacin. Advise clinician to monitor patient for clinical effect.
*Probenecid:* May increase serum norfloxacin
levels. Advise clinician to monitor patient for
toxicity.
*Warfarin:* Prolonged PT. Advise clinician to
monitor PT and INR.
*Xanthine derivatives, such as aminophylline
and theophylline:* May increase theophylline
level. Advise clinician to monitor patient for
xanthine-related toxicities.
**Drug-food.** *Any food:* Interferes with absorption of norfloxacin. Give drug 1 hour before
meals or 2 hours after meals.
**Drug-lifestyle.** *Sun exposure:* May cause photosensitivity reaction. Advise patient to take
precautions.

## Adverse reactions
**CNS:** fatigue, somnolence, headache, dizzi-
ness, *seizures,* depression, insomnia.
**GI:** nausea, constipation, flatulence, heartburn,
dry mouth, abdominal pain, diarrhea, vomit-
ing, anorexia.
**GU:** increased serum creatinine and BUN lev-
els, crystalluria.
**Hematologic:** eosinophilia, *neutropenia,* de-
creased hematocrit.
**Hepatic:** transient elevations of AST, ALT, and
alkaline phosphatase.
**Musculoskeletal:** back pain, tendinitis.
**Skin:** photosensitivity.
**Other:** hypersensitivity reactions (rash, ***anaphylactoid reaction***), fever; hyperhidrosis.

## Overdose and treatment
No information available.

## Clinical considerations
■ Culture and sensitivity tests should be obtained before therapy starts and repeated p.r.n.
throughout therapy.
■ Patient should be well hydrated before and
during therapy to avoid crystalluria.
**H** ***ALERT*** Drug may cause false-positive opiate results in urinary assays.
■ The CDC and Hawaii Department of Health
advise that fluoroquinolones not be used to
treat gonorrhea in Hawaii, or in patients who
likely acquired gonorrhea in Hawaii, Ohio, the
Pacific Islands, Asia, or Australia. This strain
of gonorrhea is resistant to fluoroquinolones.

---

### *Therapeutic monitoring*
■ Advise clinician to monitor baseline and follow-up BUN level, creatinine clearance, CBC, and liver function test results.
■ Recommend observing patient for signs and symptoms of resistant infection or reinfection.

### *Special populations*
**Breast-feeding patients.** Safety in breast-feeding women hasn't been established; an alternative to breast-feeding is recommended during treatment.
**Pediatric patients.** Contraindicated in children.

### Patient counseling
■ Instruct patient to continue taking drug as directed, even if he feels better.
■ Advise patient to take drug 1 hour before or 2 hours after meals and antacids.
■ Warn patient that drug may cause dizziness that impairs his ability to perform tasks that require alertness and coordination.
■ Instruct patient to avoid excessive exposure to sunlight.

---

# norgestrel
Ovrette

*Pharmacologic classification:* progestin
*Therapeutic classification:* contraceptive
*Pregnancy risk category X*

### Available forms
Available by prescription only
*Tablets:* 0.075 mg

### Indications and dosages
*Contraception*
*Adults:* 1 tablet P.O. daily, beginning on first day of menstruation.

### Mechanism of action
*Contraceptive action:* Norgestrel suppresses ovulation and causes thickening of cervical mucus.

### Pharmacokinetics
*Absorption:* Well absorbed.
*Distribution:* No information available.
*Metabolism:* No information available.
*Excretion:* No information available.

| Route | Onset | Peak | Duration |
|-------|-------|------|----------|
| P.O. | Unknown | Unknown | Unknown |

### Contraindications and precautions
Contraindicated in patients with thromboembolic disorders, cerebral apoplexy, or history of these conditions; breast cancer; undiagnosed abnormal vaginal bleeding; severe hepatic disease; missed abortion; during pregnancy; and in patients hypersensitive to drug.
Use cautiously in patients with renal or cardiac disease, diabetes mellitus, migraine, seizures, asthma, or mental depression.

### Interactions
**Drug-drug.** *Bromocriptine:* May cause amenorrhea or galactorrhea, interfering with the action of bromocriptine. Don't give together.

### Adverse reactions
**CNS:** *cerebral thrombosis or hemorrhage,* migraine, depression, *CVA.*
**CV:** thrombophlebitis, *pulmonary embolism,* edema, *thromboembolism.*
**EENT:** exophthalmos, diplopia.
**GU:** *breakthrough bleeding, change in menstrual flow,* dysmenorrhea, spotting, amenorrhea, cervical erosion.
**Hepatic:** cholestatic jaundice, increased serum alkaline phosphatase.
**Metabolic:** increased amino acid levels, changes in weight, decreased pregnanediol excretion, glucose tolerance.
**Skin:** melasma, rash, acne, pruritus.
**Other:** breast tenderness, enlargement, or secretion.

### Overdose and treatment
No information available.

### Clinical considerations
■ Failure rate of the progestin-only contraceptive is about three times higher than that of the combination contraceptives.
■ Ovrette tablets contain tartrazine. Use cautiously in patients with tartrazine or aspirin sensitivity.

### *Therapeutic monitoring*
■ Advise clinician to monitor liver function test results in patients with hepatic impairment or during prolonged therapy.

### *Special populations*
**Breast-feeding patients.** If possible, advise breast-feeding women not to use oral contraceptives until infant is completely weaned because drug may interfere with breast-feeding by decreasing the quantity and quality of breast milk. Recommend other means of contraception.

### Patient counseling
■ Tell patient to take drug at the same time every day, even during menstruation. Norgestrel is also known as the "minipill."
■ Advise patient of increased risk of serious adverse CV reactions from heavy smoking, especially while taking oral contraceptives.

---

■ Tell patient that risk of pregnancy increases with each tablet missed. If one tablet is missed, she should take it as soon as she remembers and then take the next tablet at the regular time. If two tablets are missed, she should take one as soon as she remembers and then take the next regular dose at the usual time; she should use a nonhormonal method of contraception in addition to norgestrel until 14 tablets have been taken. If three or more tablets are missed, she should discontinue drug and use a non-hormonal method of contraception until after her period. Instruct patient to take a pregnancy test if her menstrual period doesn't occur within 45 days.

■ Advise patient to report excessive bleeding or bleeding between menstrual cycles immediately.

■ Instruct patient to use a second method of birth control for the first cycle on norgestrel, or for 3 weeks after starting the hormonal contraceptive, to ensure full protection.

■ Advise patient who wishes to become pregnant to wait at least 3 months after discontinuing norgestrel, to prevent birth defects.

---

# nortriptyline hydrochloride
Aventyl, Pamelor

*Pharmacologic classification:* tricyclic antidepressant
*Therapeutic classification:* antidepressant
*Pregnancy risk category NR*

## Available forms
Available by prescription only
*Capsules:* 10 mg, 25 mg, 50 mg, 75 mg
*Solution:* 10 mg/5 ml (4% alcohol)

## Indications and dosages
*Depression,* ◇ *panic disorder*
Adults: 25 mg P.O. t.i.d. or q.i.d., gradually increasing to a maximum of 150 mg/day. Alternatively, entire dosage may be given h.s.
*Elderly and adolescents:* 30 to 50 mg P.O. daily or in divided doses.
◇ *Smoking cessation*
Adults: Initially, 25 mg P.O. daily; gradually increase to target dose of 75 to 100 mg P.O. daily. Therapy is continued for 12 weeks. Initiate therapy 10 to 28 days before the date set for smoking cessation.

## Mechanism of action
*Antidepressant action:* Drug is thought to exert its antidepressant effects by inhibiting reuptake of norepinephrine and serotonin in CNS nerve terminals (presynaptic neurons), which results in increased levels and enhanced activity of these neurotransmitters in the synaptic cleft. Nortriptyline inhibits reuptake of serotonin more actively than norepinephrine; it's

less likely than other tricyclic antidepressants to cause orthostatic hypotension.

## Pharmacokinetics
*Absorption:* Absorbed rapidly from the GI tract after oral administration.
*Distribution:* Distributed widely into the body, including the CNS; appears in breast milk; 95% protein-bound. Steady-state serum levels are achieved within 2 to 4 weeks. Therapeutic serum level ranges from 50 to 150 ng/ml.
*Metabolism:* Metabolized by the liver; a significant first-pass effect may account for variability of serum levels in different patients taking the same dosage.
*Excretion:* Mostly excreted in urine; some in feces, via the biliary tract.

| Route | Onset | Peak | Duration |
|-------|-------|------|----------|
| P.O. | Unknown | 7-8½ hr | Unknown |

## Contraindications and precautions
Contraindicated during acute recovery phase of MI and in patients hypersensitive to drug or those who have had MAO therapy within past 14 days. Use cautiously in patients with history of urine retention or seizures, glaucoma, suicidal tendencies, CV disease, or hyperthyroidism and in those receiving thyroid hormone.

## Interactions
**Drug-drug.** *Antiarrhythmics, such as disopyramide, procainamide and quinidine; pimozide; thyroid hormones:* May increase risk of arrhythmias and conduction defects. Use together cautiously.
*Atropine and other anticholinergics, including antihistamines, antiparkinsonians, meperidine, and phenothiazines:* Oversedation, paralytic ileus, visual changes, and severe constipation. Use together cautiously.
*Barbiturates:* Induce nortriptyline metabolism and decrease therapeutic efficacy. Advise clinician to monitor patient closely.
*Beta blockers, cimetidine, methylphenidate, oral contraceptives, propoxyphene:* May inhibit nortriptyline metabolism, increasing plasma levels. Advise clinician to monitor patient for toxicity.
*Centrally acting antihypertensives, such as clonidine, guanabenz, guanadrel, guanethidine, methyldopa, and reserpine:* Decreased hypotensive effects. Advise clinician to monitor blood pressure.
*CNS depressants, including analgesics, anesthetics (oversedation), barbiturates, narcotics, and tranquilizers:* Additive effects. Use together cautiously.
*Disulfiram, ethchlorvynol:* May cause delirium and tachycardia. Avoid use together.
*Metrizamide:* Increased risk of seizures. Avoid use together, if possible.

---

Reactions may be *common*, uncommon, ***life-threatening***, or COMMON AND LIFE-THREATENING.

*Haloperidol, phenothiazines:* Decreased nortriptyline metabolism. Advise clinician to monitor patient closely.

*Sympathomimetics, including epinephrine, phenylephrine, phenylpropanolamine, and ephedrine (often found in nasal sprays):* May increase blood pressure. Use together cautiously.

*Warfarin:* May increase PT and cause bleeding. Advise clinician to monitor PT and INR.

**Drug-herb.** *St. John's wort, SAMe, yohimbe:* Use with some tricyclic antidepressants may cause elevation of serotonin levels. Discourage concomitant use.

**Drug-lifestyle.** *Alcohol use:* Additive effects. Advise patient to avoid alcohol use.

*Heavy smoking:* Induces nortriptyline metabolism and decreases therapeutic efficacy. Advise patient to avoid smoking.

## Adverse reactions

**CNS:** *CVA, drowsiness, dizziness, seizures,* tremor, weakness, confusion, headache, nervousness, EEG changes, extrapyramidal reactions, insomnia, nightmares, hallucinations, paresthesia, ataxia, agitation.

**CV:** *tachycardia,* hypertension, hypotension, *MI, heart block,* prolonged conduction time (elongation of QT and PR intervals, flattened T waves on ECG).

**EENT:** *blurred vision,* tinnitus, mydriasis.

**GI:** dry mouth, *constipation,* nausea, vomiting, anorexia, paralytic ileus.

**GU:** *urine retention,* elevated liver function test results.

**Hematologic:** *bone marrow depression, agranulocytosis,* eosinophilia, *thrombocytopenia.*

**Metabolic:** increased serum glucose levels.

**Skin:** rash, urticaria, photosensitivity.

**Other:** *diaphoresis,* hypersensitivity reaction.

**After abrupt withdrawal of long-term therapy:** nausea, headache, malaise (doesn't indicate addiction).

## Overdose and treatment

The first 12 hours after acute ingestion are a stimulatory phase characterized by excessive anticholinergic activity, including agitation, irritation, confusion, hallucinations, hyperthermia, parkinsonian symptoms, seizures, urine retention, dry mucous membranes, pupillary dilation, constipation, and ileus. This is followed by CNS depressant effects, including hypothermia; decreased or absent reflexes; sedation; hypotension; cyanosis; and cardiac irregularities, including tachycardia, conduction disturbances, and quinidine-like effects on the ECG.

Severity of overdose is best indicated by prolonging QRS complex beyond 100 ms, which usually indicates a serum level above 1,000 ng/ml. Metabolic acidosis may follow hypotension, hypoventilation, and seizures.

Treatment is symptomatic and supportive, including maintaining a patent airway, stable body temperature, and fluid and electrolyte balance. Recommend inducing emesis with ipecac syrup if patient is conscious and following with gastric lavage and activated charcoal to prevent further absorption. Dialysis is usually ineffective. Recommend considering use of cardiac glycosides or physostigmine if serious CV abnormalities or cardiac failure occurs. Recommend treating seizures with parenteral diazepam or phenytoin; arrhythmias with parenteral phenytoin or lidocaine; and acidosis with sodium bicarbonate. Quinidine, procainamide, or disopyramide shouldn't be used to treat arrhythmias because these drugs can further depress myocardial conduction and contractility. Barbiturates shouldn't be given; these may enhance CNS and respiratory depressant effects.

## Clinical considerations

- Drug may be given at bedtime to reduce daytime sedation. Tolerance to sedative effects usually develops over the initial weeks of therapy.
- Recommend withdrawing drug gradually over a few weeks; however, it should be discontinued at least 48 hours before surgical procedures.
- Drug is available in liquid form.
- In patients with bipolar disorders, drug may cause symptoms of the manic phase to emerge.

### Therapeutic monitoring

- Advise clinician to monitor plasma notriptyline level if dose is over 100 mg/day.

### Special populations

**Breast-feeding patients.** Drug appears in breast milk in low levels; potential benefit to mother should outweigh potential harm to infant.

**Pediatric patients.** Drug isn't recommended for children. Lower dosages may be indicated for adolescents.

**Geriatric patients.** Lower dosages may be indicated. Geriatric patients are at greater risk for adverse cardiac effects. Nortriptyline is less likely to cause hypotension than other TCAs.

## Patient counseling

- Explain that patient may not see full effects of drug therapy for up to 4 weeks after start of therapy.
- Warn patient about sedative effects.
- Recommend taking full daily dose at bedtime to prevent daytime sedation.
- Instruct patient to avoid drinking alcohol, doubling doses after missing one, and discontinuing drug abruptly, unless instructed.
- Warn patient about possible dizziness. Tell patient to lie down for about 30 minutes after each dose at start of therapy and to avoid sudden orthostatic changes to prevent dizziness.

Orthostatic hypotension is usually less severe than with amitriptyline.

■ Urge patient to report unusual reactions promptly: confusion, movement disorders, fainting, rapid heartbeat, or difficulty urinating.

■ Tell patient to store drug away from children.

■ Suggest relieving dry mouth with sugarless chewing gum or candy.

■ Advise patient to avoid activities that require physical and mental alertness, such as driving a car or operating machinery.

# nystatin
Mycostatin, Nilstat

*Pharmacologic classification:* polyene macrolide
*Therapeutic classification:* antifungal
*Pregnancy risk category B*

## Available forms
Available by prescription only
*Tablets:* 500,000 units
*Suspension:* 100,000 units/ml
*Powder for suspension:* 50-, 150-, 500-million units; 1-, 2-, 5-billion units
*Vaginal suppositories:* 100,000 units
*Cream:* 100,000 units/g
*Ointment:* 100,000 units/g
*Powder:* 100,000 units/g
*Lozenges:* 200,000 units

## Indications and dosages
*GI infections*
*Adults:* 500,000 to 1 million units as oral tablets, t.i.d.
*Oropharyngeal candidiasis*
*Adults and children:* 400,000 to 600,000 units of oral suspension q.i.d. Alternatively, give 200,000 to 400,000 units (lozenges) four to five times daily for up to 14 days; allow to dissolve in mouth.
*Infants:* 200,000 units of oral suspension q.i.d.
*Neonates and premature infants:* 100,000 units of oral suspension q.i.d.
*Oropharyngeal candidiasis in HIV-infected patients*
*Adults:* 500,000 to 1,000,000 units three to five times daily as oral suspension or tablets (dissolved in mouth). Alternatively, oral lozenges may be used.
*Cutaneous or mucocutaneous candidal infections*
*Topical use:* Apply to affected areas b.i.d. or t.i.d. until healing is complete (about 2 weeks).
*Vaginal use:* 100,000 units, as vaginal tablets, inserted high into vagina daily or b.i.d. for 14 days.

For prevention of thrush in the neonate, 100,000- to 200,000-unit vaginal tablets daily for 3 to 6 weeks before delivery.

*Candidal diaper dermatitis*
*Infants:* 100,000 units of oral suspension P.O. q.i.d. as an adjunct to topical nystatin therapy.

## Mechanism of action
*Antifungal action:* Nystatin is both fungistatic and fungicidal. It binds to sterols in the fungal cell membrane, altering its permeability and allowing leakage of intracellular components. It acts against various yeasts and fungi, including *Candida albicans.*

## Pharmacokinetics
*Absorption:* Not absorbed from GI tract, nor through intact skin or mucous membranes.
*Distribution:* No detectable amount is available for tissue distribution.
*Metabolism:* No detectable amount is systemically available for metabolism.
*Excretion:* Oral nystatin is excreted almost entirely unchanged in feces.

| Route | Onset | Peak | Duration |
|-------|-------|------|----------|
| P.O., topical, intravaginal | Unknown | Unknown | Unknown |

## Contraindications and precautions
Contraindicated in patients hypersensitive to drug.

## Interactions
None reported.

## Adverse reactions
**GI:** transient nausea, diarrhea (usually with large oral dosage), vomiting (with oral administration or vaginal tablets).
**Skin:** occasional contact dermatitis from preservatives in some forms (with topical administration or vaginal tablets).

## Overdose and treatment
Overdose may result in nausea, vomiting, and diarrhea. Treatment is unnecessary because toxicity is negligible.

## Clinical considerations
■ Avoid hand contact with drug; hypersensitivity is rare but can occur.

■ For treatment of oral candidiasis, patient should have a clean mouth, and should hold suspension in mouth for several minutes before swallowing; for infant thrush, drug should be swabbed on oral mucosa.

■ May give immunosuppressed patient vaginal tablets (100,000 units) orally to provide prolonged drug contact with oral mucosa; alternatively, use clotrimazole troche.

■ For candidiasis of the feet, patient should dust powder on shoes and stockings as well as feet for maximal contact and effectiveness.

■ Avoid occlusive dressings or ointment on moist covered body areas that favor yeast growth.

■ To prevent maceration, recommend using cream on intertriginous areas, and powder on moist lesions.

■ Clean affected skin gently before topical application; cool, moist compresses applied for 15 minutes between applications help soothe dry skin.

■ Cleansing douches may be used by non-pregnant women for esthetic reasons; they should use preparations that don't contain antibacterials, which may alter flora and promote reinfection.

■ Protect drug from light, air, and heat.

■ Drug is ineffective in systemic fungal infection.

### Therapeutic monitoring
■ Advise clinician to monitor patient for proper use of drug and for clinical effect.

### Special populations
**Breast-feeding patients.** Safety in breast-feeding women hasn't been established.

## Patient counseling
■ Teach patient signs and symptoms of candidal infection. Inform patient about predisposing factors: use of antibiotics, oral contraceptives, and corticosteroids; diabetes; infected sexual partners; and tight-fitting pantyhose and undergarments.

■ Teach good oral hygiene. Explain that overuse of mouthwash and poorly fitting dentures, especially in geriatric patients, may alter flora and promote infection.

■ Tell patient to continue using vaginal cream through menstruation; emphasize importance of washing applicator thoroughly after each use.

■ Advise patient to change stockings and undergarments daily; teach good skin care.

■ Teach patient how to administer each dosage form prescribed.

■ Tell patient to continue drug for at least 48 hours after symptoms clear, to prevent reinfection.

# octreotide acetate
Sandostatin, Sandostatin LAR

*Pharmacologic classification:* synthetic octapeptide
*Therapeutic classification:* somatotropic hormone
*Pregnancy risk category B*

## Available forms
Available by prescription only
*Injection:* 0.05 mg/ml, 0.1 mg/ml, and 0.5 mg/ml in 1-ml ampules; 0.2 mg/ml and 1 mg/ml in 5-ml multidose vials
*Injection suspension, extended-release:* 10 mg/2 ml, 20 mg/2 ml, 30 mg/2 ml

## Indications and dosages
### Symptomatic treatment of flushing and diarrhea from carcinoid tumors
*Adults:* Initially, 100 to 600 mcg daily S.C. in two to four divided doses for first 2 weeks of therapy (usual daily dose, 300 mcg). Subsequent dosage based on individual response. 50 to 500 mcg I.V. and repeat, p.r.n.; prolonged I.V. infusion (such as 50 mcg/hour) infused over 8 to 24 hours also may be used. Also, 20 mg I.M. of suspension q 4 weeks for 2 months (after using injection for at least 2 weeks). Continue S.C. injection of immediate release for at least first 2 weeks of therapy with long-acting formulation. After 2 months, increase dose to 30 mg or decrease to 10 mg I.M. q 4 weeks p.r.n.
### Prevention of carcinoid crisis from surgery
*Adults:* 250 to 500 mcg S.C. 1 to 2 hours before induction of anesthesia.
### Symptomatic treatment of watery diarrhea from vasoactive intestinal peptide-secreting tumors
*Adults:* Initially, 200 to 300 mcg daily S.C. in two to four divided doses for first 2 weeks of therapy. Subsequent dosage based on individual response, but usually won't exceed 450 mcg daily. Also, 10 to 30 mg I.M. of suspension based on growth hormone concentration, insulin-like growth factor 1 (IGF-1), and symptom control q 4 weeks for 2 months (after using injection for at least 2 weeks). Continue S.C. injection of immediate release for at least first 2 weeks of therapy with long-acting formulation. After 2 months, increase dose to 30 mg or decrease to 10 mg I.M. q 4 weeks p.r.n.
### Acromegaly
*Adults:* Initially, 50 mcg t.i.d. S.C. Subsequent dosage based on individual response. Usual dosage is 100 to 200 mcg S.C. t.i.d. but some patients may require up to 500 mcg t.i.d. for maximum effectiveness. Patients currently receiving S.C. Sandostatin may be switched directly to Sandostatin LAR in a dose of 20 mg I.M. of suspension q 4 weeks for 3 months (after using S.C. injection for at least 2 weeks). After 3 months of receiving Sandostatin LAR, dosage adjustment is based on growth hormone concentration, IGF-1, and symptom control. Dose ranges from 10 to 40 mg I.M. q 4 weeks.

## I.V. administration
■ I.V. injection may be given undiluted for carcinoid crisis.
■ May be given by direct injection over 3 minutes or further diluted in 50 to 200 ml of $D_5W$ or normal saline solution and infused over 15 to 30 minutes.
■ Drug remains stable for 24 hours. Store ampules in the refrigerator. Drug may be stored at room temperature for 14 days.

### Incompatibilities
Incompatible with insulin and total parenteral nutrition solutions.

## Mechanism of action
*Antidiarrheal action:* Octreotide mimics the action of naturally occurring somatostatin and decreases the secretion of gastroenterohepatic peptides that may contribute to the adverse signs and symptoms seen in patients with metastatic carcinoid tumors and VIPomas. It isn't known if drug affects the tumor directly.

## Pharmacokinetics
*Absorption:* Administered parenterally.
*Distribution:* Distributed to the plasma, where it binds to serum lipoprotein and albumin.
*Metabolism:* Eliminated from the plasma at a slower rate than the naturally occurring hormone. Apparent half-life is about 1½ hours, with a duration of effect of up to 12 hours.
*Excretion:* About 35% appears unchanged in urine.

| Route | Onset | Peak | Duration |
|---|---|---|---|
| S.C. | ½ hr | ½ hr | < 12 hr |

or age or who are pharmacologically sensitive to drug.
- Efficacy for long-term use (longer than 6 weeks) hasn't been established.

### Therapeutic monitoring
- Advise clinician to monitor patient for signs of neuroleptic malignant syndrome (hyperpyrexia, muscle rigidity, altered mental status, autonomic instability), a rare but frequently fatal adverse reaction that may occur with the administration of antipsychotic drugs. Drug should be stopped immediately and patient monitored and treated.
- Advise clinician to monitor baseline and periodic liver function test results.

### Special populations
**Breast-feeding patients.** Drug appears in breast milk. Advise breast-feeding women to seek alternative feeding methods during therapy.
**Pediatric patients.** Safety and efficacy in children under age 18 haven't been established.
**Geriatric patients.** Drug may be initiated at lower dose because clearance may be decreased in geriatric patients. Half-life is 1½ times greater in this population.

## Patient counseling
- Warn patient to avoid hazardous tasks until adverse CNS effects of drug are known.
- Caution patient against exposure to extreme heat; drug may impair ability of the body to reduce core temperature.
- Advise patient to avoid alcohol.
- Tell patient to rise slowly to avoid orthostatic hypotension.
- Advise patient to use ice chips or sugarless candy or gum to relieve dry mouth.
- Inform patient not to take prescription or OTC drugs without medical approval because of potential drug interactions.

---

## olsalazine sodium
Dipentum

*Pharmacologic classification:* salicylate
*Therapeutic classification:* anti-inflammatory
*Pregnancy risk category C*

### Available forms
Available by prescription only
*Capsules:* 250 mg

### Indications and dosages
*Maintenance of remission of ulcerative colitis in patients intolerant of sulfasalazine*
*Adults:* 1 g P.O. daily in two divided doses.

## Mechanism of action
*Anti-inflammatory action:* Mechanism of action is unknown but appears to be topical rather than systemic. Drug is converted to mesalamine (5-aminosalicylic acid; 5-ASA) in the colon. Presumably, mesalamine diminishes inflammation by blocking cyclooxygenase and inhibiting prostaglandin production in the colon.

## Pharmacokinetics
*Absorption:* After oral administration, about 2.4% of a single dose is absorbed.
*Distribution:* Once metabolized to 5-ASA, drug is absorbed slowly from the colon, resulting in very high local levels.
*Metabolism:* 0.1% is metabolized in the liver; remainder will reach the colon, where it's rapidly converted to 5-ASA by colonic bacteria.
*Excretion:* Less than 1% is recovered in urine.

| Route | Onset | Peak | Duration |
|-------|-------|------|----------|
| P.O. | Unknown | 1 hr | Unknown |

## Contraindications and precautions
Contraindicated in patients hypersensitive to salicylates. Use cautiously in patients with existing renal disease.

## Interactions
**Drug-drug.** *Warfarin:* Increased PT. Advise clinician to monitor PT and INR.

## Adverse reactions
**CNS:** headache, depression, vertigo, dizziness, fatigue.
**GI:** *diarrhea,* nausea, *abdominal pain,* dyspepsia, bloating, anorexia, stomatitis.
**Musculoskeletal:** arthralgia.
**Skin:** rash, itching.

## Overdose and treatment
Decreased motor activity and diarrhea may occur. Overdose should be treated symptomatically and supportively.

## Clinical considerations
- Diarrhea from drug therapy is difficult to distinguish from underlying condition.

### Therapeutic monitoring
- Advise clinician to monitor CBC with differential and liver function test results periodically.

### Special populations
**Breast-feeding patients.** It's unknown if drug appears in breast milk. Use with caution in breast-feeding women.
**Pediatric patients.** Safety and efficacy in children haven't been established.

---

## Patient counseling
- Advise patient to take drug with food and in evenly divided doses.
- Inform patient to call prescriber if diarrhea develops.

---

## omeprazole
Prilosec

*Pharmacologic classification:* substituted benzimidazole
*Therapeutic classification:* gastric acid suppressant
*Pregnancy risk category C*

### Available forms
Available by prescription only
*Capsules (delayed-release):* 10 mg, 20 mg, 40 mg

### Indications and dosages
*Active duodenal ulcer*
*Adults:* 20 mg P.O. daily for 4 to 8 weeks.
**Helicobacter pylori** *eradication to reduce risk of duodenal ulcer recurrence*
**Triple therapy (omeprazole/clarithromycin/amoxicillin)**
*Adults:* 20 mg P.O. b.i.d. plus 500 mg clarithromycin P.O. b.i.d. plus 1,000 mg amoxicillin P.O. b.i.d. for 10 days. In patients with an ulcer present when therapy starts, an additional 18 days of omeprazole 20 mg once daily is recommended alone for ulcer healing and symptom relief.
**Drug-herb.** *Adults:* 40 mg q morning plus 500 mg clarithromycin t.i.d. for 14 days followed by 14 days of omeprazole 20 mg daily.
*Severe erosive esophagitis; symptomatic, poorly responsive gastroesophageal reflux disease (GERD)*
*Adults:* 20 mg P.O. daily for 4 to 12 weeks. Patients with GERD should have failed initial therapy with an H₂ antagonist. May continue with maintenance dosage of 20 mg daily for up to 1 year.
*Pathological hypersecretory conditions (such as Zollinger-Ellison syndrome)*
*Adults:* Initial dosage is 60 mg P.O. daily; adjust dosage based on patient response. Recommend giving daily doses exceeding 80 mg in divided doses. Doses up to 120 mg t.i.d. have been given. Continue therapy as long as clinically indicated.
*Gastric ulcer*
*Adults:* 40 mg P.O. daily for 4 to 8 weeks.
≡*Dosage adjustment.* Dosage adjustments aren't required for patients with impaired renal function; however, they may be needed in those with hepatic impairment. Dosage adjustments may be needed in Asian patients because of increased bioavailability of drug in this population.

## Mechanism of action
*Antisecretory action:* Omeprazole inhibits the activity of the acid (proton) pump, H⁺/K⁺ adenosine triphosphatase (ATPase), located at the secretory surface of the gastric parietal cell. This blocks the formation of gastric acid.

## Pharmacokinetics
*Absorption:* Omeprazole is acid-labile, and the formulation contains enteric-coated granules that permit absorption after drug leaves the stomach. Absorption is rapid. Bioavailability is about 40% because of instability in gastric acid as well as a substantial first-pass effect. Bioavailability increases slightly with repeated dosing, possibly because of drug's effect on gastric acidity.
*Distribution:* About 95% protein-bound.
*Metabolism:* Primarily metabolized in the liver.
*Excretion:* Primarily excreted by the kidneys. Plasma half-life is ½ to 1 hour, but drug effects may persist for days.

| Route | Onset | Peak | Duration |
|-------|-------|------|----------|
| P.O. | 1 hr | 2 hr | < 3 days |

## Contraindications and precautions
Contraindicated in patients hypersensitive to drug or its components.

## Interactions
**Drug-drug.** *Ampicillin esters, iron derivatives, itraconazole, ketoconazole:* Poor bioavailability because optimal absorption of these drugs requires a low gastric pH. Avoid use together.
*Diazepam, phenytoin, propranolol, theophylline, warfarin:* Effects may be impaired by omeprazole. Patient requires monitoring closely for decreased effect or toxicity.
**Drug-herb.** *Male fern:* Inactivated in alkaline environments. Advise patient of this effect.
*Pennyroyal:* May change the rate of formation of toxic metabolites of pennyroyal. Discourage use together.

## Adverse reactions
**CNS:** headache, dizziness, asthenia.
**GI:** diarrhea, abdominal pain, nausea, vomiting, constipation, flatulence.
**Musculoskeletal:** back pain.
**Respiratory:** cough, upper respiratory infection.
**Skin:** rash.

## Overdose and treatment
Reports of overdose are rare. Symptoms include confusion, drowsiness, blurred vision, tachycardia, nausea, vomiting, diaphoresis, dry mouth, and headache. Doses up to 360 mg daily have been well tolerated.
Dialysis is of little value because of the extent of binding to plasma proteins. Treatment should be symptomatic and supportive.

---

Reactions may be *common*, uncommon, *life-threatening*, or COMMON AND LIFE-THREATENING.

## Clinical considerations
■ Drug increases its own bioavailability with repeated administration. It is labile in gastric acid; less of it is lost to hydrolysis because drug elevates gastric pH.
■ Capsules shouldn't be crushed.

### Therapeutic monitoring
■ Advise clinician to monitor patient for clinical effects of therapy.
■ Advise clinician to monitor liver function test results in patients with hepatic impairment.

### Special populations
**Breast-feeding patients.** It isn't known if drug appears in breast milk. Avoid breast-feeding during therapy.
**Pediatric patients.** Safety in children hasn't been established.
**Geriatric patients.** No age-related differences have been reported.

## Patient counseling
■ Explain importance of taking drug exactly as prescribed.
■ Tell patient to take 30 minutes before meals and not to crush capsules.

# ondansetron hydrochloride
Zofran

*Pharmacologic classification:* serotonin (5-HT₃) receptor antagonist
*Therapeutic classification:* antiemetic
*Pregnancy risk category B*

## Available forms
Available by prescription only
*Injection:* 2 mg/ml in 20-ml multidose vials, 2-ml single-dose vials
*Injection, premixed:* 32 mg/50 ml in 5% dextrose single-dose vial
*Orally disintegrating tablets:* 4 mg, 8 mg
*Oral solution:* 4 mg/5 ml
*Tablets:* 4 mg, 8 mg

## Indications and dosages
*Prevention of nausea and vomiting from initial and repeat courses of emetogenic cancer chemotherapy, including high-dose cisplatin*
*Adults and children age 4 and older:* Three I.V. doses of 0.15 mg/kg with first dose infused over 15 minutes beginning 30 minutes before start of chemotherapy, with subsequent doses of 0.15 mg/kg given 4 and 8 hours after first dose. In adults, may also give as a single dose of 32 mg, infused over 15 minutes, 30 minutes before start of chemotherapy.
*Adults and children over age 12:* Initially, 8 mg P.O. starting 30 minutes before start of chemotherapy, with a repeat dose after the first dose,

then q 12 hours for 1 to 2 days after completion of chemotherapy.
*Children ages 4 to 11:* Initially, 4 mg given P.O. 30 minutes before start of chemotherapy with subsequent doses 4 and 8 hours after initial dose. Then 4 mg given P.O. q 8 hours for 1 to 2 days after completion of chemotherapy.
*Prevention of radiation-induced nausea and vomiting*
*Adults:* 8 mg P.O. t.i.d. First dose should be 1 to 2 hours before radiation treatment. Patients receiving single, high-dose radiation to abdomen should continue q 8-hour dosing for 1 to 2 days.
*Prevention of postoperative nausea and vomiting*
*Adults:* 16 mg P.O. 1 hour before anesthesia or 4 mg I.V. immediately before anesthesia or soon after operation. Alternatively, 4 mg I.M. undiluted as a single injection.
*Children ages 2 to 12 weighing over 40 kg (88 lb):* 4 mg I.V. as a single dose.
*Children ages 2 to 12 weighing 40 kg or less:* 0.1 mg/kg I.V. as a single dose.
≡*Dosage adjustment.* In patients with severe hepatic impairment, total daily dose shouldn't exceed 8 mg.

## I.V. administration
■ Drug may be administered I.V. undiluted over 2 to 5 minutes.
■ For infusion, dilute drug of 50 ml in compatible solution and infuse over 15 minutes.
■ Ondansetron is stable at room temperature for 48 hours after dilution with normal saline, D₅W, 5% dextrose and normal saline, 5% dextrose and 0.45% saline, or 3% saline.

### Incompatibilities
Incompatible with acyclovir sodium, allopurinol, aminophylline, amphotericin B, ampicillin sodium, ampicillin sodium and sulbactam sodium, amsacrine, cefepime, cefoperazone, fluorouracil, furosemide, ganciclovir, lorazepam, methylprednisolone sodium succinate, mezlocillin, piperacillin sodium, sargramostim, and sodium bicarbonate.

## Mechanism of action
*Antiemetic action:* Not well known. Ondansetron isn't a dopamine-receptor antagonist. Because serotonin receptors of the 5-HT₃ type occur peripherally on vagal nerve terminals and centrally in the chemoreceptor trigger zone, it's uncertain if antiemetic action is mediated centrally, peripherally, or both.

## Pharmacokinetics
*Absorption:* Absorption is variable with oral administration; bioavailability is 50% to 60%.
*Distribution:* 70% to 76% protein-bound.

*Metabolism:* Extensively metabolized by hydroxylation on the indole ring, followed by glucuronide or sulfate conjugation.
*Excretion:* 5% recovered in urine as parent compound. Half-life in adults is 3½ to 6 hours.

| Route | Onset | Peak | Duration |
|-------|-------|------|----------|
| P.O. | Unknown | 2 hr | Unknown |
| I.V. | Unknown | Unknown | Unknown |

## Contraindications and precautions
Contraindicated in patients hypersensitive to drug. Use cautiously in patients with hepatic failure. Orally disintegrating tablet contains aspartame; use cautiously in patients with phenylketonuria.

## Interactions
**Drug-herb.** *Horehound:* May enhance serotonergic effects. Discourage use together.

## Adverse reactions
**CNS:** *headache, malaise, fatigue, dizziness, sedation,* anxiety/agitation, oculogyric crisis.
**CV:** chest pain, hypotension.
**GI:** *diarrhea, constipation,* abdominal pain, xerostomia.
**GU:** urine retention, gynecologic disorders.
**Hepatic:** transient elevation of AST and ALT.
**Musculoskeletal:** *musculoskeletal pain.*
**Respiratory:** *hypoxia.*
**Skin:** rash, injection-site reaction.
**Other:** chills, fever, *anaphylaxis.*

## Overdose and treatment
Doses more than 10 times recommended dosage have been given without incident. If overdose is suspected, it should be managed with supportive therapy.

## Clinical considerations
■ Use cautiously in patients with hepatic failure.
■ Orally disintegrating tablet contains aspartame; use cautiously in patients with phenylketonuria.

### Therapeutic monitoring
■ Advise clinician to monitor liver function if giving repeated doses.
■ For patients undergoing abdominal surgery, advise clinician to monitor patient for ileus or gastric distension.

### Special populations
**Breast-feeding patients.** It's unknown if drug appears in breast milk. Use with caution in breast-feeding women.
**Pediatric patients.** Little information available for use in children age 3 and under for preventing chemotherapy-induced nausea and vomiting, and in children under age 2

for preventing postoperative nausea and vomiting.
**Geriatric patients.** No age-related problems have been reported.

## Patient counseling
■ Advise patient to report adverse effects.

# opium tincture, deodorized (laudanum)

# opium tincture, camphorated (paregoric)

*Pharmacologic classification:* opiate
*Therapeutic classification:* antidiarrheal
*Pregnancy risk category B (D for high doses or long term)*
*Controlled substance schedule II (deodorized) or III (camphorated)*

## Available forms
Available by prescription only
*Alcoholic solution:* 50 mg/5 ml, equivalent to morphine 10 mg/ml
*Alcoholic solution:* 5 ml contains: morphine, 2 mg; anise oil, 0.2 ml; benzoic acid, 20 mg; camphor, 20 mg; glycerin, 0.2 ml; and ethanol (to complete 5 ml volume)

## Indications and dosages
*Acute, nonspecific diarrhea*
Don't confuse doses of opium tincture and camphorated opium tincture.
*Adults:* 0.6 ml opium tincture (range, 0.3 to 1 ml) P.O. q.i.d. (maximum dose, 6 ml daily); or 5 to 10 ml camphorated opium tincture daily, b.i.d., t.i.d., or q.i.d. until diarrhea subsides.
*Children:* 0.25 to 0.5 ml/kg camphorated opium tincture daily, b.i.d., t.i.d., or q.i.d. until diarrhea subsides.
*Severe opiate withdrawal symptoms in neonates*
*Neonates:* Camphorated opium tincture or a 1:25 dilution of opium tincture in water, given as 0.2 ml P.O. q 3 hours. Adjust dosage to control withdrawal symptoms. Increase dosage by 0.05 ml q 3 hours until symptoms are controlled. Once symptoms are stabilized for 3 to 5 days, gradually decrease dosage over a 2- to 4-week period.

## Mechanism of action
*Antidiarrheal action:* Opium contains several ingredients. The most active, morphine, increases GI smooth-muscle tone, inhibits motility and propulsion, and diminishes secretions. By inhibiting peristalsis, the drug delays passage of intestinal contents, increasing water resorption and relieving diarrhea.

## Pharmacokinetics

*Absorption:* Absorbed variably from the gut.
*Distribution:* Although opium alkaloids are distributed widely in the body, the low doses used to treat diarrhea act primarily in the GI tract. Camphor crosses the placenta.
*Metabolism:* Metabolized rapidly in the liver.
*Excretion:* Opium is excreted in urine; opium alkaloids (especially morphine) appear in breast milk.

| Route | Onset | Peak | Duration |
|-------|-------|------|----------|
| P.O. | Unknown | Unknown | 4-5 hr |

## Contraindications and precautions

Contraindicated in patients with acute diarrhea caused by poisoning until toxic material is removed from GI tract or in those with diarrhea caused by organisms that penetrate intestinal mucosa.

Use cautiously in patients with asthma, prostatic hyperplasia, hepatic disease, and history of opium dependence.

## Interactions

**Drug-drug.** *Metoclopramide:* May antagonize the effects of metoclopramide. Avoid use together.
*Other CNS depressants:* Additive effect. Use together cautiously.

## Adverse reactions

**CNS:** dizziness, light-headedness.
**GI:** nausea, vomiting, increased serum amylase and lipase levels.
**Other:** physical dependence (after long-term use).

## Overdose and treatment

Signs and symptoms of overdose include drowsiness, hypotension, seizures, and apnea.

Stomach should be emptied by induced emesis or gastric lavage; patent airway should be maintained. Naloxone should be used to treat respiratory depression. Advise clinician to monitor patient for signs and symptoms of CNS or respiratory depression.

## Clinical considerations

■ Mix drug with sufficient water to ensure passage to stomach.
**H ALERT** Opium tincture, deodorized (laudanum) is 25 times more potent than camphorated opium tincture (paregoric); take care not to confuse these drugs. Camphorated opium tincture is more dilute, and teaspoon doses are easier to measure than dropper quantities of opium tincture.
■ When camphorated opium tincture is added to water, a milky fluid forms.
■ Risk of physical dependence on drug increases with long-term use.
■ Don't refrigerate drug.

■ Opium tincture and camphorated opium tincture may prevent delivery of technetium-99m disofenin in the small intestine during hepatobiliary imaging tests; test should be delayed until 24 hours after last dose.

### Therapeutic monitoring

■ Advise clinician to monitor patient's vital signs and bowel function.

### Special populations

**Breast-feeding patients.** Because opium alkaloids, especially morphine, appear in breast milk, possible risks must be weighed against benefits.
**Pediatric patients.** Opium tincture has been used to treat withdrawal symptoms in infants whose mothers are narcotic addicts.

## Patient counseling

■ Warn patient that physical dependence may result from long-term use.
■ Advise patient to use caution when driving a car or performing other tasks requiring alertness because drug may cause drowsiness, dizziness, and blurred vision.
■ Instruct patient to report diarrhea that persists longer than 48 hours because drug is indicated only for short-term use.
■ Advise patient to take drug with food if it causes nausea, vomiting, or constipation.
■ Instruct patient to call prescriber immediately if experiencing difficulty breathing or shortness of breath.
■ Instruct patient to drink adequate fluids while diarrhea persists.

# orlistat

Xenical

*Pharmacologic classification:* lipase inhibitor
*Therapeutic classification:* antiobesity drug
*Pregnancy risk category B*

## Available forms

Available by prescription only
*Capsules:* 120 mg

## Indications and dosages

*Management of obesity, including weight loss and weight maintenance with a reduced-calorie diet; reduction of risk of weight regain after prior weight loss*
*Adults:* 120 mg P.O. t.i.d. with each main meal containing fat (during or up to 1 hour after the meal).

## Mechanism of action

*Antiobesity action:* As a reversible inhibitor of lipases, orlistat forms a bond with the active site of gastric and pancreatic lipases. These inactivated enzymes are unavailable to hydrolyze dietary fat, in the form of triglycerides, into absorbable free fatty acids and monoglycerides. Because the undigested triglycerides aren't absorbed, the resulting caloric deficit may have a positive effect on weight control. The recommended dose of 120 mg t.i.d. inhibits dietary fat absorption by about 30%.

## Pharmacokinetics
*Absorption:* Systemic exposure to orlistat is minimal because only a small amount of the drug is absorbed.
*Distribution:* Extensively plasma protein–bound; lipoproteins and albumin are major binding proteins.
*Metabolism:* Primarily metabolized within the GI wall.
*Excretion:* Most of unabsorbed drug is excreted in feces.

| Route | Onset | Peak | Duration |
|-------|-------|------|----------|
| P.O. | Unknown | 8 hr | Unknown |

## Contraindications and precautions
Contraindicated in patients with chronic malabsorption syndrome, cholestasis, or known hypersensitivity to orlistat or to any component of this drug. Also, exclude organic causes of obesity such as hypothyroidism before starting patient on orlistat therapy.

Use cautiously in patients with a history of hyperoxaluria or calcium oxalate nephrolithiasis or a risk of anorexia nervosa or bulimia.

Use cautiously in patients receiving cyclosporine therapy because of the potential changes in cyclosporine absorption related to the variations in dietary intake.

## Interactions
**Drug-drug.** *Fat-soluble vitamins such as vitamin E and beta-carotene:* Absorption may be decreased by drug. Separate administration times by 2 hours.
*Pravastatin:* May cause slightly increased pravastatin levels and additive lipid-lowering effects of drug. Advise clinician to monitor patient carefully.
*Warfarin:* May cause possible change in coagulation parameters. Advise clinician to monitor PT and INR.

## Adverse reactions
**CNS:** *headache,* dizziness, fatigue, sleep disorder, anxiety, depression.
**CV:** pedal edema.
**EENT:** otitis.
**GI:** *oily spotting, flatus with discharge, fecal urgency, fatty or oily stool, oily evacuation, increased defecation, abdominal pain,* fecal incontinence, nausea, infectious diarrhea, rectal pain, vomiting.
**GU:** menstrual irregularity, vaginitis, urinary tract infection.

**Musculoskeletal:** *back pain,* pain in legs, arthritis, myalgia, joint disorder, tendonitis.
**Respiratory:** *influenza, upper respiratory tract infection,* lower respiratory tract infection.
**Skin:** rash, dry skin.
**Other:** tooth and gingival disorders.

## Overdose and treatment
If an overdose occurs, drug should be stopped and patient observed for 24 hours. Systemic effects attributable to the lipase-inhibiting properties of orlistat should be rapidly reversible.

## Clinical considerations
■ Drug is recommended for use in patients with an initial body mass index of 30 kg/m$^2$ or more, or 27 kg/m$^2$ or more and other risk factors, such as hypertension, diabetes, or dyslipidemia.
■ GI effects may increase when more than 30% of total daily calories come from fat.
■ Orlistat reduces absorption of some fat-soluble vitamins and beta-carotene.
■ It's unknown if orlistat is safe and effective to use in patients for longer than 2 years.

### Therapeutic monitoring
■ In diabetic patients, improved metabolic control may accompany weight loss, so the dosage of their oral antidiabetic (such as sulfonylureas and metformin) or insulin may need to be reduced. Advise clinician to monitor glucose level.

### Special populations
**Pregnant patients.** Not recommended for use in pregnant women; effects on fetus aren't known.
**Breast-feeding patients.** It's unknown if orlistat appears in breast milk; therefore, breast-feeding women shouldn't take the drug.
**Pediatric patients.** Safety and efficacy in pediatric patients haven't been established.
**Geriatric patients.** It isn't known if patients ages 65 and older respond differently to the drug than younger patients.

## Patient counseling
■ Advise patient to follow a nutritionally balanced, reduced-calorie diet that derives no more than 30% of calorie total from fat. If a meal is occasionally missed or contains no fat, instruct the patient to omit the concomitant dose.
■ Advise patient to take fat-soluble vitamins at least 2 hours before or after the administration of orlistat.
■ Tell patient with diabetes that weight loss may require dosage adjustment of oral antidiabetic or insulin.

# orphenadrine citrate
Antifles, Norflex, Orphenate

# orphenadrine hydrochloride
Disipal*

*Pharmacologic classification:* diphen-hydramine analogue
*Therapeutic classification:* skeletal muscle relaxant
*Pregnancy risk category C*

## Available forms
Available by prescription only
*Injection:* 30 mg/ml parenteral
*Tablets:* 50 mg, 100 mg
*Tablets (extended-release):* 100 mg

## Indications and dosages
**Adjunct in painful, acute musculoskeletal conditions**
*Adults:* 100 mg P.O. b.i.d., or 60 mg I.V. or I.M. q 12 hours. If used with acetylsalicylic acid and caffeine, 25 to 50 mg P.O. t.i.d. to q.i.d.
◊ **Leg cramps**
*Adults:* 100 mg P.O. h.s.

## I.V. administration
- Inject slowly over 5 minutes.
- Patient should be kept supine during and 5 to 10 minutes after injection. Paradoxical initial bradycardia may occur when giving I.V.; usually disappears in 2 minutes.

### Incompatibilities
None reported.

## Mechanism of action
*Skeletal muscle relaxant action:* Orphenadrine doesn't relax skeletal muscle directly. Atropine-like central action on cerebral motor centers or on the medulla may be the mechanism by which it reduces skeletal muscle spasm. Its reported analgesic effect may add to its skeletal muscle relaxant properties.

## Pharmacokinetics
*Absorption:* Rapidly absorbed from the GI tract.
*Distribution:* Widely distributed throughout the body.
*Metabolism:* Pathway unknown, but drug is almost completely metabolized to at least eight metabolites.
*Excretion:* Excreted in urine, mainly as its metabolites. Small amounts are excreted unchanged. Half-life is about 14 hours.

| Route | Onset | Peak | Duration |
|---|---|---|---|
| P.O. | 1 hr | 2 hr | 4-6 hr |
| I.V., I.M. | Unknown | Unknown | Unknown |

## Contraindications and precautions
Contraindicated in patients hypersensitive to drug; and those with glaucoma; prostatic hyperplasia; pyloric, duodenal, or bladder neck obstruction; myasthenia gravis; and peptic ulceration.

Use cautiously in geriatric or debilitated patients or in those with tachycardia, cardiac disease, arrhythmias, or sulfite allergy.

## Interactions
**Drug-drug.** *MAO inhibitors:* May increase CNS adverse effects. Use together cautiously.
*Other anticholinergics:* May increase anticholinergic effects. Use together cautiously.
*Propoxyphene or CNS depressants, such as antipsychotics, anxiolytics, and tricyclic antidepressants:* May produce additive CNS effects. If used together, doses of both drugs should be reduced.
**Drug-lifestyle.** *Alcohol use:* Additive CNS effects. Advise patient to avoid alcohol.

## Adverse reactions
**CNS:** weakness, *drowsiness,* light-headedness, confusion, agitation, tremor, headache, dizziness, hallucinations.
**CV:** palpitations, tachycardia, syncope.
**EENT:** dilated pupils, blurred vision, difficulty swallowing, increased intraocular pressure.
**GI:** constipation, *dry mouth,* nausea, vomiting, epigastric distress.
**GU:** urinary hesitancy, urine retention.
**Hematologic:** *aplastic anemia.*
**Skin:** urticaria, pruritus.
**Other:** *anaphylaxis.*

## Overdose and treatment
Signs and symptoms of overdose include dry mouth, blurred vision, urine retention, tachycardia, confusion, paralytic ileus, deep coma, seizures, shock, respiratory arrest, arrhythmias, and death.

Treatment includes symptomatic and supportive measures. If ingestion is recent, recommend inducing emesis or gastric lavage followed by activated charcoal. Advise clinician to monitor vital signs and fluid and electrolyte balance.

## Clinical considerations
- Some commercially available orphenadrine citrate injection formulations may contain sodium bisulfite, a sulfite that can cause allergic-type reactions, including anaphylaxis.

### Therapeutic monitoring
- Advise clinician to monitor periodic blood, urine, and liver function test results during prolonged therapy.
- Advise clinician to monitor vital signs, especially intake and output, noting urine retention.

---

* Canada only   ◊ Unlabeled clinical use

### Special populations
**Pediatric patients.** Safety and efficacy in children under age 12 haven't been established.
**Geriatric patients.** Geriatric patients may be more sensitive to effects of drug.

### Patient counseling
- Suggest ice chips, sugarless gum, hard candy, or saliva substitutes to relieve dry mouth.
- Tell patient to avoid hazardous activities that require alertness or physical coordination until CNS depressant effects can be determined.
- Warn patient to avoid alcohol and to use cough and cold preparations cautiously, because some contain alcohol.
- Tell patient to store drug away from heat and light (not in bathroom medicine cabinet) and safely out of reach of children.
- Instruct patient to take missed dose if remembered within 1 hour. Beyond 1 hour, skip the dose and return to regular schedule.

---

# oseltamivir phosphate
Tamiflu

*Pharmacologic classification:* influenza virus neuraminidase inhibitor
*Therapeutic classification:* antiviral
*Pregnancy risk category C*

### Available forms
Available by prescription only
*Capsules:* 75 mg
*Oral suspension:* 12 mg/ml after reconstitution

### Indications and dosages
*Treatment of uncomplicated, acute influenza A and B infection in adults symptomatic for 2 days or less*
*Adults:* 75 mg P.O. b.i.d. for 5 days, beginning within 2 days of symptom onset.
≡ *Dosage adjustment.* For patients with renal impairment (creatinine clearance less than 30 ml/min), 75 mg P.O. once daily for 5 days, beginning within 2 days of symptom onset.
*Prevention of influenza after close contact with infected person*
*Adults and adolescents ages 13 and older:* 75 mg P.O. once daily beginning within 2 days of exposure and lasting at least 7 days.
*Prevention of influenza during a community outbreak*
*Adults and adolescents ages 13 and older:* 75 mg P.O. once daily for up to 6 weeks.
*Treatment of influenza in children ages 1 and older*
*Children weighing 15 kg (33 lb) or less:* 30 mg oral suspension P.O. b.i.d.
*Children weighing 15 to 23 kg (33 to 51 lb):* 45 mg oral suspension P.O. b.i.d.
*Children weighing 23 to 40 kg (51 to 88 lb):* 60 mg oral suspension P.O. b.i.d.

*Children weighing over 40 kg (88 lb):* 75 mg oral suspension P.O. b.i.d.

### Mechanism of action
*Antiviral action:* Oseltamivir is hydrolyzed in the liver to its active form, oseltamivir carboxylase. Oseltamivir carboxylase inhibits the enzyme neuraminidase within the influenza virus particles. This action is thought to inhibit viral replication, possibly by interfering with viral particle aggregation and release from the host cell.

### Pharmacokinetics
*Absorption:* Well absorbed after oral administration. More than 75% of the given dose reaches the systemic circulation as oseltamivir carboxylase. Peak level of oseltamivir is 65.2 ng/ml whereas that of oseltamivir carboxylase is 348 ng/ml.
*Distribution:* Protein-binding is low for both oseltamivir (42%) and oseltamivir carboxylase (3%). Volume of distribution of oseltamivir carboxylase is 23 to 26 L.
*Metabolism:* Oseltamivir is extensively metabolized by hepatic esterases to its active component, oseltamivir carboxylase. Oseltamivir is neither a substrate nor an inhibitor of cytochrome P-450 oxidases.
*Excretion:* Oseltamivir carboxylase is almost entirely eliminated in the urine by way of glomerular filtration and tubular secretion. Less than 20% of the orally administered dose is eliminated in feces.

| Route | Onset | Peak | Duration |
|-------|-------|------|----------|
| P.O. | Unknown | Unknown | Unknown |

### Contraindications and precautions
Contraindicated in patients hypersensitive to any of the components of the formulation.

Use cautiously in patients with chronic cardiac disease, chronic respiratory disease, or any acute medical illness requiring hospitalization. The efficacy of oseltamivir hasn't been established in these settings.

### Interactions
None reported.

### Adverse reactions
**CNS:** dizziness, insomnia, headache, vertigo, fatigue.
**GI:** abdominal pain, diarrhea, nausea, vomiting.
**Respiratory:** bronchitis, cough.

### Overdose and treatment
Single doses as high as 1,000 mg have caused only nausea and vomiting. The entire 5-day course of therapy provides a total dose of 750 mg.

---

## Clinical considerations

- Oseltamivir doesn't appear to interfere with normal humoral antibody response to influenza infection.
- Consider the possibility of primary or concomitant bacterial infection when making treatment decisions.
- There's no evidence supporting prophylactic use of oseltamivir or the treatment of viral infections other than influenza virus type A and B.
- Cross-resistance between zanamivir and oseltamivir has been seen in influenza virus mutants generated in vitro; additional studies are needed.
- Nausea and vomiting are the most frequently occurring adverse effects. Administration with meals may alleviate GI symptoms.

### Therapeutic monitoring

- Advise clinician to monitor patient for adverse GI effects and clinical response of drug.

### Special populations

**Breast-feeding patients.** It's unknown if drug appears in breast milk. The potential benefits and potential risks of oseltamivir therapy on the breast-fed infant must be considered.
**Pediatric patients.** Safety and efficacy in children haven't been established.
**Geriatric patients.** Dosage reduction isn't required for geriatric patients, unless creatinine clearance is less than 30 ml/min.

## Patient counseling

- Advise patient to contact his prescriber as soon as possible to begin treatment within 2 days of onset of flu symptoms.
- Tell patient to complete the full 5 days of treatment, even when feeling better.
- Instruct patient that drug taking drug with food may help alleviate the adverse effects nausea and vomiting.
- Advise patient to take a missed dose as soon as possible; however, if the next dose is due within 2 hours, to skip the missed dose.
- Inform patient that drug is not a replacement for the influenza virus vaccine and to continue to receive vaccine each autumn.

## oxacillin sodium

Bactocill

*Pharmacologic classification:* penicillinase-resistant penicillin
*Therapeutic classification:* antibiotic
*Pregnancy risk category B*

## Available forms

Available by prescription only
*Capsules:* 250 mg, 500 mg
*Injection:* 250 mg, 500 mg, 1 g, 2 g, 4 g
*I.V. infusion:* 1 g, 2 g, 4 g

*Oral solution:* 250 mg/5 ml (after reconstitution)
*Pharmacy bulk package:* 10 g

## Indications and dosages

*Systemic infections caused by* **Staphylococcus aureus**
*Adults and children weighing over 40 kg (88 lb):* 500 mg P.O. q 4 to 6 hours for mild to moderate infections. Dose is 1 g P.O. q 4 to 6 hours when changing from I.V. to P.O. therapy. Alternatively, 250 to 500 mg I.M. or I.V. q 4 to 6 hours. For more severe infections, 1 g or more I.V. or I.M. q 4 to 6 hours. Serious infections are treated for 1 to 2 weeks.
*Children over age 1 month weighing under 40 kg:* 50 to 100 mg/kg P.O. daily, divided into doses given q 4 to 6 hours; 50 to 200 mg/kg I.M. or I.V. daily, divided into doses given q 4 to 6 hours. Doses vary based on severity of infection.
*Acute or chronic osteomyelitis caused by susceptible organisms*
*Adults:* 1.5 to 2 g I.V. q 4 hours for 4 to 8 weeks or I.V. dose for 5 to 28 days followed by P.O. dose for 3 to 6 weeks for a total of 6 weeks of therapy.
*Treatment of native valve endocarditis caused by methicillin-susceptible staphylococci*
*Adults:* 2 g I.V. q 4 hours for 4 to 6 weeks with gentamicin for the first 3 to 5 days.
*Treatment of prosthetic valve endocarditis caused by methicillin-susceptible staphylococci*
*Adults:* 2 g I.V. q 4 hours for 6 weeks or longer with gentamicin and rifampin.
≡*Dosage adjustment.* In adults with creatinine clearance below 10 ml/minute, 1 g I.M. or I.V. q 4 to 6 hours.

## I.V. administration

- For intermittent I.V. infusion, use sterile water for injection or normal saline injection; add 5 ml to 250-mg vial to equal 50 mg/ml. Add 5 ml, 10 ml, 20 ml, or 40 ml to vials containing 500 mg, 1 g, 2 g, or 4 g, respectively, and 93 ml to 10-g pharmacy bulk package to produce a concentration of 100 mg/ml. Inject slowly over 10 minutes.
- For continuous I.V. infusion, further dilute with compatible solution to 0.5 to 40 mg/ml concentration. Infuse over 30 to 60 minutes. Drug loses 10% of potency within 6 hours of dilution.

### Incompatibilities

Incompatible with acidic drugs, aminoglycosides, cytarabine, and verapamil hydrochloride.

## Mechanism of action

*Antibiotic action:* Oxacillin is bactericidal; it adheres to bacterial penicillin-binding proteins, thus inhibiting bacterial cell wall synthesis. Oxacillin resists the effects of penicillinases—enzymes that inactivate penicillin—and is thus active against many strains of penicillinase-producing bacteria; this activity is most important against penicillinase-producing staphylococci; some strains may remain resistant. Oxacillin is also active against a few gram-positive aerobic and anaerobic bacilli but has no significant effect on gram-negative bacilli.

## Pharmacokinetics

*Absorption:* Absorbed rapidly but incompletely from the GI tract; it's stable in an acid environment. Food decreases absorption.
*Distribution:* Distributed widely. CSF penetration is poor but enhanced by meningeal inflammation. Oxacillin crosses the placenta, and is 89% to 94% protein-bound.
*Metabolism:* Metabolized partially.
*Excretion:* Excreted primarily in urine by renal tubular secretion and glomerular filtration; it also appears in breast milk and is excreted in small amounts in bile. Elimination half-life in adults is ½ to 1 hour, extended to 2 hours in severe renal impairment. Dosage adjustments aren't required in patients with creatinine clearance less than 10 ml/minute.

| Route | Onset | Peak | Duration |
|---|---|---|---|
| P.O. | Unknown | ½-2 hr | Unknown |
| I.V. | Immediate | Immediate | Unknown |
| I.M. | Unknown | ½ hr | Unknown |

## Contraindications and precautions

Contraindicated in patients hypersensitive to drug or other penicillins.

Use cautiously in patients with other drug allergies (especially to cephalosporins), in neonates, and in infants.

## Interactions

**Drug-drug.** *Aminoglycosides:* Produces synergistic bactericidal effects against *S. aureus.* This is a therapeutic effect.
*Probenecid:* Blocks renal tubular secretion of penicillins, increasing their serum levels. Use together cautiously.
**Drug-food.** *Food:* Decreases absorption. Drug should be taken on an empty stomach.
*Fruit juice and carbonated beverages:* Interfere with absorption. Drug should be taken with water.

## Adverse reactions

**CNS:** neuropathy, neuromuscular irritability, *seizures,* lethargy, hallucinations, anxiety, confusion, agitation, depression, dizziness, fatigue.
**GI:** oral lesions, nausea, vomiting, diarrhea, enterocolitis, *pseudomembranous colitis.*
**GU:** interstitial nephritis, nephropathy.

**Hematologic:** *thrombocytopenia,* eosinophilia, *hemolytic anemia, neutropenia,* anemia, *agranulocytosis.*
**Hepatic:** elevated liver enzyme levels.
**Other:** hypersensitivity reactions (fever, chills, rash, urticaria, *anaphylaxis,* overgrowth of non-susceptible organisms, *thrombophlebitis*).

## Overdose and treatment

Signs of overdose include neuromuscular sensitivity or seizures. There are no specific recommendations.

Treatment is supportive. After recent ingestion (within 4 hours), recommend emptying the stomach by induced emesis or gastric lavage and following with activated charcoal to reduce absorption. Oxacillin isn't appreciably removed by peritoneal dialysis or hemodialysis.

## Clinical considerations

■ Coagulase-negative staphylococci causing prosthetic valve endocarditis is methicillin-resistant.
■ When given for group A beta-hemolytic streptococci, continue therapy for at least 10 days to decrease risk of glomerulonephritis and rheumatic fever.
■ Recommend giving oral drug with water only; acid in fruit juice or carbonated beverage may inactivate drug.
■ Recommend giving oral dose on empty stomach; food decreases absorption.
■ Except in osteomyelitis, drug shouldn't be given I.M. or I.V. unless patient can't take oral dose.
■ For oral preparation, add amount of water specified on bottle to provide a solution of 250 mg/5 ml. Add water in 2 parts and shake vigorously.
■ For I.M. preparation, add 1.4, 2.8, 5.7, 11.4, or 21.8 ml of sterile water for injection or 0.45% sodium chloride or normal saline injection to vial containing 250 mg, 500 mg, 1 g, 2 g, or 4 g, respectively. Final solution concentration is 250 mg/1.5 ml.
■ Oxacillin alters tests for urinary and serum proteins; turbidimetric urine and serum proteins are often falsely positive or elevated in tests using sulfosalicylic acid or trichloroacetic acid.
■ Oxacillin may falsely decrease serum aminoglycoside levels.

### Therapeutic monitoring

■ Advise clinician to monitor renal and hepatic function and hematologic function; recommend watching for elevated AST and ALT and report significant changes.

### Special populations

**Breast-feeding patients.** Oxacillin appears in breast milk. Use drug with caution in breast-feeding women.

**Pediatric patients.** Elimination of oxacillin is reduced in neonates. Transient hematuria, azotemia, and albuminuria have occurred in some neonates receiving oxacillin. Advise clinician to monitor renal function closely.

**Geriatric patients.** Half-life of drug may be prolonged in geriatric patients because of impaired renal function. Geriatric patients are at increased risk for thrombophlebitis during I.V. infusion.

## Patient counseling

■ Explain need to take oral preparations without food and to follow with water only, not fruit juice or carbonated beverages.

■ Tell patient to report allergic reactions or severe diarrhea promptly.

■ Emphasize importance of completing the full course of therapy.

# oxaprozin
Daypro

*Pharmacologic classification:* NSAID
*Therapeutic classification:* nonnarcotic analgesic, antipyretic, anti-inflammatory
*Pregnancy risk category C*

## Available forms
Available by prescription only
*Caplets:* 600 mg

## Indications and dosages
*Management of acute or chronic osteoarthritis or rheumatoid arthritis*
*Adults:* Initially, 1,200 mg P.O. daily. Individualize to smallest effective dosage to minimize adverse reactions. Smaller patients or those with mild symptoms may require only 600 mg daily. Maximum daily dose is 1,800 mg or 26 mg/kg, whichever is lower, in divided doses.
≡ *Dosage adjustment.* For patients with renal impairment or on hemodialysis, initial dose is 600 mg P.O. daily.

## Mechanism of action
*Analgesic, antipyretic, and anti-inflammatory actions:* Exact mechanism of action isn't clearly defined. It inhibits several steps along the arachidonic acid pathway of prostaglandin synthesis. One of the modes of action is presumed to be a result of the inhibition of cyclooxygenase activity and prostaglandin synthesis at the site of inflammation.

## Pharmacokinetics
*Absorption:* Shows high oral bioavailability (95%). Food may reduce the rate of absorption, but extent of absorption is unchanged.
*Distribution:* Bound to albumin in plasma.

*Metabolism:* Primarily metabolized in the liver by microsomal oxidation (65%) and glucuronic acid conjugation (35%).
*Excretion:* Glucuronide metabolites are excreted in urine (65%) and feces (35%). Elimination half-life in adults is 42 to 50 hours.

| Route | Onset | Peak | Duration |
|-------|-------|------|----------|
| P.O. | Unknown | 3-5 hr | Unknown |

## Contraindications and precautions
Contraindicated in patients hypersensitive to drug or with the syndrome of nasal polyps, angioedema, and bronchospastic reaction to aspirin or other NSAIDs.

Use cautiously in patients with renal or hepatic dysfunction, history of peptic ulcer, hypertension, CV disease, or conditions predisposing to fluid retention.

## Interactions
**Drug-drug.** *Aspirin:* Oxaprozin displaces salicylates from plasma protein–binding, increasing the risk of salicylate toxicity. Avoid use together.
*Beta blockers such as metoprolol:* May cause a transient increase in blood pressure after 14 days of therapy. Advise clinician to monitor blood pressure.
*Oral anticoagulants:* May increase the risk of bleeding. Advise clinician to monitor PT and INR.
**Drug-lifestyle.** *Sun exposure:* May cause photosensitivity reactions. Advise patient to use sunblock.

## Adverse reactions
**CNS:** depression, sedation, somnolence, confusion, sleep disturbances.
**EENT:** tinnitus, blurred vision.
**GI:** *nausea, dyspepsia, diarrhea, constipation,* abdominal pain or distress, anorexia, flatulence, vomiting, *hemorrhage,* stomatitis, ulcer.
**GU:** dysuria, urinary frequency.
**Hematologic:** prolonged bleeding time.
**Hepatic:** elevated liver function test results (with chronic use), *severe hepatic dysfunction.*
**Skin:** *rash,* photosensitivity.

## Overdose and treatment
No information specific to oxaprozin overdose is available. Common symptoms of acute overdose with other NSAIDs, including lethargy, drowsiness, nausea, vomiting, and epigastric pain, are generally reversible with supportive care. GI bleeding and coma have occurred after NSAID overdose. Hypertension, acute renal failure, and respiratory depression are rare.

Gut decontamination may be indicated in symptomatic patients seen within 4 hours of ingestion or after a large overdose (5 to 10 times the usual dose). This is accomplished by emesis or activated charcoal with an osmotic cathartic.

## Clinical considerations

- Serious GI toxicity, including peptic ulceration and bleeding, may occur in patients taking NSAIDs despite the absence of GI symptoms. Patients at risk for development of peptic ulceration and bleeding are those with history of serious GI events, alcoholism, smoking, or other factors that cause peptic ulcer disease.
- Dosages exceeding 1,200 mg/day should be used for patients who weigh over 50 kg (110 lb), who have normal renal and hepatic function, who are at low risk of peptic ulceration, and whose severity of disease justifies maximal therapy.
- Most patients tolerate once-daily dosing. Divided doses may be tried in patients unable to tolerate single doses.

### Therapeutic monitoring

- Elevations of liver function test results can occur after chronic use. These abnormal findings may persist, worsen, or resolve with continued therapy. Rarely, patients may progress to severe hepatic dysfunction. Periodically monitor liver function test results in patients receiving long-term therapy, and closely monitor patients with abnormal test results.
- Anemia may occur in patients receiving oxaprozin. Advise clinician to monitor hemoglobin level or hematocrit in patients with prolonged therapy at intervals appropriate for their clinical situation.

### Special populations

**Breast-feeding patients.** It's unknown if oxaprozin appears in breast milk. Use cautiously in breast-feeding women.
**Pediatric patients.** Safety and efficacy in children haven't been established.
**Geriatric patients.** Geriatric patients may need a reduced dosage because of low body weight or disorders caused by aging. Geriatric patients are less likely than younger patients to tolerate adverse reactions from oxaprozin.

## Patient counseling

- Warn patient to immediately report signs and symptoms of GI bleeding or visual or auditory adverse reactions.
- Tell patient to take drug with milk or meals if adverse GI reactions occur.
- Because photosensitivity reactions may occur, advise patient to use a sunblock, wear protective clothing, and avoid prolonged exposure to sunlight.

## oxazepam

Apo-Oxazepam\*, Novoxapam\*, Ox-pam\*, Serax

*Pharmacologic classification:* benzodiazepine
*Therapeutic classification:* anxiolytic, sedative-hypnotic
*Pregnancy risk category D*
*Controlled substance schedule IV*

## Available forms

Available by prescription only
*Capsules:* 10 mg, 15 mg, 30 mg
*Tablets:* 15 mg

## Indications and dosages

*Alcohol withdrawal, severe anxiety*
*Adults:* 15 to 30 mg P.O. t.i.d. or q.i.d.
*Tension, mild to moderate anxiety*
*Adults:* 10 to 15 mg P.O. t.i.d. or q.i.d.
≡*Dosage adjustment.* In older adults, give 10 mg P.O. t.i.d.; then increase to 15 mg t.i.d. or q.i.d., p.r.n.

## Mechanism of action

*Anxiolytic and sedative-hypnotic actions:* Oxazepam depresses the CNS at the limbic and subcortical levels of the brain. It produces an antianxiety effect by enhancing the effect of the neurotransmitter gamma-aminobutyric acid on its receptor in the ascending reticular activating system, which increases inhibition and blocks both cortical and limbic arousal.

## Pharmacokinetics

*Absorption:* When given orally, oxazepam is well absorbed through the GI tract.
*Distribution:* Distributed widely throughout the body, and is 85% to 95% protein-bound.
*Metabolism:* Metabolized in the liver to inactive metabolites.
*Excretion:* Metabolites are excreted in urine as glucuronide conjugates. Half-life of drug is 5¾ to 11 hours.

| Route | Onset | Peak | Duration |
|-------|-------|------|----------|
| P.O. | Unknown | 3 hr | Unknown |

## Contraindications and precautions

Contraindicated in patients with psychosis or those hypersensitive to drug.

Use cautiously in geriatric or debilitated patients; in those with history of drug abuse; and in those for whom a decrease in blood pressure is associated with cardiac problems.

## Interactions

**Drug-drug.** *Antacids:* May decrease rate of oxazepam absorption. Separate administration times of these drugs.
*Cimetidine and possibly disulfiram:* Diminished hepatic metabolism of oxazepam, which

increases its plasma level. Advise clinician to monitor patient carefully.

*General anesthetics, antidepressants, antihistamines, barbiturates, MAO inhibitors, narcotics, and phenothiazines:* Potentiate the CNS depressant effects of these drugs. Avoid use together, if possible.

*Levodopa:* Inhibited therapeutic effects of levodopa. Advise clinician to monitor patient closely.

**Drug-herb.** *Kava, catnip, passion flower, sassafras, skullcap, valerian:* May enhance sedative effects. Discourage use together.

**Drug-lifestyle.** *Alcohol use:* Potentiated CNS depressant effects. Avoid use together.

*Heavy smoking:* Accelerates oxazepam metabolism, lowering clinical effectiveness. Avoid use together.

## Adverse reactions
**CNS:** *drowsiness, lethargy,* dizziness, vertigo, headache, syncope, tremor, slurred speech, changes in EEG patterns.
**CV:** edema.
**GI:** nausea.
**GU:** altered libido.
**Hematologic:** *leukopenia.*
**Hepatic:** *hepatic dysfunction.*
**Skin:** rash.

## Overdose and treatment
Signs and symptoms of overdose include somnolence, confusion, coma, hypoactive reflexes, dyspnea, labored breathing, hypotension, bradycardia, slurred speech, and unsteady gait or impaired coordination.

Blood pressure and respiration should be supported until the effects of the drug have subsided; advise clinician to monitor vital signs. Mechanical ventilatory assistance via endotracheal tube may be required to maintain a patent airway and support adequate oxygenation. Flumazenil, a specific benzodiazepine antagonist, may be useful. As needed, I.V. fluids and vasopressors, such as dopamine and phenylephrine, should be used to treat hypotension. If the patient is conscious, emesis should be induced. Recommend using gastric lavage if ingestion was recent, but only if an endotracheal tube is present to prevent aspiration. After emesis or lavage, recommend giving activated charcoal with a cathartic as a single dose. Dialysis is of limited value.

## Clinical considerations
■ Oxazepam tablets contain tartrazine dye; check patient's history for allergy to this substance.
■ Store drug in a cool, dry place away from light.
■ Use of drug for longer than 4 months hasn't been established.
■ Dosage should be gradually reduced (over 8 to 12 weeks) after long-term use.

## Therapeutic monitoring
■ Advise clinician to monitor hepatic and renal function test results to ensure normal function.

## Special populations
**Breast-feeding patients.** The breast-fed infant of a woman who uses oxazepam may become sedated, have feeding difficulties, or lose weight. Avoid use in breast-feeding women.
**Pediatric patients.** Safety in children under age 6 hasn't been established. Neonates should be closely observed for withdrawal symptoms if mother took oxazepam for a prolonged period during pregnancy.
**Geriatric patients.** Geriatric patients are more susceptible to the CNS depressant effects of oxazepam. Some may require supervision with ambulation and activities of daily living during initiation of therapy or after an increase in dose. Lower doses are usually effective in geriatric patients because of decreased elimination.

## Patient counseling
■ Advise patient not to change drug regimen without medical approval.
■ Instruct patient in safety measures, such as gradual position changes and supervised ambulation, to prevent injury.
■ Because sleepiness may not occur for up to 2 hours after taking oxazepam, tell patient to wait before taking an additional dose.
■ Advise patient of potential for physical and psychological dependence with chronic use of oxazepam.
■ Tell patient not to discontinue drug suddenly.

# oxcarbazepine
Trileptal

*Pharmacologic classification:* carboxamide derivative
*Therapeutic classification:* antiepileptic
*Pregnancy risk category C*

## Available forms
Available by prescription only
*Oral suspension:* 300 mg/5 ml (60 mg/ml)
*Tablets (film-coated):* 150 mg, 300 mg, 600 mg

## Indications and dosages
*Adjunctive therapy for treatment of partial seizures in patients with epilepsy*
*Adults:* Initially, 300 mg P.O. b.i.d. Increase by a maximum of 600 mg/day (300 mg P.O. b.i.d.) at weekly intervals. Recommended daily dose is 1,200 mg P.O. divided b.i.d.
*Children ages 4 to 16:* Initially, 8 to 10 mg/kg/day P.O. divided b.i.d., not to exceed 600 mg/day. The target maintenance dose depends on patient weight, and should be divided b.i.d. If patient weighs between 20 and 29 kg, the tar-

get maintenance dose is 900 mg/day. If patient weighs between 29.1 and 39 kg, the target maintenance dose is 1,200 mg/day. If patient weighs over 39 kg, the target maintenance dose is 1,800 mg/day. Target doses should be achieved over 2 weeks.

*Conversion to monotherapy for treatment of partial seizures in patients with epilepsy*
*Adults:* Initially, 300 mg P.O. b.i.d., with simultaneous reduction in dose of concomitant antiepileptics. Increase oxcarbazepine by a maximum of 600 mg/day at weekly intervals over 2 to 4 weeks. Recommended daily dose is 2,400 mg P.O. divided b.i.d. Concomitant antiepileptics should be completely withdrawn over 3 to 6 weeks.

*Initiation of monotherapy for treatment of partial seizures in patients with epilepsy*
*Adults:* Initially, 300 mg P.O. b.i.d. Increase dosage by 300 mg/day every third day to a daily dose of 1,200 mg divided b.i.d.

## Mechanism of action

*Anticonvulsant action:* The activity of oxcarbazepine is primarily in response to its active 10-monohydroxy metabolite (MHD). The antiseizure activity of oxcarbazepine and MHD is thought to result from the blockade of voltage-sensitive sodium channels, which causes stabilization of hyperexcited neural membranes, inhibition of repetitive neuronal firing, and diminution of propagation of synaptic impulses. This activity is thought to prevent seizure spread in the brain. The anticonvulsant effects of the drug may also be attributed to increased potassium conductance and modulation of high-voltage activated calcium channels.

## Pharmacokinetics

*Absorption:* Completely absorbed after oral administration.
*Distribution:* About 40% of MHD is bound to serum proteins, mostly to albumin.
*Metabolism:* Rapidly metabolized in the liver to its MHD, which is primarily responsible for the pharmacologic effects. Minor amounts (4% of the dose) are oxidized to the pharmacologically inactive 10,11-dihydroxy metabolite (DHD).
*Excretion:* Primarily excreted by the kidneys. Greater than 95% of the dose appears in the urine, with less than 1% as unchanged oxcarbazepine. Fecal excretion accounts for less than 4% of the given dose. The half-life of the parent compound is about 2 hours, while the half-life of MHD is about 9 hours. Children under age 8 have about 30% to 40% increased clearance of drug.

| Route | Onset | Peak | Duration |
|-------|-------|------|----------|
| P.O. | Unknown | Variable | Unknown |

## Contraindications and precautions

Contraindicated in patients hypersensitive to oxcarbazepine or its components.

Use cautiously in patients who have had hypersensitivity reactions to carbamazepine.

## Interactions

**Drug-drug.** *Carbamazepine, valproic acid, verapamil:* Decreased serum levels of the active metabolite of oxcarbazepine. Advise clinician to monitor patient and serum levels closely.
*Felodipine:* Decreased felodipine level. Advise clinician to monitor patient closely.
*Hormonal contraceptives:* Decreased plasma levels of ethinylestradiol and levonorgestrel, rendering oral contraceptives less effective. Women of childbearing age should use alternative forms of contraception.
*Phenobarbital:* Decreased serum levels of the active metabolite of oxcarbazepine and increased phenobarbital level. Advise clinician to monitor patient closely.
*Phenytoin:* Decreased serum levels of the active metabolite of oxcarbazepine. May increase phenytoin level in adults receiving high doses of oxcarbazepine. Advise clinician to monitor phenytoin levels closely when initiating therapy in these patients.
**Drug-lifestyle.** *Alcohol use:* Increased CNS depression. Advise patient to avoid alcohol.

## Adverse reactions

**CNS:** *fatigue,* asthenia, feeling abnormal, *headache, dizziness, somnolence, ataxia, abnormal gait,* insomnia, *tremor,* nervousness, agitation, abnormal coordination, speech disorder, confusion, anxiety, amnesia, *aggravated seizures,* hypoesthesia, emotional lability, impaired concentration, *vertigo.*
**CV:** hypotension, edema, chest pain.
**EENT:** *nystagmus, diplopia, abnormal vision,* abnormal accommodation, rhinitis, sinusitis, pharyngitis, epistaxis, ear ache.
**GI:** *nausea, vomiting, abdominal pain,* diarrhea, dyspepsia, constipation, gastritis, anorexia, dry mouth, rectal hemorrhage, taste perversion, thirst.
**GU:** urinary tract infection, urinary frequency, vaginitis.
**Metabolic:** hyponatremia, weight increase, decreased thyroxine level.
**Musculoskeletal:** muscle weakness, back pain.
**Respiratory:** *upper respiratory tract infection,* coughing, bronchitis, chest infection.
**Skin:** acne, hot flushes, purpura, rash, bruising, increased sweating.
**Other:** fever, allergy, lymphadenopathy, toothache, infection.

## Overdose and treatment

In the event of an overdose of oxcarbazepine symptomatic and supportive treatment should be given as appropriate. There is no specific

---

Reactions may be *common,* uncommon, *life-threatening,* or COMMON AND LIFE-THREATENING.

antidote. Removal of the drug by gastric lavage or inactivation by administering activated charcoal should be considered.

## Clinical considerations

- For adults with creatinine clearance less than 30 ml/minute, therapy should start at 150 mg P.O. b.i.d. (one-half the usual starting dose), and increase slowly to achieve the desired clinical response.
- Ask patient about any history of hypersensitivity reaction to carbamazepine; 25% to 30% of these patients may develop hypersensitivities to oxcarbazepine.
- Drug should be withdrawn gradually to minimize potential for increased seizure frequency.
- Oxcarbazepine use has caused several nervous system–related adverse events, including psychomotor slowing, difficulty with concentration, speech or language problems, somnolence, fatigue, and coordination abnormalities, including ataxia and gait disturbances.
- Shake oral suspension thoroughly before administration. Suspension can be mixed with water or may be swallowed directly from the syringe.
- Oral suspension and tablets may be interchanged at equal doses.
- Can be taken without regard to food.

### Therapeutic monitoring

- Advise clinician to monitor patient for signs and symptoms of hyponatremia, including nausea, malaise, headache, lethargy, confusion, or decreased sensation.
- Advise clinician to monitor serum sodium levels in patients receiving oxcarbazepine for maintenance treatment, especially in patients who are receiving other therapies that may decrease serum sodium levels.

### Special populations

**Breast-feeding patients.** The drug and its active metabolite MHD appear in breast milk. Because of the potential for serious adverse reactions in infants, a decision must be made to either stop the drug or stop breast-feeding.
**Pediatric patients.** See pediatric dosing guidelines. Oxcarbazepine is only indicated for adjunctive therapy in children ages 4 to 16.
**Geriatric patients.** Doses may need to be adjusted in geriatric patients to compensate for age-related decreases in creatinine clearance.

## Patient counseling

- Advise patient to inform prescriber if he has ever experienced a hypersensitivity reaction to carbamazepine.
- Inform patient that drug may be taken with or without food.
- Advise patient not to interrupt or stop drug without consulting his prescriber.

- Advise patient to report signs and symptoms of hyponatremia, such as nausea, malaise, headache, lethargy, or confusion.
- Caution patient to avoid hazardous activities such as driving cars or operating machinery until the effects of the drug are known.
- Advise women using oral contraceptives for birth control to use another form of birth control while taking drug.
- Advise patient to avoid alcohol.

## oxybutynin chloride
Ditropan, Ditropan XL

*Pharmacologic classification:* synthetic tertiary amine
*Therapeutic classification:* antispasmodic
*Pregnancy risk category B*

## Available forms
Available by prescription only
*Syrup:* 5 mg/5 ml
*Tablets:* 5 mg
*Tablets (extended release):* 5 mg, 10 mg, 15 mg

## Indications and dosages
*For relief of symptoms of bladder instability associated with voiding in patients with uninhibited and reflex neurogenic bladder*
*Adults:* 5 mg P.O. b.i.d. to t.i.d. to maximum of 5 mg q.i.d.
*Children over age 5:* 5 mg P.O. b.i.d. to maximum of 5 mg t.i.d.
*For relief of symptoms of urinary frequency, urgency, or urge incontinence in patients with overactive bladder*
*Adults:* 5 mg P.O. daily, increased at 7-day intervals in increments of 5 mg up to a maximum of 30 mg daily.

## Mechanism of action
*Antispasmodic action:* Oxybutynin reduces the urge to void, increases bladder capacity, and reduces the frequency of contractions to the detrusor muscle. Drug exerts a direct spasmolytic action and an antimuscarinic action on smooth muscle.

## Pharmacokinetics
*Absorption:* Absorbed rapidly.
*Distribution:* No data available.
*Metabolism:* Metabolized by the liver.
*Excretion:* Excreted principally in urine.

| Route | Onset | Peak | Duration |
|-------|-------|------|----------|
| P.O. | ½-1 hr | 3-4 hr | 6-10 hr |

## Contraindications and precautions
Contraindicated in patients hypersensitive to drug, and those with myasthenia gravis, GI obstruction, glaucoma, adynamic ileus, megacolon, severe colitis, ulcerative colitis when

megacolon is present, or obstructive uropathy; in geriatric or debilitated patients with intestinal atony; and in hemorrhaging patients with unstable CV status.

Use cautiously in geriatric patients and in patients with impaired renal or hepatic function, autonomic neuropathy, or reflux esophagitis.

## Interactions

**Drug-drug.** *CNS depressants:* Additive sedative effects. Use together cautiously.
*Digoxin:* May increase digoxin levels. Advise clinician to monitor digoxin levels.
*Haloperidol:* Worsening of schizophrenia, decreased serum levels of haloperidol, and development of tardive dyskinesia may occur with coadministration. Use together cautiously, if at all.
*Phenothiazine:* Increased risk of anticholinergic adverse effects. Advise clinician to monitor patient closely.

## Adverse reactions

**CNS:** dizziness, insomnia, restlessness, hallucinations, asthenia.
**CV:** *palpitations, tachycardia,* vasodilation.
**EENT:** mydriasis, cycloplegia, decreased lacrimation, amblyopia.
**GI:** nausea, vomiting, *constipation, dry mouth,* decreased GI motility.
**GU:** *urinary hesitancy, urine retention,* suppressed lactation.
**Skin:** rash.
**Other:** decreased diaphoresis, fever.

## Overdose and treatment

Signs and symptoms of overdose include restlessness, excitement, psychotic behavior, flushing, hypotension, circulatory failure, and fever. In severe cases, paralysis, respiratory failure, and coma may occur.

Treatment requires gastric lavage. Activated charcoal may be given as well as a cathartic. Physostigmine may be considered to reverse symptoms of anticholinergic intoxication. Hyperpyrexia should be treated symptomatically with ice bags or other cold applications and alcohol sponges. Artificial respiration should be maintained if paralysis of respiratory muscles occurs.

## Clinical considerations

■ Drug should be stopped periodically to determine if patient still requires medication.
■ Store drug in tight, light-resistant container at 59° to 86° F (15° to 30° C); drug expires 4 years from date of manufacture.

### Therapeutic monitoring

■ Advise clinician to monitor patient with hepatic and renal disease carefully.

### Special populations

**Breast-feeding patients.** It isn't known if drug appears in breast milk. Use caution when giving to breast-feeding women.
**Pediatric patients.** Dosage guidelines haven't been established for children under age 5. Safety and efficacy of XL strength in children have not been established.
**Geriatric patients.** Geriatric patients may be more sensitive to the antimuscarinic effects. Drug is contraindicated in geriatric and debilitated patients with intestinal atony.

## Patient counseling

■ Instruct patient regarding drug and dosage schedule; tell him to take a missed dose as soon as possible and not to double the doses.
■ Tell patient not to crush or chew extended-release tablets. They may be given without regard to food. Extended-release tablets don't disintegrate and are eliminated in feces.
■ Warn patient about possibility of decreased mental alertness or visual changes.
■ Remind patient to use drug cautiously when in warm climates to minimize risk of heatstroke from decreased sweating.

# oxycodone hydrochloride

Endocodone, OxyContin, OxyFAST, Oxy IR, Roxicodone, Supeudol*

*Pharmacologic classification:* opioid
*Therapeutic classification:* analgesic
*Pregnancy risk category C*
*Controlled substance schedule II*

## Available forms

Available by prescription only
*Capsules:* 5 mg
*Oral solution:* 5 mg/ml, 20 mg/ml
*Tablets:* 5 mg, 15 mg, 30 mg
*Tablets (sustained-release):*10 mg, 20 mg, 40 mg, 80 mg, 160 mg

## Indications and dosages

*Moderate to severe pain*
*Adults:* 5 mg P.O. q 6 hours (of conventional formulation)
*Chronic pain*
*Adults:* Initially, 10-mg sustained-release tablet P.O. q 12 hours; may increase dosage q 1 to 2 days. Dosing frequency shouldn't be increased.

## Mechanism of action

*Analgesic action:* Oxycodone acts on opiate receptors, providing analgesia for moderate to moderately severe pain. Episodes of acute pain, rather than chronic pain, appear to be more responsive to treatment with oxycodone.

## Pharmacokinetics

*Absorption:* Within 15 minutes of oral administration.

*Distribution:* Rapidly distributed.
*Metabolism:* Metabolized in the liver.
*Excretion:* Excreted principally by the kidneys.

| Route | Onset | Peak | Duration |
|-------|-------|------|----------|
| P.O. | 10-15 min | 1 hr | 3-12 hr |

## Contraindications and precautions

Contraindicated in patients hypersensitive to drug.

Use cautiously in geriatric or debilitated patients and in those with head injury, increased intracranial pressure, seizures, asthma, COPD, prostatic hyperplasia, severe hepatic or renal disease, acute abdominal conditions, urethral stricture, hypothyroidism, Addison's disease, or arrhythmias.

## Interactions

**Drug-drug.** *Anticholinergics:* May cause paralytic ileus. Use together cautiously.

*Anticoagulants:* Oxycodone products containing aspirin may increase effects of anticoagulant. Advise clinician to monitor clotting times, and use together cautiously.

*Cimetidine:* May increase respiratory and CNS depression, causing confusion, disorientation, apnea, or seizures. Avoid use together.

*Digitoxin, phenytoin, rifampin:* Drug accumulation and enhanced effects may result from use with other drugs that are extensively metabolized in the liver. Advise clinician to monitor patient closely.

*General anesthetics:* Severe CV depression. Use together with extreme caution.

*Opioid agonist-antagonist or a single dose of an antagonist:* Patients who become physically dependent on oxycodone may experience acute withdrawal syndrome. Avoid use together in this situation. *Other CNS depressants, such as general anesthetics, antihistamines, barbiturates, benzodiazepines, muscle relaxants, narcotic analgesics, phenothiazines, sedative-hypnotics, and tricyclic antidepressants:* Potentiate respiratory and CNS depression, sedation, and hypotensive effects of drug. Use together with extreme caution.

**Drug-lifestyle.** *Alcohol use:* Potentiates respiratory and CNS depression, sedation, and hypotensive effects of drug. Advise patient to avoid combined use.

## Adverse reactions

**CNS:** *sedation, somnolence, clouded sensorium, euphoria, dizziness, light-headedness, seizures.*
**CV:** *hypotension,* **bradycardia.**
**GI:** *nausea, vomiting, constipation,* ileus, increased plasma amylase and lipase and liver enzyme levels.
**GU:** *urine retention.*
**Hepatic:** increased liver enzyme levels.
**Respiratory:** *respiratory depression.*
**Skin:** *diaphoresis,* pruritus, rash.
**Other:** physical dependence.

## Overdose and treatment

The most common signs and symptoms of a severe overdose are CNS depression, respiratory depression, and miosis, or pinpoint pupils. Other acute toxic effects include hypotension, bradycardia, hypothermia, shock, apnea, cardiopulmonary arrest, circulatory collapse, pulmonary edema, and convulsions.

To treat acute overdose, recommend first establishing adequate respiratory exchange via a patent airway and ventilation p.r.n.; a narcotic antagonist (naloxone) should be given to reverse respiratory depression. Because the duration of action of oxycodone is longer than that of naloxone, repeated naloxone dosing is needed. Naloxone shouldn't be given unless patient has clinically significant respiratory or CV depression. Advise clinician to monitor vital signs closely.

If patient presents within 2 hours of ingestion of an oral overdose, stomach should be immediately emptied by inducing emesis (ipecac syrup) or using gastric lavage. Use caution to avoid any risk of aspiration. Recommend giving activated charcoal via nasogastric tube for further removal of the drug in an oral overdose.

Symptomatic and supportive treatment, including continued respiratory support and correction of fluid and electrolyte imbalance, should be provided. Advise clinician to monitor laboratory values, vital signs, and neurologic status closely.

Dialysis may be helpful if combination products with aspirin or acetaminophen are involved.

## Clinical considerations

■ Some commercial preparations contain sodium metabisulfite, which may cause an allergic reaction in susceptible individuals.

■ Single-agent oxycodone solution or tablets are ideal for patients who can't take aspirin or acetaminophen.

■ The extended-release preparation isn't intended for preoperative or immediate postoperative pain in patients not already taking the drug.

**H *ALERT*** The extended-release preparation must be swallowed whole. Do not crush, break, or have patient chew the tablet because this could cause a rapid release of a potentially toxic dose.

■ Oxycodone has high abuse potential.

■ Drug may obscure signs and symptoms of an acute abdominal condition or worsen gallbladder pain.

■ A stool softener should be considered for patients on long-term therapy.

■ The 80-mg sustained-release tablets are for opioid-tolerant patients only.

■ Patients being transferred from 5 to 25 mg daily conventional dose should receive 10 to 20 mg q 12 hours of the extended-release preparation. If conventional dose is 30 to 45 mg or 50 to 60 mg daily, the extended-release dose is 20 to 30 mg q 12 hours or 30 to 40 mg q 12 hours, respectively.

### Therapeutic monitoring
■ Advise clinician to monitor patient for relief of pain and development of tolerance to drug's effects.

### Special populations
**Breast-feeding patients.** It's unknown if drug appears in breast milk. Use with caution in breast-feeding women.
**Pediatric patients.** Dosage may be individualized for children; however, safety and effectiveness in children haven't been established.
**Geriatric patients.** Lower doses are usually indicated for geriatric patients, who may be more sensitive to the therapeutic and adverse effects of drug.

### Patient counseling
■ For full analgesic effect, teach patient to take drug before onset of intense pain.
■ Warn patient about possibility of decreased alertness or visual changes.

## oxymetazoline hydrochloride
Afrin, Allerest 12 Hour Nasal Spray, Chlorphed-LA, Dristan Long Lasting, Duramist Plus, Duration, 4-Way Long Lasting Spray, Neo-Synephrine 12 Hour Nasal Spray, Nostrilla Long Acting Nasal Decongestant, NTZ Long Acting Decongestant Nasal Spray, OcuClear, Sinarest 12 Hour Nasal Spray, Sinex Long-Acting, Visine L.R.

*Pharmacologic classification:* sympathomimetic
*Therapeutic classification:* decongestant, vasoconstrictor
*Pregnancy risk category C*

### Available forms
Available without a prescription
*Nasal drops or spray:* 0.05%
*Nasal solution:* 0.025% (drops) for children
*Ophthalmic solution:* 0.025%

### Indications and dosages
*Nasal congestion*
*Adults and children over age 6:* Apply 2 to 3 drops or sprays of 0.05% solution in each nostril q 10 to 12 hours. Use no longer than 3 to 5 days. Dosage for younger children hasn't been established.
*Relief of minor eye redness*
*Adults and children over age 6:* Apply 1 to 2 drops in the conjunctival sac up to q.i.d. (space at least 6 hours apart p.r.n.).

### Mechanism of action
*Decongestant action:* Oxymetazoline produces local vasoconstriction of arterioles through alpha receptors to reduce blood flow and nasal congestion.

### Pharmacokinetics
*Absorption:* Occasional systemic absorption may occur.
*Distribution:* Unknown.
*Metabolism:* Unknown.
*Excretion:* Unknown.

| Route | Onset | Peak | Duration |
|-------|-------|------|----------|
| Ophthalmic | 5 min | Unknown | 6 hr |
| Nasal | 5-10 min | 6 hr | < 12 hr |

### Contraindications and precautions
Contraindicated in patients hypersensitive to drug. Ophthalmic form contraindicated in patients with angle-closure glaucoma.

Use cautiously in patients with hyperthyroidism, cardiac disease, or hypertension and in those receiving MAO inhibitors. Use nasal solution cautiously in patients with diabetes mellitus. Use ophthalmic form cautiously in those with eye disease, infection, or injury.

### Interactions
**Drug-drug.** *Beta blockers:* Can increase systemic adverse effects. Advise clinician to monitor patient carefully.
*Local anesthetics:* Can increase absorption of ophthalmic form. Advise clinician to monitor patient closely.
*Tricyclic antidepressants:* May potentiate the pressor effects from significant systemic absorption of the decongestant. Advise clinician to monitor patient carefully.

### Adverse reactions
**CNS:** headache, insomnia; drowsiness, dizziness, possible sedation (with nasal form); lightheadedness, nervousness (with ophthalmic form).
**CV:** palpitations; *CV collapse,* hypertension (with nasal form); tachycardia, *bradycardia,* irregular heartbeat (with ophthalmic form).
**EENT:** rebound nasal congestion or irritation with excessive or long-term use, dryness of nose and throat, increased nasal discharge, stinging, sneezing (with nasal form); *transient stinging upon instillation,* blurred vision, reactive hyperemia, keratitis, lacrimation, increased intraocular pressure (with ophthalmic form).

---

Reactions may be *common,* uncommon, *life-threatening,* or COMMON AND LIFE-THREATENING.

**Other:** systemic effects in children (with excessive or long-term use, with nasal form); trembling (with ophthalmic form).

## Overdose and treatment

Signs and symptoms of overdose include somnolence, sedation, sweating, CNS depression with hypertension, bradycardia, decreased cardiac output, rebound hypertension, CV collapse, depressed respirations, and coma.

If ingested, emesis isn't recommended, unless given early, because of rapid onset of sedation. Activated charcoal or gastric lavage may be used initially. Advise clinician to monitor vital signs and ECG. Seizures should be treated with I.V. diazepam.

## Clinical considerations

■ Excessive dosing may irritate nasal mucosa and cause rebound congestion (nasal) or rebound hyperemia (ophthalmic) and should not exceed 2 doses per day.

### Therapeutic monitoring

■ Advise clinician to monitor patient for adverse reactions in patients with CV disease, diabetes mellitus, or prostatic hypertrophy because systemic absorption can occur.

### Special populations

**Pediatric patients.** Children may exhibit increased adverse effects from systemic absorption; 0.05% nasal solution is contraindicated in children under age 6; 0.025% nasal solution should be used in children under age 2 only under medical direction and supervision.
**Geriatric patients.** Use drug with caution in geriatric patients with cardiac disease, poorly controlled hypertension, or diabetes mellitus.

## Patient counseling

■ Emphasize that only one person should use dropper bottle or nasal spray.
■ Advise patient not to exceed recommended dosage and to use drug only when needed.
■ Tell patient to discontinue drug and report symptoms that persist after 3 days of self-medication.
■ Tell patient that nasal mucosa may sting, burn, or become dry.
■ Warn patient that excessive use may cause bradycardia, hypotension, dizziness, and weakness.
■ Show patient how to apply drug. Have him bend head forward and sniff spray briskly or apply light pressure on lacrimal sac after instillation of eyedrop.

# oxymorphone hydrochloride
Numorphan

*Pharmacologic classification:* opioid
*Therapeutic classification:* analgesic
*Pregnancy risk category C*
*Controlled substance schedule II*

## Available forms

Available by prescription only
*Injection:* 1 mg/ml, 1.5 mg/ml
*Suppository:* 5 mg

## Indications and dosages

*Moderate to severe pain*
*Adults:* 1 to 1.5 mg I.M. or S.C. q 4 to 6 hours, p.r.n., or around-the-clock; 0.5 mg I.V. q 4 to 6 hours, p.r.n., or around-the-clock; or 1 suppository administered P.R. q 4 to 6 hours, p.r.n., or around-the-clock.

Note: Parenteral administration of drug is also indicated for preoperative medication, for support of anesthesia, for obstetric analgesia, and for relief of anxiety in dyspnea associated with acute left-sided HF and pulmonary edema.

## I.V. administration

■ Give drug by direct I.V. injection. If necessary, drug may be diluted in normal saline solution.
■ An opiate antagonist and oxygen should be available after I.V. administration.

### Incompatibilities

None reported.

## Mechanism of action

*Analgesic action:* Oxymorphone effectively relieves moderate to severe pain by way of agonist activity at the opiate receptors. It has little or no antitussive effect.

## Pharmacokinetics

*Absorption:* Well absorbed after P.R., S.C., I.M., or I.V. administration.
*Distribution:* Widely distributed.
*Metabolism:* Primarily metabolized in the liver.
*Excretion:* Excreted primarily in the urine as oxymorphone conjugates.

| Route | Onset | Peak | Duration |
|-------|-------|------|----------|
| I.V. | 5-10 min | 15-30 min | 3-4 hr |
| I.M. | 10-15 min | ½-1½ hr | 3-6 hr |
| S.C. | 10-20 min | 1-1½ hr | 3-6 hr |
| P.R. | 15-30 min | 2 hr | 3-6 hr |

## Contraindications and precautions

Contraindicated in patients hypersensitive to drug.

Use cautiously in geriatric or debilitated patients and in those with head injury, increased intracranial pressure, seizures, asthma, COPD, acute abdomen conditions, prostatic hyperplasia, severe renal or kidney disease, urethral stricture, respiratory depression, Addison's disease, arrhythmias, or hypothyroidism.

## Interactions

**Drug-drug.** *Anticholinergics:* May cause paralytic ileus. Use together cautiously.

*Cimetidine:* May increase respiratory and CNS depression, causing confusion, disorientation, apnea, or seizures. Avoid use together.

*CNS depressants, such as general anesthetics, antihistamines, barbiturates, benzodiazepines, muscle relaxants, opiates, phenothiazines, sedative-hypnotics, and tricyclic antidepressants:* Potentiate respiratory and CNS depression, sedation, and hypotensive effects of drug. Use together with extreme caution.

*Digitoxin, phenytoin, rifampin:* Drug accumulation and enhanced effects may result from use with other drugs that are extensively metabolized in the liver. Advise clinician to monitor patient closely.

*General anesthetics:* Severe CV depression. Use together with extreme caution.

*Opioid agonist-antagonist or a single dose of an antagonist:* Patients who become physically dependent on oxycodone may experience acute withdrawal syndrome. Avoid use together in this situation.

**Drug-lifestyle.** *Alcohol use:* Potentiates respiratory and CNS depression, sedation, and hypotensive effects of drug. Advise patient to avoid alcohol.

## Adverse reactions

**CNS:** *sedation, somnolence, clouded sensorium, euphoria,* dizziness, *seizures,* lightheadedness, headache.

**CV:** *hypotension,* **bradycardia.**

**GI:** *nausea, vomiting, constipation,* ileus, increased plasma amylase levels.

**GU:** *urine retention.*

**Respiratory:** *respiratory depression.*

**Skin:** pruritus.

**Other:** physical dependence.

## Overdose and treatment

The most common signs and symptoms of oxymorphone overdose are CNS depression, including extreme somnolence progressing to stupor and coma; respiratory depression; and miosis, or pinpoint pupils. Other acute toxic effects include hypotension, bradycardia, hypothermia, shock, apnea, cardiopulmonary arrest, circulatory collapse, pulmonary edema, and seizures.

To treat acute overdose, recommend first establishing adequate respiratory exchange via a patent airway and ventilation, p.r.n., and giving a narcotic antagonist (naloxone) to reverse respiratory depression. Because duration of action of drug is longer than that of naloxone, re-

peated naloxone dosing is needed. Naloxone shouldn't be given unless patient has clinically significant respiratory or CV depression. Advise clinician to monitor vital signs closely.

Symptomatic and supportive treatment, including continued respiratory support and correction of fluid or electrolyte imbalance, should be provided. Advise clinician to monitor laboratory values, vital signs, and neurologic status closely.

## Clinical considerations

■ Refrigerate oxymorphone suppositories.

■ Drug is well absorbed P.R. and is an alternative to opioids with more limited dosage forms.

■ Drug may worsen gallbladder pain.

### Therapeutic monitoring

■ Advise clinician to monitor vital signs and respiratory status.

### Special populations

**Breast-feeding patients.** It isn't known if drug appears in breast milk. Use with caution in breast-feeding women.

**Pediatric patients.** Don't use in children under age 12.

**Geriatric patients.** Lower doses are usually indicated for geriatric patients, who may be more sensitive to the therapeutic and adverse effects of drug.

## Patient counseling

■ Tell patient to ask for drug before pain is intense.

■ Caution ambulatory patient about getting out of bed and walking. Patient should avoid driving or other potentially hazardous activities until CNS effects are known.

■ Instruct patient to store suppositiories in the refrigerator.

■ Advise patient to avoid alcohol.

## oxytocin
Pitocin

*Pharmacologic classification:* exogenous hormone
*Therapeutic classification:* oxytocic, lactation stimulant
*Pregnancy risk category C*

## Available forms

Available by prescription only
*Injection:* 10 units/ml ampules, vials, and closed injection system

## Indications and dosages
*Induction of labor*
*Adults:* Initially, no more than 0.5 to 1 milliunits/minute I.V. infusion. Rate of infusion may be increased slowly (1 to 2 milliunits/minute at

30- to 60-minute intervals until a response is observed). Decrease rate when labor is firmly established.

*Augmentation of labor*
*Adults:* Initially, 2 milliunits/minute I.V. infusion. Rate of infusion may be increased slowly to maximum of 20 milliunits/minute.

*Reduction of postpartum bleeding after expulsion of placenta*
*Adults:* 20 to 40 milliunits/minute I.V. infusion to total of 10 units (or 10 units I.M.) after delivery of the placenta.

*To induce abortion*
*Adults:* 10 units mixed in 500 ml $D_5W$ or normal saline solution I.V. at 10 to 100 milliunits/minute (not to exceed 30 units in 12 hours).

◇ *Oxytocin challenge test to assess fetal distress in high-risk pregnancies greater than 31 weeks' gestation*
*Adults:* Prepare solution by adding 5 to 10 units oxytocin to 1 L of 5% dextrose injection, yielding a solution of 5 to 10 milliunits per ml. Infuse 0.5 milliunits/minute, gradually increasing at 15-minute intervals to maximum infusion of 20 milliunits/minute. Discontinue infusion when three moderate uterine contractions occur in a 10-minute interval. Response of fetal heart rate to test may be used to evaluate prognosis.

## I.V. administration
■ Drug must be given by I.V. infusion, not I.V. bolus injection. Use an infusion device.
■ I.V. infusion rates up to 6 milliunits/minute produce maternal plasma level similar to spontaneous labor. Rates exceeding 9 to 10 milliunits/minute are rarely needed.
■ Magnesium sulfate (20% solution) should be available for relaxation of the myometrium.
■ Solution containing 10 milliunits/ml may be prepared by adding 10 units of oxytocin to 1 L of normal saline solution or $D_5W$. Solution containing 20 milliunits/ml may be prepared by adding 10 units of oxytocin to 500 ml of normal saline solution or $D_5W$.

## Incompatibilities
Oxytocin injection is incompatible with fibrinolysin, norepinephrine bitartrate, Normosol-M with dextrose 5%, prochlorperazine edisylate, and warfarin sodium.

## Mechanism of action
*Oxytocic action:* Oxytocin increases the sodium permeability of uterine myofibrils, indirectly stimulating the contraction of uterine smooth muscle. The threshold for response is lowered in the presence of high estrogen levels. Uterine response increases with the length of the pregnancy and increases further during active labor. Response mimics labor contractions.

## Pharmacokinetics
*Absorption:* Administered parenterally.
*Distribution:* Distributed throughout the extracellular fluid; small amounts may enter the fetal circulation.
*Metabolism:* Metabolized rapidly in the kidneys and liver. In early pregnancy, a circulating enzyme, oxytocinase, can inactivate the drug.
*Excretion:* Only small amounts are excreted in the urine as oxytocin. Half-life is 3 to 5 minutes.

| Route | Onset | Peak | Duration |
|-------|-------|------|----------|
| I.V. | Immediate | Unknown | 1 hr |
| I.M. | 3-5 min | Unknown | 2-3 hr |

## Contraindications and precautions
Contraindicated when cephalopelvic disproportion is present or when delivery requires conversion, as in transverse lie; in fetal distress when delivery isn't imminent; prematurity and other obstetric emergencies; and in patients with severe toxemia, hypertonic uterine patterns, total placenta previa, and vasoprevia, and those hypersensitive to drug.

Use cautiously during first and second stages of labor and in patients with history of cervical or uterine surgery (including cesarean section), grand multiparity, uterine sepsis, traumatic delivery, overdistended uterus, and invasive cervical cancer.

## Interactions
*Drug-drug.* *Cyclopropane anesthesia:* May modify CV effects of oxytocin. Use together cautiously.
*Sympathomimetics:* May increase pressor effects, possibly resulting in postpartum hypertension. Avoid use together.
*Thiopental anesthesia:* Delays the induction of anesthesia. Use together cautiously.

## Adverse reactions
**Maternal**
CNS: *subarachnoid hemorrhage* (from hypertension), *seizures or coma* (from water intoxication).
CV: *hypertension,* increased heart rate, systemic venous return, and cardiac output, *arrhythmias.*
GI: nausea, vomiting.
GU: tetanic uterine contractions, *abruptio placentae, impaired uterine blood flow,* pelvic hematoma, *increased uterine motility, uterine rupture, postpartum hemorrhage.*
Hematologic: *afibrinogenemia* (may be related to postpartum bleeding).
Other: hypersensitivity reactions (*anaphylaxis*), water retention.
**Fetal**
CNS: *infant brain damage.*
CV: *bradycardia, premature ventricular contractions, arrhythmias.*

---

**EENT:** retinal hemorrhage.
**Hepatic:** *jaundice.*
**Respiratory:** *anoxia, asphyxia.*
**Other:** *low Apgar scores.*

## Overdose and treatment

Signs and symptoms of overdose include hyperstimulation of the uterus, causing tetanic contractions and possible uterine rupture, cervical laceration, abruptio placentae, impaired uterine blood flow, amniotic fluid embolism, and fetal trauma.

Drug has a very short half-life; recommend stopping therapy and starting supportive care.

## Clinical considerations

- When giving oxytocin challenge test, advise clinician to monitor fetal heart rate and uterine contractions immediately before and during infusion. If fetal heart rate doesn't change during test, repeat in 1 week. If late deceleration in fetal heart rate is noted, consider terminating pregnancy.
- During long infusions, recommend watching for signs of water intoxication.
- Drug isn't recommended for routine I.M. use. However, 10 units may be given I.M. after delivery of the placenta to control postpartum uterine bleeding.
- Drug should be stopped if prolonged uterine contractions are prolonged (more than 90 seconds), if intrauterine pressure rises, or if uterine motility interferes with fetal heart rate.

### Therapeutic monitoring

- Uterine contractions, heart rate, blood pressure, intrauterine pressure, fetal heart rate, and character of blood loss should be recorded every 15 minutes.
- Drug may produce an antidiuretic effect; fluid intake and output should be monitored.

### Special populations

**Breast-feeding patients.** Minimal amounts of drug appear in breast milk. Risks must be evaluated.

## Patient counseling

- Explain possible adverse effects of drug.

# paclitaxel
Taxol

*Pharmacologic classification:* novel antimicrotubule
*Therapeutic classification:* antineoplastic
*Pregnancy risk category D*

## Available forms
Available by prescription only
*Injection:* 30 mg/5 ml, 100 mg/16.7 ml, 300 mg/50 ml

## Indications and dosages
***First-line and subsequent therapy for the treatment of advanced carcinoma of the ovary***
*Adults (previously untreated):* 175 mg/m$^2$ over 3 hours every 3 weeks followed by cisplatin 75 mg/m$^2$; or, 135 mg/m$^2$ over 24 hours with cisplatin 75 mg/m$^2$ every 3 weeks. Subsequent courses shouldn't be repeated until neutrophil count is at least 1,500 cells/mm$^3$ and platelet count is at least 100,000 cells/mm$^3$.
*Adults (previously treated):* 135 or 175 mg/m$^2$ I.V. over 3 hours q 3 weeks. Subsequent courses shouldn't be repeated until neutrophil count is at least 1,500 cells/mm$^3$ and platelet count is at least 100,000 cells/mm$^3$.
***Breast carcinoma after failure of combination chemotherapy for metastatic disease or relapse within 6 months of adjuvant chemotherapy (prior therapy should have included an anthracycline unless clinically contraindicated)***
*Adults:* 175 mg/m$^2$ I.V. over 3 hours q 3 weeks. Subsequent courses shouldn't be repeated until neutrophil count is at least 1,500 cells/mm$^3$ and platelet count is at least 100,000 cells/mm$^3$.
***AIDS-related Kaposi's sarcoma***
*Adults:* 135 mg/m$^2$ I.V. over 3 hours q 3 weeks, or 100 mg/m$^2$ I.V. over 3 hours q 2 weeks. Subsequent courses shouldn't be repeated until neutrophil count is at least 1,000 cells/mm$^3$.
***Initial treatment of advanced non–small cell lung cancer for patients who are not candidates for curative surgery or radiation***
*Adults:* 135 mg/m$^2$ I.V. infusion over 24 hours or 175 mg/m$^2$ I.V. infusion over 3 hours. Follow with cisplatin 75 mg/m$^2$ or 80 mg/m$^2$, respectively. Repeat cycle every 3 weeks. Sub-

sequent courses shouldn't be repeated until neutrophil count is at least 1,500 cells/mm$^3$ and platelet count is at least 100,000 cells/mm$^3$.

## I.V. administration
■ Concentrate must be diluted before infusion. Compatible solutions include normal saline injection, $D_5W$, dextrose 5% in normal saline injection, and 5% dextrose in lactated Ringer's injection. Dilute to a final concentration of 0.3 to 1.2 mg/ml. Diluted solutions are stable for 27 hours at room temperature, 77° F (25° C).
■ Prepare and store infusion solutions in glass containers. Undiluted concentrate shouldn't contact polyvinyl chloride I.V. bags or tubing. Store diluted solution in glass or polypropylene bottles, or use polypropylene or polyolefin bags.
■ Recommend giving through polyethylene-lined administration sets and using an in-line filter with a microporous membrane not exceeding 0.22 microns.

### Incompatibilities
Incompatible with amphotericin B, chlorpromazine, hydroxyzine hydrochloride, methylprednisolone sodium succinate, and mitoxantrone.

## Mechanism of action
*Antineoplastic action:* Paclitaxel prevents depolymerization of cellular microtubules, inhibiting the normal reorganization of the microtubule network needed for mitosis and other vital cellular functions.

## Pharmacokinetics
*Absorption:* Administered I.V.
*Distribution:* About 89% to 98% of paclitaxel is serum protein–bound.
*Metabolism:* May be metabolized in the liver.
*Excretion:* Excretion isn't fully understood.

| Route | Onset | Peak | Duration |
|-------|---------|---------|----------|
| I.V. | Unknown | Unknown | Unknown |

## Contraindications and precautions
Contraindicated in patients hypersensitive to drug or polyoxyethylated castor oil, a vehicle used in drug solution, and in those with baseline neutrophil counts less than 1,500/mm$^3$.

Use cautiously in patients who have received radiation therapy.

## Interactions

**Drug-drug.** *Cisplatin:* Possible additive myelo-suppression. When given together, recommend giving paclitaxel before cisplatin.

*Cyclosporine, dexamethasone, diazepam, etoposide, ketoconazole, quinidine, teniposide, verapamil, vincristine:* May inhibit paclitaxel metabolism. Use together cautiously.

## Adverse reactions

**CNS:** *peripheral neuropathy.*
**CV:** *bradycardia, hypotension, abnormal ECG.*
**GI:** *nausea, vomiting, diarrhea, mucositis.*
**Hematologic:** NEUTROPENIA, LEUKOPENIA, THROMBOCYTOPENIA, anemia, *bleeding.*
**Hepatic:** *elevated liver enzyme levels.*
**Musculoskeletal:** *myalgia, arthralgia.*
**Skin:** *alopecia, cellulitis at injection site.*
**Other:** *hypersensitivity reactions (anaphylaxis), phlebitis, infections.*

## Overdose and treatment

Primary complications of overdose include bone marrow suppression, peripheral neurotoxicity, and mucositis and acute ethanol toxicity in pediatric patients. No specific antidote for paclitaxel overdose is known.

## Clinical considerations

■ Severe hypersensitivity reactions characterized by dyspnea, hypotension, angioedema, and generalized urticaria have occurred in 2% of patients receiving paclitaxel. To reduce the risk or severity of these reactions, recommend pretreating patient with corticosteroids such as dexamethasone; antihistamines such as diphenhydramine; and $H_2$-receptor antagonists, such as cimetidine or ranitidine.

■ Don't rechallenge patients who experience severe hypersensitivity reactions to paclitaxel.

■ In patients who experience severe neutropenia (neutrophil count less than 500 cells/mm³ for 1 week or longer) or severe peripheral neuropathy during drug therapy, recommend reducing dosage by 20% for subsequent courses. Risk and severity of neurotoxicity and hematologic toxicity increase with dose, especially more than 190 mg/m².

■ If significant conduction abnormalities develop during drug administration, recommend giving appropriate therapy and monitoring cardiac function continuously during subsequent drug therapy.

■ Use caution during preparation and administration of paclitaxel. Use of gloves is recommended. If solution contacts skin, wash skin immediately and thoroughly with soap and water. If drug contacts mucous membranes, flush membranes thoroughly with water. Mark all waste materials with CHEMOTHERAPY HAZARD labels.

**❗ALERT** Don't confuse Taxol (paclitaxel) with Taxotere (docetaxel).

## Therapeutic monitoring

■ Bone marrow toxicity is the most frequent and dose-limiting toxicity. Frequent blood count monitoring is needed during therapy. Packed RBC or platelet transfusions may be needed in severe cases. Bleeding precautions should be taken as appropriate.

■ Recommend continuously monitoring patient for 30 minutes after initiating the infusion. Close monitoring should continue throughout infusion.

## Special populations

**Pregnant patients.** Advise women of childbearing age to avoid becoming pregnant during therapy with paclitaxel because of potential harm to the fetus.

**Breast-feeding patients.** Because of potential for serious adverse reactions in breast-fed infants, breast-feeding should be discontinued during paclitaxel therapy.

**Pediatric patients.** Safety and efficacy in children haven't been established.

## Patient counseling

■ Tell patient to watch for signs and symptoms of infection, and bleeding, and to take temperature daily.

■ Teach patient to recognize and immediately report signs and symptoms of peripheral neuropathy, such as tingling, burning, or numbness in the limbs. Although mild symptoms are common, severe symptoms occur infrequently. Dosage reduction may be needed.

■ Warn patient that alopecia occurs in almost all patients.

# palivizumab
Synagis

*Pharmacologic classification:* recombinant monoclonal antibody $IgG1_K$
*Therapeutic classification:* RSV prophylaxis drug
*Pregnancy risk category C*

## Available forms

Available by prescription only
*Injection (single-use vial):* 50 mg, 100 mg

## Indications and dosages

*Prevention of serious lower respiratory tract disease caused by respiratory syncytial virus (RSV) in children at high risk*
*Children:* 15 mg/kg I.M. monthly throughout RSV season. Recommend giving first dose before beginning of RSV season.

## Mechanism of action

*RSV prophylaxis drug action:* Drug exhibits neutralizing and fusion-inhibitory activity against RSV, which inhibits RSV replication.

---

## Pharmacokinetics

*Absorption:* Not reported.
*Distribution:* Not reported.
*Metabolism:* Not reported.
*Excretion:* Half-life of drug is about 18 days.

| Route | Onset | Peak | Duration |
|-------|-------|------|----------|
| I.M. | Unknown | Unknown | Unknown |

## Contraindications and precautions

Contraindicated in children with a severe prior reaction to the drug or its components.

Give with caution in patients with thrombocytopenia or any coagulation disorder.

## Interactions

None reported.

## Adverse reactions

**CNS:** nervousness.
**EENT:** *otitis media, rhinitis,* pharyngitis, sinusitis, conjunctivitis.
**GI:** diarrhea, vomiting, gastroenteritis, oral candidiasis.
**Hematologic:** anemia.
**Hepatic:** liver function abnormality (increased ALT, AST).
**Respiratory:** *upper respiratory infection,* cough, wheeze, bronchiolitis, *apnea,* pneumonia, bronchitis, asthma, croup, dyspnea.
**Skin:** *rash,* fungal dermatitis, eczema, seborrhea.
**Other:** pain, hernia, failure to thrive, injection site reaction, viral infection, flu syndrome.

## Overdose and treatment

No information available.

## Clinical considerations

■ Patients should receive monthly doses throughout RSV season, even if RSV infection develops. In the northern hemisphere, RSV season typically lasts from November to April.
■ To reconstitute, slowly add 1 ml of sterile water for injection into a 100-mg vial. Gently swirl the vial for 30 seconds to avoid foaming. Don't shake vial. Let reconstituted solution stand at room temperature for 20 minutes.
■ Vial doesn't contain preservative and should be given within 6 hours of reconstitution.
■ Recommend giving drug in anterolateral aspect of thigh. Gluteal muscle shouldn't be used routinely as an injection site because of risk of damage to sciatic nerve. Injection volumes over 1 ml should be given as a divided dose. Drug shouldn't be administered I.V.
■ Drug is intended for prophylaxis only. Not used for treatment of present RSV infection.

### Therapeutic monitoring

■ Anaphylactoid reactions after administration of drug have not been observed, but can occur after the administration of proteins. If anaphylaxis or severe allergic reaction occurs, recommend giving epinephrine (1:1,000) and providing supportive care as required.

### Special populations

**Pregnant patients.** It isn't known if drug causes fetal harm. Not recommended for use in pregnant women.

## Patient counseling

■ Explain to parent or caregiver that drug is used to prevent RSV, not to treat it.
■ Advise parent or caregiver that monthly injections are recommended throughout RSV season (November to April in the northern hemisphere).
■ Advise parent or caregiver to report adverse reactions immediately.

# pamidronate disodium
Aredia

*Pharmacologic classification:* bisphosphonate, pyrophosphate analogue
*Therapeutic classification:* antihypercalcemic
*Pregnancy risk category C*

## Available forms

Available by prescription only
*Injection:* 30 mg/vial, 60 mg/vial, 90 mg/vial

## Indications and dosages

*Moderate to severe hypercalcemia with malignancy (with or without metastases)*
*Adults:* Dosage depends on severity of hypercalcemia. Serum calcium levels should be corrected for serum albumin. Corrected serum calcium (CCa) is calculated using the following formula:

$$\text{CCa} \atop \text{(mg/dl)} = \frac{\text{serum Ca}}{\text{(mg/dl)}} + \frac{0.8\,(4 - \text{serum albumin})}{\text{(g/dl)}}$$

*Patients with moderate hypercalcemia (CCa levels of 12 to 13.5 mg/dl):* 60 to 90 mg by I.V. infusion over 2 to 24 hours as a single dose.
*Patients with severe hypercalcemia (CCa levels of more than 13.5 mg/dl):* 90 mg over 2 to 24 hours as a single dose.
Repeat doses shouldn't be given sooner than 7 days to allow for full response of initial dose.
*Paget's disease*
*Adults:* 30 mg I.V. daily over 4 hours for 3 consecutive days for total dose of 90 mg.
*Osteolytic bone lesions of multiple myeloma*
*Adults:* 90 mg I.V. daily over 4 hours once monthly.
*Osteolytic bone lesions of breast cancer*
*Adults:* 90 mg I.V. over 2 hours q 3 to 4 weeks.

## I.V. administration

- Reconstitute vial with 10 ml sterile water for injection. Once drug is completely dissolved, add to 250 ml (2-hour infusion), 500 ml (4-hour infusion), or 1,000 ml (up to 24-hour infusion) bag of 0.45% or normal saline solution injection or D$_5$W. Don't mix with infusion solutions that contain calcium, such as Ringer's injection or lactated Ringer's injection. Recommend administering in a single I.V. solution, in a separate line from all other drugs. Visually inspect for precipitate before administering.
- Injection solution is stable for 24 hours when refrigerated. Give only by I.V. infusion. Animal studies have shown evidence of nephropathy when drug is given as a bolus.

### Incompatibilities

Don't mix with calcium-containing infusion solutions such as Ringer's injection or lactated Ringer's solution.

## Mechanism of action

*Antihypercalcemic action:* Pamidronate inhibits the resorption of bone. Drug adsorbs to hydroxyapatite crystals in bone and may directly block the dissolution of calcium phosphate. Drug apparently doesn't inhibit bone formation or mineralization.

## Pharmacokinetics

*Absorption:* Administered I.V.
*Distribution:* After I.V. administration in animals, about 50% to 60% of a dose is rapidly absorbed by bone; drug is also taken up by the kidneys, liver, spleen, teeth, and tracheal cartilage.
*Metabolism:* None.
*Excretion:* Excreted by the kidneys; an average of 51% of a dose is excreted in urine within 72 hours of administration.

| Route | Onset | Peak | Duration |
|-------|-------|------|----------|
| I.V. | Rapid | Unknown | Unknown |

## Contraindications and precautions

Contraindicated in patients hypersensitive to drug or other bisphosphonates, such as etidronate.

Use with extreme caution in patients with impaired renal function.

## Interactions

**Drug-drug.** *Solutions that contain calcium:* Pamidronate may form a precipitate when mixed together. Don't mix together.

## Adverse reactions

**CNS:** *seizures,* fatigue, headache, somnolence.
**CV:** atrial fibrillation, syncope, tachycardia, *hypertension.*
**GI:** *abdominal pain, anorexia, constipation, nausea, vomiting,* **GI hemorrhage.**

**Hematologic:** *leukopenia, thrombocytopenia, anemia.*
**Metabolic:** *hypophosphatemia, hypokalemia, hypomagnesemia, hypocalcemia.*
**Musculoskeletal:** *bone pain.*
**Other:** *fever, infusion-site reaction, generalized pain.*

## Overdose and treatment

Symptomatic hypocalcemia could result from overdose; recommend treating with I.V. calcium. In one reported case, a 95-kg (209-lb) woman who received 285 mg daily for 3 days experienced hyperpyrexia (103° F [39.4° C]), hypotension, and transient taste perversion. Fever and hypotension were rapidly corrected with corticosteroids.

## Clinical considerations

- Infusions longer than 2 hours may reduce the risk for renal toxicity.

### Therapeutic monitoring

- Because drug can cause electrolyte disturbances, careful monitoring of serum electrolytes (especially calcium, phosphate, and magnesium) is essential. Short-term administration of calcium may be needed in patients with severe hypocalcemia. Also advise clinician to monitor creatinine, CBC, differential, hematocrit, and hemoglobin levels.
- Recommend carefully monitoring patients with preexisting anemia, leukopenia, or thrombocytopenia during first 2 weeks after therapy.
- Advise clinician to monitor patient's temperature. In trials, 27% of patients experienced a slightly elevated temperature for 24 to 48 hours after therapy.

### Special populations

**Breast-feeding patients.** It's unknown if drug appears in breast milk. Use with caution in breast-feeding women.
**Pediatric patients.** Safety and efficacy in children haven't been established.

## Patient counseling

- Instruct patient to report adverse reactions immediately.

# pancuronium bromide

*Pharmacologic classification:* nondepolarizing neuromuscular blocker
*Therapeutic classification:* skeletal muscle relaxant
*Pregnancy risk category C*

## Available forms

Available by prescription only
*Injection:* 1 mg/ml, 2 mg/ml

# Indications and dosages

*Adjunct to anesthesia to induce skeletal muscle relaxation, facilitate intubation and ventilation, and weaken muscle contractions in induced seizures*
Dose depends on anesthetic used, individual needs, and response. Doses are representative and must be adjusted.
*Adults and children over age 1 month:* Initially, 0.04 to 0.1 mg/kg I.V.; then 0.01 mg/kg q 25 to 60 minutes if needed.

# I.V. administration

■ Administration requires direct medical supervision, with emergency respiratory support available.
■ Don't mix in same syringe or give through same needle with barbiturates or other alkaline solutions.
■ Store drug in refrigerator and not in plastic container or syringes. Plastic syringes may be used to administer dose.

## Incompatibilities
Incompatible with barbiturates or diazepam.

# Mechanism of action

*Skeletal muscle relaxant action:* Pancuronium prevents acetylcholine (ACh) from binding to the receptors on the motor end-plate, blocking depolarization. It may increase heart rate through direct blocking effect on the ACh receptors of the heart; increase is dose-related. Pancuronium causes little or no histamine release and no ganglionic blockade.

# Pharmacokinetics

*Absorption:* Administered I.V. Onset and duration are dose-related. After 0.06 mg/kg dose, effects begin to subside in 35 to 45 minutes. Repeated doses may increase the magnitude and duration of action.
*Distribution:* 87% plasma protein–bound.
*Metabolism:* Metabolism is unknown; small amounts may be metabolized by the liver.
*Excretion:* Mainly excreted unchanged in urine; some through biliary excretion.

| Route | Onset | Peak | Duration |
|-------|-------|------|----------|
| I.V. | 30-45 sec | 3-4½ min | 35-65 min |

# Contraindications and precautions

Contraindicated in patients hypersensitive to bromides or preexisting tachycardia and in those for whom even a minor increase in heart rate is undesirable.
Use cautiously in geriatric or debilitated patients and in those with impaired renal, pulmonary, or hepatic function; respiratory depression; myasthenia gravis; myasthenic syndrome of lung or bronchogenic cancer; dehydration; thyroid disorders; collagen diseases; porphyria; electrolyte disturbances; hyperthermia; or toxemic states. Use large doses cautiously in patients undergoing cesarean section.

# Interactions

**Drug-drug.** *Aminoglycoside antibiotics, beta blockers, clindamycin, depolarizing neuromuscular blockers, furosemide, general anesthetics, lincomycin, lithium, other nondepolarizing neuromuscular blockers, parenteral magnesium salts, polymyxin antibiotics, potassium-depleting drugs, quinidine or quinine, thiazide diuretics:* The effects of pancuronium may be potentiated. Use cautiously during surgical and postoperative periods.
*Opioid analgesics:* May increase respiratory depression. Use with extreme caution and recommend reducing dose of pancuronium.
*Succinylcholine:* May enhance and prolong neuromuscular blocking effects of pancuronium. Effects of succinylcholine should be allowed to subside before pancuronium is given.

# Adverse reactions

**CV:** tachycardia, increased blood pressure.
**GI:** excessive salivation.
**Musculoskeletal:** residual muscle weakness.
**Respiratory:** *prolonged, dose-related respiratory insufficiency or **apnea**.*
**Skin:** transient rashes.
**Other:** allergic or idiosyncratic hypersensitivity reactions.

# Overdose and treatment

Signs and symptoms of overdose include prolonged respiratory depression, apnea, and CV collapse.
Advise clinician to use a peripheral nerve stimulator to monitor response and to evaluate neuromuscular blockade. Advise clinician to maintain an adequate airway and manual or mechanical ventilation until patient can maintain adequate ventilation unassisted. Neostigmine, edrophonium, or pyridostigmine may be used to reverse effects.

# Clinical considerations

■ Dosage should be reduced when ether or other inhalation anesthetics that enhance neuromuscular blockade are used.
■ Large doses may increase frequency and severity of tachycardia.
■ Drug doesn't relieve pain or affect consciousness; recommend assessing need for analgesic or sedative.

## Therapeutic monitoring
■ Advise clinician to monitor baseline electrolyte levels, intake and output, and vital signs, especially heart rate and respiration.

## Special populations
**Breast-feeding patients.** It's unknown if drug appears in breast milk. Use with caution in breast-feeding women.

**Pediatric patients.** Dosage for neonates under age 1 month must be carefully individualized. For infants over age 1 month and children, see adult dosage.

**Geriatric patients.** The usual adult dose must be individualized depending on response.

## Patient counseling

■ Explain all events and procedures to patient because he can still hear.

---

# pantoprazole
Protonix, Protonix I.V.

*Pharmacologic classification:* substituted benzimidazole
*Therapeutic classification:* proton pump inhibitor that suppresses gastric acid production
*Pregnancy risk category B*

## Available forms
Available by prescription only
*Injection:* 40 mg per vial
*Tablet (delayed-release):* 20 mg, 40 mg

## Indications and dosages
*Treatment of erosive esophagitis with gastroesophageal reflux disease (GERD)*
*Adults:* 40 mg P.O. once daily for up to 8 weeks. For patients who haven't healed after 8 weeks, an additional 8-week course may be considered.

*Long-term maintenance of erosive esophagitis and reduction in relapse rates of day and nighttime heartburn symptoms in patients with GERD*
*Adults:* 40 mg P.O. once daily.

*Short-term treatment of GERD*
*Adults:* 40 mg I.V. every day for 7 to 10 days. Switch to oral form as soon as patient is able to take drug orally.

## I.V. administration
■ Dilute with $D_5W$, normal saline solution, or lactated Ringer's to a final concentration of 0.4 mg/ml.
■ Infuse over 15 minutes at a rate not greater than 3 mg/min (7 ml/min).
■ Do not give another infusion simultaneously through the same line.
■ The reconstituted solution may be stored for up to 2 hours at room temperature, and the admixture may be stored for up to 12 hours at room temperature.

## Incompatibilities
None reported.

## Mechanism of action
*Gastric acid suppression activity:* Pantoprazole inhibits the activity of the proton pump by binding to hydrogen-potassium adenosine triphosphatase, which is located at the secretory surface of the gastric parietal cells. This leads to suppression of gastric acid.

## Pharmacokinetics
*Absorption:* Well absorbed with an absolute bioavailability of 77%. Peak serum levels occur at 2.5 hours. Food may delay its absorption up to 2 hours; however, the extent of absorption is not affected.
*Distribution:* Distributes mainly in the extracellular fluid. Protein-binding is about 98%, mainly to albumin.
*Metabolism:* Extensively metabolized in the liver through the cytochrome P450 (CYP) system. The main metabolic pathway is demethylation by CYP2C19 with subsequent sulfation. Other pathways include oxidation by CYP3A4. There is no evidence that any of the metabolites have significant pharmacologic activity.
*Excretion:* About 71% of a dose is excreted in the urine with 18% excreted in the feces by bilary excretion. There is no renal excretion of unchanged drug.

| Route | Onset | Peak | Duration |
|-------|-------|------|----------|
| P.O. | Unknown | 2.5 hr | Unknown |
| I.V. | 15-30 min | Unknown | 24 hr |

## Contraindications and precautions
Contraindicated in patients hypersensitive to any component of the formulation.

## Interactions
**Drug-drug.** *Ketoconazole, ampicillin esters, iron salts:* May decrease absorption of these drugs. Advise clinician to monitor patient closely.
**Drug-herb.** *St. John's wort:* May cause an increased risk of sunburn. Proton pump inhibitors may increase this risk. Discourage use together.
**Drug-food.** *Food:* Delays absorption of pantoprazole for up to 2 hours; however, the extent of absorption is not affected. Can be given without regard to meals.

## Adverse reactions
**CNS:** headache, insomnia, asthenia, migraine, anxiety, dizziness.
**CV:** chest pain.
**EENT:** pharyngitis, rhinitis, sinusitis.
**GI:** diarrhea, flatulence, abdominal pain, eructation, constipation, dyspepsia, gastroenteritis, GI disorder, nausea, vomiting.
**GU:** rectal disorder, urinary frequency, urinary tract infection.
**Hepatic:** abnormal liver function test results.
**Metabolic:** hyperglycemia, hyperlipemia.
**Musculoskeletal:** back pain, neck pain, arthralgia, hypertonia.
**Respiratory:** bronchitis increased cough, dyspnea, upper respiratory tract infection.
**Skin:** rash.
**Other:** flu syndrome, infection, pain.

---

Reactions may be *common*, uncommon, *life-threatening*, or COMMON AND LIFE-THREATENING.

## Overdose and treatment
Overdose with 400 to 600 mg caused no adverse effects. Pantoprazole is not removed by hemodialysis.

## Clinical considerations
■ Can be given without regards to meals.
■ Drug is not to be used for maintenance therapy beyond 16 weeks.
■ Symptomatic response to therapy does not preclude the presence of gastric malignancy.
■ Treatment with I.V. pantoprazole should be discontinued when P.O. is warranted.
**Ⓗ ALERT** Don't confuse with Protonix tablets, Prilosec, Prozac, or Prevacid.

### Special populations
**Breast-feeding patients.** It's unknown if pantoprazole appears in breast milk. Use cautiously in nursing women.
**Pediatric patients.** Safety and effectiveness have not been established.

## Patient counseling
■ Instruct patient to take exactly as prescribed and at about the same time every day.
■ Advise patient that the drug can be taken without regard of meals.
■ Advise patient that tablet is to be swallowed whole and not crushed, split, or chewed.
■ Tell patient that antacids do not affect the absorption of pantoprazole

---

# papaverine hydrochloride
Cerespan, Genabid, Pavabid, Pavacels, Pavacot, Pavagen, Pavarine, Pavased, Pavatine, Pavatym, Paverolan

*Pharmacologic classification:* benzylisoquinoline derivative, opiate alkaloid
*Therapeutic classification:* peripheral vasodilator
*Pregnancy risk category C*

## Available forms
Available by prescription only
*Capsules (sustained-release):* 150 mg
*Injection:* 30 mg/ml

## Indications and dosages
*Relief of cerebral and peripheral ischemia from arterial spasm and myocardial ischemia; treatment of coronary occlusion and certain cerebral angiospastic states*
*Adults:* 75 to 300 mg P.O. three to five times daily or 150 to 300 mg sustained-release preparations q 8 to 12 hours; 30 to 120 mg I.M. or I.V. q 3 hours, as indicated. In treatment of extrasystoles, give two doses 10 minutes apart.
*Children:* 6 mg/kg I.M. or I.V. q.i.d.
◇ *Impotence*
*Adults:* 2.5 to 60 mg injected intracavernously.

## I.V. administration
■ Inject I.V. slowly over 1 to 2 minutes; arrhythmias and fatal apnea may follow rapid injection.

### Incompatibilities
Incompatible with lactated Ringer's injection; a precipitate will form.

## Mechanism of action
*Vasodilating action:* Papaverine relaxes smooth muscle directly by inhibiting phosphodiesterase, increasing the level of cyclic adenosine monophosphate. There's considerable controversy regarding the clinical effectiveness of papaverine. Some clinicians find little objective evidence of any clinical value.

## Pharmacokinetics
*Absorption:* About 54% of orally administered papaverine is bioavailable. Half-life varies from ½ hour to 24 hours, but levels can be maintained by giving drug at 6-hour intervals. Sustained-release forms are sometimes absorbed poorly and erratically.
*Distribution:* Tends to localize in adipose tissue and in the liver; the remainder is distributed throughout the body. About 90% of drug is protein-bound.
*Metabolism:* Metabolized by the liver.
*Excretion:* Excreted in urine as metabolites.

| Route | Onset | Peak | Duration |
|---|---|---|---|
| P.O. | Unknown | 1-2 hr | Unknown |
| I.V., I.M. | Unknown | Unknown | Unknown |

## Contraindications and precautions
I.V. use is contraindicated in patients with Parkinson's disease or complete AV block.
    Use cautiously in patients with glaucoma or hepatic dysfunction.

## Interactions
**Drug-drug.** *CNS depressants:* The effects of papaverine may be potentiated. Avoid use together.
*Levodopa:* Papaverine may decrease the antiparkinsonian effects and exacerbate such symptoms as rigidity and tremors. Don't use together.
*Morphine:* May have a synergic response. Advise clinician to monitor patient closely.
**Drug-lifestyle.** *Heavy smoking:* Interferes with the therapeutic effect of papaverine. Discourage smoking.

## Adverse reactions
**CNS:** *headache,* vertigo, drowsiness, sedation, malaise.
**CV:** *increased heart rate, increased blood pressure* (with parenteral use), depressed AV and intraventricular conduction, *arrhythmias.*
**GI:** constipation, *nausea,* anorexia, abdominal pain, diarrhea.

---

**Hepatic:** *hepatitis* (jaundice, eosinophilia, abnormal liver function test results), *cirrhosis.*
**Respiratory:** increased depth and rate of respiration.
**Skin:** *diaphoresis, flushing,* rash.

## Overdose and treatment
Signs and symptoms of overdose include drowsiness, weakness, nystagmus, diplopia, incoordination, and lassitude, progressing to coma with cyanosis and respiratory depression.

To slow drug absorption, advise clinician to give activated charcoal, tap water, or milk, then evacuate stomach contents by gastric lavage or emesis and follow with catharsis. If coma and respiratory depression occur, appropriate measures should be taken; advise clinician to maintain blood pressure. Hemodialysis may be helpful.

## Clinical considerations
■ Papaverine is an opiate; however, it has strikingly different pharmacologic properties than other drugs in this group.
■ Drug may be given orally, I.M. or, when immediate effect is needed, by slow I.V. injection.

### Therapeutic monitoring
■ When used for impotence, advise clinician to monitor patient for fibrotic changes, such as indurations and lumpy areas in the penis.

### Special populations
**Breast-feeding patients.** Safety in breast-feeding women hasn't been established.
**Pediatric patients.** Children's doses are administered parenterally.
**Geriatric patients.** Geriatric patients are at greater risk of papaverine-induced hypothermia.

## Patient counseling
■ Advise patient to avoid sudden postural changes to minimize possible orthostatic hypotension.
■ Instruct patient to report nausea, abdominal distress, anorexia, constipation, diarrhea, jaundice, rash, sweating, tiredness, or headache.

# paricalcitol
Zemplar

*Pharmacologic classification:* vitamin D analogue
*Therapeutic classification:* hyperparathyroidism drug
*Pregnancy risk category C*

## Available forms
Available by prescription only
*Injection:* 5 mcg/ml, 1-ml and 2-ml vials

## Indications and dosages
*Prevention and treatment of secondary hyperparathyroidism from chronic renal failure*
*Adults:* 0.04 to 0.1 mcg/kg (2.8 to 7 mcg) I.V. bolus no more frequently than every other day during dialysis. Doses as high as 0.24 mcg/kg (16.8 mcg) have been safely given. If satisfactory response isn't observed, dosage may be increased by 2 to 4 mcg at 2- to 4-week intervals.

## I.V. administration
■ Inspect drug for particulate matter and discoloration before use.
■ Drug is only administered as an I.V. bolus. Discard unused portion.

### Incompatibilities
None reported.

## Mechanism of action
*Parathyroid action:* A synthetic vitamin D analogue shown to reduce parathyroid hormone (PTH) levels.

## Pharmacokinetics
*Absorption:* Administered I.V.
*Distribution:* Not reported.
*Metabolism:* Not reported.
*Excretion:* Eliminated primarily by heptobiliary excretion, 74% in the feces and 16% in the urine. Half-life is about 15 hours.

| Route | Onset | Peak | Duration |
|-------|-------|------|----------|
| I.V. | Immediate | Unknown | 15 hr |

## Contraindications and precautions
Contraindicated in patients with evidence of vitamin D toxicity, hypercalcemia, and those hypersensitive to drug or its ingredients.

Use cautiously in patients taking digitalis compounds. Patients taking digoxin are at greater risk for digitalis toxicity during drug therapy secondary to potential for hypercalcemia.

## Interactions
None reported.

## Adverse reactions
**CNS:** light-headedness, malaise.
**CV:** palpitation.
**GI:** dry mouth, *GI bleeding, nausea,* vomiting.
**Hepatic:** reduced serum total alkaline phosphatase level.
**Respiratory:** pneumonia.
**Other:** chills, edema, fever, flu syndrome, *sepsis.*

## Overdose and treatment
Overdose may cause hypercalcemia. Symptoms include weakness, headache, nausea, vomiting,

constipation, anorexia, pancreatitis, ectopic calcification, cardiac arrhythmias, and death.

Treatment should include correcting electrolyte abnormalities, assessing cardiac abnormalities, and hemodialysis or peritoneal dialysis against a calcium-free dialysate.

### Clinical considerations
■ As the PTH level is decreased, paricalcitol dosage may need to be decreased. Acute overdose of paricalcitol may cause hypercalcemia, which may require emergency attention.
■ Appropriate types of phosphate-binding compounds may be needed to control serum phosphorus levels in patients with chronic renal failure; avoid excessive use of aluminum-containing compounds.
■ Store drug at a controlled room temperature (59° to 86° F [15° to 30° C]).

#### Therapeutic monitoring
■ Advise clinician to monitor patient for ECG abnormalities.
■ Advise clinician to monitor patient for symptoms of hypercalcemia and immediately notify prescriber if hypercalcemia is suspected.
■ Advise clinician to monitor serum calcium and phosphorus levels twice weekly when dosage is being adjusted, and then monitor monthly. PTH level should be measured every 3 months during therapy.

#### Special populations
**Breast-feeding patients.** It isn't known if drug appears in breast milk. Exercise caution when giving to breast-feeding women.
**Pediatric patients.** Safety and efficacy in children haven't been established.
**Geriatric patients.** No significant difference in safety and efficacy has been reported in patients over age 65.

### Patient counseling
■ Stress importance of adhering to a dietary regimen of calcium supplementation and phosphorus restriction during drug therapy.
■ Caution against use of phosphate or vitamin D–related compounds during drug therapy.
■ Instruct patient with chronic renal failure to take phosphate-binding compounds as prescribed but to avoid excessive use of aluminum-containing compounds.
■ Alert patient to early symptoms of hypercalcemia and vitamin D intoxication, such as weakness, headache, somnolence, nausea, vomiting, dry mouth, constipation, muscle pain, bone pain, and metallic taste.
■ Instruct patient to promptly report adverse reactions.
■ Remind patient taking digoxin to watch for signs of digitalis toxicity.

# paroxetine hydrochloride
Paxil

*Pharmacologic classification:* selective serotonin reuptake inhibitor
*Therapeutic classification:* antidepressant
*Pregnancy risk category C*

### Available forms
Available by prescription only
*Suspension:* 10 mg/5 ml
*Tablets:* 10 mg, 20 mg, 30 mg, 40 mg

### Indications and dosages
*Depression*
*Adults:* Initially, 20 mg P.O. daily, preferably in the morning. Increase dosage by 10 mg/day at 1-week intervals, to maximum of 50 mg daily, if needed.
*Obsessive-compulsive disorder (OCD); posttraumatic stress disorder (PTSD)*
*Adults:* Initially, 20 mg P.O. daily, preferably in the morning. May increase dosage by 10 mg/day at 1-week intervals to maximum dose of 40 mg/day for PTSD. Maximum dose, 60 mg/day for OCD.
*Generalized social phobia (social anxiety disorder)*
*Adults:* 20 mg P.O. daily.
*Panic disorder*
*Adults:* Initially, 10 mg P.O. daily, preferably in the morning. Increase dosage by 10 mg/day at 1-week intervals, to target dose of 40 mg/day. Maximum dose, 60 mg/day.
◇ *Diabetic neuropathy*
*Adults:* 10 to 60 mg P.O. daily.
◇ *Headaches*
*Adults:* 10 to 50 mg P.O. daily.
◇ *Premature ejaculation*
*Adults:* 20 mg P.O. daily.
◇ *Premenstrual dysphoric disorder*
*Adults:* 5 to 30 mg P.O. daily.
≡ *Dosage adjustment.* For geriatric or debilitated patients or patients with severe hepatic or renal disease, 10 mg P.O. daily, preferably in the morning. Increase dosage by 10 mg/day at 1-week intervals, p.r.n., to maximum of 40 mg daily.

### Mechanism of action
*Antidepressant action:* Action is presumed to be linked to potentiation of serotonergic activity in the CNS, resulting from inhibition of neuronal reuptake of serotonin.

### Pharmacokinetics
*Absorption:* Completely absorbed after oral dosing.
*Distribution:* Distributed throughout the body, including the CNS, with only 1% remaining in the plasma. About 93% to 95% of paroxetine is plasma protein–bound.

---

* Canada only    ◇ Unlabeled clinical use

*Metabolism:* About 36% is metabolized in the liver. The principal metabolites are polar and conjugated products of oxidation and methylation, which are readily cleared.

*Excretion:* About 64% is excreted in urine (2% as parent compound and 62% as metabolite).

| Route | Onset | Peak | Duration |
|-------|-------|------|----------|
| P.O. | Unknown | 2-8 hr | Unknown |

## Contraindications and precautions
Contraindicated in patients taking MAO inhibitors or within 14 days of discontinuing MAO inhibitors.

Use cautiously in patients with history of seizures or mania; in those with severe, concurrent systemic illness; or in those at risk for volume depletion and those hypersensitive to SSRIs.

## Interactions
**Drug-drug.** *Cimetidine:* Decreases hepatic metabolism of paroxetine, leading to risk of toxicity. Dosage adjustments may be needed.
*Digoxin:* Paroxetine may decrease levels. Advise clinician to monitor patient closely.
*MAO inhibitors:* May increase risk of serious, sometimes fatal, adverse reactions. Avoid use together.
*Phenobarbital, phenytoin:* Reduces plasma levels of drug. Dosage adjustment may be needed.
*Procyclidine:* Increases procyclidine levels. Advise clinician to monitor patient for excessive anticholinergic effects.
*Theophylline:* Paroxetine may increase levels. Advise clinician to monitor patient closely.
*Tryptophan:* May increase the risk of adverse reactions. Avoid use together.
*Warfarin:* Increased risk of bleeding. Advise clinician to monitor INR.
**Drug-herb.** *SAMe, St. John's wort:* May increase serotonin levels and the risk of serotonin syndrome. Discourage use together.
**Drug-lifestyle.** *Alcohol use:* May increase risk of CNS adverse effects. Advise patient to avoid alcohol during treatment.

## Adverse reactions
**CNS:** *somnolence, dizziness, insomnia, tremor, nervousness,* anxiety, paresthesia, confusion, *headache,* agitation, decreased levels, abnormal dreams, *asthenia.*
**CV:** palpitations, vasodilation, orthostatic hypotension, chest pain.
**EENT:** lump or tightness in throat, dysgeusia, visual disturbances, double vision.
**GI:** *dry mouth, nausea, constipation, diarrhea,* flatulence, vomiting, dyspepsia, increased or decreased appetite, abdominal pain.
**GU:** ejaculatory disturbances, male genital disorders (including anorgasmia, erectile difficulties, delayed ejaculation or orgasm, impotence, and sexual dysfunction), urinary frequency, other urinary disorders, female genital disorders (including anorgasmia, difficulty with orgasm).
**Musculoskeletal:** myopathy, myalgia, myasthenia.
**Skin:** *diaphoresis,* rash, pruritus.
**Other:** decreased libido, yawning.

## Overdose and treatment
Signs and symptoms of overdose may include nausea, vomiting, dizziness, sweating, facial flushing, drowsiness, sinus tachycardia, and dilated pupil.

Treatment should consist of general measures used in management of overdose with any antidepressant. Advise clinician to perform gastric evacuation by emesis, lavage, or both. In most cases, 20 to 30 g of activated charcoal may then be given every 4 to 6 hours during the first 24 to 48 hours after ingestion. Supportive care, frequent monitoring of vital signs, and careful observation are indicated. ECG and cardiac function monitoring are warranted with evidence of any abnormality.

Advise clinician to take special caution with a patient who currently receives or recently received paroxetine if the patient ingests an excessive quantity of a tricyclic antidepressant. In such cases, accumulation of the parent tricyclic and its active metabolite may increase the possibility of clinically significant sequelae and extend the time needed for close medical observation.

## Clinical considerations
■ At least 14 days should elapse between discontinuation of an MAO inhibitor and initiation of drug therapy. Similarly, at least 14 days should elapse between discontinuation of paroxetine and initiation of an MAO inhibitor.
■ If signs of psychosis occur or increase, dosage should be reduced. Advise clinician to monitor patients for suicidal tendencies and allow them only a minimum supply of drug.

### *Therapeutic monitoring*
■ Hyponatremia may occur with paroxetine use, especially in geriatric patients, those taking diuretics, and those who are otherwise volume depleted. Advise clinician to monitor serum sodium levels.

### *Special populations*
**Breast-feeding patients.** Drug appears in breast milk. Use with caution in breast-feeding women.
**Pediatric patients.** Safety and efficacy in children haven't been established.
**Geriatric patients.** Use cautiously and in lower dosages in geriatric patients.

## Patient counseling
■ Caution patient not to operate hazardous machinery, including automobiles, until reason-

ably certain that paroxetine therapy doesn't affect ability to engage in such activity.
■ Tell patient that he may notice improvement in 1 to 4 weeks but that he must continue with the prescribed regimen to obtain continued benefits.
■ Instruct patient to contact prescriber before taking other drugs, including OTC preparations, while receiving paroxetine therapy.
■ Tell patient to avoid alcohol while taking paroxetine.

## pegaspargase (PEG-L-asparaginase)
Oncaspar

*Pharmacologic classification:* modified version of the enzyme l-asparaginase
*Therapeutic classification:* antineoplastic
*Pregnancy risk category C*

### Available forms
Available by prescription only
*Injection:* 750 IU/ml in single-use vial

### Indications and dosages
**Acute lymphoblastic leukemia (ALL) in patients who require L-asparaginase but have developed hypersensitivity to the native forms of L-asparaginase**
*Adults and children with body surface area of at least 0.6 m²:* 2,500 IU/m² I.M. or I.V. q 14 days.
*Children with body surface area less than 0.6 m²:* 82.5 IU/kg I.M. or I.V. q 14 days.
Note: Moderate to life-threatening hypersensitivity reactions necessitate discontinuation of L-asparaginase treatment.

### I.V. administration
■ When administered I.V., recommend giving over 1 to 2 hours in 100 ml of normal saline solution or $D_5W$ through an infusion that is already running.
■ Avoid excessive agitation; don't shake. Keep refrigerated at 36° to 46° F (2° to 8° C). Don't use if cloudy, if precipitate is present, or if stored at room temperature for longer than 48 hours. Don't freeze. Discard unused portions. Use only one dose per vial; don't reenter the vial. Don't save unused drug for later administration.
**H ALERT** Hypersensitivity reactions to pegaspargase, including life-threatening anaphylaxis, may occur during therapy, especially in patients hypersensitive to other forms of L-asparaginase. As a precaution, observe patient for 1 hour and have resuscitation equipment and other drugs needed to treat anaphylaxis available.

### Incompatibilities
Should not be mixed with other drugs.

### Mechanism of action
*Antineoplastic action:* Pegaspargase is a modified version of the enzyme L-asparaginase, which exerts its cytotoxic activity by inactivating the amino acid asparagine. Because leukemic cells can't synthesize their own asparagine, protein synthesis and, eventually, synthesis of DNA and RNA are inhibited.

### Pharmacokinetics
No information available.

| Route | Onset | Peak | Duration |
|-------|-------|------|----------|
| I.M., I.V. | Unknown | Unknown | Unknown |

### Contraindications and precautions
Contraindicated in patients with pancreatitis or a history of pancreatitis; in those who have had significant hemorrhagic events from prior L-asparaginase therapy; and in those with previous serious allergic reactions, such as generalized urticaria, bronchospasm, laryngeal edema, hypotension, or other unacceptable adverse reactions to pegaspargase.
Use cautiously in patients with hepatic dysfunction and during pregnancy.

### Interactions
**Drug-drug.** *Aspirin, dipyridamole, heparin, NSAIDs, warfarin:* May cause imbalances in coagulation factors, predisposing the patient to bleeding or thrombosis. Use together cautiously.
*Methotrexate:* During its inhibition of protein synthesis and cell replication, pegaspargase may interfere with the action of such drugs that require cell replication for their lethal effects. Advise clinician to monitor patient for decreased effectiveness.
*Protein-bound drugs:* Depletion of serum protein by pegaspargase may increase the toxicity of these drugs. Advise clinician to monitor patient for toxicity. Pegaspargase may interfere with the enzymatic detoxification of other drugs, particularly in the liver. Use caution when giving together.

### Adverse reactions
**CNS:** *seizures,* headache, paresthesia, *status epilepticus,* somnolence, *coma,* mental status changes, dizziness, emotional lability, mood changes, parkinsonism, confusion, disorientation, fatigue, malaise.
**CV:** hypotension, tachycardia, chest pain, subacute bacterial endocarditis, hypertension, edema, peripheral edema.
**EENT:** epistaxis.
**GI:** nausea, vomiting, abdominal pain, anorexia, diarrhea, constipation, indigestion, flatulence, GI pain, mucositis, *pancreatitis (some-*

*times fulminant and fatal),* increased serum amylase and lipase levels, severe colitis, mouth tenderness.

**GU:** increased BUN level, increased creatinine level, increased urinary frequency, hematuria, severe hemorrhagic cystitis, renal dysfunction, renal failure.

**Hematologic:** *thrombosis;* prolonged PT, prolonged PTT, decreased antithrombin III; *DIC;* decreased fibrinogen; hemolytic anemia; *leukopenia; pancytopenia; agranulocytosis; thrombocytopenia;* increased thromboplastin; easy bruising; ecchymoses; *hemorrhage.*

**Hepatic:** jaundice, abnormal liver function test results, bilirubinemia, increased ALT and AST, ascites, hypoalbuminemia, fatty changes in liver, *liver failure.*

**Metabolic:** hyperuricemia, hyperglycemia, hypoglycemia, hyponatremia, uric acid nephropathy, hypoproteinemia, proteinuria, weight loss, metabolic acidosis, increased blood ammonia level.

**Musculoskeletal:** arthralgia, myalgia, musculoskeletal pain, joint stiffness, cramps.

**Respiratory:** cough, *severe bronchospasm,* upper respiratory tract infection, dyspnea, *bronchospasm.*

**Skin:** itching, alopecia, fever blister, purpura, hand whiteness, fungal changes, nail whiteness and ridging, erythema simplex, petechial rash, injection pain or reaction, localized edema, rash, erythema, urticaria.

**Other:** hypersensitivity reactions, including *anaphylaxis,* pain, fever, chills, pain in limbs, night sweats, infection; *sepsis, septic shock.*

### Overdose and treatment

Only three cases of overdose (10,000 IU/m$^2$ as an I.V. infusion) have been reported. One patient experienced a slight increase in liver enzymes, a rash developed in another, and the third experienced no adverse effects. No other information is available.

### Clinical considerations

■ I.M. is the preferred administration route because it has a lower risk of hepatotoxicity, coagulopathy, and GI and renal disorders than the I.V. route.

■ Drug shouldn't be administered if it has ever been frozen. Although there may not be an apparent change in appearance of drug, its activity is destroyed after freezing.

■ When administering I.M., limit volume at a single injection site to 2 ml. If the volume to be administered is greater than 2 ml, use multiple injection sites.

■ Pegaspargase should be the sole induction drug only when a combined regimen using other chemotherapeutic drugs is inappropriate because of toxicity or other specific patient-related factors or in patients refractory to other therapy.

■ Pegaspargase may be a contact irritant, and the solution must be handled and administered with care. Gloves are recommended. Avoid inhalation of vapors and contact with skin or mucous membranes, especially those of the eyes. In case of contact, wash with copious amounts of water for at least 15 minutes.

### Therapeutic monitoring

■ A decrease in circulating lymphoblasts is common after therapy starts. This may be accompanied by a marked increase in serum uric acid. As a guide to the effects of therapy, advise clinician to monitor patient's peripheral blood count and bone marrow.

■ Frequent serum amylase determinations should be obtained to detect early evidence of pancreatitis. Advise clinician to monitor blood glucose during therapy because hyperglycemia may occur.

■ When using pegaspargase with hepatotoxic chemotherapy, advise clinician to monitor patient for liver dysfunction.

■ Pegaspargase may affect some plasma proteins; therefore, monitoring of fibrinogen, PT, and PTT may be indicated.

### Special populations

**Breast-feeding patients.** Because of potential for serious adverse reactions in breast-fed infants, a decision must be made to stop either breast-feeding or drug, taking into account the importance of drug to the woman.

**Pediatric patients.** Safety and efficacy in infants under age 1 haven't been established.

### Patient counseling

■ Tell patient to report hypersensitivity reactions immediately.

■ Instruct patient not to take other drugs, including OTC preparations, without obtaining medical approval; pegaspargase increases the risk of bleeding when given with certain drugs, such as aspirin, and may increase the toxicity of other drugs.

■ Instruct patient to report signs and symptoms of infection (fever, chills, malaise); drug may have immunosuppressive activity.

# peginterferon alfa-2b
PEG-Intron

*Pharmacologic classification:* biological response modifier
*Therapeutic classification:* antiviral
*Pregnancy risk category C*

### Available forms

Available by prescription only
*Injection:* 100 mcg/ml, 160 mcg/ml, 240 mcg/ml, 300 mcg/ml

## Indications and dosages

*Chronic hepatitis C*

*Adults:* Give S.C. once weekly for 48 weeks on same day each week based on weight. Less than 45 kg: 40 mcg (0.4 ml) of 100-mcg/ml strength; 46 to 56 kg: 50 mcg (0.5 ml) of 100-mcg/ml strength; 57 to 72 kg: 64 mcg (0.4 ml) of 160-mcg/ml strength; 73 to 88 kg: 80 mcg (0.5 ml) of 160-mcg/ml strength; 89 to 106 kg: 96 mcg (0.4 ml) of 240-mcg/ml strength; 107 to 136 kg: 120 mcg (0.5 ml) of 240-mcg/ml strength; 137 to 160 kg: 150 mcg (0.5 ml) of 300-mcg/ml strength.

*Chronic hepatitis C in patients not previously treated with interferon alpha with Rebetol 400 mg P.O. b.i.d. with meals*

*Adults:* Give S.C. once weekly for 48 weeks on same day each week; initial dose based on weight.

Recommended regimen is 1.5 mcg/kg/week. Less than 40 kg: 50 mcg (0.5 ml) of 100-mcg/ml strength; 40 to 50 kg: 64 mcg (0.4 ml) of 160-mcg/ml strength; 51 to 60 kg: 80 mcg (0.5 ml) of 160-mcg/ml strength; 61 to 75 kg: 96 mcg (0.4 ml) of 240-mcg/ml strength; 76-85 kg: 120 mcg (0.5 ml) of 240 mcg-mcg/ml strength. Over 85 kg: 150 mcg (0.5 ml) of 300-mcg/ml strength.

≡ *Dosage adjustment.* For patients who develop a serious adverse reaction, decrease dosage to one-half starting dose. For patients with neutrophil count < 0.75 × 10⁹/L, reduce dosage. If neutrophil count is < 0.50 × 10⁹/L, discontinue drug. For patients with platelet count < 80 × 10⁹/L, reduce dosage. If platelet count is < 50 × 10⁹/L, discontinue drug.

## Mechanism of action

*Antiviral action:* Binds to specific membrane receptors on the cell surface, initiating induction of certain enzymes, suppression of cell proliferation, and immunomodulating activities and inhibition of virus replication in virus-infected cells. Increases levels of effector proteins and body temperature, and decreases leukocyte and platelet counts.

## Pharmacokinetics

*Absorption:* Serum levels peak 15 to 44 hours after dose, and last from 48 to 72 hours.
*Distribution:* Unknown.
*Metabolism:* Mean elimination half-life is about 40 hours.
*Excretion:* About 30% is excreted by the kidneys.

| Route | Onset | Peak | Duration |
|-------|-------|------|----------|
| S.C. | Unknown | 15-44 hr | Unknown |

## Contraindications and precautions

Contraindicated in patients hypersensitive to drug or any of its components. Also contraindicated in patients with autoimmune hepatitis or decompensated liver disease.

Use cautiously in patients with psychiatric disorders, diabetes mellitus, CV disease, renal failure (creatinine clearance < 50 ml/minute), pulmonary infiltrates, or pulmonary function impairment. Also use cautiously in patients with autoimmune, ischemic, and infectious disorders.

## Interactions

None reported.

## Adverse reactions

**CNS:** *dizziness,* hypertonia, *depression, insomnia, anxiety, emotional lability, irritability, headache, fatigue,* malaise, *suicidal behavior.*
**CV:** flushing.
**EENT:** *pharyngitis,* sinusitis.
**GI:** *nausea, anorexia, diarrhea, abdominal pain,* vomiting, dyspepsia, right upper quadrant pain.
**Hematologic:** *neutropenia, thrombocytopenia.*
**Hepatic:** hepatomegaly, *elevated ALT levels.*
**Metabolic:** hypothyroidism, hyperthyroidism, *weight decrease.*
**Musculoskeletal:** *musculoskeletal pain.*
**Respiratory:** cough.
**Skin:** *alopecia, pruritus, dry skin, rash, injection site inflammation or reaction, increased sweating,* injection site pain.
**Other:** *viral infection, fever, influenza-like symptoms, rigors.*

## Overdose and treatment

No serious reactions caused by overdose occurred in 13 patients given a dose greater than that prescribed. The maximum dose received was 3.45 mcg/kg weekly for about 12 weeks.

## Clinical considerations

■ Don't use drug in patients with diabetes or thyroid disorders that can't be controlled with drugs. Drug may cause or aggravate hypothyroidism, hyperthyroidism, or diabetes.
■ Don't use in patients who have failed other alpha interferon treatment or received liver or other organ transplants, or in patients with HIV or hepatitis B.
■ Advise clinician to perform ECG on patients with cardiac history before starting drug.
■ Treatment should be started in patient who is well hydrated.
■ Drug should be stopped in patients with severe neutropenia or thrombocytopenia.

### Therapeutic monitoring

■ Recommend closely monitoring patient with history of MI or arrhythmias for hypotension, arrhythmias, tachycardia, cardiomyopathy, and MI.
■ Advise clinician to monitor patient for depression and other psychiatric illness. If symp-

toms are severe, drug should be stopped and patient referred for psychiatric care.
■ Advise clinician to monitor patient for signs and symptoms of colitis, such as abdominal pain, bloody diarrhea, and fever. Drug should be stopped if colitis occurs. Symptoms should resolve within 1 to 3 weeks after discontinuing drug.
■ Advise clinician to monitor patient for signs and symptoms of pancreatitis or hypersensitivity reactions and stop drug if these occur.
■ Advise clinician to monitor patient with pulmonary disease for dyspnea, pulmonary infiltrates, pneumonitis, and pneumonia.
■ Advise clinician to perform eye examination in patient with diabetes or hypertension before starting drug. Retinal hemorrhages, cotton-wool spots, and retinal artery or vein obstruction may occur.
■ Advise clinician to monitor patient with renal disease for signs and symptoms of toxicity.
■ Advise clinician to monitor CBC count, platelets, and AST, ALT, bilirubin, and TSH levels before starting drug and periodically during treatment.

### Special populations
**Breast-feeding patients.** It's unknown if drug appears in breast milk. Because of the potential for adverse reactions in breast-feeding infants, a decision must be made to stop either breast-feeding or drug.
**Pediatric patients.** Safety and effectiveness in children under age 18 haven't been established.
**Geriatric patients.** There are no differences in pharmacokinetics in geriatric patients.

### Patient counseling
■ Advise patient on appropriate use of drug and benefits and risks of treatment. Tell patient that adverse reactions may continue for several months after treatment is stopped.
■ Advise patient to immediately report symptoms of depression or suicidal ideation.
■ Instruct patient on importance of proper disposal of needles and syringes, and caution him against reuse of old needles and syringes.
■ Tell patient that drug isn't known to prevent transmission of hepatitis C to others. It's also unknown if drug will cure hepatitis C or prevent cirrhosis, liver failure, or liver cancer that may result from hepatitis C infection.
■ Advise patient that laboratory tests are needed before therapy starts and periodically thereafter.
■ Tell patient to take drug at bedtime and to use antipyretics to decrease incidence of flu-like symptoms.

# penicillamine
Cuprimine, Depen

*Pharmacologic classification:* chelating drug
*Therapeutic classification:* heavy metal antagonist, antirheumatic
*Pregnancy risk category NR*

## Available forms
Available by prescription only
*Capsules:* 125 mg, 250 mg
*Tablets:* 250 mg

## Indications and dosages
*Wilson's disease*
*Adults:* 250 mg P.O. q.i.d. 0.5 to 1 hour before meals and at least 2 hours after evening meal. Adjust dosage to achieve urinary copper excretion of 0.5 to 1 mg daily. Dose over 2 g is seldom needed.
*Cystinuria*
*Adults:* 250 mg P.O. daily in four divided doses, then gradually increasing dosage. Usual dose, 2 g daily (range, 1 to 4 g daily). Adjust dosage to achieve urinary cystine excretion of less than 100 mg daily when renal calculi are present, or 100 to 200 mg daily when no calculi are present.
*Rheumatoid arthritis,* ◇ *Felty's syndrome*
*Adults:* Initially, 125 to 250 mg P.O. daily, with increases of 125 to 250 mg daily at 1- to 3-month intervals if needed. Maximum dose is 1.5 g daily.
◇ *Adjunctive treatment of heavy metal poisoning*
*Adults:* 500 to 1,500 mg P.O. daily for 1 to 2 months.
◇ *Primary biliary cirrhosis*
*Adults:* Initially, 250 mg P.O. daily, with increases of 250 mg q 2 weeks. Maximum dose, 1 g daily in divided doses.

## Mechanism of action
*Antirheumatic action:* Mechanism of action in rheumatoid arthritis is unknown; penicillamine depresses circulating IgM rheumatoid factor (but not total circulating immunoglobulin levels) and depresses T-cell but not B-cell activity. It also depolymerizes some macroglobulins (such as rheumatoid factor).
*Chelating drug action:* Penicillamine forms stable, soluble complexes with copper, iron, mercury, lead, and other heavy metals that are excreted in urine; it's particularly useful in chelating copper in patients with Wilson's disease. Penicillamine also combines with cystine to form a complex more soluble than cystine alone, thereby reducing free cystine below the level of urinary stone formation.

## Pharmacokinetics

*Absorption:* Well absorbed after oral administration.

*Distribution:* Limited data available.

*Metabolism:* Metabolized by liver to inactive compounds.

*Excretion:* Only small amounts of penicillamine are excreted unchanged; after 24 hours, about 50% of drug is excreted in urine and about 50% in feces.

| Route | Onset | Peak | Duration |
|-------|-------|------|----------|
| P.O. | Unknown | 3 hr | Unknown |

## Contraindications and precautions

Contraindicated in patients hypersensitive to drug, and those with history of penicillamine-related aplastic anemia or agranulocytosis, or significant renal or hepatic insufficiency; in pregnant women; and in patients receiving gold salts, immunosuppressants, antimalarials, or phenylbutazone because of the increased risk of serious hematologic effects.

Use cautiously in patients allergic to penicillin (cross-reaction is rare); in those who receive a second course of therapy and who may have become sensitized and are more likely to have allergic reactions; and in patients in whom proteinuria with Goodpasture's syndrome develops.

## Interactions

**Drug-drug.** *Antacids, iron salts:* Decrease absorption of penicillamine. Separate administration times.

*Antimalarial or cytotoxic drugs, gold therapy, oxyphenbutazone, phenylbutazone:* Serious hematologic and renal effects. Don't use together.

*Digoxin:* Levels may be decreased when given together. Advise clinician to monitor serum digoxin levels closely.

## Adverse reactions

**EENT:** oral ulcerations, glossitis, cheilosis, tinnitus, optic neuritis.

**GI:** anorexia, nausea, vomiting, dyspepsia, alteration in sense of taste (salty and sweet), metallic taste, diarrhea, dysgeusia, *hypogeusia.*

**GU:** *proteinuria.*

**Hematologic:** eosinophilia, *leukopenia, thrombocytopenia, aplastic anemia, agranulocytosis,* thrombotic *thrombocytopenic purpura,* hemolytic anemia or iron deficiency anemia, lupus-like syndrome, bone marrow suppression.

**Hepatic:** cholestatic jaundice, *pancreatitis,* hepatic dysfunction.

**Musculoskeletal:** arthralgia, myasthenia gravis (with prolonged use).

**Respiratory:** pneumonitis, Goodpasture's syndrome.

**Skin:** *pruritus; erythematous rash;* intensely pruritic rash with scaly, macular lesions on trunk; pemphigoid reactions; urticaria; *exfoliative dermatitis;* increased skin friability; purpuric or vesicular ecchymoses; wrinkling, alopecia.

**Other:** lymphadenopathy, drug fever, thyroiditis.

Note: Drug should be stopped if patient has signs of hypersensitivity or drug fever, usually with other allergic signs and symptoms (if Wilson's disease, may rechallenge); or if the following occur: rash developing 6 months or more after start of therapy; pemphigoid reaction; hematuria or proteinuria with hemoptysis or pulmonary infiltrates; gross or persistent microscopic hematuria or proteinuria greater than 2 g/day in patients with rheumatoid arthritis; platelet count less than 100,000/mm$^3$ or leukocyte count less than 3,500/mm$^3$, or if either shows three consecutive decreases, even within normal range.

## Overdose and treatment

There are no reports of significant drug overdose. Emesis should be induced unless unconscious or gag reflex is absent; otherwise advise clinician to empty stomach by gastric lavage and then give activated charcoal and sorbitol. Thereafter, treatment is supportive. Advise clinician to treat seizures with diazepam (or pyridoxine if previously successful). Hemodialysis will remove penicillamine.

## Clinical considerations

**⊞ ALERT** Beware of sound-alikes: There are various types of penicillin, plus polycillin and penicillamine. Don't confuse these various drugs.

■ About one-third of patients receiving drug experience an allergic reaction. Advise clinician to monitor patient for signs and symptoms of allergic reaction.

■ Patients with Wilson's disease or cystinuria may require daily pyridoxine (vitamin $B_6$) supplementation.

■ Prescribe drug to be taken 1 hour before or 2 hours after meals or other drugs to facilitate absorption.

■ For initial treatment of Wilson's disease, recommend giving 10 to 40 mg of sulfurated potash with each meal during penicillamine therapy for 6 months to 1 year; then it should be discontinued.

■ Drug therapy may cause positive test results for antinuclear antibody with or without clinical systemic lupus erythematosus-like syndrome.

### Therapeutic monitoring

■ Advise clinician to perform urinalyses and CBC, including differential blood count every 2 weeks for 6 months, then monthly.

---

■ Advise clinician to perform kidney and liver functions tests, usually every 6 months.
■ Fever or allergic reactions, such as rash, joint pain, and easy bruising should be reported immediately. Recommend checking routinely for proteinuria and handling patient carefully to avoid skin damage.

### Special populations

**Breast-feeding patients.** Safety hasn't been established in breast-feeding patients; alternative feeding method is recommended during therapy.

**Pediatric patients.** Recommend checking patient for possible iron deficiency resulting from chronic use. Safety and efficacy of penicillamine in juvenile rheumatoid arthritis haven't yet been established.

**Geriatric patients.** Lower doses may be indicated. Advise clinician to monitor renal and hepatic function closely. Toxicity may be more common in geriatric patients.

### Patient counseling

■ Provide health education for patients with Wilson's disease, rheumatoid arthritis, or cystinuria. Explain disease process and reason for therapy and explain that clinical results may not be evident for 3 months.
■ Stress importance of immediate reporting of fever, chills, sore throat, bruising, bleeding, or allergic reaction.
■ Tell patient to take drug on an empty stomach 30 minutes to 1 hour before meals or 2 hours after ingesting food, antacids, mineral supplements, vitamins, or other drugs. Tell patient to drink large amounts of water, especially at night.
■ Advise patient taking penicillamine for Wilson's disease to maintain a low-copper (less than 2 mg daily) diet by excluding foods with high copper content, such as chocolate, nuts, liver, and broccoli. Also, sulfurated potash may be given with meals to minimize copper absorption.
■ Advise patient receiving drug for rheumatoid arthritis that an exacerbation of disease may occur during therapy. This usually can be controlled by concurrent use of NSAIDs.

---

## penicillin G benzathine
Bicillin L-A, Megacillin, Permapen

## penicillin G benzathine and procaine
Bicillin C-R

## penicillin G potassium
Pfizerpen

## penicillin G procaine
Ayercillin*, Bicillin C-R, Crysticillin A.S., Pfizerpen-AS, Wycillin

## penicillin G sodium

*Pharmacologic classification:* natural penicillin
*Therapeutic classification:* antibiotic
*Pregnancy risk category B*

### Available forms

Available by prescription only
**penicillin G benzathine**
*Suspension:* 250,000 units/5 ml*; 500,000 units/ml*
*Injection:* 300,000 units/ml; 600,000 units/ml; 1.2 million units/2 ml; 2.4 million units/4 ml
**penicillin G benzathine and procaine**
*Injection:* 300,000 units/ml; 600,000 units/ml; 1.2 million units/2 ml; 2.4 million units/4 ml
**penicillin G potassium**
*Powder for injection:* 1 million units, 5 million units, 10 million units, 20 million units
*Injection (premixed, frozen):* 1 million units/50 ml, 2 million units/50 ml, 3 million units/50 ml
**penicillin G procaine**
*Injection:* 600,000 units/ml, 1.2 million units/2 ml, 2.4 million units/2 ml
**penicillin G sodium**
*Powder for injection:* 1 million units*, 5 million units, 10 million units*

### Indications and dosages

*Anthrax (intestinal, pulmonary, and meningeal), anthrax septicemia*
**penicillin G potassium**
*Adults:* 5 to 20 million units I.V. daily given in divided doses q 4 to 6 hours for at least 2 weeks after symptoms abate.
*Children:* 100,000 to 250,000 units/kg/day I.V. in divided doses q 4 to 6 hours for at least 2 weeks after symptoms abate.
*Anthrax from* **Bacillus anthracis,** *including inhalation anthrax (postexposure)*
**penicillin G procaine**
*Adults:* 1,200,000 units I.M. q 12 hours.
*Children:* 25,000 units/kg I.M. (maximum 1,200,000 units) q 12 hours.
*Congenital syphilis*
**penicillin G benzathine**
*Children under age 2:* 50,000 units/kg I.M. as a single injection.
*Cutaneous anthrax*
**penicillin G procaine**
*Adults:* 600,000 to 1 million units/day I.M.
*Group A streptococcal upper respiratory infections,* ◊*diphtheria,* ◊*yaws, pinta, and bejel*
**penicillin G benzathine**
*Adults:* 1.2 million units I.M. as single injection.

---

*Children weighing 27 kg (60 lb) or more:*
900,000 units I.M. in a single injection.
*Children weighing under 27 kg:* 300,000 to
600,000 units I.M. in a single injection.
*Prophylaxis of poststreptococcal rheumatic fever*
**penicillin G benzathine**
*Adults and children:* 1.2 million units I.M. once monthly.
*Syphilis of less than 1 year's duration*
**penicillin G benzathine**
*Adults:* 2.4 million units I.M. in a single dose.
*Syphilis of longer than 1 year's duration*
**penicillin G benzathine**
*Adults:* 2.4 million units I.M. weekly for 3 successive weeks.
*Moderate to severe systemic infections*
**penicillin G potassium, sodium**
*Adults:* 12 to 24 million units I.M. or I.V. daily, given in divided doses q 4 hours.
*Children:* 25,000 to 300,000 units/kg I.M. or I.V. daily, given in divided doses q 4 hours.
*Moderate to severe systemic infections, pneumococcal pneumonia*
**penicillin G procaine**
*Adults:* 600,000 to 1.2 million units I.M. daily as a single dose or q 6 to 12 hours.
*Children:* 300,000 units I.M. daily as a single dose.
*Uncomplicated gonorrhea*
**penicillin G procaine**
*Adults and children over age 12:* 1 g probenecid, P.O. then 30 minutes later, 4.8 million units of penicillin G procaine I.M., divided into two injection sites.
≣ *Dosage adjustment.* For patients with renal impairment, refer to following table.

| Creatinine clearance (ml/min) | Dosage (after full loading dose) |
|---|---|
| 10-50 | 50% of usual dose q 4-5 hr; or, give usual dose q 8-12 hr |
| < 10 | 50% of usual dose q 8-12 hr; or, give usual dose q 12-18 hr |

## I.V. administration

**⚕ ALERT** Never give penicillin G benzathine or penicillin G procaine I.V. Inadvertent I.V. administration has caused cardiac arrest and death.
**penicillin G sodium**
■ Reconstitute drug with sterile water for injection, normal saline solution for injection, or D₅W. Check manufacturer's instructions for volume of diluent necessary to produce desired drug level.
■ Give by intermittent I.V. infusion: Dilute drug in 50 to 100 ml, and give over 30 minutes to 2 hours q 4 to 6 hours.

■ In neonates and children, give divided doses over 15 to 30 minutes.
**penicillin G potassium**
■ Reconstitute drug with sterile water injection, D₅W, or normal saline solution for injection. Volume of diluent varies with manufacturer.
■ For intermittent I.V. infusion, give drug over 1 to 2 hours.
■ For continuous I.V. infusion, add reconstituted solution of drug to 1 to 2 L of compatible I.V. solution. Determine the volume of fluid and rate of administration required by the patient in a 24-hour period, and add the ordered drug dose to this fluid.

### Incompatibilities

Penicillin G potassium is incompatible with alcohol 5%, amikacin, aminoglycosides, aminophylline, amphotericin B sodium, cephalothin, heparin sodium, hydroxyzine hydrochloride, lincomycin, metaraminol, metoclopramide, pentobarbital sodium, phenytoin sodium, prochlorperazine mesylate, promazine, promethazine hydrochloride, sodium bicarbonate, thiopental, vancomycin, and vitamin B complex with C.

Penicillin G sodium is incompatible with aminoglycosides, amphotericin B, bleomycin, cephalothin, chlorpromazine, fat emulsions 10%, heparin sodium, hydroxyzine hydrochloride, invert sugar 10%, lincomycin, methylprednisolone sodium succinate, potassium chloride, prochlorperazine mesylate, and promethazine hydrochloride.

## Mechanism of action

*Antibiotic action:* Penicillin G is bactericidal; it adheres to penicillin-binding proteins, inhibiting bacterial cell wall synthesis. Penicillin G's activity includes most non–penicillinase-producing strains of gram-positive and gram-negative aerobic cocci; spirochetes, and some gram-positive aerobic and anaerobic bacilli.

## Pharmacokinetics

Penicillin G is available as four salts, each having the same bactericidal action, but designed to offer greater oral stability (potassium salt) or to prolong duration of action by slowing absorption after I.M. injection (benzathine and procaine salts).
*Absorption:* Sodium and potassium salts of penicillin G are absorbed rapidly after I.M. injection; peak serum levels occur within 15 to 30 minutes. Absorption of other salts is slower. Peak serum levels of penicillin G procaine occur at 1 to 4 hours, with drug detectable in serum for 1 to 2 days; peak serum levels of penicillin G benzathine occur at 13 to 24 hours, with serum levels detectable for 1 to 4 weeks.
*Distribution:* Distributed widely into synovial, pleural, pericardial, and ascitic fluids and bile, and into liver, skin, lungs, kidneys, muscle, in-

testines, tonsils, maxillary sinuses, saliva, and erythrocytes. CSF penetration is poor but is enhanced in patients with inflamed meninges. Penicillin G crosses the placenta; it is 45% to 68% protein-bound.

*Metabolism:* Between 16% and 30% of an I.M. dose of penicillin G is metabolized to inactive compounds.

*Excretion:* Excreted primarily in urine by tubular secretion; 20% to 60% of dose is recovered in 6 hours. Some drug appears in breast milk. Elimination half-life in adults is about ½ to 1 hour. Severe renal impairment prolongs half-life; penicillin G is removed by hemodialysis and is only minimally removed by peritoneal dialysis.

| Route | Onset | Peak | Duration |
|-------|-------|------|----------|
| I.V., I.M. | Varies | Varies | Varies |

## Contraindications and precautions

Contraindicated in patients hypersensitive to drug or other penicillins.

Use cautiously in patients with drug allergies (especially to cephalosporins or imipenem). Penicillin G potassium is contraindicated in patients with renal failure.

## Interactions

**Drug-drug.** *Aminoglycosides:* Produce synergistic therapeutic effects; however, drugs are physically and chemically incompatible and are inactivated when mixed or given together. Don't use together.

*Clavulanate:* Appears to enhance effect of penicillin G against certain beta-lactamase–producing bacteria. Advise clinician to monitor patient.

*Heparin or oral anticoagulants:* May increase the risk of bleeding. Advise clinician to monitor patient and PT and INR closely.

*Methotrexate:* Delayed elimination and elevating serum levels of methotrexate. Don't use together.

*NSAIDs:* Prolong penicillin half-life. Advise clinician to monitor patient closely.

*Oral contraceptives:* Penicillins may decrease effectiveness. Advise patient to use alternative method of birth control.

*Potassium-sparing diuretics:* Use with penicillin may cause hyperkalemia. Advise clinician to monitor patient.

*Probenecid:* Blocks tubular secretion of penicillin, increasing its serum levels. Advise clinician to monitor patient closely.

*Sulfinpyrazone:* Prolongs penicillin half-life. Advise clinician to monitor patient closely.

## Adverse reactions

**CNS:** neuropathy, *seizures* (with high doses), lethargy, hallucinations, anxiety, confusion, agitation, depression, dizziness, fatigue.

**GI:** nausea, vomiting, enterocolitis, pseudomembranous colitis.

**GU:** interstitial nephritis, nephropathy.

**Hematologic:** eosinophilia, hemolytic anemia, *thrombocytopenia, leukopenia,* anemia, *agranulocytosis.*

**Other:** hypersensitivity reactions (maculopapular and *exfoliative dermatitis,* chills, fever, edema, *anaphylaxis),* pain and sterile abscess at injection site; overgrowth of nonsusceptible organisms (with penicillin G potassium and procaine); possible severe potassium poisoning with high doses (hyperreflexia, *seizures, coma),* thrombophlebitis (with penicillin G potassium only).

## Overdose and treatment

Signs of overdose include neuromuscular irritability or seizures. No specific recommendations are available. Penicillin G can be removed by hemodialysis.

## Clinical considerations

**H ALERT** Beware of sound-alikes: There are various types of penicillin, plus polycillin and penicillamine. Don't confuse these drugs.

■ Because penicillins are dialyzable, patients undergoing hemodialysis may need dosage adjustments.

■ Recommend giving by deep I.M. injection in upper outer quadrant of buttock. In infants and small children, the midlateral aspect of thigh should be used.

■ Drug can be given as a continuous infusion for meningitis.

■ Penicillin G alters test results for urine and serum protein levels; it interferes with turbidimetric methods using sulfosalicylic acid, trichloracetic acid, acetic acid, and nitric acid. Penicillin G doesn't interfere with tests using bromophenol blue (Albustix, Albutest, Multistix).

■ Penicillin G alters urine glucose testing using cupric sulfate (Benedict's reagent); recommend using Diastix, Chemstrip uG, or glucose enzymatic test strip instead. Penicillin G may cause falsely elevated results of urine specific gravity tests in patients with low urine output and dehydration, and falsely elevated Norymberski and Zimmermann test results for 17-ketogenic steroids; it causes false-positive CSF protein test results (Folin-Ciocalteau method) and may cause positive Coombs' test results.

■ Penicillin G may falsely decrease serum aminoglycoside levels. Adding beta-lactamase to the sample inactivates the penicillin, rendering the assay more accurate. Alternatively, the sample can be spun down and frozen immediately after collection.

■ Have emergency equipment on hand to manage possible anaphylaxis.

### Therapeutic monitoring

■ Advise clinician to monitor patient closely for possible hypernatremia with sodium salt or hyperkalemia with potassium salt.

---

Reactions may be *common,* uncommon, *life-threatening,* or COMMON AND LIFE-THREATENING.

■ Patients with poor renal function are predisposed to high blood levels, which may cause seizures. Advise clinician to monitor renal function.

### Special populations
**Breast-feeding patients.** Drug appears in breast milk; use in breast-feeding women may sensitize infant to penicillin.
**Geriatric patients.** Half-life is prolonged in geriatric patients because of impaired renal function.

### Patient counseling
■ Tell patient to report adverse reactions promptly.
■ Warn patient that I.M. injection may be painful, but that ice may be applied to the site to ease discomfort.

---

## penicillin V
## penicillin V potassium
Betapen-VK, Nadopen-V*, PVF K*, V-Cillin K, Veetids

*Pharmacologic classification:* natural penicillin
*Therapeutic classification:* antibiotic
*Pregnancy risk category B*

### Available forms
Available by prescription only
**penicillin V**
*Tablets:* 250 mg, 500 mg
*Solution:* 125 mg/5 ml, 250 mg/5 ml (after reconstitution)
**penicillin V potassium**
*Tablets:* 125 mg, 250 mg, 500 mg
*Tablets (film-coated):* 250 mg, 500 mg
*Solution:* 125 mg/5 ml, 250 mg/5 ml (after reconstitution)

### Indications and dosages
*Mild to moderate susceptible infections*
*Adults and children ages 12 and older:* 125 to 500 mg (200,000 to 800,000 units) P.O. q 6 hours.
*Children ages 1 month to 12 years:* 15 to 56 mg/kg P.O. daily, divided into doses given q 6 to 8 hours.
*Endocarditis prophylaxis for dental surgery*
*Adults:* 2 g P.O. 30 to 60 minutes before procedure, then 1 g 6 hours later.
*Children weighing under 30 kg (66 lb):* Half the adult dose.
*Necrotizing ulcerative gingivitis*
*Adults:* 250 to 500 mg P.O. q 6 to 8 hours.
◇ *Lyme disease*
*Adults:* 250 to 500 mg P.O. q.i.d. for 10 to 20 days.

◇ *Prophylaxis for pneumococcal infection*
*Adults:* 250 mg P.O. b.i.d.
*Children over age 5:* 125 mg P.O. b.i.d.

### Mechanism of action
*Antibiotic action:* Penicillin V is bactericidal; it adheres to penicillin-binding proteins, inhibiting bacterial cell wall synthesis. Penicillin V's spectrum of activity includes most non–penicillinase-producing strains of gram-positive and gram-negative aerobic cocci; spirochetes; and some gram-positive aerobic and anaerobic bacilli.

### Pharmacokinetics
*Absorption:* Has greater acid stability and is absorbed more completely than penicillin G after oral administration. About 60% to 75% of an oral dose of penicillin V is absorbed.
*Distribution:* Distributed widely into synovial, pleural, pericardial, and ascitic fluids and bile, and into liver, skin, lungs, kidneys, muscle, intestines, tonsils, maxillary sinuses, saliva, and erythrocytes. CSF penetration is poor but is enhanced in patients with inflamed meninges. Penicillin V crosses the placenta, and is 75% to 89% protein-bound.
*Metabolism:* Between 35% and 70% of a dose is metabolized to inactive compounds.
*Excretion:* Excreted primarily in urine by tubular secretion; 26% to 65% of dose is recovered in 6 hours. Some drug appears in breast milk. Elimination half-life in adults is ½ hour. Severe renal impairment prolongs half-life.

| Route | Onset | Peak | Duration |
|-------|-------|------|----------|
| P.O. | Unknown | ½-1 hr | Unknown |

### Contraindications and precautions
Contraindicated in patients hypersensitive to drug or other penicillins.
    Use cautiously in patients with drug allergies (especially to cephalosporins or imipenem).

### Interactions
**Drug-drug.** *Aminoglycosides:* Drugs are physically and chemically incompatible and are inactivated when given together. Avoid use together.
*Anticoagulants and heparin:* May increase risk of bleeding. Advise clinician to monitor patient and PT and INR closely.
*Estrogen-containing oral contraceptives:* Efficacy may decrease. Recommend additional form of contraceptive during penicillin therapy.
*Probenecid:* Higher serum levels of penicillin. Probenecid may be used for this purpose.
*Sulfinpyrazone:* Prolongs penicillin half-life. Advise clinician to monitor patient closely.

### Adverse reactions
**CNS:** neuropathy.
**GI:** *epigastric distress,* vomiting, diarrhea, *nausea,* black "hairy" tongue.

---

* Canada only    ◇ Unlabeled clinical use

**GU:** nephropathy.
**Hematologic:** eosinophilia, hemolytic anemia, *leukopenia, thrombocytopenia.*
**Other:** hypersensitivity reactions (rash, urticaria, fever, laryngeal edema, *anaphylaxis),* overgrowth of nonsusceptible organisms.

## Overdose and treatment
Signs of overdose include neuromuscular sensitivity or seizures. No specific recommendations are available.

Treatment is supportive. After recent ingestion (within 4 hours), recommend emptying stomach by induced emesis or gastric lavage and following with activated charcoal to reduce absorption.

## Clinical considerations
**⚠ ALERT** Beware of sound-alikes; there are various types of penicillin, plus polycillin and penicillamine. Don't confuse these drugs.
■ Recommend giving oral dose 1 hour before or 2 hours after meals for maximum absorption.
■ After reconstitution, oral solution is stable for 14 days if refrigerated.
■ Penicillin V alters test results for urine and serum protein levels; it interferes with turbidimetric methods using sulfosalicylic acid, trichloracetic acid, acetic acid, and nitric acid. Penicillin V doesn't interfere with tests using bromophenol blue (Albustix, Albutest, Multistix). Penicillin V may falsely decrease serum aminoglycoside levels.

### Therapeutic monitoring
■ With large doses or prolonged therapy, bacterial or fungal superinfection may occur.

### Special populations
**Breast-feeding patients.** Penicillin V appears in breast milk; use in breast-feeding women may sensitize the infant to penicillins.
**Geriatric patients.** Half-life may be prolonged because of impaired renal function.

## Patient counseling
■ Instruct patient to take entire amount of drug exactly as prescribed, even if he feels better.
■ Advise patient to report rash, fever, or chills.

# pentamidine isethionate
NebuPent, Pentacarinat, Pentam 300

*Pharmacologic classification:* diamidine derivative
*Therapeutic classification:* antiprotozoal
*Pregnancy risk category C*

## Available forms
Available by prescription only
*Injection:* 300-mg vials
*Solution for inhalation:* 300 mg

## Indications and dosages
*Pneumonia caused by* **Pneumocystis** **carinii**
*Adults and children over age 4 months:* 3 to 4 mg/kg I.V. once a day for 14 to 21 days.
◊ *Primary or secondary prevention of* **P.** **carinii** *pneumonia*
*Adults and children:* 300 mg by inhalation once q 4 weeks. Aerosol form of drug should be administered by the Respirgard II jet nebulizer.
◊ *Trypanosomiasis*
*Adults:* 4 mg/kg I.M. once daily for 10 days. Alternatively, 3 to 4 mg/kg I.V. once daily or every other day, to a total of 7 to 10 doses.
◊ *Leishmaniasis*
*Adults:* 2 to 4 mg/kg I.M. daily or every other day up to 15 doses. Alternatively, 4 mg/kg I.V. 3 times weekly for 5 to 25 weeks or longer, depending on response.

## I.V. administration
■ To minimize risk of hypotensive reactions during I.V. administration, recommend giving infusions over 1 to 2 hours.
■ To prepare drug for I.V. infusion, add 3 to 5 ml of sterile water for injection or $D_5W$ at 72° to 86° F (22° to 30° C) to 300-mg vial to yield 100 mg/ml or 60 mg/ml, respectively. Withdraw desired dose and dilute further into 50 to 250 ml of $D_5W$; infuse over at least 60 minutes.
■ Diluted solution remains stable for 48 hours.

### Incompatibilities
Incompatible with fluconazole and foscarnet. Incompatible with most drugs and fluids other than $D_5W$.

## Mechanism of action
*Antiprotozoal action:* Mechanism is unknown. However, pentamidine may work by inhibiting synthesis of RNA, DNA, proteins, or phospholipids. It may also interfere with several metabolic processes, particularly certain energy-yielding reactions and reactions involving folic acid. Spectrum of activity includes *P. carinii* and *Trypanosoma* organisms.

## Pharmacokinetics
*Absorption:* Daily I.M. doses (4 mg/kg) produce surprisingly few plasma level fluctuations. Little information exists regarding pharmacokinetics with I.V. administration. Absorption is limited after aerosol administration.
*Distribution:* Appears to be extensively tissue-bound. CNS penetration is poor. Extent of plasma protein–binding is unknown.
*Metabolism:* Unknown.
*Excretion:* Mostly unchanged in urine. Tissue-binding may explain drug's appearance in urine 6 to 8 weeks after therapy ends.

| Route | Onset | Peak | Duration |
|-------|-------|------|----------|
| I.V. | Unknown | 1 hr | Unknown |
| I.M., inhalation | Unknown | ½ hr | Unknown |

## Contraindications and precautions

Contraindicated in patients hypersensitive to drug.

Use cautiously in patients with hepatic or renal dysfunction, hypertension, hypotension, hyperglycemia, hypoglycemia, hypocalcemia, leukopenia, thrombocytopenia, or anemia. Use with caution in patients with ventricular tachycardia, pancreatitis, or Stevens-Johnson syndrome.

## Interactions

**Drug-drug.** *Aminoglycosides, amphotericin B, capreomycin, cisplatin, colistin, foscarnet, methoxyflurane, polymyxin B, vancomycin:* Pentamidine may have additive nephrotoxic effects. Recommend closely monitoring patient; avoid use together if possible.

## Adverse reactions

**CNS:** confusion, hallucinations, *fatigue, dizziness,* headache.
**CV:** *hypotension, ventricular tachycardia,* chest pain, edema.
**EENT:** pharyngitis.
**GI:** nausea, metallic taste, decreased appetite, vomiting, diarrhea, abdominal pain, anorexia, bad taste in mouth.
**GU:** *elevated serum creatinine, acute renal failure.*
**Hematologic:** *leukopenia, thrombocytopenia,* anemia.
**Hepatic:** elevated liver function test results.
**Metabolic:** ketoacidosis, *hypoglycemia,* hyperglycemia, hyperkalemia, hypocalcemia, hypomagnesemia.
**Musculoskeletal:** myalgia.
**Respiratory:** *cough, bronchospasm, shortness of breath,* congestion, pneumothorax.
**Skin:** *rash, sterile abscess, Stevens-Johnson syndrome, pain or induration at injection site.*
**Other:** *anaphylactoid reaction, night sweats, chills.*

## Overdose and treatment

No information available.

## Clinical considerations

**⚠ ALERT** To minimize risk of hypotension, patient should be supine during I.V. administration. Because sudden, severe hypotension may develop after I.M. injection or during I.V. infusion, recommend closely monitoring blood pressure during infusion and several times thereafter until patient is stable.

■ Emergency drugs and equipment, including emergency airway, vasopressors, and I.V. fluids, should be kept on hand.

■ Patient should be adequately hydrated before drug is given; dehydration may lead to hypotension and renal toxicity.

■ To prepare drug for I.M. injection, add 3 ml of sterile water for injection at 72° to 86° F (22° to 30° C) to 300-mg vial to yield 100 g/ml. Withdraw desired dose and inject deep I.M.

■ When inhalation solution is used for prophylaxis against *P. carinii* pneumonia (PCP), high-risk individuals include patients infected with HIV with a history of PCP; patients who have never had an episode of PCP but whose CD4+ T cells are less than 20% of total lymphocytes; or whose CD4+ T-cell count is less than 200/mm³.

■ To administer by inhalation, dilute dose in 6 ml of sterile water and deliver at 6 L/minute from a 50-p.s.i. compressed air source until reservoir is dry. Alternate delivery systems (other than the Respirgard II) are under investigation but are currently not recommended.

■ If wheezing or cough develops during pentamidine aerosol therapy, patient may benefit by pretreatment with a bronchodilator at least 5 minutes before pentamidine administration.

### Therapeutic monitoring

■ Advise clinician to monitor daily blood glucose, BUN, and serum creatinine levels.
■ Advise clinician to monitor periodic electrolyte levels, CBC, platelet count, and liver function test results.
■ Patient should be observed for signs and symptoms of hypoglycemia.

### Special populations

**Pregnant patients.** Avoid using aerosol form in pregnant women.
**Breast-feeding patients.** It isn't known if drug appears in breast milk.
**Pediatric patients.** Safety and efficacy of inhalation therapy haven't been clearly established in children ages 16 or under.

## Patient counseling

■ Instruct patient to use aerosol device until the chamber is empty; this may take up to 45 minutes.
■ Instruct patient to complete the full course of therapy, even if he feels better.

---

# pentazocine hydrochloride
Talwin*, Talwin-Nx (with naloxone hydrochloride)

# pentazocine lactate
Talwin

*Pharmacologic classification:* narcotic agonist-antagonist, opioid partial agonist
*Therapeutic classification:* analgesic, adjunct to anesthesia
*Pregnancy risk category NR (C for Talwin-Nx)*
*Controlled substance schedule IV*

## Available forms
Available by prescription only
*Injection:* 30 mg/ml
*Tablets:* 50 mg

## Indications and dosages
*Moderate to severe pain*
*Adults:* 50 to 100 mg P.O. q 3 to 4 hours, p.r.n., or around-the-clock. Maximum oral dose, 600 mg daily. Or, 30 mg I.M., I.V., or S.C. q 3 to 4 hours, p.r.n., or around-the-clock. Maximum parenteral dose, 360 mg daily. Doses above 30 mg I.V. or 60 mg I.M. or S.C. not recommended.

For patients in labor, give 30 mg I.M. or 20 mg I.V. in 2- to 3-hour intervals.

## I.V. administration
■ No specific administration information available. I.V. opioid analgesics should generally be given slowly over several minutes.
■ Have patient lie down and remain recumbent to minimize adverse reactions like dizziness, light-headedness, or hypotension.

## Incompatibilities
Incompatible with aminophylline, amobarbital, glycopyrrolate, pentobarbital sodium, phenobarbital sodium, secobarbital, and sodium bicarbonate.

## Mechanism of action
*Analgesic action:* Exact mechanism of action is unknown. It's believed to be a competitive antagonist at some receptors, and an agonist at others, resulting in relief of moderate pain.

Pentazocine can produce respiratory depression, sedation, miosis, and antitussive effects. It also may cause psychotomimetic and dysphoric effects. In patients with coronary artery disease, it elevates mean aortic pressure, left ventricular end-diastolic pressure, and mean pulmonary artery pressure. In patients with acute MI, I.V. pentazocine increases systemic and pulmonary arterial pressures and systemic vascular resistance.

## Pharmacokinetics
*Absorption:* Well absorbed after oral or parenteral administration. However, orally administered drug undergoes first-pass metabolism in the liver, and less than 20% of a dose reaches the systemic circulation unchanged. Bioavailability is increased in patients with hepatic dysfunction; patients with cirrhosis absorb 60% to 70% of drug.
*Distribution:* Appears to be widely distributed in the body.
*Metabolism:* Metabolized in the liver, mainly by oxidation and secondarily by glucuronidation. Metabolism may be prolonged in patients with impaired hepatic function.
*Excretion:* Duration of effect is 3 hours. There's considerable interpatient variability in its urinary excretion. Small amounts of drug are excreted in feces after oral or parenteral administration.

| Route | Onset | Peak | Duration |
|---|---|---|---|
| P.O. | 15-30 min | 1-3 hr | 2-3 hr |
| I.V. | 2-3 min | 15-30 min | 2-3 hr |
| I.M., S.C. | 10-20 min | 30-60 min | 2-3 hr |

## Contraindications and precautions
Contraindicated in patients hypersensitive to drug or its components and in children under age 12.

Use cautiously in patients with impaired renal or hepatic function, acute MI, head injury, increased intracranial pressure, or respiratory depression.

## Interactions
**Drug-drug.** *Barbiturates such as thiopental:* Pentazocine may produce additive CNS and respiratory depressant effects and, possibly, apnea. Use together cautiously.
*Cimetidine:* May increase pentazocine toxicity. Advise clinician to monitor patient closely.
*General anesthetics:* May cause severe CV depression. Use together cautiously.
*Narcotic agonist-antagonists:* Patient may become physically dependent on pentazocine. Use with caution; advise clinician to monitor closely.
*Other CNS depressants, such as antihistamines, barbiturates, benzodiazepines, muscle relaxants, narcotic analgesics, phenothiazines, sedative-hypnotics, and tricyclic antidepressants:* Potentiates respiratory and CNS depression of drug; reduced doses of pentazocine usually are needed.
**Drug-lifestyle.** *Alcohol use:* Potentiates respiratory and CNS depression of drug. Advise patient to avoid alcohol.

## Adverse reactions
**CNS:** *sedation,* visual disturbances, hallucinations, drowsiness, *dizziness, light-headedness,* confusion, physical and psychological depen-

---

dence, *euphoria,* headache, syncope, psychotomimetic effects.
**CV:** circulatory depression, ***shock,*** hypertension, hypotension.
**EENT:** dry mouth, blurred vision, nystagmus.
**GI:** *nausea, vomiting,* constipation, taste alteration.
**GU:** urine retention.
**Hematologic:** WBC depression.
**Respiratory:** ***respiratory depression,*** dyspnea, ***apnea.***
**Skin:** induration, nodules, sloughing, and sclerosis of injection site; diaphoresis; pruritus.
**Other:** hypersensitivity reactions ***(anaphylaxis).***

## Overdose and treatment
The signs of pentazocine hydrochloride overdose haven't been defined because of a lack of clinical experience with overdose. If overdose should occur, recommend using all supportive measures (oxygen, I.V. fluids, vasopressors) p.r.n. Mechanical ventilation should be considered. Parenteral naloxone is an effective antagonist for respiratory depression because of pentazocine.

## Clinical considerations
■ Tablets aren't well absorbed.
■ Don't mix in same syringe with soluble barbiturates.
■ Drug possesses narcotic antagonist properties. May precipitate abstinence syndrome in narcotic-dependent patients.
■ Talwin-Nx, the available oral pentazocine, contains the narcotic antagonist naloxone, which prevents illicit I.V. use.
■ Recommend using S.C. route only when needed. Severe tissue damage is possible at injection site.

### *Therapeutic monitoring*
■ Pentazocine may obscure the signs and symptoms of an acute abdominal condition or worsen gallbladder pain.
■ Drug may cause orthostatic hypotension in ambulatory patients. Have patient sit down to relieve symptoms.

### *Special populations*
**Breast-feeding patients.** It's unknown if drug appears in breast milk; use with caution in breast-feeding women.
**Pediatric patients.** Use of drug isn't recommended in children under age 12.
**Geriatric patients.** Lower doses are usually indicated for geriatric patients, who may be more sensitive to the therapeutic and adverse effects of drug.

## Patient counseling
■ Tell patient to report rash, confusion, disorientation, or other serious adverse effects.

**◪ ALERT** Warn patient that Talwin-Nx is for oral use only. Severe reactions may result if tablets are crushed, dissolved, and injected.

# pentobarbital sodium
Nembutal

*Pharmacologic classification:* barbiturate
*Therapeutic classification:* anticonvulsant, sedative-hypnotic
*Pregnancy risk category D*
*Controlled substance schedule II (suppositories schedule III)*

## Available forms
Available by prescription only
*Capsules:* 50 mg, 100 mg
*Elixir:* 18.2 mg/5 ml
*Injection:* 50 mg/ml, 1-ml and 2-ml disposable syringes; 2-ml, 20-ml, and 50-ml vials
*Suppositories:* 30 mg, 60 mg, 120 mg, 200 mg

## Indications and dosages
### *Sedation*
*Adults:* 20 to 40 mg P.O. b.i.d., t.i.d., or q.i.d.
*Children:* 2 to 6 mg/kg P.O. daily in divided doses, to maximum of 100 mg/dose.
### *Insomnia*
*Adults:* 100 mg P.O. h.s. or 150 to 200 mg deep I.M.; 120 to 200 mg P.R.
*Children:* 2 to 6 mg/kg I.M., up to maximum of 100 mg/dose. Or 30 mg P.R. (ages 2 months to 1 year), 30 to 60 mg P.R. (ages 1 to 4), 60 mg P.R. (ages 5 to 12), 60 to 120 mg P.R. (ages 12 to 14).
### *Preanesthesia*
*Adults:* 150 to 200 mg I.M. or P.O. in two divided doses.
### *Seizures*
*Adults:* Initially, 100 mg I.V.; after 1 minute, additional doses may be given, up to a total of from 200 to 500 mg I.V. Maximum dose, 500 mg.
*Children:* 50 mg initially; after 1 minute additional small doses may be given until desired effect is obtained.

## I.V. administration
■ Avoid I.V. administration at a rate exceeding 50 mg/minute to prevent hypotension and respiratory depression.
■ Reserve I.V. injection for emergency treatment. Be prepared for emergency resuscitative measures.

### *Incompatibilities*
Incompatible with benzquinamide, butorphanol, chlorphreniramine, chlorpromazine, cimetidine, codeine phosphate, dimenhydrinate, diphenhydramine, droperidol, ephedrine, fentanyl citrate, glycopyrrolate, hydrocortisone sodium succinate, hydroxyzine hydrochloride,

meperidine, methadone, midazolam, morphine sulfate, nalbuphine, norepinephrine, opium alkaloids, penicillin G potassium, pentazocine lactate, perphenazine, phenytoin sodium, prochlorperazine edisylate, promazine, promethazine hydrochloride, ranitidine hydrochloride, regular insulin, sodium bicarbonate, streptomycin, succinylcholine triflupromazine, and vancomycin.

## Mechanism of action

*Anticonvulsant action:* Pentobarbital suppresses the spread of seizure activity produced by epileptogenic foci in the cortex, thalamus, and limbic systems by enhancing the effect of GABA. Both presynaptic and postsynaptic excitability are decreased, and the seizure threshold is raised.

*Sedative-hypnotic action:* Exact cellular site and mechanisms of action are unknown. Pentobarbital acts throughout the CNS as a nonselective depressant with a fast onset of action and short duration of action. Particularly sensitive to this drug is the reticular activating system, which controls CNS arousal. Pentobarbital decreases both presynaptic and postsynaptic membrane excitability by facilitating the action of gamma-aminobutyric acid (GABA).

## Pharmacokinetics

*Absorption:* Absorbed rapidly after oral or rectal administration. Serum levels needed for sedation and hypnosis are 1 to 5 mcg/ml and 5 to 15 mcg/ml, respectively.

*Distribution:* Distributed widely throughout the body. About 35% to 45% is protein-bound. Drug accumulates in fat with long-term use.

*Metabolism:* Metabolized in the liver by penultimate oxidation.

*Excretion:* About 99% of pentobarbital is eliminated as glucuronide conjugates and other metabolites in the urine. Terminal half-life ranges from 35 to 50 hours. Duration of action is 3 to 4 hours.

| Route | Onset | Peak | Duration |
|-------|-------|------|----------|
| P.O. | 20 min | ½–1 hr | 1-4 hr |
| I.V. | Immediate | Immediate | 15 min |
| I.M. | 10-25 min | Unknown | Unknown |
| P.R. | 20 min | Unknown | 1-4 hr |

## Contraindications and precautions

Contraindicated in patients hypersensitive to barbiturates or porphyria or those with severe respiratory disease when dyspnea or obstruction is evident.

Use cautiously in geriatric or debilitated patients and in those with acute or chronic pain, mental depression, suicidal tendencies, history of drug abuse, or impaired hepatic function.

## Interactions

**Drug-drug.** *Antidepressants, antihistamines, narcotics, sedative-hypnotics, tranquilizers:* Pentobarbital may potentiate or add to CNS and respiratory depressant effects. Use together cautiously.

*Corticosteroids, digitoxin (not digoxin), doxycycline, oral contraceptives and other estrogens, theophylline and other xanthines:* Enhanced hepatic metabolism of these drugs. Advise clinician to monitor patient closely.

*Disulfiram, MAO inhibitors, valproic acid:* Decrease metabolism of pentobarbital and increase its toxicity. Barbiturate dose may need adjustment.

*Griseofulvin:* Decreased absorption of griseofulvin. Advise clinician to monitor effectiveness of griseofulvin.

*Rifampin:* May decrease pentobarbital levels by increasing hepatic metabolism. Avoid use together.

*Warfarin and other oral anticoagulants:* Pentobarbital enhances the enzymatic degradation. Patients may require increased doses of the anticoagulants.

**Drug-herb.** *Kava:* May cause additive effects. Discourage use together.

**Drug-lifestyle.** *Alcohol use:* Pentobarbital may potentiate or add to CNS and respiratory depressant effects. Advise patient to avoid alcohol.

## Adverse reactions

**CNS:** *drowsiness, lethargy, hangover,* paradoxical excitement in geriatric patients, physical and psychological dependence, somnolence, syncope, hallucinations.

**CV:** *bradycardia,* hypotension.

**GI:** nausea, vomiting.

**Hematologic:** exacerbation of porphyria.

**Respiratory:** *respiratory depression.*

**Skin:** rash, urticaria, *Stevens-Johnson syndrome.*

**Other:** *angioedema.*

## Overdose and treatment

Signs and symptoms of overdose include unsteady gait, slurred speech, sustained nystagmus, somnolence, confusion, respiratory depression, pulmonary edema, areflexia, and coma. Typical shock syndrome with tachycardia and hypotension may occur. Jaundice, hypothermia followed by fever, and oliguria also may occur. Serum levels greater than 10 mcg/ml may produce profound coma; levels greater than 30 mcg/ml may be fatal.

To treat, recommend maintaining and support ventilation and pulmonary function p.r.n.; recommend supporting cardiac function and circulation with vasopressors and I.V. fluids, p.r.n. If patient is conscious and gag reflex is intact, emesis should be induced (if ingestion was recent) by giving ipecac syrup. If emesis is contraindicated, advise clinician to perform gastric lavage while a cuffed endotracheal tube is in place to prevent aspiration. Administration of activated charcoal or sodium chloride cathartic should follow. Recommend measuring intake and output, vital signs, and laboratory parameters. Body temperature should be maintained.

Alkalinization of urine may be helpful in removing drug from the body. Hemodialysis may be useful in severe overdose.

## Clinical considerations

■ High-dose therapy for elevated intracranial pressure may require mechanically assisted ventilation.
■ Recommend giving I.M. dose deep into large muscle mass. Don't administer more than 5 ml into any one site.
■ Discard solution that's discolored or contains precipitate.
■ Administration of full loading doses over short periods of time to treat status epilepticus will require ventilatory support in adults.
■ To ensure accuracy of dosage, don't divide suppositories.
■ Nembutal tablets contain tartrazine dye, which may cause allergic reactions in susceptible persons.
■ To prevent rebound of rapid-eye-movement sleep after prolonged therapy, recommend stopping gradually over 5 to 6 days.
■ Pentobarbital may cause a false-positive phentolamine test. Physiologic effects of drug may impair the absorption of cyanocobalamin $^{57}Co$; it may decrease serum bilirubin levels in neonates, epileptic patients, and patients with congenital nonhemolytic unconjugated hyperbilirubinemia. EEG patterns show a change in low-voltage, fast activity; changes persist for a time after discontinuation of therapy.

### Therapeutic monitoring

■ Patient's skin should be inspected. Skin eruptions may precede potentially fatal reactions to barbiturate therapy.
■ In some patients, high fever, stomatitis, headache or rhinitis may precede skin eruptions.

### Special populations

**Pregnant patients.** Advise pregnant women of potential hazard to fetus or neonate when taking pentobarbital late in pregnancy. Withdrawal symptoms can occur.
**Breast-feeding patients.** Pentobarbital appears in breast milk. Don't give to breast-feeding women.
**Pediatric patients.** Barbiturates may cause paradoxical excitement in children. Use with caution.
**Geriatric patients.** Usually require lower doses because of increased susceptibility to CNS depressant effects of pentobarbital. Confusion, disorientation, and excitability may occur in geriatric patients. Use with caution.

## Patient counseling

■ Tell patient not to take drug continuously for longer than 2 weeks.
■ Drug has no analgesic effect and may cause restlessness or delirium in patients with pain.
■ Caution patient about performing activities that require mental alertness or physical coordination.

# pentostatin
# (2'-deoxycoformycin; DCF)
Nipent

*Pharmacologic classification:* antimetabolite (adenosine deaminase inhibitor)
*Therapeutic classification:* antineoplastic
*Pregnancy risk category D*

## Available forms
Available by prescription only
*Powder for injection:* 10 mg/vial

## Indications and dosages
*Alpha-interferon-refractory hairy cell leukemia*
Adults: 4 mg/m$^2$ I.V. every other week.

## I.V. administration
■ Follow appropriate guidelines for proper handling, administration, and disposal of chemotherapeutic drugs. Treat all spills and waste products with 5% sodium hypochlorite solution. Wear protective clothing and polyethylene gloves.
■ Add 5 ml sterile water for injection to the vial containing pentostatin powder for injection. Mix thoroughly to make a solution of 5 mg/ml.
■ Recommend giving drug by I.V. bolus injection, or dilute further in 25 or 50 ml of $D_5W$ or normal saline injection and infuse over 20 to 30 minutes.
■ Make sure patient is adequately hydrated before therapy. Recommend giving 500 to 1,000 ml of $D_5W$ in 0.45% saline injection. Recommend giving 500 ml of $D_5W$ after drug is given.

### Incompatibilities
Don't mix with other drugs unless specific compatibility data are available.

## Mechanism of action
*Antileukemic action:* Pentostatin inhibits the enzyme adenosine deaminase (ADA), causing an increase in intracellular levels of deoxyadenosine triphosphate. This increase leads to cell damage and death. Because ADA is most active in cells of the lymphoid system (espe-

cially malignant T cells), drug is useful in treating leukemias.

## Pharmacokinetics
*Absorption:* Achieves response in 3 to 24 months; duration of pharmacologic action is more than 1 week after a single dose.
*Distribution:* Plasma protein–binding is low (about 4%); distribution half-life is about 11 minutes.
*Metabolism:* Unknown.
*Excretion:* More than 90% is excreted in urine. Clearance depends on renal function; mean terminal half-life is about 6 hours in patients with normal renal function; increases to 18 hours or longer in patients with renal impairment (creatinine clearance less than 50 ml/minute).

| Route | Onset | Peak | Duration |
|-------|-------|------|----------|
| I.V. | Unknown | Unknown | Unknown |

## Contraindications and precautions
Contraindicated in patients hypersensitive to drug.

## Interactions
**Drug-drug.** *Fludarabine:* Increases the risk of severe or fatal pulmonary toxicity. Don't use together.
*Vidarabine:* Increases the risk or severity of adverse effects from either drug. Don't use together.

## Adverse reactions
**CNS:** *headache, neurologic symptoms,* anxiety, confusion, depression, dizziness, insomnia, nervousness, paresthesia, somnolence, abnormal thinking, *fatigue,* malaise.
**CV:** **ARRHYTHMIAS,** abnormal ECG, thrombophlebitis, peripheral edema, **HEMORRHAGE,** chest pain.
**EENT:** abnormal vision, conjunctivitis, ear pain, eye pain, epistaxis, pharyngitis, rhinitis, sinusitis.
**GI:** *nausea, vomiting, anorexia, diarrhea,* constipation, flatulence, stomatitis, abdominal pain.
**GU:** hematuria, dysuria, increased BUN and creatinine levels.
**Hematologic:** *myelosuppression,* **LEUKOPENIA,** *anemia,* **THROMBOCYTOPENIA,** lymphadenopathy.
**Hepatic:** *elevated liver enzyme levels.*
**Metabolic:** weight loss.
**Musculoskeletal:** myalgia, arthralgia, asthenia, back pain.
**Respiratory:** *cough, bronchitis,* dyspnea, lung edema, pneumonia.
**Skin:** ecchymosis, petechiae, *rash,* eczema, dry skin, maculopapular rash, vesiculobullous rash, pruritus, seborrhea, discoloration, diaphoresis.

**Other:** *fever,* **INFECTION,** *pain, hypersensitivity reactions, chills,* **sepsis, neoplasm,** herpes simplex or zoster, flulike syndrome.

## Overdose and treatment
High dosage of pentostatin (20 to 50 mg/m² in divided doses over 5 days) has caused deaths from severe CNS, hepatic, pulmonary, and renal toxicity. No specific antidote is known. If overdose occurs, recommend treating symptoms and providing supportive care.

## Clinical considerations
■ Use drug only in patients who have hairy cell leukemia refractory to alpha interferon, and when disease progresses after a minimum of 3 months of treatment with alpha interferon or doesn't respond after 6 months of therapy.
■ Optimal duration of therapy is unknown. Current recommendations call for two additional courses of therapy after a complete response. If patient hasn't had a partial response after 6 months of therapy, discontinue drug. If patient has had only a partial response, drug should be continued for another 6 months; if patient has had a complete response, drug should be continued for two courses of therapy.
■ Store powder for injection in the refrigerator (36° to 46° F [2° to 8° C]). Use reconstituted and diluted solutions within 8 hours because drug contains no preservative.

### Therapeutic monitoring
■ Before therapy, recommend assessing renal function with a serum creatinine or creatinine clearance assay; determinations should be repeated periodically.
■ Baseline and periodic determinations of CBC should be made.
■ Bone marrow aspirates and biopsies may be required at 2- to 3-month intervals to assess response to treatment.

### Special populations
**Breast-feeding patients.** It isn't known if drug appears in breast milk. Because of the risk of serious toxicity to the breast-feeding infant, either the drug or breast-feeding should be discontinued.
**Pediatric patients.** Safety in children and adolescents hasn't been established.

## Patient counseling
■ Warn patient to avoid contact with infected persons.
■ Tell patient to immediately report signs of infection or unusual bleeding.

---

Reactions may be *common,* uncommon, *life-threatening,* or COMMON AND LIFE-THREATENING.

# pentoxifylline

Pentoxil, Trental

*Pharmacologic classification:* xanthine derivative
*Therapeutic classification:* hemorrheologic
*Pregnancy risk category C*

## Available forms

Available by prescription only
*Tablets (extended-release):* 400 mg

## Indications and dosages

**Intermittent claudication from chronic occlusive vascular disease**
*Adults:* 400 mg P.O. t.i.d. with meals.

## Mechanism of action

*Hemorrheologic action:* Pentoxifylline improves capillary blood flow by increasing erythrocyte flexibility and reducing blood viscosity.

## Pharmacokinetics

*Absorption:* Absorbed almost completely from the GI tract but undergoes first-pass hepatic metabolism. Absorption is slowed by food.
*Distribution:* Unknown; drug is bound to erythrocyte membrane.
*Metabolism:* Metabolized extensively by erythrocytes and the liver.
*Excretion:* Metabolites are excreted principally in urine; less than 4% of drug is excreted in feces. Half-life of unchanged drug is about ½ to ¾ hour; half-life of metabolites is about 1 to 1½ hours.

| Route | Onset | Peak | Duration |
|-------|-------|------|----------|
| P.O. | Unknown | 1 hr | Unknown |

## Contraindications and precautions

Contraindicated in patients who are intolerant to pentoxifylline or methylxanthines, such as caffeine, theophylline, and theobromine, and in patients with recent cerebral or retinal hemorrhage.

Use cautiously in geriatric patients.

## Interactions

**Drug-drug.** *Antihypertensives:* May increase hypotensive response; blood pressure must be monitored closely.
*Oral anticoagulants such as warfarin or drugs that inhibit platelet aggregation:* When used with pentoxifylline, may have bleeding abnormalities. Advise clinician to monitor PT and INR.
*Theophylline:* Levels may increase when given with pentoxifylline. Advise clinician to monitor patient closely.

**Drug-lifestyle.** *Smoking:* Vasoconstriction may result. Advise patient to avoid smoking, as it may worsen his condition.

## Adverse reactions

**CNS:** headache, dizziness.
**CV:** angina, chest pain.
**GI:** dyspepsia, nausea, vomiting, flatus, bloating.

## Overdose and treatment

Signs of overdose include flushing, hypotension, seizures, somnolence, loss of consciousness, fever, and agitation. There's no known antidote. Recommend emptying stomach by gastric lavage and using activated charcoal; recommend treating symptoms and supporting respiration and blood pressure.

## Clinical considerations

■ If GI and CNS adverse effects occur, dosage should be decreased to b.i.d. If adverse effects persist, drug should be stopped.
■ Drug is useful in patients who aren't good candidates for surgery.
■ Don't crush or break extended-release tablets; make sure patient swallows them whole.

### Therapeutic monitoring

■ Advise clinician to monitor blood pressure regularly, especially in patients taking antihypertensives, and monitor INR, especially in patients taking anticoagulants such as warfarin.

### Special populations

**Breast-feeding patients.** Pentoxifylline appears in breast milk. Alternative feeding method is recommended during therapy.
**Pediatric patients.** Safety and efficacy haven't been established for children under age 18.
**Geriatric patients.** Geriatric patients may have increased bioavailability and decreased excretion of drug and are at higher risk for toxicity; adverse reactions may be more common in geriatric patients.

## Patient counseling

■ Explain need for continuing therapy for at least 8 weeks; warn patient not to discontinue drug during this period without medical approval.
■ Advise patient to take drug with meals to minimize GI distress.
■ Tell patient to report GI or CNS adverse reactions; they may require dosage reduction.

# pergolide mesylate
Permax

*Pharmacologic classification:*
dopaminergic agonist
*Therapeutic classification:* antiparkinsonian
*Pregnancy risk category B*

## Available forms
Available by prescription only
*Tablets:* 0.05 mg, 0.25 mg, 1 mg

## Indications and dosages
**Adjunct to levodopa-carbidopa in the management of Parkinson's disease**
*Adults:* Initially, 0.05 mg P.O. daily for first 2 days. Gradually increase dosage by 0.1 to 0.15 mg every third day over next 12 days of therapy. Subsequent dosage can be increased by 0.25 mg every third day until optimum response occurs. Mean therapeutic daily dose is 3 mg.

Drug is usually given in divided doses t.i.d. Gradual reductions in levodopa-carbidopa dosage may be made during dosage adjustment.

## Mechanism of action
*Antiparkinsonian action:* Pergolide stimulates dopamine receptors at both $D_1$ and $D_2$ sites. It acts by directly stimulating postsynaptic receptors in the nigrostriatal system.

## Pharmacokinetics
*Absorption:* Well absorbed after oral administration. Half-life is about 24 hours.
*Distribution:* About 90% plasma protein-bound.
*Metabolism:* Metabolized to at least 10 different compounds, some of which retain some pharmacologic activity.
*Excretion:* Excreted primarily by the kidneys.

| Route | Onset | Peak | Duration |
|-------|-------|------|----------|
| P.O. | Unknown | Unknown | Unknown |

## Contraindications and precautions
Contraindicated in patients hypersensitive to drug or to ergot alkaloids.

Use cautiously in patients susceptible to arrhythmias and underlying psychiatric disorders.

## Interactions
**Drug-drug.** *Dopamine antagonists, including butyrophenones, metoclopramide, phenothiazines, and thioxanthines:* May antagonize the effects of pergolide. Advise clinician to monitor patient closely.
*Drugs known to affect protein-binding:* Pergolide is extensively protein-bound; use caution if pergolide is coadministered.

## Adverse reactions
**CNS:** headache, asthenia, *dyskinesia, dizziness, hallucinations, dystonia, confusion, somnolence,* insomnia, anxiety, depression, tremor, abnormal dreams, personality disorder, psychosis, abnormal gait, akathisia, extrapyramidal syndrome, incoordination, akinesia, hypertonia, neuralgia, speech disorder, twitching, paresthesia.
**CV:** *orthostatic hypotension,* vasodilation, palpitations, hypotension, syncope, hypertension, *arrhythmias, MI.*
**EENT:** *rhinitis,* epistaxis, abnormal vision, diplopia, eye disorder.
**GI:** dry mouth, taste perversion, abdominal pain, *nausea, constipation,* diarrhea, dyspepsia, anorexia, vomiting.
**GU:** urinary frequency, urinary tract infection, hematuria.
**Hematologic:** anemia.
**Metabolic:** weight gain.
**Musculoskeletal:** chest, neck, and back pain, arthralgia; bursitis; myalgia.
**Respiratory:** dyspnea.
**Skin:** rash, diaphoresis.
**Other:** flulike syndrome; chills; infection; facial, peripheral, or generalized edema.

## Overdose and treatment
Some cases of overdose revealed symptoms of hallucinations, involuntary movements, palpitations, and arrhythmias.

Supportive treatment should be provided. Advise clinician to monitor cardiac function and protect the patient's airway. Antiarrhythmics and sympathomimetics may be needed to support CV function. Adverse CNS effects may be treated with dopaminergic antagonists such as phenothiazines. If indicated, gastric lavage or induced emesis may be used to empty the stomach of its contents. Orally administered activated charcoal may be useful in attenuating absorption.

## Clinical considerations
■ In early clinical trials, 27% of patients who attempted pergolide therapy didn't finish the trial because of adverse effects (primarily hallucinations and confusion).

### Therapeutic monitoring
■ Advise clinician to monitor blood pressure. Symptomatic orthostatic or sustained hypotension may occur especially at the start of therapy.

### Special populations
**Breast-feeding patients.** Safety in breast-feeding women hasn't been established.
**Pediatric patients.** Safety in children hasn't been established.

---

## Patient counseling
- Inform patient of potential for adverse effects. Warn patient to avoid activities that could expose him to injury secondary to orthostatic hypotension and syncope.
- Caution patient to rise slowly to avoid orthostatic hypotension, especially when therapy starts.

# perindopril erbumine
Aceon

*Pharmacologic classification:* angiotensin converting enzyme (ACE) inhibitor
*Therapeutic classification:* antihypertensive
*Pregnancy risk category C (first trimester) and D (second and third trimesters)*

## Available forms
Available by prescription only
*Tablets:* 2 mg, 4 mg, 8 mg

## Indications and dosages
*Treatment of essential hypertension*
*Adults:* Initially, 4 mg P.O. once daily. Increase dosage until blood pressure is controlled or to a maximum of 16 mg per day; usual maintenance dose, 4 to 8 mg once daily; may be given en two divided doses.
*Elderly:* Initially, 4 mg P.O. daily as one dose or in two divided doses. Dosage increases exceeding 8 mg per day should only be made under close medical supervision.
≡ *Dosage adjustment.* For renally impaired patients, initially, 2 mg P.O. daily with a maximum maintenance dose of 8 mg/day.
≡ *Dosage adjustment.* For patients taking diuretics, initially, 2 to 4 mg P.O. daily as one dose or in two divided doses with close medical supervision for several hours and until blood pressure has stabilized. Adjust dosage based on patient's blood pressure response.

## Mechanism of action
*Antihypertensive action:* Perindopril erbumine is a prodrug that's converted by the liver to the active metabolite perindoprilat. Perindoprilat is thought to lower blood pressure through inhibition of angiotensin-converting enzyme (ACE) activity, thereby preventing the conversion of angiotensin I to angiotensin II, a potent vasoconstrictor. Inhibition of ACE results in decreased vasoconstriction, and decreased aldosterone, reducing sodium and water retention and lowering blood pressure.

## Pharmacokinetics
*Absorption:* Rapidly absorbed after oral administration. The absolute oral bioavailability of perindopril is around 75%. Plasma level of perindopril and perindoprilat are increased about twofold in geriatric patients.
*Distribution:* Perindopril and perindoprilat are about 60% and 10% to 20% plasma protein–bound, respectively. Therefore, drug interactions resulting from effects on protein-binding aren't anticipated.
*Metabolism:* Extensively metabolized by the liver to the active ACE inhibitor perindoprilat.
*Excretion:* About 4% to 12% of a given dose of perindopril is excreted in the urine as unchanged drug. Clearance of the drug is reduced in geriatric patients, and patients with HF or renal insufficiency.

| Route | Onset | Peak | Duration |
|-------|-------|------|----------|
| P.O. | Unknown | 1 hr | Unknown |

## Contraindications and precautions
Contraindicated in patients hypersensitive to perindopril or to any other ACE inhibitor. Also contraindicated in patients with a history of angioedema secondary to ACE inhibitors. Don't use drug in pregnant women.

Use cautiously in patients with a history of angioedema unrelated to ACE inhibitor therapy. Also use cautiously in patients with impaired renal function, HF, ischemic heart disease, cerebrovascular disease or renal artery stenosis, and in patients with collagen vascular disease, such as systemic lupus erythematosus or scleroderma.

## Interactions
**Drug-drug.** *Diuretics:* Additive hypotensive effect. Advise clinician to monitor patient closely.
*Lithium:* Increased serum lithium levels; symptoms of lithium toxicity can occur. Use together cautiously and recommend monitoring serum lithium level. Use of a diuretic may further increase the risk of lithium toxicity.
*Potassium-sparing diuretics, such as amiloride, spironolactone, and triamterene; potassium supplements; other drugs capable of increasing serum potassium, such as cyclosporine, heparin, and indomethacin:* Additive hyperkalemic effect. Use together cautiously and recommend monitoring serum potassium frequently.
**Drug-herb.** *Capsaicin:* Increased risk of cough. Discourage use together.
*Licorice:* Can cause sodium retention and increase blood pressure interfering with the therapeutic effects of ACE inhibitors. Discourage use together.
**Drug-food.** *Salt substitutes containing potassium:* May increase risk of hyperkalemia. Use together cautiously.

## Adverse reactions
**CNS:** dizziness, asthenia, sleep disorder, paresthesia, depression, somnolence, nervousness, *headache.*

---

* Canada only    ◇ Unlabeled clinical use

**CV:** palpitation, edema, chest pain, abnormal ECG.
**EENT:** rhinitis, sinusitis, ear infection, pharyngitis, tinnitus.
**GI:** dyspepsia, diarrhea, abdominal pain, nausea, vomiting, flatulence.
**GU:** proteinuria, urinary tract infection, male sexual dysfunction, menstrual disorder.
**Hepatic:** increased ALT.
**Metabolic:** increased triglycerides.
**Musculoskeletal:** back pain, hypertonia, neck pain, joint pain, myalgia, arthritis, low or upper extremity pain.
**Respiratory:** cough, upper respiratory infection.
**Skin:** rash.
**Other:** viral infection, fever, injury, seasonal allergy, *angioedema*.

## Overdose and treatment
Hypotension would be the most likely manifestation of perindopril overdose. Treatment should be symptomatic and supportive. Perindopril should be stopped and patient observed closely. Advise clinician to treat dehydration, electrolyte imbalances, and hypotension using established protocols.

## Clinical considerations
**◆ ALERT** Angioedema involving the face, limbs, lips, tongue, glottis, and larynx has been reported in patients treated with perindopril. Recommend stopping drug and observing patient until the swelling disappears. If swelling is confined to the face and lips, it will probably resolve without treatment, but antihistamines may be useful in relieving symptoms. Angioedema with involvement of the tongue, glottis, or larynx may cause fatal airway obstruction. Appropriate therapy, such as subcutaneous epinephrine solution should be promptly given.
■ Patients with a history of angioedema unrelated to ACE inhibitor therapy may be at increased risk of angioedema while receiving an ACE inhibitor.
■ Excessive hypotension may occur when drug is given with diuretics. If possible, recommend stopping diuretic therapy 2 to 3 days before starting perindopril to decrease potential for excessive hypotensive response. If it isn't possible to discontinue the diuretic, recommend starting with a lower dose of perindopril or decreasing the dose of diuretic.
■ Although ACE inhibitors reduce blood pressure in many races, African-Americans who receive these drugs as monotherapy have a relatively weaker response. Including a thiazide diuretic leads to a more favorable response.
■ Advise clinician to monitor patients at risk for hypotension closely when therapy starts and for the first 2 weeks of treatment, and whenever the dose of perindopril or concomitant diuretic is increased.

■ If severe hypotension occurs, recommend placing patient in supine position and treating symptomatically.
■ Hypotension may also occur when therapy starts or changes in patients who have been volume- or salt-depleted as a result of prolonged diuretic therapy, dietary salt restriction, dialysis, diarrhea, or vomiting. Volume and salt depletion should be corrected before treatment starts.
■ ACE inhibitors have rarely caused a syndrome of cholestatic jaundice, fulminant hepatic necrosis, and death. Drug should be stopped in patients for whom jaundice or marked elevations of hepatic enzyme levels develop during therapy.

### Therapeutic monitoring
■ Advise clinician to monitor CBC with differential before therapy, especially in renally impaired patients with systemic lupus erythematosus or scleroderma.
■ Advise clinician to monitor renal function before and periodically throughout therapy. Drug shouldn't be used in patients with a creatinine clearance less than 30 ml/minute.
■ Advise clinician to monitor serum potassium levels closely.

### Special populations
**Pregnant patients.** Advise women of childbearing age of the consequences of second- and third-trimester exposure to drug. Advise them to notify prescriber immediately if pregnancy is suspected.
**Breast-feeding patients.** It isn't known if drug appears in breast milk. Use with caution in breast-feeding women.
**Pediatric patients.** Safety and efficacy in children haven't been established.
**Geriatric patients.** Plasma levels of both perindopril and perindoprilat in patients over age 70 are about twice those observed in younger patients. With the exception of dizziness and possibly rash, adverse effects don't appear to be increased in geriatric patients. Recommend giving doses above 8 mg/day with caution and under close medical supervision.

## Patient counseling
■ Inform patient that angioedema, including laryngeal edema, may occur during therapy, especially with the first dose. Advise patient to stop taking the drug and immediately report any signs or symptoms suggestive of angioedema, such as swelling of face, limbs, eyes, lips, tongue, hoarseness, or difficulty in swallowing or breathing.
■ Advise patient to promptly report to prescriber any sign of infection, such as sore throat or fever, or jaundice (yellowing of eyes or skin).
■ Caution patient that light-headedness may occur, especially during the first few days of ther-

apy. Advise patient to report light-headedness and, if fainting occurs, to discontinue the drug and consult a prescriber promptly.

■ Caution patient that inadequate fluid intake or excessive perspiration, diarrhea, or vomiting can lead to an excessive decrease in blood pressure.

# permethrin
Acticin, Elimite, Nix

*Pharmacologic classification:* synthetic pyrethroid
*Therapeutic classification:* scabicide, pediculocide
*Pregnancy risk category B*

## Available forms
Available by prescription only
**Elimite**
*Cream:* 5%
Available without a prescription
**Acticin, Nix**
*Lotion:* 1%

## Indications and dosages
*Pediculosis*
*Adults and children:* Apply sufficient volume to saturate the hair and scalp. Allow drug to remain on the hair for 10 minutes before rinsing.
*Scabies*
*Adults and children:* Thoroughly massage into skin from head to soles. Treat infants on the hairline, neck, scalp, temple, and forehead. Remove cream by washing after 8 to 14 hours. One application usually is curative.

## Mechanism of action
*Scabicidal action:* Permethrin acts on the parasites' nerve cell membranes to disrupt the sodium channel current and thereby paralyze them.

## Pharmacokinetics
*Absorption:* Not entirely investigated but probably less than 2% of the amount applied.
*Distribution:* Systemic distribution is unknown.
*Metabolism:* Rapidly metabolized by ester hydrolysis to inactive metabolites.
*Excretion:* Metabolites are excreted in urine. Residue on hair is detectable for up to 10 days.

| Route | Onset | Peak | Duration |
|---|---|---|---|
| Topical | 10-15 min | Unknown | 10 days |

## Contraindications and precautions
Contraindicated in patients hypersensitive to pyrethrins or chrysanthemums.

## Interactions
None reported.

## Adverse reactions
**Skin:** pruritus, *burning, stinging,* edema, tingling, numbness or scalp discomfort, mild erythema, scalp rash.

## Overdose and treatment
For accidental ingestion, advise clinician to perform gastric lavage and use general supportive measures.

## Clinical considerations
■ A single treatment is usually effective. Although combing of nits isn't required for effectiveness, drug package supplies a fine-toothed comb.
■ Permethrin is at least as effective as lindane (Kwell) in treating head lice.

### Therapeutic monitoring
■ A second application may be needed if lice are observed 7 days after the initial application.

### Special populations
**Breast-feeding patients.** It isn't known if permethrin appears in breast milk. Advise patient to stop breast-feeding temporarily or not use the drug.
**Pediatric patients.** Safety and efficacy for use in children under age 2 haven't been established.

## Patient counseling
■ Tell patient or caregiver to wash hair with shampoo, rinse it thoroughly, and then towel dry.
■ Tell patient or caregiver to apply sufficient volume to saturate the hair and scalp.
■ Instruct patient to report itching, redness, or swelling of the scalp.
■ Advise patient that drug is for external use only and to avoid contact with mucous membranes.

# perphenazine
Apo-Perphenazine*, Trilafon

*Pharmacologic classification:* phenothiazine (piperazine derivative)
*Therapeutic classification:* antipsychotic; antiemetic
*Pregnancy risk category NR*

## Available forms
Available by prescription only
*Injection:* 5 mg/ml
*Oral concentrate:* 16 mg/5 ml
*Tablets:* 2 mg, 4 mg, 8 mg, 16 mg

## Indications and dosages
*Psychosis*
*Adults:* Initially, 8 to 16 mg P.O. b.i.d., t.i.d., or q.i.d., increasing to 64 mg daily. Alterna-

tively, administer 5 to 10 mg I.M.; change to P.O. as soon as possible. Oral preparation may be given 8 to 16 mg P.O. b.i.d. for outpatients; 8 to 32 mg P.O. b.i.d. for inpatients.

*Mental disturbances, acute alcoholism, nausea, vomiting, hiccups*

*Adults:* 5 to 10 mg I.M., p.r.n. Maximum dose is 15 mg daily in ambulatory patients; 30 mg daily in hospitalized patients; or 8 to 16 mg P.O. daily in divided doses. A maximum of 5 mg I.V. diluted to 0.5 mg/ml with normal saline solution may be given for severe hiccups or vomiting.

## I.V. administration

■ Perphenazine may be given slowly by I.V. drip at 1 mg/2 minutes with continuous blood pressure monitoring.

### Incompatibilities

Incompatible with aminophylline, cefoperazone, midazolam hydrochloride, opium alkaloid hydrochlorides, oxytocin, pentobarbital sodium, and thiethylperazine.

## Mechanism of action

*Antipsychotic action:* Perphenazine is thought to exert its antipsychotic effects by postsynaptic blockade of CNS dopamine receptors, thus inhibiting dopamine-mediated effects; antiemetic effects are attributed to dopamine receptor blockade in the medullary chemoreceptor trigger zone. Perphenazine has many other central and peripheral effects: it produces both alpha and ganglionic blockade and counteracts histamine- and serotonin-mediated activity. Its most serious adverse reactions are extrapyramidal.

## Pharmacokinetics

*Absorption:* Rate and extent of absorption vary with administration route: oral tablet absorption is erratic and variable; oral concentrate absorption is much more predictable. I.M. drug is absorbed rapidly.

*Distribution:* Distributed widely into the body; appears in breast milk. Drug is 91% to 99% protein-bound.

*Metabolism:* Metabolized extensively by the liver, but no active metabolites are formed.

*Excretion:* Mostly excreted in urine via the kidneys; some in feces via the biliary tract.

| Route | Onset | Peak | Duration |
|-------|-------|------|----------|
| P.O., I.M., I.V. | ½-1 hr | 2-4 hr | Unknown |

## Contraindications and precautions

Contraindicated in patients hypersensitive to drug; in patients experiencing coma; in those with CNS depression, blood dyscrasia, bone marrow depression, liver damage, or subcortical damage; and in those receiving large doses of CNS depressants.

Use cautiously in geriatric or debilitated patients; in those with alcohol withdrawal, psychic depression, suicidal tendencies, adverse reaction to other phenothiazines, impaired renal function, respiratory disorders; and in patients receiving other CNS depressants or anticholinergics.

## Interactions

**Drug-drug.** *Aluminum- and magnesium-containing antacids and antidiarrheals, phenobarbital:* Pharmacokinetic alterations and subsequent decreased therapeutic response to perphenazine. Don't use together.

*Antiarrhythmics, disopyramide, procainamide, quinidine:* Increased risk of arrhythmias and conduction defects. Don't use together.

*Appetite suppressants; sympathomimetics, such as ephedrine, epinephrine, phenylephrine:* May decrease their stimulatory and pressor effects. Advise clinician to monitor patient closely.

*Atropine or other anticholinergics:* Oversedation, paralytic ileus, visual changes, and severe constipation. Avoid use together.

*Beta blockers:* May inhibit perphenazine metabolism, increasing plasma levels and toxicity. Don't use together.

*Bromocriptine:* Perphenazine may antagonize therapeutic effect. Avoid use together.

*Centrally acting antihypertensive drugs, such as clonidine, guanabenz, guanadrel, guanethidine, methyldopa, and reserpine:* Perphenazine may inhibit blood pressure response. Avoid use together.

*CNS depressants, general, spinal, or epidural anesthetics, or parenteral magnesium sulfate:* Additive effects are likely if perphenazine is used. Avoid use together.

*High-dose dopamine:* Decreased vasoconstricting effects. Don't use together.

*Levodopa:* Decreased effectiveness and increased toxicity. Don't use together.

*Lithium:* May result in severe neurologic toxicity with an encephalitis-like syndrome, and a decreased therapeutic response to perphenazine. Don't use together.

*Metrizamide:* Increased risk of seizures. Don't use together.

*Nitrates:* Hypotension. Advise clinician to monitor blood pressure.

*Phenytoin:* Perphenazine may inhibit metabolism and increase toxicity. Don't use together.

*Propylthiouracil:* Increases risk of agranulocytosis. Advise clinician to monitor CBC results.

**Drug-herb.** *Kava:* Increased risk or severity of dystonic reactions. Discourage concomitant use.

*Yohimbe:* Increased the risk of toxicity. Discourage concomitant use.

**Drug-food.** *Caffeine:* Decreases therapeutic response to perphenazine. Instruct patient to avoid foods and beverages that contain caffeine.

---

**Drug-lifestyle.** *Alcohol use:* Additive effects are likely. Advise patient to avoid alcohol.
*Heavy smoking:* Decreased therapeutic response to perphenazine. Discourage smoking.
*Sun exposure:* Photosensitivity reactions may occur. Advise patient to use sunblock.

## Adverse reactions
**CNS:** *extrapyramidal reactions, tardive dyskinesia,* sedation, pseudoparkinsonism, EEG changes, dizziness, adverse behavioral effects, *seizures,* drowsiness, *neuroleptic malignant syndrome.*
**CV:** *orthostatic hypotension,* tachycardia, ECG changes, *cardiac arrest.*
**EENT:** ocular changes, *blurred vision,* nasal congestion.
**GI:** *dry mouth, constipation,* nausea, vomiting, diarrhea, ileus.
**GU:** *urine retention,* dark urine, menstrual irregularities, inhibited ejaculation.
**Hematologic:** *leukopenia,* galactorrhea, hyperglycemia, hypoglycemia, *agranulocytosis,* eosinophilia, *hemolytic anemia, thrombocytopenia.*
**Hepatic:** jaundice, abnormal liver function test results.
**Metabolic:** weight gain, SIADH.
**Skin:** *mild photosensitivity,* allergic reactions, pain at I.M. injection site, sterile abscess.
**Other:** gynecomastia.
**After abrupt withdrawal of long-term therapy:** gastritis, nausea, vomiting, dizziness, tremor, feeling of warmth or cold, diaphoresis, tachycardia, headache, insomnia.

## Overdose and treatment
CNS depression is characterized by deep, unarousable sleep and possible coma, hypotension, or hypertension, extrapyramidal symptoms, dystonia, abnormal involuntary muscle movements, agitation, seizures, arrhythmias, ECG changes, hypothermia or hyperthermia, and autonomic nervous system dysfunction.

Treatment is symptomatic and supportive, including maintaining vital signs, airway, stable body temperature, and fluid and electrolyte balance.

Vomiting should be induced in a conscious patient with ipecac syrup even if spontaneous vomiting has occurred. Vomiting shouldn't be induced in patients with impaired consciousness. Advise clinician to use gastric lavage, then activated charcoal and sodium chloride cathartics; dialysis is usually ineffective. Advise clinician to regulate body temperature p.r.n. Hypotension should be treated with I.V. fluids; epinephrine shouldn't be given. Seizures should be treated with parenteral diazepam or barbiturates; arrhythmias with parenteral phenytoin (1 mg/kg with rate titrated to blood pressure); and extrapyramidal reactions with benztropine at 1 to 2 mg or parenteral diphenhydramine at 10 to 50 mg.

## Clinical considerations
■ Oral formulations may cause stomach upset; recommend giving with food or fluid.
■ Dilute the concentrate in 2 to 4 ounces (60 to 120 ml) of liquid (water, caffeine-free carbonated drinks, fruit juice [not apple], tomato juice, milk, or puddings). Dilute every 5 ml of concentrate with 60 ml of suitable fluid. Shake oral concentrate before administration.
■ Liquid formulation may cause rash upon contact with skin.
■ I.M. injection may cause skin necrosis; avoid extravasation.
■ Recommend giving I.M. injection deep into upper outer quadrant of buttocks. Massaging the injection site may prevent formation of abscesses.
■ Drug shouldn't be administered for injection if it's excessively discolored or contains precipitate.
■ Perphenazine causes false-positive test results for urinary porphyrins, urobilinogen, amylase, and 5-hydroxyindoleacetic acid because of darkening of urine by metabolites; it also causes false-positive urine pregnancy test results using human chorionic gonadotropin.

### Therapeutic monitoring
■ Advise clinician to monitor blood pressure before and after parenteral administration.

### Special populations
**Breast-feeding patients.** Drug is widely distributed and appears in breast milk; use with caution. Potential benefits to the woman should outweigh the potential harm to the infant.
**Pediatric patients.** Drug isn't recommended for children under age 12.
**Geriatric patients.** Lower doses should be used in geriatric patients. Dose must be titrated to effects; 30% to 50% of the usual dose may be effective. Geriatric patients are at greater risk for adverse effects, especially tardive dyskinesia and other extrapyramidal effects.

## Patient counseling
■ Explain the risks of dystonic reactions and tardive dyskinesia, and tell patient to report abnormal body movements.
■ Tell patient to avoid spilling the liquid; contact with skin may cause rash and irritation.
■ Warn patient not to take extremely hot or cold baths and to avoid exposure to temperature extremes, sun lamps, or tanning beds; drug may cause thermoregulatory changes.
■ Advise patient to take drug exactly as prescribed and not to double the dose for missed doses.
■ Instruct patient not to stop taking drug suddenly; any adverse reactions may be alleviated by a dosage reduction. Patient should promptly report difficulty urinating, sore throat, dizziness, or fainting.

■ Tell patient to avoid hazardous activities that require alertness until effect of drug is established. Reassure patient that sedative effects of drug should become tolerable in several weeks.
■ Explain which fluids are appropriate for diluting the concentrate (not apple juice or caffeine-containing drinks); explain dropper technique of measuring dose.
■ Recommend sugarless hard candy or chewing gum, ice chips, or artificial saliva to relieve dry mouth.

# phenazopyridine hydrochloride

Azo-dine, Azo-Gesic, Azo-Standard, Baridium, Phenazo*, Prodium, Pyridium, Pyridium Plus, Re-Azo, UTI Relief

*Pharmacologic classification:* azo dye
*Therapeutic classification:* urinary analgesic
*Pregnancy risk category B*

## Available forms
Available by prescription only
*Tablets:* 97.2 mg, 100 mg, 150 mg, 200 mg
Available without prescription
*Tablets:* 95 mg, 97 mg, 100 mg

## Indications and dosages
*Pain with urinary tract irritation or infection*
*Adults:* 200 mg P.O. t.i.d. Give drug after meals.

## Mechanism of action
*Analgesic action:* Phenazopyridine has a local anesthetic effect on urinary tract mucosa via an unknown mechanism.

## Pharmacokinetics
*Absorption:* Not described.
*Distribution:* Traces of drug are thought to enter CSF and cross the placenta.
*Metabolism:* Metabolized in the liver.
*Excretion:* Excreted by the kidneys; 65% is excreted unchanged in urine. Average time of total excretion of drug is 20½ hours.

| Route | Onset | Peak | Duration |
|-------|-------|------|----------|
| P.O. | Unknown | Unknown | Unknown |

## Contraindications and precautions
Contraindicated in patients hypersensitive to drug, and those with glomerulonephritis, severe hepatitis, uremia, pyelonephritis during pregnancy, or renal insufficiency.

## Interactions
None significant.

## Adverse reactions
**CNS:** headache.
**GI:** nausea, GI disturbances.
**Hematologic:** hemolytic anemia, methemoglobinemia.
**Skin:** rash, pruritus.
**Other:** *anaphylactoid reactions.*

## Overdose and treatment
Signs and symptoms of overdose include methemoglobinemia (most obvious as cyanosis), along with renal and hepatic impairment and failure.

To treat overdose of phenazopyridine, advise clinician to empty stomach immediately by inducing emesis with ipecac syrup or by gastric lavage. Recommend giving methylene blue, 1 to 2 mg/kg I.V., or 100 to 200 mg ascorbic acid P.O. to reverse methemoglobinemia. Symptomatic and supportive measures (respiratory support and correction of fluid and electrolyte imbalances) should be provided. Advise clinician to monitor laboratory effects and vital signs closely. Contact local or regional poison information center for specific instructions.

## Clinical considerations
■ Drug colors urine red or orange; it may stain fabrics.
■ Use only as an analgesic.
■ May be used with an antibiotic to treat urinary tract infections.
■ Advise clinician to stop drug in 2 days with concurrent antibiotic use.
■ Drug may alter results of Diastix, Chemstrip uG, glucose enzymatic test strip, Acetest, and Ketostix. Clinitest should be used to obtain accurate urine glucose test results.
■ Drug may also interfere with Ehrlich's test for urine urobilinogen; phenolsulfonphthalein excretion tests of kidney function; sulfobromophthalein excretion tests of liver function; and urine tests for protein, steroids, or bilirubin.

### Therapeutic monitoring
■ Advise clinician to monitor patient for anaphlyactic reactions.
■ Advise clinician to evaluate response to drug therapy and assessing urinary function, such as output, complaints of burning, pain, and frequency.
■ Advise clinician to monitor vital signs, especially temperature.

### Special populations
**Breast-feeding patients.** Safety in breast-feeding women hasn't been established.
**Geriatric patients.** Use with caution in geriatric patients because of possible decreased renal function.

## Patient counseling
- Instruct patient in measures to prevent urinary tract infection.
- Tell patient that stains on clothing may be removed with a 0.25% solution of sodium dithionate or hydrosulfite.
- Advise patient to take a missed dose as soon as possible and not to double the doses.
- Instruct patient to report symptoms that worsen or don't resolve.
- Encourage patient to force fluids (if not contraindicated). Advise clinician to monitor intake and output.

# phenobarbital
Barbita

# phenobarbital sodium
Luminal

*Pharmacologic classification:* barbiturate
*Therapeutic classification:* anticonvulsant, sedative-hypnotic
*Pregnancy risk category D*
*Controlled substance schedule IV*

## Available forms
Available by prescription only
*Elixir:* 15 mg/5 ml; 20 mg/5 ml
*Injection:* 30 mg/ml, 60 mg/ml, 65 mg/ml, 130 mg/ml
*Tablets:* 15 mg, 16 mg, 30 mg, 32 mg, 60 mg, 65 mg, 100 mg

## Indications and dosages
*All forms of epilepsy except absence seizures, febrile seizures in children*
*Adults:* 60 to 100 mg P.O. daily, divided t.i.d. or given as single dose h.s. Alternatively, give 200 to 300 mg I.M. or I.V. and repeat q 6 hours, p.r.n.
*Children:* 1 to 6 mg/kg P.O. daily, usually divided q 12 hours. It can, however, be given once daily. Alternatively, give 4 to 6 mg/kg I.V. or I.M. daily and monitor patient's blood levels.
*Status epilepticus*
*Adults and children:* 10 to 20 mg/kg I.V. over 10 to 15 minutes; don't exceed 60 mg/min. Repeat if needed.
*Sedation*
*Adults:* 30 to 120 mg P.O., I.M., or I.V. daily in two or three divided doses. Maximum dose, 400 mg/24 hours.
*Children:* 8 to 32 mg P.O. daily.
*Insomnia*
*Adults:* 100 to 200 mg P.O. or 100 to 320 mg I.M.
*Preoperative sedation*
*Adults:* 100 to 200 mg I.M. 60 to 90 minutes before surgery.

*Children:* 1 to 3 mg/kg I.V. or I.M. 60 to 90 minutes before surgery.

## I.V. administration
- Reconstitute powder for injection with 2.5 to 5 ml sterile water for injection. Roll vial in hands; don't shake.
- A larger vein should be used for I.V. administration to prevent extravasation.
- Avoid I.V. administration at a rate exceeding 60 mg/minute to prevent hypotension and respiratory depression. It may take up to 30 minutes after I.V. administration to achieve maximum effect.
- Recommend giving a parenteral dose within 30 minutes of reconstitution because phenobarbital hydrolyzes both in solution and on exposure to air.

### Incompatibilities
Incompatible with alcohol-dextrose solutions, cephalothin, chlorpromazine, codeine phosphate, ephedrine, hydralazine, hydrocortisone sodium succinate, levorphanol, meperidine, morphine, norepinephrine, pentazocine lactate, prochlorperazine mesylate, promazine, promethazine hydrochloride, ranitidine hydrochloride, regular insulin, streptomycin, and vancomycin.

## Mechanism of action
*Anticonvulsant action:* Phenobarbital suppresses the spread of seizure activity produced by epileptogenic foci in the cortex, thalamus, and limbic systems by enhancing the effect of gamma-aminobutyric acid (GABA). Both presynaptic and postsynaptic excitability are decreased; also, phenobarbital raises the seizure threshold.
*Sedative-hypnotic action:* Phenobarbital acts throughout the CNS as a nonselective depressant with a slow onset of action and a long duration of action. Particularly sensitive to this drug is the reticular-activating system, which controls CNS arousal. Phenobarbital decreases both presynaptic and postsynaptic membrane excitability by facilitating the action of GABA. The exact cellular site and mechanisms of action are unknown.

## Pharmacokinetics
*Absorption:* Well absorbed after oral and rectal administration, with 70% to 90% reaching the bloodstream. Absorption after I.M. administration is 100%. After oral administration peak levels in the CNS are achieved at 1 to 3 hours. A serum level of 10 mcg/ml is needed to produce sedation; 40 mcg/ml usually produces sleep. Levels of 20 to 40 mcg/ml are considered therapeutic for anticonvulsant therapy.
*Distribution:* Distributed widely throughout the body. Phenobarbital is about 25% to 30% protein-bound.

*Metabolism:* Metabolized by the hepatic microsomal enzyme system.

*Excretion:* About 25% to 50% of a phenobarbital dose is eliminated unchanged in urine; remainder is excreted as metabolites of glucuronic acid. Half-life of drug is 5 to 7 days.

| Route | Onset | Peak | Duration |
|-------|-------|------|----------|
| P.O. | 1 hr | 8-12 hr | 10-12 hr |
| I.V. | 5 min | ½ hr | 4-10 hr |
| I.M. | > 5 min | > ½ hr | 4-10 hr |

## Contraindications and precautions

Contraindicated in patients hypersensitive to barbiturates, and those with history of manifest or latent porphyria, hepatic dysfunction, respiratory disease with dyspnea or obstruction, and nephritis.

Use cautiously in geriatric or debilitated patients and in those with acute or chronic pain, depression, suicidal tendencies, history of drug abuse, blood pressure alterations, CV disease, shock, or uremia.

## Interactions

**Drug-drug.** *Antidepressants, antihistamines, narcotics, phenothiazines, sedative-hypnotics, tranquilizers:* Phenobarbital may add to or potentiate CNS and respiratory depressant effects. Don't use together.

*Corticosteroids, digitoxin (not digoxin), doxycycline, oral contraceptives and other estrogens, theophylline and other xanthines:* Drug enhances hepatic metabolism. Avoid use together; advise clinician to monitor patient closely.

*Disulfiram, MAO inhibitors, valproic acid:* Decrease the metabolism of phenobarbital and can increase its toxicity. Advise clinician to monitor patient for toxicity.

*Griseofulvin:* Phenobarbital impairs the effectiveness of griseofulvin by decreasing absorption from the GI tract. Recommend giving drugs at separate times.

*Rifampin:* May decrease phenobarbital levels by increasing hepatic metabolism. Advise clinician to monitor levels closely.

*Warfarin and other oral anticoagulants:* Phenobarbital enhances the enzymatic degradation. May require increased doses of the anticoagulant.

**Drug-herb.** *Evening primrose oil:* Possible increase in anticonvulsant dosage requirement. Discourage use together.

**Drug-lifestyle.** *Alcohol use:* Phenobarbital may add to or potentiate CNS and respiratory depressant effects. Advise patient to avoid alcohol.

## Adverse reactions

**CNS:** *drowsiness, lethargy, hangover,* paradoxical excitement in geriatric patients, phys-

ical and psychological dependence, somnolence.

**CV:** *bradycardia,* hypotension.

**GI:** nausea, vomiting.

**Hematologic:** exacerbation of porphyria.

**Respiratory:** *respiratory depression, apnea.*

**Skin:** rash, *erythema multiforme, Stevens-Johnson syndrome,* urticaria; pain, swelling, thrombophlebitis, necrosis, nerve injury at injection site.

**Other:** *angioedema.*

## Overdose and treatment

Signs and symptoms of phenobarbital overdose include unsteady gait, slurred speech, sustained nystagmus, somnolence, confusion, respiratory depression, pulmonary edema, areflexia, and coma. Typical shock syndrome with tachycardia and hypotension along with jaundice, oliguria, and chills followed by fever may occur.

Treatment aims to maintain and support ventilation and pulmonary function p.r.n.; and to support cardiac function and circulation with vasopressors and I.V. fluids p.r.n. If patient is conscious and gag reflex is intact, recommend inducing emesis (if ingestion was recent) by giving ipecac syrup. If emesis is contraindicated, gastric lavage should be performed while a cuffed endotracheal tube is in place to prevent aspiration. Recommend following with administration of activated charcoal or sodium chloride cathartic. Recommend measuring intake and output, vital signs, and laboratory parameters. Body temperature should be maintained.

Alkalinization of urine may be helpful in removing drug from the body; hemodialysis may be useful in severe overdose. Oral activated charcoal may enhance phenobarbital elimination regardless of its route of administration.

## Clinical considerations

■ Oral solution may be mixed with water or juice to improve taste.

■ Recommend giving I.M. dose deep into a large muscle mass to prevent tissue injury.

■ Don't use injectable solution if it contains a precipitate.

■ Administration of full loading doses over short periods of time to treat status epilepticus will require ventilatory support in adults.

■ Phenobarbital may cause a false-positive phentolamine test. The physiologic effects of drug may impair the absorption of cyanocobalamin $^{57}Co$; it may decrease serum bilirubin levels in neonates and epileptics, and in patients with congenital nonhemolytic unconjugated hyperbilirubinemia. Barbiturates may increase sulfobromophthalein retention. EEG patterns show a change in low-voltage, fast ac-

---

Reactions may be *common,* uncommon, *life-threatening,* or COMMON AND LIFE-THREATENING.

tivity; changes persist for a time after discontinuation of therapy.

### Therapeutic monitoring
■ Recommend keeping emergency resuscitation equipment on hand when giving phenobarbital intravenously.
■ Full therapeutic effects aren't seen for 2 to 3 weeks, except when loading dose is used.

### Special populations
**Breast-feeding patients.** Phenobarbital appears in breast milk; avoid giving to breast-feeding women.
**Pediatric patients.** Paradoxical hyperexcitability may occur in children. Use with caution.
**Geriatric patients.** Geriatric patients are more sensitive to effects of drug and usually require lower doses. Confusion, disorientation, and excitability may occur in geriatric patients.

### Patient counseling
■ Advise patient of the potential for physical and psychological dependence with prolonged use.
■ Caution patient not to stop taking drug suddenly because this could cause a withdrawal reaction.
■ Advise patient to avoid driving and other hazardous activities that require alertness until the adverse CNS effects of drug are known.

# phentermine hydrochloride
Adipex-P, Anoxine-AM, Dapex, Ionamin, Obe-Nix, Obephen, Obermine, Obestin-30, Parmine, Phentrol

*Pharmacologic classification:* amphetamine congener
*Therapeutic classification:* short-term adjunctive anorexigenic, indirect-acting sympathomimetic amine
*Pregnancy risk category X*
*Controlled substance schedule IV*

### Available forms
Available by prescription only
*Capsules:* 8 mg, 18.75 mg, 30 mg, 37.5 mg
*Capsules (resin complex):* 15 mg, 30 mg, 37.5 mg
*Tablets:* 8 mg, 37.5 mg

### Indications and dosages
*Short-term adjunct in exogenous obesity*
Adults: 8 mg P.O. t.i.d. ½ hour before meals; or 15 to 37.5 mg P.O. daily before breakfast; or 15 to 30 mg P.O. daily before breakfast (resin complex).

### Mechanism of action
*Anorexigenic action:* Phentermine is an indirect-acting sympathomimetic amine; it causes fewer and less severe adverse reactions from CNS stimulation than do amphetamines, and its potential for addiction is lower. Anorexigenic effects are thought to follow direct stimulation of the hypothalamus; they may involve other CNS and metabolic effects.

### Pharmacokinetics
*Absorption:* Absorbed readily after oral administration.
*Distribution:* Distributed widely throughout the body.
*Metabolism:* Unknown.
*Excretion:* Excreted in urine.

| Route | Onset | Peak | Duration |
|-------|-------|------|----------|
| P.O. | Unknown | Unknown | 12-14 hr |

### Contraindications and precautions
Contraindicated in patients with hyperthyroidism, moderate to severe hypertension, advanced arteriosclerosis, symptomatic CV disease, glaucoma, or hypersensitivity or idiosyncrasy to sympathomimetic amines; within 14 days of MAO inhibitor therapy; and in agitated patients.
Use cautiously in patients with mild hypertension.

### Interactions
**Drug-drug.** *Acetazolamide, antacids, sodium bicarbonate:* Increase renal reabsorption of phentermine and prolong its duration of action. Advise clinician to monitor patient closely.
*General anesthetics:* May result in arrhythmias. Advise clinician to monitor patient closely.
*Guanethidine and other antihypertensives:* Phentermine may decrease hypotensive effect. Don't use together.
*Haloperidol and phenothiazines:* Decrease phentermine effects. Avoid use together.
*Insulin:* Phentermine may alter requirements in diabetic patients. Advise clinician to monitor serum glucose levels and patient closely.
*MAO inhibitors:* May cause hypertensive crisis. Don't use together or within 14 days after MAO inhibitor has been discontinued.
**Drug-food.** *Caffeine:* May cause additive CNS stimulation. Discourage use together.

### Adverse reactions
**CNS:** overstimulation, headache, euphoria, dysphoria, dizziness, *insomnia.*
**CV:** *palpitations, tachycardia,* increased blood pressure.
**GI:** dry mouth, dysgeusia, constipation, diarrhea, other GI disturbances.

**GU:** impotence, dysuria, polyuria, urinary frequency.
**Skin:** urticaria.
**Other:** altered libido.

## Overdose and treatment
Signs and symptoms of acute overdose include restlessness, tremor, hyperreflexia, fever, tachypnea, dizziness, confusion, aggressive behavior, hallucinations, blood pressure changes, arrhythmias, nausea, vomiting, diarrhea, and cramps. Fatigue and depression usually follow CNS stimulation; seizures, coma, and death may follow.

Recommend treating overdose symptomatically and supportively; sedation may be needed. Chlorpromazine may antagonize CNS stimulation. Acidification of urine may hasten excretion. Advise clinician to monitor vital signs and fluid and electrolyte balance.

## Clinical considerations
■ Intermittent courses of treatment (6 weeks on, followed by 4 weeks off) are as effective as continuous use.
■ Greatest weight loss occurs in the first weeks of therapy and diminishes in succeeding weeks. When such tolerance to drug effect develops, drug should be stopped instead of increasing the dosage.

### Therapeutic monitoring
■ Advise clinician to monitor patient for tolerance and dependence.

### Special populations
**Pregnant patients.** Safety hasn't been established for use in pregnant women; drug should be given to pregnant women only if clearly needed.
**Pediatric patients.** Phentermine isn't recommended for children under age 12.

## Patient counseling
■ Advise patient to avoid caffeine-containing drinks.
■ Tell patient to take last daily dose at least 6 hours before bedtime to prevent insomnia.
■ Warn patient not to take drug more frequently than prescribed.
■ Advise patient that drug may produce dizziness, fatigue, or drowsiness.
■ Tell patient to contact prescriber if palpitations occur.

# phentolamine mesylate
Regitine

*Pharmacologic classification:* alpha
adrenergic blocker
*Therapeutic classification:* antihypertensive for pheochromocytoma, cutaneous vasodilator
*Pregnancy risk category C*

## Available forms
Available by prescription only
*Injection:* 5 mg/ml in 1-ml vials

## Indications and dosages
**Aid for diagnosis of pheochromocytoma**
*Adults:* 5 mg I.V. or I.M.
*Children:* 1 mg I.V., or 3 mg I.M.
***Control or prevention of paroxysmal hypertension immediately before or during pheochromocytomectomy***
*Adults:* 5 mg I.M. or I.V. 1 to 2 hours preoperatively, repeated p.r.n.; 5 mg I.V. during surgery if indicated.
*Children:* 1 mg I.M. or I.V. 1 to 2 hours preoperatively, repeated p.r.n.; 1 mg I.V. during surgery if indicated.
***Prevention or treatment of dermal necrosis and sloughing of extravasation after I.V. administration of norepinephrine or ◇dopamine***
*Adults:* Inject 5 to 10 mg in 10 ml of normal saline solution into the affected area, or add 10 mg to each L of I.V. fluids containing norepinephrine.
*Children:* 0.1 to 0.2 mg/kg injected into affected area, up to a maximum of 10 mg per dose, after extravasation of dopamine.
***◇Adjunctive treatment of left-sided heart failure secondary to acute MI***
*Adults:* 0.17 to 0.4 mg/minute by I.V. infusion.
***◇Treatment adjunct for males with impotence (neurogenic or vascular)***
*Adults:* 0.5 to 1 mg by intracavernosal injection. Usually given with 30 mg papaverine injection.
***◇Hypertensive crisis from sympathomimetic amines***
*Adults:* 5 to 15 mg I.V.
***◇Cocaine-induced acute coronary syndrome***
*Adults:* 2.5 to 5 mg, repeat every 5 to 10 minutes until blood pressure is controlled.
*Children:* 0.05 to 0.1 mg/kg, repeat every 5 to 10 minutes until blood pressure is controlled, to a maximum total dose of 2.5 to 5 mg.

## I.V. administration
■ Before test for pheochromocytoma, have patient rest in supine position until blood pressure is stabilized.
■ When phentolamine is administered I.V., advise clinician to inject dose rapidly after ef-

fects of the venipuncture on the blood pressure have passed. A marked decrease in blood pressure is seen immediately, with the maximum effect seen within 2 minutes. Blood pressure should be recorded immediately after the injection, at 30-second intervals for the first 3 minutes, and at 1-minute intervals for the next 7 minutes.

■ When drug is administered I.M., maximum effect occurs within 20 minutes. Blood pressure should be recorded every 5 minutes for 30 to 45 minutes after injection.

### Incompatibilities
None reported.

### Mechanism of action
*Antihypertensive action:* Phentolamine competitively antagonizes endogenous and exogenous amines at presynaptic and postsynaptic alpha-adrenergic receptors, decreasing both preload and afterload.

*Cutaneous vasodilation action:* Phentolamine blocks epinephrine- and norepinephrine-induced vasoconstriction.

### Pharmacokinetics
*Absorption:* Unknown.
*Distribution:* Unknown.
*Metabolism:* Unknown.
*Excretion:* About 10% of a given dose is excreted unchanged in urine; excretion of remainder is unknown. Drug has a short duration of action; plasma half-life is 19 minutes after I.V. administration.

| Route | Onset | Peak | Duration |
|-------|-------|------|----------|
| I.V. | Immediate | Unknown | Unknown |
| I.M. | Unknown | Unknown | Unknown |

### Contraindications and precautions
Contraindicated in patients with angina, coronary artery disease, MI or history of MI, or those hypersensitive to drug.

Use cautiously in patients with peptic ulcer or gastritis.

### Interactions
**Drug-drug.** *Ephedrine and epinephrine:* Phentolamine antagonizes vasoconstrictor and hypertensive effects. Don't use together.

### Adverse reactions
**CNS:** *dizziness, weakness, flushing, **cerebrovascular occlusion,** cerebrovascular spasm.*
**CV:** *hypotension, **shock, arrhythmias,** tachycardia, **MI.***
**EENT:** *nasal congestion.*
**GI:** *diarrhea, nausea, vomiting.*

### Overdose and treatment
Signs and symptoms of overdose include hypotension, dizziness, fainting, tachycardia, vomiting, lethargy, and shock.

Advise clinician to treat supportively and symptomatically. Norepinephrine should be used if needed to increase the blood pressure. Epinephrine shouldn't be given; it stimulates both alpha and beta receptors and causes vasodilation and a further decrease in blood pressure.

### Clinical considerations
■ Usual doses of phentolamine have little effect on the blood pressure of normal individuals or patients with essential hypertension.

■ A positive test response occurs when patient's blood pressure decreases at least 35 mm Hg systolic and 25 mm Hg diastolic; a negative test response occurs when the patient's blood pressure remains unchanged, is elevated, or decreases less than 35 mm Hg systolic and 25 mm Hg diastolic.

■ When possible, recommend withdrawing sedatives, analgesics, and all other drugs at least 24 hours (preferably 48 to 72 hours) before the phentolamine test. Recommend withdrawing antihypertensives; test shouldn't be performed until blood pressure returns to pretreatment levels. Rauwolfia drugs should be withdrawn at least 4 weeks before test.

■ Drug has been used to treat hypertension resulting from clonidine withdrawal and to treat the reaction to sympathetic amines or other drugs or foods in patients taking MAO inhibitors.

■ Drug has also been used in patients with MI from left-sided HF in an attempt to reduce infarct size and decrease left ventricular ejection impedance. It also has been used to treat supraventricular premature contractions.

### Therapeutic monitoring
■ Advise clinician to monitor vital signs closely.

### Special populations
**Breast-feeding patients.** It isn't known if drug appears in breast milk. Because of possible adverse reactions in the infant, recommend stopping either breast-feeding or drug based on the importance of drug to the woman.

### Patient counseling
■ Teach patient about phentolamine test, if indicated.
■ Tell patient to report adverse effects at once.
■ Tell patient not to take sedatives or narcotics for at least 24 hours before phentolamine test.

# phenylephrine hydrochloride

*Nasal products*
Alconefrin 12, Alconefrin 25,
Neo-Synephrine, Nostril, Rhinall,
Sinex

*Parenteral*
Neo-Synephrine

*Ophthalmic*
AK-Dilate, AK-Nefrin, Isopto Frin,
Mydfrin, Neo-Synephrine, Prefrin
Liquifilm, Relief Phenoptic

*Pharmacologic classification:* adrenergic
*Therapeutic classification:* vasoconstrictor
*Pregnancy risk category C*

## Available forms

Available by prescription only
*Injection:* 10 mg/ml parenteral
*Ophthalmic solution:* 0.12%, 2.5%, 10%
Available without a prescription
*Nasal solution:* 0.125%, 0.16%, 0.25%,
0.5%, 1%
*Nasal spray:* 0.25%, 0.5%, 1%

## Indications and dosages

*Hypotensive emergencies during spinal
anesthesia*
*Adults:* Initially, 0.1 to 0.2 mg I.V.; subsequent
doses should also be low (0.1 mg).
*Prevention of hypotension during spinal
or inhalation anesthesia*
*Adults:* 2 to 3 mg S.C. or I.M. 3 to 4 minutes
before anesthesia.
*Mild to moderate hypotension*
*Adults:* 1 to 10 mg S.C. or I.M.; initial dose
shouldn't exceed 5 mg. Additional doses may
be given in 1 to 2 hours if needed. Or, 0.1 to
0.5 mg slow I.V. injection; initial dose shouldn't
exceed 0.5 mg. Additional doses may be giv-
en q 10 to 15 minutes.
*Children:* 0.1 mg/kg or 3 mg/m² I.M. or S.C.
*Paroxysmal supraventricular tachycardia*
*Adults:* Initially, 0.5 mg rapid I.V.; subsequent
doses may be increased in increments of 0.1
to 0.2 mg. Maximum dose shouldn't exceed
1 mg.
*Prolongation of spinal anesthesia*
*Adults:* 2 to 5 mg added to anesthetic solution.
*Adjunct in the treatment of severe
hypotension or shock*
*Adults:* 0.1 to 0.18 mg/minute I.V. infusion.
After blood pressure stabilizes, maintain at 0.04
to 0.06 mg/minute, adjusted to patient response.
*Vasoconstrictor for regional anesthesia*
*Adults:* 1 mg phenylephrine added to 20 ml lo-
cal anesthetic.

*Mydriasis (without cycloplegia)*
*Adults:* Instill one or two drops 2.5% or 10%
solution in eye before procedure. May be repeated in 10 to 60 minutes if needed.
*Posterior synechia (adhesion of iris)*
*Adults:* Instill one drop of 10% solution in eye
three or more times daily with atropine sulfate.
*Diagnosis of Horner's or Raeder's
syndrome*
*Adults:* Instill a 1% or 10% solution in both
eyes.
*Initial treatment of postoperative
malignant glaucoma*
*Adults:* Instill one drop of a 10% solution with
one drop of a 1% to 4% atropine sulfate solution three or more times daily.
*Nasal, ◇ sinus, or eustachian tube
congestion*
*Adults and children over age 12:* Apply two to
three drops or one to two sprays of 0.25% to
1% solution instilled in each nostril; or a small
quantity of 0.5% nasal jelly applied into each
nostril. Apply jelly or spray to nasal mucosa.
*Children ages 6 to 12:* Apply two to three drops
or one to two sprays in each nostril.
*Children under age 6:* Apply two to three drops
or sprays of 0.125% or 0.16% solution in each
nostril.
    Note: Drops, spray, or jelly can be given q
4 hours, p.r.n.
*Conjunctival congestion*
*Adults:* 1 to 2 drops of 0.08% to 0.25% solution applied to conjunctiva q 3 to 4 hours, p.r.n.

## I.V. administration

■ Recommend giving I.V. through large veins
and monitoring flow rate. To treat extravasation ischemia, recommend infiltrating site
promptly and liberally with 10 to 15 ml of normal saline solution containing 5 to 10 mg of
phentolamine through fine needle. Topical nitroglycerin has also been used.
■ During I.V. administration, pulse, blood pressure, and central venous pressure should be
monitored every 2 to 5 minutes. Recommend
controlling flow rate and dosage to prevent excessive increases. I.V. overdoses may induce
ventricular arrhythmias.

### Incompatibilities

Phenylephrine is chemically incompatible with
butacaine, sulfate, alkalies, ferric salts, and oxidizing agents and metals.

## Mechanism of action

*Vasopressor action:* Phenylephrine acts predominantly by direct stimulation of alpha-
adrenergic receptors, which constrict resistance
and capacitance blood vessels, resulting in increased total peripheral resistance; increased
systolic and diastolic blood pressure; decreased
blood flow to vital organs, skin, and skeletal
muscle; and constriction of renal blood ves-

---

Reactions may be *common*, uncommon, *life-threatening*, or COMMON AND LIFE-THREATENING.

sels, reducing renal blood flow. Its main therapeutic effect is vasoconstriction.

It may also act indirectly by releasing norepinephrine from its storage sites. Phenylephrine doesn't stimulate beta receptors except in large doses, when it activates beta$_1$ receptors. Tachyphylaxis (tolerance) may follow repeated injections.

Other alpha-adrenergic effects include action on the dilator muscle of the pupil (producing contraction) and local decongestant action in the arterioles of the conjunctiva (producing constriction).

Phenylephrine acts directly on alpha-adrenergic receptors in the arterioles of conjunctiva nasal mucosa, producing constriction. Its vasoconstricting action on skin, mucous membranes, and viscera slows the vascular absorption rate of local anesthetics, which prolongs their action, localizes anesthesia, and decreases the risk of toxicity.

Phenylephrine may cause contraction of pregnant uterus and constriction of uterine blood vessels.

## Pharmacokinetics
*Absorption:* Variable depending on route of administration.
*Distribution:* Unknown.
*Metabolism:* Metabolized in the liver and intestine by MAO.
*Excretion:* Unknown.

| Route | Onset | Peak | Duration |
|---|---|---|---|
| I.V. | Immediate | Unknown | 15-20 min |
| I.M. | 10-15 min | Unknown | ½-2 hr |
| S.C. | 10-15 min | Unknown | 50-60 min |
| Ophthalmic | Rapid | 10-90 min | 3-7 hr |
| Nasal | Rapid | Unknown | ½-4 hr |

## Contraindications and precautions
All forms are contraindicated in patients hypersensitive to drug. Injected form is also contraindicated in those with severe hypertension or ventricular tachycardia. Ophthalmic form is also contraindicated in patients with angle-closure glaucoma and in those who wear soft contact lenses.

Use all forms cautiously in geriatric patients and in patients with hyperthyroidism or cardiac disease. Use nasal and ophthalmic forms cautiously in patients with type I diabetes mellitus, hypertension, or advanced arteriosclerotic changes and in children who have low body weight. Use injectable form cautiously in patients with severe atherosclerosis, bradycardia, partial heart block, myocardial disease, or allergy to sulfites.

## Interactions
**Drug-drug.** *Alpha adrenergic blockers, antihypertensives, diuretics used as antihypertensives, guanadrel or guanethidine, nitrates, rau-*

*wolfia alkaloids:* Decreased pressor response (hypotension). Advise clinician to monitor blood pressure closely.
*Cardiac glycosides; epinephrine or other sympathomimetics; general anesthetics, such as cycloproprane and halothane, guanadrel or guanethidine, levodopa, MAO inhibitors, tricyclic antidepressants:* Phenylephrine may increase risk of arrhythmias, including tachycardia. Advise clinician to monitor patient closely.
*Cycloplegic antimuscarinic drugs:* Mydriatic response to phenylephrine is increased. Avoid use together.
*Doxapram, ergot alkaloids, MAO inhibitors, mazindol, methyldopa, oxytocics:* Pressor effects are potentiated when phenylephrine is used concomitantly. Advise clinician to monitor patient closely.
*Levodopa:* The mydriatic response to phenylephrine is decreased. Avoid use together.
*Nitrates:* May reduce antianginal effects. Avoid use together.
*Thyroid hormones:* May increase effects of either drug. Avoid use together.

## Adverse reactions
**CNS:** *headache;* excitability (with injected form); brow ache (with ophthalmic form); tremor, dizziness, nervousness (with nasal form).
**CV:** *bradycardia, arrhythmias,* hypertension (with injected form); *hypertension* (with 10% solution), tachycardia, palpitations, PVCs, *MI* (with ophthalmic form); *palpitations, tachycardia,* PVCs, hypertension, pallor (with nasal form).
**EENT:** transient eye burning or stinging on instillation, blurred vision, increased intraocular pressure, keratitis, lacrimation, reactive hyperemia of eye, allergic conjunctivitis, rebound miosis (with ophthalmic form); transient burning or stinging, dryness of nasal mucosa, rebound nasal congestion with continued use (with nasal form).
**GI:** nausea (with nasal form).
**Skin:** pallor, dermatitis (with ophthalmic form); tissue sloughing with extravasation (with injected form); diaphoresis (with ophthalmic form).
**Other:** tachyphylaxis (may occur with continued use), *anaphylaxis, asthmatic episodes,* decreased organ perfusion (with prolonged use); trembling (with ophthalmic form).

## Overdose and treatment
Signs and symptoms of overdose include exaggeration of common adverse reactions, palpitations, paresthesia, vomiting, arrhythmias, and hypertension.

To treat, advise clinician to stop drug and provide symptomatic and supportive measures. Advise clinician to monitor vital signs closely. Recommend using atropine sulfate to block reflex bradycardia; phentolamine to treat excessive hypertension; and propranolol to treat cardiac arrhythmias, or levodopa to reduce an excessive mydriatic effect of an ophthalmic preparation p.r.n.

## Clinical considerations
■ Hypovolemic states should be corrected before administration of drug; phenylephrine shouldn't be used in place of fluid, blood, plasma, and electrolyte replacement.
■ Drug may cause false-normal tonometry readings.

**Ophthalmic**
■ Recommend applying digital pressure to lacrimal sac during and for 1 to 2 minutes after instillation to prevent systemic absorption.
■ Prolonged exposure to air or strong light may cause oxidation and discoloration. Don't use if solution is brown or contains precipitate.
■ To prevent contamination, don't touch applicator tip to any surface. Instruct patient in proper technique.

**Nasal**
■ After use, rinse tip of spray bottle or dropper with hot water and dry with clean tissue. Wipe tip of nasal jelly container with clean, damp tissues.

## Therapeutic monitoring
■ Prolonged or chronic use may result in rebound congestion and chronic swelling of nasal mucosa.
■ To reduce risk of rebound congestion, recommend using weakest effective dose.

## Special populations
**Breast-feeding patients.** It isn't known if drug appears in breast milk; use with caution in breast-feeding women.
**Pediatric patients.** Infants and children may be more susceptible than adults to effects of drug. Because of the risk of precipitating severe hypertension, only ophthalmic solutions containing 0.5% or less should be used in infants under age 1. The 10% ophthalmic solution is contraindicated in infants. Most manufacturers recommend that the 0.5% nasal solution not be used in children under age 12 except under medical supervision, and the 0.25% nasal solution shouldn't be used in children under age 6 except under medical supervision.
**Geriatric patients.** Effects may be exaggerated in geriatric patients. In patients over age 50, phenylephrine (ophthalmic solution) appears to alter the response of the dilator muscle of the pupil; rebound miosis may occur the day after drug is given.

## Patient counseling
■ Tell patient to store away from heat, light, and humidity (not in bathroom medicine cabinet) and out of children's reach.

■ Warn patient to use only as directed. If using OTC product, patient should follow directions on label and not use more often or in larger doses than prescribed or recommended.
■ Caution patient not to exceed recommended dosage regardless of formulation; patient shouldn't double, decrease, or omit doses, or change dosage intervals, unless so instructed.
■ Tell patient to contact prescriber if drug provides no relief in 2 days after using phenylephrine ophthalmic solution or 3 days after using the nasal solution.
■ Explain that systemic absorption from nasal and conjunctival membranes may occur. Patient should report systemic reactions, such as dizziness and chest pain, and discontinue drug.

**Ophthalmic**
■ Instruct patient not to use if solution is brown or contains a precipitate.
■ Tell patient to wash hands before applying and to use finger to apply pressure to lacrimal sac during and for 1 to 2 minutes after instillation to decrease systemic absorption.
■ Inform patient that after applying drops, pupils will become unusually large. Advise patient to use sunglasses to protect eyes from sunlight and other bright lights, and to report if effects persist 12 hours or longer.

**Nasal**
■ After use, tell patient to rinse tip of spray bottle or dropper with hot water and dry with clean tissue or wipe tip of nasal jelly container with clean, damp tissues.
■ Instruct patient to blow nose gently (with both nostrils open) to clear nasal passages well, before using drug.
■ Teach patient correct method of instillation:
– Drops: Tilt head back while sitting or standing up, or lie on bed and hang head over side. Stay in position a few minutes to permit drug to spread through nose.
– Spray: With head upright, squeeze bottle quickly and firmly to produce 1 or 2 sprays into each nostril; wait 3 to 5 minutes, blow nose and repeat dose.
– Jelly: Place in each nostril and sniff it well back into nose.
■ Tell patient that increased fluid intake helps keep secretions liquid.
■ Warn patient to avoid using nonprescription drugs with phenylephrine to prevent possible hazardous interactions.

# phenytoin, phenytoin sodium, phenytoin sodium (extended)
Dilantin, Dilantin Infatab, Dilantin Kapseals, Dilantin-125

# phenytoin sodium (prompt)

*Pharmacologic classification:* hydantoin derivative
*Therapeutic classification:* anticonvulsant
*Pregnancy risk category D*

## Available forms
Available by prescription only
**phenytoin**
*Tablets (chewable):* 50 mg
*Oral suspension:* 30 mg/5 ml,* 125 mg/5 ml
**phenytoin sodium**
*Injection:* 50 mg/ml
**phenytoin sodium (extended)**
*Capsules:* 30 mg, 100 mg
**phenytoin sodium (prompt)**
*Capsules:* 100 mg

## Indications and dosages
***Generalized tonic-clonic seizures, status epilepticus, nonepileptic seizures (post-head trauma, Reye's syndrome)***
*Adults:* Loading dose is 10 to 15 mg/kg I.V. slowly, not to exceed 50 mg/minute; oral loading dose consists of 1 g divided into three doses (400 mg, 300 mg, 300 mg) given at 2-hour intervals. Maintenance dosage once controlled is 300 mg P.O. daily (extended only); initially use a dose divided t.i.d. (extended or prompt).
*Children:* Loading dose is 15 to 20 mg/kg I.V. at 50 mg/minute, or P.O. divided q 8 to 12 hours; then start maintenance dosage of 4 to 8 mg/kg P.O. or I.V. daily, divided q 12 hours.
***Neuritic pain (migraine, trigeminal neuralgia, and Bell's palsy)***
*Adults:* 200 to 600 mg P.O. daily in divided doses.
***Skeletal muscle relaxant***
*Adults:* 200 to 600 mg P.O. daily, p.r.n.
***◇ Ventricular arrhythmias unresponsive to lidocaine or procainamide, and arrhythmias induced by cardiac glycosides***
*Adults:* 50 to 100 mg I.V. q 10 to 15 minutes, p.r.n., not to exceed 15 mg/kg. Infusion rate should never exceed 50 mg/minute (slow I.V. push).
*Alternate method:* 100 mg I.V. q 15 minutes until adverse effects develop, arrhythmias are controlled, or 1 g has been given. Also may administer entire loading dose of 1 g I.V. slowly at 25 mg/minute. Can be diluted in normal saline solution. I.M. dosage isn't recommended because of pain and erratic absorption.

***Prophylactic control of seizures during neurosurgery***
*Adults:* 100 to 200 mg I.V. at intervals of about 4 hours during perioperative and postoperative periods.

## I.V. administration
■ If using I.V. bolus, recommend using slow (50 mg/minute) I.V. push or constant infusion; too-rapid I.V. injection may cause hypotension and circulatory collapse. Don't use I.V. push in veins on back of hand; larger veins are needed to prevent discoloration from purple glove syndrome.
■ Mix I.V. doses in normal saline solution and use within 30 minutes; mixtures with D₅W will precipitate. Don't refrigerate solution; don't mix with other drugs. In-line filter is recommended.
■ Abrupt withdrawal may precipitate status epilepticus.

### Incompatibilities
Incompatible with amikacin, aminophylline, bretylium, cephapirin, clindamycin, codeine phosphate, $D_5W$, dobutamine, fat emulsions, levorphanol, lidocaine, lincomycin, meperidine, metaraminol, methadone, morphine sulfate, nitroglycerin, norepinephrine, pentobarbital sodium, procaine regular insulin, secobarbital, and streptomycin.

## Mechanism of action
*Anticonvulsant action:* Like other hydantoin derivatives, phenytoin stabilizes neuronal membranes and limits seizure activity by either increasing efflux or decreasing influx of sodium ions across cell membranes in the motor cortex during generation of nerve impulses. Phenytoin exerts its antiarrhythmic effects by normalizing sodium influx to Purkinje's fibers in patients with cardiac glycoside-induced arrhythmias. It's indicated for generalized tonic-clonic (grand mal) and partial seizures.
*Other actions:* Phenytoin inhibits excessive collagenase activity in patients with epidermolysis bullosa.

## Pharmacokinetics
*Absorption:* Absorbed slowly from the small intestine; absorption is formulation-dependent, and bioavailability may differ among products. Extended-release capsules give peak serum levels at 4 to 12 hours; prompt-release products peak at 1½ to 3 hours. I.M. doses are absorbed erratically; about 50% to 75% of I.M. dose is absorbed in 24 hours.
*Distribution:* Distributed widely throughout the body; therapeutic plasma levels are 10 to 20 mcg/ml, although in some patients, they occur at 5 to 10 mcg/ml. Lateral nystagmus may occur at levels above 20 mcg/ml; ataxia usually occurs at levels above 30 mcg/ml; significantly decreased mental capacity occurs at

---

* Canada only    ◇ Unlabeled clinical use

40 mcg/ml. Phenytoin is about 90% protein-bound, less so in uremic patients.

*Metabolism:* Metabolized by the liver to inactive metabolites.

*Excretion:* Excreted in urine and exhibits dose-dependent (zero-order) elimination kinetics; above a certain dosage level, small increases in dosage disproportionately increase serum levels.

| Route | Onset | Peak | Duration |
|-------|-------|------|----------|
| P.O. | Unknown | 1½-12 hr | Unknown |
| I.V. | Immediate | 1-2 hr | Unknown |
| I.M. | Unknown | Unknown | Unknown |

## Contraindications and precautions

Contraindicated in patients hypersensitive to hydantoin, and those with sinus bradycardia, SA block, second- or third-degree AV block, or Adams-Stokes syndrome.

Use cautiously in geriatric or debilitated patients; in those with hepatic dysfunction, hypotension, myocardial insufficiency, diabetes, or respiratory depression; and in those receiving hydantoin derivatives.

## Interactions

**Drug-drug.** *Allopurinol, amiodarone, benzodiazepines, chloramphenicol, chlorpheniramine, cimetidine, diazepam, disulfiram, fluconazole, ibuprofen, imipramine, isoniazid, metronidazole, miconazole, omeprazole, phenacemide, phenylbutazone, salicylates, succinimides, trimethoprim, or valproic acid:* Therapeutic effects of phenytoin may be increased. Advise clinician to monitor patient carefully.

*Antacids, antineoplastics, barbiturates, calcium, calcium gluconate, carbamazepine, charcoal, diazoxide, folic acid, loxapine, nitrofurantoin, pyridoxine, rifampin, sucralfate, or theophylline:* Therapeutic effects of phenytoin may be decreased. Advise clinician to monitor levels.

*Antipsychotic drugs:* May attenuate therapeutic effects of phenytoin. Advise clinician to monitor patient closely.

*APAP, amiodarone, carbamazepine, corticosteroids, cyclosporine, dicumarol, digitoxin, disopyramide, dopamine, doxycycline, estrogens, furosemide, haloperidol, levodopa, mebendazole, meperidine, methadone, metyrapone, oral contraceptives, phenothiazines, quinidine, or sulfonylureas:* Phenytoin may decrease the effects of these drugs by stimulating hepatic metabolism. Advise clinician to monitor patient.

**Drug-food.** *Enteral tube feedings:* May interfere with absorption of oral phenytoin. Enteral feedings should be stopped for 2 hours before and 2 hours after phenytoin administration.

**Drug-lifestyle.** *Alcohol use:* Therapeutic effects of phenytoin may be decreased. Don't use together.

## Adverse reactions

**CNS:** *ataxia, slurred speech,* dizziness, insomnia, nervousness, twitching, headache, *mental confusion, decreased coordination.*

**CV:** periarteritis nodosa, hypotension.

**EENT:** *nystagmus, diplopia,* blurred vision, *gingival hyperplasia* (especially in children).

**GI:** *nausea, vomiting,* constipation.

**Hematologic:** ***thrombocytopenia, leukopenia, agranulocytosis, pancytopenia,*** macrocythemia, megaloblastic anemia.

**Hepatic:** *toxic hepatitis.*

**Metabolic:** hyperglycemia.

**Skin:** scarlatiniform or morbilliform rash; bullous, *exfoliative,* or purpuric dermatitis; ***Stevens-Johnson syndrome;*** lupus erythematosus; *hirsutism; **toxic epidermal necrolysis;*** photosensitivity; pain, necrosis, and inflammation at injection site; discoloration of skin ("purple glove syndrome") if given by I.V. push in back of hand.

**Other:** lymphadenopathy, osteomalacia, hypertrichosis.

## Overdose and treatment

Early signs and symptoms of overdose may include drowsiness, nausea, vomiting, nystagmus, ataxia, dysarthria, tremor, and slurred speech; hypotension, arrhythmias, respiratory depression, and coma may follow. Death is caused by respiratory and circulatory depression. Estimated lethal dose in adults is 2 to 5 g.

Recommend treating overdose with gastric lavage or emesis and following with supportive treatment. Recommend carefully monitoring vital signs and fluid and electrolyte balance. Forced diuresis is of little or no value. Hemodialysis or peritoneal dialysis may be helpful.

## Clinical considerations

- Only extended-release capsules are approved for once-daily dosing; all other forms are given in divided doses every 8 to 12 hours.
- If suspension is used, shake well.
- Avoid I.M. administration; it's painful and drug absorption is erratic.
- Phenytoin may raise blood glucose levels by inhibiting pancreatic insulin release; it may decrease serum levels of protein-bound iodine and may interfere with the 1-mg dexamethasone suppression test.

### *Therapeutic monitoring*

- Monitoring of serum levels is essential because of dose-dependent excretion.
- When giving I.V., continuous monitoring of ECG, blood pressure, and respiratory status is essential.

---

### Special populations
**Breast-feeding patients.** Drug appears in breast milk; an alternative feeding method is recommended during therapy.
**Pediatric patients.** Special pediatric-strength suspension (30 mg/5 ml) is available in Canada only. Take extreme care to use correct strength. Don't confuse with adult strength (125 mg/5 ml).
**Geriatric patients.** Geriatric patients metabolize and excrete phenytoin slowly; therefore, they may require lower doses.

### Patient counseling
■ Tell patient to use same brand of phenytoin consistently. Changing brands may change therapeutic effect.
■ Instruct patient to take drug with food or milk to minimize GI distress.
■ Warn patient not to discontinue drug, except with medical supervision; to avoid hazardous activities that require alertness until CNS effect is determined; and to avoid alcohol.
■ Encourage patient to wear a medical identification bracelet or necklace.
■ Stress good oral hygiene to minimize overgrowth and sensitivity of gums.

# physostigmine salicylate
Antilirium

# physostigmine sulfate
Eserine, Isopto Eserine

*Pharmacologic classification:*
cholinesterase inhibitor
*Therapeutic classification:* antimuscarinic antidote, antiglaucoma
*Pregnancy risk category C*

### Available forms
Available by prescription only
*Injection:* 1 mg/ml
*Ophthalmic ointment:* 0.25%

### Indications and dosages
*Anticholinergic toxicity from drugs and plants*
*Adults:* 0.5 to 2 mg I.M. or I.V. given slowly (not to exceed 1 mg/minute I.V.). Dosage individualized and repeated, p.r.n., q 20 minutes until response or adverse effects occur.
*Children:* Reserve for life-threatening situations only. Initial pediatric I.V. or I.M. dose of physostigmine salicylate is 0.02 mg/kg. Dosage may be repeated at 5- to 10-minute intervals to maximum of 2 mg if no adverse cholinergic signs are present.
*Postanesthesia care*
*Adults:* 0.5 to 1 mg I.M. or I.V. given slowly (not to exceed 1 mg/minute I.V.). Dosage individualized and repeated, p.r.n., q 10 to 30 minutes.
*Open-angle glaucoma*
*Adults:* Instill 2 drops into eye up to q.i.d., or apply ointment to lower fornix up to t.i.d.

### I.V. administration
■ Give I.V. at controlled rate; use direct injection at no more than 1 mg/minute in adults or 0.5 mg/minute in children.
■ Monitor vital signs frequently, especially respirations. Position patient to ease breathing. Keep atropine injection available, and be prepared to give 0.5 mg S.C. or by slow I.V. push, as ordered. Provide respiratory support p.r.n.
■ Observe solution for discoloration. Don't use if darkened.

### Incompatibilities
None reported.

### Mechanism of action
*Antimuscarinic action:* Physostigmine competitively blocks acetylcholine hydrolysis by cholinesterase, resulting in acetylcholine accumulation at cholinergic synapses; that antagonizes the muscarinic effects of overdose with antidepressants and anticholinergics. With ophthalmic use, miosis and ciliary muscle contraction increase aqueous humor outflow and decrease intraocular pressure.

### Pharmacokinetics
*Absorption:* Well absorbed from the GI tract, mucous membranes, and S.C. tissues when given I.M. or I.V., with effects peaking within 5 minutes. After ophthalmic use, drug may be absorbed orally after passage through the nasolacrimal duct.
*Distribution:* Distributed widely and crosses the blood-brain barrier.
*Metabolism:* Cholinesterase hydrolyzes physostigmine relatively quickly. Duration of effect is 1 to 2 hours after I.V. administration, 12 to 48 hours after ophthalmic use.
*Excretion:* Only a small amount of drug is excreted in urine. Exact mode of excretion is unknown.

| Route | Onset | Peak | Duration |
|---|---|---|---|
| Ophthalmic | 10-30 min | Unknown | 12-48 hr |

### Contraindications and precautions
Injected form contraindicated in patients with mechanical obstruction of the intestine or urogenital tract, asthma, gangrene, diabetes, CV disease, or vagotonia and in those receiving choline esters or depolarizing neuromuscular blockers.
   Ophthalmic form is contraindicated in patients with intolerance to physostigmine, active uveitis, or corneal injury. Use injectable form cautiously during pregnancy.

## Interactions
**Drug-drug.** *Succinylcholine:* May prolong respiratory depression. Advise clinician to monitor patient closely.
*Systemic cholinergics:* May cause additive toxicity. Advise clinician to monitor patient closely.
**Drug-herb.** *Jaborandi tree and pill-bearing spurge:* May have additive effect when used together. Use with caution to avoid risk of toxicity.

## Adverse reactions
**CNS:** weakness; headache (with ophthalmic form); *seizures, restlessness, excitability* (with injected form).
**CV:** slow or irregular heartbeat (with ophthalmic form); *bradycardia,* hypotension (with injected form).
**EENT:** blurred vision, eye pain, burning, redness, stinging, eye irritation, twitching of eyelids, watering of eyes (with ophthalmic form); miosis (with injected form).
**GI:** nausea, vomiting, diarrhea; epigastric pain, *excessive salivation* (with injected form).
**GU:** loss of bladder control (with ophthalmic form); urinary urgency (with injected form).
**Respiratory:** *bronchospasm,* bronchial constriction, dyspnea (with injected form).
**Skin:** diaphoresis.

## Overdose and treatment
Signs and symptoms of overdose include headache, nausea, vomiting, diarrhea, blurred vision, miosis, myopia, excessive tearing, bronchospasm, increased bronchial secretions, hypotension, incoordination, excessive sweating, muscle weakness, bradycardia, excessive salivation, restlessness or agitation, and confusion.

Recommend supporting respiration; bronchial suctioning may be performed. Drug should be stopped immediately. Atropine may be given to block muscarinic effects of physostigmine. Avoid atropine overdose because it may cause bronchial plug formation.

## Clinical considerations
■ The commercially available formulation of physostigmine salicylate injection contains sodium bisulfite, a sulfite that can cause allergic-type reactions, including anaphylaxis and life-threatening or less severe asthmatic episodes in certain susceptible individuals.
**Ophthalmic**
■ Have patient lie down or tilt his head back to facilitate administration of eyedrops.
■ Wait at least 5 minutes before administering any other eyedrops.
■ Gently pinch patient's nasal bridge for 1 to 2 minutes after administering each dose of eyedrops to minimize systemic absorption.
■ After applying ointment, have patient close eyelids and roll eyes.

## Therapeutic monitoring
■ Advise clinician to monitor vital signs; patient should be observed for evidence of bronchoconstriction.
■ Advise clinician to monitor patient for tolerance to drug.
■ Cardiac monitoring is recommended.

## Special populations
**Breast-feeding patients.** Safety and efficacy in breast-feeding women haven't been established.
**Geriatric patients.** Use caution when giving to geriatric patients because they may be more sensitive to effects of drug.

## Patient counseling
**Ophthalmic**
■ Teach patient how to administer ophthalmic ointment or solution.
■ Instruct patient not to close his eyes tightly or blink unnecessarily after instilling the ophthalmic solution.
■ Warn patient that he may experience blurred vision and difficulty seeing after initial doses.
■ Instruct patient to report abdominal cramps, diarrhea, or excessive salivation.

# pilocarpine hydrochloride
Adsorbocarpine, Akarpine, Isopto Carpine, Minims Pilocarpine*, Miocarpine*, Ocusert Pilo, Pilocar, Pilopine HS

# pilocarpine nitrate
P.V. Carpine Liquifilm

*Pharmacologic classification:* cholinergic agonist
*Therapeutic classification:* miotic
*Pregnancy risk category C*

## Available forms
Available by prescription only
**pilocarpine hydrochloride**
*Ophthalmic solution:* 0.25%, 0.5%, 1%, 2%, 3%, 4%, 5%, 6%, 8%, 10%
*Gel:* 4%
*Releasing-system insert:* 20 mcg/hour, 40 mcg/hour
**pilocarpine nitrate**
*Solution:* 1%, 2%, 4%

## Indications and dosages
*Chronic open-angle glaucoma; before, or instead of, emergency surgery in acute narrow-angle glaucoma*
*Adults and children:* Instill 1 or 2 drops of a 1% to 4% solution in the lower conjunctival sac q 4 to 12 hours (dosage should be based on periodic tonometric readings) or apply ½ inch ribbon of 4% gel (Pilopine HS) h.s.

Alternatively, apply one Ocusert Pilo System (20 or 40 mcg/hour) q 7 days.
**Emergency treatment of acute narrow-angle glaucoma**
*Adults and children:* 1 drop of 2% solution q 5 minutes for three to six doses, followed by 1 drop q 1 to 3 hours until pressure is controlled.
*To counteract mydriatic effects of sympathomimetics*
*Adults:* 1 drop of 1% solution in affected eye.

## Mechanism of action
*Miotic action:* Pilocarpine stimulates cholinergic receptors of the sphincter muscles of the iris, resulting in miosis. It also produces ciliary muscle contraction, resulting in accommodation with deepening of the anterior chamber, and vasodilation of conjunctival vessels of the outflow tract.

## Pharmacokinetics
*Absorption:* With the Ocusert Pilo System, 0.3 to 7 mg of pilocarpine are released during the initial 6-hour period; during the remainder of the 1-week insertion period, the release rate is within ± 20% of the rated value.
*Distribution:* Unknown.
*Metabolism:* Unknown.
*Excretion:* Duration of effect of pilocarpine drops is 4 to 6 hours.

| Route | Onset | Peak | Duration |
|-------|-------|------|----------|
| Ophthalmic | 10-30 min | 30-85 min | 4-8 hr |

## Contraindications and precautions
Contraindicated in patients hypersensitive to drug or when cholinergic effects such as constriction are undesirable (such as acute iritis, some forms of secondary glaucoma, pupillary block glaucoma, acute inflammatory disease of the anterior chamber).

Use cautiously in patients with acute cardiac failure, bronchial asthma, peptic ulcer, hyperthyroidism, GI spasm, urinary obstruction, and Parkinson's disease.

## Interactions
**Drug-drug.** *Demecarium, echothiophate, isoflurophate:* Decrease the pharmacologic effects of pilocarpine. Avoid use together.
*Epinephrine derivatives and timolol:* Pilocarpine can enhance reductions in intraocular pressure. Advise clinician to monitor patient closely.

## Adverse reactions
**CV:** hypertension, tachycardia.
**EENT:** periorbital or supraorbital headache, *myopia,* ciliary spasm, *blurred vision,* conjunctival irritation, transient stinging and burning, keratitis, lens opacity, retinal detachment, lacrimation, changes in visual field, *brow pain.*
**GI:** nausea, vomiting, diarrhea, salivation.

**Respiratory:** *bronchoconstriction, pulmonary edema.*
**Skin:** diaphoresis.
**Other:** hypersensitivity reactions.

## Overdose and treatment
Signs and symptoms of overdose include flushing, vomiting, bradycardia, bronchospasm, increased bronchial secretion, sweating, tearing, involuntary urination, hypotension, and tremors. Vomiting is usually spontaneous with accidental ingestion; if not, emesis should be induced and followed with activated charcoal or a cathartic.

Recommend treating dermal exposure by washing the areas twice with water. Epinephrine should be used to treat the CV responses. Atropine sulfate is the antidote of choice. The eye should be flushed with water or sodium chloride to treat a local overdose. Doses up to 20 mg are generally considered nontoxic.

## Clinical considerations
- Drug may be used alone or with mannitol, urea, glycerol, or acetazolamide. It also may be used to counteract effects of mydriatic and cycloplegic drugs after surgery or ophthalmoscopic examination and may be used alternately with atropine to break adhesions.

### Therapeutic monitoring
- Patients with dark eyes may require stronger solutions or more frequent installation because eye pigment may absorb drug.

## Patient counseling
- Warn patient that vision will be temporarily blurred, that miotic pupil may make surroundings appear dim and reduce peripheral field of vision, and that transient brow ache and myopia are common at first; assure patient that adverse effects subside 10 to 14 days after therapy begins.
- Instruct patient to check for the presence of the pilocarpine ocular system at bedtime and upon rising.
- Tell patient that if systems in both eyes are lost, they should be replaced as soon as possible. If one system is lost, it may either be replaced with a fresh system or the system remaining in the other eye may be removed and both replaced with fresh systems so that both systems will subsequently be replaced on the same schedule.
- Instruct patient that if the Ocusert System falls out of the eye during sleep, he should wash hands, then rinse Ocusert in cool tap water and reposition it in the eye. Don't use the insert if it's deformed.
- Inform patient that systems should be replaced every 7 days.
- Tell patient to use caution in night driving and other activities in poor illumination be-

---

* Canada only    ◇ Unlabeled clinical use

cause miotic pupil diminishes side vision and illumination.

■ Teach patient the correct way to instill drops and to apply light finger pressure on lacrimal sac for 1 minute after administration to minimize systemic absorption.

■ Instruct patient to apply gel at bedtime because it will cause blurred vision.

# pilocarpine hydrochloride
Salagen

*Pharmacologic classification:* cholinergic agonist
*Therapeutic classification:* antixerostomia drug
*Pregnancy risk category C*

## Available forms
Available by prescription only
*Tablets:* 5 mg

## Indications and dosages
***Treatment of symptoms of xerostomia from salivary gland hypofunction caused by radiotherapy for cancer of the head and neck***
*Adults:* 5 mg P.O. t.i.d. Dosage may be increased to 10 mg P.O. t.i.d., p.r.n.

## Mechanism of action
*Antixerostomia action:* Oral pilocarpine increases secretion of the salivary glands, which eliminates dryness.

## Pharmacokinetics
*Absorption:* Pilocarpine is absorbed in the GI tract. A high-fat meal may decrease rate of absorption.
*Distribution:* Unknown.
*Metabolism:* Inactivation of pilocarpine is believed to occur at neuronal synapses and probably in plasma.
*Excretion:* Drug and its minimally active or inactive degradation products are excreted in urine.

| Route | Onset | Peak | Duration |
|-------|-------|------|----------|
| P.O. | 20 min | 1 hr | 3-5 hr |

## Contraindications and precautions
Contraindicated in patients with uncontrolled asthma, those hypersensitive to pilocarpine, and when miosis is undesirable, such as in acute iritis and narrow-angle glaucoma.

Use cautiously in patients with CV disease, controlled asthma, chronic bronchitis, COPD, cholelithiasis, biliary tract disease, nephrolithiasis, and cognitive or psychiatric disturbances.

## Interactions
**Drug-drug.** *Beta blockers:* May increase risk of conduction disturbances. Use together cautiously.
*Drugs with anticholinergic effects:* May antagonize anticholinergic effects of oral pilocarpine. Use together cautiously.
*Drugs with parasympathomimetic effects:* May result in additive pharmacologic effects. Advise clinician to monitor patient closely.

## Adverse reactions
**CNS:** *dizziness, headache,* tremor.
**CV:** hypertension, tachycardia, edema.
**EENT:** *rhinitis,* lacrimation, amblyopia, pharyngitis, voice alteration, conjunctivitis, epistaxis, sinusitis, abnormal vision.
**GI:** *nausea,* dyspepsia, diarrhea, abdominal pain, vomiting, dysphagia, taste perversion.
**GU:** *urinary frequency.*
**Musculoskeletal:** *asthenia,* myalgia.
**Skin:** *flushing,* rash, pruritis, *sweating.*
**Other:** *chills.*

## Overdose and treatment
Taking 100 mg of oral pilocarpine is considered potentially fatal. Treatment is with atropine titration (0.5 mg to 1 mg S.C. or I.V.) and supportive measures to maintain respiration and circulation. Epinephrine (0.3 mg to 1 mg S.C. or I.M.) may also be useful during severe CV depression or bronchoconstriction. It isn't known if pilocarpine is dialyzable.

## Clinical considerations
■ Patient should undergo careful examination of the fundus before therapy starts because retinal detachment has been reported with pilocarpine use in patients with preexisting retinal disease.

### Therapeutic monitoring
■ Advise clinician to monitor patient for signs and symptoms of pilocarpine toxicity characterized by an exaggeration of its parasympathomimetic effects; these include headache, visual disturbance, lacrimation, sweating, respiratory distress, GI spasm, nausea, vomiting, diarrhea, AV block, tachycardia, bradycardia, hypotension, hypertension, shock, mental confusion, cardiac arrhythmia, and tremors.

### Special populations
**Breast-feeding patients.** It's unknown if drug appears in breast milk. Because of the potential for serious adverse reactions in nursing infants, a decision should be made to stop either breast-feeding or drug, taking into account the importance of drug to the woman.
**Pediatric patients.** Safety and efficacy in children haven't been established.

## Patient counseling
- Warn patient that drug may cause visual disturbances, especially at night, that could impair his ability to drive safely.
- Tell patient to drink plenty of fluids to prevent dehydration if drug causes excessive sweating. If adequate fluid intake can't be maintained, tell patient to notify prescriber.

# pimozide
Orap

*Pharmacologic classification:* diphenylbutylpiperidine
*Therapeutic classification:* antipsychotic
*Pregnancy risk category C*

## Available forms
Available by prescription only
*Tablets:* 1 mg, 2 mg

## Indications and dosages
**Suppression of severe motor and phonic tics in patients with Tourette syndrome**
*Adults:* Initially, 1 to 2 mg/day P.O. in divided doses. Then, increase dosage, p.r.n., every other day. Maximum dose 0.2 mg/kg/day or 10 mg/day.
*Children over age 12:* 0.05 mg/kg P.O. h.s.; increase at 3-day intervals to maximum of 0.2 mg/kg. Maximum dose, 10 mg/day.

## Mechanism of action
*Antipsychotic action:* Mechanism of action in Tourette syndrome is unknown; it's thought to exert its effects by postsynaptic or presynaptic blockade, or both, of CNS dopamine receptors, inhibiting dopamine-mediated effects. Pimozide also has anticholinergic, antiemetic, and anxiolytic effects and produces mild alpha blockade.

## Pharmacokinetics
*Absorption:* Absorbed slowly and incompletely from the GI tract; bioavailability is about 50%.
*Distribution:* Distributed widely into the body.
*Metabolism:* Metabolized by the liver, mainly by cytochrome P-450 3A and to a lesser extent 1A2; a significant first-pass effect exists.
*Excretion:* About 40% of a given dose is excreted in urine as parent drug and metabolites in 3 to 4 days; about 15% is excreted in feces via the biliary tract within 3 to 6 days.

| Route | Onset | Peak | Duration |
|---|---|---|---|
| P.O. | Unknown | 4-12 hr | Unknown |

## Contraindications and precautions
Contraindicated in patients hypersensitive to drug, in treating simple tics or tics other than those associated with Tourette syndrome, and in patients with concurrent drug therapy known to cause motor and phonic tics, congenital long QT syndrome or history of arrhythmias, severe toxic CNS depression, or those experiencing coma.

Use cautiously in patients with impaired renal or hepatic function, glaucoma, prostatic hyperplasia, seizure disorders, or EEG abnormalities.

## Interactions
**Drug-drug.** *Amphetamines, methylphenidate, pemoline:* May induce Tourette-like tic and may exacerbate existing tics. Avoid use together.
*Anticonvulsants, such as carbamazepine, phenobarbital, and phenytoin:* May induce seizures; an anticonvulsant dosage increase may be required.
*Antidepressants, disopyramide, other antiarrhythmics, other antipsychotics, phenothiazines, procainamide, quinidine:* May further depress cardiac conduction and prolong QT interval, resulting in serious arrhythmias. Use with caution and recommend monitoring patient closely.
*CNS depressants:* May cause additive CNS depressant effects. Avoid use together.
*Drugs that inhibit CYP-450 isoenzyme 3A (azole fungal drugs, macrolide antibiotics, protease inhibitors):* Inhibit metabolism of pimozide. Don't use together.
**Drug-food.** *Grapefruit juice:* May inhibit metabolism of pimozide. Don't use together.
**Drug-lifestyle.** *Alcohol use:* Additive CNS depressant effects. Advise patient to avoid alcohol.

## Adverse reactions
**CNS:** *parkinsonian-like symptoms,* drowsiness, headache, insomnia, **neuroleptic malignant syndrome,** extrapyramidal reactions, *tardive dyskinesia, sedation, adverse behavioral effects.*
**CV:** *ECG changes (prolonged QT interval),* hypotension, hypertension, tachycardia.
**EENT:** visual disturbances.
**GI:** *dry mouth, constipation.*
**GU:** impotence, urinary frequency.
**Musculoskeletal:** muscle rigidity.
**Skin:** rash, diaphoresis.

## Overdose and treatment
Signs of overdose include severe extrapyramidal reactions, hypotension, respiratory depression, coma, and ECG abnormalities, including prolongation of QT interval, inversion or flattening of T waves, and new appearance of U waves.

Recommend treating with gastric lavage and maintaining blood pressure with I.V. fluids, plasma expanders, or norepinephrine. Epinephrine shouldn't be used. Vomiting shouldn't be induced because of the potential for aspiration. Recommend treating extrapyramidal symptoms with parenteral diphenhydramine.

Advise clinician to monitor patient for adverse effects for at least 4 days because of prolonged half-life (55 hours) of drug.

## Clinical considerations
■ Advise clinician to obtain baseline ECG before therapy begins and then periodically to monitor CV effects.
■ Patient should be assessed periodically for abnormal body movement.
■ Extrapyramidal reactions develop in about 10% to 15% of patients at normal doses. They're especially likely to occur during early days of therapy.
■ If excessive restlessness and agitation occur, therapy with a beta blocker, such as propranolol or metoprolol, may be helpful.
■ Pimozide causes quinidine-like ECG effects, including prolongation of QT interval and flattened T waves.

### Therapeutic monitoring
■ Maintain patient's serum potassium level within normal range; decreased potassium levels increase risk of arrhythmias. Advise clinician to monitor potassium level in patients with diarrhea and those taking diuretics.

### Special populations
**Pediatric patients.** Use and efficacy in children under age 12 are limited. Dosage should be kept at the lowest possible level. Use of drug in children for any disorder other than Tourette syndrome isn't recommended.
**Geriatric patients.** Cardiac toxicity and tardive dyskinesia are more likely to develop in geriatric patients, even at normal doses.

## Patient counseling
■ Inform patient of risks, signs, and symptoms of dystonic reactions and tardive dyskinesia.
■ Advise patient to take pimozide exactly as prescribed, not to double dose for missed doses, not to share drug with others, and not to stop taking it suddenly.
■ Explain that therapeutic effect of drug may not be apparent for several weeks.
■ Urge patient to report unusual effects promptly.
■ Recommend use of sugarless hard candy or chewing gum, ice chips, or artificial saliva to relieve dry mouth.
■ To prevent dizziness at start of therapy, tell patient to lie down for 30 minutes after taking each dose and to avoid sudden changes in posture, especially when rising to upright position.
■ To minimize daytime sedation, suggest taking entire daily dose at bedtime.
■ Warn patient to avoid hazardous activities that require alertness until effects of drug are known.

# pindolol
Visken

*Pharmacologic classification:* beta blocker
*Therapeutic classification:* antihypertensive
*Pregnancy risk category B*

## Available forms
Available by prescription only
*Tablets:* 5 mg, 10 mg

## Indications and dosages
### Hypertension
*Adults:* Initially, 5 mg P.O. b.i.d. increased by 10 mg/day q 3 to 4 weeks up to maximum of 60 mg/day. Usual dosage is 10 to 30 mg daily, given in two or three divided doses. In some patients, once-daily dosing may be possible.
◇*Angina*
*Adults:* 15 to 40 mg daily P.O. in three or four divided doses.

## Mechanism of action
*Antihypertensive action:* Exact mechanism of antihypertensive action is unknown. Pindolol doesn't consistently affect cardiac output or renin release, and its other mechanisms such as decreased peripheral resistance probably contribute to its hypotensive effect. Because pindolol has some intrinsic sympathomimetic activity (beta-agonist sympathomimetic activity), it may be useful in patients in whom bradycardia develops with other beta blockers. It's a nonselective beta blocker, inhibiting both $beta_1$ and $beta_2$ receptors.

## Pharmacokinetics
*Absorption:* After oral administration, pindolol is absorbed rapidly from the GI tract. Food doesn't reduce bioavailability but may increase the rate of GI absorption.
*Distribution:* Distributed widely throughout the body and is 40% to 60% protein-bound.
*Metabolism:* About 60% to 65% of a given dose of pindolol is metabolized by the liver.
*Excretion:* In adults with normal renal function, 35% to 50% of a given dose is excreted unchanged in urine; half-life is about 3 to 4 hours.

| Route | Onset | Peak | Duration |
|-------|---------|--------|----------|
| P.O. | Unknown | 1-2 hr | 24 hr |

## Contraindications and precautions
Contraindicated in patients hypersensitive to drug, and those with bronchial asthma, severe bradycardia, heart block greater than first degree, cardiogenic shock, or overt cardiac failure. Also contraindicated in patients taking thioridazine.

---

Use cautiously in patients with HF, nonallergic bronchospastic disease, diabetes, hyperthyroidism, and impaired renal or hepatic function.

## Interactions

**Drug-drug.** *Antihypertensives:* Pindolol may potentiate the antihypertensive effects. Advise clinician to monitor patient closely.
*Thioridazine:* May prolong QTc interval and increase the risk of potentially fatal cardiac arrythmias. Also, may increase pindolol serum levels. Avoid use.

## Adverse reactions

**CNS:** *insomnia, fatigue, dizziness, nervousness,* vivid dreams, weakness, paresthesia.
**CV:** *edema,* **bradycardia, HF,** chest pain.
**GI:** *nausea,* abdominal discomfort.
**Hepatic:** elevated serum transaminase, alkaline phosphatase, lactic dehydrogenase.
**Musculoskeletal:** *muscle pain, joint pain.*
**Respiratory:** *increased airway resistance,* dyspnea.
**Skin:** rash, pruritus.
**Other:** elevated uric acid levels.

## Overdose and treatment

Signs of overdose include severe hypotension, bradycardia, HF, and bronchospasm.

After acute ingestion, advise clinician to empty stomach by induced emesis or gastric lavage; activated charcoal should be given to reduce absorption. Subsequent treatment is usually symptomatic and supportive.

## Clinical considerations

■ Maximum therapeutic response may not be seen for 2 weeks or longer.

### *Therapeutic monitoring*

■ Patient's apical pulse rate should always be checked before drug is given. Drug should be withheld and prescriber notified if pulse rate extremes are found.
■ Advise clinician to monitor blood pressure frequently.

### *Special populations*

**Breast-feeding patients.** Pindolol appears in breast milk; an alternative feeding method is recommended during therapy.
**Pediatric patients.** Safety and efficacy of pindolol in children haven't been established; use only if potential benefit outweighs risk.
**Geriatric patients.** Geriatric patients may require lower maintenance dosages of pindolol because of increased bioavailability or delayed metabolism; they also may experience enhanced adverse effects. Half-life of drug may be increased in geriatric patients.

## Patient counseling

■ Instruct patient to take drug exactly as prescribed.
■ Advise patient not to stop drug abruptly and to report adverse effects.

# pioglitazone hydrochloride
Actos

*Pharmacologic classification:* thiazolidinedione
*Therapeutic classification:* antidiabetic
*Pregnancy risk category C*

## Available forms

Available by prescription only
*Tablets:* 15 mg, 30 mg, 45 mg

## Indications and dosages

*Monotherapy adjunct to diet and exercise to improve glycemic control in patients with type 2 diabetes mellitus, or combination therapy with a sulfonylurea, metformin, or insulin when diet and exercise plus the single drug doesn't result in adequate glycemic control*
*Adults:* Initially, 15 or 30 mg P.O. once daily. For patients who respond inadequately to the initial dose, dosage may be increased in increments; maximum dose is 45 mg/day. If used in combination therapy, maximum dose shouldn't exceed 30 mg/day.

## Mechanism of action

*Antidiabetic action:* Pioglitazone lowers blood glucose levels by decreasing insulin resistance in the periphery and in the liver, resulting in increased insulin-dependent glucose disposal and decreased glucose output by the liver. Pioglitazone is a potent and highly selective agonist for receptors found in insulin-sensitive tissues, such as adipose tissue, skeletal muscle, and liver. Activation of these receptors modulates the transcription of a number of insulin-responsive genes involved in the control of glucose and lipid metabolism.

## Pharmacokinetics

*Absorption:* When taken on an empty stomach, pioglitazone is rapidly absorbed and is measurable in the serum within 30 minutes. Food delays the time to peak serum levels slightly (to 3 to 4 hours), but doesn't affect the overall extent of absorption.
*Distribution:* Pioglitazone and its metabolites are extensively protein-bound (more than 98%), primarily to serum albumin.
*Metabolism:* Extensively metabolized by the liver. Three metabolites, M-II, M-III, and M-IV, are pharmacologically active.
*Excretion:* About 15% to 30% of the dose is recovered in the urine, primarily as metabolites and their conjugates. The majority of an

oral dose is excreted into the bile and eliminated in the feces. The half-life of pioglitazone ranges from 3 to 7 hours.

| Route | Onset | Peak | Duration |
|-------|-------|------|----------|
| P.O. | Unknown | 2 hr | Unknown |

## Contraindications and precautions

Contraindicated in patients hypersensitive to pioglitazone or its components. Drug shouldn't be used in patients with type 1 diabetes mellitus or for the treatment of diabetic ketoacidosis, in patients with clinical evidence of active liver disease or serum ALT levels greater than 2½ times the upper limit of normal, or in those who experienced jaundice while taking troglitazone. Don't use in patients with New York Heart Association Class III or IV HF.

Use cautiously in patients with edema or HF.

## Interactions

**Drug-drug.** *Ketoconazole:* May inhibit the metabolism of pioglitazone. Advise clinician to monitor patient's blood glucose levels more frequently.

*Oral contraceptives:* May reduce plasma levels of oral contraceptives, resulting in less effective contraception. Advise patients taking pioglitazone and oral contraceptives to consider additional birth control measures.

## Adverse reactions

**CNS:** headache.
**CV:** *edema* (with insulin).
**EENT:** sinusitis, pharyngitis.
**Hematologic:** anemia.
**Metabolic:** hypoglycemia (with combination therapy), aggravated diabetes mellitus, weight gain, decreased triglycerides, increased high-density lipoprotein cholesterol.
**Musculoskeletal:** myalgia.
**Respiratory:** upper respiratory infection.
**Other:** tooth disorder.

## Overdose and treatment

In the event of overdose, recommend supportive treatment appropriate to patient's clinical signs and symptoms to reverse hypoglycemia.

## Clinical considerations

■ Because ovulation may resume in premenopausal, anovulatory women with insulin resistance, contraceptive measures may need to be considered.

■ Patients with normal liver enzyme levels who are switched from troglitazone to pioglitazone should undergo a 1-week washout period before starting pioglitazone.

■ Management of type 2 diabetes should include diet control. Because caloric restrictions, weight loss, and exercise help improve insulin sensitivity and help make drug therapy effec-

tive, these measures are essential for proper diabetes management.

### Therapeutic monitoring

■ Advise clinician to monitor patient for hypoglycemia in patients receiving pioglitazone with insulin or a sulfonylurea and adjust dosage of these drugs p.r.n.

■ Besides having blood glucose levels checked regularly, patients should also have glycosylated hemoglobin checked periodically to evaluate therapeutic response to drug.

■ Liver enzyme levels should be measured at the start of therapy, every 2 months for the first year of therapy, and periodically thereafter. Liver function tests also should be performed in patients for whom signs and symptoms of liver dysfunction, such as nausea, vomiting, abdominal pain, fatigue, anorexia, or dark urine develop. Drug should be stopped if jaundice develops or if results of liver functions tests show ALT elevations greater than three times the upper limit of normal.

■ Patients with HF should be monitored for increased edema during pioglitazone therapy.

■ Hemoglobin levels and hematocrit may decrease, usually during the first 4 to 12 weeks of therapy.

### Special populations

**Pregnant patients.** Use drug in pregnancy only if the benefit justifies the risk to the fetus. Insulin is the preferred antidiabetic for use during pregnancy.

**Breast-feeding patients.** It isn't known if drug appears in breast milk. Pioglitazone shouldn't be given to breast-feeding women.

**Pediatric patients.** Safety and efficacy of pioglitazone in children haven't been evaluated.

**Geriatric patients.** No significant differences in safety and efficacy of pioglitazone have been seen between patients ages 65 and older and younger patients.

## Patient counseling

■ Instruct patient to adhere to dietary instructions and to have blood glucose levels and glycosylated hemoglobin tested regularly.

■ Inform patient taking pioglitazone with insulin or oral antidiabetics of the signs and symptoms of hypoglycemia.

■ Advise patient to notify prescriber during periods of stress, such as during fever, trauma, infection, or surgery, because drug requirements may change.

■ Tell patient to report unexplained nausea, vomiting, abdominal pain, fatigue, anorexia, or dark urine immediately because these may indicate potential liver problems.

■ Inform patient that pioglitazone can be taken with or without meals. If a dose is missed, the dose shouldn't be doubled the next day.

■ Advise anovulatory, premenopausal women with insulin resistance that therapy with pioglitazone may cause resumption of ovulation and contraceptive measures may need to be considered.

# piperacillin sodium
Pipracil

*Pharmacologic classification:* extended-spectrum penicillin, acyl-aminopenicillin
*Therapeutic classification:* antibiotic
*Pregnancy risk category B*

## Available forms
Available by prescription only
*Infusion:* 2 g, 3 g, 4 g
*Injection:* 2 g, 3 g, 4 g
*Pharmacy bulk package:* 40 g

## Indications and dosages
*Infections caused by susceptible organisms*
*Adults and children over age 12:* Serious infection: 12 to 18 g/day I.V. in divided doses q 4 to 6 hours; uncomplicated urinary tract infection (UTI) and community-acquired pneumonia: 6 to 8 g/day I.V. in divided doses q 6 to 12 hours; complicated UTI: 8 to 16 g/day I.V. in divided doses q 6 to 8 hours; uncomplicated gonorrhea: 2 g I.M. as a single dose. Maximum daily dose, 24 g.
*Prophylaxis of surgical infections*
*Adults:* Intra-abdominal surgery: 2 g I.V. before surgery, 2 g during surgery, and 2 g q 6 hours after surgery for no longer than 24 hours; vaginal hysterectomy: 2 g I.V. before surgery, 2 g 6 hours after first dose then 2 g 12 hours after second dose; cesarean section: 2 g I.V. after cord is clamped, then 2 g q 4 hours for two doses; abdominal hysterectomy: 2 g I.V. before surgery, 2 g in postanesthesia care unit, and 2 g after 6 hours.
≡ *Dosage adjustment.* For adult patients with renal impairment, refer to the following table.

| Creatinine clearance (ml/min) | Urinary tract infection | | Serious systemic infection |
| | Uncom-plicated | Compli-cated | |
|---|---|---|---|
| 20-40 | * | 3 g q 8 hr | 4 g q 8 hr |
| < 20 | 3 g q 12 hr | 3 g q 12 hr | 4 g q 12 hr |

*No dosage adjustment needed.

## I.V. administration
■ Drug may be administered by direct I.V. injection, given slowly over at least 5 minutes; chest discomfort occurs if injection is given too rapidly.

## Incompatibilities
Incompatible with fluconazole.

## Mechanism of action
*Antibiotic action:* Piperacillin is bactericidal; it adheres to bacterial penicillin-binding proteins, inhibiting bacterial cell wall synthesis.
    Extended-spectrum penicillins are more resistant to inactivation by certain beta-lactamases, especially those produced by gram-negative organisms, but are still liable to inactivation by certain others. Because of the potential for rapid development of bacterial resistance, it shouldn't be used as a sole drug in the treatment of an infection.
    The spectrum of activity of piperacillin includes many gram-negative aerobic and anaerobic bacilli, many gram-positive and gram-negative aerobic cocci, and some gram-positive aerobic and anaerobic bacilli. Piperacillin may be effective against some strains of carbenicillin-resistant and ticarcillin-resistant gram-negative bacilli. Piperacillin is more active against *Pseudomonas aeruginosa* than are other extended-spectrum penicillins.

## Pharmacokinetics
*Absorption:* Peak plasma levels occur 30 to 50 minutes after an I.M. dose.
*Distribution:* Distributed widely after parenteral administration. It penetrates minimally into uninflamed meninges and slightly into bone and sputum. Piperacillin is 16% to 22% protein-bound; it crosses the placenta.
*Metabolism:* None significant.
*Excretion:* Excreted primarily (42% to 90%) in urine by renal tubular secretion and glomerular filtration; it's also excreted in bile and appears in breast milk. Elimination half-life in adults is about ½ to 1½ hours; in extensive renal impairment, half-life is extended to about 2 to 6 hours; in combined hepatorenal dysfunction, half-life may extend from 11 to 32 hours. Drug is removed by hemodialysis but not by peritoneal dialysis.

| Route | Onset | Peak | Duration |
|---|---|---|---|
| I.V. | Immediate | Immediate | Unknown |
| I.M. | Unknown | 30-50 min | Unknown |

## Contraindications and precautions
Contraindicated in patients hypersensitive to drug or other penicillins.
    Use cautiously in patients with other drug allergies (especially to cephalosporins), bleeding tendencies, uremia, or hypokalemia.

## Interactions
*Drug-drug. Aminoglycoside antibiotics:* Synergistic bactericidal effects against *Pseudomonas aeruginosa, Escherichia coli, Citrobacter, Enterobacter, Klebsiella, Serratia,* and *Proteus mirabilis.* The drugs are physically and chemically incompatible and are in-

activated when mixed or given together. Don't administer together.

*Clavulanic acid, sulbactam, tazobactam:* Synergistic bactericidal effect against certain beta-lactamase–producing bacteria. May be used for this advantage.

*Methotrexate:* Large doses of penicillins may interfere with renal tubular secretion, delaying elimination and elevating serum levels of methotrexate. Advise clinician to monitor patient closely.

*Oral contraceptives:* Penicillins may decrease efficacy. Recommend additional form of contraceptive while on penicillin therapy.

*Probenecid:* Blocks tubular secretion of piperacillin, raising serum levels of drug. Probenecid may be used for this purpose.

## Adverse reactions

**CNS:** *seizures,* headache, dizziness, fatigue.
**GI:** nausea, diarrhea, vomiting, pseudomembranous colitis, elevations in liver function studies.
**GU:** interstitial nephritis.
**Hematologic:** *bleeding* (with high doses), *neutropenia,* eosinophilia, *leukopenia, thrombocytopenia.*
**Metabolic:** *hypokalemia,* hypernatremia.
**Musculoskeletal:** prolonged muscle relaxation.
**Skin:** pain at injection site.
**Other:** hypersensitivity reactions (edema, fever, chills, rash, pruritus, urticaria, *anaphylaxis),* overgrowth of nonsusceptible organisms, vein irritation, phlebitis.

## Overdose and treatment

Signs of overdose include neuromuscular hypersensitivity or seizures resulting from CNS irritation by high drug levels. A 4- to 6-hour session of hemodialysis removes 10% to 50% of piperacillin.

## Clinical considerations

■ Piperacillin is almost always used with another antibiotic such as an aminoglycoside in life-threatening situations.
■ Patients with cystic fibrosis are most susceptible to fever or rash from piperacillin.
■ Because drug is dialyzable, patients undergoing hemodialysis may need dosage adjustments.
■ Reduced dosage should be used in patients with creatinine clearance less than 40 ml/minute.
■ Piperacillin may falsely decrease serum aminoglycoside levels. Piperacillin may cause positive Coombs' tests.

### Therapeutic monitoring

■ Advise clinician to monitor serum electrolyte levels, especially potassium.

■ Advise clinician to monitor neurologic status. High serum levels of this drug may cause seizures.
■ Advise clinician to monitor CBC, differential, and platelets. Drug may cause thrombocytopenia. Patient should be observed carefully for signs of occult bleeding.

### Special populations

**Breast-feeding patients.** Drug appears in breast milk; use with caution in breast-feeding women.
**Pediatric patients.** Safety of piperacillin in children under age 12 hasn't been established.
**Geriatric patients.** Half-life may be prolonged in geriatric patients because of impaired renal function.

### Patient counseling

■ Tell patient to report adverse effects or discomfort at I.V. site.
■ Instruct patient to limit salt intake while on therapy.
■ Drug may be more suitable than carbenicillin or ticarcillin for patients on salt-free diets; piperacillin contains only 1.85 mEq of sodium per gram.

# piperacillin sodium and tazobactam sodium

Zosyn

*Pharmacologic classification:* extended-spectrum penicillin/beta-lactamase inhibitor
*Therapeutic classification:* antibiotic
*Pregnancy risk category B*

## Available forms

Available by prescription only
*Powder for injection (equivalent to piperacillin/tazobactam in a ratio of 8 to 1):* 2.25 g, 3.375 g, 4.5 g

## Indications and dosages

*Treatment of moderate to severe infections caused by piperacillin-resistant, piperacillin/tazobactam-susceptible, beta-lactamase-producing strains of microorganisms in the following conditions: appendicitis (complicated by rupture or abscess) and peritonitis caused by* Escherichia coli, Bacteroides fragilis, B. ovatus, B. thetaiotaomicron, B. vulgatus; *skin and skin structure infections caused by* Staphylococcus aureus; *postpartum endometritis or pelvic inflammatory disease caused by* E. coli; *moderately severe community-acquired pneumonia caused by* Haemophilus influenzae
*Adults:* 3.375 g (3.0 g piperacillin/0.375 g tazobactam) q 6 hours as a 30-minute I.V. infusion.

---

≡ *Dosage adjustment.* For patients with renal impairment, refer to the following table.

| Creatinine clearance (ml/min) | Recommended dosage |
|---|---|
| > 40 | 12 g/1.5 g/day in divided doses of 3.375 g q 6 hr |
| 20-40 | 8 g/1 g/day in divided doses of 2.25 g q 6 hr |
| < 20 | 6 g/0.75 g/day in divided doses of 2.25 g q 8 hr |

## I.V. administration

■ Reconstitute piperacillin/tazobactam with 5 ml of diluent per 1 g of piperacillin. Appropriate diluents include sterile or bacteriostatic water for injection, normal saline injection, bacteriostatic normal saline injection, $D_5W$, dextrose 5% in normal saline solution injection, or dextran 6% in normal saline injection. Don't use lactated Ringer's injection. Shake until dissolved. Further dilution can be made to a final desired volume.
■ Infuse over at least 30 minutes. Primary infusion should be stopped during administration if possible. Don't mix with other drugs.
■ Use single-dose vials immediately after reconstitution. Discard unused drug after 24 hours if held at room temperature; 48 hours if refrigerated. Once diluted, drug is stable in I.V. bags for 24 hours at room temperature or 1 week if refrigerated.

### Incompatibilities
Don't reconstitute with lactated Ringer's because drug degrades over 8 hours, decreasing its potency. Incompatible with acyclovir sodium, amphotericin B, chlorpromazine, dacarbazine, daunorubicin, dobutamine, doxorubicin, doxycycline hyclate, droperidol, famotidine, ganciclovir, haloperidol lactate, hydroxyzine hydrochloride, idarubicin, miconazole, minocycline, mitomycin, mitoxantrone, nalbuphine, prochlorperazine edisylate, promethazine hydrochloride, streptozocin, and vancomycin.

## Mechanism of action
*Antibiotic action:* Piperacillin is an extended-spectrum penicillin that inhibits cell wall synthesis during microorganism multiplication; tazobactam increases piperacillin effectiveness by inactivating beta-lactamases, which destroy penicillins.

## Pharmacokinetics
*Absorption:* Unknown.
*Distribution:* Both piperacillin and tazobactam are about 30% plasma protein–bound.

*Metabolism:* Piperacillin is metabolized to a minor microbiologically active desethyl metabolite. Tazobactam is metabolized to a single metabolite that lacks pharmacologic and antibacterial activities.
*Excretion:* Both piperacillin and tazobactam are eliminated via the kidneys by glomerular filtration and tubular secretion. Piperacillin is excreted rapidly as unchanged drug (68% of dose) and tazobactam is excreted as unchanged drug (80%) in the urine. Piperacillin, tazobactam, and desethyl piperacillin also are secreted into the bile.

| Route | Onset | Peak | Duration |
|---|---|---|---|
| I.V. | Immediate | Immediate | Unknown |

## Contraindications and precautions
Contraindicated in patients hypersensitive to drug or other penicillins.
Use cautiously in patients with drug allergies (especially to cephalosporins), bleeding tendencies, uremia, or hypokalemia.

## Interactions
**Drug-drug.** *Aminoglycosides:* May result in substantial inactivation of the aminoglycoside. Don't mix in the same I.V. container.
*Heparin, oral anticoagulants, and other drugs that may affect the blood coagulation system or the thrombocyte function:* Prolonged effectiveness. Advise clinician to monitor PT and INR closely.
*Probenecid:* Increases blood levels of piperacillin/tazobactam. Probenecid may be used for this reason.
*Vecuronium:* Prolonged neuromuscular blockade of vecuronium. Advise clinician to monitor patient closely.

## Adverse reactions
**CNS:** *headache, insomnia,* agitation, dizziness, anxiety.
**CV:** hypertension, tachycardia, chest pain, edema.
**EENT:** rhinitis.
**GI:** *diarrhea, nausea, constipation,* vomiting, dyspepsia, stool changes, abdominal pain.
**GU:** interstitial nephritis, candidiasis.
**Hematologic:** *leukopenia,* anemia, eosinophilia, *thrombocytopenia.*
**Respiratory:** dyspnea.
**Skin:** rash (including maculopapular, bullous, urticarial, and eczematoid), pruritus, inflammation.
**Other:** fever; pain; phlebitis at I.V. site; *anaphylaxis.*

## Overdose and treatment
No information available.

---

## Clinical considerations

■ Specimen for culture and sensitivity tests should be obtained before giving first dose. Therapy may begin pending results.

■ Pseudomembranous colitis has been reported with nearly all antibacterial drugs, including piperacillin/tazobactam, and may range in severity from mild to life-threatening. Therefore, consider this diagnosis in patients presenting with diarrhea after piperacillin/tazobactam administration.

■ Bacterial and fungal superinfection may occur and warrants appropriate measures.

■ Recommend using piperacillin/tazobactam with an aminoglycoside to treat infections caused by *Pseudomonas aeruginosa*.

■ Piperacillin/tazobactam contains 2.35 mEq (54 mg) of sodium per gram of piperacillin in the combination product. This should be considered in patients who require restricted sodium intake.

■ As with other penicillins, piperacillin/tazobactam may result in a false-positive reaction for urine glucose using a copper-reduction method such as Clinitest. Glucose tests based on enzymatic glucose oxidase reactions (such as Diastix or glucose enzymatic test strip) are recommended.

■ Therapy should be stopped if hypersensitivity reactions or bleeding signs and symptoms occur.

### Therapeutic monitoring

■ Periodic electrolyte determinations should be performed in patients with low potassium reserves; hypokalemia can occur when patient with potentially low potassium reserves receives cytotoxic therapy or diuretics.

■ As with other semisynthetic penicillins, piperacillin has caused an increased risk of fever and rash in patients with cystic fibrosis.

### Special populations

**Pregnant patients.** Safety for use during pregnancy hasn't been established.

**Breast-feeding patients.** Piperacillin appears in low levels in breast milk; tazobactam levels haven't been studied. Use with caution when giving piperacillin/tazobactam to breast-feeding women.

**Pediatric patients.** Safety and efficacy in children under age 12 haven't been established.

### Patient counseling

■ Instruct patient to report adverse effects.

■ Advise patient to report discomfort at I.V. site. Inform patient that I.V. site will need to be changed every 48 hours.

# pirbuterol acetate
Maxair

*Pharmacologic classification:* beta-adrenergic agonist
*Therapeutic classification:* bronchodilator
*Pregnancy risk category C*

## Available forms

Available by prescription only
*Inhaler:* 0.2 mg per inhalation

## Indications and dosages

*Prevention and reversal of bronchospasm; asthma*

Adults and children ages 12 and over: 1 or 2 inhalations (0.2 to 0.4 mg) repeated q 4 to 6 hours. Not to exceed 12 inhalations daily.

## Mechanism of action

*Bronchodilating action:* Pirbuterol stimulates beta$_2$-adrenergic receptors and increases the activity of intracellular adenylate cyclase, an enzyme that catalyzes the conversion of adenosine triphosphate to cyclic adenosine monophosphate (cAMP). Elevated cellular cAMP is associated with bronchodilation and inhibition of the cellular release of mediators of immediate hypersensitivity.

## Pharmacokinetics

*Absorption:* Negligible serum levels are achieved after inhalation of the usual dose.
*Distribution:* Pirbuterol acts locally.
*Metabolism:* Metabolized in the liver.
*Excretion:* About 50% of an inhaled dose is recovered in urine as the parent drug and metabolites.

| Route | Onset | Peak | Duration |
|-------|-------|------|----------|
| Inhalation | 5 min | ½-1 hr | 5 hr |

## Contraindications and precautions

Contraindicated in patients hypersensitive to pirbuterol.

Use cautiously in patients with CV disorders, hyperthyroidism, diabetes, or seizure disorders and in those sensitive to sympathomimetic amines.

## Interactions

**Drug-drug.** *MAO inhibitors or tricyclic antidepressants:* May enhance the vascular effects of beta-adrenergic agonists. *Propranolol and other beta blockers:* May decrease the bronchodilating effects of beta agonists. Avoid use together.

## Adverse reactions

**CNS:** tremor, nervousness, dizziness, insomnia, headache, vertigo.
**CV:** tachycardia, palpitations, chest tightness.

---

**EENT:** dry or irritated throat.
**GI:** nausea, vomiting, dry mouth, diarrhea.
**Respiratory:** cough.

## Overdose and treatment
Anginal pain, hypertension, and tachycardia may result from overdose. Treatment is generally supportive. Sedatives or barbiturates may be needed to counter any adverse CNS effects; cautious use of beta blockers may be useful to counter cardiac effects.

## Clinical considerations
■ Drug shouldn't be given to patients who are receiving other beta-adrenergic bronchodilators.

### Therapeutic monitoring
■ Advise clinician to monitor patient for adverse effects, and lack of effectiveness of drug.

### Special populations
**Breast-feeding patients.** It isn't known if pirbuterol appears in breast milk. Use with caution in breast-feeding women.
**Pediatric patients.** Use in children under age 12 isn't recommended.

## Patient counseling
■ Warn patient not to exceed recommended maximum dose of 12 inhalations daily. He should seek medical attention if a previously effective dosage doesn't control symptoms because this may signify a worsening of disease.
■ Tell patient to promptly report increased bronchospasm after using drug.
■ Teach patient how to use metered dose inhaler correctly. Have him shake container, exhale through the nose; administer aerosol while inhaling deeply on mouthpiece of inhaler; hold breath for a few seconds, then exhale slowly. Tell him to allow at least 2 minutes between inhalations and to wait at least 5 minutes before using his steroid inhalant, if he's also taking inhalational corticosteroids.

# piroxicam
Apo-Piroxicam*, Feldene, Novo-Pirocam*

*Pharmacologic classification:* NSAID
*Therapeutic classification:* nonnarcotic analgesic, anti-inflammatory, antipyretic
*Pregnancy risk category B (D in third trimester or near delivery)*

## Available forms
Available by prescription only
*Capsules:* 10 mg, 20 mg

## Indications and dosages
*Osteoarthritis and rheumatoid arthritis*
*Adults:* 20 mg P.O. once daily. If desired, the dose may be divided.
◇ *Juvenile rheumatoid arthritis*
*Children weighing 15 to 30 kg (33 to 67 lb):* 5 mg P.O.
*Children weighing 31 to 45 kg (68 to 100 lb):* 10 mg P.O.
*Children weighing 46 to 55 kg (101 to 121 lb):* 15 mg P.O.

## Mechanism of action
*Analgesic, antipyretic, and anti-inflammatory actions:* Exact mechanisms of action are unknown, but piroxicam is thought to inhibit prostaglandin synthesis.

## Pharmacokinetics
*Absorption:* Absorbed rapidly from the GI tract. Food delays absorption.
*Distribution:* Highly protein-bound.
*Metabolism:* Metabolized in the liver.
*Excretion:* Excreted in urine. Its long half-life (about 50 hours) allows for once-daily dosing.

| Route | Onset | Peak | Duration |
|-------|-------|------|----------|
| P.O. | 1 hr | 3-5 hr | 48-72 hr |

## Contraindications and precautions
Contraindicated in patients hypersensitive to drug or with bronchospasm or angioedema precipitated by aspirin or NSAIDs, and in pregnant or breast-feeding women.

Use cautiously in geriatric patients and in patients with GI disorders, history of renal, peptic ulcer, or cardiac disease, hypertension, or conditions predisposing to fluid retention.

## Interactions
**Drug-drug.** *Acetaminophen, diuretics, gold compounds, or other anti-inflammatory drugs:* Increased nephrotoxicity may occur. Avoid use together.
*Anticoagulants and thrombolytics, such as coumarin derivatives, heparin, and other highly protein-bound drugs:* May potentiate anticoagulant effects. Advise clinician to monitor PT, INR, and patient closely.
*Antihypertensives and diuretics:* Piroxicam may decrease effectiveness. Advise clinician to monitor patient closely.
*Anti-inflammatory drugs, corticosteroids, corticotropin, salicylates:* May cause increased GI adverse effects. Avoid use together.
*Aspirin, cefamandole, cefoperazone, dextran, dipyridamole, mezlocillin, piperacillin, plicamycin, salicylates, sulfinpyrazone, ticarcillin, valproic acid, and other anti-inflammatory drugs:* Increased risk of bleeding. Advise clinician to monitor PT, INR, and patient closely.
*Nifedipine, phenytoin, verapamil:* Toxicity may occur. Avoid use together.

*Insulin or oral antidiabetics:* May potentiate hypoglycemic effects. Advise clinician to monitor glucose levels closely.
*Lithium, methotrexate:* Increased plasma lithium and methotrexate levels. Advise clinician to monitor patient for toxicity.
**Drug-herb.** *Dong quai, feverfew, garlic, ginger, horse chestnut, red clover:* Possible increased risk of bleeding. Discourage use together.
*St. John's wort, dong quai:* Increased risk of photosensitivity. Advise patient to avoid unprotected exposure to sunlight.
**Drug-lifestyle.** *Alcohol use:* Increased GI toxicity. Decreased plasma levels of piroxicam. Advise patient to avoid alcohol.
*Sun exposure:* May cause photosensitivity reaction. Advise patient to use sunblock.

## Adverse reactions
**CNS:** headache, drowsiness, dizziness, somnolence, vertigo.
**CV:** peripheral edema.
**EENT:** auditory disturbances.
**GI:** *epigastric distress, nausea, occult blood loss, peptic ulceration, severe GI bleeding,* diarrhea, constipation, abdominal pain, dyspepsia, flatulence, anorexia, stomatitis.
**GU:** *nephrotoxicity,* elevated BUN level.
**Hematologic:** prolonged bleeding time, anemia, *leukopenia, aplastic anemia, agranulocytosis,* eosinophilia, *thrombocytopenia.*
**Hepatic:** elevated liver enzyme levels.
**Skin:** pruritus, rash, urticaria, *photosensitivity.*

## Overdose and treatment
To treat piroxicam overdose, recommend emptying stomach immediately by inducing emesis with ipecac syrup or by gastric lavage. Recommend giving activated charcoal via nasogastric tube. Symptomatic and supportive measures, such as respiratory support and correction of fluid and electrolyte imbalances, should be provided. Advise clinician to monitor laboratory effects and vital signs closely.

## Clinical considerations
■ Drug is usually given as a single dose.
■ Adverse skin reactions are more common with piroxicam than with other NSAIDs; photosensitivity reactions are the most common.
■ Disease-modifying antirheumatic drugs should be considered in patients nonresponsive to NSAID therapy.

### Therapeutic monitoring
■ Effectiveness of piroxicam usually isn't seen for at least 2 weeks after therapy begins. Recommend evaluating response to drug as evidenced by reduced symptoms.
■ Advise clinician to check renal, hepatic, and auditory functions and CBC periodically during prolonged therapy. Drug should be stopped if abnormalities are found.

### Special populations
**Pregnant patients.** Drug hasn't been proven safe to the fetus.
**Breast-feeding patients.** Piroxicam may inhibit lactation. Because piroxicam appears in breast milk at 1% of maternal serum levels, recommend using an alternative feeding method during drug therapy. Avoid use in breast-feeding women.
**Pediatric patients.** Safety of long-term piroxicam in children hasn't been established.
**Geriatric patients.** Patients over age 60 are more sensitive to the adverse effects of piroxicam. Use with caution. Through its effect on renal prostaglandins, piroxicam may cause fluid retention and edema. This may be significant in geriatric patients and those with HF.

## Patient counseling
■ Advise patient to seek medical approval before taking OTC drugs.
■ Caution patient to avoid hazardous activities requiring alertness until CNS effects are known. Instruct patient in safety measures to prevent injury.
■ Instruct patient in signs and symptoms of adverse effects. Tell patient to report them immediately.
■ Encourage patient to comply with recommended medical follow-up.

# plasma protein fraction
Plasmanate, Plasma-Plex, Plasmatein, Protenate

*Pharmacologic classification:* blood derivative
*Therapeutic classification:* plasma volume expander
*Pregnancy risk category C*

## Available forms
Available by prescription only
*Injection:* 50 mg/ml (5% solution in 50-ml, 250-ml, 500-ml vials)

## Indications and dosages
*Shock*
*Adults:* Varies with patient's condition and response, but usually 250 to 500 ml (12.5 to 25 g protein) I.V., not to exceed 10 ml/minute.
*Infants and young children:* Initially, 6.6 to 33 ml/kg (0.33 to 1.65 g/kg of protein) infused at up to 5 to 10 ml/minute. Subsequent dosage is based on patient's condition.
*Hypoproteinemia*
*Adults:* 1,000 to 1,500 ml I.V. daily. Maximum infusion rate, 8 ml/minute (500 ml infused in 30 to 45 minutes).

## I.V. administration
■ Don't use solution that's cloudy, contains sediment, or has been frozen. Store at room

temperature; freezing may break bottle and allow bacterial contamination.
- Use opened solution promptly, discarding unused portion after 4 hours; solution contains no preservatives and becomes unstable.
- One unit is usually considered to be 250 ml of the 5% concentration.
- Avoid rapid I.V. infusion. Rate is individualized according to patient's age, condition, and diagnosis. Maximum dose is 250 g/48 hours; don't give faster than 10 ml/minute. Decrease infusion rate to 5 to 8 ml/minute as plasma volume approaches normal.

### Incompatibilities
Incompatible with alcohol-containing solutions, norepinephrine, and protein hydrolysates.

### Mechanism of action
*Plasma-expanding action:* Plasma protein fraction (PPF) supplies colloid to the blood and expands plasma volume. It causes fluid to shift from interstitial spaces into the circulation and slightly increases the plasma protein level. It's comprised mostly of albumin, but may contain up to 17% alpha and beta globulins and not more than 1% gamma globulin.

### Pharmacokinetics
The pharmacokinetics of PPF are similar to its chief constituent, albumin (about 83% to 90%).
*Absorption:* Administered I.V.
*Distribution:* Albumin accounts for about 50% of plasma proteins. It's distributed into the intravascular space and extravascular sites, including skin, muscle, and lungs. In patients with reduced circulating blood volumes, hemodilution secondary to albumin administration persists for many hours; in patients with normal blood volume, excess fluid and protein are lost from the intravascular space within a few hours.
*Metabolism:* Although albumin is synthesized in the liver, the liver isn't involved in clearance of albumin from the plasma in healthy individuals.
*Excretion:* Little is known about albumin excretion in healthy individuals. Administration of albumin decreases hepatic albumin synthesis and increases albumin clearance if plasma oncotic pressure is high. In certain pathologic states, the liver, kidneys, or intestines may provide elimination mechanisms.

| Route | Onset | Peak | Duration |
|-------|-------|------|----------|
| I.V. | Immediate | Immediate | Unknown |

### Contraindications and precautions
Contraindicated in patients with severe anemia or HF and in those undergoing cardiac bypass.
Use cautiously in patients with impaired renal or hepatic function, low cardiac reserve, or restricted salt intake.

### Interactions
None significant.

### Adverse reactions
**CNS:** headache.
**CV:** hypotension (after rapid infusion or intra-arterial administration), *vascular overload* (after rapid infusion), tachycardia.
**GI:** nausea, vomiting, hypersalivation.
**Musculoskeletal:** back pain.
**Respiratory:** dyspnea, *pulmonary edema.*
**Skin:** rash, flushing.
**Other:** chills, fever, increased plasma protein levels.

### Overdose and treatment
Rapid infusion may cause circulatory overload and pulmonary edema. Advise clinician to watch patient for signs of hypervolemia and monitor blood pressure and central venous pressure. Treatment is symptomatic.

### Clinical considerations
- PPF is also used in treatment of shock resulting from burns; dosage depends on the extent and severity of burn.
- No cross-matching is required.
- If patient is dehydrated, additional fluids should be given either P.O. or I.V.
- Each L contains 130 to 160 mEq of sodium before dilution with any additional I.V. fluids; a 250-ml container of the 5% concentration contains about 33 to 40 mEq sodium.

### Therapeutic monitoring
- Advise clinician to monitor blood pressure frequently and slow or stop infusion if hypotension suddenly occurs. Vital signs should return to normal gradually.
- Patient should be observed for signs of vascular overload, such as HF, pulmonary edema, and widening pulse pressure indicating increased cardiac output, and signs of hemorrhage or shock after surgery or trauma; advise clinician to be alert for bleeding sites not evident at lower blood pressure.
- Advise clinician to monitor intake and output (watch especially for decreased output), hemoglobin, hematocrit, and serum protein and electrolyte levels to help determine ongoing dosage.

### Patient counseling
- Explain use and administration to patient and family.
- Instruct patient to report adverse effects.

---

# plicamycin
Mithracin

*Pharmacologic classification:* antibiotic antineoplastic (cell cycle–phase nonspecific)
*Therapeutic classification:* antineoplastic, hypocalcemic
*Pregnancy risk category X*

## Available forms
Available by prescription only
*Injection:* 2,500-mcg vials

## Indications and dosages
Dosage and indications may vary. Check current literature for recommended protocol.
*Hypercalcemia*
*Adults:* 25 mcg/kg I.V. daily over 4 to 6 hours for 3 to 4 days. Repeat at intervals of 1 week, p.r.n.
*Testicular cancer*
*Adults:* 25 to 30 mcg/kg I.V. daily over 4 to 6 hours for up to 10 days (based on ideal body weight or actual weight, whichever is less).
◇ *Paget's disease*
*Adults:* 15 mcg/kg I.V. daily over 4 to 6 hours for up to 10 days.

## I.V. administration
■ To reconstitute drug, use 4.9 ml of sterile water to give a concentration of 500 mcg/ml. Reconstitute drug immediately before administration, and discard unused solution.
■ Drug may be further diluted with normal saline solution or $D_5W$ to a volume of 1,000 ml and administered as an I.V. infusion over 4 to 6 hours.
■ Although drug may be administered by I.V. push injection, it's discouraged because of the higher risk and greater severity of GI toxicity. Nausea and vomiting are greatly diminished as infusion rate is decreased.
■ Infusions of plicamycin in 1,000 ml $D_5W$ are stable for up to 24 hours.
■ If I.V. infiltrates, recommend stopping infusion immediately and applying ice packs before restarting an I.V. in other arm.

## Incompatibilities
None reported. However, drug may form a complex with metal ions such as iron and readily hydrolyzes in acidic solutions—those with pH below 4.

## Mechanism of action
*Antineoplastic action:* Plicamycin exerts its cytotoxic activity by intercalating between DNA base pairs and also binding to the outside of the DNA molecule. The result is inhibition of DNA-dependent RNA synthesis.
*Hypocalcemic action:* The exact mechanism by which plicamycin lowers serum calcium levels is unknown. Plicamycin may block the hypercalcemic effect of vitamin D or may inhibit the effect of parathyroid hormone upon osteoclasts, preventing osteolysis. Both mechanisms reduce serum calcium levels.

## Pharmacokinetics
*Absorption:* Administered I.V.
*Distribution:* Distributed mainly into the Kupffer's cells of the liver, into renal tubular cells, and along formed bone surfaces. Drug also crosses the blood-brain barrier and achieves appreciable levels in the CSF.
*Metabolism:* Poorly understood.
*Excretion:* Eliminated primarily through the kidneys.

| Route | Onset | Peak | Duration |
|-------|-------|------|----------|
| I.V. | 1-2 days | 3 days | 7-10 days |

## Contraindications and precautions
Contraindicated in patients with thrombocytopenia, bone marrow suppression, or coagulation and bleeding disorders and in women who are or who may become pregnant.
   Use cautiously in patients with impaired renal or hepatic function.

## Interactions
None reported.

## Adverse reactions
**CNS:** drowsiness, weakness, lethargy, headache, malaise.
**GI:** *nausea, vomiting,* anorexia, diarrhea, stomatitis.
**GU:** increased BUN and serum creatinine levels.
**Hematologic:** *leukopenia, thrombocytopenia; bleeding syndrome* (from epistaxis to generalized hemorrhage).
**Hepatic:** *elevated liver enzymes levels, hepatotoxicity.*
**Metabolic:** *decreased serum calcium,* potassium, and phosphorus levels.
**Skin:** facial flushing, rash, cellulitis with extravasation.
**Other:** fever; phlebitis.

## Overdose and treatment
Signs of overdose include myelosuppression, electrolyte imbalance, and coagulation disorders. Treatment is usually supportive and includes transfusion of blood components and appropriate symptomatic therapy. Advise clinician to monitor patient's renal and hepatic status closely.

## Clinical considerations
■ Facial flushing is an early indication of bleeding. The first evidence of bleeding may manifest in epistaxis.
■ Recommend giving antiemetics before administering drug, to reduce nausea.

- Therapeutic effect in hypercalcemia may not be seen for 24 to 48 hours, and may last 3 to 15 days.
- Avoid drug contact with skin or mucous membranes.
- Store lyophilized powder in refrigerator.

### Therapeutic monitoring
- Advise clinician to monitor LDH, AST, ALT, alkaline phosphatase, BUN, creatinine, potassium, calcium, and phosphorus levels.
- Advise clinician to monitor platelet count and PT before and during therapy.
- Recommend checking serum calcium levels. Advise clinician to monitor patient for tetany, carpopedal spasm, Chvostek's sign, and muscle cramps because a sharp drop in calcium levels is possible.
- Patient should be observed for signs of bleeding.

### Special populations
**Pregnant patients.** Drug may cause fetal toxicity. Drug is contraindicated for use during pregnancy. Advise patient to use contraceptive measures during therapy and to notify prescriber immediately if she becomes pregnant or suspects she is pregnant.
**Breast-feeding patients.** It isn't known if drug appears in breast milk. However, because of potential for serious adverse reactions, mutagenicity, and carcinogenicity in the infant, breast-feeding isn't recommended.

### Patient counseling
- Tell patient to use salicylate-free drug for pain relief or fever reduction.
- Instruct patient to avoid exposure to people with infections and to immediately report signs of infection or unusual bleeding.
- Inform patient that he and household members shouldn't receive immunizations during therapy and for several weeks after therapy.

## pneumococcal vaccine, polyvalent
Pneumovax 23, Pnu-Imune 23

*Pharmacologic classification:* vaccine
*Therapeutic classification:* bacterial vaccine
*Pregnancy risk category C*

### Available forms
Available by prescription only
*Injection:* 25 mcg each of 23 polysaccharide isolates of *Streptococcus pneumoniae* per 0.5-ml dose, in 1-ml and 5-ml vials and disposable syringes.

## Indications and dosages
*Pneumococcal immunization*
*Adults and children over age 2:* 0.5 ml I.M. or S.C. as a one-time dose.

## Mechanism of action
*Pneumonia prophylaxis:* Pneumococcal vaccine promotes active immunity against the 23 most prevalent pneumococcal types.

## Pharmacokinetics
*Absorption:* Protective antibodies are produced within 3 weeks after injection.
*Distribution:* No information available.
*Metabolism:* No information available.
*Excretion:* No information available.

| Route | Onset | Peak | Duration |
|-------|-------|------|----------|
| I.M., S.C. | 2-3 wk | Unknown | 5 yr |

## Contraindications and precautions
Contraindicated in patients hypersensitive to drug or its components (phenol). Also contraindicated in patients with Hodgkin's disease who have received extensive chemotherapy or nodal irradiation.

## Interactions
**Drug-drug.** *Corticosteroids, other immunosuppressants:* May impair the immune response to vaccine; therefore, vaccination should be avoided.

## Adverse reactions
**CNS:** headache, general weakness.
**GI:** nausea, vomiting.
**Musculoskeletal:** myalgia, arthralgia.
**Respiratory:** difficulty breathing.
**Skin:** rash, itching, *soreness at injection site.*
**Other:** adenitis, *anaphylaxis,* serum sickness, *slight fever,* severe local reaction associated with revaccination within 3 years.

## Overdose and treatment
No information available.

## Clinical considerations
- Revaccination is not recommended except for high-risk patients and healthy patients over age 65 for whom at least 5 years have elapsed since the first dose.
- Persons with asplenia who received the 14-valent vaccine should be revaccinated with the 23-valent vaccine.
- Epinephrine solution 1:1,000 should be available to treat allergic reactions.
- Recommend using the deltoid or midlateral thigh. Don't inject I.V. Avoid intradermal administration because this may cause severe local reactions.
- Polyvalent pneumococcal vaccine also may be given to children to prevent pneumococcal otitis media.

- Candidates for pneumococcal vaccine include adults and children ages 2 or older with chronic illness, asplenia, or splenic dysfunction; and those with sickle-cell anemia and HIV infection.
- Vaccine also is recommended for patients awaiting organ transplants, those receiving radiation therapy or cancer chemotherapy, persons in nursing homes and orphanages, and bedridden individuals.
- If different sites and separate syringes are used, pneumococcal vaccine may be administered simultaneously with influenza, DTP, poliovirus, or *Haemophilus* b polysaccharide vaccines.
- Store vaccine at 36° to 46° F (2° to 8° C). Reconstitution or dilution is unnecessary.

### *Therapeutic monitoring*
- Check immunization history to avoid revaccination within 3 years.
- Severe local reaction has been caused by revaccination done within a 3-year period.

### *Special populations*
**Breast-feeding patients.** It's unknown if vaccine appears in breast milk. Use with caution in breast-feeding women.
**Pediatric patients.** Children under age 2 don't respond satisfactorily to pneumococcal vaccine. Safety and efficacy of vaccine haven't been established.
**Geriatric patients.** Vaccine is recommended for all adults over age 65.

### Patient counseling
- Tell patient to expect redness, soreness, swelling, and pain at the injection site after vaccination. Fever, joint or muscle aches and pains, rash, itching, general weakness, or difficulty breathing may also develop.
- Encourage patient to report distressing adverse reactions promptly.
- Advise patient to use acetaminophen to relieve adverse reactions.

---

# poliovirus vaccine, live, oral, trivalent (Sabin vaccine, TOPV)
Orimune

# poliovirus vaccine, inactivated (IPV)
IPOL

---

*Pharmacologic classification:* vaccine
*Therapeutic classification:* viral vaccine
*Pregnancy risk category C*

### Available forms
Available by prescription only

**Orimune**
*Oral vaccine:* Mixture of three viruses (types 1, 2, and 3), grown in monkey kidney tissue culture, in 0.5-ml single-dose Dispettes.
**IPOL**
*Injectable suspension:* 40 D antigen units of type 1 (Mahoney), 8D antigen units of type 2 (MEF-1), and 32 D antigen units of type 3 (Saukett) per 0.5 ml.

### Indications and dosages
*Poliovirus immunization (primary series)*
*IPOL*
*Adults (at increased risk of exposure to poliovirus):* 0.5 ml I.M. or S.C. at 4- to 8-week intervals for two doses; third dose is given 6 to 12 months after second dose; total of three 0.5-ml doses are given. Booster vaccination of one additional dose may be given to adults who have completed the three-dose primary series of IPV or OPV or combination of IPV and OPV, and who are at a high risk for exposure to poliovirus.
*Infants and children:* 0.5 ml I.M. or S.C. at age 2 months and 4 months; third dose is given at ages 6 to 18 months; and fourth dose at ages 4 to 6 years.
*Poliovirus immunization (primary series)*
*Orimune*
*Infants and children ages 6 weeks and older:* 0.5-ml doses P.O. at ages 2, 4, and 6 to 18 months. A fourth dose at age 4 to 6 years or before entering school may be given unless third primary dose was given on or after fourth birthday.
*Adults ages 18 and older:* Use IPV whenever possible. If fewer than 4 weeks are available before prevention is needed, a single dose of OPV or IPV may be given.
*IPV/OPV regimen for primary immunization when IPV cannot be given*
*Infants and children:* Two doses of IPV given I.M. or S.C. at ages 2 and 4 months, and OPV given P.O. at ages 12 to 18 months and 4 to 6 years.

### Mechanism of action
*Polio prophylaxis:* TOPV promotes immunity to poliomyelitis by inducing humoral and secretory antibodies and antibodies in the lymphatic tissue of the GI tract.

### Pharmacokinetics
*Absorption:* Immunity is thought to be lifelong.
*Distribution:* No information available.
*Metabolism:* No information available.
*Excretion:* No information available.

| Route | Onset | Peak | Duration |
|-------|-------|------|----------|
| P.O. | 7-10 days | 21 days | Years |
| S.C., I.M. | Unknown | Unknown | Years |

## Contraindications and precautions
Oral vaccine is contraindicated in immuno-suppressed patients, in those with cancer or immunoglobulin abnormalities, and in those receiving radiation, antimetabolite, alkylating drug, or corticosteroid therapy. These patients should receive IPV. OPV is also contraindicated in patients with a history of anaphylactic reaction to the vaccine, and in patients who are allergic to neomycin and streptomycin. Injectable vaccine is contraindicated in patients hypersensitive to neomycin, streptomycin, or polymyxin B.

Use cautiously in siblings of children with known immunodeficiency syndrome.

## Interactions
**Drug-drug.** *Corticosteroids, other immuno-suppressants:* Use of OPV with these drugs may impair the immune response to the vaccine. Vaccination with OPV should be deferred until the immunosuppressant is stopped or, alternatively, inactivated poliovirus vaccine may be used.
*Immune serum globulin and transfusions of blood or blood products:* May also interfere with the immune response to poliovirus vaccine. Vaccination should be deferred for 3 months in these situations.

## Adverse reactions
**Other:** crying, decreased appetite, *fever,* hypersensitivity reactions, ***poliomyelitis,*** sleepiness, erythema, induration, *pain* (at injection site).

## Overdose and treatment
No information available.

## Clinical considerations
**ⓗ ALERT** Parenteral form should be given to immunodeficient patients or those with altered immune status because they may be at risk for development of the disease if live virus vaccine is administered.
■ Obtain a thorough history of patient's allergies, especially to antibiotics, and of reactions to immunizations.
■ IPV regimen is currently recommended for routine primary immunization in healthy infants.
■ OPV is no longer recommended for routine immunizations but is recommended for outbreak control.
■ Vaccine isn't effective in modifying or preventing existing or incubating poliomyelitis.
■ OPV isn't for parenteral use. Dose may be given directly or mixed with distilled water, chlorine-free tap water, simple syrup USP, or milk. It also may be placed on bread, cake, or a sugar cube.
■ Keep vaccine frozen until used. It may be refrigerated up to 30 days once thawed, if unopened. Opened vials may be refrigerated up to 7 days.
■ Color change from pink to yellow has no effect on the efficacy of the vaccine as long as the vaccine remains clear. Yellow color results from storage at low temperatures.
■ OPV may temporarily decrease the response to tuberculin skin testing. If a tuberculin test is needed, recommend giving either before, simultaneously with, or at least 8 weeks after OPV.

### Therapeutic monitoring
■ Recommend having epinephrine 1:1,000 nearby in case of a rapid allergic reaction.
■ Advise clinician to check parents' immunization history when they bring in a child for the vaccine; this is an excellent time for parents to receive booster immunizations.

### Special populations
**Breast-feeding patients.** Breast-feeding doesn't interfere with successful immunization; no interruption in the feeding schedule is needed.
**Pediatric patients.** Poliovirus vaccine shouldn't be given to neonates under age 6 weeks.

## Patient counseling
■ Inform patient that risk of vaccine-associated paralysis is extremely small for vaccines, susceptible family members, and other close contacts (about 1 case per 2.6 million patients receiving the vaccines).
■ Encourage patient to report distressing adverse reactions promptly.

# polyethylene glycol-electrolyte solution (PEG-ES)
Colovage, CoLyte, GoLYTELY, NuLytely, OCL

*Pharmacologic classification:* polyethylene glycol 3350 nonabsorbable solution
*Therapeutic classification:* laxative and bowel evacuant
*Pregnancy risk category C*

## Available forms
Available by prescription only
*Powder for oral solution:* Polyethylene glycol (PEG) 3350 (6 g), anhydrous sodium sulfate (568 mg), sodium chloride (146 mg), potassium chloride (74.5 mg/100 ml) (Colovage); PEG 3350 (120 g), sodium sulfate (3.36 g), sodium chloride (2.92 g), potassium chloride (1.49 g/2 L) (CoLyte); PEG 3350 (236 g), sodium sulfate (22.74 g), sodium bicarbonate (6.74 g), sodium chloride (5.86 g), potassium chloride (2.97 g/4.8 L) (GoLYTELY); PEG 3350 (420 g), sodium bicarbonate (5.72 g),

sodium chloride (11.2 g), potassium chloride (1.48 g/4 L) (NuLytely); PEG 3350 (6 g), sodium sulfate decahydrate (1.29 g), sodium chloride (146 mg), potassium chloride (75 mg), polysorbate-80 (30 mg/100 ml) (OCL)

## Indications and dosages

**Bowel preparation before GI examination**
*Adults:* 240 ml P.O. q 10 minutes until 4 L are consumed or the rectal effluent is clear. Typically, administer 4 hours before examination, allowing 3 hours for drinking and 1 hour for bowel evacuation.
*Children ages 3 weeks to 18 years:* 25 to 40 ml/kg for 4 to 10 hours.
◇ **Management of acute iron overdose**
*Children under age 3:* 0.5 L/hour.
Note: If a patient experiences severe bloating, distention, or abdominal pain, slow or temporarily discontinue administration until symptoms abate.

## Mechanism of action

*Laxative and bowel evacuant actions:* PEG-ES acts as an osmotic drug. With sodium sulfate as the major sodium source, active sodium absorption is markedly reduced. Diarrhea results, which rapidly cleans the bowel, usually within 4 hours.

## Pharmacokinetics

*Absorption:* PEG-ES is a nonabsorbable solution.
*Distribution:* Not applicable because drug isn't absorbed.
*Metabolism:* Not applicable because drug isn't absorbed.
*Excretion:* Excreted via the GI tract.

| Route | Onset | Peak | Duration |
|-------|-------|------|----------|
| P.O. | 1 hr | Variable | Variable |

## Contraindications and precautions

Contraindicated in patients with GI obstruction or perforation, gastric retention, toxic colitis, ileus, or megacolon.

## Interactions

**Drug-drug.** *Oral medication given within 1 hour before start of therapy:* May be flushed from the GI tract and not absorbed. Drugs shouldn't be given during this time period.

## Adverse reactions

**EENT:** rhinorrhea.
**GI:** *nausea, bloating, cramps, vomiting, abdominal fullness,* anal irritation.
**Skin:** urticaria, dermatitis.
**Other:** *anaphylaxis.*

## Overdose and treatment

No information available.

## Clinical considerations

■ Drug may be given via a nasogastric tube (at 20 to 30 ml/minute, or 1.2 to 1.8 L/hour) to patients unwilling or unable to drink the preparation. The first bowel movement should occur within 1 hour.
■ Tap water may be used to reconstitute the solution. Shake container vigorously several times to ensure powder is completely dissolved. After reconstitution to 4 L with water, the solution contains PEG 3350 17.6 mmol/L, sodium 125 mmol/L, sulfate 40 mmol/L (Colyte 80 mmol/L), chloride 35 mmol/L, bicarbonate 20 mmol/L, and potassium 10 mmol/L (1 mmol/L = 1 mEq/L).
■ Store reconstituted solution in refrigerator (chilling before administration improves palatability); use within 48 hours.
■ Don't add flavorings or additional ingredients to solution before use.
■ Patient preparation for barium enema may be less satisfactory with this solution because it may interfere with the barium coating of the colonic mucosa using the double-contrast technique.

### Therapeutic monitoring

■ If given to semiconscious patient or to patients with impaired gag reflex, caution should be used to prevent aspiration.
■ Advise clinician to monitor intake and output. No major shifts in fluid or electrolyte balance have been reported.

### Special populations

**Pediatric patients.** Consult prescriber; no dosing information is available for pediatric patients.

## Patient counseling

■ Instruct patient to fast about 3 to 4 hours before ingesting the solution.
■ Tell patient never to take solid foods less than 2 hours before solution is administered. Also inform him that no foods except clear liquids are permitted after administration of solution until the examination is completed.

---

# polysaccharide-iron complex

Ferrex-150, Fe-Tinic 150, Hytinic, Niferex, Niferex-150, Nu-Iron, Nu-Iron 150

*Pharmacologic classification:* oral iron supplement
*Therapeutic classification:* hematinic
*Pregnancy risk category NR*

## Available forms

Available without a prescription
*Capsules:* 150 mg

*Solution:* 100 mg/5 ml
*Tablets (film-coated):* 50 mg

## Indications and dosages
### Treatment of uncomplicated iron-deficiency anemia
*Adults and children ages 12 and older:* 150 to 300 mg P.O. daily as capsules or tablets or 1 to 2 teaspoonfuls of elixir P.O. daily.
*Children ages 6 to 12:* 150 mg to 300 mg P.O. daily as tablets or 1 teaspoonful of elixir P.O. daily.
*Children ages 2 to 6:* ½ teaspoonful of elixir P.O. daily.

## Mechanism of action
*Hematinic action:* Polysaccharide-iron complex provides elemental iron, an essential component in the formation of hemoglobin.

## Pharmacokinetics
*Absorption:* Although iron is absorbed from entire length of GI tract, the duodenum and proximal jejunum are the primary absorption sites. Up to 10% of iron is absorbed by healthy individuals; patients with iron-deficiency anemia may absorb up to 60%. Enteric coating has decreased absorption because they're designed to release iron past points in GI tract of highest absorption. Food may decrease absorption by 33% to 50%.
*Distribution:* Iron is transported through GI mucosal cells directly into the blood where it's immediately bound to a carrier protein, transferrin, and transported to the bone marrow for incorporation into hemoglobin. Iron is highly protein-bound.
*Metabolism:* Iron is liberated by the destruction of hemoglobin, but is conserved and reused by the body.
*Excretion:* Healthy individuals lose only small amounts of iron each day. Men and postmenopausal women lose about 1 mg/day and premenopausal women about 1.5 mg/day. Loss usually occurs in nails, hair, feces, and urine; trace amounts are lost in bile and sweat.

| Route | Onset | Peak | Duration |
|-------|-------|------|----------|
| P.O. | Few days | 2-10 days | 2 mo |

## Contraindications and precautions
Contraindicated in patients hypersensitive to any component of drug and in those with hemochromatosis and hemosiderosis.

## Interactions
**Drug-drug.** *Antacids, cholestyramine resin, cimetidine, tetracycline, vitamin E:* Decrease iron absorption. Separate doses by 2 to 4 hours.
*Chloramphenicol:* Causes a delayed response to iron therapy. Advise clinician to monitor patient carefully.
*Fluoroquinolones, levodopa, methyldopa, penicillamine:* Iron decreases absorption of these drugs, possibly resulting in decreased serum levels or efficacy. Advise clinician to monitor patient.
*Vitamin C:* May increase iron absorption. Drugs may be given together.
**Drug-herb.** *Black cohosh, chamomile, feverfew, gossypol, hawthorn, nettle, plantain, St. John's wort:* Decreased iron absorption. Discourage use together.
*Oregano:* May reduce iron absorption. Oregano and iron supplements or iron-containing foods should be taken at least 2 hours apart.
**Drug-food.** *Dairy products, eggs, whole-grain breads and cereals, tea, and coffee:* Decrease iron absorption. Separate doses by 2 to 4 hours.
*Foods high in vitamin C:* May increase iron absorption. May be taken with these foods.

## Adverse reactions
Although nausea, constipation, black stools, and epigastric pain are common adverse reactions from iron therapy, few, if any, occur with polysaccharide-iron complex. Iron-containing liquids may cause temporary staining of teeth.

## Overdose and treatment
The lethal dose of iron is between 200 and 250 mg/kg; fatalities have occurred with lower doses. Symptoms may follow ingestion of 20 to 60 mg/kg. Clinical signs of acute overdose may occur as follows:

Between ½ and 8 hours after ingestion, patient may experience lethargy, nausea and vomiting, green then tarry stools, weak and rapid pulse, hypotension, dehydration, acidosis, and coma. If death doesn't immediately ensue, symptoms may clear for about 24 hours.

At 12 to 48 hours, symptoms may return, accompanied by diffuse vascular congestion, pulmonary edema, shock, seizures, anuria, and hyperthermia. Death may follow.

Treatment requires immediate support of airway, respiration, and circulation. Recommend inducing emesis with ipecac in conscious patients with intact gag reflex; for unconscious patients, stomach should be emptied by gastric lavage. Emesis should be followed by lavage, using 1% sodium bicarbonate solution, to convert iron to less irritating, poorly absorbed form. (Phosphate solutions have been used, but carry risk of other adverse effects.) Advise clinician to perform radiographic evaluation of abdomen to determine continued presence of excess iron; if serum iron levels exceed 350 mg/dl, deferoxamine may be used for systemic chelation.

Survivors are likely to sustain organ damage, including pyloric or antral stenosis, hepatic cirrhosis, CNS damage, and intestinal obstruction.

## Clinical considerations

▪ Recommend giving iron with juice (preferably orange juice) or water, but not with milk or antacids.

▪ Polysaccharide-iron complex is nontoxic and there are relatively few, if any, of the GI adverse effects associated with other iron preparations.

▪ Oral iron may turn stools black. This unabsorbed iron is harmless; however, it could mask melena.

▪ Iron overload may decrease uptake of technetium-99m and, thus, interfere with skeletal imaging. Polysaccharide iron complex may interfere with test for occult blood in stool; guaiac and orthotoluidine tests may yield false-positive results.

### Therapeutic monitoring

▪ Advise clinician to monitor hemoglobin level, hematocrit, and reticulocyte counts during therapy.

### Special populations

**Breast-feeding patients.** Iron supplements are often recommended for breast-feeding women; no adverse effects have been documented.
**Pediatric patients.** Overdose of iron may be fatal in children; patient should be treated immediately.
**Geriatric patients.** Because iron-induced constipation is common in geriatric patients, stress proper diet to minimize this adverse effect. Geriatric patients may need higher doses of iron because reduced gastric secretions and achlorhydria may lower capacity for iron absorption.

## Patient counseling

▪ Inform parents that as few as three or four tablets may cause serious iron poisoning in children.

▪ If patient misses a dose, tell him to take it as soon as he remembers but not to double the dose.

▪ Advise patient to separate iron from certain foods that may impair oral iron absorption, including yogurt, cheese, eggs, milk, whole-grain breads and cereals, tea, and coffee.

▪ Teach patient dietary measures to follow for preventing constipation.

---

# potassium salts, oral

# potassium acetate

# potassium bicarbonate

K+ Care ET, K-Electrolyte, Klor-Con/EF, K-Lyte, K-Vescent, Quick-K

# potassium chloride

Apo-K*, Cena-K, K-8, K-10*, Kalium Durules*, Kaochlor, Kaon-Cl, Kaon-Cl-10, Kato, Kay Ciel, K+ Care, KCL*, K-Dur, K-Lease, K-Long*, K-Lor, Klor-Con, Klotrix, K-Lyte/Cl Powder, K-Med 900*, K-Norm, K-Sol, K-Tab, Micro-K Extencaps, Micro-K 10 Extencaps, Potasalan, Rum-K, Slow-K

# potassium gluconate

Glu-K, Kaon

*Pharmacologic classification:* potassium supplement
*Therapeutic classification:* therapeutic drug for electrolyte balance
*Pregnancy risk category C*

---

## Available forms

Available by prescription only
**potassium bicarbonate**
*Tablets (effervescent):* 6.5 mEq, 25 mEq
**potassium acetate**
*Vials:* 2 mEq/ml, 4 mEq/ml in 20-ml vials
**potassium chloride**
*Capsules:* 8 mEq, 10 mEq
*Injection:* 1.5 mEq/ml, 2 mEq/ml
*Liquid:* 0.1mEq/ml, 0.2 mEq/ml, 0.3 mEq/ml, 0.4 mEq/ml
*Powder:* 15 mEq/package, 20 mEq/package, and 25 mEq/package
*Tablets (extended-release):* 8 mEq, 10 mEq, 20 mEq
**potassium gluconate**
*Liquid:* 20 mEq/15 ml
*Tablets:* 2 mEq, 500 mg, 595 mg

## Indications and dosages

*Hypokalemia*
*Adults and children:* 40- to 100-mEq tablets divided into 2 to 4 doses daily. Use I.V. potassium chloride when oral replacement isn't feasible or when hypokalemia is life-threatening. Dosage up to 20 mEq/hour in concentration of 60 mEq/L or less. Further dose based on serum potassium determinations. Don't exceed total daily dose of 150 mEq (3 mEq/kg in children).

Further doses are based on serum potassium levels and blood pH. I.V. potassium replacement should be carried out only with ECG monitoring and frequent serum potassium determinations.
*Prevention of hypokalemia*
*Adults and children:* Initially, 20 mEq of potassium supplement P.O. daily, in divided doses. Adjust dosage, p.r.n., based on serum potassium levels.
*Potassium replacement*
*Adults and children:* Potassium chloride should be diluted in a suitable I.V. solution (not more than 40 mEq/L) and administered at rate not exceeding 20 mEq/hour. Don't exceed total dose of 400 mEq/day (3 mEq/kg/day or 40 mEq/m²/day for children). I.V. potassium replacement should be carried out only with

---

**Metabolic:** abnormal thyroid function test results.
**Musculoskeletal:** myositis, myopathy, *localized muscle pain*, myalgia, **rhabdomyolysis.**
**Respiratory:** cough.
**Skin:** rash, photosensitivity.
**Other:** flulike symptoms; CK, alkaline phosphatase increased; influenza, common cold.

## Overdose and treatment
No information available. Treatment is symptomatic.

## Clinical considerations
■ Drug should be stopped temporarily in patient with an acute condition that suggests a developing myopathy or in patient with risk factors that may predispose him to development of renal failure secondary to rhabdomyolysis, including severe acute infection; severe endocrine, metabolic, or electrolyte disorders; hypotension; major surgery; or uncontrolled seizures.
■ Drug therapy should be started only after diet and other nonpharmacologic therapies have proved ineffective. Patients should continue a cholesterol-lowering diet during therapy.
■ Recommend giving drug in the evening, preferably at bedtime. Drug may be given without regard to meals.
■ Dosage adjustments should be made about every 4 weeks. May reduce dosage if cholesterol levels fall below target range.

### *Therapeutic monitoring*
■ Advise clinician to watch for signs of myositis. Rarely, myopathy and marked elevations of CK, possibly leading to rhabdomyolysis and renal failure secondary to myoglobinuria, have been reported.

### *Special populations*
**Breast-feeding patients.** Drug appears in breast milk. Women shouldn't breast-feed while taking pravastatin.
**Pediatric patients.** Safety and efficacy in children under age 18 haven't been established.
**Geriatric patients.** Maximum effectiveness is usually evident with daily doses of 20 mg or less.

## Patient counseling
■ Teach patient appropriate dietary management (restricting total fat and cholesterol intake), weight control, and exercise. Explain importance of these interventions in controlling serum lipids.
■ Tell patient to report adverse reactions, particularly muscle aches and pains.

# prazosin hydrochloride
Minipress

*Pharmacologic classification:* alpha-adrenergic blocker
*Therapeutic classification:* antihypertensive
*Pregnancy risk category C*

## Available forms
Available by prescription only
*Capsules:* 1 mg, 2 mg, 5 mg

## Indications and dosages
### *Hypertension*
*Adults:* Initially, 1 mg P.O. b.i.d. or t.i.d.; gradually increased to maximum of 20 mg daily. Usual maintenance dosage is 6 to 15 mg daily in divided doses. If other antihypertensives or diuretics are added to prazosin therapy, reduce dose of prazosin to 1 or 2 mg t.i.d. and then gradually increase p.r.n.
◊ *Benign prostatic hyperplasia (BPH)*
*Adults:* Initially, 2 mg P.O. b.i.d. Dosage may range from 1 to 9 mg/day.

## Mechanism of action
*Antihypertensive action:* Prazosin selectively and competitively inhibits alpha-adrenergic receptors, causing arterial and venous dilation, reducing peripheral vascular resistance and blood pressure.
*Hypertrophic action:* Alpha blockade of prazosin in nonvascular smooth muscle causes relaxation, notably in prostatic tissue, reducing urinary symptoms in men with BPH.

## Pharmacokinetics
*Absorption:* Absorption from the GI tract is variable. Full antihypertensive effect may not occur for 4 to 6 weeks.
*Distribution:* Distributed throughout the body and is highly protein-bound (about 97%).
*Metabolism:* Metabolized extensively in the liver.
*Excretion:* Over 90% of a given dose is excreted in feces via bile; remainder is excreted in urine. Plasma half-life is 2 to 4 hours. Antihypertensive effect lasts less than 24 hours.

| Route | Onset | Peak | Duration |
|-------|-------|------|----------|
| P.O. | ½-1½ hr | 2-4 hr | 7-10 hr |

## Contraindications and precautions
No known contraindications. Use cautiously in patients receiving antihypertensives and in those with chronic renal failure.

## Interactions
**Drug-drug.** *Diuretics or other antihypertensives:* Hypotensive effects of prazosin may be increased when given concurrently. Avoid use together.

---

*Highly protein-bound drugs:* Because prazosin is highly bound to plasma proteins, it may interact with other highly protein-bound drugs. Advise clinician to monitor patient.
**Drug-herb.** *Butcher's broom:* May cause reduction of drug effects. Don't use together.

### Adverse reactions

**CNS:** *dizziness,* headache, drowsiness, nervousness, paresthesia, weakness, *"first-dose syncope,"* depression.
**CV:** orthostatic hypotension, *palpitations,* edema.
**EENT:** blurred vision, tinnitus, conjunctivitis, nasal congestion, epistaxis.
**GI:** vomiting, diarrhea, abdominal cramps, constipation, *nausea.*
**GU:** priapism, impotence, urinary frequency, incontinence, increased BUN levels.
**Hematologic:** *transient leukopenia.*
**Hepatic:** liver function test abnormalities.
**Metabolic:** increased serum uric acid.
**Musculoskeletal:** arthralgia, myalgia.
**Respiratory:** dyspnea.
**Skin:** pruritus.
**Other:** fever.

### Overdose and treatment

Overdose is manifested by hypotension and drowsiness.

After acute ingestion, advise clinician to empty stomach by induced emesis or gastric lavage and give activated charcoal to reduce absorption. Further treatment is usually symptomatic and supportive. Prazosin isn't dialyzable.

### Clinical considerations

■ First-dose syncope (dizziness, light-headedness, and syncope) may occur within ½ to 1 hour after initial dose; it may be severe, with loss of consciousness, if initial dose exceeds 2 mg. Effect is transient and may be diminished by giving drug at bedtime, by limiting the initial dose of prazosin to 1 mg, by subsequently increasing the dosage gradually, and by introducing other antihypertensives into the patient's regimen cautiously; it's more common during febrile illness and more severe if patient has hyponatremia. Recommend always increasing dosage gradually and having patient sit or lie down if he experiences dizziness.
■ Drug has been used to treat vasospasm from Raynaud's syndrome. It also has been used with diuretics and cardiac glycosides to treat severe HF, to manage the signs and symptoms of pheochromocytoma preoperatively, and to treat ergotamine-induced peripheral ischemia.
■ Prazosin alters results of screening tests for pheochromocytoma and causes increases in levels of the urinary metabolite of norepinephrine and vanillylmandelic acid.

### Therapeutic monitoring

■ Advise clinician to monitor patient's blood pressure and heart rate frequently.

### Special populations

**Pregnant patients.** Use only when potential benefits outweigh risks to fetus. Safety hasn't been established for use during pregnancy.
**Breast-feeding patients.** Small amounts of prazosin appear in breast milk; an alternative feeding method is recommended during therapy.
**Pediatric patients.** Safety and efficacy in children haven't been established; use only when potential benefit outweighs risk.
**Geriatric patients.** Geriatric patients may be more sensitive to hypotensive effects and may require lower doses because of altered drug metabolism.

### Patient counseling

■ Teach patient about his disease and therapy, and explain that he must take drug exactly as prescribed, even when feeling well; advise him never to discontinue drug suddenly because severe rebound hypertension may occur.
■ Advise patient to promptly report malaise or unusual adverse effects.
■ Tell patient to avoid hazardous activities that require mental alertness until tolerance develops to sedation, drowsiness, and other CNS effects; to avoid sudden position changes to minimize orthostatic hypotension; and to use ice chips, candy, or gum to relieve dry mouth.
■ Warn patient to seek medical approval before taking OTC cold preparations.

## prednisolone (systemic)
Delta-Cortef, Prelone

## prednisolone acetate
Key-Pred-25, Predacort 50, Predalone-50, Predate, Predatone, Predcor-50

## prednisolone sodium phosphate
Orapred, Pediapred

## prednisolone tebutate
Hydeltra-TBA, Nor-Pred TBA, Predate TBA, Predcor-TBA, Prednisol TBA

*Pharmacologic classification:* glucocorticoid, mineralocorticoid
*Therapeutic classification:* anti-inflammatory, immunosuppressant
*Pregnancy risk category C*

### Available forms
Available by prescription only
**prednisolone**
*Tablets:* 5 mg

*Syrup:* 15 mg/5 ml
**prednisolone acetate**
*Injection:* 25 mg/ml, 50 mg/ml suspension
**prednisolone sodium phosphate**
*Oral liquid:* 6.7 mg (5 mg base)/5 ml, 20.2 mg
(15 mg base)/5 ml
**prednisolone tebutate**
*Injection:* 20 mg/ml suspension

## Indications and dosages
*Severe inflammation, modification of body's immune response to disease*
**prednisolone**
*Adults:* 2.5 to 15 mg P.O. b.i.d., t.i.d., or q.i.d.
*Children:* 0.14 to 2 mg/kg or 4 to 60 mg/m$^2$
P.O. daily in divided doses.
**prednisolone acetate**
*Adults:* 4 to 60 mg I.M. q 12 hours.
*Children:* 0.04 to 0.25 mg/kg or 1.5 to
7.5 mg/m$^2$ I.M. once or twice daily.
**prednisolone sodium phosphate**
*Adults:* 5 to 60 mg I.M., I.V., or P.O.
*Children:* 0.14 to 2 mg/kg or 4 to 60 mg/m$^2$
daily in divided doses I.M., I.V., or P.O.
**prednisolone tebutate**
*Adults:* 4 to 40 mg into joints and lesions, p.r.n.
*Acute exacerbations of multiple sclerosis*
**prednisolone sodium phosphate**
*Children:* 200 mg/day for a week followed by
80 mg every other day.
*Nephrotic syndrome*
**prednisolone sodium phosphate**
*Children:* 60 mg/m$^2$/day in three divided doses for 4 weeks, followed by 4 weeks of single dose alternate-day therapy at 40 mg/m$^2$/day.
*Uncontrolled asthma in those taking inhaled corticosteroids and long-acting bronchodilators*
**prednisolone sodium phosphate**
*Children:* 1 to 2 mg/kg/day in single or divided doses. It is further recommended that short-course ("burst") therapy be continued until a child achieves a peak expiratory flow rate of 80% of his or her personal best or symptoms resolve. This usually requires 3 to 10 days of treatment, although it can take longer. There is no evidence that tapering the dose after improvement will prevent a relapse.

## I.V. administration
■ Use only prednisolone sodium phosphate.
■ When administering as intermittent or continuous infusion, dilute solution according to manufacturer's instructions, and give over prescribed duration.
■ Use D$_5$W or normal saline solution as diluent for I.V. infusion.

### Incompatibilities
Incompatible with calcium gluceptate or gluconate, dimenhydrinate, metaraminol, methotrexate sodium, polymyxin B, prochlorperazine edisylate, promazine, and promethazine hydrochloride.

## Mechanism of action
*Anti-inflammatory action:* Prednisolone stimulates the synthesis of enzymes needed to decrease the inflammatory response. It suppresses the immune system by reducing activity and volume of the lymphatic system, thus producing lymphocytopenia (primarily of T-lymphocytes), decreasing immunoglobulin and complement levels, decreasing passage of immune complexes through basement membranes, and possibly by depressing reactivity of tissue to antigen-antibody interactions.

The mineralocorticoids regulate electrolyte homeostasis by acting renally at the distal tubules to enhance the reabsorption of sodium ions (and thus water) from the tubular fluid into the plasma and enhance the excretion of both potassium and hydrogen ions.

Prednisolone is an adrenocorticoid with both glucocorticoid and mineralocorticoid properties. It's a weak mineralocorticoid with only half the potency of hydrocortisone but is a more potent glucocorticoid, having four times the potency of equal weight of hydrocortisone. It's used primarily as an anti-inflammatory and an immunosuppressant. It isn't used for mineralocorticoid replacement therapy because of the availability of more specific and potent drugs.

Prednisolone and prednisolone sodium phosphate may be administered orally. Prednisolone acetate and tebutate are suspensions that may be administered by intra-articular, intrasynovial, intrabursal, intralesional, or soft-tissue injection. They have a slow onset but a long duration of action.

## Pharmacokinetics
*Absorption:* Absorbed readily after oral administration. Acetate and tebutate suspensions for injection have a variable absorption, depending on whether they're injected into an intra-articular space or a muscle. Systemic absorption occurs slowly after intra-articular injection.
*Distribution:* Removed rapidly from the blood and distributed to muscle, liver, skin, intestines, and kidneys. Drug is extensively bound to plasma proteins (transcortin and albumin). Only the unbound portion is active. Adrenocorticoids appear in breast milk and through the placenta.
*Metabolism:* Metabolized in the liver to inactive glucuronide and sulfate metabolites.
*Excretion:* The inactive metabolites, and small amounts of unmetabolized drug, are excreted in urine. Insignificant quantities of drug are excreted in feces. Biologic half-life of prednisolone is 18 to 36 hours.

| Route | Onset | Peak | Duration |
|---|---|---|---|
| P.O. | Rapid | 1-2 hr | 3-36 hr |
| I.V. | Rapid | 1 hr | Unknown |
| I.M. | Rapid | 1 hr | 4 wk |

\* Canada only   ◇ Unlabeled clinical use

## Contraindications and precautions

Contraindicated in patients hypersensitive to drug or its ingredients and those with systemic fungal infections.

Use cautiously in patients with a recent MI, GI ulcer, renal disease, hypertension, osteoporosis, diabetes mellitus, hypothyroidism, cirrhosis, diverticulitis, nonspecific ulcerative colitis, recent intestinal anastamoses, thromboembolic disorders, seizures, myasthenia gravis, HF, tuberculosis, ocular herpes simplex, emotional instability, or psychotic tendencies.

## Interactions

**Drug-drug.** *Amphotericin B or diuretics:* May enhance hypokalemia, which may increase the risk of toxicity in patients also receiving cardiac glycosides. Advise clinician to monitor patient closely.

*Antacids, cholestyramine, colestipol:* Decrease effect of prednisolone. Avoid use together.

*Barbiturates, phenytoin, and rifampin:* May cause decreased corticosteroid effects. Corticosteroid dose should be increased p.r.n.

*Estrogens:* May reduce the metabolism of prednisolone. Advise clinician to monitor patient closely.

*Insulin or oral antidiabetics:* Hyperglycemia may occur. May require dosage adjustment in diabetic patients.

*Isoniazid and salicylates:* Increased metabolism of these drugs. Advise clinician to monitor patient closely.

*NSAIDs:* May increase risk of GI ulceration. Give together cautiously.

*Oral anticoagulants:* Prednisolone rarely may decrease the effects of oral anticoagulants. Advise clinician to monitor PT and INR closely.

## Adverse reactions

Most adverse reactions to corticosteroids are dose- or duration-dependent.

**CNS:** *euphoria, insomnia,* psychotic behavior, pseudotumor cerebri, vertigo, headache, paresthesia, *seizures.*

**CV:** *HF, thromboembolism,* hypertension, edema, *arrhythmias,* thrombophlebitis.

**EENT:** cataracts, glaucoma.

**GI:** *peptic ulceration,* GI irritation, increased appetite, *pancreatitis,* nausea, vomiting.

**GU:** menstrual irregularities, increased urine glucose.

**Metabolic:** altered thyroid studies, hypocalcemia, increased serum cholesterol levels, hypokalemia, hyperglycemia, and carbohydrate intolerance.

**Musculoskeletal:** muscle weakness, osteoporosis, growth suppression in children.

**Skin:** delayed wound healing, acne, various skin eruptions, hirsutism.

**Other:** susceptibility to infections; *acute adrenal insufficiency with increased stress (infection, surgery, or trauma) or abrupt withdrawal after long-term therapy,* cushingoid state (moonface, buffalo hump, central obesity). **After abrupt withdrawal:** rebound inflammation, fatigue, weakness, arthralgia, fever, dizziness, lethargy, depression, fainting, orthostatic hypotension, dyspnea, anorexia, hypoglycemia. *After prolonged use, sudden withdrawal may be fatal.*

## Overdose and treatment

Acute ingestion, even in massive doses, is rarely a clinical problem. Toxic signs and symptoms rarely occur if drug is used for less than 3 weeks, even at large dosage ranges. However, chronic use causes adverse physiologic effects, including suppression of the hypothalamic-pituitary-adrenal axis, cushingoid appearance, muscle weakness, and osteoporosis.

## Clinical considerations

**H ALERT** Don't confuse prednisolone with prednisone.

■ Determine if patient is sensitive to other corticosteroid drugs.

■ Recommend always adjusting to lowest effective dose.

■ Store Orapred in the refrigerator.

■ Prednisolone suppresses reactions to skin tests and causes false-negative results in the nitroblue tetrazolium test for systemic bacterial infections.

### Therapeutic monitoring

■ Advise clinician to monitor patient's weight, blood pressure, and serum electrolytes.

■ Advise clinician to watch patient for signs of depression or psychotic episodes, especially in high-dose therapy.

### Special populations

**Pediatric patients.** Chronic use of adrenocorticoids or corticotropin may suppress growth and maturation in children and adolescents.

**Geriatric patients.** Geriatric patients may be more susceptible to osteoporosis with long-term use.

## Patient counseling

■ Instruct patient not to abruptly discontinue drug.

■ Teach patient the signs of early adrenal insufficiency: fatigue, muscular weakness, joint pain, fever, anorexia, nausea, dyspnea, dizziness, and fainting.

■ Patient should carry a medical identification card.

■ Unless contraindicated, patient should follow low-sodium diet that's high in potassium and protein.

■ Advise patient to store Orapred in the refrigerator.

---

Reactions may be *common*, uncommon, *life-threatening*, or COMMON AND LIFE-THREATENING.

# prednisolone acetate (ophthalmic)

AK-Tate, Econopred Ophthalmic,
Ocu-Pred-A, Predair A, Pred Forte,
Pred Mild Ophthalmic

# prednisolone sodium phosphate

AK-Pred, Inflamase Forte, Inflamase
Mild Ophthalmic, I-Pred, Ocu-Pred,
Predair

*Pharmacologic classification:* corticosteroid
*Therapeutic classification:* ophthalmic
anti-inflammatory
*Pregnancy risk category C*

## Available forms

Available by prescription only
**prednisolone acetate**
*Suspension:* 0.12%, 0.125%, 1%
**prednisolone sodium phosphate**
*Solution:* 0.125%, 0.5%, 1%

## Indications and dosages

*Inflammation of palpebral and bulbar
conjunctiva, cornea, and anterior segment
of globe; corneal injury; graft rejection*
Adults and children: Instill 1 or 2 drops in eye.
In severe conditions, may be used hourly, tapering to discontinuation as inflammation subsides. In mild conditions, may be used four to
six times daily.

## Mechanism of action

*Anti-inflammatory action:* Corticosteroids stimulate the synthesis of enzymes needed to decrease the inflammatory response. Prednisolone, a synthetic corticosteroid, has about
four times the anti-inflammatory potency of
an equal weight of hydrocortisone. Prednisolone
acetate is poorly soluble and therefore has a
slower onset of action, but a longer duration
of action, when applied in a liquid suspension.
The sodium phosphate salt is highly soluble
and has a rapid onset but short duration of
action.

## Pharmacokinetics

*Absorption:* After ophthalmic administration,
drug is absorbed through the aqueous humor.
Systemic absorption rarely occurs.
*Distribution:* After ophthalmic application,
drug is distributed throughout local tissue layers. Any drug that's absorbed into circulation
is rapidly removed from the blood and distributed into muscle, liver, skin, intestines, and
kidneys.
*Metabolism:* After ophthalmic administration,
corticosteroids are primarily metabolized locally. The small amount that's absorbed into

systemic circulation is metabolized primarily
in the liver to inactive compounds.
*Excretion:* Inactive metabolites are excreted
by the kidneys, primarily as glucuronides and
sulfates, but also as unconjugated products.
Small amounts of metabolites are excreted in
feces.

| Route | Onset | Peak | Duration |
|-------|-------|------|----------|
| Ophthalmic | Unknown | Unknown | Unknown |

## Contraindications and precautions

Contraindicated in patients with acute, untreated, purulent ocular infections; acute superficial herpes simplex (dendritic keratitis);
vaccinia, varicella, or other viral or fungal eye
diseases; or ocular tuberculosis.
    Use cautiously in patients with corneal abra-
sions that may be contaminated (especially
with herpes).

## Interactions

None reported.

## Adverse reactions

**EENT:** increased intraocular pressure; thinning of cornea, interference with corneal wound
healing, increased susceptibility to viral or fungal corneal infection, corneal ulceration; with
excessive or long-term use: discharge, discomfort, foreign body sensation, glaucoma exacerbation, cataracts, visual acuity and visual
field defects, optic nerve damage.
**Other:** systemic effects and adrenal suppression with excessive or long-term use.

## Overdose and treatment

No information available.

## Clinical considerations

■ Shake suspension and check dosage before
administering. Store in tightly covered
container.

### Therapeutic monitoring

■ Patients on long-term therapy should have
frequent tonometric examinations.

## Patient counseling

■ Teach patient correct way to instill drug.
■ Advise patient to wash hands before and after applying, and warn him not to touch tip of
dropper to eye or surrounding area.
■ Advise patient to apply light pressure on
lacrimal sac for 1 minute after instillation.
■ Warn patient not to share drug or towels with
family members.
■ Tell patient to report if no improvement occurs within several days or if he experiences
pain, itching, or swelling of the eye.

# prednisone acetate

Apo-Prednisone*, Deltasone,
Meticorten, Sterapred, Winpred*

*Pharmacologic classification:* adrenocorticoid
*Therapeutic classification:* anti-
inflammatory, immunosuppressant
*Pregnancy risk category C*

## Available forms

Available by prescription only
*Oral solution:* 5 mg/5 ml
*Oral solution (concentrate):* 5 mg/ml
*Tablets:* 1 mg, 2.5 mg, 5 mg, 10 mg, 20 mg,
25 mg, 50 mg
*Tablets (film-coated):* 5 mg

## Indications and dosages

*Severe inflammation, modification of
body's immune response to disease*
*Adults:* 5 to 60 mg P.O. daily in single dose or
divided doses. Maximum daily dose, 250 mg.
Maintenance dosage given once daily or every
other day. Dosage must be individualized.
*Children:* 0.14 mg/kg or 4 to 6 mg/m$^2$ P.O. dai-
ly in divided doses; alternatively, may use the
following dosage schedule:
*Children ages 11 to 18:* 20 mg P.O. q.i.d.
*Children ages 5 to 10:* 15 mg P.O. q.i.d.
*Children age 18 months to 4 years:* 7.5 to 10 mg
P.O. q.i.d.
*Acute exacerbations of multiple sclerosis*
*Adults:* 200 mg P.O. daily for 1 week, then
80 mg every other day for 1 month.
*Advanced pulmonary or extrapulmonary
tuberculosis*
*Adults:* 40 to 60 mg P.O. daily, tapered over 4
to 8 weeks.
◊ *Adjunct to anti-infective therapy in the
treatment of moderate to severe* **Pneumocystis carinii** *pneumonia*
*Adults or children over age 13 with AIDS:*
40 mg P.O. b.i.d. for 5 days; then 40 mg. P.O.
once daily for 5 days; then 20 mg P.O. once
daily for 11 days (or until completion of the
concurrent anti-infective regimen).

## Mechanism of action

*Anti-inflammatory action:* Prednisone is one
of the intermediate-acting glucocorticoids, with
greater glucocorticoid activity than cortisone
and hydrocortisone, but less anti-inflammatory
activity than betamethasone, dexamethasone,
and paramethasone. Prednisone is about four to
five times more potent as an anti-inflammatory
than hydrocortisone, but it has only half the
mineralocorticoid activity of an equal weight
of hydrocortisone. Prednisone is the oral glucocorticoid of choice for anti-inflammatory or
immunosuppressant effects.

*Immunosuppressant action:* Prednisone stimulates the synthesis of enzymes needed to decrease the inflammatory response. It suppresses
the immune system by reducing activity and
volume of the lymphatic system, producing
lymphocytopenia (primarily of T-lymphocytes),
decreasing immunoglobulin and complement
levels, decreasing passage of immune complexes through basement membranes, and
possibly by depressing reactivity of tissue to
antigen-antibody interactions.

For patients who can't swallow tablets, liquid forms are available. The oral concentrate
(5 mg/ml) may be diluted in juice or another
flavored diluent or mixed in semisolid food
such as applesauce before administration.

## Pharmacokinetics

*Absorption:* Absorbed readily after oral administration.
*Distribution:* Distributed rapidly to muscle,
liver, skin, intestines, and kidneys. Prednisone
is extensively bound to plasma proteins
(transcortin and albumin). Only the unbound
portion is active. Adrenocorticoids appear in
breast milk and through the placenta.
*Metabolism:* Metabolized in the liver to the
active metabolite prednisolone, which, in turn,
is then metabolized to inactive glucuronide and
sulfate metabolites.
*Excretion:* The inactive metabolites and small
amounts of unmetabolized drug are excreted
by the kidneys. Insignificant quantities of drug
are also excreted in feces. Biologic half-life of
prednisone is 18 to 36 hours.

| Route | Onset | Peak | Duration |
|-------|-------|------|----------|
| P.O. | Variable | 1-2 hr | Variable |

## Contraindications and precautions

Contraindicated in patients hypersensitive to
drug or those with systemic fungal infections.

Use cautiously in patients with GI ulcer, renal disease, hypertension, osteoporosis, diabetes mellitus, hypothyroidism, cirrhosis, diverticulitis, nonspecific ulcerative colitis, recent
intestinal anastamoses, thromboembolic disorders, seizures, myasthenia gravis, HF, tuberculosis, ocular herpes simplex, emotional
instability, and psychotic tendencies.

## Interactions

**Drug-drug.** *Amphotericin B or diuretic therapy:* Prednisone may enhance hypokalemia.
Advise clinician to monitor serum potassium
levels.
*Antacids, cholestyramine, colestipol:* Decrease
the amount of prednisone absorbed. Advise
clinician to monitor patient closely.
*Barbiturates, phenytoin, rifampin:* May cause
decreased effects because of increased hepatic metabolism. Advise clinician to monitor patient closely.

*Cardiac glycosides:* Increase the risk of toxicity in patients concurrently receiving cardiac glycosides. Advise clinician to monitor patient closely.

*Estrogens:* May reduce the metabolism of prednisone by increasing the level of transcortin. Advise clinician to monitor patient closely.

*Insulin or oral antidiabetics:* Causes hyperglycemia. Dosage adjustment is needed.

*Isoniazid and salicylates:* Prednisone increases the metabolism of isoniazid and salicylates. Advise clinician to monitor patient for lack of effect.

*NSAIDs:* May increase the risk of GI ulceration. Give together cautiously.

*Oral anticoagulants:* Use of prednisone may decrease clotting factors. Advise clinician to monitor PT and INR closely.

**Drug-herb.** *Alfalfa sprouts, astragulus, echinacea, licorice:* Possible interference with immunosuppressive effect of the drug. Discourage use together.

## Adverse reactions

Most adverse reactions to corticosteroids are dose- or duration-dependent.

**CNS:** *euphoria, insomnia,* psychotic behavior, pseudotumor cerebri, vertigo, headache, paresthesia, *seizures.*

**CV:** hypertension, edema, *arrhythmias,* thrombophlebitis, *thromboembolism, HF.*

**EENT:** cataracts, glaucoma.

**GI:** *peptic ulceration,* GI irritation, increased appetite, *pancreatitis,* nausea, vomiting.

**GU:** menstrual irregularities, increased urine glucose.

**Musculoskeletal:** muscle weakness, osteoporosis, growth suppression in children.

**Skin:** delayed wound healing, acne, various skin eruptions, hirsutism.

**Other:** altered thyroid tests, elevated serum cholesterol; hypocalcemia; susceptibility to infections; hypokalemia, hyperglycemia, and carbohydrate intolerance; *acute adrenal insufficiency may occur with increased stress (infection, surgery, or trauma) or abrupt withdrawal after long-term therapy,* cushingoid state (moonface, buffalo hump, central obesity).

**After abrupt withdrawal:** rebound inflammation, fatigue, weakness, arthralgia, fever, dizziness, lethargy, depression, fainting, orthostatic hypotension, dyspnea, anorexia, hypoglycemia. *After prolonged use, sudden withdrawal may be fatal.*

## Overdose and treatment

Acute ingestion, even in massive doses, is rarely a clinical problem. Toxic signs and symptoms rarely occur if drug is used for less than 3 weeks, even at large dosage ranges. However, chronic use causes adverse physiologic effects, including suppression of the hypothalamic-pituitary-adrenal axis, cushingoid appearance, muscle weakness, and osteoporosis.

## Clinical considerations

■ Determine if patient is sensitive to other corticosteroid drugs.
■ For better results and less toxicity, recommend giving a once-daily dose in the morning.
■ Prednisone suppresses reactions to skin tests and causes false-negative results in the nitroblue tetrazolium test for systemic bacterial infections.

### Therapeutic monitoring

■ Advise clinician to monitor patient's blood pressure, sleep patterns, and serum potassium levels.
■ Advise clinician to weigh patient daily.
■ Advise clinician to watch patient for depression or psychotic episodes, especially in high-dose therapy.

### Special populations

**Pediatric patients.** Chronic use of prednisone in drug or adolescents may delay growth and maturation.

**Geriatric patients.** Geriatric patients may be more susceptible to osteoporosis with long-term therapy.

## Patient counseling

■ Tell patient not to stop drug abruptly or without prescriber's consent.
■ Instruct patient to take drug with food or milk.
■ Instruct patient to carry a card identifying his need for supplemental systemic glucocorticosteroids during stress.

# primaquine phosphate

*Pharmacologic classification:* 8-aminoquinoline
*Therapeutic classification:* antimalarial
*Pregnancy risk category C*

## Available forms

Available by prescription only
*Tablets:* 26.3 mg (15-mg base)

## Indications and dosages

*Radical cure of relapsing vivax malaria, eliminating symptoms and infection completely, and prevention of relapse*
*Adults:* 15 mg (base) P.O. daily for 14 days (26.3-mg tablet equals 15 mg of base), or 79 mg (45-mg base) once weekly for 8 weeks.
*Children:* 0.3 mg (base)/kg/day for 14 days, or 0.9 mg (base)/kg/day once weekly for 8 weeks.
◇ **Pneumocystis carinii** *pneumonia*
*Adults:* 15 to 30 mg (base) P.O. daily.

## Mechanism of action

*Antimalarial action:* Primaquine disrupts the parasitic mitochondria, thereby interrupting metabolic processes requiring energy.

Spectrum of activity includes preerythrocytic and exoerythrocytic forms of *Plasmodium falciparum, P. malariae, P. ovale,* and *P. vivax.* Nifurtimox (Lampit), an investigational drug available from the Centers for Disease Control and Prevention, is preferred for intracellular parasites.

## Pharmacokinetics
*Absorption:* Well absorbed from the GI tract.
*Distribution:* Distributed widely into the liver, lungs, heart, brain, skeletal muscle, and other tissues.
*Metabolism:* Carboxylated rapidly in the liver.
*Excretion:* Only a small amount is excreted unchanged in urine. Plasma half-life is 4 to 10 hours.

| Route | Onset | Peak | Duration |
|-------|-------|------|----------|
| P.O. | Unknown | 1-3 hr | Unknown |

## Contraindications and precautions
Contraindicated in patients with systemic diseases in which granulocytopenia may develop (such as lupus erythematosus or rheumatoid arthritis) and in those taking bone marrow suppressants and potentially hemolytic drugs.

Use cautiously in patients with previous idiosyncratic reaction (manifested by hemolytic anemia, methemoglobinemia, or leukopenia) and in those with family or personal history of favism, erythrocytic G6PD deficiency, or nicotinamide adenine dinucleotide (NADH) methemoglobin reductase deficiency.

## Interactions
**Drug-drug.** *Magnesium and aluminum salts:* May decrease GI absorption. Recommend giving drugs at separate times.
*Quinacrine:* May potentiate the toxic effects of primaquine. Don't use together.

## Adverse reactions
**GI:** nausea, vomiting, epigastric distress, abdominal cramps.
**Hematologic:** *leukopenia, hemolytic anemia in G6PD deficiency,* methemoglobinemia in NADH methemoglobin reductase deficiency.

## Overdose and treatment
Signs and symptoms of overdose include abdominal distress, vomiting, CNS and CV disturbances, cyanosis, methemoglobinemia, leukocytosis, leukopenia, and anemia. Treatment is symptomatic.

## Clinical considerations
**⚠ ALERT** Drug dosage may be discussed in mg or mg-base. Be aware of the difference.
■ Primaquine is often used with a fast-acting antimalarial, such as chloroquine.
■ Before therapy starts, patients should be screened for possible G6PD deficiency.

■ Light-skinned patients taking more than 30 mg daily, dark-skinned patients taking more than 15 mg daily, and patients with severe anemia or suspected sensitivity should have frequent blood studies and urine examinations. A sudden decrease in hemoglobin levels or erythrocyte or leukocyte counts, or a marked darkening of the urine suggests impending hemolytic reaction.

### Therapeutic monitoring
■ Advise clinician to perform periodic blood tests and urinalyses to monitor for impending hemolytic reactions.

### Special populations
**Pregnant patients.** Safety for use during pregnancy hasn't been established.
**Breast-feeding patients.** Safety in breast-feeding women hasn't been established.

## Patient counseling
■ Teach patient signs and symptoms of adverse reactions and to report them if they occur.
■ Advise patient to check urine color at each voiding and to report if urine darkens, becomes tinged with red, or decreases in volume.
■ Tell patient to take drug with meals to minimize gastric irritation and not to take with antacids, which may decrease absorption.
■ Advise patient to complete entire course of therapy.

# primidone
Myidone, Mysoline, Sertan

*Pharmacologic classification:* barbiturate analogue
*Therapeutic classification:* anticonvulsant
*Pregnancy risk category NR*

## Available forms
Available by prescription only
*Suspension:* 250 mg/5 ml
*Tablets:* 50 mg, 250 mg

## Indications and dosages
*Generalized tonic-clonic seizures, focal seizures, complex-partial (psychomotor) seizures*
*Adults and children ages 8 and older:* 100 to 125 mg P.O. h.s. on days 1 to 3; 100 to 125 mg P.O. b.i.d. on days 4 to 6; 100 to 125 mg P.O. t.i.d. on days 7 to 9; and maintenance dosage of 250 mg P.O. t.i.d. on day 10. May require up to 2 g/day.
*Children under age 8:* 50 mg P.O. h.s. on days 1 to 3; 50 mg P.O. b.i.d. on days 4 to 6; 100 mg P.O. t.i.d. on days 7 to 9; and maintenance dosage of 125 to 250 mg P.O. t.i.d. on day 10.
*Benign familial tremor (essential tremor)*
*Adults:* 750 mg P.O. daily.

---

## Mechanism of action

*Anticonvulsant action:* Primidone acts as a non-specific CNS depressant used alone or with other anticonvulsants to control refractory tonic-clonic seizures and to treat psychomotor or focal seizures. Mechanism of action is unknown; some activity may be from phenobarbital, an active metabolite.

## Pharmacokinetics

*Absorption:* Absorbed readily from the GI tract. Phenobarbital appears in plasma after several days of continuous therapy; most laboratory assays detect both phenobarbital and primidone. Therapeutic levels are 5 to 12 mcg/ml for primidone and 10 to 30 mcg/ml for phenobarbital.
*Distribution:* Distributed widely throughout the body.
*Metabolism:* Metabolized slowly by the liver to phenylethylmalonamide (PEMA) and phenobarbital; PEMA is the major metabolite.
*Excretion:* Excreted in urine; substantial amounts appear in breast milk.

| Route | Onset | Peak | Duration |
|-------|-------|------|----------|
| P.O. | Unknown | 3-4 hr | Unknown |

## Contraindications and precautions

Contraindicated in patients with phenobarbital hypersensitivity or porphyria.

## Interactions

**Drug-drug.** *Acetazolamide and succinimides:* Coadministration may decrease levels of primidone. Advise clinician to monitor levels.
*Carbamazepine, phenytoin:* May decrease effects of primidone and increase its conversion to phenobarbital. Advise clinician to monitor serum levels to prevent toxicity.
*CNS depressants:* Cause excessive depression in patients taking primidone. Don't use together.
**Drug-lifestyle.** *Alcohol use:* Causes excessive depression in patients taking primidone. Advise patient to avoid alcohol.

## Adverse reactions

**CNS:** *drowsiness, ataxia,* emotional disturbances, vertigo, hyperirritability, fatigue, paranoia.
**EENT:** *diplopia,* nystagmus.
**GI:** anorexia, nausea, vomiting.
**GU:** impotence, polyuria.
**Hematologic:** megaloblastic anemia, *thrombocytopenia.*
**Hepatic:** abnormalities in liver function test results.
**Skin:** morbilliform rash.

## Overdose and treatment

Signs and symptoms of overdose resemble those of barbiturate intoxication; they include CNS and respiratory depression, areflexia, olig-uria, tachycardia, hypotension, hypothermia, and coma. Shock may occur.

Overdose should be treated supportively. In conscious patient with intact gag reflex, emesis should be induced with ipecac, followed in 30 minutes with repeated doses of activated charcoal. Lavage should be used if emesis isn't feasible. Alkalinization of urine and forced diuresis may hasten excretion. Hemodialysis may be needed. Advise clinician to monitor vital signs and fluid and electrolyte balance.

## Clinical considerations

■ Abrupt withdrawal of drug may cause status epilepticus; dosage should be reduced gradually.
■ Barbiturates impair ability to perform tasks requiring mental alertness, such as driving a car.

### Therapeutic monitoring

■ Advise clinician to perform a CBC and liver function tests every 6 months.

### Special populations

**Breast-feeding patients.** Considerable amounts of drug appear in breast milk; recommend using an alternative feeding method during therapy.
**Pediatric patients.** Primidone may cause hyperexcitability in children under age 6.
**Geriatric patients.** Reduce dose in geriatric patients; many have decreased renal function.

## Patient counseling

■ Explain reason for therapy and the potential risks and benefits.
■ Teach patient signs and symptoms of adverse reactions.
■ Instruct patient not to stop drug or alter dosage without medical approval.
■ Explain that barbiturates may render oral contraceptives ineffective; advise patient to consider a different birth control method.
■ Advise patient to avoid hazardous tasks that require mental alertness until degree of sedative effect is determined. Tell the patient that dizziness and incoordination are common at first but will disappear.
■ Recommend that patient wear a medical identification bracelet or necklace identifying him as having a seizure disorder and listing drug.
■ Tell patient to shake oral suspension well before use.

# probenecid

Benemid, Probalan

*Pharmacologic classification:*
sulfonamide-derivative
*Therapeutic classification:* uricosuric
*Pregnancy risk category NR*

## Available forms

Available by prescription only
*Tablets:* 500 mg
*Tablets (film-coated):* 500 mg

## Indications and dosages

*Adjunct to penicillin therapy*
*Adults and children over age 14 or weighing over 50 kg (110 lb):* 500 mg P.O. q.i.d.
*Children ages 2 to 14 or weighing under 50 kg:* Initially, 25 mg/kg or 700 mg/m² daily, then 40 mg/kg or 1.2 g/m² divided q.i.d.
*Single-dose penicillin treatment of gonorrhea*
*Adults:* 1 g P.O. given together with penicillin treatment, or 1 g P.O. 30 minutes before I.M. dose of penicillin.
*Hyperuricemia with gout*
*Adults:* 250 mg P.O. b.i.d. for first week, then 500 mg b.i.d., to maximum of 2 to 3 g daily.
◇ *To diagnose parkinsonian syndrome or mental depression*
*Adults:* 500 mg P.O. q 12 hours for five doses.

## Mechanism of action

*Adjunctive action in antibiotic therapy:* Probenecid competitively inhibits secretion of weak organic acids, including penicillins, cephalosporins, and other beta-lactam antibiotics, increasing serum levels of these drugs.
*Uricosuric action:* Probenecid competitively inhibits the active reabsorption of uric acid at the proximal convoluted tubule, increasing urinary excretion of uric acid.

## Pharmacokinetics

*Absorption:* Completely absorbed after oral administration.
*Distribution:* Distributed throughout the body; drug is about 75% protein-bound. CSF levels are about 2% of serum levels.
*Metabolism:* Metabolized in the liver to active metabolites, with some uricosuric effect.
*Excretion:* Drug and metabolites are excreted in urine; probenecid (but not metabolites) is actively reabsorbed.

| Route | Onset | Peak | Duration |
|-------|-------|------|----------|
| P.O. | Unknown | 2-4 hr | Unknown |

## Contraindications and precautions

Contraindicated in patients hypersensitive to drug, and those with uric acid kidney stones or blood dyscrasias; in acute gout attack; and in children under age 2.

Use cautiously in patients with impaired renal function or peptic ulcer.

## Interactions

**Drug-drug.** *Aminosalicylic acid, dapsone, methotrexate, nitrofurantoin:* Increased serum levels of these drugs, which increase risk of toxicity. Altered doses may be needed.
*Cephalosporins, penicillins, and other beta-lactam antibiotics, sulfonamides, and possibly ketamine and thiopental:* Probenecid significantly increases or prolongs effects of these drugs. Use together cautiously.
*Chlorpropamide and other oral sulfonylureas:* Enhanced hypoglycemic effects. Advise clinician to monitor blood glucose levels.
*Diuretics and pyrazinamide:* Decrease uric acid levels of probenecid; increased doses of probenecid may be required.
*Indomethacin, naproxen:* Decreased excretion of these drugs. Use of lower doses may be possible.
*Salicylates:* Inhibit the uricosuric effect of probenecid only in doses that achieve levels of 50 mcg/ml or more. Don't use together.
*Zidovudine:* Cutaneous eruptions accompanied by systemic symptoms, including malaise, myalgia, or fever. Advise clinician to monitor patient.
**Drug-lifestyle.** *Alcohol use:* Decreases uric acid levels of probenecid; increased doses of probenecid may be required.

## Adverse reactions

**CNS:** *headache,* dizziness.
**GI:** anorexia, nausea, vomiting, sore gums.
**GU:** urinary frequency, renal colic, nephrotic syndrome.
**Hematologic:** *hemolytic anemia, aplastic anemia,* anemia.
**Hepatic:** *hepatic necrosis.*
**Skin:** dermatitis, pruritus, flushing.
**Other:** fever, exacerbation of gout, hypersensitivity reactions (including *anaphylaxis).*

## Overdose and treatment

Signs and symptoms include nausea, copious vomiting, stupor, coma, and tonic-clonic seizures. Recommend treating supportively, using mechanical ventilation, if needed; recommend inducing emesis or using gastric lavage, as appropriate. Seizures should be controlled with I.V. phenobarbital and phenytoin.

## Clinical considerations

■ When used for hyperuricemia with gout, probenecid has no analgesic or anti-inflammatory actions, and no effect on acute attacks; therapy should be started after attack subsides. Because drug may increase the frequency of acute attacks during the first 6 to 12 months of therapy, prophylactic doses of colchicine or an NSAID should be given dur-

ing the first 3 to 6 months of probenecid therapy.
- Recommend giving with food, milk, or prescribed antacids to lessen GI upset.
- Recommend maintaining adequate hydration with high fluid intake to prevent formation of uric acid stones. Alkalinization of urine
should also be maintained.
- Drug has been used in the diagnosis of parkinsonian syndrome and mental depression.
- Probenecid causes false-positive test results
for urinary glucose with tests using cupric sulfate reagent (Benedict's reagent, Clinitest, and
Fehling's test); perform tests with glucose oxidase reagent (Diastix, Chemstrip uG, or glucose enzymatic test strip) instead.

### Therapeutic monitoring
- Advise clinician to monitor BUN and serum
creatinine levels closely; drug is ineffective in
severe renal insufficiency.
- Advise clinician to monitor uric acid levels
and adjusting dose to the lowest dose that maintains normal uric acid levels.

### Special populations
**Breast-feeding patients.** It's unknown if drug
appears in breast milk. An alternative feeding
method is recommended during therapy.
**Pediatric patients.** Drug is contraindicated in
infants under age 2.
**Geriatric patients.** Lower doses are indicated in geriatric patients.

### Patient counseling
- Instruct patient not to discontinue drug without medical approval.
- Warn patient not to use drug for pain or inflammation and not to increase dose during
gouty attack.
- Tell patient to drink 8 to 10 glasses of fluid
daily and to take drug with food to minimize
GI upset.

# procainamide hydrochloride
Procanbid, Promine, Pronestyl,
Pronestyl-SR

*Pharmacologic classification:* procaine
derivative
*Therapeutic classification:* ventricular
antiarrhythmic, supraventricular antiarrhythmic
*Pregnancy risk category C*

### Available forms
Available by prescription only
*Capsules:* 250 mg, 375 mg, 500 mg
*Injection:* 100 mg/ml, 500 mg/ml
*Tablets (film-coated):* 250 mg, 375 mg, 500 mg
*Tablets (extended-release, film-coated):* 250 mg,
500 mg, 750 mg, 1 g

## Indications and dosages
*Symptomatic PVCs, life-threatening
ventricular tachycardia*
*Adults:* 100 mg q 5 minutes by slow I.V. push,
no faster than 25 to 50 mg/minute, until arrhythmias disappear, adverse effects develop,
or 500 mg has been given. When arrhythmias
disappear, give continuous infusion of 2 to
6 mg/minute. Usual effective loading dose is
500 to 600 mg. If arrhythmias recur, repeat bolus as above and increase infusion rate. For
I.M. administration, give 50 mg/kg divided q
3 to 6 hours; arrythmias during surgery, 100 to
500 mg I.M. For oral therapy, initiate dosage
at 50 mg/kg P.O. in divided doses q 3 hours
until therapeutic levels are reached. For the
maintenance dose, substitute sustained-release
form q 6 hours or extended-release form (Procanbid) at dose of 50 mg/kg in two divided
doses q 12 hours.
◇ *Maintainance of normal sinus rhythm
after conversion of atrial flutter*
*Adults:* 0.5 to 1 g P.O. every 4 to 6 hours.
◇ *Loading dose to prevent atrial fibrillation or paroxysmal atrial tachycardia*
*Adults:* 1.25 g P.O. If arrhythmias persist after
1 hour, give additional 750 mg. If no change
occurs, give 500 mg to 1 g P.O. q 2 hours until arrhythmias disappear or adverse effects occur. Maintenance dose is 1 g every 6 hours.
◇ *Treatment of malignant hyperthermia*
*Adults:* 200 to 900 mg I.V., followed by an infusion.

## I.V. administration
- Dilute with $D_5W$ and administer to patient
in a supine position at a rate not exceeding
50 mg/minute.
- Advise clinician to monitor patient receiving infusions at all times.
- Advise clinician to monitor blood presser
and ECG, and adjust the rate of infusion accordingly.
- Recommend using infusion pump or microdrip system and timer to monitor infusion precisely.
- Closely follow manufacturer's instructions.

### Incompatibilities
Incompatible with bretylium, esmolol, ethacrynate, milrinone, and phenytoin sodium.

## Mechanism of action
*Antiarrhythmic action:* A class IA antiarrhythmic, procainamide depresses phase 0 of the action potential. It's considered a myocardial depressant because it decreases myocardial
excitability and conduction velocity and may
depress myocardial contractility. It also possesses anticholinergic activity, which may modify its direct myocardial effects. In therapeutic doses, it reduces conduction velocity in the
atria, ventricles, and His-Purkinje system. Its
effectiveness in controlling atrial tachyarrhyth-

mias stems from its ability to prolong the effective refractory period (ERP) and increase the action potential duration in the atria, ventricles, and His-Purkinje system. Because ERP prolongation exceeds action potential duration, tissue remains refractory even after returning to resting membrane potential (membrane-stabilizing effect).

Procainamide shortens the effective refractory period of the AV node. Anticholinergic action of drug also may increase AV node conductivity. Suppression of automaticity in the His-Purkinje system and ectopic pacemakers accounts for effectiveness of drug in treating ventricular premature beats. At therapeutic doses, procainamide prolongs the PR and QT intervals. (This effect may be used as an index of drug effectiveness and toxicity.) The QRS interval usually isn't prolonged beyond normal range; the QT interval isn't prolonged to the extent achieved with quinidine.

Procainamide exerts a peripheral vasodilatory effect; with I.V. administration, it may cause hypotension, which limits the administration rate and amount of drug deliverable.

## Pharmacokinetics

*Absorption:* Rate and extent of absorption from the intestines vary; usually, 75% to 95% of an orally given dose is absorbed. Extended-release tablets are formulated to provide a sustained and relatively constant rate of release and absorption throughout the small intestine. After release of drug, extended wax matrix isn't absorbed and may appear in feces after 15 minutes to 1 hour.

*Distribution:* Distributed widely in most body tissues, including CSF, liver, spleen, kidneys, lungs, muscles, brain, and heart. Only about 15% plasma protein–bound. Usual therapeutic range for serum procainamide levels is 4 to 8 mcg/ml. Some experts suggest that a range of 10 to 30 mcg/ml for the sum of procainamide and N-acetyl procainamide (NAPA) serum levels are therapeutic.

*Metabolism:* Acetylated in the liver to form NAPA. Acetylation rate is determined genetically and affects NAPA formation. NAPA also exerts antiarrhythmic activity.

*Excretion:* Procainamide and NAPA metabolite are excreted in the urine. Half-life of procainamide is about 2½ to 4¾ hours. Half-life of NAPA is about 6 hours. In patients with HF or renal dysfunction, half-life increases; therefore, in such patients, dosage reduction is required to avoid toxicity.

| Route | Onset | Peak | Duration |
|-------|-------|------|----------|
| P.O. | 1-2 hr | ½-1½ hr | Unknown |
| I.V. | Immediate | Immediate | Unknown |
| I.M. | 10-30 min | 15-60 min | Unknown |

## Contraindications and precautions

Contraindicated in patients hypersensitive to procaine and related drugs; in those with complete, second-, or third-degree heart block in the absence of an artificial pacemaker; and in patients with myasthenia gravis or systemic lupus erythematosus. Also contraindicated in patients with atypical ventricular tachycardia (torsades de pointes) because procainamide may aggravate this condition.

Use cautiously in patients with ventricular tachycardia during coronary occlusion; HF or other conduction disturbances, such as bundle-branch heart block, sinus bradycardia, and cardiac glycoside intoxication; impaired renal or hepatic function; preexisting blood dyscrasia; or bone marrow suppression.

## Interactions

**Drug-drug.** *Anticholinergics, such as atropine, diphenhydramine, and tricyclic antidepressants:* May cause additive anticholinergic effects. Limit concomitant use as much as possible. Advise clinician to monitor patient closely.
*Antihypertensives:* May cause additive hypotensive effects (most common with I.V. procainamide). Advise clinician to monitor blood pressure closely.
*Cholinergics, such as neostigmine and pyridostigmine:* May negate the effects of these drugs, requiring increased dosage.
*Cimetidine:* May result in impaired renal clearance of procainamide and NAPA, with elevated serum drug levels. Advise clinician to monitor patient for toxicity.
*Neuromuscular blockers, such as decamethonium bromide, gallium triethiodide, metocurine iodide, pancuronium bromide, succinylcholine chloride, and tubocurarine chloride:* May potentiate the effects of the neuromuscular blockers. Advise clinician to monitor patient closely.
*Other antiarrhythmics:* May result in additive or antagonistic cardiac effects and with possible additive toxic effects. Use cautiously.
**Drug-herb.** *Jimsonweed:* May adversely affect the function of the CV system. Discourage use together.
*Licorice:* May prolong the QT interval and be potentially additive. Discourage use together.
**Drug-lifestyle.** *Alcohol use:* Reduced drug levels. Advise patient to avoid alcohol.

## Adverse reactions

**CNS:** hallucinations, confusion, *seizures,* depression, dizziness.
**CV:** *hypotension, ventricular asystole, bradycardia,* AV block, *ventricular fibrillation* (after parenteral use).
**GI:** nausea, vomiting, anorexia, diarrhea, bitter taste.
**Hematologic:** *thrombocytopenia, neutropenia* (especially with sustained-release forms), *agranulocytosis, hemolytic anemia.*
**Hepatic:** elevated liver function test results.

**Skin:** *maculopapular rash, urticaria, pruritus, flushing, angioneurotic edema.*
**Other:** *fever, lupuslike syndrome* (especially after prolonged administration) positive antinuclear antibody (ANA) titers, positive direct antiglobulin (Coombs') tests.

## Overdose and treatment

Effects of overdose include severe hypotension, widening QRS complex, junctional tachycardia, intraventricular conduction delay, ventricular fibrillation, oliguria, confusion and lethargy, and nausea and vomiting.

Treatment involves general supportive measures, including respiratory and CV support, with hemodynamic and ECG monitoring. After recent ingestion of oral form, gastric lavage, emesis, and activated charcoal may be used to decrease absorption. Phenylephrine or norepinephrine may be used to treat hypotension after adequate hydration has been ensured. Hemodialysis may be effective in removing procainamide and NAPA. A 1/6 M solution of sodium lactate may reduce cardiotoxic effect of procainamide.

## Clinical considerations

■ In treating atrial fibrillation and flutter, ventricular rate may accelerate from vagolytic effects on the AV node; to prevent this effect, a cardiac glycoside may be given before procainamide therapy begins.
■ Baseline and periodic determinations of ANA titers, lupus erythematosus cell preparations, and CBCs may be indicated because procainamide therapy (usually long-term) has caused a syndrome resembling systemic lupus erythematosus.
■ For initial oral therapy, recommend using conventional capsules and tablets; extended-release tablets should only be used for maintenance therapy.
■ I.V. drug form is more likely to cause adverse cardiac effects, possibly resulting in severe hypotension.
■ In prolonged use of oral form, perform ECGs occasionally to determine continued need for drug.
■ Procainamide invalidates bentiromide test results; drug should be stopped at least 3 days before bentiromide test. Procainamide may alter edrophonium test results.

### Therapeutic monitoring

■ Advise clinician to monitor blood pressure and ECG continuously during I.V. administration and watch for prolonged QT and QRS intervals (50% or greater widening), heart block, or increased arrhythmias. When these ECG signs appear, procainamide should be discontinued and the patient monitored closely.
■ Advise clinician to monitor therapeutic serum levels of procainamide: 3 to 10 mcg/ml (most patients are controlled at 4 to 8 mcg/ml and

may exhibit toxicity at levels greater than 16 mcg/ml). Advise clinician to monitor NAPA levels as well; some clinicians believe that procainamide and NAPA levels should be 10 to 30 mcg/ml.
■ Advise clinician to monitor renal function.

### Special populations

**Breast-feeding patients.** Because procainamide and NAPA appear in breast milk, an alternative feeding method is recommended for women receiving procainamide.
**Pediatric patients.** Manufacturer hasn't established dosage guidelines for pediatric patients because safety in children hasn't been established. For treating arrhythmias, the suggested dosage 2 to 5 mg/kg (not exceeding 100 mg) I.V. Repeat every 5 to 10 minutes. Don't exceed 15 mg/kg/day or 500 mg/30 minutes. For I.M. administration, give 20 to 30 mg/kg/day I.M. divided every 4 to 6 hours. Maximum 4 g/day.
**Geriatric patients.** Geriatric patients may require reduced dosage. Take into consideration their hepatic, renal, and cardiac function, concomitant disease states and drugs.

## Patient counseling

■ Stress importance of taking drug exactly as prescribed.
■ Instruct patient to report fever, rash, muscle pain, diarrhea, bruises, or pleuritic chest pain.

# procarbazine hydrochloride
Matulane, Natulan*

*Pharmacologic classification*: antibiotic antineoplastic (cell cycle-phase specific, S phase)
*Therapeutic classification:* antineoplastic
*Pregnancy risk category D*

## Available forms

Available by prescription only
*Capsules:* 50 mg

## Indications and dosages

Dosage and indications may vary. Check current literature for recommended protocol.
***Hodgkin's disease, lymphomas, brain and lung cancer***
*Adults:* 2 to 4 mg/kg/day P.O. in single or divided doses for the first week, followed by 4 to 6 mg/kg/day until response or toxicity occurs. Maintenance dose is 1 to 2 mg/kg/day.
*Children:* 50 mg/m$^2$ daily P.O. for first week, then 100 mg/m$^2$ daily until response or toxicity occurs. Maintenance dose is 50 mg/m$^2$ P.O. daily after bone marrow recovery.

## Mechanism of action
*Antineoplastic action:* Exact mechanism of cytotoxic activity of procarbazine is unknown. Drug appears to have several sites of action; the result is inhibition of DNA, RNA, and protein synthesis. Procarbazine has also been reported to damage DNA directly and to inhibit the mitotic S phase of cell division.

## Pharmacokinetics
*Absorption:* Rapidly and completely absorbed after oral administration.
*Distribution:* Distributed widely into body tissues, with the highest levels found in the liver, kidneys, intestinal wall, and skin. Drug crosses the blood-brain barrier.
*Metabolism:* Extensively metabolized in the liver. Some metabolites have cytotoxic activity.
*Excretion:* Excreted primarily in urine.

| Route | Onset | Peak | Duration |
|-------|-------|------|----------|
| P.O. | Unknown | Unknown | Unknown |

## Contraindications and precautions
Contraindicated in patients hypersensitive to drug and in those with inadequate bone marrow reserve as shown by bone marrow aspiration.

Use cautiously in patients with impaired renal or hepatic function.

## Interactions
**Drug-drug.** *CNS depressants:* Enhanced CNS depression through an additive mechanism. Avoid use together.
*Digoxin:* Serum digoxin levels may be decreased. Advise clinician to monitor patient closely.
*Levodopa:* May cause flushing and a significant increase in blood pressure. Advise clinician to monitor patient closely.
*MAO inhibitors, selective serotonin reuptake inhibitors, sympathomimetics, or tricyclic antidepressants:* May cause a hypertensive crisis, tremors, excitation, and cardiac palpitations. Advise clinician to monitor patient closely.
*Meperidine:* May result in severe hypotension and death. Avoid use together.
**Drug-food.** *Tyramine-containing foods:* May cause a hypertensive crisis, tremors, excitation, and cardiac palpitations. Don't give together.
**Drug-lifestyle.** *Alcohol use:* May cause a disulfiram-like reaction. Advise patient to avoid alcohol.
*Sun exposure:* May cause photosensitivity reactions. Advise patient to use sunblock.

## Adverse reactions
**CNS:** nervousness, depression, headache, dizziness, *coma, seizures,* insomnia, nightmares, paresthesia, neuropathy, *hallucinations,* confusion.
**CV:** hypotension, tachycardia, syncope.

**EENT:** retinal hemorrhage, nystagmus, photophobia.
**GI:** *nausea, vomiting,* anorexia, stomatitis, dry mouth, dysphagia, diarrhea, constipation.
**GU:** hematuria, urinary frequency, nocturia.
**Hematologic:** *bleeding tendency, thrombocytopenia, leukopenia, anemia,* hemolytic anemia.
**Respiratory:** *pleural effusion,* pneumonitis, cough.
**Skin:** dermatitis, pruritus, rash, reversible alopecia.
**Other:** allergic reactions, gynecomastia.

## Overdose and treatment
Signs and symptoms of overdose include myalgia, arthralgia, fever, weakness, dermatitis, alopecia, paresthesia, hallucinations, tremors, seizures, coma, myelosuppression, nausea, and vomiting.

Treatment is usually supportive and includes transfusion of blood components, antiemetics, antipyretics, and appropriate antianxiety drugs.

## Clinical considerations
■ Nausea and vomiting may be decreased if drug is taken h.s. and in divided doses.
■ Drug should be used cautiously in inadequate bone marrow reserve, leukopenia, thrombocytopenia, anemia, and impaired hepatic or renal function.
■ Store capsules in dry environment.

### Therapeutic monitoring
■ Patient should be observed for signs of bleeding.
■ Advise clinician to monitor CBC and platelet counts.

### Special populations
**Pregnant patients.** Drug causes fetal toxicity and teratogenicity in laboratory studies. Advise patient not to become pregnant while on drug therapy and to consult prescriber before becoming pregnant.
**Breast-feeding patients.** It isn't known if drug appears in breast milk. However, because of potential for serious adverse reactions, mutagenicity, and carcinogenicity in the infant, breast-feeding isn't recommended.
**Pediatric patients.** Severe reactions, such as tremors, seizures, and coma, have occurred in children after administration of procarbazine.

## Patient counseling
■ Emphasize importance of continuing drug despite nausea and vomiting.
■ Advise patient to immediately report if vomiting occurs shortly after taking dose.
■ Warn patient that drowsiness may occur, so patient should avoid hazardous activities that require alertness until effect of drug is established.

---

■ Instruct patient to stop drug and immediately report disulfiram-like reactions, such as chest pains, rapid or irregular heartbeat, severe headache, or stiff neck, that may occur.

■ Tell patient to avoid exposure to people with infections.

■ Tell patient to contact prescriber if a sore throat or fever or unusual bruising or bleeding occurs.

# prochlorperazine
Compazine, Compro, Stemetil*

# prochlorperazine edisylate
Compazine

# prochlorperazine maleate
Compazine, Compazine Spansule, Stemetil*

*Pharmacologic classification:* phenothiazine (piperazine derivative)
*Therapeutic classification:* antipsychotic, antiemetic, antianxiety
*Pregnancy risk category C*

## Available forms
Available by prescription only
**prochlorperazine edisylate**
*Spansules (sustained-release):* 10 mg, 15 mg
*Syrup:* 5 mg/ml
*Injection:* 10 mg/2 ml
**prochlorperazine maleate**
*Tablets:* 5 mg, 10 mg
*Suppositories:* 2.5 mg, 5 mg, 25 mg

## Indications and dosages
*Preoperative nausea control*
*Adults:* 5 to 10 mg I.M. 1 to 2 hours before induction of anesthesia, repeated once in 30 minutes, if needed; or 5 to 10 mg I.V. 15 to 30 minutes before induction of anesthesia, repeated once, if needed; or 20 mg/L D₅W and normal saline solution by I.V. infusion, added to infusion 15 to 30 minutes before induction. Maximum parenteral dose is 40 mg daily.
*Severe nausea, vomiting*
*Adults:* 5 to 10 mg P.O. t.i.d. or q.i.d.; or 15 mg of sustained-release form P.O. on arising; or 10 mg of sustained-release form P.O. q 12 hours; or 25 mg P.R. b.i.d.; or 5 to 10 mg I.M. injected deeply into upper outer quadrant of gluteal region. Repeat q 3 to 4 hours, p.r.n. May be given I.V. Maximum parenteral dose, 40 mg daily.
*Children weighing 18 to 39 kg (39 to 86 lb):* 2.5 mg P.O. or rectally t.i.d.; or 5 mg P.O. or P.R. b.i.d.; or 0.132 mg/kg deep I.M. injection (control usually obtained with one dose). Maximum dose is 15 mg daily.
*Children weighing 14 to 17 kg (31 to 38 lb):* 2.5 mg P.O. or P.R. b.i.d. or t.i.d.; or 0.132 mg/kg

deep I.M. injection (control usually is obtained with one dose). Maximum dose, 10 mg daily.
*Children weighing 9 to 14 kg (20 to 30 lb):* 2.5 mg P.O. or P.R. daily or b.i.d.; or 0.132 mg/kg deep I.M. injection (control usually is obtained with one dose). Maximum dose, 7.5 mg daily.
*Anxiety*
*Adults:* 5 mg P.O. t.i.d. or q.i.d.
*Psychotic disorders*
*Adults:* 5 to 10 mg P.O. or 10 to 20 mg I.M. t.i.d. or q.i.d.; up to 150 mg daily P.O. for hospitalized patients.

## I.V. administration
■ Dilute the concentrate in 60 to 120 ml (2 to 4 ounces) of water. Store the suppository form in a cool place.

■ Recommend giving I.V. dose slowly (5 mg/minute). I.M. injection may cause skin necrosis; take care to prevent extravasation. Don't mix with other drugs in the syringe. Don't administer S.C.

### Incompatibilities
Incompatible with aminophylline, amphotericin B, ampicillin sodium, calcium gluceptate and gluconate, cephalothin sodium, chloramphenicol sodium succinate, chlorothiazide, dexamethasone sodium phosphate, dimenhydrinate, heparin sodium, hydrocortisone sodium succinate, hydromorphonemethicillin, methotrexate sodium, midazolam hydrochloride, penicillin G potassium and sodium, phenobarbital sodium, phenytoin sodium, prednisolone sodium phosphate, thiopental, and vitamin B complex with C. Also incompatible with solutions containing methylparabens or propylparabens.

Don't mix prochlorperazine in the same syringe with other drugs.

## Mechanism of action
*Antiemetic action:* Antiemetic effects are attributed to dopamine receptor blockade in the medullary chemoreceptor trigger zone.
*Antipsychotic action:* Prochlorperazine is thought to exert its antipsychotic effects by postsynaptic blockade of CNS dopamine receptors, inhibiting dopamine-mediated effects.

Prochlorperazine has many other central and peripheral effects: It produces alpha and ganglionic blockade and counteracts histamine- and serotonin-mediated activity. Its most prevalent adverse reactions are extrapyramidal. It's used primarily as an antiemetic, and is ineffective against motion sickness.

## Pharmacokinetics
*Absorption:* Rate and extent of absorption vary with administration route.
*Distribution:* Distributed widely into the body; appears in breast milk. Drug is 91% to 99% protein-bound. Peak effect occurs at 2 to 4 hours; steady-state serum levels are achieved within 4 to 7 days.

---

*Metabolism:* Metabolized extensively by the liver, but no active metabolites are formed; duration of action is about 3 to 4 hours and 10 to 12 hours for the extended-release form.

*Excretion:* Mostly excreted in urine via the kidneys; some is excreted in feces via the biliary tract.

| Route | Onset | Peak | Duration |
|-------|-------|------|----------|
| P.O. | 30-40 min | Unknown | 3-12 hr |
| I.V. | Unknown | Unknown | Unknown |
| I.M. | 10-20 min | Unknown | 3-4 hr |
| P.R. | 1 hr | Unknown | 3-4 hr |

## Contraindications and precautions
Contraindicated in patients hypersensitive to phenothiazines and in those with CNS depression including coma; during pediatric surgery; when using spinal or epidural anesthetic, adrenergic blockers, or ethanol; and in infants under age 2.

Use cautiously in patients with impaired CV function, glaucoma, or seizure disorders; in those who have been exposed to extreme heat; and in children with acute illness.

## Interactions
**Drug-drug.** *Aluminum- and magnesium-containing antacids and antidiarrheals:* Decreased absorption. Don't give together.

*Anesthetics (general, spinal, epidural), CNS depressants, parenteral magnesium sulfate:* Additive effects are likely. Avoid use together.

*Antiarrhythmics, disopyramide, procainamide, quinidine:* Increased risk of arrhythmias and conduction defects. Advise clinician to monitor patient closely.

*Appetite suppressants; sympathomimetics, such as ephedrine, epinephrine, phenylephrine:* May decrease their stimulatory and pressor effects and may cause epinephrine reversal (hypotensive response to epinephrine). Use cautiously.

*Atropine, other anticholinergics, antihistamines, antiparkinsonians, MAO inhibitors, meperidine, phenothiazines:* Oversedation, paralytic ileus, visual changes, and severe constipation. Advise clinician to monitor patient closely.

*Beta blockers:* May inhibit prochlorperazine metabolism, increasing plasma levels and toxicity. Advise clinician to monitor patient for toxicity.

*Bromocriptine:* Prochlorperazine may antagonize therapeutic effect of bromocriptine on prolactin secretion. Advise clinician to monitor patient closely.

*Clonidine, guanabenz, guanadrel, guanethidine, methyldopa, reserpine:* Prochlorperazine may inhibit blood pressure response. Advise clinician to monitor patient closely.

*High-dose dopamine:* Decreases the vasoconstricting effects of dopamine. Advise clinician to monitor patient.

*Levodopa:* Decreases effectiveness and increases toxicity (by dopamine blockade). Advise clinician to monitor patient closely.

*Lithium:* May result in severe neurologic toxicity with an encephalitis-like syndrome and in decreased therapeutic response to prochlorperazine. Advise clinician to monitor patient closely.

*Metrizamide:* Increased risk of seizures. Patient requires careful observation.

*Nitrates:* May cause hypotension. Advise clinician to monitor blood pressure.

*Phenobarbital:* Enhanced renal excretion. Advise clinician to monitor patient for lack of drug effect.

*Phenytoin:* Prochlorperazine may inhibit metabolism and increase toxicity of phenytoin. Advise clinician to monitor patient closely.

*Propylthiouracil:* Increases risk of agranulocytosis. Advise clinician to monitor CBC.

**Drug-herb.** *Kava:* Increased risk or severity of dystonic reactions. Discourage use together.

*Yohimbe:* Increased the risk of toxicity. Discourage use together.

**Drug-food.** *Caffeine:* Increases prochlorperazine metabolism. Discourage use together.

**Drug-lifestyle.** *Alcohol use:* Additive effects are likely. Advise patient to avoid alcohol.

*Heavy smoking:* Increases prochlorperazine metabolism. Discourage smoking.

*Sun exposure:* May cause photosensitivity reactions. Advise patient to use sunblock.

## Adverse reactions
**CNS:** *extrapyramidal reactions,* sedation, pseudoparkinsonism, EEG changes, dizziness.
**CV:** *orthostatic hypotension,* tachycardia, ECG changes.
**EENT:** *ocular changes, blurred vision.*
**GI:** *dry mouth, constipation,* ileus, increased appetite.
**GU:** *urine retention,* dark urine, menstrual irregularities, inhibited ejaculation.
**Hematologic:** *transient leukopenia, agranulocytosis, thrombocytopenia, hemolytic anemia.*
**Hepatic:** *cholestatic jaundice.*
**Metabolic:** weight gain, hyperglycemia or hypoglycemia.
**Skin:** mild photosensitivity, allergic reactions, *exfoliative dermatitis.*
**Other:** hyperprolactinemia, gynecomastia.

## Overdose and treatment
CNS depression is characterized by deep, unarousable sleep and possible coma, hypotension or hypertension, extrapyramidal symptoms, dystonia, abnormal involuntary muscle movements, agitation, seizures, arrhythmias, ECG changes, hypothermia or hyperthermia, and autonomic nervous system dysfunction.

Treatment is symptomatic and supportive and includes maintaining vital signs, airway,

---

Reactions may be *common*, uncommon, *life-threatening*, or COMMON AND LIFE-THREATENING.

stable body temperature, and fluid and electrolyte balance.

Vomiting shouldn't be induced. Drug inhibits cough reflex, and aspiration may occur. Gastric lavage should be used, then activated charcoal and saline cathartics; dialysis doesn't help. Body temperature should be regulated p.r.n. Hypotension should be treated with I.V. fluids; epinephrine shouldn't be given. Recommend treating seizures with parenteral diazepam or barbiturates; arrhythmias with parenteral phenytoin (1 mg/kg with rate titrated to blood pressure); and extrapyramidal reactions with benztropine or parenteral diphenhydramine 2 mg/kg/minute.

## Clinical considerations

■ Liquid and injectable formulations may cause a rash after contact with skin.
■ Drug causes a high risk of extrapyramidal effects.
■ Recommend giving I.M. injection deep into the upper outer quadrant of the buttock. Massaging the area after administration may prevent formation of abscesses.
■ Solution for injection may be slightly discolored. Don't use if excessively discolored or if a precipitate is evident.
■ Drug is ineffective in treating motion sickness.
■ Protect the liquid formulation from light.
■ Prochlorperazine causes false-positive test results for urinary porphyrins, urobilinogen, amylase, and 5-hydroxyindoleacetic acid because of darkening of urine by metabolites; it also causes false-positive urine pregnancy results in tests using human chorionic gonadotropin as the indicator.

### Therapeutic monitoring

■ Advise clinician to monitor patient's blood pressure before and after parenteral administration.
■ Advise patient that drug may cause a pink to brown discoloration of urine.

### Special populations

**Breast-feeding patients.** Drug appears in breast milk; use with caution. Potential benefits to the woman should outweigh potential harm to the infant.
**Pediatric patients.** Prochlorperazine is contraindicated in infants under age 2 or weighing under 9 kg (20 lb). Don't give sustained-release form to children.
**Geriatric patients.** Geriatric patients tend to require lower doses, adjusted to individual effects. These patients are at greater risk for adverse reactions, especially tardive dyskinesia, other extrapyramidal effects, and hypotension.

## Patient counseling

■ Explain risks of dystonic reactions and tardive dyskinesia. Tell patient to report abnormal body movements promptly.
■ Tell patient to avoid spilling the liquid form. Contact with skin may cause rash and irritation.
■ Warn patient to avoid extremely hot or cold baths and exposure to temperature extremes, sunlamps, or tanning beds; drug may cause thermoregulatory changes.
■ Advise patient to take drug exactly as prescribed, not to double the doses after missing one, and not to share drug with others.
■ Oral formulations may cause stomach upset. Recommend giving with food or fluid.
■ Tell patient to dilute the concentrate in water; explain the dropper technique of measuring dose; teach correct use of suppository.
■ Tell patient that hard candy, chewing gum, or ice chips can alleviate dry mouth.
■ Warn patient not to stop taking drug suddenly and to promptly report difficulty urinating, sore throat, dizziness, or fainting. Reassure patient that most reactions can be relieved by reducing dose.
■ Caution patient to avoid hazardous activities that require alertness until effect of drug is established. Reassure patient that sedative effects subside and become tolerable in several weeks.

# progesterone

Crinone, Gesterol 50, Progestasert, Prometrium

*Pharmacologic classification:* progestin
*Therapeutic classification:* progestin, contraceptive
*Pregnancy risk category X*

## Available forms

Available by prescription only
*Capsules:* 100 mg
*Gel:* 4% (45 mg), 8% (90 mg)
*Injection:* 25 mg, 50 mg, and 100 mg/ml (in oil); 25 mg and 50 mg/ml (aqueous)
*Intrauterine device:* 38 mg (with barium sulfate, dispersed in silicone fluid)

## Indications and dosages

*Amenorrhea*
*Adults:* 5 to 10 mg I.M. daily for 6 to 8 days. Or, for secondary amenorrhea, one application of 4% gel vaginally every other day up to a total of six doses. If no response, may use Crinone 8% every other day up to a total of six doses.
*Secondary amenorrhea*
*Adults:* 400 mg (Prometrium) P.O. daily, in the evening, for 10 days.
*Dysfunctional uterine bleeding*
*Adults:* 5 to 10 mg I.M. daily for 6 days. Alternatively, a single 50- to 100-mg I.M. dose.

*Corpus luteum insufficiency*
*Adults:* 12.5 mg I.M. initiated within several days of ovulation and continuing for 2 weeks. May continue for up to 11th week of gestation. Or, for infertility, one application of 8% gel vaginally, daily or b.i.d. If pregnancy occurs, treatment may be continued until placental autonomy is achieved up to 10 to 12 weeks.
*Contraception (as an intrauterine device [IUD])*
*Adults:* Progestasert system inserted into uterine cavity; replaced after 1 year.

## Mechanism of action
*Contraceptive action:* Progesterone suppresses ovulation, thickens cervical mucus, and induces sloughing of the endometrium.

## Pharmacokinetics
*Absorption:* Must be administered parenterally because it's inactivated by the liver after oral administration.
*Distribution:* Little information available.
*Metabolism:* Reduced to pregnanediol in the liver, then conjugated with glucuronic acid. Plasma half-life of progesterone is short (several minutes).
*Excretion:* Glucuronide-conjugated pregnanediol is excreted in urine.

| Route | Onset | Peak | Duration |
|---|---|---|---|
| I.M., P.O. | Unknown | Unknown | Unknown |
| Intrauterine | Unknown | Unknown | Unknown |
| Intravaginal | Unknown | Unknown | Unknown |

## Contraindications and precautions
Contraindicated in patients with thromboembolic disorders or cerebral apoplexy (or history of these conditions), breast cancer, undiagnosed abnormal vaginal bleeding, severe hepatic disease, missed abortion, and in breast-feeding women and those hypersensitive to drug.

Use cautiously in patients with diabetes mellitus, seizures, migraines, cardiac or renal disease, asthma, or mental depression.

## Interactions
**Drug-drug.** *Bromocriptine:* Progesterone may cause amenorrhea or galactorrhea, interfering with the action of bromocriptine. Use together isn't recommended. Use IUD with caution in patients receiving anticoagulants.
**Drug-herb.** *Red clover:* May interfere with hormonal therapies. Discourage use together.

## Adverse reactions
**CNS:** depression, somnolence, headache (Crinone).
**CV:** thrombophlebitis, *thromboembolism, CVA, pulmonary embolism,* edema.
**GI:** nausea, constipation, diarrhea, vomiting (Crinone).

**GU:** breakthrough bleeding, dysmenorrhea, amenorrhea, cervical erosion, abnormal secretions, nocturia (Crinone).
**Hepatic:** cholestatic jaundice.
**Skin:** melasma, rash, acne, pruritus, pain at injection site.
**Other:** breast tenderness, enlargement, or secretion; pregnanediol excretion may decrease; serum alkaline phosphatase and amino acid levels may increase.

## Overdose and treatment
No information available.

## Clinical considerations
■ Parenteral form for I.M. administration only. Drug should be injected deep into large muscle mass, preferably the gluteal muscle. Sites should be checked for irritation.
■ Large doses of progesterone may cause a moderate catabolic effect and a transient increase in sodium and chloride excretion.

### Therapeutic monitoring
■ Be alert for signs and symptoms of increased depression.

### Special populations
**Breast-feeding patients.** Drug is contraindicated in breast-feeding women.
**Pregnant patients.** Potential exists for fetal harm, especially during first 4 months of pregnancy. Instruct patient to promptly report if she suspects pregnancy while receiving progestin therapy.

## Patient counseling
■ Advise patient that withdrawal bleeding usually occurs 2 to 3 days after discontinuing drug.
**For patient using Progestasert**
■ Inform patient that bleeding and cramping may occur for a few weeks after insertion.
■ Advise patient to contact prescriber if abnormal or excessive bleeding, severe cramping, abnormal vaginal discharge, fever, or flu-like syndrome occurs.
■ Teach patient how to check for proper placement of IUD.
■ Tell patient with Progestasert IUD that the progesterone supply is depleted in 1 year and the device must be changed at that time. Pregnancy risk increases after 1 year if patient relies on progesterone-depleted device for contraception.
■ Inform patient of adverse effects, including uterine perforation, increased risk of infection, pelvic inflammatory disease, ectopic pregnancy, abdominal cramping, increased menstrual flow, and expulsion of the device.
**For patient using Crinone gel**
■ Inform patient not to use the gel concurrently with other local intravaginal therapy. If other local intravaginal therapy is used concurrent-

---

Reactions may be *common,* uncommon, *life-threatening,* or COMMON AND LIFE-THREATENING.

ly, there should be at least a 6-hour period before or after gel administration.

# promethazine hydrochloride

Antinaus 50, Histantil*, Pentazine, Phenazine 50, Phencen-50, Phenergan, Phenergan Fortis, Phenergan Plain, Phenoject-50, Promacot, Prorex, Prorex-25, Prorex-50, Prothazine, Prothazine Plain, V-Gan-25, V-Gan-50

*Pharmacologic classification:* phenothiazine derivative
*Therapeutic classification:* antiemetic, antivertigo, antihistamine ($H_1$-receptor antagonist), preoperative, postoperative, or obstetric sedative and adjunct to analgesics
*Pregnancy risk category NR*

## Available forms
Available by prescription only
*Injection:* 25 mg/ml, 50 mg/ml
*Suppositories:* 12.5 mg, 25 mg, 50 mg
*Syrup:* 6.25 mg/5 ml, 25 mg/5 ml
*Tablets:* 12.5 mg, 25 mg, 50 mg

## Indications and dosages
*Motion sickness*
*Adults:* 25 mg P.O. b.i.d.
*Children:* 12.5 to 25 mg P.O., I.M., or P.R. b.i.d.
*Nausea*
*Adults:* 12.5 to 25 mg P.O., I.M., or P.R. q 4 to 6 hours, p.r.n.
*Children:* 0.25 to 0.5 mg/kg I.M. or P.R. q 4 to 6 hours, p.r.n.
*Rhinitis, allergy symptoms*
*Adults:* 12.5 to 25 mg P.O. before meals and h.s.; or 25 mg P.O. h.s.
*Children:* 6.25 to 12.5 mg P.O. t.i.d., or 25 mg P.O. or P.R. h.s.
*Sedation*
*Adults:* 25 to 50 mg P.O. or I.M. h.s., or P.R., p.r.n.
*Children:* 12.5 to 25 mg P.O., I.M., or P.R. h.s.
*Routine preoperative or postoperative sedation or as an adjunct to analgesics*
*Adults:* 25 to 50 mg I.M., I.V., or P.O.
*Children:* 12.5 to 25 mg I.M., I.V., or P.O.
*Obstetric sedation*
*Women:* 25 to 50 mg I.M. or I.V. in early stages of labor, and 25 to 75 mg after labor is established; repeat q 2 to 4 hours, p.r.n. Maximum daily dose, 100 mg.

## I.V. administration
▪ Drug may be administered I.V. in concentrations not to exceed 25 mg/ml and at a rate not to exceed 25 mg/minute.
▪ When using I.V. drip, wrap in aluminum foil to protect drug from light.

## Incompatibilities
Incompatible with aminophylline, chloramphenicol sodium succinate, chlorothiazide, diatrizoate meglumine and diatrizoate sodium, diatrizoate meglumine, iothalamate meglumine, iothalamate sodium, methicillin, methohexital, morphine, penicillin G potassium and sodium, pentobarbital sodium, phenytoin sodium, prednisolone sodium phosphate, thiopental, and vitamin B complex.

## Mechanism of action
*Antiemetic and antivertigo actions:* The central antimuscarinic actions of antihistamines probably are responsible for their antivertigo and antiemetic effects; promethazine also is believed to inhibit the medullary chemoreceptor trigger zone.
*Antihistamine action:* Promethazine competes with histamine for the $H_1$-receptor, thereby suppressing allergic rhinitis and urticaria; drug doesn't prevent the release of histamine.
*Sedative action:* CNS depressant mechanism of promethazine is unknown; phenothiazines probably cause sedation by reducing stimuli to the brain-stem reticular system.

## Pharmacokinetics
*Absorption:* Well absorbed from the GI tract.
*Distribution:* Distributed widely throughout the body; it crosses the placenta.
*Metabolism:* Metabolized in the liver.
*Excretion:* Metabolites are excreted in urine and feces.

| Route | Onset | Peak | Duration |
|---|---|---|---|
| P.O. | 15-60 min | Unknown | < 12 hr |
| I.V. | 3-5 min | Unknown | < 12 hr |
| I.M., P.R. | 20 min | Unknown | < 12 hr |

## Contraindications and precautions
Contraindicated in patients hypersensitive to drug; in those with intestinal obstruction, prostatic hyperplasia, bladder neck obstruction, seizure disorders, coma, CNS depression, and stenosing peptic ulcerations; in newborns, premature neonates, and breastfeeding women; and in acutely ill or dehydrated children.
    Use cautiously in patients with asthma or cardiac, pulmonary, or hepatic disease.

## Interactions
**Drug-drug.** *CNS depressants, such as antianxiety drugs, barbiturates, sleeping aids, and tranquilizers; other antihistamines:* Additive CNS depression may occur. Use together cautiously.
*Epinephrine:* Use may result in partial adrenergic blockade, producing further hypotension. Don't give together.

---

*Levodopa:* Promethazine may block the antiparkinsonian action of levodopa. Avoid use together.

*MAO inhibitors:* Interfere with the detoxification of antihistamines and phenothiazines and thus prolong and intensify their sedative and anticholinergic effects. Don't use together.

**Drug-herb.** *Kava:* Increased risk for development or worsening of dystonic reactions. Discourage use together.

*Yohimbe:* Increased risk of toxicity. Discourage use together.

**Drug-lifestyle.** *Alcohol use:* Additive CNS depression may occur. Advise patient to avoid alcohol.

*Sun exposure:* May cause photosensitivity reactions. Advise patient to use sunblock.

### Adverse reactions

**CNS:** *sedation,* confusion, sleepiness, dizziness, disorientation, extrapyramidal symptoms, *drowsiness.*
**CV:** hypotension, hypertension.
**EENT:** blurred vision.
**GI:** nausea, vomiting, *dry mouth.*
**GU:** urine retention.
**Hematologic:** *leukopenia, agranulocytosis, thrombocytopenia.*
**Metabolic:** hyperglycemia.
**Skin:** photosensitivity, rash.

### Overdose and treatment

Signs and symptoms of overdose may include either CNS depression (sedation, reduced mental alertness, apnea, and CV collapse) or CNS stimulation (insomnia, hallucinations, tremors, or seizures). Atropine-like signs and symptoms, such as dry mouth, flushed skin, fixed and dilated pupils, and GI symptoms, are common, especially in children.

Advise clinician to empty stomach by gastric lavage; vomiting shouldn't be induced. Advise clinician to treat hypotension with vasopressors and control seizures with diazepam or phenytoin; acidosis and electrolyte imbalance should be corrected. Urinary acidification promotes excretion of drug. Stimulants shouldn't be given.

### Clinical considerations

■ Pronounced sedative effects may limit use in some ambulatory patients.
■ The 50-mg/ml concentration is for I.M. use only; inject deep into large muscle mass. Don't administer drug S.C.; this may cause chemical irritation and necrosis.
■ Promethazine and meperidine (Demerol) may be mixed in the same syringe.
■ Recommend stopping drug 4 days before diagnostic skin tests to avoid preventing, reducing, or masking test response. Promethazine may cause either false-positive or false-negative pregnancy test results. It also may interfere with blood grouping in the ABO system.

### Therapeutic monitoring

■ Advise clinician to monitor CBC.
■ There may be a pronounced sedative effect. Take precautions for patient's safety.

### Special populations

**Breast-feeding patients.** Antihistamines such as promethazine shouldn't be used during breast-feeding. Many of these drugs appear in breast milk, exposing the infant to risks of unusual excitability, especially premature infants and other neonates, who may experience seizures.

**Pediatric patients.** Use cautiously in children with respiratory dysfunction. Safety and efficacy in children under age 2 haven't been established; don't give promethazine to infants under age 3 months.

**Geriatric patients.** Geriatric patients are usually more sensitive to adverse effects of antihistamines and are especially likely to experience a greater degree of dizziness, sedation, hyperexcitability, dry mouth, and urine retention than younger patients. Symptoms usually respond to a decrease in dosage.

### Patient counseling

■ When treating motion sickness, tell patient to take first dose 30 to 60 minutes before travel; on succeeding days, he should take dose upon arising and with evening meal.
■ Tell patient that coffee or tea may reduce drowsiness.
■ Suggest sugarless gum, sugarless sour hard candy, or ice chips to relieve dry mouth.
■ Tell patient to take oral form with food or milk.

## propantheline bromide
Pro-Banthine, Propanthel*

*Pharmacologic classification:* anticholinergic
*Therapeutic classification:* antimuscarinic, GI antispasmodic
*Pregnancy risk category C*

### Available forms

Available by prescription only
*Tablets:* 7.5 mg, 15 mg

### Indications and dosages

***Adjunctive treatment of peptic ulcer, irritable bowel syndrome, and other GI disorders; to reduce duodenal motility during diagnostic radiologic procedures***
*Adults:* 15 mg P.O. t.i.d. before meals, and 30 mg h.s. up to 60 mg q.i.d.
*Geriatric patients:* 7.5 mg P.O. t.i.d. before meals.
*Children:* Antispasmodic dose 2 to 3 mg/kg/day P.O. divided q 4 hours to q 6 hours and h.s.

---

Antisecretory dose 1.5 mg/kg/day P.O. divided q 6 hours to q 8 hours.

## Mechanism of action

*Anticholinergic action:* Propantheline competitively blocks actions of acetylcholine at cholinergic neuroeffector sites, decreasing GI motility and inhibiting gastric acid secretion.

## Pharmacokinetics

*Absorption:* Only about 10% to 25% is absorbed (absorption varies among patients).
*Distribution:* Doesn't cross the blood-brain barrier; little else is known about its distribution.
*Metabolism:* Appears to undergo considerable metabolism in the upper small intestine and liver.
*Excretion:* Absorbed drug is excreted in urine as metabolites and unchanged drug.

| Route | Onset | Peak | Duration |
|-------|-------|------|----------|
| P.O. | 1½ hr | 2-6 hr | 6 hr |

## Contraindications and precautions

Contraindicated in patients with angle-closure glaucoma, obstructive uropathy, obstructive disease of the GI tract, severe ulcerative colitis, myasthenia gravis, hypersensitivity to anticholinergics, paralytic ileus, intestinal atony, unstable CV status in acute hemorrhage, or toxic megacolon.

Use cautiously in patients with impaired renal or hepatic function, autonomic neuropathy, hyperthyroidism, coronary artery disease, arrhythmias, HF, hypertension, hiatal hernia with gastric reflux, or ulcerative colitis and in those living in a hot or humid environment.

## Interactions

**Drug-drug.** *Antacids:* Decrease oral absorption of anticholinergics. Recommend giving propantheline at least 1 hour before antacids.
*Atenolol:* Propantheline may increase atenolol absorption, thereby enhancing effects of atenolol. Advise clinician to monitor patient closely.
*Digoxin (slowly dissolving tablets):* May yield higher serum digoxin levels when given with anticholinergics. Advise clinician to monitor patient closely for digitalis toxicity.
*Drugs with anticholinergic effects:* May cause additive toxicity. Avoid use together.
*Ketoconazole, levodopa:* Decreased GI absorption. Separate administration times by 2 to 3 hours.
*Oral potassium supplements, especially wax-matrix formulations:* Risk of potassium-induced GI ulcerations may be increased. Avoid use together.

## Adverse reactions

**CNS:** headache, insomnia, drowsiness, dizziness, *confusion or excitement in geriatric patients,* nervousness, weakness.
**CV:** *palpitations,* tachycardia.
**EENT:** *blurred vision,* mydriasis, increased intraocular pressure, cycloplegia.
**GI:** *dry mouth,* constipation, loss of taste, nausea, vomiting, paralytic ileus, bloated feeling, drying of salivary secretions.
**GU:** *urinary hesitancy, urine retention,* impotence.
**Skin:** urticaria, decreased sweating or possible anhidrosis, other dermal signs and symptoms.
**Other:** allergic reactions *(anaphylaxis).*

## Overdose and treatment

Signs and symptoms of overdose include curare-like symptoms, such as respiratory paralysis, and such peripheral effects as headache; dilated, nonreactive pupils; blurred vision; flushed, hot, dry skin; dryness of mucous membranes; dysphagia; decreased or absent bowel sounds; urine retention; hyperthermia; tachycardia; hypertension; and increased respirations.

Treatment is primarily symptomatic and supportive, p.r.n. If patient is alert, recommend inducing emesis (or using gastric lavage), followed with a NaCl cathartic and activated charcoal to prevent further drug absorption. In severe cases, physostigmine may be given to block antimuscarinic effects of propantheline. Fluids should be given, p.r.n., to treat shock. If urine retention develops, catheterization may be needed.

## Clinical considerations

■ Consider the recommendations relevant to all anticholinergics.
■ Drug may be used with histamine-2 receptor to treat Zollinger-Ellison syndrome as an unlabeled use.

### Therapeutic monitoring

■ Drug should be adjusted until therapeutic effect is obtained or adverse effects become intolerable.
■ Advise clinician to monitor urine output and vital signs carefully.

### Special populations

**Breast-feeding patients.** Drug may appear in breast milk, possibly resulting in infant toxicity. Don't use in breast-feeding women. Propantheline may decrease milk production.
**Geriatric patients.** Give drug cautiously to geriatric patients. Lower doses are recommended.

## Patient counseling

■ Instruct patient to swallow tablets whole rather than chewing or crushing them.

---

- Advise patient to avoid driving and other activities that require alertness if drowsiness, dizziness, or blurred vision occur.
- Encourage patient to increase fluid intake to avoid constipation.

# propofol
Diprivan

*Pharmacologic classification:* phenol derivative
*Therapeutic classification:* anesthetic
*Pregnancy risk category B*

## Available forms
Available by prescription only
*Injection:* 10 mg/ml in 20-ml ampules and 50-ml and 100-ml infusion vials

## Indications and dosages
***Induction and maintenance of sedation in mechanically ventilated intensive care unit patients***
*Adults:* Initially, 5 mcg/kg/minute I.V. for 5 minutes (0.3 mg/kg/hour). Subsequent increments of 5 to 10 mcg/kg/minute (0.3 to 0.6 mg/kg/hour) over 5 to 10 minutes until desired level of sedation is achieved. Maintenance rates of 5 to 50 mcg/kg/minute (0.3 to 3 mg/kg/hour) or higher may be required. Use minimum amount needed. Lower dosages are required for patients over age 55.
***Induction of anesthesia***
*Adults:* Individualize doses based on patient's condition and age. Most patients classified as American Society of Anesthesiologists (ASA) Physical Status (PS) category I or II under age 55 require 2 to 2.5 mg/kg I.V. Drug is usually administered in a 40-mg bolus q 10 seconds until desired response is obtained.
*Children ages 3 to 16:* 2.5 to 3.5 mg/kg I.V. over 20 to 30 seconds.
*Geriatric, debilitated, or hypovolemic patients or patients in ASA PS III or IV:* Half of the usual induction dose (20-mg bolus q 10 seconds).
***Maintenance of anesthesia***
*Adults:* May give as a variable rate infusion, titrated to clinical effect. Most patients may be maintained with 0.1 to 0.2 mg/kg/minute (6 to 12 mg/kg/hour).
*Geriatric, debilitated, or hypovolemic patients or patients in ASA PS III or IV:* Half the usual maintenance dose (0.05 to 0.1 mg/kg/minute or 3 to 6 mg/kg/hour).
*Children ages 3 to 16:* 0.125 to 0.3 mg/kg/minute I.V.

## I.V. administration
- When administered into a running I.V. catheter, emulsion is compatible with D₅W, lactated Ringer's injection, lactated Ringer's and 5% dextrose injection, 5% dextrose and

0.45% saline injection, and 5% dextrose and 0.2% saline injection.

## Incompatibilities
**⚠ ALERT** Don't mix propofol with other drugs or blood products. If it's to be diluted before infusion, use only D₅W and don't dilute to a concentration less than 2 mg/ml. After dilution, drug appears to be more stable in glass containers than in plastic.

## Mechanism of action
*Anesthetic action:* Propofol produces a dose-dependent CNS depression similar to benzodiazepines and barbiturates. However, it can be used to maintain anesthesia through careful titration of infusion rate.

## Pharmacokinetics
*Absorption:* Administered I.V.
*Distribution:* Terminal half-life of 1 to 3 days.
*Metabolism:* Metabolized within liver and tissues. Metabolites aren't fully characterized.
*Excretion:* Excreted through the kidneys. However, termination of drug action is probably caused by redistribution out of the CNS as well as metabolism.

| Route | Onset | Peak | Duration |
|-------|-------|------|----------|
| I.V. | < 40 sec | Unknown | 10-15 min |

## Contraindications and precautions
Contraindicated in patients hypersensitive to propofol or components of the emulsion, including soybean oil, egg lecithin, and glycerol. Don't use drug in obstetric anesthesia because safety to fetus hasn't been established. Also avoid in patients with increased intracranial pressure or impaired cerebral circulation because the reduction in systemic arterial pressure caused by drug may substantially reduce cerebral perfusion pressure. Don't use drug in children under age 3 and in those in intensive care units or under monitored anesthesia care sedation.

Because drug is administered as an emulsion, give with caution to patients with a disorder of lipid metabolism, such as pancreatitis, primary hyperlipoproteinemia, and diabetic hyperlipidemia. Use cautiously if patient is receiving lipids as part of a total parenteral nutrition infusion; I.V. lipid dose may need to be reduced. Use cautiously in geriatric or debilitated patients and in those with circulatory disorders. Although the hemodynamic effects of drug can vary, its major effect in patients maintaining spontaneous ventilation is arterial hypotension (arterial pressure can decrease as much as 30%) with little or no change in heart rate and cardiac output. However, significant depression of cardiac output may occur in patients undergoing assisted or controlled positive pressure ventilation.

Administer drug under direct medical supervision by persons familiar with airway management and the administration of I.V. anesthetics.

## Interactions
**Drug-drug.** *Inhalational anesthetics, such as enflurane, halothane, and isoflurane; supplemental anesthetics, such as nitrous oxide and opiates:* May be expected to enhance the anesthetic and CV actions of propofol. Advise clinician to monitor patient closely.
*Opiate analgesics or sedatives:* May intensify the reduction of systolic, diastolic, mean arterial pressure, and cardiac output and may decrease induction dose requirements. Advise clinician to monitor patient closely.

## Adverse reactions
**CNS:** *movement,* headache, dizziness, twitching, clonic-myoclonic movement.
**CV:** *hypotension,* **bradycardia,** hypertension.
**GI:** nausea, vomiting, abdominal cramping.
**GU:** discolored urine
**Metabolic:** hyperlipidemia.
**Respiratory:** *apnea,* cough, hiccups.
**Skin:** flushing.
**Other:** fever, *injection site burning or stinging, pain,* tingling or numbness, coldness.

## Overdose and treatment
Specific information not available. However, treatment of overdose may include support of respiration and administration of fluids, pressor agents, and anticholinergics as indicated.

## Clinical considerations
- Drug has no vagolytic activity. Premedication with anticholinergics, such as glycopyrrolate or atropine, may help manage potential increases in vagal tone caused by other drugs or surgical manipulations.
- Store emulsion in temperatures more than 40° F (4° C) and less than 72° F (22° C). Refrigeration isn't recommended.
- If used for sedation of mechanically ventilated patients, wake patient every 24 hours.
- Use strict aseptic technique when administering drug; discard unused drug after 12 hours.
- This drug is not approved for sedation in pediatric intensive care unit patients in the United States and should not be used for this purpose. The results of a study involving 327 pediatric patients showed an increase in the number of deaths in patients treated with propofol versus other standard sedative drugs.

### Therapeutic monitoring
- Advise clinician to monitor patients receiving drug for signs of significant hypotension or bradycardia. Treatment may include increased rate of fluid administration, pressor agents, elevation of legs, or atropine. Apnea may occur during induction and may persist

for longer than 60 seconds. Ventilatory support may be required.

### Special populations
**Breast-feeding patients.** Propofol appears in breast milk and shouldn't be used by breast-feeding women.
**Pediatric patients.** Safety in children hasn't been established.
**Geriatric patients.** Pharmacokinetics of propofol aren't influenced by chronic hepatic cirrhosis, chronic renal failure, or gender.

## Patient counseling
- Advise patient that performance of activities that require mental alertness, such as operating a motor vehicle or hazardous machinery, may be impaired for some time after drug use.

# propoxyphene hydrochloride, propoxyphene hydrochloride with acetaminophen, propoxyphene with aspirin and caffeine
Darvon, Darvon Compound-65, Dolene, Wygesic

# propoxyphene napsylate
Darvon-N, Propocet 100 (with acetaminophen)

*Pharmacologic classification:* opioid
*Therapeutic classification:* analgesic
*Pregnancy risk category NR*
*Controlled substance schedule IV*

## Available forms
Available by prescription only
**propoxyphene hydrochloride**
*Capsules:* 65 mg
*Tablets:* 65 mg
**propoxyphene hydrochloride and acetaminophen**
*Tablets:* 65 mg propoxyphene hydrochloride, 650 mg acetaminophen
**propoxyphene hydrochloride, aspirin, and caffeine**
*Capsules:* 65 mg propoxyphene hydrochloride, 389 mg aspirin, 32.4 mg caffeine
**propoxyphene napsylate**
*Capsules:* 50 mg, 100 mg
*Suspension:* 50 mg/5 ml
*Tablets:* 50 mg, 100 mg
**propoxyphene napsylate and acetaminophen**
*Tablets:* 50 mg propoxyphene napsylate, 325 mg acetaminophen; 100 mg propoxyphene napsylate, 650 mg acetaminophen

---

## Indications and dosages

*Mild to moderate pain*
*Adults:* 65 mg (hydrochloride) P.O. q 4 hours, p.r.n., or 100 mg (napsylate) P.O. q 4 hours, p.r.n.

## Mechanism of action

*Analgesic action:* Propoxyphene exerts its analgesic effect by way of opiate agonist activity and alters the patient's response to painful stimuli, particularly those causing mild to moderate pain.

## Pharmacokinetics

*Absorption:* After oral administration, drug is absorbed primarily in the upper small intestine. Equimolar doses of the hydrochloride and napsylate salts provide similar plasma levels.
*Distribution:* Enters the CSF. It's assumed that it crosses the placental barrier; however, placental fluid and fetal blood levels haven't been determined.
*Metabolism:* Degraded mainly in the liver; about one-fourth of a dose is metabolized to norpropoxyphene, an active metabolite.
*Excretion:* Excreted in the urine. Duration of effect is 4 to 6 hours.

| Route | Onset | Peak | Duration |
|-------|-------|------|----------|
| P.O. | 15-60 min | 2-2½ hr | 4-6 hr |

## Contraindications and precautions

Contraindicated in patients hypersensitive to drug.
Use cautiously in patients with impaired renal or hepatic function, emotional instability, or history of drug or alcohol abuse.

## Interactions

**Drug-drug.** *Antagonists:* Patients who become physically dependent on propoxyphene may experience acute withdrawal syndrome when given a single dose of an antagonist. Use with caution and recommend monitoring patient closely.
*Antidepressants:* Propoxyphene may inhibit the metabolism of these drugs. A lower dose of antidepressant may be needed.
*Carbamazepine:* Increased effects of carbamazepine. Advise clinician to monitor patient for adverse reactions.
*Cimetidine:* May enhance respiratory and CNS depression. Avoid use together.
*CNS depressants, such as antidepressants, antihistamines, barbiturates, benzodiazepines, general anesthetics, narcotic analgesics, muscle relaxants, phenothiazines, and sedative-hypnotics:* Potentiation of adverse effects (respiratory depression, sedation, hypotension). Reduced doses of propoxyphene are usually needed.
*Digitoxin, phenytoin, rifampin:* Accumulation of either drug may occur. Advise clinician to monitor patient closely.

*General anesthetics:* Severe CV depression may result from use with these drugs. Advise clinician to monitor patient closely and use with caution.
**Drug-lifestyle.** *Alcohol use:* Potentiated CNS depressant effects of propoxyphene. Advise patient to avoid alcohol.
*Smoking:* Increased metabolism of propoxyphene. Advise clinician to monitor patient closely.

## Adverse reactions

**CNS:** *dizziness, sedation,* headache, euphoria, light-headedness, weakness, hallucinations, psychological and physical dependence.
**GI:** *nausea, vomiting,* constipation, abdominal pain.
**Hepatic:** abnormal liver function test results.
**Respiratory:** *respiratory depression.*

## Overdose and treatment

The most common signs and symptoms of overdose are CNS depression, respiratory depression, and miosis (pinpoint pupils). Others include hypotension, bradycardia, hypothermia, shock, apnea, cardiopulmonary arrest, circulatory collapse, pulmonary edema, and seizures.

Drug is known to cause ECG changes (prolonged QRS complex) and nephrogenic diabetes insipidus in acute toxic doses. Death from an acute overdose is most likely to occur within the first hour. Signs and symptoms of overdose with propoxyphene combination products may include salicylism from aspirin or acetaminophen toxicity.

To treat an acute overdose, first establish adequate respiratory exchange by way of a patent airway and ventilation p.r.n.; administer a narcotic antagonist (naloxone) to reverse respiratory depression. (Because the duration of action of drug is longer than naloxone, repeated dosing is needed.) Don't give naloxone in the absence of clinically significant respiratory or CV depression. Advise clinician to monitor vital signs closely.

If patient shows symptoms within 2 hours of ingestion of an oral overdose, the stomach should be induced immediately by induced emesis (ipecac syrup) or gastric lavage. Use caution to avoid risk of aspiration. Recommend giving activated charcoal via nasogastric tube for further removal of drug in an oral overdose.

Symptomatic and supportive treatment (continued respiratory support, correction of fluid or electrolyte imbalance) should be provided. Anticonvulsants may be needed; advise clinician to monitor laboratory parameters, vital signs, and neurologic status closely. Dialysis may be helpful in the treatment of overdose with propoxyphene combination products containing aspirin or acetaminophen.

---

## Clinical considerations
- Propoxyphene may obscure the signs and symptoms of an acute abdominal condition or worsen gallbladder pain.
- Don't prescribe drug for maintenance purposes in narcotic addiction.
- Propoxyphene can be considered a mild narcotic analgesic, but pain relief is equivalent to that of aspirin.
- Drug may cause false decrease in test results for urinary steroid excretion.

### Therapeutic monitoring
- Recommend closely monitoring patient's response to pain relief.

### Special populations
**Breast-feeding patients.** Drug appears in breast milk; use with caution in breast-feeding women.
**Geriatric patients.** Lower doses are usually indicated for geriatric patients because they may be more sensitive to therapeutic and adverse effects of drug.

## Patient counseling
- Advise patient not to exceed recommended dosage.
- Warn patient of additive depressant effect that can occur if drug is prescribed for medical conditions requiring use of sedatives, tranquilizers, muscle relaxants, antidepressants, or other CNS-depressant drugs.
- Tell patient to take drug with food if GI upset occurs.

## propranolol hydrochloride
Inderal, Inderal LA

*Pharmacologic classification:* beta blocker
*Therapeutic classification:* antihypertensive, antianginal, antiarrhythmic, adjunctive therapy of migraine, adjunctive therapy of MI
*Pregnancy risk category C*

## Available forms
Available by prescription only
*Capsules (extended-release):* 60 mg, 80 mg, 120 mg, 160 mg
*Injection:* 1 mg/ml
*Solution:* 4 mg/ml, 8 mg/ml, 80 mg/ml (concentrated)
*Tablets:* 10 mg, 20 mg, 40 mg, 60 mg, 80 mg

## Indications and dosages
*Hypertension*
*Adults:* Initially, 20 to 40 mg P.O. b.i.d. or 60 to 80 mg once daily (extended-release). Increase at 3- to 7-day intervals until optimum blood pressure response is achieved. Usual maintenance dose is 160 to 480 mg daily. Or,

120 to 160 mg P.O. once daily (extended release). Maximum daily dose 640 mg.
◇ *Children:* 1 mg/kg P.O. daily (maximum daily dose is 16 mg/kg).
*Management of angina pectoris*
*Adults:* 10 to 20 mg P.O. t.i.d. or q.i.d., or one 80-mg extended-release capsule daily. Dosage may be increased at 3- to 7-day intervals. Average optimum dose is 160 to 240 mg daily.
*Supraventricular, ventricular, and atrial arrhythmias; tachyarrhythmias caused by excessive catecholamine action during anesthesia, hyperthyroidism, and pheochromocytoma*
*Adults:* 1 to 3 mg I.V. diluted in 50 ml D₅W or normal saline solution infused slowly, not to exceed 1 mg/minute. After 3 mg have been infused, another dose may be given in 2 minutes; subsequent doses no sooner than q 4 hours. Usual maintenance dose is 10 to 30 mg P.O. t.i.d. or q.i.d.
*Prevention of frequent, severe, uncontrollable, or disabling migraine or vascular headache*
*Adults:* Initially, 80 mg P.O. daily in divided doses or one extended-release capsule once daily. Usual maintenance dose is 160 to 240 mg daily, divided t.i.d. or q.i.d.
*To reduce risk of death after MI*
*Adults:* 180 to 240 mg P.O. daily in divided doses. Usually given in three to four doses daily, beginning 5 to 21 days after infarct.
*Hypertrophic subaortic stenosis*
*Adults:* 20 to 40 mg P.O. t.i.d. or q.i.d. Or, 80 to 160 mg once daily (extended release).
*Preoperative pheochromocytoma*
*Adults:* 60 mg P.O. daily in divided doses with alpha blocker for 3 days before surgery.
◇ *Adjunctive treatment of anxiety*
*Adults:* 10 to 80 mg P.O. 1 hour before anxiety-provoking activity.
◇ *Treatment of essential, familial, or senile movement tremors*
*Adults:* 40 mg P.O. b.i.d., p.r.n.

## I.V. administration
- For life-threatening arrythmias or those that occur during anesthesia, I.V. injection should be administered at a rate not exceeding 1 mg/min.

### Incompatibilities
Incompatible with diazoxide.

## Mechanism of action
*Antianginal action:* Propranolol decreases myocardial oxygen consumption by blocking catecholamine access to beta-adrenergic receptors, relieving angina.
*Antiarrhythmic action:* Propranolol decreases heart rate and prevents exercise-induced increases in heart rate. It also decreases myocardial contractility, cardiac output, and SA and AV nodal conduction velocity.

---

* Canada only    ◇ Unlabeled clinical use

*Antihypertensive action:* Exact mechanism of antihypertensive effect is unknown; drug may reduce blood pressure by blocking adrenergic receptors (decreasing cardiac output), by decreasing sympathetic outflow from the CNS, and by suppressing renin release.

*Migraine prophylactic action:* Migraine-preventive effect of propranolol is thought to result from inhibition of vasodilation.

*MI prophylactic action:* Mechanism by which drug reduces risk of death after MI is unknown.

## Pharmacokinetics

*Absorption:* Absorbed almost completely from the GI tract, especially when given with food.

*Distribution:* Distributed widely throughout the body; drug is more than 90% protein-bound.

*Metabolism:* Hepatic metabolism is almost total; oral dosage form undergoes extensive first-pass metabolism.

*Excretion:* About 96% to 99% of a given dose of propranolol is excreted in urine as metabolites; remainder is excreted in feces as unchanged drug and metabolites. Biologic half-life is about 4 hours.

| Route | Onset | Peak | Duration |
|-------|-------|------|----------|
| P.O. | 30 min | 1-1½ hr | 12 hr |
| I.V. | 1 min | Immediate | 5 min |

## Contraindications and precautions

Contraindicated in patients with bronchial asthma, sinus bradycardia and heart block greater than first-degree, cardiogenic shock, and HF (unless failure is secondary to a tachyarrhythmia that can be treated with propranolol).

Use cautiously in geriatric patients; in patients with impaired renal or hepatic function, nonallergic bronchospastic diseases, diabetes mellitus, or thyrotoxicosis; and in those receiving other antihypertensives.

## Interactions

**Drug-drug.** *Aluminum hydroxide antacid:* Decreases GI absorption. Don't give together.

*Antihypertensives:* Propranolol may potentiate antihypertensive effects. Advise clinician to monitor patient closely.

*Atropine, tricyclic antidepressants, and other drugs with anticholinergic effects:* May antagonize propranolol-induced bradycardia. Advise clinician to monitor ECG.

*Calcium channel blockers, especially I.V. verapamil:* May depress myocardial contractility or AV conduction. Use together cautiously.

*Cimetidine:* May decrease clearance of propranolol. Advise clinician to monitor patient for increased beta-blocking effects.

*Epinephrine:* Causes severe vasoconstriction. Advise clinician to monitor blood pressure and patient closely.

*Insulin or antidiabetics:* Can alter dosage requirements in previously stable diabetic patients. Advise clinician to monitor patient for hypoglycemia.

*NSAIDs:* May antagonize hypotensive effects. Advise clinician to monitor blood pressure closely.

*Phenytoin, rifampin:* Accelerate clearance of propranolol. Advise clinician to monitor patient closely.

*Sympathomimetics, such as isoproterenol and MAO inhibitors:* Propranolol may antagonize beta-adrenergic-stimulating effects. Advise clinician to monitor patient closely. May be used therapeutically and in emergencies.

*Tubocurarine:* High doses of propranolol may potentiate neuromuscular blocking effect. Advise clinician to monitor patient closely.

**Drug-herb.** *Betel palm:* Reduces temperature-elevating effects and enhanced CNS effects of arecoline in betel palm. Discourage use together.

**Drug-lifestyle.** *Cocaine use:* Increased angina-inducing potential of cocaine. Advise clinician to monitor patient closely.

## Adverse reactions

**CNS:** *fatigue, lethargy,* vivid dreams, hallucinations, mental depression, light-headedness, insomnia.

**CV:** *bradycardia,* hypotension, **HF,** intermittent claudication, *intensification of AV block.*

**GI:** nausea, vomiting, diarrhea, abdominal cramping.

**GU:** elevated BUN levels.

**Hematologic:** *agranulocytosis.*

**Hepatic:** elevated serum transaminase, alkaline phosphatase, and LDH levels.

**Respiratory:** *bronchospasm.*

**Skin:** rash.

**Other:** fever.

## Overdose and treatment

Signs of overdose include severe hypotension, bradycardia, HF, and bronchospasm.

After acute ingestion, recommend inducing emesis or emptying stomach by gastric lavage, followed with activated charcoal to reduce absorption; care should be symptomatic and supportive. Bradycardia should be treated with atropine (0.25 to 1 mg); if no response, isoproterenol should be given cautiously. Recommend treating cardiac failure with cardiac glycosides and diuretics and treating hypotension with glucagon, vasopressors, or both; epinephrine is preferred. Bronchospasm should be treated with isoproteronol and aminophylline.

## Clinical considerations

■ Propranolol also has been used to treat aggression and rage, stage fright, recurrent GI bleeding in cirrhotic patients, and menopausal symptoms.

- Never administer propranolol as an adjunct in treatment of pheochromocytoma unless patient has had pretreatment with alpha blockers.

### Therapeutic monitoring
- Patient's apical rate should always be checked before drug is given. If extremes in pulse rates are detected, drug should be withheld and prescriber contacted immediately.

### Special populations
**Breast-feeding patients.** Drug appears in breast milk; an alternative feeding method is recommended during therapy.
**Pediatric patients.** Safety and efficacy of propranolol in children haven't been established; use only if potential benefit outweighs risk.
**Geriatric patients.** Geriatric patients may require lower maintenance dosages of propranolol because of increased bioavailability or delayed metabolism; they also may experience enhanced adverse effects.

### Patient counseling
- Warn patient not to abruptly stop taking propranolol because this can exacerbate angina and precipitate MI.
- Instruct patient on proper use, dosage, and potential adverse effects of propranolol.
- Tell patient to contact prescriber before taking OTC drugs that may interact with propranolol, such as nasal decongestants or cold preparations.

## propylthiouracil (PTU)
Propyl-Thyracil*

*Pharmacologic classification:* thyroid hormone antagonist
*Therapeutic classification:* antihyperthyroid
*Pregnancy risk category D*

### Available forms
Available by prescription only
*Tablets:* 50 mg

### Indications and dosages
*Hyperthyroidism*
*Adults:* 300 to 450 mg P.O. daily in divided doses. Continue until patient is euthyroid; then start maintenance dose of 100 mg daily to t.i.d.
*Neonates and children:* 5 to 7 mg/kg P.O. daily in divided doses q 8 hours. Alternatively, give according to age.
*Children ages 6 to 10:* 50 to 150 mg P.O. daily in divided doses q 8 hours.
*Children over age 10:* 100 mg P.O. t.i.d. Continue until patient is euthyroid; then start maintenance dose of 25 mg t.i.d. to 100 mg b.i.d.

## Mechanism of action
*Antithyroid action:* Used to treat hyperthyroidism, PTU inhibits synthesis of thyroid hormone by interfering with the incorporation of iodine into thyroglobulin; it also inhibits the formation of iodothyronine. Besides blocking hormone synthesis, it also inhibits the peripheral deiodination of thyroxine to triiodothyronine (liothyronine). Clinical effects become evident only when the preformed hormone is depleted and circulating hormone levels decline.

As preparation for thyroidectomy, PTU inhibits synthesis of the thyroid hormone and causes a euthyroid state, reducing surgical problems during thyroidectomy; as a result, the risk of death for a single-stage thyroidectomy is low. Iodide reduces the vascularity of the gland and makes it less friable.

Used in treating thyrotoxic crisis, PTU inhibits peripheral deiodination of thyroxine to triiodothyronine. Theoretically, it's preferred over methimazole in thyroid storm because of its peripheral action.

### Pharmacokinetics
*Absorption:* Absorbed rapidly and readily (about 80%) from the GI tract.
*Distribution:* PTU appears to be concentrated in the thyroid gland. PTU readily crosses the placenta and appears in breast milk. Drug is 75% to 80% protein-bound.
*Metabolism:* Metabolized rapidly in the liver.
*Excretion:* About 35% of a dose is excreted in urine. Half-life is 1 to 2 hours in patients with normal renal function and 8½ hours in anuric patients.

| Route | Onset | Peak | Duration |
| --- | --- | --- | --- |
| P.O. | Unknown | 1-1½ hr | Unknown |

### Contraindications and precautions
Contraindicated in patients hypersensitive to drug and in breast-feeding women. Use cautiously in pregnant women.

### Interactions
**Drug-drug.** *Adrenocorticoids, corticotropin:* May require a dosage adjustment of the steroid when thyroid status changes.
*Bone marrow depressants:* Increases the risk of agranulocytosis. Advise clinician to monitor patient closely.
*Hepatotoxic drugs:* Increased risk of hepatotoxicity. Advise clinician to monitor patient closely.
*Iodinated glycerol, lithium, potassium iodide:* May potentiate hypothyroid effects. Dosage adjustment may be needed.
*Oral anticoagulants:* May be potentiated by the anti-vitamin K activity attributed to PTU. Advise clinician to monitor PT and INR.

## Adverse reactions
**CNS:** headache, drowsiness, vertigo, paresthesia, neuritis, neuropathies, CNS stimulation, depression.
**CV:** vasculitis.
**EENT:** visual disturbances.
**GI:** diarrhea, *nausea, vomiting* (may be dose-related), epigastric distress, salivary gland enlargement, loss of taste.
**GU:** nephritis.
**Hematologic:** *agranulocytosis, thrombocytopenia, aplastic anemia,* leukopenia.
**Hepatic:** jaundice, *hepatotoxicity.*
**Musculoskeletal:** arthralgia, myalgia.
**Skin:** rash, urticaria, skin discoloration, pruritus, erythema nodosum, exfoliative dermatitis, lupuslike syndrome.
**Other:** fever, lymphadenopathy; dose-related hypothyroidism (mental depression; hypoprothrombinemia and bleeding; cold intolerance; hard, nonpitting edema).

## Overdose and treatment
Signs and symptoms of overdose include nausea, vomiting, epigastric distress, fever, headache, arthralgia, pruritus, edema, and pancytopenia.

Treatment includes withdrawal of drug in the presence of agranulocytosis, pancytopenia, hepatitis, fever, or exfoliative dermatitis. For depression of bone marrow, treatment may require antibiotics and transfusions of fresh whole blood. For hepatitis, treatment includes rest, adequate diet, and symptomatic support, including analgesics, gastric lavage, I.V. fluids, and mild sedation.

## Clinical considerations
■ Best response occurs when drug is given around-the-clock and given at the same time each day in respect to meals.
■ A beta blocker, usually propranolol, commonly is given to manage the peripheral signs of hyperthyroidism, which are primarily cardiac related (tachycardia).
■ PTU therapy alters selenomethionine levels and INR; it also alters AST, ALT, and LDH levels, as well as liothyronine uptake.

### Therapeutic monitoring
■ Patient should be observed for signs and symptoms of hypothyroidism (mental depression; cold intolerance; hard, nonpitting edema; hair loss).
■ Drug should be stopped if severe rash or enlarged cervical lymph nodes develop.

### Special populations
**Pregnant patients.** Potential exists for harm to the fetus. If drug must be used, recommend giving the lowest possible dose.
**Breast-feeding patients.** Because PTU appears in breast milk, advise patient to avoid breast-feeding during treatment. However, if

it's necessary, PTU is the preferred antithyroid hormone.

## Patient counseling
■ Warn patient to avoid using self-prescribed cough medicines; many contain iodine.
■ Suggest taking drug with meals to reduce GI adverse effects.
■ Instruct patient to store drug in a light-resistant container. Warn patient not to store drug in the bathroom; heat and humidity may cause drug to deteriorate.
■ Tell patient to promptly report fever, sore throat, malaise, unusual bleeding, yellowing of eyes, nausea, or vomiting.
■ Advise patient to have medical review of thyroid status before undergoing surgery, including dental surgery.
■ Teach patient how to recognize the signs of hyperthyroidism and hypothyroidism and what to do if they occur.

# protamine sulfate

*Pharmacologic classification:* antidote
*Therapeutic classification:* heparin antagonist
*Pregnancy risk category C*

## Available forms
Available by prescription only
*Injection:* 10 mg/ml in 5-ml ampule, 25-ml ampule, 5-ml vial, 10-ml vial, 25-ml vial

## Indications and dosages
### Heparin overdose
*Adults and children:* Dosage based on venous blood coagulation studies, usually 1 mg for each 90 units of heparin derived from lung tissue or 1 mg for each 115 units of heparin derived from intestinal mucosa. Give by slow I.V. injection over 1 to 3 minutes. Maximum dose, 50 mg in any 10-minute period.

## I.V. administration
■ Reconstitute powder by adding 5 ml sterile water to 50-mg vial (25 ml to 250-mg vial); discard unused solution.
■ Slow I.V. administration (over 1 to 3 minutes) decreases adverse effects; antishock equipment should be available.

### Incompatibilities
Incompatible with cephalosporins, diatrizoate meglumine, diatrizoate sodium, ioxaglate meglumine, ioxaglate sodium, and penicillins. Don't mix with other drugs.

## Mechanism of action
*Heparin antagonism:* Protamine has weak anticoagulant activity; however, when given in the presence of heparin, it forms a salt that neutralizes anticoagulant effects of both drugs.

---

Reactions may be *common*, uncommon, *life-threatening*, or COMMON AND LIFE-THREATENING.

## Pharmacokinetics

*Absorption:* Administered I.V.
*Distribution:* Unknown.
*Metabolism:* Fate of the heparin-protamine complex is unknown; however, it appears to be partially degraded, with release of some heparin.
*Excretion:* Binding action lasts about 2 hours.

| Route | Onset | Peak | Duration |
|-------|-------|------|----------|
| I.V. | 30-60 sec | Unknown | 2 hr |

## Contraindications and precautions

Contraindicated in patients hypersensitive to drug. Use cautiously after cardiac surgery.

## Interactions

None significant.

## Adverse reactions

**CNS:** lassitude.
**CV:** decrease in blood pressure, ***bradycardia, circulatory collapse.***
**GI:** nausea, vomiting.
**Respiratory:** dyspnea, ***pulmonary edema, acute pulmonary hypertension.***
**Skin:** transitory flushing.
**Other:** feeling of warmth, ***anaphylaxis, anaphylactoid reactions.***

## Overdose and treatment

Overdose may cause bleeding secondary to interaction with platelets and proteins including fibrinogen. Recommend replacing blood loss with blood transfusions or fresh frozen plasma. If hypotension occurs, treatment with fluids, epinephrine, dobutamine, or dopamine should be considered.

## Clinical considerations

■ Check for possible fish allergy.
■ Drug shortens heparin-prolonged PTT.

### *Therapeutic monitoring*

■ Advise clinician to monitor patient continually and check vital signs frequently; blood pressure may fall suddenly.
■ Dosage is based on blood coagulation studies as well as on route of administration of heparin and time elapsed since heparin was given.

### *Special populations*

**Pregnant patients.** Use only when clearly needed; it isn't known if drug will cause harm to the fetus.
**Pediatric patients.** Safety and efficacy haven't been established for children.

## Patient counseling

■ Advise patient that he may experience transitory flushing or feel warm after I.V. administration.

# pseudoephedrine hydrochloride

Allermed, Cenafed, Decofed, Dimetapp Decongestant, Efidac 24, Novafed, PediaCare Infants' Decongestant Drops, Pseudogest, Sinufed Timecelles, Sudafed, Suphedrin, Triaminic

# pseudoephedrine sulfate

Afrin, Drixoral, Duration

*Pharmacologic classification:* adrenergic
*Therapeutic classification:* decongestant
*Pregnancy risk category B*

## Available forms

Available without a prescription
*Capsules:* 30 mg, 60 mg
*Oral solution:* 7.5 mg/0.8 ml, 15 mg/5 ml, 30 mg/5 ml
*Tablets:* 30 mg, 60 mg
*Tablets (chewable):* 15 mg
*Tablets (extended-release):* 120 mg, 240 mg
*Tablets (extended-release, film-coated):* 120 mg

## Indications and dosages

***Nasal and eustachian tube decongestant***
*Adults and children ages 12 and older:* 60 mg P.O. q 4 to 6 hours. Maximum dose, 240 mg daily, or 120 mg P.O. extended-release tablet q 12 hours.
*Children ages 6 to 11:* Administer 30 mg P.O. q 4 to 6 hours. Maximum dose, 120 mg daily.
*Children ages 2 to 5:* 15 mg P.O. q 4 to 6 hours. Maximum dose, 60 mg/day, or 4 mg/kg or 125 mg/m² P.O. divided q.i.d.

## Mechanism of action

*Decongestant action:* Pseudoephedrine directly stimulates alpha-adrenergic receptors of respiratory mucosa to produce vasoconstriction; shrinkage of swollen nasal mucous membranes; reduction of tissue hyperemia, edema, and nasal congestion; an increase in airway (nasal) patency and drainage of sinus excretions; and opening of obstructed eustachian ostia. Relaxation of bronchial smooth muscle may result from direct stimulation of beta-adrenergic receptors. Mild CNS stimulation may also occur.

## Pharmacokinetics

*Absorption:* Nasal decongestion occurs within 30 minutes and persists 4 to 6 hours after oral dose of 60-mg tablet or oral solution. Effects persist 8 hours after 60-mg dose and up to 12 hours after 120-mg dose of extended-release form.

*Distribution:* Widely distributed throughout the body.
*Metabolism:* Incompletely metabolized in liver by *N*-demethylation to inactive compounds.
*Excretion:* 55% to 75% of a dose is excreted unchanged in urine; remainder is excreted as unchanged drug and metabolites.

| Route | Onset | Peak | Duration |
|-------|-------|------|----------|
| P.O. | ½ hr | ½-1 hr | 4-12 hr |

## Contraindications and precautions
Contraindicated in patients with severe hypertension or severe coronary artery disease; in those receiving MAO inhibitors; and in breast-feeding women. Extended-release preparations are contraindicated in children under age 12.

Use cautiously in geriatric patients and in patients with hypertension, cardiac disease, diabetes, glaucoma, hyperthyroidism, or prostatic hyperplasia.

## Interactions
**Drug-drug.** *Beta blockers:* May increase pressor effects of pseudoephedrine. Advise clinician to monitor patient closely.
*MAO inhibitors:* Potentiate pressor effects of pseudoephedrine. Avoid use together.
*Methyldopa, reserpine:* May reduce their antihypertensive effects. Advise clinician to monitor patient closely.
*Sympathomimetics:* May produce additive effects and toxicity. Advise clinician to monitor patient closely and give with extreme caution.
*Tricyclic antidepressants:* May antagonize effects of pseudoephedrine. Use cautiously.

## Adverse reactions
**CNS:** *anxiety,* transient stimulation, tremor, dizziness, headache, insomnia, *nervousness.*
**CV:** *arrhythmias, palpitations,* tachycardia.
**GI:** anorexia, nausea, vomiting, dry mouth.
**GU:** difficulty urinating.
**Respiratory:** respiratory difficulties.
**Skin:** pallor.

## Overdose and treatment
Signs and symptoms of overdose include exaggeration of common adverse reactions, particularly seizures, arrhythmias, and nausea and vomiting.

Treatment may include an emetic and gastric lavage within 4 hours of ingestion. Charcoal is effective only if given within 1 hour, unless extended-release form was used. If renal function is adequate, forced diuresis will increase elimination. Don't force diuresis in severe overdose. Advise clinician to monitor vital signs, cardiac state, and electrolyte levels. I.V. propranolol may control cardiac toxicity; I.V. diazepam may help manage delirium or seizures; diluted I.V. potassium chloride solutions may be given for hypokalemia.

## Clinical considerations
■ Recommend giving last daily dose several hours before bedtime to minimize insomnia.
■ If symptoms persist longer than 5 days or fever is present, reevaluate therapy.

### Therapeutic monitoring
■ Patient should be observed for complaints of headache or dizziness.
■ Blood pressure should be monitored.

### Special populations
**Breast-feeding patients.** Drug may appear in breast milk; avoid use in breast-feeding women.
**Pediatric patients.** Don't use extended-release form in children under age 12.
**Geriatric patients.** Geriatric patients may be sensitive to effects of drug; lower dose may be needed. Overdose may cause hallucinations, CNS depression, seizures, and death in patients over age 60. Use extended-release preparations with caution in geriatric patients.

## Patient counseling
■ If it's difficult for patient to swallow drug, suggest opening capsules and mixing contents with applesauce, jelly, honey, or syrup. Mixture must be swallowed without chewing.
■ Suggest using ice chips, sugarless gum, or hard candy for relief of dry mouth.
■ Instruct patient to take missed dose if remembered within 1 hour. If beyond 1 hour, patient should skip dose and resume regular schedule; patient shouldn't double the dose.
■ Tell patient to store drug away from heat and light (not in bathroom medicine cabinet) and safely out of reach of children.
■ Caution patient that many OTC preparations may contain sympathomimetics, which can cause additive, hazardous reactions.
■ Advise patient to take last dose at least 2 to 3 hours before bedtime to avoid insomnia.

## psyllium
Cillium, Hydrocil Instant, Konsyl, Konsyl-D, Metamucil, Modane, Naturacil, Peridiem, Reguloid, Serutan, Syllact

*Pharmacologic classification:* adsorbent
*Therapeutic classification:* bulk laxative
*Pregnancy risk category C*

### Available forms
Available without a prescription
*Powder:* 250 mg/g, 273 mg/g, 390 mg/g, 429 mg/g, 500 mg/g, 517 mg/g, 555 mg/g, 672 mg/g, 946 mg/g, 1,000 mg/g
*Wafers:* 3.4 g/wafer

## Indications and dosages
*Constipation, bowel management, irritable bowel syndrome*
*Adults:* 1 to 2 rounded tsp P.O. in full glass of liquid daily, b.i.d. or t.i.d., followed by second glass of liquid; or 1 packet P.O. dissolved in water daily; or 2 wafers b.i.d. or t.i.d.
*Children over age 6:* 1 level tsp P.O. in ½ glass of liquid h.s.

## Mechanism of action
*Laxative action:* Psyllium adsorbs water in the gut; it also serves as a source of indigestible fiber, increasing stool bulk and moisture, stimulating peristaltic activity and bowel evacuation.

## Pharmacokinetics
*Absorption:* None; onset of action varies from 12 hours to 3 days.
*Distribution:* Distributed locally in the gut.
*Metabolism:* Not metabolized.
*Excretion:* Excreted in feces.

| Route | Onset | Peak | Duration |
|-------|-------|------|----------|
| P.O. | 12-24 hr | 3 days | Variable |

## Contraindications and precautions
Contraindicated in patients hypersensitive to drug, those with abdominal pain, nausea, vomiting, or other symptoms of appendicitis and in those with intestinal obstruction or ulceration, disabling adhesions, or difficulty swallowing.

## Interactions
None reported.

## Adverse reactions
**GI:** nausea, vomiting, diarrhea (with excessive use); esophageal, gastric, small intestinal, and rectal obstruction when drug is taken in dry form; abdominal cramps, especially in severe constipation.

## Overdose and treatment
No cases of overdose have been reported; probable clinical effects include abdominal pain and diarrhea.

## Clinical considerations
■ Before administering drug, add at least 8 ounces (240 ml) of water or juice and stir for a few seconds to improve taste. Have patient drink mixture immediately to prevent it from congealing; then have him drink another glass of fluid.
■ Separate administration of psyllium and oral anticoagulants, cardiac glycosides, and salicylates by at least 2 hours.
■ Drug may reduce appetite if given before meals.

■ Psyllium and other bulk laxatives most closely mimic natural bowel function and don't cause laxative dependence; they're especially useful for patients with postpartum constipation or diverticular disease, for debilitated patients, for irritable bowel syndrome, and for chronic laxative users.

## Therapeutic monitoring
■ Inform patient that laxative effect usually occurs in 12 to 24 hours but may be delayed 3 days.

## Special populations
**Breast-feeding patients.** Because drug isn't absorbed, it presumably is safe for use in breast-feeding women.

## Patient counseling
■ Warn patient not to swallow drug in dry form; he should mix it with at least 8 ounces (240 ml) of fluid, stir briefly, drink immediately (to prevent mixture from congealing), and follow it with another 8 oz of fluid.
■ Explain that drug may reduce appetite if taken before meals; recommend taking drug 2 hours after meals and any other oral drugs.
■ Advise diabetic patients and those with restricted sodium or sugar intake to avoid psyllium products containing salt or sugar. Advise patients who must restrict phenylalanine intake to avoid psyllium products containing aspartame.

---

# pyrazinamide
PMS-Pyrazinamide*, Tebrazid*

*Pharmacologic classification:* synthetic pyrazine analogue of nicotinamide
*Therapeutic classification:* antituberculotic
*Pregnancy risk category C*

## Available forms
Available by prescription only
*Tablets:* 500 mg

## Indications and dosages
*Adjunctive treatment of tuberculosis (when primary and secondary antitubercular drugs can't be used or have failed)*
*Adults:* 15 to 30 mg/kg P.O. daily, in one or more doses. Maximum dose is 2 g daily. Alternatively, a twice-weekly dose of 50 to 70 mg/kg (up to 4 g) (based on lean body weight) has been developed to promote patient compliance. Lower dosage is recommended in decreased renal function.

## Mechanism of action
*Antibiotic action:* Mechanism of action is unknown; drug may be bactericidal or bacterio-

static depending on organism susceptibility and drug concentration at infection site. Pyrazinamide is active only against *Mycobacterium tuberculosis*. Pyrazinamide is considered adjunctive in tuberculosis therapy and is given with other drugs to prevent or delay development of resistance to pyrazinamide by *M. tuberculosis*.

## Pharmacokinetics
*Absorption:* Well absorbed after oral administration.
*Distribution:* Distributed widely into body tissues and fluids, including lungs, liver, and CSF; drug is 50% protein-bound. It isn't known if it crosses the placenta.
*Metabolism:* Hydrolyzed in the liver; some hydrolysis occurs in stomach.
*Excretion:* Excreted almost completely in urine by glomerular filtration. It isn't known if drug appears in breast milk. Elimination half-life in adults is 9 to 10 hours. Half-life is prolonged in renal and hepatic impairment.

| Route | Onset | Peak | Duration |
|-------|-------|------|----------|
| P.O. | Unknown | 1-2 hr | Unknown |

## Contraindications and precautions
Contraindicated in patients hypersensitive to drug, and those with severe hepatic disease or acute gout.

Use cautiously in patients with diabetes mellitus, renal failure, or gout.

## Interactions
**Drug-drug.** *Rifampin:* May cause severe hepatitis. Advise clinician to monitor patient closely. Discontinue immediately if symptoms of hepatic injury occur.
**Drug-lifestyle.** *Sun exposure:* May cause photosensitivity reactions. Advise patient to use sunblock.

## Adverse reactions
**CNS:** malaise.
**GI:** anorexia, nausea, vomiting.
**GU:** dysuria, interstitial nephritis.
**Hematologic:** sideroblastic anemia, ***thrombocytopenia***, porphyria.
**Hepatic:** *hepatitis*.
**Metabolic:** hyperuricemia and gout.
**Musculoskeletal:** *arthralgia, myalgia.*
**Skin:** rash, urticaria, pruritus, photosensitivity.
**Other:** fever.

## Overdose and treatment
No specific recommendations are available. Treatment is supportive. After recent ingestion (4 hours or less), stomach should be emptied by induced emesis or gastric lavage. Follow with activated charcoal to decrease absorption.

## Clinical considerations
■ In patients with diabetes mellitus, pyrazinamide therapy may hinder stabilization of serum glucose levels.
■ In many cases, drug elevates serum uric acid levels. Although usually asymptomatic, a uricosuric drug, such as probenecid or allopurinol, may be needed.
■ Patients with HIV infection may require a longer course of treatment.
■ Pyrazinamide may interfere with urine ketone determinations. Systemic effects of drug may temporarily decrease 17-ketosteroid levels; it may increase protein-bound iodine and urate levels and results of liver enzyme tests.

### Therapeutic monitoring
■ Advise clinician to monitor liver function, especially enzyme and bilirubin levels, and renal function, especially serum uric acid levels, before therapy and thereafter at 2- to 4-week intervals; patient should be observed for signs of liver damage or decreased renal function.

### Special populations
**Breast-feeding patients.** Safety in breast-feeding women hasn't been established. Alternative feeding method is recommended during therapy.
**Pediatric patients.** Use cautiously. Dosage not exceeding 30 mg/kg (up to 2 g per day) is well tolerated and is seldom hepatotoxic.
**Geriatric patients.** Because geriatric patients commonly have diminished renal function, which decreases drug excretion, use pyrazinamide with caution.

## Patient counseling
■ Explain disease process and reason for long-term therapy.
■ Teach signs and symptoms of hypersensitivity and other adverse reactions, and emphasize need to report them; urge patient to report unusual reactions, especially signs of gout.
■ Make sure patient understands how and when to take drugs; urge patient to complete entire prescribed regimen, to comply with instructions for around-the-clock dosage, and to keep follow-up appointments.

# pyridostigmine bromide
Mestinon, Regonol

*Pharmacologic classification:* cholinesterase inhibitor
*Therapeutic classification:* muscle stimulant
*Pregnancy risk category NR*

## Available forms
Available by prescription only
*Injection:* 5 mg/ml in 2-ml ampule or 5-ml vial

*Syrup:* 60 mg/5 ml
*Tablets:* 60 mg
*Tablets (sustained-release):* 180 mg

## Indications and dosages
### Reversal of the effects of nondepolarizing drugs, curariform antagonist (postoperatively)
*Adults:* 10 to 20 mg I.V. preceded by atropine sulfate 0.6 to 1.2 mg I.V.
### Myasthenia gravis
*Adults:* 60 to 180 mg P.O. b.i.d. or q.i.d. Usual dose 600 mg daily, but higher doses may be needed (up to 1,500 mg daily). Give ⅓₀ of oral dose I.M. or I.V. Adjust dosage based on patient response and tolerance of adverse effects. Sustained-release and rapid-release forms are often used together depending on patient's symptoms.
*Children:* 7 mg/kg/24 hours P.O. divided into five or six doses.
*Neonates of myasthenic mothers:* 0.05 to 0.15 mg/kg I.M.

## I.V. administration
**ℍ ALERT** Administer I.V. injection no faster than 1 mg/minute. Rapid I.V. infusion may cause bradycardia and seizures. Monitor vital signs frequently, especially respirations. Position patient to ease breathing. Keep atropine injection available, and be prepared to give it, as ordered; provide respiratory support p.r.n.
■ If patient's muscle weakness is severe, prescriber will determine whether severity is caused by drug-induced toxicity or worsening of myasthenia gravis. Test dose of edrophonium I.V. will aggravate drug-induced weakness, but will temporarily relieve disease-induced weakness.

### Incompatibilities
Unstable in alkaline solutions.

## Mechanism of action
*Muscle stimulant action:* Pyridostigmine blocks hydrolysis of acetylcholine by cholinesterase, resulting in acetylcholine accumulation at cholinergic synapses, increasing stimulation of cholinergic receptors at the myoneural junction.

## Pharmacokinetics
*Absorption:* Poorly absorbed from the GI tract.
*Distribution:* Little is known; however, drug may cross the placenta, especially when given in large doses.
*Metabolism:* Exact metabolic fate is unknown. Duration of effect is usually 3 to 6 hours after oral dose and 2 to 3 hours after I.V. dose, depending on patient's physical and emotional status and disease severity. Pyridostigmine is hydrolyzed by cholinesterase.

*Excretion:* Excreted in urine.

| Route | Onset | Peak | Duration |
|---|---|---|---|
| P.O. | 20-30 min | 1-2 hr | 3-6 hr |
| P.O. (extended) | 30-60 min | 1-2 hr | 6-12 hr |
| I.V. | 2-5 min | Unknown | 2-4 hr |
| I.M. | 15 min | Unknown | 2-4 hr |

## Contraindications and precautions
Contraindicated in patients hypersensitive to anticholinesterase drugs and in those with mechanical obstruction of the intestine or urinary tract.
Use cautiously in patients with bronchial asthma, bradycardia, and arrhythmias.

## Interactions
**Drug-drug.** *Aminoglycoside antibiotics:* Have a mild but definite nondepolarizing blocking action that may accentuate neuromuscular block. Use together cautiously.
*Corticosteroids:* May decrease cholinergic effect of pyridostigmine; when corticosteroids are stopped, this effect may increase, possibly affecting muscle strength. Advise clinician to monitor patient closely.
*Ganglionic blockers:* May critically decrease blood pressure; effect is usually preceded by abdominal symptoms. Advise clinician to monitor patient closely.
*Magnesium:* Has a direct depressant effect on skeletal muscle and may antagonize beneficial effects of pyridostigmine. Use together cautiously. Advise clinician to monitor patient closely.
*Procainamide, quinidine:* May reverse cholinergic effect of pyridostigmine on muscle. Advise clinician to monitor patient for drug effect.
*Succinylcholine:* May result in prolonged respiratory depression from plasma esterase inhibition, delaying succinylcholine hydrolysis. Use together cautiously.

## Adverse reactions
**CNS:** headache (with high doses), weakness.
**CV:** *bradycardia,* hypotension, thrombophlebitis.
**EENT:** miosis.
**GI:** abdominal cramps, nausea, vomiting, diarrhea, excessive salivation, increased peristalsis.
**Musculoskeletal:** muscle cramps, muscle fasciculations.
**Respiratory:** *bronchospasm, bronchoconstriction,* increased bronchial secretions.
**Skin:** rash, diaphoresis.

## Overdose and treatment
Clinical effects of overdose include nausea, vomiting, diarrhea, blurred vision, miosis, excessive tearing, bronchospasm, increased

bronchial secretions, hypotension, incoordination, excessive sweating, muscle weakness, cramps, fasciculations, paralysis, bradycardia or tachycardia, excessive salivation, and restlessness or agitation.

Respiration should be supported; bronchial suctioning may be performed. Drug should be stopped immediately. Atropine may be given to block muscarinic effects of pyridostigmine; however, it won't counter skeletal muscle paralysis. Avoid atropine overdose because it may lead to bronchial plug formation.

### Clinical considerations
■ If muscle weakness is severe, determine whether this effect stems from drug toxicity or exacerbation of myasthenia gravis. A test dose of edrophonium I.V. will aggravate drug-induced weakness but will temporarily relieve weakness that results from the disease.
■ Avoid giving large doses to patients with decreased GI motility because toxicity may result once motility has been restored.
■ Recommend giving drug with food or milk to reduce risk of muscarinic adverse effects.
■ Atropine sulfate should always be readily available as an antagonist for the muscarinic effects of pyridostigmine.

### *Therapeutic monitoring*
■ Patients may develop resistance to drug. Advise clinician to monitor patient closely.

### *Special populations*
**Breast-feeding patients.** It isn't known if drug appears in breast milk. Because of the potential for serious adverse reactions in the breast-fed infant, either breast-feeding or drug should be discontinued, taking into account the importance of drug to the woman.

### Patient counseling
■ When drug is used in patient with myasthenia gravis, stress importance of taking drug exactly as ordered, on time, and in evenly spaced doses.
■ If patient is taking sustained-release tablets, explain how these work and instruct him to take them at the same time each day and to swallow these tablets whole rather than crushing them.
■ Teach patient how to evaluate muscle strength; instruct him to observe changes in muscle strength and to report muscle cramps, rash, or fatigue.

# pyridoxine hydrochloride (vitamin B₆)
Aminoxin, Hexa-Betalin, Nestrex, Rodex

*Pharmacologic classification:* water-soluble vitamin
*Therapeutic classification:* nutritional supplement
*Pregnancy risk category A (C if greater than RDA)*

## Available forms
Available by prescription only
*Injection:* 10-ml vial (100 mg/ml), 30-ml vial (100 mg/ml), 10-ml vial (100 mg/ml, with 1.5% benzyl alcohol), 30-ml vial (100 mg/ml, with 1.5% benzyl alcohol), 10-ml vial (100 mg/ml, with 0.5% chlorobutanol), 1-ml vial (100 mg/ml)
Available without a prescription
*Tablets:* 10 mg, 20 mg (enteric-coated), 25 mg, 50 mg, 100 mg, 200 mg, 250 mg, 500 mg, 500 mg extended-release

## Indications and dosages
*RDA*
*Neonates and infants to age 6 months:* 0.3 mg daily.
*Infants ages 6 months to 1 year:* 0.6 mg daily.
*Children ages 1 to 3:* 1 mg daily.
*Children ages 4 to 6:* 1.1 mg daily.
*Children ages 7 to 10:* 1.4 mg daily.
*Girls ages 11 to 14:* 1.4 mg daily.
*Girls ages 15 to 18:* 1.5 mg daily.
*Women ages 19 and older:* 1.6 mg daily.
*Women during pregnancy:* 2.2 mg daily.
*Breast-feeding women:* 2.1 mg daily.
*Boys ages 11 to 14:* 1.7 mg daily.
*Men ages 15 and older:* 2 mg daily.
*Dietary vitamin B₆ deficiency*
*Adults:* 2.5 to 10 mg P.O. daily until signs of deficiency are corrected, then 2 to 5 mg daily as a multivitamin preparation for several weeks.
*Drug-induced deficiency anemia or neuritis*
*Adults:* 100 to 200 mg P.O. daily for 3 weeks. Then 25 to 100 mg daily.
*Pyridoxine-dependent seizures*
*Neonates and infants:* 10 to 100 mg I.M. or I.V.
◊ *Premenstrual syndrome*
*Adults:* 40 to 500 mg P.O., I.M., or I.V. daily.
◊ *Hyperoxaluria type I*
*Adults:* 25 to 300 mg P.O., I.M., or I.V. daily.
*Seizures secondary to isoniazid overdose*
*Adults and children:* A dose of pyridoxine hydrochloride equal to the amount of isoniazid ingested is usually given; generally, 1 to 4 g I.V. initially and then 1 g I.M. every 30 minutes until the entire dosage has been given.

## I.V. administration
■ Inject undiluted drug into I.V. line of free-flowing compatible solution. Or, infuse diluted drug over prescribed duration for intermittent infusion. Don't use for continous infusion.

### Incompatibilities
Incompatible with alkaline solutions, erythromycin estolate, iron salts, kanamycin, oxidizers, riboflavin, sodium phosphate, and streptomycin.

## Mechanism of action
*Metabolic action:* Natural vitamin $B_6$ contained in plant and animal foodstuffs is converted to physiologically active forms of vitamin $B_6$, pyridoxal phosphate, and pyridoxamine phosphate. Exogenous forms of the vitamin are metabolized. Vitamin $B_6$ acts as a coenzyme in protein, carbohydrate, and fat metabolism and participates in the decarboxylation of amino acids in protein metabolism. Vitamin $B_6$ also helps convert tryptophan to niacin as well as facilitate the deamination, transamination, and transulfuration of amino acids. Finally, vitamin $B_6$ is responsible for the breakdown of glycogen to glucose-1-phosphate in carbohydrate metabolism. The total adult body store consists of 16 to 27 mg of pyridoxine. The need for pyridoxine increases with the amount of protein in the diet.

## Pharmacokinetics
*Absorption:* After oral administration, pyridoxine and its substituents are absorbed readily from the GI tract. GI absorption may be diminished in patients with malabsorption syndromes or following gastric resection. Normal serum levels of pyridoxine are 30 to 80 ng/ml.
*Distribution:* Stored mainly in the liver. The total body store is about 16 to 27 mg. Pyridoxal and pyridoxal phosphate are the most common forms found in the blood and are highly protein-bound. Pyridoxal crosses the placenta; fetal plasma levels are five times greater than maternal plasma levels. After maternal intake of 2.5 to 5 mg/day of pyridoxine, the level of the vitamin in breast milk is about 240 ng/ml.
*Metabolism:* Degraded to 4-pyridoxic acid in the liver.
*Excretion:* In erythrocytes, pyridoxine is converted to pyridoxal phosphate, and pyridoxamine is converted to pyridoxamine phosphate. The phosphorylated form of pyridoxine is transaminated to pyridoxal and pyridoxamine, which is phosphorylated rapidly. The conversion of pyridoxine phosphate to pyridoxal phosphate requires riboflavin. Biologic half-life is 15 to 20 days.

| Route | Onset | Peak | Duration |
|---|---|---|---|
| P.O., I.V., I.M. | Unknown | Unknown | Unknown |

## Contraindications and precautions
Contraindicated in patients hypersensitive to pyridoxine.

## Interactions
**Drug-drug.** *Cycloserine, hydralazine, isoniazid, oral contraceptives, penicillamine:* May increase pyridoxine requirements. Advise clinician to monitor patient closely.
*Levodopa:* Pyridoxine reverses the therapeutic effects of levodopa. Avoid use together.
*Phenobarbital, phenytoin:* May cause a 50% decrease in serum levels of these anticonvulsants. Avoid use together.

## Adverse reactions
**CNS:** paresthesia, unsteady gait, numbness, somnolence.

## Overdose and treatment
Signs of overdose include ataxia and severe sensory neuropathy after chronic consumption of high daily doses of pyridoxine (2 to 6 g). These neurologic deficits usually resolve after pyridoxine is discontinued.

## Clinical considerations
■ Prepare a dietary history. A single vitamin deficiency is unusual; lack of one vitamin often indicates a deficiency of others.
■ Don't mix with sodium bicarbonate in the same syringe.
■ Store in a tight, light-resistant container.
■ Don't use injection solution if it contains precipitate. Slight darkening is acceptable.
■ Pyridoxine is sometimes useful for treating nausea and vomiting during pregnancy.
■ Pyridoxine therapy alters determinations for urobilinogen in the spot test using Ehrlich's reagent, resulting in a false-positive reaction.

### Therapeutic monitoring
■ Advise clinician to monitor protein intake; excessive protein intake increases pyridoxine requirements.
■ A dosage of 25 mg/kg/day is well tolerated. Adults consuming 200 mg/day for 33 days and on a normal dietary intake develop vitamin $B_6$ dependency.

### Special populations
**Breast-feeding patients.** It's unknown if drug appears in breast milk. Use caution when giving to breast-feeding women. Pyridoxine may inhibit lactation by suppression of prolactin.
**Pediatric patients.** Safety and efficacy in children haven't been established. The use of large doses of pyridoxine during pregnancy has been implicated in pyridoxine-dependency seizures in neonates.

## Patient counseling
■ Teach patient about dietary sources of vitamin B$_6$, such as yeast, wheat germ, liver, whole grain cereals, bananas, and legumes.

# pyrimethamine
Daraprim

*Pharmacologic classification:* aminopyrimidine derivative (folic acid antagonist)
*Therapeutic classification:* antimalarial
*Pregnancy risk category C*

## Available forms
Available by prescription only
*Tablets:* 25 mg

## Indications and dosages
*Chemoprophylaxis of malaria*
*Adults and children over age 10:* 25 mg P.O. weekly.
*Children ages 4 to 10:* 12.5 mg P.O. weekly.
*Children under age 4:* 6.25 mg P.O. weekly.
    Dosage should be continued for all agegroups for at least 10 weeks after leaving endemic areas.
*Treatment of acute malaria*
Not recommended alone for treatment. 25 mg P.O. once daily for 2 days with a sulfonamide to initiate transmission control and suppression of non-*falciparum* malaria. If drug must be used alone in semi-immune patients:
*Adults:* 50 mg P.O. daily for 2 days followed by 25 mg once weekly for at least 10 weeks.
*Children ages 4 to 10:* 25 mg P.O. once daily for 2 days followed by 12.5 mg once weekly for at least 10 weeks.
*Toxoplasmosis*
*Adults:* Initially, 50 to 75 mg P.O. daily with sulfonamide 1 to 4 g P.O. daily for 1 to 3 weeks. Then may decrease dose of each drug 50% and continue for an additional 4 to 5 weeks.
*Children:* 1 mg/kg/day P.O. divided in 2 equal doses. After 2 to 4 days may decrease dose 50% to 0.5 mg/kg/day and continue treatment for 1 month.
◊ *Primary prophylaxis against toxoplasmosis in patients with HIV infection*
*Adults and adolescents:* 50 mg P.O. once weekly with leucovorin and dapsone. Or, 25 mg P.O. once daily with leucovorin and atovaquone.
◊ *Secondary prophylaxis of toxoplasmosis in patients with HIV infection*
*Adults and adolescents:* 25 to 75 mg P.O. once daily with leucovorin and sulfadiazine. Or, 25 mg P.O. daily with leucovorin and atovaquone.
◊ *Isosporiasis*
*Adults:* 50 to 75 mg P.O. daily.

## Mechanism of action
*Antimalarial action:* Pyrimethamine inhibits the reduction of dihydrofolate to tetrahydrofolate, blocking folic acid metabolism needed for survival of susceptible organisms. This mechanism is distinct from sulfonamide-induced folic acid antagonism. Pyrimethamine is active against the asexual erythrocytic forms of susceptible plasmodia and against *Toxoplasma gondii.*

## Pharmacokinetics
*Absorption:* Well absorbed from the intestinal tract.
*Distribution:* Distributed to the kidneys, liver, spleen, and lungs; drug is about 80% bound to plasma proteins.
*Metabolism:* Metabolized to several unidentified compounds.
*Excretion:* Excreted in the urine and appears in breast milk; elimination half-life is 2 to 6 days. Its half-life isn't changed in end-stage renal disease.

| Route | Onset | Peak | Duration |
|-------|-------|------|----------|
| P.O. | Unknown | 1½-8 hr | 2 wk |

## Contraindications and precautions
Contraindicated in patients hypersensitive to drug and in those with megaloblastic anemia caused by folic acid deficiency.
    Use cautiously in patients with impaired renal or hepatic function, severe allergy or bronchial asthma, G6PD deficiency, or seizure disorders and in those after treatment with chloroquine.

## Interactions
**Drug-drug.** *Co-trimoxazole, sulfonamides:* Act synergistically against some organisms because each inhibits folic acid synthesis at a different level. Advise clinician to monitor patient for adverse reactions.
*Folic acid, para-aminobenzoic acid:* Reduce the antitoxoplasmic effects of pyrimethamine and may require higher dosage of the latter drug.
*Lorazepam:* Mild hepatotoxicity has been reported in patients who were also given lorazepam. Advise clinician to monitor patient closely.

## Adverse reactions
**GI:** anorexia, vomiting, atrophic glossitis.
**Hematologic:** *aplastic anemia,* megaloblastic anemia, *leukopenia, thrombocytopenia, pancytopenia.*

## Overdose and treatment
Overdose is marked by anorexia, vomiting, and CNS stimulation, including seizures. Megaloblastic anemia, thrombocytopenia, leukopenia, glossitis, and crystalluria may also occur.

---

Reactions may be *common,* uncommon, *life-threatening,* or COMMON AND LIFE-THREATENING.

Treatment of overdose consists of gastric lavage followed by a cathartic; barbiturates may help to control seizures. Leucovorin (folinic acid) in a dosage of 5 to 15 mg/day P.O., I.M., or I.V. for 3 days or longer is used to restore decreased platelet or leukocyte counts.

## Clinical considerations

■ No longer considered a first-line antimalarial drug. Other antimalarial drugs, such as mefloquine, chloroquine, and sulfadoxine, are generally preferred.
■ Drug should be given with meals to minimize GI distress.
■ Because severe reactions may occur, pyrimethamine with sulfadoxine should be given only in unusual situations in which the recommended drugs cannot be used.
■ Adverse drug reactions related to sulfadiazine are similar to those related to sulfonamides.

### Therapeutic monitoring

■ Advise clinician to monitor CBC, including platelet counts, twice weekly.
■ Advise clinician to monitor patient for signs of folate deficiency or bleeding when platelet count is low; if abnormalities appear, advise clinician to decrease dosage or stop drug. Leucovorin (folinic acid) may be prescribed to raise blood counts during reduced dosage or after drug is discontinued.

### Special populations

**Breast-feeding patients.** Pyrimethamine and sulfadoxine combination is contraindicated in breast-feeding women because it contains a sulfonamide.
**Pediatric patients.** Use with caution in children.

## Patient counseling

■ Teach patient how to recognize signs and symptoms of adverse blood reactions and tell him to report them immediately. Teach emergency measures to control overt bleeding.
■ Teach patient signs and symptoms of folate deficiency.
■ Counsel patient about need to report adverse effects and to keep follow-up medical appointments.
■ Tell patient to keep drug out of reach of children.

# quetiapine fumarate
Seroquel

*Pharmacologic classification:* dibenzo-thiazepine derivative
*Therapeutic classification:* antipsychotic
*Pregnancy risk category C*

## Available forms
Available by prescription only
*Tablets:* 25 mg, 100 mg, 200 mg, 300 mg

## Indications and dosages
***Management of signs and symptoms of psychotic disorders***
*Adults:* Initially, 25 mg P.O. b.i.d., with increases in increments of 25 to 50 mg b.i.d. or t.i.d. on days 2 and 3, as tolerated to a target dosage range of 300 to 400 mg daily by day 4, divided into two or three doses. Further dosage adjustments, if indicated, should generally occur at intervals of not less than 2 days. Dosages can be increased or decreased by 25 to 50 mg b.i.d. Antipsychotic efficacy is generally in dosage range of 150 to 750 mg/day. Safety of doses above 800 mg/day hasn't been evaluated.
≡ *Dosage adjustment.* In geriatric or debilitated patients or those who have hepatic impairment or a predisposition to hypotensive reactions, consider lower doses, slower dosage adjustment, and careful monitoring during initial dosing period. No specific dosing recommendations are given.

## Mechanism of action
*Antipsychotic action:* Exact mechanism of action is unknown. Quetiapine is a dibenzo-thiazepine derivative that is thought to exert antipsychotic activity through antagonism of dopamine type 2 ($D_2$) and serotonin type 2 ($5\text{-}HT_2$) receptors. Antagonism at serotonin $5\text{-}HT_{1A}$, $D_1$, $H_1$, and alpha$_1$- and alpha$_2$-adrenergic receptors may explain other effects.

## Pharmacokinetics
*Absorption:* Rapidly absorbed after oral administration. Absorption is affected by food, with maximum level increasing 25% and bioavailability increasing 15%.
*Distribution:* Apparent volume of distribution is 10 ± 4 L/kg. Drug is 83% plasma protein–bound. Steady-state levels are reached within 2 days.
*Metabolism:* Extensively metabolized by the liver via sulfoxidation and oxidation. Cytochrome P-450 3A4 is the major isoenzyme involved.
*Excretion:* Less than 1% of dose is excreted as unchanged drug. About 73% is recovered in urine and 20% in feces. Mean terminal half-life is about 6 hours.

| Route | Onset | Peak | Duration |
|-------|-------|------|----------|
| P.O. | Unknown | 1½ hr | Unknown |

## Contraindications and precautions
Contraindicated in patients hypersensitive to drug or its ingredients.

Use cautiously in patients with known CV or cerebrovascular disease or conditions that would predispose patient to hypotension, in patients with history of seizures or with conditions that potentially lower the seizure threshold, and in those at risk for aspiration pneumonia because of associated esophageal dysmotility and aspiration. Also use with caution in patients with conditions that may contribute to an elevation in core body temperature.

## Interactions
**Drug-drug.** *Antihypertensives:* May potentiate the hypotensive effect of both drugs. Advise clinician to monitor blood pressure.
*Cimetidine, phenytoin, thioridazine:* Increased clearance of quetiapine. Quetiapine dose may need adjustment.
*CNS depressants:* Increased CNS effects. Use cautiously.
*Dopamine agonists, levodopa:* Quetiapine may antagonize the effect of these drugs. Advise clinician to monitor patient closely.
*Erythromycin, fluconazole, itraconazole, ketoconazole:* Decreased quetiapine clearance. Use with caution.
*Lorazepam:* Reduced clearance when coadministered with quetiapine. Advise clinician to monitor patient.
**Drug-lifestyle.** *Alcohol use:* May cause potentiated cognitive and motor effects. Advise patient to avoid alcohol during quetiapine therapy.

---

Reactions may be *common*, uncommon, *life-threatening*, or **COMMON AND LIFE-THREATENING**.

## Adverse reactions

**CNS:** *dizziness, headache, somnolence,* hypertonia, asthenia, dysarthria.
**CV:** orthostatic hypotension, tachycardia, palpitations, peripheral edema.
**EENT:** pharyngitis, rhinitis, ear pain.
**GI:** dry mouth, dyspepsia, abdominal pain, constipation, anorexia.
**Hematologic:** *leukopenia.*
**Metabolic:** *weight gain.*
**Musculoskeletal:** back pain.
**Respiratory:** increased cough, dyspnea.
**Skin:** rash, diaphoresis.
**Other:** fever, flulike syndrome.

## Overdose and treatment

Usually exaggeration of pharmacologic effects of drug is seen (drowsiness, sedation, tachycardia, hypotension). Hypokalemia and first-degree heart block may also occur.

For acute overdose, treatment includes establishing and maintaining an airway to ensure adequate oxygenation and ventilation. Gastric lavage and administration of activated charcoal or a laxative should be considered. CV monitoring, including ECG monitoring, should begin immediately. Avoid use of disopyramide, procainamide, quinidine, and bretylium if antiarrhythmic therapy is indicated. Recommend giving I.V. fluids or sympathomimetics (not epinephrine or dopamine) to treat hypotension and circulatory collapse. For severe extrapyramidal symptoms, recommend giving anticholinergics.

## Clinical considerations

■ A decrease in total and free $T_4$ may occur; this is usually not clinically significant. Although rare, some patients experience increased thyroid-stimulating hormone levels and require thyroid replacement.
■ Increases in cholesterol and triglycerides have been observed.
■ Asymptomatic, transient, and reversible increases in serum transaminases (primarily ALT) have been reported. These elevations usually occur within the first 3 weeks of therapy and promptly return to pretreatment levels with continued use.
■ Neuroleptic malignant syndrome, a potentially fatal syndrome, has been reported with use of antipsychotic drugs. Signs and symptoms include hyperpyrexia, muscle rigidity, altered mental status, and evidence of autonomic instability. Recommend carefully monitoring at-risk patients.
■ Smallest effective dose should be used for shortest duration to minimize risk of tardive dyskinesia.

### Therapeutic monitoring

■ Recommend examining patient's lens before therapy begins or shortly thereafter, and at 6-month intervals during chronic treatment for possible cataract formation.
■ Schizophrenic patient should be closely supervised during drug therapy because of the inherent risk of a suicide attempt.

### Special populations

**Pregnant patients.** Instruct women to report if pregnancy is being planned or is suspected.
**Breast-feeding patients.** Breast-feeding isn't recommended during quetiapine therapy.
**Pediatric patients.** Safety and efficacy in children haven't been established.
**Geriatric patients.** There appears to be no difference in tolerability in patients ages 65 or older. However, factors that may decrease pharmacokinetic clearance, increase pharmacodynamic response to the drug, or cause poorer tolerance or orthostasis should indicate use of a lower starting dose, slower dosage adjustment, and careful monitoring during the initial dosing period.

### Patient counseling

■ Advise patient of risk of orthostatic hypotension, especially during the 3- to 5-day period of initial dosage adjustment and when dose is increased or treatment reinitiated.
■ Tell patient to avoid becoming overheated or dehydrated.
■ During initial dosage adjustment period or dosage increases, warn patient to avoid activities that require mental alertness, such as driving a car or operating hazardous machinery until CNS effects of drug are known.
■ Remind patient to have an initial eye examination at beginning of drug therapy and every 6 months during treatment period to monitor for cataract formation.
■ Tell patient to contact his prescriber before taking other prescription or OTC drugs.

# quinapril hydrochloride
Accupril

*Pharmacologic classification:* ACE inhibitor
*Therapeutic classification:* antihypertensive
*Pregnancy risk category C (D second and third trimesters)*

## Available forms

Available by prescription only
*Tablets:* 5 mg, 10 mg, 20 mg, 40 mg

## Indications and dosages

*Heart failure*
*Adults:* Initially, 5 mg P.O. b.i.d., given with a cardiac glycoside, diuretic, and a beta blocker. Adjust dosage weekly based on response. Usual dose is 20 to 40 mg P.O. daily in two equally divided doses.

### Hypertension in patients not receiving a diuretic

*Adults:* Initially, 10 mg P.O. daily. Adjust dosage based on response at intervals of about 2 weeks. Most patients are controlled at 20, 40, or 80 mg daily, as a single dose or in two divided doses.
≡ *Dosage adjustment.* In adults with renal impairment, initial dose is 10 mg P.O. daily if creatinine clearance exceeds 60 ml/minute; 5 mg if it's 30 to 60 ml/minute; and 2.5 mg if it's 10 to 30 ml/minute. No dose recommendations are available for creatinine clearance less than 10 ml/minute.

## Mechanism of action

*Antihypertensive action:* Quinapril and its active metabolite, quinaprilat, inhibit ACE, preventing conversion of angiotensin I to angiotensin II, a potent vasoconstrictor. Reduced formation of angiotensin II decreases peripheral arterial resistance, decreases aldosterone secretion, reduces sodium and water retention, and lowers blood pressure. Quinapril also has antihypertensive activity in patients with low-renin hypertension.

## Pharmacokinetics

*Absorption:* At least 60% of drug is absorbed. Rate and extent of absorption are decreased 25% to 30% when drug is given during a high-fat meal.
*Distribution:* About 97% of drug and active metabolite are plasma protein–bound.
*Metabolism:* About 38% of an oral dose is de-esterified in the liver to quinaprilat, the active metabolite.
*Excretion:* Primarily excreted in urine; terminal elimination half-life is about 25 hours.

| Route | Onset | Peak | Duration |
|-------|-------|------|----------|
| P.O. | 1 hr | 2-6 hr | 24 hr |

## Contraindications and precautions

Contraindicated in patients hypersensitive to ACE inhibitors or who have a history of angioedema related to treatment with an ACE inhibitor. Use cautiously in patients with impaired renal function. Also contraindicated in patients at immediate risk for cardiogenic shock.

## Interactions

**Drug-drug.** *Diuretics, other antihypertensives:* Increase risk of excessive hypotension. Recommend stopping diuretic or lowering dose of quinapril p.r.n.
*Lithium:* Increased serum lithium levels and lithium toxicity. Advise clinician to monitor serum lithium levels.
*Potassium-sparing diuretics and potassium supplements:* May increase risk of hyperkalemia. Don't use together.
*Tetracycline:* Significantly impairs absorption of tetracycline. Avoid use together.

**Drug-herb.** *Capsaicin:* Increased risk of cough. Discourage use together.
*Licorice:* May cause sodium retention and increase blood pressure, interfering with the therapeutic effects of ACE inhibitors. Discourage use together.
**Drug-food.** *Potassium-containing salt-substitutes:* Can cause hyperkalemia. Don't use together.

## Adverse reactions

**CNS:** somnolence, vertigo, nervousness, headache, dizziness, fatigue, depression.
**CV:** palpitations, tachycardia, angina, hypertensive crisis, orthostatic hypotension, chest pain, *rhythm disturbances.*
**GI:** dry mouth, abdominal pain, constipation, vomiting, nausea, *hemorrhage.*
**Hematologic:** *thrombocytopenia, agranulocytosis.*
**Hepatic:** elevated liver enzyme levels.
**Metabolic:** hyperkalemia.
**Respiratory:** *dry, persistent, tickling, nonproductive cough.*
**Skin:** pruritus, *exfoliative dermatitis,* photosensitivity, diaphoresis.
**Other:** *angioedema.*

## Overdose and treatment

No information is available regarding overdose. The most likely symptom is hypotension.
Peritoneal dialysis or hemodialysis isn't beneficial. No data are available to support use of certain physiologic maneuvers such as acidification of urine. Treatment is symptomatic. Infusions of normal saline solution have been suggested to treat hypotension.

## Clinical considerations

■ Because administration with diuretics is linked to a risk of excessive hypotension, diuretic therapy should be stopped 2 to 3 days before start of quinapril, if possible. If quinapril alone doesn't adequately control blood pressure, a diuretic may be carefully added to the regimen.
■ Like other ACE inhibitors, drug may cause a dry, persistent, tickling cough; it's reversible when therapy is discontinued.
■ Each tablet of quinapril contains magnesium carbonate and magnesium stearate.

### Therapeutic monitoring

■ Blood pressure measurements should be made when drug levels are at their peak (2 to 6 hours after dosing) and at their trough (just before a dose) to verify adequate blood pressure control.
■ Renal and hepatic function should be assessed before and periodically throughout therapy. Also, CBC and serum potassium levels should be monitored.

## Special populations

**Breast-feeding patients.** It's unknown if drug appears in breast milk. Use with caution in breast-feeding women.

**Pediatric patients.** Safety and efficacy in children haven't been established.

**Geriatric patients.** Geriatric patients have shown higher peak plasma levels and slower elimination of drug; these changes were related to decreased renal function that often occurs in geriatric patients. No overall differences in safety or efficacy have been seen in geriatric patients.

## Patient counseling

- Tell patient that drug should be taken on an empty stomach because meals, particularly high-fat meals, can impair absorption.

**H ALERT** Advise patient to immediately report signs or symptoms of angioedema: swelling of face, eyes, lips, tongue, or difficulty in breathing. If these occur, patient should stop taking drug and seek immediate medical attention.

- Warn patient that light-headedness may occur, especially during first few days of therapy. Tell him to arise slowly to minimize this effect and to report persistent or severe symptoms. If syncope (fainting) occurs, patient should stop taking drug and report immediately.
- Inadequate fluid intake, vomiting, diarrhea, and excessive perspiration can lead to light-headedness and syncope. Patient should take care in hot weather and during periods of exercise to avoid dehydration and overheating.
- Tell patient to immediately report signs or symptoms of infection (sore throat, fever) or of easy bruising or bleeding. Other ACE inhibitors have caused the development of agranulocytosis and neutropenia.

# quinidine gluconate
Quinaglute Dura-Tabs, Quinalan

# quinidine polygalacturonate
Cardioquin

# quinidine sulfate
Apo-Quinidine*, Quinidex Extentabs

*Pharmacologic classification:* cinchona alkaloid
*Therapeutic classification:* ventricular antiarrhythmic, supraventricular antiarrhythmic, atrial antitachyarrhythmic
*Pregnancy risk category C*

## Available forms

Available by prescription only
*Injection:* 80 mg/ml (gluconate)

*Tablets:* 275 mg (polygalacturonate); 200 mg, 300 mg (sulfate); 300 mg (extended-release, sulfate); 324 mg (extended-release, gluconate)

## Indications and dosages

### Atrial flutter or fibrillation

*Adults:* 200 mg (sulfate or equivalent base) P.O. q 2 to 3 hours for five to eight doses with subsequent daily increases until sinus rhythm is restored or toxic effects develop. Administer quinidine only after digitalization, to avoid increasing AV conduction. Maximum dose, 3 to 4 g daily.

Maintenance dose, 200 to 400 mg P.O. t.i.d. or q.i.d., or 600 mg P.O. q 8 to 12 hours daily (extended-release).

### Paroxysmal supraventricular tachycardia

*Adults:* 400 to 600 mg (sulfate) P.O. q 2 to 3 hours until toxic effects develop or arrhythmia subsides.

### Premature atrial contractions, PVCs, paroxysmal AV junctional rhythm or atrial or ventricular tachycardia, maintenance of cardioversion

*Adults:* Give test dose of 50 to 200 mg P.O. of sulfate (or 200 mg gluconate I.M.); then monitor vital signs before beginning therapy: 200 to 400 mg P.O. sulfate or equivalent base q 4 to 6 hours; or initially, 600 mg of gluconate I.M., then up to 400 mg q 2 hours, p.r.n.; or 800 mg I.V. gluconate diluted in 40 ml of D$_5$W, infused at 16 mg (1 ml)/minute. Alternatively, give 300 to 600 mg of sulfate (extended-release), or 324 to 648 mg of gluconate (extended-release), q 8 to 12 hours.

*Children:* Give test dose of 2 mg/kg, then 30 mg/kg/day P.O. or 900 mg/m$^2$/day P.O. in five divided doses.

### ◇ Malaria

*Adults:* Administer quinidine gluconate by continuous I.V. infusion. Initial loading dose of 10 mg/kg diluted in 250 ml of normal saline injection and infused over 1 to 2 hours, followed by a continuous maintenance infusion of 0.02 mg/kg/minute (20 mcg/kg/minute) for 72 hours or until parasitemia is reduced to less than 1% or oral therapy can be started; or 10 mg/kg or 300 to 600 mg quinidine sulfate P.O. q 8 hours for 5 to 7 days. Contact the Centers for Disease Control and Prevention (CDC) Malaria Branch for protocol instructions for recommendations at 1-707-488-7788 (weekdays) or 1-404-639-2888 (evenings, weekends, holidays), if using regimen.

## I.V. administration

- Administer following current CDC regimen guidelines. Contact the CDC Malaria Branch for protocol instructions at 1-707-488-7788 (weekdays) or 1-404-639-2888 (evenings, weekends, holidays), if using regimen.

## Incompatibilities

Incompatible with alkalies, amiodarone, furosemide, heparin sodium, and iodides.

## Mechanism of action

*Antiarrhythmic action:* A class IA antiarrhythmic, quinidine depresses phase 0 of the action potential. It's considered a myocardial depressant because it decreases myocardial excitability and conduction velocity and may depress myocardial contractility. It also exerts anticholinergic activity, which may modify its direct myocardial effects. In therapeutic doses, quinidine reduces conduction velocity in the atria, ventricles, and His-Purkinje system. It helps control atrial tachyarrhythmias by prolonging the effective refractory period (ERP) and increasing the action potential duration in the atria, ventricles, and His-Purkinje system. Because ERP prolongation exceeds action potential duration, tissue remains refractory even after returning to resting membrane potential (membrane-stabilizing effect).

Quinidine shortens the effective refractory period of the AV node. Because anticholinergic action of quinidine may increase AV node conductivity, a cardiac glycoside should be given for atrial tachyarrhythmias before quinidine therapy begins, to prevent ventricular tachyarrhythmias. Quinidine also suppresses automaticity in the His-Purkinje system and ectopic pacemakers, making it useful in treating PVCs. At therapeutic doses, quinidine prolongs the QRS complex and QT interval; these ECG effects may be used as an index of drug effectiveness and toxicity.

## Pharmacokinetics

*Absorption:* Although all quinidine salts are well absorbed from the GI tract, individual serum drug levels vary greatly. For extended-release forms, onset of action may be slightly slower but duration of effect is longer because drug delivery system allows longer-than-usual dosing intervals.

*Distribution:* Well distributed in all tissues except the brain, and concentrates in the heart, liver, kidneys, and skeletal muscle. Distribution volume decreases in patients with heart failure, possibly requiring reduction in maintenance dosage. About 80% of drug is plasma protein–bound; the unbound (active) fraction may increase in patients with hypoalbuminemia from various causes, including hepatic insufficiency. Usual therapeutic serum levels depend on assay method and ranges as follows:
—Specific assay (enzyme multiplied immunoassay technique, high-performance liquid chromatography, fluorescence polarization): 2 to 5 mcg/ml.
—Nonspecific assay (fluorometric): 4 to 8 mcg/ml.

*Metabolism:* About 60% to 80% of drug is metabolized in the liver to two metabolites that may have some pharmacologic activity.

*Excretion:* About 10% to 30% of given dose is excreted in the urine within 24 hours as unchanged drug. Urine acidification increases quinidine excretion; alkalinization decreases excretion. Most of an administered dose is eliminated in the urine as metabolites; elimination half-life ranges from 5 to 12 hours (usual half-life is about 6½ hours). Duration of effect ranges from 6 to 8 hours.

| Route | Onset | Peak | Duration |
|-------|-------|------|----------|
| P.O. | 1-3 hr | 1-6 hr | 6-8 hr |
| I.V. | Immediate | Immediate | Unknown |
| I.M. | ½-1½ min | Unknown | Unknown |

## Contraindications and precautions

Contraindicated in patients with idiosyncrasy or hypersensitivity to quinidine or related cinchona derivatives, intraventricular conduction defects, cardiac glycoside toxicity when AV conduction is grossly impaired, abnormal rhythms from escape mechanisms, and history of drug-induced torsades de pointes or QT syndrome.

Use cautiously in patients with impaired renal or hepatic function, asthma, muscle weakness, or infection accompanied by a fever because hypersensitivity reactions may be masked.

## Interactions

**Drug-drug.** *Antacids, sodium bicarbonate, thiazide diuretics:* May decrease quinidine elimination when urine pH increases, requiring close monitoring of therapy.

*Anticholinergics:* May lead to additive anticholinergic effects. Use with caution.

*Anticonvulsants, such as phenobarbital and phenytoin:* Increases the rate of quinidine metabolism; this leads to decreased quinidine levels. Advise clinician to monitor patient closely.

*Cholinergics:* May fail to terminate paroxysmal supraventricular tachycardia. Also, anticholinergic effects of quinidine may negate the effects of these drugs when these drugs are used to treat myasthenia gravis. Use with caution.

*Coumarin:* May potentiate anticoagulant effect of coumarin, possibly leading to hypoprothrombinemic hemorrhage. Advise clinician to monitor patient closely.

*Digitoxin or digoxin:* May cause increased (possibly toxic) serum digoxin levels. Some experts recommend a 50% reduction in digoxin dosage when quinidine therapy starts, with subsequent monitoring of serum levels.

*Hypotensives:* May cause additive hypotensive effects, mainly when administered I.V. Advise clinician to monitor blood pressure closely.

*Neuromuscular blockers, such as metocurine iodide, pancuronium bromide, succinylcholine chloride, and tubocurarine chloride:* May potentiate anticholinergic effects. Use of quinidine should be avoided immediately after use of these drugs; if quinidine must be used, respiratory support may be needed.

*Nifedipine:* May result in decreased quinidine levels. Advise clinician to monitor closely.

*Other antiarrhythmics, such as amiodarone, lidocaine, phenytoin, procainamide, and propranolol:* May cause additive or antagonistic cardiac effects and additive toxic effects. Use together cautiously.

*Phenothiazines, reserpine:* May cause additive cardiac depressant effects. Avoid use together.

*Rifampin:* May increase quinidine metabolism and decrease serum quinidine levels, possibly necessitating dosage adjustment when rifampin therapy starts or stops.

*Verapamil:* May result in significant hypotension in some patients with hypertrophic cardiomyopathy. Advise clinician to monitor patient closely.

**Drug-herb.** *Jimsonweed:* May adversely affect CV function. Discourage use together.

*Licorice:* May prolong the QT interval and be potentially additive. Discourage use together.

**Drug-food.** *Grapefruit juice:* Delayed onset of quinidine effect. Advise patient to take with liquid other than grapefruit juice.

## Adverse reactions

**CNS:** *vertigo, headache, light-headedness,* confusion, ataxia, depression, dementia.

**CV:** *PVCs; ventricular tachycardia; atypical ventricular tachycardia (torsades de pointes);* hypotension; *complete AV block, tachycardia; ECG changes (particularly widening of QRS complex, widened QT and PR intervals).*

**EENT:** *tinnitus,* blurred vision, diplopia, photophobia.

**GI:** *diarrhea, nausea, vomiting,* anorexia, abdominal pain, excessive salivation.

**Hematologic:** *hemolytic anemia, thrombocytopenia, agranulocytosis.*

**Hepatic:** *hepatotoxicity.*

**Respiratory:** *acute asthmatic attack, respiratory arrest.*

**Skin:** rash, petechial hemorrhage of buccal mucosa, pruritus, urticaria, photosensitivity.

**Other:** *angioedema, fever, cinchonism,* lupus erythematosus.

## Overdose and treatment

The most serious clinical effects of overdose include severe hypotension, ventricular arrhythmias (including torsades de pointes), and seizures. QRS complexes and QT and PR intervals may be prolonged, and ataxia, anuria, respiratory distress, irritability, and hallucinations may develop. If ingestion was recent, gastric lavage, emesis, and activated charcoal may be used to decrease absorption. Urine acidifi-

cation may be used to help increase quinidine elimination.

Treatment involves general supportive measures (including CV and respiratory support) with hemodynamic and ECG monitoring. Metaraminol or norepinephrine may be used to reverse hypotension (after adequate hydration has been ensured). Avoid CNS depressants because CNS depression may occur, possibly with seizures. Cardiac pacing may be needed. Isoproterenol or ventricular pacing possibly may be used to treat torsades de pointes tachycardia.

I.V. infusion of 1/6 M sodium lactate solution reduces cardiotoxic effect of quinidine. Hemodialysis, although rarely warranted, also may be effective.

## Clinical considerations

**◢ ALERT** When changing route of administration or oral salt form, be aware that dosage needs to be altered to compensate for variations in quinidine base content.

■ Use of I.V. route is generally avoided because of the potential for severe hypotension.

■ Dosage should be decreased in patients with HF and hepatic disease.

■ When drug is used to treat atrial tachyarrhythmias, ventricular rate may be accelerated from anticholinergic effects of drug on AV node. This can be prevented by previous treatment with a digitalis glycoside.

■ Because conversion of chronic atrial fibrillation may be linked to embolism, recommend giving anticoagulant for several weeks before quinidine therapy begins.

■ Lidocaine may be effective in treating quinidine-induced arrhythmias because it increases AV conduction.

■ For maintenance, give only by oral or I.M. route. Dosage requirements vary. Some patients may require drug q 4 hours, others q 6 hours. Titrate dose by both clinical response and blood levels.

■ When changing administration route, dosage should be altered to compensate for variations in quinidine base content.

■ Drug may increase toxicity of cardiac glycoside derivatives. Use cautiously in patients receiving cardiac glycosides. Advise clinician to monitor digoxin levels and expect to reduce dosage of cardiac glycoside derivatives. Many clinicians recommend that digoxin dosage be reduced by 50% when quinidine therapy starts.

■ Quinidine may cause hemolysis in patients with G6PD deficiency.

■ Small amounts of quinidine are removed by hemodialysis; drug isn't removed by peritoneal dialysis.

■ Amount of quinidine in the various salt forms varies as follows:

—Gluconate: 62% quinidine (324 mg of gluconate, 202 mg sulfate).

—Polygalacturonate: 60% quinidine (275 mg polygalacturonate, 166 mg sulfate).
—Sulfate: 83% quinidine. The sulfate form is considered the standard dosage preparation.
■ Quinidine gluconate is reported to be as or more active in vitro against *Plasmodium falciparum* than quinine dihydrochloride. Because the latter drug is only available through the CDC, quinidine gluconate may be useful in the treatment of severe malaria when delay of therapy may be life-threatening. The current CDC protocol involves follow-up treatment with either tetracycline or sulfadoxine and pyrimethamine.
**H ALERT** Don't confuse drug with Quinamm, quinine, or clonidine.

### Therapeutic monitoring
■ Recommend checking apical pulse rate, blood pressure, and ECG tracing, before therapy starts.
■ Advise clinician to monitor ECG, especially when large doses of drug are being given. Quinidine-induced cardiotoxicity is evidenced by conduction defects (50% widening of the QRS complex), ventricular tachycardia or flutter, frequent PVCs, and complete AV block. When these ECG signs appear, recommend stopping drug and monitoring patient closely.
■ Advise clinician to monitor liver function test results during first 4 to 8 weeks of therapy.
■ GI adverse effects, especially diarrhea, are signs of toxicity. Advise clinician to check quinidine blood levels; suspect toxicity when they exceed 8 mcg/ml. GI symptoms may be minimized by giving drug with meals.

### Special populations
**Pregnant patients.** The drug has some oxytocic properties. Safety for use during pregnancy and labor and delivery hasn't been established.
**Breast-feeding patients.** Because drug appears in breast milk, alternative feeding method is recommended during therapy with quinidine.
**Pediatric patients.** Safety and efficacy haven't been established for use in children. Quinidine sulfate has been used in cardiac arrythmias at 30 mg/kg/day or 900 mg/m²/day P.O. in 5 divided doses; or quinidine gluconate 30 mg/kg/day or 900 mg/m²/day I.V. or I.M. For malaria in children, quinidine gluconate adult doses have been used.
**Geriatric patients.** Dosage reduction may be needed in geriatric patients. Because of highly variable metabolism, advise clinician to monitor serum levels.

### Patient counseling
■ Instruct patient to report rash, fever, unusual bleeding, bruising, ringing in ears, or visual disturbance.
■ Stress importance of taking drug exactly as prescribed.

# quinine sulfate

*Pharmacologic classification:* cinchona alkaloid
*Therapeutic classification:* antimalarial
*Pregnancy risk category D*

## Available forms
Available by prescription only
*Capsules:* 260 mg
*Tablets:* 260 mg, 325 mg

## Indications and dosages
*Malaria (chloroquine-resistant)*
*Adults:* 650 mg P.O. q 8 hours for 3 to 7 days, with 25 mg pyrimethamine q 12 hours for 3 days and with 500 mg sulfadiazine q.i.d. for 5 days.
*Children:* 25 to 30 mg/kg/day P.O. divided into three doses for 3 to 7 days.
◊ **Babesia microti** *infections*
*Adults:* 650 mg P.O. q 8 hours for 7 days.
*Children:* 25 mg/kg/day P.O. divided into three doses for 7 days.
◊ *Nocturnal recumbency leg muscle cramps*
*Adults:* 200 to 300 mg P.O. h.s. Discontinue if leg cramps don't occur after several days to determine if continued therapy is needed.
◊ *Suppression or chemoprophylaxis of malaria*
*Adults:* 325 mg P.O. b.i.d. for 6 weeks after exposure. May use with primaquine phosphate.

## Mechanism of action
*Antimalarial action:* Quinine intercalates into DNA, disrupting the parasite's replication and transcription; it also depresses its oxygen uptake and carbohydrate metabolism. It's active against the asexual erythrocytic forms of *Plasmodium falciparum, P. malariae, P. ovale,* and *P. vivax* and is used for chloroquine-resistant malaria.
*Skeletal muscle relaxant action:* Quinine increases the refractory period, decreases excitability of the motor end plate, and affects calcium distribution within muscle fibers.

## Pharmacokinetics
*Absorption:* Almost completely absorbed.
*Distribution:* Distributed widely into the liver, lungs, kidneys, and spleen; CSF levels reach 2% to 5% of serum levels. Quinine is about 70% plasma protein–bound and readily crosses the placenta.
*Metabolism:* Metabolized in the liver.
*Excretion:* Less than 5% of a single dose is excreted unchanged in the urine; small amounts of metabolites appear in the feces, gastric juice, bile, saliva, and breast milk. Half-life is 7 to 21 hours in healthy or convalescing persons;

it's longer in patients with malaria. Urine acidification hastens elimination.

| Route | Onset | Peak | Duration |
|-------|-------|------|----------|
| P.O. | Unknown | 1-3 hr | Unknown |

## Contraindications and precautions
Contraindicated during pregnancy, in patients hypersensitive to drug, and those with G6PD deficiency, optic neuritis, tinnitus, or history of blackwater fever or thrombocytopenic purpura from previous quinine ingestion.

Use cautiously in patients with arrhythmias and in those taking sodium bicarbonate together.

## Interactions
**Drug-drug.** *Acetazolamide or sodium bicarbonate:* May increase the level of quinine by decreasing urinary excretion. Advise clinician to monitor level closely.
*Aluminum-containing antacids:* May delay or decrease absorption of quinine. Avoid use together.
*Digitoxin and digoxin:* Increased plasma levels of these drugs. Advise clinician to monitor levels closely.
*Mefloquine:* May cause additive cardiac effects. Don't use together.
*Neuromuscular blockers:* May potentiate the effects of these drugs. Advise clinician to monitor patient closely.
*Warfarin:* May potentiate the action by depressing synthesis of vitamin K–dependent clotting factors. Advise clinician to monitor PT and INR closely.

## Adverse reactions
**CNS:** severe headache, apprehension, excitement, confusion, delirium, syncope, hypothermia, vertigo, *seizures* (with toxic doses).
**CV:** hypotension, *CV collapse* (with overdose or rapid I.V. administration), conduction disturbances.
**EENT:** altered color perception, photophobia, blurred vision, night blindness, amblyopia, scotoma, diplopia, mydriasis, optic atrophy, tinnitus, impaired hearing.
**GI:** epigastric distress, diarrhea, nausea, vomiting.
**GU:** renal tubular damage, anuria.
**Hematologic:** hemolytic anemia, *thrombocytopenia, agranulocytosis,* hypoprothrombinemia, thrombosis at infusion site.
**Metabolic:** hypoglycemia.
**Respiratory:** asthma, dyspnea.
**Skin:** rash, pruritus.
**Other:** flushing, fever, facial edema.

## Overdose and treatment
Signs and symptoms of overdose include tinnitus, vertigo, headache, fever, rash, CV effects, GI distress (including vomiting), blindness, apprehension, confusion, and seizures.

Treatment includes gastric lavage followed by supportive measures, which may include fluid and electrolyte replacement, artificial respiration, and stabilization of blood pressure and renal function.

Anaphylactic reactions may require epinephrine, corticosteroids, or antihistamines. Urinary acidification may increase elimination of quinine but will also augment renal obstruction. Hemodialysis or hemoperfusion may be helpful. Vasodilator therapy or stellate blockage may relieve visual disturbances.

## Clinical considerations
■ Recommend giving quinine after meals to minimize gastric distress; don't crush tablets, as drug irritates gastric mucosa.
■ Quinine is no longer used for acute malarial attack by *P. vivax* or for suppression of malaria from resistant organisms.
■ Drug causes false elevations of urinary catecholamines and may interfere with 17-hydroxycorticosteroid and 17-ketogenic steroid tests.

### Therapeutic monitoring
■ Drug should be stopped if signs of idiosyncrasy or toxicity occur.
■ Serum levels of 10 mcg/ml or more may confirm toxicity as the cause of tinnitus or hearing loss.

### Special populations
**Breast-feeding patients.** Before drug is given to a breast-feeding woman, the infant should be evaluated for possible G6PD deficiency.
**Geriatric patients.** Use with caution in patients with conduction disturbances.

## Patient counseling
■ Teach patient about adverse reactions and need to report these immediately, especially tinnitus and hearing impairment.
■ Tell patient to avoid concurrent use of aluminum-containing antacids because these may alter drug absorption.
■ Instruct patient to keep drug out of reach of children.

# quinupristin/dalfopristin
Synercid

*Pharmacologic classification:* streptogramin
*Therapeutic classification:* antibiotic
*Pregnancy risk category B*

## Available forms
Available by prescription only
*Injection:* 500 mg/10 ml (150 mg quinupristin and 350 mg dalfopristin)

## Indications and dosages

**Serious or life-threatening infections from vancomycin-resistant Enterococcus faecium (VREF) bacteremia**
*Adults and adolescents ages 16 and older:* 7.5 mg/kg I.V. infusion over 1 hour q 8 hours. Treatment duration should be determined by the site and severity of the infection.

**Complicated skin and skin structure infections caused by Staphylococcus aureus (methicillin susceptible) or Streptococcus pyogenes**
*Adults and adolescents ages 16 and older:* 7.5 mg/kg by I.V. infusion over 1 hour q 12 hours for at least 7 days.

## I. V. administration

■ Reconstitute powder for injection by adding 5 ml of either sterile water for injection or D5W and gently swirling vial by manual rotation to ensure dissolution; avoid shaking to limit foaming. Reconstituted solutions must be further diluted within 30 minutes.

■ The appropriate dose, according to patient's weight, of reconstituted solution should be added to 250 ml of D5W to make a final concentration of no more than 2 mg/ml. This diluted solution is stable for 5 hours at room temperature or 54 hours if refrigerated.

■ Don't dilute drug with saline-containing solutions or infuse into lines that contain saline or heparin. Flush line with D5W before and after each dose.

■ Recommend giving all doses by I.V. infusion over 1 hour. An infusion pump or device may be used to control rate of infusion.

### Incompatibilities

Incompatible with saline and heparin solutions.

## Mechanism of action

*Antibiotic action:* The two antibacterial drugs that make up quinupristin/dalfopristin work synergistically to inhibit or destroy susceptible bacteria through combined inhibition on protein synthesis in bacterial cells. Dalfopristin has been shown to inhibit the early phase of protein synthesis in the bacterial ribosome while quinupristin inhibits the late phase of protein synthesis. Without the ability to manufacture new proteins, the bacterial cells are inactivated or die.

## Pharmacokinetics

*Absorption:* Administered I.V. Quinupristin and dalfopristin have different pharmacokinetic profiles. After multiple infusion doses of 7.5 mg/kg every 8 hours, peak levels of quinupristin and metabolites are 3.2 mcg/ml; peak dalfopristin levels are 8.0 mcg/ml.
*Distribution:* Protein-binding is moderate.
*Metabolism:* Quinupristin and dalfopristin are converted to several active major metabolites by nonenzymatic reactions.

*Excretion:* Biliary excretion with resultant fecal elimination accounts for about 75% of elimination of both drugs and their metabolites. Urinary excretion accounts for about 15% of a quinupristin dose and 19% of a dalfopristin dose. The elimination half-lives of quinupristin and dalfopristin are about 0.85 and 0.70 hours, respectively.

| Route | Onset | Peak | Duration |
| --- | --- | --- | --- |
| I.V. | Unknown | Variable | Unknown |

## Contraindications and precautions

Contraindicated in patients hypersensitive to drug or other streptogramin antibiotics.

## Interactions

**Drug-drug.** *Calcium channel blockers, such as diltiazem, nifedipine, or verapamil; carbamazepine; diazepam; disopyramide; docetaxel; drugs metabolized by cytochrome P-450 3A4, including protease inhibitors such as delavirdine, indinavir, lidocaine; nevirapine, and ritonavir; lovastatin; methylprednisolone; midazolam; paclitaxel, tacrolimus; vinblastine:* Increased plasma levels of these drugs that could increase their therapeutic effects and adverse reactions. Use together cautiously.
*Cyclosporine:* Metabolism is reduced and levels may be increased. Advise clinician to monitor cyclosporine levels.
*Drugs metabolized by cytochrome P-450 3A4 that increase the QTc interval on the ECG (quinidine and others):* Decreased metabolism of these drugs resulting in QTc prolongation. Avoid use together.

## Adverse reactions

**CNS:** headache, pain.
**CV:** thrombophlebitis.
**GI:** nausea, diarrhea, vomiting.
**Hepatic:** *elevated total and conjugated bilirubin,* altered liver function test results.
**Musculoskeletal:** arthralgia, myalgia.
**Skin:** rash, pruritus, *inflammation, pain, edema at infusion site.*
**Other:** *infusion site reaction.*

## Overdose and treatment

Patients given an overdose should be observed and given supportive care. Drug isn't removed by peritoneal or hemodialysis.

## Clinical considerations

■ Quinupristin/dalfopristin isn't active against *Enterococcus faecalis.* Appropriate blood cultures are needed to avoid misidentifying *E. faecalis* as *E. faecium.*
■ Because mild to life-threatening pseudomembranous colitis has been reported with use of quinupristin/dalfopristin, consider this diagnosis in patients who develop diarrhea during or after therapy with drug.

- Adverse reactions, such as arthralgia and myalgia, may be reduced by decreasing dosage interval to every 12 hours.
- Fluid-restricted patients with a central venous catheter may receive dose in 100 ml of $D_5W$. This concentration isn't recommended for peripheral venous administration.
- If moderate to severe peripheral venous irritation occurs, consider increasing infusion volume to 500 or 750 ml, changing injection site, or infusing by a central venous catheter.

### Therapeutic monitoring
- Advise clinician to monitor I.V. site closely.
- Advise clinician to monitor blood work and vital signs frequently.
- Because overgrowth of nonsusceptible organisms may occur, advise clinician to monitor patient closely for signs and symptoms of superinfection.
- Advise clinician to monitor liver function test results during therapy.

### Special populations
**Pregnant patients.** Safety hasn't been established for use during pregnancy.
**Breast-feeding patients.** It isn't known if drug appears in breast milk. Use caution in breast-feeding women.
**Pediatric patients.** Safety and efficacy in patients under age 16 haven't been established. Limited clinical trials in pediatric patients used a dosage of 7.5 mg every 8 or 12 hours.
**Geriatric patients.** No dosage adjustment is required in geriatric patients.

### Patient counseling
- Advise patient to report irritation at I.V. site, pain in joints or muscles, and diarrhea immediately.
- Tell patient about the importance of reporting persistent or worsening symptoms of infection, such as pain or erythema.

---

# rabeprazole sodium
Aciphex

*Pharmacologic classification:* proton pump inhibitor
*Therapeutic classification:* antiulcerative
*Pregnancy risk category B*

### Available forms
Available by prescription only
*Tablets (delayed-release):* 20 mg

### Indications and dosages
*Healing of erosive or ulcerative gastroesophageal reflux disease (GERD)*
*Adults:* 20 mg P.O. daily for 4 to 8 weeks. Additional 8-week course may be considered, if needed.

*Maintenance of healing of erosive or ulcerative GERD*
*Adults:* 20 mg P.O. daily.
*Healing of duodenal ulcers*
*Adults:* 20 mg P.O. daily after morning meal for up to 4 weeks.
*Treatment of pathological hypersecretory conditions including Zollinger-Ellison syndrome*
*Adults:* 60 mg P.O. daily; may be increased, p.r.n., to 100 mg P.O. daily or 60 mg P.O. b.i.d.

### Mechanism of action
*Antiulcerative action:* Rabeprazole blocks activity of the acid (proton) pump by inhibiting gastric hydrogen-potassium adenosine triphosphatase at the secretory surface of the gastric parietal cell, blocking gastric acid secretion.

### Pharmacokinetics
*Absorption:* Drug is acid-labile because enteric coating allows it to pass through the stomach relatively intact.
*Distribution:* 96.3% plasma protein–bound.
*Metabolism:* Extensively metabolized by the liver to inactive compounds.
*Excretion:* 90% is eliminated in urine as metabolites. Remaining 10% of metabolites are eliminated in feces. Plasma half-life is 1 to 2 hours.

| Route | Onset | Peak | Duration |
|-------|-------|------|----------|
| P.O. | Unknown | 2-5 hr | > 24 hr |

### Contraindications and precautions
Contraindicated in patients hypersensitive to rabeprazole, other benzimidazoles (lansoprazole, omeprazole), or components in these formulations.

Use cautiously in patients with severe hepatic impairment.

### Interactions
**Drug-drug.** *Cyclosporine:* May inhibit cyclosporine metabolism. Use together cautiously.
*Digoxin, ketoconazole, other gastric pH-dependent drugs:* Decreased or increased drug absorption at increased pH values. Advise clinician to monitor patient closely during use with rabeprazole.
**Drug-herb.** *St. John's wort:* Increased risk of photosensitivity reactions. Advise patient to use sunblock.

### Adverse reactions
**CNS:** headache.

### Overdose and treatment
Treatment is supportive and symptomatic. There's no specific antidote for rabeprazole overdose, and drug isn't dialyzable because of extensive protein-binding.

---

## Clinical considerations
■ Consider additional courses of therapy when duodenal ulcers or GERD isn't healed after first course of therapy.
■ Symptomatic response to therapy doesn't preclude presence of GI cancer.

### Therapeutic monitoring
■ Advise clinician to monitor patient's response to drug therapy.

### Special populations
**Breast-feeding patients.** It's unknown if drug appears in breast milk. Taking into account importance of drug to woman, recommend either stopping drug or advise patient to stop breast-feeding.
**Pediatric patients.** Safety and efficacy haven't been established in pediatric patients.
**Geriatric patients.** No differences in safety and efficacy have been observed in geriatric patients.

## Patient counseling
■ Explain importance of taking drug exactly as prescribed for treatment course.
■ Advise patient that rabeprazole delayed-release tablets should be swallowed whole. Tablets shouldn't be crushed, chewed, or split.
■ Advise patient that drug may be taken without regard to meals.

---

# rabies immune globulin, human (RIG)
Hyperab, Imogam Rabies Immune Globulin

*Pharmacologic classification:* immune serum
*Therapeutic classification:* rabies prophylaxis
*Pregnancy risk category C*

## Available forms
Available by prescription only
*Injection:* 150 IU/ml in 2-ml and 10-ml vials

## Indications and dosages
### Rabies exposure
*Adults and children:* 20 IU/kg at time of first dose of rabies vaccine. Use half dose to infiltrate wound area. Give remainder I.M. (gluteal area preferred). Don't give rabies vaccine and RIG in same syringe or at same site.

## Mechanism of action
*Postexposure rabies prophylaxis:* RIG provides passive immunity to rabies.

## Pharmacokinetics
*Absorption:* After slow I.M. absorption, rabies antibody appears in serum within 24 hours and peaks within 2 to 13 days.
*Distribution:* Probably crosses the placenta and appears in breast milk.
*Metabolism:* No information available.
*Excretion:* Serum half-life for rabies antibody titer is about 24 days.

| Route | Onset | Peak | Duration |
|-------|-------|------|----------|
| I.M. | 24 hr | Unknown | Unknown |

## Contraindications and precautions
Repeated doses shouldn't be given once vaccine treatment has been started.

Use cautiously in patients with immunoglobulin A deficiency or history of prior systemic allergic reactions after administration of human immunoglobulin preparations and in those hypersensitive to thimerosal.

## Interactions
**Drug-drug.** *Corticosteroids, immunosuppressant drugs:* May interfere with the immune response to RIG. Whenever possible, avoid using these drugs during the postexposure immunization period. Because antirabies serum may partially suppress the antibody response to rabies vaccine, use only the recommended dose of antirabies vaccine.
*Live virus vaccine, such as measles, mumps, and rubella:* RIG may interfere with the immune response to these live viruses. Don't administer live virus vaccines within 3 months of administering RIG.

## Adverse reactions
**GU:** *nephrotic syndrome.*
**Skin:** *rash,* pain, redness, induration at injection site.
**Other:** slight fever, *anaphylaxis, angioedema.*

## Overdose and treatment
No information available.

## Clinical considerations
■ Obtain a thorough history of the animal bite, allergies, and reactions to immunizations.
■ Epinephrine solution 1:1,000 should be available to treat allergic reactions.
■ Don't administer more than 5 ml I.M. at one injection site; divide I.M. doses exceeding 5 ml and administer them at different sites.
■ Ask patient when he received his last tetanus immunization; a booster may be indicated.
■ Patients previously immunized with a tissue culture-derived rabies vaccine and those who have confirmed adequate rabies antibody titers should receive only the vaccine.
■ RIG hasn't caused an increased frequency of AIDS. The immune globulin is devoid of HIV. Immune globulin recipients don't develop antibodies to HIV.

---

Reactions may be *common*, uncommon, *life-threatening*, or COMMON AND LIFE-THREATENING.

■ Store between 36° and 46° F (2° and 8° C). Don't freeze.

**H ALERT** Don't confuse drug with rabies vaccine, which is a suspension of attenuated or killed microorganisms used to confer active immunity. These two drugs are commonly given together prophylactically after exposure to known or suspected rabid animals.

### Therapeutic monitoring

■ Repeated doses of RIG shouldn't be given after rabies vaccine is started.
■ Reactions to antirabies serum may occur up to 12 days after product is given.

### Special populations

**Pregnant patients.** Because rabies can be fatal if untreated, use of RIG during pregnancy appears justified. No fetal risk from RIG use has been reported to date.

**Breast-feeding patients.** Safety in breast-feeding women hasn't been established. RIG probably appears in breast milk. An alternative feeding method is recommended.

### Patient counseling

■ Explain that the body needs about 1 week to develop immunity to rabies after vaccine is given. Therefore, patients receive RIG to provide antibodies in their blood for immediate protection against rabies.
■ Advise patient to report skin changes, difficulty breathing, or headache.
■ Tell patient that local pain, swelling, and tenderness at injection site may occur. Recommend acetaminophen to alleviate these minor effects.

## rabies vaccine, adsorbed

*Pharmacologic classification:* vaccine
*Therapeutic classification:* viral vaccine
*Pregnancy risk category C*

### Available forms

Available by prescription only
*Injection:* 1 ml single-dose vial

### Indications and dosages

*Preexposure prophylaxis rabies immunization for patients in high-risk groups*
*Adults and children:* 1 ml I.M. at 0, 7, and 21 or 28 days for a total of three injections. Patients at increased risk for rabies should be checked every 6 months and given a booster vaccination, 1 ml I.M., p.r.n., to maintain adequate serum titer.

*Postexposure rabies prophylaxis*
*Adults and children not previously vaccinated against rabies:* 20 IU/kg of human rabies immune globulin (HRIG) I.M. and five 1-ml injections of rabies vaccine, adsorbed, I.M. given one each on days 0, 3, 7, 14, and 28.

*Adults and children previously vaccinated against rabies:* Two 1-ml injections of rabies vaccine, adsorbed, I.M. given one each on days 0 and 3. HRIG shouldn't be given.

### Mechanism of action

*Vaccine action:* Promotes active immunity to rabies.

### Pharmacokinetics

*Absorption:* People at high risk should be retested for rabies antibody titer every 6 months.
*Distribution:* No information available.
*Metabolism:* No information available.
*Excretion:* No information available.

| Route | Onset | Peak | Duration |
|-------|-------|------|----------|
| I.M. | Unknown | 2 wk after 3 doses | Unknown |

### Contraindications and precautions

Contraindicated in patients who have experienced life-threatening allergic reactions to previous injections of vaccine or its components, including thimerosal.

Use cautiously in patients with history of non–life-threatening allergic reactions to previous injections of vaccine or those hypersensitive to monkey proteins.

### Interactions

**Drug-drug.** *Antimalarial drugs, corticosteroids, and immunosuppressives:* Decrease response to rabies vaccine. Don't use together.

### Adverse reactions

**CNS:** *headache, fatigue, dizziness.*
**GI:** *abdominal pain, nausea.*
**Musculoskeletal:** aching of injected muscle, *myalgia.*
**Skin:** transient pain, erythema, swelling, itching, mild inflammatory reaction at injection site.
**Other:** *anaphylaxis, slight fever,* serum sickness-like reactions.

### Overdose and treatment

No information available.

### Clinical considerations

■ Recommend keeping epinephrine 1:1,000 readily available.
■ Recommend giving I.M. into deltoid region in adults and older children; midanterolateral aspect of the thigh is acceptable for younger children. Vaccine shouldn't be used by intradermal route. Vaccine shouldn't be injected in close approximation to a peripheral nerve or in adipose and S.C. tissue.
■ Vaccine is normally a light pink color because of presence of phenol red in the suspension.

- Recommend delaying preexposure immunization in patient with acute intercurrent illness.

### Therapeutic monitoring
- If patient experiences a serious adverse reaction to the vaccine, report this promptly to the manufacturer.

### Special populations
**Pregnant patients.** Administration isn't contraindicated because of the potential harm from rabies exposure.
**Pediatric patients.** Use caution when giving vaccine because of limited experience in children.

## Patient counseling
- Tell patient that pain, swelling, and itching at injection site; headache; stomach upset; or fever may occur.
- Recommend acetaminophen to alleviate headache, fever, and muscle aches.

---

# rabies vaccine, human diploid cell (HDCV)
Imovax Rabies I.D. Vaccine (inactivated whole virus), Imovax Rabies Vaccine

*Pharmacologic classification:* vaccine
*Therapeutic classification:* viral vaccine
*Pregnancy risk category C*

## Available forms
Available by prescription only
*I.D. injection:* 0.25 IU rabies antigen per dose
*I.M. injection:* 2.5 IU of rabies antigen/ml, in single-dose vial with diluent

## Indications and dosages
*Preexposure prophylaxis immunization for persons in high-risk groups*
*Adults and children:* Three 0.1-ml injections intradermally or three 1-ml injections I.M. Give first dose on day 0 (first-day vaccination), second dose on day 7, and third dose on day 21 or 28.
*Booster:* Persons exposed to rabies virus at their workplace should have antibody titers checked q 6 months. Those persons with continued risk of exposure should have antibody titers checked q 2 years. When the titers are inadequate, recommend giving a booster dose.
*Primary postexposure dosage*
*Adults and children:* Five 1-ml doses I.M. on days 3, 7, 14, and 28 (with rabies immune globulin on day 0). A sixth dose may be given on day 90. For patients who previously received the full HDCV vaccination regimen or who

have shown rabies antibody, give two 1-ml doses I.M. Give first dose on day 0 and the second 3 days later. Rabies immune globulin (RIG) shouldn't be given.

## Mechanism of action
*Rabies prophylaxis:* Vaccine promotes active immunity to rabies.

## Pharmacokinetics
*Absorption:* After I.D. injection, rabies antibodies appear in the serum within 7 to 10 days.
*Distribution:* No information available.
*Metabolism:* No information available.
*Excretion:* No information available.

| Route | Onset | Peak | Duration |
|-------|-------|------|----------|
| I.M., I.D. | 1 wk | 1-2 mo | > 2 yr |

## Contraindications and precautions
No contraindications reported for persons after exposure. An acute febrile illness contraindicates use of vaccine for persons previously exposed.
Use cautiously in patients with history of hypersensitivity.

## Interactions
**Drug-drug.** *Corticosteroids, immunosuppressants:* May interfere with the development of active immunity to rabies vaccine. Avoid use whenever possible.

## Adverse reactions
**CNS:** *headache,* dizziness, *fatigue.*
**GI:** abdominal pain, diarrhea, *nausea.*
**Musculoskeletal:** muscle aches.
**Skin:** *pain, erythema, swelling, itching at injection site.*
**Other:** *anaphylaxis, fever, serum sickness.*

## Overdose and treatment
No information available.

## Clinical considerations
**ℍ ALERT** I.D. form is for preexposure use only.
- Obtain a thorough history of allergies, especially to antibiotics, and of reactions to immunizations.
- Epinephrine solution 1:1,000 should be available to treat allergic reactions.
- I.M. injections should be made in the deltoid or upper outer quadrant of the gluteus muscle in adults and children. In infants and young children, the midlateral aspect of the thigh should be used.
- Reconstitute with diluent provided. Gently shake vial until vaccine is completely dissolved.
- Store vaccine at 36° to 46° F (2° to 8° C). Don't freeze.

---

### Therapeutic monitoring
- Advise clinician to watch patient for signs of serum sickness–like hypersensitivity reactions. Antihistamine treatment may be needed in these patients.

### Special populations
**Pregnant patients.** It's recommended that treatment be given to pregnant women, because of the possible harm of rabies exposure. Preexposure immunization may also be indicated for a pregnant woman at high exposure risk for rabies.

**Breast-feeding patients.** It's unknown if HDCV appears in breast milk or if transmission to breast-feeding infant presents risk. Breast-feeding women should choose an alternative feeding method.

### Patient counseling
- Tell patient that pain, swelling, and itching at injection site as well as headache, stomach upset, or fever may occur after vaccination.
- Recommend acetaminophen to alleviate headache, fever, and muscle aches.

# raloxifene hydrochloride
Evista

*Pharmacologic classification:* selective estrogen receptor modulator (SERM)
*Therapeutic classification:* antiosteoporotic
*Pregnancy risk category X*

### Available forms
Available by prescription only
*Tablets:* 60 mg

### Indications and dosages
*Prevention and treatment of osteoporosis in postmenopausal women*
*Adults:* One 60-mg tablet P.O. once daily.

### Mechanism of action
*Antiosteoporotic action:* Decreases bone turnover and reduces bone resorption, manifested as reduced serum and urine levels of bone turnover markers and increased bone mineral density. Biologic actions of drug are mediated through binding to estrogen receptors resulting in differential expression of multiple estrogen-regulated genes in different tissues.

### Pharmacokinetics
*Absorption:* Rapidly absorbed. Peak levels depend on systemic interconversion and enterohepatic cycling of drug and its metabolites. After oral administration, about 60% of raloxifene is absorbed. Absolute bioavailability is 2%.
*Distribution:* Apparent volume of distribution is 2,348 L/kg and doesn't depend on dose given. Drug is highly bound to plasma proteins,

both albumin and alpha-1 acid glycoprotein, but it doesn't appear to interact with the binding of warfarin, phenytoin, or tamoxifen to plasma proteins.
*Metabolism:* Undergoes extensive first-pass metabolism to glucuronide conjugates.
*Excretion:* Primarily excreted in the feces with less than 6% of dose eliminated as glucuronide conjugates in the urine. Less than 0.2% of dose is excreted unchanged in urine.

| Route | Onset | Peak | Duration |
|-------|-------|------|----------|
| P.O. | Unknown | Unknown | 24 hr |

### Contraindications and precautions
Contraindicated in patients hypersensitive to drug or constituents of tablet. Also contraindicated in pregnant women or those planning pregnancy and in women with past history of or currently active venous thromboembolic events, including pulmonary embolism, retinal vein thrombosis, and deep vein thrombosis. Use with hormone replacement therapy or systemic estrogen hasn't been evaluated and isn't recommended.

Use with caution in patients with severe hepatic impairment. Potential risk-benefit should be assessed in women at high risk for thromboembolic disease secondary to HF, superficial thrombophlebitis, or active malignancy.

### Interactions
**Drug-drug.** *Cholestyramine:* Causes a significant reduction in absorption of raloxifene; don't use these drugs together.
*Other highly protein-bound drugs, such as clofibrate, diazepam, diazoxide, ibuprofen, indomethacin, and naproxen:* May interfere with binding sites. Use together cautiously.
*Warfarin:* Decreases PT. Advise clinician to monitor PT and INR.

### Adverse reactions
**CNS:** depression, insomnia, headache, migraine.
**CV:** *hot flashes,* chest pain, peripheral edema.
**EENT:** *sinusitis,* pharyngitis, laryngitis.
**GI:** nausea, dyspepsia, vomiting, flatulence, GI disorder, gastroenteritis, diarrhea, abdominal pain.
**GU:** vaginitis, urinary tract infection, cystitis, leukorrhea, endometrial disorder, vaginal bleeding.
**Hematologic:** increased fibrinogen.
**Metabolic:** weight gain, increased apolipoprotein A-I and reduced serum total cholesterol, low-density lipoprotein cholesterol, apolipoprotein B, and lipoprotein.
**Musculoskeletal:** *arthralgia,* myalgia, arthritis, leg cramps.
**Respiratory:** increased cough, pneumonia.
**Skin:** rash, sweating.
**Other:** *infection, flu syndrome,* fever, increased hormone-binding globulin levels, breast pain.

---

## Overdose and treatment
There have been no reports of overdose. No specific antidote for raloxifene overdose exists. In one study, a dose of 600 mg/day was safely tolerated.

## Clinical considerations
- Drug should be stopped at least 72 hours before prolonged immobilization.
- Endometrial proliferation hasn't been linked to drug use. Unexplained uterine bleeding should be evaluated.
- A decrease in total and low-density lipoprotein cholesterol by 6% and 11% respectively has been reported. No effect on high-density lipoprotein or triglycerides has been shown.
- There are no data to support drug use in premenopausal women; avoid use in this population.
- Effect on bone mineral density beyond 2 years of drug treatment isn't known. Safety and efficacy haven't been established beyond 2 years.

### Therapeutic monitoring
- The greatest risk for thromboembolic events (deep vein thrombosis, pulmonary embolism, retinal vein thrombosis) occurs during first 4 months of treatment.
- No association between breast enlargement, breast pain, or an increased risk of breast cancer has been shown. Breast abnormalities that occur during treatment should be evaluated.

### Special populations
**Breast-feeding patients.** It's unknown if drug appears in breast milk. Don't use in breast-feeding women.
**Pediatric patients.** Drug hasn't been evaluated in children; don't use in this population.
**Geriatric patients.** No age-related differences have been observed in patients ages 42 to 84.

## Patient counseling
- Tell patient to avoid long periods of restricted movement (such as during traveling) because of an increased risk of venous thromboembolic events, such as deep vein thrombosis and pulmonary embolism.
- Inform patient that hot flashes or flushing may occur and don't disappear with drug use.
- Tell patient to take supplemental calcium and vitamin D if dietary intake is inadequate.
- Encourage patient to perform weight-bearing exercises. Also advise her to stop alcohol consumption and smoking.
- Tell patient that drug may be taken without regard for food.

# ramipril
Altace

*Pharmacologic classification:* ACE inhibitor
*Therapeutic classification:* antihypertensive
*Pregnancy risk category C (D second and third trimesters)*

## Available forms
Available by prescription only
*Capsules:* 1.25 mg, 2.5 mg, 5 mg, 10 mg

## Indications and dosages
*Treatment of hypertension either alone or with thiazide diuretics*
*Adults:* Initially, 2.5 mg P.O. daily in patients not receiving concomitant diuretic therapy. Adjust dosage based on blood pressure response. Usual maintenance dose is 2.5 to 20 mg daily as a single dose or in two equal doses.
   In patients receiving diuretic therapy, symptomatic hypotension may occur. To minimize this, discontinue diuretic, if possible, 2 to 3 days before starting ramipril. When this isn't possible, initial dose of ramipril should be 1.25 mg.
≡*Dosage adjustment.* In renally impaired patients with creatinine clearance below 40 ml/minute (serum creatinine above 2.5 mg/dl), recommended initial dose is 1.25 mg daily, adjusted upward to maximum dose of 5 mg based on blood pressure response.
*Heart failure post-MI*
*Adults:* Initially, 2.5 mg P.O. b.i.d. Adjust to target dose of 5 mg P.O. b.i.d.
*Risk reduction for major CV events in patients with a history of CV event and at least one other risk factor*
*Adults ages 55 years and older:* Initially, 2.5 mg P.O. daily for 1 week, then 5 mg daily P.O. for 3 weeks, then increase as tolerated to 10 mg daily P.O.
≡*Dosage adjustment.* In patients who are hypertensive or recently post-MI, daily dose may be divided.

## Mechanism of action
*Antihypertensive action:* Ramipril and its active metabolite, ramiprilat, inhibit angiotensin-converting enzyme (ACE), preventing conversion of angiotensin I to angiotensin II, a potent vasoconstrictor. Reduced formation of angiotensin II decreases peripheral arterial resistance and, in turn, decreases aldosterone secretion, reduces sodium and water retention, and lowers blood pressure. Ramipril also has antihypertensive activity in patients with low-renin hypertension.

---

Reactions may be *common*, uncommon, *life-threatening*, or COMMON AND LIFE-THREATENING.

## Pharmacokinetics

*Absorption:* 50% to 60% is absorbed after oral administration.

*Distribution:* Ramipril is 73% serum protein–bound; ramiprilat, 56%.

*Metabolism:* Ramipril is almost completely metabolized to ramiprilat, which has six times more ACE-inhibitory effects than parent drug.

*Excretion:* 60% is excreted in urine; 40% in feces. Less than 2% of given dose is excreted in urine as unchanged drug.

| Route | Onset | Peak | Duration |
|-------|-------|------|----------|
| P.O. | 1-2 hr | 1-3 hr | 24 hr |

## Contraindications and precautions

Contraindicated in patients hypersensitive to ACE inhibitors or those with history of angioedema related to treatment with an ACE inhibitor.

Use cautiously in patients with impaired renal function.

## Interactions

**Drug-drug.** *Diuretics:* Excessive hypotension may result if used together. Recommend stopping diuretic or lowering dosage of ramipril p.r.n.

*Lithium:* Increased serum lithium levels and lithium toxicity have been reported when used together. Advise clinician to monitor levels closely.

*Potassium-sparing diuretics or potassium supplements:* May result in hyperkalemia. Advise clinician to monitor serum potassium levels.

**Drug-herb.** *Capsaicin:* Increased risk of cough. Discourage use together.*Licorice:* May cause sodium retention and increase blood pressure, interfering with the therapeutic effects of ACE inhibitors. Discourage use together.

**Drug-food.** *Potassium-containing salt substitutes:* May cause hyperkalemia. Discourage use together.

**Drug-lifestyle.** *Sun exposure:* May cause photosensitivity reaction. Advise patient to use sunblock.

## Adverse reactions

**CNS:** asthenia, dizziness, fatigue, headache, malaise, light-headedness, anxiety, amnesia, *seizures,* depression, insomnia, nervousness, neuralgia, neuropathy, paresthesia, somnolence, tremor, vertigo.

**CV:** orthostatic hypotension, syncope, angina, *arrhythmias, MI,* chest pain, palpitations, edema.

**EENT:** epistaxis, tinnitus.

**GI:** nausea, vomiting, abdominal pain, anorexia, constipation, diarrhea, dyspepsia, dry mouth, gastroenteritis, *hepatitis.*

**GU:** impotence, increased BUN and creatinine levels.

**Hematologic:** hemolytic anemia, *pancytopenia, neutropenia, thrombocytopenia,* decreased hemoglobin levels and hematocrit.

**Hepatic:** elevations of liver enzyme levels and serum bilirubin.

**Metabolic:** hyperkalemia, weight gain, elevated uric acid and blood glucose levels.

**Musculoskeletal:** arthralgia, arthritis, myalgia.

**Respiratory:** *dry, persistent, tickling, nonproductive cough;* dyspnea.

**Skin:** hypersensitivity reactions, rash, dermatitis, pruritus, photosensitivity, increased diaphoresis.

**Other:** *angioedema.*

## Overdose and treatment

The most common sign is expected to be hypotension. No cases of overdose have been reported; specific management of ramipril overdose hasn't been established. Supportive care should be provided.

## Clinical considerations

■ Like other ACE inhibitors, ramipril may cause a dry, persistent, tickling, nonproductive cough, which is reversible when drug is stopped.

### Therapeutic monitoring

■ Advise clinician to monitor blood pressure regularly.

■ Advise clinician to monitor CBC and differential counts before and during therapy.

■ Assess renal and hepatic function before and periodically throughout therapy.

■ Advise clinician to monitor serum potassium levels.

### Special populations

**Breast-feeding patients.** Drug shouldn't be given to breast-feeding women.

**Pediatric patients.** Safety and efficacy in children haven't been established.

**Geriatric patients.** No age-related differences in safety or efficacy have been observed.

## Patient counseling

■ Tell patient to report signs or symptoms of angioedema immediately: swelling of face, eyes, lips, or tongue or difficulty in breathing. Tell him to stop taking drug and seek medical attention.

■ Warn patient that light-headedness may occur, especially during first few days of therapy. Tell him to change positions slowly to reduce hypotensive effect and to report these symptoms. If syncope occurs, instruct patient to stop taking drug and call prescriber immediately.

■ Warn patient that inadequate fluid intake, vomiting, diarrhea, or excessive perspiration can lead to light-headedness and syncope. Advise patient to use caution in excessive heat and during exercise.

■ Tell patient to immediately report signs of infection, such as sore throat or fever.

---

# ranitidine
Zantac, Zantac 75, Zantac EFFERdose, Zantac GELdose

*Pharmacologic classification:* H$_2$-receptor antagonist
*Therapeutic classification:* antiulcer
*Pregnancy risk category B*

## Available forms
Available by prescription only
*Capsules:* 150 mg, 300 mg
*Granules (effervescent):* 150 mg
*Injection:* 25 mg/ml
*Injection (premixed):* 50 mg/50 ml, 50 mg/100 ml
*Syrup:* 15 mg/ml
*Tablets:* 150 mg, 300 mg
*Tablets (effervescent):* 150 mg
Available without a prescription
*Tablets:* 75 mg

## Indications and dosages
*Duodenal and gastric ulcer (short-term treatment); pathologic hypersecretory conditions such as Zollinger-Ellison syndrome*
*Adults:* 150 mg P.O. b.i.d. or 300 mg after evening meal or h.s. Doses up to 6 g/day may be given in patients with Zollinger-Ellison syndrome. May give drug parenterally: 50 mg I.V. or I.M. q 6 to 8 hours. Maximum dose is 400 mg/day. For Zollinger-Ellison syndrome, continuous I.V. infusion has been started at 1 mg/kg/hr and increased up to 2.5 mg/kg/hr (200 mg/hr).
*Children ages 1 month to 16 years:* 2 to 4 mg/kg b.i.d. Maximum dose not to exceed 300 mg.
*Maintenance therapy in duodenal or gastric ulcer and erosive esophagitis*
*Adults:* 150 mg P.O. h.s.
*Children ages 1 month to 16 years:* 2 to 4 mg/kg b.i.d. Maximum dose not to exceed 150 mg.
*Prophylaxis of stress ulcer*
*Adults:* Continuous I.V. infusion of 150 mg in 250 ml compatible solution delivered at 6.25 mg/hour using an infusion pump.
*Gastroesophageal reflux disease*
*Adults:* 150 mg P.O. b.i.d.
*Children ages 1 month to 16 years:* 5 to 10 mg/kg/day in 2 divided doses.
*Erosive esophagitis*
*Adults:* 150 mg or 10 ml (2 tsp equivalent to 150 mg of ranitidine) P.O. q.i.d.
*Children ages 1 month to 16 years:* 5 to 10 mg/kg/day in 2 divided doses.

*Self-medication for relief of occasional heartburn, acid indigestion, and sour stomach*
*Adults and adolescents ages 12 and older:* 75 mg P.O. once or twice daily; maximum dose, 150 mg in 24 hours. Don't exceed 2 weeks of continuous use unless otherwise recommended by a prescriber.
≡ *Dosage adjustment.* If patient's creatinine clearance is less than 50 ml/minute, decrease the dose to 150 mg daily P.O. and 50 mg every 18 to 24 hours for I.M. or intermittent I.V.

## I.V. administration
■ When administering I.V. push, dilute to a total volume of 20 ml and inject over 5 minutes.
■ When administering by intermittent I.V. infusion, dilute 50 mg ranitidine in 100 ml of D$_5$W and infuse over 15 to 20 minutes.

## Incompatibilities
Incompatible with amphotericin B, chlorpromazine, clindamycin, phosphate, methotrimeprazine, midazolam, opium alkaloid hydrochlorides, and pentobarbital sodium.

## Mechanism of action
*Antiulcer action:* Ranitidine competitively inhibits action of histamine at H$_2$-receptors in gastric parietal cells. This reduces basal and nocturnal gastric acid secretion as well as that caused by histamine, food, amino acids, insulin, and pentagastrin.

## Pharmacokinetics
*Absorption:* About 50% to 60% of an oral dose is absorbed; food doesn't significantly affect absorption. After I.M. injection, drug is absorbed rapidly from parenteral sites.
*Distribution:* Distributed to many body tissues and appears in CSF and breast milk. Drug is about 10% to 19% protein-bound.
*Metabolism:* Metabolized in the liver.
*Excretion:* Excreted in urine and feces. Half-life is 2 to 3 hours.

| Route | Onset | Peak | Duration |
|---|---|---|---|
| P.O. | 1 hr | 1-3 hr | 13 hr |
| I.V., I.M. | Unknown | Unknown | Unknown |

## Contraindications and precautions
Contraindicated in patients hypersensitive to drug or in those with history of acute porphyria.
    Use cautiously in patients with impaired renal or hepatic function.

## Interactions
**Drug-drug.** *Antacids:* Decrease ranitidine absorption. Give drugs at least 1 hour apart.
*Diazepam:* Concurrent use decreases diazepam absorption. Advise clinician to monitor patient closely.

---

*Glipizide:* May increase hypoglycemic effect. Dosage adjustment of glipizide may be needed.
*Procainamide:* Drug may decrease renal clearance of procainamide. Advise clinician to monitor patient closely for toxicity.
*Warfarin:* May interfere with clearance of warfarin. Advise clinician to monitor patient closely.

## Adverse reactions
**CNS:** malaise, vertigo.
**EENT:** blurred vision.
**GU:** increased serum creatinine.
**Hematologic:** *reversible leukopenia, pancytopenia, granulocytopenia, thrombocytopenia.*
**Hepatic:** elevated liver enzyme levels, *hepatic failure,* jaundice.
**Skin:** burning, itching (at injection site).
**Other:** *anaphylaxis,* angioneurotic edema.

## Overdose and treatment
No cases of overdose have been reported. However, treatment would involve emesis or gastric lavage and supportive measures p.r.n. Drug is removed by hemodialysis.

## Clinical considerations
▪ Dosage adjustment may be required in patients with impaired renal function.
▪ Discontinue immediately if patient develops hepatitis.
▪ Dialysis removes ranitidine; recommend giving drug after treatment.
▪ Ranitidine may cause false-positive results in urine protein tests using Multistix.
**H ALERT** Don't confuse Zantac (ranitidine) and Zyrtec (certirizine).

### Therapeutic monitoring
▪ Recommend assessing patient for abdominal pain and noting presence of blood in emesis, stool, or gastric aspirate.

### Special populations
**Breast-feeding patients.** Drug appears in breast milk; use cautiously in breast-feeding women.

## Patient counseling
▪ Instruct patient to take drug as directed, even after pain subsides, to ensure proper healing.
▪ If patient is taking a single daily dose, advise him to take it h.s.
▪ Instruct patient not to take OTC preparations continuously for longer than 2 weeks without medical supervision.
▪ Tell patient to swallow oral drug whole with water and not to chew tablets.

# ranitidine bismuth citrate
Tritec

*Pharmacologic classification:* H$_2$-receptor antagonist, antimicrobial
*Therapeutic classification:* antiulcer
*Pregnancy risk category C*

## Available forms
Available by prescription only
*Tablets:* 400 mg

## Indications and dosages
**With clarithromycin for treatment of active duodenal ulcer from Helicobacter pylori infection**
*Adults:* 400 mg P.O. b.i.d for 28 days with clarithromycin 500 mg P.O. t.i.d. for first 14 days.

## Mechanism of action
*Antiulcer activity:* Ranitidine reduces gastric acid secretion by competitively inhibiting histamine at the H$_2$-receptor of the gastric parietal cells. Bismuth is a topical drug that disrupts the integrity of bacterial cell walls, prevents adhesion of *H. pylori* to gastric epithelium, decreases the development of resistance, and inhibits *H. pylori's* urease, phospholipase, and proteolytic activity.

## Pharmacokinetics
*Absorption:* Dissociates to ranitidine and bismuth after ingestion. Oral bioavailability of bismuth is variable.
*Distribution:* Volume of distribution of ranitidine is 1.7 L/kg. Ranitidine and bismuth are 15% and 98% protein-bound, respectively.
*Metabolism:* Metabolized by the liver. It's unknown if bismuth undergoes biotransformation.
*Excretion:* Primarily eliminated by the kidney. Elimination half-life of ranitidine is about 3 hours. Bismuth is excreted primarily in feces. Bismuth also undergoes minor excretion in the bile and urine. Terminal elimination half-life of bismuth is 11 to 28 days.

| Route | Onset | Peak | Duration |
|-------|-------|------|----------|
| P.O. | Unknown | Variable | Variable |

## Contraindications and precautions
Contraindicated in patients hypersensitive to drug or its components.

## Interactions
**Drug-drug.** *Clarithromycin:* Combination of these drugs shouldn't be used in patients with history of acute porphyria. Also, this combination isn't recommended in patients with creatinine clearance below 25 ml/minute.
*Diazepam:* Decreased absorption. Separate administration times.

*Glipizide:* Ranitidine may increase the hypoglycemic effects of glipizide. Advise clinician to monitor glucose levels.

*High-dose antacids (170 mEq):* May decrease plasma level of ranitidine and bismuth. Advise clinician to monitor levels closely.

*Procainamide:* Ranitidine may increase plasma levels of procainamide. Advise clinician to monitor levels closely.

*Warfarin:* May increase hypoprothrombinemic effects. Advise clinician to monitor PT and INR and adjust dosage p.r.n.

## Adverse reactions
**CNS:** headache.
**GI:** constipation, diarrhea.

## Overdose and treatment
There has been limited experience with overdose. If overdose occurs, measures should be taken to remove unabsorbed drug from GI tract. Advise clinician to monitor symptoms and use other supportive measures if needed.

## Clinical considerations
■ Drug shouldn't be prescribed alone for treatment of active duodenal ulcers.
■ If drug therapy with clarithromycin isn't successful, patient is considered to have clarithromycin-resistant *H. pylori* and shouldn't be retreated with another regimen containing clarithromycin.
■ Dialysis removes ranitidine; recommend giving drug after treatment.
■ Drug may cause false-positive results in urine protein tests using Multistix; advise clinician to test with sulfosalicylic acid if needed.

### *Therapeutic monitoring*
■ Advise clinician to monitor patient for abdominal pain, blood in stool, or emesis. Drug may cause a temporary and harmless darkening of the tongue or stool.

### *Special populations*
**Breast-feeding patients.** Ranitidine appears in breast milk; use caution when giving drug to breast-feeding women.
**Pediatric patients.** Safety and efficacy haven't been established in children.
**Geriatric patients.** Serum drug levels may be increased in geriatric patients.

## Patient counseling
■ Inform patient that drug may be given without regard to food.
■ Instruct patient to take drug as directed, even after pain has subsided.
■ Stress importance of taking clarithromycin with drug for specified length of time.

# remifentanil hydrochloride
Ultiva

*Pharmacologic classification:* μ-opioid agonist
*Therapeutic classification:* analgesic, anesthetic
*Pregnancy risk category C*
*Controlled substance schedule II*

## Available forms
Available by prescription only
*Injection:* 1 mg/3 ml, 2 mg/5 ml, 5 mg/10 ml vials

## Indications and dosages
### *Induction of anesthesia through intubation*
*Adults:* 0.5 to 1 mcg/kg/minute with hypnotic or volatile drug; may load with 1 mcg/kg over 30 to 60 seconds if endotracheal intubation is to occur less than 8 minutes after start of remifentanil infusion.

### *Maintenance of anesthesia*
*Adults:* 0.25 to 0.4 mcg/kg/minute, based on concurrent anesthetics (nitrous oxide, isoflurane, propofol). Increase doses by 25% to 100% and decrease by 25% to 50% q 2 to 5 minutes, p.r.n. If rate exceeds 1 mcg/kg/minute, consider increases in concurrent anesthetics. May supplement with 1 mcg/kg boluses over 30 to 60 seconds q 2 to 5 minutes, p.r.n.

### *Continuation as analgesic immediately postoperatively*
*Adults:* 0.1 mcg/kg/minute, followed by infusion rate of 0.025 to 0.2 mcg/kg/minute. Adjust rate by 0.025-mcg/kg/minute increments q 5 minutes. Rates over 0.2 mcg/kg/minute cause respiratory depression (under 8 breaths/minute).

### *Dosing for monitored anesthesia care*
*Adults:* As single I.V. dose: administer 0.5 to 1 mcg/kg over 30 to 60 seconds starting 90 seconds before placement of local or regional anesthetic. Decrease dosage by 50% if given with 2 mg midazolam.

As continuous I.V. infusion: 0.1 mcg/kg/minute beginning 5 minutes before local anesthetic given; after placement of local anesthetic, adjust rate to 0.05 mcg/kg/minute. Adjust rate by 0.025 mcg/kg/minute q 5 minutes, p.r.n. Rates over 0.2 mcg/kg/minute are associated with respiratory depression (less than 8 breaths/minute). Decrease dosage by 50% if given with 2 mg midazolam. Bolus doses administered simultaneously with continuously infusing remifentanil to spontaneously breathing patients aren't recommended.

≡ *Dosage adjustment.* In obese patients, base starting dose on ideal body weight.

In patients over age 65, decrease starting dose by 50%. Cautiously titrate to effect.

## I.V. administration
■ Continuous infusions of drug must be given by infusion device; use I.V. bolus administration only during maintenance of general anesthesia. In nonintubated patients, recommend giving single doses over 30 to 60 seconds.
■ Interruption of drug infusion results in rapid reversal (no residual opioid effects within 5 to 10 minutes of infusion discontinuation) of effects; first establish adequate postoperative anesthesia.
■ Upon discontinuation of drug, clear I.V. tubing to avoid inadvertent administration of drug at a later time.

### Incompatibilities
Incompatible with blood products. Don't mix with lactated Ringer's or dextrose 5% in lactated Ringer's solutions, but can coadminister with the above two diluents in a running I.V. administration set.

## Mechanism of action
*Analgesic action:* Drug binds to μ-opiate receptors throughout the CNS, resulting in analgesia.

## Pharmacokinetics
*Absorption:* Administered I.V.
*Distribution:* Initially, drug is distributed throughout the blood and rapidly perfused tissues; then moves into peripheral tissues. Drug is about 70% plasma protein–bound, of which two-thirds is bound to alpha$_1$-acid-glycoprotein.
*Metabolism:* Rapidly metabolized by hydrolysis via blood and tissue esterases, resulting in an inactive carboxylic acid metabolite. Drug isn't metabolized by plasma cholinesterase and isn't appreciably metabolized by the liver or lungs.
*Excretion:* After hydrolysis, inactive metabolite is excreted by the kidneys with an elimination half-life of about 90 minutes. Clearance of active drug is high; elimination half-life is 3 to 10 minutes.

| Route | Onset | Peak | Duration |
|-------|-------|------|----------|
| I.V. | Immediate | Unknown | 5-10 min |

## Contraindications and precautions
Don't use via epidural or intrathecal routes because of presence of glycine in preparation. Contraindicated in patients hypersensitive to fentanyl analogues.

## Interactions
**Drug-drug.** *Inhaled anesthetics, benzodiazepines, and hypnotics:* Produces a synergistic effect. Advise clinician to monitor patient closely.

## Adverse reactions
**CNS:** agitation, chills, dizziness, *headache.*

**CV:** *bradycardia,* hypertension, *hypotension,* tachycardia.
**EENT:** visual disturbances.
**GI:** *nausea, vomiting.*
**Musculoskeletal:** *muscle rigidity.*
**Respiratory:** *apnea, hypoxia, respiratory depression.*
**Skin:** flushing, pain at injection site, *pruritus,* sweating.
**Other:** chills, fever, postoperative pain, shivering, warm sensation.

## Overdose and treatment
Signs of overdose include apnea, chest wall rigidity, hypoxemia, hypotension, seizures, or bradycardia.

If these signs occur, recommend stopping drug, maintaining patent airway, starting assisted or controlled ventilation with oxygen, and maintaining CV function. Recommend giving a neuromuscular blocker or opioid antagonist if decreased respiration accompanies muscle rigidity. Recommend giving I.V. fluids and vasopressors for hypotension and glycopyrrolate or atropine for bradycardia. Naloxone may be used to manage severe respiratory depression. Other supportive measures should be used as appropriate.

## Clinical considerations
■ Don't use as a single drug in general anesthesia.
■ Effects of long-term (over 16 hours) use in intensive care settings aren't known.
■ Bradycardia has been reported and is responsive to ephedrine, atropine, and glycopyrrolate.
■ Drug shouldn't be used outside the monitored anesthesia care setting.
■ Obtain history from patient regarding previous adverse anesthesia reactions in patient or patient's family.

### Therapeutic monitoring
■ Advise clinician to monitor vital signs and oxygenation continually throughout drug administration.
■ If respiratory depression occurs in a spontaneously breathing patient, infusion rate should be decreased by 50% or the infusion temporarily stopped.
■ If skeletal muscle rigidity occurs in a spontaneously breathing patient, recommend stopping infusion or decreasing rate.
■ If hypotension occurs, it should be treated by decreasing administration rate, I.V. fluids, or catecholamine administration.

### Special populations
**Breast-feeding patients.** Because fentanyl analogues appear in breast milk, use with caution in breast-feeding women.
**Pediatric patients.** Use in children under age 2 hasn't been studied.

**Geriatric patients.** Recommend decreasing initial doses by 50% in geriatric patients and titrating to desired effect.

## Patient counseling

■ Reassure patient that appropriate monitoring will occur during anesthesia administration.

---

# repaglinide
Prandin

*Pharmacologic classification:* meglitinide
*Therapeutic classification:* antidiabetic
*Pregnancy risk category C*

## Available forms
Available by prescription only
*Tablets:* 0.5 mg, 1 mg, 2 mg

## Indications and dosages
***Adjunct to diet and exercise in lowering blood glucose levels in patients with type 2 (non–insulin-dependent) diabetes mellitus whose hyperglycemia can't be controlled by diet and exercise alone***
*Adults:* For patients not previously treated or whose HbA$_{1c}$ is below 8%, starting dose is 0.5 mg P.O. with each meal given 15 minutes before meal; however, time may vary from immediately before to as long as 30 minutes before meal. For patients previously treated with glucose-lowering drugs and whose HbA$_{1c}$ is 8% or more, initial dose is 1 to 2 mg P.O. with each meal. Recommended dosage range is 0.5 to 4 mg with meals b.i.d., t.i.d., or q.i.d. Maximum daily dose is 16 mg.

Dosage should be determined by blood glucose response. May double dosage up to 4 mg with each meal until satisfactory blood glucose response is achieved. At least 1 week should elapse between dosage adjustments to assess response to each dose.

Metformin may be added if repaglinide monotherapy is inadequate.

## Mechanism of action
*Antidiabetic action:* Stimulates the release of insulin from the beta cells in the pancreas. Repaglinide closes ATP-dependent potassium channels in the beta cell membrane, which causes depolarization of the B-cell and opening of the calcium channels. The increased calcium influx induces insulin secretion; the overall effect is to lower the blood glucose level.

## Pharmacokinetics
*Absorption:* Rapidly and completely absorbed with oral administration.
*Distribution:* Mean volume of distribution after I.V. administration is 31 L; protein-binding to albumin exceeds 98%.

*Metabolism:* Completely metabolized by oxidative biotransformation and conjugation with glucuronic acid. The P-450 isoenzyme system (specifically CYP 3A4) has also been shown to be involved in N-dealkylation of repaglinide. All metabolites are inactive and don't contribute to the blood glucose-lowering effect.
*Excretion:* About 90% of dose occurs in the feces as metabolites. About 8% of a dose is recovered in the urine as metabolites and less than 0.1% as parent drug. Half-life is about 1 hour.

| Route | Onset | Peak | Duration |
|-------|-------|------|----------|
| P.O. | Unknown | 1 hr | Unknown |

## Contraindications and precautions
Contraindicated in patients hypersensitive to drug or its inactive ingredients and in those with insulin-dependent diabetes mellitus or ketoacidosis.

Use cautiously in patients with hepatic insufficiency in whom reduced metabolism could cause elevated blood levels of repaglinide and hypoglycemia.

## Interactions
**Drug-drug.** *Barbiturates, carbamazepine, rifampin:* May increase the metabolism of repaglinide. Advise clinician to monitor glucose levels.
*Beta blockers, chloramphenicol, coumarin, MAO inhibitors, NSAIDs, other drugs that are highly protein-bound, probenecid, salicylates, and sulfonamides:* May potentiate the hypoglycemic action of repaglinide. Advise clinician to monitor glucose levels.
*Calcium channel blockers, corticosteroids, estrogens, isoniazid, nicotinic acid, oral contraceptives, phenothiazines, phenytoin, sympathomimetics, thiazides and other diuretics, thyroid hormones:* May produce hyperglycemia. Advise clinician to monitor glucose levels.
*Erythromycin, ketoconazole, miconazole, and similar inhibitors of the P-450 cytochrome system 3A4:* Repaglinide metabolism may be inhibited. Advise clinician to monitor glucose levels.
**Drug-herb.** *Aloe, bitter melon, bilberry leaf, burdock, dandelion, fenugreek, garlic, and ginseng:* Concomitant use may improve blood sugar control requiring a reduction of antidiabetic drugs. Advise patient to discuss the use of herbal medicines with his prescriber before use.

## Adverse reactions
**CNS:** headache.
**CV:** chest pain, angina.
**EENT:** rhinitis, sinusitis.
**GI:** nausea, diarrhea, constipation, vomiting, dyspepsia.
**GU:** urinary tract infection.
**Metabolic:** HYPOGLYCEMIA.

---

Reactions may be *common,* uncommon, *life-threatening,* or COMMON AND LIFE-THREATENING.

**Musculoskeletal:** arthralgia, back pain.
**Respiratory:** bronchitis, *upper respiratory infection.*
**Other:** tooth disorder.

## Overdose and treatment
Overdose causes few adverse effects other than those related to the intended effect of lowering blood glucose levels. Advise clinician to treat hypoglycemic symptoms without loss of consciousness or neurologic findings aggressively with oral glucose and dosage or meal pattern adjustments. Advise clinician to monitor patient closely for minimum of 24 to 48 hours because hypoglycemia may recur after apparent clinical recovery. Advise clinician to treat severe hypoglycemic reactions with coma, seizure, or other neurologic impairment immediately with I.V. dextrose 50% solution followed by a continuous infusion of glucose 10% solution. Careful blood sugar monitoring must occur.

## Clinical considerations
- Be aware that administration of other oral antidiabetics has been reported to cause increased CV mortality compared with diet treatment alone. Although not specifically evaluated for repaglinide, this warning may also apply.
- Loss of glycemic control may occur during stress, such as fever, trauma, infection, or surgery. If this occurs, recommend stopping drug and giving insulin.
- Be aware that hypoglycemia may be difficult to recognize in geriatric patients and in patients taking beta blockers.

### *Therapeutic monitoring*
- Use caution when increasing drug dosage in patients with impaired renal function or renal failure requiring dialysis.
- Advise clinician to monitor patient's blood glucose periodically to determine minimum effective dose.
- Advise clinician to monitor long-term efficacy by measuring $HbA_{1c}$ levels every 3 months.

### *Special populations*
**Breast-feeding patients.** Although it isn't known if drug appears in breast milk, studies in animals have indicated excretion similar to other glucose-lowering drugs. Because the potential for hypoglycemia in a breast-fed infant exists, a decision should be made to either stop drug or breast-feeding.
**Pediatric patients.** No studies have been performed in pediatric patients to determine safety and efficacy.
**Geriatric patients.** In clinical studies there was no increase in the frequency or severity of hypoglycemia in older patients.

## Patient counseling
- Instruct patient on importance of diet and exercise with drug therapy.
- Discuss symptoms of hypoglycemia with patient and family.
- Tell patient to take drug before meals, usually 15 minutes before start of meal; however, time can vary from immediately preceding meal to up to 30 minutes before meal.
- Tell patient that if a meal is skipped or an extra meal added, he should skip the dose or add an extra dose of drug for that meal.

# reteplase, recombinant
Retavase

*Pharmacologic classification:* tissue-plasminogen activator
*Therapeutic classification:* thrombolytic enzyme
*Pregnancy risk category C*

## Available forms
Available by prescription only
*Injection:* 10.8 units (18.8 mg)/vial (supplied in kit with components for reconstitution and administration of two single-use vials)

## Indications and dosages
*Management of acute MI*
*Adults:* Double-bolus injection of 10 + 10 units. Give each bolus I.V. over 2 minutes. If no complications occur after first bolus, such as serious bleeding or anaphylactoid reactions, give second bolus 30 minutes after start of first bolus. Initiate treatment soon after onset of symptoms of acute MI. There's no experience of repeat courses with reteplase.

## I.V. administration
- Reconstitute drug according to manufacturer's instructions using items provided in the kit.
- Don't administer drug with other I.V. drugs through same I.V. line.
- Drug is administered I.V. as a double-bolus injection. If bleeding or anaphylactoid reactions occur after first bolus, second bolus may be withheld.

### *Incompatibilities*
No other drug should be added to the injection solution containing drug. Heparin and reteplase are incompatible in solution.

## Mechanism of action
*Thrombolytic action:* Drug catalyzes the cleavage of plasminogen to generate plasmin, which leads to fibrinolysis.

## Pharmacokinetics
*Absorption:* Administered I.V.

*Distribution:* Cleared from plasma at 250 to 450 ml/minute.
*Metabolism:* Metabolized primarily by the liver and kidney.
*Excretion:* Plasma half-life of drug is 13 to 16 minutes.

| Route | Onset | Peak | Duration |
|-------|-------|------|----------|
| I.V. | Unknown | Unknown | Unknown |

## Contraindications and precautions

Contraindicated in patients with active internal bleeding, known bleeding diathesis, history of CVA, recent intracranial or intraspinal surgery or trauma, severe uncontrolled hypertension, intracranial neoplasm, arteriovenous malformation, or aneurysm.

Use cautiously in patients with recent (within 10 days) major surgery, obstetric delivery, organ biopsy, or trauma; previous puncture of noncompressible vessels; cerebrovascular disease; recent GI or GU bleeding; hypertension (systolic pressure 180 mm Hg or more or diastolic pressure 110 mm Hg or more); likelihood of left-sided heart thrombus; subacute bacterial endocarditis; acute pericarditis; hemostatic defects; diabetic hemorrhagic retinopathy; septic thrombophlebitis; other conditions in which bleeding would be difficult to manage; pregnancy; and in patients ages 75 or older.

## Interactions

**Drug-drug.** *Heparin, oral anticoagulants, platelet inhibitors, such as abciximab, aspirin, and dipyridamole, and vitamin K antagonists:* May increase risk of bleeding. Use together cautiously.

## Adverse reactions

**CNS:** *intracranial hemorrhage.*
**CV:** *arrhythmias, cholesterol embolization.*
**GI:** *hemorrhage.*
**GU:** hematuria.
**Hematologic:** *anemia, bleeding tendency, hemorrhage.*
**Other:** *bleeding* (at puncture site).

## Overdose and treatment

No information available. Advise clinician to monitor patient for increased bleeding.

## Clinical considerations

■ Be aware that potency is expressed in terms of units specific for reteplase and not comparable to other thrombolytics.
■ Avoid use of noncompressible pressure sites during therapy. If an arterial puncture is needed, recommend using an upper extremity vessel. Pressure should be applied for at least 30 minutes; then, a pressure dressing should be applied. Recommend checking site frequently.
■ Drug may alter coagulation studies; it remains active in vitro and can lead to degradation of fibrinogen in sample. Recommend collecting blood samples in the presence of PPACK (chloromethylketone) at 2-μM concentrations.

### Therapeutic monitoring

■ Recommend carefully monitoring ECG during treatment. Coronary thrombolysis may cause arrhythmias with reperfusion. Be prepared to treat bradycardia or ventricular irritability.
■ Advise clinician to monitor patient for bleeding. Avoid I.M. injections, invasive procedures, and nonessential handling of patient. Bleeding is the most common adverse reaction and may occur internally or at external puncture sites. If local measures don't control serious bleeding, concurrent anticoagulation therapy should be stopped. Second bolus of reteplase should be withheld.

### Special populations

**Breast-feeding patients.** It's unknown if drug appears in breast milk. Use caution.
**Pediatric patients.** Safety and efficacy in children haven't been established.
**Geriatric patients.** Use cautiously in geriatric patients. Risk of intracranial hemorrhage increases with age.

## Patient counseling

■ Explain to patient and family about use and administration of reteplase.
■ Tell patient to report adverse reactions such as signs and symptoms of bleeding or allergic reaction immediately.
■ Advise patient about proper dental care to avoid excessive gum trauma.

# ribavirin
Virazole

*Pharmacologic classification:* synthetic nucleoside
*Therapeutic classification:* antiviral
*Pregnancy risk category X*

## Available forms

Available by prescription only
*Powder to be reconstituted for inhalation:* 6 g in 100-ml glass vial

## Indications and dosages

**Treatment of hospitalized infants and young children infected by respiratory syncytial virus (RSV)**
*Infants and young children:* Solution in concentration of 20 mg/ml delivered via the Viratek Small Particle Aerosol Generator (SPAG-2) results in a mist with a concentration of 190 mcg/L. Treatment is carried out for 12 to 18 hours/day for at least 3, and no longer than 7, days with a flow rate of 12.5 L of mist per minute.

For ventilated patients, use same dose with a pressure- or volume-cycled ventilator with SPAG-2. Patient should be suctioned q 1 to 2 hours and pulmonary pressures checked q 2 to 4 hours.

## Mechanism of action
*Antiviral action:* Drug action probably involves inhibition of RNA and DNA synthesis, inhibition of RNA polymerase, and interference with completion of viral polypeptide coat.

## Pharmacokinetics
*Absorption:* Some ribavirin is absorbed systemically.
*Distribution:* Concentrates in bronchial secretions; plasma levels are subtherapeutic for plaque inhibition.
*Metabolism:* Metabolized to 1,2,4-triazole-3-carboxamide (deribosylated ribavirin).
*Excretion:* Mostly excreted renally. First phase of drug's plasma half-life is 9½ hours; second phase has extended half-life of 40 hours (from slow drug release from RBC binding sites).

| Route | Onset | Peak | Duration |
|-------|-------|------|----------|
| Inhalation | Unknown | Unknown | Unknown |

## Contraindications and precautions
Contraindicated in patients hypersensitive to drug and in women who are or may become pregnant during treatment. Contraindicated in women of childbearing age and their male partners when used with interferon alfa-2b. Women of childbearing age and men must use two forms of contraception during therapy and 6 months after.

## Interactions
None reported.

## Adverse reactions
**CV:** *cardiac arrest,* hypotension.
**EENT:** conjunctivitis, erythema of eyelids.
**Hematologic:** anemia, reticulocytosis.
**Respiratory:** worsening respiratory state, *apnea,* bacterial pneumonia, pneumothorax, *bronchospasm.*
**Skin:** rash.

## Overdose and treatment
Unknown in humans; high doses in animals have produced GI symptoms.

## Clinical considerations
■ Ribavirin aerosol is indicated for use only for lower respiratory tract infection caused by RSV. Although treatment may begin before test results are available, RSV infection must eventually be confirmed.
■ Ribavirin aerosol should be administered only by SPAG-2. Other aerosol-generating devices shouldn't be used.

■ Reconstitute solution with USP sterile water for injection or inhalation, then transfer aseptically to sterile 500-ml Erlenmeyer flask. Dilute further with sterile water to 300 ml to yield final level of 20 mg/ml. Solution remains stable for 24 hours at room temperature.
■ Don't use bacteriostatic water (or any other water containing antimicrobial drug) to reconstitute drug.
■ Discard unused solution in SPAG-2 unit before adding newly reconstituted solution. Change solution at least every 24 hours.

### Therapeutic monitoring
■ Advise clinician to monitor ventilator-dependent patients carefully because drug may precipitate in ventilatory apparatus. Change heated wire connective tubing and bacteria filters in series in expiratory limb of the system frequently (such as every 4 hours).
■ Drug is most useful for infants with most severe RSV form, typically premature infants and those with underlying disorders such as cardiopulmonary disease. Most other infants and children with RSV infection don't require treatment because disease is self-limiting.
■ Drug therapy must be accompanied by appropriate respiratory and fluid therapy.

### Special populations
**Pregnant patients.** May cause fetal toxicity.
**Breast-feeding patients.** It's unknown if drug appears in breast milk. Not recommended for use in breast-feeding women.

## Patient counseling
■ Inform parents of need for drug and answer any questions they may have.
■ Parents should report any change in child immediately.
■ Inform patient that drug may be taken without regard to meals but should be given in a consistent manner.

# riboflavin (vitamin B₂)

*Pharmacologic classification:* water-soluble vitamin
*Therapeutic classification:* vitamin B complex vitamin
*Pregnancy risk category A (C if more than the RDA)*

## Available forms
Available without a prescription
*Tablets:* 25 mg, 50 mg, 100 mg

## Indications and dosages
*Riboflavin deficiency or adjunct to thiamine treatment for polyneuritis or cheilosis secondary to pellagra*
*Adults and adolescents over age 12:* 5 to 30 mg P.O. daily, depending on severity.

*Children under age 12:* 3 to 10 mg P.O. daily, depending on severity.

**Microcytic anemia with splenomegaly and glutathione reductase deficiency**
*Adults:* 10 mg P.O. daily for 10 days.

**Dietary supplementation**
*Adults:* 1 to 4 mg P.O. daily. For maintenance, increase nutritional intake and supplement with vitamin B complex.

## Mechanism of action

*Metabolic action:* Riboflavin, a coenzyme, functions in the forms of flavin adenine dinucleotide (FAD) and flavin mononucleotide (FMN) and plays a vital metabolic role in numerous tissue respiration systems. FAD and FMN act as hydrogen-carrier molecules for several flavoproteins involved in intermediary metabolism. Riboflavin is also directly involved in maintaining erythrocyte integrity.

Riboflavin deficiency causes a clinical syndrome with the following symptoms: cheilosis, angular stomatitis, glossitis, keratitis, scrotal skin changes, ocular changes, and seborrheic dermatitis. In severe deficiency, normochromic, normocytic anemia and neuropathy may occur. Clinical signs may become evident after 3 to 8 months of inadequate riboflavin intake. Administration of riboflavin reverses signs of deficiency. Riboflavin deficiency rarely occurs alone and commonly accompanies deficiency of other B vitamins and protein.

## Pharmacokinetics

*Absorption:* Although riboflavin is absorbed readily from the GI tract, extent of absorption is limited. Absorption occurs at a specialized segment of the mucosa; drug absorption is limited by duration of drug's contact with this area. Before being absorbed, riboflavin-5-phosphate is rapidly dephosphorylated in the GI lumen. GI absorption increases when drug is given with food and decreases when hepatitis, cirrhosis, biliary obstruction, or probenecid administration is present.

*Distribution:* FAD and FMN are distributed widely to body tissues. Free riboflavin is present in the retina. Riboflavin is stored in limited amounts in the liver, spleen, kidneys, and heart, mainly in the form of FAD. FAD and FMN are about 60% protein-bound in blood. Drug crosses the placenta, and breast milk contains about 400 ng/ml.

*Metabolism:* Metabolized in the liver.

*Excretion:* After a single oral dose, biologic half-life is about 66 to 84 minutes in healthy individuals. Drug is metabolized to FMN in erythrocytes, GI mucosal cells, and the liver; FMN is converted to FAD in the liver. About 9% of drug is excreted unchanged in the urine after normal ingestion. Excretion involves renal tubular secretion and glomerular filtration. Amount renally excreted unchanged is directly proportional to the dose. Drug removal by hemodialysis is slower than by natural renal excretion.

| Route | Onset | Peak | Duration |
|-------|-------|------|----------|
| P.O. | Unknown | Unknown | Unknown |

## Contraindications and precautions

No known contraindications.

## Interactions

**Drug-drug.** *Oral contraceptives:* Riboflavin dose may need to be increased.
*Propantheline bromide:* Delays absorption rate of riboflavin but increases total amount absorbed. Advise clinician to monitor closely.
**Drug-lifestyle.** *Alcohol use:* Impairs intestinal absorption of riboflavin. Advise patient to avoid alcohol.

## Adverse reactions

**GU:** bright yellow urine with high doses.

## Overdose and treatment

No information available.

## Clinical considerations

■ RDA of riboflavin is 0.4 to 1.8 mg/day in children, 1.2 to 1.7 mg/day in adults, and 1.6 to 1.8 mg/day in pregnant and breast-feeding women.
■ Recommend giving oral preparation of riboflavin with food to increase absorption.
■ Riboflavin therapy alters urinalysis based on spectrophotometry or color reactions. Riboflavin produces fluorescent substances in urine and plasma, which can falsely elevate fluorometric determinations of catecholamines and urobilinogen.

### Therapeutic monitoring

■ Obtain patient's dietary history because other vitamin deficiencies may coexist.

### Special populations

**Breast-feeding patients.** Drug crosses the placenta; during pregnancy and lactation, riboflavin requirements are increased. Increased food intake during this time usually provides adequate amounts of the vitamin. The National Research Council recommends daily intake of 1.8 mg/day during first 6 months of breast-feeding.

## Patient counseling

■ Teach patient about good dietary sources of riboflavin, such as whole grain cereals and green vegetables. Liver, kidney, heart, eggs, and dairy products are also dietary sources but may not be appropriate, based on patient's serum cholesterol and triglyceride levels.
■ Advise patient to store riboflavin in a tight, light-resistant container.

# rifabutin
Mycobutin

*Pharmacologic classification:* semisynthetic ansamycin
*Therapeutic classification:* antibiotic
*Pregnancy risk category B*

## Available forms
Available by prescription only
*Capsules:* 150 mg

## Indications and dosages
**Primary prevention of disseminated**
**Mycobacterium avium** *complex (MAC) in*
*patients with advanced HIV infection*
*Adults:* 300 mg P.O. daily as a single dose or divided b.i.d. with food.

## Mechanism of action
*Antibiotic action:* Rifabutin inhibits DNA-dependent RNA polymerase in susceptible strains of *Escherichia coli* and *Bacillus subtilis,* but not in mammalian cells. It isn't known whether rifabutin inhibits this enzyme in *M. avium* or in *M. intracellulare,* which compose MAC.

## Pharmacokinetics
*Absorption:* Readily absorbed from the GI tract.
*Distribution:* Because of its high lipophilicity, rifabutin shows a high propensity for distribution and intracellular tissue uptake. About 85% of drug is bound in a concentration-independent manner to plasma proteins.
*Metabolism:* Metabolized in the liver to five identified metabolites. The 25-0-desacetyl metabolite has an activity equal to parent drug and contributes up to 10% of total antimicrobial activity.
*Excretion:* Less than 10% is excreted in urine as unchanged drug. About 53% of the oral dose is excreted in urine, primarily as metabolites. About 30% is excreted in feces.

| Route | Onset | Peak | Duration |
|-------|-------|------|----------|
| P.O. | Unknown | 2-4 hr | Unknown |

## Contraindications and precautions
Contraindicated in patients hypersensitive to drug or other rifamycin derivatives such as rifampin, and in patients with active tuberculosis because single-agent therapy with rifabutin increases the risk of inducing bacterial resistance to both rifabutin and rifampin.

Use cautiously in patients with preexisting neutropenia and thrombocytopenia.

## Interactions
**Drug-drug.** *Drugs metabolized by the liver, zidovudine:* Rifabutin may decrease the serum levels, although it doesn't affect zidovudine's

inhibition of HIV. Dosage adjustments may be needed.
*Oral contraceptives:* Rifabutin decreases the effectiveness. Instruct patient to use nonhormonal forms of birth control.

## Adverse reactions
**CNS:** headache, insomnia.
**GI:** dyspepsia, eructation, flatulence, diarrhea, nausea, vomiting, abdominal pain, altered taste.
**GU:** *discolored urine* (brown-orange).
**Hematologic:** NEUTROPENIA, LEUKOPENIA, *thrombocytopenia,* eosinophilia.
**Skin:** *rash.*
**Other:** fever, myalgia.

## Overdose and treatment
Although there's no experience in the treatment of drug overdose, clinical experience with rifamycins suggests that gastric lavage to evacuate gastric contents (within a few hours of overdose), followed by instillation of an activated charcoal slurry into the stomach, may help absorb any remaining drug from the GI tract. Hemodialysis or forced diuresis isn't expected to enhance systemic elimination of unchanged rifabutin.

## Clinical considerations
■ High-fat meals slow rate but not extent of drug absorption.
**⚠ ALERT** Don't confuse similar-sounding drugs like rifampin and rifapentine with rifabutin.

### Therapeutic monitoring
■ Patient who develops complaints consistent with active tuberculosis during rifabutin prophylaxis should be evaluated immediately, so active disease may be given an effective combination regimen of antituberculosis drugs. Administration of single-agent rifabutin to patients with active tuberculosis likely leads to development of tuberculosis that is resistant to rifabutin and rifampin.
■ Because rifabutin may cause neutropenia, and more rarely thrombocytopenia, hematologic test results should be obtained periodically in patients receiving rifabutin prophylaxis.

### Special populations
**Breast-feeding patients.** It's unknown if drug appears in breast milk. Because of potential for serious adverse effects in breast-fed infants, either breast-feeding or drug should be discontinued, depending on importance of drug to woman.
**Pediatric patients.** Although safety and efficacy in children haven't been fully established, several studies indicate that drug may be helpful in children at maximum daily dose of 5 mg/kg.

## Patient counseling

- Tell patient with swallowing difficulty to mix drug with soft foods such as applesauce.
- Advise patient with nausea, vomiting, or other GI upset to take drug with food, in two divided doses.
- Warn patient that urine and other body fluids may become discolored (brown-orange). Clothes and soft contact lenses may become permanently discolored.

# rifampin
Rifadin, Rimactane

*Pharmacologic classification:* semisynthetic rifamycin B derivative (macrocyclic antibiotic)
*Therapeutic classification:* antituberculotic
*Pregnancy risk category C*

## Available forms
Available by prescription only
*Capsules:* 150 mg, 300 mg
*Injection:* 600 mg/vial

## Indications and dosages
***Primary treatment in pulmonary tuberculosis***
*Adults:* 10 mg/kg (up to 600 mg) P.O. or I.V. daily as a single dose (give P.O. dose 1 hour before or 2 hours after meals).
*Children:* 10 to 20 mg/kg P.O. or I.V. daily as a single dose (give P.O. dose 1 hour before or 2 hours after meals). Maximum daily dose, 600 mg. Concurrent administration of other effective antitubercular drugs is recommended. Treatment usually lasts 6 to 9 months.
***Asymptomatic meningococcal carriers***
*Adults:* 600 mg P.O. b.i.d. for 2 days.
*Infants and children over 1 month:* 10 mg/kg P.O. b.i.d. for 2 days.
*Neonates under age 1 month:* 5 mg/kg P.O. b.i.d. for 2 days.
≡ *Dosage adjustment.* Reduce dosage in patients with hepatic dysfunction.
***Prophylaxis of Haemophilus influenzae type B***
*Adults and children:* 20 mg/kg (up to 600 mg) once daily for 4 consecutive days.
◊ *Leprosy*
*Adults:* 600 mg P.O. once monthly, usually used with other drugs.

## I.V. administration
- Reconstitute drug with 10 ml of sterile water for injection to make a solution containing 60 mg/ml. Add to 100 ml of $D_5W$ and infuse over 30 minutes, or add to 500 ml of $D_5W$ and infuse over 3 hours.
- Prepare and use solution within a 4-hour period. When dextrose is contraindicated, drug may be diluted with normal saline solution for injection.
- Don't use other I.V. solutions.

### Incompatibilities
Incompatible with minocycline and many solutions. Use only $D_5W$ or sterile saline as infusion solutions.

## Mechanism of action
*Antibiotic action:* Rifampin impairs RNA synthesis by inhibiting DNA-dependent RNA polymerase. Rifampin may be bacteriostatic or bactericidal, depending on organism susceptibility and drug level at infection site.

Rifampin acts against *Mycobacterium bovis, M. kansasii, M. marinum,* and *M. tuberculosis,* some strains of *M. avium, M. aviumintracellulare,* and *M. fortuitum,* and many gram-positive and some gram-negative bacteria. Resistance to rifampin by *M. tuberculosis* can develop rapidly; rifampin is usually given with other antituberculosis drugs to prevent or delay resistance.

## Pharmacokinetics
*Absorption:* Absorbed completely from the GI tract after oral administration. Food delays absorption.
*Distribution:* Distributed widely into body tissues and fluids, including ascitic, pleural, seminal, and cerebrospinal fluids, tears, and saliva; and into liver, prostate, lungs, and bone. Drug crosses the placenta, and is 84% to 91% protein-bound.
*Metabolism:* Metabolized extensively in the liver by deacetylation. It undergoes enterohepatic circulation.
*Excretion:* Undergoes enterohepatic circulation, and drug and metabolite are excreted primarily in bile; drug, but not metabolite, is reabsorbed. From 6% to 30% of rifampin and metabolite appear unchanged in urine in 24 hours; about 60% is excreted in feces. Some drug appears in breast milk. Plasma half-life in adults is 1½ to 5 hours; serum levels rise in obstructive jaundice. Dosage adjustment isn't needed for patients with renal failure. Rifampin isn't removed by either hemodialysis or peritoneal dialysis.

| Route | Onset | Peak | Duration |
|-------|-------|------|----------|
| P.O. | Unknown | 2-4 hr | Unknown |
| I.V. | Unknown | Unknown | Unknown |

## Contraindications and precautions
Contraindicated in patients hypersensitive to drug. Use cautiously in patients with hepatic disease.

## Interactions
**Drug-drug.** *Anticoagulants, barbiturates, beta blockers, cardiac glycoside derivatives, chloramphenicol, clofibrate, corticosteroids, cy-*

*closporine, dapsone, disopyramide, estrogens, methadone, oral contraceptives, oral sulfonylureas, phenytoin, quinidine, tocainide, and verapamil:* Decreased effectiveness of these drugs. Advise clinician to monitor patient closely; may need dosage adjustment.

*Isoniazid:* Increased hazard of isoniazid hepatotoxicity. Advise clinician to monitor patient closely.

*Oral contraceptives:* Rifampin inactivates such drugs and may alter menstrual patterns. Advise oral contraceptive users to use other methods of birth control.

*Para-aminosalicylate:* May decrease oral absorption of rifampin, lowering serum levels. Recommend giving drugs 8 to 12 hours apart.

**Drug-lifestyle.** *Alcohol use:* May increase risk of hepatotoxicity. Advise patient to avoid alcohol use during drug therapy.

## Adverse reactions

**CNS:** headache, fatigue, drowsiness, behavioral changes, dizziness, ataxia, mental confusion, generalized numbness.
**EENT:** visual disturbances, exudative conjunctivitis.
**GI:** epigastric distress, anorexia, nausea, vomiting, abdominal pain, diarrhea, flatulence, sore mouth and tongue, pseudomembranous colitis, *pancreatitis.*
**GU:** hemoglobinuria, hematuria, menstrual disturbances, *acute renal failure.*
**Hematologic:** eosinophilia, *thrombocytopenia, transient leukopenia,* hemolytic anemia, porphyria exacerbation.
**Hepatic:** *hepatotoxicity, transient abnormalities in liver function test results.*
**Metabolic:** hyperuricemia.
**Musculoskeletal:** osteomalacia.
**Respiratory:** shortness of breath, wheezing.
**Skin:** pruritus, urticaria, rash.
**Other:** flulike syndrome, discoloration of body fluids, *shock.*

## Overdose and treatment

Signs of overdose include lethargy, nausea, and vomiting; hepatotoxicity from massive overdose includes hepatomegaly, jaundice, elevated liver function test results and bilirubin levels, and loss of consciousness. Red-orange discoloration of the skin, urine, sweat, saliva, tears, and feces may occur.

Treatment should be with gastric lavage, followed by activated charcoal; if needed, advise clinician to force diuresis. Bile drainage should be performed if hepatic dysfunction persists beyond 24 to 48 hours.

## Clinical considerations

■ Drug should be given 1 hour before or 2 hours after meals for maximum absorption; capsule contents may be mixed with food or fluid to enhance swallowing.

■ Specimens for culture and sensitivity testing will be obtained before giving first dose but don't delay therapy; repeat periodically to detect drug resistance.

■ Increased liver enzyme activity inactivates certain drugs, especially warfarin, corticosteroids, and oral hypoglycemics, requiring dosage adjustments.

■ Rifampin alters standard serum folate and vitamin $B_{12}$ assays.

■ Rifampin may cause temporary retention of sulfobromophthalein in the liver excretion test; it may also interfere with contrast material in gallbladder studies and urinalysis based on spectrophotometry.

**Ⓗ ALERT** Don't confuse similar-sounding drugs like rifabutin and rifapentine with rifampin.

### Therapeutic monitoring

■ Patient should be observed for adverse reactions, and hematologic, renal and liver function test results, and serum electrolytes should be monitored to minimize toxicity. Recommend watching for signs and symptoms of hepatic impairment, such as anorexia, fatigue, malaise, jaundice, dark urine, and liver tenderness.

### Special populations

**Breast-feeding patients.** Drug may appear in breast milk. Use with caution in breast-feeding women.
**Pediatric patients.** Safety in children under age 5 hasn't been established.
**Geriatric patients.** Usual dose in geriatric and debilitated patients is 10 mg/kg once daily. Advise clinician to monitor renal function closely, as geriatric patients may be more susceptible to toxic effects.

### Patient counseling

■ Explain disease process and reason for long-term therapy.

■ Teach signs and symptoms of hypersensitivity and other adverse reactions, and emphasize need to call if these occur; urge patient to report any unusual reactions.

■ Urge patient to comply with prescribed regimen, not to miss doses, and not to discontinue drug without medical approval. Explain importance of follow-up appointments.

■ Encourage patient to promptly report any flulike signs or symptoms, weakness, sore throat, loss of appetite, unusual bruising, rash, itching, tea-colored urine, clay-colored stools, or yellow discoloration of eyes or skin.

■ Explain that drug turns all body fluids red-orange color; advise patient of possible permanent stains on clothes and soft contact lenses.

# rifapentine
Priftin

*Pharmacologic classification:* cyclopentyl rifamycin
*Therapeutic classification:* antibiotic
*Pregnancy risk category C*

## Available forms
Available by prescription only
*Tablets (film-coated):* 150 mg

## Indications and dosages
*Pulmonary tuberculosis, with at least one other antitubercular drug to which the isolate is susceptible*
*Adults:* During the intensive phase of short-course therapy, 600 mg P.O. twice weekly for 2 months, with an interval between doses of not less than 3 days (72 hours).

During the continuation phase of short-course therapy, 600 mg P.O. once weekly for 4 months with isoniazid or another drug to which the isolate is susceptible.

## Mechanism of action
*Antibiotic action:* Rifapentine inhibits DNA-dependent RNA polymerase in susceptible strains of *Mycobacterium tuberculosis*. It has bactericidal activity against the organism both intra- and extracellularly. Rifapentine and rifampin share similar antimicrobial action.

## Pharmacokinetics
*Absorption:* Relative bioavailablity after oral absorption is 70%.
*Distribution:* Bound primarily to albumin.
*Metabolism:* Unknown.
*Excretion:* Appears to be excreted through the urine and feces.

| Route | Onset | Peak | Duration |
|-------|-------|------|----------|
| P.O. | Unknown | 5-6 hr | Unknown |

## Contraindications and precautions
Contraindicated in patients with history of porphyria and those hypersensitive to a rifamycin (rifapentine, rifampin, or rifabutin).

Use drug cautiously and with frequent monitoring in patients with liver disease.

## Interactions
**Drug-drug.** *Anticonvulsants; antiarrhythmics; antibiotics; antifungals; barbiturates; benzodiazepines; beta blockers; calcium channel blockers; cardiac glycosides; corticosteroids; clofibrate; haloperidol; HIV protease inhibitors; oral anticoagulants; immunosuppressants; levothyroxine; narcotic; oral or other systemic hormonal contraceptives; oral hypoglycemics; progestins; quinine; reverse transcriptase inhibitors; sildenafil; theophylline; tricyclic antidepressants:* Rifapentine decreases

the activity of these drugs. Dosage adjustments may be needed.

## Adverse reactions
**CNS:** headache, dizziness.
**CV:** hypertension.
**GI:** anorexia, nausea, vomiting, dyspepsia, diarrhea.
**GU:** pyuria, proteinuria, hematuria, urinary casts.
**Hematologic:** *neutropenia,* lymphopenia, anemia, *leukopenia,* thrombocytosis.
**Hepatic:** elevated AST and ALT.
**Metabolic:** *hyperuricemia.*
**Musculoskeletal:** arthralgia.
**Respiratory:** hemoptysis.
**Skin:** rash, pruritus, acne, maculopapular rash.
**Other:** pain.

## Overdose and treatment
Use of gastric lavage followed by activated charcoal may help after rifapentine overdose. Neither hemodialysis or forced diuresis is suggested. Supportive care and close monitoring of the patient should be initiated.

## Clinical considerations
■ Coadministration of pyridoxine (vitamin $B_6$) is recommended in malnourished patients, in those predisposed to neuropathy (alcoholics, diabetics), and in adolescents.
■ Drug must be given with appropriate daily companion drugs. Compliance with all drugs, especially with daily companion drugs on the days when rifapentine isn't given, is crucial for early sputum conversion and protection from relapse of tuberculosis.
■ Rifapentine can turn body tissues and fluids red-orange. This can lead to permanent staining of contact lenses.
**⚠ ALERT** Don't confuse similar-sounding drugs like rifabutin and rifampin with rifapentine.

### Therapeutic monitoring
■ Rifamycin antibiotics have caused hepatotoxicity. Advise clinician to monitor liver function test results before beginning drug therapy.
■ Drug therapy may affect liver function test results, CBC, and platelet counts; advise clinician to monitor carefully.
■ Notify prescriber of persistent or severe diarrhea.

### Special populations
**Pregnant patients.** Administration of drug during the last 2 weeks of pregnancy may lead to postnatal hemorrhage in the woman or infant. Advise clinician to monitor clotting parameters closely if drug is given.
**Breast-feeding patients.** Because rifapentine may appear in breast milk, it isn't recommended for breast-feeding women.

---

**Pediatric patients.** Safety and efficacy in children under age 12 haven't been established.
**Geriatric patients.** Careful titration is recommended because of potential for decreased hepatic, renal and cardiac function.

## Patient counseling

■ Stress importance of strict compliance with drug and daily companion drugs, as well as needed follow-up visits and laboratory tests.
■ Advise patient to use nonhormonal methods of birth control.
■ Tell patient to take drug with food if nausea, vomiting, or GI upset occurs.
■ Instruct patient to notify prescriber if the following occur: fever, loss of appetite, malaise, nausea, vomiting, darkened urine, yellowish discoloration of the skin and eyes, pain or swelling of the joints, and excessive loose stools or diarrhea.
■ Instruct patient to protect pills from excessive heat.

# riluzole
Rilutek

*Pharmacologic classification:* benzothiazole
*Therapeutic classification:* neuroprotector
*Pregnancy risk category C*

## Available forms
Available by prescription only
*Tablets:* 50 mg

## Indications and dosages
*Amyotrophic lateral sclerosis (ALS)*
*Adults:* 50 mg P.O. q 12 hours on an empty stomach.

## Mechanism of action
*Neuroprotector action:* Unknown.

## Pharmacokinetics
*Absorption:* Well absorbed from GI tract (about 90%) with average absolute oral bioavailability of about 60%. A high-fat meal decreases absorption.
*Distribution:* 96% protein-bound.
*Metabolism:* Extensively metabolized in the liver to six major and several minor metabolites, not all of which have been identified.
*Excretion:* Excreted primarily in urine and a small amount in feces. Half-life is 12 hours with repeated doses.

| Route | Onset | Peak | Duration |
|-------|-------|------|----------|
| P.O. | Unknown | Unknown | Unknown |

## Contraindications and precautions
Contraindicated in patients severely hypersensitive to drug or components in its tablets.

Use cautiously in patients with hepatic or renal dysfunction and in geriatric patients. Also use cautiously in women and Japanese patients who may possess a lower metabolic capacity to eliminate drug compared with men and white patients, respectively.

## Interactions
**Drug-drug.** *Allopurinol, methyldopa, or sulfasalazine:* Increased potential for hepatotoxicity. Use caution when giving together.
**Drug-food.** *Any food:* Decreased bioavailability. Drug should be given 1 hour before or 2 hours after meals.
*Charbroiled foods:* May increase riluzole elimination. Advise patient to avoid charbroiled foods.
**Drug-lifestyle.** *Alcohol use:* May increase risk of hepatotoxicity. Advise patient to avoid alcohol.
*Smoking:* May increase riluzole elimination. Discourage smoking.

## Adverse reactions
**CNS:** *asthenia,* headache, aggravation reaction, hypertonia, malaise, depression, dizziness, insomnia, somnolence, vertigo, circumoral paresthesia.
**CV:** hypertension, tachycardia, palpitation, orthostatic hypotension, peripheral edema.
**EENT:** rhinitis, sinusitis.
**GI:** abdominal pain, *nausea,* vomiting, dyspepsia, anorexia, diarrhea, flatulence, stomatitis, oral candidiasis, dry mouth.
**GU:** urinary tract infection, dysuria.
**Metabolic:** weight loss.
**Musculoskeletal:** back pain, arthralgia.
**Respiratory:** *decreased lung function,* increased cough.
**Skin:** pruritus, eczema, alopecia, exfoliative dermatitis.
**Other:** phlebitis, tooth disorder.

## Overdose and treatment
No information available. In the event of an overdose, therapy should be stopped immediately and supportive measures implemented.

## Clinical considerations
■ Use cautiously in patients with hepatic or renal dysfunction; and in geriatric patients, women, and Japanese patients who may have a lower metabolic capacity to eliminate drug.

### Therapeutic monitoring
■ Baseline elevations in liver function test results, especially elevated bilirubin, should preclude riluzole use.
■ Liver function tests should be performed periodically during therapy. In many patients, drug may cause serum aminotransferase elevations; drug should be stopped if levels exceed 10 times upper limit of normal range or if clinical jaundice develops.

## Special populations

**Breast-feeding patients.** It's unknown if drug appears in breast milk. Because of potential for serious adverse reactions in infants, use of drug in breast-feeding women isn't recommended.

**Pediatric patients.** Safety and efficacy in children haven't been established.

**Geriatric patients.** Age-related decreased renal and hepatic function may cause a decrease in clearance of riluzole. Give drug cautiously to this age group.

## Patient counseling

■ Tell patient or caregiver that drug must be taken regularly and at the same time each day. If a dose is missed, tell patient to take the next tablet as originally planned.

■ Instruct patient to report febrile illness; the patient's WBC count should be checked.

■ Warn patient to avoid hazardous activities until CNS effects of drug are known.

■ Tell patient to store drug at room temperature and protect it from bright light.

■ Stress importance of keeping drug out of reach of children.

# rimantadine hydrochloride

Flumadine

*Pharmacologic classification:* adamantine
*Therapeutic classification:* antiviral
*Pregnancy risk category C*

## Available forms

Available by prescription only
*Syrup:* 50 mg/5 ml
*Tablets:* 100 mg

## Indications and dosages

*Prophylaxis against influenza A virus*
*Adults and children ages 10 and older:* 100 mg P.O. b.i.d.; for patients with severe hepatic dysfunction or renal failure (creatinine clearance 10 ml/minute or less) and for geriatric nursing home patients, a dosage reduction to 100 mg P.O. daily is recommended.
*Children under age 10:* 5 mg/kg P.O. once daily. Maximum dose, 150 mg.
*Treatment of illness caused by various strains of influenza A virus*
*Adults:* 100 mg P.O. b.i.d. for 7 days from initial onset of symptoms; for patients with severe hepatic dysfunction or renal failure (creatinine clearance 10 ml/minute or less) and for geriatric nursing home patients, a dosage reduction to 100 mg P.O. daily is recommended.

## Mechanism of action

*Antiviral action:* Mechanism of action isn't fully understood. It appears to exert its inhibitory effect early in the viral replicative cycle, possibly inhibiting the uncoating of the virus. Genetic studies suggest that a virus protein specified by the virion $M^2$ gene plays an important role in the susceptibility of influenza A virus to inhibition by rimantadine.

## Pharmacokinetics

*Absorption:* Tablet and syrup formulations are equally absorbed after oral administration.
*Distribution:* Plasma protein–binding is about 40% for rimantadine.
*Metabolism:* Extensively metabolized in the liver.
*Excretion:* Less than 25% is excreted in urine as unchanged drug. Elimination half-life of drug is about 25½ to 32 hours. Hemodialysis doesn't contribute to drug clearance.

| Route | Onset | Peak | Duration |
|-------|---------|------|----------|
| P.O. | Unknown | 6 hr | Unknown |

## Contraindications and precautions

Contraindicated in patients hypersensitive to drug or to amantadine.

Use cautiously during pregnancy and in patients with impaired renal or hepatic function or seizure disorders (especially epilepsy).

## Interactions

**Drug-drug.** *Acetaminophen, aspirin:* Reduced level of rimantadine. Advise clinician to monitor patient for drug effect.
*Cimetidine:* May decrease total rimantadine clearance by about 16%. Advise clinician to monitor patient for adverse effects.

## Adverse reactions

**CNS:** insomnia, headache, dizziness, nervousness, fatigue, asthenia.
**GI:** nausea, vomiting, anorexia, dry mouth, abdominal pain.

## Overdose and treatment

Information specific to rimantadine overdose isn't available. As with any overdose, recommend giving supportive therapy as indicated. Overdoses of a related drug, amantadine, have been reported, with reactions ranging from agitation to hallucinations, cardiac arrhythmia, and death. Administration of I.V. physostigmine (1 to 2 mg in adults and 0.5 mg in children; repeated p.r.n. but not to exceed 2 mg/hour) has been reported anecdotally to benefit patients with CNS effects from overdose of amantadine.

## Clinical considerations

■ Consider the possibility of primary or concomitant bacterial infection.

■ For illnesses from various strains of influenza A, treatment should begin as soon as possible, preferably within 48 hours after onset of signs and symptoms, to reduce duration of fever and systemic symptoms.

■ An increased incidence of seizures has been observed in some patients with history of seizures who weren't taking an anticonvulsant during rimantadine therapy. If seizures develop, drug should be stopped.

■ Influenza A–resistant strains can emerge during therapy. Patients taking drug may still be able to spread the disease.

■ If seizures develop, discontinue rimantadine.

**⊬ ALERT** Don't confuse this drug with amantadine.

### Therapeutic monitoring

■ Because of risk of drug metabolites accumulation during multiple dosing, advise clinician to monitor patient with any degree of renal insufficiency for adverse effects and adjust dosage p.r.n.

### Special populations

**Breast-feeding patients.** Drug shouldn't be given to breast-feeding women because of the potential adverse effects to the infant.

**Pediatric patients.** Drug is recommended for prophylaxis of influenza A. Safety and efficacy of drug in treating symptomatic influenza infection in children haven't been established. Prophylaxis studies with rimantadine haven't been performed in those under age 1.

**Geriatric patients.** Adverse reactions from drug occur more frequently in geriatric patients than in general population. Advise clinician to monitor these patients closely.

### Patient counseling

■ Advise patient to take drug several hours before bedtime to prevent insomnia.

■ Inform patient that taking drug doesn't prevent him from spreading the disease and that he should limit contact with others until fully recovered.

■ Warn patient that drug may cause adverse CNS effects; he shouldn't drive or perform activities that require mental alertness until these effects are known.

---

# risperidone
Risperdal

*Pharmacologic classification:* benzisoxazole derivative
*Therapeutic classification:* antipsychotic
*Pregnancy risk category C*

## Available forms

Available by prescription only
*Solution:* 1 mg/ml
*Tablets:* 0.25 mg, 0.5 mg, 1 mg, 2 mg, 3 mg, 4 mg

## Indications and dosages
### Psychosis

*Adults:* Initially, 1 mg P.O. b.i.d. Increase in increments of 1 mg b.i.d. on days 2 and 3 of treatment to a target dose of 3 mg b.i.d. Wait at least 1 week before adjusting dosage further. Doses above 6 mg/day weren't more effective than lower doses and caused more extrapyramidal reactions.

**≡ Dosage adjustment.** Geriatric or debilitated patients, hypotensive patients, or patients with severe renal or hepatic impairment should initially receive 0.5 mg P.O. b.i.d. Increase dosage in increments of 0.5 mg b.i.d. on second and third days of treatment to target dose of 1.5 mg P.O. b.i.d. Wait at least 1 week before increasing dosage further.

## Mechanism of action

*Antipsychotic action:* Exact mechanism of action is unknown. Its antipsychotic activity may be mediated through a combination of dopamine type 2 (D2) and serotonin type 2 (5-HT$_2$) antagonism. Antagonism at receptors other than D2 and 5-HT$_2$ may explain other effects of drug.

## Pharmacokinetics

*Absorption:* Well absorbed after oral administration. Absolute oral bioavailability is 70%. Food doesn't affect rate or extent of absorption.

*Distribution:* Plasma protein–binding is about 90% for drug and 77% for its major active metabolite, 9-hydroxyrisperidone.

*Metabolism:* Extensively metabolized in the liver to 9-hydroxyrisperidone, which is the predominant circulating species and appears about equi-effective with risperidone with respect to receptor binding activity. About 6% to 8% of whites and a low percentage of Asians show little or no receptor binding activity and are "poor metabolizers."

*Excretion:* Metabolite is excreted by the kidney. Clearance of drug and its metabolite is reduced in renally impaired patients.

| Route | Onset | Peak | Duration |
|-------|-------|------|----------|
| P.O. | Unknown | 1 hr | Unknown |

## Contraindications and precautions

Contraindicated in patients hypersensitive to drug and in breast-feeding women.

Use cautiously in patients with prolonged QT interval, CV disease, cerebrovascular disease, dehydration, hypovolemia, history of seizures, or exposure to extreme heat or conditions that could affect metabolism or hemodynamic responses.

## Interactions

**Drug-drug.** *Antihypertensives:* May enhance the effects of certain antihypertensives. Advise clinician to monitor patient closely.

*Carbamazepine:* May increase risperidone clearance, decreasing the effectiveness of carbamazepine. Advise clinician to monitor patient closely.

*Clozapine:* May decrease risperidone clearance, increasing the risk of toxicity. Advise clinician to monitor patient closely.

*CNS depressants:* May cause additive CNS depression when given together. Give together with caution.

*Levodopa and dopamine agonists:* Risperidone may antagonize the effects of these drugs. Avoid use together.

**Drug-lifestyle.** *Alcohol use:* Additive CNS depression. Advise patient to avoid alcohol.

*Sun exposure:* May cause photosensitivity reactions. Advise patient to use sunblock.

## Adverse reactions

**CNS:** *somnolence, extrapyramidal reactions, headache, insomnia, agitation, anxiety,* tardive dyskinesia, aggressiveness, ***neuroleptic malignant syndrome.***

**CV:** tachycardia, chest pain, orthostatic hypotension, prolonged QT interval.

**EENT:** *rhinitis,* sinusitis, pharyngitis, abnormal vision.

**GI:** *constipation, nausea, vomiting, dyspepsia.*

**Musculoskeletal:** arthralgia, back pain.

**Respiratory:** coughing, upper respiratory infection.

**Skin:** rash, dry skin, photosensitivity.

**Other:** fever, increase serum prolactin levels.

## Overdose and treatment

Signs and symptoms of overdose result from an exaggeration of the known pharmacologic effects of risperidone, such as drowsiness and sedation, tachycardia and hypotension, and extrapyramidal symptoms. Hyponatremia, hypokalemia, prolonged QT interval, widened QRS complex, and seizures also have been reported.

There's no specific antidote to risperidone overdose; recommend appropriate supportive measures. Consider gastric lavage (after intubation, if patient is unconscious) and administration of activated charcoal with a laxative. CV monitoring is essential to detect possible arrhythmias. If antiarrhythmic therapy is given, disopyramide, procainamide, and quinidine carry a theoretical hazard of QT-prolonging effects that might be additive to those of risperidone. Similarly, it's reasonable to expect that the alpha-blocking properties of bretylium might be additive to those of risperidone, resulting in problematic hypotension.

## Clinical considerations

■ Risperidone and 9-hydroxyrisperidone appear to lengthen the QT interval in some patients, although there's no average increase in treated patients, even at 12 to 16 mg/day (well above recommended dose). Other drugs that prolong the QT interval have been associated with torsades de pointes, a life-threatening arrhythmia. Bradycardia, electrolyte imbalance, use with other drugs that prolong the QT interval, or congenital prolongation of the QT interval may increase risk for occurrence of this arrhythmia.

■ Drug has an antiemetic effect in animals; this may occur in humans, masking signs and symptoms of overdose or of such conditions as intestinal obstruction, Reye's syndrome, and brain tumor.

■ When restarting drug therapy for patients who have been off drug, initial 3-day dose initiation schedule should be followed.

■ Advise clinician to immediately stop any other antipsychotic drug on initiation of risperidone therapy when medically appropriate.

### Therapeutic monitoring

■ Tardive dyskinesia may occur after prolonged risperidone therapy. It may not appear until months or years later and may disappear spontaneously or persist for life despite discontinuation of drug.

■ Neuroleptic malignant syndrome is rare, but in many cases fatal. It isn't necessarily related to length of drug use or type of neuroleptic. Advise clinician to monitor patient closely for symptoms, including hyperpyrexia, muscle rigidity, altered mental status, irregular pulse, alteration in blood pressure, and diaphoresis.

### Special populations

**Pregnant patients.** Instruct women to call prescriber if pregnancy is being planned or is suspected.

**Breast-feeding patients.** Advise patient to stop breast-feeding.

**Pediatric patients.** Safety and efficacy in children haven't been established.

**Geriatric patients.** A lower starting dose is recommended for geriatric patients because they have decreased pharmacokinetic clearance; a greater risk of hepatic, renal, or cardiac dysfunction; and a greater tendency toward orthostatic hypotension.

## Patient counseling

■ Advise patient to rise slowly from a recumbent or seated position to minimize lightheadedness.

■ Warn patient not to operate hazardous machinery, including driving a car, until effects of drug are known.

■ Tell patient to call before taking new drugs, including OTC drugs, because of potential for interactions.

---

# ritonavir

Norvir

*Pharmacologic classification:* HIV
protease inhibitor
*Therapeutic classification:* antiviral
*Pregnancy risk category B*

## Available forms

Available by prescription only
*Capsules:* 100 mg
*Oral solution:* 80 mg/ml

## Indications and dosages

**Treatment of HIV infection when anti-
retroviral therapy is warranted**
*Adults:* 600 mg P.O. b.i.d. with meals. If nausea occurs, this schedule may provide some relief: 300 mg b.i.d., increased at 2- to 3-day intervals by 100 mg b.i.d., up to 600 mg b.i.d.
*Children ages 2 and older:* 400 mg/m$^2$ P.O.
b.i.d. with other antiretroviral drugs. To minimize nausea, initially 250 mg/m$^2$ b.i.d. May
increase by 50 mg/m$^2$ b.i.d. at 2- to 3-day intervals.

## Mechanism of action

*Antiviral action:* Ritonavir is an HIV protease
inhibitor. HIV protease is an enzyme required
for the proteolytic cleavage of the viral polyprotein precursors into the individual functional
proteins found in infectious HIV. Ritonavir
binds to the protease active site and inhibits the
activity of the enzyme. This inhibition prevents
cleavage of the viral polyproteins, resulting in
the formation of immature noninfectious viral
particles.

## Pharmacokinetics

*Absorption:* Absorbed better when taken with
food; its absolute bioavailability hasn't been
determined.
*Distribution:* 98% to 99% plasma protein–
bound.
*Metabolism:* Metabolized in the liver; P-450
3A (CYP3A) is the major isoform involved in
ritonavir metabolism.
*Excretion:* Primarily excreted in feces, although
a small amount has been found in the urine.
Half-life is 3 to 5 hours.

| Route | Onset | Peak | Duration |
|-------|-------|------|----------|
| P.O. | Unknown | 2-4 hr | Unknown |

## Contraindications and precautions

Contraindicated in patients hypersensitive to
any components of drug.
    Use cautiously in patients with hepatic in-
sufficiency.

## Interactions

**Drug-drug.** *Drugs that increase CYP3A activity, such as carbamazepine, dexamethasone,*
*phenobarbital, phenytoin, rifabutin, and ri-
fampin:* Increase ritonavir clearance resulting
in decreased ritonavir plasma levels. Advise
clinician to monitor patient closely. Advise
clinician to monitor anticonvulsant drug levels. May reduce rifabutin dosage if needed.
*Alprazolam, clorazepate, diazepam, estazo-
lam, flurazepam, midazolam, triazolam, and
zolpidem:* Potential for extreme sedation and
respiratory depression from these drugs. Don't
co-administer with ritonavir.
*Alprazolam, methadone:* Decreased levels of
these drugs. Use together cautiously.
*Amiodarone, bepridil, bupropion, clozapine,
encainide, flecainide, meperidine, piroxicam,
propafenone, propoxyphene, quinidine, rifabutin:* Significant increases in the plasma levels of these drugs, thus increasing the patient's
risk of arrhythmias, hematologic abnormalities, seizures, or other potentially serious adverse effects. Don't use together.
*Amprenavir:* Increased AUC of amprenavir.
There are limited data in adjusting the dosage
to amprenavir 600 to 1,200 mg bid and ritonavir 100 to 200 mg b.i.d.
*Clarithromycin:* Increased clarithromycin level. Patients with impaired renal function receiving drug with ritonavir require a 50% reduction in their clarithromycin if creatinine
clearance is 30 to 60 ml/minute and a 75% reduction if it's below 30 ml/minute.
*Desipramine:* Increased overall serum levels
of desipramine. May require dosage adjustment.
*Disopyramide:* Cardiac and neurologic events
may occur. Use together with caution.
*Disulfiram or other drugs that produce disul-
firam-like reactions, such as metronidazole:*
Increased risk of disulfiram-like reactions. Ritonavir formulations contain alcohol that can
produce reactions when co-administered. Advise clinician to monitor patient.
*Efavirenz:* Increased plasma levels of both
drugs. Leave the dose at 600 mg b.i.d., or may
reduce dosage of ritonavir to 500 mg b.i.d. if
intolerance occurs.
*Ethinyl estradiol:* Decreased ethinyl estradiol
plasma levels. Advise patient to use an alternative or additional method of birth control.
*Glucuronosyltransferases, including oral an-
ticoagulants or immunosuppressants:* Loss of
therapeutic effects from directly glucuronidated
drugs. May need dosage alteration of these
drugs; advise clinician to monitor drug levels
and drug effects. A dosage reduction greater
than 50% may be required for those drugs extensively metabolized by CYP3A.
*HMG CoA reductase inhibitors:* Large increase
in statin levels, causing myopathy. Avoid concomitant use.
*Ketoconazole:* Increased level of ritonavir. Use
together cautiously and recommend monitoring patient carefully.

*Ketoconazole, sildenafil:* Increased levels of these drugs. Use together cautiously. Don't exceed 25 mg of sildenafil in a 48-hour period.
*Nelfinavir:* Increased nelfinavir plasma levels. Adjust dosage by taking ritonavir 400 mg b.i.d. and nelfinavir 500 to 750 mg b.i.d.
*Nevirapine, delaviridine:* Altered plasma levels of ritonavir. No dosage adjustment is needed.
*Oral contraceptives:* Decreased overall serum levels of the contraceptive. May require a dosage increase in the oral contraceptive or alternate contraceptive measures.
*Saquinavir:* Increased saquinavir plasma levels. Adjust dosage by taking saquinavir 400 mg b.i.d. and ritonavir 400 mg b.i.d.
*Theophylline:* Decreased overall serum levels of theophylline. Increased dosage may be required.
**Drug-herb.** *St. John's wort:* May substantially reduce blood levels of the drug that could cause loss of therapeutic effects. Advise patient against using together.
**Drug-food.** *Any food:* Increased absorption. Drug should be taken with food.
**Drug-lifestyle.** *Smoking:* Decrease in serum levels of ritonavir. Discourage smoking.

## Adverse reactions

**CNS:** *asthenia,* headache, malaise, circumoral paresthesia, dizziness, insomnia, paresthesia, peripheral paresthesia, somnolence, thinking abnormality, migraine headache, abnormal dreams, abnormal gait, agitation, amnesia, anxiety, aphasia, ataxia, confusion, depression, diplopia, emotional lability, euphoria, *generalized tonic-clonic seizure,* hallucinations, hyperesthesia, incoordination, nervousness, neuralgia, neuropathy, paralysis, peripheral neuropathy, peripheral sensory neuropathy, personality disorder, tremor, vertigo.
**CV:** vasodilation, hypertension, palpation, peripheral vascular disorder, syncope, orthostatic hypotension, tachycardia, chest pain.
**EENT:** abnormal electrooculogram, abnormal electroretinogram, abnormal vision, amblyopia, blurred vision, blepharitis, ear pain, epistaxis, eye pain, hearing impairment, increased cerumen, iritis, parosmia, pharyngitis, photophobia, rhinitis, tinnitus, uveitis, visual field defect.
**GI:** abdominal pain, anorexia, constipation, *diarrhea, nausea, vomiting,* dyspepsia, flatulence, enlarged abdomen, abnormal stools, bloody diarrhea, cheilitis, cholangitis, colitis, dry mouth, dysphagia, eructation, esophagitis, gastritis, gastroenteritis, GI disorder, *GI hemorrhage,* gingivitis, ileitis, mouth ulcer, oral candidiasis, *pancreatitis,* periodontal abscess, rectal disorder, tenesmus, thirst, *taste perversion,* taste loss.
**GU:** kidney pain, dysuria, hematuria, impotence, renal calculus, renal failure, nocturia, penis disorder, polyuria, pyelonephritis, ure-thritis, urine retention, urinary frequency, glycosuria.
**Hematologic:** anemia, ecchymosis, *leukopenia,* hemorrhage, lymphadenopathy, lymphocytosis, *thrombocytopenia.*
**Hepatic:** *hepatitis,* hepatomegaly, liver damage, and abnormal liver function test results.
**Metabolic:** altered hormonal levels, diabetes mellitus, avitaminosis, gout, hyperlipidemia, hypercholesteremia.
**Musculoskeletal:** arthralgia, arthrosis, joint disorder, muscle cramps, muscle weakness, myalgia, myositis, and twitching, back pain, neck pain, neck rigidity.
**Respiratory:** asthma, dyspnea, hiccups, hypoventilation, increased cough, interstitial pneumonia, lung disorder.
**Skin:** rash, sweating, photosensitivity reaction, acne, contact dermatitis, dry skin, eczema, folliculitis, maculopapular rash, molluscum contagiosum, pruritus, psoriasis, seborrhea, urticaria, vesiculobullous rash.
**Other:** fever, local throat irritation, increased CK level, allergic reaction, cachexia, chills, facial edema, facial pain, flu syndrome, hypothermia, decreased libido, pain (unspecified, substernal chest pain, peripheral edema, dehydration, edema).

## Overdose and treatment

Information is limited to one patient who reported paresthesia, which resolved after the dosage was decreased. Treatment consists of general supportive measures. Emesis or gastric lavage may be used as well as activated charcoal. Dialysis isn't likely to be beneficial.

## Clinical considerations

■ Drug may be given alone or with nucleoside analogues.
■ GI tolerance may be improved in patients starting combination regimens with ritonavir and nucleosides by initiating ritonavir alone and subsequently adding nucleosides before completing 2 weeks of ritonavir monotherapy.

### Therapeutic monitoring

■ Advise clinician to monitor patient's response to drug therapy.
■ Plasma HIV-1 RNA levels and CD4+ T-cell counts should be measured to determine disease progression and when to modify therapy.

### Special populations

**Breast-feeding patients.** It's unknown if ritonavir appears in breast milk. However, HIV-positive women shouldn't breast-feed to prevent transmission of infection.
**Pregnant patients.** Potential adverse effect on fetus. Cases of exposure of pregnant women exposed to antiretroviral drugs can be reported to the Antiretroviral Pregnancy Registry for monitoring maternal-fetal outcomes (1-800-258-4263).

---

**Pediatric patients.** Safety and efficacy in children under age 12 haven't been established.

## Patient counseling
■ Inform patient that drug isn't a cure for HIV infection. He may continue to develop opportunistic infections and other complications from HIV infection. Drug has also not been shown to reduce risk of transmitting HIV to others through sexual contact or blood contamination.
■ Caution patient not to adjust dosage or stop ritonavir therapy without medical approval.
■ Tell patient that he may improve taste of oral solution by mixing with chocolate milk, Ensure, or Advera.
■ Tell patient that if a dose is missed, he should take the next dose as soon as possible. However, if a dose is skipped, he shouldn't double the next dose.
■ Advise patients receiving sildenafil that there is an increased risk of adverse events, including hypotension, visual changes, and priapism. They should promptly report any symptoms to their prescriber. Tell them not to exceed 25 mg in a 48-hour period.

# rivastigmine tartrate
Exelon

*Pharmacologic classification:*
cholinesterase inhibitor
*Therapeutic classification:* drug for Alzheimer's disease
*Pregnancy risk category B*

## Available forms
Available by prescription only
*Capsules:* 1.5 mg, 3 mg, 4.5 mg, 6 mg

## Indications and dosages
*Symptomatic treatment of patients with mild to moderate Alzheimer's disease*
*Adults:* Initially, 1.5 mg P.O. b.i.d. with food. If tolerated, dosage may be increased to 3 mg b.i.d. after 2 weeks of treatment. Further increases to 4.5 mg b.i.d. and 6 mg b.i.d. may be implemented as tolerated after 2 weeks on the previous dose. The effective dosage range is 6 to 12 mg daily with a maximum recommended dose of 12 mg daily.

## Mechanism of action
*Anticholinesterase action:* The drug is thought to increase acetylcholine level through reversible inhibition of its hydrolysis by cholinesterase. It is thought that acetylcholine is the primary neurotransmitter that is depleted in Alzheimer's disease. By increasing acetylcholine activity, symptomatic improvement in cognitive function may be seen.

## Pharmacokinetics
*Absorption:* Rapidly absorbed and reaches peak serum levels in about 1 hour. Although it should be taken with food, the time to reach peak levels is delayed by about 1½ hours. Absolute bioavailability is 36%.
*Distribution:* Widely distributed throughout the body and crosses the blood brain barrier. Protein-binding is about 40%.
*Metabolism:* Rapidly and extensively metabolized.
*Excretion:* Elimination is primarily through the kidneys. Half-life is about 1½ hours in patients with normal renal function.

| Route | Onset | Peak | Duration |
|-------|-------|------|----------|
| P.O. | Unknown | 1 hr | 12 hr |

## Contraindications and precautions
Contraindicated in patients hypersensitive to drug or its components or to other carbamate derivatives.

Use cautiously in patients with history of ulcers or GI bleeding, sick sinus syndrome or other supraventricular cardiac conditions, asthma or obstructive pulmonary disease, seizures, and in those taking nonsteroidal anti-inflammatory drugs.

## Interactions
**Drug-drug.** *Anticholinergics:* Rivastigmine may interfere with activity of anticholinergics. Advise clinician to monitor patient closely.
*Bethanechol, succinylcholine, other neuromuscular blockers or cholinergic antagonists:* May have a synergistic effect on rivastigmine. Advise clinician to monitor patient closely.
**Drug-lifestyle.** *Nicotine:* Increased clearance of rivastgimine. Advise clinician to monitor patient closely.

## Adverse reactions
**CNS:** fatigue, asthenia, malaise, *dizziness, headache,* somnolence, tremor, insomnia, confusion, depression, anxiety, hallucination, aggressive reaction, vertigo, agitation, nervousness, delusion, paranoid reaction.
**CV:** syncope, hypertension, chest pain, peripheral edema.
**EENT:** rhinitis, pharyngitis.
**GI:** *nausea, vomiting, diarrhea, anorexia, abdominal pain,* dyspepsia, constipation, flatulence, eructation.
**GU:** urinary tract infection, urinary incontinence.
**Metabolic:** weight loss.
**Musculoskeletal:** back pain, arthralgia, bone fracture.
**Respiratory:** upper respiratory infection, cough, bronchitis.
**Skin:** increased sweating, rash.
**Other:** *accidental trauma,* flulike symptoms, pain.

## Overdose and treatment

Symptoms of overdose are cholinergic in nature and may include severe nausea, vomiting, salivation, sweating, bradycardia, hypotension, muscle weakness, respiratory depression, respiratory collapse, and seizures.

If these occur, withhold additional doses of Exelon for 24 hours. Administration of antiemetics may be considered if severe nausea and vomiting occur. Dialysis is not recommended because of the short half-life.

## Clinical considerations

■ Significant GI adverse effects, such as nausea, vomiting, anorexia, and weight loss are to be expected. Risk is less common while on maintenance doses.

**H ALERT** The manufacturer has issued a warning that severe vomiting has occurred among patients who resumed rivastigmine therapy after an interruption. Revised package labeling states that therapy should resume at the recommended starting dosage (1.5 mg b.i.d.) if therapy is interrupted for longer than several days. The dosage should then be adjusted upward to maintenance levels.

■ Advise clinician to monitor patient for symptoms of active or occult GI bleeding.

■ Dramatic memory improvement is unlikely. As disease progresses, the benefits of rivastigmine may decline.

■ Advise clinician to monitor patient for severe nausea, vomiting, and diarrhea, which may lead to dehydration and weight loss.

■ Recommend carefully monitoring patient with a history of GI bleeding, NSAID use, arrhythmias, seizures, or pulmonary conditions for adverse effects.

### Special populations

**Breast-feeding patients.** It's not known if rivastigmine appears in breast milk. There is no indication for use in nursing mothers.

**Pediatric patients.** Safety and effectiveness have not been evaluated.

## Patient counseling

■ Advise patient to report any episodes of nausea, vomiting, or diarrhea.

■ Advise patient and caregiver that improvement in memory may be subtle and that a more likely result of taking rivastigmine will be a slower decline in memory loss.

■ Advise patient to take rivastigmine with food in the morning and evening.

■ Advise patient to consult a prescriber before taking OTC drugs.

# rizatriptan benzoate
Maxalt, Maxalt-MLT

*Pharmacologic classification:* selective 5-hydroxytryptamine ($5\text{-HT}_{1b/1d}$) receptor agonist
*Therapeutic classification:* antimigraine
*Pregnancy risk category C*

## Available forms

Available by prescription only
*Tablets:* 5 mg, 10 mg
*Tablets (orally disintegrating):* 5 mg, 10 mg

## Indications and dosages

*Treatment of acute migraine headaches with or without aura*

**Adults:** Initially, 5 or 10 mg P.O. If first dose is ineffective, another dose can be given at least 2 hours after first dose. Maximum dose is 30 mg within a 24-hour period. For patients receiving propranolol, 5 mg P.O. up to maximum of three doses (15 mg) in 24 hours.

## Mechanism of action

*Vasoconstricting action:* Rizatriptan is believed to exert its effect by acting as an agonist at serotonin receptors on the extracerebral intracranial blood vessels, which results in vasoconstriction of the affected vessels, inhibition of neuropeptide release, and reduction of pain transmission in the trigeminal pathways.

## Pharmacokinetics

*Absorption:* Bioavailablity after oral administration is 45%.
*Distribution:* Minimally plasma-bound.
*Metabolism:* Primary metabolism takes place via oxidative deamination by monoamine oxidase-A to the indole acetic acid metabolite.
*Excretion:* 82% excreted in urine, 12% in feces, after oral administration.

| Route | Onset | Peak | Duration |
|-------|-------|------|----------|
| P.O. | Unknown | 1½ hr | Unknown |

## Contraindications and precautions

Contraindicated in patients with ischemic heart disease (angina pectoris, history of MI, or documented silent ischemia) or in those with symptoms or findings consistent with ischemic heart disease, coronary artery vasospasm (Prinzmetal's variant angina), or other significant underlying CV disease. Also contraindicated in patients with uncontrolled hypertension or within 24 hours of treatment with another 5-HT agonist, or an ergotamine-containing or ergot-type drug like dihydroergotamine or methysergide. Don't use within 2 weeks of discontinuation of MAO inhibitor. Also contraindicated in patients hypersensitive to drug or its inactive ingredients.

Use cautiously in patients with hepatic or renal impairment. Use with caution in patients with risk factors for coronary artery disease, such as hypertension, hypercholesterolemia, smoking, obesity, diabetes, strong family history of coronary artery disease, women with surgical or physiologic menopause, or men over 40 years, unless a cardiac evaluation provides evidence that patient is free from cardiac disease.

## Interactions
**Drug-drug.** *Ergot-containing or ergot-type drugs, such as dihydroergotamine and methysergide; other 5-HT$_1$ agonists:* May cause prolonged vasospastic reactions. Shouldn't be used within 24 hours of rizatriptan.
*MAO inhibitors (isocarboxazid, moclobemidepargyline, phenelzine, tranylcypromine):* May cause increased plasma levels of rizatriptan. Avoid use together and allow at least 14 days to elapse between discontinuation of an MAO inhibitor and administration of rizatriptan.
*Propranolol:* May cause increased rizatriptan levels. Dosage reduction may be needed.
*Selective serotonin reuptake inhibitors, such as fluoxetine, fluvoxamine, paroxetine, and sertraline:* May cause weakness, hyperreflexia, and incoordination. Advise clinician to monitor patient closely.

## Adverse reactions
**CNS:** dizziness, headache, somnolence, paresthesia, asthenia, fatigue, hypesthesia, decreased mental acuity, euphoria, tremor.
**CV:** chest pain, pressure or heaviness, palpitations.
**EENT:** neck, throat, and jaw pain, pressure or heaviness.
**GI:** dry mouth, nausea, diarrhea, vomiting.
**Respiratory:** dyspnea.
**Skin:** flushing.
**Other:** pain, warm or cold sensations, hot flashes.

## Clinical considerations
■ Drug should be used only after a definite diagnosis of migraine is established.
■ Drug shouldn't be used for prophylactic therapy of migraines or in patients with hemiplegic or basilar migraine or cluster headaches.
■ Safety of treating, on average, more than four headaches in a 30-day period hasn't been established.
■ Orally disintegrating tablets contain phenylalanine.

### Therapeutic monitoring
■ For patients with risk factors that have a satisfactory cardiac evaluation, advise clinician to monitor closely after first dose.

■ CV status should be assessed in patients who develop risk factors for coronary artery disease during treatment.

### Special populations
**Pregnant patients.** Advise women to immediately notify prescriber if pregnancy occurs or is suspected.
**Breast-feeding patients.** Instruct women not to breast-feed because the effects on infants are unknown.
**Pediatric patients.** Safety and efficacy in children under age 18 haven't been established.

## Patient counseling
■ Inform patient that drug doesn't prevent migraine headache from occurring.
■ For Maxalt-MLT, tell patient to remove blister pack from pouch, then remove drug from blister pack immediately before use. Tablet shouldn't be popped out of blister pack, but pack should be carefully peeled away with dry hands, and tablet placed on tongue and allowed to dissolve. Tablet is then swallowed with the saliva. No water is needed or recommended. Tell patient that orally dissolving tablet doesn't provide more rapid headache relief.
■ Advise patient that if headache returns after initial dose, a second dose may be taken with medical approval at least 2 hours after the first dose. Don't take more than 30 mg in a 24-hour period.
■ Inform patient that drug may cause somnolence and dizziness and warn him to avoid hazardous activities until effects are known.
■ Tell patient that food may delay onset of action of drug.

# rocuronium bromide
Zemuron

*Pharmacologic classification:* nondepolarizing neuromuscular blocker
*Therapeutic classification:* skeletal muscle relaxant
*Pregnancy risk category B*

## Available forms
Available by prescription only
*Injection:* 10 mg/ml

## Indications and dosages
*Adjunct to general anesthesia, facilitation of endotracheal intubation, or skeletal muscle relaxation during surgery or mechanical ventilation*
*Adults and children ages 3 months or older:* Initially, 0.6 to 1.2 mg/kg I.V. bolus. In most patients, tracheal intubation may be performed within 2 minutes; muscle paralysis should last about 30 minutes. Maintenance dose of 0.1 mg/kg should provide an additional 12 min-

utes of muscle relaxation (0.15 mg/kg will add 17 minutes; 0.2 mg/kg will add 24 minutes).

Note: Dosage depends on anesthetic used, individual needs, and response. Dosages are representative and must be adjusted.

## I.V. administration
■ Administer sedatives or general anesthetics before neuromuscular blockers. Neuromuscular blockers don't obtund consciousness or alter the pain threshold.
■ Administer by rapid I.V. injection. Or, give by continuous I.V. infusion. Infusion rates are highly individualized. Compatible solutions include $D_5W$, normal saline solution for injection, dextrose 5% in normal saline solution for injection, sterile water for injection, and lactated Ringer's injection.
■ Store vials at room temperature for up to 30 days. Use diluted infusion solutions within 24 hours.

### Incompatibilities
Incompatible with alkaline solutions. Don't mix with other drugs.

## Mechanism of action
*Skeletal muscle relaxation action:* Rocuronium acts by competing for cholinergic receptors at the motor end plate. This action is antagonized by acetylcholinesterase inhibitors, such as neostigmine and edrophonium.

## Pharmacokinetics
*Absorption:* Administered I.V.
*Distribution:* Rapid distribution half-life is 1 to 2 minutes; slower distribution half-life is 14 to 18 minutes. Drug is about 30% plasma protein–bound.
*Metabolism:* No information available, but hepatic clearance could be significant. The rocuronium analogue 17-desacetyl-rocuronium, a metabolite, has rarely been observed in plasma or urine.
*Excretion:* About 33% of given dose is recovered in urine within 24 hours.

| Route | Onset | Peak | Duration |
|-------|-------|------|----------|
| I.V. | 1 min | 2 min | 22-67 min |

## Contraindications and precautions
Contraindicated in patients hypersensitive to bromides.

Use cautiously in patients with hepatic disease, severe obesity, bronchogenic carcinoma, electrolyte disturbances, neuromuscular disease, or altered circulation time caused by CV, age, or edematous states.

## Interactions
**Drug-drug.** *Antibiotics, such as aminoglycosides, bacitracin, colistimethate sodium, colistin, polymyxins, tetracylines, and vancomycin:* May enhance neuromuscular blocking action of rocuronium. Use cautiously.
*Anticonvulsant therapy, such as carbamazepine or phenytoin:* May develop a form of diminished magnitude of neuromuscular block or shortened clinical duration. Use cautiously.
*Enflurane, isoflurane:* May prolong duration of action of initial and maintenance dosages of rocuronium. Use cautiously during surgical and postoperative periods.
*Quinidine:* An injection of quinidine during recovery from rocuronium may cause recurrent paralysis. Avoid use together.

## Adverse reactions
**CV:** tachycardia, abnormal ECG, *arrhythmias,* transient hypotension and hypertension.
**GI:** nausea, vomiting.
**Respiratory:** hiccups, asthma.
**Skin:** rash, edema, pruritus.

## Overdose and treatment
No cases of rocuronium overdose have been reported. Overdose with neuromuscular blockers may result in neuromuscular block beyond the time needed for surgery and anesthesia.

Primary treatment is maintenance of a patent airway and controlled ventilation until patient recovers normal neuromuscular function. After initial evidence of such recovery is observed, further recovery may be facilitated by administration of an anticholinesterase drug, such as neostigmine or edrophonium, with an appropriate anticholinergic.

## Clinical considerations
■ Drug should be used only by personnel experienced in airway management.
■ Airway should be kept clear. Emergency respiratory support equipment (endotracheal equipment, ventilator, oxygen, atropine, edrophonium, epinephrine, and neostigmine) should be available.
■ Neuromuscular blockers don't obtund consciousness or alter the pain threshold. Patients should receive sedatives or general anesthetics before neuromuscular blockers are given.
■ Drug is well tolerated in patients with renal failure.
■ In obese patients, initial dose should be based on patient's actual body weight.

### Therapeutic monitoring
■ A peripheral nerve stimulator should be used to measure neuromuscular function during drug administration to monitor drug effect, determine need for additional doses, and confirm recovery from neuromuscular block. Once spontaneous recovery starts, drug-induced neuromuscular blockade may be reversed with an anticholinesterase drug.

---

## Special populations
**Pediatric patients.** Use of rocuronium in children under age 3 months hasn't been studied.

## Patient counseling
■ Explain all events and procedures to patient because he can still hear.

# rofecoxib
Vioxx

*Pharmacologic classification:* cyclo-oxygenase-2 (COX-2) inhibitor
*Therapeutic classification:* nonnarcotic analgesic, anti-inflammatory
*Pregnancy risk category C*

## Available forms
Available by prescription only
*Oral suspension:* 12.5 mg/5 ml, 25 mg/5 ml
*Tablets:* 12.5 mg, 25 mg, 50 mg

## Indications and dosages
*Relief of signs and symptoms of osteo-arthritis*
*Adults:* Initially, 12.5 mg P.O. once daily, increased p.r.n. to a maximum of 25 mg P.O. once daily.
*Management of acute pain and treatment of primary dysmenorrhea*
*Adults:* 50 mg P.O. once daily p.r.n. for up to 5 days.
*◇ Rheumatoid arthritis*
*Adults:* Initially, 25 to 50 mg P.O. once daily.

## Mechanism of action
*Analgesic and anti-inflammatory actions:* The exact mechanism of action of rofecoxib is unknown. Its anti-inflammatory and analgesic effects along with its antipyretic activity may come from its ability to inhibit prostaglandin synthesis, which it does by inhibiting the COX-2 isoenzyme. At therapeutic serum levels, rofecoxib doesn't inhibit the cyclooxygenase-1 (COX-1) isoenzyme.

## Pharmacokinetics
*Absorption:* Well absorbed, with a mean bioavailability of 93%. The median time for serum levels to peak is 2 to 3 hours.
*Distribution:* About 87% protein-bound.
*Metabolism:* The liver metabolizes the drug to inactive metabolites.
*Excretion:* Eliminated predominantly through hepatic metabolism. Less than 1% of the drug is eliminated from the kidneys as unchanged drug. Half-life is about 17 hours.

| Route | Onset | Peak | Duration |
|-------|-------|------|----------|
| P.O. | Unknown | 2-9 hr | Unknown |

## Contraindications and precautions
Contraindicated in patients hypersensitive to rofecoxib or any of its components, and in patients who have experienced asthma, urticaria, or allergic-type reactions after taking aspirin or other NSAIDs. Avoid use in patients with advanced kidney disease or moderate or severe hepatic insufficiency and in pregnant women because it may cause the ductus arteriosus to close prematurely.

Use cautiously in patients with preexisting asthma, renal disease, liver dysfunction, or abnormal liver function test results. Also use cautiously in patients with a history of ulcer disease or GI bleeding. Use cautiously in patients being treated with oral corticosteroids or anticoagulants, in patients with a history of smoking or alcoholism, and in geriatric or debilitated patients because of the increased risk of GI bleeding.

Use cautiously in patients with considerable dehydration. Rehydration is recommended before therapy begins. Use cautiously, and initiate therapy at the lowest recommended dosage in patients with fluid retention, hypertension, or HF.

## Interactions
**Drug-drug.** *ACE inhibitors:* Decreased antihypertensive effects of ACE inhibitors. Advise clinician to monitor patient closely.
*Aspirin:* Increased rate of GI ulceration and other complications. Don't use together, if possible. If used together, advise clinician to monitor patient closely for GI bleeding.
*Furosemide, thiazide diuretics:* Potentially reduced efficacy of these drugs. Advise clinician to monitor patient closely.
*Lithium:* Increased plasma lithium levels and decreased lithium clearance. Advise clinician to monitor patient closely for toxic reaction to lithium.
*Methotrexate:* Increased plasma methotrexate levels. Advise clinician to monitor patient closely for toxic reaction to methotrexate.
*Rifampin:* Decreased rofecoxib levels by about 50%. Therapy should be started with a higher dosage of rofecoxib.
*Warfarin:* Increased effects of warfarin. Advise clinician to monitor INR frequently in the first few days after therapy with rofecoxib starts or changes.
**Drug-herb.** *Dong quai, feverfew, garlic, ginger, horse chestnut, red clover:* Possible increased risk of bleeding. Discourage use together.
*St. John's wort, dong quai:* Increased risk of photosensitivity. Advise patient to avoid unprotected exposure to sunlight.
**Drug-lifestyle.** *Long-term alcohol use, smoking:* Increased risk of GI bleeding. Advise clinician to monitor patient closely.

## Adverse reactions

**CNS:** headache, asthenia, fatigue, dizziness.
**CV:** hypertension, leg edema.
**EENT:** sinusitis.
**GI:** diarrhea, dyspepsia, epigastric discomfort, heartburn, nausea, abdominal pain.
**GU:** urinary tract infection.
**Musculoskeletal:** back pain.
**Respiratory:** bronchitis, upper respiratory tract infection.
**Other:** flulike syndrome.

## Overdose and treatment

In an overdose, unabsorbed drug should be removed from GI tract, patient monitored, and supportive therapy provided p.r.n. Hemodialysis doesn't remove drug; it's unknown if peritoneal dialysis removes it.

## Clinical considerations

**⚠ ALERT** Patient may be allergic to rofecoxib if he has an allergy to aspirin or other NSAIDs.

■ Advise clinician to rehydrate patients who are dehydrated before starting treatment with rofecoxib.

■ Rofecoxib may be hepatotoxic. Advise clinician to monitor patient for signs and symptoms of hepatotoxicity. Drug should be stopped p.r.n. if any signs and symptoms consistent with liver disease develop.

■ Fluid retention and edema have occurred in patients taking rofecoxib. Use the lowest recommended dose cautiously in patients with fluid retention, hypertension, or HF.

**⚠ ALERT** A study concluded that patients taking Vioxx had more than twice as many heart attacks, strokes, and other cardiac events as patients taking naproxen. More studies have to be performed to make clinical judgments.

### *Therapeutic monitoring*

■ NSAIDs may cause serious GI toxicity. Signs and symptoms include bleeding, ulceration, and perforation of the stomach, small intestine, and large intestine. Such toxicity can occur any time, with or without warning. To minimize the risk of an adverse GI event, use the lowest effective dosage of rofecoxib for the shortest possible duration. Advise clinician to monitor patient closely for GI bleeding.

■ Patients undergoing long-term treatment should have their hemoglobin level and hematocrit checked if they experience signs or symptoms of anemia or blood loss.

### *Special populations*

**Pregnant patients.** Instruct women to inform prescriber if pregnancy is suspected or planned while taking this drug.
**Breast-feeding patients.** It's unknown if rofecoxib appears in breast milk. However, because breast-fed infants are at risk for serious adverse reactions, women taking this drug shouldn't breast-feed.
**Pediatric patients.** The safety and efficacy of rofecoxib in pediatric patients under age 18 haven't been evaluated.
**Geriatric patients.** No substantial differences in safety and effectiveness exist between geriatric and younger patients. Although dosage doesn't need to be adjusted in geriatric patients, rofecoxib should be initiated at the lowest recommended dosage.

## Patient counseling

■ Warn patient that he may experience GI bleeding. Signs and symptoms include bloody vomitus, blood in urine and stool, and black, tarry stools. Advise patient to seek medical advice if he experiences any of these signs or symptoms.

■ Advise patient to report rash, unexplained weight gain, or edema.

■ Tell patient that drug may be taken without regard to food, though taking the drug with food may decrease GI upset.

■ Tell patient that the most common minor adverse effects are dyspepsia, epigastric discomfort, heartburn, and nausea. Taking drug with food may help minimize these effects.

■ Tell patient to avoid aspirin and aspirin-containing products unless his prescriber has instructed him otherwise.

■ Inform patient to avoid OTC anti-inflammatory drugs such as ibuprofen (Advil) unless his prescriber has instructed him otherwise.

■ Tell patient that all NSAIDs, including rofecoxib, may adversely affect the liver. Signs and symptoms of liver toxicity include nausea, fatigue, lethargy, itching, jaundice, right upper quadrant tenderness, and flulike symptoms. Advise patient to stop therapy and seek immediate medical advice if he experiences any of these signs or symptoms.

# ropinirole hydrochloride
Requip

*Pharmacologic classification:* non-ergoline dopamine agonist
*Therapeutic classification:* antiparkinsonian
*Pregnancy risk category C*

## Available forms

Available by prescription only
*Tablets:* 0.25 mg, 0.5 mg, 1 mg, 2 mg, 4 mg, 5 mg

## Indications and dosages

*Treatment of signs and symptoms of idiopathic Parkinson's disease*
*Adults:* Initially, 0.25 mg P.O. t.i.d. Based on patient response, dosage should then be adjusted at weekly intervals: 0.5 mg t.i.d. after

week 1, 0.75 mg t.i.d. after week 2, and 1 mg t.i.d. after week 3. After week 4, dosage may be increased by 1.5 mg/day on a weekly basis up to a dose of 9 mg/day and then increased weekly by up to 3 mg/day to maximum dose of 24 mg/day.

## Mechanism of action
*Antiparkinsonian action:* Exact mechanism of action is unknown. Ropinirole is a nonergoline dopamine agonist thought to stimulate postsynaptic dopamine $D_2$ receptors within the caudate-putamen in the brain.

## Pharmacokinetics
*Absorption:* Rapidly absorbed. Absolute bioavailability is 55%.
*Distribution:* Widely distributed throughout the body, with an apparent volume of distribution of 7.5 L/kg. Up to 40% plasma protein–bound.
*Metabolism:* Extensively metabolized by cytochrome P-450 CYP1A2 isoenzyme to inactive metabolites.
*Excretion:* Less than 10% of the given dose is excreted unchanged in the urine. Elimination half-life is 6 hours.

| Route | Onset | Peak | Duration |
|-------|-------|------|----------|
| P.O. | Unknown | 1-2 hr | 6 hr |

## Contraindications and precautions
Contraindicated in patients hypersensitive to drug or its components.
    Use cautiously in patients with severe renal or hepatic impairment.

## Interactions
**Drug-drug.** *CNS depressants, including antipsychotics and benzodiazepines:* Increase CNS effects. Use cautiously.
*Dopamine antagonists, including butyrophenones, metoclopramide, phenothiazines, and thioxanthenes:* May decrease effectiveness of ropinirole when given together. Avoid use together.
*Estrogens:* Reduce clearance of ropinirole. Dosage adjustment of ropinirole may be needed.
*Inhibitors or substrates of cytochrome P-450 CYP1A2, such as ciprofloxacin, fluvoxamine, mexiletine, and norfloxacin:* Alter clearance. Dosage adjustment of ropinirole may be required.
**Drug-lifestyle.** *Alcohol use:* Increases CNS effects. Advise patient to use cautiously.
*Smoking:* May increase clearance of ropinirole. Advise clinician to monitor closely.

## Adverse reactions
**Early Parkinson's disease (without levodopa)**
**CNS:** asthenia, hallucinations, *dizziness,* aggravated Parkinson's disease, *somnolence, fatigue,* headache, confusion, hyperkinesia, hy-

pesthesia, vertigo, amnesia, impaired concentration, malaise.
**CV:** orthostatic hypotension, orthostatic symptoms, hypertension, *syncope,* edema, chest pain, extrasystoles, *atrial fibrillation,* palpitation, tachycardia.
**EENT:** pharyngitis, dry mouth, abnormal vision, eye abnormality, xerophthalmia, rhinitis, sinusitis.
**GI:** *nausea, vomiting, dyspepsia,* flatulence, abdominal pain, anorexia, abdominal pain.
**GU:** urinary tract infection, impotence.
**Respiratory:** bronchitis; dyspnea.
**Skin:** flushing, increased sweating.
**Other:** *viral infection,* pain, yawning, peripheral ischemia.
**Advanced Parkinson's disease (with levodopa)**
**CNS:** *dizziness,* aggravated parkinsonism, *somnolence, headache,* insomnia, *hallucinations,* abnormal dreaming, confusion, tremor, *dyskinesia,* anxiety, nervousness, amnesia, hypokinesia, paresthesia, paresis.
**CV:** hypotension, syncope.
**EENT:** diplopia, dry mouth.
**GI:** *nausea,* abdominal pain, vomiting, constipation, diarrhea, dysphagia, flatulence, increased saliva.
**GU:** urinary tract infection, pyuria, urinary incontinence.
**Hematologic:** anemia.
**Metabolic:** weight decrease.
**Musculoskeletal:** arthralgia, arthritis.
**Respiratory:** upper respiratory infection, dyspnea.
**Skin:** increased sweating.
**Other:** injury, *falls,* viral infection, increased drug level, pain.

## Overdose and treatment
There are reports of 10 patients ingesting more than 24 mg/day. Symptoms of overdose include mild or facial dyskinesia, agitation, increased dyskinesia, grogginess, sedation, orthostatic hypotension, chest pain, confusion, vomiting, and nausea.
    Treatment involves general supportive measures and removal of unabsorbed drug.

## Clinical considerations
■ Dosage adjustment isn't needed in patients with mild to moderate renal impairment.
■ Drug should be adjusted with caution in patients with severe renal or hepatic impairment.
■ Although not reported with ropinirole, a symptom complex resembling neuroleptic malignant syndrome (elevated temperature, muscular rigidity, altered consciousness, and autonomic instability) has been reported with rapid dose reduction or withdrawal of antiparkinsonians. If this occurs, recommend stopping drug gradually over 7 days and reducing frequency of administration to b.i.d. for 4 days and then once daily over the remaining 3 days.

---

■ Other adverse events reported with dopaminergic therapy may occur with ropinirole, including withdrawal emergent hyperpyrexia and confusion, and fibrotic complications.

■ Ropinirole can potentiate the dopaminergic adverse effects of levodopa and may cause or exacerbate existing dyskinesia. If this occurs, the levodopa dose may need to be decreased.

■ After reviewing data from several studies, prescribers now recommend the use of dopamine agonists (such as Larodopa), rather than levodopa, as first-line treatments for early Parkinson's disease. A revised treatment algorithm recommends delaying the use of levodopa while starting treatment with dopamine agonists, such as pramipexole (Mirapex) or ropinirole (Requip). The drugs treat the stiffness caused by the disease while reducing the risk of developing dyskinesia, which is caused by levodopa. After 5 years of dopamine agonist therapy, patients would need to start levodopa.

### Therapeutic monitoring
■ Drug may cause increased alkaline phosphatase and BUN levels. Advise clinician to monitor these levels.

■ Symptomatic hypotension may occur because of dopamine agonists' impairment of systemic regulation of blood pressure. Advise clinician to monitor patient carefully for orthostatic hypotension, especially during dose escalation.

■ Syncope, with or without bradycardia, has been reported. Advise clinician to monitor patient carefully, especially 4 weeks after therapy starts and with dosage increases.

### Special populations
**Breast-feeding patients.** Drug inhibits prolactin secretion and could potentially inhibit lactation. It's unknown if drug appears in breast milk. A decision should be made to discontinue either the drug or breast-feeding, taking into account the importance of drug to the woman. **Pediatric patients.** Safety and efficacy in children haven't been established.
**Geriatric patients.** Dosage adjustments aren't needed.

### Patient counseling
■ Inform patient to take drug with food to reduce nausea.

■ Advise patient that hallucinations may occur. Geriatric patients are at greater risk than younger patients with Parkinson's disease.

■ Instruct patient to rise slowly after sitting or lying down because of risk of orthostatic hypotension, which may occur when therapy starts or changes.

■ Advise patient to use caution when driving or operating machinery until CNS effects of drug are known.

# ropivacaine hydrochloride
Naropin

*Pharmacologic classification:*
aminoamide
*Therapeutic classification:* local
anesthetic
*Pregnancy risk category B*

## Available forms
Available by prescription only
*E-Z off single-dose vials:* 7.5 mg/ml, 10 mg/ml
in 10-ml vials
*Infusion bottles:* 2 mg/ml in 100-ml and 200-ml
bottles
*Single-dose vials:* 2 mg/ml, 7.5 mg/ml,
10 mg/ml in 20-ml vials; 5 mg/ml in 30-ml
vials
*Single-dose ampules:* 2 mg/ml, 7.5 mg/ml,
10 mg/ml in 20-ml ampules; 5 mg/ml in 30-ml
ampules
*Sterile-pak single-dose vials:* 2 mg/ml,
7.5 mg/ml, 10 mg/ml in 20-ml vials; 5 mg/ml
in 30-ml vials

## Indications and dosages
### Surgical anesthesia
*Adults:* Lumbar epidural administration in surgery: 75 to 200 mg doses (duration, 2 to 5 hours). Lumbar epidural administration for cesarean section: 100 to 150 mg (duration, 2 to 5 hours). Thoracic epidural administration: 25 to 113 mg doses to establish block for postoperative pain relief. Major nerve block (for example, brachial plexus block): 175 to 300 mg (duration, 5 to 10 hours). Field block (such as minor nerve blocks and infiltration): 5 to 200 mg (duration, 2 to 6 hours).
### Labor pain management
*Adults:* Lumbar epidural administration: Initially, 20 to 40 mg (duration, ½ to 1½ hours), then 12 to 28 mg/hour as continuous infusion or 20 to 30 mg/hour as incremental "top-up" injections.
### Postoperative pain management
*Adults:* Lumbar epidural administration: 12 to 28 mg/hour as continuous infusion. Thoracic epidural administration: 12 to 28 mg/hour as continuous infusion. For infiltration (minor nerve block): 2 to 200 mg (duration, 2 to 6 hours).

## Mechanism of action
*Anesthetic action:* Drug blocks the generation and conduction of nerve impulses, presumably by increasing the threshold for electrical excitation in the nerve by slowing the propagation of the nerve impulse and by reducing the rate of the action potential. Generally, progression of anesthesia is related to the diameter, myelination, and conduction velocity of affected nerve fibers. Clinically, the order of loss of

---

nerve function is as follows: pain, temperature, touch, proprioception, and skeletal muscle tone.

## Pharmacokinetics

*Absorption:* Absorption depends on total dose and concentration of administered drug, route of administration, patient's hemodynamic or circulatory condition, and vascularity of administration site. From the epidural space, drug shows complete and biphasic absorption; mean half-lives of two phases are 14 minutes and 4½ hours, respectively. The slow absorption is a rate-limiting factor in elimination of drug. Terminal half-life is longer after epidural than after I.V. administration.

*Distribution:* After intravascular infusion, drug has steady-state volume of distribution of 41 ± 7 L. Drug is 94% protein-bound, mainly to alpha₁ acid glycoprotein. An increase in total plasma levels during continuous epidural infusion has been observed, secondary to a postoperative increase in alpha₁ acid glycoprotein.

*Metabolism:* Extensively metabolized in the liver, via cytochrome P-4501A to 3-hydroxy ropivacaine. About 37% of dose is excreted in the urine as free drug and as conjugated metabolites. Urinary excretion of metabolites accounts for only 3% of dose.

*Excretion:* Primarily excreted by the kidneys; 86% of the dose appears in urine after I.V. administration, of which only 1% relates to unchanged drug.

| Route | Onset | Peak | Duration |
|---|---|---|---|
| Epidural | Unknown | Unknown | Unknown |

## Contraindications and precautions

Contraindicated in patients hypersensitive to drug or local anesthetics of amide type.

Use with caution in debilitated, geriatric, and acutely ill patients because accumulation may result. Also use cautiously in patients with hypotension, hypovolemia, impaired CV function, or heart block and in those with hepatic disease, especially repeat doses of drug.

## Interactions

**Drug-drug.** *Amide-type anesthetics:* Effects are additive if given with ropivacaine. Use with caution.

*Fluvoxamine, imipramine, theophylline, verapamil:* May result in competitive inhibition of ropivacaine. Use with caution.

## Adverse reactions

**CNS:** anxiety, dizziness, headache, hypesthesia, pain, paresthesia.

**CV:** *bradycardia,* chest pain, *hypotension,* hypertension, tachycardia, FETAL BRADYCARDIA, *fetal tachycardia.*

**GI:** *nausea,* neonatal vomiting, vomiting.

**GU:** oliguria, urine retention.

**Hematologic:** anemia.

**Hepatic:** neonatal jaundice.

**Musculoskeletal:** back pain.

**Respiratory:** *neonatal tachypnea, respiratory distress.*

**Skin:** pruritus.

**Other:** FETAL DISTRESS, fever, neonatal fever, postoperative complications, rigors.

## Overdose and treatment

Treatment should be supportive and symptomatic. Drug should be discontinued. In case of unintentional subarachnoid injection of drug, recommend establishing a patent airway and giving 100% oxygen. This may prevent seizures if they haven't already occurred. Recommend giving drug to control seizures as appropriate.

## Clinical considerations

**H** *ALERT* Don't inject drug rapidly. Emergency equipment and personnel should be immediately available.

■ Drug should only be used by personnel familiar with its use.

■ Doses should be increased in incremental steps.

■ Don't use in emergency situations where a rapid onset of surgical anesthesia is needed. Drug shouldn't be used for production of obstetric paracervical block anesthesia, retrobulbar block, or spinal anesthesia (subarachnoid block) because of insufficient data to support use. I.V. regional anesthesia (bier block) shouldn't be performed because of lack of clinical experience and risk of obtaining toxic blood levels of ropivacaine.

■ To reduce risk of potentially serious adverse reactions, attempts should be made to optimize patient who may be at risk, such as those with complete heart block, and hepatic or renal impairment.

■ Recommend using an adequate test dose (3 to 5 ml of short-acting local anesthetic solution containing epinephrine) before induction of complete block.

■ Drug shouldn't be used in ophthalmic surgery.

### Therapeutic monitoring

■ Early signs of CNS toxicity include restlessness, anxiety, incoherent speech, lightheadedness, numbness and tingling of mouth and lips, metallic taste, tinnitus, dizziness, blurred vision, tremors, twitching, depression, or drowsiness.

### Special populations

**Breast-feeding patients.** It's unknown if drug appears in breast milk; use with caution.

**Pediatric patients.** Don't use in children under age 12.

## Patient counseling

■ Tell patient that he may experience a temporary loss of sensation and motor activity in the anesthetized body part after proper administration of lumbar epidural anesthesia. Also explain adverse reactions that may occur.

# rosiglitazone maleate
Avandia

*Pharmacologic classification:* thiazolidinedione
*Therapeutic classification:* antidiabetic
*Pregnancy risk category C*

## Available forms
Available by prescription only
*Tablets:* 2 mg, 4 mg, 8 mg

## Indications and dosages
*Monotherapy adjunct to diet and exercise to improve glycemic control in patients with type 2 diabetes mellitus or combination therapy with metformin or sulfonaureas when diet, exercise, and rosiglitazone alone or diet, exercise, and metformin alone don't provide adequate glycemic control in patients with type 2 diabetes mellitus*
*Adults:* Initially, 4 mg P.O. daily in the morning or in divided doses b.i.d. in the morning and evening. Dosage may be increased to 8 mg P.O. daily or in divided doses b.i.d. if fasting plasma glucose level doesn't improve after 12 weeks of treatment.

## Mechanism of action
*Antidiabetic action:* Rosiglitazone lowers blood glucose levels by improving insulin sensitivity. Rosiglitazone is a highly selective and potent agonist for the receptors, which are found in key target areas for insulin action, such as adipose tissue, skeletal muscle, and liver.

## Pharmacokinetics
*Absorption:* Plasma levels peak about 1 hour after dosing. The absolute bioavailability is 99%.
*Distribution:* About 99.8% bound to plasma proteins, primarily albumin.
*Metabolism:* Extensively metabolized, with no unchanged drug excreted in the urine. Primarily metabolized through *N*-demethylation and hydroxylation.
*Excretion:* After oral administration, about 64% and 23% of dose is eliminated in urine and feces, respectively. The elimination half-life is 3 to 4 hours.

| Route | Onset | Peak | Duration |
|-------|-------|------|----------|
| P.O. | Unknown | 1 hr | Unknown |

## Contraindications and precautions
Contraindicated in patients hypersensitive to rosiglitazone or any of its components and in patients with New York Heart Association Class III and IV cardiac status unless the expected

benefits outweigh the potential risks. Don't use in patients with active liver disease, increased baseline liver enzyme levels (ALT level is greater than 2½ times the upper limit of normal), type 1 diabetes, or diabetic ketoacidosis or in patients who experienced jaundice while taking troglitazone. Because metformin is contraindicated in patients with renal impairment, combination therapy with metformin and rosiglitazone is also contraindicated in such patients.

Rosiglitazone can be used as monotherapy in patients with renal impairment. Use cautiously in patients with edema or HF.

## Interactions
**Drug-drug.** *Insulin:* May increase the risk of HF and other CV effects in patients. Advise clinician to monitor patient closely.
**Drug-herb.** *Aloe, bitter melon, bilberry leaf, burdock, dandelion, fenugreek, garlic, ginseng:* Use together may improve blood sugar control, requiring a reduction of antidiabetics. Advise patient to discuss the use of herbal medicines with his prescriber before use.

## Adverse reactions
**CNS:** headache, fatigue.
**CV:** edema.
**EENT:** sinusitis.
**GI:** diarrhea.
**Hematologic:** anemia.
**Metabolic:** hyperglycemia.
**Musculoskeletal:** back pain.
**Respiratory:** upper respiratory tract infection.
**Other:** injury.

## Overdose and treatment
In an overdose, recommend supportive treatment appropriate to patient's condition.

## Clinical considerations
■ Management of type 2 diabetes should include diet control. Because caloric restriction, weight loss, and exercise help improve insulin sensitivity and help make drug therapy effective, these measures are essential to proper diabetes treatment.
■ Patients with normal hepatic enzyme levels who are switched from troglitazone to rosiglitazone should undergo a 1-week washout before starting rosiglitazone.
■ For patients whose blood glucose levels are inadequately controlled with metformin, rosiglitazone should be added to—not substituted for—metformin.

### Therapeutic monitoring
■ Liver enzyme levels should be checked before therapy starts, every 2 months for the first 12 months of treatment, and then periodically afterward. If ALT level is elevated during treatment, levels should be rechecked as soon as

possible. Drug should be stopped if levels remain elevated.

■ Hemoglobin level and hematocrit may decrease while patient is receiving this drug, usually during the first 4 to 8 weeks of therapy. Increases in total cholesterol, low-density lipoprotein, and high-density lipoprotein levels and decreases in free fatty acid levels may also occur.

### Special populations
**Breast-feeding patients.** It's unknown if rosiglitazone appears in breast milk. Rosiglitazone shouldn't be given to breast-feeding women.
**Pediatric patients.** The safety and efficacy of rosiglitazone in pediatric patients haven't been established.
**Geriatric patients.** No substantial differences in safety and efficacy exist between patients over age 65 and younger patients. No dosage adjustments are required for geriatric patients.

### Patient counseling
■ Advise patient that rosiglitazone can be taken with or without food.
■ Tell patient to immediately report unexplained signs and symptoms, such as nausea, vomiting, abdominal pain, fatigue, anorexia, or dark urine, to his prescriber because these may indicate potential liver problems.
■ Inform premenopausal, anovulatory women with insulin resistance that ovulation may resume and contraceptive measures may need to be considered.
■ Advise patient that management of diabetes should include diet control. Because caloric restriction, weight loss, and exercise help improve insulin sensitivity and help make drug therapy effective, these measures are essential to proper diabetes treatment.

---

# rubella and mumps virus vaccine, live
Biavax II

*Pharmacologic classification:* vaccine
*Therapeutic classification:* viral vaccine
*Pregnancy risk category C*

### Available forms
Available by prescription only
*Injection:* Single-dose vial containing not less than 1,000 $TCID_{50}$ (tissue culture infective doses) of the Wistar RA 27/3 rubella virus (propagated in human diploid cell culture) and not less than 20,000 $TCID_{50}$ of the Jeryl Lynn mumps strain (grown in chick embryo cell culture)

### Indications and dosages
*Rubella (German measles) and mumps immunization*
*Adults and children over age 1:* 1 vial (0.5 ml) S.C. in outer aspect of the upper arm.

### Mechanism of action
*Live rubella and mumps prophylaxis:* Vaccine promotes active immunity to rubella and mumps viruses by inducing production of antibodies.

### Pharmacokinetics
*Absorption:* Antibodies are usually detectable within 2 to 6 weeks; duration of vaccine-induced immunity is expected to be lifelong.
*Distribution:* No information available.
*Metabolism:* No information available.
*Excretion:* No information available.

| Route | Onset | Peak | Duration |
|---|---|---|---|
| S.C. | Unknown | Unknown | 10½ yr |

### Contraindications and precautions
Contraindicated in pregnant women or immunosuppressed patients; in those with cancer, blood dyscrasia, gamma globulin disorders, fever, active untreated tuberculosis, or history of anaphylaxis or anaphylactoid reactions to neomycin or eggs; and in those receiving corticosteroids (except those receiving corticosteroids as replacement therapy) or radiation therapy.

### Interactions
**Drug-drug.** *Immune serum globulin or transfusions of blood and blood products:* May impair the immune response to the vaccine. Vaccination should be deferred for 3 months in these situations.
*Immunosuppressive drugs:* May interfere with the response to vaccine. Advise clinician to monitor patient closely.

### Adverse reactions
**GI:** diarrhea.
**Musculoskeletal:** arthritis, arthralgia.
**Skin:** rash, urticaria, pain, erythema, induration (at injection site).
**Other:** polyneuritis, thrombocytopenic purpura, fever, *anaphylaxis*, lymphadenopathy.

### Overdose and treatment
No information available.

### Clinical considerations
■ Obtain a thorough history of allergies (especially to antibiotics, eggs, chicken, or chicken feathers) and of reactions to immunizations.
■ Recommend performing skin testing first to assess vaccine sensitivity (against a control of normal saline solution in the opposite arm) in patients with history of anaphylactoid reactions to egg ingestion. Recommend giving I.D.

or scratch test with a 1:10 dilution. Read results after 5 to 30 minutes. Positive reaction is a wheal with or without pseudopodia and surrounding erythema.
- Epinephrine solution 1:1,000 should be available to treat allergic reactions.
- Rubella and mumps vaccine shouldn't be given less than 1 month before or after immunization with other live virus vaccines, except for monovalent or trivalent live poliovirus vaccine or live, attenuated measles virus vaccine, which may be given simultaneously.
- Use only the diluent supplied. Discard reconstituted vaccine after 8 hours.
- Drug should be injected S.C. (not I.M.) into the outer aspect of the upper arm.
- Women who have rubella antibody titers of 1:8 or greater (by hemagglutination inhibition) need not be vaccinated with the rubella vaccine component.
- Although rubella vaccine administration should be deferred in patients with febrile illness, it may be given to susceptible children with mild illness such as upper respiratory infection.
- According to Centers for Disease Control and Prevention recommendations, measles, mumps, and rubella is the preferred vaccine.
- Women who aren't immune to rubella are at risk for congenital rubella injury to the fetus if exposed to rubella during pregnancy.
- Store vaccine at 36° to 46° F (2° to 8° C) and protect from light. Solution may be used if red, pink, or yellow, but it must be clear.
- Rubella and mumps vaccine may temporarily decrease the response to tuberculin skin testing. Should a tuberculin skin test be needed, recommend giving it either before or simultaneously with rubella and mumps vaccine.

### Therapeutic monitoring
- Revaccination or booster isn't required if patient was previously vaccinated at age 1 or older; however, there's no conclusive evidence of an increased risk of adverse reactions for persons who are already immune when vaccinated.
- Vaccine won't offer protection when given after exposure to natural rubella or mumps, but there's no evidence that it would be harmful.

### Special populations
**Pregnant patients.** Tell women of childbearing age to avoid pregnancy for 3 months after immunization. Provide contraceptive information if needed.
**Breast-feeding patients.** Some reports have shown transfer of rubella virus or virus antigen into breast milk in about 68% of patients. Few adverse effects have been linked to breast-feeding after immunization with rubella-containing vaccines. Use caution when giving vaccine to breast-feeding women.

**Pediatric patients.** Live rubella and mumps virus vaccine isn't recommended for children under age 1 because retained maternal antibodies may interfere with immune response.

## Patient counseling
- Tell patient that tingling sensations in the limbs or joint aches and pains that may resemble arthritis may occur beginning several days to several weeks after vaccination. These symptoms usually resolve within 1 week. Pain and inflammation at injection site and low-grade fever, rash, or breathing difficulties may also occur. Encourage patient to report distressing adverse reactions.
- Recommend acetaminophen to relieve fever or other minor discomfort.

## rubella virus vaccine, live
Meruvax II

*Pharmacologic classification:* vaccine
*Therapeutic classification:* viral vaccine
*Pregnancy risk category C*

### Available forms
Available by prescription only
*Injection:* Single-dose vial containing not less than 1,000 TCID$_{50}$ (tissue culture infective doses) of the Wistar RA 27/3 strain of rubella virus propagated in human diploid cell culture

### Indications and dosages
**Rubella (German measles) immunization**
*Adults and children over age 1:* One vial (0.5 ml) S.C.

### Mechanism of action
*Rubella prophylaxis:* Vaccine promotes active immunity to rubella by inducing production of antibodies.

### Pharmacokinetics
*Absorption:* Antibodies are usually detectable 2 to 6 weeks after injection; duration of vaccine-induced immunity is expected to be lifelong.
*Distribution:* No information available.
*Metabolism:* No information available.
*Excretion:* No information available.

| Route | Onset | Peak | Duration |
|-------|-------|------|----------|
| S.C. | 2-6 wk | Unknown | > 10 yr |

### Contraindications and precautions
Contraindicated in pregnant women or immunosuppressed patients; in those with cancer, blood dyscrasia, gamma globulin disorders, fever, active untreated tuberculosis, or history of hypersensitivity to neomycin; and in patients receiving corticosteroids (except those receiving corticosteroids as replacement therapy) or radiation therapy.

---

## Interactions

**Drug-drug.** *Immune serum globulin or transfusions of blood and blood products:* May impair the immune response to the vaccine. If possible, defer vaccination for 3 months in these situations.

*Immunosuppressants:* May have reduced response to vaccine. Advise clinician to monitor patient closely. Vaccination should be deferred until immunosuppressant is discontinued, if possible.

## Adverse reactions

**CNS:** polyneuritis, malaise, headache.
**EENT:** sore throat.
**Musculoskeletal:** arthralgia, arthritis.
**Skin:** rash, urticaria, pain, erythema, induration (at injection site).
**Other:** thrombocytopenic purpura, fever, *anaphylaxis,* lymphadenopathy.

## Overdose and treatment

No information available.

## Clinical considerations

■ Obtain a thorough history of allergies, especially to antibiotics, and of reactions to immunizations.

■ Epinephrine solution 1:1,000 should be available to treat allergic reactions.

■ Don't give rubella vaccine less than 1 month before or after immunization with other live virus vaccines, except for monovalent or trivalent live poliovirus vaccine; live, attenuated measles virus vaccine; or live mumps virus vaccine, which may be given simultaneously.

■ Vaccine shouldn't be injected I.M. Recommend injecting S.C. into the outer aspect of the upper arm.

■ Use only diluent supplied. Discard 8 hours after reconstituting.

■ Store vaccine at 36° to 46° F (2° to 8° C), and protect from light. Solution may be used if red, pink, or yellow, but it must be clear.

■ Vaccine won't offer protection when given after exposure to natural rubella, although there's no evidence that it would be harmful.

■ Although rubella vaccine administration should be deferred in patients with febrile illness, it may be given to susceptible children with mild illnesses such as upper respiratory tract infection.

■ Rubella vaccine may temporarily decrease response to tuberculin skin testing. If a tuberculin test is needed, recommend giving it either before, simultaneously with, or at least 8 weeks after rubella vaccine.

### Therapeutic monitoring

■ Women who have rubella antibody titers of 1:8 or greater (by hemagglutination inhibition) need not be vaccinated with rubella virus vaccine.

■ Revaccination or booster dose is required if patient was previously vaccinated under age 1. The Advisory Committee on Immunization Practices and the American Academy of Pediatrics currently recommend that a second dose be routinely given at ages 4 to 6 or 11 to 12. It may be given at any other time provided at least 1 month has elapsed since the first dose. There's no conclusive evidence of an increased risk of adverse reactions for persons who are already immune when revaccinated.

### Special populations

**Pregnant patients.** Women who aren't immune to rubella are at risk for congenital rubella injury to the fetus if exposed to rubella during pregnancy. Tell women of childbearing age to avoid pregnancy for 3 months after rubella immunization. Provide contraceptive information if needed.

**Breast-feeding patients.** Although early studies failed to show evidence of attenuated rubella virus in breast milk, subsequent reports showed transfer of rubella virus or virus antigen into breast milk in about 68% of patients. Few adverse effects have been linked to breast-feeding after immunization with rubella-containing vaccines. Risk-benefit ratio suggests that breast-feeding women may be immunized, if needed.

**Pediatric patients.** Live, attenuated rubella virus vaccine isn't recommended for children under age 1 because retained maternal antibodies may impair immune response.

## Patient counseling

■ Tell patient to expect tingling sensations in the limbs or joint aches and pains that may resemble arthritis to occur beginning several days to several weeks after vaccination. The symptoms usually resolve within 1 week. Pain and inflammation at injection site and low-grade fever, rash, or breathing difficulties may also occur. Encourage patient to report distressing reactions.

■ Recommend acetaminophen to relieve fever or other minor discomfort after vaccination.

## salmeterol xinafoate
Serevent

*Pharmacologic classification:* selective
beta$_2$-adrenergic stimulating agonist
*Therapeutic classification:* bronchodilator
*Pregnancy risk category C*

### Available forms
Available by prescription only
*Inhalation aerosol:* 25 mcg per activation in
6.5-g canister (60 activations), 25 mcg per ac-
tivation in 13-g canister (120 activations)
*Inhalation powder:* 50 mcg/blister

### Indications and dosages
***Long-term maintenance treatment of
asthma; prevention of bronchospasm in
patients with nocturnal asthma or reversible obstructive airway disease who
require regular treatment with short-
acting beta agonists***
*Adults and children over age 12:* Two inhalations b.i.d. in the morning and evening.
***Prevention of exercise-induced broncho-
spasm***
*Adults and children over age 12:* Two inhalations at least 30 to 60 minutes before exercise.
Note: Paradoxical bronchospasms (which
can be life-threatening) have been reported after use of salmeterol. If they occur, discontinue salmeterol immediately and institute alternative therapy.
◊ *COPD or emphysema*
*Adults and children over age 12:* Single oral
inhalation of 42 to 63 mcg.

### Mechanism of action
*Bronchodilator action:* Salmeterol selectively
stimulates beta$_2$-adrenergic receptors, resulting in bronchodilation. Drug also blocks the
release of histamine from mast cells lining the
respiratory tract, which produces vasodilation
and increases ciliary motility.

### Pharmacokinetics
*Absorption:* Because of the low therapeutic
dose, systemic levels of salmeterol are low or
undetectable after inhalation.
*Distribution:* Highly bound to human plasma
proteins (94% to 99%).

*Metabolism:* Extensively metabolized by hydroxylation.
*Excretion:* Excreted primarily in the feces.

| Route | Onset | Peak | Duration |
|-------|-------|------|----------|
| Inhalation | 10-20 min | 3 hr | 12 hr |

### Contraindications and precautions
Contraindicated in patients hypersensitive to
drug or its formulation.
Use cautiously in patients with coronary insufficiency, arrhythmias, hypertension, other
CV disorders, thyrotoxicosis, or seizure disorders and in those unusually responsive to
sympathomimetics.

### Interactions
**Drug-drug.** *Beta-adrenergic agonists, theophylline, or other methylxanthines:* May result in
possible adverse cardiac effects with excessive
use of salmeterol. Advise clinician to monitor
patient closely.
*MAO inhibitors or tricyclic antidepressants:*
Risk of severe adverse CV effects. Avoid use
of salmeterol within 14 days of MAO therapy.

### Adverse reactions
**CNS:** *headache,* sinus headache, tremor, ner-
vousness, giddiness.
**CV:** tachycardia, palpitations, ***ventricular ar-
rhythmias.***
**EENT:** *upper respiratory infection, naso-
pharyngitis,* nasal cavity or sinus disorder.
**GI:** nausea, vomiting, diarrhea, heartburn.
**Musculoskeletal:** joint and back pain, myal-
gia.
**Respiratory:** cough, lower respiratory infec-
tion, ***bronchospasm.***
**Skin:** hypersensitivity reactions (rash, urticaria).

### Overdose and treatment
Overdose may result in exaggerated adverse
pharmacologic effects caused by beta-adreno-
ceptor agonists: tachycardia, arrhythmias,
tremor, headache, and muscle cramps. Overdose can lead to clinically significant prolongation of the QT interval, which can produce
ventricular arrhythmias. Cardiac arrest and
death may be associated with abuse of salmeterol. Other signs of overdose may include
hypokalemia and hyperglycemia.
In these cases, therapy with salmeterol and
all beta-adrenergic-stimulant drugs should be
stopped, supportive therapy provided, and ju-

dicious use of a beta blocker should be considered, bearing in mind the possibility that such drugs may produce bronchospasm. Cardiac monitoring is recommended in cases of salmeterol overdose. Dialysis isn't appropriate treatment.

## Clinical considerations
■ Drug shouldn't be used in patients whose asthma can be managed by occasional use of a short-acting, inhaled beta₂-agonist such as albuterol.
■ Salmeterol inhalation shouldn't be used more than b.i.d. (morning and evening) at the recommended dose. Provide patient with a short-acting inhaled beta₂-agonist for treatment of symptoms that occur despite regular twice-daily use of salmeterol.
■ Patients taking a short-acting inhaled beta₂-agonist daily should be advised to use it only p.r.n. if they develop asthma symptoms while taking salmeterol.
■ Salmeterol isn't a substitute for oral or inhaled corticosteroids.
■ Products containing drug in fixed combination with fluticasone propionate should be considered when disease severity warrants two maintenance therapies.

### Therapeutic monitoring
■ Advise clinician to monitor patient's response to drug therapy.
■ Tell patient to call if the short-acting agonist no longer provides sufficient relief or if more than four inhalations are being used daily. This may be a sign that asthma symptoms are worsening.
■ Patients receiving drug b.i.d. shouldn't use additional doses for prevention of exercise-induced bronchospasm.

### Special populations
**Breast-feeding patients.** Give drug cautiously to breast-feeding women because it isn't known if drug appears in breast milk.
**Pediatric patients.** Safety and efficacy in children under age 12 haven't been established.
**Geriatric patients.** As with other beta₂-agonists, use with extreme caution when using drug in geriatric patients who have CV disease and who could be adversely affected by this class of drugs.

## Patient counseling
■ Instruct patient on the proper use of the salmeterol inhalation device and tell him to review the illustrated instructions in the package insert.
■ Tell patient to shake the container well before using.
■ Remind patient to take drug at 12-hour intervals for optimum effect and to take it even when he's feeling better.

■ Inform patient that drug isn't meant to relieve acute asthmatic symptoms. Instead, acute symptoms should be treated with an inhaled, short-acting bronchodilator that has been prescribed for symptomatic relief.
■ Instruct patient already receiving short-acting beta₂-agonist to discontinue the regular daily-dosing regimen for drug and to use the short-acting drug only if asthma symptoms are experienced while taking salmeterol.
■ Tell patient taking an inhaled corticosteroid to continue to use it regularly. Warn patient not to take other drugs without medical approval.
■ If drug is being used to prevent exercise-induced bronchospasm, tell patient to take it 30 to 60 minutes before exercise.

# saquinavir
Fortovase

# saquinavir mesylate
Invirase

*Pharmacologic classification:* HIV-1 and HIV-2 protease inhibitor
*Therapeutic classification:* antiviral
*Pregnancy risk category B*

## Available forms
Available by prescription only
**saquinavir**
*Capsules (soft gelatin):* 200 mg
**saquinavir mesylate**
*Capsules (hard gelatin):* 200 mg

## Indications and dosages
*Adjunct treatment of advanced HIV infection in selected patients*
*Adults:* 600 mg (Invirase, three 200-mg capsules) P.O. t.i.d. taken within 2 hours after a full meal and with a nucleoside analogue such as zalcitabine at a dose of 0.75 mg P.O. t.i.d. or 200 mg zidovudine P.O. t.i.d. Or, 1,200 mg (Fortovase, six 200-mg capsules) t.i.d. within 2 hours after a full meal with a nucleoside analogue.
≡*Dosage adjustment.* If toxicity develops with saquinavir or saquinavir mesylate, interrupt drug therapy. In combination therapy with nucleoside analogues, base dosage adjustments of the nucleoside analogue on the known toxicity profile of specific drug.

## Mechanism of action
*Antiviral action:* Saquinavir inhibits the activity of HIV protease and prevents the cleavage of HIV polyproteins, which are essential for the maturation of HIV.

## Pharmacokinetics
*Absorption:* Poorly absorbed from the GI tract. Higher saquinavir levels are achieved with For-

tovase compared with Invirase. Fortovase has a relative bioavailability of 331% of Invirase.
*Distribution:* About 98% plasma protein–bound.
*Metabolism:* Rapidly metabolized.
*Excretion:* Excreted mainly in feces.

| Route | Onset | Peak | Duration |
|-------|-------|------|----------|
| P.O. | Unknown | Unknown | Unknown |

## Contraindications and precautions

Contraindicated in patients hypersensitive to drug or the components contained in the capsule. Safety of drug hasn't been established in pregnant women.

## Interactions

**Drug-drug.** *Amprenavir:* Decreased plasma levels of amprenavir. Use together cautiously.
*Delavirdine:* Increased saquinavir plasma level. Use cautiously and recommend monitoring hepatic enzymes. Dose should be decreased.
*Dexamethasone:* Decreased saquinavir levels. Avoid use together.
*Efavirenz:* Decreased levels of both drugs. Use together is not recommended.
*HMG-CoA reductase inhibitors:* Increased levels of these drugs, causing increased risk of myopathy, including rhabdomyolysis. Avoid use together.
*Indinavir, lopinavir/ritonavir combination, nelfinavir, ritonavir:* Increased plasma levels of saquinavir. Use together cautiously.
*Ketoconazole:* Coadministration may increase saquinavir levels. No dosage adjustment needed.
*Macrolide antibiotics such as clarithromycin:* Increased plasma levels of both drugs. Use together cautiously.
*Nevirapine:* Decreased saquinavir levels. Advise clinician to monitor patient.
*Phenobarbital, phenytoin, carbamazepine:* May decrease saquinavir levels. Avoid use together.
*Rifabutin, rifampin:* Reduce the steady-state concentration of saquinavir. Use rifabutin and saquinavir together cautiously. Don't use with rifampin.
*Sildenafil:* Increased peak plasma levels and sildenafil-associated adverse effects of hypotension, visual changes, and priapism. Patient should not exceed 25 mg of sildenafil in 48 hours.
**Drug-herb.** *Garlic, St. John's wort:* May substantially reduce blood levels of the drug that could cause loss of therapeutic effects. Warn against use together.
**Drug-food.** *Any food:* Increases drug absorption. Advise patient to take drug with food.
*Grapefruit juice:* Increases drug levels. Recommend taking with liquid other than grapefruit juice.

## Adverse reactions

**CNS:** paresthesia, headache.
**EENT:** pharyngitis, rhinitis, epistaxis.
**GI:** diarrhea, ulcerated buccal mucosa, abdominal pain, nausea, *pancreatitis.*
**Hepatic:** increased liver function test results.
**Musculoskeletal:** asthenia, musculoskeletal pain.
**Respiratory:** bronchitis, dyspnea, hemoptysis, upper respiratory tract disorder, cough.
**Skin:** rash.

## Overdose and treatment

Limited information available. One patient in clinical studies ingested 8 g as a single dose without showing evidence of acute toxicity. Emesis was induced in the patient within 2 to 4 hours after ingestion.

## Clinical considerations

■ If a serious or severe toxicity occurs during treatment, drug should be stopped until the cause is identified or the toxicity resolves. Dose modification isn't needed when drug is resumed.
■ Invirase will be phased out and replaced by Fortovase. Be aware of the dosing differences.
■ Prolonged prior therapy with saquinavir monotherapy may result in mutations that are cross-resistant to ritonavir.
**H** *ALERT* Soft gelatin capsules and hard gelatin capsules are not bioequivalent and cannot be used interchangeably.

### Therapeutic monitoring

■ Evaluate CBC, platelets, electrolytes, uric acid, liver enzymes, and bilirubin before therapy is begun and then at appropriate intervals during therapy.
■ Advise clinician to monitor plasma HIV-1 RNA levels and CD4+ T-cell counts to determine risk of disease progression and when to modify antiretroviral therapy.

### Special populations

**Pregnant patients.** Safety is not established for use during pregnancy. Clinicians are encouraged to enroll patients exposed to drug during pregnancy in the Pregnancy Registry (1-800-258-4263).
**Breast-feeding patients.** Although safety of drug hasn't been established in breast-feeding women, women with HIV infection shouldn't breast-feed to avoid transmitting virus to infant.
**Pediatric patients.** Safety and efficacy in children under age 16 haven't been established.
**Geriatric patients.** Because risk of decreased hepatic, renal, and cardiac function is higher in this population, dosage should be selected carefully.

## Patient counseling

■ Warn patient of adipogenic effects such as redistribution or accumulation of body fat.
■ Inform patient that drug should be taken within 2 hours after a full meal.
■ Tell patient to report adverse reactions.
■ Inform patient that drug is usually given together with other AIDS-related antiviral drugs.
■ Tell patient to use Fortovase within 3 months when stored at room temperature or refer to expiration date on the label if capsules are refrigerated.
■ Advise patients receiving sildenafil that there is an increased risk of sildenafil-associated adverse events, including hypotension, visual changes, and priapism. They should promptly report any symptoms to their prescriber. Tell them not to exceed 25 mg in a 48-hour period.

## sargramostim (granulocyte macrophage-colony stimulating factor [GM-CSF])

Leukine

*Pharmacologic classification:* biologic response modifier
*Therapeutic classification:* colony-stimulating factor
*Pregnancy risk category C*

## Available forms

Available by prescription only
*Injection (preservative-free):* 250 mcg, 500 mcg (as lyophilized powder) in single-dose vials

## Indications and dosages

*Acceleration of hematopoietic reconstitution after autologous bone marrow transplantation in patients with malignant lymphoma, acute lymphoblastic leukemia, or Hodgkin's disease*
*Adults:* 250 mcg/m² daily for 21 consecutive days given as a 2-hour I.V. infusion daily, beginning 2 to 4 hours after the bone marrow transplant. Don't administer within 24 hours of last dose of chemotherapy or within 12 hours after last dose of radiotherapy because of potential sensitivity of rapidly dividing progenitor cells to cytotoxic chemotherapeutic or radiologic therapies.
≣ *Dosage adjustment.* Reduce dosage by half or temporarily discontinue if severe adverse reactions occur. Therapy may be resumed when reaction abates. If blast cells appear or increase to 10% or more of the WBC count or if progression of the underlying disease occurs, discontinue therapy. If absolute neutrophil count is more than 20,000 cells/mm³ or if WBC counts are more than 50,000 cells/mm³, discontinue therapy temporarily or reduce the dosage by half.

*Bone marrow transplantation failure or engraftment delay*
*Adults:* 250 mcg/m² daily for 14 days as a 2-hour I.V. infusion. Same course may be repeated after 7 days off therapy if engraftment hasn't occurred. Third course of 500 mcg/m² daily for 14 days may be given after another 7 days off therapy if engraftment hasn't occurred.
*Acute myelogenous leukemia*
*Adults:* 250 mcg/m² daily by I.V. infusion over 4 hours. Start therapy about day 11 or 4 days after completion of induction therapy. Use only if bone marrow is hypoplastic (fewer than 5% blasts on day 10). Continue until absolute neutrophil count exceeds 1,500/mm³ for 3 consecutive days or for a maximum of 42 days.
◊ *Myelodysplastic syndromes*
*Adults:* 15 to 500 mcg/m² daily by I.V. infusion over 1 to 12 hours.
◊ *Aplastic anemia*
*Adults:* 15 to 480 mcg/m² daily by I.V. infusion over 1 to 12 hours.

## I.V. administration

■ To prepare, reconstitute with 1 ml sterile water for injection. Don't reenter or reuse the single-dose vial. Discard unused portion.
■ Direct stream of sterile water against side of vial and gently swirl contents to minimize foaming. Avoid excessive or vigorous agitation or shaking.
■ Dilute in normal saline. If final concentration is less than 10 mcg/ml, add albumin (human) at a final concentration of 0.1% to the saline before addition of sargramostim to prevent adsorption to components of the delivery system. For a final concentration of 0.1% human albumin, add 1 mg human albumin per milliliter normal saline.
■ Recommend giving as soon as possible after admixture, because sargramostim has no preservative. Discard unused solution after 6 hours of reconstitution or dilution.
■ Don't infuse drug using an in-line membrane filter because absorption of drug could occur.

## Incompatibilities

Don't add other drugs unless specific compatibility data are available.

## Mechanism of action

*Immunostimulant action:* Sargramostim is a 127-amino acid glycoprotein manufactured by recombinant DNA technology in a yeast expression system. It differs from the natural human GM-CSF by the substitution of leucine for arginine at position 23. The carbohydrate moiety may also be different. Sargramostim induces cellular responses by binding to specific receptors on cell surfaces of target cells. Blood counts return to normal or baseline levels within 2 to 10 days after stopping treatment.

## Pharmacokinetics

*Absorption:* Blood levels detectable within 5 minutes after S.C. administration.
*Distribution:* Bound to specific receptors on target cells.
*Metabolism:* Unknown.
*Excretion:* Unknown.

| Route | Onset | Peak | Duration |
|---|---|---|---|
| I.V., S.C. | 15 min | 2-4 hr | Unknown |

## Contraindications and precautions

Contraindicated in patients with excessive leukemic myeloid blasts in bone marrow or peripheral blood and in those hypersensitive to drug or its components or to yeast-derived products. Also contraindicated in patients receiving chemotherapy or radiotherapy.

Use cautiously in patients with impaired renal or hepatic function, preexisting cardiac disease or fluid retention, hypoxia, pulmonary infiltrates, or HF.

## Interactions

**Drug-drug.** *Corticosteroids, lithium:* May potentiate the myeloproliferative effects of sargramostim. Use with caution.

## Adverse reactions

**CNS:** *malaise, CNS disorders, asthenia.*
**CV:** *edema,* supraventricular arrhythmia, pericardial effusion, *peripheral edema.*
**GI:** *nausea, vomiting, diarrhea, anorexia, hemorrhage, GI disorders, stomatitis.*
**GU:** *urinary tract disorder,* abnormal kidney function.
**Hematologic:** stimulation of hematopoiesis, *hemorrhage, blood dyscrasias.*
**Hepatic:** *liver damage.*
**Musculoskeletal:** *bone pain.*
**Respiratory:** *dyspnea, lung disorders,* pleural effusion.
**Skin:** *alopecia, rash.*
**Other:** *fever, mucous membrane disorder,* SEPSIS.

## Overdose and treatment

Doses up to 16 times the recommended dose have been given with the following reversible adverse reactions: WBC counts up to 200,000/mm³, dyspnea, malaise, nausea, fever, rash, sinus tachycardia, headache, and chills. The maximum dose that can be given safely has yet to be determined. If overdose is suspected, advise clinician to monitor WBC count increase and respiratory symptoms.

## Clinical considerations

▪ Transient rash and local injection site reactions may occur; no serious allergic or anaphylactic reactions have been reported.
▪ Drug can act as a growth factor for any tumor type, particularly myeloid malignancies.

▪ Unlabeled indications include use to increase WBC counts in patients with myelodysplastic syndromes and in patients with AIDS on zidovudine; to decrease nadir of leukopenia secondary to myelosuppressive chemotherapy; to decrease myelosuppression in preleukemic patients; to correct neutropenia in patients with aplastic anemia; and to decrease transplant-associated organ system damage, particularly of the liver and kidneys.
▪ When used in neutropenic HIV patients to reduce the risk of bacterial infections (unlabeled), some clinicians recommend a dosage of 250 mcg/m², I.V. daily infused over 2 hours, for 2 to 4 weeks.
▪ Drug is effective in accelerating myeloid recovery in patients receiving bone marrow purged from monoclonal antibodies.
▪ Refrigerate the sterile powder, reconstituted solution, and diluted solution for injection. Don't freeze or shake. Don't use after expiration date.

### Therapeutic monitoring

▪ Stimulation of marrow precursors may result in rapid elevation of WBC count; biweekly monitoring of CBC count with differential, including examination for blast cells, is recommended.
▪ The effect of drug may be limited in patients who have received extensive radiotherapy to hematopoietic sites for treatment of primary disease in the abdomen or chest or have been exposed to several drugs (alkylating agents, anthracycline antibiotics, antimetabolites) before autologous bone marrow transplant.

### Special populations

**Breast-feeding patients.** It isn't known if drug appears in breast milk; use with caution.
**Pediatric patients.** Safety and efficacy in children haven't been established; however, available data suggest that no differences in toxicity exist. The type and frequency of adverse reactions were comparable with those seen in adults.

## Patient counseling

▪ Review administration schedule with patient and caregivers. Answer any questions and address concerns.

# scopolamine hydrobromide

Isopto Hyoscine, Scopace, Transderm-Scop

*Pharmacologic classification:* anticholinergic
*Therapeutic classification:* antimuscarinic, cycloplegic mydriatic
*Pregnancy risk category C*

## Available forms

Available by prescription only
*Injection:* 0.3 and 1 mg/ml in 1-ml vials; 0.4 mg/ml, 0.86 mg/ml in 0.5-ml ampules
*Ophthalmic solution:* 0.25%
*Oral:* Soluble tablets 0.4 mg
*Topical:* Transdermal system 1.5 mg

## Indications and dosages

***Antimuscarinic, adjunct to anesthesia, prevention of nausea and vomiting***
*Adults:* 0.3 to 0.6 mg I.M., S.C., or I.V. as a single dose. Apply transdermal system the evening before surgery. In cesarean section, apply 1 hour before surgery.
*Children:* 0.006 mg/kg I.M., S.C., or I.V. as a single daily dose; maximum dose, 0.3 mg.
***Prevention of nausea and vomiting from motion sickness***
*Adults:* One transdermal patch applied behind the ear 4 hours before anticipated exposure to motion, or 0.25 to 0.8 mg P.O. 1 hour before exposure to motion, then t.i.d., p.r.n.
***Cycloplegic refraction***
*Adults:* One to two drops 0.25% solution in eye 1 hour before refraction.
*Children:* One drop 0.25% solution b.i.d. for 2 days before refraction.
***Iritis, uveitis***
*Adults:* One to two drops of 0.25% solution daily or up to t.i.d.
*Children:* One drop of 0.25% solution up to t.i.d.

## I.V. administration

- Dilute with sterile water for injection.
- Give by direct I.V. injection.

### *Incompatibilities*

Incompatible with alkalies, anticholinergics, and methohexital.

## Mechanism of action

*Antimuscarinic action:* Scopolamine inhibits muscarinic action of acetylcholine on autonomic effectors, decreasing secretions and GI motility; blocks vagal inhibition of SA node.
*Mydriatic action:* Scopolamine competitively blocks acetylcholine at cholinergic neuroeffector sites, antagonizing effects of acetylcholine on the sphincter muscle and ciliary body, producing mydriasis and cycloplegia.

## Pharmacokinetics

*Absorption:* Rapidly absorbed when administered I.M. or S.C. Systemic drug absorption may occur from drug passage through the nasolacrimal duct.
*Distribution:* Distributed widely throughout body tissues. Drug crosses the placenta and probably the blood-brain barrier.
*Metabolism:* Probably metabolized completely in the liver; however, its exact metabolic fate is unknown. Mydriatic and cycloplegic effects persist for 3 to 7 days.
*Excretion:* Probably in urine as metabolites.

| Route | Onset | Peak | Duration |
|---|---|---|---|
| P.O. | Unknown | 1 hr | Unknown |
| I.M., I.V., S.C. | Varies | Varies | Varies |
| Ophthalmic | Rapid | 15-45 min | < 1 wk |
| Transdermal | 4 hr | 24 hr | 72 hr |

## Contraindications and precautions

Scopolamine is contraindicated in patients hypersensitive to the drug, to any other belladonna alkaloid, or to any ingredient or component in the formulation or administration system.

Systemic form is contraindicated in patients with angle-closure glaucoma, obstructive uropathy, obstructive disease of the GI tract, asthma, chronic pulmonary disease, myasthenia gravis, paralytic ileus, intestinal atony, unstable CV status in acute hemorrhage, or toxic megacolon. Ophthalmic form is contraindicated in patients with shallow anterior chamber and angle-closure glaucoma.

Soluble tablets are contraindicated in patients with prostatic hyperplasia or impaired renal or hepatic function, and should be used cautiously in patients with cardiac disease.

Use systemic form cautiously in patients with autonomic neuropathy, hyperthyroidism, coronary artery disease, arrhythmias, HF, hypertension, hiatal hernia associated with reflux esophagitis, hepatic or renal disease, or ulcerative colitis; or in patients in a hot or humid environment. Use ophthalmic form cautiously in geriatric patients, in infants and children, and in those with cardiac disease.

Use transdermal form cautiously in patients with history of seizures or psychosis.

## Interactions

**Drug-drug.** *Anticholinergics, such as ketoconazole and levodopa:* Decreased GI absorption has been reported. Separate administration times by 2 to 3 hours.
*CNS depressants, including sedative-hypnotics and tranquilizers:* May increase CNS depression. Advise clinician to monitor patient closely.
*Digoxin:* Higher serum digoxin levels when given with anticholinergics. Advise clinician to monitor patient for digitalis toxicity.
*Drugs having anticholinergic effects:* May cause additive toxicity. Avoid use together.
*Oral potassium supplements, especially waxmatrix formulations:* Potassium-induced GI ulcerations may be increased. Use cautiously.
**Drug-herb.** *Jaborandi tree and pill-bearing spurge:* May have decreased effects. Advise clinician to monitor patient closely.
*Squaw vine:* Tannic acid may decrease metabolic breakdown. Advise clinician to monitor patient.

**Drug-lifestyle.** *Alcohol use:* May increase the risk of CNS depression. Advise patient to avoid alcohol.
*Sun exposure:* With ophthalmic form, photophobia may occur. Take precautions.

## Adverse reactions

**CNS:** disorientation, restlessness, irritability, dizziness, drowsiness, headache, confusion, hallucinations, delirium.
**CV:** tachycardia; palpitations, *paradoxical bradycardia* (with systemic form).
**EENT:** blurred vision, photophobia, increased intraocular pressure; dilated pupils (with systemic form); ocular congestion (with prolonged use), conjunctivitis, eye dryness, eye pruritus, transient stinging and burning, edema (with ophthalmic form).
**GI:** dry mouth; *constipation, nausea, vomiting,* difficulty swallowing, *epigastric distress* (with systemic form).
**GU:** urinary hesitancy, urine retention (with systemic form).
**Respiratory:** bronchial plugging, depressed respirations (with systemic form).
**Skin:** rash, flushing (with systemic form); dryness or contact dermatitis (with ophthalmic form).
**Other:** fever (with systemic form).

## Overdose and treatment

Effects of overdose include excitability, seizures, CNS stimulation followed by depression, and such psychotic symptoms as disorientation, confusion, hallucinations, delusions, anxiety, agitation, delirium, and restlessness. Peripheral effects include dilated, nonreactive pupils; blurred vision; flushed, hot, dry skin; dryness of mucous membranes; dysphagia; decreased or absent bowel sounds; urine retention; hyperthermia; tachycardia; hypertension; and increased respiration.

Treatment is primarily symptomatic and supportive, p.r.n. Advise clinician to maintain patent airway and remove transdermal system. If patient is awake and alert, advise clinician to induce emesis (or use gastric lavage) and follow with a sodium chloride cathartic and activated charcoal to prevent further drug absorption. In severe life-threatening cases, physostigmine may be given to block the antimuscarinic effects of scopolamine. Fluids should be given, p.r.n., to treat shock; diazepam to control psychotic symptoms; and pilocarpine (instilled into the eyes) to relieve mydriasis. If urine retention develops, catheterization may be needed.

## Clinical considerations

■ Intermittent and continuous I.V. infusions aren't recommended.
■ Some patients, especially geriatric patients, may experience transient excitement or disorientation.

■ Scopolamine may interfere with the gastric secretion test.
**Ophthalmic**
■ Advise clinician to apply pressure to the lacrimal sac for 1 minute after instillation to reduce the risk of systemic drug absorption.
■ Have patient lie down, tilt head back, or look at ceiling to aid instillation.

### Therapeutic monitoring

■ Therapeutic doses may produce amnesia, drowsiness, and euphoria (desired effects for use as an adjunct to anesthesia). Advise clinician to reorient patient p.r.n.

### Special populations

**Breast-feeding patients.** Scopolamine appears in breast milk. Use cautiously in nursing women.
**Pediatric patients.** Safety and efficacy of soluble tablets or transdermal system have not been established in children. Use ophthalmic form cautiously, if at all, in infants and young children.
**Geriatric patients.** Use caution when giving drug to geriatric patients. Lower doses are indicated.

## Patient counseling
**Ophthalmic**
■ Instruct patient to apply pressure to bridge of nose for about 1 minute after instillation.
■ Advise patient not to close eyes tightly or blink for about 1 minute after instillation.
**Topical**
■ Tell patient to wash hands after applying the patch.
■ Instruct patient to use only one patch at a time.
■ Patch delivers about 1 mg in 72 hours. Advise clinician to remove the patch when antiemetic effect is no longer needed.

# secobarbital sodium
Novosecobarb*, Seconal

*Pharmacologic classification:* barbiturate
*Therapeutic classification:* sedative-hypnotic, anticonvulsant
*Pregnancy risk category D*
*Controlled substance schedule II*

## Available forms
Available by prescription only
*Capsules:* 100 mg

## Indications and dosages
*Preoperative sedation*
*Adults:* 200 to 300 mg P.O. 1 to 2 hours before surgery
*Children:* 2 to 6 mg/kg P.O. (maximum dose, 100 mg)
*Insomnia*
*Adults:* 100 mg P.O.

---

Reactions may be *common*, uncommon, **life-threatening**, or COMMON AND LIFE-THREATENING.

## Mechanism of action
*Sedative-hypnotic action:* Secobarbital acts throughout the CNS as a nonselective depressant with a rapid onset and short duration of action. Particularly sensitive to this drug is the reticular activating system, which controls CNS arousal. Secobarbital decreases both presynaptic and postsynaptic membrane excitability by facilitating the action of gamma-aminobutyric acid. The exact cellular site and mechanisms of action are unknown.

## Pharmacokinetics
*Absorption:* After oral administration, 90% is absorbed rapidly. Levels of 1 to 5 mcg/ml are needed to produce sedation; 5 to 15 mcg/ml are needed for hypnosis.
*Distribution:* Distributed rapidly throughout body tissues and fluids; about 30% to 45% is protein-bound.
*Metabolism:* Oxidized in the liver to inactive metabolites. Duration of action is 3 to 4 hours.
*Excretion:* About 95% of a dose is eliminated as glucuronide conjugates and other metabolites in urine. Drug has an elimination half-life of about 30 hours.

| Route | Onset | Peak | Duration |
|-------|-------|------|----------|
| P.O. | 15 min | 15-30 min | 1-4 hr |

## Contraindications and precautions
Contraindicated in patients with respiratory disease in which dyspnea or obstruction is evident, or there's hypersensitivity to barbiturates or porphyria.
    Use cautiously in patients with acute or chronic pain, depression, suicidal tendencies, history of drug abuse, or impaired hepatic or renal function.

## Interactions
**Drug-drug.** *Antidepressants, antihistamines, narcotics, sedative-hypnotics, tranquilizers:* Secobarbital may add to or potentiate CNS and respiratory depressant effects. Use together cautiously.
*Corticosteroids, digitoxin (not digoxin), doxycycline, oral contraceptives and other estrogens, theophylline and other xanthines, warfarin and other oral anticoagulants:* Secobarbital enhances the metabolism of these drugs. Advise clinician to monitor patient for lack of effect.
*Disulfiram, MAO inhibitors, valproic acid:* Decrease the metabolism of secobarbital and can increase its toxicity. Reduce barbiturate dosage.
*Griseofulvin:* Secobarbital impairs the effectiveness of griseofulvin by decreasing absorption from the GI tract. Advise clinician to monitor effectiveness of griseofulvin.
*Rifampin:* May decrease secobarbital levels by increasing metabolism. Advise clinician to monitor patient for decreased effect.

**Drug-lifestyle.** *Alcohol use:* May potentiate CNS depressant effects. Advise patient to avoid alcohol.

## Adverse reactions
**CNS:** *drowsiness, lethargy, hangover,* paradoxical excitement in geriatric patients, somnolence, physical and psychological dependence, change in EEG patterns.
**GI:** nausea, vomiting.
**Hematologic:** exacerbation of porphyria.
**Hepatic:** decreased serum bilirubin levels.
**Respiratory:** *respiratory depression.*
**Skin:** rash, urticaria, *Stevens-Johnson syndrome,* tissue reactions, injection-site pain.
**Other:** *angioedema.*

## Overdose and treatment
Signs and symptoms of overdose include unsteady gait, slurred speech, sustained nystagmus, somnolence, confusion, respiratory depression, pulmonary edema, areflexia, and coma. Typical shock syndrome with tachycardia and hypotension, jaundice, hypothermia followed by fever, and oliguria may occur.
    Advise clinician to maintain and support ventilation and pulmonary function p.r.n.; advise clinician to support cardiac function and circulation with vasopressors and I.V. fluids p.r.n. If patient is conscious and gag reflex is intact, emesis should be induced (if ingestion was recent) by giving ipecac syrup. If emesis is contraindicated, advise clinician to perform gastric lavage while a cuffed endotracheal tube is in place to prevent aspiration. Follow with administration of activated charcoal or sodium chloride cathartic. Advise clinician to measure intake and output, vital signs, and laboratory parameters, and maintain body temperature. Roll patient from side to side every 30 minutes to avoid pulmonary congestion.
    Alkalinization of urine may be helpful in removing drug from the body; hemodialysis may be useful in severe overdose.

## Clinical considerations
■ Secobarbital may cause a false-positive phentolamine test. The physiologic effects of the drug may impair the absorption of cyanocobalamin $^{57}$Co.

### Therapeutic monitoring
■ Advise clinician to watch for signs of barbiturate toxicity: coma, pupillary constriction, cyanosis, clammy skin, and hypotension. Overdose may be fatal.
■ Advise clinician to monitor hepatic and renal tests frequently to prevent possible toxicity.

### Special populations
**Breast-feeding patients.** Because drug appears in breast milk, don't give to breast-feeding women.

**Pediatric patients.** Drug may cause paradoxical excitement in children; use cautiously.
**Geriatric patients.** Geriatric patients are more susceptible to effects of drug and usually require lower doses. Confusion, disorientation, and excitability may occur in geriatric patients.

## Patient counseling
■ Inform patient the morning "hangover" is common after hypnotic dose, which suppresses REM sleep.
■ Caution patient about performing activities that require mental alertness or physical coordination.

## selegiline hydrochloride (L-deprenyl hydrochloride)
Atapryl, Carbex, Eldepryl, Selpak

*Pharmacologic classification:* MAO inhibitor
*Therapeutic classification:* antiparkinsonian
*Pregnancy risk category C*

## Available forms
Available by prescription only
*Capsules:* 5 mg
*Tablets:* 5 mg

## Indications and dosages
*Adjunctive treatment to levodopa-carbidopa in the management of symptoms associated with Parkinson's disease*
Adults: 10 mg P.O. daily, taken as 5 mg at breakfast and 5 mg at lunch. After 2 or 3 days of therapy, begin gradual decrease of levodopa-carbidopa dose.

## Mechanism of action
*Antiparkinsonian action:* Probably acts by selectively inhibiting MAO type B (found mostly in the brain). At higher-than-recommended doses, it's a nonselective inhibitor of MAO, including MAO type A found in the GI tract. It may also directly increase dopaminergic activity by decreasing the reuptake of dopamine into nerve cells. It has pharmacologically active metabolites (amphetamine and methamphetamine) that may contribute to this effect.

## Pharmacokinetics
*Absorption:* Rapidly absorbed; about 73% of dose is absorbed.
*Distribution:* After a single dose, plasma levels are below detectable levels (less than 10 ng/ml).
*Metabolism:* Three metabolites have been detected in the serum and urine: N-desmethyldeprenyl, amphetamine, and methamphetamine.

*Excretion:* About 45% appears as a metabolite in urine after 48 hours.

| Route | Onset | Peak | Duration |
|-------|-------|------|----------|
| P.O. | Unknown | ½-2 hr | Unknown |

## Contraindications and precautions
Contraindicated in patients hypersensitive to drug and in those receiving meperidine and other opioids.

## Interactions
**Drug-drug.** *Adrenergics:* May increase the pressor response. Use together cautiously.
*Meperidine:* Fatal interactions have been reported. Don't use together.
**Drug-herb.** *Ginseng:* May cause headache, tremors, mania. Discourage use together.
**Drug-food.** *Cacao:* May cause potential vasopressor effects if used together. Discourage use together.
*Foods high in tyramine:* May cause possible hypertensive crisis. Advise clinician to monitor blood pressure.
**Drug-lifestyle.** *Alcohol use:* Excessive depressant effect is possible. Advise patient to avoid alcohol.

## Adverse reactions
**CNS:** malaise, *dizziness,* increased tremor, chorea, loss of balance, restlessness, increased bradykinesia, facial grimacing, stiff neck, dyskinesia, involuntary movements, twitching, increased apraxia, behavioral changes, fatigue, headache, confusion, hallucinations, vivid dreams, anxiety, insomnia, lethargy.
**CV:** orthostatic hypotension, hypertension, hypotension, *arrhythmias,* palpitations, new or increased anginal pain, tachycardia, peripheral edema, syncope.
**EENT:** blepharospasm.
**GI:** dry mouth, *nausea,* vomiting, constipation, abdominal pain, anorexia or poor appetite, dysphagia, diarrhea, heartburn.
**GU:** slow urination, transient nocturia, prostatic hyperplasia, urinary hesitancy, urinary frequency, urine retention, sexual dysfunction.
**Metabolic:** weight loss.
**Skin:** rash, hair loss, diaphoresis.

## Overdose and treatment
Limited experience with overdose suggests that symptoms may include hypotension and psychomotor agitation. Because selegiline becomes a nonselective MAO inhibitor in high doses, consider the possibility of symptoms of MAO inhibitor poisoning: drowsiness, dizziness, hyperactivity, agitation, seizures, coma, hypertension, hypotension, cardiac conduction disturbances, and CV collapse. These symptoms may not develop immediately after ingestion; delays of 12 hours or more are possible.

Advise clinician to provide supportive treatment and closely monitor the patient for worsening of symptoms. Emesis or lavage may be helpful in the early stages of overdose treatment. Avoid phenothiazine derivatives and CNS stimulants; adrenergics may provoke an exaggerated response. Diazepam may be useful in treating seizures.

## Clinical considerations
■ In some patients who experience an increase of adverse reactions from levodopa (including dyskinesias), reduction of levodopa-carbidopas needed. Most of these patients require a levodopa-carbidopa dosage reduction of 10% to 30%.

### Therapeutic monitoring
■ Advise clinician to monitor patient's response to drug therapy.

### Special populations
**Breast-feeding patients.** It isn't known if drug appears in breast milk. Use with caution in breast-feeding women.

## Patient counseling
■ Advise patient not to take more than 10 mg daily. There's no evidence that higher doses improve efficacy and it may increase adverse reactions.
■ Tell patient to move about cautiously at the start of therapy because dizziness may occur, which can cause falls.
■ Because drug is an MAO inhibitor, tell patient about the possibility of an interaction with tyramine-containing foods. Tell patient to immediately report signs or symptoms of hypertension, including severe headache. Reportedly, however, this interaction doesn't occur at the recommended dose; at 10 mg daily, drug inhibits only MAO type B. Therefore, dietary restrictions appear unnecessary, provided that patient doesn't exceed the recommended dose.
■ Advise patient to take second dose with lunch to avoid nighttime sedation.

---

## senna
Black-Draught, Ex-lax Chocolated, Fletcher's Castoria, Nytilax, Senexon, Senokot, Senolax, X-Prep

*Pharmacologic classification:* anthraquinone derivative
*Therapeutic classification:* stimulant laxative
*Pregnancy risk category C*

---

## Available forms
Available without a prescription
(Dosages expressed as sennosides [active principle])
*Chewable pieces:* 15 mg
*Granules:* 15 mg/tsp, 20 mg/5 ml
*Liquid:* 3 mg/ml

*Powder:* 15 mg/3g
*Suppositories:* 30 mg
*Syrup:* 8.8 mg/5 ml
*Tablets:* 6 mg, 8.6 mg, 15 mg, 17 mg, 25 mg

## Indications and dosages
***Acute constipation, preparation for bowel examination***
**Black-Draught**
*Adults:* 2 tablets or ¼ to ½ level tsp of granules mixed with water. Not for children.
**Other preparations**
*Adults and children ages 12 and older:* Usual dose is 2 tablets, 1 tsp of granules dissolved in water, or 10 to 15 ml syrup h.s. Maximum dose varies with preparation used.
*Children ages 6 to 11:* 1 tablet, ¼ tsp of granules dissolved in water, ¼ suppository h.s., or 5 to 10 ml syrup. Maximum dose is 2 tablets b.i.d. or 1 tsp of granules b.i.d.
*Children ages 2 to 5:* ¼ tablet, or ¼ tsp of granules dissolved in water. Maximum dose is 1 tablet b.i.d. or ½ tsp of granules b.i.d.
*Children ages 1 to 5:* 2.5 to 5 ml syrup h.s.
*Children ages 1 to 12 months:* Consult prescriber.

## Mechanism of action
*Laxative action:* Senna has a local irritant effect on the colon, which promotes peristalsis and bowel evacuation. It also enhances intestinal fluid accumulation, thereby increasing the moisture content of the stool.

## Pharmacokinetics
*Absorption:* Absorbed minimally.
*Distribution:* May be distributed in bile, saliva and the colonic mucosa, and may appear in breast milk.
*Metabolism:* Absorbed portion is metabolized in the liver.
*Excretion:* Unabsorbed senna is excreted mainly in feces; absorbed drug is excreted in urine and feces.

| Route | Onset | Peak | Duration |
|---|---|---|---|
| P.O. | 6-10 hr | Variable | Variable |
| P.R. | ½-2 hr | Unknown | Unknown |

## Contraindications and precautions
Contraindicated in patients with ulcerative bowel lesions; nausea, vomiting, abdominal pain, or other symptoms of appendicitis or acute surgical abdomen; fecal impaction; or intestinal obstruction or perforation.

## Interactions
None reported.

## Adverse reactions
**GI:** *nausea,* vomiting, diarrhea, loss of normal bowel function with excessive use, *abdominal cramps* (especially in severe constipation), malabsorption of nutrients, "cathartic colon"

(syndrome resembling ulcerative colitis radiologically) with chronic misuse, possible constipation after catharsis, yellow or yellow-green cast to feces, diarrhea in breast-feeding infants of mothers receiving senna, darkened pigmentation of rectal mucosa with long-term use (usually reversible within 4 to 12 months after stopping drug), laxative dependence with excessive use.

**GU:** red-pink discoloration in alkaline urine; yellow-brown color to acidic urine.

**Metabolic:** protein-losing enteropathy, electrolyte imbalance such as hypokalemia.

## Overdose and treatment
No information available.

## Clinical considerations
- Protect drug from excessive heat or light.
- Drug is for short-term treatment.

### Therapeutic monitoring
- Before giving drug, determine if patient has adequate fluid intake, exercise, and diet. Also, stress importance of maintaining these during drug therapy.

### Special populations
**Breast-feeding patients.** Senna appears in breast milk; diarrhea has been reported in breast-feeding infants.

**Pediatric patients.** Senna and other stimulant laxatives are used infrequently in children.

**Geriatric patients.** Geriatric patients often overuse laxatives and may be more susceptible to laxative dependency.

## Patient counseling
- In the phenolsulfonphthalein excretion test, senna may turn urine pink to red, red to violet, or red to brown.
- Instruct patient that laxative use shouldn't exceed 1 week. Excessive use may result in dependence or electrolyte imbalance.
- Tell patient that bowel movement may have a yellow or yellow-green cast.
- Teach patient about dietary sources of bulk, including bran and other cereals, fresh fruit and vegetables.

# sertraline hydrochloride
Zoloft

*Pharmacologic classification:* selective serotonin reuptake inhibitor
*Therapeutic classification:* antidepressant
*Pregnancy risk category C*

## Available forms
Available by prescription only
*Oral solution:* 20 mg/ml
*Tablets (film-coated):* 25 mg, 50 mg, 100 mg

## Indications and dosages
*Posttraumatic stress disorder or panic disorder*
*Adults:* 25 mg P.O. daily. Increase to 50 mg P.O. daily after 1 week. If no improvement, dose may be increased up to a maximum of 200 mg P.O. daily.

*Depression, obsessive-compulsive disorder*
*Adults:* 50 mg P.O. daily. Adjust dosage p.r.n. and as tolerated; clinical trials involved doses of 50 to 200 mg daily. Dosage adjustments should be made at intervals of no less than 1 week.

*Children ages 6 to 12 (OCD only):* Initially, 25 mg P.O. once daily. Increase dosage at intervals no less than 1 week. Maximum dose 200 mg/day.

*Children ages 13 to 17 (OCD only):* Initially, 50 mg P.O. once daily. Increase dosage at intervals no less than 1 week. Maximum dose 200 mg/day.

≡*Dosage adjustment.* Use a lower or less-frequent dosage in patients with hepatic impairment. Use particular care in patients with renal failure.

◇*Premenstrual disphoric disorder*
*Adults:* 50 to 150 mg P.O. daily.
◇*Premature ejaculation*
*Adults:* 25 to 50 mg P.O. daily or p.r.n.

## Mechanism of action
*Antidepressant action:* Sertraline probably acts by blocking the reuptake of serotonin (5-hydroxy-tryptamine; 5-HT) into presynaptic neurons in the CNS, prolonging the action of 5-HT.

## Pharmacokinetics
*Absorption:* Well absorbed after oral administration; absorption rate and extent are enhanced when taken with food.

*Distribution:* In vitro studies indicate that drug is highly protein-bound (more than 98%).

*Metabolism:* Metabolism is probably hepatic; drug undergoes significant first-pass metabolism. N-desmethylsertraline is substantially less active than the parent compound.

*Excretion:* Excreted mostly as metabolites in the urine and feces. Mean elimination half-life is 26 hours. Steady-state levels are reached within 1 week of daily dosing in young, healthy patients.

| Route | Onset | Peak | Duration |
|-------|-------|------|----------|
| P.O. | Unknown | 4½-8½ hr | Unknown |

## Contraindications and precautions
Contraindicated in patients receiving MAO inhibitors.

Use cautiously in patients at risk for suicide and in those with seizure disorders, major affective disorder, or diseases or conditions that affect metabolism or hemodynamic responses.

---

## Interactions

**Drug-drug.** *Cimetidine:* Increased sertraline bioavailability, peak plasma levels, and half-life. Advise clinician to monitor patient closely.
*Diazepam, tolbutamide:* Clearance of these drugs is decreased by sertraline. Advise clinician to monitor patient for increased drug effects.
*Disulfiram:* Oral concentrate contains alcohol that could cause a reaction. Avoid use.
*MAO inhibitors:* Serious mental status changes, hyperthermia, autonomic instability, rapid fluctuations of vital signs, delirium, coma, and death. Drug must not be given within 14 days of an MAO inhibitor.
*Warfarin, other highly protein-bound drugs:* May cause interactions, increasing the plasma levels of sertraline or the other highly bound drug. Advise clinician to monitor patient closely.
**Drug-herb.** *St. John's wort:* Serotonin levels may rise too high, causing serotonin syndrome. Discourage use together.

## Adverse reactions

**CNS:** *headache, tremor, dizziness, insomnia, somnolence,* paresthesia, hypoesthesia, *fatigue,* nervousness, anxiety, agitation, hypertonia, twitching, confusion.
**CV:** palpitations, chest pain, hot flashes.
**GI:** *dry mouth, nausea, diarrhea, loose stools, dyspepsia,* vomiting, constipation, thirst, flatulence, anorexia, abdominal pain, increased appetite.
**GU:** *sexual dysfunction in men,* polyuria, nocturia, dysuria.
**Hepatic:** elevated liver enzyme levels.
**Metabolic:** minor increases in serum cholesterol and triglyceride levels; decreased uric acid.
**Musculoskeletal:** myalgia.
**Skin:** rash, pruritus, *diaphoresis.*

## Overdose and treatment

Clinical experience with sertraline overdose is limited. Treatment is supportive. Advise clinician to establish an airway and maintain adequate ventilation. Because recent studies question the value of forced emesis or lavage, consider the use of activated charcoal in sorbitol to bind drug in the GI tract.

There's no specific antidote for sertraline. Advise clinician to monitor vital signs closely. Because drug has a large volume of distribution, hemodialysis, peritoneal dialysis, or forced diuresis probably isn't useful.

## Clinical considerations

■ Drug may activate mania or hypomania in patients with cyclic disorders.
■ Avoid using the oral concentrate dropper, which is made of rubber, in a patient with a latex allergy.

## Therapeutic monitoring

■ Patients who respond during the first 8 weeks of therapy will probably continue to respond to drug, although there are limited studies of drug in depressed patients for periods longer than 16 weeks. If patients are continued on drug for prolonged therapy, periodically monitor the effectiveness of drug. It's unknown if periodic dosage adjustments are needed to maintain effectiveness.
■ Advise clinician to record mood changes and monitor patient for suicidal tendencies.

## Special populations

**Breast-feeding patients.** It isn't known if drug appears in breast milk. Use with caution.
**Pediatric patients.** Safety and efficacy in children haven't been established.
**Geriatric patients.** Plasma clearance of drug is slower in geriatric patients. Studies indicate that it may take 2 to 3 weeks of daily dosing before steady-state levels are reached. Advise clinician to monitor patient closely for dose-related side effects.

## Patient counseling

■ Tell patient to take drug once daily, either in the morning or evening, with or without food.
■ Advise patient to avoid alcohol while taking drug and to call before taking OTC drugs.
■ Although problems haven't been reported to date, advise patient to use caution when performing hazardous tasks that require alertness, such as driving and operating heavy machinery. Drugs that influence the CNS may impair judgment.
■ Advise patient to mix the oral concentrate with 4 ounces (½ cup) of water, ginger ale, lemon or lime soda only, and to take the dose right away.

# sibutramine hydrochloride monohydrate
Meridia

*Pharmacologic classification:* norepinephrine, serotonin, and dopamine re-uptake inhibitor
*Therapeutic classification:* antiobesity
*Pregnancy risk category C*
*Controlled substance schedule IV*

## Available forms

Available by prescription only
*Capsules:* 5 mg, 10 mg, 15 mg

## Indications and dosages

***Management of obesity, including weight loss and maintenance of weight loss; should be used with a reduced-calorie diet***
*Adults:* 10 mg P.O. once daily with or without food. May increase dosage to 15 mg daily af-

ter 4 weeks if there is inadequate weight loss. Patients who don't tolerate the 10-mg dose may receive 5 mg daily. Doses above 15 mg daily aren't recommended.

## Mechanism of action
*Antiobesity action:* Sibutramine produces its therapeutic effects by inhibiting the reuptake of norepinephrine, serotonin, and dopamine.

## Pharmacokinetics
*Absorption:* Rapidly absorbed from the GI tract. On average, at least 77% of a single oral dose of sibutramine is absorbed.
*Distribution:* Distributed extensively into tissues, especially the liver and kidney with relatively low transfer to the fetus. In vitro, sibutramine, $M_1$, and $M_2$ are extensively bound (97%, 94%, and 94%, respectively) to human plasma proteins.
*Metabolism:* Undergoes extensive first-pass metabolism by the cytochrome P-450 3A4 isoenzyme to active desmethyl metabolites $M_1$ and $M_2$; elimination half-lives of $M_1$ and $M_2$ are 14 and 16 hours, respectively.
*Excretion:* About 77% of a single oral dose is excreted in the urine.

| Route | Onset | Peak | Duration |
|-------|-------|------|----------|
| P.O. | Unknown | 3-4 hr | Unknown |

## Contraindications and precautions
Contraindicated in patients taking MAO inhibitors or other centrally acting appetite-suppressant drugs. Also contraindicated in patients hypersensitive to drug or its inactive ingredients and in those with anorexia nervosa. Don't use drug in patients with history of coronary artery disease, HF, arrhythmias, CVA, severe renal failure, hepatic dysfunction, or a history of seizures.

Use cautiously in patients with narrow angle glaucoma.

## Interactions
**Drug-drug.** *CNS depressants:* May enhance CNS depression. Use with caution.
*Dextromethorphan, dihydroergotamine, fentanyl, fluoxetine, fluvoxamine, lithium, MAO inhibitors, meperidine, paroxetine, pentazocine, sertraline, sumatriptan, tryptophan, venlafaxine:* May cause hyperthermia, tachycardia, and loss of consciousness. Don't use together. At least 2 weeks should elapse between stopping an MAO inhibitor and starting sibutramine, and vice versa.
*Drugs that inhibit cytochrome P-450 3A4 metabolism, such as erythromycin and ketoconazole:* Dose of sibutramine may need to be reduced when given together.
*Ephedrine, pseudoephedrine:* May increase blood pressure or heart rate. Advise clinician to monitor patient carefully.

**Drug-herb.** *L-tryptophan:* Possible additive effect leading to serotonin syndrome. Concomitant use is not recommended.
**Drug-lifestyle.** *Alcohol use:* May enhance CNS depression. Discourage use.

## Adverse reactions
**CNS:** *headache, insomnia,* dizziness, nervousness, anxiety, depression, paresthesia, somnolence, CNS stimulation, emotional lability, migraine.
**CV:** tachycardia, vasodilation, hypertension, palpitation, chest pain, generalized edema.
**EENT:** thirst, *dry mouth, rhinitis, pharyngitis,* laryngitis, sinusitis, ear disorder, ear pain.
**GI:** *anorexia, constipation,* increased appetite, nausea, dyspepsia, gastritis, vomiting, abdominal pain, rectal disorder, taste perversion.
**GU:** dysmenorrhea, urinary tract infection, vaginal candidiasis, metrorrhagia.
**Hepatic:** elevated liver function test results.
**Musculoskeletal:** arthralgia, myalgia, asthenia, tenosynovitis, joint disorder, neck or back pain.
**Respiratory:** cough increase.
**Skin:** rash, sweating, acne.
**Other:** flu syndrome, herpes simplex, *allergic reaction.*

## Overdose and treatment
There's no specific antidote to sibutramine. Treatment should consist of general measures used in the management of overdose. Advise clinician to establish an airway, monitor cardiac and vital signs, and institute general symptomatic and supportive measures. Cautious use of beta blockers may be indicated to control elevated blood pressure or tachycardia. The benefits of forced diuresis and hemodialysis are unknown.

## Clinical considerations
■ Drug is recommended for obese patients with an initial body mass index of 30 kg/m$^2$ or more or 27 kg/m$^2$ or more in the presence of other risk factors, such as hypertension, diabetes, or dyslipidemia.
■ Organic causes of obesity should be ruled out before therapy starts.
■ Weight loss can precipitate or exacerbate gallstone formation.
■ Although not reported with sibutramine, some centrally acting weight-loss drugs have caused a rare but fatal condition known as primary pulmonary hypertension.

### *Therapeutic monitoring*
■ Advise clinician to measure blood pressure and heart rate before therapy starts, with dose changes, and at regular intervals during therapy because drug is known to increase both blood pressure and heart rate.

---

■ If a patient has not lost at least 4 lb in the first 4 weeks of treatment, therapy should be reevaluated to consider dose increase or discontinuation of drug.

### Special populations
**Breast-feeding patients.** It isn't known if drug or its metabolites appear in breast milk. Avoid use of drug in breast-feeding women.
**Pediatric patients.** Safety and efficacy in children under age 16 haven't been established.
**Geriatric patients.** Dose selection for a geriatric patient should be cautious, reflecting the greater frequency of decreased hepatic, renal, or cardiac function, and of concomitant disease or other drug therapy.

### Patient counseling
■ Advise patient to read the package insert before therapy starts and to review again each time the prescription is renewed.
■ Instruct patient to report rash, hives, or other allergic reactions immediately.
■ Inform patient to inform prescriber of other prescription or OTC drugs being taken, especially other weight-reducing drugs, decongestants, antidepressants, cough suppressants, lithium, dihydroergotamine, sumatriptan, or tryptophan, as there is a potential for drug interactions.
■ Emphasize importance of regular follow-up visits with prescriber.
■ Advise patient to use drug with a reduced-calorie diet.

---

# sildenafil citrate
Viagra

*Pharmacologic classification:* selective inhibitor of cyclic guanosine monophosphate-specific phosphodiesterase type 5
*Therapeutic classification:* therapy for erectile dysfunction
*Pregnancy risk category B*

---

### Available forms
Available by prescription only
*Tablets:* 25 mg, 50 mg, 100 mg

### Indications and dosages
*Treatment of erectile dysfunction*
*Adults:* 50 mg P.O. as a single dose, p.r.n., 1 hour before sexual activity. However, may take drug 30 minutes to 4 hours before sexual activity. Based on effectiveness and tolerance by patient, may increase dose to maximum single dose of 100 mg or decrease dose to 25 mg. A maximum recommended dosing frequency is once daily.
≡ *Dosage adjustment.* For geriatric patients with hepatic impairment or severe renal im-

pairment, and those taking potent cytochrome P-450 3A4 inhibitors, a starting dose of 25 mg should be considered.

### Mechanism of action
*Erectile action:* Sildenafil has no direct relaxant effect on isolated human corpus cavernosum, but enhances the effect of nitric oxide (NO) by inhibiting phosphodiesterase type 5 (PDE5), which is responsible for degradation of cyclic guanosine monophosphate (cGMP) in the corpus cavernosum. When sexual stimulation causes local release of NO, inhibition of PDE5 by sildenafil causes increased levels of cGMP in the corpus cavernosum, resulting in smooth-muscle relaxation and inflow of blood to the corpus cavernosum.

### Pharmacokinetics
*Absorption:* Rapidly absorbed after oral administration. A high-fat meal delays the rate of absorption by about 1 hour and reduces peak levels by one third. Absolute bioavailability of sildenafil is about 40%.
*Distribution:* Widely distributed to body tissues with a mean steady-state volume of distribution of 105 L. Both drug and its major active metabolite are 96% plasma protein–bound. Protein-binding is independent of drug levels.
*Metabolism:* The primary pathway for sildenafil elimination is metabolism by the CYP 3A4 and CYP 2C9 hepatic microsomal isoenzymes. N-desmethylation converts sildenafil into the major circulating metabolite, which accounts for about 20% of the pharmacologic effects of sildenafil.
*Excretion:* About 80% of an oral dose is metabolized and excreted in the feces, and about 13% is excreted in the urine.

| Route | Onset | Peak | Duration |
|-------|-------|------|----------|
| P.O. | Unknown | ½-2 hr | 4 hr |

### Contraindications and precautions
Contraindicated in patients also using organic nitrates and in those hypersensitive to drug or its components.

Use with caution in patients who have had an MI, CVA, or life-threatening arrhythmias within the past 6 months; have a history of cardiac failure, coronary artery disease, or uncontrolled high or low blood pressure; in those with anatomic deformation of the penis; and in those predisposed to priapism (sickle cell anemia, multiple myeloma, leukemia), retinitis pigmentosa, bleeding disorders, or active peptic ulcers.

### Interactions
**Drug-drug.** *Inhibitors of cytochrome P-450 isoforms 3A4, such as cimetidine, erythromycin, itraconazole, and ketoconazole:* May reduce the clearance of sildenafil. Avoid use together.

---

*Nitrates:* Sildenafil enhances the hypotensive effects of nitrates. Don't use together.

*Protease inhibitors, delavirdine:* Increased sildenafil plasma levels and may result in an increase in sildenafil-associated adverse events, including hypotension, visual changes, and priapism. Patient shouldn't exceed 25 mg of sildenafil in a 48-hour period.

*Rifampin:* May reduce sildenafil plasma levels. Advise clinician to monitor effect closely.

**Drug-food.** *High-fat meals:* May delay absorption of drug and onset of action by 1 hour. Separate administration time from meals.

## Adverse reactions
**CNS:** *headache,* dizziness.
**CV:** *flushing.*
**EENT:** nasal congestion, abnormal vision (photophobia, color blindness).
**GI:** dyspepsia, diarrhea.
**GU:** urinary tract infection.
**Skin:** rash.

## Overdose and treatment
In healthy volunteers, doses up to 800 mg produced adverse events similar to those seen at lower doses, but at an increased rate. Advise clinician to use standard supportive measures to treat overdose. Renal dialysis isn't expected to increase clearance.

## Clinical considerations
■ Because cardiac risk is related to sexual activity, advise clinician to evaluate patient's CV status before therapy starts.
■ Drug seems to have favorable teratogenic, embryotoxic, and fetotoxic profiles, and isn't readily distributed into semen; it isn't expected to be harmful to pregnant women.

### Therapeutic monitoring
■ Advise clinician to monitor patient's compliance with drug regimen.

### Special populations
**Breast-feeding patients.** Drug isn't indicated for use in women.
**Pediatric patients.** Drug shouldn't be used in children or neonates.
**Geriatric patients.** Reduced drug clearance is seen in healthy geriatric patients ages 65 or older. This reduction results in plasma levels about 40% greater than those in younger subjects.

## Patient counseling
■ Tell patient that drug doesn't protect against sexually transmitted diseases and that he should use protective measures to prevent infection.
■ Advise patient that drug is most rapidly absorbed if taken on an empty stomach.
■ Tell patient to notify prescriber of visual changes.

■ Urge patient to seek medical attention if erection persists for longer than 4 hours.
■ Advise patient that drug has no effect in the absence of sexual stimulation.
■ Advise patient receiving HIV drugs that there is an increased risk of sildenafil-associated adverse events, including hypotension, visual changes, and priapism, and that he should promptly report any symptoms to his prescribers. Tell him not to exceed 25 mg of sildenafil in a 48-hour period.

# simethicone
Alka-Seltzer, Flatulex, Gas-X, Maalox, Mylanta, Mylicon, Phazyme

*Pharmacologic classification:* dispersant
*Therapeutic classification:* antiflatulent
*Pregnancy risk category C*

## Available forms
Available without a prescription
*Capsules:* 125 mg, 166 mg
*Suspension:* 40 mg/0.6 ml, 50 mg/5 ml
*Tablets:* 62.5 mg
*Tablets (chewable):* 40 mg, 80 mg, 125 mg, 150 mg, 166 mg

## Indications and dosages
*Flatulence, functional gastric bloating*
*Adults and children ages 12 and older:* 40 to 125 mg P.O. after each meal and h.s.
*Children ages 2 to 12:* 40 mg (drops) P.O. q.i.d.
*Children under age 2:* 20 mg (drops) P.O. q.i.d., up to 240 mg/day.

## Mechanism of action
*Antiflatulent action:* Simethicone acts as a defoaming agent by decreasing the surface tension of gas bubbles, preventing the formation of mucous-coated gas bubbles.

## Pharmacokinetics
**Absorption:** None.
**Distribution:** None.
**Metabolism:** None.
**Excretion:** Excreted in feces.

| Route | Onset | Peak | Duration |
|-------|-------|------|----------|
| P.O. | Immediate | Unknown | Unknown |

## Contraindications and precautions
Contraindicated in patients hypersensitive to drug.

## Interactions
**Drug-drug.** *Alginic acid:* Decreased effectiveness of alginic acid. Advise clinician to monitor patient closely.

## Adverse reactions

**GI:** expulsion of excessive liberated gas as belching, rectal flatus.

## Overdose and treatment

No information available.

## Clinical considerations

- Simethicone is found in many combination antacid products.
- This drug doesn't prevent formation of gas.

### Therapeutic monitoring

- Advise clinician to monitor patient's response to drug therapy.

### Special populations

**Pediatric patients.** Simethicone isn't recommended as treatment for infant colic; it has limited use in children.

## Patient counseling

- Tell patient to chew tablets thoroughly or to shake suspension well before using. Advise patient that liquid-filled capsules should not be chewed.
- Encourage patient to change positions frequently and ambulate to aid flatus passage.

# simvastatin

Zocor

*Pharmacologic classification:* HMG-CoA reductase inhibitor
*Therapeutic classification:* antilipemic, cholesterol-lowering drug
*Pregnancy risk category X*

## Available forms

Available by prescription only
*Tablets:* 5 mg, 10 mg, 20 mg, 40 mg, 80 mg

## Indications and dosages

*Adjunct to diet for reduction of low-density lipoprotein (LDL) and total cholesterol levels in patients with primary hypercholesterolemia (types IIa and IIb) and mixed dyslipidemia and in patients with coronary heart disease and hypercholesterolemia to reduce the risk of coronary death, nonfatal MI, CVA, transient ischemic attack, and undergoing myocardial revascularization procedures; to increase high-density lipoprotein cholesterol levels in patients with primary hypercholesterolemia and mixed dyslipidemia (Fredrickson types IIa and IIb); as an adjunct to diet to reduce elevated total cholesterol, low-density lipoprotein-cholesterol (LDL-C), apolipoprotein B, and triglyceride levels in patients with primary hypercholesterolemia and mixed dyslipidemia; hypertriglyc-*
eridemia (Fredrickson type IV hyperlipidemia), primary dysbetalipoproteinemia (Fredrickson type III hyperlipidemia)
*Adults:* Initially, 20 mg P.O. daily in the evening. Dosage adjusted q 4 weeks based on patient tolerance and response. Maintenance dose is usually 5 to 80 mg daily.
*Geriatric patients:* Initially, 5 mg P.O. daily in the evening. Maximum, 20 mg daily.
***Reduction of total cholesterol and LDL in patients with homozygous familial hypercholesterolemia***
*Adults:* 40 mg daily in the evening or 80 mg daily given in three divided doses of 20 mg, 20 mg, and 40 mg in the evening.
≣*Dosage adjustment.* For patients receiving immunosuppressants, start with 5 mg/day; maximum daily dose, 10 mg. For patients with mild to moderate renal insufficiency, give usual daily dose; in those with severe renal impairment, start therapy with 5 mg P.O. daily and closely monitor patient.

## Mechanism of action

*Antilipemic action:* Simvastatin inhibits the enzyme 3-hydroxy-3-methylglutaryl-coenzyme A (HMG-CoA) reductase. This hepatic enzyme is an early (and rate-limiting) step in the synthetic pathway of cholesterol.

## Pharmacokinetics

*Absorption:* Readily absorbed; however, extensive hepatic extraction limits the plasma availability of active inhibitors to 5% of a dose or less. Individual absorption varies considerably.
*Distribution:* Parent drug and active metabolites are more than 95% plasma protein–bound.
*Metabolism:* Hydrolysis occurs in the plasma; at least three major metabolites have been identified.
*Excretion:* Excreted primarily in bile.

| Route | Onset | Peak | Duration |
|-------|-------|------|----------|
| P.O. | Unknown | 1⅓-½ hr | Unknown |

## Contraindications and precautions

Contraindicated in patients hypersensitive to drug and in those with active hepatic disease or conditions that cause unexplained persistent elevations of serum transaminase; in pregnant and breast-feeding women; and in women of childbearing age unless there's no risk of pregnancy.

Use cautiously in patients with history of liver disease or who consume excessive amounts of alcohol.

## Interactions

**Drug-drug.** *Cimetidine, ketoconazole, spironolactone:* May increase the risk of development of endocrine dysfunction. No intervention appears needed; obtain complete drug history in patients for whom endocrine dysfunction develops.

*Digoxin:* Simvastatin may slightly elevate levels. Recommend closely monitoring plasma digoxin levels at the start of simvastatin therapy.

*Erythromycin; fibric acid derivatives such as clofibrate and gemfibrozil; high doses of niacin (nicotinic acid; 1 g or more daily); immunosuppressive drugs such as cyclosporine:* May increase risk of rhabdomyolysis. Advise clinician to monitor patient closely if use together can't be avoided. Limit daily dose of simvastatin to 10 mg if patient must take cyclosporine.

*Hepatotoxic drugs:* Increased risk for hepatotoxicity. Avoid use together.

*Warfarin:* Simvastatin may slightly enhance the anticoagulant effect. Advise clinician to monitor PT and INR at the start of therapy and during dosage adjustment.

**Drug-herb.** *Red yeast rice:* Contains similar components to those of statin drugs, increasing the risk of adverse events or toxicity. Discourage use together.

**Drug-food.** *Grapefruit juice:* Elevated levels of drug increasing the risk of side effects. Drug should be taken with liquid other than grapefruit juice.

**Drug-lifestyle.** *Alcohol use:* May increase the risk of hepatotoxicity. Advise patient to avoid alcohol.

### Adverse reactions
**CNS:** headache, asthenia.
**GI:** abdominal pain, constipation, diarrhea, dyspepsia, flatulence, nausea, vomiting.
**Hepatic:** elevated liver enzyme levels.
**Respiratory:** upper respiratory tract infection.

### Overdose and treatment
There has been no experience with simvastatin overdose. No specific antidote is known. Treatment is symptomatic.

### Clinical considerations
■ Simvastatin should be started only after diet and other nonpharmacologic therapies have proved ineffective. Patient should continue a cholesterol-lowering diet during therapy.

#### Therapeutic monitoring
■ Dosage adjustments should be made about every 4 weeks. If the cholesterol levels decrease below the target range, dose may be reduced.
■ Perform liver function tests frequently when therapy starts and periodically thereafter.

#### Special populations
**Pregnant patients.** Safety hasn't been established. Patient should immediately notify prescriber if pregnancy occurs or is suspected.

**Breast-feeding patients.** It isn't known if drug appears in breast milk. Because of the risk to infants, avoid breast-feeding during therapy.
**Pediatric patients.** Safety and efficacy in children haven't been established.
**Geriatric patients.** Most geriatric patients respond to daily dose of 20 mg or less.

### Patient counseling
■ Tell patient that drug should be taken in the evening and may be taken without regard to meals.
■ Tell patient to report adverse reactions, particularly muscle aches and pains.
■ Explain importance of controlling serum lipids to CV health. Teach appropriate dietary management (restricting total fat and cholesterol intake), weight control, and exercise.

## sirolimus
Rapamune

*Pharmacologic classification:* macrocyclic lactone
*Therapeutic classification:* immunosuppressant
*Pregnancy risk category C*

### Available forms
Available by prescription only
*Oral solution:* 1 mg/ml
*Tablet:* 1 mg

### Indications and dosages
***Prophylaxis, with cyclosporine and corticosteroids, of organ rejection in patients receiving renal transplants***
*Adults and adolescents ages 13 and older who weigh 40 kg (88 lb) or more:* Initially, 6 mg P.O. as a one-time loading dose as soon as possible after transplantation; then maintenance dose of 2 mg P.O. once daily.
*Adolescents ages 13 and older who weigh less than 40 kg:* Initially, 3 mg/m$^2$ P.O. as a one-time loading dose after transplantation; then maintenance dose of 1 mg/m$^2$ P.O. once daily.
**≡ *Dosage adjustment.*** In patients with mild to moderate hepatic impairment, reduce maintenance dose by about one-third. It isn't necessary to reduce loading dose.

### Mechanism of action
*Immunosuppressant action:* Sirolimus is an immunosuppressant that inhibits T-lymphocyte activation and proliferation that occur in response to antigenic and cytokine stimulation. Drug also inhibits antibody formation.

### Pharmacokinetics
*Absorption:* Rapidly absorbed from GI tract, with mean peak levels occurring in about 1 to 3 hours. Oral bioavailability of the solution is about 14%, and even higher with the tablets.

*Severe metabolic acidosis*
*Adults:* Dose depends on blood carbon dioxide content, pH, and patient's clinical condition. Generally, administer 90 to 180 mEq/L I.V. during first hour, then adjust, p.r.n.
*Less urgent metabolic acidosis*
*Adults and adolescents:* 2 to 5 mEq/kg as a 4 to 8 hour I.V. infusion.
*Urinary alkalization*
*Adults:* 48 mEq (4 g) P.O. initially, then 12 to 24 mEq (1 to 2 g) every 4 hours. May need doses of 30 to 48 mEq (2.5 to 4 g) every 4 hours, up to 192 mEq (16 g) daily.
*Children:* 1 to 10 mEq (84 to 840 mg)/kg P.O. daily.
*Antacid*
*Adults:* 300 mg to 2 g P.O. one to four times daily.

## I.V. administration
■ Administer by rapid, direct I.V. injection.
■ Carefully irrigate I.V. tubing with 5 to 10 ml bolus of normal saline solution after administration of sodium bicarbonate.

### Incompatibilities
Incompatible with alcohol 5% in dextrose 5%, amino acids, ascorbic acid injection, calcium salts, carmustine, cisplatin, codeine phosphate, corticotropin, dextrose 5% in lactated Ringer's injection, dobutamine, dopamine, epinephrine hydrochloride, fat emulsion 10% glycopyrrolate, hydromorphone, ionosol B, D, or G with invert sugar 10%, isoproterenol, labetalol, lactated Ringer's injection, levorphanol, magnesium sulfate, meperidine, methadone, methicillin, methylprednisolone sodium succinate, metoclopramide, morphine sulfate, norepinephrine bitartrate, penicillin G potassium, pentazocine lactate, pentobarbital sodium, phenobarbital sodium, procaine, promazine regular insulin, Ringer's injection, secobarbital, sodium lactate (1/6 M), streptomycin, succinylcholine, thiopental, vancomycin, and vitamin B complex with vitamin C.

## Mechanism of action
*Alkalizing buffering action:* Sodium bicarbonate is an alkalinizing agent that dissociates to provide bicarbonate ion. Bicarbonate in excess of that needed to buffer hydrogen ions causes systemic alkalinization and, when excreted, urinary alkalinization as well.
*Oral antacid action:* Taken orally, sodium bicarbonate neutralizes stomach acid by the above mechanism.

## Pharmacokinetics
*Absorption:* Well absorbed after oral administration as sodium ion and bicarbonate.
*Distribution:* Occurs naturally and is confined to the systemic circulation.
*Metabolism:* None.

*Excretion:* Filtered and reabsorbed by the kidney; less than 1% of filtered bicarbonate is excreted.

| Route | Onset | Peak | Duration |
|-------|-------|------|----------|
| P.O. | Unknown | Unknown | Unknown |
| I.V. | Immediate | Immediate | Unknown |

## Contraindications and precautions
Contraindicated in patients with metabolic or respiratory alkalosis; in those who are losing chlorides by vomiting or from continuous GI suction; in those receiving diuretics known to produce hypochloremic alkalosis; and in patients with hypocalcemia in which alkalosis may produce tetany, hypertension, seizures, or HF. Orally administered sodium bicarbonate is contraindicated in patients with acute ingestion of strong mineral acids.

Use with extreme caution in patients with HF, renal insufficiency, or other edematous or sodium-retaining conditions.

## Interactions
**Drug-drug.** *Amphetamines, ephedrine, pseudoephedrine, quinidine:* If urinary alkalinization occurs, sodium bicarbonate increases half-life of these drugs. Advise clinician to monitor patient closely.
*Chlorpropamide, lithium, salicylates, tetracyclines:* Increased urinary excretion of these drugs. Advise clinician to monitor patient closely.
*Corticosteroids:* May increase sodium retention. Advise clinician to monitor patient closely.

## Adverse reactions
**GI:** gastric distention, belching, flatulence.
**Metabolic:** *metabolic alkalosis,* hypernatremia, increased serum lactate levels, hyperosmolarity (with overdose).
**Skin:** local pain and irritation at injection site.

## Overdose and treatment
Signs of overdose include depressed consciousness and obtundation from hypernatremia, tetany from hypocalcemia, arrhythmias from hypokalemia, and seizures from alkalosis. Recommend correcting fluid, electrolyte, and pH abnormalities. Advise clinician to monitor vital signs and fluid and electrolytes closely.

## Clinical considerations
**◄ ALERT** Sodium bicarbonate isn't routinely recommended for use in cardiac arrest because it may produce a paradoxical acidosis from carbon dioxide production.
■ Advise clinician to monitor blood gases and adjust dosage p.r.n.
■ Extravasation of I.V. solutions should be avoided. Addition of calcium salts may cause precipitate; bicarbonate may inactivate cate-

---

cholamines in solution (epinephrine, phenylephrine, and dopamine).

■ Discourage use as an oral antacid because of hazardous excessive systemic absorption.

■ Drug may be used as an adjunct to treat hyperkalemia (with dextrose and insulin).

### Therapeutic monitoring

■ Advise clinician to monitor blood pH, partial pressure of arterial oxygen, partial pressure of arterial carbon dioxide and serum electrolytes.

■ Patient should be assessed for milk-alkali syndrome if drug use is long-term.

■ Advise clinician to monitor vital signs regularly and, when drug is used as urinary alkalinizer, monitor urine pH.

### Special populations

**Pregnant patients.** Safety hasn't been established for use during pregnancy.

**Breast-feeding patients.** It isn't known if sodium bicarbonate appears in breast milk. Use cautiously when giving to breast-feeding women.

**Pediatric patients.** Treatment of metabolic acidosis after cardiac arrest in children has not been fully evaluated. Avoid rapid infusion (10 ml/minute) of hypertonic solutions in children under age 2.

**Geriatric patients.** Geriatric patients with HF or other fluid-retaining conditions are at greater risk for increased fluid retention; therefore, use drug with caution.

### Patient counseling

■ Advise patient not to take drug with milk. Drug may cause hypercalcemia, alkalosis, and possibly renal calculi.

■ If patient takes an oral dose form, tell patient to take drug 1 hour before or 2 hours after taking enteric-coated drugs because drug may cause enteric-coated products to dissolve in the stomach.

---

# sodium ferric gluconate complex

Ferrlecit

*Pharmacologic classification:* macro-molecular iron complex
*Therapeutic classification:* hematinic
*Pregnancy risk category B*

### Available forms

Available by prescription only
*Injection:* 62.5 mg elemental iron (12.5 mg/ml) in 5-ml ampules

### Indications and dosages

*Treatment of iron deficiency anemia in patients undergoing chronic hemodialysis*

*who are receiving supplemental erythro-poietin therapy*

*Adults:* Before initiating therapeutic doses, administer a test dose of 2 ml sodium ferric gluconate complex (25 mg elemental iron) diluted in 50 ml normal saline and given I.V. over 1 hour. If test dose is tolerated, give therapeutic dose of 10 ml (125 mg elemental iron) diluted in 100 ml normal saline and given I.V. over 1 hour. Most patients require a minimum cumulative dose of 1 g elemental iron administered at more than eight sequential dialysis treatments to achieve a favorable hemoglobin or hematocrit response.

### I.V. administration

■ Dilute test dose of sodium ferric gluconate complex in 50 ml normal saline and recommend giving over 1 hour. Dilute therapeutic doses of drug in 100 ml normal saline and recommend giving over 1 hour.

■ Don't mix sodium ferric gluconate complex with other drugs, or add to parenteral nutrition solutions for I.V. infusion. Use immediately after dilution in normal saline.

### Incompatibilities

Don't mix sodium ferric gluconate complex with other drugs or add to parenteral nutrition solutions for I.V. infusion. Use immediately after dilution in normal saline.

### Mechanism of action

*Hematinic action:* Sodium ferric gluconate complex restores total body iron content, which is critical for normal hemoglobin synthesis and oxygen transport. Iron deficiency in hemodialysis patients can be caused by increased iron utilization (such as from erythropoietin therapy), blood loss (such as from fistula, retention in dialyzer, hematologic testing, menses), decreased dietary intake or absorption, surgery, iron sequestration resulting from inflammatory process, and malignancy.

### Pharmacokinetics

No information available.

| Route | Onset | Peak | Duration |
|-------|-------|------|----------|
| I.V. | Unknown | Unknown | Unknown |

### Contraindications and precautions

Contraindicated in patients hypersensitive to sodium ferric gluconate complex or its components (such as benzyl alcohol). Also contraindicated in patients with anemias not related to iron deficiency. Don't give to patients with iron overload.

Use cautiously in geriatric patients.

### Interactions

None reported.

---

## Adverse reactions

**CNS:** asthenia, headache, fatigue, malaise, dizziness, paresthesia, agitation, insomnia, somnolence, syncope.

**CV:** hypotension, hypertension, tachycardia, *bradycardia,* angina, chest pain, *MI,* edema.

**EENT:** conjunctivitis, abnormal vision, rhinitis.

**GI:** nausea, vomiting, diarrhea, rectal disorder, dyspepsia, eructation, flatulence, melena, abdominal pain.

**GU:** urinary tract infection.

**Hematologic:** abnormal erythrocytes, anemia.

**Metabolic:** hyperkalemia, hypoglycemia, hypokalemia, hypervolemia.

**Musculoskeletal:** myalgia, arthralgia, back pain, arm pain, cramps.

**Respiratory:** dyspnea, coughing, upper respiratory tract infections, pneumonia, pulmonary edema.

**Skin:** pruritus, increased sweating, rash, flushing.

**Other:** injection site reaction, pain, fever, infection, rigors, chills, flulike syndrome, sepsis, *carcinoma,* hypersensitivity reactions, lymphadenopathy.

## Overdose and treatment

Serum iron levels greater than 300 mcg/dl (with transferrin oversaturation) may indicate iron poisoning. Symptoms include abdominal pain, diarrhea, or vomiting that progresses to pallor or cyanosis; lassitude; drowsiness; hyperventilation resulting from acidosis; and CV collapse. Treatment consists of supportive measures. Drug isn't dialyzable.

## Clinical considerations

**H ALERT** Dosage is expressed in milligrams of elemental iron.

■ Drug shouldn't be given to patients with iron overload, which generally occurs in hemoglobinopathies and other refractory anemias.

**H ALERT** Potentially life-threatening hypersensitivity reactions, characterized by CV collapse, cardiac arrest, bronchospasm, oral or pharyngeal edema, dyspnea, angioedema, urticaria, or pruritus sometimes associated with pain and muscle spasm of chest or back, may occur during infusion. Have adequate supportive measures readily available. Advise clinician to monitor patient closely during infusion.

■ Some adverse reactions in hemodialysis patients may be related to dialysis itself or to chronic renal failure.

■ Profound hypotension associated with flushing, light-headedness, malaise, fatigue, weakness, or severe chest, back, flank, or groin pain has been reported after rapid I.V. administration of iron. These reactions aren't associated with hypersensitivity reactions and may be caused by too-rapid administration of drug. Don't exceed recommended rate of adminis-

tration (2.1 mg/min). Advise clinician to monitor patient closely during infusion.

### Therapeutic monitoring

■ Advise clinician to monitor hematocrit and hemoglobin, serum ferritin, and iron saturation levels during therapy, p.r.n.

■ Check with patient about other potential sources of iron, such as nonprescription iron preparations and iron-containing multiple vitamins with minerals.

### Special populations

**Breast-feeding patients.** It's unknown if drug appears in breast milk. Use caution when giving drug to breast-feeding women.

**Pediatric patients.** Safety and efficacy of drug haven't been established in children.

**Geriatric patients.** It's unknown if patients ages 65 and older respond differently than younger patients. In general, use cautiously in geriatric patients because they may be taking other drugs or may have concomitant disease or decreased hepatic, renal, or cardiac function.

## Patient counseling

■ Advise patient to immediately report these symptoms of iron poisoning: abdominal pain, diarrhea, vomiting, drowsiness, and hyperventilation.

# sodium fluoride

ACT, Fluorigard, Fluorinse, Fluoritab, Flura-Drops, Flura-Loz, Karidium, Karigel, Karigel-N, Listermint with Fluoride, Luride, Luride Lozi-Tabs, Luride-SF Lozi-Tabs, Pediaflor, Phos-Flur, Point-Two, Prevident, Thera-Flur, Thera-Flur-N

*Pharmacologic classification:* trace mineral
*Therapeutic classification:* dental caries prophylactic
*Pregnancy risk category C*

## Available forms

Available by prescription only
*Drops:* 0.125 mg/drop (30 ml), 0.125 mg/drop (60 ml, sugar-free), 0.25 mg/drop (19 ml), 0.25 mg/drop (24 ml, sugar-free), 0.5 mg/ml (50 ml)
*Gel:* 0.1% (65 g, 105 g, 122 g), 0.5% (24 g, 30 g, 60 g, 120 g, 130 g, 250 g), 1.23% (480 ml)
*Gel drops:* 0.5% (24 ml)
*Rinse:* 0.09% (240 ml, 480 ml), 0.09% (480 ml, sugar-free)
*Tablets:* 1 mg (sugar-free)
*Tablets (chewable):* 0.5 mg, 1 mg (sugar-free)
Available without a prescription
*Gel:* 0.1%
*Rinse:* 0.02%; 0.04%; 0.08%; 0.2%

## Indications and dosages

*Aid in the prevention of dental caries*

**Oral**

*Children ages 6 months to 2 years:* 0.25 mg daily.

*Children ages 3 to 5:* 0.5 mg daily.

*Children ages 6 to 16:* 1 mg daily.

≡ *Dosage adjustment.* If fluoride in the drinking water is less than 0.3 parts per million (ppm), use dosage listed; if fluoride content is 0.3 to 0.7 ppm, use one half of dosage; if fluoride content exceeds 0.7 ppm, don't use.

**Topical**

*Adults and children over age 12:* 10 ml of 0.09% (0.2% fluoride ion) rinse. Use once daily after thoroughly brushing teeth and rinsing mouth. Rinse around and between teeth for 1 minute, then spit out.

*Children ages 6 to 12:* 5 ml of 0.09% (0.2% fluoride ion) solution.

## Mechanism of action

*Dental caries prophylactic action:* Sodium fluoride acts systemically before tooth eruption and topically afterward by increasing tooth resistance to acid dissolution, by promoting remineralization, and by inhibiting the cariogenic microbial process. Acidulation provides greater topical fluoride uptake by dental enamel than neutral solutions. When topical fluoride is applied to hypersensitive exposed dentin, the formation of insoluble materials within the dentinal tubules blocks transmission of painful stimuli.

## Pharmacokinetics

*Absorption:* Absorbed readily and almost completely from the GI tract. A large amount of an oral dose may be absorbed in the stomach; rate of absorption may depend on the gastric pH. Normal total plasma fluoride levels range from 0.14 to 0.19 mcg/ml.

*Distribution:* Stored in bones and developing teeth after absorption. Skeletal tissue also has a high storage capacity for fluoride ions. Because of the storage-mobilization mechanism in skeletal tissue, a constant fluoride supply may be provided. Fluoride has been found in all organs and tissues with a low accumulation in noncalcified tissues. Fluoride is distributed into sweat, tears, hair, and saliva. Fluoride crosses the placenta and appears in breast milk. Fluoride levels in milk range from about 0.05 to 0.13 ppm and remain fairly constant.

*Metabolism:* Not metabolized.

*Excretion:* Excreted rapidly, mainly in urine. About 90% of fluoride is filtered by the glomerulus and reabsorbed by the renal tubules.

| Route | Onset | Peak | Duration |
|-------|-------|------|----------|
| P.O. | Unknown | 30-60 min | Unknown |

## Contraindications and precautions

Contraindicated in patients hypersensitive to fluoride or when intake from drinking water exceeds 0.6 ppm.

## Interactions

**Drug-drug.** *Aluminum hydroxide or magnesium:* May impair the absorption of sodium fluoride. Recommend giving drugs at separate times.

**Drug-food.** *Dairy foods:* Incompatibility may occur because of the formation of calcium fluoride, which is poorly absorbed. Avoid use together.

## Adverse reactions

**CNS:** headache, weakness.

**GI:** gastric distress, staining of teeth.

**Skin:** hypersensitivity reactions (atopic dermatitis, eczema, urticaria).

## Overdose and treatment

In children, acute ingestion of 10 to 20 mg of sodium fluoride may cause excessive salivation and GI disturbances; 500 mg may be fatal. GI disturbances include salivation, nausea, abdominal pain, vomiting, and diarrhea. CNS disturbances include CNS irritability, paresthesia, tetany, hyperactive reflexes, seizures, and respiratory or cardiac failure (from the calcium-binding effect of fluoride). Hypoglycemia and hypocalcemia are frequent laboratory findings.

By using gastric lavage with 1% to 5% calcium chloride solution, the fluoride may be precipitated. Recommend giving glucose I.V. in saline solution; parenteral calcium administration may be indicated for tetany. Recommend maintaining adequate urine output.

## Clinical considerations

■ Recommended doses are currently under study. Some evidence suggests that considerably less fluoride is needed for adequate supplementation.

■ Tablets can be dissolved in the mouth, chewed, swallowed whole, added to drinking water or fruit juice, or added to water in infant formula or other foods.

■ Drops may be administered orally undiluted or added to fluids or food.

■ Sodium fluoride may be preferred to stannous fluoride to avoid staining tooth surfaces. Neutral sodium fluoride may also be preferred to acidulated fluoride to avoid dulling of porcelain and ceramic restorations.

■ Prolonged intake of drinking water containing a fluoride ion concentration of 0.4 to 0.8 ppm may result in increased density of bone mineral and fluoride osteosclerosis.

■ An oral sodium fluoride dose of 40 to 65 mg/day has resulted in adverse rheumatic effects.

■ Drug is used investigationally to treat osteoporosis.

### Therapeutic monitoring
■ Fluoride supplementation must be continuous from infancy to age 14 to be effective.
■ Review dietary history with the family. A diet that includes large amounts of fish, mineral water, and tea provides about 5 mg/day of fluoride.

### Special populations
**Breast-feeding patients.** Very little sodium fluoride appears in breast milk. The fluoride levels in breast milk increase only when daily intake exceeds 1.5 mg.
**Pediatric patients.** Young children usually can't perform the rinse process needed with oral solutions. Because prolonged ingestion or improper techniques may result in dental fluorosis and osseous changes, the dose must be carefully adjusted according to the amount of fluoride ion in drinking water.

### Patient counseling
■ Tell patient that sodium fluoride tablets and drops should be taken with meals, but not with dairy products.
■ Advise patient that rinse and gel are most effective if used immediately after brushing or flossing and when taken just before retiring to bed.
■ Tell patient to expectorate (and not swallow) excess liquid or gel.
■ Warn patient not to eat, drink, or rinse mouth for 15 to 30 minutes after application. Tell patient to use a plastic container—not glass—to dilute drops or rinse, because the fluoride interacts with glass.
■ Encourage patient to notify dentist if mottling of teeth occurs.
■ Advise patient that if there is a change in water supply or if the patient moves to another area, then a dentist should be contacted because excessive fluoride causes mottled tooth enamel. If patient uses a private well, the water should be tested for fluoride.
■ Warn parents to treat fluoride tablets as a drug and to keep them away from children.

# sodium phosphates (sodium phosphate and sodium biphosphate)
Fleet Phospho-soda

*Pharmacologic classification:* acid salt
*Therapeutic classification:* NaCl laxative
*Pregnancy risk category C*

### Available forms
Available without a prescription

*Solution:* 2.4 g monobasic sodium phosphate and 0.9 g dibasic sodium biphosphate/5 ml

## Indications and dosages
### Constipation
*Adults:* 20 to 45 ml solution daily, mixed with 4 ounces (120 ml) cold water.
*Children ages 10 to 11:* 10 to 20 ml solution daily mixed with 4 ounces cold water.
*Children ages 5 to 9:* 5 to 10 ml solution daily mixed with 4 ounces cold water.
### Purgative action
*Adults:* 45 ml solution mixed with 4 ounces cold water.

## Mechanism of action
*Laxative action:* Sodium phosphate and sodium biphosphate exert an osmotic effect in the small intestine by drawing water into the intestinal lumen, producing distention that promotes peristalsis and bowel evacuation.

## Pharmacokinetics
*Absorption:* About 1% to 20% of an oral dose of sodium and phosphate is absorbed. With oral administration, action begins in 3 to 6 hours.
*Distribution:* Unknown.
*Metabolism:* Unknown.
*Excretion:* Unknown; probably in feces and urine.

| Route | Onset | Peak | Duration |
|-------|-------|------|----------|
| P.O. | Variable | Variable | Variable |

## Contraindications and precautions
Contraindicated in patients with abdominal pain, nausea, vomiting, or other symptoms of appendicitis or acute surgical abdomen; intestinal obstruction or perforation; edema; HF; megacolon; or impaired renal function and in patients on sodium-restricted diets.

Use cautiously in patients with large hemorrhoids or anal excoriations.

## Interactions
**Drug-drug.** *Antacids:* May cause inactivation of both. Don't use together.

## Adverse reactions
**GI:** *abdominal cramping.*
**Metabolic:** fluid and electrolyte disturbances (hypernatremia, hyperphosphatemia) with daily use.
**Other:** laxative dependence with long-term or excessive use.

## Overdose and treatment
No information available; probable clinical effects include abdominal pain and diarrhea.

## Clinical considerations
■ Dilute drug with water before giving orally (add 30 ml of drug to 120 ml of water). Fol-

---

low drug administration with full glass of water.
- Drug isn't routinely used to treat constipation but is commonly used to evacuate the bowel.

### Therapeutic monitoring
- Advise clinician to monitor serum electrolyte levels; when drug is given as NaCl laxative, up to 10% of sodium content may be absorbed.

### Special populations
**Breast-feeding patients.** It's not known if drug appears in breast milk. Use cautiously in nursing women.

### Patient counseling
- Instruct patient on how to mix the drug.
- Instruct patient on dose schedule.
- Warn patient that frequent or prolonged use of drug may lead to laxative dependence.
- Teach patient about dietary sources of bulk, which include bran and other cereals, fresh fruit, and vegetables.
- Tell patient to drink 8 ounces of cool water after taking Fleet Phospho-soda.
- For children under age 5, parent should contact prescriber.

---

# sodium polystyrene sulfonate
Kayexalate, Kionex, SPS

*Pharmacologic classification:* cation-exchange resin
*Therapeutic classification:* potassium-removing resin
*Pregnancy risk category C*

## Available forms
Available by prescription only
*Oral powder:* 1.25 g/5 ml suspension
*Powder for oral or rectal administration:* 454 g in 1-lb jar
*Rectal administration:* 1.25 g/5 ml, 15 g/60 ml suspension

## Indications and dosages
### Hyperkalemia
*Adults:* 15 g P.O. daily to q.i.d. in water or sorbitol. Alternatively, give 30 to 50 g q.i.d. or q 6 hours as a retention enema.

## Mechanism of action
*Potassium-removing action:* Sodium polystyrene sulfonate is a cation-exchange resin that releases sodium in exchange for other cations in the GI tract. High levels of potassium ion are found in the large intestine and therefore are exchanged and eliminated.

## Pharmacokinetics
*Absorption:* Not absorbed. The onset of action varies from hours to days.
*Distribution:* None.
*Metabolism:* None.
*Excretion:* Excreted unchanged in feces.

| Route | Onset | Peak | Duration |
|-------|-------|------|----------|
| P.O., P.R. | Unknown | Unknown | Unknown |

## Contraindications and precautions
Contraindicated in patients with hypokalemia or those hypersensitive to drug.
  Use cautiously in patients with marked edema or severe HF or hypertension.

## Interactions
**Drug-drug.** *Cardiac glycosides:* Toxic effects are exaggerated by hypokalemia, even when serum digoxin levels are in the normal range. Don't use together.
*Magnesium- and calcium-containing antacids:* Metabolic alkalosis in patients with renal impairment. Don't use together.

## Adverse reactions
**GI:** *constipation,* fecal impaction (in geriatric patients), anorexia, gastric irritation, nausea, vomiting, *diarrhea* (with sorbitol emulsions).
**Metabolic:** *hypokalemia,* hypocalcemia, sodium retention, altered serum magnesium level.

## Overdose and treatment
Signs and symptoms of overdose include signs and symptoms of hypokalemia, such as irritability, confusion, arrhythmias, ECG changes, severe muscle weakness, and sometimes paralysis; and digitalis toxicity in digitalized patients. Drug may be discontinued or dose lowered when serum potassium level decreases to the 4 to 5 mEq/L range.

## Clinical considerations
- For oral administration: mix resin only with water or sorbitol; never mix with orange juice because of its high potassium content.
- Chill oral suspension to increase palatability; don't heat because that inactivates resin.
- Recommend using P.R. route when vomiting, P.O. restrictions, or upper GI tract problems are present.
- Fecal impaction can be prevented in geriatric patients by giving resin P.R. Cleaning enema should precede rectal administration.
- For rectal administration, mix polystyrene resin only with water and sorbitol for rectal use. Don't use other vehicles such as mineral oil for rectal administration to prevent impactions. Ion exchange requires aqueous medium. Sorbitol content prevents impaction. Prepare rectal dose at room temperature. Stir emulsion gently during administration.

---

■ Constipation is more likely when drug is given with phosphate binders such as aluminum hydroxide. Advise clinician to monitor patient's bowel habits.

### Therapeutic monitoring
■ Advise clinician to monitor serum potassium at least once daily and watch for other signs of hypokalemia.
■ Advise clinician to monitor patient for symptoms of other electrolyte deficiencies (magnesium, calcium) because drug is nonselective. Advise clinician to monitor serum calcium determination in patients receiving sodium polystyrene therapy for longer than 3 days. Supplementary calcium may be needed.
■ If hyperkalemia is severe, more drastic modalities should be added; for example, dextrose 50% with regular insulin I.V. push. Don't depend solely on polystyrene resin to lower serum potassium levels in severe hyperkalemia.

### Special populations
**Pediatric patients.** Dosage should be adjusted in children based on a calculation of 1 mEq of potassium bound for each 1 g of resin.
**Geriatric patients.** Fecal impaction is more likely in geriatric patients.

### Patient counseling
■ Instruct patient in the importance of following a prescribed low-potassium diet.
■ Explain necessity of retaining enema to patient. Retention for 6 to 10 hours is ideal, but 30 to 60 minutes is acceptable.

# somatropin
Genotropin, Humatrope, Nutropin

*Pharmacologic classification:* anterior pituitary hormone
*Therapeutic classification:* purified growth hormone (GH)
*Pregnancy risk category C*

### Available forms
Available by prescription only
*Injection:* 10 mg (30 IU)/2-ml vial
*Powder for injection:* 5 mg (15 IU)/vial with 5-ml diluent

### Indications and dosages
*Long-term treatment of growth failure in children with inadequate secretion of endogenous GH*
*Children:* 0.18 mg/kg of body weight of Humatrope S.C. or I.M. weekly divided equally and given on either 3 alternate days or six times per week; or 0.3 mg/kg of body weight of Nutropin S.C. weekly in daily divided doses. Alternatively, 0.16 to 0.24 mg/kg/week of Genotropin, divided into 5 to 7 doses S.C.

*Growth failure in children from chronic renal insufficiency up to time of renal transplantation*
*Children:* Administer 0.35 mg/kg of body weight of Nutropin S.C. weekly in daily divided doses.
*Long-term treatment of growth failure in children with Prader-Willi syndrome diagnosed by genetic testing*
*Children:* 0.24 mg/kg/week of Genotropin, divided into 5 to 7 doses S.C.
*Long-term replacement therapy in adults with GH deficiency of either childhood- or adult-onset etiology and confirmed by appropriate GH stimulation tests*
*Adults:* Starting dose is not more than 0.04 mg/kg/week of Genotropin, divided into 5 to 7 doses S.C. Dosage may be increased at 4- to 8-week intervals to a maximum dose 0.08 mg/kg/week, divided into 5 to 7 doses S.C.
*Long-term treatment of growth failure in children born small for gestational age who do not achieve catch-up growth by 2 years of age*
*Children:* 0.48 mg/kg/week of Genotropin, divided into 5 to 7 doses S.C.

### Mechanism of action
*Growth-stimulating action:* Somatropin is a purified GH of recombinant DNA origin that stimulates skeletal, linear bone, muscle, and organ growth.

### Pharmacokinetics
*Absorption:* Absorbed from the injection site in a similar fashion as somatrem (human GH).
*Distribution:* Localizes to highly perfused organs, notably the liver and kidney.
*Metabolism:* Metabolized in the liver.
*Excretion:* Returned to the systemic circulation as amino acids.

| Route | Onset | Peak | Duration |
|-------|-------|------|----------|
| I.M., S.C. | Unknown | 3-5 hr | 12-48 hr |

### Contraindications and precautions
Contraindicated in patients with closed epiphyses or an active underlying intracranial lesion. Humatrope shouldn't be reconstituted with the supplied diluent for patients with known sensitivity to either m-Cresol or glycerin.

Use cautiously in children with hypothyroidism and in those whose GH deficiency results from an intracranial lesion; these children should be examined frequently for progression or recurrence of underlying disease.

### Interactions
None reported.

---

## Adverse reactions

**CNS:** headache, weakness.
**CV:** mild, transient edema.
**Hematologic:** *leukemia.*
**Metabolic:** mild hyperglycemia, hypothyroidism; inorganic phosphorus, alkaline phosphatase, and parathyroid hormone levels may increase.
**Other:** injection site pain, localized muscle pain, antibody formation to GH.

## Overdose and treatment

Long-term overdose may cause signs and symptoms of gigantism or acromegaly consistent with the known effects of excess human GH.

## Clinical considerations

- To prepare solution, inject the supplied diluent into the vial containing the drug by aiming the stream of the liquid against the glass wall of the vial. Swirl the vial with a gentle rotary motion until the contents are completely dissolved. Don't shake the vial.
- After reconstitution, vial solution should be clear. Don't use if it's cloudy or contains particles.
- Store reconstituted vial in refrigerator; use within 14 days.
- If sensitivity to diluent occurs, vial may be reconstituted with sterile water for injection. When drug is reconstituted in this manner, use only one reconstituted dose per vial and refrigerate the solution if it isn't used immediately after reconstitution. Use reconstituted dose within 24 hours, and discard unused portion.

### Therapeutic monitoring

- Advise clinician to monitor child's height regularly. Regular monitoring of blood and radiologic studies is also needed.
- Advise clinician to monitor patient's blood glucose levels regularly because GH may induce a state of insulin resistance.
- Excessive glucocorticoid therapy inhibits the growth-promoting effect of somatropin. Advise clinician to adjust glucocorticoid replacement dose in patients with a coexisting corticotropin deficiency to avoid an inhibitory effect on growth.
- Periodically monitor thyroid function test results for hypothyroidism, which may require treatment with a thyroid hormone.

## Patient counseling

- Inform parents that children with endocrine disorders including GH deficiency are more likely to develop slipped capital epiphyses. Tell them to call if they notice their child limping.
- Stress to parents importance of close follow-up care.

# sotalol

Betapace, Betapace AF

*Pharmacologic classification:* beta blocker
*Therapeutic classification:* anti-arrhythmic
*Pregnancy risk category B*

## Available forms

Available by prescription only
*Tablets:* 80 mg, 120 mg, 160 mg, 240 mg

## Indications and dosages

*Documented, life-threatening ventricular arrhythmias*
*Adults:* Initially, 80 mg P.O. b.i.d. Increase dose q 3 days p.r.n. and as tolerated. Most patients respond to daily dose of 160 to 320 mg. A few patients with refractory arrhythmias have received as much as 640 mg daily.
≡*Dosage adjustment.* For adults with renal impairment and creatinine clearance above 60 ml/minute, no adjustment in dosage interval is needed. If creatinine clearance is 30 to 60 ml/minute, give q 24 hours; 10 to 30 ml/minute, q 36 to 48 hours; and if it is less than 10 ml/minute, individualize dosage.
*Maintenance of normal sinus rhythm (delay in time to recurrence of atrial fibrillation/atrial flutter [AFIB/AFL]) in patients with symptomatic AFIB/AFL who are currently in sinus rhythm*
*Adults:* (Betapace AF only) Initially, 80 mg P.O. b.i.d. If initial dose does not reduce the frequency of relapses of AFIB/AFL and is tolerated without excessive QT interval prolongation (such as ≥ 520 msec), the dose level may be increased after 3 days to 120 mg P.O. b.i.d. Maximum dose is 160 mg P.O. b.i.d.
≡*Dosage adjustment.* In patients with creatinine clearance of 40 to 60 ml/min, dose once daily. Do not give to patients with a creatinine clearance less than 40 ml/min.

## Mechanism of action

*Antiarrhythmic action:* Sotalol is a nonselective beta blocker that depresses sinus heart rate, slows AV conduction, increases AV nodal refractoriness, prolongs the refractory period of atrial and ventricular muscle and AV accessory pathways in anterograde and retrograde directions, decreases cardiac output, and lowers systolic and diastolic blood pressure.

## Pharmacokinetics

*Absorption:* Well absorbed after oral administration, with a bioavailability of 90% to 100%. After oral administration, steady-state plasma levels are attained in 2 to 3 days (after five to six doses when given b.i.d.).

---

*Distribution:* Doesn't bind to plasma proteins and crosses the blood-brain barrier poorly.
*Metabolism:* Not metabolized.
*Excretion:* Excreted primarily in urine unchanged.

| Route | Onset | Peak | Duration |
|-------|-------|------|----------|
| P.O. | Unknown | 2½-4 hr | Unknown |

## Contraindications and precautions

Contraindicated in patients hypersensitive to drug and those with severe sinus node dysfunction, sinus bradycardia, second- and third-degree AV block in the absence of an artificial pacemaker, congenital or acquired long QT syndrome, cardiogenic shock, uncontrolled HF, and bronchial asthma.

Use cautiously in patients with impaired renal function or diabetes mellitus.

## Interactions

**Drug-drug.** *Antacids:* Decreased effects of sotalol. Advise patient to take 2 hours apart.
*Antiarrhythmics:* Cause additive effects when given with sotalol. Avoid use together.
*Calcium channel antagonists:* Enhance myocardial depression. Don't give with sotalol.
*Catecholamine-depleting drugs, such as guanethidine and reserpine:* Enhance the hypotensive effects of sotalol. Advise clinician to monitor patient closely.
*Clonidine:* Sotalol may enhance the rebound hypertensive effect seen after withdrawal of clonidine. Discontinue sotalol several days before withdrawing clonidine.
*Insulin, oral antidiabetics:* Increase blood glucose levels; may mask symptoms of hypoglycemia. Sotalol may require dosage adjustments with these drugs.
**Drug-food.** *Any food:* Decreases absorption. Drug should be given on an empty stomach.

## Adverse reactions

**CNS:** asthenia, light-headedness, headache, dizziness, weakness, fatigue, sleep problems.
**CV:** *bradycardia, palpitations, chest pain, arrhythmias, HF, AV block, proarrhythmic events (ventricular tachycardia, PVCs, ventricular fibrillation),* edema, ECG abnormalities, hypotension.
**GI:** *nausea, vomiting,* diarrhea, dyspepsia.
**Hepatic:** elevated liver enzyme levels.
**Metabolic:** increased serum glucose levels.
**Respiratory:** *dyspnea, bronchospasm.*

## Overdose and treatment

The most common signs of overdose are bradycardia, HF, hypotension, bronchospasm, and hypoglycemia. If overdose occurs, sotalol should be stopped and the patient observed closely. Because of the lack of protein binding, hemodialysis is useful in reducing sotalol plasma levels. Advise clinician to observe pa-

tient carefully until QT intervals are normalized.

Atropine, another anticholinergic, a beta-adrenergic agonist, or transvenous cardiac pacing may also be used to treat bradycardia; transvenous cardiac pacing to treat second- or third-degree heart block; epinephrine to treat hypotension (depending on associated factors); aminophylline or an aerosol beta₂-receptor stimulant to treat bronchospasm; and electric cardioversion, transvenous cardiac pacing, epinephrine, or magnesium sulfate to treat torsades de pointes.

## Clinical considerations

■ Because proarrhythmic events, such as sustained ventricular tachycardia or ventricular fibrillation, may occur at start of therapy and during dosage adjustments, patient should be hospitalized. Facilities and personnel should be available for cardiac rhythm monitoring and ECG interpretation.
■ Although patients receiving I.V. lidocaine have begun sotalol therapy without ill effect, other antiarrhythmics should be withdrawn before sotalol therapy begins. Sotalol therapy typically is delayed until two or three half-lives of the withdrawn drug have elapsed. After withdrawal of amiodarone, sotalol shouldn't be given until the QT interval normalizes.
■ The baseline QT interval must be ≤ 450 msec to start a patient on Betapace AF. During initiation and titration, advise clinician to monitor QT interval 2 to 4 hours after each dose. If the QT interval prolongs ≥ 500 msec, the dosage must be reduced or the drug discontinued.

### *Therapeutic monitoring*

■ Make dosage adjustments slowly, allowing 2 to 3 days between dose increments for adequate monitoring of QT intervals and for drug plasma levels to reach steady state.
■ Advise clinician to monitor serum electrolytes regularly, especially if patient is receiving diuretics. Electrolyte imbalances, such as hypokalemia or hypomagnesemia, may enhance QT prolongation and increase risk of serious arrhythmias, such as torsades de pointes.

### *Special populations*

**Pregnant patients.** Safety hasn't been established. Use only when potential benefits outweigh the risks to the fetus.
**Breast-feeding patients.** Because drug may appear in breast milk, either breast-feeding or sotalol may be discontinued depending on importance of drug to woman's health.
**Pediatric patients.** Safety and efficacy in children haven't been established.

## Patient counseling
■ Explain importance of taking sotalol as prescribed, even when feeling well.
■ Caution patient not to discontinue drug suddenly.
■ Tell patient not to take antacids within 2 hours of taking sotalol.

# sparfloxacin
Zagam

*Pharmacologic classification:* fluorinated quinolone
*Therapeutic classification:* broadspectrum antibacterial
*Pregnancy risk category C*

## Available forms
Available by prescription only
*Tablets:* 200 mg

## Indications and dosages
*Acute bacterial exacerbation of chronic bronchitis caused by* Staphylococcus aureus, Streptococcus pneumoniae, Chlamydia pneumoniae, Enterobacter cloacae, Klebsiella pneumoniae, Moraxella catarrhalis, Haemophilus influenzae, *or* H. parainfluenzae; *community-acquired pneumonia caused by* S. pneumoniae, M. catarrhalis, H. influenzae, H. parainfluenzae, C. pneumoniae, *or* Mycoplasma pneumoniae
*Adults over age 18:* 400 mg P.O. on first day as a loading dose, then 200 mg daily for total of 10 days of therapy (total, 11 tablets).
≡ *Dosage adjustment.* In patients with renal impairment, if creatinine clearance is less than 50 ml/minute, give a loading dose of 400 mg P.O.; thereafter, 200 mg P.O. q 48 hours for a total of 9 days of therapy (total, six tablets).

## Mechanism of action
*Antibactericidal action:* Inhibits bacterial DNA gyrase and prevents DNA replication, transcription, repair, and deactivation in susceptible bacteria.

## Pharmacokinetics
*Absorption:* Well absorbed after oral administration with an absolute bioavailability of 92%.
*Distribution:* Volume of distribution is about 3.9 L/kg, indicating distribution well into the tissues. Level of drug in respiratory tissues at 2 to 6 hours after dosing is about three to six times greater than plasma.
*Metabolism:* Metabolized by the liver, primarily by phase II glucuronidation. Its metabolism doesn't interfere with or use the cytochrome P-450 system.
*Excretion:* Excreted in both the urine (50%) and feces (50%). Terminal elimination half-

life varies between 16 and 30 hours; mean, 20 hours.

| Route | Onset | Peak | Duration |
|-------|-------|------|----------|
| P.O. | Unknown | 3-6 hr | Unknown |

## Contraindications and precautions
Contraindicated in patients with history of hypersensitivity or photosensitivity reactions to drugs and those who can't stay out of the sun. Don't use in patients with cardiac conditions that predispose them to arrhythmias. Contraindicated in patients taking drugs that prolong the QTc interval.

Use with caution in patients with known or suspected CNS disorders, such as seizures, toxic psychoses, or tremors.

## Interactions
**Drug-drug.** *Antacids containing aluminum or magnesium, iron salts, zinc, or sucralfate:* May interfere with GI absorption of sparfloxacin. Recommend giving at least 4 hours apart.
*Drugs that prolong the QTc interval, including amiodarone, bepridil, disopyramide, class Ia antiarrhythmics (procainamide, quinidine), class III drugs (sotalol); erythromycin, pentamidine, tricyclic antidepressants, and some antipsychotics including phenothiazines:* May cause torsades de pointes. Don't give together.
**Drug-lifestyle.** *Sun exposure:* May cause photosensitivity reactions. Advise patient to take precautions.

## Adverse reactions
**CNS:** asthenia, dizziness, headache, insomnia, *seizures,* somnolence.
**CV:** *QT interval prolongation,* vasodilatation.
**GI:** abdominal pain, diarrhea, dyspepsia, flatulence, nausea, pseudomembranous colitis, dry mouth, taste perversion, vomiting.
**GU:** vaginal candidiasis.
**Hematologic:** elevated WBC.
**Hepatic:** elevated liver enzyme levels.
**Musculoskeletal:** tendon rupture.
**Skin:** photosensitivity, pruritus, rash.
**Other:** hypersensitivity reactions.

## Overdose and treatment
If overdose is suspected, have patient avoid sunlight exposure for 5 days. Advise clinician to monitor ECG for possible QTc prolongation. It isn't known if drug is dialyzable.

## Clinical considerations
■ Use cautiously in patients with a history of seizure disorder or other CNS diseases, such as cerebral arteriosclerosis.
■ Acute hypersensitivity reactions may require treatment with epinephrine, oxygen, I.V. fluids, antihistamines, corticosteroids, pressor amines, and airway management.
■ Drug may produce false-negative culture results for *Mycobacterium tuberculosis.*

### Therapeutic monitoring
- Advise clinician to monitor renal function.
- Specimen for culture and sensitivity should be obtained before therapy starts and p.r.n. to determine if bacterial resistance has occurred.

### Special populations
**Breast-feeding patients.** Because drug appears in breast milk, recommend stopping either breast-feeding or drug.
**Pediatric patients.** Safety and efficacy of children and adolescents under age 18 haven't been established. Benefit-risk balance should be carefully considered. Quinolones, including sparfloxacin, cause arthropathy and osteochondrosis in juvenile animals of several species.
**Geriatric patients.** Pharmacokinetics of drug aren't altered in geriatric patients with normal renal function. Advise clinician to monitor renal function carefully and adjust doses p.r.n.

### Patient counseling
- Inform patient that drug may be taken with food, milk, or products that contain caffeine.
- Tell patient to take drug as prescribed, even if symptoms disappear.
- Advise patient to take drug with plenty of fluids and to avoid antacids, sucralfate, and products containing iron or zinc for at least 4 hours after each dose.
- Warn patient to avoid hazardous tasks until adverse CNS effects of drug are known.
- Tell patient to discontinue drug and report pain or inflammation; tendon rupture may occur with drug. Tell patient to rest and refrain from exercise until a diagnosis is made.

---

# spironolactone
Aldactone

*Pharmacologic classification:* potassium-sparing diuretic
*Therapeutic classification:* management of edema; antihypertensive; diagnosis of primary hyperaldosteronism; treatment of diuretic-induced hypokalemia
*Pregnancy risk category NR*

### Available forms
Available by prescription only
*Tablets:* 25 mg
*Tablets (film-coated):* 25 mg, 50 mg, 100 mg

### Indications and dosages
**Edema**
*Adults:* 25 to 200 mg P.O. daily in divided doses.
*Children:* Initially, 3.3 mg/kg or 60 mg/m$^2$ P.O. daily in divided doses.

**Hypertension**
*Adults:* 25 to 100 mg P.O. daily as a single dose or in divided doses.
*Children:* 1 to 2 mg/kg P.O. b.i.d. has been used.
**Diuretic-induced hypokalemia**
*Adults:* 25 to 100 mg P.O. daily when oral potassium supplements are considered inappropriate or inadequate.
**Detection of primary hyperaldosteronism**
*Adults:* 400 mg P.O. daily for 4 days (short test) or for 3 to 4 weeks (long test). If hypokalemia and hypertension are corrected, a presumptive diagnosis of primary hyperaldosteronism is made.
◇ **Hirsutism**
*Adults:* 50 to 200 mg P.O. daily.
◇ **Premenstrual syndrome**
*Adults:* 25 mg q.i.d. P.O. on day 14 of menstrual cycle.
◇ **Heart failure in patients receiving an angiotensin-converting enzyme (ACE) inhibitor and a loop diuretic with or without a cardiac glycoside**
*Adults:* Initially, 12.5 to 25 mg P.O. daily. May increase to 50 mg daily after 8 weeks of treatment for those patients with progressive HF with no hyperkalemia.
◇ **To decrease risk of metrorrhagia**
*Adults:* 50 mg b.i.d. P.O. on days 4 through 21 of menstrual cycle.
◇ **Acne vulgaris**
*Adults:* 100 mg P.O. daily.

### Mechanism of action
*Antihypertensive action:* The mechanism of action is unknown; spironolactone may block the effect of aldosterone on arteriolar smooth muscle.
*Diagnosis of primary hyperaldosteronism:* Spironolactone inhibits the effects of aldosterone; therefore, correction of hypokalemia and hypertension is presumptive evidence of primary hyperaldosteronism.
*Diuretic and potassium-sparing actions:* Spironolactone competitively inhibits aldosterone effects on the distal renal tubules, increasing sodium and water excretion and decreasing potassium excretion.

Spironolactone is used to treat edema caused by excessive aldosterone secretion, such as that from hepatic cirrhosis, nephrotic syndrome, and HF. It's also used to treat diuretic-induced hypokalemia.

### Pharmacokinetics
*Absorption:* About 90% is absorbed after oral administration.
*Distribution:* Drug and its major metabolite, canrenone, are more than 90% plasma protein–bound.
*Metabolism:* Rapidly and extensively metabolized to canrenone.
*Excretion:* Canrenone and other metabolites are excreted primarily in urine, and a small

---

amount is excreted in feces via the biliary tract; half-life of canrenone is 13 to 24 hours. Half-life of parent compound is 1 to 2 hours.

| Route | Onset | Peak | Duration |
|-------|-------|------|----------|
| P.O. | 1-2 days | 2-3 days | 2-3 days |

## Contraindications and precautions

Contraindicated in patients with anuria, acute or progressive renal insufficiency, or hyperkalemia.

Use cautiously in patients with impaired renal function, hepatic disease, or fluid and electrolyte imbalances.

## Interactions

**Drug-drug.** *Anesthetics, norepinephrine:* Reduced response to these drugs. Use together cautiously.

*Aspirin:* May slightly decrease the clinical response to spironolactone. Advise clinician to watch for diminished effect.

*Cardiac glycosides:* Increased serum digoxin levels and subsequent toxicity. Advise clinician to monitor drug levels of digoxin.

*NSAIDs, such as ibuprofen or indomethacin:* May impair renal function and thus affect potassium excretion. Use together cautiously.

*Other antihypertensives:* Spironolactone may potentiate the hypotensive effects. May be used to therapeutic advantage.

*Other potassium-sparing diuretics, ACE inhibitors, potassium supplements, potassium-containing drugs such as parenteral penicillin G:* Spironolactone increases the risk of hyperkalemia when given with these drugs. Use together cautiously, especially in patients with renal impairment.

**Drug-herb.** *Licorice:* Antiulcer and aldosterone-like effects of herb may be blocked. There is also an increased risk of hypokalemia. Discourage concomitant use.

**Drug-food.** *Potassium-containing salt substitutes, potassium-rich foods, such as citrus fruit and tomatoes:* Increase the risk of hyperkalemia. Low-potassium salt substitutes and high-potassium foods should be ingested cautiously.

## Adverse reactions

**CNS:** headache, drowsiness, lethargy, confusion, ataxia.

**GI:** diarrhea, gastric bleeding, ulceration, cramping, gastritis, vomiting.

**GU:** inability to maintain erection, menstrual disturbances.

**Hematologic:** *agranulocytosis.*

**Metabolic:** *hyperkalemia,* dehydration, hyponatremia, transient elevation in BUN, *metabolic acidosis.*

**Skin:** urticaria, maculopapular eruptions, hirsutism.

**Other:** drug fever, gynecomastia, breast soreness in women.

## Overdose and treatment

Signs of overdose are consistent with dehydration and electrolyte disturbance.

Treatment is supportive and symptomatic. In acute ingestion, recommend emptying stomach by emesis or lavage. In severe hyperkalemia (more than 6.5 mEq/L), recommend reducing serum potassium levels with I.V. sodium bicarbonate or glucose with insulin. A cation exchange resin, sodium polystyrene sulfonate (Kayexalate), given orally or as a retention enema, may also reduce serum potassium levels.

## Clinical considerations

- Recommend giving drug with meals to enhance absorption.
- Protect drug from light.
- Spironolactone is antiandrogenic and has been used to treat hirsutism in doses of 200 mg/day.
- Avoid unnecessary use of drug. Drug has been shown to induce tumors in laboratory animals.
- Spironolactone therapy alters fluorometric determinations of plasma and urinary 17-hydroxycorticosteroid levels and may cause false elevations on radioimmunoassay of serum digoxin.

### Therapeutic monitoring

- Diuretic effect may be delayed 2 to 3 days if drug is used alone; maximum antihypertensive effect may be delayed 2 to 3 weeks.
- Adverse reactions are related to dose levels and duration of therapy and usually disappear with withdrawal of drug; however, gynecomastia may persist.
- Advise clinician to watch for hyperchloremic metabolic acidosis.

### Special populations

**Breast-feeding patients.** Safety during breast-feeding hasn't been established. Canrenone, a metabolite, appears in breast milk. Alternative feeding method is recommended during therapy with spironolactone.

**Pediatric patients.** When giving drug to children, recommend crushing tablets and giving them in cherry syrup as an oral suspension.

**Geriatric patients.** Geriatric patients are more susceptible to diuretic effects and may require lower doses to prevent excessive diuresis.

## Patient counseling

- Instruct patient to report mental confusion or lethargy immediately.
- Explain that adverse reactions usually disappear after drug is discontinued; gynecomastia, however, may persist.
- Caution patient to avoid such hazardous activities as driving until response to drug is known.

---

# stavudine (d4T)
Zerit

*Pharmacologic classification:* synthetic
thymidine nucleoside analogue
*Therapeutic classification:* antiviral
*Pregnancy risk category C*

## Available forms
Available by prescription only
*Capsules:* 15 mg, 20 mg, 30 mg, 40 mg
*Oral solution:* 1 mg/ml

## Indications and dosages
*Treatment of patients with HIV infection
who have received prolonged prior zidovudine therapy*
*Adults and children weighing 60 kg (132 lb)
or more:* 40 mg P.O. q 12 hours.
*Adults and children weighing over 30 kg (66 lb)
but under 60 kg (132 lb):* 30 mg P.O. q 12 hours.
*Children weighing under 30 kg (66 lb):*
1 mg/kg q 12 hours.
≡ *Dosage adjustment.* For adults with renal
impairment, refer to the table below.

| Creatinine clearance (ml/min) | Dosage for patients weighing ≥ 60 kg | Dosage for patients weighing < 60 kg |
|---|---|---|
| 26-50 | 20 mg q 12 hours | 15 mg q 12 hours |
| 10-25 | 20 mg q 24 hours | 15 mg q 24 hours |

*Adults undergoing hemodialysis:* 20 mg q 24
hours for patients weighing 132 lb or more and
15 mg q 24 hours for patients weighing under
60 kg.

## Mechanism of action
*Antiviral action:* Stavudine is phosphorylated
by cellular kinases to stavudine triphosphate,
which slows HIV replication by inhibiting HIV
reverse transcriptase and inhibiting viral DNA
synthesis. The triphosphate also inhibits cellular DNA polymerase beta and gamma and
reduces mitochondrial DNA synthesis.

## Pharmacokinetics
*Absorption:* Rapidly absorbed with a mean absolute bioavailability of 86.4%.
*Distribution:* Mean volume of distribution is
58 L, suggesting distribution into extravascular space. Drug is distributed equally between
RBCs and plasma. It binds poorly to plasma
proteins.
*Metabolism:* Not clearly defined.
*Excretion:* Renal elimination accounts for
about 40% of overall clearance, regardless of

administration route; there's active tubular secretion in addition to glomerular filtration.

## Contraindications and precautions
Contraindicated in patients hypersensitive to
drug.
    Use cautiously in patients with impaired re-
nal function or history of peripheral neuropathy and in pregnant women.

## Interactions
**Drug-drug.** *Didanosine and hydroxyurea:* Increased risk of hepatotoxicity and pancreatitis. Advise clinician to monitor closely.

## Adverse reactions
**CNS:** *peripheral neuropathy, headache,
malaise, insomnia, anxiety, depression, ner-
vousness, asthenia,* dizziness.
**CV:** chest pain.
**EENT:** conjunctivitis.
**GI:** *abdominal pain, diarrhea, nausea, vom-
iting, anorexia,* dyspepsia, constipation.
**Hematologic:** *neutropenia, thrombocytope-
nia,* anemia.
**Hepatic:** elevated liver enzyme levels, *hepa-
totoxicity.*
**Metabolic:** weight loss.
**Musculoskeletal:** *myalgia, back pain, arthral-
gia.*
**Respiratory:** *dyspnea.*
**Skin:** *rash, diaphoresis, pruritus,* macu-
lopapular rash.
**Other:** *chills, fever,* **lactic acidosis.**

## Overdose and treatment
Experience with adults who had received 12
to 24 times the recommended daily dose revealed no acute toxicity. Complications of
chronic overdose include peripheral neuropathy and hepatic toxicity. It isn't known if drug
is eliminated by peritoneal dialysis or hemodialysis.

## Clinical considerations
■ Use cautiously in patients with renal impairment or history of peripheral neuropathy.
Dosage adjustment may be needed.
■ Advise clinician to monitor patient for development of peripheral neuropathy, usually
characterized by numbness, tingling, or pain
in the feet or hands. If symptoms develop, drug
therapy should be interrupted. Symptoms may
resolve if therapy is withdrawn promptly. Sometimes symptoms may worsen temporarily after drug discontinuation. If symptoms resolve
completely, treatment should be resumed using the following dosage schedule: patients
weighing 132 lb or more should receive 20 mg
b.i.d.; patients weighing under 132 lb should
receive 15 mg b.i.d. Clinically significant elevations of hepatic transaminase levels should
be managed in the same way.

■ If neuropathy recurs after restarting drug, consideration should be given to permanently discontinuing drug.

■ Use with other antiretroviral drugs.

**ℍ ALERT** Don't confuse this drug with other antivirals that may use initials for identification.

### Therapeutic monitoring

■ Advise clinician to monitor CBC and serum levels of creatinine, AST, ALT, and alkaline phosphatase.

### Special populations

**Pregnant patients.** Avoid use; benefits should clearly outweigh risk to patient and fetus.

**Breast-feeding patients.** It isn't known if drug appears in breast milk. Because of the potential for adverse reactions from stavudine in breast-fed infants, breast-feeding should be stopped during therapy.

### Patient counseling

■ Inform patient that stavudine isn't a cure for HIV infection and that the patient may continue to acquire illnesses related to AIDS or AIDS-related complex, including opportunistic infections.

■ Inform patient that drug doesn't reduce risk of transmitting HIV to others through sexual contact or blood contamination.

■ Instruct patient to report signs of peripheral neuropathy, such as tingling, burning, pain, or numbness in the hands or feet, because dosage adjustments may be needed.

■ Advise patient not to use other drugs, including OTC preparations, without contacting prescriber first.

■ Explain that long-term effects of drug are currently unknown.

## streptokinase

Kabikinase, Streptase

*Pharmacologic classification:* plasminogen activator
*Therapeutic classification:* thrombolytic enzyme
*Pregnancy risk category C*

### Available forms

Available by prescription only
*Injection:* 250,000 IU, 750,000 IU, 1,500,000 IU in vials for reconstitution

### Indications and dosages

**Lysis of coronary artery thrombi after acute MI**

*Adults:* 1,500,000 IU by I.V. infusion over 60 minutes; intracoronary loading dose of 15,000 to 20,000 IU in a small amount of diluent, via coronary catheter, followed by a maintenance dose of 2,000 to 4,000 IU/minute for 60 minutes as an infusion.

**Venous thrombosis, pulmonary embolism, and arterial thrombosis and embolism**

*Adults:* Loading dose of 250,000 IU I.V. infusion over 30 minutes. Sustaining dose: 100,000 IU/hour I.V. infusion for 72 hours for deep vein thrombosis and 100,000 IU/hour over 24 hours by I.V. infusion pump for pulmonary embolism.

**Arteriovenous cannula occlusion**

*Adults:* 250,000 IU in 2 ml I.V. solution by I.V. infusion pump into each occluded limb of the cannula over 25 to 35 minutes. Clamp off cannula for 2 hours, then aspirate contents of cannula, flush with saline solution, and reconnect. The manufacturer doesn't recommend using drug to restore patency of occluded I.V. catheters.

◇ **Arterial occlusion in children**

*Children:* Loading dose of 1,000 to 3,000 IU/kg I.V., then a maintenance infusion of 1,000 to 1,500 IU/kg/hour up to 24 hours.

### I.V. administration

■ Reconstitute vial with 5 ml normal saline injection, and further dilute to 45 ml; roll gently to mix. Don't shake. Use immediately; refrigerate remainder and discard after 8 hours. Store powder at room temperature.

■ Rate of I.V. infusion depends on thrombin time and streptokinase resistance; higher loading dose may be needed in patients with recent streptococcal infection or recent treatment with streptokinase, to compensate for antibody drug neutralization.

### Incompatibilities

Incompatible with dextrans. Don't mix with other drugs.

### Mechanism of action

*Thrombolytic action:* Streptokinase promotes thrombolysis by activating plasminogen in two steps. First, plasminogen and streptokinase form a complex, exposing plasminogen-activating site, and second, cleavage of peptide bond converts plasminogen to plasmin.

In treatment of acute MI, streptokinase prevents primary or secondary thrombus formation in microcirculation surrounding the necrotic area.

### Pharmacokinetics

*Absorption:* Administered I.V. Plasminogen activation begins promptly after infusion or instillation of streptokinase.

*Distribution:* Doesn't cross placenta, but antibodies do.

*Metabolism:* Insignificant.

*Excretion:* Removed from circulation by antibodies and reticuloendothelial system. Half-life is biphasic; initially it's 18 minutes (from antibody action) and then extends up to 83 minutes. Anticoagulant effect may persist for 12 to 24 hours after infusion is discontinued.

| Route | Onset | Peak | Duration |
|-------|-------|------|----------|
| I.V. | Immediate | 20 min-2 hr | 4 hr |

## Contraindications and precautions
Contraindicated in patients with ulcerative wounds, active internal bleeding, and recent CVA; recent trauma with possible internal injuries; visceral or intracranial malignant neoplasms; ulcerative colitis; diverticulitis; severe hypertension; acute or chronic hepatic or renal insufficiency; uncontrolled hypocoagulation; chronic pulmonary disease with cavitation; subacute bacterial endocarditis or rheumatic valvular disease; or recent cerebral embolism, thrombosis, or hemorrhage.

Also contraindicated within 10 days after intra-arterial diagnostic procedure or any surgery, including liver or kidney biopsy, lumbar puncture, thoracentesis, paracentesis, or extensive or several cutdowns. I.M. injections and other invasive procedures are contraindicated during streptokinase therapy.

Use cautiously in patients with arterial embolism that originates from the left side of the heart.

Not recommended by manufacturer to restore patency of occluded I.V. catheters, because of the risk of life-threatening reactions.

## Interactions
**Drug-drug.** *Aminocaproic acid:* Inhibits streptokinase-induced activation of plasminogen. Don't use together.
*Anticoagulants:* May cause hemorrhage. It may also be needed to reverse effects of oral anticoagulants before beginning therapy. Advise clinician to monitor patient closely.
*Aspirin, indomethacin, phenylbutazone, or other drugs affecting platelet activity:* Increase risk of bleeding. Advise clinician to monitor patient closely.

## Adverse reactions
**CNS:** polyradiculoneuropathy, headache.
**CV:** reperfusion arrhythmias, *hypotension,* vasculitis.
**EENT:** periorbital edema.
**GI:** nausea.
**Hematologic:** *bleeding.*
**Musculoskeletal:** musculoskeletal pain.
**Respiratory:** minor breathing difficulty, *bronchospasm, apnea.*
**Skin:** urticaria, pruritus, flushing.
**Other:** phlebitis at injection site, hypersensitivity reactions *(anaphylaxis),* delayed hypersensitivity reactions (interstitial nephritis, serum sickness-like reactions), *angioedema, fever.*

## Overdose and treatment
Symptoms of overdose include signs of potentially serious bleeding: bleeding gums, epis-

taxis, hematoma, spontaneous ecchymoses, oozing at catheter site, increased pulse, and pain from internal bleeding. Recommend stopping drug and restarting when bleeding stops.

## Clinical considerations
■ Don't discontinue therapy for minor allergic reactions that can be treated with antihistamines or corticosteroids; about one third of patients experience a slight temperature elevation, and some have chills. Symptomatic treatment with acetaminophen (but not aspirin or other salicylates) is indicated if temperature reaches 104° F (40° C). Patients may be pretreated with corticosteroids, repeating doses during therapy, to minimize pyrogenic or allergic reactions.
■ Death of patient has occurred when pancreatitis symptoms were misindentified as MI symptoms and drug therapy was given.

### Therapeutic monitoring
■ Advise clinician to monitor pulse, color, and sensation of limbs every hour.
■ If minor bleeding can be controlled by local pressure, don't decrease dose so more plasminogen is available for conversion to plasmin.
■ Antibodies to streptokinase can persist for 3 to 6 months or longer after the initial dose; if further thrombolytic therapy is needed, urokinase should be considered.

### Special populations
**Pediatric patients.** Safety and efficacy in children haven't been established. Adverse effects have been noted to be similar to that experienced by adults. Advise clinician to monitor patient closely for bleeding.
**Geriatric patients.** Patients ages 75 or older have a greater risk of cerebral hemorrhage because they're likely to have preexisting cerebrovascular disease.

## Patient counseling
■ Explain use and administration to patient and family.

# streptomycin sulfate

*Pharmacologic classification:* aminoglycoside
*Therapeutic classification:* antibiotic
*Pregnancy risk category D*

## Available forms
Available by prescription only
*Injection:* 400 mg/ml

## Indications and dosages
*Primary and adjunctive treatment in tuberculosis*
*Adults with normal renal function:* 1 g or 15 mg/kg I.M. daily for 2 to 3 months, then

1 g two or three times weekly. Inject deeply into upper outer quadrant of buttocks or midlateral thigh. Maximum daily dose, 1 g.

*Children with normal renal function:* 20 to 40 mg/kg I.M. daily in divided doses injected deeply into large muscle mass, preferably in the midlateral muscles of the thigh. Give with other antitubercular drugs, but not with capreomycin, and continue until sputum specimen becomes negative. Maximum daily dose, 1 g.

≣*Dosage adjustment.* Doses in geriatric patients should depend on age, renal function, and eighth cranial nerve function. Use up to 10 mg/kg (750 mg) daily I.M.

*Enterococcal endocarditis*
*Adults:* 1 g I.M. q 12 hours for 2 weeks, then 500 mg I.M. q 12 hours for 4 weeks with penicillin.

*Tularemia*
*Adults:* 1 to 2 g I.M. daily in divided doses injected deep into upper outer quadrant of buttocks. Continue until patient is afebrile for 5 to 7 days.

*Plague*
*Adults:* 2 g or 30 mg/kg I.M. daily in divided doses injected deep into upper outer quadrant of buttocks for a minimum of 10 days.
*Children:* 30 mg/kg/day I.M. in two to three divided doses for 10 days.

≣*Dosage adjustment.* In adults and children with renal impairment, initial dose is same as for those with normal renal function. Subsequent doses and frequency determined by renal function study results and blood serum levels; peak serum levels shouldn't exceed 20 to 25 mcg/ml, and trough levels should be 5 mcg/ml or less. Patients with a creatinine clearance of more than 50 ml/minute usually can tolerate drug daily; if creatinine clearance is 10 to 50 ml/minute, increase administration interval to q 24 to 72 hours. Patients with a creatinine clearance less than 10 ml/minute may require 72 to 96 hours between doses.

## Mechanism of action
*Antibiotic action:* Streptomycin is bactericidal; it binds directly to the 30S ribosomal subunit, inhibiting bacterial protein synthesis. Its spectrum of activity includes many aerobic gram-negative organisms and some aerobic gram-positive organisms. Streptomycin is generally less active against many gram-negative organisms than is tobramycin, gentamicin, amikacin, or netilmicin. Streptomycin is also active against *Mycobacterium* and *Brucella* organisms.

## Pharmacokinetics
*Absorption:* Absorbed poorly after oral administration and usually is given by deep I.M. injection.
*Distribution:* Widely distributed after parenteral administration; intraocular penetration is poor. CSF penetration is low, even in patients with

inflamed meninges. Streptomycin crosses the placenta, and is 36% protein-bound.
*Metabolism:* Not metabolized.
*Excretion:* Excreted primarily in urine by glomerular filtration; small amounts may be excreted in bile and breast milk. Elimination half-life in adults is 2 to 3 hours. In severe renal damage, half-life may extend to 110 hours.

| Route | Onset | Peak | Duration |
|-------|-------|------|----------|
| I.M. | Unknown | 1-2 hr | Unknown |

## Contraindications and precautions
Contraindicated in patients hypersensitive to drug or other aminoglycosides and in those with labyrinthine disease. Drug should never be administered I.V.

Use cautiously in patients with impaired renal function or neuromuscular disorders and in geriatric patients.

## Interactions
**Drug-drug.** *Amphotericin B, capreomycin, cephalosporins, cisplatin, methoxyflurane, polymyxin B, vancomycin, and other aminoglycosides:* Use with these drugs may increase the hazard of nephrotoxicity, ototoxicity, and neurotoxicity. Use together cautiously.
*Bumetanide, ethacrynic acid, furosemide, mannitol, urea:* Hazard of ototoxicity is increased during use together. Use together cautiously.
*Dimenhydrinate, other antiemetic and antivertigo drugs:* May mask streptomycin-induced ototoxicity. Use together cautiously.
*General anesthetics or neuromuscular blockers, such as succinylcholine and tubocurarine:* Streptomycin may potentiate neuromuscular blockade. Advise clinician to monitor patient closely.
*Penicillin:* Results in synergistic bactericidal effect against *Pseudomonas aeruginosa, Escherichia coli, Klebsiella, Citrobacter, Enterobacter, Proteus mirabilis,* and *Serratia;* however, the drugs are physically and chemically incompatible and are inactivated when mixed or given together. Don't use together.

## Adverse reactions
**CNS:** *neuromuscular blockade.*
**EENT:** *ototoxicity.*
**GI:** vomiting, nausea.
**GU:** some *nephrotoxicity* (not as frequently as with other aminoglycosides).
**Hematologic:** eosinophilia, *leukopenia, thrombocytopenia.*
**Respiratory:** *apnea.*
**Skin:** *exfoliative dermatitis.*
**Other:** hypersensitivity reactions (rash, fever, urticaria, *angioedema), anaphylaxis.*

## Overdose and treatment
Signs of overdose include ototoxicity, nephrotoxicity, and neuromuscular toxicity. Advise clinician to remove drug by hemodialysis or

peritoneal dialysis. Treatment with calcium salts or anticholinesterases reverses neuromuscular blockade.

## Clinical considerations
- Protect hands when preparing drug; drug irritates skin.
- In primary tuberculosis therapy, streptomycin should be stopped when sputum culture is negative.
- Because streptomycin is dialyzable, patients undergoing hemodialysis may need dosage adjustments.
- Streptomycin may cause false-positive reaction in copper sulfate test for urine glucose (Benedict's reagent or Clinitest).

### Therapeutic monitoring
- Check blood for peak streptomycin level 1 to 2 hours after I.M. injection; for trough levels, blood should be drawn just before next dose. Heparinized tube shouldn't be used because heparin is incompatible with aminoglycosides.

### Special populations
**Pregnant patients.** Aminoglycosides have caused fetal harm.
**Pediatric patients.** Use with caution and at reduced doses in premature and full-term neonates because of renal immaturity.

## Patient counseling
- Instruct patient to report adverse reactions promptly.
- Encourage adequate fluid intake.
- Emphasize the need for blood tests to monitor streptomycin levels and determine the effectiveness of therapy.

---

# streptozocin
Zanosar

*Pharmacologic classification:* antibiotic antineoplastic nitrosourea (cell cycle–phase nonspecific)
*Therapeutic classification:* antineoplastic
*Pregnancy risk category C*

## Available forms
Available by prescription only
*Injection:* 1-g vials

## Indications and dosages
Dosage and indications may vary. Check current literature for recommended protocol.
*Metastatic islet cell carcinoma of the pancreas*
*Adults and children:* 500 mg/m$^2$ I.V. for 5 consecutive days q 6 weeks until maximum benefit or toxicity is observed. Alternatively, 1,000 mg/m$^2$ at weekly intervals for first 2 weeks; may be increased to a maximum single dose of 1,500 mg/m$^2$. Usual course of therapy is 4 to 6 weeks.
≡*Dosage adjustment.* In patients with impaired renal function, give 75% of dose if creatinine clearance is 10 to 50 ml/minute and 50% of dose if it's less than 10 ml/minute.

## I.V. administration
- To reconstitute drug, use 9.5 ml of normal saline injection to yield a level of 100 mg/ml.
- Drug may be further diluted in 10 to 200 ml of D$_5$W to infuse over 10 to 15 minutes. It can also be infused over 6 hours.
- Drug may be administered by rapid I.V. push injection.
- Wear gloves to protect the skin from contact during preparation or administration. If contact occurs, wash solution off immediately with soap and water. Follow recommended procedures for the safe preparation, administration, and disposal of chemotherapeutic drugs.

### Incompatibilities
Incompatible with allopurinol, aztreonam, cefepime, piperacillin, and tazobactam.

## Mechanism of action
*Antineoplastic action:* Streptozocin exerts its cytotoxic activity by selectively inhibiting DNA synthesis. The drug also causes cross-linking of DNA strands through an alkylation mechanism.

## Pharmacokinetics
*Absorption:* Administered I.V.
*Distribution:* After an I.V. dose, drug and its metabolites distribute mainly into the liver, kidneys, intestines, and pancreas. Drug hasn't been shown to cross the blood-brain barrier; however, its metabolites achieve levels in the CSF equivalent to the level in the plasma.
*Metabolism:* Extensively metabolized in the liver and kidneys.
*Excretion:* Elimination of drug from the plasma is biphasic, with an initial half-life of 5 minutes and a terminal phase half-life of 35 to 40 minutes. Plasma half-life of metabolites is longer than parent drug. Drug and its metabolites are excreted primarily in urine and a small amount of dose may also be excreted in expired air.

| Route | Onset | Peak | Duration |
|-------|-------|------|----------|
| I.V. | Unknown | Unknown | Unknown |

## Contraindications and precautions
No known contraindications. Use cautiously in patients with preexisting renal and hepatic disease.

## Interactions
**Drug-drug.** *Doxorubicin:* Prolongs elimination half-life of doxorubicin. Reduced dosage of doxorubicin is needed.

---

*Other nephrotoxic drugs:* May potentiate nephrotoxicity caused by streptozocin. Use cautiously.

*Phenytoin:* May decrease effects of streptozocin on the pancreas. Advise clinician to monitor patient carefully.

### Adverse reactions
**CNS:** confusion, lethargy, depression.
**GI:** *nausea, vomiting,* diarrhea.
**GU:** *renal toxicity* (evidenced by azotemia, glycosuria, and renal tubular acidosis), mild proteinuria.
**Hematologic:** *anemia, leukopenia, thrombocytopenia.*
**Hepatic:** elevated liver enzyme levels, jaundice, *liver dysfunction, hepatotoxicity.*
**Metabolic:** hyperglycemia, hypoglycemia, diabetes mellitus.

### Overdose and treatment
Signs and symptoms of overdose include myelosuppression, nausea, and vomiting. Treatment is usually supportive and includes transfusion of blood components and antiemetics.

### Clinical considerations
■ Use drug within 12 hours of reconstitution. Reconstituted solution is a golden color that changes to dark brown upon decomposition.
■ Product contains no preservatives and isn't intended as a multiple-dose vial.
■ Extravasation may cause ulceration and tissue necrosis.
■ Keep dextrose 50% at bedside because of risk of hypoglycemia from sudden release of insulin.
■ Drug has also been used in the treatment of colon cancer, pancreatic adenocarcinoma, and carcinoid tumors. These uses are unlabeled, and dosing schedules and protocols vary.

### Therapeutic monitoring
■ Nausea and vomiting occur in almost all patients within 1 to 4 hours. Make sure patient is being treated with an antiemetic.
■ Mild proteinuria is one of the first signs of renal toxicity and may necessitate dosage reduction.
■ Test urine regularly for protein and glucose.
■ Advise clinician to monitor CBC and liver function test results at least weekly.
■ Renal toxicity resulting from therapy is dose related and cumulative. Advise clinician to monitor renal function before and after each course of therapy. Urinalysis, BUN levels, and creatinine clearance should be obtained before therapy and at least weekly during drug administration. Weekly monitoring should continue for 4 weeks after each course.

### Special populations
**Breast-feeding patients.** It isn't known if drug appears in breast milk. However, because of the potential for serious adverse reactions, mutagenicity, and carcinogenicity in the infant, breast-feeding isn't recommended.

### Patient counseling
■ Encourage adequate fluid intake to increase urine output and reduce potential for renal toxicity.
■ Remind diabetic patients that intensive monitoring of blood glucose levels is needed.
■ Tell patient to report symptoms of anemia, infection, or bleeding immediately.
■ Warn patient that bruising may occur easily because of effect of drug on blood count.

## succimer
Chemet

*Pharmacologic classification:* heavy metal
*Therapeutic classification:* chelating drug
*Pregnancy risk category C*

### Available forms
Available by prescription only
*Capsules:* 100 mg

### Indications and dosages
***Treatment of lead poisoning in children with blood lead levels greater than 45 mcg/dl***
*Children:* Initially, 10 mg/kg or 350 mg/m$^2$ P.O. q 8 hours for 5 days. Higher starting doses aren't recommended. Frequency of administration may be reduced to 10 mg/kg or 350 mg/m$^2$ q 12 hours for an additional 2 weeks of therapy. A course of treatment lasts 19 days and repeated courses may be needed if indicated by weekly monitoring of blood lead levels. A minimum of 2 weeks between courses is recommended unless blood lead levels mandate more prompt action.
≣*Dosage adjustment.* Dose is to be given q 8 hours for 5 days, followed by same dose q 12 hours for 14 days.

| PEDIATRIC DOSES | | | |
|---|---|---|---|
| **Weight** | | **Dose (mg)** | **No. of capsules** |
| **(lb)** | **(kg)** | | |
| 18-35 | 8-15 | 100 | 1 |
| 36-55 | 16-23 | 200 | 2 |
| 56-75 | 24-34 | 300 | 3 |
| 76-100 | 35-44 | 400 | 4 |
| > 100 | > 45 | 500 | 5 |

## Mechanism of action

*Antidote action:* Succimer forms water-soluble chelates and increases the urinary excretion of lead.

## Pharmacokinetics

*Absorption:* Rapidly but variably absorbed after oral administration.
*Distribution:* Unknown.
*Metabolism:* Rapidly and extensively metabolized.
*Excretion:* Excreted 39% in feces as nonabsorbed drug; 9% in urine; 1% as carbon dioxide from the lungs. About 90% of absorbed drug is excreted in urine.

| Route | Onset | Peak | Duration |
|---|---|---|---|
| P.O. | Unknown | 1-2 hr | Unknown |

## Contraindications and precautions

Contraindicated in patients hypersensitive to drug. Use cautiously in patients with impaired renal function.

## Interactions

**Drug-drug.** *Other chelating drugs:* Concurrent administration of succimer with other chelating drugs isn't recommended. Interactions haven't been systematically studied. Avoid use together.

## Adverse reactions

**CNS:** *drowsiness, dizziness, sensory motor neuropathy, sleepiness, paresthesia, headache.*
**CV:** *arrhythmias.*
**EENT:** plugged ears, cloudy film in eyes, otitis media, watery eyes, sore throat, rhinorrhea, nasal congestion.
**GI:** *nausea, vomiting, diarrhea, loss of appetite, abdominal cramps, hemorrhoidal symptoms, metallic taste in mouth, loose stools.*
**GU:** decreased urination, difficult urination, proteinuria, candidiasis.
**Hematologic:** increased platelet count, intermittent eosinophilia.
**Hepatic:** *elevated serum AST, ALT, alkaline phosphatase levels.*
**Metabolic:** *elevated cholesterol levels.*
**Musculoskeletal:** *leg, kneecap, back, stomach, rib, or flank pain.*
**Respiratory:** cough, head cold.
**Skin:** papular rash, herpetic rash, mucocutaneous eruptions, pruritus.
**Other:** *flulike symptoms.*

## Overdose and treatment

No cases of overdose have been reported. In cases of acute overdose, recommend inducing vomiting with ipecac syrup or performing gastric lavage, followed by administration of activated charcoal slurry and appropriate supportive therapy.

## Clinical considerations

■ Identification and abatement of lead sources in child's environment are critical to successful therapy. Chelation therapy isn't a substitute for preventing further exposure and shouldn't be used to permit continued exposure.
■ Don't use drug for treatment of lead poisoning.
■ Patients who have received ethylenediaminetetraacetic acid, with or without dimercaprol, may use succimer as subsequent therapy after an interval of 4 weeks. Use with other chelating drugs isn't recommended.
■ Consider the possibility of allergic or other mucocutaneous reactions each time drug is used, including during the initial course.
■ False-positive results for ketones in urine using nitroprusside reagents (Ketostix) and false decreased levels of serum uric acid and CK have been reported.

### Therapeutic monitoring

■ Advise clinician to monitor serum transaminase levels before and at least weekly during therapy. Patients with a history of hepatic disease should be monitored more closely.
■ Elevated blood lead levels and associated symptoms may return rapidly after drug is discontinued because of redistribution of lead from bone to soft tissues and blood. Advise clinician to monitor patients at least once weekly for rebound blood lead levels.
■ The severity of lead intoxication should be used as a guide for more frequent blood lead monitoring. This is measured by the initial blood lead level and the rate and degree of rebound of blood lead.

### Special populations

**Pediatric patients.** For young children who can't swallow capsules, succimer capsule may be opened and sprinkled on a small amount of soft food, or medicated beads from the capsules may be poured onto a spoon for administration and followed with a fruit drink.

## Patient counseling

■ Instruct parents to maintain child's adequate fluid intake.
■ Tell parents to report rash.
■ Urge parents to identify and remove source of lead in environment.
■ Tell parents to store capsules at room temperature, out of reach of children.

# succinylcholine chloride (suxamethonium chloride)

Anectine, Anectine Flo-Pack, Quelicin, Sucostrin

*Pharmacologic classification:* depolarizing neuromuscular blocker
*Therapeutic classification:* skeletal muscle relaxant
*Pregnancy risk category C*

## Available forms

Available by prescription only
*Injection:* 20 mg/ml, 50 mg/ml, 100 mg/ml (parenteral); 500 mg, 1 g (sterile for I.V. infusion)

## Indications and dosages

*To induce skeletal muscle relaxation; facilitate intubation, ventilation, or orthopedic manipulations; and lessen muscle contractions in induced seizures*
Dosage depends on the anesthetic used, patient's needs, and response. Doses are representative and must be adjusted. Paralysis is induced after inducing hypnosis with thiopental or other appropriate drug.
*Adults:* For short procedures, 0.6 mg/kg (range, 0.3 to 1.1 mg/kg) I.V. over 10 to 30 seconds; additional doses may be given if needed. For long procedures, 2.5 mg/minute (range, 0.5 to 10 mg/minute) continuous I.V. infusion, or alternatively, 0.3 to 1.1 mg/kg by intermittent I.V. injection, followed by additional doses of 0.04 to 0.07 mg/kg, p.r.n.
*Children:* Administer 2 mg/kg I.V. for infants; for older children and adolescents, give 1 mg/kg I.V. or 3 to 4 mg/kg I.M. Don't exceed 150 mg.

## I.V. administration

■ Administration requires direct medical supervision by trained anesthesia personnel.
■ Usually administered I.V., succinylcholine may be administered I.M. if suitable vein is inaccessible. Give deep I.M., preferably high into the deltoid muscle.
■ Store injectable form in refrigerator. Store powder form at room temperature and keep tightly closed. Use immediately after reconstitution.

## Incompatibilities

Don't mix drug with alkaline solutions, such as thiopental, nafcillin, sodium bicarbonate, and barbiturates.

## Mechanism of action

*Skeletal muscle relaxant action:* Similar to acetylcholine (ACh), succinylcholine produces depolarization of the motor end-plate at the myoneural junction. Drug has a high affinity for ACh receptor sites and is resistant to acetyl-cholinesterase, producing a more prolonged depolarization at the motor end-plate. It also possesses histamine-releasing properties and reportedly stimulates the cardiac vagus and sympathetic ganglia.
A transient increase in intraocular pressure occurs immediately after injection and may persist after the onset of complete paralysis.

## Pharmacokinetics

*Absorption:* After I.V. administration, drug has a rapid onset of action.
*Distribution:* After I.V. administration, drug is distributed in extracellular fluid and rapidly reaches its site of action. It crosses the placenta.
*Metabolism:* Rapidly metabolized by plasma pseudocholinesterase.
*Excretion:* About 10% is excreted unchanged in urine.

| Route | Onset | Peak | Duration |
|-------|-------|------|----------|
| I.V. | ½-1 sec | 1-2 min | 4-10 min |
| I.M. | 2-3 min | Unknown | 10-30 min |

## Contraindications and precautions

Contraindicated in patients hypersensitive to drug and in those with abnormally low plasma pseudocholinesterase, angle-closure glaucoma, malignant hyperthermia, or penetrating eye injuries.

Use cautiously in geriatric or debilitated patients; in those receiving quinidine or cardiac glycoside therapy; in those undergoing a cesarean section; and in patients with respiratory depression, severe burns or trauma, electrolyte imbalances, hyperkalemia, paraplegia, spinal neuraxis injury, CVA, degenerative or dystrophic neuromuscular disease, myasthenia gravis, myasthenic syndrome of lung or bronchiogenic cancer, dehydration, thyroid disorders, collagen diseases, porphyria, fractures, muscle spasms, eye surgery, pheochromocytoma, or impaired renal, pulmonary, or hepatic function.

## Interactions

**Drug-drug.** *Aminoglycoside antibiotics, including amikacin, gentamicin, kanamycin, neomycin, and streptomycin; polymyxin antibiotics, such as colistin and polymyxin B sulfate; clindamycin, lincomycin; general anesthetics; local anesthetics; antimalarial drugs; cholinesterase inhibitors, such as demecarium, echothiophate and isofluran; cyclophosphamide; oral contraceptives; nondepolarizing neuromuscular blockers; parenteral magnesium salts; lithium, phenelzine; quinidine; quinine; pancuronium; phenothiazines; thiotepa; and exposure to neurotoxic insecticides:* Enhance or prolong neuromuscular blocking effects of succinylcholine. Use drugs cautiously during surgical and postoperative periods.
*Cardiac glycosides:* Produces possible arrhythmias. Use together cautiously.

---

**Drug-herb.** *Melatonin:* Potentiates blocking properties of succinylcholine. Discourage use together.

## Adverse reactions
**CV:** *bradycardia,* tachycardia, hypertension, hypotension, *arrhythmias,* flushing, *cardiac arrest.*
**EENT:** increased intraocular pressure.
**Hematologic:** myoglobinemia.
**Metabolic:** hyperkalemia.
**Musculoskeletal:** muscle fasciculation, *postoperative muscle pain.*
**Respiratory:** *prolonged respiratory depression, apnea, bronchospasm.*
**Other:** *malignant hyperthermia,* allergic or idiosyncratic hypersensitivity reactions *(anaphylaxis).*

## Overdose and treatment
Signs and symptoms of overdose include apnea or prolonged muscle paralysis, which may be treated with controlled respiration. Recommend using a peripheral nerve stimulator to monitor effects and degree of blockade.

## Clinical considerations
■ Succinylcholine is drug of choice for short procedures (less than 3 minutes) and for orthopedic manipulations; use cautiously in fractures or dislocations.
■ Duration of action is prolonged to 20 minutes with continuous I.V. infusion or when given with hexafluorenium bromide.
■ Some clinicians advocate pretreating adult patients with tubocurarine (3 to 6 mg) to minimize muscle fasciculations.
■ Repeated fractional doses of succinylcholine alone aren't advised; they may cause reduced response or prolonged apnea.

### Therapeutic monitoring
■ Advise clinician to monitor baseline electrolyte determinations and vital signs, and check respirations every 5 to 10 minutes during infusion.
■ Airway should be kept clear. Emergency respiratory support (endotracheal equipment, ventilator, oxygen, atropine, neostigmine) should be on hand.
■ Tachyphylaxis may occur.

### Special populations
**Breast-feeding patients.** Use cautiously in breast-feeding women because it isn't known if drug appears in breast milk.
**Geriatric patients.** Use with caution in geriatric patients.

## Patient counseling
■ Reassure patient that postoperative stiffness is normal and will soon subside. Advise clinician to monitor for residual muscle weakness.

■ Explain all procedures and events to patient because he can still hear.

# sucralfate
Carafate

*Pharmacologic classification:* pepsin inhibitor
*Therapeutic classification:* antiulcer
*Pregnancy risk category B*

## Available forms
Available by prescription only
*Suspension:* 1 g/10 ml
*Tablets:* 1 g

## Indications and dosages
*Short-term (up to 8 weeks) treatment of duodenal ulcer,* ◇*aspirin-induced gastric erosion*
*Adults:* 1 g P.O. q.i.d. 1 hour before meals and h.s.
*Maintenance therapy of duodenal ulcer*
*Adults:* 1 g P.O. b.i.d.

## Mechanism of action
*Antiulcer action:* Sucralfate has a unique mechanism of action. It adheres to proteins at the ulcer site, forming a protective coating against gastric acid, pepsin, and bile salts. It also inhibits pepsin, exhibits a cytoprotective effect, and forms a viscous, adhesive barrier on the surface of the intact intestinal mucosa and the stomach.

## Pharmacokinetics
*Absorption:* Only about 3% to 5% of a dose is absorbed. Drug activity isn't related to the amount absorbed.
*Distribution:* Acts locally, at the ulcer site. Absorbed drug is distributed to many body tissues, including the liver and kidneys.
*Metabolism:* None.
*Excretion:* About 90% of a dose is excreted in feces; absorbed drug is excreted unchanged in urine.

| Route | Onset | Peak | Duration |
|-------|-------|------|----------|
| P.O. | Unknown | Unknown | 6 hr |

## Contraindications and precautions
No known contraindications. Use cautiously in patients with chronic renal failure.

## Interactions
**Drug-drug.** *Antacids:* May decrease binding of drug to gastroduodenal mucosa, impairing effectiveness. Separate dosing of sucralfate and antacids by 30 minutes.
*Cimetidine, digoxin, phenytoin, quinidine, quinolones, ranitidine, tetracycline, theophylline, and fat-soluble vitamins A, D, E, and K:* Sucralfate decreases absorption of these drugs.

Separate administration times by at least 2 hours.

## Adverse reactions
**CNS:** dizziness, sleepiness, headache, vertigo.
**GI:** *constipation,* nausea, gastric discomfort, diarrhea, bezoar formation, vomiting, flatulence, dry mouth, indigestion.
**Musculoskeletal:** back pain.
**Skin:** rash, pruritus.

## Overdose and treatment
No information available.

## Clinical considerations
■ Drug is poorly water-soluble. For administration by nasogastric tube, prepare water-sorbitol suspension of sucralfate. Alternatively, place tablet in 60-ml syringe; add 20 ml water. Let stand with tip up for about 5 minutes, occasionally shaking gently. The resultant suspension may be administered from the syringe. After administration, flush tube several times to ensure that the patient receives the entire dose.
■ Patients who have difficulty swallowing tablet may place it in 15 to 30 ml of water at room temperature, allow it to disintegrate, and then ingest the resulting suspension. This is particularly useful for patients with esophagitis and painful swallowing.
■ Some experts believe that 2 g given b.i.d. is as effective as the standard regimen.
■ Drug treats ulcers as effectively as $H_2$-receptor antagonists.

### Therapeutic monitoring
■ Advise clinician to monitor patient for constipation.
■ Therapy exceeding 8 weeks isn't recommended.

### Special populations
**Breast-feeding patients.** The risks to breast-feeding infants must be weighed against benefits.
**Pediatric patients.** Safety and efficacy in children haven't been established.

## Patient counseling
■ Remind patient to take drug on an empty stomach and at least 1 hour before meals.
■ Advise patient to continue taking drug as directed, even after pain begins to subside, to ensure adequate healing.
■ Warn patient not to take drug for longer than 8 weeks.

# sufentanil citrate
Sufenta

*Pharmacologic classification:* opioid
*Therapeutic classification:* analgesic, adjunct to anesthesia, anesthetic
*Pregnancy risk category C*
*Controlled substance schedule II*

## Available forms
Available by prescription only
*Injection:* 50 mcg/ml

## Indications and dosages
### Adjunct to general anesthetic
*Adults:* 1 to 8 mcg/kg I.V. given with nitrous oxide and oxygen. Maintenance dose, 10 to 50 mcg.
### Primary anesthetic
*Adults:* 8 to 30 mcg/kg I.V. given with 100% oxygen and a muscle relaxant. Maintenance dose, 25 to 50 mcg.
*Children:* 10 to 25 mcg/kg I.V. given with 100% oxygen and a muscle relaxant. Maintenance dose, up to 25 to 50 mcg.

## I.V. administration
■ Sufentanil should only be given by persons specifically trained in the use of I.V. anesthetics.

### Incompatibilities
None reported.

## Mechanism of action
*Analgesic action:* Sufentanil has a high affinity for the opiate receptors, exerting an agonistic effect to provide analgesia. It's also used as an adjunct to anesthesia or as a primary anesthetic because of its potent CNS depressant effects.

## Pharmacokinetics
*Absorption:* Administered I.V.
*Distribution:* Highly lipophilic and is rapidly and extensively distributed in animals. It's highly protein-bound (greater than 90%) and redistributed rapidly.
*Metabolism:* Appears to be metabolized mainly in the liver and small intestine. Relatively little accumulation occurs. Drug has an elimination half-life of about 2½ hours.
*Excretion:* Drug and its metabolites are excreted primarily in urine.

| Route | Onset | Peak | Duration |
|-------|-------|------|----------|
| I.V. | 1 min | 1 min | 5 min |

## Contraindications and precautions
Contraindicated in patients hypersensitive to drug. Use cautiously in geriatric or debilitated patients and in those with decreased respira-

tory reserve, head injuries, or renal, pulmonary, or hepatic disease.

## Interactions
**Drug-drug.** *Anticholinergics:* Use together may cause paralytic ileus. Advise clinician to monitor patient closely.

*Beta blockers:* If beta blockers have been used preoperatively, recommend decreasing dose of sufentanil.

*Cimetidine:* Increased respiratory and CNS depression. Reduced dose of sufentanil is usually needed.

*Digitoxin, phenytoin, rifampin:* Drug accumulation and enhanced effects may result from use together. Advise clinician to monitor patient closely.

*General anesthetics:* Severe CV depression may result from use together. Advise clinician to monitor patient closely.

*Narcotic agonist-antagonist or a single dose of an antagonist:* Patient who becomes physically dependent on drug may experience acute withdrawal syndrome if given high doses of these drugs. Avoid this use.

*Nitrous oxide:* May produce CV depression when given with high doses of sufentanil. Advise clinician to monitor patient closely.

*Other CNS depressants, such as antihistamines, barbiturates, benzodiazepines, general anesthetics, muscle relaxants, narcotic analgesics, phenothiazines, sedative-hypnotics, and tricyclic antidepressants:* Additive CNS depression. Use together cautiously.

*Pancuronium:* May produce a dose-dependent elevation in heart rate during sufentanil and oxygen anesthesia. Recommend using moderate doses of pancuronium or a less vagolytic neuromuscular blocker. The vagolytic effect of pancuronium may be reduced in patients given nitrous oxide with sufentanil.

## Adverse reactions
**CNS:** chills, somnolence.
**CV:** *hypotension, **bradycardia**,* hypertension, ***arrhythmias,*** tachycardia.
**GI:** nausea, vomiting.
**Metabolic:** increased plasma amylase, lipase and serum prolactin levels.
**Musculoskeletal:** intraoperative muscle movement.
**Respiratory:** *chest wall rigidity, apnea, bronchospasm.*
**Skin:** *pruritus,* erythema.

## Overdose and treatment
There's no clinical experience with acute overdose of sufentanil, but signs and symptoms are expected to be similar to those occurring with other opioids, with less CV toxicity. The most common signs and symptoms of acute opiate overdose are CNS depression, respiratory depression, and miosis (pinpoint pupils). Other

acute toxic effects include hypotension, bradycardia, hypothermia, shock, apnea, cardiopulmonary arrest, circulatory collapse, pulmonary edema, and seizures.

To treat acute overdose, recommend establishing adequate respiratory exchange via a patent airway and ventilation, p.r.n., and giving a narcotic antagonist (naloxone) to reverse respiratory depression. (Because the duration of action of sufentanil is longer than that of naloxone, repeated naloxone dosing is needed.) Naloxone shouldn't be given unless the patient has clinically significant respiratory or CV depression. Advise clinician to monitor vital signs closely.

Symptomatic and supportive treatment (continued respiratory support, correction of fluid or electrolyte imbalance) should be provided. Advise clinician to monitor laboratory parameters, vital signs, and neurologic status closely.

## Clinical considerations
■ Compared with fentanyl and morphine, sufentanil has a more rapid onset and shorter duration of action.

### Therapeutic monitoring
■ When used at doses exceeding 8 mcg/kg, postoperative mechanical ventilation and observation are essential because of extended postoperative respiratory depression.
■ Sufentanil may produce muscle rigidity involving all the skeletal muscles (risk and severity are dose-related). Recommend choosing a neuromuscular blocker appropriate for the patient's CV status.
■ In patients weighing over 20% above ideal body weight, determine dose based on ideal body weight.

### Special populations
**Pediatric patients.** Safety and efficacy in children under age 2 have been documented in only a limited number of patients (who were undergoing CV surgery).
**Geriatric patients.** Lower doses are usually indicated for geriatric patients, who may be more sensitive to the therapeutic and adverse effects of drug.

## Patient counseling
■ Assure patient and family that he'll be monitored continuously.
■ Answer questions and concerns regarding drug.

# sulfadiazine

*Pharmacologic classification:* sulfonamide
*Therapeutic classification:* antibiotic
*Pregnancy risk category NR*

## Available forms
Available by prescription only
*Tablets:* 500 mg

## Indications and dosages
*Urinary tract infection*
*Adults:* Initially, 2 to 4 g P.O.; then 2 to 4 g/day in three to six divided doses.
*Children ages 2 months or older:* Initially, 75 mg/kg or 2 g/m² P.O.; then 150 mg/kg/day P.O. in four to six divided doses. Maximum daily dose, 6 g.
*Rheumatic fever prophylaxis, as an alternative to penicillin*
*Children weighing over 30 kg (66 lb):* 1 g P.O. daily.
*Children weighing under 30 kg:* 500 mg P.O. daily.
*Adjunctive treatment in toxoplasmosis*
*Adults:* 1 to 1.5 g P.O. q.i.d. for 3 to 4 weeks; given with pyrimethamine.
*Children:* 100 to 200 mg/kg P.O. daily in divided doses q 6 hours for 3 to 4 weeks; given with pyrimethamine.
*Nocardiasis*
*Adults:* 4 to 8 g P.O. daily in divided doses q 6 hours for 6 weeks.
*Asymptomatic meningococcal carrier*
*Adults:* 1 g P.O. b.i.d. for 2 days.
*Children ages 1 to 12:* 500 mg P.O. b.i.d. for 2 days.
*Children ages 2 to 12 months:* 500 mg P.O. daily for 2 days.

## Mechanism of action
*Antibacterial action:* Sulfadiazine is bacteriostatic. It inhibits formation of tetrahydrofolic acid from para-aminobenzoic acid (PABA), preventing bacterial cell synthesis of folic acid.

Sulfadiazine is active against many gram-positive bacteria, *Chlamydia trachomatis,* many enterobacteriaceae, and some strains of *Toxoplasma gondii* and *Plasmodium falciparum.*

## Pharmacokinetics
*Absorption:* Absorbed from the GI tract after oral administration.
*Distribution:* Distributed widely into most body tissues and fluids, including synovial, pleural, amniotic, prostatic, peritoneal, and seminal fluids; CSF penetration, however, is poor. Drug crosses the placenta, and is 32% to 56% protein-bound.
*Metabolism:* Metabolized partially in the liver.

*Excretion:* Both unchanged drug and metabolites are excreted primarily in urine by glomerular filtration and, to a lesser extent, renal tubular secretion; some drug appears in breast milk. Urine solubility of unchanged drug increases as urine pH increases.

| Route | Onset | Peak | Duration |
|-------|-------|------|----------|
| P.O. | Unknown | 4-6 hr | Unknown |

## Contraindications and precautions
Contraindicated in patients hypersensitive to sulfonamides, in those with porphyria, in infants under age 2 months (except in congenital toxoplasmosis), in pregnant women at term, and during breast-feeding.

Use cautiously in patients with impaired renal or hepatic function, bronchial asthma, multiple allergies, G6PD deficiency, or blood dyscrasia.

## Interactions
**Drug-drug.** *Oral anticoagulants:* Sulfadiazine may inhibit hepatic metabolism of these drugs and enhance anticoagulant effects. Advise clinician to monitor PT, INR blood levels, and patient for bleeding.
*Oral antidiabetics including sulfonylureas:* Enhances their hypoglycemic effects. Advise clinician to monitor blood glucose levels.
*PABA:* Antagonizes effects of sulfonamides. Don't use together.
*Trimethoprim or pyrimethamine (folic acid antagonists with different mechanisms of action):* Results in synergistic antibacterial effects and delays or prevents bacterial resistance. Don't use together.
**Drug-lifestyle.** *Sun exposure:* May cause photosensitivity reactions. Advise patient to take precautions.

## Adverse reactions
**CNS:** headache, mental depression, *seizures,* hallucinations.
**GI:** *nausea, vomiting, diarrhea,* abdominal pain, anorexia, stomatitis.
**GU:** elevated serum creatinine, *toxic nephrosis* with oliguria and anuria, crystalluria, hematuria.
**Hematologic:** *agranulocytosis, aplastic anemia, hemolytic anemia, thrombocytopenia,* megaloblastic anemia, *leukopenia.*
**Hepatic:** elevated liver enzyme levels, jaundice.
**Skin:** *erythema multiforme (Stevens-Johnson syndrome),* generalized skin eruption, *epidermal necrolysis, exfoliative dermatitis,* photosensitivity, urticaria, pruritus.
**Other:** hypersensitivity reactions (serum sickness, drug fever, *anaphylaxis),* local irritation, extravasation.

---

## Overdose and treatment
Signs and symptoms of overdose include dizziness, drowsiness, headache, unconsciousness, anorexia, abdominal pain, nausea, and vomiting. More severe complications, including hemolytic anemia, agranulocytosis, dermatitis, acidosis, sensitivity reactions, and jaundice, may be fatal.

Treatment includes gastric lavage if ingestion has occurred within the preceding 4 hours followed by correction of acidosis, forced fluids, and urinary alkalinization to enhance solubility and excretion. Treatment of renal failure and transfusion of appropriate blood products (in severe hematologic toxicity) may be required.

## Clinical considerations
▪ Sulfadiazine is a less-soluble sulfonamide; therefore, it's more likely to cause crystalluria. Avoid using drug with urine acidifiers and ensure adequate fluid intake. If adequate fluid intake can't be ensured, recommend sodium bicarbonate to reduce risk of crystalluria.
▪ Sulfadiazine alters urine glucose tests using cupric sulfate (Benedict's reagent or Clinitest).
**◪ ALERT** Beware of sound-alikes: sulfadiazine and sulfasalazine. Don't confuse the sulfonamide drugs.

### Therapeutic monitoring
▪ Advise clinician to monitor renal and liver function test results.
▪ Advise clinician to monitor patient for signs of blood dyscrasia.
▪ Advise clinician to monitor urine cultures and CBCs, and conduct urinalyses before and during therapy.

### Special populations
**Breast-feeding patients.** Drug appears in breast milk and shouldn't be used.
**Pediatric patients.** Contraindicated in children under age 2 months.

## Patient counseling
▪ Instruct patient to report adverse reactions promptly.
▪ Patient should drink a glass of water with each dose and extra water daily as tolerated to prevent crystalluria.

## sulfamethoxazole
Gantanol

*Pharmacologic classification:* sulfonamide
*Therapeutic classification:* antibiotic
*Pregnancy risk category C*

## Available forms
Available by prescription only
*Tablets:* 500 mg

## Indications and dosages
*Urinary tract and systemic infections*
*Adults:* Initially, 2 g P.O.; then 1 g P.O. b.i.d., up to t.i.d. for severe infections.
*Children and infants over age 2 months:* Initially, 50 to 60 mg/kg P.O., then 25 to 30 mg/kg b.i.d. Maximum dose shouldn't exceed 75 mg/kg daily.

## Mechanism of action
*Antibacterial action:* Sulfamethoxazole is bacteriostatic. It acts by inhibiting formation of tetrahydrofolic acid from para-aminobenzoic acid (PABA), thus preventing bacterial cell synthesis of folic acid.

Spectrum of action includes some gram-positive bacteria, *Chlamydia trachomatis,* many enterobacteriaceae, and some strains of *Toxoplasma* and *Plasmodium.*

## Pharmacokinetics
*Absorption:* Absorbed from the GI tract after oral administration.
*Distribution:* Distributed widely into most body tissues and fluids, including cerebrospinal, synovial, pleural, amniotic, prostatic, peritoneal, and seminal fluids. Sulfamethoxazole crosses the placenta, and is 50% to 70% protein-bound.
*Metabolism:* Metabolized partially in the liver.
*Excretion:* Both unchanged drug and metabolites are excreted primarily in urine by glomerular filtration and, to a lesser extent, renal tubular secretion; some drug appears in breast milk. Urinary solubility of unchanged drug increases as urine pH increases. Elimination half-life in patients with normal renal function is 7 to 12 hours.

| Route | Onset | Peak | Duration |
|---|---|---|---|
| P.O. | Unknown | 2 hr | Unknown |

## Contraindications and precautions
Contraindicated in patients with porphyria or hypersensitivity to sulfonamides, in infants under age 2 months (except in congenital toxoplasmosis), in pregnant women at term, and during breast-feeding.

Use cautiously in patients with renal or hepatic impairment, bronchial asthma, severe allergies, G6PD deficiency, or blood dyscrasia.

## Interactions
**Drug-drug.** *Oral anticoagulants:* Enhanced anticoagulant effects. Advise clinician to monitor patient for bleeding.
*Oral antidiabetics including sulfonylureas:* Enhanced hypoglycemic effects. Advise clinician to monitor blood sugar.
*PABA:* Antagonizes sulfonamide effects. Don't use together.
*Trimethoprim or pyrimethamine (folic acid antagonists with different mechanisms of action):* Results in synergistic antibacterial effects and

delays or prevents bacterial resistance. Don't use together.
**Drug-lifestyle.** *Sun exposure:* May cause photosensitivity reactions. Advise patient to take precautions.

## Adverse reactions
**CNS:** headache, mental depression, *seizures,* hallucinations, aseptic meningitis, apathy.
**EENT:** tinnitus.
**GI:** nausea, vomiting, diarrhea, abdominal pain, anorexia, stomatitis, *pancreatitis,* pseudomembranous colitis.
**GU:** *toxic nephrosis* with oliguria and anuria, crystalluria, hematuria, interstitial nephritis.
**Hematologic:** *agranulocytosis, hemolytic anemia, aplastic anemia,* megaloblastic anemia, *thrombocytopenia, leukopenia.*
**Hepatic:** elevated liver enzyme levels, jaundice.
**Skin:** *erythema multiforme, Stevens-Johnson syndrome,* generalized skin eruption, *epidermal necrolysis, exfoliative dermatitis,* photosensitivity, urticaria, pruritus.
**Other:** hypersensitivity reactions (serum sickness, drug fever, *anaphylaxis).*

## Overdose and treatment
Signs and symptoms of overdose include dizziness, drowsiness, headache, unconsciousness, anorexia, abdominal pain, nausea, and vomiting. More severe complications, including hemolytic anemia, agranulocytosis, dermatitis, acidosis, sensitivity reactions, and jaundice, may be fatal.

Treat by gastric lavage if ingestion has occurred within the preceding 4 hours, followed by correction of acidosis, forced fluids, and I.V. fluids if urine output is low and renal function is normal. Treatment of renal failure and transfusion of appropriate blood products (in severe hematologic toxicity) may be required.

## Clinical considerations
■ Sulfamethoxazole alters results of urine glucose tests using cupric sulfate (Benedict's reagent or Clinitest).
**H ALERT** Beware of sound-alikes: sulfamethoxazole and sulfamethizole. Don't confuse the combination products with sulfamethoxazole alone (such as Azo-gantanol and Gantanol).

### Therapeutic monitoring
■ Advise clinician to monitor urine cultures and CBCs and conduct urinalyses before and during therapy.
■ Advise clinician to monitor fluid intake and output.

### Special populations
**Breast-feeding patients.** Sulfamethoxazole appears in breast milk and shouldn't be given to breast-feeding women.

**Pediatric patients.** Sulfamethoxazole is contraindicated in children under age 2 months.

## Patient counseling
■ Instruct patient to take drug exactly as prescribed, even if he feels better.
■ Tell patient to drink a glass of water with each dose, and extra water daily as tolerated to prevent crystalluria.
■ Advise patient to use precautions and avoid sun exposure.

## sulfasalazine
Azulfidine, Azulfidine En-tabs

*Pharmacologic classification:* sulfonamide
*Therapeutic classification:* antibiotic
*Pregnancy risk category B*

## Available forms
Available by prescription only
*Suspension:* 250 mg/5 ml
*Tablets (with or without enteric coating):* 500 mg

## Indications and dosages
*Mild to moderate ulcerative colitis, adjunctive therapy in severe ulcerative colitis (conventional or enteric-coated tablets)*
*Adults:* Initially, 3 to 4 g P.O. daily in evenly divided doses. Maintenance dose is 2 g P.O. daily in divided doses q 6 hours. May need to start with 1 to 2 g initially, with a gradual increase in dosage to minimize adverse reactions.
*Children over age 2:* Initially, 40 to 60 mg/kg P.O. daily, divided into three to six doses; then 30 mg/kg daily in four doses. Maximum daily dose, 2 g. May need to start at lower dose if GI intolerance occurs.
*Rheumatoid arthritis (enteric-coated tablets)*
*Adults:* 2 to 3 g P.O. daily in two evenly divided doses. Initiate at lower dosage (suggested below) to minimize GI side effects.
0.5 g q evening during the first week
0.5 g b.i.d. during the second week
0.5 g q morning, 1 g q evening during the third week
1 g b.i.d. thereafter
*Juvenile rheumatoid arthritis polyarticular course (enteric-coated tablets)*
*Children ages 6 and older:* 30 to 50 mg/kg daily in two evenly divided doses. Maximum dose is 2 g/day. To reduce GI side effects begin with one-quarter to one-third of the planned maintenance dose and increase weekly until reaching the maintenance dose at 1 month.

## Mechanism of action
*Antibacterial and anti-inflammatory action:* Exact mechanism of action of the drug in ulcerative colitis is unknown; it's believed to be

---

a prodrug metabolized by intestinal flora in the colon. One metabolite (5-aminosalicylic acid or mesalamine) is responsible for the anti-inflammatory effect; the other metabolite (sulfapyridine) may be responsible for antibacterial action and for some adverse effects.

## Pharmacokinetics

*Absorption:* Absorbed poorly from the GI tract after oral administration; 70% to 90% is transported to the colon where intestinal flora metabolize drug to its active ingredients—sulfapyridine (antibacterial) and 5-aminosalicylic acid (anti-inflammatory)—which exert their effects locally. Sulfapyridine is absorbed from the colon, but only a small portion of 5-aminosalicylic acid is absorbed.

*Distribution:* Human data on sulfasalazine distribution are lacking; animal studies have identified drug and metabolites in sera, liver, and intestinal walls. Parent drug and both metabolites cross the placenta.

*Metabolism:* Cleaved by intestinal flora in the colon.

*Excretion:* Systemically absorbed sulfasalazine is excreted chiefly in urine; some parent drug and metabolites appear in breast milk. Plasma half-life is about 6 to 8 hours.

| Route | Onset | Peak | Duration |
|-------|-------|------|----------|
| P.O. | Unknown | 3-12 hr | Unknown |

## Contraindications and precautions

Contraindicated in patients hypersensitive to salicylates or sulfonamides or to other drugs containing sulfur, such as thiazides, furosemide, or oral sulfonylureas; in those with porphyria or severe renal or hepatic dysfunction; during pregnancy and at term; in breast-feeding women; and in infants and children under age 2. Sulfasalazine is also contraindicated in patients with intestinal or urinary tract obstructions because of the risk of local GI irritation and crystalluria.

Use cautiously in patients with mild to moderate renal or hepatic dysfunction, severe allergies, asthma, blood dyscrasia, or G6PD deficiency.

## Interactions

**Drug-drug.** *Antacids:* Increased systemic absorption and hazard of toxicity. Advise clinician to monitor patient closely.

*Antibiotics that alter intestinal flora:* May interfere with conversion of sulfasalazine to sulfapyridine and 5-aminosalicylic acid, decreasing its effectiveness. Advise clinician to monitor closely.

*Digoxin and folic acid:* Sulfasalazine may reduce GI absorption of these drugs. Advise clinician to monitor patient closely.

*Oral anticoagulants:* Enhanced anticoagulant effects. Advise clinician to monitor patient for bleeding.

*Oral antidiabetics including sulfonylureas:* Enhanced hypoglycemic effects. Advise clinician to monitor blood glucose levels.

*Urine acidifying drugs, such as ammonium chloride and ascorbic acid:* Increasing risk of crystalluria. Advise clinician to monitor closely.

**Drug-lifestyle.** *Sun exposure:* Photosensitivity may occur. Advise patient to take precautions.

## Adverse reactions

**CNS:** headache, mental depression, *seizures,* hallucinations.

**EENT:** tinnitus.

**GI:** nausea, vomiting, diarrhea, abdominal pain, anorexia, stomatitis.

**GU:** toxic nephrosis with oliguria and anuria, crystalluria, hematuria, oligospermia, infertility.

**Hematologic:** *agranulocytosis, aplastic anemia,* megaloblastic anemia, *thrombocytopenia, leukopenia, hemolytic anemia.*

**Hepatic:** jaundice, elevated liver enzyme levels.

**Skin:** *erythema multiforme, Stevens-Johnson syndrome,* generalized skin eruption, *epidermal necrolysis, exfoliative dermatitis,* photosensitivity, urticaria, pruritus.

**Other:** hypersensitivity reactions, serum sickness, drug fever, *anaphylaxis,* bacterial and fungal superinfection.

## Overdose and treatment

Signs and symptoms of overdose include dizziness, drowsiness, headache, unconsciousness, anorexia, abdominal pain, nausea, and vomiting. More severe complications, including hemolytic anemia, agranulocytosis, dermatitis, acidosis, sensitivity reactions, and jaundice, may be fatal.

Recommend treating by gastric lavage, if ingestion has occurred within the preceding 4 hours, followed by correction of acidosis, forced fluids, and urinary alkalinization to enhance solubility and excretion. Treatment of renal failure and transfusion of appropriate blood products (in severe hematologic toxicity) may be required.

## Clinical considerations

■ Most adverse effects involve the GI tract; recommend minimizing reactions and facilitating absorption by spacing doses evenly and giving drug after food.

■ Drug colors urine orange-yellow; may also color patient's skin orange-yellow.

■ Don't give antacids together with enteric-coated sulfasalazine; they may alter absorption.

■ Sulfasalazine alters results of urine glucose tests using cupric sulfate (Benedict's reagent or Clinitest).

---

* Canada only    ◊ Unlabeled clinical use

### Therapeutic monitoring

■ Drug should be stopped if signs of toxicity or hypersensitivity occur; if hematologic abnormalities are accompanied by sore throat, pallor, fever, jaundice, purpura, or weakness; if crystalluria is accompanied by renal colic, hematuria, oliguria, proteinuria, urinary obstruction, urolithiasis, increased BUN levels, or anuria; if severe diarrhea indicates pseudomembranous colitis; or if severe nausea, vomiting, or diarrhea persists.

### Special populations

**Breast-feeding patients.** Drug appears in breast milk; use with caution.

**Pediatric patients.** Contraindicated in patients under age 2 months.

### Patient counseling

■ Tell patient that sulfasalazine normally turns urine orange-yellow. Warn him that skin may also turn orange-yellow and that drug may permanently stain soft contact lenses yellow.

■ Advise patient to take drug after meals to reduce GI distress and to facilitate passage into intestines.

## sulfinpyrazone

Anturane

*Pharmacologic classification:* uricosuric
*Therapeutic classification:* renal tubular-blocker, platelet aggregation inhibitor
*Pregnancy risk category NR*

### Available forms

Available by prescription only
*Capsules:* 200 mg
*Tablets:* 100 mg

### Indications and dosages

***Chronic gouty arthritis and intermittent gouty arthritis, or hyperuricemia with gout***
Adults: Initially, 200 to 400 mg P.O. daily in two divided doses, gradually increasing to maintenance dose in 1 week. Maintenance dose is 400 mg P.O. daily in two divided doses; may increase to 800 mg daily or decrease to 200 mg daily.

◇***Prophylaxis of thromboembolic disorders, including angina, MI, and transient (cerebral) ischemic attacks, and in patients with prosthetic heart valves***
Adults: 600 to 800 mg P.O. daily in divided doses to decrease platelet aggregation.

### Mechanism of action

*Uricosuric action:* Sulfinpyrazone competitively inhibits renal tubule reabsorption of uric acid. Sulfinpyrazone inhibits adenosine diphosphate and 5-HT, resulting in decreased platelet adhesiveness and increased platelet survival time.

### Pharmacokinetics

*Absorption:* Absorbed completely after oral administration.
*Distribution:* 98% to 99% protein-bound.
*Metabolism:* Metabolized rapidly in the liver.
*Excretion:* Drug and its metabolites are eliminated in urine; about 50% is excreted unchanged.

| Route | Onset | Peak | Duration |
|-------|-------|------|----------|
| P.O. | Unknown | 1-2 hr | 4-6 hr |

### Contraindications and precautions

Contraindicated in patients hypersensitive to pyrazolone derivatives (including oxyphenbutazone and phenylbutazone), and those with blood dyscrasia, active peptic ulcer, or symptoms of GI inflammation or ulceration.

Use cautiously in patients with healed peptic ulcer and during pregnancy.

### Interactions

**Drug-drug.** *Cholestyramine:* Decreases absorption of sulfinpyrazone. Sulfinpyrazone should be taken 1 hour before or 4 to 6 hours after cholestyramine.

*Diazoxide, diuretics, pyrazinamide:* Increase serum uric acid. Increased sulfinpyrazone dose requirements.

*Oral antidiabetics:* Increased effects. Advise clinician to monitor blood glucose levels.

*Penicillin, other beta-lactam antibiotics, nitrofurantoin, and sulfonylureas:* Reduced excretion of nitrofurantoin, decreasing the efficacy of sulfinpyrazone in urinary tract infections and increasing systemic toxicity; may cause hypoglycemia. Advise clinician to monitor closely.

*Probenecid:* Inhibits renal excretion of sulfinpyrazone. Use together cautiously.

*Salicylates:* Block the uricosuric effects of sulfinpyrazone only in high doses. Avoid use together.

*Warfarin:* Enhanced hypoprothrombinemic effect and risk of bleeding; increased bleeding in these patients also may result from the antiplatelet effect of sulfinpyrazone. Use together cautiously.

**Drug-lifestyle.** *Alcohol use:* May decrease effectiveness of drug. Advise patient to avoid alcohol.

### Adverse reactions

**GI:** nausea, dyspepsia, epigastric pain, reactivation of peptic ulcerations.
**GU:** altered renal function test results, decreased urinary excretion of aminohippuric acid and phenolsulfonphthalein.
**Hematologic:** *blood dyscrasias* (such as anemia, *leukopenia, agranulocytosis, thrombocytopenia, aplastic anemia).*
**Respiratory:** *bronchoconstriction* in patients with aspirin-induced asthma.
**Skin:** rash.

---

## Overdose and treatment
Signs and symptoms of overdose include nausea, vomiting, epigastric pain, ataxia, labored breathing, seizures, and coma. Treatment is supportive; recommend inducing emesis or using gastric lavage as appropriate. Seizures should be treated with diazepam or phenytoin or both.

## Clinical considerations
- Drug doesn't accumulate and tolerance to it doesn't develop; it's suitable for long-term use.
- Drug has no analgesic or anti-inflammatory actions.
- Recommend giving with food, milk, or prescribed antacids to lessen GI upset.
- Sulfinpyrazone is used investigationally to increase platelet survival time, to treat thromboembolic phenomena, and to prevent MI recurrence.

### Therapeutic monitoring
- Drug may not be effective and should be avoided when creatinine clearance is less than 50 ml/minute.
- Advise clinician to monitor renal function and CBC routinely.
- Advise clinician to monitor serum uric acid levels and adjust dosage accordingly.
- Advise clinician to maintain adequate hydration with high fluid intake to prevent formation of uric acid kidney stones.

### Special populations
**Breast-feeding patients.** Safety in breast-feeding women hasn't been established. An alternative feeding method is recommended during therapy.
**Geriatric patients.** Geriatric patients are more likely to have glomerular filtration rates less than 50 ml/minute; sulfinpyrazone may be ineffective.

## Patient counseling
- Explain that gouty attacks may increase during first 6 to 12 months of therapy; patient shouldn't discontinue drug without medical approval.
- Encourage patient to comply with dose regimen and to keep scheduled follow-up visits.
- Tell patient to drink 8 to 10 glasses of fluid each day and to take drug with food to minimize GI upset; warn patient to avoid alcohol, which decreases the therapeutic effect of sulfinpyrazone.

# sulfisoxazole
Gantrisin

# sulfisoxazole diolamine
Gantrisin (Ophthalmic Solution)

*Pharmacologic classification:* sulfonamide
*Therapeutic classification:* antibiotic
*Pregnancy risk category C*

## Available forms
Available by prescription only
*Liquid:* 500 mg/5 ml (sulfisoxazole acetyl)
*Ophthalmic solution:* 4%
*Tablets:* 500 mg

## Indications and dosages
*Urinary tract and systemic infections*
*Adults:* Initially, 2 to 4 g P.O. then 4 to 8 g P.O. daily in divided doses q 4 to 6 hours.
*Children and infants over age 2 months:* Initially, 75 mg/kg P.O., then 150 mg/kg (or 4 g/m$^2$) P.O. daily in divided doses q 4 to 6 hours. Maximum dose shouldn't exceed 6 g/24 hours.
*Conjunctivitis, corneal ulcer, superficial ocular infections; adjunct in systemic treatment of trachoma*
*Adults:* Instill 1 to 2 drops in the lower conjuctival sac of affected eye daily q 1 to 4 hours.

## Mechanism of action
*Antibacterial action:* Sulfisoxazole is bacteriostatic. It acts by inhibiting formation of tetrahydrofolic acid from para-aminobenzoic acid (PABA), preventing bacterial cell synthesis of folic acid. It acts synergistically with folic acid antagonists such as trimethoprim, which block folic acid synthesis at a later stage, thus delaying or preventing bacterial resistance.
Sulfisoxazole is active against some gram-positive bacteria, *Chlamydia trachomatis,* many *Enterobacteriaceae,* and some strains of *Toxoplasma* and *Plasmodium.*

## Pharmacokinetics
*Absorption:* Absorbed readily from the GI tract after oral administration.
*Distribution:* Distributed into extracellular compartments; CSF penetration is 8% to 57% of blood levels in uninflamed meninges. Sulfisoxazole crosses the placenta, and is 85% protein-bound.
*Metabolism:* Metabolized partially in the liver.
*Excretion:* Both unchanged drug and metabolites are excreted primarily in urine by glomerular filtration and, to a lesser extent, renal tubular secretion; some drug appears in breast milk. Urinary solubility of unchanged drug increases as urine pH increases. Plasma half-life in

patients with normal renal function is about 4½ to 8 hours.

| Route | Onset | Peak | Duration |
|---|---|---|---|
| P.O. | Unknown | 1-4 hr | Unknown |
| Ophthalmic | Unknown | Unknown | Unknown |

## Contraindications and precautions

Contraindicated in patients hypersensitive to sulfonamines, in infants under age 2 months (except in congenital toxoplasmosis [with oral form only]), in pregnant women at term, and during breast-feeding.

Recommend using oral form cautiously in patients with impaired renal or hepatic function, severe allergies, bronchial asthma, or G6PD deficiency. Recommend using ophthalmic form cautiously in patients with severely dry eyes.

## Interactions

**Drug-drug.** *Oral anticoagulants:* Exaggerated anticoagulant effects. Advise clinician to monitor patient for bleeding.
*Oral antidiabetics including sulfonylureas:* Enhance hypoglycemic effects. Advise clinician to monitor blood glucose levels.
*PABA:* Antagonizes effects of sulfonamides. Don't use together.
*Trimethoprim or pyrimethamine (folic acid antagonists with different mechanisms of action):* Results in synergistic antibacterial effects and delays or prevents bacterial resistance. Don't use together.
*Urine acidifying drugs, such as ammonium chloride and ascorbic acid:* Increased risk of crystalluria. Advise clinician to monitor closely.
**Drug-lifestyle.** *Sun exposure:* Photosensitivity reaction may occur. Advise patient to take precautions.

## Adverse reactions

**CNS:** headache; mental depression, hallucinations, *seizures* (with oral administration).
**CV:** tachycardia, palpitations, syncope, cyanosis (with oral administration).
**EENT:** ocular irritation, itching, chemosis, periorbital edema (with ophthalmic form).
**GI:** nausea, vomiting, diarrhea, abdominal pain, anorexia, stomatitis, pseudomembranous colitis (with oral administration).
**GU:** toxic nephrosis with oliguria and anuria, acute renal failure, crystalluria, hematuria (with oral administration).
**Hematologic:** *agranulocytosis, aplastic anemia, thrombocytopenia, hemolytic anemia,* megaloblastic anemia, *leukopenia* (with oral administration).
**Hepatic:** elevated liver enzyme levels, jaundice (with oral administration), *hepatitis.*
**Skin:** *erythema multiforme, epidermal necrolysis, exfoliative dermatitis,* generalized skin eruption, photosensitivity, urticaria, pruritus (with oral administration).

**Other:** hypersensitivity reactions (serum sickness, drug fever, *anaphylaxis), Stevens-Johnson syndrome,* overgrowth of nonsusceptible organisms (with ophthalmic form).

## Overdose and treatment

Signs and symptoms of overdose include dizziness, drowsiness, headache, unconsciousness, anorexia, abdominal pain, nausea, and vomiting. More severe complications, including hemolytic anemia, agranulocytosis, dermatitis, acidosis, sensitivity reactions, and jaundice, may be fatal.

Treatment requires gastric lavage, if ingestion has occurred within the preceding 4 hours, followed by correction of acidosis, and forced fluids and urinary alkalinization to enhance solubility and excretion. Treatment of renal failure and transfusion of appropriate blood products (in severe hematologic toxicity) may be required.

## Clinical considerations

■ Sulfisoxazole-pyrimethamine is used to treat toxoplasmosis.
■ Sulfisoxazole alters results of urine glucose tests using cupric sulfate (Benedict's reagent or Clinitest).
**ℍALERT** Don't confuse the combination products with sulfamethoxazole alone (such as Azogantrisin and Gantrisin). Beware of sound-alike names, such as sulfisoxazole and sulfasalazine.

### Therapeutic monitoring

■ Advise clinician to monitor urine cultures, CBCs, and PT, and conduct urinalyses before and during therapy.
■ Advise clinician to monitor renal and liver function test results.

### Special populations

**Breast-feeding patients.** Drug appears in breast milk and shouldn't be given to breast-feeding women.
**Pediatric patients.** Contraindicated in children under age 2 months.

## Patient counseling

■ Tell patient to drink 8 ounces (240 ml) of water with each oral dose and to take drug on an empty stomach.
■ Tell patient to complete prescribed drug.
■ Teach patient how to use ophthalmic preparations. Warn patient not to touch tip of dropper or tube to any surface.
■ Warn patient that ophthalmic solution may cause blurred vision immediately after application. Tell patient to gently close eyes and keep closed for 1 to 2 minutes.

---

# sulindac
Clinoril

*Pharmacologic classification:* NSAID
*Therapeutic classification:* nonnarcotic
analgesic, anti-inflammatory, antipyretic
*Pregnancy risk category NR*

## Available forms
Available by prescription only
*Tablets:* 150 mg, 200 mg

## Indications and dosages
**Osteoarthritis, rheumatoid arthritis, anky-
losing spondylitis**
*Adults:* 150 mg P.O. b.i.d. initially; may in-
crease to 200 mg P.O. b.i.d.
**Acute subacromial bursitis or supraspina-
tus tendinitis, acute gouty arthritis**
*Adults:* 200 mg P.O. b.i.d. for 7 to 14 days.
Dosage may be reduced as symptoms subside.

## Mechanism of action
*Analgesic, antipyretic, and anti-inflammatory
actions:* Mechanisms of action are unknown
but are thought to inhibit prostaglandin synthesis.

## Pharmacokinetics
*Absorption:* Rapidly and completely absorbed
from the GI tract.
*Distribution:* Highly protein-bound.
*Metabolism:* Inactive and metabolized hepatically to the active sulfide metabolite.
*Excretion:* Excreted in urine. Half-life of parent drug is about 8 hours; half-life of active
metabolite is about 16 hours.

| Route | Onset | Peak | Duration |
|-------|-------|------|----------|
| P.O. | Unknown | 2-4 hr | Unknown |

## Contraindications and precautions
Contraindicated in patients hypersensitive to
drug or for whom acute asthmatic attacks, urticaria, or rhinitis is precipitated by use of aspirin or NSAIDs. Avoid use during pregnancy.
    Use cautiously in patients with history of
ulcer or GI bleeding, renal dysfunction, compromised cardiac function, hypertension, or
conditions predisposing to fluid retention.

## Interactions
**Drug-drug.** *Antacids:* Delay and decrease the
absorption of sulindac. Give drugs at separate
times.
*Anticoagulants, thrombolytics:* May be potentiated by the platelet-inhibiting effect of sulindac. Advise clinician to monitor PT closely.
*Diflunisal, aspirin:* Cause decreased plasma
levels of the active sulfide metabolite. Don't
use together.
*Dimethyl sulfoxide:* May cause decreased plasma levels of the active sulfide metabolite. Pe-

ripheral neuropathies have also been reported
with this combination. Advise clinician to monitor closely.
*GI-irritating drugs, including antibiotics,
NSAIDs, and steroids:* May potentiate the adverse GI effects of sulindac. Use together with
caution.
*Highly protein-bound drugs, such as pheny-
toin, sulfonylureas and warfarin:* May cause
displacement of either drug, and adverse effects. Advise clinician to monitor therapy closely for both drugs.
*Lithium carbonate:* NSAIDs are known to decrease renal clearance of this drug, thus increasing lithium serum levels and risks of adverse effects. Avoid use together.
*Probenecid:* Increases plasma levels of sulindac; sulindac may decrease the uricosuric effect of probenecid. Advise clinician to monitor patient for toxicity.
**Drug-herb.** *Dong quai, feverfew, garlic, ginger, horse chestnut, red clover:* Possible increased risk of bleeding. Discourage use together.
*St. John's wort, dong quai:* Increased risk of
photosensitivity. Advise patient to use sunblock
and avoid unprotected exposure to sunlight.

## Adverse reactions
**CNS:** dizziness, headache, nervousness, psychosis.
**CV:** hypertension, *HF,* palpitations, edema.
**EENT:** tinnitus, transient visual disturbances.
**GI:** epigastric distress, *peptic ulceration, GI
bleeding, pancreatitis,* occult blood loss, nau-
sea, constipation, dyspepsia, flatulence, anorex-
ia, vomiting, diarrhea.
**GU:** increased BUN, serum creatinine; inter-
stitial nephritis, *nephrotic syndrome, renal
failure.*
**Hematologic:** prolonged bleeding time, *aplas-
tic anemia, thrombocytopenia, agranulocytosis, neutropenia, hemolytic anemia.*
**Hepatic:** elevated liver enzyme levels.
**Metabolic:** hyperkalemia.
**Skin:** rash, pruritus.
**Other:** drug fever, *anaphylaxis, hypersensitivity syndrome, angioedema.*

## Overdose and treatment
Signs and symptoms of overdose include dizziness, drowsiness, mental confusion, disorientation, lethargy, paresthesias, numbness, vomiting, gastric irritation, nausea, abdominal pain,
headache, stupor, coma, and hypotension.
    To treat overdose of sulindac, advise clini-
cian to empty stomach immediately by inducing emesis with ipecac syrup or by gastric
lavage. Recommend giving activated charcoal
via nasogastric tube. Symptomatic and supportive measures (respiratory support and correction of fluid and electrolyte imbalances)
should be provided. Dialysis is thought to be
of minimal value because sulindac is highly

protein-bound. Advise clinician to monitor laboratory parameters and vital signs closely.

## Clinical considerations

■ Sulindac may be the safest NSAID for patients with mild renal impairment. It may also be less likely to cause further renal toxicity.

■ Impose safety measures to prevent injury, such as using raised side rails and supervised ambulation.

■ Disease modifying antirheumatic drugs should be considered in patient not responding adequately to NSAIDs.

■ Misoprostol should be considered in patients at high risk for complications from NSAID-induced GI ulceration.

### Therapeutic monitoring

■ Cardiopulmonary status should be assessed frequently. Advise clinician to monitor vital signs, especially heart rate and blood pressure, to detect abnormalities.

■ Fluid balance status should be assessed. Advise clinician to monitor intake and output and daily weight. Advise clinician to observe patient for presence and amount of edema.

■ Symptomatic improvement may take 7 days or longer.

### Special populations

**Breast-feeding patients.** Safe use of sulindac during breast-feeding hasn't been established. Avoid use of drug in breast-feeding women.
**Pediatric patients.** Safety of long-term drug use in children hasn't been established.
**Geriatric patients.** Patients over age 60 are more sensitive to the adverse effects of sulindac. Use with caution. Because of its effect on renal prostaglandins, drug may cause fluid retention and edema. This may be significant in geriatric patients and in those with HF.

## Patient counseling

■ Caution patient to avoid use of OTC drugs unless medically approved.

■ Teach patient how to recognize signs and symptoms of possible adverse reactions; instruct patient to report such adverse reactions.

■ Instruct patient to check weight two or three times weekly and to report weight gain of 1.4 kg (3 lb) or more within 1 week, to prescriber.

■ Advise patient to report edema and have blood pressure checked routinely.

■ Instruct patient in safety measures; advise him to avoid hazardous activities that require alertness until CNS effects of drug are known.

# sumatriptan succinate
Imitrex

*Pharmacologic classification:* selective 5-hydroxytryptamine ($5HT_1$)-receptor agonist
*Therapeutic classification:* antimigraine drug
*Pregnancy risk category C*

## Available forms

Available by prescription only
*Injection:* 12 mg/ml (0.5 ml in 1-ml prefilled syringe), 6-mg single-dose (0.5 ml in 2 ml) vial, and stat dose system
*Nasal spray:* 5 mg/0.1 ml, 20 mg/0.1 ml
*Tablets:* 25 mg, 50 mg, 100 mg

## Indications and dosages
### Acute migraine attacks (with or without aura)

**Adults:** 6 mg S.C. Maximum recommended dose is two 6-mg injections in 24 hours, separated by at least 1 hour, or 25 to 100 mg P.O. initially. If response isn't achieved in 2 hours, may give second dose of 25 to 100 mg. Additional doses may be used in at least 2-hour intervals. Maximum daily dose, 300 mg.

For nasal spray, recommend giving single dose of 5 mg, 10 mg, or 20 mg once in one nostril; may repeat once after 2 hours under prescriber's guidance for maximum daily dose of 40 mg. A 10-mg dose may be achieved by the administration of a single 5-mg dose in each nostril.

## Mechanism of action

*Antimigraine action:* Sumatriptan selectively binds to a $5\text{-HT}_1$ receptor subtype found in the basilar artery and vasculature of dura mater, where it presumably exerts its antimigraine effect. In these tissues, sumatriptan activates the receptor to cause vasoconstriction, an action correlating with the relief of migraine.

## Pharmacokinetics

*Absorption:* Bioavailability via S.C. injection is 97% of that obtained via I.V. injection.
*Distribution:* Has a low protein-binding capacity (about 14% to 21%).
*Metabolism:* About 80% is metabolized in the liver, primarily to an inactive indoleacetic acid metabolite.
*Excretion:* Excreted primarily in urine, partly (20%) as unchanged drug and partly as the indoleacetic acid metabolite. Elimination half-life is about 2 hours.

| Route | Onset | Peak | Duration |
|-------|-------|------|----------|
| P.O. | ½ hr | 1½ hr | Unknown |
| S.C. | 10-20 min | 12 min | Unknown |
| Nasal | Unknown | Unknown | Unknown |

---

Reactions may be *common*, uncommon, *life-threatening*, or COMMON AND LIFE-THREATENING.

## Contraindications and precautions

Contraindicated in patients hypersensitive to drug; in those with uncontrolled hypertension; ischemic heart disease, such as angina pectoris, Prinzmetal's angina, history of MI, or documented silent ischemia; or hemiplegic or basilar migraine; within 14 days of MAO therapy; and in patients taking ergotamine.

Use cautiously in patients who may be at risk for coronary artery disease (CAD) (such as postmenopausal women or men over age 40) or those with risk factors such as hypertension, hypercholesterolemia, obesity, diabetes, smoking, or family history. Use cautiously in women of childbearing age and during pregnancy.

## Interactions

**Drug-drug.** *Ergot and ergot derivatives:* Prolongs vasospastic effects when given with sumatriptan. These drugs shouldn't be used within 24 hours of sumatriptan therapy.
*MAO inhibitors:* Increased effects of sumatriptan. Avoid use within 2 weeks of discontinuing MAO inhibitor therapy.
**Drug-herb.** *Horehound:* May enhance serotonergic effects. Discourage use together.

## Adverse reactions

**CNS:** dizziness, vertigo, drowsiness, headache, anxiety, malaise, fatigue.
**CV:** atrial fibrillation, *ventricular fibrillation, ventricular tachycardia, MI,* ECG changes, pressure or tightness in chest.
**EENT:** discomfort of throat, nasal cavity or sinus, mouth, jaw, or tongue; altered vision.
**GI:** abdominal discomfort, dysphagia.
**Musculoskeletal:** myalgia, muscle cramps, neck pain.
**Skin:** flushing.
**Other:** tingling; warm or hot sensation; burning sensation; heaviness, pressure or tightness; anxious feeling; tight feeling in head; cold sensation; diaphoresis; injection site reaction.

## Overdose and treatment

No specific information available. However, it would be expected to cause seizures, tremor, inactivity, erythema of the limbs, reduced respiratory rate, cyanosis, ataxia, mydriasis, injection site reactions, and paralysis.

Patient should be continually monitored while signs and symptoms persist and for at least 10 hours thereafter. Effect of hemodialysis or peritoneal dialysis on serum levels of sumatriptan is unknown.

## Clinical considerations

■ Drug shouldn't be used for management of hemiplegic or basilar migraine. Safety and effectiveness also haven't been established for cluster headache, which occurs in an older, predominantly male population.

■ Drug shouldn't be given I.V. because coronary vasospasm may occur.
■ Nasal spray is generally well tolerated; however, adverse reactions seen with the other forms of the drug can still occur.
■ Clinical data on sumatriptan injection include rare reports of serious or life-threatening arrhythmias, such as atrial and ventricular fibrillation, ventricular tachycardia, MI, and marked ischemic ST-segment elevations. Data also include rare, but more frequent, reports of chest and arm discomfort thought to represent angina pectoris. Because such coronary events can occur, consider administering first dose in an outpatient setting to patients for whom unrecognized CAD is comparatively likely (postmenopausal women; men over age 40; and patients with risk factors for CAD, such as hypertension, hypercholesterolemia, obesity, diabetes, smoking, and strong family history of CAD).

### Therapeutic monitoring

■ Patient response to nasal spray may be varied. The choice of dose should be made individually, weighing the possible benefit of the 20-mg dose with the potential for a greater risk of adverse events.

### Special populations

**Pregnant patients.** Potential for harm to fetus. Use only when benefits outweigh risks to fetus. Tell pregnant women or those who intend to become pregnant during therapy to consult prescriber and discuss risks and benefits of drug use.
**Breast-feeding patients.** Drug appears in breast milk. Use caution when giving to breast-feeding women.
**Pediatric patients.** Safety and efficacy in children haven't been established.
**Geriatric patients.** No longer recommended. This population is reported to be more susceptible to decreased hepatic function, higher risk of coronary artery disease, and increased blood pressure when treated with the drug.

## Patient counseling

■ Tell patient that drug may be given at any time during a migraine attack, but preferably as soon as symptoms begin. A second injection may be given if symptoms recur. Tell patient not to use more than two injections in 24 hours and to allow at least 1 hour between doses. Pain or redness at the injection site may occur but usually lasts less than 1 hour.
■ Explain that drug is intended to relieve migraine, not to prevent or reduce the number of attacks.
■ Tell patient not to use a second nasal spray dose if there was no response to the initial dose unless the prescriber is first contacted.

---

■ Explain that drug is available in a spring-loaded injector system that facilitates self-administration. Review detailed information with patient. Make sure he understands how to load the injector, administer the injection, and dispose of the used syringes.

■ Tell patient who feels persistent or severe chest pain to call the prescriber immediately. Tell patient who experiences pain or tightness in the throat, wheezing, heart throbbing, rash, lumps, hives, or swollen eyelids, face, or lips to stop using the drug and call prescriber immediately.

# tacrine hydrochloride
Cognex

*Pharmacologic classification:* centrally acting reversible cholinesterase inhibitor
*Therapeutic classification:* psychotherapeutic drug (for Alzheimer's disease)
*Pregnancy risk category C*

## Available forms
Available by prescription only
*Capsules:* 10 mg, 20 mg, 30 mg, 40 mg

## Indications and dosages
*Mild to moderate dementia of the Alzheimer's type*
*Adults:* Initially, 10 mg P.O. q.i.d. Maintain dose for at least 4 weeks, with every-other-week monitoring of transaminase levels beginning at week 4 of therapy. If patient tolerates treatment and transaminase levels remain normal, increase to 20 mg P.O. q.i.d. After 4 weeks, adjust dosage to 30 mg P.O. q.i.d. If still tolerated, increase to 40 mg P.O. q.i.d. after another 4 weeks.
≡ *Dosage adjustment.* For patients with ALT level two to three times the upper limit of normal, advise clinician to monitor ALT level weekly. If ALT level is three to five times the upper limit of normal, advise clinician to reduce daily dose by 40 mg/day and monitor ALT level weekly. Dosage adjustment and every-other-week monitoring should be resumed when ALT level returns to normal. If ALT level is above five times the upper limit of normal, advise clinician to stop treatment and monitor ALT level. Advise clinician to monitor patient for signs and symptoms of hepatitis. Advise clinician to rechallenge when ALT level is normal and to monitor weekly.

## Mechanism of action
*Psychotherapeutic action:* Tacrine presumably slows degradation of acetylcholine released by still-intact cholinergic neurons, thereby elevating acetylcholine levels in the cerebral cortex. If this theory is correct, the effects of tacrine may lessen as the disease process advances and fewer cholinergic neurons remain functionally intact. No evidence suggests that tacrine alters the course of the underlying dementia.

## Pharmacokinetics
*Absorption:* Rapidly absorbed after oral administration. Absolute bioavailability of tacrine is about 17%. Food reduces tacrine bioavailability by about 30% to 40% if taken less than 1 hour before a meal.
*Distribution:* About 55% plasma protein–bound.
*Metabolism:* Undergoes first-pass metabolism, which is dose-dependent. It's extensively metabolized by the cytochrome P-450 system to multiple metabolites, not all of which have been identified.
*Excretion:* Elimination half-life is about 2 to 4 hours.

| Route | Onset | Peak | Duration |
|-------|-------|------|----------|
| P.O. | Unknown | ½-3 hr | Unknown |

## Contraindications and precautions
Contraindicated in patients hypersensitive to drug or acridine derivatives. Also contraindicated in patients with tacrine-related jaundice that's been confirmed with an elevated total bilirubin level of more than 3 mg/dl and in patients hypersensitive to ALT elevations.

Use cautiously in patients with sick sinus syndrome, bradycardia, history of hepatic disease, renal disease, Parkinson's disease, asthma, prostatic hyperplasia, or other urinary outflow impairment and in those at risk for peptic ulcer.

## Interactions
**Drug-drug.** *Anticholinergics:* Decreased effectiveness of anticholinergics. Advise clinician to monitor patient closely.
*Cholinergics, cholinesterase inhibitors:* Additive effects. Advise clinician to monitor patient for signs of toxicity.
*Cimetidine:* Increases the plasma level of tacrine. Advise clinician to monitor patient.
*Drugs that undergo extensive metabolism via cytochrome P-450:* Drug interactions may occur. Use cautiously.
*NSAIDs:* May contribute to GI irritation and gastric bleeding. Advise clinician to monitor patient carefully.
*Theophylline:* Increased theophylline elimination half-life and average plasma levels. Advise clinician to monitor theophylline levels.
**Drug-food.** *Any food:* Possible delayed absorption of drug. Drug should be given 1 hour before meals.

**Drug-lifestyle.** *Smoking:* Decreased plasma levels of drug. Discourage smoking.

## Adverse reactions

**CNS:** agitation, ataxia, insomnia, abnormal thinking, somnolence, depression, anxiety, *headache, dizziness,* fatigue, confusion, *seizures.*
**CV:** *bradycardia,* hypertension, palpitations, chest pain.
**EENT:** rhinitis.
**GI:** *nausea, vomiting, diarrhea,* dyspepsia, loose stools, changes in stool color, anorexia, abdominal pain, flatulence, constipation.
**Hepatic:** elevated liver enzyme levels, jaundice.
**Metabolic:** weight loss.
**Musculoskeletal:** myalgia.
**Respiratory:** upper respiratory tract infection, cough.
**Skin:** rash, facial flushing, increased sweating.

## Overdose and treatment

Overdose with cholinesterase inhibitors may cause a cholinergic crisis characterized by severe nausea, vomiting, salivation, sweating, bradycardia, hypotension, and seizures. Increasing muscle weakness may occur and can result in death if respiratory muscles are involved.

Advise clinician to use general supportive measures. Tertiary anticholinergics, such as atropine, may be used as an antidote for tacrine overdose. I.V. atropine sulfate titrated to effect is recommended (initial dose of 1 to 2 mg I.V., with subsequent doses based on clinical response). It isn't known if tacrine or its metabolites can be eliminated by dialysis.

## Clinical considerations

■ Tacrine as a cholinesterase inhibitor is likely to exaggerate succinylcholine-type muscle relaxation during anesthesia.
■ Drug may have vagotonic effects on the heart rate, such as bradycardia. Use with caution in patients with sick sinus syndrome.
■ Rate of dose escalation may be slowed if patient is intolerant to recommended titration schedule. Acceleration of titration schedule is never recommended.
■ Cognitive function may worsen after abrupt discontinuation of tacrine or after a reduction in total daily dose of 80 mg per day or more.
■ If drug is discontinued for 4 weeks or longer, full-dose titration and monitoring of schedule should be resumed.
■ The incidence of elevations in transaminase level is higher among women. There are no other known predictors of risk of hepatocellular injury.

### Therapeutic monitoring

■ Advise clinician to monitor ALT levels every other week from at least week 4 to week 16 following start of therapy, after which monitoring

may be decreased to every 3 months if ALT level is less than or equal to two times the upper limit of normal. After each dosage adjustment, schedule monitoring should be resumed.
■ Advise clinician to monitor patient for dose tolerance and cognitive changes.

## Patient counseling

■ Instruct caregiver to give drug between meals. If GI upset occurs, drug may be taken with food but plasma levels may be reduced.
■ Inform caregiver that drug can alleviate symptoms but doesn't alter the underlying degenerative disease.
■ Inform caregiver that effectiveness of therapy depends on drug administration at regular intervals.
■ Caution caregiver that dosage adjustment is an integral part of the safe use of drug. Abrupt discontinuation or a large reduction in daily dose (80 mg per day or more) may precipitate behavioral disturbances and a decline in cognitive function.
■ Advise caregiver to promptly report significant adverse effects or changes in status.

# tacrolimus
Prograf

*Pharmacologic classification:* bacteria-derived macrolide
*Therapeutic classification:* immuno-suppressant
*Pregnancy risk category C*

## Available forms

Available by prescription only
*Capsules:* 0.5 mg, 1 mg, 5 mg
*Injection:* 5 mg/ml

## Indications and dosages

*Prophylaxis of organ rejection in allogenic liver or kidney transplants*
*Adults:* 0.03 to 0.05 mg/kg/day I.V. as continuous infusion administered no sooner than 6 hours after transplantation. Substitute P.O. therapy as soon as possible, with first oral dose given 8 to 12 hours after discontinuing I.V. infusion. Or, administer P.O. dose within 24 hours of transplantation after renal function has recovered. Recommended initial P.O. dose for allogenic liver transplants is 0.1 to 0.15 mg/kg/day P.O. in two divided doses q 12 hours. Recommended initial P.O. dose for allogenic kidney transplants is 0.2 mg/kg/day in two divided doses q 12 hours. Adjust dosages based on clinical response.
*Children:* Initially, 0.03 to 0.05 mg/kg/day I.V.; then 0.15 to 0.2 mg/kg/day P.O. on schedule similar to adults adjusted, p.r.n.
≡ *Dosage adjustment.* For patients with renal or hepatic impairment, use lowest recommended I.V. and P.O. dosages.

## I.V. administration

■ Dilute I.V. form with normal saline injection or $D_5W$ injection to a level between 0.004 and 0.02 mg/ml before use.
■ Store diluted infusion solution in glass or polyethylene container and discard after 24 hours.
■ Advise clinician to continuously observe patient receiving drug I.V. for at least 30 minutes after start of infusion and frequently thereafter. Advise clinician to stop infusion if signs or symptoms of anaphylaxis occur and have an aqueous solution of epinephrine 1:1,000 and a source of oxygen available at patient's bedside.

### Incompatibilities

Don't mix or infuse with solutions or drugs that have a pH above 9, such as acyclovir and ganciclovir. Don't store in polyvinyl chloride container because of decreased stability and potential for extraction of phthalates.

## Mechanism of action

*Immunosuppressant action:* Exact mechanism is unknown. Inhibits T-lymphocyte activation. Evidence suggests that drug binds to an intracellular protein, FKBP-12. A complex of tacrolimus-FKBP-12, calcium, calmodulin, and calcineurin then forms, inhibiting the phosphatase activity of calcineurin. This effect may prevent the generation of nuclear factor of activated T cells, a nuclear component thought to initiate gene transcription for the formation of lymphocyte activation and, therefore, to cause immunosuppression.

## Pharmacokinetics

*Absorption:* Absorption of oral drug from the GI tract varies. Absorption half-life in liver transplant patients is about 5½ hours. Levels in blood and plasma peak in 1½ to 3½ hours. Absolute bioavailability is 14% to 17%. Food reduces absorption and bioavailability.
*Distribution:* Bound to proteins, mainly albumin and alpha$_1$-acid glycoprotein, and is highly bound to erythrocytes. Protein-binding between 75% and 99%. Distribution of drug between whole blood and plasma depends on several factors, such as hematocrit, temperature of separation of plasma, drug level, and plasma protein level.
*Metabolism:* Extensively metabolized by mixed-function oxidase system, primarily cytochrome P-450.
*Excretion:* Less than 1% of dose excreted unchanged in urine. Ten possible metabolites identified in human plasma. Two metabolites, a demethylated and a double demethylated tacrolimus, retain 10% and 7%, respectively, of inhibitory effect of tacrolimus on T-lymphocyte activation.

| Route | Onset | Peak | Duration |
|---|---|---|---|
| P.O., I.V. | Unknown | 1½-3½ hr | Unknown |

## Contraindications and precautions

Contraindicated in patients hypersensitive to drug. Injection form is contraindicated in those hypersensitive to castor oil derivatives. Use cautiously in patients with impaired renal and hepatic function.

## Interactions

**Drug-drug.** *Antifungals, bromocriptine, calcium channel blockers, cimetidine, clarithromycin, danazol, diltiazem, erythromycin, methylprednisolone, metoclopramide:* Possible interference with tacrolimus metabolism. Reduced tacrolimus dosage may be needed.
*Carbamazepine, phenobarbital, phenytoin, rifamycins:* Decreased tacrolimus blood level. Increase tacrolimus dosage.
*Live vaccines:* Active infection. Avoid concomitant use.
*Nephrotoxic drugs (aminoglycosides, amphotericin B, cisplatin, cyclosporine):* Increased risk of nephrotoxicity. Avoid use of tacrolimus and cyclosporine; stop one at least 24 hours before starting other. With elevated tacrolimus or cyclosporine levels, further dosing with other drug is usually delayed.
*Other immunosuppressants (except adrenal corticosteroids):* Increased susceptibility to infection. Avoid use together.
**Drug-food.** *Any food:* Inhibited drug absorption. Drug should be taken on empty stomach.
*Grapefruit juice:* Increased drug blood levels in liver transplant patients. Don't use together.

## Adverse reactions

**CNS:** *headache, tremor, insomnia, paresthesia, asthenia.*
**CV:** *hypertension, peripheral edema.*
**GI:** *diarrhea, nausea, constipation, anorexia, vomiting, abdominal pain.*
**GU:** *abnormal renal function, increased creatinine or BUN levels, urinary tract infection, oliguria.*
**Hematologic:** *anemia, leukocytosis,* THROMBOCYTOPENIA.
**Hepatic:** *abnormal liver function test results.*
**Metabolic:** *hyperkalemia, hypokalemia, hyperglycemia, hypomagnesemia.*
**Musculoskeletal:** *back pain.*
**Respiratory:** *pleural effusion, atelectasis, dyspnea.*
**Skin:** *pruritus, rash.*
**Other:** *pain, fever, ascites,* **anaphylaxis.**

## Overdose and treatment

There is minimal experience with overdose. Patients who inadvertently received an overdose experienced adverse reactions no different from those occurring in patients receiving therapeutic doses. Follow general supportive measures and systemic treatment in all cases

---

* Canada only    ◇ Unlabeled clinical use

of overdose. Because of its poor aqueous solubility and extensive erythrocyte and plasma protein–binding, tacrolimus probably isn't significantly dialyzable.

## Clinical considerations
■ Adult patients should be given doses at lower end of dosing range. Dosage adjustment should be based on assessment of rejection and tolerance. Lower doses may be sufficient as maintenance therapy. Use tacrolimus with adrenal corticosteroids in early posttransplant period.
■ Because of risk of anaphylaxis, reserve injection for patients unable to take capsules.
■ Drug is being investigated for use in bone marrow, cardiac, pancreas, pancreatic island cell, and small bowel transplantation. It also may be used to treat autoimmune disease and severe recalcitrant psoriasis.
■ Tacrolimus therapy is usually delayed 48 hours or longer in patients with postoperative oliguria.
■ Because mild to severe hyperkalemia has been noted in 10% to 44% of liver transplant recipients given tacrolimus, advise clinician to monitor serum potassium level; potassium-sparing diuretics shouldn't be used.
**◄ ALERT** Patients receiving drug are at increased risk for developing lymphomas and other malignancies, particularly of skin. Risk appears to be related to intensity and duration of immunosuppression rather than to use of any specific drug.
■ A lymphoproliferative disorder (LPD) related to Epstein-Barr virus (EBV) has been reported in immunosuppressed organ transplant recipients. LPD risk appears greatest in young children who are at risk for primary EBV infection while immunosuppressed or who are switched to tacrolimus after long-term immunosuppressive therapy.
■ Antihypertensive therapy may be needed to control blood pressure elevations caused by drug use. Likewise, therapy may be needed to control elevations in blood glucose level caused by drug use.
■ Black renal transplant patients may need higher doses to maintain comparable whole blood trough drug levels.

### Therapeutic monitoring
■ In both adult and pediatric liver transplant patients, the typical trough whole blood tacrolimus level should be 5 to 20 mg/ml at months 1 to 12 posttransplant. In renal transplant patients, the whole blood tacrolimus level should be 7 to 20 ng/ml and 5 to 15 ng/ml at 1 to 3 or 4 to 12 months posttransplant, respectively.
■ Advise clinician to closely monitor patient with impaired renal function; dosage may need to be reduced. In patients with persistent elevations of serum creatinine level who are

unresponsive to dosage adjustments, advise clinician to consider changing to another immunosuppressive therapy.
■ Advise clinician to closely monitor patient experiencing posttransplant hepatic impairment because of increased risk of renal insufficiency related to high whole blood levels of tacrolimus. Dosage adjustments may be needed.

### Special populations
**Breast-feeding patients.** Drug appears in breast milk. Avoid use in breast-feeding women.
**Pediatric patients.** Children without preexisting renal or hepatic dysfunction have needed and tolerated higher doses than adults to achieve similar levels. Children should receive high end of recommended adult I.V. and oral dosing ranges (0.1 mg/kg/day I.V. and 0.3 mg/kg/day P.O.). Dosage adjustments may be needed. Experience with renal transplants is limited.
**Geriatric patients.** Advise clinician to evaluate renal function before therapy with tacrolimus starts and subsequently thereafter.

### Patient counseling
■ Tell patient to take capsules on empty stomach because food affects drug absorption.
■ Inform patient of need for repeated laboratory tests during therapy to watch for adverse reactions and to monitor drug effectiveness.
■ Advise a woman of childbearing age to call prescriber if she becomes pregnant or plans to become pregnant.

## tamoxifen citrate
Nolvadex, Nolvadex-D*, Tamofen*

*Pharmacologic classification:* nonsteroidal antiestrogen
*Therapeutic classification:* antineoplastic
*Pregnancy risk category D*

### Available forms
Available by prescription only
*Tablets:* 10 mg, 20 mg
*Tablets (enteric-coated):* 20 mg*

### Indications and dosages
Dosage and indications may vary. Check current literature for recommended protocol.
***Advanced breast cancer (men and postmenopausal women)***
*Adults:* 20 to 40 mg P.O. daily. Doses greater than 20 mg should be given b.i.d.
***Adjunct treatment for breast cancer (with radiation and surgery)***
*Adults:* 20 to 40 mg P.O. daily. Doses greater than 20 mg should be given b.i.d. Therapy should continue for no longer than 5 years.

## Patient counseling

- Instruct patient not to crush, chew, or open capsules and to take drug at the same time each day 30 minutes after eating.
- Tell patient to get up slowly from chair or bed during initiation of therapy and to avoid situations in which injury could occur as a result of syncope.
- Instruct patient not to drive or perform hazardous tasks during initiation of therapy and for 12 hours after therapy starts or changes until response can be monitored.

# telmisartan

Micardis

*Pharmacologic classification:* angiotensin II antagonist
*Therapeutic classification:* antihypertensive
*Pregnancy risk category C (D in second and third trimesters)*

## Available forms

Available by prescription only
*Tablets:* 40 mg, 80 mg

## Indications and dosages

*Hypertension (used alone or with other antihypertensives)*
*Adults:* 40 mg P.O. once daily. Blood pressure response is dose-related over a range of 20 to 80 mg daily.

## Mechanism of action

*Antihypertensive action:* Inhibits vasoconstriction and aldosterone production by selectively blocking the binding of angiotensin II to its receptors.

## Pharmacokinetics

*Absorption:* Absolute bioavailability is about 42% for a 40-mg dose. Plasma levels peak in ½ to 1 hour following oral administration.
*Distribution:* Extensively plasma protein–bound.
*Metabolism:* Metabolized by glucuronide conjugation to an inactive metabolite.
*Excretion:* Half-life is about 24 hours. Majority is excreted unchanged in the feces via biliary excretion.

| Route | Onset | Peak | Duration |
|-------|-------|------|----------|
| P.O. | Unknown | ½-1 hr | 24 hr |

## Contraindications and precautions

Contraindicated in patients hypersensitive to drug or its components and during pregnancy.

Use cautiously in patients with biliary obstruction disorders, renal stenosis, or renal or hepatic insufficiency and in those with an activated renin-angiotensin system, such as volume- or salt-depleted patients (such as those receiving high doses of diuretics).

## Interactions

**Drug-drug.** *Digoxin:* Increased digoxin levels. Advise clinician to monitor level closely.
*Warfarin:* Decreased plasma warfarin levels. Advise clinician to monitor level closely.
**Drug-lifestyle.** *Alcohol use:* Enhanced hypotensive effects of drug. Advise patient to avoid alcohol.

## Adverse reactions

**CNS:** dizziness, pain, fatigue, headache.
**CV:** chest pain, hypertension, peripheral edema.
**EENT:** pharyngitis, sinusitis.
**GI:** abdominal pain, diarrhea, dyspepsia, nausea.
**GU:** urinary tract infection.
**Hepatic:** elevated liver enzyme levels.
**Musculoskeletal:** back pain, myalgia.
**Respiratory:** cough, upper respiratory tract infection.
**Other:** flulike symptoms.

## Overdose and treatment

Limited data exist. Most likely, symptoms include hypotension, tachycardia, dizziness, and possibly bradycardia. Treatment should involve supportive care. Telmisartan isn't removed by hemodialysis.

## Clinical considerations

- Blood pressure response in black patients is less than in white patients.
- Most of the antihypertensive effect is present within 2 weeks. Maximal blood pressure reduction is generally attained after 4 weeks.
- Diuretic may be added if blood pressure isn't controlled by drug alone.
- Orthostatic hypotension may develop in patients undergoing dialysis.

### Therapeutic monitoring

- Advise clinician to monitor patient for hypotension following initiation of drug. Advise clinician to place patient in supine position if hypotension occurs and administer I.V. normal saline as indicated.
- Advise clinician to closely monitor blood pressure throughout therapy.

### Special populations

**Pregnant patients.** Use of drug is contraindicated during pregnancy because of potential risk of fetal and neonatal morbidity and death.
**Breast-feeding patients.** It isn't known if drug appears in breast milk. Risks and benefits should be assessed before drug is continued in breast-feeding women.
**Pediatric patients.** Safety and efficacy in children haven't been established.

**Geriatric patients.** No significant difference has been reported compared to younger patients.

### Patient counseling

- Inform patient that drug shouldn't be removed from blister-sealed packet until immediately before use.
- Inform women of childbearing age of the consequences of second- and third-trimester exposure to drug.
- Inform patient that transient hypotension may occur.

# temazepam
Restoril

*Pharmacologic classification:* benzodiazepine
*Therapeutic classification:* sedative-hypnotic
*Pregnancy risk category X*
*Controlled substance schedule IV*

### Available forms
Available by prescription only
*Capsules:* 7.5 mg, 15 mg, 30 mg

### Indications and dosages
*Insomnia*
*Adults:* 7.5 to 30 mg P.O. 30 minutes before bedtime. Usual adult dose is 15 mg daily.
≡*Dosage adjustment.* For elderly or debilitated patients, initiate at 7.5 mg P.O. h.s. until individual response is determined.

### Mechanism of action
*Sedative-hypnotic action:* Temazepam depresses the CNS at the limbic and subcortical levels of the brain. It produces a sedative-hypnotic effect by potentiating the effect of the neurotransmitter gamma-aminobutyric acid on its receptor in the ascending reticular activating system, which increases inhibition and blocks both cortical and limbic arousal.

### Pharmacokinetics
*Absorption:* Well absorbed through the GI tract when administered orally.
*Distribution:* Widely distributed throughout the body. Drug is 96% protein-bound.
*Metabolism:* Metabolized in the liver primarily to inactive metabolites.
*Excretion:* Metabolites are excreted in urine as glucuronide conjugates. Half-life of drug is 4 to 20 hours.

| Route | Onset | Peak | Duration |
|-------|-------|------|----------|
| P.O. | ½-1 hr | 1¼-1½ hr | Unknown |

### Contraindications and precautions
Contraindicated in patients hypersensitive to drug or other benzodiazepines and during pregnancy.

Use cautiously in patients with impaired renal or hepatic function, chronic pulmonary insufficiency, severe or latent mental depression, suicidal tendencies, or history of drug abuse.

### Interactions
**Drug-drug.** *Antidepressants, antihistamines, barbiturates, general anesthetics, MAO inhibitors, narcotics, phenothiazines:* Enhanced CNS depressant effects. Use together cautiously.
*Haloperidol:* Increased serum haloperidol level. Advise clinician to monitor patient closely.
*Levodopa:* Reduced levodopa therapeutic effect. Use together cautiously.
**Drug-herb.** *Catnip, kava, lady's slipper, lemon balm, passion flower, sassafras, skullcap, valerian:* Possible enhanced sedative effects. Discourage using together.
**Drug-lifestyle.** *Alcohol use:* Increased CNS depression. Advise patient to avoid alcohol.
*Smoking:* Accelerated temazepam metabolism, which lowers clinical effectiveness. Discourage smoking.

### Adverse reactions
**CNS:** *drowsiness, dizziness, lethargy,* disturbed coordination, daytime sedation, confusion, nightmares, vertigo, euphoria, weakness, headache, fatigue, nervousness, anxiety, depression, physical and psychological dependence, minor changes in EEG patterns.
**EENT:** blurred vision.
**GI:** diarrhea, nausea, dry mouth.
**Hepatic:** elevated liver enzyme levels.

### Overdose and treatment
Signs and symptoms of overdose include somnolence, confusion, hypoactive or absent reflexes, dyspnea, labored breathing, hypotension, bradycardia, slurred speech, unsteady gait or impaired coordination and, ultimately, coma.

Advise clinician to support blood pressure and respiration until drug effects subside and monitor vital signs. Mechanical ventilatory assistance via endotracheal tube may be required to maintain a patent airway and support adequate oxygenation. Flumazenil, a specific benzodiazepine antagonist, may be useful. Advise clinician to use I.V. fluids and vasopressors, such as dopamine and phenylephrine, to treat hypotension p.r.n. If patient is conscious, induce emesis. Gastric lavage should be used if ingestion was recent, but only if an endotracheal tube is present to prevent aspiration. After emesis or lavage, activated charcoal with a cathartic should be given as a single dose. Barbiturates shouldn't be used if excitation occurs. Dialysis is of limited value.

## Clinical considerations

■ Drug is useful for patients who have difficulty falling asleep or who awaken frequently in the night.

■ Prolonged use isn't recommended; however, drug has proved effective for up to 4 weeks of continuous use.

■ After long-term use, avoid abrupt withdrawal and follow a gradual tapering dose schedule.

### Therapeutic monitoring

■ To prevent toxicity, advise clinician to monitor liver function test results; lower doses are indicated for patients with hepatic dysfunction.

### Special populations

**Pregnant patients.** Use is contraindicated during pregnancy because of potential risk of harm to fetus.

**Breast-feeding patients.** Drug appears in breast milk. A breast-fed infant may become sedated, have feeding difficulties, or lose weight. Avoid use in breast-feeding women.

**Pediatric patients.** Safe use in patients under age 18 hasn't been established.

**Geriatric patients.** Geriatric patients are more susceptible to the CNS depressant effects of temazepam. Use with caution.

## Patient counseling

■ Instruct patient to seek medical approval before making changes in drug regimen.

■ Inform patient of the risk of physical and psychological dependence with long-term use.

■ Caution women about risks to fetus.

■ Warn patient about potential CNS depression with alcohol use and the decreased therapeutic benefits from heavy smoking.

## temozolomide

Temodar

*Pharmacologic classification:* alkylating drug
*Therapeutic classification:* antineoplastic
*Pregnancy risk category D*

### Available forms

Available by prescription only
*Capsules:* 5 mg, 20 mg, 100 mg, 250 mg

### Indications and dosages

**Refractory anaplastic astrocytoma that has relapsed following chemotherapy regimen containing a nitrosourea and procarbazine**
*Adults:* Initial cycle: 150 mg/m² P.O. once daily for first 5 days of 28-day treatment cycle. Timing and dosage of subsequent cycles must be adjusted according to the absolute neutrophil count (ANC) and platelet count measured on cycle day 22 (expected nadir) and cycle day 29 (initiation of next cycle).

Dosage adjustments are based on the lowest of these ANC and platelet results. For ANC less than 1,000/mm³ or platelets less than 50,000/mm³: Hold therapy until ANC is greater than 1,500/mm³ and platelets greater than 100,000/mm³. Reduce dosage by 50 mg/m² for subsequent cycle. Minimum dose is 100 mg/m².

For ANC 1,000 to 1,500/mm³ or platelets 50,000 to 100,000/mm³: Hold therapy until ANC is greater than 1,500/mm³ and platelets greater than 100,000/mm³. Subsequent cycle administer 150 mg/m².

For ANC greater than 1,500/mm³ and platelets greater than 100,000/mm³: Increase dosage to, or maintain at, 200 mg/m² for first 5 days of subsequent cycle.

### Mechanism of action

*Antineoplastic action:* Temozolomide is a prodrug that's rapidly hydrolyzed to the active agent. It's thought to interfere with DNA replication in rapidly dividing tissues, primarily through alkylation (methylation) of guanine nucleotides in the DNA structure.

### Pharmacokinetics

*Absorption:* Rapidly and completely absorbed from the GI tract following oral administration, with plasma levels peaking in 1 hour.
*Distribution:* 15% plasma protein–bound.
*Metabolism:* Undergoes spontaneous hydrolysis to its active form and other metabolites. After 7 days, 38% of given dose is recovered in urine and 0.8% in feces.
*Excretion:* Rapidly eliminated, with an elimination half-life of 1¾ hours.

| Route | Onset | Peak | Duration |
|-------|-------|------|----------|
| P.O. | Unknown | Unknown | Unknown |

### Contraindications and precautions

Contraindicated in patients hypersensitive to temozolomide or its components, in those allergic to dacarbazine, which is structurally similar to temozolomide, and in pregnancy.

### Interactions

**Drug-drug.** *Valproic acid:* Decreased oral clearance of temozolomide by about 5%. Use cautiously.
**Drug-food.** *Any food:* Reduced rate and extent of drug absorption; however, there are no dietary restrictions with drug administration. Advise clinician to give drug on an empty stomach to reduce nausea and vomiting.

### Adverse reactions

**CNS:** *amnesia,* anxiety, *asthenia,* ataxia, confusion, **seizures,** *coordination abnormality,* depression, *dizziness, fatigue,* gait abnormality, *headache, hemiparesis,* insomnia, **local seizures,** paresis, *paresthesia, somnolence.*
**CV:** *peripheral edema.*

---

* Canada only    ◇ Unlabeled clinical use

**EENT:** abnormal vision, diplopia, pharyngitis, sinusitis.
**GI:** *abdominal pain, anorexia, constipation, diarrhea, nausea, vomiting,* dysphasia.
**GU:** increased urinary frequency, urinary incontinence, urinary tract infection.
**Hematologic:** anemia, *leukopenia, neutropenia, thrombocytopenia.*
**Metabolic:** weight increase.
**Musculoskeletal:** back pain, myalgia.
**Respiratory:** coughing, upper respiratory tract infection.
**Skin:** pruritus, rash.
**Other:** breast pain (female), *fever,* hyperadrenocorticism, *viral infection.*

## Overdose and treatment
Neutropenia and thrombocytopenia occurred following a single dose of 1,000 mg/m². Advise clinician to closely monitor patient's hematologic status and give supportive therapies, p.r.n.

## Clinical considerations
■ Store capsules at 59° to 86° F (15° to 30° C).
■ Avoid skin contact with, or inhalation of, capsule contents if capsule is accidentally opened or damaged. Follow procedures for safe handling and disposal of antineoplastics.

### Therapeutic monitoring
■ A CBC should be drawn on day 22 and then weekly until ANC is greater than 1,500/mm³ and platelet count is greater than 100,000/mm³.

### Special populations
**Pregnant patients.** Drug shouldn't be used during pregnancy because of risk of harm to fetus, unless potential benefit outweighs fetal risk.
**Breast-feeding patients.** It's unknown if temozolomide appears in breast milk; patient should discontinue breast-feeding while receiving drug.
**Pediatric patients.** Safety and efficacy in children haven't been evaluated.
**Geriatric patients.** Severe neutropenia and thrombocytopenia are more common following first treatment cycle in patients ages 70 and older.

## Patient counseling
■ Emphasize importance of taking dose exactly as prescribed, to swallow capsules, and to take drug on an empty stomach or h.s.
■ Stress importance of continuing drug even when suffering nausea and vomiting.
■ Tell patient to call prescriber immediately if vomiting (dose loss) occurs shortly after a dose is taken.
■ Tell patient to promptly report sore throat, fever, unusual bruising or bleeding, rash, or seizures.
■ Advise patient to avoid exposure to people with infections.

■ Advise patient that drug may cause birth defects.

# tenecteplase
TNKase

*Pharmacologic classification:* recombinant tissue plasminogen activator
*Therapeutic classification:* thrombolytic
*Pregnancy risk category C*

## Available forms
*Injection:* 50 mg

## Indications and dosages
*Reduction of mortality from acute MI—*
*Adults weighing under 60 kg (132 lb):* 30 mg (6 ml) by I.V. bolus over 5 seconds.
*Adults weighing 60 to 69 kg (132 to 152 lb):* 35 mg (7 ml) by I.V. bolus over 5 seconds.
*Adults weighing 70 to 79 kg (154 to 174 lb):* 40 mg (8 ml) by I.V. bolus over 5 seconds.
*Adults weighing 80 to 89 kg (176 to 196 lb):* 45 mg (9 ml) by I.V. bolus over 5 seconds.
*Adults weighing 90 kg (198 lb) or more:* 50 mg (10 ml) by I.V. bolus over 5 seconds.
   Maximum dose is 50 mg.

## I.V. administration
■ Use syringe prefilled with sterile water for injection and inject 10 ml into the 50-mg vial.
**ALERT** Gently swirl solution once mixed; don't shake it.
■ Draw up the appropriate dose needed from the reconstituted vial with the syringe and discard any unused portion.
■ Visually inspect product for particulate matter before administration.
■ Drug is given rapidly over 5 seconds via a designated line.
■ Give drug immediately once reconstituted, or refrigerate and use within 8 hours.

### Incompatibilities
Don't give tenecteplase in the same I.V. line as dextrose. Flush lines containing dextrose with normal saline before administration.

## Mechanism of action
*Thrombolytic action:* Tenecteplase is a human tissue plasminogen activator that binds to fibrin and converts plasminogen to plasmin. The specificity to fibrin decreases systemic activation of plasminogen and the resulting breakdown of circulating fibrinogen.

## Pharmacokinetics
*Absorption:* Administered I.V.
*Distribution:* Distribution is related to weight and is an approximation of plasma volume.
*Metabolism:* Metabolized primarily in the liver.

---

*Excretion:* Initial half-life is 20 to 24 minutes with a terminal half-life of 90 to 130 minutes.

| Route | Onset | Peak | Duration |
|-------|-------|------|----------|
| I.V. | Immediate | Immediate | 20-24 min |

## Contraindications and precautions

Contraindicated in patients with active internal bleeding; history of CVA; intracranial or intraspinal surgery or trauma within the previous 2 months; intracranial neoplasm, aneurysm, or arteriovenous malformation; severe uncontrolled hypertension; or known bleeding diathesis.

Use with caution in patients who have had recent major surgery, such as coronary artery bypass graft (CABG), organ biopsy, obstetric delivery, or previous puncture of noncompressible vessels. Also use cautiously in patients with recent trauma; recent GI or GU bleeding; high risk of left ventricular thrombus; acute pericarditis; hypertension (systolic blood pressure ≥ 180 mm Hg or diastolic blood pressure ≥ 110 mm Hg); severe hepatic dysfunction; hemostatic defects; subacute bacterial endocarditis; septic thrombophlebitis; diabetic hemorrhagic retinopathy; cerebrovascular disease; during pregnancy; and in patients ages 75 and older.

## Interactions

**Drug-drug.** *Anticoagulants (heparin, vitamin K antagonists), drugs that alter platelet function (acetylsalicylic acid, dipyridamole, glycoprotein IIb/IIIa inhibitors):* Increased risk of bleeding when used before, during, or after therapy with tenecteplase. Use cautiously.

## Adverse reactions

**CNS:** *intracranial hemorrhage, CVA.*
**EENT:** pharyngeal bleed, epistaxis.
**GI:** *GI bleeding.*
**GU:** hematuria.
**Skin:** *hematoma,* bleeding at puncture site.

## Overdose and treatment

No data are available regarding overdose. Advise clinician to monitor patient for increased bleeding.

## Clinical considerations

■ Advise clinician to begin therapy as soon as possible after onset of MI symptoms.
■ Advise clinician to minimize arterial and venous punctures during treatment.
■ Avoid noncompressible arterial punctures and internal jugular and subclavian venous punctures.
■ Give heparin with tenecteplase, but not in the same I.V. line.

### Therapeutic monitoring

■ Advise clinician to monitor patient for bleeding. If serious bleeding occurs, heparin and an-

tiplatelet drugs should be stopped immediately.
■ Advise clinician to monitor ECG for reperfusion arrhythmias.
■ Cholesterol embolism is rarely caused by thrombolytic use, but may be lethal. Signs and symptoms include livedo reticularis "purple toe" syndrome, acute renal failure, gangrenous fingers or toes, hypertension, pancreatitis, MI, cerebral infarction, spinal cord infarction, retinal artery occlusion, bowel infarction, and rhabdomyolysis.

### Special populations

**Breast-feeding patients.** It's unknown if drug appears in breast milk. Use with caution in breast-feeding women.
**Pediatric patients.** Safety and efficacy in children haven't been established.
**Geriatric patients.** Use caution when giving tenecteplase to patients ages 75 and older. Benefits should be weighed against the risk of increased adverse events.

## Patient counseling

■ Advise patient about proper dental care to avoid excessive gum bleeding.
■ Advise patient to report any adverse events or excess bleeding immediately.
■ Explain to patient and family the use of tenecteplase

# teniposide
Vumon

*Pharmacologic classification:*
podophyllotoxin (cell cycle–phase specific, $G_2$ and late S phase)
*Therapeutic classification:* antineoplastic
*Pregnancy risk category D*

## Available forms

Available by prescription only
*Injection:* 50 mg/5-ml ampules

## Indications and dosages

Dosage and indications may vary. Check current literature for recommended protocol.
*Acute lymphoblastic leukemia induction therapy in childhood*
*Children:* Optimum dose hasn't been established. One protocol reported by manufacturer is 165 mg/m$^2$ I.V. teniposide with cytarabine 300 mg/m$^2$ I.V. twice weekly for eight or nine doses. Another protocol suggests 250 mg/m$^2$ I.V. teniposide with 1.5 mg/m$^2$ I.V. vincristine weekly for 4 to 8 weeks, along with prednisone 40 mg/day for 28 days for patients refractory to regimens containing vincristine and prednisone.

## I.V. administration

- Use glass or polyolefin plastic bags or containers for infusion. Don't use polyvinyl chloride containers.
- Dilute with $D_5W$ or normal saline solution to give final teniposide levels of 0.1 mg/ml, 0.2 mg/ml, 0.4 mg/ml, or 1 mg/ml.
- Solutions containing levels of 0.1 mg/ml, 0.2 mg/ml, or 0.4 mg/ml are stable at room temperature for 24 hours. Administer solutions with a final level of 1 mg/ml within 4 hours of preparation.
- Give I.V. infusion over 30 to 60 minutes to prevent hypotension. Avoid I.V. push because of increased risk of hypotension.

### Incompatibilities
Incompatible with heparin and idarubicin.

## Mechanism of action
*Antineoplastic action:* Teniposide causes single- and double-stranded breaks in DNA and DNA protein cross-links, preventing cells from entering mitosis.

## Pharmacokinetics
*Absorption:* Not administered orally.
*Distribution:* More than 99% plasma protein–bound. Teniposide crosses the blood-brain barrier to a limited extent.
*Metabolism:* Metabolized extensively in the liver.
*Excretion:* About 4% to 12% of a dose is eliminated through the kidneys as unchanged drug or metabolites. Terminal half-life of drug is 5 hours.

| Route | Onset | Peak | Duration |
|-------|-------|------|----------|
| I.V. | Unknown | Unknown | Unknown |

## Contraindications and precautions
Contraindicated in patients hypersensitive to drug or to polyoxyethylated castor oil, an injection vehicle.

## Interactions
**Drug-drug.** *Methotrexate:* Possible increased clearance and intracellular levels of methotrexate. Avoid use together.
*Sodium salicylate, sulfamethizole, tolbutamide:* Possible displacement of teniposide from protein-binding sites and increased toxicity. Don't administer together.

## Adverse reactions
**CV:** hypotension from rapid infusion.
**GI:** *nausea, vomiting, mucositis, diarrhea.*
**Hematologic:** LEUKOPENIA, NEUTROPENIA, THROMBOCYTOPENIA, MYELOSUPPRESSION (dose-limiting), *anemia.*
**Metabolic:** elevated uric acid levels in blood and urine.
**Skin:** rash, alopecia, *phlebitis and extravasation* (at injection site).

**Other:** *anaphylaxis, infection,* bleeding, hypersensitivity reactions (chills, fever, urticaria, tachycardia, *bronchospasm,* dyspnea, hypotension, flushing).

## Overdose and treatment
Signs and symptoms of overdose include myelosuppression, nausea, and vomiting. Treatment is usually supportive and includes transfusion of blood components, antiemetics, and antibiotics for infections that may develop.

## Clinical considerations
- Use caution when handling and preparing solution. The use of gloves is recommended.
- If teniposide solution contacts skin, immediately wash with soap and water. If drug makes contact with mucous membranes, immediately flush with water.
- Don't administer drug through a membrane-type in-line filter because the diluent may dissolve the filter.
**H ALERT** Diphenhydramine, hydrocortisone, epinephrine, and oral airway should be available in case of an anaphylactic reaction.
- Advise clinician to decrease dose in patients with renal or hepatic insufficiency and in patients with Down syndrome.

### Therapeutic monitoring
- Advise clinician to monitor patient for chemical phlebitis at injection site.
- Advise clinician to monitor blood pressure before infusion and at 30-minute intervals during infusion. If systolic blood pressure decreases below 90 mm Hg, infusion should be stopped.
- Advise clinician to monitor CBC and observe patient for signs of bone marrow depression.
- Advise clinician to monitor renal and hepatic function during therapy.

### Special populations
**Pregnant patients.** Use of drug during pregnancy may cause fetal harm. Use during pregnancy only when expected benefits justify risk to fetus.
**Breast-feeding patients.** It isn't known if drug appears in breast milk. However, because of the risk of serious adverse reactions, mutagenicity, and carcinogenicity in the infant, breast-feeding isn't recommended.

## Patient counseling
- Encourage adequate fluid intake to increase urine output and facilitate excretion of uric acid.
- Caution patient to avoid exposure to people with infections.
- Caution patient of potential for harm to fetus.
- Advise patient that hair should grow back after treatment is discontinued.

Reactions may be *common,* uncommon, *life-threatening,* or COMMON AND LIFE-THREATENING.

■ Tell patient to call prescriber promptly if a sore throat or fever develops or if unusual bruising or bleeding occurs.

# terazosin hydrochloride
Hytrin

*Pharmacologic classification:* selective alpha₁ blocker
*Therapeutic classification:* antihypertensive
*Pregnancy risk category C*

## Available forms
Available by prescription only
*Capsules:* 1 mg, 2 mg, 5 mg, 10 mg
*Tablets:* 1 mg, 2 mg, 5 mg, 10 mg

## Indications and dosages
*Mild to moderate hypertension*
*Adults:* Initially, 1 mg P.O. h.s. Adjust dosage and schedule according to patient response at an interval of no less than every 2 weeks. Recommended range, 1 to 5 mg daily or divided b.i.d.

If therapy is discontinued for several days or longer, reinstitute using the initial dosing regimen of 1 mg P.O. h.s. Slowly increase dosage until desired blood pressure is attained. Doses of more than 20 mg don't appear to further affect blood pressure.
*BPH*
*Adults:* Initially, 1 mg P.O. h.s. Dosage may be adjusted upward based on patient response. Increase in a stepwise manner to 2 mg, 5 mg, and 10 mg. A daily dose of 10 mg may be needed.

## Mechanism of action
*Antihypertensive action:* Terazosin reduces blood pressure by selectively inhibiting alpha₁ receptors in vascular smooth muscle, reducing peripheral vascular resistance. Because of its selectivity for alpha₁ receptors, heart rate increases minimally. Significant decreases in serum cholesterol, low-density lipoprotein, and very-low-density lipoprotein cholesterol fractions occur during therapy; the significance of these changes is unknown, as is the mechanism by which they occur.

Terazosin administration doesn't significantly alter potassium or glucose levels; it has been used successfully with diuretics, beta blockers, and a combination of other antihypertensive regimens.
*Hypertrophic action:* Alpha blockade in nonvascular smooth muscle causes relaxation, notably in prostatic tissue, reducing urinary symptoms in men with BPH.

## Pharmacokinetics
*Absorption:* Rapidly absorbed after oral administration. About 90% of oral dose is bioavail-able; ingestion of food doesn't appear to alter bioavailability.
*Distribution:* About 90% to 94% is plasma protein–bound.
*Metabolism:* Metabolized in the liver. Mechanism of action of drug doesn't appear to be affected by hypertension, HF, or age.
*Excretion:* About 40% is excreted in urine, 60% in feces, mostly as metabolites. Up to 30% may be excreted unchanged. Elimination half-life is about 12 hours.

| Route | Onset | Peak | Duration |
|-------|-------|------|----------|
| P.O. | 15 min | 2-3 hr | 24 hr |

## Contraindications and precautions
Contraindicated in patients hypersensitive to drug.

## Interactions
**Drug-drug.** *Antihypertensives:* Excessive hypotension. Use together cautiously.
*Clonidine:* Decreased antihypertensive effect of clonidine. Advise clinician to monitor patient closely.
**Drug-herb.** *Butcher's broom:* Possible reduction in effects. Don't use together.

## Adverse reactions
**CNS:** *asthenia, dizziness, headache,* nervousness, paresthesia, somnolence.
**CV:** *palpitations, peripheral edema,* orthostatic hypotension, tachycardia, syncope.
**EENT:** *nasal congestion,* sinusitis, blurred vision.
**GI:** *nausea.*
**GU:** impotence.
**Musculoskeletal:** back pain, muscle pain.
**Respiratory:** dyspnea.

## Overdose and treatment
Signs of overdose are exaggerated adverse reactions, particularly hypotension and shock. In case of overdose, treatment is symptomatic and supportive. Dialysis may not be helpful because drug is highly protein-bound.

## Clinical considerations
■ Terazosin may cause marked hypotension, especially orthostatic hypotension, and syncope with the first dose or during the first few days of therapy. A similar response occurs if therapy is interrupted for longer than a few doses.
■ Terazosin therapy causes small but significant decreases in hematocrit, WBC count, and hemoglobin, total protein, and albumin levels; the magnitude of these decreases hasn't been shown to worsen with time, suggesting the possibility of hemodilution.

### Therapeutic monitoring
■ Advise clinician to monitor blood pressure closely.

## Special populations

**Pregnant patients.** Safety during pregnancy hasn't been established.

**Breast-feeding patients.** It isn't known if drug appears in breast milk. Avoid use in breast-feeding women.

**Pediatric patients.** Safety and efficacy in patients under age 21 haven't been established.

**Geriatric patients.** Patients over age 65 may be particularly susceptible to adverse effects of drug.

## Patient counseling

■ Instruct patient to take first dose h.s.

■ Warn patient to avoid hazardous tasks that require alertness for 12 hours following the first dose, dose increases, or when restarting dose after interruption of therapy.

■ Caution patient to rise carefully and slowly from sitting and supine positions and to report dizziness, light-headedness, or palpitations. Dosage adjustment may be needed.

# terbinafine hydrochloride

Lamisil, Lamisil AT, Lamisil AT Spray Pump

*Pharmacologic classification:* synthetic allylamine derivative
*Therapeutic classification:* antifungal
*Pregnancy risk category B*

## Available forms

Available by prescription only
*Tablets:* 250 mg
Available without a prescription
*Cream:* 1%
*Solution:* 1 %

## Indications and dosages

*Interdigital tinea pedis*

*Adults and children over age 12:* Apply a sufficient amount of cream to the affected and surrounding areas and rub in gently b.i.d. in the morning and evening for a minimum of 1 week. For plantar or moccasin type, therapy should last 2 weeks. Alternatively, apply solution b.i.d. for 1 week.

*Tinea corporis, tinea cruris*

*Adults and children over age 12:* Apply a sufficient amount of cream to the affected and surrounding areas and rub in gently b.i.d. in the morning and evening for a minimum of 1 week. Or, apply solution once daily for 1 week.

*Pityriasis (tinea) versicolor*

*Adults and children over age 12:* Apply solution b.i.d. for 1 week.

Note: Manufacturer states that therapy with topical terbinafine should continue until improvement occurs, for at least 1 week and not to exceed 4 weeks.

*Onychomycosis of fingernails or toenails caused by dermatophytes (tinea unguium)*

*Adults and children over age 18:* For treatment of fingernails, give 250 mg/day P.O. for 6 weeks; for toenails, give 250 mg/day P.O. for 12 weeks. Before initiating treatment, obtain appropriate nail specimens for laboratory testing (KOH preparation, fungal culture, or nail biopsy) to confirm the diagnosis of onychomycosis.

## Mechanism of action

*Antifungal action:* Terbinafine exerts its antifungal effect by inhibiting squalene epoxidase, a key enzyme in sterol biosynthesis in fungi. This action results in a deficiency in ergosterol and a corresponding accumulation of squalene within the fungal cell and causes fungal cell death.

## Pharmacokinetics

**Topical**

*Absorption:* Systemic absorption of terbinafine is highly variable.

*Distribution:* None reported.

*Metabolism:* None reported.

*Excretion:* About 75% of cutaneously absorbed terbinafine is eliminated in urine, predominantly as metabolites.

**Oral**

*Absorption:* More than 70% of drug is absorbed; food enhances absorption.

*Distribution:* Distributed to serum and skin. Plasma half-life is about 36 hours; half-life in tissue is 200 to 400 hours. More than 99% of drug is plasma protein–bound.

*Metabolism:* First-pass metabolism is about 40%.

*Excretion:* About 70% of dose is eliminated in urine; clearance is decreased by 50% in patients with hepatic cirrhosis and impaired renal function.

| Route | Onset | Peak | Duration |
|---------|---------|---------|----------|
| P.O. | Unknown | 2 hr | Unknown |
| Topical | Unknown | Unknown | Unknown |

## Contraindications and precautions

Contraindicated in patients hypersensitive to drug. Oral form is also contraindicated in patients with preexisting hepatic disease or impaired renal function (creatinine clearance of 50 ml/minute or less) and during pregnancy. Rare cases of liver failure, some leading to death or liver transplant, may occur with the use of tablets in individuals with and without preexisting liver disease. Tablets not recommended for patients with chronic or active liver disease. Pretreatment serum transaminase (ALT, AST) tests are advised for all patients.

## Interactions

None reported for topical form.

---

**Drug-drug.** *I.V. caffeine:* Decreased caffeine clearance. Advise clinician to monitor patient closely.
*Cimetidine:* Decreased terbinafine clearance by 33%. Avoid use together.
*Cyclosporine:* Increased cyclosporine clearance. Advise clinician to monitor levels carefully.
*Rifampin:* Increased terbinafine clearance by 100%. Advise clinician to monitor patient closely.

## Adverse reactions
**CNS:** *headache.*
**EENT:** visual disturbances.
**GI:** diarrhea, dyspepsia, abdominal pain, nausea, flatulence, taste disturbances.
**Hematologic:** decreased absolute lymphocyte count, *neutropenia.*
**Hepatic:** elevated liver enzyme levels.
**Skin:** *Stevens-Johnson syndrome, toxic epidermal necrolysis,* irritation, burning, pruritus, dryness.

## Overdose and treatment
Acute overdose with topical application is unlikely because of the limited absorption of topically applied drug and wouldn't be expected to lead to a life-threatening situation.

## Clinical considerations
■ Diagnosis should be confirmed either by direct microscopic examination of scrapings from infected tissue mounted in a solution of potassium hydroxide or by culture.
■ Topical form of drug is for topical use only; it isn't for oral, ophthalmic, or intravaginal use.
■ Before topical application, the affected skin and surrounding areas should be washed with soap and water and dried completely.
■ Tablets are not recommended for patients with chronic or active liver disease. Pretreatment serum transaminase (ALT, AST) tests are advised for all patients.
■ Report symptoms of persistent nausea, anorexia, fatigue, vomiting, right upper abdominal pain or jaundice, dark urine, or pale stools. Advise clinician to discontinue therapy with tablets and have liver test results evaluated.
**❗ALERT** Be aware of soundalikes: terbinafine and terbutaline; lamisil and lamictal.

### Therapeutic monitoring
■ Many patients given shorter durations of therapy (1 to 2 weeks) continue to improve during the 2 to 4 weeks after drug therapy has been completed. As a consequence, patients shouldn't be considered therapeutic failures until they've been observed for a period of 2 to 4 weeks off therapy. If successful outcome isn't achieved during the posttreatment observation period, the diagnosis should be reviewed.

■ Advise clinician to monitor patient for irritation or sensitivity to drug. Advise clinician to discontinue therapy if irritation or sensitivity is present and institute appropriate treatment measures.
■ Advise clinician to perform liver function tests for patients receiving oral treatment for longer than 6 weeks.

### Special populations
**Pregnant patients.** Not recommended for use during pregnancy.
**Breast-feeding patients.** Drug appears in breast milk. A decision to discontinue either breast-feeding or drug must be made, taking into account the importance of drug to the woman. Women who are breast-feeding should avoid application of terbinafine cream to the breast.
**Pediatric patients.** Safety and efficacy in children under age 18 haven't been established.

## Patient counseling
■ Advise patient to use drug as directed and to avoid contact with eyes, nose, mouth, or other mucous membranes.
■ Stress importance of using drug for recommended treatment time.
■ Tell patient to call his prescriber if the area of application shows signs or symptoms of increased irritation or possible sensitization, such as redness, itching, burning, blistering, swelling, or oozing.
■ Instruct patient not to use occlusive dressings unless directed.

# terbutaline sulfate
Brethine

*Pharmacologic classification:* adrenergic (beta$_2$ agonist)
*Therapeutic classification:* bronchodilator, premature labor inhibitor (tocolytic)
*Pregnancy risk category B*

## Available forms
Available by prescription only
*Tablets:* 2.5 mg, 5 mg
*Injection:* 1 mg/ml parenteral

## Indications and dosages
*Relief of bronchospasm in patients with reversible obstructive airway disease*
*Adults and adolescents ages 15 and older:* Administer 5 mg P.O. t.i.d. at 6-hour intervals. Reduce dosage to 2.5 mg P.O. t.i.d. if adverse effects occur. Maximum daily dose, 15 mg. Alternatively, 0.25 mg S.C.; may repeat 0.25 mg S.C. in 15 to 30 minutes. No more than 0.5 mg should be given in a 4-hour period.
*Children ages 12 to 15:* 2.5 mg P.O. t.i.d. Maximum daily dose, 7.5 mg.

◇ *Premature labor*
*Adults:* Initially, 2.5 to 10 mcg/minute I.V. Titrate at 10- to 20-minute intervals to maximum dose of 80 mcg/minute. Maintain I.V. dosage at minimum effective dose for 12 hours after uterine contractions have stopped. Maintainance therapy until term is 2.5 to 10 mg P.O. q 4 to 6 hours.

## I.V. administration
■ The infusion rate and duration should be carefully adjusted according to maternal blood pressure, maternal and fetal heart rates, and uterine response.
■ Store injection solution away from light. Don't use if discolored.

### Incompatibilities
Incompatible with bleomycin.

## Mechanism of action
*Bronchodilator action:* Terbutaline acts directly on beta$_2$-adrenergic receptors to relax bronchial smooth muscle, relieving bronchospasm and reducing airway resistance. Cardiac and CNS stimulation may occur with high doses.
*Tocolytic action:* When used in premature labor, terbutaline relaxes uterine smooth muscle, which inhibits uterine contractions.

## Pharmacokinetics
*Absorption:* About 33% to 50% of an oral dose is absorbed through the GI tract.
*Distribution:* Distributed widely throughout the body.
*Metabolism:* Partially metabolized in liver to inactive compounds.
*Excretion:* After parenteral administration, 60% of drug is excreted unchanged in urine, 3% in feces through bile, and the remainder in urine as metabolites. After oral administration, most drug is excreted as metabolites.

| Route | Onset | Peak | Duration |
|---|---|---|---|
| P.O. | 30 min | 2-3 hr | 4-8 hr |
| S.C. | 15 min | ½ hr | 1½-4 hr |
| Inhalation | 5-30 min | 1-2 hr | 3-6 hr |

## Contraindications and precautions
Contraindicated in patients hypersensitive to drug or sympathomimetic amines. Use cautiously in patients with CV disorders, hyperthyroidism, diabetes, or seizure disorders.

## Interactions
**Drug-drug.** *Cardiac glycosides, cyclopropane, halogenated inhalation anesthetics, levodopa:* Increased risk of arrhythmias. Advise clinician to monitor patient closely. Avoid use with levodopa.
*CNS stimulants:* Increased CNS stimulation. Avoid use together.

*MAO inhibitors:* Potential for hypertensive crisis. Give together with caution.
*Propranolol, other beta blockers:* Blocked bronchodilation effects of terbutaline. Avoid use together.

## Adverse reactions
**CNS:** *nervousness, tremor, drowsiness, dizziness, headache,* weakness.
**CV:** *palpitations,* tachycardia, **arrhythmias,** flushing.
**GI:** *vomiting, nausea,* heartburn.
**Metabolic:** hypokalemia (with high doses).
**Respiratory:** *paradoxical bronchospasm with prolonged usage,* dyspnea.
**Skin:** diaphoresis.

## Overdose and treatment
Signs and symptoms of overdose include exaggeration of common adverse reactions, particularly arrhythmias, seizures, nausea, and vomiting.

Treatment requires supportive measures. If patient is conscious and ingestion was recent, advise clinician to induce emesis and follow with gastric lavage. If patient is comatose, after endotracheal tube is in place with cuff inflated, advise clinician to perform gastric lavage; then give activated charcoal to reduce drug absorption. Advise clinician to maintain adequate airway, provide cardiac and respiratory support, and monitor vital signs closely.

## Clinical considerations
■ CV effects are more likely with S.C. route and when patient has arrhythmias.
■ Most adverse reactions are transient; however, tachycardia may persist for a relatively long time.
■ Terbutaline may reduce the sensitivity of spirometry for diagnosis of bronchospasm.
**◖ ALERT** Be aware of soundalikes: terbinafine and terbutaline.

### Therapeutic monitoring
■ Advise clinician to carefully monitor patient for toxicity.
■ When drug is used for tocolytic therapy, advise clinician to monitor patient for CV effects, including tachycardia, for 12 hours after discontinuation of drug. Advise clinician to monitor intake and output; fluid restriction may be needed. Muscle tremor is common but may subside with continued use. Periodic monitoring of oral glucose tolerance is recommended.
■ Advise clinician to monitor neonate for hypoglycemia if the mother used terbutaline during pregnancy.

### Special populations
**Pregnant patients.** Manufacturers state that drug shouldn't be used to treat preterm labor. Use drug during pregnancy only when expected benefits justify risk to fetus.

**Breast-feeding patients.** Drug appears in breast milk in minute amounts. Use drug with caution in breast-feeding women.

**Pediatric patients.** Drug isn't recommended for use in children under age 12.

**Geriatric patients.** Geriatric patients are more sensitive to effects of terbutaline; a lower dose may be required.

## Patient counseling

■ Instruct patient to avoid simultaneous administration with adrenocorticoid aerosol. Separate administration time by 15 minutes.

■ Instruct patient to use terbutaline only as directed. If drug produces no relief or if condition worsens, he should call his prescriber promptly.

■ Advise patient to take a missed dose within 1 hour, and if remembered longer than 1 hour after missed dose, to skip and not double the dose.

■ Caution patient that many OTC cold and allergy remedies contain a sympathomimetic that may be harmful when combined with terbutaline.

---

# terconazole
Terazol 3, Terazol 7

*Pharmacologic classification:* triazole derivative
*Therapeutic classification:* antifungal
*Pregnancy risk category C*

## Available forms

Available by prescription only
*Vaginal cream:* 0.4% in 45-g tube, 0.8% in 20-g tube with applicator
*Vaginal suppositories:* 80 mg

## Indications and dosages
*Local treatment of vulvovaginal candidiasis*

*Adults:* 0.4%: 1 full applicatorful (5 g) intravaginally once daily h.s. for 7 consecutive days. 0.8%: 1 full applicatorful (5 g) intravaginally once daily h.s. for 3 consecutive days. Alternatively, insert 1 suppository vaginally h.s. for 3 consecutive days.

## Mechanism of action
*Antifungal action:* Exact mechanism of action is unknown. Terconazole may disrupt fungal cell membrane permeability.

## Pharmacokinetics
*Absorption:* Minimally absorbed, about 5% to 16%.
*Distribution:* Effect is mainly local.
*Metabolism:* Metabolized mainly by oxidative *N*- and *O*-dealkylation, dioxolane ring cleavage, and conjugation pathways.

*Excretion:* Following oral administration of terconazole, 32% to 56% of dose is excreted in urine and 47% to 52% is excreted in feces within 24 hours.

| Route | Onset | Peak | Duration |
|---|---|---|---|
| Intravaginal | Unknown | Unknown | Unknown |

## Contraindications and precautions
Contraindicated in patients sensitive to terconazole or its inactive ingredients.

## Interactions
None reported.

## Adverse reactions
**CNS:** *headache.*
**GU:** dysmenorrhea, genitalia pain, vulvovaginal burning.
**Skin:** irritation, *pruritus,* photosensitivity.
**Other:** fever, chills, body aches.

## Overdose and treatment
None reported.

## Clinical considerations
■ Drug is only effective against vulvovaginitis caused by *Candida* organisms. Diagnosis should be confirmed by cultures or potassium hydroxide smears.

■ A persistent infection may be caused by reinfection. Patient should be evaluated for possible sources.

### Therapeutic monitoring
■ Intractable candidiasis may be a sign of diabetes mellitus. Advise clinician to perform blood and urine glucose determinations to rule out undiagnosed diabetes mellitus.

### Special populations
**Pregnant patients.** There are no adequate and controlled studies regarding use of drug during first trimester. Drug was used during second and third trimesters in at least 100 women without adversely affecting the outcome of pregnancy.

**Breast-feeding patients.** Safety hasn't been established. Breast-feeding isn't recommended during therapy with terconazole.

## Patient counseling
■ Instruct patient to insert cream high into the vagina.

■ Tell patient to complete full course of therapy and to use it continuously, even during menstrual period. The therapeutic effect of terconazole isn't affected by menstruation.

■ Inform patient to report if drug causes burning or irritation.

---

# testosterone

Histerone 100, Malogen in Oil\*,
Testamone, Testandro, Testaqua

# testosterone cypionate

depAndro 100, depAndro 200,
Depotest 100, Depotest 200, Depo-
Testosterone, Duratest-100, Duratest-
200, T-Cypionate, Testred Cypionate
200, Virilon IM

# testosterone enanthate

Andro L.A. 200, Andropository 200,
Delatestryl, Durathate-200, Everone
200, Testrin-P.A.

# testosterone propionate

Malogen in Oil\*, Testex

*Pharmacologic classification:* androgen
*Therapeutic classification:* androgen
replacement, antineoplastic
*Pregnancy risk category X*
*Controlled substance schedule III*

## Available forms

Available by prescription only
**testosterone**
*Injection (aqueous suspension):* 25 mg/ml, 50
mg/ml, 100 mg/ml
**testosterone cypionate (in oil)**
*Injection:* 100 mg/ml, 200 mg/ml
**testosterone enanthate (in oil)**
*Injection:* 100 mg/ml, 200 mg/ml
**testosterone propionate (in oil)**
*Injection:* 50 mg/ml, 100 mg/ml

## Indications and dosages

*Male hypogonadism*
**testosterone or testosterone propionate**
*Adults:* 10 to 25 mg I.M. two or three times
weekly.
**testosterone cypionate or enanthate**
*Adults:* 50 to 400 mg I.M. q 2 to 4 weeks.
*Delayed puberty in males*
**testosterone or testosterone propionate**
*Children:* 25 to 50 mg I.M. two or three times
weekly for up to 6 months.
**testosterone cypionate or enanthate**
*Children:* 50 to 200 mg I.M. q 2 to 4 weeks for
up to 6 months.
*Postpartum breast pain and engorgement*
**testosterone or testosterone propionate**
*Adults:* 25 to 50 mg I.M. daily for 3 to 4 days.
*Inoperable breast cancer*
**testosterone**
*Adults:* 100 mg I.M. three times weekly.
**testosterone cypionate or enanthate**
*Adults:* 200 to 400 mg I.M. q 2 to 4 weeks.
**testosterone propionate**
*Adults:* 50 to 100 mg I.M. three times weekly.

*Postpubertal cryptorchidism*
**testosterone or testosterone propionate**
*Adults:* 10 to 25 mg I.M. two or three times
weekly.
*Growth stimulation in Turner's syndrome*
**testosterone propionate**
*Adults:* 40 to 50 mg/m$^2$ I.M. once monthly for
6 months.

## Mechanism of action

*Androgenic action:* Testosterone is the endogenous androgen that stimulates receptors
in androgen-responsive organs and tissues to
promote growth and development of male sexual organs and secondary sexual characteristics.
*Antineoplastic action:* Testosterone exerts inhibitory, antiestrogenic effects on hormone-
responsive breast tumors and metastases.

## Pharmacokinetics

*Absorption:* Testosterone and its esters must
be administered parenterally because they're
inactivated rapidly by the liver when given orally. The onset of action of cypionate and enanthate esters of testosterone is somewhat slower than that of testosterone itself.
*Distribution:* Normally 98% to 99% plasma
protein–bound, primarily to the testosterone-
estradiol binding globulin.
*Metabolism:* Metabolized to several 17-ke-
tosteroids by two main pathways in the liver.
A large portion of these metabolites then form
glucuronide and sulfate conjugates. Plasma
half-life of testosterone ranges from 10 to 100
minutes. The cypionate and enanthate esters
of testosterone have longer durations of action
than testosterone.
*Excretion:* Very little unchanged testosterone
appears in urine or feces. About 90% of metabolized testosterone is excreted in urine in
the form of sulfate and glucuronide conjugates.

| Route | Onset | Peak | Duration |
|-------|-------|------|----------|
| I.M. | Unknown | 10-100 min | Unknown |

## Contraindications and precautions

Contraindicated in men with breast or prostate
cancer; in patients with hypercalcemia or cardiac, hepatic, or renal decompensation; during
pregnancy; and in breast-feeding women.
Use cautiously in geriatric patients and in
women of childbearing age.

## Interactions

**Drug-drug.** *Hepatotoxic drugs:* Increased risk
of hepatotoxicity. Advise clinician to monitor
patient closely.
*Insulin, oral antidiabetics:* Decreased serum
glucose; altered glucose levels in diabetic patient. Advise clinician to monitor patient closely. Dosage may require adjustment.
*Oral anticoagulants:* Prolonged PT and INR.
Advise clinician to monitor patient closely.

*Oxyphenbutazone:* Possible increased serum oxyphenbutazone level. Advise clinician to monitor patient closely.

## Adverse reactions

**CNS:** headache, anxiety, depression, paresthesia, sleep apnea syndrome.
**CV:** edema.
**GI:** nausea.
**GU:** increased serum creatinine.
**Hematologic:** elevated PT and INR, polycythemia, suppression of clotting factors.
**Hepatic:** reversible jaundice, cholestatic hepatitis, abnormal liver enzyme levels.
**Metabolic:** hypercalcemia; hypernatremia; hyperkalemia; hyperphosphatemia; hypercholesteremia; abnormal results of glucose tolerance tests; decreased thyroid function test results and serum 17-ketosteroid levels.
**Skin:** pain and induration at injection site, local edema, hypersensitivity manifestations.
**Other:** hypoestrogenic effects in women (flushing; diaphoresis; vaginitis, including itching, drying, and burning; vaginal bleeding; menstrual irregularities); androgenic effects in women *(acne, edema, oily skin, weight gain, hirsutism, hoarseness,* clitoral enlargement, deepening voice, decreased or increased libido); excessive hormonal effects in men (prepubertal—premature epiphyseal closure, *acne,* priapism, *growth of body and facial hair,* phallic enlargement; postpubertal—testicular atrophy, oligospermia, decreased ejaculatory volume, impotence, gynecomastia, epididymitis).

## Overdose and treatment

None reported.

## Clinical considerations

■ When used to treat male hypogonadism, therapy should be started with full therapeutic doses and tapered according to patient tolerance and response. Administering long-acting esters (enanthate or cypionate) at intervals greater than every 2 to 3 weeks may cause hormone levels to fall below those found in normal adults.
■ Testosterone enanthate has been used for postmenopausal osteoporosis and to stimulate erythropoiesis.

## Therapeutic monitoring

■ Advise clinician to carefully observe women for signs of excessive virilization. If possible, therapy should be stopped at first sign of virilization because some adverse effects, such as deepening of voice and clitoral enlargement, are irreversible.
■ Patients with metastatic breast cancer should have regular determinations of serum calcium level to avoid serious hypercalcemia.

### Special populations

**Pregnant patients.** Drug isn't indicated for use during pregnancy.
**Breast-feeding patients.** It's unknown if drug appears in breast milk. An alternative to breast-feeding is recommended because of potential for severe adverse effects of androgens on infant.
**Pediatric patients.** Use with extreme caution in children to avoid precocious puberty and premature closure of the epiphyses. Advise clinician to obtain X-ray examinations every 6 months to assess skeletal maturation.
**Geriatric patients.** Advise clinician to observe elderly men for prostatic hyperplasia. Development of symptomatic prostatic hyperplasia or prostatic carcinoma mandates the discontinuation of drug.

## Patient counseling

■ Explain to women that virilization may occur and to report androgenic effects immediately. Stopping drug prevents further androgenic changes but probably won't reverse those already present.
■ Tell women to report menstrual irregularities; drug may be discontinued pending determination of the cause.
■ Inform men to report too frequent or persistent penile erections.
■ Advise patient to report persistent GI distress, diarrhea, or the onset of jaundice.

# testosterone transdermal system

Androderm, Testoderm

*Pharmacologic classification:* androgen
*Therapeutic classification:* androgen replacement
*Pregnancy risk category X*
*Controlled substance schedule III*

## Available forms

Available by prescription only
*Transdermal system:* 2.5 mg/day (Androderm), 4 mg/day (Testoderm), 6 mg/day (Testoderm)

## Indications and dosages

*Primary or hypogonadotropic hypogonadism*
**Androderm**
*Adult men ages 18 and older:* Two systems applied nightly for 24 hours, providing a total dose of 5 mg/day. Apply on dry area of skin on back, abdomen, upper arms, or thighs. Don't apply to scrotum.
**Testoderm**
*Adult men ages 18 and older:* Apply one 6-mg/day patch to scrotal area daily for 22 to 24

hours. If scrotal area is too small for 6-mg/day patch, start therapy with 4-mg/day patch.

Note: Discontinue testosterone transdermal system if edema occurs.

## Mechanism of action
*Androgenic action:* Testosterone transdermal system releases testosterone, the endogenous androgen that stimulates receptors in androgen-responsive organs and tissues to promote growth and development of male sex organs and secondary sex characteristics.

## Pharmacokinetics
*Absorption:* Occurs after placement of a testosterone transdermal system on scrotal skin. Daily application of two Androderm systems at bedtime results in a serum testosterone concentration profile that mimics the normal circadian variation observed in healthy young men.
*Distribution:* Circulating testosterone is chiefly bound in the serum to sex hormone-binding globulin and albumin.
*Metabolism:* Metabolized to various 17-ketosteroids through two different pathways; the major active metabolites are estradiol and dihydrotestosterone.
*Excretion:* Little unchanged testosterone appears in urine or feces.

| Route | Onset | Peak | Duration |
|-------|-------|------|----------|
| Transdermal | Unknown | 2-4 hr | 2 hr after removal |

## Contraindications and precautions
Contraindicated in patients hypersensitive to drug, in women, and in men with known or suspected breast or prostate cancer.

Use cautiously in patients with preexisting renal, cardiac, or hepatic disease and in elderly men.

## Interactions
**Drug-drug.** *Hepatotoxic drugs:* Increased risk of hepatotoxicity. Advise clinician to monitor patient closely.
*Insulin, oral antidiabetics:* Decreased serum glucose level; altered glucose levels in diabetic patient. Advise clinician to monitor patient closely. Dosage may require adjustment.
*Oral anticoagulants:* Prolonged PT and INR. Advise clinician to monitor patient closely.
*Oxyphenbutazone:* Possible increased serum oxyphenbutazone level. Advise clinician to monitor patient closely.

## Adverse reactions
**CNS:** *CVA.*
**GU:** prostatitis, urinary tract infection.
**Metabolic:** altered thyroid function test results.
**Skin:** acne, *pruritus.*

**Other:** discomfort, irritation, *gynecomastia,* breast tenderness.

## Overdose and treatment
Testosterone levels of up to 11,400 ng/dl have been implicated in CVA. No other information is available.

## Clinical considerations
■ Testoderm form of testosterone transdermal system doesn't produce adequate serum testosterone level if applied to nongenital skin.
■ Gynecomastia commonly develops and occasionally persists in patients receiving treatment for hypogonadism.
■ Topical adverse reactions decrease with duration of use.
■ Store testosterone transdermal system at room temperature.

### Therapeutic monitoring
■ Advise clinician to check hemoglobin level and hematocrit periodically (to detect polycythemia) in patients on long-term androgen therapy.
■ Advise clinician to check liver function, prostatic acid phosphatase, prostatic specific antigen, cholesterol, and high-density lipoproteins periodically.
■ After 3 to 4 weeks of daily system use in patients receiving Testoderm, draw blood 2 to 4 hours after system application for determination of serum total testosterone. For patients receiving Androderm, advise clinician to monitor serum testosterone level the morning following regular evening application. Because of variability in analytical values among diagnostic laboratories, this laboratory work and later analyses for assessing the effect of testosterone transdermal system should be performed at the same laboratory.
■ If patient hasn't achieved desired results within 8 weeks, another form of testosterone replacement therapy should be considered.

### Special populations
**Pediatric patients.** Testosterone transdermal system hasn't been evaluated in males under age 18.
**Geriatric patients.** Geriatric patients given androgens may be at increased risk for development of prostatic hyperplasia and prostatic carcinoma. Use cautiously.

## Patient counseling
■ Instruct patient regarding proper administration technique.
■ Advise patient to report if nausea, vomiting, skin color changes, ankle edema, or too-frequent or persistent penile erections occurs.
■ Inform patient that topical testosterone preparations used by men have caused virilization in female partners. Changes in body hair dis-

## Available forms
Available by prescription only
*Capsules:* 100 mg, 250 mg, 500 mg
*Tablets:* 250 mg, 500 mg
*Suspension:* 125 mg/5 ml
Available without a prescription
*Topical ointment:* 3%

## Indications and dosages
*Infections caused by sensitive organisms*
*Adults:* 1 to 2 g P.O. divided into two to four doses.
*Children over age 8:* 25 to 50 mg/kg P.O. daily, divided into two to four doses. Alternatively, 0.6 to 1.2 g/m² daily.
*Uncomplicated urethral, endocervical, or rectal infection caused by Chlamydia trachomatis*
*Adults:* 500 mg P.O. q.i.d. for at least 7 days.
*Brucellosis*
*Adults and children ages 8 and older:* 500 mg P.O. q 6 hours for 3 to 6 weeks with streptomycin 1 g I.M. q 12 hours during week 1, then once daily during week 2.
*Gonorrhea in patients sensitive to penicillin*
*Adults:* Initially, 1.5 g P.O.; then 500 mg q 6 hours for 4 days.
*Syphilis in nonpregnant patients sensitive to penicillin*
*Adults:* 500 mg P.O. q.i.d. for 14 days.
*Acne*
*Adults and adolescents:* Initially, 500 to 1,000 mg P.O. divided q.i.d. for 1 to 2 weeks; then 125 to 500 mg P.O. daily. Apply topical ointment generously to affected areas b.i.d. until skin is thoroughly wet.
◇ *Lyme disease*
*Adults:* 250 to 500 mg P.O. q.i.d. for 10 to 30 days.
◇ *Acute transmitted epididymitis (children over age 8);* ◇ *pelvic inflammatory disease;* ◇ *infection with Helicobacter pylori (all these indications use tetracycline as adjunctive therapy)*
*Adults:* 500 mg P.O. q.i.d. for 10 to 14 days.
*Infection prophylaxis in minor skin abrasions and treatment of superficial infections caused by susceptible organisms*
*Adults and children:* Apply topical ointment to infected area one to three times daily.

## Mechanism of action
*Antibacterial action:* Tetracycline is bacteriostatic; it binds reversibly to ribosomal subunits, inhibiting bacterial protein synthesis. Its spectrum of action includes many gram-negative and gram-positive organisms, *Mycoplasma*, *Rickettsia*, *Chlamydia*, and spirochetes.

Tetracycline is useful against brucellosis, glanders, mycoplasma pneumonia infections (some clinicians prefer erythromycin), leptospirosis, early stages of Lyme disease, rickettsial infections (such as Rocky Mountain spotted fever, Q fever, and typhus fever), and chlamydial infections. It's an alternative to penicillin for infection with *Neisseria gonorrhoeae,* but because of a high level of resistance in the United States, other alternative drugs should be considered.

## Pharmacokinetics
*Absorption:* 75% to 80% absorbed after oral administration. Food or milk products significantly reduce oral absorption.
*Distribution:* Widely distributed into body tissues and fluids, including synovial, pleural, prostatic, and seminal fluids, bronchial secretions, saliva, and aqueous humor; CSF penetration is poor. Drug crosses the placental barrier, and is 20% to 67% protein-bound.
*Metabolism:* Not metabolized.
*Excretion:* Excreted primarily unchanged in urine by glomerular filtration; plasma half-life is 6 to 12 hours in adults with normal renal function. Some drug appears in breast milk. Only minimal amounts of tetracycline are removed by hemodialysis or peritoneal dialysis.

| Route | Onset | Peak | Duration |
|---|---|---|---|
| P.O. | Unknown | 2-4 hr | Unknown |
| Topical | Unknown | Unknown | Unknown |

## Contraindications and precautions
Contraindicated in patients hypersensitive to tetracyclines. Use cautiously in patients with impaired renal or hepatic function. Use oral form cautiously in last half of pregnancy and in children under age 8.

## Interactions
**Drug-drug.** *Antacids containing aluminum, calcium, magnesium; laxatives containing magnesium, oral iron, sodium bicarbonate:* Decreased absorption of tetracycline. Avoid use together.
*Anticoagulants:* Enhanced anticoagulation effects; advise clinician to monitor effects closely. Dosage adjustment may be needed.
*Cimetidine:* Possible decreased GI absorption of tetracycline. Avoid use together.
*Digoxin:* Increased bioavailability. Dosage adjustment may be needed. Advise clinician to monitor patient closely.
*Methoxyflurane:* Increased risk of nephrotoxicity. Avoid use together.
*Oral contraceptives:* Decreased contraceptive effect. Advise patient to use another contraceptive method.
*Penicillin:* Inhibited cell growth from bacteriostatic action. Advise clinician to give penicillin 2 to 3 hours before tetracycline.
**Drug-food.** *Milk, dairy products, other foods:* Decreased antibiotic absorption. Advise clinician to give antibiotic 1 hour before or 2 hours after ingesting such foods.

---

**Drug-lifestyle.** *Sun exposure:* Enhanced photosensitivity reactions. Advise patient to use sunblock.

## Adverse reactions
Unless otherwise noted, the following adverse reactions refer to oral form of drug.
**CNS:** dizziness, headache, *intracranial hypertension (pseudotumor cerebri).*
**CV:** *cardiac arrest, arrhythmias,* pericarditis.
**EENT:** sore throat, glossitis.
**GI:** anorexia, *epigastric distress, nausea,* vomiting, *diarrhea,* esophagitis, oral candidiasis, stomatitis, enterocolitis, inflammatory lesions in anogenital region, dysphagia.
**GU:** elevated BUN level.
**Hematologic:** *neutropenia,* eosinophilia, *thrombocytopenia.*
**Hepatic:** elevated liver enzyme levels.
**Respiratory:** *status asthmaticus, respiratory arrest.*
**Skin:** *candidal superinfection, maculopapular and erythematous rashes, urticaria, photosensitivity, increased pigmentation;* temporary stinging or burning on application; slight yellowing of treated skin, especially in patients with light complexions; severe dermatitis (with topical administration).
**Other:** *anaphylactoid reactions,* hypersensitivity reactions; when used in children under age 8, *permanent discoloration of teeth, enamel defects,* and *retardation of bone growth.*

## Overdose and treatment
Signs of overdose are usually limited to GI tract; recommend giving antacids or emptying stomach by gastric lavage if ingestion occurs within the preceding 4 hours.

## Clinical considerations
**◪ ALERT** Check expiration date. Outdated or deteriorated tetracyclines have caused reversible nephrotoxicity (Fanconi's syndrome).
**Topical use**
■ Avoid contact with eyes, nose, and mouth.
■ Tetracycline causes false-negative results in urine tests using glucose oxidase reagent (Diastix, Chemstrip uG, or glucose enzymatic test strip) and false elevations in fluorometric tests for urinary catecholamines.

### *Therapeutic monitoring*
■ Advise clinician to monitor patient for hypersensitivity reactions.
■ Advise clinician to monitor patient for resolution of symptoms.
■ If condition persists or worsens, drug use should be stopped.

### *Special populations*
**Pregnant patients.** Drug causes fetal harm and should be given during pregnancy only when expected benefits justify risk to fetus.

**Breast-feeding patients.** Because drug appears in breast milk, don't use in breast-feeding women.
**Pediatric patients.** Don't use in children under age 8.

## Patient counseling
■ Inform patient using topical form that normal use of cosmetics may continue.
■ Tell patient that stinging may occur with topical use but resolves quickly.
■ Inform patient that tetracycline may stain clothing.
■ Warn patient to avoid prolonged exposure to sunlight.
■ Tell patient to report persistent nausea or vomiting, or yellowing of skin or eyes.

# tetrahydrozoline hydrochloride
Collyrium Fresh, Eyesine, Geneye, Mallazine Eye Drops, Murine Plus, Optigene 3, Tetrasine, Tyzine, Tyzine Pediatric, Visine

*Pharmacologic classification:* sympathomimetic
*Therapeutic classification:* vasoconstrictor, decongestant
*Pregnancy risk category C*

## Available forms
Available by prescription only
*Nasal solution:* 0.05%, 0.1%
Available without a prescription
*Ophthalmic solution:* 0.05%

## Indications and dosages
*Nasal congestion*
*Adults and children over age 6:* Apply 2 to 4 drops or sprays of 0.1% nasal solution in each nostril q 4 to 8 hours, p.r.n. Don't use for longer than 3 to 5 days.
*Children ages 2 to 6:* Apply 2 or 3 drops of 0.05% solution in each nostril q 4 to 6 hours, p.r.n. Don't use for longer than 3 to 5 days.
*Conjunctival congestion*
*Adults:* 1 or 2 drops of ophthalmic solution in each eye b.i.d. to q.i.d. Don't use for longer than 3 to 4 days without consulting an ophthalmologist.

## Mechanism of action
*Vasoconstrictor and decongestant action:* In ocular use, vasoconstriction is produced by local adrenergic action on the blood vessels of the conjunctiva. After nasal application, drug acts on alpha-adrenergic receptors in nasal mucosa to produce constriction, decreasing blood flow and nasal congestion.

---

## Pharmacokinetics
None reported.

| Route | Onset | Peak | Duration |
|-------|-------|------|----------|
| Ophthalmic | Few min | Unknown | 1-4 hr |

## Contraindications and precautions
Contraindicated in patients hypersensitive to drug or its components, in those with angle-closure glaucoma or other serious eye diseases, and in patients on MAO inhibitor therapy. Nasal solution is contraindicated in children under age 2; 0.1% solution is contraindicated in children under age 6.

Use cautiously in patients with hyperthyroidism, hypertension, and diabetes mellitus. Use ophthalmic form cautiously in patients with cardiac disease.

## Interactions
**Drug-drug.** *Guanethidine, MAO inhibitors, tricyclic antidepressants:* Increased adrenergic response and hypertensive crisis. Avoid use together.

## Adverse reactions
**CNS:** headache, drowsiness, insomnia, dizziness, tremor (with ophthalmic form).
**CV:** *arrhythmias* (with ophthalmic form), tachycardia, palpitations.
**EENT:** transient eye stinging, pupillary dilation, increased intraocular pressure, keratitis, lacrimation, eye irritation (with ophthalmic form); transient burning, stinging; sneezing, rebound nasal congestion with excessive or long-term use (with nasal form).

## Overdose and treatment
Signs and symptoms of accidental overdose include bradycardia, decreased body temperature, shocklike hypotension, apnea, drowsiness, CNS depression, and coma.

Because of rapid onset of sedation, emesis isn't recommended unless induced early. Activated charcoal or gastric lavage may be used initially. Advise clinician to monitor vital signs and ECG and treat seizures with I.V. diazepam.

## Clinical considerations
■ Excessive use of either preparation may cause rebound effect.
■ Drug shouldn't be used for longer than 3 to 4 days.
■ Don't use in geriatric patients to treat redness and inflammation, which may indicate more serious eye conditions.
■ Use in glaucoma requires close medical supervision.

### Therapeutic monitoring
■ Advise clinician to monitor cardiac status (ophthalmic solution only).
■ Advise clinician to monitor patient for resolution of symptoms.

## Special populations
**Pregnant patients.** It isn't known if drug causes fetal harm. Give drug during pregnancy only when clearly indicated.
**Pediatric patients.** The 0.1% nasal solution is contraindicated in children under age 6. All uses are contraindicated in children under age 2.
**Geriatric patients.** Geriatric patients are more likely to experience adverse reactions to sympathomimetics.

## Patient counseling
■ Instruct patient on proper administration technique.
■ Advise patient not to exceed recommended dose and to use drug only when needed.
■ Tell patient to remove contact lenses before using drug.

# thalidomide
Thalomid

*Pharmacologic classification:* immunomodulator
*Therapeutic classification:* antileprotic
*Pregnancy risk category X*

## Available forms
Available by prescription only
*Capsules:* 50 mg

## Indications and dosages
*Acute treatment of cutaneous manifestations of moderate to severe erythema nodosum leprosum (ENL)*
*Adults:* 100 to 300 mg P.O. daily h.s. If patient weighs under 50 kg (110 lb), start dosing at the lower end of range.
*Maintenance therapy for prevention and suppression of cutaneous manifestations of ENL recurrence*
*Adults:* Up to 400 mg P.O. daily h.s. or in divided doses at least 1 hour after meals.
◊ *Recurrent aphthous stomatitis*
*Adults:* 100 to 600 mg P.O. daily.
◊ *Treatment of graft versus host disease*
*Adults:* 800 to 1,600 mg P.O. daily.

## Mechanism of action
*Antileprotic action:* Mechanism of action in patients with ENL isn't fully known.

## Pharmacokinetics
*Absorption:* Slowly absorbed from GI tract.
*Distribution:* Not reported.
*Metabolism:* Exact metabolic fate isn't known.
*Excretion:* Mean half-life is 5 to 7 hours. Route of elimination isn't fully understood.

| Route | Onset | Peak | Duration |
|-------|-------|------|----------|
| P.O. | Unknown | 3-6 hr | Unknown |

## Contraindications and precautions

Contraindicated in patients hypersensitive to drug or its components; in pregnant women, and in those capable of becoming pregnant, except when alternative therapies are inappropriate and patient meets all conditions listed in the System for Thalidomide Education and Prescribing Safety (S.T.E.P.S.) program.

## Interactions

**Drug-drug.** *Barbiturates, chlorpromazine, reserpine:* Possible enhanced sedative activity. Use together with caution.
*Drugs associated with peripheral neuropathy:* Increased risk of peripheral neuropathy. Use together cautiously.
**Drug-food.** *Any food:* Decreased absorption of drug. Drug should be given at least 1 hour after meals at h.s.
**Drug-lifestyle.** *Alcohol use:* Increased sedation. Advise patient to avoid alcohol.

## Adverse reactions

**CNS:** *asthenia, drowsiness, somnolence, dizziness,* peripheral neuropathy, *headache,* agitation, insomnia, malaise, nervousness, *paresthesia,* tremor, vertigo.
**CV:** orthostatic hypotension, **bradycardia,** peripheral edema.
**EENT:** pharyngitis, sinusitis.
**GI:** abdominal pain, anorexia, constipation, *diarrhea,* flatulence, *nausea,* dry mouth, oral candidiasis.
**GU:** albuminuria, *hematuria,* impotence.
**Hematologic: neutropenia, increased HIV viral load,** anemia, *lymphadenopathy,* LEUKOPE-NIA.
**Hepatic:** abnormal liver function test results, increased AST level.
**Metabolic:** hyperlipidemia.
**Musculoskeletal:** back pain, neck pain, neck rigidity.
**Skin:** acne, fungal dermatitis, nail disorder, pruritus, *rash, maculopapular rash,* sweating.
**Other: *human teratogenicity, hypersensitivity reactions,*** facial edema, lymphadenopathy, fever, chills, accidental injury, infection, pain.

## Overdose and treatment

There have been three reported cases of overdose, none of which resulted in fatality.

## Clinical considerations

**◪ ALERT** Thalidomide must only be given in compliance with all of the terms outlined in the S.T.E.P.S. program; may only be prescribed by prescribers registered with the S.T.E.P.S. program; and may only be dispensed by pharmacists registered with the S.T.E.P.S. program.
■ All sexually mature patients, men or women, capable of reproduction must meet rigid S.T.E.P.S. program requirements including ability to understand and carry out instructions, ability and willingness to comply with manda-

tory contraceptive measures (concurrent use of at least two highly effective means of contraception), and a written acknowledgment of understanding of all warnings concerning the hazards of fetal exposure to thalidomide and the risk of contraception failure.
■ Sexually mature women who haven't undergone a hysterectomy or who haven't been postmenopausal for at least 24 consecutive months (who have had menses at some time in the preceding 24 consecutive months) are considered to be women of childbearing potential even with history of infertility.
■ Pregnancy test is mandatory within 24 hours before thalidomide therapy for women of childbearing potential, then weekly during first month of therapy, then monthly for women with regular menstrual cycles. If menstrual cycles are irregular, pregnancy testing continues every 2 weeks during therapy. Retesting is performed if menstrual changes occur, including missed menses.
■ Corticosteroids may be given with drug in patients with moderate to severe neuritis associated with severe ENL reaction. Corticosteroids can be tapered and discontinued when neuritis improves.
■ A patient with a history of requiring prolonged treatment to prevent recurrence of cutaneous ENL or who experiences flare during tapering, should use minimum effective dose. Tapering should be attempted every 3 to 6 months at a dose reduction rate of 50 mg every 2 to 4 weeks.
■ An unlabeled use for this drug is multiple myeloma.

### Therapeutic monitoring

■ Immediately report suspected fetal exposure to FDA via MedWATCH at 1-800-FDA-1088 and report to manufacturer.
■ Advise clinician to perform CBC and differential before initiating therapy and periodically thereafter, p.r.n. Patients with an absolute neutrophil count below 750/mm³ while on treatment should be reevaluated.
■ Advise clinician to monitor patient for signs and symptoms of neuropathy, such as numbness, tingling, or pain in hands or feet, at least once monthly during first 3 months of drug therapy, then periodically.

### Special populations

**Pregnant patients.** Drug is highly dangerous to fetus in any amount. At least two highly reliable means of contraception must be used simultaneously and continuously from at least 1 month before thalidomide therapy until 1 month following completion of therapy.
**Breast-feeding patients.** It isn't known if drug appears in breast milk. A decision should be made to discontinue either drug or breast-feeding, depending on the importance of drug to the mother.

**Pediatric patients.** Safety and efficacy in children under age 12 aren't known.
**Geriatric patients.** Safety and efficacy in geriatric patients aren't significantly different from those in younger patients.

## Patient counseling

- Warn patient of dangers of fetal exposure to any amount of thalidomide and that blood and sperm donations are prohibited while taking thalidomide.
- Explain that at least two highly reliable means of contraception must be used simultaneously and continuously from at least 1 month before thalidomide therapy until 1 month following completion of therapy.
- Instruct patient to report signs or symptoms of pregnancy immediately without regard to probability or improbability of pregnancy.
- Inform women with childbearing potential of mandatory pregnancy testing schedule.
- Inform patient that, if pregnancy occurs, drug must be discontinued immediately.
- Caution patient that it isn't known if drug is present in ejaculate of men receiving drug, and that men receiving thalidomide must always use a latex condom when engaging in sexual activity with women of childbearing potential.
- Advise patient to read package insert carefully.
- Caution patient about potential for dizziness and orthostatic hypotension; instruct patient to change position slowly when rising.
- Inform patient that drug frequently causes drowsiness and somnolence. Advise patient to avoid hazardous activities and the use of alcohol or other drugs that might cause drowsiness.
- Tell patient to take drug h.s. with a glass of water, at least 1 hour after the evening meal.
- Tell patient drug has caused hypersensitivity reactions and to notify prescriber if erythematous macular rash, fever, tachycardia, hypotension, or other adverse reactions occurs.

---

# theophylline

Accurbron, Aerolate, Aquaphyllin, Asmalix, Bronkodyl, Constant-T, Elixophyllin, Lanophyllin, Quibron-T, Respbid, Slo-bid Gyrocaps, Slo-Phyllin, Sustaire, Theobid Duracaps, Theochron, Theo-Dur, Theolair, Theo-24, Theospan-SR, Theostat 80, Theovent, Theo-X, T-Phyl, Uniphyl

*Pharmacologic classification:* xanthine derivative
*Therapeutic classification:* bronchodilator
*Pregnancy risk category C*

## Available forms

Available by prescription only
*Capsules:* 100 mg, 200 mg
*Capsules (extended-release):* 50 mg, 60 mg, 65 mg, 75 mg, 100 mg, 125 mg, 130 mg, 200 mg, 250 mg, 260 mg, 300 mg
*Tablets:* 100 mg, 125 mg, 200 mg, 250 mg, 300 mg
*Tablets (extended-release):* 100 mg, 200 mg, 250 mg, 300 mg, 400 mg, 450 mg, 500 mg
*Elixir:* 50 mg/5 ml, 80 mg/15 ml
*Syrup:* 50 mg/5 ml, 80 mg/15 ml, 150 mg/15 ml
*$D_5W$ injection:* 200 mg in 50 ml or 100 ml; 400 mg in 100 ml, 250 ml, or 1,000 ml; 800 mg in 500 ml or 1,000 ml

## Indications and dosages

*Symptomatic relief of bronchospasm in patients not currently receiving theophylline who require rapid relief of acute symptoms*
*Loading dose:* 6 mg/kg anhydrous theophylline, then:
*Adults (nonsmokers):* 3 mg/kg P.O. q 6 hours for two doses; then 3 mg/kg q 8 hours.
*Older adults and patients with cor pulmonale:* 2 mg/kg P.O. q 6 hours for two doses; then 2 mg/kg q 8 hours.
*Adults with HF:* 2 mg/kg P.O. q 8 hours for two doses; then 1 to 2 mg/kg q 12 hours.
*Children and adolescents ages 9 to 16 and young adult smokers:* 3 mg/kg P.O. q 4 hours for three doses; then 3 mg/kg q 6 hours.
*Neonates and children ages 6 months to 9 years:* 4 mg/kg P.O. q 4 hours for three doses; then 4 mg/kg q 6 hours.
◊ *Neonates and infants under age 6 months:* Dose highly individualized. Serum theophylline level should be maintained at less than 10 mcg/ml in neonates and less than 20 mcg/ml in older infants.
*Loading dose:* 1 mg/kg P.O. or I.V. for each 2-mcg/ml increase in theophylline level, then:
*Infants over 8 weeks to 6 months:* 1 to 3 mg/kg q 6 hours.
*Infants ages 4 to 8 weeks:* 1 to 2 mg/kg q 8 hours.
*Neonates under 4 weeks:* 1 to 2 mg/kg q 12 hours.
*Premature neonates (less than 40 weeks' gestational age):* 1 mg/kg q 12 hours.
*Parenteral theophylline for patients not currently receiving theophylline*
*Loading dose:* 4.7 mg/kg (equivalent to 6 mg/kg anhydrous aminophylline) I.V. slowly; then maintenance infusion.
*Adults (nonsmokers):* 0.55 mg/kg/hour (equivalent to 0.7 mg/kg/hour anhydrous aminophylline) for 12 hours, then 0.39 mg/kg/hour (equivalent to 0.5 mg/kg/hour anhydrous aminophylline).
*Older adults and patients with cor pulmonale:* 0.47 mg/kg/hour (equivalent to 0.6 mg/kg/hour anhydrous aminophylline) for 12 hours; then 0.24 mg/kg/hour (equivalent to 0.3 mg/kg/hour anhydrous aminophylline).

*Adults with HF or liver disease:* 0.39 mg/kg/hour (equivalent to 0.5 mg/kg/hour anhydrous aminophylline) for 12 hours; then 0.08 to 0.16 mg/kg/hour (equivalent to 0.1 to 0.2 mg/kg/hour anhydrous aminophylline).

*Children ages 9 to 16:* 0.79 mg/kg/hour (equivalent to 1 mg/kg/hour anhydrous aminophylline) for 12 hours; then 0.63 mg/kg/hour (equivalent to 0.8 mg/kg/hour anhydrous aminophylline).

*Infants and children ages 6 months to 9 years:* 0.95 mg/kg/hour (equivalent to 1.2 mg/kg/hour anhydrous aminophylline) for 12 hours; then 0.79 mg/kg/hour (equivalent to 1 mg/kg/hour anhydrous aminophylline).

Switch to oral theophylline as soon as patient shows adequate improvement.

***Symptomatic relief of bronchospasm in patients currently receiving theophylline***
*Adults and children:* Each 0.5 mg/kg I.V. or P.O. (loading dose) increases plasma levels by 1 mcg/ml. Ideally, dose is based on current theophylline level and lean body weight. In emergency situations, may use a 2.5-mg/kg P.O. dose of rapidly absorbed form if no obvious signs of theophylline toxicity are present.

***Prophylaxis of bronchial asthma, bronchospasm of chronic bronchitis, emphysema***
*Adults and children:* Using rapidly absorbed forms, initial dose is 16 mg/kg or 400 mg P.O. daily (whichever is less) divided q 6 to 8 hours; dose may be increased in approximate increments of 25% at 2- to 3-day intervals. Using extended-release forms, initial dose is 12 mg/kg or 400 mg P.O. daily (whichever is less) divided q 8 to 12 hours; dose may be increased, if tolerated, by 2 to 3 mg/kg daily at 3-day intervals. Regardless of form used, dose may be increased, if tolerated, to the following maximum daily doses, without measurements of serum theophylline level:
*Adults and adolescents ages 16 and older:* 13 mg/kg P.O. or 900 mg P.O. whichever is less, daily in divided doses.
*Adolescents ages 12 to 16:* 18 mg/kg P.O. daily in divided doses.
*Children ages 9 to 12:* 20 mg/kg P.O. daily in divided doses.
*Children under age 9:* 24 mg/kg P.O. daily in divided doses.

Note: Dose individualization is needed. Use peak plasma and trough levels to estimate dose. Therapeutic range is 10 to 20 mcg/ml. All doses are based on theophylline anhydrous and lean body weight.
◊ ***Cystic fibrosis***
*Infants:* 10 to 20 mg/kg I.V. daily.
◊ ***Promotion of diuresis;*** ◊ ***treatment of Cheyne-Stokes respirations;*** ◊ ***paroxysmal nocturnal dyspnea***
*Adults:* 200 to 400 mg I.V. bolus (single dose).

## I.V. administration
■ Drug may be administered undiluted.
■ Drug may be given by slow I.V. injection or, preferably, in large volume parenteral fluids by slow I.V. infusion.
■ Loading doses are usually given over 20 to 30 minutes at a rate not exceeding 20 mg/minute.

### Incompatibilities
Incompatible with ascorbic acid, ceftriaxone, cimetidine, hetastarch, and phenytoin.

## Mechanism of action
*Bronchodilator action:* Drug may act by inhibiting phosphodiesterase, elevating cellular cAMP levels, or antagonizing adenosine receptors in the bronchi, resulting in relaxation of the smooth muscle.

Drug also increases sensitivity of the medullary respiratory center to carbon dioxide, to reduce apneic episodes. It prevents muscle fatigue, especially that of the diaphragm. It also causes diuresis and cardiac and CNS stimulation.

## Pharmacokinetics
*Absorption:* Well absorbed. Rate and onset of action depend on the dose form; food may further alter rate of absorption, especially of some extended-release preparations.
*Distribution:* Distributed throughout the extracellular fluids; equilibrium between fluid and tissues occurs within an hour of an I.V. loading dose. Therapeutic plasma levels are 10 to 20 mcg/ml, but many patients respond to lower levels.
*Metabolism:* Metabolized in the liver to inactive compounds. Half-life is 7 to 9 hours in adults, 4 to 5 hours in smokers, 20 to 30 hours in premature infants, and 3 to 5 hours in children.
*Excretion:* About 10% of dose is excreted in urine unchanged. The other metabolites include 1,3-dimethyluric acid, 1-methyluric acid, and 3-methylxanthine.

| Route | Onset | Peak | Duration |
|---|---|---|---|
| P.O. | 15-60 min | 1-2 hr | Unknown |
| P.O. (extended) | 15-60 min | 4-7 hr | Unknown |
| I.V. | 15 min | 15-30 min | Unknown |

## Contraindications and precautions
Contraindicated in patients hypersensitive to xanthine compounds, such as caffeine and theobromine, and in those with active peptic ulcer or seizure disorders.

Use cautiously in geriatric patients; in neonates, infants under age 1, and young children; and in patients with COPD, cardiac failure, cor pulmonale, renal or hepatic disease, peptic ulcer, hyperthyroidism, diabetes mellitus, glaucoma, severe hypoxemia, hypertension, compromised cardiac or circulatory function, angina, acute MI, or sulfite sensitivity.

## Interactions

**Drug-drug.** *Activated charcoal, barbiturates, ketoconazole, phenytoin, rifampin:* Decreased plasma theophylline levels. Advise clinician to monitor patient closely. Dosage adjustment may be needed if use together can't be avoided.

*Allopurinol (high dose), calcium channel blockers, cimetidine, corticosteroids, erythromycin, interferon, mexiletine, oral contraceptives, propranolol, quinolones, troleandomycin:* Possible increased serum levels of theophylline. Advise clinician to monitor patient closely. Dosage adjustment may be needed if use together can't be avoided.

*Beta blockers:* Antagonistic pharmacologic effect. Avoid use together.

*Carbamazepine, isoniazid, loop diuretics:* Possible increased or decreased theophylline levels. Advise clinician to monitor patient closely. Dosage adjustment may be needed if use together can't be avoided.

*Lithium:* Increased excretion of lithium. Lithium dosage may require adjustment. Advise clinician to monitor patient carefully.

**Drug-herb.** *Cacao tree:* Possible inhibition of theophylline metabolism. Patient should avoid ingesting large amounts of cocoa when using theophylline.

*Caffeine, guarana:* Additive CNS and CV effects. Discourage use together.

*Ephedra:* Possible increased risk of adverse reactions. Discourage use together.

*St. John's wort:* Decreased theophylline levels and efficacy. Discourage use together, if possible. If not, advise clinician to monitor theophylline levels and adjust dose p.r.n.

**Drug-food.** *Any food:* Accelerated absorption. Advise patient to take drug on an empty stomach.

**Drug-lifestyle.** *Smoking (cigarettes, marijuana):* Increased elimination of theophylline. Advise clinician to monitor theophylline response and serum level. Dosage adjustment may be needed.

## Adverse reactions

**CNS:** *restlessness, dizziness, insomnia,* headache, irritability, *seizures,* muscle twitching.
**CV:** *palpitations, sinus tachycardia, extrasystoles,* marked hypotension, *arrhythmias.*
**GI:** *nausea, vomiting,* diarrhea, epigastric pain.
**Respiratory:** tachypnea, *respiratory arrest.*
**Skin:** flushing.

## Overdose and treatment

Signs and symptoms of overdose include nausea, vomiting, insomnia, irritability, tachycardia, extrasystoles, tachypnea, or tonic-clonic seizures. The onset of toxicity may be sudden and severe, with arrhythmias and seizures as the first signs. Advise clinician to induce emesis except in convulsing patients, then use activated charcoal and cathartics. Advise clinician to treat arrhythmias with lidocaine and seizures with I.V. diazepam and support respiratory and CV systems.

## Clinical considerations

■ Theophylline has a low therapeutic index.
■ Dosage is determined by monitoring response, tolerance, pulmonary function, and serum theophylline level. Target range is 10 to 20 mcg/ml.
■ Use cautiously in young children, infants, neonates and geriatric patients.
■ Depending on assay used, theophylline level may be falsely elevated in the presence of furosemide, phenylbutazone, probenecid, theobromine, caffeine, tea, chocolate, cola beverages, and acetaminophen.

### Therapeutic monitoring

■ Advise clinician to monitor vital signs and observe for signs and symptoms of toxicity.
■ Advise clinician to obtain serum theophylline measurements in patients receiving long-term therapy. Ideal levels are between 10 and 20 mcg/ml, although some patients may respond adequately with lower serum levels. Check every 6 months. If levels are less than 10 mcg/ml, dose should be increased by about 25% each day. If levels are 20 to 25 mcg/ml, dose should be decreased by about 10% each day. If levels are 25 to 30 mcg/ml, skip next dose and decrease by 25% each day. If levels are more than 30 mcg/ml, advise clinician to skip patient's next two doses and decrease by 50% each day. Serum level determination should be repeated.

### Special populations

**Breast-feeding patients.** Drug appears in breast milk and may cause irritability, insomnia, or fretfulness in the breast-fed infant. A decision must be made to stop either breast-feeding or drug therapy.

**Pediatric patients.** Use with caution in neonates. Children usually require higher doses (on a mg/kg basis) than adults. Maximum recommended doses are 24 mg/kg/day in children under age 9; 20 mg/kg/day in children ages 9 to 12; 18 mg/kg/day in adolescents ages 12 to 16; 13 mg/kg/day or 900 mg (whichever is less) in adolescents and adults ages 16 and older.

## Patient counseling

■ Instruct patient regarding drug and dosing schedule; if a dose is missed, he should take it as soon as possible, but he shouldn't double the dose.
■ Advise patient to take drug at regular intervals as instructed, around-the-clock.

- Inform patient of adverse effects and possible signs of toxicity.
- Tell patient to take drug with food if GI upset occurs with liquid preparations or non–sustained-release forms.
- Instruct patient to continue to use the same brand of theophylline.
- Advise patient who smokes to notify prescriber if he quits. The dose of theophylline will probably need to be reduced to avoid toxicity.

# thiamine hydrochloride (vitamin B₁)
Biamine, Thiamilate

*Pharmacologic classification:* water-soluble vitamin
*Therapeutic classification:* nutritional supplement
*Pregnancy risk category A (C if more than RDA)*

## Available forms
Available by prescription only
*Injection:* 1-ml ampules (100 mg/ml), 1-ml vials (100 mg/ml), 2-ml vials (100 mg/ml), 10-ml vials (100 mg/ml), 30-ml vials (100 mg/ml)
Available without a prescription
*Tablets:* 25 mg, 50 mg, 100 mg, 250 mg, 500 mg
*Tablets (enteric-coated):* 20 mg

## Indications and dosages
### Beriberi
*Adults:* 10 to 20 mg I.M., depending on severity (can receive up to 100 mg I.M. or I.V. for severe cases), t.i.d. for 2 weeks, followed by dietary correction and multivitamin supplement containing 5 to 30 mg thiamine daily in single or three divided doses for 1 month.
*Children:* 10 to 25 mg, depending on severity, I.M. daily for several weeks with adequate dietary intake.
### Anemia secondary to thiamine deficiency; polyneuritis secondary to alcoholism, pregnancy, or pellagra
*Adults and children:* P.O. dosage is based on RDA for age group.
### Wernicke's encephalopathy
*Adults:* Initially, 100 mg I.V., followed by 50 to 100 mg I.M. or I.V. daily.
### Wet beriberi with heart failure
*Adults and children:* 10 to 30 mg I.V. for emergency treatment.

## I.V. administration
- Store thiamine in light-resistant, nonmetallic container.
- An intradermal skin test should be performed before I.V. thiamine administration if sensitivity is suspected.

- Advise clinician to keep epinephrine available when administering large parenteral doses.

## Incompatibilities
Incompatible with alkali carbonates, amobarbital, barbiturates, citrates, erythromycin estolate, kanamycin, phenobarbital, streptomycin, and sulfites.

## Mechanism of action
*Metabolic action:* Exogenous thiamine is required for carbohydrate metabolism. Thiamine combines with ATP to form thiamine pyrophosphate, a coenzyme in carbohydrate metabolism and transketolation reactions. This coenzyme is also necessary in the hexose monophosphate shunt during pentose utilization. One sign of thiamine deficiency is an increase in pyruvic acid. The body's need for thiamine is greater when the carbohydrate content of the diet is high. Within 3 weeks of total absence of dietary thiamine, significant vitamin depletion may occur. Thiamine deficiency may cause beriberi.

## Pharmacokinetics
*Absorption:* Absorbed readily after oral administration of small doses; after oral administration of a large dose, the total amount absorbed is limited to 4 to 8 mg. In alcoholics and in patients with cirrhosis or malabsorption, GI absorption of thiamine is decreased. When given with meals, GI rate of drug absorption decreases, but total absorption remains the same. After I.M. administration, drug is absorbed rapidly and completely.
*Distribution:* Distributed widely into body tissues. When intake exceeds the minimal requirements, tissue stores become saturated. About 100 to 200 mcg/day of thiamine appears in the milk of breast-feeding women on a normal diet.
*Metabolism:* Metabolized in the liver.
*Excretion:* Excess thiamine is excreted in urine. After administration of large doses (more than 10 mg), both unchanged thiamine and metabolites are excreted in urine after tissue stores become saturated.

| Route | Onset | Peak | Duration |
|---|---|---|---|
| P.O., I.V., I.M. | Unknown | Unknown | Unknown |

## Contraindications and precautions
Contraindicated in patients hypersensitive to thiamine products.

## Interactions
**Drug-drug.** *Neuromuscular blockers:* Possible enhanced effects of these drugs. Monitor patient closely.

## Adverse reactions
**CNS:** restlessness.

---

**CV:** *CV collapse,* cyanosis.
**EENT:** tightness of throat (allergic reaction).
**GI:** nausea, *hemorrhage.*
**Respiratory:** pulmonary edema.
**Skin:** feeling of warmth, pruritus, urticaria, diaphoresis.
**Other:** *angioedema,* weakness; tenderness and induration following I.M. administration.

## Overdose and treatment
Very large doses of thiamine administered parenterally may produce neuromuscular and ganglionic blockade and neurologic symptoms. Treatment is supportive.

## Clinical considerations
■ The RDA of thiamine is as follows:
*Neonates and infants up to age 6 months:* 0.2 mg daily.
*Infants ages 6 months to 1 year:* 0.3 mg daily.
*Children ages 1 to 3:* 0.5 mg daily.
*Children ages 4 to 8:* 0.6 mg daily.
*Children ages 9 to 13:* 0.9 mg daily.
*Males ages 14 and older:* 1.2 mg daily.
*Females ages 14 to 18:* 1 mg daily.
*Females ages 19 and older:* 1.1 mg daily.
*Pregnant women:* 1.4 mg daily.
*Breast-feeding women:* 1.5 mg daily.
■ I.M. injection may be painful. Injection site rotation is recommended.
■ Total absence of dietary thiamine can produce a deficiency state in about 3 weeks.
■ Accurate dietary history is important during vitamin replacement therapy.
■ Many clinicians recommend administration of at least 1 dose of I.V. or I.M. thiamine to all alcoholic patients with altered sensorium (such as delirium) who are admitted to the hospital.
■ Drug therapy may produce false-positive results in the phosphotungstate method for determination of uric acid and in urine spot tests with Ehrlich's reagent for urobilinogen.
■ Large doses of thiamine interfere with the Schack and Waxler spectrophotometric determination of serum theophylline levels.

### Therapeutic monitoring
■ Advise clinician to monitor patient for adverse reactions including injection site reactions.
■ Advise clinician to monitor patient for symptom relief.

### Special populations
**Breast-feeding patients.** Thiamine, in amounts that don't exceed the RDA, is safe to use in breast-feeding women. It appears in breast milk and fulfills a nutritional requirement of the infant.

## Patient counseling
■ Inform patient of potential adverse reactions.

# thioguanine (6-thioguanine, 6-TG)

*Pharmacologic classification:* antimetabolite (cell cycle–phase specific, S phase)
*Therapeutic classification:* antineoplastic
*Pregnancy risk category D*

## Available forms
Available by prescription only
*Tablets (scored):* 40 mg

## Indications and dosages
Dosage and indications may vary. Check current literature for recommended protocol.
*Acute nonlymphocytic leukemias*
*Adults and children:* Initially, 2 mg/kg/day P.O. (usually calculated to nearest 20 mg); then, if no toxic effects occur, increase dose gradually over 3 to 4 weeks to 3 mg/kg/day. Maintenance dosage, 2 to 3 mg/kg/day P.O.

## Mechanism of action
*Antineoplastic action:* Thioguanine requires conversion intracellularly to its active form to exert its cytotoxic activity. Acting as a false metabolite, thioguanine inhibits purine synthesis. Cross-resistance exists between mercaptopurine and thioguanine.

## Pharmacokinetics
*Absorption:* After an oral dose, absorption is incomplete and variable. The average bioavailability is 30%.
*Distribution:* Well distributed into bone marrow cells. It doesn't cross the blood-brain barrier to any appreciable extent.
*Metabolism:* Extensively metabolized to a less active form in the liver and other tissues.
*Excretion:* Plasma levels of thioguanine decrease in a biphasic manner, with a half-life of 15 minutes in the initial phase and 11 hours in the terminal phase. Drug is excreted in the urine, mainly as metabolites.

| Route | Onset | Peak | Duration |
|-------|-------|------|----------|
| P.O. | Unknown | Unknown | Unknown |

## Contraindications and precautions
Contraindicated in patients whose disease has shown resistance to drug and in those hypersensitive to drug or mercaptopurine. Use cautiously in patients with renal or hepatic dysfunction.

## Interactions
**Drug-drug.** *Busulfan:* Risk of hepatotoxicity, esophageal varices, portal hypertension. Avoid prolonged use together.

---

## Adverse reactions
**GI:** nausea, vomiting, stomatitis, diarrhea, anorexia.
**Hematologic:** *leukopenia,* anemia, *thrombocytopenia* (occurs slowly over 2 to 4 weeks).
**Hepatic:** *hepatotoxicity,* jaundice.
**Metabolic:** hyperuricemia.
**Skin:** rash.

## Overdose and treatment
Signs and symptoms of overdose include myelosuppression, nausea, vomiting, malaise, hypertension, and diaphoresis.

Treatment is usually supportive and includes transfusion of blood components and antiemetics. Induction of emesis may be helpful if performed soon after ingestion.

## Clinical considerations
- Total daily dose can be given at one time.
- Dosage modification may be required in renal or hepatic dysfunction.
- Drug is sometimes ordered as 6-thioguanine.
- Avoid all I.M. injections when platelet count is less than 100,000/mm³.

### Therapeutic monitoring
- Advise clinician to monitor serum uric acid level. Alkalinize urine if serum uric acid level is elevated.
- Advise clinician to monitor liver function test results.
- Advise clinician to watch for jaundice, which may reverse if drug is stopped promptly.
- CBC should be conducted daily during induction, then weekly during maintenance therapy.

### Special populations
**Pregnant patients.** Use drug during pregnancy only in life-threatening situations or severe disease for which safer drugs can't be used or are ineffective.
**Breast-feeding patients.** It isn't known if drug appears in breast milk. However, because of risk of serious adverse reactions, mutagenicity, and carcinogenicity in the infant, breast-feeding isn't recommended.

## Patient counseling
- Emphasize importance of continuing drug despite occurrence of nausea and vomiting.
- Tell patient to report promptly if vomiting (dose loss) occurs shortly after a dose is taken.
- Advise avoiding exposure to people with infections and to promptly report signs of infection or unusual bleeding.
- Encourage adequate fluid intake to increase urine output and facilitate excretion of uric acid.

# thiopental sodium
Pentothal

*Pharmacologic classification:* barbiturate
*Therapeutic classification:* anesthetic
*Pregnancy risk category C*
*Controlled substance schedule III*

## Available forms
Available by prescription only
*Injection:* 250-mg (2.5%), 400-mg (2% or 2.5%), 500-mg (2.5%) syringes; 500-mg (2.5%), 1-g (2.5%), 2.5-g (2.5%), 5-g (2.5%), 1-g (2%), 2.5-g (2%), 5-g (2%) kits
*Rectal suspension:* 2-g disposable syringe (400 mg/g of suspension)

## Indications and dosages
**General anesthetic for short-term procedures**
*Adults and children:* 2 to 4 ml 2.5% solution (50 to 100 mg) administered I.V. for induction and repeated as a maintenance dose; dosage is individualized.
**Convulsive states following anesthesia**
*Adults:* 50 to 125 mg (2 to 5 ml 2.5% solution) I.V.
**Basal anesthesia by rectal administration**
*Adults and children:* 30 mg/kg P.R.

## I.V. administration
- May give a small test dose of 25 to 75 mg to assess tolerance or unusual sensitivity.
- Administer slowly because onset of action is immediate.
- Advise clinician to monitor patient closely during and after administration.

### Incompatibilities
Incompatible with amikacin, benzquinamide, cephapirin, chlorpromazine, codeine phosphate, dextrose 10% in water or normal saline, dimenhydrinate, diphenhydramine, ephedrine, fructose 10% glycopyrrolate, human fibrinolysin, hydromorphone, invert sugar 5% and 10% in normal saline, lactated Ringer's solution, levorphanol, meperidine, metaraminol, methadone, morphine, norepinephrine, Normosol solutions except Normosol-R, penicillin G potassium, prochlorperazine edisylate, promazine, promethazine hydrochloride, regular insulin, Ringer's injection, sodium bicarbonate, and succinylcholine.

## Mechanism of action
*Anesthetic action:* Thiopental produces anesthesia by direct depression of the polysynaptic midbrain reticular activating system. Thiopental decreases presynaptic (by way of decreased neurotransmitter release) and postsynaptic excitation. These effects may be subsequent to increased gamma-aminobutyric acid

---

*Sun exposure:* Potentiation of photosensitivity reactions. Advise patient to use sunblock.

## Adverse reactions

**CNS:** extrapyramidal reactions, *tardive dyskinesia, sedation,* EEG changes, dizziness, *neuroleptic malignant syndrome.*
**CV:** *orthostatic hypotension,* tachycardia, ECG changes, *arrhythmias.*
**EENT:** *ocular changes, blurred vision,* retinitis pigmentosa.
**GI:** *dry mouth, constipation,* increased appetite.
**GU:** *urine retention,* dark urine, menstrual irregularities, inhibited ejaculation.
**Hematologic:** *transient leukopenia, agranulocytosis,* hyperprolactinemia.
**Hepatic:** cholestatic jaundice, elevated liver enzyme levels.
**Metabolic:** weight gain.
**Skin:** *mild photosensitivity,* allergic reactions.
**Other:** gynecomastia.
**After abrupt withdrawal of long-term therapy:** gastritis, nausea, vomiting, dizziness, tremor, feeling of warmth or cold, diaphoresis, tachycardia, headache, insomnia.

## Overdose and treatment

CNS depression is characterized by deep, unarousable sleep and possible coma, hypotension or hypertension, extrapyramidal symptoms, abnormal involuntary muscle movements, agitation, seizures, arrhythmias, ECG changes, hypothermia or hyperthermia, and autonomic nervous system dysfunction.

Treatment is symptomatic and supportive and includes maintaining vital signs, airway, stable body temperature, and fluid and electrolyte balance.

Don't induce vomiting; drug inhibits cough reflex, and aspiration may occur. Advise clinician to use gastric lavage, then activated charcoal and sodium chloride cathartics; dialysis doesn't help. Body temperature should be regulated p.r.n. Advise clinician to treat hypotension with I.V. fluids; epinephrine shouldn't be given. Advise clinician to treat seizures with parenteral diazepam or barbiturates; arrhythmias with parenteral phenytoin (1 mg/kg with rate adjusted to blood pressure); and extrapyramidal reactions with benztropine at 1 to 2 mg or parenteral diphenhydramine at 10 to 50 mg. Contact local or regional poison information center for specific instructions.

Patients who have overdosed should receive immediate CV monitoring, including continuos ECG to detect arrhythmias. Drugs that may produce additive QT prolongation effects, such as disopyramide, procainamide, and quinidine, should also be avoided.

## Clinical considerations

■ Before treatment starts, advise clinician to perform baseline ECG and measure serum potassium level. Patients with a QTc interval above 450 msec should not receive Mellaril. Patients with a QTc over 500 msec should discontinue use.
■ All liquid formulations must be protected from light.
**ALERT** Different liquid formulations have different concentrations. Check dosage carefully.
■ Dilute concentrate in 2 to 4 ounces (60 to 120 ml) of liquid, preferably water, carbonated drinks, fruit juice, tomato juice, milk, or pudding.
■ Oral formulations may cause stomach upset. Advise clinician to give with food or fluid.
■ Doses of more than 300 mg per day are usually reserved for adults with severe psychosis. Don't exceed 800 mg daily because ophthalmic toxicity may result.
■ Liquid formulations may cause a rash if skin contact occurs.
■ Drug can cause pink to brown discoloration of patient's urine.
■ Thioridazine causes a high risk of sedation, anticholinergic effects, orthostatic hypotension, photosensitivity reactions, and delayed or absent ejaculation. It has the lowest potential for extrapyramidal reactions of all phenothiazines.
■ Thioridazine causes false-positive test results for urinary porphyrins, urobilinogen, amylase, and 5-hydroxyindoleacetic acid because of darkening of urine by metabolites; it also causes false-positive urine pregnancy results in tests using human chorionic gonadotropin as the indicator.

### Therapeutic monitoring

■ Advise clinician to check patient regularly for abnormal body movements (at least once every 6 months).

### Special populations

**Breast-feeding patients.** Thioridazine may appear in breast milk. Potential benefits to the woman should outweigh the potential harm to the infant.
**Pediatric patients.** Drug isn't recommended for children under age 2. For children over age 2, dosage is 0.5 mg/kg/day in divided doses.
**Geriatric patients.** Geriatric patients tend to require lower doses, adjusted to individual response. Such patients also are more likely to develop adverse reactions, especially tardive dyskinesia and other extrapyramidal effects.

## Patient counseling

■ Explain risks of dystonic reactions and tardive dyskinesia, and tell patient to report abnormal body movements.
■ Tell patient to avoid sun exposure and to wear sunblock when going outdoors to prevent photosensitivity reactions. (Heat lamps and tanning beds also may cause burning of the skin or skin discoloration.)

■ Warn patient not to spill the liquid on the skin; rash and irritation may result.

■ Warn patient to avoid extremely hot or cold baths or exposure to temperature extremes, sunlamps, or tanning beds; drug may cause thermoregulatory changes.

■ Advise patient to take drug exactly as prescribed and not to double doses that are missed.

■ Explain that many drug interactions are possible. Patient should seek medical approval before taking any OTC drugs.

■ Tell patient not to stop taking drug suddenly; most adverse reactions may be relieved by dose reduction. However, patient should call prescriber if he experiences difficulty urinating, sore throat, dizziness, or fainting, or if visual changes develop.

■ Warn patient to avoid hazardous activities that require alertness until the effect of drug is established. Reassure patient that excessive sedation usually subsides after several weeks.

■ Tell patient not to drink alcohol or take other drugs that may cause excessive sedation.

■ Advise patient to maintain adequate hydration.

■ Explain which fluids are appropriate for diluting the concentrate and the dropper technique of measuring dose.

■ Tell patient to store drug safely away from children.

## thiotepa
Thioplex

*Pharmacologic classification:* alkylating (cell cycle–phase nonspecific)
*Therapeutic classification:* antineoplastic
*Pregnancy risk category D*

### Available forms
Available by prescription only
*Injection:* 15-mg vials

### Indications and dosages
Dosage and indications may vary. Check current literature for recommended protocol.
**Breast and ovarian cancer, Hodgkin's disease, lymphomas**
*Adults and children ages 12 and older:* 0.2 mg/kg I.V. daily for 4 to 5 days, repeated q 2 to 4 weeks; or 0.3 to 0.4 mg/kg I.V. q 1 to 4 weeks.
**Bladder tumor**
*Adults and children ages 12 and older:* 60 mg in 30 to 60 ml of normal saline solution (thiotepa in distilled water) instilled in bladder once weekly for 4 weeks.
**Neoplastic effusions**
*Adults and children ages 12 and older:* 0.6 to 0.8 mg/kg intracavity or intratumor. Maintenance doses of 0.07 to 0.8 mg/kg intratumor at 1- to 4-week intervals.

◇**Malignant meningeal neoplasm**
*Adults:* 1 to 10 mg/m$^2$ intrathecally, once to twice weekly.

### I.V. administration
**H ALERT** Follow institutional policy to minimize risks. Preparation and administration of parenteral form of drug are linked with mutagenic, teratogenic, and carcinogenic risks to personnel.

■ Reconstitute with 1.5 ml of sterile water for injection. Don't use other solutions. Further dilute with normal saline solution for injection, $D_5W$, $D_5W$ in normal saline, Ringer's injection, or lactated Ringer's injection. Use within 8 hours.

■ Discard if solution appears grossly opaque or has a precipitate. Solutions should be clear to slightly opaque.

■ To eliminate haze, filter solutions through a 0.22-micron filter before use.

■ If pain occurs at insertion site, drug may be further diluted or use a local anesthetic to reduce pain.

■ Avoid infiltration.

■ Refrigerate dry powder; protect from light.

### Incompatibilities
Incompatible with cisplatin.

### Mechanism of action
*Antineoplastic action:* Thiotepa exerts its cytotoxic activity as an alkylating drug, cross-linking strands of DNA and RNA and inhibiting protein synthesis, resulting in cell death.

### Pharmacokinetics
*Absorption:* Incompletely absorbed across the GI tract; absorption from the bladder is variable, ranging from 10% to 100% of an instilled dose. Absorption is increased by certain pathologic conditions. I.M. and pleural membrane absorption of thiotepa is also variable.
*Distribution:* It isn't known if drug or its metabolites appear in breast milk.
*Metabolism:* Metabolized extensively in the liver.
*Excretion:* Drug and its metabolites are excreted in urine. Half-life is 2½ hours.

| Route | Onset | Peak | Duration |
|---|---|---|---|
| I.V., intrathecal, intracavitary | Unknown | Unknown | Unknown |

### Contraindications and precautions
Contraindicated in patients hypersensitive to drug and in those with severe bone marrow, hepatic, or renal dysfunction. Use cautiously in patients with impaired renal or hepatic function or bone marrow suppression.

### Interactions
**Drug-drug.** *Anticoagulants, aspirin:* Increased risk of bleeding. Avoid use together.

*Myelosuppressives:* Additive myelosuppression. Advise clinician to monitor patient closely.
*Neuromuscular blockers:* Prolonged muscular paralysis. Advise clinician to monitor patient closely.
*Other alkylating drugs, irradiation therapy:* Toxicity. Avoid use together.
*Succinylcholine:* Prolonged respirations and apnea. Advise clinician to monitor patient closely. Avoid use together.

### Adverse reactions
**CNS:** headache, dizziness, blurred vision, fatigue, weakness.
**EENT:** *laryngeal edema,* conjunctivitis.
**GI:** *nausea, vomiting,* abdominal pain, anorexia.
**GU:** amenorrhea, decreased spermatogenesis, dysuria, urine retention, hemorrhagic cystitis.
**Hematologic:** *leukopenia* (begins within 5 to 10 days), *thrombocytopenia, neutropenia,* anemia.
**Metabolic:** hyperuricemia, decreased plasma pseudocholinesterase level.
**Respiratory:** asthma.
**Skin:** hives, rash, dermatitis, alopecia.
**Other:** fever, hypersensitivity, *anaphylactic shock.*

### Overdose and treatment
Signs and symptoms of overdose include nausea, vomiting, and precipitation of uric acid in the renal tubules. Treatment is usually supportive and includes transfusion of blood components, antiemetics, hydration, and allopurinol.

### Clinical considerations
■ Drug can be given by all parenteral routes, including direct injection into the tumor.
■ To prevent hyperuricemia with resulting uric acid nephropathy, allopurinol may be given; advise clinician to keep patient well hydrated.
■ Avoid all I.M. injections when platelet count is less than 100,000/mm³.
■ Toxicity may be delayed and prolonged because drug binds to tissues and stays in body several hours.

#### Therapeutic monitoring
■ Stop drug or decrease dosage if WBC count decreases to less than 4,000/mm³ or if platelet count decreases to less than 150,000/mm³.
■ Advise clinician to monitor uric acid level.
■ Advise clinician to monitor CBC weekly for at least 3 weeks after last dose. Warn patient to report even mild infections.

#### Special populations
**Pregnant patients.** Drug shouldn't be used during pregnancy.
**Breast-feeding patients.** It isn't known if drug appears in breast milk. However, because of risk of serious adverse reactions, mutagenici-

ty, and carcinogenicity in the infant, breast-feeding isn't recommended.

### Patient counseling
■ Encourage patient to maintain an adequate fluid intake to facilitate the excretion of uric acid.
■ Instruct patient to avoid OTC products containing aspirin.
■ Tell patient to avoid exposure to people with infections.
■ Advise patient that hair should grow back after therapy has ended.
■ Tell patient to report sore throat, fever, or unusual bruising or bleeding.
■ Instruct patient to use effective contraception measures and to notify prescriber immediately if she becomes pregnant.

# thiothixene
# thiothixene hydrochloride
Navane

*Pharmacologic classification:* thioxanthene
*Therapeutic classification:* antipsychotic
*Pregnancy risk category C*

### Available forms
Available by prescription only
*Capsules:* 1 mg, 2 mg, 5 mg, 10 mg, 20 mg
*Oral concentrate:* 5 mg/ml (7% alcohol)
*Injection:* 2 mg/ml, 5 mg/ml

### Indications and dosages
*Acute agitation*
*Adults:* 4 mg I.M. b.i.d. to q.i.d.; maximum dose, 30 mg I.M. daily. Change to P.O. form as soon as possible (may need to adjust dosage); I.M. dosage form is irritating.
*Mild to moderate psychosis*
*Adults:* Initially, 2 mg P.O. t.i.d.; may increase gradually to 15 mg daily.
*Severe psychosis*
*Adults:* Initially, 5 mg P.O. b.i.d.; may increase gradually to 20 to 30 mg daily. Maximum recommended daily dose, 60 mg.

### Mechanism of action
*Antipsychotic action:* Thiothixene is thought to exert its antipsychotic effects by postsynaptic blockade of CNS dopamine receptors, thereby inhibiting dopamine-mediated effects.
　　Thiothixene has many other central and peripheral effects; it also acts as an alpha blocker. Its most prominent adverse reactions are extrapyramidal.

### Pharmacokinetics
*Absorption:* Rapidly absorbed.
*Distribution:* Widely distributed into the body. Drug is 91% to 99% protein-bound.

*Metabolism:* Metabolized in the liver.
*Excretion:* Mostly excreted as parent drug in feces by way of the biliary tract.

| Route | Onset | Peak | Duration |
|---|---|---|---|
| P.O., I.M. | 10-30 min | 1-6 hr | Unknown |

## Contraindications and precautions

Contraindicated in patients hypersensitive to drug and in those experiencing circulatory collapse, coma, CNS depression, or blood dyscrasia.

Use cautiously in geriatric or debilitated patients; in those with history of seizure disorders, CV disease, heat exposure, glaucoma, or prostatic hyperplasia; and in those in a state of alcohol withdrawal.

## Interactions

**Drug-drug.** *CNS depressants:* Increased CNS depression. Avoid use together.
**Drug-herb.** *Nutmeg:* Possible loss of symptom control. Discourage use together.
**Drug-food.** *Caffeine:* Increased metabolism of drug. Advise patient to avoid caffeine.
**Drug-lifestyle.** *Alcohol use:* Increased CNS depression. Advise patient to avoid alcohol.
*Smoking (heavy):* Increased metabolism of drug. Discourage smoking.
*Sun exposure:* Possible potentiation of photosensitivity reactions. Advise patient to use sunblock.

## Adverse reactions

**CNS:** *extrapyramidal reactions,* drowsiness, restlessness, agitation, insomnia, *tardive dyskinesia,* sedation, pseudoparkinsonism, EEG changes, dizziness, **neuroleptic malignant syndrome.**
**CV:** *hypotension,* tachycardia, ECG changes.
**EENT:** ocular changes, *blurred vision,* nasal congestion.
**GI:** *dry mouth, constipation.*
**GU:** *urine retention,* menstrual irregularities, inhibited ejaculation.
**Hematologic:** *transient leukopenia, leukocytosis, agranulocytosis.*
**Hepatic:** jaundice, elevated liver enzyme levels.
**Metabolic:** weight gain.
**Skin:** *mild photosensitivity,* allergic reactions, pain at I.M. injection site, sterile abscess.
**Other:** gynecomastia.
**After abrupt withdrawal of long-term therapy:** gastritis, nausea, vomiting, dizziness, tremor, feeling of warmth or cold, diaphoresis, tachycardia, headache, insomnia.

## Overdose and treatment

CNS depression is characterized by deep, unarousable sleep and possible coma, hypotension or hypertension, extrapyramidal symptoms, abnormal involuntary muscle movements, agitation, seizures, arrhythmias, ECG changes, hypothermia or hyperthermia, and autonomic nervous system dysfunction.

Treatment is symptomatic and supportive and includes maintaining vital signs, airway, stable body temperature, and fluid and electrolyte balance.

Don't induce vomiting; drug inhibits cough reflex, and aspiration may occur. Advise clinician to use gastric lavage, then activated charcoal and sodium chloride cathartics; dialysis doesn't help. Advise clinician to regulate body temperature p.r.n. and treat hypotension with I.V. fluids; epinephrine shouldn't be given. Seizures may be treated with parenteral diazepam or barbiturates; arrhythmias with parenteral phenytoin (1 mg/kg with rate titrated to blood pressure); and extrapyramidal reactions with benztropine at 1 to 2 mg or parenteral diphenhydramine at 10 to 50 mg.

## Clinical considerations

- Protect liquid formulation from light.
- Solution for injection may be slightly discolored. Don't use if excessively discolored or if a precipitate is evident.
- Drug is stable after reconstitution for 48 hours at room temperature.
- Dilute concentrate in 2 to 4 ounces (60 to 120 ml) of liquid, preferably water, carbonated drinks, fruit juice, tomato juice, milk, or pudding.
- Because stomach upset may occur, advise clinician to give oral form with food or fluid.
- Drug causes a high risk of extrapyramidal effects.
- Liquid and injectable formulations may cause a rash if skin contact occurs.
- Photosensitivity reactions may occur; advise patient to avoid exposure to sunlight or heat lamps.
- I.M. injection may cause skin necrosis.
- Drug causes false-positive test results for urinary porphyrins, urobilinogen, amylase, and 5-hydroxyindoleacetic acid because of darkening of urine by metabolites; it also causes false-positive urine pregnancy results in tests using human chorionic gonadotropin as the indicator.

### Therapeutic monitoring

- Advise clinician to monitor blood pressure before and after parenteral administration.
- Check patient regularly for abnormal body movements (at least once every 6 months).

### Special populations

**Pregnant patients.** Hyperreflexia has been reported in infants following in utero exposure. Use drug during pregnancy only when potential benefit justifies risk to fetus.
**Pediatric patients.** Drug isn't recommended for children under age 12.
**Geriatric patients.** Geriatric patients tend to require lower doses, adjusted to individual re-

sponse. Adverse reactions are more likely to develop in such patients, especially tardive dyskinesia and other extrapyramidal effects.

## Patient counseling

■ Explain risks of dystonic reactions and tardive dyskinesia, and tell patient to report abnormal body movements.

■ Tell patient to avoid sun exposure and to wear sunblock when going outdoors to prevent photosensitivity reactions. Remind him that heat lamps and tanning beds also may cause burning of the skin or skin discoloration.

■ Instruct patient not to spill the liquid on skin. Contact with skin may cause rash and irritation.

■ Tell patient to take drug exactly as prescribed, not to double doses for missed doses, and not to share drug with others.

■ Explain that many drug interactions are possible. Tell patient to seek medical approval before taking any OTC drugs.

■ Tell patient not to stop taking drug suddenly; most adverse reactions may be relieved by reducing the dose. However, patient should call if difficulty urinating, sore throat, dizziness, or fainting develops.

■ Warn patient against hazardous activities that require alertness until effect of drug is established. Reassure patient that sedation usually subsides after several weeks.

■ Tell patient not to drink alcohol or take other drugs that may cause excessive sedation.

■ Explain which fluids are appropriate for diluting the concentrate and the dropper technique of measuring dose.

■ Tell patient to shake concentrate before administration.

■ Instruct patient to store drug away from children.

---

# tiagabine hydrochloride
Gabitril

*Pharmacologic classification:* gamma aminobutyric acid (GABA) enhancer
*Therapeutic classification:* anticonvulsant
*Pregnancy risk category C*

## Available forms

Available by prescription only
*Tablets:* 2 mg, 4 mg, 12 mg, 16 mg, 20 mg

## Indications and dosages

*Adjunctive therapy in treatment of partial seizures*
*Adults:* Initially, 4 mg P.O. once daily. May increase total daily dose by 4 to 8 mg at weekly intervals until clinical response occurs or to maximum of 56 mg/day. Give total daily dose in divided doses b.i.d. to q.i.d.

*Adolescents ages 12 to 18:* Initially, 4 mg P.O. once daily. May increase total daily dose by 4 mg beginning of week 2 and thereafter by 4 to 8 mg/week at weekly intervals until clinical response is seen or to maximum of 32 mg/day. Give total daily dose in divided doses b.i.d. to q.i.d.

≣*Dosage adjustment.* For patients with impaired liver function, initial and maintenance dosages may be reduced or dosing intervals increased.

## Mechanism of action

*Anticonvulsant action:* Exact mechanism unknown. Tiagabine is thought to act by enhancing the activity of GABA, the major inhibitory neurotransmitter in the CNS. It binds to recognition sites associated with the GABA uptake carrier and may thus permit more GABA to be available for binding to receptors on postsynaptic cells.

## Pharmacokinetics

*Absorption:* Rapidly and nearly completely absorbed (more than 95%). Absolute bioavailability is about 90%.
*Distribution:* About 96% is bound to plasma proteins, mainly to serum albumin and alpha-1 acid glycoprotein.
*Metabolism:* Likely to be metabolized by the cytochrome P-450 3A isoenzymes.
*Excretion:* About 2% is excreted unchanged, with 25% and 63% of dose excreted into urine and feces, respectively. Half-life is about 7 to 9 hours.

| Route | Onset | Peak | Duration |
|-------|-------|------|----------|
| P.O. | Rapid | 45 min | 7-9 hr |

## Contraindications and precautions

Contraindicated in patients hypersensitive to drug or its ingredients. Use cautiously in breast-feeding women.

## Interactions

**Drug-drug.** *Carbamazepine, phenobarbital, phenytoin:* Increased tiagabine clearance. Advise clinician to monitor patient closely.
*CNS depressants:* Enhanced CNS effects. Use cautiously.
*Valproate:* Decreased valproate level. Advise clinician to monitor patient closely.
**Drug-lifestyle.** *Alcohol use:* Enhanced CNS effects. Advise patient to avoid alcohol.

## Adverse reactions

**CNS:** *dizziness, asthenia, somnolence, nervousness,* tremor, difficulty with concentration and attention, insomnia, ataxia, confusion, speech disorder, difficulty with memory, paresthesia, depression, emotional lability, abnormal gait, hostility, language problems, agitation.
**CV:** vasodilation.
**EENT:** amblyopia, nystagmus, pharyngitis.

**GI:** abdominal pain, *nausea,* diarrhea, vomiting, increased appetite, mouth ulceration.
**GU:** urinary tract infection.
**Musculoskeletal:** myalgia, myasthenia.
**Respiratory:** increased cough.
**Skin:** rash, pruritus.
**Other:** flu syndrome.

## Overdose and treatment
Common symptoms reported after an overdose include somnolence, impaired consciousness, impaired speech, agitation, confusion, speech difficulty, hostility, depression, weakness, and myoclonus.

There's no specific antidote for overdose. If indicated, elimination of unabsorbed drug should be achieved by emesis or gastric lavage. Advise clinician to observe usual precautions to maintain the airway, and provide general supportive care.

## Clinical considerations
■ A therapeutic range for plasma drug levels hasn't been established.
■ Status epilepticus and sudden unexpected death in epilepsy have occurred in patients receiving tiagabine. Patients who aren't receiving at least one other enzyme-inducing antiepilepsy drug at the time of tiagabine initiation may require lower doses or a slower dosage adjustment.
■ Never withdraw drug suddenly because seizure frequency may increase. Tiagabine should be withdrawn gradually unless safety concerns require a more rapid withdrawal.

### Therapeutic monitoring
■ Because of the potential for pharmacokinetic interactions between tiagabine and drugs that induce or inhibit hepatic metabolizing enzymes, advise clinician to obtain plasma levels of tiagabine before and after changes are made in the therapeutic regimen.

### Special populations
**Pregnant patients.** Drug shouldn't be used during pregnancy unless potential benefit justifies potential risk.
**Breast-feeding patients.** Tiagabine and its metabolites appear in breast milk. Use in breast-feeding women only if the benefits clearly outweigh the risks.
**Pediatric patients.** Drug hasn't been investigated in adequate and well-controlled trials in children under age 12.
**Geriatric patients.** Because few patients over age 65 were exposed to tiagabine hydrochloride during its clinical evaluation, safety or efficacy in this age-group isn't clear.

## Patient counseling
■ Advise patient to take drug only as prescribed and to take tiagabine with food.

■ Warn patient that drug may cause dizziness, somnolence, and other signs and symptoms of CNS depression.
■ Advise patient to avoid driving and other potentially hazardous activities that require mental alertness until CNS effects of drug are known.

# ticarcillin disodium/ clavulanate potassium
Timentin

*Pharmacologic classification:* extended-spectrum penicillin, beta-lactamase inhibitor
*Therapeutic classification:* antibiotic
*Pregnancy risk category B*

## Available forms
Available by prescription only
*Injection:* 3 g ticarcillin and 100 mg clavulanic acid

## Indications and dosages
*Infections of the lower respiratory tract, urinary tract, bones and joints, skin and skin structure, and septicemia when caused by susceptible organisms*
*Adults:* 3.1 g (contains 3 g ticarcillin and 0.1 g clavulanate) I.V. q 4 to 6 hours.
*Children ages 3 months to 16 years weighing under 60 kg (133 lb):* For mild to moderate infections, 200 mg/kg/day (contains 3 g ticarcillin and 0.1 g clavulanate potassium) I.V. infusion given in divided doses q 6 hours. For severe infections, 300 mg/kg/day (contains 3 g ticarcillin and 0.1 g clavulanate potassium) I.V. given in divided doses q 4 hours.
≡*Dosage adjustment.* For patients with renal impairment, give loading dose of 3.1 g (3 g ticarcillin and 0.1 g clavulanate) then refer to the table.

| Creatinine clearance (ml/min) | Adult dosage |
|---|---|
| 30-60 | 2 g I.V. q 4 hours |
| 10-30 | 2 g I.V. q 8 hours |
| < 10 | 2 g I.V. q 12 hours |
| < 10 with hepatic failure | 2 g I.V. q 24 hours |

## I.V. administration
■ Reconstitute with 13 ml of sterile water or normal saline solution for injection.
■ Further dilute to a maximum of 10 to 100 mg/ml (based on ticarcillin component) and infuse over 30 minutes.
■ In fluid-restricted patients, dilute to a maximum of 48 mg/ml if using $D_5W$, 43 mg/ml if

using normal saline solution for injection, or 86 mg/ml if using sterile water for injection.

### Incompatibilities
Incompatible with aminoglycosides, doxapram, fluconazole, and gentamicin.

### Mechanism of action
*Antibiotic action:* Ticarcillin is bactericidal; it adheres to bacterial penicillin-binding proteins, inhibiting bacterial cell-wall synthesis. Extended-spectrum penicillins are more resistant to inactivation by certain beta-lactamases, especially those produced by gram-negative organisms, but are still liable to inactivation by certain others.

Clavulanic acid has only weak antibacterial activity and doesn't affect the action of ticarcillin. However, clavulanic acid has a beta-lactam ring and is structurally similar to penicillin and cephalosporins; it binds irreversibly with certain beta-lactamases, preventing inactivation of ticarcillin and broadening its bactericidal spectrum.

Spectrum of activity of ticarcillin includes many gram-negative aerobic and anaerobic bacilli, many gram-positive and gram-negative aerobic cocci, and some gram-positive aerobic and anaerobic bacilli. The combination of ticarcillin and clavulanate potassium is also effective against many beta-lactamase-producing strains, including *Staphylococcus aureus, Haemophilus influenzae, Neisseria gonorrhoeae, Escherichia coli, Klebsiella,* and *Providencia* organisms, and *Bacteroides fragilis,* but not *Pseudomonas aeruginosa.*

### Pharmacokinetics
*Absorption:* Administered I.V.
*Distribution:* Distributed widely. Penetrates minimally into CSF with uninflamed meninges; clavulanic acid penetrates into pleural fluid, lungs, and peritoneal fluid. Ticarcillin achieves high levels in urine. Protein-binding is 45% to 65% for ticarcillin and 22% to 30% for clavulanic acid; both cross the placental barrier.
*Metabolism:* About 13% of a ticarcillin dose is metabolized by hydrolysis to inactive compounds; clavulanic acid is thought to undergo extensive metabolism, but its fate is as yet unknown.
*Excretion:* Ticarcillin is excreted primarily (83% to 90%) in urine by renal tubular secretion and glomerular filtration; it's also excreted in bile and in breast milk. Metabolites of clavulanate are excreted in urine by glomerular filtration and appears in breast milk. Elimination half-life of ticarcillin in adults is about 1 hour and that of clavulanate is about 1 hour; in severe renal impairment, half-life of ticarcillin is extended to about 8 hours and that of clavulanate to about 3 hours. Both drugs are

removed by hemodialysis but only slightly by peritoneal dialysis.

| Route | Onset | Peak | Duration |
|-------|-------|------|----------|
| I.V. | Unknown | Immediate | Unknown |

### Contraindications and precautions
Contraindicated in patients hypersensitive to drug or other penicillins. Use cautiously in patients with other drug allergies, especially to cephalosporins, impaired renal function, hemorrhagic conditions, hypokalemia, or sodium restrictions.

### Interactions
**Drug-drug.** *Oral contraceptives:* Decreased efficacy of contraceptive. Advise patient to use another contraceptive method.
*Probenecid:* Elevated serum ticarcillin level. Advise clinician to monitor patient carefully.

### Adverse reactions
**CNS:** *seizures,* neuromuscular excitability, headache, giddiness.
**EENT:** smell disturbances.
**GI:** nausea, diarrhea, stomatitis, vomiting, epigastric pain, flatulence, pseudomembranous colitis, taste disturbances.
**Hematologic:** *leukopenia, neutropenia,* eosinophilia, *thrombocytopenia,* hemolytic anemia, anemia, positive Coombs' test, prolonged PT and INR.
**Hepatic:** elevated liver enzyme levels.
**Metabolic:** hypokalemia, hypernatremia.
**Other:** hypersensitivity reactions (rash, pruritus, urticaria, chills, fever, edema, *anaphylaxis*), overgrowth of nonsusceptible organisms, pain at injection site, vein irritation, phlebitis.

### Overdose and treatment
Signs of overdose include neuromuscular hypersensitivity or seizures; ticarcillin and clavulanate potassium can be removed by hemodialysis.

### Clinical considerations
■ Ticarcillin disodium/clavulanate potassium is almost always used with another antibiotic such as an aminoglycoside in life-threatening situations.
■ Advise clinician to give aminoglycosides 1 hour before or after administration of ticarcillin disodium/clavulanate potassium.
■ Ticarcillin contains 5.2 mEq of sodium per gram of drug. Use with caution in patients with sodium restriction.
■ Because ticarcillin disodium/clavulanate potassium is dialyzable, patients undergoing hemodialysis may need dosage adjustments.
■ Ticarcillin disodium/clavulanate potassium alters tests for urinary or serum proteins; it interferes with turbidimetric methods that use sulfosalicylic acid, trichloroacetic acid, acetic

acid, or nitric acid. Ticarcillin disodium/clavulanate potassium doesn't interfere with tests using bromophenol blue (Albustix, Albutest, MultiStix). It may falsely decrease serum aminoglycoside level.

### Therapeutic monitoring
■ Advise clinician to monitor serum electrolyte levels and observe for signs of hypernatremia and hypokalemia.
■ Advise clinician to monitor neurologic status. High blood levels may cause seizures.

### Special populations
**Pregnant patients.** Use drug during pregnancy only when clearly needed.
**Breast-feeding patients.** Ticarcillin and clavulanate potassium appear in breast milk; use with caution in breast-feeding women.
**Geriatric patients.** Half-life may be prolonged in geriatric patients because of impaired renal function.

### Patient counseling
■ Advise patient of adverse experiences and advise him to limit salt intake during drug therapy.

## ticlopidine hydrochloride
Ticlid

*Pharmacologic classification:* platelet aggregation inhibitor
*Therapeutic classification:* antithrombotic
*Pregnancy risk category B*

### Available forms
Available by prescription only
*Tablets (film-coated):* 250 mg

### Indications and dosages
**Reduction of risk of thrombotic CVA in patients with history of CVA, in those who have experienced CVA precursors, or in those who are intolerant to aspirin therapy**
*Adults:* 250 mg P.O. b.i.d. with meals.

### Mechanism of action
*Antithrombotic action:* Ticlopidine blocks adenosine diphosphate–induced platelet-fibrinogen and platelet-platelet binding.

### Pharmacokinetics
*Absorption:* Rapidly and extensively (more than 80%) absorbed after oral administration. Absorption is enhanced by food.
*Distribution:* 98% bound to serum proteins and lipoproteins.
*Metabolism:* Extensively metabolized by the liver. It's unknown if parent drug or active metabolites are responsible for pharmacologic activity.

*Excretion:* About 60% is excreted in urine and 23% in feces; only trace amounts of intact drug are found in urine. After one dose, half-life is 12½ hours; with repeat dosing, half-life increases to 4 to 5 days.

| Route | Onset | Peak | Duration |
|-------|-------|------|----------|
| P.O. | Unknown | 2 hr | Unknown |

### Contraindications and precautions
Contraindicated in patients hypersensitive to drug; and those with hematopoietic disorders, such as neutropenia, thrombocytopenia, or disorders of hemostasis; active pathologic bleeding from peptic ulceration or active intracranial bleeding; or severe liver dysfunction.

### Interactions
**Drug-drug.** *Antacids:* Decreased plasma levels of ticlopidine. Separate administration times by at least 2 hours.
*Aspirin:* Potentiated effects of aspirin on platelets. Avoid use together.
*Cimetidine:* Decreased clearance of ticlopidine; increased toxicity risk. Don't use together.
*Digoxin:* Slightly decreased serum digoxin level. Advise clinician to monitor serum digoxin level.
*Theophylline:* Increased risk of theophylline toxicity. Advise clinician to monitor patient closely and adjust theophylline dose p.r.n.
**Drug-herb.** *Red clover:* Increased risk of bleeding. Discourage use together.

### Adverse reactions
**CNS:** dizziness, *intracerebral bleeding,* peripheral neuropathy.
**CV:** vasculitis.
**EENT:** epistaxis, conjunctival hemorrhage.
**GI:** *diarrhea, nausea, dyspepsia, abdominal pain,* anorexia, vomiting, flatulence, bleeding, light-colored stools.
**GU:** hematuria, *nephrotic syndrome,* dark-colored urine.
**Hematologic:** prolonged bleeding time, *neutropenia, pancytopenia, agranulocytosis, immune thrombocytopenia.*
**Hepatic:** hepatitis, cholestatic jaundice, abnormal liver function test results.
**Metabolic:** *hyponatremia, increased serum cholesterol levels.*
**Musculoskeletal:** arthropathy, myositis.
**Respiratory:** *allergic pneumonitis.*
**Skin:** *rash,* pruritus, ecchymoses, maculopapular rash, urticaria, *thrombocytopenic purpura.*
**Other:** hypersensitivity reactions, postoperative bleeding, systemic lupus erythematosus, *serum sickness.*

### Overdose and treatment
Only one case of overdose has been reported. The patient, who ingested more than 6 g of drug, showed increased bleeding time and in-

---

Reactions may be *common,* uncommon, *life-threatening,* or COMMON AND LIFE-THREATENING.

creased ALT level. The patient recovered with supportive therapy alone.

## Clinical considerations

■ If drug is being substituted for a fibrinolytic or anticoagulant drug, advise clinician to discontinue previous drug before starting ticlopidine therapy.

■ If needed, methylprednisolone 20 mg I.V. has been shown to normalize the bleeding time within 2 hours. Platelet transfusions may also be needed.

■ Drug has been used investigationally for many conditions, including intermittent claudication, chronic arterial occlusion, subarachnoid hemorrhage, primary glomerulonephritis, sickle cell disease, and uremic patients with AV shunts. When used preoperatively, it may decrease risk of graft occlusion in patients receiving coronary artery bypass grafts and reduce severity of decreased platelet count in patients receiving extracorporeal hemoperfusion during open heart surgery.

■ Unlabeled uses include unstable angina, rheumatic mitral valve disease, and treatment for patients undergoing coronary angioplasty when aspirin therapy has failed or cannot be used.

### Therapeutic monitoring

■ Advise clinician to perform baseline liver function tests and repeat whenever liver dysfunction is suspected. Advise clinician to monitor patient closely, especially during the first 4 months of treatment.

■ Advise clinician to monitor CBC and WBC differential every 2 weeks for the first 3 months of therapy. Severe hematologic adverse events may occur with ticlopidine.

■ After the first 3 months of therapy, advise clinician to perform CBC and WBC differential determinations in patients showing signs of infection.

### Special populations

**Pregnant patients.** Use drug during pregnancy only when clearly needed.

**Breast-feeding patients.** It isn't known if drug appears in breast milk. Breast-feeding isn't recommended.

**Pediatric patients.** Safety and efficacy in children under age 18 haven't been established.

### Patient counseling

■ Tell patient to take drug with meals because food substantially increases bioavailability and improves GI tolerance.

■ Emphasize that drug prolongs bleeding time. Tell patient to report unusual bleeding and to inform dentists and other prescribers that he's taking ticlopidine.

■ Be sure patient understands the need to report for regular blood tests. Neutropenia can result in an increased risk of infection. Tell pa-

tient to report signs and symptoms of infection, such as fever, chills, or sore throat, immediately.

■ Warn patient to avoid aspirin and aspirin-containing products, which may prolong bleeding. Instruct him to call before taking OTC drugs because many contain aspirin.

■ Tell patient to report yellow skin or sclera, severe or persistent diarrhea, rash, S.C. bleeding, light-colored stools, dark urine.

## tiludronate disodium
Skelid

*Pharmacologic classification:* bisphosphonate analogue
*Therapeutic classification:* antihypercalcemic
*Pregnancy risk category C*

### Available forms

Available by prescription only
*Tablets:* 200 mg

### Indications and dosages

*Paget's disease*
*Adults:* 400 mg P.O. once daily taken with 6 to 8 ounces (180 to 240 ml) of plain water for 3 months, given 2 hours before or after meals.

### Mechanism of action

*Antihypercalcemic action:* Tiludronate is thought to suppress bone resorption by reducing osteoclastic activity through inhibition of the osteoclastic proton pump and through disruption of the cytoskeletal ring structure, possibly by inhibiting protein-tyrosine-phosphatase, leading to detachment of osteoclasts from the bone surface.

### Pharmacokinetics

*Absorption:* Bioavailability of drug on an empty stomach is 8%. Food and beverages other than water can reduce bioavailability by up to 90%.

*Distribution:* Widely distributed in bone and soft tissue. Protein-binding is about 90% (mainly albumin).

*Metabolism:* Probably not metabolized.

*Excretion:* Principally excreted in urine. Mean plasma half-life is 150 hours.

| Route | Onset | Peak | Duration |
|-------|-------|------|----------|
| P.O. | Unknown | 2 hr | Unknown |

### Contraindications and precautions

Contraindicated in patients hypersensitive to any component of drug and in patients with creatinine clearance below 30 ml/minute. Use cautiously in patients with upper GI disease, such as dysphagia, esophagitis, esophageal ulcer, or gastric ulcer.

## Interactions
**Drug-drug.** *Aluminum antacids, aspirin, calcium supplements, indomethacin, magnesium antacids:* Reduced bioavailability of tiludronate. Advise clinician to monitor patient closely and adjust dosage p.r.n.
**Drug-food.** *Any food:* Delayed drug absorption. Don't give drug within 2 hours of meals. *Beverages other than plain water:* Reduced drug absorption. Don't give with drug.

## Adverse reactions
**CNS:** anxiety, dizziness, headache, insomnia, involuntary muscle contractions, paresthesia, somnolence, vertigo.
**CV:** chest pain, hypertension, edema.
**EENT:** cataracts, conjunctivitis, glaucoma, pharyngitis, sinusitis, rhinitis.
**GI:** anorexia, constipation, diarrhea, dry mouth, dyspepsia, flatulence, gastritis, nausea, vomiting.
**Metabolic:** hyperparathyroidism, vitamin D deficiency.
**Musculoskeletal:** arthralgia, arthrosis, back pain.
**Respiratory:** bronchitis, coughing, crackles.
**Skin:** pruritus, sweating.
**Other:** *whole body pain,* tooth disorder.

## Overdose and treatment
No specific information available. Use standard treatment for hypocalcemia or renal insufficiency, if they occur. Dialysis isn't beneficial.

## Clinical considerations
■ Use drug in patients with Paget's disease who have serum alkaline phosphatase level at least twice the upper limit of normal or who are symptomatic or at risk for future complications of disease.
■ Drug should be given for 3 months to assess response.
■ Hypocalcemia and other disturbances of mineral metabolism such as vitamin D deficiency should be corrected before therapy starts.

### Therapeutic monitoring
■ Advise clinician to monitor symptom control.
■ Advise clinician to monitor patient for adverse reaction.

### Special populations
**Breast-feeding patients.** It isn't known if drug appears in breast milk. Use cautiously in breast-feeding women.
**Pediatric patients.** Safety and efficacy in children haven't been established.
**Geriatric patients.** Plasma levels may be higher in geriatric patients. However, dosage adjustment isn't needed.

## Patient counseling
■ Instruct patient to take drug with 6 to 8 ounces (180 to 240 ml) of plain water and not to take it within 2 hours of food.
■ Advise patient to maintain adequate vitamin D and calcium intake.
■ Inform patient that calcium supplements, aspirin, and indomethacin shouldn't be taken within 2 hours before or after tiludronate.
■ Tell patient that aluminum- and magnesium-containing antacids can be taken 2 hours after taking tiludronate.

# timolol maleate
Blocadren, Timoptic, Timoptic-XE

*Pharmacologic classification:* beta blocker
*Therapeutic classification:* antihypertensive, adjunct in MI, antiglaucoma drug
*Pregnancy risk category C*

## Available forms
Available by prescription only
*Tablets:* 5 mg, 10 mg, 20 mg
*Ophthalmic gel-forming solution:* 0.25%, 0.5%
*Ophthalmic solution:* 0.25%, 0.5%

## Indications and dosages
### Hypertension
*Adults:* Initially, 10 mg P.O. b.i.d. Usual maintenance dosage, 20 to 40 mg/day. Maximum dose, 60 mg/day. There should be an interval of at least 7 days between dose increases.
### Reduction of risk of CV mortality and reinfarction after MI
*Adults:* 10 mg P.O. b.i.d. initiated within 1 to 4 weeks after infarction.
### Migraine headache
*Adults:* 10 mg P.O. daily b.i.d., then increase up to 20 or 30 mg daily (10 mg P.O. in the morning and 20 mg P.O. in the evening).
### Glaucoma
*Adults:* 1 drop of 0.25% or 0.5% solution to the conjunctiva once or twice daily; or 1 drop of 0.25% or 0.5% gel to the conjunctiva once daily.
### ◊Angina
*Adults:* 15 to 45 mg P.O. daily given in three or four divided doses. Adjust dosage to maintain a resting heart rate of 55 to 60 beats per minute.

## Mechanism of action
*Antihypertensive action:* Exact mechanism is unknown. Timolol may reduce blood pressure by blocking adrenergic receptors (decreasing cardiac output), by decreasing sympathetic outflow from the CNS, and by suppressing renin release.
*MI prophylactic action:* Exact mechanism by which timolol decreases risk of mortality after MI is unknown. Timolol produces a nega-

tive chronotropic and inotropic activity. This decrease in heart rate and myocardial contractility results in reduced myocardial oxygen consumption.

*Antiglaucoma action:* Beta-blocking action of timolol decreases the production of aqueous humor, decreasing intraocular pressure.

## Pharmacokinetics
*Absorption:* About 90% of an oral dose is absorbed from the GI tract.
*Distribution:* After oral administration, timolol is distributed throughout the body; depending on assay method, drug is 10% to 60% protein-bound.
*Metabolism:* About 80% of a given dose is metabolized in the liver to inactive metabolites.
*Excretion:* Drug and its metabolites are excreted primarily in urine; half-life is about 4 hours.

| Route | Onset | Peak | Duration |
|---|---|---|---|
| P.O. | 15-30 min | 1-2 hr | 6-12 hr |
| Ophthalmic | 30 min | 1-2 hr | 12-24 hr |

## Contraindications and precautions
Contraindicated in patients with bronchial asthma, severe COPD, sinus bradycardia and heart block greater than first degree, cardiogenic shock, HF, or those hypersensitive to drug.

Use cautiously in patients with diabetes, hyperthyroidism, or respiratory disease (especially nonallergic bronchospasm or emphysema). Use oral form cautiously in patients with compensated HF and hepatic or renal disease. Use ophthalmic form cautiously in patients with cerebrovascular insufficiency.

## Interactions
**Drug-drug.** *Cardiac glycosides, diltiazem, verapamil:* Excessive bradycardia and increased depressant effect on myocardium. Use together cautiously.
*Fentanyl, general anesthetics, NSAIDs, other antihypertensives:* Hypotension. Advise clinician to monitor patient closely.
*Indomethacin:* Decreased antihypertensive effect. Advise clinician to monitor patient closely; dosage may need adjustment.
*Insulin, oral antidiabetics:* Altered requirements for these drugs. Advise clinician to monitor glucose level; dosage may need adjustment.
*Quinidine:* Decreased heart rate. Advise clinician to monitor patient.

## Adverse reactions
**CNS:** *CVA,* fatigue, lethargy, dizziness; depression, hallucinations, confusion, insomnia, nightmares, memory loss (with ophthalmic form).
**CV:** *arrhythmias, bradycardia,* hypotension, *HF,* peripheral vascular disease (with oral administration); *cardiac arrest, heart block,* palpitations, edema, claudication, Raynaud's phenomenon, cold hands and feet (with ophthalmic form).
**EENT:** minor eye irritation, decreased corneal sensitivity with long-term use, conjunctivitis, blepharitis, keratitis, visual disturbances, diplopia, ptosis (with ophthalmic form).
**GI:** nausea, vomiting, diarrhea (with oral administration).
**GU:** increased BUN level.
**Hematologic:** decreased hemoglobin level and hematocrit.
**Metabolic:** hyperkalemia, hyperuricemia, hyperglycemia.
**Respiratory:** dyspnea, *bronchospasm,* increased airway resistance, *pulmonary edema* (with oral administration); *asthmatic attacks in patients with history of asthma* (with ophthalmic form).
**Skin:** pruritus (with oral administration).

## Overdose and treatment
Signs of overdose include severe hypotension, bradycardia, HF, and bronchospasm.

After acute ingestion, advise clinician to empty stomach by induced emesis or gastric lavage and give activated charcoal to reduce absorption. Subsequent treatment is usually symptomatic and supportive.

## Clinical considerations
■ Dosage adjustment may be needed for patient with renal or hepatic impairment.
■ Although controversial, drug may need to be discontinued 48 hours before surgery in patients receiving ophthalmic timolol because systemic absorption occurs.
■ Drug may mask signs of hypoglycemia.
■ Systolic blood pressure is primary clinical endpoint.
■ Drug therapy may slightly increase BUN, serum potassium, uric acid, and blood glucose levels and may slightly decrease hemoglobin level and hematocrit.

### Therapeutic monitoring
■ Advise clinician to monitor patient for cardiac and respiratory symptoms.

### Special populations
**Pregnant patients.** Use drug during pregnancy only when potential benefits justify possible risk to fetus.
**Breast-feeding patients.** Drug appears in breast milk. Because of the potential for serious adverse reactions in breast-fed infants, an alternative to breast-feeding is recommended during therapy.
**Pediatric patients.** Safety and efficacy in children haven't been established; use only if potential benefit outweighs risk.
**Geriatric patients.** Geriatric patients may require lower oral maintenance doses of timolol because of increased bioavailability or delayed

metabolism; they also may experience enhanced adverse effects. Use cautiously because half-life may be prolonged in geriatric patients.

## Patient counseling

■ For ophthalmic form of timolol, teach patient proper method of eye drop administration. Warn patient not to touch dropper to eye or surrounding tissue; lightly press lacrimal sac with finger after administration to decrease systemic absorption.

■ Instruct patient to invert ophthalmic gel container once before each use.

■ Instruct patient to administer other ophthalmic drugs at least 10 minutes before the ophthalmic gel.

---

# tinzaparin sodium

Innohep

*Pharmacologic classification:* low–molecular weight heparin
*Therapeutic classification:* anticoagulant
*Pregnancy risk category B*

## Available forms

Available by prescription only
*Injection:* 20,000 anti-Xa IU/ml in 2-ml vials

## Indications and dosages

*Symptomatic deep vein thrombosis with or without pulmonary embolism with warfarin sodium*
*Adults:* 175 anti-Xa IU/kg of body weight S.C. once daily for at least 6 days and until patient is adequately anticoagulated with warfarin sodium (INR of at least 2.0) for 2 consecutive days. Initiate warfarin sodium therapy when appropriate, usually within 1 to 3 days of tinzaparin initiation. Volume of dose to be given may be calculated as follows:
Patient weight in kg × 0.00875 ml/kg = volume to be given in ml.
◇ *Prophylaxis of postoperative deep vein thrombosis*
*Adults:* 3,500 units or 50 units/kg S.C. daily for patients at moderate or high risk, respectively. Begin treatment 1 to 2 hours before surgery and continue for 5 to 10 days.

## Mechanism of action

*Anticoagulant action:* Tinzaparin is a low–molecular weight heparin that inhibits reactions that lead to the clotting of blood, including the formation of fibrin clots. It also acts as a potent co-inhibitor of several activated coagulation factors, especially factors Xa and IIa (thrombin). The primary inhibitory activity is activated by binding with the plasma protease inhibitor, antithrombin. By binding with antithrombin, drug causes an increased ability to inactivate coagulation enzymes factor Xa and thrombin. Tinzaparin also induces release of tissue factor pathway inhibitor, which may contribute to the antithrombotic effect.

## Pharmacokinetics

*Absorption:* Plasma levels peak in 4 to 5 hours.
*Distribution:* Volume of distribution is similar in magnitude to that of blood volume, which suggests that distribution is limited to the central compartment.
*Metabolism:* Partially metabolized by desulfation and depolymerization, similar to that seen with other low–molecular weight heparins.
*Excretion:* Primarily eliminated renally. Elimination half-life is about 3 to 4 hours.

| Route | Onset | Peak | Duration |
|-------|-------|------|----------|
| S.C. | 2-3 hr | 4-5 hr | 18-24 hr |

## Contraindications and precautions

Contraindicated in patients hypersensitive to tinzaparin, heparin, sulfites, benzyl alcohol, or pork products. Also contraindicated in patients with active major bleeding and in those with a known history of heparin-induced thrombocytopenia.

Use cautiously in patients with increased risk of hemorrhage, such as those with bacterial endocarditis, uncontrolled hypertension, diabetic retinopathy, congenital or acquired bleeding disorders such as hepatic failure and amyloidosis, GI ulceration, or hemorrhagic CVA. Also use cautiously in patients who have recently undergone brain, spinal, or ophthalmologic surgery and in patients being treated with platelet inhibitors. Use cautiously in geriatric patients and in patients with renal insufficiency.

## Interactions

**Drug-drug.** *Oral anticoagulants, platelet inhibitors (such as dextran, dipyridamole, NSAIDs, salicylates, sulfinpyrazone), thrombolytics:* Possible increased risk of bleeding. Use together cautiously. If drugs must be given together, advise clinician to monitor patient for signs and symptoms of bleeding.

## Adverse reactions

**CNS:** headache, dizziness, insomnia, confusion, *cerebral or intracranial bleeding.*
**CV:** *arrhythmias,* chest pain, hypotension, hypertension, *MI, thromboembolism,* tachycardia, dependent edema, angina pectoris.
**EENT:** epistaxis, ocular hemorrhage.
**GI:** anorectal bleeding, constipation, flatulence, hematemesis, hemarthrosis, *GI hemorrhage,* nausea, vomiting, dyspepsia, retroperitoneal or intra-abdominal bleeding, melena.
**GU:** dysuria, hematuria, urinary tract infection, urine retention, vaginal hemorrhage.

**Hematologic:** granulocytopenia, *thrombocytopenia,* anemia, *agranulocytosis, pancytopenia, hemorrhage.*
**Hepatic:** elevated AST and ALT levels.
**Musculoskeletal:** back pain.
**Respiratory:** pneumonia, respiratory disorder, *pulmonary embolism,* dyspnea.
**Skin:** bullous eruption, cellulitis, *injection site hematoma,* pruritus, purpura, rash, skin necrosis, wound hematoma, bullous eruption.
**Other:** hypersensitivity reactions, *spinal or epidural hematoma,* fever, pain, infection, impaired healing, allergic reaction, congenital anomaly, *fetal death, fetal distress.*

## Overdose and treatment

Tinzaparin overdose may lead to bleeding complications. The first signs of bleeding may be nosebleeds, hematuria, or tarry stools. Easy bruising or petechial hemorrhages may precede frank bleeding.

If minor bleeding occurs, advise clinician to discontinue drug, apply pressure to the site, and monitor patient for signs and symptoms of more severe bleeding. In the case of serious bleeding or large overdoses, advise clinician to replace volume and hemostatic blood elements (such as RBCs, fresh frozen plasma, and platelets) p.r.n. If this is ineffective, protamine sulfate can be given.

## Clinical considerations

■ Store tinzaparin at room temperature.
■ Drug isn't intended for I.M. or I.V. administration nor should it be mixed with other injections or infusions.
■ Drug shouldn't be interchanged (unit to unit) with heparin or other low–molecular weight heparins.
■ Advise clinician to have patient lie or sit down during drug administration. Advise clinician to give by deep S.C. injection into the abdominal wall with the following recommendations: Introduce whole length of needle into skin fold held between thumb and forefinger. Make sure to hold skin fold throughout injection. Rotate injection sites between the right and left anterolateral and posterolateral abdominal wall. To minimize bruising, don't rub injection site after administration.
■ Use an appropriately calibrated syringe to ensure withdrawal of correct volume of drug from vials.
■ Drug contains sodium metabisulfite, which may cause allergic reactions in susceptible people.
■ **ALERT** When neuraxial anesthesia (epidural or spinal anesthesia) or spinal puncture is used, the patient is at risk for developing spinal hematoma, which can result in long-term or permanent paralysis. Monitor patient for signs and symptoms of neurologic impairment. Consider the risk versus benefit of neuraxial inter-

vention in patients receiving low–molecular weight heparins or heparinoids.
■ If patient becomes pregnant while taking tinzaparin, notify her about the potential hazards to the fetus. Cases of "gasping syndrome" have occurred in premature infants when large amounts of benzyl alcohol have been given.

### *Therapeutic monitoring*

■ Advise clinician to monitor platelet count during therapy. Drug should be stopped if platelet count falls below 100,000/mm³.
■ Advise clinician to periodically monitor CBC and stool tests for occult blood during treatment.
■ Drug may affect PT and INR levels. For patients also receiving warfarin, advise clinician to draw blood for PT and INR just before next scheduled dose of tinzaparin.

### *Special populations*

**Breast-feeding patients.** It isn't known if drug appears in breast milk; use cautiously in breast-feeding women.
**Pediatric patients.** Safety and efficacy in children haven't been established.
**Geriatric patients.** Elderly patients and patients with renal insufficiency may show reduced elimination of tinzaparin. Use drug with care in these patients.

## Patient counseling

■ Explain to patient importance of laboratory monitoring to ensure effectiveness of drugs while maintaining safety.
■ Teach patient warning signs of bleeding and instruct him to report these signs immediately.
■ Caution patient to take such safety measures as using soft toothbrush and electric razor to prevent cuts and bruises.
■ Instruct patient that concomitant warfarin therapy will be started when appropriate, within 1 to 3 days of tinzaparin administration. Explain importance of warfarin therapy and monitoring to ensure safety and efficacy.

# tirofiban hydrochloride
Aggrastat

*Pharmacologic classification:* GP IIb/IIIa receptor antagonist
*Therapeutic classification:* platelet aggregation inhibitor
*Pregnancy risk category B*

## Available forms

Available by prescription only
*Injection:* 50-ml vials (250 mcg/ml), 500-ml premixed vials (50 mcg/ml)

## Indications and dosages

*Treatment of acute coronary syndrome,*
*with heparin, including patients who are*
*to be managed medically and those under-*
*going percutaneous transluminal coro-*
*nary angioplasty (PTCA) or atherectomy*
*Adults:* I.V. loading dose of 0.4 mcg/kg/minute
for 30 minutes followed by a continuous I.V.
infusion of 0.1 mcg/kg/minute. Continue infusion through angiography and for 12 to 24
hours after angioplasty or atherectomy.

≡ *Dosage adjustment.* For patients with renal
insufficiency (creatinine clearance less than 30
ml/minute), use a loading dose of 0.2 mcg/kg/
minute for 30 minutes followed by a continuous infusion of 0.05 mcg/kg/minute. Continue infusion through angiography and for 12 to
24 hours after angioplasty or atherectomy.

## I.V. administration

■ Dilute 50-ml vial (250 mcg/ml) to same
strength as 500-ml premixed vials (50 mcg/ml)
as follows: Withdraw and discard 100 ml from
a 500-ml bag of sterile normal saline solution
or D₅W and replace this volume with 100 ml
of tirofiban injection (from two 50-ml vials);
or withdraw 50 ml from a 250-ml bag of sterile normal saline solution or D₅W and replace
this volume with 50 ml of tirofiban injection
to yield 50 mcg/ml.
■ Firmly squeeze inner bag to check for leaks
and look for particulate matter. If either is present, discard solution.
■ Store drug at 59° to 86° F (15° to 30° C) and
protect from light.
■ May administer drug through same line as
heparin.
■ Discard unused solution 24 hours after the
start of infusion.

### Incompatibilities
Incompatibile with diazepam.

## Mechanism of action

*Platelet-inhibiting action:* Drug is a reversible
antagonist of fibrinogen binding to the GP
IIb/IIIa receptor on human platelets producing
a dose-dependent inhibition of platelet aggregation.

## Pharmacokinetics

*Absorption:* Not reported.
*Distribution:* 65% protein-bound. Volume of
distribution ranges from 22 to 42 L.
*Metabolism:* Metabolism is limited. Half-life
is about 2 hours.
*Excretion:* Renal clearance accounts for 39%
to 69% of elimination; feces accounts for 25%.

| Route | Onset | Peak | Duration |
|-------|-------|------|----------|
| I.V. | Immediate | Immediate | 4-8 hr after end of infusion |

## Contraindications and precautions

Contraindicated in patients hypersensitive to
drug or its components; and those with active
internal bleeding or history of bleeding diathesis within the previous 30 days; history of intracranial hemorrhage, intracranial neoplasm,
arteriovenous malformation, or aneurysm;
thrombocytopenia following prior exposure to
drug; CVA within 30 days or history of hemorrhagic CVA; symptoms or findings suggestive of aortic dissection; severe hypertension
(systolic blood pressure greater than 180 mm
Hg or diastolic blood pressure greater than 110
mm Hg); or acute pericarditis. Also contraindicated in patients who have experienced a major surgical procedure or severe physical trauma within previous month; and in use with
another parenteral GP IIb/IIIa inhibitor.

Use with caution in patients with platelet
count less than 150,000/mm³ and in patients
with hemorrhagic retinopathy.

## Interactions

**Drug-drug.** *Anticoagulants such as warfarin,*
*clopidogrel, dipyridamole, NSAIDs, thrombly-*
*tics, ticlopidine:* Increased risk of bleeding.
Advise clinician to monitor patient closely.
*Levothyroxine, omeprazole:* Increased renal
clearance of tirofiban. Advise clinician to monitor patient carefully.

## Adverse reactions

**CNS:** dizziness, headache.
**CV:** *bradycardia, coronary artery dissection,*
edema, vasovagal reaction.
**GI:** nausea, *occult bleeding.*
**GU:** pelvic pain.
**Hematologic:** *bleeding, thrombocytopenia,*
decreased hemoglobin and hematocrit.
**Musculoskeletal:** leg pain.
**Skin:** sweating.
**Other:** fever, bleeding at arterial access site.

## Overdose and treatment

Advise clinician to treat overdose by assessing patient's condition and by stopping or adjusting infusion. Drug is removed by dialysis.

## Clinical considerations

■ Don't infuse at levels greater than 50 mcg/ml.
■ Minimize use of arterial and venous punctures, I.M. injections, urinary catheters, nasotracheal intubation, and nasogastric tubes. Avoid
noncompressible I.V. access sites, such as subclavian or jugular veins.
■ Use of concomitant aspirin or low–molecular weight heparin is recommended for patients
with non–ST-segment elevation MI who have
high risk characteristics or refractory ischemia.
**H** **ALERT** Don't confuse Aggrastat (tirofiban)
with Acova (argatroban).

### Therapeutic monitoring

■ Drug causes increases in bleeding rates, particularly at the site of arterial access for femoral sheath placement. Before the sheath is pulled, advise clinician to discontinue heparin for 3 to 4 hours and document activated clotting time less than 180 seconds or aPTT less than 45 seconds. Sheath hemostasis should be achieved at least 4 hours before hospital discharge.

■ Advise clinician to monitor hemoglobin level, hematocrit, and platelet count before starting therapy, 6 hours following loading dose, and at least daily during therapy.

### Special populations
**Pregnant patients.** Use drug during pregnancy only if expected benefit justifies potential risk.
**Breast-feeding patients.** It isn't known if drug appears in breast milk. Depending on the importance of the drug to the mother, either breast-feeding or drug should be discontinued.
**Pediatric patients.** Safety and efficacy in patients under age 18 haven't been established.

### Patient counseling
■ Instruct patient to report chest discomfort or other adverse events immediately.
■ Inform patient that frequent blood sampling may be needed to evaluate therapy.

# tobramycin
# tobramycin ophthalmic
Aktob, Tobrasol, Tobrex, Tomycine

# tobramycin sulfate
Nebcin

# tobramycin solution for inhalation
TOBI

*Pharmacologic classification:* aminoglycoside
*Therapeutic classification:* antibiotic
*Pregnancy risk category D*

### Available forms
Available by prescription only
*Injection:* 40 mg/ml, 10 mg/ml (pediatric)
*Ophthalmic solution:* 0.3%
*Ophthalmic ointment:* 0.3%
*Nebulizer solution for inhalation:* Single-use 5-ml (300-mg) ampule

### Indications and dosages
*Serious infections caused by sensitive* **Escherichia coli, Proteus, Klebsiella, Enterobacter, Serratia, Staphylococcus aureus, Pseudomonas, Citrobacter, or Providencia organisms**
*Adults and children with normal renal function:* 3 mg/kg I.M. or I.V. daily, divided q 8

hours. Up to 5 mg/kg I.M. or I.V. daily, divided q 6 to 8 hours for life-threatening infections.
*Neonates under age 1 week:* Up to 4 mg/kg I.M. or I.V. daily, divided q 12 hours. For I.V. use, dilute in 50 to 100 ml normal saline solution or $D_5W$ for adults and in less volume for children. Infuse over 20 to 60 minutes.
≡*Dosage adjustment.* Advise clinician of the following recommendations: For patients with impaired renal function, initial dosage is same as for those with normal renal function. Subsequent doses and frequency are determined by renal function study results and blood levels; keep peak serum levels between 4 and 10 mcg/ml and trough serum levels between 1 and 2 mcg/ml. Several methods have been used to calculate dosage in renal failure.

After a 1 mg/kg loading dose, adjust subsequent dosage by reducing doses given at 8-hour intervals or by prolonging the interval between normal doses. Both of these methods are useful when serum levels of tobramycin can't be measured directly. They're based on either creatinine clearance (preferred) or serum creatinine because these values correlate with half-life of drug.

To calculate reduced dosage for 8-hour intervals, use available nomograms; or, if patient's steady-state serum creatinine level is known, divide the normally recommended dose by patient's serum creatinine level. To determine frequency in hours for normal dosage (if creatinine clearance rate isn't available), divide the normal dose by patient's serum creatinine level. Dosage schedules derived from either method require careful clinical and laboratory observations of patient and should be adjusted as appropriate. These methods of calculation may be misleading in geriatric patients and in those with severe wasting; neither should be used when dialysis is performed.

Hemodialysis removes 50% to 75% of a dose in 6 hours. In anephric patients maintained by dialysis, 1.5 to 2 mg/kg after each dialysis usually maintains therapeutic, nontoxic serum levels. Patients receiving peritoneal dialysis twice a week should receive a 1.5- to 2-mg/kg loading dose followed by 1 mg/kg q 3 days. Those receiving dialysis q 2 days should receive a 1.5-mg/kg loading dose after first dialysis and 0.75 mg/kg after each subsequent dialysis.

◊*Intrathecally or intraventricularly, in conjunction with I.M. or I.V. administration*
*Adults:* 3 to 8 mg q 18 to 48 hours.
*Management of cystic fibrosis patients with Pseudomonas aeruginosa infection*
*Adults and children over age 6:* 1 single-use ampule (300 mg) given q 12 hours for 28 days, then off for 28 days, then on for 28 days as advised by prescriber. There's no dosage adjustment for age or renal failure.

*Treatment of external ocular infection caused by susceptible gram-negative bacteria*
*Adults and children:* In mild to moderate infections, instill 1 or 2 drops into affected eye q 4 to 6 hours. In severe infections, instill 2 drops into affected eye hourly or apply a small amount of ointment into conjunctival sac t.i.d. or q.i.d.

## I.V. administration

- For adults, dilute in 50 to 100 ml of normal saline solution or $D_5W$. For children, the volume should be proportionately less. Infuse over 20 to 60 minutes. Flush line with normal saline solution or $D_5W$ post infusion.
- Don't premix tobramycin with other drugs; administer separately at least 1 hour apart.

### Incompatibilities
Incompatible with penicillins; allopurinol; cefamandole; cefoperazone; cefotaxine; dextrose 5% in Isolyte E, M, or P; heparin sodium; hetastarch; indomethacin; propofol; and I.V. solutions containing alcohol. Because of other potential incompatibilities, manufacturer recommends that other drugs not be mixed with tobramycin.

## Mechanism of action
*Antibiotic action:* Tobramycin is bactericidal; it binds directly to the 30S ribosomal subunit, thereby inhibiting bacterial protein synthesis. Its spectrum of activity includes many aerobic gram-negative organisms, including most strains of *P. aeruginosa* and some aerobic gram-positive organisms. Tobramycin may act against some bacterial strains resistant to other aminoglycosides; many strains resistant to tobramycin are susceptible to amikacin, gentamicin, or netilmicin.

## Pharmacokinetics
*Absorption:* Absorbed poorly after oral administration and usually is given parenterally. Inhaled drug remains concentrated in the airway, with serum level after 20 weeks of therapy being 1.05 mcg/ml 1 hour after dosing.
*Distribution:* Distributed widely after parenteral administration; intraocular penetration is poor. CSF penetration is low, even in patients with inflamed meninges. Protein-binding is minimal; tobramycin crosses the placental barrier. Inhaled drug remains primarily concentrated in the airway.
*Metabolism:* Not metabolized.
*Excretion:* Excreted primarily in urine by glomerular filtration; small amounts may be excreted in bile and breast milk. Elimination half-life in adults is 2 to 3 hours. In severe renal damage, half-life may extend to 24 to 60 hours. With inhalation use, unabsorbed tobramycin is probably eliminated in the sputum.

| Route | Onset | Peak | Duration |
|---|---|---|---|
| I.V. | Immediate | Immediate | 8 hr |
| I.M. | Unknown | 30-90 min | 8 hr |
| Ophthalmic, inhalation | Unknown | Unknown | Unknown |

## Contraindications and precautions
Contraindicated in patients hypersensitive to drug or other aminoglycosides. Use injectable form cautiously in patients with impaired renal function or neuromuscular disorders and in geriatric patients.

## Interactions
**Drug-drug.** *Amphotericin B, capreomycin, cephalosporins, cisplatin, methoxyflurane, polymyxin B, vancomycin, other aminoglycosides:* Increased hazard of nephrotoxicity, ototoxicity, and neurotoxicity. Advise clinician to monitor patient carefully.
*Antiemetics, antivertigo drugs, dimenhydrinate:* Possible masked tobramycin-induced ototoxicity. Advise clinician to monitor patient closely.
*Bumetanide, ethacrynic acid, furosemide, mannitol, urea:* Increased hazard of ototoxicity. Advise clinician to monitor patient's hearing closely.
*General anesthetics, neuromuscular blockers, succinylcholine, tubocurarine:* Potentiation of neuromuscular blockade. Advise clinician to monitor patient closely.

## Adverse reactions
**CNS:** headache, lethargy, confusion, *seizures,* disorientation (with injectable form).
**EENT:** *ototoxicity* (with injectable form); blurred vision (with ophthalmic ointment); burning or stinging on instillation, lid itching or swelling, conjunctival erythema (with ophthalmic administration).
**GI:** vomiting, nausea, diarrhea (with injectable form).
**GU:** elevated BUN, nonprotein nitrogen, and serum creatinine levels; increased urinary excretion of casts; *nephrotoxicity* (with injectable form).
**Hematologic:** anemia, eosinophilia, *leukopenia, thrombocytopenia, granulocytopenia* (with injectable form).
**Respiratory:** BRONCHOSPASM (with inhalation form).
**Skin:** rash, urticaria, pruritus (with injectable form).
**Other:** fever, hypersensitivity reactions, overgrowth of nonsusceptible organisms (with ophthalmic administration).

## Overdose and treatment
Signs and symptoms of overdose include ototoxicity, nephrotoxicity, and neuromuscular toxicity. Advise clinician to remove drug by hemodialysis or peritoneal dialysis. Treatment

---

Reactions may be *common*, uncommon, *life-threatening*, or COMMON AND LIFE-THREATENING.

with calcium salts or anticholinesterases reverses neuromuscular blockade.

## Clinical considerations
- Ophthalmic preparation should be stopped if keratitis, erythema, lacrimation, edema, or lid itching occurs.
- Because tobramycin is dialyzable, patients undergoing hemodialysis may need dosage adjustments.
- Inhalation form of tobramycin is an orphan drug used specifically for management of cystic fibrosis patients with *P. aeruginosa* infection.
**◢ALERT** Don't confuse tobramycin with Trobicin.

### Therapeutic monitoring
- Advise clinician to monitor patient for symptoms of toxicity.

### Special populations
**Pregnant patients.** Use drug during pregnancy only when clearly indicated.
**Breast-feeding patients.** Drug may appear in breast milk. A decision should be made to discontinue either breast-feeding or drug.

## Patient counseling
- Tell patient to take inhalation doses as close to 12 hours apart as possible and no less than 6 hours apart.
- Instruct patient on proper administration (inhalation).

# tocainide hydrochloride
Tonocard

*Pharmacologic classification:* local anesthetic (amide type)
*Therapeutic classification:* ventricular antiarrhythmic
*Pregnancy risk category C*

## Available forms
Available by prescription only
*Tablets:* 400 mg, 600 mg

## Indications and dosages
*Suppression of symptomatic ventricular arrhythmias, including frequent PVCs*
Dosage must be individualized based on antiarrhythmic response and tolerance.
*Adults:* Initially, 400 mg P.O. q 8 hours. Usual dose is between 1,200 and 1,800 mg/day divided into three doses. Drug may be given on a twice-daily regimen if patient is able to tolerate the t.i.d. regimen. Maximum dose is 2,400 mg/day.
≡ *Dosage adjustment.* Patients with impaired renal or hepatic function may be adequately treated with less than 1,200 mg/day.

◊ *Myotonic dystrophy*
*Adults:* 800 to 1,200 mg P.O. daily.
◊ *Trigeminal neuralgia*
*Adults:* 20 mg/kg/day P.O. divided t.i.d.

## Mechanism of action
*Antiarrhythmic action:* Tocainide is structurally similar to lidocaine and possesses similar electrophysiologic and hemodynamic effects. A class IB antiarrhythmic, it suppresses automaticity and shortens the effective refractory period and action potential duration of His-Purkinje fibers and suppresses spontaneous ventricular depolarization during diastole. Conductive atrial tissue and AV conduction aren't affected significantly at therapeutic levels. Unlike quinidine and procainamide, tocainide doesn't significantly alter hemodynamics when given in usual doses. Tocainide exerts its effects on the conduction system, causing inhibition of reentry mechanisms and cessation of ventricular arrhythmias; these effects may be more pronounced in ischemic tissue. Tocainide doesn't cause a significant negative inotropic effect. Its direct cardiac effects are less potent than those of lidocaine.

## Pharmacokinetics
*Absorption:* Rapidly and completely absorbed from the GI tract; unlike lidocaine, it undergoes negligible first-pass effect in the liver. Bioavailability is nearly 100%.
*Distribution:* Distribution is only partially known; however, it appears to be distributed widely and apparently crosses the blood-brain barrier and placental barrier in animals (it is, however, less lipophilic than lidocaine). Only about 10% to 20% is plasma protein–bound.
*Metabolism:* Apparently metabolized in the liver to inactive metabolites.
*Excretion:* Excreted in urine as unchanged drug and inactive metabolites. About 30% to 50% of an orally given dose is excreted in urine as metabolites. Elimination half-life is about 11 to 23 hours, with an initial biphasic plasma level decline similar to that of lidocaine. Half-life may be prolonged in patients with renal or hepatic insufficiency. Urine alkalinization may substantially decrease the amount of unchanged drug excreted in urine.

| Route | Onset | Peak | Duration |
|-------|-------|------|----------|
| P.O. | Unknown | 1½-2 hr | 8 hr |

## Contraindications and precautions
Contraindicated in patients hypersensitive to lidocaine or other amide-type local anesthetics and in those with second- or third-degree AV block in the absence of an artificial pacemaker.

Use cautiously in patients with HF, diminished cardiac reserve, preexisting bone marrow failure, cytopenia, or impaired renal or hepatic function.

## Interactions
**Drug-drug.** *Allopurinol:* Increased effects of this drug. Advise clinician to monitor patient carefully.
*Cimetidine, rifampin:* Decreased elimination half-life and bioavailability of tocainide. Advise clinician to monitor patient carefully. Dosage adjustment may be needed.
*Lidocaine:* Possible CNS toxicity. Advise clinician to monitor patient closely.
*Metoprolol:* Decreased myocardial contractility and bradycardia. Advise clinician to monitor patient's cardiac status.
*Other antiarrhythmics:* Additive, synergistic, or antagonistic effects. Advise clinician to monitor patient's cardiac status closely.

## Adverse reactions
**CNS:** *light-headedness, tremor,* paresthesia, *dizziness, vertigo,* drowsiness, fatigue, confusion, headache.
**CV:** hypotension, **new or worsened arrhythmias, HF, bradycardia,** palpitations.
**EENT:** blurred vision, tinnitus.
**GI:** *nausea, vomiting,* diarrhea, anorexia.
**Hematologic:** *blood dyscrasia.*
**Hepatic:** abnormal liver function test results, hepatitis.
**Skin:** rash, diaphoresis.

## Overdose and treatment
Effects of overdose include extensions of common adverse reactions, particularly those associated with the CNS or GI tract.

Treatment generally involves symptomatic and supportive care. In acute overdose, advise clinician to perform gastric emptying by inducing emesis or gastric lavage. Respiratory depression necessitates immediate attention and maintenance of a patent airway with ventilatory assistance, if required. Seizures may be treated with small incremental doses of a benzodiazepine, such as diazepam, or a short- or ultrashort-acting barbiturate, such as pentobarbital or thiopental.

## Clinical considerations
■ Drug is considered an oral lidocaine and may be used to ease transition from I.V. lidocaine to oral antiarrhythmic therapy.
■ Use cautiously and with lower doses in patients with hepatic or renal impairment.
■ Advise clinician to obtain a chest radiograph if pulmonary symptoms exist.
■ Adverse effects tend to be frequent and problematic.

### Therapeutic monitoring
■ Advise clinician to monitor blood levels; therapeutic levels range from 4 to 10 mcg/ml.
■ Advise clinician to monitor periodic blood counts for the first 3 months of therapy and frequently thereafter. CBC should be performed promptly if signs of infection develop.

■ Advise clinician to observe patient for tremors, a possible sign that maximum safe dose has been reached.

### Special populations
**Pregnant patients.** Use drug during pregnancy only when potential benefits justify possible risks to fetus.
**Breast-feeding patients.** Safety in breast-feeding women hasn't been established. An alternative to breast-feeding is recommended.
**Pediatric patients.** Safety and efficacy in children haven't been established.
**Geriatric patients.** Use with caution in geriatric patients; increased serum drug levels and toxicity are more likely. Advise clinician to monitor patients carefully. Geriatric patients are more likely to experience dizziness and may require assistance while walking.

## Patient counseling
■ Instruct patient to report unusual bleeding or bruising; signs or symptoms of infection, such as fever, sore throat, stomatitis, or chills; or pulmonary symptoms, such as cough, wheezing, or exertional dyspnea.
■ Tell patient he may take tocainide with food to lessen GI upset.
■ Tell patient that tocainide may cause drowsiness or dizziness and to be careful while performing tasks that require alertness.

---

# tolazamide
Tolinase

*Pharmacologic classification:* sulfonylurea
*Therapeutic classification:* antidiabetic
*Pregnancy risk category C*

## Available forms
Available by prescription only
*Tablets:* 100 mg, 250 mg, 500 mg

## Indications and dosages
*Adjunct to diet to lower blood glucose levels in patients with type 2 diabetes*
*Adults:* Initially, 100 mg P.O. daily with breakfast if fasting blood sugar (FBS) is less than 200 mg/dl; or 250 mg P.O. daily if FBS is more than 200 mg/dl. May adjust dosage at weekly intervals in increments of 100 to 250 mg based on blood glucose response. Maximum dose is 500 mg P.O. b.i.d. before meals.
*Elderly:* Initially, 100 mg P.O. daily.
≡*Dosage adjustment.* Initially, malnourished or underweight patients may be given 100 mg P.O. daily.

## Mechanism of action
*Antidiabetic action:* Tolazamide lowers blood glucose levels by stimulating insulin release from functioning beta cells of the pancreas. Af-

ter prolonged administration, the hypoglycemic effects of drug appear to reflect extrapancreatic effects, possibly including reduction of basal hepatic glucose production and enhanced peripheral sensitivity to insulin.

## Pharmacokinetics

*Absorption:* Absorbed well from the GI tract.
*Distribution:* Probably distributed into the extracellular fluid.
*Metabolism:* Metabolized probably by the liver to several mildly active metabolites.
*Excretion:* Excreted in urine primarily as metabolites, with small amounts excreted as unchanged drug. Half-life is 7 hours.

| Route | Onset | Peak | Duration |
|-------|-------|------|----------|
| P.O. | Unknown | 3-4 hr | Unknown |

## Contraindications and precautions

Contraindicated in patients hypersensitive to drug or other sulfonylureas; type 1 diabetes or diabetes that can be adequately controlled by diet; in patients with type 2 diabetes complicated by ketosis, acidosis, coma, or other acute complications such as major surgery, severe infection, or severe trauma; in patients with uremia; and in pregnant or breast-feeding women.

Use cautiously in geriatric, debilitated, or malnourished patients, in those with impaired renal or hepatic function, and in those with adrenal or pituitary insufficiency.

## Interactions

**Drug-drug.** *Beta blockers, including ophthalmics:* Increased risk of hypoglycemia; masked hypoglycemic symptoms (increasing pulse rate and blood pressure); prolonged hypoglycemia effect from blocked gluconeogenesis. Use together cautiously.
*Calcium channel blockers, corticosteroids, estrogens, isoniazid, oral contraceptives, phenothiazines, phenytoin, sympathomimetics, thiazide diuretics, triamterene, thyroid hormones:* Decreased hypoglycemic effect. Advise clinician to monitor blood glucose level and adjust dosage accordingly.
*Chloramphenicol, insulin, MAO inhibitors, NSAIDs, probenecid, salicylates, sulfonamides:* Enhanced hypoglycemic effect. Advise clinician to monitor blood glucose level closely.
*Oral anticoagulants:* Possible increased hypoglycemic activity or enhanced anticoagulant effect. Advise clinician to monitor blood glucose level and PT and INR.
**Drug-herb.** *Aloe, bitter melon, bilberry leaf, burdock, dandelion, fenugreek, garlic, ginseng:* Possible improved blood glucose control requiring reduction of antidiabetics with concomitant use. Advise patient to discuss the use of herbal medicines with prescriber before taking them.

**Drug-lifestyle.** *Alcohol use:* Disulfiram-like reaction (nausea, vomiting, abdominal cramps, headaches). Advise patient to avoid alcohol.

## Adverse reactions

**CNS:** weakness, fatigue, dizziness, vertigo, malaise, headache.
**GI:** nausea, vomiting, epigastric distress, heartburn.
**Hematologic:** *leukopenia,* hemolytic anemia, *thrombocytopenia, aplastic anemia, agranulocytosis,* pancytopenia.
**Metabolic:** *hyponatremia, hypoglycemia.*
**Skin:** photosensitivity reactions.

## Overdose and treatment

Signs and symptoms of overdose include low blood glucose level, tingling of lips and tongue, hunger, nausea, decreased cerebral function (lethargy, yawning, confusion, agitation, nervousness), increased sympathetic activity (tachycardia, sweating, tremor) and ultimately, seizures, stupor, and coma.

Mild hypoglycemia, without loss of consciousness or neurologic findings, responds to treatment with oral glucose and adjustments in drug dosages and meal patterns. If patient loses consciousness or neurologic findings develop, advise clinician to give rapid injection of dextrose 50%, followed by a continuous infusion of dextrose 10% at a rate to maintain blood glucose levels greater than 100 mg/dl. Advise clinician to monitor patient for 24 to 48 hours.

## Clinical considerations

■ Over time, patients may become unresponsive (uncontrolled blood glucose level) to therapy with this drug as well as other sulfonylureas; advise clinician to monitor patient appropriately.
■ To avoid GI intolerance for those patients receiving doses of 500 mg per day or more and to improve control of hyperglycemia, divided doses are recommended; these are given before the morning and evening meals.
■ Tablets may be crushed to ease administration.
■ Use with caution in women of childbearing age. Tolazamide isn't recommended for treatment of diabetes from pregnancy.
■ Oral antidiabetics have caused an increased risk of CV mortality as compared with diet or diet and insulin therapy.
**To change from insulin to tolazamide:**
■ If insulin dose is less than 20 units daily, insulin may be stopped and oral therapy started at 100 mg P.O. daily in the morning. If insulin dose is 20 to 40 units daily, insulin may be stopped and oral therapy started at 250 mg P.O. daily in the morning. If insulin dose is more than 40 units daily, advise clinician to decrease insulin dosage by 50% and start oral therapy at

---

250 mg P.O. daily with breakfast. Doses should be increased as appropriate based on blood glucose response.

■ Maintenance dose of drug should be conservative in debilitated, malnourished, or geriatric patients or in patients with impaired renal or hepatic function because of increased risk of hypoglycemia.

### Therapeutic monitoring

■ When substituting tolazamide for chlorpropamide therapy, advise clinician to monitor patient closely for 1 to 2 weeks because of prolonged retention of chlorpropamide in the body, which may result in hypoglycemia.

### Special populations

**Pregnant patients.** Use with caution in pregnant women.

**Breast-feeding patients.** Because of the risk of hypoglycemia in breast-fed infant, a risk-benefit decision should be made to discontinue either drug or breast-feeding.

**Pediatric patients.** Tolazamide is ineffective in type 1 and juvenile-onset diabetes. Safety and efficacy in children haven't been established.

**Geriatric patients.** Geriatric patients may be more sensitive to effects of drug because of reduced metabolism and elimination. Hypoglycemia causes more neurologic symptoms in these patients. Geriatric patients usually require a lower initial dose.

### Patient counseling

■ Advise patient to take drug at the same time each day. If he misses a dose, tell him to take the missed dose immediately unless it's almost time to take the next dose; warn him not to double the dose.

■ Warn patient to avoid alcohol when taking tolazamide.

■ Recommend that patient take drug with food if it causes GI upset.

## tolbutamide

Orinase

*Pharmacologic classification:* sulfonylurea
*Therapeutic classification:* antidiabetic
*Pregnancy risk category C*

### Available forms

Available by prescription only
*Tablets:* 500 mg

### Indications and dosages

*Adjunct to diet to lower blood glucose levels in patients with type 2 diabetes*
*Adults:* Usual dose is 1 to 2 g P.O. daily as single dose or divided b.i.d. or t.i.d. May adjust dosage to maximum of 3 g P.O. daily.

## Mechanism of action

*Antidiabetic action:* Tolbutamide lowers blood glucose level by stimulating insulin release from functioning beta cells of the pancreas. After prolonged administration, hypoglycemic effects of drug appear to reflect extrapancreatic effects, possibly including reduction of basal hepatic glucose production and enhanced peripheral sensitivity to insulin.

## Pharmacokinetics

*Absorption:* Absorbed readily from the GI tract with peak levels occurring at 3 to 4 hours.
*Distribution:* Probably distributed into extracellular fluid. Drug is 95% plasma protein–bound.
*Metabolism:* Metabolized in the liver to inactive metabolites.
*Excretion:* Drug and its metabolites are excreted in urine and feces. Half-life is 4½ to 6½ hours.

| Route | Onset | Peak | Duration |
|-------|-------|------|----------|
| P.O. | ½-1 hr | 3-5 hr | 24 hr |

## Contraindications and precautions

Contraindicated in patients hypersensitive to drug or other sulfonylureas; in patients with type 1 diabetes or diabetes that can be adequately controlled by diet; in patients with type 2 diabetes complicated by fever, ketosis, acidosis, coma, or other acute complications such as major surgery, severe infection, or severe trauma; in patients with severe renal insufficiency; and in pregnant or breast-feeding women.

Use cautiously in geriatric, debilitated, or malnourished patients and in those with impaired renal or hepatic function or porphyria.

## Interactions

**Drug-drug.** *Anticoagulants:* Increased hypoglycemic activity, enhanced anticoagulant effect. Advise clinician to monitor blood glucose level, PT, and INR. Dosage adjustment may be needed.

*Beta blockers, including ophthalmics:* Masked symptoms of hypoglycemia; possible prolonged hypoglycemic effect. Use together cautiously.

*Calcium channel blockers, corticosteroids, estrogens, isoniazid, oral contraceptives, phenothiazines, phenytoin, sympathomimetics, thiazide diuretics, triamterene, thyroid products:* Decreased hypoglycemic effect. Advise clinician to monitor blood glucose level; dosage adjustment may be needed.

*Chloramphenicol, insulin, MAO inhibitors, NSAIDs, probenecid, salicylates, sulfonamides:* Enhanced hypoglycemic effect. Advise clinician to monitor blood glucose level closely.

**Drug-herb.** *Aloe, bitter melon, bilberry leaf, burdock, dandelion, fenugreek, garlic, ginseng:* Possible improved blood glucose control requiring reduction of antidiabetics with concomitant use. Advise patient to discuss the use of herbal medicines with prescriber before taking them.

**Drug-lifestyle.** *Alcohol use:* Possible disulfiram-like reaction with nausea, vomiting, abdominal cramps, and headaches. Advise patient to avoid alcohol.

## Adverse reactions

**CNS:** headache.

**GI:** nausea, heartburn, epigastric distress, taste alterations.

**Hematologic:** *leukopenia,* hemolytic anemia, *thrombocytopenia, aplastic anemia, agranulocytosis,* pancytopenia.

**Hepatic:** hepatic porphyria.

**Metabolic:** *hypoglycemia, dilutional hyponatremia,* SIADH, weight gain.

**Skin:** rash, pruritus, erythema, urticaria.

**Other:** hypersensitivity reactions, *disulfiram-like reactions.*

## Overdose and treatment

Signs and symptoms of overdose include low blood glucose level, tingling of lips and tongue, hunger, nausea, decreased cerebral function (lethargy, yawning, confusion, agitation, nervousness), increased sympathetic activity (tachycardia, sweating, tremor) and ultimately, seizures, stupor, and coma.

Mild hypoglycemia, without loss of consciousness or neurologic findings, responds to treatment with oral glucose and dosage adjustments. If patient loses consciousness or develops neurologic findings, advise clinician to give rapid injection of dextrose 50%, followed by a continuous infusion of dextrose 10% at a rate to maintain blood glucose level greater than 100 mg/dl. Advise clinician to monitor patient for 24 to 48 hours.

## Clinical considerations

■ To avoid GI intolerance for those patients on larger doses and to improve control of hyperglycemia, divided doses given before the morning and evening meals are recommended.

■ Patients should avoid taking tolbutamide at h.s. because of the potential for nocturnal hypoglycemia.

■ Tolbutamide may give a false-positive reading for albumin in urine if measured by the acidification-after-boiling test. There's no interference with the sulfosalicylic acid test.

**To change from insulin to tolbutamide:**

■ If insulin dose is less than 20 units daily, insulin may be stopped and oral therapy started at 1 to 2 g daily. If insulin dose is 20 to 40 units daily, insulin dose is reduced 30% to 50% and oral therapy started as above. If insulin dose is more than 40 units daily, insulin dose is decreased 20% and oral therapy started as above. Further reductions in insulin dosage are based on patient's response to oral therapy.

### Therapeutic monitoring

■ When substituting tolbutamide for chlorpropamide therapy, advise clinician to monitor patient closely for the first 2 weeks because of prolonged retention of chlorpropamide in the body, which may result in hypoglycemia.

### Special populations

**Pregnant patients.** Use with caution in women of childbearing age. Tolbutamide isn't recommended for treatment of diabetes from pregnancy.

**Breast-feeding patients.** Tolbutamide appears in breast milk. Because of the risk of hypoglycemia in the breast-fed infant, a decision should be made to discontinue either drug or breast-feeding.

**Pediatric patients.** Tolbutamide is ineffective in type 1 and juvenile-onset diabetes. Safety and efficacy in children haven't been established.

**Geriatric patients.** Geriatric patients may be more sensitive to the effects of drug because of reduced metabolism and elimination. Hypoglycemia causes more neurologic symptoms in these patients. Geriatric patients usually require a lower initial dose.

## Patient counseling

■ Emphasize to patient the importance of following prescribed diet, exercise, and medical regimen.

■ Instruct patient to take drug at the same time each day.

■ Inform patient that, if a dose is missed, it should be taken immediately, unless it's almost time to take the next dose. Tell patient not to double the dose.

■ Advise patient to avoid products containing alcohol while taking tolbutamide because of prolonged hypoglycemic effect.

# tolcapone

Tasmar

*Pharmacologic classification:* catechol-*O*-methyltransferase (COMT) inhibitor
*Therapeutic classification:* antiparkinsonian
*Pregnancy risk category C*

## Available forms

Available by prescription only
*Tablets:* 100 mg, 200 mg

## Indications and dosages

*Adjunct to levodopa and carbidopa for treatment of signs and symptoms of idiopathic Parkinson's disease*

*Adults:* Recommended initial dosage is 100 mg (preferred) or 200 mg P.O. t.i.d. If initiating treatment with 200 mg t.i.d. and dyskinesias occur, then a decrease in dose of levodopa may be needed. Maximum daily dose is 600 mg daily. Always give with levodopa/carbidopa. The first tolcapone dose of the day should always be taken with the first levodopa/carbidopa dose of the day.

≡ *Dosage adjustment.* Don't use doses over 100 mg t.i.d. in patients with severe hepatic or renal dysfunction.

## Mechanism of action
*Antiparkinsonian action:* Exact mechanism of action isn't known. It's thought to reversibly inhibit human erythrocyte COMT when given with levodopa/carbidopa, resulting in a decrease in the clearance of levodopa and a twofold increase in the bioavailability of levodopa. The decrease in clearance of levodopa prolongs the elimination half-life of levodopa from 2 to 3½ hours.

## Pharmacokinetics
*Absorption:* Rapidly absorbed; plasma levels peak within 2 hours. Following oral administration, absolute bioavailability is 65%. Onset of effect occurs following administration of first dose. Absorption of tolcapone decreases when given within 1 hour before or 2 hours after food; however, drug can be given without regard to meals.
*Distribution:* Highly bound to plasma proteins (greater than 99.9%), primarily to albumin. The steady-state volume of distribution is small.
*Metabolism:* Completely metabolized before excretion. The main mechanism of metabolism is glucuronidation.
*Excretion:* Only 0.5% of dose is found unchanged in urine. Tolcapone is a low-extraction-ratio drug with a systemic clearance of 7 L/hour. Elimination half-life is 2 to 3 hours. Dialysis isn't expected to affect clearance because of the high protein-binding.

| Route | Onset | Peak | Duration |
|-------|-------|------|----------|
| P.O. | Unknown | 2 hr | Unknown |

## Contraindications and precautions
Contraindicated in patients hypersensitive to drug or its components; in those with liver disease or ALT or AST levels exceeding the upper limit of normal; in patients withdrawn from therapy because of drug-induced hepatocellular injury; and in patients with history of nontraumatic rhabdomyolysis or hyperpyrexia and confusion, possibly related to drug.

Use cautiously in patients with Parkinson's disease because syncope and orthostatic hypotension may worsen.

## Interactions
**Drug-drug.** *Anticoagulants:* Possible increased plasma levels of anticoagulants. Advise clinician to monitor PT and INR.
*Desipramine:* Increased risk of adverse effects. Use together cautiously.

*MAO inhibitors:* Possible hypertensive crisis. Avoid use together.

## Adverse reactions
**CNS:** *dyskinesia, sleep disorder, dystonia, excessive dreaming, somnolence, dizziness, confusion, headache, hallucinations,* hyperkinesia, fatigue, falling, syncope, balance loss, depression, tremor, speech disorder, paresthesia.
**CV:** *orthostatic complaints,* chest pain, chest discomfort, palpitation, hypotension.
**EENT:** pharyngitis, tinnitus.
**GI:** *nausea, anorexia, diarrhea,* flatulence, *vomiting,* constipation, abdominal pain, dyspepsia, dry mouth.
**GU:** urinary tract infection, urine discoloration, hematuria, urinary incontinence, impotence.
**Musculoskeletal:** *muscle cramps,* myalgia, stiffness, arthritis, neck pain.
**Respiratory:** bronchitis, dyspnea, upper respiratory tract infections.
**Skin:** increased sweating, rash.

## Overdose and treatment
The highest dosage used is 800 mg t.i.d.; nausea, vomiting, and dizziness were noted. Advise clinician to provide supportive care and hospitalize, if indicated.

## Clinical considerations
■ Because of the risk of potentially fatal, acute fulminant liver failure, use drug only in patients on levodopa/carbidopa who don't respond to or who aren't suitable for other adjunctive therapy.
■ Diarrhea occurs commonly in patients taking tolcapone. It may occur 2 weeks after therapy begins or after 6 to 12 weeks. Although it usually resolves with discontinuation of drug, hospitalization may be required in rare cases.
■ Dosage adjustments aren't needed in patients with mild to moderate renal dysfunction; use cautiously in patients with severe renal impairment.
■ Advise clinician to withdraw drug in patients who fail to show clinical benefit within 3 weeks of treatment.

### Therapeutic monitoring
■ Advise clinician to monitor liver enzyme levels every 2 weeks for the first year of therapy, and then every 8 weeks. Drug should be stopped if hepatic transaminase levels exceed the upper limits of normal or if patient appears jaundiced.
■ Advise clinician to monitor patient for improvement, which should occur within 3 weeks.

### Special populations
**Pregnant patients.** Use drug during pregnancy only when potential benefits justify risk to fetus.

---

Reactions may be *common,* uncommon, *life-threatening,* or COMMON AND LIFE-THREATENING.

**Breast-feeding patients.** Because drug may appear in breast milk, use with caution in breast-feeding women.

**Pediatric patients.** There's no identified potential use in children.

**Geriatric patients.** Patients ages 75 and older are more likely to develop hallucinations but less likely to develop dystonia than younger patients.

### Patient counseling

■ Advise patient to take drug exactly as prescribed.

■ Warn patient about risk of orthostatic hypotension; tell him to use caution when rising from a seated or recumbent position.

■ Caution patient to avoid hazardous activities until CNS effects of drug are known.

■ Tell patient that nausea may occur and to report signs of liver injury immediately.

■ Advise patient about risk of increased dyskinesia or dystonia.

■ Inform patient that hallucinations may occur.

■ Tell patient to report if pregnancy is being planned or suspected during therapy.

# tolmetin sodium
Tolectin, Tolectin DS

*Pharmacologic classification:* NSAID
*Therapeutic classification:* nonnarcotic analgesic, anti-inflammatory
*Pregnancy risk category C*

### Available forms
Available by prescription only
*Tablets:* 200 mg, 600 mg
*Capsules:* 400 mg

### Indications and dosages
*Rheumatoid arthritis and osteoarthritis, juvenile rheumatoid arthritis*
*Adults:* Initially, 400 mg P.O. t.i.d.; maximum dose is 1,800 mg/day; usual dose ranges from 600 to 1,800 mg daily in three divided doses. *Children ages 2 and older:* Initially, 20 mg/kg/day P.O. in three or four divided doses; usual dose ranges from 15 to 30 mg/kg/day in three or four divided doses.

◇*Ankylosing spondylitis*
*Adults:* 600 to 1,600 mg P.O. daily.

◇*Adhesive capsulitis shoulder (frozen shoulder), radiohumeral bursitis (tennis elbow), local trauma (such as recent sprains)*
*Adults:* 600 mg or 1,200 mg P.O. daily.

### Mechanism of action
*Analgesic and anti-inflammatory actions:* Although exact mechanism of action is unknown, inhibition of prostaglandin synthesis may be responsible for the anti-inflammatory effects

of tolmetin. Drug also seems to possess analgesic and antipyretic activity.

### Pharmacokinetics
*Absorption:* Absorbed rapidly from GI tract.
*Distribution:* Highly protein-bound.
*Metabolism:* Metabolized in the liver.
*Excretion:* Excreted in urine as an inactive metabolite or conjugates of tolmetin. Elimination is biphasic, consisting of a rapid phase with a half-life of 1 to 2 hours followed by a slower phase with a half-life of about 5 hours.

| Route | Onset | Peak | Duration |
|-------|-------|------|----------|
| P.O. | Unknown | ½-1½ hr | 24 hr |

### Contraindications and precautions
Contraindicated in patients hypersensitive to drug and for whom acute asthmatic attacks, urticaria, or rhinitis is precipitated by aspirin or NSAIDs. Also contraindicated in breast-feeding women.

Use cautiously in patients with renal or cardiac disease, GI bleeding, history of peptic ulcer, hypertension, or conditions predisposing to fluid retention.

### Interactions
**Drug-drug.** *Anticoagulants, thrombolytics:* Increased risk of bleeding. Use together cautiously.

*Aspirin:* Decreased plasma levels of tolmetin. Advise clinician to monitor patient closely. Dosage adjustment may be required.

*Highly protein-bound drugs, such as phenytoin, salicylates, sulfonamides, sulfonylureas, and warfarin:* Increased adverse effects. Advise clinician to monitor patient closely.

*Methotrexate:* Increased risk of methotrexate toxicity. Avoid use together. If given together, advise clinician to monitor patient closely.

*Other GI irritating drugs, such as antibiotics, corticosteroids, and other NSAIDs:* Potentiate adverse GI effects. Use together cautiously.

**Drug-herb.** *Dong quai, feverfew, garlic, ginger, horse chestnut, red clover:* Possible increased risk of bleeding. Discourage use together.

*Dong quai, St. John's wort:* Increased risk of photosensitivity. Advise patient to use sunblock.

**Drug-food.** *Any food:* Delayed and decreased absorption of tolmetin. Separate administration times.

### Adverse reactions
**CNS:** headache, dizziness, drowsiness, asthenia, depression.
**CV:** chest pain, hypertension, edema.
**EENT:** tinnitus, visual disturbances.
**GI:** epigastric distress, peptic ulceration, occult blood loss, *nausea,* vomiting, abdominal pain, diarrhea, constipation, dyspepsia, flatulence, anorexia.

**GU:** elevated BUN level, urinary tract infection.
**Hematologic:** decreased hemoglobin level and hematocrit.
**Metabolic:** weight gain, weight loss.
**Skin:** irritation.
**Other:** *anaphylaxis.*

## Overdose and treatment
Signs and symptoms of overdose include dizziness, drowsiness, mental confusion, and lethargy. To treat tolmetin overdose, advise clinician to empty stomach immediately by inducing emesis or by gastric lavage followed by administration of activated charcoal. Symptomatic and supportive measures (respiratory support and correction of fluid and electrolyte imbalances) should be provided. Advise clinician to monitor laboratory parameters and vital signs closely. Alkalinization of urine by sodium bicarbonate ingestion may enhance renal excretion of tolmetin.

## Clinical considerations
■ Advise clinician to assess cardiopulmonary status closely.
■ Therapeutic effect usually occurs within a few days to 1 week of therapy. Advise clinician to evaluate patient's response to drug as evidenced by relief of symptoms.
■ Advise clinician to give drug on empty stomach for maximum absorption. However, it may be given with meals to lessen GI upset.
■ For patients who don't have adequate response to NSAIDs, advise clinician to consider therapy with a disease-modifying antirheumatic.
■ Concomitant use with misoprostol may be considered in patients at increased risk for NSAID-induced ulcers.
■ Tolmetin falsely elevates results of urinary protein (pseudoproteinuria) in tests that rely on acid precipitation, such as those using sulfosalicylic acid.

### Therapeutic monitoring
■ Advise clinician to monitor vital signs closely, especially heart rate and blood pressure.
■ Advise clinician to assess renal function periodically during therapy and monitor fluid intake and output and daily weight.
■ Advise clinician to monitor patient for presence and amount of edema.

### Special populations
**Pregnant patients.** Use drug during pregnancy only when clearly needed.
**Breast-feeding patients.** Because drug appears in breast milk, it may adversely affect neonates. Avoid use in breast-feeding women.
**Pediatric patients.** Safety and efficacy in children under age 2 haven't been established.

## Patient counseling
■ Explain that therapeutic effects may occur in 1 week but could take 2 to 4 weeks.
■ Advise patient to avoid use of OTC drugs, such as NSAIDs, unless medically approved.
■ Instruct patient to follow prescribed regimen and recommended schedule of follow up.
■ Advise patient to report signs of edema or other adverse reactions.

# tolterodine tartrate
Detrol, Detrol LA

*Pharmacologic classification:* muscarinic receptor antagonist
*Therapeutic classification:* anticholinergic
*Pregnancy risk category C*

## Available forms
Available by prescription only
*Tablets:* 1 mg, 2 mg
*Capsules (extended-release):* 2 mg, 4 mg

## Indications and dosages
*Treatment of patients with overactive bladder with symptoms of urinary frequency, urgency, or urge incontinence*
*Adults:* Initially, 2 mg P.O. b.i.d. May lower to 1 mg b.i.d. based on response and tolerance. Or, for extended-release capsules, 4 mg P.O. daily. May lower to 2 mg P.O. daily based on response and tolerance.
≡ *Dosage adjustment.* For patients who have significantly reduced hepatic function or who are currently taking a drug that inhibits the cytochrome P-450 3A4 isoenzyme system, recommended dose is 1 mg b.i.d.

## Mechanism of action
*Anticholinergic action:* Tolterodine is a competitive muscarinic receptor antagonist. Both urinary bladder contraction and salivation are mediated by cholinergic muscarinic receptors.

## Pharmacokinetics
*Absorption:* Well absorbed with about 77% bioavailability. Food increases bioavailability by 53%.
*Distribution:* Volume of distribution is about 113 L. Tolterodine is 96% protein-bound.
*Metabolism:* Metabolized by the liver primarily by oxidation by the cytochrome P-450 2D6 pathway; leads to formation of a pharmacologically active 5-hydroxymethyl metabolite.
*Excretion:* Excreted mostly via urine; the rest in feces. Less than 1% of a dose is recovered as unchanged drug and 5% to 14% is recovered as the active metabolite. Half-life is 2 to 3½ hours.

| Route | Onset | Peak | Duration |
|-------|-------|------|----------|
| P.O. | Unknown | 1-2 hr | Unknown |

## Contraindications and precautions
Contraindicated in patients with urine or gastric retention and uncontrolled angle-closure glaucoma. Also contraindicated in patients hypersensitive to tolterodine or its ingredients.

Use with caution in patients with significantly reduced hepatic or renal function.

## Interactions
**Drug-drug.** *Antifungals, such as itraconazole, ketoconazole, and miconazole; cytochrome P-450 3A4 inhibitors such as macrolide antibiotics, including clarithromycin and erythromycin:* Effects haven't been studied. Tolterodine doses of more than 1 mg b.i.d. shouldn't be given with these drugs.
**Drug-food.** *Any food:* Increased tolterodine absorption. May be used for this effect.

## Adverse reactions
**CNS:** paresthesia, vertigo, dizziness, *headache,* nervousness, somnolence, fatigue.
**CV:** hypertension, chest pain.
**EENT:** abnormal vision (including accommodation), xerophthalmia, pharyngitis, rhinitis, sinusitis.
**GI:** *dry mouth,* abdominal pain, constipation, diarrhea, dyspepsia, flatulence, nausea, vomiting.
**GU:** dysuria, micturition frequency, urine retention, urinary tract infection.
**Metabolic:** weight gain.
**Musculoskeletal:** arthalgia, back pain.
**Respiratory:** bronchitis, coughing, upper respiratory infection.
**Skin:** pruritis, rash, erythema, dry skin.
**Other:** flulike symptoms.

## Overdose and treatment
Overdoses may potentially result in severe central anticholinergic effects and should be treated accordingly. Advise clinician to perform ECG monitoring if an overdose occurs.

## Clinical considerations
■ Food increases the absorption of tolterodine, but no dosage adjustment is needed.
■ Dry mouth is the most frequently reported adverse event.

### Therapeutic monitoring
■ Advise clinician to monitor patient for urinary symptoms and adverse reactions.

### Special populations
**Pregnant patients.** Use drug during pregnancy only when clearly needed.
**Breast-feeding patients.** It's unknown if drug appears in breast milk. Drug isn't recommended for use in breast-feeding women.
**Pediatric patients.** Safety and efficacy in children haven't been established.

**Geriatric patients.** No overall differences in safety have been observed between older and younger patients.

## Patient counseling
■ Inform patient that antimuscarinics such as tolterodine may produce blurred vision.
■ Caution patient to avoid hazardous activities until effects of drug are known.

# topiramate
Topamax

*Pharmacologic classification:*
sulfamate-substituted monosaccharide
*Therapeutic classification:* anticonvulsant
*Pregnancy risk category C*

## Available forms
Available by prescription only
*Capsules:* 15 mg, 25 mg
*Tablets:* 25 mg, 100 mg, 200 mg

## Indications and dosages
**Adjunctive therapy of partial onset seizures or primary generalized tonic-clonic seizures**
*Adults:* Initially, 50 mg P.O. daily in two divided doses for the first week, followed by an increase of 50 mg increments at weekly intervals. Maximum daily dose is 400 mg in two divided doses.
**Adjunctive therapy for partial seizures, primary generalized tonic-clonic seizures, or Lennox-Gestaut syndrome**
*Children ages 2 to 16:* 5 to 9 mg/kg P.O. daily in two divided doses. Dosage adjustment should begin at 1 to 3 mg/kg nightly for 1 week. Then increase at 1- to 2-week intervals by 1 to 3 mg/kg daily to achieve optimal response. Dosage adjustment should be guided by clinical outcome.
≡ *Dosage adjustment.* For patients with moderate to severe renal impairment, reduce dosage by 50%. A supplemental dose may be required during hemodialysis.

## Mechanism of action
*Anticonvulsant action:* Mechanism of action is unknown. Thought to block action potential, suggestive of a sodium channel-blocking action. Drug may potentiate activity of gamma-aminobutyric acid (GABA) and antagonize the ability of kainate to activate the kainate/AMPA subtype of excitatory amino acid (glutamate) receptor. Topiramate also has weak carbonic anhydrase inhibitor activity, which is unrelated to its anticonvulsant properties.

## Pharmacokinetics

*Absorption:* Rapidly absorbed. Relative bioavailability of drug is about 80% compared with a solution and isn't affected by food.
*Distribution:* Plasma levels increase proportionately with dose; mean elimination half-life is 21 hours. Steady state is reached in 4 days in patients with normal renal function. Drug is 13% to 17% plasma protein–bound.
*Metabolism:* Not extensively metabolized.
*Excretion:* Primarily eliminated unchanged in urine (about 70% of a given dose). Mean plasma half-life is 21 hours.

| Route | Onset | Peak | Duration |
|-------|-------|------|----------|
| P.O. | Unknown | 2 hr | Unknown |

## Contraindications and precautions

Contraindicated in patients hypersensitive to drug or its components.

## Interactions

**Drug-drug.** *Carbamazepine, phenytoin:* Decreased topiramate levels. Advise clinician to monitor patient closely.
*Carbonic anhydrase inhibitors, such as acetazolamide and dichlorphenamide:* Possible increased risk of renal stone formation. Avoid use together.
*CNS depressants:* Effects haven't been evaluated. Because of risk of topiramate-induced CNS depression or other adverse cognitive and neuropsychiatric events, use together cautiously.
*Oral contraceptives:* Decreased contraceptive effect. Advise patient to use another method of contraception.
*Phenobarbital, primidone, valproic acid:* Increased phenytoin levels. Advise clinician to monitor patient closely.
**Drug-lifestyle.** *Alcohol use:* CNS depression, as well as other adverse cognitive and neuropsychiatric events. Advise patient to avoid alcohol.

## Adverse reactions

**CNS:** *fatigue,* abnormal coordination, agitation, apathy, asthenia, *ataxia, confusion,* depression, difficulty with concentration, attention, language, or memory, *dizziness,* emotional lability, euphoria, *generalized tonic-clonic seizures,* hallucinations, hyperkinesia, hypertonia, hypoesthesia, hypokinesia, insomnia, malaise, mood problems, *nervousness, nystagmus, paresthesia,* psychomotor slowing, psychosis, *somnolence, speech disorders,* stupor, *suicide attempt, tremor,* vertigo.
**CV:** chest pain, palpitations, edema.
**EENT:** *abnormal vision,* conjunctivitis, *diplopia,* eye pain, epistaxis, hearing or vestibular problems, pharyngitis, sinusitis, tinnitus.
**GI:** abdominal pain, anorexia, constipation, diarrhea, dry mouth, dyspepsia, flatulence, gastroenteritis, gingivitis, *nausea,* vomiting, taste perversion.
**GU:** amenorrhea, dysuria, dysmenorrhea, leukorrhea, hematuria, impotence, intermenstrual bleeding, menstrual disorder, menorrhagia, micturition frequency, renal calculus, urinary incontinence, urinary tract infection, vaginitis.
**Hematologic:** anemia, *leukopenia.*
**Metabolic:** weight gain or loss.
**Musculoskeletal:** back pain, leg pain, myalgia.
**Respiratory:** bronchitis, coughing, dyspnea, *upper respiratory tract infection.*
**Skin:** acne, alopecia, aggressive reaction, increased sweating, pruritus, rash.
**Other:** body odor, fever, flulike symptoms, hot flashes, rigors.

## Overdose and treatment

In acute overdose after recent ingestion, advise clinician to institute gastric lavage or emesis. Activated charcoal isn't recommended. Advise clinician to institute supportive treatment. Hemodialysis is an effective means of removing drug.

## Clinical considerations

■ Because of the bitter taste, tablets shouldn't be broken.
■ Capsules can be opened and contents sprinkled on soft food.
■ If needed, withdraw anticonvulsants gradually to minimize risk of increased seizure activity.
■ Drug should be stopped if an ocular adverse event occurs, characterized by acute myopia and secondary angle-closure glaucoma.

### Therapeutic monitoring

■ Advise clinician to monitor CBC.
■ Advise clinician to monitor patient for seizure activity.

### Special populations

**Breast-feeding patients.** It isn't known if drug appears in breast milk. Use with caution in breast-feeding women.
**Pediatric patients.** Safety and efficacy in children under age 2 haven't been established.
**Geriatric patients.** No age-related problems have been seen in geriatric patients; however, age-related renal abnormalities should be considered.

## Patient counseling

■ Carefully review dosing schedule with patient to avoid undermedication or overmedication.
■ Tell patient to maintain adequate fluid intake during therapy because of potential for renal stone formation.
■ Advise patient to avoid hazardous activities until effects of drug are known.

---

*Reactions may be* common, uncommon, *life-threatening,* or **COMMON AND LIFE-THREATENING.**

■ Tell patient to notify prescriber immediately if he experiences changes in vision.

# topotecan hydrochloride
Hycamtin

*Pharmacologic classification:* semisynthetic camptothecin derivative
*Therapeutic classification:* antineoplastic
*Pregnancy risk category D*

## Available forms
Available by prescription only
*Injection:* 4-mg single-dose vial

## Indications and dosages
*Metastatic carcinoma of the ovary after failure of initial or subsequent chemotherapy*
Adults: 1.5 mg/m²/day as I.V. infusion given over 30 minutes for 5 consecutive days, starting on day 1 of a 21-day cycle. Minimum of four cycles should be given.
*Treatment of small-cell lung cancer sensitive disease after failure of first-line chemotherapy*
Adults: 1.5 mg/m² I.V. infusion given over 30 minutes daily for 5 consecutive days, followed by a 16-day rest period for a 21-day treatment course. Minimum of four cycles should be given.
≡*Dosage adjustment.* For adults with renal impairment and creatinine clearance of 20 to 39 ml/minute, dosage should be adjusted to 0.75 mg/m². For patients with mild renal impairment (creatinine clearance, 40 to 60 ml/minute), adjustment isn't needed. There are insufficient data available for a dosage recommendation for patients with creatinine clearance less than 20 ml/minute. If severe neutropenia occurs during any course, advise clinician to reduce dosage by 0.25 mg/m² for subsequent courses. Alternatively, advise clinician to give granulocyte-colony stimulating factor (G-CSF) starting from day 6 of subsequent courses (24 hours after completion of topotecan) before resorting to dosage reduction.

## I.V. administration
■ Prepare drug under a vertical laminar flow hood wearing gloves and protective clothing. If drug solution contacts the skin, wash the skin immediately and thoroughly with soap and water. If mucous membranes are affected, flush areas thoroughly with water.
■ Reconstitute each 4-mg vial with 4 ml sterile water for injection. Then dilute appropriate volume of reconstituted solution in either normal saline solution or D₅W before use.
■ Use reconstituted product immediately.

■ Protect unopened vials of drug from light. Reconstituted vials are stable at 68° to 77° F (20° to 25° C) with ambient lighting conditions for 24 hours.
■ Drug extravasation may cause mild local reactions such as erythema and bruising.

## Incompatibilities
None reported.

## Mechanism of action
*Antineoplastic action:* Topotecan relieves torsional strain in DNA by inducing reversible single-strand breaks. It binds to the topoisomerase I-DNA complex and prevents religation of these single-strand breaks. The cytotoxicity of topotecan is thought to be from double-strand DNA damage produced during DNA synthesis when replication enzymes interact with the ternary complex formed by topotecan, topoisomerase I, and DNA.

## Pharmacokinetics
*Absorption:* Administered I.V.
*Distribution:* About 35% is plasma protein–bound.
*Metabolism:* Undergoes a reversible pH-dependent hydrolysis of its lactone moiety; the lactone form is pharmacologically active.
*Excretion:* About 30% is excreted in the urine. Terminal half-life is 2 to 3 hours.

| Route | Onset | Peak | Duration |
|-------|-------|------|----------|
| I.V. | Unknown | Unknown | Unknown |

## Contraindications and precautions
Contraindicated in patients hypersensitive to drug or its components, in those with severe bone marrow depression, and in pregnant or breast-feeding women.

## Interactions
**Drug-drug.** *Cisplatin:* Increased severity of myelosuppression. Use together with extreme caution.
*G-CSF:* Prolonged duration of neutropenia. Don't initiate G-CSF until day 6 of the course of therapy, 24 hours after completion of treatment with topotecan.

## Adverse reactions
**CNS:** *fatigue, asthenia, headache,* paresthesia.
**GI:** *nausea, vomiting, diarrhea, constipation, abdominal pain, stomatitis, anorexia.*
**Hematologic:** NEUTROPENIA, LEUKOPENIA, THROMBOCYTOPENIA, anemia.
**Hepatic:** transient elevations of liver enzyme levels.
**Respiratory:** *dyspnea.*
**Skin:** *alopecia.*
**Other:** *sepsis,* fever.

## Overdose and treatment

The primary adverse effect of topotecan overdose is thought to be bone marrow suppression. Treatment should be supportive. There's no known antidote.

## Clinical considerations

■ Before administration of the first course, baseline neutrophil count should exceed 1,500 cells/mm³ and platelet count of more than 100,000 cells/mm³.

■ Bone marrow suppression (primarily neutropenia) is the dose-limiting toxicity of topotecan. The nadir occurs at about 11 days. If severe neutropenia occurs during therapy, advise clinician to reduce dosage by 0.25 mg/m² for subsequent courses. Alternatively, advise clinician to give G-CSF after the subsequent course (before dosage is reduced) starting from day 6 (24 hours after completion of topotecan administration). Neutropenia isn't cumulative over time.

■ Thrombocytopenia occurred with a median duration of 5 days and platelet nadir at a median of 15 days; anemia occurred with a median nadir at day 15. Blood or platelet (or both) transfusions may be needed.

■ Inadvertent extravasation with topotecan has caused only mild local reactions, such as erythema and bruising.

### Therapeutic monitoring

■ Frequent monitoring of peripheral blood cell counts is needed. Don't give patients subsequent courses of topotecan until neutrophil counts exceed 1,000 cells/mm³, platelet counts are more than 100,000 cells/mm³, and hemoglobin levels are 9 mg/dl (with transfusion if needed).

### Special populations

**Pregnant patients.** Contraindicated during pregnancy.
**Breast-feeding patients.** Because it isn't known if drug appears in breast milk, avoid use of drug in breast-feeding women.
**Pediatric patients.** Safety and efficacy in children haven't been established.

## Patient counseling

■ Instruct patient to promptly report sore throat, fever, chills, bruising, or unusual bleeding.
■ Inform patient of need for frequent blood work to identify potential bone marrow suppression.

---

# toremifene citrate
Fareston

*Pharmacologic classification:* nonsteroidal antiestrogen
*Therapeutic classification:* antineoplastic
*Pregnancy risk category D*

## Available forms

Available by prescription only
*Tablets:* 60 mg

## Indications and dosages

***For treatment of metastatic breast cancer in postmenopausal women with estrogen receptor–positive or unknown tumors***
*Adults:* 60 mg P.O. once daily. Treatment is usually continued until disease progression is observed.

## Mechanism of action

*Antineoplastic action:* Toremifene is a nonsteroidal triphenylethylene derivative that exerts its antitumor effect by competing with estrogen for binding sites in the tumor. This blocks the growth-stimulating effects of endogenous estrogen in the tumor, causing an antiestrogenic effect.

## Pharmacokinetics

*Absorption:* Well absorbed after oral administration and not influenced by food. Plasma levels peak within 3 hours. Steady-state levels are reached in about 4 to 6 weeks.
*Distribution:* Apparent volume of distribution is 580 L; drug binds extensively to serum proteins, mainly albumin.
*Metabolism:* Extensively metabolized in liver, mainly by CYP3A4, to *N*-demethyltoremifene, which is also antiestrogenic but with weak in vivo antitumor potency. Elimination half-life is about 5 days.
*Excretion:* Eliminated in feces, with about 10% excreted unchanged in urine. Elimination is slow because of enterohepatic circulation.

| Route | Onset | Peak | Duration |
|-------|-------|------|----------|
| P.O. | Unknown | 3 hr | Unknown |

## Contraindications and precautions

Contraindicated in patients hypersensitive to drug. Avoid use in patients with history of thromboembolic diseases. Don't use drug long-term in patients with preexisting endometrial hyperplasia.

## Interactions

**Drug-drug.** *Drugs that decrease renal calcium excretion such as thiazide diuretics:* Increased risk of hypercalcemia. Advise clinician to monitor calcium levels closely.

---

*Coumarin-like anticoagulants such as warfarin:* Prolonged PT and INR. Advise clinician to monitor PT and INR closely.

*Cytochrome P-450 3A4 enzyme inducers, such as carbamazepine, phenobarbital, and phenytoin:* Increased toremifene metabolism. Advise clinician to monitor patient closely; dosage adjustment may be needed.

*Cytochrome P-450 3A4-6 enzyme inhibitors, such as erythromycin and ketoconazole:* Decreased toremifene metabolism. Advise clinician to monitor patient closely; dosage adjustment may be needed.

### Adverse reactions
**CNS:** dizziness, fatigue, depression.
**CV:** edema, *thromboembolism, HF, MI, pulmonary embolism.*
**EENT:** visual disturbances, glaucoma, ocular changes (such as dry eyes), *cataracts, abnormal visual fields.*
**GI:** *nausea,* vomiting.
**GU:** *vaginal discharge,* vaginal bleeding.
**Hepatic:** *elevated levels of AST, alkaline phosphatase,* and bilirubin.
**Metabolic:** hypercalcemia.
**Skin:** *sweating.*
**Other:** *hot flashes.*

### Overdose and treatment
Theoretically, overdose may cause an increase of antiestrogenic effects (hot flashes), estrogenic effects (vaginal bleeding), or nervous system disorders (vertigo, dizziness, ataxia, and nausea). There's no specific antidote; treatment is symptomatic.

### Clinical considerations
■ Disease flare-up may occur during first weeks of therapy. This doesn't indicate treatment failure.
■ Drug causes fetal harm; indicated only for postmenopausal women.

#### Therapeutic monitoring
■ Advise clinician to obtain periodic CBC, calcium levels, and liver function test results.
■ Advise clinician to monitor calcium levels closely for first weeks of treatment in patients with bone metastases because of increased risk of hypercalcemia and tumor flare.

#### Special populations
**Pregnant patients.** Drug is contraindicated during pregnancy because of potential for fetal harm.
**Breast-feeding patients.** It's unknown if drug appears in breast milk. Use with caution in breast-feeding women.
**Geriatric patients.** No significant age-related differences in drug's efficacy or safety were noted.

### Patient counseling
■ Instruct patient to take drug exactly as prescribed.
■ Warn patient not to discontinue therapy without consulting prescriber.
■ Inform patient to report vaginal bleeding and other adverse effects.
■ Warn patient that a disease flare-up may occur during first weeks of therapy. Reassure patient that this doesn't indicate treatment failure.

## torsemide
Demadex

*Pharmacologic classification:* loop diuretic
*Therapeutic classification:* diuretic, antihypertensive
*Pregnancy risk category B*

### Available forms
Available by prescription only
*Tablets:* 5 mg, 10 mg, 20 mg, 100 mg
*Injection:* 2-ml ampule (10 mg/ml), 5-ml ampule (10 mg/ml)

### Indications and dosages
*Diuresis in patients with heart failure*
*Adults:* Initially, 10 to 20 mg P.O. or I.V. once daily. If response is inadequate, double the dose until response is obtained. Maximum dose, 200 mg daily.
*Diuresis in patients with chronic renal failure*
*Adults:* Initially, 20 mg P.O. or I.V. once daily. If response is inadequate, double the dose until response is obtained. Maximum dose, 200 mg daily.
*Diuresis in patients with hepatic cirrhosis*
*Adults:* Initially, 5 to 10 mg P.O. or I.V. once daily with an aldosterone antagonist or a potassium-sparing diuretic. If response is inadequate, double the dose until response is obtained. Maximum dose, 40 mg daily.
*Hypertension*
*Adults:* Initially, 5 mg P.O. daily. Increase to 10 mg once daily in 4 to 6 weeks, if needed and tolerated. If response is still inadequate, add another antihypertensive or increase torsemide up to 100 mg daily in one or two divided doses.

### I.V. administration
■ Inject drug slowly over 2 minutes; single doses shouldn't exceed 200 mg.

#### Incompatibilities
None reported.

### Mechanism of action
*Diuretic and antihypertensive actions:* Loop diuretics such as torsemide enhance excretion

of sodium, chloride, and water by acting on the ascending portion of the loop of Henle. Torsemide doesn't significantly alter glomerular filtration rate, renal plasma flow, or acid-base balance.

## Pharmacokinetics
*Absorption:* Absorbed with little first-pass metabolism; serum level peaks within 1 hour after oral administration.
*Distribution:* Volume of distribution is 12 to 15 L in healthy patients and in those with mild to moderate renal failure or HF. In patients with hepatic cirrhosis, volume of distribution is about doubled. Drug is extensively plasma protein–bound (97% to 99%).
*Metabolism:* Metabolized in the liver to an inactive major metabolite and to two lesser metabolites that have some diuretic activity; for practical purposes, metabolism terminates action of drug. Duration of action is 6 to 8 hours after oral or I.V. use.
*Excretion:* From 22% to 34% of dose is excreted unchanged in urine via active secretion of drug by the proximal tubules.

| Route | Onset | Peak | Duration |
|-------|-------|------|----------|
| P.O. | 1 hr | 1-2 hr | 6-8 hr |
| I.V. | 10 min | 1 hr | 6-8 hr |

## Contraindications and precautions
Contraindicated in patients with anuria or those hypersensitive to drug or other sulfonylurea derivatives. Use cautiously in patients with hepatic disease and associated cirrhosis and ascites.

## Interactions
**Drug-drug.** *Aminoglycosides, other ototoxic drugs:* Auditory toxicity. Advise clinician to monitor patient carefully.
*Cholestyramine:* Decreased torsemide absorption. Separate administration by at least 3 hours.
*Indomethacin, probenecid:* Decreased diuretic effect. Avoid use together.
*Lithium:* Lithium toxicity. Advise clinician to monitor patient and lithium levels closely.
*NSAIDs:* Renal dysfunction. Use together cautiously.
*Salicylates:* Reduced excretion of salicylate. Avoid use together.
**Drug-herb.** *Dandelion:* Possible interference with diuretic activity. Discourage use together.

## Adverse reactions
**CNS:** asthenia, dizziness, headache, nervousness, insomnia, syncope.
**CV:** ECG abnormalities, chest pain, edema, *dehydration.*
**EENT:** rhinitis, cough, sore throat.
**GI:** diarrhea, constipation, nausea, dyspepsia, *hemorrhage.*

**GU:** *excessive urination,* altered renal function test results.
**Metabolic:** altered electrolyte balance.
**Musculoskeletal:** arthralgia, myalgia.

## Overdose and treatment
Although data specific to torsemide overdose are lacking, signs and symptoms would probably reflect excessive pharmacologic effect: dehydration, hypovolemia, hypotension, hyponatremia, hypokalemia, hypochloremic alkalosis, and hemoconcentration. Treatment should consist of fluid and electrolyte replacement.

## Clinical considerations
■ Oral and I.V. doses of drug are therapeutically equivalent.
■ Tinnitus and hearing loss (usually reversible) have been observed after rapid I.V. injection of other loop diuretics and have been noted after oral torsemide administration.
■ CV disease (especially in patients receiving cardiac glycosides) and diuretic-induced hypokalemia may be risk factors for the development of arrhythmias.
■ The risk of hypokalemia is greatest in patients with hepatic cirrhosis, brisk diuresis, inadequate oral intake of electrolytes, or concurrent therapy with corticosteroids or corticotropin. Advise clinician to perform periodic monitoring of serum potassium and other electrolytes.
■ Excessive diuresis may cause dehydration, blood-volume reduction, and possibly thrombosis and embolism, especially in geriatric patients.

### Therapeutic monitoring
■ Advise clinician to monitor fluid intake and output, serum electrolyte levels, blood pressure, weight, and pulse rate during rapid diuresis and routinely with long-term use.
■ If fluid and electrolyte imbalances occur, drug should be stopped until the imbalances are corrected. Drug may then be restarted at a lower dose.

### Special populations
**Breast-feeding patients.** It isn't known if drug appears in breast milk. Use caution when giving drug to breast-feeding women.
**Pediatric patients.** Safety and efficacy in children under age 18 haven't been established.
**Geriatric patients.** Special dosage adjustment usually isn't needed. However, geriatric patients are at greater risk for dehydration, blood-volume reduction, and possibly thrombosis and embolism with excessive diuresis.

## Patient counseling
■ Instruct patient to take torsemide in the morning to prevent nocturia and to change positions slowly to prevent dizziness.

---

Reactions may be *common,* uncommon, *life-threatening,* or COMMON AND LIFE-THREATENING.

■ Instruct patient to report ringing in ears immediately because this may indicate toxicity.

# tramadol hydrochloride
Ultram

*Pharmacologic classification:* synthetic derivative
*Therapeutic classification:* analgesic
*Pregnancy risk category C*

## Available forms
Available by prescription only
*Tablets:* 50 mg

## Indications and dosages
**Moderate to moderately severe pain**
*Adults and children ages 16 and older:* 50 to 100 mg P.O. q 4 to 6 hours, p.r.n. Maximum dose, 400 mg/day.
≡*Dosage adjustment.* For patients with creatinine clearance less than 30 ml/minute, advise clinician to increase dosing interval to q 12 hours; maximum daily dose, 200 mg. For patients with cirrhosis, recommended dosage is 50 mg q 12 hours.

## Mechanism of action
*Analgesic action:* Mechanism of action is unknown. Drug is a centrally acting synthetic analgesic compound that isn't chemically related to opiates but is thought to bind to opioid receptors and inhibit reuptake of norepinephrine and serotonin.

## Pharmacokinetics
*Absorption:* Almost completely absorbed. Mean absolute bioavailability of a 100-mg dose is about 75%.
*Distribution:* About 20% plasma protein–bound; it may cross the blood-brain barrier.
*Metabolism:* Extensively metabolized.
*Excretion:* About 30% of a dose is excreted unchanged in urine and 60% as metabolites. Half-life of drug is about 6 to 7 hours.

| Route | Onset | Peak | Duration |
|---|---|---|---|
| P.O. | Unknown | 2 hr | Unknown |

## Contraindications and precautions
Contraindicated in patients hypersensitive to drug or in those with acute intoxication with alcohol, hypnotics, centrally acting analgesics, opioids, or psychotropic drugs.

Use cautiously in patients at risk for seizures or respiratory depression; in those with increased intracranial pressure or head injury, acute abdominal conditions, or impaired renal or hepatic function; and in patients physically dependent on opioids.

## Interactions
**Drug-drug.** *Carbamazepine:* Increased tramadol metabolism. Advise clinician to monitor patient closely. Tramadol dose may need to be increased.
*CNS depressants:* Additive effects. Use together cautiously. Tramadol dose may need to be reduced.
*MAO inhibitors, neuroleptic drugs:* Increased risk of seizures. Advise clinician to monitor patient closely.
**Drug-lifestyle.** *Alcohol use:* Increased CNS depression. Advise patient to avoid alcohol.

## Adverse reactions
**CNS:** *dizziness, vertigo, headache, somnolence, CNS stimulation, asthenia,* anxiety, confusion, coordination disturbance, euphoria, nervousness, sleep disorder, *seizures,* malaise.
**CV:** vasodilation.
**EENT:** visual disturbances.
**GI:** *nausea, constipation, vomiting,* dyspepsia, dry mouth, diarrhea, abdominal pain, anorexia, flatulence.
**GU:** urine retention, urinary frequency, increased creatinine clearance, proteinuria, menopausal symptoms.
**Hematologic:** decreased hemoglobin levels.
**Hepatic:** elevated liver enzyme levels.
**Musculoskeletal:** hypertonia.
**Respiratory:** *respiratory depression.*
**Skin:** *pruritus,* diaphoresis, rash.

## Overdose and treatment
Serious potential consequences of overdose are respiratory depression and seizures. Because naloxone will reverse some, but not all, of the symptoms caused by tramalol overdose, supportive therapy is recommended. Hemodialysis removes only a small percentage of drug.

## Clinical considerations
■ Drug has been reported to reduce seizure threshold.
■ Serious and rarely fatal anaphylactoid reactions have been reported.

### Therapeutic monitoring
■ Advise clinician to monitor patient closely for seizures.
■ Advise clinician to monitor patient's CV and respiratory status and stop drug if respirations decrease or rate is less than 12 breaths per minute or if patient exhibits signs of respiratory depression.
■ Advise clinician to monitor patient for drug dependence. Because drug dependence similar to codeine or dextropropoxyphene may occur, the potential for abuse exists.

### Special populations
**Pregnant patients.** Safe use during pregnancy hasn't been established.

**Breast-feeding patients.** Use of drug in breast-feeding women isn't recommended.
**Pediatric patients.** Safety and efficacy in children under age 16 haven't been established.
**Geriatric patients.** Use cautiously because serum levels are slightly elevated and the elimination half-life of drug is prolonged. Don't exceed daily dose of 300 mg.

## Patient counseling
■ Instruct patient to take drug only as prescribed.
■ Caution patient to avoid potentially hazardous activities that require mental alertness until adverse CNS effects of drug are known.

# trandolapril
Mavik

*Pharmacologic classification:* ACE inhibitor
*Therapeutic classification:* antihypertensive
*Pregnancy risk category C (D second and third trimesters)*

## Available forms
Available by prescription only
*Tablets:* 1 mg, 2 mg, 4 mg

## Indications and dosages
*Hypertension*
**Adults:** For patient not taking a diuretic, initially 1 mg for a nonblack patient and 2 mg for a black patient P.O. once daily. If control isn't adequate, dosage can be increased at intervals of at least 1 week. Maintenance dose ranges from 2 to 4 mg daily for most patients; there's little experience with doses of more than 8 mg. Patients receiving once-daily dosing at 4 mg may use b.i.d. dosing.

For patient receiving a diuretic, initially 0.5 mg P.O. once daily. Subsequent dosage adjustment made should be based on blood pressure response.
*Heart failure post-MI or left ventricular dysfunction post-MI*
**Adults:** Initially, 1 mg P.O. daily, adjusted to 4 mg P.O. daily. Begin therapy 3 to 5 days post-MI. If patient can't tolerate 4 mg, continue at highest tolerated dose.
≡*Dosage adjustment.* For patients with hepatic impairment or for patients with renal insufficiency and a creatinine clearance less than 30 ml/minute, advise clinician to give 0.5 mg/day initially, then increase p.r.n. to maximum of 4 mg/day.

## Mechanism of action
*Antihypertensive action:* Unknown. Drug action is thought to result primarily from inhibition of circulating and tissue ACE activity, reducing angiotensin II formation, decreasing vasoconstriction, decreasing aldosterone secretion, and increasing plasma renin. Decreased aldosterone secretion leads to diuresis, natriuresis, and a small increase in serum potassium.

## Pharmacokinetics
*Absorption:* Absolute bioavailability after oral administration of trandolapril is about 10% for trandolapril and 70% for its metabolite, trandolaprilat.
*Distribution:* About 80% protein-bound.
*Metabolism:* Metabolized by the liver to the active metabolite, trandolaprilat, and at least seven other metabolites.
*Excretion:* About 66% excreted in feces; 33% in urine. Elimination half-lives of trandolapril and trandolaprilat are about 6 and 10 hours, respectively, but like all ACE inhibitors, trandolaprilat also has a prolonged terminal elimination phase.

| Route | Onset | Peak | Duration |
|-------|-------|------|----------|
| P.O. | Unknown | 1-10 hr | 24 hr |

## Contraindications and precautions
Contraindicated in patients hypersensitive to drug and those with a history of angioedema related to previous treatment with an ACE inhibitor. Drug isn't recommended for use in pregnant women.
Use cautiously in patients with impaired renal function, HF, or renal artery stenosis.

## Interactions
**Drug-drug.** *Diuretics:* Increased risk of excessive hypotension. Advise clinician to stop diuretic or lower dose of trandolapril.
*Lithium:* Potential for lithium toxicity. Monitor lithium levels closely.
*Potassium-sparing diuretics, potassium supplements:* Increased risk of hyperkalemia. Advise clinician to monitor serum potassium level closely.
**Drug-herb.** *Licorice:* Possible sodium retention and increased blood pressure interfering with therapeutic effects of ACE inhibitors. Discourage concomitant use.
*Capsaicin:* Increased risk of cough. Discourage concomitant use.
**Drug-food.** *Salt substitutes containing potassium:* Increased risk of hyperkalemia. Advise patient to avoid these substitutes.

## Adverse reactions
**CNS:** dizziness, headache, fatigue, drowsiness, insomnia, paresthesia, vertigo, anxiety.
**CV:** chest pain, first-degree AV block, *brady-cardia,* edema, hypotension, palpitations.
**EENT:** epistaxis, throat inflammation.
**GI:** diarrhea, dyspepsia, abdominal distention, abdominal pain or cramps, constipation, vomiting, *pancreatitis.*

---

GU: urinary frequency, increased creatinine clearance and BUN, impotence.
Hepatic: elevated liver enzyme levels.
Hematologic: *neutropenia, leukopenia.*
Metabolic: hyperkalemia, hyponatremia, hyperuricemia.
Respiratory: dry, persistent, tickling, nonproductive cough, upper respiratory tract infection, dyspnea.
Skin: rash, pruritus, pemphigus, flushing.
Other: *anaphylactoid reactions, angioedema,* decreased libido.

## Overdose and treatment
It's thought that the effects of overdose are similar to those seen in other ACE inhibitor overdose, with hypotension being the main adverse reaction. Because the hypotensive effect of trandolapril is achieved through vasodilation and effective hypovolemia, it's reasonable to treat trandolapril overdose by infusion of normal saline solution. In addition, renal function and serum potassium level should be monitored. Trandolaprilat is removed by hemodialysis.

## Clinical considerations
■ Advise clinician to obtain baseline CBC with differential counts before therapy, especially in patients who have collagen vascular disease with impaired renal function.
■ Other ACE inhibitors have caused agranulocytosis and neutropenia.
■ Angioedema with involvement of the tongue, glottis, or larynx may be fatal because of airway obstruction. Appropriate therapy, such as S.C. epinephrine 1:1,000 (0.3 to 0.5 ml) and equipment to ensure a patent airway, should be readily available.
■ If jaundice develops, advise clinician to discontinue drug; although rare, ACE inhibitors have caused a syndrome of cholestatic jaundice, fulminant hepatic necrosis, and death.

### Therapeutic monitoring
■ Advise clinician to assess patient's renal function before and periodically throughout therapy and monitor serum potassium levels.
■ Advise clinician to monitor patient for hypotension. Excessive hypotension may occur when drug is given with diuretics. If possible, diuretic therapy should be stopped 2 to 3 days before trandolapril starts, to decrease potential for excessive hypotensive response. If trandolapril doesn't adequately control blood pressure, diuretic therapy may be reinstituted with care.

### Special populations
Pregnant patients. Drug is contraindicated for use during pregnancy.

Breast-feeding patients. It isn't known if drug appears in breast milk; avoid use in breast-feeding women.
Pediatric patients. Safety and efficacy in children haven't been established.

## Patient counseling
■ Advise patient to report signs of infection, easy bruising, or bleeding; swelling of tongue, lips, face, eyes, mucous membranes, or limbs; difficulty swallowing or breathing; and hoarseness.
■ Instruct patient to avoid products containing potassium, such as sodium substitutes.
■ If syncope occurs, instruct patient to stop taking drug and notify prescriber immediately.

# trastuzumab
Herceptin

*Pharmacologic classification:* monoclonal antibody to human epidermal growth factor receptor 2 protein (HER2)
*Therapeutic classification:* antineoplastic
*Pregnancy risk category B*

## Available forms
Available by prescription only
*Injection:* lyophilized sterile powder containing 440 mg/vial

## Indications and dosages
*Single-drug treatment of metastatic breast cancer in patients whose tumors overexpress the HER2 protein and who have received one or more chemotherapy regimen for their metastatic disease, or with paclitaxel for metastatic breast cancer in patients whose tumors overexpress the HER2 protein and who haven't received chemotherapy for their metastatic disease*
Adults: Initial loading dose 4 mg/kg I.V. over 90 minutes. Maintenance dose is 2 mg/kg I.V. weekly as a 30-minute I.V. infusion if initial loading dose is well tolerated.

## I.V. administration
■ Reconstitute drug in each vial with 20 ml of bacteriostatic water for injection, 1.1% benzyl alcohol preserved, as supplied, to yield a multidose solution containing 21 mg/ml. Immediately after reconstitution, label vial with expiration 28 days from date of reconstitution.
**ALERT** If patient is hypersensitive to benzyl alcohol, reconstitute drug with sterile water for injection, use immediately, and discard unused portion. Avoid use of other reconstitution diluents.
■ Don't mix or administer with solutions that contain dextrose.

- Determine dose (mg) of drug needed, based on loading dose of 4 mg/kg or maintenance dose of 2 mg/kg. Calculate volume of 21-mg/ml solution and withdraw this amount from vial and add it to an infusion bag containing 250 ml of normal saline solution. Gently invert bag to mix solution.
- Infuse loading dose over 90 minutes. If well tolerated, infuse maintenance doses over 30 minutes.
- Vials of drug are stable at 36° to 46° F (2° to 8° C) before reconstitution. Discard reconstituted solution after 28 days. Don't freeze drug that has been reconstituted. Solution of drug diluted in normal saline solution for injection should be stored at 36° to 46° F (2° to 8° C) before use; it's stable for up to 24 hours.

### Incompatibilities

Don't mix or dilute drug with other drugs. Don't use $D_5W$ solution for reconstitution.

## Mechanism of action

*Antineoplastic action:* Protein overexpression is observed in 25% to 30% of primary breast cancers. Drug is a recombinant DNA-derived monoclonal antibody that selectively binds to HER2, inhibiting the proliferation of human tumor cells that overexpress HER2.

## Pharmacokinetics

*Absorption:* Not reported.
*Distribution:* Volume of distribution is about that of serum volume (44 ml/kg). Between weeks 16 and 32, serum levels reach steady state with a mean trough of 79 mcg/ml and peak of 123 mcg/ml.
*Metabolism:* Not reported.
*Excretion:* Half-life and clearance are dose-dependent. At the recommended dosage, a mean half-life of 5¾ days (range 1 to 32 days) has been observed.

| Route | Onset | Peak | Duration |
|-------|-------|------|----------|
| I.V. | Unknown | Unknown | Unknown |

## Contraindications and precautions

Use with extreme caution in patients with pre-existing pulmonary compromise; weigh risks and benefits carefully. Use cautiously in patients hypersensitive to drug or its components, in those with preexisting cardiac dysfunction, and in geriatric patients.

## Interactions

**Drug-drug.** *Anthracyclines:* Increased risk of cardiotoxicity. Avoid use together.
*Paclitaxel:* Increased trastuzumab serum level. Advise clinician to monitor patient closely.

## Adverse reactions

**CNS:** depression, *headache, dizziness, insomnia, asthenia,* neuropathy, paresthesia, peripheral neuritis.

**CV:** *HF, peripheral edema,* tachycardia, paroxysmal nocturnal dyspnea, cardiomyopathy, decreased ejection fraction, edema.
**EENT:** *rhinitis, pharyngitis, sinusitis.*
**GI:** *anorexia, abdominal pain, diarrhea, nausea, vomiting.*
**GU:** urinary tract infection.
**Hematologic:** *leukopenia,* anemia.
**Musculoskeletal:** arthralgia, *back pain,* bone pain.
**Respiratory:** *dyspnea, increased cough,* acute respiratory distress syndrome.
**Skin:** acne, rash.
**Other:** *allergic reaction,* chills, *fever, flu syndrome,* herpes simplex, *infection, pain.*

## Overdose and treatment

None reported.

## Clinical considerations

- Before therapy starts, patients should undergo a thorough baseline cardiac assessment, including history and physical examination and other evaluation methods to identify those at risk for development of cardiotoxicity.
- Drug should be used only in patients with metastatic breast cancer whose tumors have HER2 protein overexpression.
- A first-infusion symptom complex (chills or fever) occurred in about 40% of patients. Advise clinician to treat with acetaminophen, diphenhydramine, and meperidine (with or without reducing infusion rate). Other signs or symptoms may include nausea, vomiting, pain, rigors, headache, dizziness, dyspnea, hypotension, rash, and asthenia. These symptoms occur infrequently with subsequent infusions.
- Advise clinician to strongly consider stopping drug in patients for whom a significant decrease in left ventricular function develops.

### Therapeutic monitoring

- Advise clinician to monitor patient for dyspnea, increased cough, paroxysmal nocturnal dyspnea, peripheral edema, or $S_3$ gallop, especially if patient is receiving drug with anthracyclines and cyclophosphamide.

### Special populations

**Breast-feeding patients.** Because immunoglobulin G appears in breast milk and because the potential for adverse effects on the infant is unknown, advise women to discontinue breast-feeding during and for 6 months following therapy.
**Pediatric patients.** Safety and efficacy in children haven't been established
**Geriatric patients.** Risk of cardiac dysfunction may increase in geriatric patients.

## Patient counseling

- Tell patient about risk of first-dose, infusion-associated adverse effects.

■ Instruct patient to notify prescriber immediately if signs or symptoms of cardiac dysfunction occur, such as shortness of breath, increased cough, or peripheral edema.

# travoprost
Travatan

*Pharmacologic classification:* prostaglandin analogue
*Therapeutic classification:* antiglaucoma drug, ocular antihypertensive
*Pregnancy risk category C*

## Available forms
Available by prescription only
*Ophthalmic solution:* 0.004%

## Indications and dosages
*Reduction of elevated intraocular pressure (IOP) in patients with open-angle glaucoma or ocular hypertension who are intolerant of other IOP-lowering drugs, and in patients who have had insufficient responses to other IOP-lowering drugs*
*Adults:* 1 drop in conjunctival sac of affected eye once daily in evening.

## Mechanism of action
*Antiglaucoma and ocular antihypertensive actions:* Exact mechanism of action is unknown. Drug is thought to reduce IOP by increasing uveoscleral outflow.

## Pharmacokinetics
*Absorption:* Absorbed through the cornea.
*Distribution:* Plasma levels peak within 30 minutes following topical ocular administration.
*Metabolism:* Drug is an isopropyl ester prodrug, which is hydrolyzed by esterases in the cornea to its biologically active free acid. The active acid of drug reaching the systemic circulation is primarily metabolized by the liver.
*Excretion:* Following ocular administration, travoprost-free acid is rapidly eliminated from plasma within 1 hour.

| Route | Onset | Peak | Duration |
|-------|-------|------|----------|
| Ophthalmic | Unknown | 30 min | Unknown |

## Contraindications and precautions
Contraindicated in patients hypersensitive to travoprost, benzalkonium chloride, or other components. Not recommended for pregnant women or for women attempting to become pregnant.

Use cautiously in patients with renal or hepatic impairment, active intraocular inflammation (iritis, uveitis), or risk factors for macular edema. Also use cautiously in aphakic patients and pseudophakic patients with a torn posterior lens capsule.

## Interactions
**Drug-herb.** *Areca, jaborandi:* Possible additive effects. Discourage use together.

## Adverse reactions
**CNS:** anxiety, depression, headache, pain.
**CV:** angina pectoris, ***bradycardia***, chest pain, hypertension, hypotension.
**EENT:** *ocular hyperemia, decreased visual acuity, eye discomfort, foreign body sensation, eye pain, eye pruritus,* conjunctival hyperemia, abnormal vision, blepharitis, blurred vision, cataract, conjunctivitis, dry eye, eye disorder, iris discoloration, keratitis, lid margin crusting, photophobia, subconjunctival hemorrhage, tearing, sinusitis.
**GI:** dyspepsia, GI disorder.
**GU:** prostate disorder, urinary incontinence, urinary tract infection.
**Metabolic:** hypercholesterolemia.
**Respiratory:** bronchitis.
**Musculoskeletal:** arthritis, back pain.
**Other:** accidental injury, cold syndrome, infection.

## Overdose and treatment
Aside from ocular irritation and conjunctival hyperemia, ocular effects of drug at high doses aren't known. Treatment should be symptomatic if overdose occurs.

## Clinical considerations
■ Store drug between 36° and 77° F (2° and 25° C).
■ Don't use in patients with angle-closure glaucoma or inflammatory or neovascular glaucoma.
■ Patient should remove contact lenses before administration of drug. Lenses may be reinserted 15 minutes after administration.
■ If more than one ophthalmic drug is being used, advise clinician to give drugs at least 5 minutes apart.

### Therapeutic monitoring
■ Advise clinician to monitor patient for temporary or permanent increased pigmentation of the iris and eyelid as well as increased pigmentation and growth of eyelashes.

### Special populations
**Breast-feeding patients.** It's unknown if drug appears in breast milk. Use cautiously in breast-feeding women.
**Pediatric patients.** Safety and efficacy in children haven't been established.
**Geriatric patients.** No overall differences in safety or effectiveness have been observed between geriatric and other adult patients.

## Patient counseling
■ Teach patient to instill drops and advise him to wash hands before and after instilling solu-

---

tion. Warn him not to touch dropper or tip to eye or surrounding tissue.
■ Tell patient receiving treatment in only one eye about the potential for increased brown pigmentation of the iris, eyelid skin darkening, and increased length, thickness, pigmentation, or number of lashes in the treated eye.
■ Tell patient that, if eye trauma or infection occurs or if eye surgery is needed, he should seek medical advice before continuing to use multidose container.
■ Advise patient to immediately report conjunctivitis or lid reactions.
■ Advise patient to apply light pressure on lacrimal sac for 1 minute after instillation to minimize systemic absorption of drug.
■ Tell patient to remove contact lenses before administration of solution and that he can reinsert them 15 minutes after administration.
■ Advise patient that, if more than one ophthalmic drug is being used, the drugs should be given at least 5 minutes apart.
■ Stress importance of compliance with recommended therapy.
■ Tell patient to discard container within 6 weeks of removing it from sealed pouch.
■ If a pregnant woman or a woman attempting to become pregnant accidentally comes in contact with drug, tell her to thoroughly cleanse the exposed area with soap and water immediately.

---

# trazodone hydrochloride
Desyrel

*Pharmacologic classification:* triazolopyridine derivative
*Therapeutic classification:* antidepressant
*Pregnancy risk category C*

## Available forms
Available by prescription only
*Tablets (film-coated):* 50 mg, 100 mg, 150 mg
*Dividose tablets:* 150 mg, 300 mg

## Indications and dosages
*Depression*
*Adults:* Initially, 150 mg daily in divided doses, which can be increased by 50 mg/day q 3 to 4 days. Average dose ranges from 150 to 400 mg/day. Maximum dose, 400 mg/day in outpatients; 600 mg/day in hospitalized patients.
◊*Aggressive behavior*
*Adults:* 50 mg P.O. b.i.d.
◊*Panic disorder*
*Adults:* 300 mg P.O. daily.

## Mechanism of action
*Antidepressant action:* Trazodone is thought to exert its antidepressant effects by inhibiting reuptake of norepinephrine and serotonin in

CNS nerve terminals (presynaptic neurons), which results in increased level and enhanced activity of these neurotransmitters in the synaptic cleft. Trazodone shares some properties with tricyclic antidepressants: it has antihistaminic, alpha-adrenergic–blocking, analgesic, and sedative effects as well as relaxant effects on skeletal muscle. Unlike tricyclic antidepressants, however, trazodone counteracts the pressor effects of norepinephrine, has limited effects on the CV system and, in particular, has no direct quinidine-like effects on cardiac tissue; it also causes relatively fewer anticholinergic effects. Trazodone has been used in patients with alcohol dependence to decrease tremors and to alleviate anxiety and depression. Adverse reactions somewhat dose-related; risk increases with higher dose levels.

## Pharmacokinetics
*Absorption:* Well absorbed from GI tract after oral administration. Taking drug with food delays absorption and increases amount absorbed by 20%.
*Distribution:* Widely distributed in the body; drug doesn't concentrate in any particular tissue, but small amounts may appear in breast milk. About 90% is protein-bound. Proposed therapeutic drug levels haven't been established. Steady-state plasma levels are reached in 3 to 7 days, and onset of therapeutic activity occurs in 7 days.
*Metabolism:* Metabolized by the liver; more than 75% of metabolites are excreted within 3 days.
*Excretion:* Mostly excreted in urine; the rest is excreted in feces via the biliary tract.

| Route | Onset | Peak | Duration |
|-------|-------|------|----------|
| P.O. | Unknown | 1-2 hr | Unknown |

## Contraindications and precautions
Contraindicated during initial recovery phase of MI and in patients hypersensitive to drug. Use cautiously in patients with cardiac disease and in those at risk for suicide.

## Interactions
**Drug-drug.** *Antihypertensives, CNS depressants:* Additive effects of antihypertensives and CNS depressants. Advise clinician to monitor patient closely. Dosage adjustment may be needed.
*Digoxin, phenytoin:* Increased serum levels of digoxin and phenytoin. Advise clinician to monitor blood levels closely.
**Drug-herb.** *Ginkgo biloba:* Increased risk of sedation. Discourage concomitant use.
*St. John's wort:* Serotonin syndrome. Discourage use together.
**Drug-lifestyle.** *Alcohol use:* Exacerbated CNS depression. Advise patient to avoid alcohol.

---

*Reactions may be common, uncommon, **life-threatening**, or COMMON AND LIFE-THREATENING.*

## Adverse reactions

**CNS:** *drowsiness, dizziness,* nervousness, fatigue, confusion, tremor, weakness, hostility, anger, nightmares, vivid dreams, headache, insomnia, *generalized tonic-clonic seizures.*
**CV:** orthostatic hypotension, tachycardia, hypertension, prolonged conduction time on ECG, syncope.
**EENT:** blurred vision, tinnitus, nasal congestion.
**GI:** dry mouth, dysgeusia, constipation, nausea, vomiting, anorexia.
**GU:** urine retention; priapism, possibly leading to impotence; hematuria.
**Hematologic:** anemia, decreased WBC counts.
**Hepatic:** elevated liver function test results.
**Metabolic:** altered serum glucose levels.
**Respiratory:** shortness of breath.
**Skin:** rash, urticaria, diaphoresis.
**Other:** decreased libido.

## Overdose and treatment

The most common signs and symptoms of drug overdose are drowsiness and vomiting; other signs and symptoms include orthostatic hypotension, tachycardia, headache, shortness of breath, dry mouth, and incontinence. Coma may occur.

Treatment is symptomatic and supportive and includes maintaining airway and stabilizing vital signs and fluid and electrolyte balance. Advise clinician to induce emesis if gag reflex is intact and follow with gastric lavage (begin with lavage if emesis is unfeasible) and activated charcoal to prevent further absorption. Forced diuresis may aid elimination. Dialysis is usually ineffective.

## Clinical considerations

■ Drug has fewer adverse cardiac and anticholinergic effects than tricyclic antidepressants.
■ Consider the inherent risk of suicide until significant improvement of depressive state occurs.
■ Tolerance to adverse effects (especially sedative effects) usually develops after 1 to 2 weeks of treatment.
■ Drug may cause prolonged, painful erections that may require surgical correction. An involuntary erection lasting longer than 1 hour should be considered a medical emergency.
■ Adverse effects are more common when doses exceed 300 mg per day.
■ Don't withdraw drug abruptly.
■ Discontinue drug at least 48 hours before surgical procedures.

### Therapeutic monitoring

■ Advise clinician to closely monitor patients at high risk for suicide, especially during initial stage of drug therapy.
■ Advise clinician to monitor blood pressure because hypotension may occur.

### Special populations

**Pregnant patients.** Use drug during pregnancy only when potential benefits justify risk to fetus.
**Breast-feeding patients.** Drug appears in breast milk; use with caution in breast-feeding women.
**Pediatric patients.** Drug isn't recommended for children under age 18.
**Geriatric patients.** Geriatric patients usually require lower initial doses because adverse reactions are more likely to develop. However, drug may be preferred in geriatric patients because it has fewer adverse cardiac effects.

### Patient counseling

■ Tell patient that full effects of drug may not become apparent for up to 2 weeks after therapy begins.
■ Tell patient to take drug exactly as prescribed.
■ Instruct patient not to participate in activities that require mental alertness until full effects of drug are known.
■ Tell patient to avoid alcoholic beverages and medicinal elixirs while taking drug.
■ Advise patient to promptly report adverse reactions, including prolonged, painful erections, sexual dysfunction, dizziness, fainting, and rapid heartbeat.

## tretinoin (systemic)
Vesanoid

*Pharmacologic classification:* retinoid
*Therapeutic classification:* antineoplastic
*Pregnancy risk category D*

### Available forms
Available by prescription only
*Capsules:* 10 mg

### Indications and dosages
*Induction of remission in patients with acute promyelocytic leukemia (APL), French-American-British classification M³ (including the M³ variant), characterized by the presence of the t(15,17) translocation or the presence of PML/RAR alpha gene, who are refractory to, or who have relapsed from, anthracycline chemotherapy or for whom anthracycline-based chemotherapy is contraindicated*
Adults and children ages 1 and older: 45 mg/m²/day P.O. divided b.i.d. until complete remission is documented. Discontinue therapy 30 days after achievement of complete remission or after 90 days of treatment, whichever occurs first.

### Mechanism of action
*Antineoplastic action:* Exact mechanism of action is unknown. Tretinoin produces an initial maturation of primitive promyelocytes derived

from the leukemic clone, followed by a repopulation of bone marrow and peripheral blood by normal, polyclonal hematopoietic cells.

## Pharmacokinetics

**Absorption:** Well absorbed from the GI tract.
**Distribution:** About 95% plasma protein–bound.
**Metabolism:** May induce its own metabolism.
**Excretion:** Excreted in urine and feces.

| Route | Onset | Peak | Duration |
|-------|-------|------|----------|
| P.O. | Unknown | 1-2 hr | Unknown |

## Contraindications and precautions

Contraindicated in patients hypersensitive to retinoids or parabens, which are used as preservatives in the gelatin capsule. Don't use in pregnant or breast-feeding women.

## Interactions

**Drug-drug.** *Ketoconazole:* Increased tretinoin plasma level. Use together cautiously.

## Adverse reactions

**CNS:** *CVA, malaise,* dizziness, *paresthesia, headache,* anxiety, insomnia, *depression, confusion,* **cerebral hemorrhage,** intracranial hypertension, agitation, hallucination, abnormal gait, agnosia, aphasia, asterixis, cerebellar edema, cerebellar disorders, *seizures, coma,* CNS depression, dysarthria, encephalopathy, facial paralysis, hemiplegia, hyporeflexia, hypotaxia, no light reflex neurologic reaction, spinal cord disorder, tremor, leg weakness, unconsciousness, dementia, forgetfulness, somnolence, slow speech.
**CV:** *chest discomfort,* **arrhythmias, HF,** *hypotension,* hypertension, *peripheral edema, phlebitis, edema,* **cardiac failure, cardiac arrest, MI,** enlarged heart, heart murmur, ischemia, myocarditis, pericarditis, secondary cardiomyopathy.
**EENT:** *ear fullness, visual disturbances, ocular disorders,* hearing loss, *mucositis.*
**GI:** **GI hemorrhage,** nausea, vomiting, anorexia, *abdominal pain,* GI disorders, *diarrhea,* constipation, dyspepsia, abdominal distention, hepatosplenomegaly, ulcer.
**GU:** *renal insufficiency,* **acute renal failure,** micturition frequency, dysuria, renal tubular necrosis, enlarged prostate.
**Hematologic:** leukocytosis, **hemorrhage, DIC.**
**Hepatic:** elevated liver function results, **hepatitis,** unspecified liver disorder.
**Metabolic:** acidosis, hypothermia, fluid imbalance, hypercholesterolemia, hypertriglyceridemia, *weight increase, weight decrease.*
**Musculoskeletal:** flank pain, *myalgia, bone pain,* bone inflammation.
**Respiratory:** *pneumonia, upper respiratory tract disorders, dyspnea, respiratory insufficiency, pleural effusion, crackles, expiratory wheezing,* lower respiratory tract disorders, pulmonary infiltrate, bronchial asthma, pulmonary or larynx edema, unspecified pulmonary disease, pulmonary hypertension.
**Skin:** *flushing, skin mucous membrane dryness, pruritus, decreased sweating, alopecia, skin changes,* cellulitis.
**Other:** *fever, infections, shivering, pain, injection site reactions,* **retinoic acid-APL syndrome, septicemia, multiorgan failure,** facial edema, pallor, lymph disorder, ascites.

## Overdose and treatment

None reported. Overdose with other retinoids has caused transient headache, facial flushing, cheilosis, abdominal pain, dizziness, and ataxia. These signs and symptoms have quickly resolved without apparent residual effects.

## Clinical considerations

■ Drug must be administered in a facility with laboratory and supportive services sufficient to monitor drug tolerance and protect and maintain patients compromised by drug toxicity.
■ For women, a pregnancy test is required within 1 week before tretinoin therapy. When possible, therapy is delayed until a negative result is obtained.
■ Patients with high WBC counts at diagnosis are at greater risk for rapid increases in WBC counts. Rapidly evolving leukocytosis has with it a higher risk of life-threatening complications.
■ About 25% of patients given drug during clinical studies have experienced retinoic acid-APL syndrome, characterized by fever, dyspnea, weight gain, radiographic pulmonary infiltrates, and pleural or pericardial effusions. This syndrome has occasionally been accompanied by impaired myocardial contractility and episodic hypotension with or without leukocytosis. Some patients have died because of progressive hypoxemia and multiorgan failure. The syndrome generally occurs during the first month of therapy. Treatment with high-dose steroids at the first signs of the syndrome appears to reduce morbidity and mortality risk.

### Therapeutic monitoring

■ Advise clinician to monitor CBC and platelet counts regularly.
■ Advise clinician to monitor patients, especially children, for symptoms of pseudotumor cerebri, such as papilledema, headache, nausea, vomiting, and visual disturbances.
■ Advise clinician to monitor cholesterol and triglyceride levels and liver function test results.

### Special populations

**Breast-feeding patients.** It isn't known if drug appears in breast milk. Because of the potential for serious adverse reactions in breast-fed

---

infants, don't give drug to breast-feeding women.

**Pediatric patients.** Safety and efficacy in children under age 1 haven't been established.

### Patient counseling

■ Instruct patient to report signs or symptoms of infection, (fever, sore throat, fatigue) or bleeding (easy bruising, nosebleeds, bleeding gums, melena).

■ Tell patient to record his temperature daily.

## tretinoin (topical)

Avita, Renova, Retin-A, Retin-A Micro

*Pharmacologic classification:* vitamin A derivative
*Therapeutic classification:* antiacne drug
*Pregnancy risk category C*

### Available forms

Available by prescription only
*Cream:* 0.02%, 0.025%, 0.05%, 0.1%
*Gel:* 0.01%, 0.025%
*Solution:* 0.05%
*Microsphere gel:* 0.1%

### Indications and dosages

*Acne vulgaris (especially grades I, II, and III)*
*Adults and children:* Clean affected area and lightly apply solution, cream, or gel once daily h.s. or as directed.
*Treatment of photodamaged skin (wrinkles)*
*Adults:* 0.05% solution or 0.02% to 0.1% cream in pearl-sized amount to cover affected area applied daily at h.s. for at least 4 months.

### Mechanism of action

*Antiacne action:* Mechanism of action is unknown; however, it appears that tretinoin acts as a follicular epithelium irritant, preventing horny cells from sticking together and inhibiting the formation of additional comedones.

### Pharmacokinetics

*Absorption:* Limited with topical use.
*Distribution:* None.
*Metabolism:* None.
*Excretion:* Minimal amount is excreted in the urine.

| Route | Onset | Peak | Duration |
|-------|-------|------|----------|
| Topical | Unknown | Unknown | Unknown |

### Contraindications and precautions

Contraindicated in patients hypersensitive to vitamin A or retinoic acid, and in pregnancy.

Use cautiously in patients with eczema. Avoid contact of drug with eyes, mouth, angles of the nose, mucous membranes, or open wounds. Avoid use of topical preparations containing high levels of alcohol, menthol, spices, or lime because they may cause skin irritation. Avoid use of medicated cosmetics on treated skin.

### Interactions

**Drug-drug.** *Topical agents:* Risk of skin irritation. Avoid use together.
**Drug-lifestyle.** *Abrasive cleaners, medicated cosmetics, and skin preparations containing alcohol:* Increased risk of skin irritation. Avoid use together.
*Sun exposure:* Potentiation of photosensitivity reactions. Advise patient to use sunblock.

### Adverse reactions

**Skin:** peeling, erythema, blisters, crusting, hyperpigmentation and hypopigmentation, contact dermatitis.

### Overdose and treatment

None reported. Advise clinician to stop use and rinse area thoroughly. Oral ingestion of drug may lead to the same adverse effects as those from excessive oral intake of vitamin A.

### Clinical considerations

■ Don't use drug in patients who can't or won't minimize sun exposure.

■ Although tretinoin microsphere gel was developed to minimize dermal irritation, the skin of some individuals may become excessively dry, red, swollen, blistered, or crusted.

■ Drug should be stopped if sensitization or extreme redness and blistering of skin occurs.

*Therapeutic monitoring*

■ Advise clinician to monitor patient for improvement. Therapeutic effect normally occurs in 2 to 3 weeks but may take 6 weeks or longer. Relapses generally occur within 3 to 6 weeks of stopping drug.

*Special populations*

**Breast-feeding patients.** It isn't known if drug appears in breast milk. Because of the potential for serious adverse reactions in breast-fed infants, don't give drug to breast-feeding women.

**Pediatric patients.** Safety and efficacy in children under age 1 haven't been established.

### Patient counseling

■ Advise patient on proper application technique. Stress importance of thorough removal of dirt and makeup before application and of hand washing after each use.

■ Inform patient that application of drug may cause a temporary feeling of warmth and, if discomfort occurs, to promptly report to prescriber.

■ Advise patient that initial exacerbation of inflammatory lesions is common and that redness and scaling (usually occurring in 7 to 10 days) are normal skin responses that disappear when therapy is discontinued.

- Caution patient to minimize exposure to sunlight or ultraviolet rays.
- Advise patient to keep drug away from eyes, mouth, angles of nose, and mucous membranes or open wounds.
- Tell patient that therapeutic effect normally occurs in 2 to 3 weeks but may take 6 weeks or longer and that relapses generally occur within 3 to 6 weeks of stopping drug.

---

# triamcinolone (systemic)
Aristocort, Aristo-Pak, Kenacort

# triamcinolone acetonide
Kenaject, Kenalog, Tac, Triam-A

# triamcinolone diacetate
Amcort, Aristocort, Aristocort Forte, Aristocort Intralesional, Articulose-L.A., Cenocort Forte, Kenacort, Triam-Forte, Triamolone 40, Tristoject

# triamcinolone hexacetonide
Aristospan Intra-articular, Aristospan Intralesional

*Pharmacologic classification:* glucocorticoid
*Therapeutic classification:* anti-inflammatory, immunosuppressant
*Pregnancy risk category C*

## Available forms
Available by prescription only
**triamcinolone**
*Tablets:* 4 mg
*Syrup:* 2 mg/ml, 4 mg/ml
**triamcinolone acetonide**
*Injection:* 10 mg/ml, 40 mg/ml suspension
**triamcinolone diacetate**
*Injection:* 25 mg/ml, 40 mg/ml suspension
**triamcinolone hexacetonide**
*Injection:* 5 mg/ml, 20 mg/ml suspension

## Indications and dosages
*Adrenal insufficiency*
**triamcinolone**
*Adults:* 4 to 12 mg P.O. daily, in single or divided doses.
*Children:* 117 mcg/kg or 3.3 mg/m² P.O. daily, in single or divided doses.
*Severe inflammation or immunosuppression*
**triamcinolone**
*Adults:* 8 to 16 mg P.O. daily, in single or divided doses.
*Children:* 416 mcg to 1.7 mg/kg or 12.5 to 50 mg/m² P.O. daily, in single or divided doses.

**triamcinolone acetonide**
*Adults:* Initially, 60 mg I.M. Additional doses of 20 to 100 mg may be given, p.r.n., at 6-week intervals. Alternatively, 2.5 to 15 mg intra-articularly, or up to 1 mg intralesionally, p.r.n.
*Children ages 6 to 12:* 0.03 to 0.2 mg/kg I.M. at 1- to 7-day intervals.
**triamcinolone diacetate**
*Adults:* 40 mg I.M. once weekly; or 2 to 40 mg intra-articularly, intrasynovially, or intralesionally q 1 to 8 weeks; or 4 to 48 mg P.O. divided q.i.d.
*Children:* 0.117 to 1.66 mg/kg/day P.O. divided q.i.d.
**triamcinolone hexacetonide**
*Adults:* 2 to 20 mg intra-articularly q 3 to 4 weeks, p.r.n.; or up to 0.5 mg intralesionally per square inch of skin.
*Tuberculous meningitis*
**triamcinolone**
*Adults:* 32 to 48 mg P.O. daily.
*Edematous states*
**triamcinolone**
*Adults:* 16 to 48 mg P.O. daily.
*Collagen diseases*
**triamcinolone**
*Adults:* 30 to 48 mg P.O. daily.
*Dermatologic disorders*
**triamcinolone**
*Adults:* 8 to 16 mg P.O. daily.
*Allergic states*
**triamcinolone**
*Adults:* 8 to 12 mg P.O. daily.
*Ophthalmic diseases*
**triamcinolone**
*Adults:* 12 to 40 mg P.O. daily.
*Respiratory diseases*
**triamcinolone**
*Adults:* 16 to 48 mg P.O. daily.
*Hematologic diseases*
**triamcinolone**
*Adults:* 16 to 60 mg P.O. daily.
*Neoplastic diseases*
**triamcinolone**
*Adults:* 16 to 100 mg P.O. daily.

## Mechanism of action
*Anti-inflammatory and immunosuppressant actions:* Triamcinolone stimulates the synthesis of enzymes needed to decrease the inflammatory response. It suppresses the immune system by reducing activity and volume of the lymphatic system, producing lymphocytopenia (primarily of T lymphocytes), decreasing immunoglobulin and complement levels, decreasing passage of immune complexes through basement membranes, and possibly depressing reactivity of tissue to antigen-antibody interactions.

Triamcinolone is an intermediate-acting glucocorticoid. The addition of a fluorine group in the molecule increases the anti-inflammatory activity, which is five times more potent

---

Reactions may be *common*, uncommon, *life-threatening*, or COMMON AND LIFE-THREATENING.

than an equal weight of hydrocortisone. It has essentially no mineralocorticoid activity.

Triamcinolone may be administered orally. The diacetate and acetonide salts may be administered by I.M., intra-articular, intrasynovial, intralesional or sublesional, and soft-tissue injection. The diacetate suspension is slightly soluble, providing a prompt onset of action and a longer duration of effect (1 to 2 weeks). Triamcinolone acetonide is relatively insoluble and slowly absorbed. Its extended duration of action lasts for several weeks. Triamcinolone hexacetonide is relatively insoluble, is absorbed slowly, and has a prolonged action of 3 to 4 weeks. Don't administer any of the parenteral suspensions I.V.

## Pharmacokinetics

*Absorption:* Absorbed readily after oral administration, levels peak in about 1 to 2 hours. The suspensions for injection have variable onset and duration of action, depending on whether they're injected into an intra-articular space or a muscle, and on the blood supply to that muscle.

*Distribution:* Removed rapidly from the blood and distributed to muscle, liver, skin, intestines, and kidneys. Drug is extensively bound to plasma proteins (transcortin and albumin). Only the unbound portion is active. Adrenocorticoids appear in breast milk and through the placental barrier.

*Metabolism:* Metabolized in the liver to inactive glucuronide and sulfate metabolites.

*Excretion:* Inactive metabolites and small amounts of unmetabolized drug are excreted by the kidneys. Insignificant quantities of drug are also excreted in feces. Biologic half-life of triamcinolone is 18 to 36 hours.

| Route | Onset | Peak | Duration |
|---|---|---|---|
| P.O., I.M., intralesion, intra-articular | Variable | Variable | Variable |

## Contraindications and precautions

Contraindicated in patients hypersensitive to drug or its components and in those with systemic fungal infections.

Use cautiously in patients with GI ulcer, renal disease, hypertension, osteoporosis, diabetes mellitus, hypothyroidism, cirrhosis, diverticulitis, nonspecific ulcerative colitis, recent intestinal anastomosis, thromboembolic disorders, seizures, myasthenia gravis, HF, tuberculosis, ocular herpes simplex, emotional instability, or psychotic tendencies.

## Interactions

**Drug-drug.** *Amphotericin B, diuretics:* Enhanced hypokalemia. Advise clinician to monitor electrolyte levels closely.

*Antacids, cholestyramine, colestipol:* Decreased effect of triamcinolone. Dosage adjustment may be needed.

*Barbiturates, phenytoin, rifampin:* Decreased corticosteroid effects. Dosage adjustment may be needed.

*Cardiac glycosides:* Increased toxicity. Advise clinician to monitor patient closely.

*Estrogens:* Reduced metabolism of triamcinolone. Dosage may need adjustment.

*Isoniazid, salicylates:* Hyperglycemia. Dosage adjustment may be needed.

*NSAIDs, ulcerogenic drugs:* Increased risk of GI ulceration. Avoid use together.

*Oral anticoagulants:* Decreased anticoagulation. Advise clinician to monitor patient closely; dosage adjustment may be needed.

## Adverse reactions

**CNS:** *euphoria, insomnia,* psychotic behavior, pseudotumor cerebri, vertigo, headache, paresthesia, *seizures.*

**CV:** *HF, thromboembolism,* hypertension, edema, *arrhythmias,* thrombophlebitis.

**EENT:** cataracts, glaucoma.

**GI:** *peptic ulceration,* GI irritation, increased appetite, *pancreatitis,* nausea, vomiting.

**GU:** increased urine glucose levels, menstrual irregularities.

**Metabolic:** hypokalemia, hyperglycemia, hypocalcemia, decreased $T_3$ and $T_4$ levels, hypercholesterolemia, and carbohydrate intolerance.

**Musculoskeletal:** muscle weakness, osteoporosis, growth suppression in children.

**Skin:** delayed wound healing, acne, various skin eruptions, hirsutism.

**Other:** susceptibility to infections; *acute adrenal insufficiency with increased stress (infection, surgery, or trauma) or abrupt withdrawal after long-term therapy,* cushingoid state (moonface, buffalo hump, central obesity).

**After abrupt withdrawal:** rebound inflammation, fatigue, weakness, arthralgia, fever, dizziness, lethargy, depression, fainting, orthostatic hypotension, dyspnea, anorexia, hypoglycemia. *After prolonged use, sudden withdrawal may be fatal.*

## Overdose and treatment

Acute ingestion, even in massive doses, is rarely a clinical problem. Toxic signs and symptoms rarely occur if drug is used for less than 3 weeks, even at large doses. However, long-term use causes adverse physiologic effects, including suppression of the hypothalamic-pituitary-adrenal axis, cushingoid appearance, muscle weakness, and osteoporosis.

## Clinical considerations

■ Triamcinolone suppresses reactions to skin tests, causes false-negative results in the nitroblue tetrazolium test for systemic bacterial infections, and decreases [131]I uptake and protein-bound iodine levels in thyroid function test results.

■ Most adverse reactions to corticosteroids are dose- or duration-dependent.

### Therapeutic monitoring

■ Advise clinician to monitor patient for allergic reactions, adrenal insufficiency, and seizure activity.
■ Advise clinician to monitor cardiac status.

### Special populations

**Breast-feeding patients.** Use drug with caution in breast-feeding women.
**Pediatric patients.** Long-term use of drug in children and adolescents may delay growth and maturation.

### Patient counseling

■ Instruct patient to take drug exactly as prescribed and not to suddenly stop drug.
■ Instruct patient to promptly report any adverse reactions or unusual symptoms.

---

## triamcinolone acetonide (oral and nasal inhalant)

Azmacort, Nasacort, Nasacort AQ

*Pharmacologic classification:* glucocorticoid
*Therapeutic classification:* anti-inflammatory, antasthmatic
*Pregnancy risk category C*

### Available forms

Available by prescription only
*Oral inhalation aerosol:* 100 mcg/metered spray, 240 doses/inhaler
*Nasal aerosol:* 55 mcg/metered spray

### Indications and dosages

**Steroid-dependent asthma**
*Adults:* 2 inhalations t.i.d. or q.i.d. Maximum dose, 16 inhalations daily.
*Children ages 6 to 12:* 1 or 2 inhalations t.i.d. or q.i.d. Maximum dose, 12 inhalations daily.
**Rhinitis, allergic disorders, inflammatory conditions, nasal polyps**
*Adults:* 2 sprays (Nasacort) in each nostril daily; may increase dose to maximum of 4 sprays per nostril daily, if needed. Or 2 sprays (Nasacort AQ) in each nostril daily; may decrease to 1 spray in each nostril daily for allergic disorders.
*Children ages 6 to 12:* 2 sprays (Nasacort) in each nostril daily. Or, 1 spray (Nasacort AQ) in each nostril daily. Maximum 2 sprays in each nostril daily.

### Mechanism of action

*Anti-inflammatory and antasthmatic actions:* Glucocorticoids stimulate the synthesis of en-

zymes needed to decrease the inflammatory response. Triamcinolone acetonide is used as an oral inhalant to treat bronchial asthma in patients who require corticosteroids to control symptoms.

### Pharmacokinetics

*Absorption:* Systemic absorption from the lungs is similar to oral administration.
*Distribution:* After oral inhalation, 10% to 25% is distributed to the lungs; the rest is swallowed or deposited within the mouth. After nasal use, only a small amount reaches systemic circulation.
*Metabolism:* Metabolized mainly by the liver. Some of drug that reaches the lungs may be metabolized locally.
*Excretion:* Major portion of dose is eliminated in feces. Biologic half-life is 18 to 36 hours.

| Route | Onset | Peak | Duration |
|---|---|---|---|
| Inhalation | Unknown | 1-2 hours | Unknown |

### Contraindications and precautions

Oral form is contraindicated in patients hypersensitive to drug or its components and in those with status asthmaticus. Nasal form is contraindicated in patients with hypersensitivity or untreated localized infections.

Use oral form cautiously in patients with tuberculosis of the respiratory tract; untreated fungal, bacterial, or systemic viral infections; or ocular herpes simplex and in those receiving corticosteroids. Use both forms with caution in breast-feeding women.

### Interactions

None reported.

### Adverse reactions

**EENT:** dry or irritated tongue, dry or irritated nose or throat, hoarseness.
**GI:** *oral candidiasis,* dry or irritated mouth.
**Respiratory:** cough, wheezing (with oral form).
**Other:** facial edema (with oral form).

### Overdose and treatment

None reported.

### Clinical considerations

■ Most adverse reactions to corticosteroids are dose- or duration-dependent.
■ When excessive doses are used, signs and symptoms of hyperadrenocorticism and adrenal axis suppression may occur; drug should be discontinued slowly.
**H ALERT** Don't confuse triamcinolone with Triaminicin.

### Therapeutic monitoring

■ Advise clinician to monitor patient for symptom resolution.
■ Advise clinician to monitor respiratory status.

---

## Special populations
**Breast-feeding patients.** Use drug with caution in breast-feeding women.
**Pediatric patients.** Safety and efficacy haven't been established for children under age 12 for nasal aerosol and under age 6 for oral aerosol.

## Patient counseling
■ Instruct patient to rinse mouth or gargle after oral inhaler use.
■ Instruct patient to report lack of therapeutic effect or any adverse events.

# triamcinolone acetonide (topical)
Aristocort, Kenalog, Kenalog in Orabase, Triacet, Triaderm*

*Pharmacologic classification:* topical adrenocorticoid
*Therapeutic classification:* anti-inflammatory
*Pregnancy risk category C*

## Available forms
Available by prescription only
*Cream, ointment:* 0.025%, 0.1%, 0.5%
*Lotion:* 0.025%, 0.1%
*Paste:* 0.1%

## Indications and dosages
*Inflammation of corticosteroid-responsive dermatoses*
*Adults and children:* Apply cream, ointment, or lotion sparingly once to four times daily. Apply paste to oral lesions by pressing a small amount into lesion without rubbing until thin film develops. Apply b.i.d. or t.i.d. after meals and h.s.

## Mechanism of action
*Anti-inflammatory action:* Glucocorticoids stimulate the synthesis of enzymes needed to decrease the inflammatory response. Triamcinolone acetonide is a synthetic fluorinated corticosteroid. The 0.5% cream and ointment are recommended only for dermatoses refractory to treatment with lower levels.

## Pharmacokinetics
*Absorption:* Absorption depends on potency of preparation, amount applied, and nature of skin at application site. It ranges from about 1% in areas with a thick stratum corneum, such as the palms, soles, elbows, and knees, to as high as 36% in areas of the thinnest stratum corneum, such as the face, eyelids, and genitals. Absorption increases in areas of skin damage, inflammation, or occlusion. Some systemic absorption of steroids occurs, especially through the oral mucosa.

*Distribution:* After topical application, drug is distributed throughout the local skin layer. Drug absorbed into circulation is rapidly distributed into muscle, liver, skin, intestines, and kidneys.
*Metabolism:* After topical administration, drug is metabolized primarily in the skin. The small amount that's absorbed into systemic circulation is metabolized primarily in the liver to inactive compounds.
*Excretion:* Inactive metabolites are excreted by the kidneys, primarily as glucuronides and sulfates, but also as unconjugated products. Small amounts of the metabolites are also excreted in feces.

| Route | Onset | Peak | Duration |
|-------|-------|------|----------|
| Topical | Unknown | Unknown | Unknown |

## Contraindications and precautions
Contraindicated in patients hypersensitive to drug.

## Interactions
None reported.

## Adverse reactions
**GU:** glycosuria.
**Metabolic:** hyperglycemia.
**Skin:** burning, pruritus, irritation, dryness, erythema, folliculitis, hypertrichosis, hypopigmentation, acneiform eruptions, perioral dermatitis, allergic contact dermatitis, *maceration, secondary infection, atrophy, striae, miliaria* (with occlusive dressings).
**Other:** *hypothalamic-pituitary-adrenal axis suppression,* Cushing's syndrome.

## Overdose and treatment
None reported.

## Clinical considerations
■ Skin should be washed gently before applying a thin coat.
■ Hairy sites should be parted so drug can be directly applied to lesions.
■ Don't apply near eyes or ear canal.
■ If antibiotics or antifungals are used concurrently, corticosteroid should be stopped until infection is under control.

### Therapeutic monitoring
■ Advise clinician to monitor patient for symptom resolution.
■ Advise clinician to monitor respiratory status.

## Patient counseling
■ Advise patient or family members of proper administration technique.
■ If an occlusive dressing is ordered, advise patient not to leave it in place longer than 12 hours each day and not to use occlusive dressings on infected or exudative lesions.

■ Tell patient to promptly report signs of systemic absorption, skin irritation or ulceration, hypersensitivity, infection, or no improvement.

# triamterene
Dyrenium

*Pharmacologic classification:* potassium-sparing diuretic
*Therapeutic classification:* diuretic
*Pregnancy risk category B*

## Available forms
Available by prescription only
*Capsules:* 50 mg, 100 mg

## Indications and dosages
*Edema*
*Adults:* Initially, 100 mg P.O. b.i.d. after meals. Total daily dose shouldn't exceed 300 mg.

## Mechanism of action
*Diuretic action:* Triamterene acts directly on the distal renal tubules to inhibit sodium reabsorption and potassium excretion, reducing the potassium loss associated with other diuretic therapy.

Triamterene is commonly used with other more effective diuretics to treat edema from excessive aldosterone secretion, hepatic cirrhosis, nephrotic syndrome, and HF.

## Pharmacokinetics
*Absorption:* Absorbed rapidly after oral administration, but the extent varies. Diuretic effect may be delayed 2 to 3 days if used alone; maximum antihypertensive effect may be delayed 2 to 3 weeks.
*Distribution:* About 67% protein-bound.
*Metabolism:* Metabolized by hydroxylation and sulfation.
*Excretion:* Excreted in urine; half-life of triamterene is 100 to 150 minutes.

| Route | Onset | Peak | Duration |
|-------|-------|------|----------|
| P.O. | 2-4 hr | 2-4 hr | 7-9 hr |

## Contraindications and precautions
Contraindicated in patients receiving other potassium-sparing drugs, such as spirolactone or amiloride hydrochloride, in those hypersensitive to drug, and in those with anuria, severe or progressive renal disease or dysfunction, severe hepatic disease, or hyperkalemia.

Use cautiously in patients with impaired hepatic function or diabetes mellitus and in geriatric or debilitated patients.

## Interactions
**Drug-drug.** *ACE inhibitors, such as captopril and enalapril; potassium-containing drugs such as parenteral penicillin G; other potassium-sparing diuretics; potassium supplements:*
Increased risk of hyperkalemia. Advise clinician to monitor patient closely.
*Antihypertensives:* Enhanced hypoglycemia. Advise clinician to monitor patient closely. May be a therapeutic advantage.
*Cimetidine:* Increased bioavailability of triamterene. Advise clinician to monitor patient closely.
*Lithium:* Decreased lithium clearance. Avoid use together.
*NSAIDs:* Altered potassium excretion. Advise clinician to monitor patient closely.
**Drug-herb.** *Licorice:* Increased risk of hypokalemia. Discourage concomitant use.
**Drug-food.** *Potassium-containing salt substitutes, potassium-rich foods:* Increased risk of hyperkalemia. Avoid use together.
**Drug-lifestyle.** *Sun exposure:* Possible photosensitivity reactions. Advise patient to use sunblock.

## Adverse reactions
**CNS:** dizziness, weakness, fatigue, headache.
**CV:** hypotension.
**GI:** dry mouth, nausea, vomiting, diarrhea.
**GU:** transient elevation in BUN or creatinine levels, interstitial nephritis.
**Hematologic:** megaloblastic anemia related to low folic acid levels, *agranulocytosis, thrombocytopenia.*
**Hepatic:** jaundice, increased liver enzyme levels.
**Metabolic:** *hyperkalemia,* acidosis, hypokalemia, azotemia.
**Musculoskeletal:** muscle cramps.
**Skin:** photosensitivity, rash.
**Other:** *anaphylaxis.*

## Overdose and treatment
Signs and symptoms include those indicative of dehydration and electrolyte disturbance.

Treatment is supportive and symptomatic. For recent ingestion (less than 4 hours), advise clinician to empty stomach by induced emesis or gastric lavage. In severe hyperkalemia (more than 6.5 mEq/L), serum potassium levels should be reduced with I.V. sodium bicarbonate or glucose with insulin. A cation exchange resin, sodium polystyrene sulfonate (Kayexalate), given orally or as a retention enema, may also reduce serum potassium levels.

## Clinical considerations
■ Drug is less potent than thiazides and loop diuretics and is useful as an adjunct to other diuretic therapy. Usually used with potassium-wasting diuretics. Full effect is delayed 2 to 3 days when used alone.
■ To minimize excessive rebound potassium excretion, drug should be withdrawn gradually.
■ Drug therapy may interfere with enzyme assays that use fluorometry, such as serum quinidine determinations.

---

### Therapeutic monitoring
■ Advise clinician to monitor blood pressure, CBC, and uric acid, glucose, BUN, and electrolyte levels.
■ Advise clinician to watch for blood dyscrasia.

### Special populations
**Pregnant patients.** Use drug during pregnancy only when potential benefits justify possible risk to fetus.
**Breast-feeding patients.** Drug may appear in breast milk; safety during breast-feeding hasn't been established.
**Pediatric patients.** Use with caution; children are more susceptible to hyperkalemia.
**Geriatric patients.** Geriatric and debilitated patients require close observation because they're more susceptible to drug-induced diuresis and hyperkalemia. Reduced doses may be indicated.

### Patient counseling
■ Warn patient to avoid excessive ingestion of potassium-rich foods, such as citrus fruits, tomatoes, bananas, dates, and apricots; potassium-containing salt substitutes; and potassium supplements to prevent serious hyperkalemia.
■ Advise patient to avoid direct sunlight, wear protective clothing, and use a sunblock to prevent photosensitivity reactions.
■ Tell patient his urine may turn blue.
■ Tell patient to promptly report weakness, sore throat, headache, fever, bruising, bleeding, mouth sores, nausea, vomiting, or dry mouth.

---

## triazolam
Halcion

*Pharmacologic classification:* benzodiazepine
*Therapeutic classification:* sedative-hypnotic
*Pregnancy risk category X*
*Controlled substance schedule IV*

### Available forms
Available by prescription only
*Tablets:* 0.125 mg, 0.25 mg

### Indications and dosages
*Insomnia*
*Adults:* 0.125 to 0.25 mg P.O. h.s. (0.5 mg P.O. h.s. only in exceptional patients; maximum dose, 0.5 mg).
*Elderly:* 0.125 mg P.O. h.s. May give up to 0.25 mg.

### Mechanism of action
*Sedative-hypnotic action:* Triazolam depresses the CNS at the limbic and subcortical levels of the brain. It produces a sedative-hypnotic effect by potentiating the effect of the neurotransmitter gamma-aminobutyric acid on its receptor in the ascending reticular activating system, which increases inhibition and blocks both cortical and limbic arousal.

### Pharmacokinetics
*Absorption:* Well absorbed through the GI tract after oral administration.
*Distribution:* Distributed widely throughout the body. Drug is 90% protein-bound.
*Metabolism:* Metabolized in the liver primarily to inactive metabolites.
*Excretion:* Metabolites are excreted in urine. Half-life of triazolam ranges from about 1½ to 5½ hours.

| Route | Onset | Peak | Duration |
|-------|-------|------|----------|
| P.O. | 15-20 min | 1-2 hr | Unknown |

### Contraindications and precautions
Contraindicated in patients hypersensitive to benzodiazepines and during pregnancy. Also contraindicated in patients taking ketoconazole, itraconazole, nefazodone, or other drugs that impair the oxidative metabolism of triazolam by cytochrome P-450 3A.
  Use cautiously in patients with impaired renal or hepatic function, chronic pulmonary insufficiency, sleep apnea, mental depression, suicidal tendencies, or history of drug abuse.

### Interactions
**Drug-drug.** *Antidepressants, antihistamines, barbiturates, general anesthetics, MAO inhibitors, narcotics, phenothiazines:* Enhanced CNS depressant effects. Avoid use together.
*Cimetidine, disulfiram, isoniazid, oral contraceptives:* Increased plasma triazolam level. Advise clinician to monitor patient carefully.
*Drugs that inhibit the CYP3A isoenzymes:* Increased plasma triazolam levels. Use caution with concomitant use; dosage adjustment may be needed.
*Erythromycin:* Decreased triazolam clearance. Advise clinician to monitor patient closely.
*Haloperidol:* Decreased serum levels of haloperidol. Advise clinician to monitor patient closely.
*Levodopa:* Decreased therapeutic effects of levodopa. Avoid use together.
**Drug-herb.** *Catnip, kava, lady's slipper, lemon balm, passion flower, sassafras, skullcap, valerian:* Possible enhanced sedative effects. Discourage use together.
**Drug-food.** *Grapefruit juice:* Increased triazolam levels. Advise patient not to take with grapefruit juice.
**Drug-lifestyle.** *Alcohol use:* Enhanced amnesia, excessive CNS depression. Advise patient to avoid alcohol.
*Smoking (heavy):* Lowered triazolam effectiveness. Discourage smoking.

---

\* Canada only    ◇ Unlabeled clinical use

## Adverse reactions

**CNS:** *drowsiness, dizziness, headache,* rebound insomnia, amnesia, light-headedness, lack of coordination, mental confusion, depression, nervousness, physical or psychological dependence, ataxia, minor changes in EEG patterns.
**GI:** nausea, vomiting.
**Hepatic:** elevated liver enzyme levels.

## Overdose and treatment

Signs and symptoms of overdose include somnolence, confusion, hypoactive reflexes, dyspnea, labored breathing, hypotension, bradycardia, slurred speech, unsteady gait or impaired coordination and, ultimately, coma.

Advise clinician to support blood pressure and respiration until drug effects subside and monitor vital signs. Flumazenil, a specific benzodiazepine antagonist, may be useful. Mechanical ventilatory assistance via endotracheal tube may be required to maintain a patent airway and support adequate oxygenation. Recommend using I.V. fluids and vasopressors, such as dopamine and phenylephrine, to treat hypotension if appropriate. If patient is conscious, advise clinician to induce emesis. Gastric lavage should be used if ingestion was recent, but only if an endotracheal tube is present to prevent aspiration. After emesis or lavage, recommend giving activated charcoal with a cathartic as a single dose. Don't use barbiturates if excitation occurs. Dialysis is of limited value.

## Clinical considerations

■ Prevent hoarding or overdosing by patients who are depressed, suicidal, or drug-dependent or have a history of drug abuse.
**H ALERT** Don't confuse Halcion with Haldol or halcinonide.
■ Onset of sedation or hypnosis is rapid; patient should be in bed when taking triazolam.

### Therapeutic monitoring

■ Advise clinician to monitor hepatic function test results to prevent toxicity.

### Special populations

**Breast-feeding patients.** Triazolam appears in breast milk. A breast-fed infant may become sedated, have feeding difficulties, or lose weight. Avoid use in breast-feeding women.
**Pediatric patients.** Safety in children under age 18 hasn't been established.
**Geriatric patients.** Geriatric patients are more susceptible to CNS-depressant effects of drug and require supervision during initiation and after dosage increases.

## Patient counseling

■ Advise patient of potential for physical and psychological dependence.

■ Instruct patient not to take OTC drugs or change drug regimen without medical approval.
■ Tell patient that rebound insomnia may occur after drug is stopped.
■ Advise women to report suspected pregnancy immediately.
■ Caution patient not to take triazolam when a full night's sleep and clearance of the drug from the body isn't possible before normal daily activities resume.

# trifluoperazine hydrochloride

Apo-Trifluoperazine*, Novo-Flurazine*, Solazine*, Stelazine, Terfluzine*

*Pharmacologic classification:* phenothiazine (piperazine derivative)
*Therapeutic classification:* antipsychotic, antiemetic
*Pregnancy risk category C*

## Available forms

Available by prescription only
*Tablets (regular and film-coated):* 1 mg, 2 mg, 5 mg, 10 mg
*Oral concentrate:* 10 mg/ml
*Injection:* 2 mg/ml

## Indications and dosages

*Anxiety states*
*Adults:* 1 to 2 mg P.O. b.i.d. Increase dosage, p.r.n., but don't exceed 6 mg/day.
*Schizophrenia and other psychotic disorders*
*Adults:* For outpatients, 1 to 2 mg P.O. b.i.d., increased, p.r.n. For hospitalized patients, 2 to 5 mg P.O. b.i.d.; may increase gradually to 40 mg daily. For I.M. injection, 1 to 2 mg q 4 to 6 hours, p.r.n.
*Children ages 6 to 12 (hospitalized or under close supervision):* 1 mg P.O. daily or b.i.d.; may increase dosage gradually to 15 mg daily. Alternatively, administer 1 mg I.M. once or twice daily.

## Mechanism of action

*Antipsychotic and antiemetic actions:* Trifluoperazine is thought to exert its antipsychotic effects by postsynaptic blockade of CNS dopamine receptors, inhibiting dopamine-mediated effects; antiemetic effects are attributed to dopamine receptor blockade in the medullary chemoreceptor trigger zone. Trifluoperazine has many other central and peripheral effects; it produces alpha and ganglionic blockade and counteracts histamine- and serotonin-mediated activity. Its most prevalent adverse reactions are extrapyramidal; it has less sedative and autonomic activity than aliphatic and piperidine phenothiazines.

## Pharmacokinetics

*Absorption:* Rate and extent of absorption vary with route of administration: Oral tablet absorption is erratic and variable, with onset of action ranging from ½ to 1 hour; oral concentrate absorption is much more predictable. I.M. drug is absorbed rapidly.

*Distribution:* Distributed widely in the body; drug appears in breast milk. Drug is 91% to 99% protein-bound; steady-state serum levels are achieved within 4 to 7 days.

*Metabolism:* Metabolized extensively by the liver, but no active metabolites are formed.

*Excretion:* Mostly excreted in urine via the kidneys; some is excreted in feces by way of the biliary tract.

| Route | Onset | Peak | Duration |
|-------|-------|------|----------|
| P.O., I.M. | Unknown | 2-4 hr | 4-6 hr |

## Contraindications and precautions

Contraindicated in patients hypersensitive to phenothiazines and in patients with coma, CNS depression, bone marrow suppression, or liver damage.

Use cautiously in geriatric or debilitated patients; in those exposed to extreme heat; and in patients with CV disease, seizure disorders, glaucoma, or prostatic hyperplasia.

## Interactions

**Drug-drug.** *Barbiturates, lithium:* Decreased phenothiazine effect. Advise clinician to monitor patient closely.

*Beta blockers:* Increased trifluoperazine levels and toxicity. Advise clinician to monitor patient closely.

*Centrally acting antihypertensives, such as clonidine, guanabenz, guanadrel, guanethidine, methyldopa, and reserpine:* Inhibition of blood pressure response. Monitor patient closely.

*CNS depressants:* Enhanced CNS depression. Avoid use together.

*Epinephrine:* Further lowering of blood pressure. Advise clinician to monitor patient closely. Dosage adjustment may be needed.

*Lithium:* Severe neurologic toxicity with an encephalitis-like syndrome, decreased therapeutic response to trifluoperazine. Avoid use together.

*Propylthiouracil:* Increased risk of agranulocytosis. Advise clinician to monitor patient closely.

*Sympathomimetics:* Decreased stimulatory and pressor effects. Advise clinician to monitor patient carefully.

**Drug-herb.** *Kava:* Increased risk or severity of dystonic reactions. Discourage concomitant use.

*Yohimbe:* Increased risk of toxicity. Discourage concomitant use.

**Drug-food.** *Caffeine:* Decreased therapeutic effects. Dosage adjustment may be needed.

**Drug-lifestyle.** *Alcohol use:* Additive effects. Advise patient to avoid alcohol.

*Smoking:* Decreased therapeutic effects. Encourage smoking cessation.

*Sun exposure:* Increased photosensitivity reactions. Advise patient to use sunblock.

## Adverse reactions

**CNS:** *extrapyramidal reactions,* **neuroleptic malignant syndrome** (fever, tachycardia, tachypnea, profuse diaphoresis), *tardive dyskinesia,* pseudoparkinsonism, dizziness, drowsiness, insomnia, fatigue, headache.

**CV:** *orthostatic hypotension,* tachycardia, ECG changes.

**EENT:** ocular changes, *blurred vision.*

**GI:** *dry mouth, constipation,* nausea.

**GU:** *urine retention,* menstrual irregularities.

**Hematologic:** *transient leukopenia, agranulocytosis.*

**Hepatic:** cholestatic jaundice, elevated liver function test results.

**Metabolic:** weight gain.

**Skin:** *photosensitivity,* allergic reactions, pain at I.M. injection site, sterile abscess, rash.

**Other:** inhibited lactation, gynecomastia.

**After abrupt withdrawal of long-term therapy:** gastritis, nausea, vomiting, dizziness, tremor, feeling of warmth or cold, diaphoresis, tachycardia, headache, insomnia, anorexia, muscle rigidity, altered mental status, and evidence of autonomic instability.

## Overdose and treatment

CNS depression is characterized by deep, unarousable sleep and possible coma, hypotension or hypertension, extrapyramidal symptoms, dystonia, abnormal involuntary muscle movements, agitation, seizures, arrhythmias, ECG changes, hypothermia or hyperthermia, and autonomic nervous system dysfunction.

Treatment is symptomatic and supportive and includes maintaining vital signs, airway, stable body temperature, and fluid and electrolyte balance.

Don't induce vomiting. Drug inhibits cough reflex, and aspiration may occur. Advise clinician to use gastric lavage, then activated charcoal and sodium chloride cathartics; dialysis is usually ineffective. Advise clinician to regulate body temperature p.r.n. and treat hypotension with I.V. fluids. Don't give epinephrine. Recommend treating seizures with parenteral diazepam or barbiturates; arrhythmias with parenteral phenytoin (1 mg/kg with rate titrated to blood pressure); extrapyramidal reactions with benztropine at 1 to 2 mg or parenteral diphenhydramine at 10 to 50 mg.

## Clinical considerations

■ Other drugs, such as benzodiazepines, are preferred for the treatment of anxiety. When

---

drug is given for anxiety, don't exceed 6 mg daily for longer than 12 weeks.

■ Drug causes a high risk of extrapyramidal symptoms and photosensitivity reactions.

■ Worsening anginal pain has been reported in patients receiving trifluoperazine; however, ECG reactions are less common with drug than with other phenothiazines.

■ Liquid and injectable formulations may cause rash after contact with skin.

■ Drug may cause pink to brown discoloration of urine or blue-gray skin.

■ Drug causes false-positive test results for urine porphyrins, urobilinogen, amylase, and 5-hydroxyindoleacetic acid levels from darkening of urine by metabolites; it also causes false-positive urine pregnancy results in tests using human chorionic gonadotropin as the indicator.

### Therapeutic monitoring

■ Advise clinician to monitor blood pressure before and after parenteral administration.

■ Advise clinician to monitor patient regularly for abnormal body movements (at least once every 6 months).

### Special populations

**Breast-feeding patients.** Drug may appear in breast milk. Potential benefits to the mother should outweigh potential harm to the infant.

**Pediatric patients.** Not recommended for children under age 6.

**Geriatric patients.** Geriatric patients tend to require lower doses, adjusted to effect. Adverse effects, especially tardive dyskinesia and other extrapyramidal effects and hypotension, are more likely to develop in such patients.

### Patient counseling

■ Explain risks of dystonic reactions, akathisia, and tardive dyskinesia, and tell patient to report abnormal body movements.

■ Explain that many drug interactions are possible. Tell patient to seek medical approval before taking self-prescribed drugs.

■ Warn patient against hazardous activities that require alertness until effect of drug is established.

■ Tell patient to avoid sun exposure and exposure to temperature extremes because drug may cause thermoregulatory changes.

■ Tell patient to take drug exactly as prescribed and to avoid alcohol and other drugs that may cause excessive sedation.

# trihexyphenidyl hydrochloride

Apo-Trihex*, Artane, Artane Sequels, Trihexane, Trihexy-2, Trihexy-5

*Pharmacologic classification:* anticholinergic
*Therapeutic classification:* antiparkinsonian
*Pregnancy risk category C*

## Available forms

Available by prescription only
*Tablets:* 2 mg, 5 mg
*Capsules (sustained-release):* 5 mg
*Elixir:* 2 mg/5 ml

## Indications and dosages

*Idiopathic parkinsonism*

*Adults:* 1 mg P.O. on first day, 2 mg on second day, then increase 2 mg q 3 to 5 days until total of 6 to 10 mg is given daily. Usually given t.i.d. with meals and, if needed, q.i.d. (last dose should be before bedtime). Postencephalitic parkinsonism may require 12 to 15 mg total daily dose. Patients receiving levodopa may need 3 to 6 mg daily. Sustained-release capsules shouldn't be used as initial therapy, but after the patient has been stabilized on the conventional dose forms. Sustained-release capsules can be dosed on a mg per mg of total daily dose and given as a single dose after breakfast or in two divided doses 12 hours apart.

*Drug-induced parkinsonism*

*Adults:* 5 to 15 mg daily.

## Mechanism of action

*Antiparkinsonian action:* Trihexyphenidyl blocks central cholinergic receptors, helping to balance cholinergic activity in the basal ganglia. It may also prolong the effects of dopamine by blocking dopamine reuptake and storage at central receptor sites.

## Pharmacokinetics

*Absorption:* Rapidly absorbed after oral administration.

*Distribution:* Crosses the blood-brain barrier; little else is known about its distribution.

*Metabolism:* Exact metabolic fate is unknown.

*Excretion:* Excreted in urine as unchanged drug and metabolites.

| Route | Onset | Peak | Duration |
|-------|-------|------|----------|
| P.O. | 1 hr | Unknown | 6-12 hr |

## Contraindications and precautions

Contraindicated in patients hypersensitive to drug. Use cautiously in patients with impaired renal, cardiac, or hepatic function; glaucoma; obstructive disease of the GI or GU tract; or prostatic hyperplasia.

## Interactions
**Drug-drug.** *Amantadine:* Amplified anticholinergic adverse effects, including confusion and hallucinations. Trihexyphenidyl dose should be reduced before amantadine is given.
*Antacids, antidiarrheals:* Possible decreased absorption of trihexyphenidyl. Advise clinician to monitor patient closely. Dosage adjustment may be needed.
*CNS depressants, including tranquilizers and sedative-hypnotics:* Increased sedative effects. Avoid use together.
*Haloperidol, phenothiazines:* Decreased antipsychotic effectiveness. Dosage adjustment may be needed.
*Levodopa:* Synergistic anticholinergic effects, enhanced GI metabolism of levodopa. Advise clinician to monitor patient closely. Dosage adjustment may be needed
*Phenothiazine:* Increased risk of anticholinergic adverse effects. Advise clinician to monitor patient.
**Drug-lifestyle.** *Alcohol use:* Increased sedative effects. Advise patient to avoid alcohol.

## Adverse reactions
**CNS:** nervousness, dizziness, headache, hallucinations, drowsiness, weakness.
**CV:** tachycardia.
**EENT:** blurred vision, mydriasis, increased intraocular pressure.
**GI:** *dry mouth, nausea,* constipation, vomiting.
**GU:** urinary hesitancy, urine retention.

## Overdose and treatment
Effects of overdose include central stimulation followed by depression, with such psychotic symptoms as disorientation, confusion, hallucinations, delusions, anxiety, agitation, and restlessness. Peripheral effects may include dilated, nonreactive pupils; blurred vision; flushed, dry, hot skin; dry mucous membranes; dysphagia; decreased or absent bowel sounds; urine retention; hyperthermia; headache; tachycardia; hypertension; and increased respiration.

Treatment is primarily symptomatic and supportive, p.r.n. Patent airway should be maintained. If patient is alert, advise clinician to induce emesis (or use gastric lavage) and follow with sodium chloride cathartic and activated charcoal to prevent further drug absorption. In severe cases, physostigmine may be given to block antimuscarinic effects of trihexyphenidyl. Advise clinician to give fluids, p.r.n., to treat shock; diazepam to control psychotic symptoms; and pilocarpine (instilled into the eyes) to relieve mydriasis. If urine retention occurs, catheterization may be needed.

## Clinical considerations
■ Tolerance may develop to drug, necessitating higher doses.
■ Use drug with caution in hot weather because of the increased risk of heat prostration.

### Therapeutic monitoring
■ Advise clinician to monitor patient for urinary hesitancy.
■ Advise clinician to obtain gonioscopic evaluation and close intraocular pressure monitoring, especially in patients over age 40.

### Special populations
**Breast-feeding patients.** Drug may appear in breast milk, possibly resulting in infant toxicity. It may also decrease milk production.
**Geriatric patients.** Use caution when giving drug to geriatric patients. Lower doses are indicated.

## Patient counseling
■ Tell patient to avoid activities that require alertness until CNS effects of drug are known.
■ Advise patient to report signs of urinary hesitation or urine retention.
■ Tell patient to take drug with food if GI upset occurs.

---

# trimethobenzamide hydrochloride
Arrestin, Tebamide, Ticon, Tigan

*Pharmacologic classification:*
ethanolamine-related antihistamine
*Therapeutic classification:* antiemetic
*Pregnancy risk category C*

## Available forms
Available by prescription only
*Capsules:* 100 mg, 250 mg
*Suppositories:* 100 mg, 200 mg
*Injection:* 100 mg/ml

## Indications and dosages
*Nausea and vomiting (treatment)*
*Adults:* 250 mg P.O. t.i.d. or q.i.d.; or 200 mg I.M. or P.R. t.i.d. or q.i.d.
*Children weighing 13 to 45 kg (29 to 88 lb):* 100 or 200 mg P.O. t.i.d. or q.i.d. Or, 100 to 200 mg P.R. t.i.d. or q.i.d.
*Children weighing under 13 kg (29 lb):* 100 mg P.R. t.i.d. or q.i.d. Alternatively, children may receive 15 mg/kg or 400 mg/m$^2$ daily P.R. or 20 mg/kg or 500 mg/m$^2$ daily P.O., divided t.i.d. or q.i.d.

## Mechanism of action
*Antiemetic action:* Exact mechanism of action is unknown. Trimethobenzamide is a weak antihistamine with limited antiemetic properties. Drug effects may occur in the chemoreceptor

trigger zone of the brain; however, drug apparently doesn't inhibit direct impulses to the vomiting center.

## Pharmacokinetics
*Absorption:* About 60% of an oral dose is absorbed.
*Distribution:* Unknown.
*Metabolism:* About 50% to 70% of dose is metabolized, probably in the liver.
*Excretion:* Excreted in urine and feces.

| Route | Onset | Peak | Duration |
|-------|-------|------|----------|
| P.O. | 10-20 min | Unknown | 3-4 hr |
| I.M. | 15-35 min | Unknown | 2-3 hr |
| P.R. | Unknown | Unknown | Unknown |

## Contraindications and precautions
Contraindicated in patients hypersensitive to drug. Suppositories are contraindicated in patients hypersensitive to benzocaine hydrochloride or similar local anesthetic. Parenteral form is contraindicated in children and suppositories are contraindicated in premature infants and neonates. Use cautiously in children.

## Interactions
**Drug-drug.** *Other CNS depressants, including antihypertensives, belladonna alkaloids, phenothiazines, and tricyclic antidepressants:* Increased trimethobenzamide toxicity. Avoid use together.
**Drug-lifestyle.** *Alcohol use:* Increased sedative effects. Avoid use together.

## Adverse reactions
**CNS:** *drowsiness,* dizziness (in large doses), headache, disorientation, depression, parkinsonian-like symptoms, ***coma, seizures.***
**CV:** hypotension.
**EENT:** blurred vision.
**GI:** diarrhea.
**Hepatic:** jaundice.
**Musculoskeletal:** muscle cramps.
**Skin:** hypersensitivity reactions (pain, stinging, burning, redness, swelling at I.M. injection site).

## Overdose and treatment
Signs and symptoms of overdose may include severe neurologic reactions, such as opisthotonos, seizures, coma, and extrapyramidal reactions. Advise clinician to discontinue drug and provide supportive care.

## Clinical considerations
■ Drug may be less effective against severe vomiting than other drugs.
■ Drug has little or no value in treating motion sickness.

## Therapeutic monitoring
■ Advise clinician to monitor patient for hypersensitivity reactions.
■ Advise clinician to monitor patient for relief from symptoms.

## Special populations
**Pregnant patients.** Safety during pregnancy hasn't been established.
**Breast-feeding patients.** Safety in breast-feeding women hasn't been established.
**Pediatric patients.** Use drug with caution in children. Don't give to children with viral illness because drug may contribute to development of Reye's syndrome. Don't use in newborn or premature infants.
**Geriatric patients.** Use drug with caution in geriatric patients because they may be more susceptible to adverse CNS effects.

## Patient counseling
■ Warn patient to avoid hazardous activities that require alertness because drug may cause drowsiness, and to avoid consuming alcohol to prevent additive sedation.
■ Instruct patient to report persistent vomiting.
■ Instruct patient on proper administration and storage of suppositories.

# trimethoprim
Primsol, Proloprim, Trimpex

*Pharmacologic classification:* synthetic folate antagonist
*Therapeutic classification:* antibiotic
*Pregnancy risk category C*

## Available forms
Available by prescription only
*Tablets:* 100 mg, 200 mg
*Solution:* 50 mg/5 ml

## Indications and dosages
*Treatment of uncomplicated urinary tract infections*
*Adults:* 100 mg P.O. (tablets or solution) q 12 hours or 200 mg q 24 hours for 10 days.
*Acute otitis media caused by susceptible strains of Streptococcus pneumoniae and Haemophilus influenzae*
*Children ages 6 months and older:* 10 mg/kg/day of solution, given in divided doses every 12 hours for 10 days.
◊ *Prophylaxis of chronic and recurrent urinary tract infections*
*Adults:* 100 mg P.O. h.s. for 6 weeks to 6 months.
◊ *Traveler's diarrhea*
*Adults:* 200 mg P.O. b.i.d. for 3 to 5 days.
◊ *Pneumocystis carinii pneumonia*
*Adults:* 5 mg/kg P.O. t.i.d. in conjunction with dapsone 100 mg daily for 21 days.

---

≡ *Dosage adjustment.* If creatinine clearance is 15 to 30 ml/minute, give one-half the normal dose. If creatinine clearance is less than 15 ml/minute, manufacturer doesn't recommend use of this drug.

## Mechanism of action
*Antibacterial action:* By interfering with action of dihydrofolate reductase, drug inhibits bacterial synthesis of folic acid. Drug is effective against many gram-positive and gram-negative organisms, including most Enterobacteriaceae organisms (except *Pseudomonas*), *Proteus mirabilis, Klebsiella,* and *Escherichia coli.* Trimethoprim is usually bactericidal.

## Pharmacokinetics
*Absorption:* Absorbed quickly and completely.
*Distribution:* Widely distributed. About 42% to 46% of dose is plasma protein–bound.
*Metabolism:* Less than 20% of dose is metabolized in the liver.
*Excretion:* Most of dose is excreted in urine via filtration and secretion. In patients with normal renal function, elimination half-life is 8 to 11 hours; in patients with impaired renal function, half-life is prolonged.

| Route | Onset | Peak | Duration |
|-------|-------|------|----------|
| P.O. | Unknown | 1-4 hr | Unknown |

## Contraindications and precautions
Contraindicated in patients hypersensitive to drug and in those with documented megaloblastic anemia caused by folate deficiency. Use cautiously in patients with folate deficiency and impaired hepatic or renal function, especially those with creatinine clearance of 15 ml/minute or less.

## Interactions
**Drug-drug.** *Phenytoin:* Increased serum phenytoin levels. Advise clinician to monitor patient closely.

## Adverse reactions
**GI:** *epigastric distress, nausea, vomiting,* glossitis, diarrhea.
**GU:** increased BUN and serum creatinine levels.
**Hematologic:** *thrombocytopenia, leukopenia,* megaloblastic anemia, methemoglobinemia.
**Hepatic:** elevated liver enzyme levels.
**Skin:** *rash, pruritus,* exfoliative dermatitis.
**Other:** fever.

## Overdose and treatment
Effects of acute overdose include nausea, vomiting, dizziness, headache, confusion, and bone marrow depression. Treatment includes gastric lavage and supportive measures. Urine may be acidified to enhance drug elimination.

Effects of chronic toxicity caused by prolonged high-dose therapy include bone marrow depression, leukopenia, thrombocytopenia, and megaloblastic anemia. Treatment includes drug discontinuation and administration of leucovorin, 3 to 6 mg I.M. daily for 3 days or 5 to 15 mg P.O. daily until normal hematopoiesis returns.

## Clinical considerations
■ Advise clinician to obtain urine specimen for culture and sensitivity tests before starting therapy.
■ Drug is usually used with other antibiotics, especially sulfamethoxazole, because resistance develops rapidly when used alone.
■ Advanced age, malnourishment, pregnancy, debilitation, renal impairment, and prolonged high-dose therapy increase risk of hematologic toxicity, as does use of drug with folate antagonistic drugs, such as phenytoin.
**◪ ALERT** Trimethoprim is also used with sulfamethoxazole. Don't confuse the two products.

### Therapeutic monitoring
■ If patient is receiving drug with phenytoin, advise clinician to monitor serum phenytoin levels.
■ Sore throat, fever, pallor, and purpura may be early signs and symptoms of serious blood disorders. Advise clinician to monitor blood counts regularly.

### Special populations
**Pregnant patients.** Use drug during pregnancy only when benefits justify risk to fetus.
**Breast-feeding patients.** Drug appears in breast milk; an alternative to breast-feeding is recommended during trimethoprim therapy.
**Pediatric patients.** Safety in children under age 2 months hasn't been established; efficacy in children under age 6 months hasn't been established.
**Geriatric patients.** Geriatric patients may be more susceptible to hematologic toxicity.

## Patient counseling
■ Instruct patient to continue taking drug as directed until course of therapy is completed.
■ Advise patient to report signs or symptoms of blood disorders.

---

# trimipramine maleate
Surmontil

*Pharmacologic classification:* tricyclic antidepressant
*Therapeutic classification:* antidepressant, anxiolytic
*Pregnancy risk category C*

## Available forms
Available by prescription only
*Capsules:* 25 mg, 50 mg, 100 mg

## Indications and dosages
*Depression*
*Adults:* Initially, give 75 to 100 mg/day P.O. in divided doses and increase to 200 mg/day. Dosage for inpatients may range up to 300 mg/day. Maintenance dose, 50 to 150 mg/day.
*Elderly:* 50 to 100 mg/day P.O.
*Adolescents:* 50 to 100 mg/day P.O.
◊ *Duodenal ulcers*
*Adults:* 50 mg P.O. h.s. for 4 weeks.

## Mechanism of action
*Antidepressant and anxiolytic actions:* Trimipramine is thought to exert its antidepressant effects by equally inhibiting reuptake of norepinephrine and serotonin in CNS nerve terminals (presynaptic neurons), which results in increased concentration and enhanced activity of these neurotransmitters in the synaptic cleft. Trimipramine also has anxiolytic effects and inhibits gastric acid secretion.

## Pharmacokinetics
*Absorption:* Absorbed rapidly from the GI tract after oral administration.
*Distribution:* Distributed widely in the body. Drug is 90% protein-bound; steady state occurs within 7 days.
*Metabolism:* Metabolized by the liver; a significant first-pass effect may explain variability of serum levels in different patients taking the same dose.
*Excretion:* Mostly excreted in urine; some is excreted in feces by way of the biliary tract.

| Route | Onset | Peak | Duration |
|-------|-------|------|----------|
| P.O. | Unknown | 2 hr | Unknown |

## Contraindications and precautions
Contraindicated during acute recovery phase of MI, in patients hypersensitive to drug, and in those receiving MAO inhibitor therapy within 14 days.
    Use cautiously in adolescents; in geriatric or debilitated patients; in those receiving thyroid hormones; and in those with CV disease, increased intraocular pressure, hyperthyroidism, impaired hepatic function, or history of seizures, urine retention, or angle-closure glaucoma.

## Interactions
**Drug-drug.** *Antiarrhythmics, such as disopyramide, procainamide, and quinidine; pimozide, thyroid hormones:* Increased risk of cardiac arrhythmias and conduction defects. Advise clinician to monitor patient closely.
*Atropine and other anticholinergics, including antihistamines, antiparkinsonians, meperidine, and phenothiazines:* Possible oversedation, paralytic ileus, visual changes, and severe constipation. Advise clinician to monitor patient.
*Barbiturates:* Decreased trimipramine therapeutic efficacy. Dosage adjustment may be needed.
*Beta blockers, cimetidine, methylphenidate, oral contraceptives, propoxyphene:* Increased trimipramine plasma levels and toxicity. Advise clinician to monitor patient closely.
*Centrally acting antihypertensives, including clonidine, guanabenz, guanadrel, guanethidine, methyldopa, and reserpine:* Decreased hypotensive effects. Advise clinician to monitor patient carefully.
*CNS depressants, including analgesics, anesthetics, barbiturates, narcotics, and tranquilizers:* Possible oversedation. Advise clinician to monitor patient.
*Disulfiram, etchlorvynol:* Possible delirium and tachycardia. Advise clinician to monitor patient carefully.
*Haloperidol, phenothiazines:* Decreased trimipramine metabolism, decreased therapeutic efficacy. Dosage adjustment may be needed.
*Metrizamide:* Increased risk of seizures. Advise clinician to monitor patient closely.
*SSRIs, including fluoxetine, paroxetine, and sertraline:* Increased pharmacologic and toxic effects of trimipramine. Advise clinician to monitor patient closely. Dosage adjustment may be needed.
*Sympathomimetics, including ephedrine, epinephrine, and phenylephrine:* Increased blood pressure. Advise clinician to monitor patient closely.
*Warfarin:* Increased PT and INR with resultant bleeding. Advise clinician to monitor PT and INR. Dosage adjustment may be needed.
**Drug-herb.** *St. John's wort, SAMe, yohimbe:* Possible elevation of serotonin levels when used with some tricyclic antidepressants. Discourage concomitant use.
**Drug-lifestyle.** *Alcohol use:* Additive trimipramine effects. Advise patient to avoid alcohol.
*Smoking (heavy):* Decreased therapeutic efficacy. Discourage smoking.
*Sun exposure:* Increased risk of photosensitivity reactions. Advise patient to use sunblock.

## Adverse reactions
**CNS:** *drowsiness, dizziness,* paresthesia, ataxia, hallucinations, delusions, anxiety, agitation, insomnia, tremor, weakness, confusion, head-

ache, EEG changes, *seizures,* extrapyramidal reactions.
**CV:** *orthostatic hypotension,* tachycardia, hypertension, *arrhythmias, heart block, MI, CVA,* prolonged conduction time on ECG.
**EENT:** *blurred vision,* tinnitus, mydriasis.
**GI:** *dry mouth, constipation,* nausea, vomiting, anorexia, paralytic ileus.
**GU:** *urine retention.*
**Hematologic:** decreased WBC counts, altered PT and INR.
**Hepatic:** elevated liver enzyme levels.
**Metabolic:** altered serum glucose levels.
**Skin:** rash, urticaria, photosensitivity, *diaphoresis.*
**Other:** hypersensitivity reaction.
**After abrupt withdrawal of long-term therapy:** nausea, headache, malaise (doesn't indicate addiction).

### Overdose and treatment
The first 12 hours after acute ingestion are a stimulatory phase characterized by excessive anticholinergic activity, including agitation, irritation, confusion, hallucinations, parkinsonian symptoms, seizure, urine retention, dry mucous membranes, pupillary dilation, constipation, and ileus. This is followed by CNS depressant effects, including hypothermia, decreased or absent reflexes, sedation, hypotension, cyanosis, and cardiac irregularities, including tachycardia, conduction disturbances, and quinidine-like effects on the ECG.

Severity of overdose is best indicated by prolongation of QRS interval beyond 100 msec, which usually represents a serum level in excess of 1,000 ng/ml; serum levels are generally not helpful. Metabolic acidosis may follow hypotension, hypoventilation, and seizures.

Treatment is symptomatic and supportive and includes maintaining airway, stable body temperature, and fluid and electrolyte balance. Advise clinician to induce emesis with ipecac if patient is conscious and follow with gastric lavage and activated charcoal to prevent further absorption. Dialysis is of little use. Physostigmine given I.V. slowly has been used to reverse most CV and CNS effects of overdose. Seizures should be treated with parenteral diazepam or phenytoin; arrhythmias with parenteral phenytoin or lidocaine; and acidosis with sodium bicarbonate. Don't give barbiturates; these may enhance CNS and respiratory depressant effects.

### Clinical considerations
■ Consider the inherent risk of suicide until significant improvement of depressive state occurs.
■ Tolerance generally develops to the sedative effects of drug.
■ Maintenance therapy should be given at bedtime as a single dose.

■ Therapy should be continued for at least 3 months to prevent relapse.

### Therapeutic monitoring
■ Advise clinician to watch for bleeding because drug may cause alterations in PT and INR.
■ Advise clinician to closely monitor high-risk patients during initial drug therapy.

### Special populations
**Geriatric patients.** Geriatric patients may be more vulnerable to adverse cardiac effects.

### Patient counseling
■ Explain that full effects of drug may not become apparent for up to 2 to 6 weeks after therapy begins.
■ Tell patient to take drug exactly as prescribed.
■ Warn patient that drug may cause drowsiness or dizziness and to avoid activities that require mental alertness until the full effects of drug are known.
■ Warn patient not to drink alcoholic beverages or medicinal elixirs while taking drug.
■ Suggest taking drug with food or milk if it causes stomach upset and to ease dry mouth with sugarless chewing gum, hard candy, or ice.
■ Tell patient to report adverse reactions promptly, especially confusion, movement disorders, rapid heartbeat, dizziness, fainting, or difficulty urinating.

# troleandomycin
Tao

*Pharmacologic classification:*
macrolide antibiotic
*Therapeutic classification:* antibiotic
*Pregnancy risk category C*

### Available forms
Available by prescription only
*Capsules:* 250 mg

### Indications and dosages
*Pneumonia or respiratory tract infection caused by sensitive pneumococci or group A beta-hemolytic streptococci*
*Adults:* 250 to 500 mg P.O. q 6 hours for 10 days.
*Children:* 125 to 250 mg P.O. q 6 hours for 10 days. Alternatively, 6.6 to 11 mg/kg every 6 hours for 10 days.

### Mechanism of action
*Antibacterial action:* Drug inhibits bacterial protein synthesis by binding to 50S ribosomal subunit. It produces bacteriostatic effects on susceptible bacteria, including gram-positive cocci and bacilli and a few gram-negative or-

ganisms, including *Haemophilus influenzae*, *Neisseria gonorrhoeae*, and *N. meningitidis*.

## Pharmacokinetics
***Absorption:*** Absorbed rapidly but incompletely.
***Distribution:*** Distributed widely to body fluids, except to CSF.
***Metabolism:*** Metabolized in the liver.
***Excretion:*** Excreted in bile, feces, and urine (10% to 25%).

| Route | Onset | Peak | Duration |
|-------|-------|------|----------|
| P.O. | Unknown | 2 hr | Unknown |

## Contraindications and precautions
Contraindicated in patients hypersensitive to drug. Use cautiously in patients with hepatic dysfunction.

## Interactions
**Drug-drug.** *Carbamazepine, methylprednisolone, theophylline:* Increased toxicity of drugs. Avoid use together.
*Ergotamine:* Possible precipitation of severe ischemic reactions and peripheral vasospasms. Advise clinician to monitor patient closely.
*Oral contraceptives:* Possible marked cholestatic jaundice. Advise clinician to monitor patient closely.

## Adverse reactions
**GI:** *abdominal cramps, discomfort,* vomiting, diarrhea.
**Hematologic:** eosinophilia, leukocytosis.
**Hepatic:** elevated liver enzyme levels, cholestatic jaundice.
**Skin:** urticaria, rash.
**Other:** *anaphylaxis.*

## Overdose and treatment
None reported.

## Clinical considerations
■ Advise clinician to obtain culture and sensitivity tests before starting therapy.
■ Repeated courses of therapy or therapy exceeding 2 weeks may lead to allergic cholestatic hepatitis, as indicated by jaundice, right upper abdominal quadrant pain, fever, nausea, vomiting, eosinophilia, and leukocytosis.
■ Advise clinician to discontinue drug if liver function test values increase or if signs or symptoms of cholestatic hepatitis occur.

### *Therapeutic monitoring*
■ If patient is receiving drug with theophylline or carbamazepine, advise clinician to closely monitor theophylline or carbamazepine levels and assess patient frequently for signs and symptoms of theophylline or carbamazepine toxicity.
■ Advise clinician to monitor total serum bilirubin and AST, ALT, and serum alkaline phosphatase levels.

## Patient counseling
■ Instruct patient to continue taking drug as prescribed, even if he's feeling better.
■ For best absorption, advise patient to take drug on an empty stomach 1 hour before or 2 hours after meals, with full glass of water.
■ Instruct patient to report abdominal pain or nausea immediately.

# trovafloxacin mesylate
Trovan

# alatrofloxacin mesylate
Trovan I.V.

*Pharmacologic classification:* fluoroquinolone derivative
*Therapeutic classification:* antibiotic
*Pregnancy risk category C*

## Available forms
Available by prescription only
*Tablets:* 100 mg, 200 mg
*Injection:* 5 mg/ml, in 40-ml (200 mg) and 60-ml (300 mg) vials

## Indications and dosages
***Gynecologic and pelvic infections, complicated intra-abdominal and postsurgical infections***
*Adults:* 300 mg I.V. daily followed by 200 mg P.O. daily for 7 to 14 days.
***Nosocomial pneumonia***
*Adults:* 300 mg I.V. daily followed by 200 mg P.O. daily for 10 to 14 days.
***Community-acquired pneumonia***
*Adults:* 200 mg P.O. or I.V. daily followed by 200 mg P.O. daily for 7 to 14 days.
***Complicated skin and diabetic foot infections***
*Adults:* 200 mg P.O. or I.V. daily followed by 200 mg P.O. daily for 10 to 14 days.
**≡*Dosage adjustment.*** Dosage adjustments are unnecessary when switching from I.V. to oral forms. An adjustment in dose isn't needed for patients with renal impairment; however, for patients with mild to moderate hepatic disease (cirrhosis), the following dosage reductions are recommended: Reduce 300 mg I.V. to 200 mg I.V., reduce 200 mg I.V. or P.O. to 100 mg I.V. or P.O.; no reduction needed for 100 mg P.O.

## I.V. administration
■ Alatrofloxacin mesylate is supplied in single-use vials that must be further diluted with a compatible solution, such as $D_5W$ or half-normal saline, before administration.
■ After dilution, administer I.V. drug as a 60-minute infusion.

## Incompatibilities

Don't administer simultaneously through same I.V. line with other additives or drugs. Don't administer through same I.V. line with solutions containing multivalent cations, such as magnesium. Don't dilute drug with normal saline solution or lactated Ringer's solution.

## Mechanism of action

*Antibiotic action:* Trovafloxacin is related to the fluoroquinolones with in vitro activity against a wide range of gram-positive and gram-negative aerobic and anaerobic microorganisms. The bactericidal action of trovafloxacin results from inhibition of DNA gyrase and topoisomerase IV, two enzymes involved in bacterial replication.

## Pharmacokinetics

*Absorption:* Well absorbed after oral administration with an absolute bioavailability of about 88%. Steady-state levels are obtained by the third day of oral or I.V. administration.
*Distribution:* Widely and rapidly distributed throughout the body, resulting in significantly higher tissue levels than in plasma or serum. Mean plasma protein–bound fraction is about 76%. Trovafloxacin appears in breast milk.
*Metabolism:* Primarily metabolized by conjugation although there is minimal oxidative metabolism by cytochrome P-450. About 13% of a dose occurs in urine as the glucuronide ester and 9% as the *N*-acetyl metabolite.
*Excretion:* Primary route of elimination is fecal. About 50% of an oral dose (43% in feces and 6% in urine) is excreted as unchanged drug.

| Route | Onset | Peak | Duration |
|---|---|---|---|
| P.O., I.V. | Unknown | 1 hr | Unknown |

## Contraindications and precautions

Contraindicated in patients hypersensitive to trovafloxacin, alatrovafloxacin, or other quinolone antimicrobials. Use cautiously in patients with history of seizures, psychosis, or increased intracranial pressure.

## Interactions

**Drug-drug.** *Aluminum-, magnesium-, and iron-containing preparations, such as antacids and vitamin-minerals; divalent and trivalent cations such as didanosine:* Decreased absorption of antibiotic. Don't take trovafloxacin and alatrofloxacin mesylate 2 hours before or 6 hours after these products.
*I.V. morphine, sucralfate:* Reduced trovafloxacin plasma levels. Advise clinician to give I.V. morphine at least 2 hours after oral trovafloxacin

in fasting state and at least 4 hours after oral trovafloxacin is taken with food.
*Warfarin:* Enhanced anticoagulation effect. Advise clinician to monitor PT and INR.
**Drug-lifestyle.** *Sun exposure:* Photosensitivity reaction. Advise patient to use sunblock.

## Adverse reactions

**CNS:** *dizziness,* light-headedness, headache, *seizures.*
**GI:** diarrhea, nausea, vomiting, abdominal pain, pseudomembranous colitis.
**GU:** vaginitis.
**Hematologic:** *bone marrow aplasia (anemia, thrombocytopenia, leukopenia).*
**Hepatic:** elevated hepatic transaminase levels, *hepatitis,* jaundice, *liver failure.*
**Musculoskeletal:** arthralgia, arthropathy, myalgia.
**Skin:** pruritus, rash, injection site reaction (I.V.), photosensitivity.

## Overdose and treatment

Trovafloxacin has a low order of acute toxicity. Signs of overdose include decreased activity and respiration, ataxia, ptosis, tremors, and seizures.
   Advise clinician to treat by emptying the stomach and providing symptomatic and supportive treatment. Drug isn't efficiently removed by hemodialysis.

## Clinical considerations

■ Oral form is more cost-effective and carries less risk; both forms have similar clinical efficacy and pharmacokinetics. Patients started with I.V. therapy may be switched to oral therapy when clinically indicated and at the discretion of the prescriber.
**⚠ ALERT** Short- and long-term drug exposure is associated with serious liver injury leading to organ transplant or death. Drug use longer than 2 weeks significantly increases this risk.
■ Don't use if a safer, alternative antibiotic is available.

### Therapeutic monitoring

■ Advise clinician to perform periodic assessment of liver function because drug increases ALT, AST, and alkaline phosphatase levels.
■ Advise clinician to monitor patient for neurologic complications.

### Special populations

**Breast-feeding patients.** Drug appears in breast milk. Because of unknown effects in infants, the risks of therapy and breast-feeding should be evaluated.
**Pediatric patients.** Safety and efficacy in children under age 18 haven't been established.
**Geriatric patients.** The pharmacokinetics don't differ between ages 19 and 78.

## Patient counseling

- Inform patient that drug may be taken without regard to meals; however, tell him to take vitamins, minerals, and antacids at least 2 hours before or after a trovafloxacin dose.
- Warn patient to avoid excessive sunlight or artificial ultraviolet light.
- Instruct patient to discontinue treatment, refrain from exercise, and seek medical advice if pain, inflammation, or rupture of a tendon occurs.
- Advise patient to promptly report symptoms of allergic reaction or diarrhea.
- Advise patient to promptly report signs of liver dysfunction (nausea, vomiting, abdominal pain, jaundice, dark urine, anorexia, pale stools, or fatigue) to prescriber and to stop drug.

---

# tuberculosis skin test antigens

## tuberculin purified protein derivative (PPD)

Aplisol, Tubersol

## tuberculin cutaneous multiple-puncture device

Aplitest (PPD), Mono-Vacc Test (Old Tuberculin), Sclavo-Test PPD, Tine Test (Old Tuberculin), Tine Test PPD

*Pharmacologic classification: Mycobacterium tuberculosis* and *Mycobacterium bovis* antigen
*Therapeutic classification:* diagnostic skin test antigen
*Pregnancy risk category C*

## Available forms

Available by prescription only
**tuberculin PPD**
*Injection (intradermal):* 1 tuberculin unit/0.1 ml, 5 tuberculin units/0.1 ml, 250 tuberculin units/0.1 ml
**tuberculin cutaneous multiple-puncture device**
*Test:* 25 devices/pack

## Indications and dosages

*Diagnosis of tuberculosis; evaluation of immunocompetence in patients with cancer or malnutrition*
*Adults and children:* Intradermal injection of 5 tuberculin units/0.1 ml.

A single-use, multiple-puncture device is used for determining tuberculin sensitivity. All multiple-puncture tests are equivalent to or more potent than 5 tuberculin units of PPD.

*Adults and children:* Apply unit firmly and without any twisting to the upper one-third of the forearm for about 3 seconds; this ensures stabilizing the dried tuberculin B in the tissue lymph. Exert enough pressure to ensure that all four tines have entered the skin of the test area and a circular depression is visible.

## Mechanism of action

*Diagnosis of tuberculosis:* Administration to a patient who is naturally infected with *M. tuberculosis* usually results in sensitivity to tuberculin and a delayed hypersensitivity reaction (after administration of old tuberculin or PPD). The cell-mediated immune reaction to tuberculin in tuberculin-sensitive individuals, which results mainly from cellular infiltrates of the dermis of the skin, usually causes local edema.

*Evaluation of immunocompetence in patients with cancer or malnutrition:* PPD is given intradermally with three or more antigens to detect anergy, the absence of an immune response to the test. The reaction may not be evident. Injection into a site subject to excessive exposure to sunlight may cause a false-negative reaction.

## Pharmacokinetics

*Absorption:* Local.
*Distribution:* Local.
*Metabolism:* None reported.
*Excretion:* None reported.

| Route | Onset | Peak | Duration |
|-------|-------|------|----------|
| Intradermal | 5-6 hr | 48-72 hr | Unknown |

## Contraindications and precautions

Severe reactions to tuberculin PPD are rare and usually result from extreme sensitivity to the tuberculin. Inadvertent S.C. administration of PPD may result in a febrile reaction in highly sensitized patients. Old tubercular lesions aren't activated by administration of PPD.

## Interactions

**Drug-drug.** *Aminocaproic acid, systemic corticosteroids:* Possible false-negative reactions. Don't use together.
*Live or inactivated viral vaccines:* Suppressed reaction. PPD antigen is used 4 to 6 weeks after immunization.
*Topical alcohol:* Possible inactivation of the PPD antigen and invalidation of test. Avoid use together.

## Adverse reactions

**Other:** local pain, pruritus, vesiculation, ulceration, or necrosis, hypersensitivity, *anaphylaxis,* Arthus reaction (type III hypersensitivity reaction).

---

## Overdose and treatment
None reported.

## Clinical considerations
■ *Positive reaction:* Induration greater than 2 mm, but consider further diagnostic procedures.
*Negative reaction:* Induration less than 2 mm.
**Tuberculin PPD**
■ Injection must be given intradermally or by skin puncture; an S.C. injection invalidates the test.
**Multiple-puncture device**
■ Reaction may be depressed in patients with malnutrition, immunosuppression, or miliary tuberculosis.

### *Therapeutic monitoring*
**Tuberculin PPD**
■ Read test in 48 to 72 hours. An induration of 10 mm or greater is a significant reaction in patients who aren't suspected to have tuberculosis and who haven't been exposed to active tuberculosis, indicating present or past infection. An induration of 5 mm or more is significant in patients with AIDS or in those suspected to have tuberculosis or who have recently been exposed to active tuberculosis. An induration of 5 to 9 mm is inconclusive in patients not suspected of having been exposed or having tuberculosis infection; therefore, test should be repeated if there's more than 10 mm of erythema without induration. The amount of induration at the site, not the erythema, determines the significance of the reaction.
**Multiple-puncture device**
■ Read test at 48 to 72 hours. Positive reactions may persist for up to 1 week.

### *Special populations*
**Pregnant patients.** Use during pregnancy only when clearly needed and with the understanding that result can be falsely insignificant reaction (Old Tuberculin multiple-puncture test).
**Breast-feeding patients.** There appears to be no risk to breast-feeding infants.
**Geriatric patients.** Geriatric patients not having a cell-mediated immune reaction to the test may be anergic or they may test negative.

## Patient counseling
■ Advise patient that test must be read in 48 to 72 hours.
■ Instruct patient to promptly report any unexpected adverse events.

# tubocurarine chloride
*Pharmacologic classification:* nondepolarizing neuromuscular blocker
*Therapeutic classification:* skeletal muscle relaxant
*Pregnancy risk category C*

## Available forms
Available by prescription only
*Injection:* 3 mg/ml parenteral

## Indications and dosages
*Adjunct to general anesthesia to induce skeletal muscle relaxation, facilitate intubation, and reduce fractures and dislocations*
Dose depends on anesthetic used, individual needs, and response. Doses listed are representative and must be adjusted. Dose may be calculated on the basis of 0.165 mg/kg.
*Adults:* Initially, 6 to 9 mg I.V. or I.M., followed by 3 to 4.5 mg in 3 to 5 minutes if needed. Additional doses of 3 mg may be given, if needed, during prolonged anesthesia.
*To assist with mechanical ventilation*
*Adults:* Initially, 0.0165 mg/kg I.V. or I.M. (average 1 mg), then adjust subsequent doses to patient's response.
*To weaken muscle contractions in pharmacologically or electrically induced seizures*
*Adults:* Initially, 0.165 mg/kg I.V. or I.M. slowly. As a precaution, 3 mg less than the calculated dose should be given initially.
*Diagnosis of myasthenia gravis*
*Adults:* Single I.V. or I.M. dose of 0.004 to 0.033 mg/kg.

## I.V. administration
■ I.V. administration requires direct medical supervision. Give drug I.V. slowly over 60 to 90 seconds or I.M. by deep injection in deltoid muscle.
■ Tubocurarine is usually administered by I.V. injection, but if patient's veins are inaccessible, drug may be given I.M. in same dose as given I.V.

### *Incompatibilities*
Incompatible with alkaline solutions, including barbiturates, sodium bicarbonate, and other drugs with high pH. Also incompatible with trimethaphan.

## Mechanism of action
*Skeletal muscle relaxant action:* Tubocurarine prevents acetylcholine from binding to receptors on motor end-plate, blocking depolarization. Tubocurarine has histamine-releasing and ganglionic-blocking properties, and is usually antagonized by anticholinesterase drugs.

## Pharmacokinetics
*Absorption:* Administered I.V. or I.M.
*Distribution:* After I.V. injection, drug is distributed in extracellular fluid and rapidly reaches its site of action. After tissue compartment is saturated, drug may persist in tissues for up to 24 hours; 40% to 45% bound to plasma proteins, mainly globulins.
*Metabolism:* Undergoes *N*-demethylation in the liver.
*Excretion:* About 33% to 75% of a dose is excreted unchanged in urine in 24 hours; up to 11% is excreted in bile.

| Route | Onset | Peak | Duration |
|-------|-------|------|----------|
| I.V. | 1 min | 2-5 min | 25-90 min (first dose; longer for subsequent doses) |
| I.M. | 10-25 min | Unknown | Unknown |

## Contraindications and precautions
Contraindicated in patients hypersensitive to drug and in those for whom histamine release is a hazard (asthmatic patients).

Use cautiously in geriatric or debilitated patients; in those with impaired hepatic or pulmonary function, hypothermia, respiratory depression, myasthenia gravis, myasthenic syndrome of lung cancer or bronchiogenic carcinoma, dehydration, thyroid disorders, collagen diseases, porphyria, electrolyte disturbances, fractures, or muscle spasms; and in women undergoing cesarean section.

## Interactions
**Drug-drug.** *Aminoglycoside antibiotics, beta blockers, calcium salts, clindamycin, depolarizing neuromuscular blockers, furosemide, general anesthetics, lincomycin, local anesthetics, other nondepolarizing neuromuscular blockers, other potassium-depleting drugs, parenteral magnesium salts, polymyxin antibiotics, quinidine or quinine, thiazide diuretics:* Enhanced or prolonged tubocurarine-induced neuromuscular blockade. Use cautiously. Advise clinician to monitor patient closely.
*Opioid analgesics, quinidine, quinine:* Increased respiratory depression. Advise clinician to monitor patient closely. Use cautiously.

## Adverse reactions
**CV:** hypotension, *arrhythmias, cardiac arrest, bradycardia.*
**GI:** increased salivation.
**Musculoskeletal:** profound and prolonged muscle relaxation, idiosyncrasy, residual muscle weakness.
**Respiratory:** *respiratory depression or apnea, bronchospasm.*
**Other:** hypersensitivity reactions.

## Overdose and treatment
Signs of overdose include apnea or prolonged muscle paralysis, which can be treated with controlled ventilation. Advise clinician to use a peripheral nerve stimulator to monitor effects and to determine nature and degree of blockade. Anticholinesterases may antagonize tubocurarine. Atropine given before or with the antagonist counteracts its muscarinic effects.

## Clinical considerations
■ The margin of safety between therapeutic dose and dose causing respiratory paralysis is small.
■ Drug doesn't affect consciousness or relieve pain.
■ Don't mix with barbiturates or other alkaline solutions in same syringe.
■ Renal dysfunction prolongs drug action.

### Therapeutic monitoring
■ Advise clinician to assess baseline tests of renal function and serum electrolyte levels before drug administration. Electrolyte imbalance, particularly potassium and magnesium, can potentiate effects of drug.
■ Advise clinician to monitor respirations closely for early symptoms of paralysis.
■ A nerve stimulator may be used to evaluate recovery from neuromuscular blockade.
■ Advise clinician to monitor blood pressure, vital signs, and airway until patient recovers from drug effects. Ganglionic blockade (hypotension), histamine liberation (increased salivation, bronchospasm), and neuromuscular blockade (respiratory depression) are known effects of tubocurarine.
■ After neuromuscular blockade dissipates, advise clinician to watch for residual muscle weakness.

### Special populations
**Breast-feeding patients.** It isn't known if drug appears in breast milk. Use with caution.
**Pediatric patients.** Give drug cautiously.
**Geriatric patients.** Give drug cautiously.

## Patient counseling
■ Reassure patient that he will be closely monitored throughout anesthesia.

# typhoid vaccine
Vivotif Berna

*Pharmacologic classification:* vaccine
*Therapeutic classification:* bacterial vaccine
*Pregnancy risk category C*

## Available forms
Available by prescription only
*Oral vaccine:* Enteric-coated capsules of 2 to $6 \times 10^9$ colony-forming units of viable *Sal-*

*monella typhi* Ty-21a and 5 to 10 × 10⁹ bacterial cells of nonviable *S. typhi* Ty-21a
*Injection:* Suspension of killed Ty-2 strain of *S. typhi;* provides 8 units/ml in 5-ml, 10-ml, and 20-ml vials
*Powder for suspension:* Killed Ty-2 strain of *S. typhi;* provides 8 units/ml in 50-dose vial with 20 ml diluent/dose

## Indications and dosages
*Primary immunization (exposure to typhoid carrier or foreign travel planned to area endemic for typhoid fever)*
**Parenteral**
*Adults and children over age 9:* 0.5 ml S.C.; repeat in 4 or more weeks.
*Infants and children ages 6 months to 9 years:* 0.25 ml S.C.; repeat in 4 or more weeks.
**Booster**
*Adults and children over age 10:* 0.5 ml S.C. or 0.1 ml intradermally q 3 years.
*Infants and children ages 6 months to 10 years:* 0.25 ml S.C. or 0.1 ml intradermally q 3 years.
**Oral**
*Adults and children over age 6:* Primary immunization—1 capsule on alternate days (such as days 1, 3, 5, 7) for four doses. Booster—repeat primary immunization regimen q 5 years.

## Mechanism of action
*Typhoid fever prophylaxis action:* Vaccine promotes active immunity to typhoid fever in 70% to 90% of patients vaccinated.

## Pharmacokinetics
None reported.

| Route | Onset | Peak | Duration |
|---|---|---|---|
| P.O., S.C., intradermal | After final dose | Unknown | 3-5 yr |

## Contraindications and precautions
Contraindicated in immunosuppressed patients and in those hypersensitive to vaccine. Advise clinician to defer vaccination in patients with acute illness. Oral vaccine shouldn't be given to patients with acute GI distress, such as diarrhea or vomiting.

## Interactions
**Drug-drug.** *Corticosteroids, immunosuppressants, sulfonamides, other anti-infectives active against* S. typhi, *phenytoin:* Possible impaired immune response to this vaccine. Avoid use together.

## Adverse reactions
**CNS:** malaise, headache.
**GI:** nausea, abdominal cramps, vomiting.
**Musculoskeletal:** myalgia.
**Skin:** rash, urticaria, swelling, pain, inflammation (at injection site).
**Other:** *fever, anaphylaxis.*

## Overdose and treatment
None reported.

## Clinical considerations
- Store injection at 36° to 50° F (2° to 10° C). Don't freeze.
- Store enteric-coated capsules at 36° to 46° F (2° to 8° C).
- It's essential that all four doses of oral vaccine be taken at the prescribed alternate-day interval to obtain a maximal protective immune response.

### Therapeutic monitoring
- Advise clinician to monitor patient for adverse reactions.

### Special populations
**Pregnant patients.** Use in pregnancy only when clearly needed.
**Breast-feeding patients.** It isn't known if typhoid vaccine appears in breast milk. Use with caution in breast-feeding women.
**Pediatric patients.** Parenteral typhoid vaccine isn't indicated for children under age 6 months. Oral typhoid vaccine isn't indicated for children under age 6.

## Patient counseling
- Advise patient that it's essential that all four doses of oral vaccine be taken at the prescribed alternate-day interval to obtain a maximal protective immune response.
- Tell patient to take oral vaccine capsule about 1 hour before a meal with a cold or lukewarm drink (not exceeding body temperature) and to swallow the capsule as soon as possible after placement in the mouth. Remind patient not to chew the capsule.
- Tell patient to expect the following after vaccination: pain and inflammation at the injection site, fever, malaise, headache, nausea, or difficulty breathing. These reactions occur in most patients within 24 hours and may persist for 1 to 2 days. Recommend acetaminophen for fever.
- Encourage patient to report adverse reactions.
- Inform patient that not all recipients of typhoid vaccine are fully protected. Travelers should take all necessary precautions to avoid infection.

---

\* Canada only  ◇ Unlabeled clinical use

# typhoid Vi polysaccharide vaccine
Typhim Vi

*Pharmacologic classification:* vaccine
*Therapeutic classification:* bacterial vaccine
*Pregnancy risk category C*

## Available forms
Available by prescription only
*Injection:* 0.5-ml syringe, 20-dose vial, 50-dose vial

## Indications and dosages
*Active immunization against typhoid fever*
*Adults and children ages 2 and older:* 0.5 ml I.M. as a single dose. Reimmunization is recommended q 2 years with 0.5 ml I.M. as a single dose, if needed.

## Mechanism of action
*Antibacterial vaccine action:* Typhoid Vi polysaccharide vaccine promotes active immunity to typhoid fever.

## Pharmacokinetics
*Absorption:* Antibody levels usually remain elevated for 12 months after vaccination. Because of the low incidence of typhoid fever in the United States, efficacy studies haven't been feasible.
*Distribution:* None reported.
*Metabolism:* None reported.
*Excretion:* None reported.

| Route | Onset | Peak | Duration |
|-------|-------|------|----------|
| I.M. | 2 wk | Unknown | 2 yr |

## Contraindications and precautions
Contraindicated in patients hypersensitive to any component of vaccine. Don't use to treat typhoid fever or give to those who are chronic typhoid carriers. Use cautiously in patients with thrombocytopenia or bleeding disorders and in those taking an anticoagulant because bleeding may occur following an I.M. injection in these individuals.

## Interactions
None significant.

## Adverse reactions
**CNS:** *headache, malaise.*
**GI:** nausea, diarrhea, vomiting.
**Musculoskeletal:** myalgia.
**Skin:** *local injection site pain or tenderness, induration, erythema at injection site.*
**Other:** *anaphylaxis;* fever.

## Overdose and treatment
None reported.

## Clinical considerations
■ Patients who should receive the vaccine include those traveling to or living in areas of higher endemicity for typhoid fever.
■ Although anaphylaxis is rare, advise clinician to keep epinephrine readily available to treat anaphylactoid reactions.
■ Delay administration of vaccine, if possible, in patients with febrile illnesses.
■ If vaccine is given to immunosuppressed patients or those receiving immunosuppressive therapy, the expected immune response may not be obtained.

### Therapeutic monitoring
■ Advise clinician to monitor patient for anaphylaxis and other adverse reactions.

### Special populations
**Pregnant patients.** Use in pregnancy only when clearly needed.
**Pediatric patients.** Safety and efficacy in patients under age 2 haven't been established.

## Patient counseling
■ Inform patient that immunization should be given at least 2 weeks before expected exposure. Tell him that, although an optimal reimmunization schedule hasn't been established, reimmunization with a single dose for United States travelers every 2 years, if exposure to typhoid fever is possible, is recommended at this time.

# urokinase

Abbokinase, Abbokinase Open-Cath

*Pharmacologic classification:* thrombolytic enzyme
*Therapeutic classification:* thrombolytic enzyme
*Pregnancy risk category B*

## Available forms

Available by prescription only
*Injection:* 5,000 IU/ml unit-dose vial; 250,000-IU/vial

## Indications and dosages

**Lysis of acute massive pulmonary emboli and of pulmonary emboli accompanied by unstable hemodynamics**
*Adults:* For I.V. infusion only by constant infusion pump; priming dose: 4,400 IU/kg over 10 minutes, followed with 4,400 IU/kg hourly for 12 hours.
**Coronary artery thrombosis**
*Adults:* 6,000 IU/minute of urokinase intra-arterial via a coronary artery catheter until artery is maximally opened, usually within 15 to 30 minutes; however, drug has been given for up to 2 hours. Average total dose, 500,000 IU.
**Venous catheter occlusion**
*Adults:* Instill 5,000 IU into occluded line.

## I.V. administration

■ Reconstitute drug by adding sterile water for injection to a concentration of 50,000 IU/ml.
■ Reconstitute drug immediately before use and discard any unused drug.
■ Reconstituted drug should be gently rolled and tilted, not shaken.
■ Further dilute the needed dose with normal saline solution or D₅W. The total volume of fluid administered should not exceed 200 ml.

### Incompatibilities

None reported; however, manufacturer recommends that urokinase not be mixed with other drugs.

## Mechanism of action

*Thrombolytic action:* Urokinase promotes thrombolysis by directly activating conversion of plasminogen to plasmin.

## Pharmacokinetics

*Absorption:* Administered I.V.
*Distribution:* Rapidly cleared from circulation; most drug accumulates in the kidneys and liver.
*Metabolism:* Rapidly metabolized by the liver.
*Excretion:* Small amount is eliminated in urine and bile. Half-life is 10 to 20 minutes; longer in patients with hepatic dysfunction.

| Route | Onset | Peak | Duration |
|-------|-------|------|----------|
| I.V. | Immediate | 20 min-4 hr | 4 hr |

## Contraindications and precautions

Contraindicated in patients with active internal bleeding, history of CVA, aneurysm, arteriovenous malformation, known bleeding diathesis, recent trauma with possible internal injuries, visceral or intracranial malignancy, ulcerative colitis, diverticulitis, severe hypertension, hemostatic defects including those resulting from severe hepatic or renal insufficiency, uncontrolled hypocoagulation, chronic pulmonary disease with cavitation, subacute bacterial endocarditis or rheumatic valvular disease, and recent cerebral embolism, thrombosis, or hemorrhage.

Also contraindicated during pregnancy and first 10 days postpartum; within 10 days after intra-arterial diagnostic procedure or any surgery (liver or kidney biopsy, lumbar puncture, thoracentesis, paracentesis, or extensive or multiple cutdowns); or within 2 months after intracranial or intraspinal surgery.

I.M. injections and other invasive procedures are contraindicated during urokinase therapy.

## Interactions

**Drug-drug.** *Aminocaproic acid:* Inhibited urokinase-induced activation of plasminogen. Avoid use together.
*Anticoagulants, including heparin and oral anticoagulants:* Increased risk of hemorrhage. Heparin must be stopped and its effects allowed to diminish. It may also be necessary to reverse effects of oral anticoagulants before beginning therapy.
*Aspirin, indomethacin, phenylbutazone, other drugs affecting platelet activity:* Increased risk of bleeding. Avoid use together.

## Adverse reactions

**CV:** *reperfusion arrhythmias,* tachycardia, transient hypotension or hypertension.
**GI:** nausea, vomiting.
**Hematologic:** *bleeding;* increased thrombin time, PTT, PT, and INR; decreased hematocrit.
**Respiratory:** *bronchospasm,* minor breathing difficulties.
**Other:** phlebitis at injection site, fever, *anaphylaxis,* chills.
**Skin:** rash.

## Overdose and treatment

Signs and symptoms of overdose include the following signs of potentially serious bleeding: bleeding gums, epistaxis, hematoma, spontaneous ecchymoses, oozing at catheter site, increased pulse, and pain from internal bleeding. Advise clinician to stop drug and restart when bleeding stops.

## Clinical considerations

■ Don't use bacteriostatic water to reconstitute.
■ Product contains no preservatives; discard unused portion.
■ Concurrent use of heparin may be indicated during intracoronary administration of drug. Advise clinician to monitor patient carefully for excessive bleeding.

### Therapeutic monitoring

■ Inform prescriber that drug may affect platelet function.
■ Patient should be monitored for signs of hemorrhage.

### Special populations

**Pregnant patients.** There are no adequate or controlled studies using urokinase in pregnant women. The drug shouldn't be used during pregnancy unless clearly needed.
**Breast-feeding patients.** It isn't known if drug appears in breast milk; use drug with caution in breast-feeding women.
**Pediatric patients.** Safety and efficacy in children haven't been established.
**Geriatric patients.** Patients ages 75 and older have a greater risk of cerebral hemorrhage because they're more apt to have preexisting cerebrovascular disease.

## Patient counseling

■ Explain use and administration of urokinase to patient and family.
■ Instruct patient to report adverse reactions promptly.

# valacyclovir hydrochloride
Valtrex

*Pharmacologic classification:* synthetic purine nucleoside
*Therapeutic classification:* antiviral
*Pregnancy risk category B*

## Available forms

Available by prescription only
*Caplets:* 500 mg, 1 g

## Indications and dosages

*Treatment of herpes zoster in immunocompetent patients*
*Adults:* 1 g P.O. t.i.d. daily for 7 days.
*Treatment of initial episode of genital herpes*
*Adults:* 1 g P.O. b.i.d. for 10 days.
*Treatment of recurrent genital herpes in immunocompetent patients*
*Adults:* 500 mg P.O. b.i.d. for 3 days.
*Chronic suppressive therapy of recurrent genital herpes in immunocompetent patients*
*Adults:* 1 g P.O. once daily. In patients with a history of 9 or fewer recurrences per year, an alternative dose is 500 mg once daily.
◊ *Chronic suppressive or maintenance prophylaxis of herpes simplex virus infections in patients infected with HIV*
*Adults and adolescents:* 500 mg P.O. b.i.d.
≡ *Dosage adjustment.* Dosage adjustments in renally impaired patients should be based on creatinine clearance levels.

## Mechanism of action

*Antiviral action:* Valacyclovir rapidly becomes converted to acyclovir. Acyclovir becomes incorporated into viral DNA and inhibits viral DNA polymerase, inhibiting viral multiplication.

## Pharmacokinetics

*Absorption:* Rapidly absorbed from GI tract. Absolute bioavailability of drug is 54.5%.
*Distribution:* 13.5% to 17.9% protein-bound.
*Metabolism:* Rapidly and nearly completely converted to acyclovir and L-valine by first-pass intestinal or hepatic metabolism.
*Excretion:* Excreted in urine and feces. Half-life of drug is about 1½ to 3⅓ hours.

| Route | Onset | Peak | Duration |
|-------|-------|------|----------|
| P.O. | 30 min | Unknown | Unknown |

## Contraindications and precautions

Contraindicated in patients with hypersensitivity or intolerance to valacyclovir, acyclovir, or components of the formulation and in immunocompromised patients.

Use cautiously in patients with impaired renal function and in those receiving other nephrotoxic drugs.

Thrombotic thrombocytopenic purpura and hemolytic uremic syndrome have occurred, resulting in death in some patients with advanced HIV infection, and in bone marrow transplant and renal transplant recipients participating in clinical trials of valacyclovir.

### Interactions
**Drug-drug.** *Cimetidine, probenecid:* Increased acyclovir blood levels. Advise clinician to monitor patient for possible toxicity.

### Adverse reactions
**CNS:** *headache,* dizziness, asthenia.
**GI:** *nausea,* vomiting, diarrhea, constipation, abdominal pain, anorexia.

### Overdose and treatment
There are no reports of overdose. However, precipitation of acyclovir in renal tubules may occur when the solubility (2.5 mg/ml) is exceeded in the intratubular fluid. If acute renal failure and anuria occur, hemodialysis may be helpful until renal function is restored.

### Clinical considerations
■ Initiate treatment as soon as possible after symptoms appear. Drug is most effective when initiated within 48 hours of the onset of zoster rash.
**⛌ALERT** Don't confuse valacyclovir with valganciclovir.

### Therapeutic monitoring
■ Advise clinician to monitor symptoms to determine success of therapeutic effect.

### Special populations
**Pregnant patients.** GlaxoSmithKline, the manufacturer, maintains an ongoing registry of women exposed to valacyclovir during pregnancy. Follow-up studies to date haven't shown an increased risk of birth defects in infants born to women exposed to this drug during pregnancy. Prescribers are encouraged to report such exposures to the manufacturer.
**Breast-feeding patients.** It isn't known if drug appears in breast milk. Use in breast-feeding women isn't recommended.
**Pediatric patients.** Safety and efficacy in children hasn't been established.
**Geriatric patients.** Dosage adjustment may be needed in geriatric patients based on underlying renal status.

### Patient counseling
■ Tell patient that valacyclovir may be taken without regard to meals.
■ Inform patient that valacyclovir isn't a cure for herpes but it may decrease the length and severity of symptoms.

■ Instruct patient to report adverse events promptly.

# valganciclovir
Valcyte

*Pharmacologic classification:* synthetic nucleoside
*Therapeutic classification:* antiviral
*Pregnancy risk category C*

### Available forms
*Tablets:* 450 mg

### Indications and dosages
***Active cytomegalovirus (CMV) retinitis in patients with AIDS***
*Adults:* 900 mg P.O. b.i.d. with food for 21 days; maintenance dose: 900 mg P.O. once daily with food.
***Inactive CMV retinitis***
*Adults:* 900 mg P.O. once daily with food.
**≡Dosage adjustment.** For patients with impaired renal function, if creatinine clearance (CrCl) is 40 to 59 ml/minute, induction dose is 450 mg P.O. b.i.d.; maintenance dose is 450 mg P.O. daily. If CrCl is 25 to 39 ml/minute, induction dose is 450 mg P.O. daily; maintenance dose is 450 mg P.O. every 2 days. If CrCl is 10 to 24 ml/minute, induction dose is 450 mg P.O. every 2 days; maintenance dose is 450 mg P.O. twice weekly.

### Mechanism of action
*Antiviral action:* Drug is a prodrug that is converted to ganciclovir, which inhibits replication of viral DNA synthesis of CMV.

### Pharmacokinetics
*Absorption:* Well absorbed from GI tract. Has higher absorption when taken with food.
*Distribution:* Minimal binding to plasma proteins.
*Metabolism:* Metabolized in intestinal wall and liver to ganciclovir.
*Excretion:* Eliminated renally.

| Route | Onset | Peak | Duration |
|-------|-------|------|----------|
| P.O. | Unknown | 1-3 hr | Unknown |

### Contraindications and precautions
Contraindicated in patients hypersensitive to valganciclovir or ganciclovir. Don't use in patients receiving hemodialysis. Use cautiously in patients with preexisting cytopenias and in those who have received immunosuppressants or radiation.

### Interactions
**Drug-drug.** *Didanosine:* Possible increased absorption of didanosine. Advise clinician to monitor patient closely for didanosine toxicity.

*Immunosuppressants, zidovudine:* Possible enhanced neutropenia, anemia, thrombocytopenia, and bone marrow depression when used concomitantly. Advise clinician to monitor CBC.
*Mycophenolate mofetil:* Possible increased levels of both drugs in renally impaired patients. Use together carefully.
*Probenecid:* Decreased renal clearance of ganciclovir. Advise clinician to monitor patient for ganciclovir toxicity.
**Drug-food.** *Any food:* Increased absorption of drug. Drug should be given with food.

### Adverse reactions
**CNS:** *headache, insomnia,* peripheral neuropathy, paresthesia, *seizures,* psychosis, hallucinations, confusion, agitation.
**EENT:** *retinal detachment.*
**GI:** *diarrhea, nausea, vomiting, abdominal pain.*
**GU:** *decreased creatinine clearance.*
**Hematologic:** NEUTROPENIA, *anemia, thrombocytopenia, pancytopenia, bone marrow depression, aplastic anemia.*
**Other:** catheter-related infection, *sepsis,* local or systemic infections, *pyrexia,* hypersensitivity reactions.

### Overdose and treatment
Overdose may cause severe, fatal bone marrow depression and renal toxicity. Treatment should include maintenance of adequate hydration and consideration of hematopoietic growth factors. Dialysis may be useful in reducing serum levels.

### Clinical considerations
■ Make sure to adhere to dosing guidelines for valganciclovir because ganciclovir and valganciclovir aren't interchangeable, and overdose may occur.
**◪ ALERT** Don't confuse valganciclovir with valacyclovir.
■ Cytopenia may occur at any time during treatment and increase with continued dosing. Cell counts usually recover 3 to 7 days after stopping drug.
■ No drug interaction studies have been conducted with valganciclovir; however, because drug is converted to ganciclovir, it can be assumed that drug interactions would be similar.
■ Drug may cause temporary or permanent inhibition of spermatogenesis.
■ Women of childbearing potential must use contraception during treatment. Men should use barrier contraception during and for 90 days after treatment.

#### Therapeutic monitoring
■ Toxicities include severe leukopenia, neutropenia, anemia, pancytopenia, bone marrow depression, aplastic anemia, and thrombocytopenia. Don't use if patient's absolute neutrophil count is less than 500 cells/mm³,

platelets are less than 25,000/mm³, or hemoglobin is less than 8 g/dl.
■ Advise clinician to monitor CBC, platelet counts, and serum creatinine levels or creatinine clearance values frequently.

### Special populations
**Breast-feeding patients.** It's unknown if drug appears in breast milk. Because of the possibility of serious adverse reactions in infants who are breast-fed, don't use in breast-feeding women.
**Pediatric patients.** Safety and effectiveness in children haven't been established.
**Geriatric patients.** Advise clinician to carefully monitor renal function before and during treatment. Use cautiously, keeping in mind the increased frequency of decreased hepatic, renal, or cardiac function; concomitant disease; or other drug therapy.

### Patient counseling
■ Inform patient to use contraception during treatment with this drug.
■ Advise patient to report any adverse effects.
■ Tell patient to take drug with food.

# valproic acid
Depakene

# divalproex sodium
Depakote, Depakote ER, Depakote Sprinkle

# valproate sodium
Depacon, Depakene

*Pharmacologic classification:* carboxylic acid derivative
*Therapeutic classification:* anticonvulsant
*Pregnancy risk category D*

### Available forms
Available by prescription only
**valproic acid**
*Capsules:* 250 mg
**divalproex sodium**
*Tablets (enteric-coated):* 125 mg, 250 mg, 500 mg
*Capsules (sprinkle):* 125 mg
*Tablets (extended-release):* 500 mg
**valproate sodium**
*Injection:* 5 ml single-dose vials
*Oral solution:* 250 mg/ml

### Indications and dosages
*Simple and complex absence seizures and mixed seizure types,* ◇ *tonic-clonic seizures*
*Adults and children ages 10 and older:* Initially, 15 mg/kg P.O. daily, divided b.i.d. or t.i.d.; may

increase by 5 to 10 mg/kg daily at weekly intervals up to a maximum of 60 mg/kg daily, divided b.i.d. or t.i.d. The b.i.d. dose is recommended for the enteric-coated tablets.

Note: Doses of divalproex sodium (Depakote) are expressed as valproic acid.
*Adults and children:* Initially, 10 to 15 mg/kg/day I.V. The dosage may increase by 5 to 10 mg/kg daily at weekly intervals up to a maximum of 60 mg/kg daily.
*Mania*
*Adults:* 750 mg P.O. in divided doses (divalproex sodium). Maximum dose is 60 mg/kg daily.
*Migraine prophylaxis*
*Adults:* 250 mg P.O. b.i.d. Some patients may benefit from doses up to 1 g daily. Or, 500 mg P.O. once daily of extended-release tablets for 1 week, then increased to 1 g once daily.
◇ *Status epilepticus refractory to I.V. diazepam*
*Adults:* 400 to 600 mg P.R. by enema or wax base suppository at 6-hour intervals.
≡*Dosage adjustment.* Reduce starting doses in geriatric patients and increase doses more slowly.

## I.V. administration
■ I.V. use is indicated only in patients who are unable to take drug orally.
■ Dilute drug in at least 50 ml of compatible diluent ($D_5W$, normal saline, or lactated Ringers).
■ Give drug as a 60-minute I.V. infusion (rate 20 mg/minute or less).

### Incompatibilities
None reported.

## Mechanism of action
*Anticonvulsant action:* Mechanism of action is unknown; effects may be from increased brain levels of gamma-aminobutyric acid (GABA), an inhibitory transmitter. Valproic acid also may decrease GABA's enzymatic catabolism. Onset of therapeutic effects may require a week or longer. Valproic acid may be used with other anticonvulsants.

## Pharmacokinetics
*Absorption:* Valproate sodium and divalproex sodium quickly convert to valproic acid after administration of oral dose; bioavailability of drug is same for all dose forms.
*Distribution:* Distributed rapidly throughout the body; drug is 80% to 95% protein-bound.
*Metabolism:* Metabolized by the liver.
*Excretion:* Excreted in urine; some drug is excreted in feces and exhaled air. Breast milk levels are 1% to 10% of serum levels.

| Route | Onset | Peak | Duration |
|-------|-------|------|----------|
| P.O. | Unknown | 15 min-4 hr | Unknown |
| I.V. | Unknown | 1 hr | Unknown |

## Contraindications and precautions
Contraindicated in patients hypersensitive to drug. Use cautiously in patients with history of hepatic dysfunction, and in children under age 2.

Don't give valproate sodium injection to patients with hepatic disease or significant hepatic dysfunction.

## Interactions
**Drug-drug.** *Clonazepam:* Absence seizures. Avoid use together.
*Felbamate, lamotrigine, salicylates:* Increased valproate levels. Advise clinician to monitor patient closely.
*MAO inhibitors, oral anticoagulants, other CNS antidepressants:* Potentiated actions of these drugs. Advise clinician to monitor patient closely.
*Phenobarbital, phenytoin, primidone:* Excessive somnolence. Advise clinician to monitor patient closely.
**Drug-lifestyle.** *Alcohol use:* Possible decreased valproic acid effectiveness and increased CNS adverse effects. Advise clinician to monitor patient closely.

## Adverse reactions
Because drug usually is used with other anticonvulsants, adverse reactions reported may not be caused by valproic acid alone.
**CNS:** *sedation,* emotional upset, depression, psychosis, aggressiveness, hyperactivity, behavioral deterioration, muscle weakness, tremor, ataxia, headache, dizziness, incoordination, hallucinations, abnormal dreams, amnesia, confusion, hostility, nervousness, speech disorder, abnormal gait, agitation, hypertonia, hypokinesia, insomnia, increased reflexes, paresthesia, myasthenia, tardive dyskinesia, thinking abnormalities, personality disorder, vertigo, malaise.
**CV:** chest pain, tachycardia, hypertension, palpitations, edema.
**EENT:** nystagmus, diplopia, abnormal vision, amblyopia, conjunctivitis, ocular pain, dry eyes, deafness, otic disorder, otic pain, tinnitus, rhinitis, sinusitis.
**GI:** *nausea, vomiting, indigestion,* diarrhea, abdominal cramps, constipation, increased appetite, anorexia, *pancreatitis,* fecal incontinence, flatulence, eructation, gastroenteritis, unspecified GI disorder, stomatitis, hematemesis, glossitis, dry mouth, periodontal abscess.
**GU:** dysmenorrhea, amenorrhea, vaginitis, metrorrhaggia, vaginal hemorrhage, dysuris, urinary incontinence, cystitis, urinary frequency.
**Hematologic:** *thrombocytopenia,* increased bleeding time, petechiae, bruising, eosinophilia, *hemorrhage, leukopenia, bone marrow suppression.*
**Hepatic:** *elevated liver enzyme levels, toxic hepatitis.*

---

**Metabolic:** weight gain.
**Respiratory:** increased cough, dyspnea, pneumonia.
**Skin:** rash, alopecia, pruritus, photosensitivity, erythema multiforme, seborrhea, dry skin, furunculosis, discoid lupus erythematous.
**Other:** fever, chills, injection site reactions, back pain, *allergic reaction.*

## Overdose and treatment
Symptoms of overdose include somnolence and coma. Overdose should be treated supportively; advise clinician to maintain adequate urinary output and monitor vital signs, fluid, and electrolyte balance carefully. Naloxone reverses CNS and respiratory depression but also may reverse anticonvulsant effects of valproic acid. Hemodialysis and hemoperfusion have been used.

## Clinical considerations
■ Therapeutic range of drug is 50 to 100 mcg/ml.
■ Drug shouldn't be withdrawn abruptly.
■ Advise clinician to give drug with food to minimize GI irritation. Enteric-coated formulation may be better tolerated.
■ Use of valproate sodium injection for periods of longer than 14 days hasn't been studied. Patients should be switched to oral products as soon as is clinically feasible. When switching from I.V. to oral therapy or from oral to I.V. therapy, the total daily dose should be equivalent and given with the same frequency.
■ Valproic acid may cause false-positive test results for urinary ketones.

### Therapeutic monitoring
■ Evaluate liver function, platelet count, and PT at baseline and at monthly intervals, especially during first 6 months of therapy.
■ Advise clinician to monitor plasma level and make dosage adjustments p.r.n.
■ Advise clinician to monitor patient for tremors, which may indicate need for dosage reduction.

### Special populations
**Pregnant patients.** Safe use during pregnancy hasn't been established; drug may cause teratogenic effects.
**Breast-feeding patients.** Valproic acid appears in breast milk in serum levels from 1% to 10%. An alternative to breast-feeding is recommended during therapy.
**Pediatric patients.** Children under age 2 are at higher risk for development of fatal hepatotoxicity. Use drug with extreme caution in children; benefits should be weighed against the risks.
**Geriatric patients.** Geriatric patients eliminate drug more slowly; lower doses are recommended. The safety and efficacy in patients ages 65 and older for the treatment of manic episodes from bipolar disorder or prevention of migraine headaches haven't been established.

## Patient counseling
■ Tell patient to report promptly any adverse events.
■ Instruct patient to take with food to reduce GI irritation.
■ Advise patient to avoid activities requiring mental alertness.

# valrubicin
Valstar

*Pharmacologic classification:* anthracycline
*Therapeutic classification:* antineoplastic
*Pregnancy risk category C*

## Available forms
Available by prescription only
*Solution for intravesical instillation:* 200 mg/5 ml

## Indication and dosages
*Intravesical therapy of bacillus Calmette-Guérin carcinoma in situ (CIS) of the urinary bladder in patients for whom immediate cystectomy would cause unacceptable morbidity or mortality risks*
*Adults:* 800 mg intravesically once weekly for 6 weeks.

## Mechanism of action
*Antineoplastic action:* Valrubicin is an anthracycline that exerts its cytotoxic activity by penetrating into cells, where it inhibits the incorporation of nucleosides into nucleic acids, causes extensive chromosomal damage, and arrests cell cycle in $G_2$. It also interferes with the normal DNA breaking-resealing action of DNA topoisomerase II, inhibiting DNA synthesis.

## Pharmacokinetics
*Absorption:* Only small quantities are absorbed into the plasma after intravesical administration.
*Distribution:* Penetrates into the bladder wall after intravesical administration. Systemic exposure is dependent on the condition of the bladder wall.
*Metabolism:* Metabolites of valrubicin were found in the blood.
*Excretion:* After retention, drug is almost completely excreted by voiding the instillate.

| Route | Onset | Peak | Duration |
|---|---|---|---|
| Intravesical | Unknown | Unknown | Unknown |

## Contraindications and precautions

Contraindicated in patients hypersensitive to drug or other anthracyclines or Cremophor EL (polyoxyethyleneglycol triricinoleate). Also contraindicated in pregnant patients and in patients with concurrent urinary tract infections, patients with a small bladder capacity (patients unable to tolerate a 75-ml instillation), and patients with a perforated bladder or patients for whom the integrity of the bladder mucosa has been compromised.

Use cautiously in patients with severe irritable bladder symptoms.

## Interactions

None reported.

## Adverse reactions

**CNS:** asthenia, headache, malaise, dizziness.
**CV:** vasodilation, chest pain, peripheral edema.
**GI:** diarrhea, flatulence, nausea, vomiting, abdominal pain.
**GU:** urine retention, *urinary tract infection, urinary frequency, dysuria, urinary urgency, bladder spasm, hematuria, bladder pain, urinary incontinence,* pelvic pain, urethral pain, nocturia, *cystitis,* local burning symptoms, *bladder irritation,* pelvic pain.
**Hematologic:** anemia.
**Metabolic:** hyperglycemia.
**Musculoskeletal:** myalgia, back pain.
**Respiratory:** pneumonia.
**Skin:** rash.
**Other:** fever.

## Overdose and treatment

There is no known antidote for overdoses of valrubicin. The primary anticipated complications of overdose associated with intravesical administration would be consistent with irritable bladder symptoms.

## Clinical considerations

■ Advise clinician to give drug no sooner than 2 weeks following transurethral resection or fulguration.
■ Drug has been shown to induce complete response in only about one in five patients with refractory CIS.
■ Use procedures for proper handling and disposal of antineoplastics.
■ Store unopened vials under refrigeration at 36° to 46° F (2° to 8° C). Diluted valrubicin is stable for 12 hours at temperatures up to 77° F (25° C).
■ Prepare and store solution in glass, polypropylene, or polyolefin containers and tubing. It's recommended that polyethylene-lined administration sets be used. Don't use polyvinyl chloride I.V. bags and tubing.
■ Recommend giving drug intravesically only, and only under the supervision of clinicians

experienced in the use of intravesical antineoplastics.
■ Aseptic techniques must be used during administration to avoid introducing contaminants into the urinary tract or traumatizing the urinary mucosa.
■ In patients with severe irritable bladder symptoms, bladder spasm and spontaneous discharge of the intravesical instillate may occur. Clamping of the urinary catheter isn't advised and, if performed, should be executed cautiously under medical supervision.

### Therapeutic monitoring

■ If there isn't a complete response of CIS to valrubicin treatment after 3 months or if CIS recurs, cystectomy must be reconsidered because delaying cystectomy could lead to the development of metastatic bladder cancer.
■ Myelosuppression is possible if drug is inadvertently administered systemically or if significant systemic exposure occurs following intravesical administration, such as in patients with bladder rupture or perforation. If valrubicin is given when bladder rupture or perforation is suspected, weekly monitoring of CBCs should be performed for 3 weeks. Myelosuppression begins during the first week, with the nadir by the second week, and recovery by the third week.
■ Advise clinician to monitor patient closely for disease recurrence or progression by cystoscopy, biopsy, and urine cytology every 3 months.

### Special populations

**Pregnant patients.** Women of childbearing age and men and their partners should be advised to avoid pregnancy during treatment. Effective contraception should be used during the treatment period.
**Breast-feeding patients.** It isn't known if valrubicin appears in breast milk, but because this drug is highly lipophilic and exposure of infants to the drug could cause serious health risks, women should discontinue breast-feeding before valrubicin therapy starts.
**Pediatric patients.** Safety and efficacy in children haven't been established.
**Geriatric patients.** There are no specific precautions regarding the use of valrubicin in geriatric patients who are otherwise in good health.

## Patient counseling

■ Inform patient that drug has been shown to induce complete response in only about 1 in 5 patients with refractory CIS. If there isn't a complete response of CIS to treatment after 3 months or if CIS recurs, tell patient to discuss with prescriber the risks for cystectomy versus the risks of metastatic bladder cancer.
■ Advise patient to retain drug for 2 hours before voiding, if possible. Instruct patient to void at the end of 2 hours.

- Instruct patient to maintain adequate hydration following treatment.
- Inform patient that the major adverse reactions are related to irritable bladder symptoms that may occur during instillation and retention of drug and for a limited period following voiding. For the first 24 hours following administration, red-tinged urine is typical. Tell patient to report prolonged irritable bladder symptoms or prolonged passage of red-colored urine immediately.
- Advise women of childbearing age and men and their partners to avoid pregnancy and to use effective contraception during the treatment period.

## valsartan
Diovan

*Pharmacologic classification:* angiotensin II antagonist
*Therapeutic classification:* antihypertensive
*Pregnancy risk category C (D in second and third trimesters)*

### Available forms
Available by prescription only
*Capsules:* 80 mg, 160 mg

### Indications and dosages
*Hypertension, used alone or with other antihypertensives*
*Adults:* Initially, 80 mg P.O. once daily as monotherapy in patients who aren't volume-depleted. Blood pressure reduction should occur in 2 to 4 weeks. If additional antihypertensive effect is needed, dosage may be increased to 160 or 320 mg daily or diuretic may be added. (Addition of diuretic has greater effect than dosage increases beyond 80 mg.) Usual dose range, 80 to 320 mg daily.

### Mechanism of action
*Antihypertensive action:* Blocks the binding of angiotensin II to receptor sites in vascular smooth muscle and the adrenal gland, which inhibits the pressor effects of the renin-angiotensin system.

### Pharmacokinetics
*Absorption:* Absolute bioavailability is about 25%.
*Distribution:* Doesn't distribute extensively into tissues; drug is 95% bound to serum proteins, mainly to serum albumin.
*Metabolism:* Only about 20% is metabolized. The enzymes responsible for valsartan metabolism haven't been identified, but they don't appear to be cytochrome P-450 enzymes.

*Excretion:* Excreted primarily through feces (83% of dose) and about 13% in urine. Average elimination half-life is about 6 hours.

| Route | Onset | Peak | Duration |
|-------|-------|------|----------|
| P.O. | 2 hr | 2-4 hr | 24 hr |

### Contraindications and precautions
Contraindicated in patients hypersensitive to drug. Also contraindicated in the second and third trimesters of pregnancy. Use cautiously in patients with renal or hepatic disease.

### Interactions
*Drug-drug. Diuretics:* Increased risk of excessive hypotension. Advise clinician to assess fluid status before using together and monitor patient carefully.

### Adverse reactions
**CNS:** fatigue, dizziness, headache.
**EENT:** pharyngitis, rhinitis, sinusitis.
**GI:** abdominal pain, diarrhea, nausea.
**Hematologic:** *neutropenia.*
**Metabolic:** hyperkalemia.
**Musculoskeletal:** arthralgia.
**Respiratory:** cough, upper respiratory tract infection.
**Other:** edema, viral infection.

### Overdose and treatment
Limited data are available. The most likely symptoms are hypotension and tachycardia; bradycardia could occur from parasympathetic (vagal) stimulation. If symptomatic hypotension occurs, institute supportive treatment.

### Clinical considerations
- Excessive hypotension may occur when drug is given with high doses of diuretics.
- Volume depletion and salt depletion should be corrected before therapy starts.

### *Therapeutic monitoring*
- Advise clinician to monitor patient for therapeutic effect and for excessive hypotension.
- Systolic blood pressure is considered the primary clinical endpoint.

### *Special populations*
**Pregnant patients.** Drug may cause fetal or neonatal morbidity and death if given during the second or third trimester.
**Breast-feeding patients.** Drug shouldn't be used in breast-feeding women.
**Pediatric patients.** Safety and efficacy in children haven't been established.
**Geriatric patients.** Although no overall difference in efficacy or safety was observed, greater sensitivity of some older individuals can't be ruled out.

---

## Patient counseling
- Inform women of fetal risk; advise patient to inform prescriber immediately if pregnancy occurs.

# vancomycin hydrochloride
Lyphocin, Vancocin, Vancoled

*Pharmacologic classification:* glyco-peptide
*Therapeutic classification:* antibiotic
*Pregnancy risk category C*

## Available forms
Available by prescription only
*Pulvules:* 125 mg, 250 mg
*Powder for oral solution:* 1-g, 10-g bottles
*Powder for injection:* 500-mg, 1-g, 5-g vials; 10-g pharmacy bulk package

## Indications and dosages
*Severe staphylococcal infections when other antibiotics are ineffective or contraindicated*
*Adults:* 500 mg I.V. q 6 hours, or 1 g I.V. q 12 hours.
*Children:* 40 mg/kg I.V. daily, divided q 6 hours.
*Neonates:* Initially, 15 mg/kg; then 10 mg/kg I.V. q 12 hours for first week of life; then q 8 hours up to age 1 month.

Note: The American Academy of Pediatrics (AAP) recommends that neonates less than 1 week of age receive 10 to 15 mg/kg every 12 to 18 hours (those weighing 2 kg or less) or every 8 to 12 hours (those weighing over 2 kg) and that neonates 1 week of age or older receive 10 to 15 mg/kg every 8 to 12 hours (those weighing 2 kg or less) or every 6 to 8 hours (those weighing over 2 kg). The AAP suggests that a dosing interval of 18 to 24 hours may be appropriate for very low birth weight infants (under 1.2 kg) during the first week of life, and recommends that neonates 4 weeks of age or younger weighing under 1.2 kg receive 15 mg/kg once every 24 hours.

The AAP suggests that children 1 month of age or older with mild to moderate infections receive 40 mg/kg I.V. daily in 3 or 4 divided doses and those with severe infections receive 40 to 60 mg/kg I.V. daily in 4 divided doses. For treatment of meningitis in children 1 month of age or older, 60 mg/kg daily (maximum 2 g daily) in divided doses every 6 hours.
*Antibiotic-associated pseudomembranous and staphylococcal enterocolitis*
*Adults:* 0.5 to 2 g P.O. daily in three to four divided doses for 7 to 10 days.
*Children:* 40 mg/kg P.O. daily, divided q 6 to 8 hours for 7 to 10 days. Don't exceed 2 g/day in children.
*Treatment of bacterial endocarditis caused by methicillin-resistant Staphylococcus*

*aureus or methicillin-susceptible staphylococci in patients with native cardiac valves*
*Adults:* 30 mg/kg daily I.V. in two equally divided doses (maximum dose is 2 g daily unless serum levels are monitored) for 4 to 6 weeks.
*Treatment of bacterial endocarditis caused by methicillin-resistant Staphylococcus aureus or methicillin-susceptible staphylococci in patients with prosthetic valve or other prosthetic material*
*Adults:* 30 mg/kg daily I.V. in two to four equally divided doses (maximum dose is 2 g daily unless serum levels are monitored) for 6 weeks or longer with oral rifampin and I.M. or I.V. gentamicin.
*Treatment of endocarditis caused by viridans streptococci or Streptococcus bovis*
*Adults:* 30 mg/kg daily I.V. in two equally divided doses (maximum dose is 2 g daily unless serum levels are monitored) for 4 weeks.
*Treatment of enterococcal endocarditis*
*Adults:* 30 mg/kg daily I.V. in two equally divided doses (maximum dose is 2 g daily unless serum levels are monitored) for 4 to 6 weeks in conjunction with I.M. or I.V. gentamicin for 4 to 6 weeks.
*Perioperative prophylaxis in patients undergoing surgery*
*Adults:* 1 g I.V. for one dose, just before procedures. If surgery is prolonged, additional intraoperative doses should be given every 4 to 8 hours for the duration of the procedure; additional doses are also advisable if substantial blood loss occurs.
◇ *Endocarditis prophylaxis for dental, GI, biliary, and GU tract surgery, or instrumentation procedures*
*Adults:* 1 g I.V.
*Children:* 20 mg/kg I.V.

Note: For both adults and children, give dose over 1 to 2 hours with the infusion completed within 30 minutes of the start of the procedure. High risk patients should also receive a single 1.5 mg/kg (maximum 120 mg) of gentamicin I.M. or I.V. within 30 minutes of the start of the procedure.
≡ *Dosage adjustment.* For patients with renal failure, adjust dosage based on degree of renal impairment, severity of infection, and susceptibility of causative organism. Base dosage on serum levels of drug.

Recommended initial dose is 15 mg/kg. Adjust subsequent doses, p.r.n. Some clinicians use the following schedule.

| Serum creatinine level (mg/dl) | Adult dosage |
|---|---|
| < 1.5 | 1 g q 12 hours |
| 1.5-5 | 1 g q 3-6 days |
| > 5 | 1 g q 10-14 days |

---

## I.V. administration
■ For intermittent infusion, reconstituted solutions containing 500 mg or 1 g of drug must be further diluted with at least 100 ml or at least 200 ml, respectively, or a compatible I.V. solution and given over at least 1 hour.
■ Thawed solutions of the commercially available frozen drug should be administered by I.V. infusion only. Thaw at room temperature or under refrigeration.
■ Rapid I.V. administration of drug should be avoided.
■ Advise clinician to monitor patient for hypotensive reaction.

### Incompatibilities
Incompatible with alkaline solutions, aminophylline, amobarbital, chloramphenicol, chlorothiazide, corticosteroids, heavy metals, heparin, methicillin, pentobarbital, phenobarbital, secobarbital, and sodium bicarbonate.

## Mechanism of action
*Antibacterial action:* Vancomycin is bactericidal by hindering cell-wall synthesis and blocking glycopeptide polymerization. Its spectrum of activity includes many gram-positive organisms, including those resistant to other antibiotics. It's useful for *Staphylococcus epidermidis* and methicillin-resistant *S. aureus.* It's also useful for penicillin-resistant *S. pneumococcus.*

## Pharmacokinetics
*Absorption:* Minimal systemic absorption occurs with oral administration; however, drug may accumulate in patients with colitis or renal failure.
*Distribution:* Distributed widely in body fluids, including pericardial, pleural, ascitic, synovial, and placental fluid. It will achieve therapeutic levels in CSF in patients with inflamed meninges. Therapeutic drug levels are 18 to 26 mcg/ml for 2-hour, postinfusion peaks; 5 to 10 mcg/ml for preinfusion troughs (however, these values may vary, depending on laboratory and sampling time).
*Metabolism:* Unknown.
*Excretion:* When administered parenterally, drug is excreted renally, mainly by filtration. When administered orally, drug is excreted in feces. In patients with normal renal function, plasma half-life is 6 hours; in those with creatinine clearance of 10 to 30 ml/minute, plasma half-life is about 32 hours; if creatinine clearance is less than 10 ml/minute, plasma half-life is 146 hours.

| Route | Onset | Peak | Duration |
|-------|-------|------|----------|
| P.O. | Unknown | Unknown | Unknown |
| I.V. | Unknown | Immediate | Unknown |

## Contraindications and precautions
Contraindicated in patients hypersensitive to drug. Use cautiously in patients with impaired renal or hepatic function, preexisting hearing loss, or allergies to other antibiotics; in those receiving other neurotoxic, nephrotoxic, or ototoxic drugs; and in patients over age 60.

## Interactions
**Drug-drug.** *Aminoglycosides, amphotericin B, capreomycin, cisplatin, colistin, methoxyflurane, polymyxin B:* Increased nephrotoxic effects. Advise clinician to monitor renal function.
*Nondepolarizing muscle relaxants:* Increased neuromuscular blockade. Avoid use together.

## Adverse reactions
**CV:** hypotension.
**EENT:** tinnitus, ototoxicity.
**GI:** nausea.
**GU:** increased BUN and serum creatinine levels, *nephrotoxicity.*
**Hematologic:** *neutropenia, leukopenia,* eosinophilia.
**Respiratory:** wheezing, dyspnea.
**Skin:** maculopapular rash on face, neck, trunk, and limbs (with rapid I.V. infusion), pain or thrombophlebitis at injection site.
**Other:** chills, fever, *anaphylaxis,* superinfection.

## Overdose and treatment
Little information is available on acute toxicity of vancomycin. Treatment includes providing supportive care and maintaining glomerular filtration rate. Hemodialysis and hemoperfusion have been used.

## Clinical considerations
**H *ALERT*** Oral administration is ineffective for systemic infections, and I.V. administration is ineffective for pseudomembranous (*Clostridium difficile*) diarrhea.
■ Instruct prescriber to obtain culture and sensitivity tests before starting therapy (unless drug is being used for prophylaxis).
■ I.M. administration is contraindicated because drug is highly irritating.
■ Hemodialysis and peritoneal dialysis remove only minimal drug amounts. Patients receiving these treatments require usual dose only once every 5 to 7 days; however, some dialysis centers use high-flux hemodialysis, which can remove up to 50% of vancomycin, creating a need for supplemental doses. Dose should be based on serum level of drug.

### Therapeutic monitoring
■ Advise clinician to monitor blood counts and BUN, serum creatinine, and drug levels.
■ If maculopapular rash develops on patient's face, neck, abdomen, and arms, infusion rate should be slowed.

---

■ If patient has preexisting auditory dysfunction or requires prolonged therapy, auditory function tests may be indicated before and during therapy.

### Special populations
**Pregnant patients.** It isn't known if vancomycin can cause fetal harm; avoid use during pregnancy and use only when clearly needed.
**Breast-feeding patients.** Drug appears in breast milk. Use with caution in breast-feeding women.
**Geriatric patients.** Geriatric patients may be more susceptible to ototoxic effects of drug. Advise clinician to monitor serum levels closely and adjust dosage p.r.n.

### Patient counseling
■ Instruct patient to take entire amount of drug, exactly as directed, for the full length of prescription.
■ Inform patient that relief from symptoms shouldn't be used as a guide for discontinuing therapy.

# varicella virus vaccine, live
Varivax

*Pharmacologic classification:* vaccine
*Therapeutic classification:* viral vaccine
*Pregnancy risk category C*

### Available forms
Available by prescription only
*Injection:* Single-dose vial containing 1,350 plaque-forming units of Oka/Merck varicella virus

### Indications and dosages
*Prevention of varicella-zoster (chickenpox) infections*
*Adults and children ages 13 and older:* Administer 0.5 ml S.C. followed by a second dose of 0.5 ml 4 to 8 weeks later.
*Children ages 1 to 12:* 0.5 ml S.C. as a single dose.

### Mechanism of action
*Antiviral vaccine action:* Varicella virus vaccine prevents chickenpox by inducing the production of antibodies to varicella-zoster virus.

### Pharmacokinetics
None reported.

| Route | Onset | Peak | Duration |
|-------|-------|------|----------|
| S.C. | 4-6 wk | Unknown | > 2 yr |

### Contraindications and precautions
Contraindicated in patients hypersensitive to drug, in pregnant women, and in those with history of anaphylactoid reaction to neomycin, blood dyscrasia, leukemia, lymphomas, neoplasms affecting bone marrow or lymphatic system, primary and acquired immunosuppressive states, active untreated tuberculosis, or any febrile respiratory illness or other active febrile infection.

### Interactions
**Drug-drug.** *Blood products, immune globulin:* Inactivate vaccine. Advise clinician to defer vaccination for at least 5 months following blood or plasma transfusions or administration of immune globulin or varicella-zoster immune globulin.
*Immunosuppressants:* Increased risk of severe reactions to live-virus vaccines. Routine vaccination should be postponed.
*Salicylates:* Reye's syndrome. Avoid use of salicylates for 6 weeks after varicella infections.

### Adverse reactions
**Other:** *anaphylaxis, fever, injection site reactions (swelling, redness, pain, rash),* varicella-like rash.

### Overdose and treatment
None reported.

### Clinical considerations
**◪ALERT** Administer immediately after reconstitution. Discard if not used within 30 minutes.
■ Advise clinician to have epinephrine available.
■ Vaccine has been safely and effectively used with measles, mumps, and rubella vaccine.
■ Vaccine appears to be less effective in adults compared with children.
■ Vaccine contains live attenuated virus. Children for whom a rash develops may be capable of transmitting the virus.
■ Primary immunization may be integrated with primary immunization against diphtheria, tetanus, pertussis, *Haemophilus influenzae* type B, and poliomyelitis. However, the vaccines should be administered at separate sites and with separate syringes.

### Therapeutic monitoring
■ Advise clinician to monitor patient for postadministration anaphylaxis.

### Special populations
**Pregnant patients.** Pregnancy should be avoided for 3 months after receiving vaccine.
**Breast-feeding patients.** It isn't known if varicella vaccine appears in breast milk. Use cautiously in breast-feeding women.
**Pediatric patients.** An investigational protocol program is available for children and adolescents with acute lymphoblastic leukemia in remission. Clinicians can contact the Varivax

---

coordinating center at 215-283-0897. Safety and efficacy haven't been established for children under age 1.

## Patient counseling

- Caution women of childbearing age to notify prescriber of suspected pregnancy before administration and to avoid pregnancy for 3 months after administration.
- Instruct patient to avoid salicylate use for 6 weeks after administration to prevent Reye's syndrome.
- Warn patient to avoid close contact with susceptible high-risk individuals during postinjection period.

---

# varicella-zoster immune globulin (VZIG)

*Pharmacologic classification:* immune serum
*Therapeutic classification:* varicella-zoster prophylaxis
*Pregnancy risk category D*

## Available forms

Available by prescription only
*Injection:* 10% to 18% solution of the globulin fraction of human plasma containing 125 units of varicella-zoster virus antibody in 2.5 ml or less

## Indications and dosages

**Passive immunization of susceptible patients, primarily immunocompromised patients after exposure to varicella (chickenpox or herpes zoster)**
*Adults and children:* 125 units per 10 kg of body weight I.M., to a maximum of 625 units. Higher doses may be needed in immunocompromised adults.

## Mechanism of action

*Postexposure prophylaxis:* This drug provides passive immunity to varicella-zoster virus.

## Pharmacokinetics

None reported.

| Route | Onset | Peak | Duration |
|-------|---------|---------|----------|
| I.M. | Unknown | Unknown | 1 mo |

## Contraindications and precautions

Contraindicated in patients with thrombocytopenia, coagulation disorders, immunoglobulin A deficiency, or history of severe reaction to human immune serum globulin or thimerosal.

## Interactions

**Drug-drug.** *Corticosteroids, immunosuppressants:* Possible interference with immune response to this immune globulin. Whenever possible, avoid using these drugs during the post-exposure immunization period.
*Live virus vaccines, such as measles, mumps, and rubella:* Reduced immune response. Don't administer live virus vaccines within 2 weeks before or 3 months after administering VZIG. If it becomes necessary to administer VZIG together with a live virus vaccine, advise clinician to confirm seroconversion with follow-up serologic testing.

## Adverse reactions

**CNS:** malaise, headache.
**CV:** chest tightness.
**GI:** GI distress.
**GU:** *nephrotic syndrome.*
**Musculoskeletal:** myalgia.
**Respiratory:** respiratory distress.
**Skin:** rash.
**Other:** *anaphylaxis,* discomfort at injection site, *angioedema,* angioneurotic edema, fever.

## Overdose and treatment

None reported.

## Clinical considerations

- VZIG is recommended primarily for immunodeficient children under age 15 and certain infants exposed in utero, although use in other patients (especially immunocompromised patients of any age, normal adults, pregnant women, and premature and full-term infants) should be considered on a case-by-case basis. It isn't routinely recommended for use in immunocompetent pregnant women because chickenpox is much less severe than in immunosuppressed patients. Moreover, it won't protect the fetus. VZIG isn't for use in immunodeficient patients with history of varicella, unless there's immunosuppression caused by bone marrow transplantation.
- For maximum benefit, VZIG should be given within 96 hours of presumed exposure.
- The chance of AIDS or hepatitis developing from VZIG is very small.

**H ALERT** Have epinephrine solution 1:1,000 available to treat allergic reactions.
- Recommend that clinician give only by deep I.M. injection. Never administer I.V. Advise clinician to use the gluteal muscle in infants and small children and the deltoid or anterolateral thigh in adults and larger children. For patients weighing over 10 kg (22 lb), give no more than 2.5 ml at a single injection site.
- False-positive results to serologic test for immunity to varicella-zoster virus may occur for a period of about 2 months after administration.

### Therapeutic monitoring

- Advise clinician to monitor patient for postadministration anaphylaxis, injection site reaction, and other adverse reactions.

## Special populations
**Pregnant patients.** Use drug during pregnancy only when clearly indicated. Exposure to varicella has caused congenital abnormalities (congenital varicella syndrome). Postexposure administration of VZIG during pregnancy may prevent or suppress clinical disease in the woman without preventing fetal infection.
**Breast-feeding patients.** It's unknown if VZIG appears in breast milk. Use cautiously in breast-feeding women.

## Patient counseling
■ Warn patient about local adverse reactions caused by drug administration; discuss use of acetaminophen for fever reductions and cool compresses for injection site discomfort.
■ Instruct patient to report serious adverse events promptly.

# vasopressin (antidiuretic hormone [ADH])
Pitressin Synthetic

*Pharmacologic classification:* posterior pituitary hormone
*Therapeutic classification:* antidiuretic hormone, peristaltic stimulant, hemostatic
*Pregnancy risk category C*

## Available forms
Available by prescription only
*Injection:* 0.5-ml and 1-ml ampules and vials, 20 units/ml

## Indications and dosages
*Nonnephrogenic, nonpsychogenic diabetes insipidus*
*Adults:* 5 to 10 units I.M. or S.C. b.i.d. to q.i.d., p.r.n.
*Children:* 2.5 to 10 units I.M. or S.C. b.i.d. to q.i.d., p.r.n.
*Postoperative abdominal distention*
*Adults:* 5 units I.M. initially, then q 3 to 4 hours, increasing dose to 10 units, if needed. Reduce dose for children proportionately.
*To expel gas before abdominal radiographic examination or kidney biopsy*
*Adults:* Inject 5 to 15 units S.C. at 2 hours, then again at 30 minutes before X-ray study. Enema before first dose may also help to eliminate gas.
◇ *Upper GI tract hemorrhage*
*Adults:* 0.2 to 0.4 units/minute I.V. or 0.1 to 0.5 units/minute intra-arterially. Dosage can be increased up to 0.9 units/minute, if needed.
◇ *Provocative testing for growth hormone and corticotropin release*
*Adults:* 10 units I.M.
*Children:* 0.3 units/kg I.M.
◇ *Cardiopulmonary resuscitation*
*Adults:* 40 units I.V. as a single dose.

◇ *Vasodilatory shock*
*Adults:* 0.02-0.1 units/minute as a continuous I.V. infusion.

## I.V. administration
■ Dilute to a concentration of 0.1 to 1 unit/ml using $D_5W$ or normal saline solution.
■ Give by continuous I.V. using a controlled infusion device.
■ Store drug at 59° to 86° F (15° to 30° C); don't freeze.

## Incompatibilities
None reported.

## Mechanism of action
*Antidiuretic action:* Vasopressin is used as an antidiuretic to control or prevent signs and complications of neurogenic diabetes insipidus. Acting primarily at the renal tubular level, vasopressin increases cAMP, which increases water permeability at the renal tubule and collecting duct, resulting in increased urine osmolality and decreased urinary flow rate.
*Hemostatic action:* In patients with GI hemorrhage, vasopressin, administered I.V. or intra-arterially into the superior mesenteric artery, controls bleeding of esophageal varices by directly stimulating vasoconstriction of capillaries and small arterioles.
*Peristaltic stimulant action:* Used to treat postoperative abdominal distention and to facilitate abdominal radiographic procedures, vasopressin induces peristalsis by directly stimulating contraction of smooth muscle in the GI tract.

## Pharmacokinetics
*Absorption:* Destroyed by trypsin in the GI tract and must be administered intranasally or parenterally.
*Distribution:* Distributed throughout the extracellular fluid, with no evidence of protein-binding.
*Metabolism:* Most of dose is destroyed rapidly in the liver and kidneys.
*Excretion:* About 5% of an S.C. dose is excreted unchanged in urine after 4 hours.

| Route | Onset | Peak | Duration |
|-------|-------|------|----------|
| I.M., S.C. | 2-8 hr | Unknown | Unknown |
| I.V. | Unknown | Unknown | Unknown |

## Contraindications and precautions
Contraindicated in patients with known anaphylaxis or those hypersensitive to vasopressin or its components. Also, contraindicated in patients with chronic nephritis accompanied by nitrogen retention.
    Use cautiously in patients with seizure disorders, migraine headache, asthma, CV or renal disease, HF, goiter with cardiac complications, arteriosclerosis, or fluid overload; in children, geriatric patients, and pregnant women;

and in preoperative or postoperative patients who are polyuric.

## Interactions

**Drug-drug.** *Carbamazepine, chlorpropamide, clofibrate:* Possible potentiation of antidiuretic effect of vasopressin. Advise clinician to monitor fluid balance and renal function.

*Demeclocycline, epinephrine, heparin, lithium, norepinephrine:* Decreased antidiuretic effect. Advise clinician to monitor fluid balance and renal function.

**Drug-lifestyle.** *Alcohol use:* Reduced antidiuretic activity. Advise patient to avoid alcohol.

## Adverse reactions

**CNS:** tremor, headache, vertigo.
**CV:** angina in patients with vascular disease; vasoconstriction, *arrhythmias, cardiac arrest,* myocardial ischemia, circumoral pallor, decreased cardiac output.
**GI:** abdominal cramps, nausea, vomiting, flatulence.
**Skin:** *cutaneous gangrene,* diaphoresis.
**Other:** *water intoxication* (drowsiness, listlessness, headache, confusion, weight gain, *seizures, coma),* hypersensitivity reactions (urticaria, *angioedema, bronchoconstriction, anaphylaxis).*

## Overdose and treatment

Signs and symptoms of overdose include drowsiness, listlessness, headache, confusion, anuria, and weight gain (water intoxication). Treatment requires water restriction and temporary withdrawal of vasopressin until polyuria occurs. Severe water intoxication may require osmotic diuresis with mannitol, hypertonic dextrose, or urea, either alone or with furosemide.

## Clinical considerations

- Administration during first stage of labor may cause ruptured uterus.
- Extravasation carries the risk of necrosis and gangrene.

### Therapeutic monitoring

- Advise clinician to establish baseline vital signs and intake and output ratio when therapy starts.
- Advise clinician to monitor patient's blood pressure b.i.d. and watch for excessively elevated blood pressure or lack of response to drug, which may be indicated by hypotension. Also advise clinician to monitor fluid intake and output and daily weight.
- Advise clinician to monitor patient for signs of water intoxication and hypersensitivity reactions.

### Special populations

**Pregnant patients.** Use drug during pregnancy only when clearly indicated because of its potential for producing tonic uterine contractions.
**Breast-feeding patients.** Use caution.
**Pediatric patients.** Children show increased sensitivity to the effects of vasopressin. Use with caution. Safety and efficacy in pediatric advanced life support haven't been established.
**Geriatric patients.** Geriatric patients show increased sensitivity to the effects of vasopressin. Use with caution.

## Patient counseling

- Advise patient that rotation of injection sites reduces risk of tissue damage.
- Instruct patient to report serious adverse events promptly.

# vecuronium bromide

Norcuron

*Pharmacologic classification:* nondepolarizing neuromuscular blocker
*Therapeutic classification:* skeletal muscle relaxant
*Pregnancy risk category C*

## Available forms

Available by prescription only
*Injection:* 10 mg (with or without diluent), 20 mg (without diluent)

## Indications and dosages

*Adjunct to anesthesia, to facilitate intubation, and to provide skeletal muscle relaxation during surgery or mechanical ventilation*

Dose depends on anesthetic used, individual needs, and response. Doses are representative and must be adjusted.

*Adults and children ages 10 and older:* Initially, 0.08 to 0.10 mg/kg I.V. bolus. Higher initial doses (up to 0.3 mg/kg) may be used for rapid onset. Maintenance doses of 0.010 to 0.015 mg/kg within 25 to 40 minutes of initial dose should be given during prolonged surgical procedures. Maintenance doses may be given q 12 to 15 minutes in patients receiving balanced anesthetic.

Alternatively, after the initial dosing of 0.08 to 0.10 mg/kg, a continuous infusion of 1 mcg/kg/minute may be initiated 20 to 40 minutes later.

## I.V. administration

- Diluent supplied by manufacturer contains benzyl alcohol, which isn't intended for use in neonates.
- Reconstitute using diluent supplied by manufacturer (bacteriostatic water for injection) or a compatible solution, such as normal saline, $D_5W$, sterile water for injection, 5% dextrose in normal saline, or lactated Ringer's, to produce a solution containing 1 mg/ml or 2 mg/ml.

- Protect solution from light.
- After reconstitution, store solution in refrigerator or at room temperature not exceeding 86° F (30° C). Don't use if discolored.
- Advise clinician to give only by rapid I.V. injection or I.V. infusion and accompany with adequate anesthesia.

### Incompatibilities
**H ALERT** Drug must not be mixed in same syringe or given through same needle as barbiturates or other alkaline solutions.

### Mechanism of action
*Skeletal muscle relaxant action:* Vecuronium prevents acetylcholine from binding to receptors on motor end-plate, blocking depolarization. Vecuronium exhibits minimal CV effects and doesn't appear to alter heart rate or rhythm, systolic or diastolic blood pressure, cardiac output, systemic vascular resistance, or mean arterial pressure. It has little or no histamine-releasing properties.

### Pharmacokinetics
*Absorption:* Administered I.V.
*Distribution:* After I.V. administration, drug is distributed in extracellular fluid and rapidly reaches its site of action. It is 60% to 90% plasma protein–bound. Volume of distribution is decreased in children under age 1 and may be decreased in geriatric patients.
*Metabolism:* Undergoes rapid and extensive hepatic metabolism.
*Excretion:* Drug and its metabolites appear to be primarily excreted in feces by biliary elimination; it's also excreted in urine.

| Route | Onset | Peak | Duration |
|-------|-------|------|----------|
| I.V. | 1 min | 3-5 min | 15-25 min |

### Contraindications and precautions
Contraindicated in patients hypersensitive to vecuronium and bromides. Use cautiously in patients with altered circulation caused by CV disease and edematous states, hepatic disease, severe obesity, bronchogenic carcinoma, electrolyte disturbances, or neuromuscular diseases and in geriatric patients.

### Interactions
**Drug-drug.** *Aminoglycosides, clindamycin, depolarizing neuromuscular blockers, furosemide, general anesthetics (decrease dose by 15%, especially with enflurane and isoflurane), lincomycin, other nondepolarizing neuromuscular blockers, other potassium-depleting drugs, parenteral magnesium salts, polymyxin antibiotics, quinidine or quinine, thiazide diuretics:* Increased vecuronium-induced neuromuscular blockade. Use cautiously during and after surgery.

*Anticholinesterases:* Antagonized effects of vecuronium. Use with extreme caution. Advise clinician to monitor patient closely.
*Narcotic (opioid) analgesics:* Increased central respiratory depression. Use with extreme caution. Advise clinician to monitor patient closely.

### Adverse reactions
**Respiratory:** *prolonged, dose-related respiratory insufficiency or apnea.*
**Other:** skeletal muscle weakness.

### Overdose and treatment
Signs and symptoms of overdose include prolonged duration of neuromuscular blockade, skeletal muscle weakness, decreased respiratory reserve, low tidal volume, and apnea. Treatment is supportive and symptomatic. Advise clinician to keep airway clear and maintain adequate ventilation.

Advise clinician to use peripheral nerve stimulator to determine and monitor the degree of blockade. Advise clinician to give an anticholinesterase, such as edrophonium, neostigmine, or pyridostigmine, to reverse neuromuscular blockade and atropine or glycopyrrolate to overcome muscarinic effects.

### Clinical considerations
- Drug doesn't relieve pain or affect consciousness.
**H ALERT** Apply a bright label with WARNING: PARALYTIC AGENT if drug is prepared ahead of time as a premixed syringe. Store in a safe place. Be aware of careful drug calculation. Always verify with a second individual.
- Emergency respiratory support equipment should be immediately available.

### Therapeutic monitoring
- Advise clinician to assess baseline serum electrolyte levels, acid-base balance, and renal and hepatic function before administration.
- Peripheral nerve stimulator may be used to identify residual paralysis during recovery and is especially useful during administration to high-risk patients.
- After procedure, advise clinician to monitor vital signs at least every 15 minutes until patient is stable, then every 30 minutes for next 2 hours. Advise clinician to monitor airway and pattern of respirations until patient has recovered from drug effects. Anticipate problems with ventilation in obese patients and those with myasthenia gravis or other neuromuscular disease.
- Recovery from neuromuscular blockade is evaluated by checking strength of hand grip and by patient's ability to breathe naturally, to take deep breaths and cough, to keep eyes open, and to lift head, keeping mouth closed.

### Special populations
**Pregnant patients.** Use drug during pregnancy only when clearly indicated.
**Breast-feeding patients.** It isn't known if drug appears in breast milk. Use with caution.
**Pediatric patients.** Safety and efficacy haven't been established in infants under age 7 weeks. Infants ages 7 weeks to 1 year are more sensitive to neuromuscular blocking effects; less frequent administration may be needed. Higher doses may be needed in children ages 1 to 9.
**Geriatric patients.** Use caution.

### Patient counseling
- Reassure patient that he will be carefully monitored during anesthesia.

---

# venlafaxine hydrochloride
Effexor, Effexor XR

*Pharmacologic classification:* neuronal serotonin, norepinephrine, dopamine reuptake inhibitor
*Therapeutic classification:* antidepressant
*Pregnancy risk category C*

### Available forms
Available by prescription only
*Capsules (extended-release):* 37.5 mg, 75 mg, 150 mg
*Tablets:* 25 mg, 37.5 mg, 50 mg, 75 mg, 100 mg

### Indications and dosages
*Depression*
*Adults:* Initially, 75 mg P.O. daily, in two or three divided doses with food. Increase dosage as tolerated and needed in increments of 75 mg/day at intervals of no less than 4 days. For moderately depressed outpatients, usual maximum dose is 225 mg/day; in certain severely depressed patients, dose may be as high as 375 mg/day divided into three doses. For extended-release capsules, 75 mg P.O. daily, in a single dose. For some patients, it may be desirable to start at 37.5 mg P.O. daily for 4 to 7 days before increasing to 75 mg daily. Dosage may be increased at increments of 75 mg/day q 4 days to a maximum of 225 mg/day.
*Generalized anxiety disorder*
*Adults:* 75 mg P.O. once daily (extended-release capsules). For some patients, it may be desirable to start at 37.5 mg P.O. daily for 4 to 7 days before increasing to 75 mg daily. Dosage may be increased at increments of 75 mg/day q 4 days to a maximum of 225 mg/day.
*Prevention of major depressive disorder relapse*
*Adults:* 75 to 225 mg/day P.O. (Effexor), or 75 to 150 mg/day P.O. (Effexor XR).
≡ *Dosage adjustment.* Reduce dosage by 50% in patients with moderately impaired hepatic

function. For patients with moderate renal impairment (glomerular filtration rate of 10 to 70 ml/minute), reduce total daily dose by 25%. For hemodialysis patients, reduce dosage by 50% and withhold drug until after dialysis treatment.

### Mechanism of action
*Antidepressant action:* Venlafaxine is thought to potentiate neurotransmitter activity in the CNS. Venlafaxine and its active metabolite, O-desmethylvenlafaxine (ODV), are potent inhibitors of neuronal serotonin and norepinephrine reuptake and weak inhibitors of dopamine reuptake.

### Pharmacokinetics
*Absorption:* About 92% is absorbed after oral administration.
*Distribution:* 25% to 29% plasma protein–bound.
*Metabolism:* Extensively metabolized in the liver, with ODV being the only major active metabolite.
*Excretion:* About 87% of dose is recovered in urine within 48 hours (5% as unchanged venlafaxine, 29% as unconjugated ODV, 26% as conjugated ODV, and 27% as minor inactive metabolites).

| Route | Onset | Peak | Duration |
|-------|-------|------|----------|
| P.O. | Unknown | Unknown | Unknown |

### Contraindications and precautions
Contraindicated in patients hypersensitive to drug and within 14 days of MAO inhibitor therapy. Use cautiously in patients with impaired renal or hepatic function, diseases or conditions that could affect hemodynamic responses or metabolism, or history of seizures or mania.

### Interactions
**Drug-drug.** *Cimetidine:* Increased in venlafaxine level. Use with caution. Advise clinician to monitor patient closely.
*MAO inhibitors:* Possible precipitation of syndrome similar to neuroleptic malignant syndrome when used with venlafaxine. Don't start venlafaxine within 14 days of discontinuing therapy with an MAO inhibitor, and don't start MAO inhibitor therapy within 7 days of stopping venlafaxine.
**Drug-herb.** *Yohimbe:* Possible additive stimulation. Use together cautiously.

### Adverse reactions
**CNS:** *headache, somnolence, dizziness, nervousness, insomnia,* anxiety, tremor, abnormal dreams, paresthesia, agitation, *asthenia.*
**CV:** hypertension, vasodilation.
**EENT:** blurred vision.
**GI:** *nausea, constipation,* vomiting, *dry mouth, anorexia,* diarrhea, dyspepsia, flatulence.
**GU:** *abnormal ejaculation,* impotence, urinary frequency, impaired urination.

---

Reactions may be *common*, uncommon, *life-threatening*, or COMMON AND LIFE-THREATENING.

**Metabolic:** weight loss.
**Skin:** *diaphoresis,* rash.
**Other:** yawning, chills, infection.

## Overdose and treatment
Symptoms may range from none (most commonly) to somnolence, generalized seizures, and prolongation of the QT interval.

Treatment should consist of general measures used in managing any antidepressant overdose (ensuring an adequate airway, providing oxygenation and ventilation, monitoring cardiac rhythm and vital signs). General supportive and symptomatic measures also are recommended. Use of activated charcoal, induction of emesis, or gastric lavage should be considered. No specific antidotes are known for venlafaxine overdose.

## Clinical considerations
■ Drug causes sustained increases in blood pressure.
■ Drug may activate mania or hypomania.
■ When discontinuing drug therapy after more than 1 week, advise clinician to taper dose; when discontinuing after at least 6 weeks, advise clinician to gradually taper dose over 2 weeks.
■ Drug should be stopped in patient who develops seizures.

### Therapeutic monitoring
■ Regular monitoring of blood pressure is recommended. For patients who experience a sustained increase in blood pressure while receiving venlafaxine, either dose reduction or discontinuation should be considered.
■ Advise clinician to monitor patient for signs of mania, hypomania, and seizure activity.

### Special populations
**Pregnant patients.** Use drug during pregnancy only when clearly indicated.
**Breast-feeding patients.** Use cautiously in breast-feeding women.
**Pediatric patients.** Safety and effectiveness in children under age 18 haven't been established.
**Geriatric patients.** Patients may be more sensitive to drug's effects. Dosage should be initiated and adjusted cautiously.

## Patient counseling
■ Caution patient not to operate hazardous machinery until effects of drug are known.
■ Advise a woman to call prescriber if pregnancy is planned or suspected during therapy.
■ Instruct patient to call prescriber before taking other drugs, including OTC preparations, because of potential interactions.
■ Advise patient to avoid alcohol while taking venlafaxine.
■ Instruct patient to report rash, hives, or related allergic reaction.

# verapamil hydrochloride
Calan, Calan SR, Covera-HS, Isoptin,
Isoptin SR, Verelan, Verelan PM

*Pharmacologic classification:* calcium channel blocker
*Therapeutic classification:* antianginal, antihypertensive, antiarrhythmic
*Pregnancy risk category C*

## Available forms
Available by prescription only
*Tablets:* 40 mg, 80 mg, 120 mg
*Tablets (sustained-release):* 120 mg, 180 mg, 240 mg
*Tablets (extended-release):* 120 mg, 180 mg, 240 mg
*Capsules (sustained-release):* 100 mg, 120 mg, 180 mg, 200 mg, 240 mg, 300 mg, 360 mg
*Capsules (extended-release):* 120 mg, 180 mg, 240 mg
*Injection:* 2.5 mg/ml

## Indications and dosages
*Management of Prinzmetal's variant angina, unstable angina, and chronic stable angina pectoris*
*Adults:* Initial dose of 80 mg P.O. every 6 to 8 hours. Dosage may be increased by 80-mg increments at weekly intervals. Some patients may require up to 480 mg daily. Or, 180 mg P.O. h.s. of Covera-HS (maximum dose 480 mg daily).
*Supraventricular tachyarrhythmias*
*Adults:* 0.075 to 0.15 mg/kg (5 to 10 mg) I.V. push over 2 minutes. Some clinicians recommend 2.5 to 5 mg (0.0375 to 0.075 mg/kg). If no response occurs, give a second dose of 10 mg (0.15 mg/kg) 30 minutes after the initial dose. Some experts recommend 5 to 10 mg I.V. every 15 to 30 minutes p.r.n. (maximum dose 20 mg).
*Children ages 1 to 15:* 0.1 to 0.3 mg/kg (2 to 5 mg) as I.V. bolus over 2 minutes. Dose shouldn't exceed 5 mg. Dose may be repeated in 30 minutes if no response occurs. The repeat dose shouldn't exceed 10 mg.
*Children under age 1:* 0.1 to 0.2 mg/kg (0.75 to 2 mg) as I.V. bolus over 2 minutes. Dose may be repeated in 30 minutes if no response occurs.
*Control of ventricular rate in digitalized patients with chronic atrial flutter or fibrillation*
*Adults:* 240 to 320 mg P.O. daily in three to four divided doses.
*Prophylaxis of repetitive paroxysmal supraventricular tachycardia (PSVT)*
*Adults:* 240 to 480 mg/day given in three to four divided doses.
*Hypertension*
*Adults:* 120 to 240 mg P.O. daily of extended-release capsules or tablets in the morning.

Dosage may be increased by 120 mg increments. Or, 180 mg P.O. daily h.s. of extended-release core tablets (Covera-HS). Dosage may be increased to 240 mg P.O. daily. Dosage may be further increased by 120-mg increments to maximum dose of 480 mg. Or, 200 mg P.O. daily of controlled extended-release capsules (Verelan-PM). Dosage may be increased to 300 to 400 mg P.O. daily h.s. Or, 40 mg P.O. b.i.d. to 80 mg P.O. t.i.d. of immediate-release preparation. Maximum dosage is 360 to 480 mg P.O. daily.

## I.V. administration
■ Drug should be given over a period not less than 2 minutes; or, in geriatric patients, not less than 3 minutes.
■ Drug should be given under continuous ECG and blood pressure monitoring.
■ Store injection at 59° to 86° F (15° to 30° C) and should be protected from light.

### Incompatibilities
Incompatible with albumin, aminophylline, amphotericin B, ampicillin sodium, cotrimoxazole, dobutamine, floxacillin, hydralazine, mezlocillin, nafcillin, oxacillin, sodium bicarbonate, and trimethoprim.

## Mechanism of action
*Antianginal action:* Verapamil manages unstable and chronic stable angina by reducing afterload, both at rest and with exercise, decreasing oxygen consumption. It also decreases myocardial oxygen demand and cardiac work by exerting a negative inotropic effect, reducing heart rate, relieving coronary artery spasm (via coronary artery vasodilation), and dilating peripheral vessels. The net result of these effects is relief of angina-related ischemia and pain. In patients with Prinzmetal's variant angina, verapamil inhibits coronary artery spasm, resulting in increased myocardial oxygen delivery.
*Antiarrhythmic action:* Combined effects of verapamil on the SA and AV nodes help manage arrhythmias. Primary effect of drug is on the AV node; slowed conduction reduces the ventricular rate in atrial tachyarrhythmias and blocks reentry paths in paroxysmal supraventricular arrhythmias.
*Antihypertensive action:* Verapamil reduces blood pressure, mainly by dilating peripheral vessels. Its negative inotropic effect blocks reflex mechanisms that lead to increased blood pressure.

## Pharmacokinetics
*Absorption:* Absorbed rapidly and completely from GI tract after oral administration; however, only about 20% to 35% of drug reaches systemic circulation because of first-pass effect.

*Distribution:* Steady-state distribution volume in healthy adults ranges from about 4.5 to 7 L/kg but may increase to 12 L/kg in patients with hepatic cirrhosis. About 90% of circulating drug is plasma protein–bound.
*Metabolism:* Metabolized in the liver.
*Excretion:* Excreted in urine as unchanged drug and active metabolites. Elimination half-life is normally 6 to 12 hours and increases to as much as 16 hours in patients with hepatic cirrhosis. In infants, elimination half-life may be 5 to 7 hours.

| Route | Onset | Peak | Duration |
|---|---|---|---|
| P.O. | ½ hr | 1-2 hr | 8-10 hr |
| P.O. (extended) | ½ hr | 5-9 hr | 24 hr |
| I.V. | 1-5 min | Immediate | 1-6 hr |

## Contraindications and precautions
Contraindicated in patients hypersensitive to drug, severe left ventricular dysfunction, cardiogenic shock, second- or third-degree AV block or sick sinus syndrome except in presence of functioning pacemaker, atrial flutter or fibrillation and accessory bypass tract syndrome, severe HF (unless secondary to verapamil therapy), and severe hypotension. In addition, I.V. verapamil is contraindicated in patients receiving I.V. beta blockers and in those with ventricular tachycardia.

Use cautiously in geriatric patients and in patients with impaired renal or hepatic function or increased intracranial pressure.

## Interactions
**Drug-drug.** *Antihypertensives, quinidine:* Possible hypotension. Advise clinician to monitor blood pressure closely.
*Carbamazepine, cardiac glycosides, cyclosporine:* Possible increased serum levels of these drugs. Advise clinician to monitor serum levels. Digoxin dose should be reduced by 50%.
*Disopyramide, flecainide, propranolol, other beta blockers, including ophthalmic timolol:* Possible HF. Use together cautiously.
*Lithium:* Possible decreased or increased serum lithium levels. Advise clinician to monitor patient closely.
*Rifampin:* Possible decreased oral bioavailability of verapamil. Advise clinician to monitor patient for lack of effect.
**Drug-herb.** *Black catechu:* Possible additive effects. Discourage use together.
*Yerba maté:* Possible decreased clearance of yerba maté methylxanthines, causing toxicity. Discourage use together.
**Drug-food.** *Any food:* Increased absorption. Advise patient to take drug with food.
**Drug-lifestyle.** *Alcohol use:* Possible prolonged intoxicating effects of alcohol. Advise patient to avoid alcohol.

## Adverse reactions

**CNS:** dizziness, headache, asthenia.
**CV:** *transient hypotension, HF, bradycardia, AV block, ventricular asystole, ventricular fibrillation,* peripheral edema.
**GI:** *constipation,* nausea.
**Hepatic:** elevated liver enzyme levels.
**Respiratory:** *pulmonary edema.*
**Skin:** rash.

## Overdose and treatment

Effects of overdose are primarily extensions of adverse reactions. Heart block, asystole, and hypotension are the most serious reactions and require immediate attention.

Treatment may include administering I.V. isoproterenol, norepinephrine, epinephrine, atropine, or calcium gluconate in usual doses. Advise clinician to ensure adequate hydration.

For patients with hypertrophic cardiomyopathy, alpha-adrenergic drugs, including methoxamine, phenylephrine, and metaraminol, should be used to maintain blood pressure. (Avoid isoproterenol and norepinephrine.) Inotropic drugs, including dobutamine and dopamine, may be used if needed.

If severe conduction disturbances, such as heart block and asystole, occur with hypotension that doesn't respond to drug therapy, advise clinician to initiate cardiac pacing immediately, with CPR measures as indicated.

For patients with Wolff-Parkinson-White or Lown-Ganong-Levine syndrome and a rapid ventricular rate caused by hemodynamically significant antegrade conduction, synchronized cardioversion may be used. Lidocaine and procainamide may be used as adjuncts.

## Clinical considerations

■ Generic sustained-release verapamil tablets may be substituted only for Isoptin SR and Calan SR, not Verelan capsules. Capsule formulation should be given only once daily. When using sustained-release tablets, doses of more than 240 mg b.i.d. should be given.

■ Advise clinician to discontinue disopyramide 48 hours before starting verapamil therapy; don't reinstitute until 24 hours after verapamil has been discontinued.

■ Dosage should be reduced in patients with renal or hepatic impairment.

■ Reduced doses should be used in patients with severely compromised cardiac function and in those receiving beta blockers.

### Therapeutic monitoring

■ Advise clinician to monitor patient closely for signs of toxicity.

■ If patient is receiving I.V. verapamil, advise clinician to monitor ECG and blood pressure continuously.

■ During long-term combination therapy with verapamil and digoxin, advise clinician to monitor ECG periodically to observe for AV block and bradycardia.

■ Advise clinician to obtain periodic liver function test results.

■ Systolic blood pressure is considered the primary clinical endpoint.

### Special populations

**Pregnant patients.** Use drug during pregnancy only when clearly indicated.
**Breast-feeding patients.** Drug appears in breast milk. Breast-feeding should be discontinued during therapy.
**Pediatric patients.** Currently, only the I.V. form is indicated for use in children to treat supraventricular tachyarrhythmias.
**Geriatric patients.** Geriatric patients may require lower doses. Advise clinician to give I.V. doses over at least 3 minutes to minimize risk of adverse effects.

## Patient counseling

■ Instruct patient to report signs of HF, such as swelling of hands and feet or shortness of breath.

## vidarabine (adenine arabinoside)
Vira-A

*Pharmacologic classification:* purine nucleoside
*Therapeutic classification:* antiviral
*Pregnancy risk category C*

## Available forms

Available by prescription only
*Ophthalmic ointment:* 3% in 3.5-g tube (equivalent to 2.8% vidarabine)

## Indications and dosages

***Acute keratoconjunctivitis and recurrent epithelial keratitis caused by herpes simplex virus types 1 and 2***
*Adults and children:* Administer ½ inch (1.3 cm) ointment into lower conjunctival sac five times daily at 3-hour intervals.

## Mechanism of action

*Antiviral action:* Vidarabine is an adenine analogue. Its exact mechanism of action is unknown; presumably it involves inhibition of DNA polymerase and viral replication by incorporation into viral DNA.

## Pharmacokinetics

*Absorption:* No systemic absorption occurs with ophthalmic use.
*Distribution:* Only trace amounts are detected in the aqueous humor if the cornea is intact.
*Metabolism:* Metabolized into the active metabolite arabinosyl-hypoxanthine.

---

*Excretion:* Unknown.

| Route | Onset | Peak | Duration |
|-------|-------|------|----------|
| Ophthalmic | Unknown | Unknown | Unknown |

## Contraindications and precautions
Contraindicated in patients hypersensitive to drug or with sterile trophic ulcers. Use cautiously in patients receiving corticosteroids.

## Interactions
None reported.

## Adverse reactions
**EENT:** temporary burning, itching, mild irritation, pain, lacrimation, foreign body sensation, conjunctival injection, punctal occlusion, sensitivity, superficial punctate keratitis, photophobia.
**Other:** hypersensitivity reactions.

## Overdose and treatment
None reported.

## Clinical considerations
▪ Drug is effective only if patient has at least minimal immunocompetence.
▪ If there are no signs of improvement after 7 days or if reepithelialization hasn't occurred in 21 days, advise clinician to consider other forms of therapy. However, severe cases may require longer treatment. Advise clinician to continue drug for 5 to 7 days, b.i.d., to prevent recurrence.
▪ Definitive diagnosis of herpes simplex conjunctivitis should be made before administration of ophthalmic form.

### Therapeutic monitoring
▪ Advise clinician to monitor patient for signs of improvement and reepithelialization.

### Special populations
**Pregnant patients.** Use drug during pregnancy only when potential benefits justify possible risks to the fetus.
**Breast-feeding patients.** Because vidarabine has been shown to be tumorigenic, breast-feeding should be discontinued during drug therapy.

## Patient counseling
▪ Warn patient who is receiving ophthalmic ointment not to exceed recommended frequency or duration of therapy. Instruct him to wash hands before and after applying ointment.
▪ Warn patient against allowing tip of tube to touch eye or surrounding area.
▪ Advise patient to wear sunglasses if photosensitivity occurs.
▪ Instruct patient to store ophthalmic ointment in tightly sealed, light-resistant container.

# vinblastine sulfate (VLB)
Velban, Velbe*

*Pharmacologic classification:* vinca alkaloid (cell cycle–phase specific, M phase)
*Therapeutic classification:* antineoplastic
*Pregnancy risk category D*

## Available forms
Available by prescription only
*Injection:* 10-mg vials (lyophilized powder), 10 mg/10 ml vials

## Indications and dosages
Dosage and indications may vary. Check current literature for recommended protocol.
*Breast or testicular cancer, Hodgkin's and malignant lymphomas, choriocarcinoma, lymphosarcoma, neuroblastoma, lung cancer, mycosis fungoides, histiocytosis, Kaposi's sarcoma*
*Adults:* 0.1 mg/kg or 3.7 mg/m$^2$ I.V. weekly or q 2 weeks. May be increased in weekly increments of 50 mcg/kg or 1.8 to 1.9 mg/m$^2$ to maximum dose of 0.5 mg/kg or 18.5 mg/m$^2$ I.V. weekly, based on response. Dose shouldn't be repeated if WBC count goes to less than 4,000/mm$^3$.
*Children:* 2.5 mg/m$^2$ I.V. as a single dose every week, increased weekly in increments of 1.25 mg/m$^2$ to maximum of 7.5 mg/m$^2$.

## I.V. administration
▪ Follow institutional policy to reduce risks. Preparation and administration of parenteral form of drug are linked to carcinogenic, mutagenic, and teratogenic risks for personnel.
**◪ ALERT** Drug is fatal if given intrathecally; it's for I.V. use only.
▪ Inject drug directly into vein or tubing of running I.V. line over 1 minute. Drug is a vesicant; if extravasation occurs, stop infusion immediately and notify prescriber. The manufacturer recommends that moderate heat be applied to area of leakage. Local injection of hyaluronidase may help disperse drug, as ordered. Moderate heat may be applied on and off every 2 hours for 24 hours, with local injection of hydrocortisone or normal saline solution.
▪ Reconstitute drug in 10-mg vial with 10 ml of saline solution for injection. This yields 1 mg/ml. Refrigerate reconstituted solution. Protect solution from light and discard after 28 days.

## Incompatibilities
Incompatible with cefepime, furosemide, and heparin.

---

## Mechanism of action
*Antineoplastic action:* Vinblastine exerts its cytotoxic activity by arresting the cell cycle in the metaphase portion of cell division, resulting in a blockade of mitosis. Drug also inhibits DNA-dependent RNA synthesis and interferes with amino acid metabolism, inhibiting purine synthesis.

## Pharmacokinetics
*Absorption:* Administered I.V.
*Distribution:* Distributed widely into body tissues. Drug crosses the blood-brain barrier but doesn't achieve therapeutic levels in the CSF.
*Metabolism:* Metabolized partially in the liver to an active metabolite.
*Excretion:* Excreted primarily in bile as unchanged drug. A smaller portion is excreted in urine. Plasma elimination of vinblastine is described as triphasic, with half-lives of 3½ minutes, 1½ hours, and 24¾ hours for the alpha, beta, and terminal phases, respectively.

| Route | Onset | Peak | Duration |
|-------|---------|---------|----------|
| I.V. | Unknown | Unknown | Unknown |

## Contraindications and precautions
Contraindicated in patients with severe leukopenia, granulocytopenia (unless result of disease being treated), or bacterial infection. Use cautiously in patients with hepatic dysfunction.

## Interactions
**Drug-drug.** *Erythromycin:* Vinblastine toxicity. Use with caution. Advise clinician to monitor patient for signs of toxicity.
*Mitomycin:* Acute shortness of breath and severe bronchospasm. Advise clinician to monitor respiratory status closely.
*Phenytoin:* Possible decreased plasma phenytoin levels, requiring increased doses of phenytoin. Advise clinician to monitor phenytoin plasma level.

## Adverse reactions
**CNS:** *CVA,* depression, *paresthesia, peripheral neuropathy and neuritis, numbness, loss of deep tendon reflexes, muscle pain and weakness, seizures,* headache.
**CV:** hypertension, *MI.*
**EENT:** pharyngitis.
**GI:** *nausea, vomiting,* ulcer, bleeding, *constipation, ileus, anorexia,* diarrhea, abdominal pain, *stomatitis.*
**Hematologic:** *anemia, leukopenia* (nadir occurs days 4 to 10 and lasts another 7 to 14 days), *thrombocytopenia.*
**Metabolic:** *weight loss,* hyperuricemia.
**Respiratory:** *acute bronchospasm,* shortness of breath.
**Skin:** vesiculation, reversible alopecia; *irritation, phlebitis,* cellulitis, necrosis with extravasation.

## Overdose and treatment
Signs and symptoms of overdose include stomatitis, ileus, mental depression, paresthesia, loss of deep reflexes, permanent CNS damage, and myelosuppression.
    Treatment is usually supportive and includes transfusion of blood components and appropriate symptomatic therapy.

## Clinical considerations
**◨ ALERT** Don't confuse vinblastine with vincristine or vindesine.
■ Peripheral infusion increases risk of extravasation. Drug may be administered as an I.V. infusion through a central venous catheter.
■ Drug shouldn't be given more frequently than every 7 days to allow for review of effect on leukocytes.
■ Patients with liver disease may need reduced doses.
■ Risk of uric acid nephropathy can be reduced with generous oral fluid intake and administration of allopurinol.
■ Drug is less neurotoxic than vincristine.
■ Unlabeled use of drug is with cisplatin and mitomycin as an alternative for the treatment of non–small-cell lung cancer.

### Therapeutic monitoring
■ Review effect on leukocytes before administration of each dose.
■ Advise clinician to monitor patient for life-threatening acute bronchospasm reaction. This reaction is most likely to occur in patients also receiving mitomycin.

### Special populations
**Pregnant patients.** Drug may cause fetal toxicity when given during pregnancy.
**Breast-feeding patients.** It isn't known if drug appears in breast milk. However, because of risk of serious adverse reactions, mutagenicity, and carcinogenicity in infants, breast-feeding isn't recommended.
**Geriatric patients.** Patients with cachexia or ulceration of the skin (which is more common in geriatric patients) may be more susceptible to leukopenic effect of drug.

## Patient counseling
■ Inform women of childbearing age of the potential risks to pregnancy.
■ Encourage adequate fluid intake to increase urine output and facilitate excretion of uric acid.
■ Reassure patient that therapeutic response isn't immediate. Adequate trial is 12 weeks.
■ Advise patient to avoid exposure to people with infections and to report signs of infection or unusual bleeding immediately.
■ Reassure patient that hair should grow back after treatment has ended.

## vincristine sulfate
Oncovin, Vincasar PFS

*Pharmacologic classification:* vinca alkaloid (cell cycle–phase specific, M phase)
*Therapeutic classification:* antineoplastic
*Pregnancy risk category D*

### Available forms
Available by prescription only
*Injection:* 1 mg/1 ml, 2 mg/2 ml, 5 mg/5 ml multiple-dose vials; 1 mg/1 ml, 2 mg/2 ml preservative-free vials

### Indications and dosages
Dosage and indications may vary. Check current literature for recommended protocol.
*Acute lymphoblastic and other leukemias; Hodgkin's disease; lymphosarcoma; reticulum cell, osteogenic, and other sarcomas; neuroblastoma; rhabdomyosarcoma; Wilms' tumor; lung and* ◇ *breast cancer*
*Adults:* 10 to 30 mcg/kg I.V. or 0.4 to 1.4 mg/m² I.V. weekly.
*Children:* 1.5 to 2 mg/m² I.V. weekly. Maximum single dose (adults and children), 2 mg.
*Children weighing under 10 kg (22 lb) or body surface area less than 1 m²:* 0.05 mg/kg once weekly.
≡*Dosage adjustment.* Reduce dosage by 50% in patients with direct serum bilirubin level exceeding 3 ml/dl or other evidence of significant hepatic impairment.

### I.V. administration
■ Follow facility policy to reduce risks. Preparation and administration of parenteral form of drug are linked to carcinogenic, mutagenic, and teratogenic risks for staff.
■ Inject directly into vein or tubing of running I.V. line slowly over 1 minute. Vincristine is a vesicant; if it extravasates, stop infusion immediately and notify prescriber. Apply heat on and off every 2 hours for 24 hours. Administer 150 units hyaluronidase, as ordered, to area of infiltrate.
■ Protect solution from light.
■ Refrigerate injection at 36° to 46° F (2° to 8° C).

### Incompatibilities
Incompatible with cefepime, furosemide, idarubicin, and sodium bicarbonate.

### Mechanism of action
*Antineoplastic action:* Vincristine exerts its cytotoxic activity by arresting the cell cycle in the metaphase portion of cell division, resulting in a blockade of mitosis. Drug also inhibits DNA-dependent RNA synthesis and interferes with amino acid metabolites, inhibiting purine synthesis.

### Pharmacokinetics
*Absorption:* Administered I.V.
*Distribution:* Rapidly and widely distributed into body tissues and is bound to erythrocytes and platelets. Drug crosses blood-brain barrier but doesn't achieve therapeutic levels in CSF.
*Metabolism:* Largely metabolized in the liver.
*Excretion:* Drug and its metabolites are primarily excreted into bile. A smaller portion is eliminated through the kidneys. The plasma elimination of vincristine is described as triphasic, with half-lives of about 4 minutes, 2¼ hours, and 85 hours for the distribution, second, and terminal phases, respectively.

| Route | Onset | Peak | Duration |
|-------|-------|------|----------|
| I.V. | Unknown | Unknown | Unknown |

### Contraindications and precautions
Contraindicated in patients hypersensitive to drug or who have the demyelinating form of Charcot-Marie-Tooth syndrome. Don't give to patients who are also receiving radiation therapy through ports that include the liver.

Use cautiously in patients with hepatic dysfunction, neuromuscular disease, or infection.

### Interactions
**Drug-drug.** *Asparaginase:* Decreased hepatic clearance of vincristine. Advise clinician to monitor patient for toxicity.
*Calcium channel blockers:* Enhanced vincristine accumulation in cells. Advise clinician to monitor patient closely.
*Digoxin:* Decreased digoxin levels. Advise clinician to monitor serum digoxin levels.
*Methotrexate:* Increased therapeutic effect of methotrexate. This interaction may be used to therapeutic advantage; it allows a lower dose of methotrexate, reducing the potential for methotrexate toxicity. Advise clinician to monitor patient closely.
*Mitomycin:* Possible increased frequency of bronchospasm and acute pulmonary reactions. Advise clinician to monitor respiratory status.
*Other neurotoxic drugs:* Increased neurotoxicity through an additive effect. Use with caution. Advise clinician to monitor patient for toxicity.
*Phenytoin:* Possible decreased plasma phenytoin levels. Dosage adjustments may be needed. Advise clinician to monitor patient closely.

### Adverse reactions
**CNS:** *peripheral neuropathy,* sensory loss, *loss of deep tendon reflexes, paresthesia, wristdrop and footdrop,* **seizures,** **coma,** headache, ataxia, cranial nerve palsies, *jaw pain,* hoarseness, vocal cord paralysis, *muscle weakness and*

---

*cramps* (some neurotoxicities may be permanent).
**CV:** hypotension, hypertension.
**EENT:** diplopia, optic and extraocular neuropathy, hearing impairment, ptosis, photophobia, transient cortical blindness, optical atrophy.
**GI:** diarrhea, *constipation, cramps,* ileus that mimics surgical abdomen, paralytic ileus, *nausea, vomiting,* anorexia, dysphagia, *intestinal necrosis, stomatitis.*
**GU:** urine retention, dysuria, acute uric acid neuropathy, polyuria.
**Hematologic:** anemia, *leukopenia, thrombocytopenia.*
**Metabolic:** weight loss, *hyperuricemia,* hyponatremia, SIADH.
**Respiratory:** *acute bronchospasm,* dyspnea.
**Skin:** *reversible alopecia,* severe local reaction with extravasation, *phlebitis,* cellulitis at injection site.
**Other:** fever.

### Overdose and treatment

Signs and symptoms of overdose include alopecia, myelosuppression, paresthesia, neuritic pain, motor difficulties, loss of deep tendon reflexes, nausea, vomiting, and ileus.

Treatment is usually supportive and includes transfusion of blood components, antiemetics, enemas for ileus, phenobarbital for seizures, and other appropriate symptomatic therapy. Administration of calcium leucovorin at a dosage of 15 mg I.V. every 3 hours for 24 hours, then every 6 hours for 48 hours may help protect cells from the toxic effects of vincristine.

### Clinical considerations

◪ *ALERT* Don't confuse vincristine with vinblastine or vindesine.
■ Necrosis may result from extravasation.
■ Drug may be administered by I.V. push injection over 1 minute into the tubing of a freely flowing I.V. infusion.
■ Neurotoxicity is dose-related and usually reversible.
■ Risk of uric acid nephropathy is reduced with generous oral fluid intake and administration of allopurinol. Alkalinization of urine may be required if serum uric acid level increases.
■ Patients with obstructive jaundice or liver disease may need reduced dosage.

### Therapeutic monitoring

■ Advise clinician to monitor patient for neurotoxicity.
■ Advise clinician to monitor patient for life-threatening bronchospasm reaction.
■ Advise clinician to monitor patient for leukopenia and thrombocytopenia.

### Special populations

**Pregnant patients.** Vincristine may cause fetal toxicity and should be used during pregnancy only in life-threatening situations or in severe circumstances in which safer drugs aren't available.
**Breast-feeding patients.** It isn't known if drug appears in breast milk. However, because of risk of serious adverse reactions, mutagenicity, and carcinogenicity in the infant, breast-feeding isn't recommended.
**Geriatric patients.** Geriatric patients who are weak or bedridden may be more susceptible to neurotoxic effects. Use cautiously.

### Patient counseling

■ Inform women of childbearing potential of the possibility of fetal harm.
■ Encourage adequate fluid intake to increase urine output and facilitate excretion of uric acid.
■ Assure patient that hair growth should resume after treatment is discontinued.

# vinorelbine tartrate

Navelbine

*Pharmacologic classification:* semisynthetic vinca alkaloid
*Therapeutic classification:* antineoplastic
*Pregnancy risk category D*

### Available forms

Available by prescription only
*Injection:* 10 mg/ml in 1-ml and 5-ml single-use vials

### Indications and dosages

*Alone or as adjunct therapy with cisplatin for first-line treatment of ambulatory patients with nonresectable advanced non-small-cell lung cancer (NSCLC); alone or with cisplatin in stage IV of NSCLC; with cisplatin in stage III of NSCLC*
*Adults:* 30 mg/m$^2$ I.V. weekly. In combination treatment, same dosage used along with 120 mg/m$^2$ of cisplatin, given on days 1 and 29, then q 6 weeks.
≣*Dosage adjustment.* Adjust dosage based on hematologic toxicity or hepatic insufficiency.

### I.V. administration

■ Dilute concentrate with normal saline or D$_5$W to a final concentration of 1.5 to 3 mg/ml or in I.V. bag of normal saline, 0.45% normal saline, D$_5$W, 5% dextrose in half-normal saline solution, Ringer's injection, or lactated Ringer's to concentration of 0.5 to 2 mg/ml.
■ Administer by I.V. injection into a free-flowing I.V. over 6 to 10 minutes.

■ Flush after administration with at least 75 to 125 ml of normal saline or D₅W over 10 minutes.

## Incompatibilities
Incompatible with acyclovir, allopurinol, aminophylline, amphotericin b, ampicillin, cefazolin, cefoperazone, cefotetan, ceftizoxime, ceftriaxone, cefuroxime, fluorouracil, furosemide, ganciclovir, methylprednisolone, mitomycin, piperacillin, sodium bicarbonate, thiotepa, and TMP-SMZ.

## Mechanism of action
*Antineoplastic action:* Vinorelbine exerts its antineoplastic effect by disrupting microtubule assembly, which disrupts spindle formation and prevents mitosis.

## Pharmacokinetics
*Absorption:* Administered I.V.
*Distribution:* Binding to plasma constituents ranges from 79.6% to 91.2%. It shows high binding to human platelets and lymphocytes.
*Metabolism:* Undergoes substantial hepatic metabolism.
*Excretion:* About 18% is excreted in urine and 46% is excreted in feces. Terminal phase half-life averages 27½ to 43½ hours.

| Route | Onset | Peak | Duration |
|-------|-------|------|----------|
| I.V. | Unknown | Unknown | Unknown |

## Contraindications and precautions
Contraindicated in patients with pretreatment granulocyte counts less than 1,000 cells/mm³. Use with extreme caution in patients whose bone marrow may have been compromised by previous exposure to radiation or chemotherapy or whose bone marrow is still recovering from previous chemotherapy. Also use cautiously in patients with impaired hepatic function. Use in pregnancy only if benefit outweighs risk to fetus.

## Interactions
**Drug-drug.** *Cisplatin:* Increased risk of bone marrow depression. Advise clinician to monitor hematologic status closely.
*Mitomycin:* Possible pulmonary reactions. Advise clinician to monitor respiratory status closely.

## Adverse reactions
**CNS:** *fatigue, peripheral neuropathy, asthenia.*
**CV:** *chest pain.*
**GI:** *nausea, vomiting, anorexia, diarrhea, constipation, stomatitis.*
**Hematologic:** **bone marrow suppression** (*agranulocytosis,* LEUKOPENIA, *thrombocytopenia,* anemia).
**Hepatic:** *abnormal liver function test results, bilirubinemia.*

**Metabolic:** SIADH.
**Musculoskeletal:** jaw pain, myalgia, arthralgia.
**Respiratory:** dyspnea.
**Skin:** *alopecia,* rash, *injection pain or reaction.*

## Overdose and treatment
The primary anticipated complications of overdose are bone marrow suppression and peripheral neurotoxicity. Treatment includes general supportive measures and appropriate blood transfusions and antibiotics p.r.n. There's no known antidote.

## Clinical considerations
■ Drug may cause considerable irritation, localized tissue necrosis, and thrombophlebitis.
■ Drug may be a contact irritant and the solution must be handled and given with care. Use gloves. Avoid inhalation of vapors and contact with skin or mucous membranes, especially the eyes. If contact occurs, wash area with copious amounts of water for at least 15 minutes.
■ Dosage adjustment should be based on hematologic toxicity or hepatic insufficiency, whichever results in a lower dose. Dosage should be reduced by 50% if patient's granulocyte count goes to less than 1,500 cells/mm³ but exceeds 1,000 cells/mm³. If three consecutive doses are skipped because of granulocytopenia, drug therapy should be stopped.

### Therapeutic monitoring
■ Advise clinician to check patient's granulocyte count before initiating therapy. It should be 1,000 cells/mm³ or more for drug to be administered.
■ Advise clinician to monitor patient closely for hypersensitivity reactions.
■ Advise clinician to monitor patient's peripheral blood count and bone marrow to guide effects of therapy.

### Special populations
**Pregnant patients.** Drug may cause fetal toxicity and should be used during pregnancy only in life-threatening situations or severe conditions for which safer drugs aren't available.
**Breast-feeding patients.** It isn't known if drug appears in breast milk. Because of risk of adverse effects in breast-fed infant, don't use drug in breast-feeding women.
**Pediatric patients.** Safety and effectiveness in children haven't been established.

## Patient counseling
■ Instruct patient not to take other drugs, including OTC preparations, unless instructed.
■ Tell patient to report signs and symptoms of infection (fever, chills, malaise) because drug has immunosuppressive activity.
■ Inform patient of the risk of fetal toxicity.

---

Reactions may be *common,* uncommon, *life-threatening,* or COMMON AND LIFE-THREATENING.

# vitamin A (retinol)

Aquasol A, Del-Vi-A, Palmitate-A 5000

*Pharmacologic classification:* fat-soluble vitamin
*Therapeutic classification:* vitamin
*Pregnancy risk category A (X if dose exceeds RDA)*

## Available forms

Available by prescription only
*Tablets:* 10,000 IU
*Capsules:* 25,000 IU, 50,000 IU
*Injection:* 2-ml vials (50,000 IU/ml with 0.5% chlorobutanol, polysorbate 80, butylated hydroxyanisole, and butylated hydroxytoluene)
Available without a prescription, as appropriate
*Drops:* 30 ml with dropper (5,000 IU/0.1 ml)
*Capsules:* 10,000 IU
*Tablets:* 5,000 IU

## Indications and dosages

*Severe vitamin A deficiency with xerophthalmia*
*Adults and children over age 8:* 500,000 IU P.O. daily for 3 days, then 50,000 IU P.O. daily for 14 days, then maintenance dose of 10,000 to 20,000 IU P.O. daily for 2 months, followed by adequate dietary nutrition and RDA vitamin A supplements.
*Severe vitamin A deficiency*
*Adults and children over age 8:* 100,000 IU P.O. or I.M. daily for 3 days, then 50,000 IU P.O. or I.M. daily for 14 days, then maintenance dose of 10,000 to 20,000 IU P.O. daily for 2 months, followed by adequate dietary nutrition and RDA vitamin A supplements.
*Children ages 1 to 8:* 17,500 to 35,000 IU I.M. daily for 10 days.
*Infants under age 1:* 7,500 to 15,000 IU I.M. daily for 10 days.
　　The RDA for vitamin A is as follows.

| | Vitamin A RDA | Vitamin A and beta-carotene RDA |
|---|---|---|
| **Infants** | | |
| birth-12 months | 375 RE | 1,875 IU |
| **Children** | | |
| ages 1-3 | 400 RE | 2,000 IU |
| ages 4-6 | 500 RE | 2,500 IU |
| ages 7-10 | 700 RE | 3,500 IU |

RE = retinol equivalents; IU = combination of retinol and beta-carotene.

| | Vitamin A RDA | Vitamin A and beta-carotene RDA |
|---|---|---|
| **Males** | | |
| ages 11 and older | 1,000 RE | 4,000 IU |
| **Females** | | 4,000 IU |
| ages 11 and older | 800 RE | 6,500 IU |
| pregnant | 800 RE | 6,000 IU |
| breast-feeding | 1,300 RE (1st 6 months) | |
| | 1,200 RE (2nd 6 months) | |

RE = retinol equivalents; IU = combination of retinol and beta-carotene.

## Mechanism of action

*Metabolic action:* One IU of vitamin A is equivalent to 0.3 mcg of retinol or 0.6 mcg of beta-carotene. Beta-carotene, or provitamin A, yields retinol after absorption from the intestinal tract. Use of retinol with opsin, the red pigment in the retina, helps form rhodopsin, which is needed for visual adaptation to darkness. Vitamin A prevents growth retardation and preserves the integrity of the epithelial cells. Vitamin A deficiency is characterized by nyctalopia (night blindness), keratomalacia (necrosis of the cornea), keratinization and drying of the skin, low resistance to infection, growth retardation, bone thickening, diminished cortical steroid production, and fetal malformations.

## Pharmacokinetics

*Absorption:* Absorbed readily and completely in normal doses if fat absorption is normal. Larger doses, or regular doses in patients with fat malabsorption, low protein intake, or hepatic or pancreatic disease, may be absorbed incompletely. Because vitamin A is fat-soluble, absorption requires bile salts, pancreatic lipase, and dietary fat.
*Distribution:* Stored (primarily as palmitate) in Kupffer's cells of the liver. Normal adult liver stores are sufficient to provide vitamin A requirements for 2 years. Lesser amounts of retinyl palmitate are stored in the kidneys, lungs, adrenal glands, retinas, and intraperitoneal fat. Vitamin A circulates bound to a specific alpha$_1$ protein, retinol-binding protein (RBP). Blood level assays may not reflect liver storage of vitamin A because serum levels depend partly on circulating RBP. Liver storage should be adequate before therapy stops. Vitamin A appears in breast milk. It doesn't readily cross the placental barrier.

*Metabolism:* Vitamin A is metabolized in the liver.

*Excretion:* Retinol (fat-soluble) is conjugated with glucuronic acid and then further metabolized to retinal and retinoic acid. Retinoic acid is excreted in feces via biliary elimination. Retinal, retinoic acid, and other water-soluble metabolites are excreted in urine and feces. Normally, no unchanged retinol is excreted in urine, except in patients with pneumonia or chronic nephritis.

| Route | Onset | Peak | Duration |
|-------|-------|------|----------|
| P.O. | Unknown | 3-5 hr | Unknown |
| I.M. | Unknown | Unknown | Unknown |

## Contraindications and precautions

Oral form is contraindicated in patients with malabsorption syndrome; if malabsorption is from inadequate bile secretion, oral route may be used with concurrent administration of bile salts (dehydrocholic acid). Also contraindicated in those with hypervitaminosis A and those hypersensitive to ingredients in product. I.V. route is contraindicated except for special water-miscible forms intended for infusion with large parenteral volumes. I.V. push of vitamin A of any type is also contraindicated; anaphylaxis or anaphylactoid reactions and death may occur.

Use cautiously in pregnant women.

## Interactions

**Drug-drug.** *Cholestyramine:* Possible decreased absorption of vitamin A. Daily vitamin A supplements are recommended during long-term cholestyramine therapy.

*Mineral oil (prolonged use):* Possible interference with intestinal absorption of vitamin A. Avoid use together.

*Neomycin:* Possible decreased vitamin A absorption. Avoid use together.

*Oral contraceptives:* Significantly increased vitamin A plasma levels. Advise clinician to monitor patient closely.

*Orlistat:* Possible decreased vitamin A absorption. Advise clinician to give drugs at least 2 hours apart.

*Retinoids, such as etretinate or isotretinoin:* Increased risk of adverse drug events resulting from potentiation. Avoid use together.

*Warfarin:* Decreased anticoagulation effect. Advise clinician to monitor PT and INR closely.

## Adverse reactions

**CNS:** irritability, headache, *increased intracranial pressure,* fatigue, lethargy, malaise.
**EENT:** papilledema, exophthalmos.
**GI:** anorexia, epigastric pain, vomiting, polydipsia.
**GU:** hypomenorrhea, polyuria.
**Hepatic:** jaundice, hepatomegaly, *cirrhosis,* elevated liver enzyme levels.

**Musculoskeletal:** slow growth, decalcification, hypercalcemia, periostitis, premature closure of epiphyses, migratory arthralgia, cortical thickening over the radius and tibia.
**Skin:** alopecia; dry, cracked, scaly skin; pruritus; lip fissures; erythema; inflamed tongue, lips, and gums; massive desquamation; increased pigmentation; night sweats.
**Other:** splenomegaly, *anaphylactic shock, death* (reported with I.V. use).

## Overdose and treatment

In cases of acute toxicity, increased intracranial pressure develops within 8 to 12 hours; cutaneous desquamation follows in a few days. Toxicity may follow a single dose of 25,000 IU/kg, which in infants would represent about 75,000 IU and in adults over 2 million IU.

Chronic toxicity results from administration of 4,000 IU/kg for 6 to 15 months. In infants (ages 3 to 6 months), this represents about 18,500 IU/day for 1 to 3 months; in adults, 1 million IU/day for 3 days, 50,000 IU/day for longer than 18 months, or 500,000 IU/day for 2 months.

To treat toxicity, advise clinician to discontinue vitamin A administration if hypercalcemia persists and give I.V. saline solution, prednisone, and calcitonin, if indicated. Advise clinician to perform liver function tests to detect possible liver damage.

## Clinical considerations

■ Adverse reactions usually occur only with toxic drug levels.
■ In any dietary deficiency, multiple vitamin deficiency should be suspected.
■ It's recommended that vitamin A be given with bile salts to patients with malabsorption caused by inadequate bile secretion.
■ Vitamin A given by I.V. push is contraindicated because of the risk of anaphylaxis and death.
■ Special water-miscible forms of vitamin A are available for use when adding to large parenteral volumes.
■ Vitamin A therapy may falsely increase serum cholesterol level readings by interfering with the Zlatkis-Zak reaction. Vitamin A has also been reported to falsely elevate bilirubin determinations.

### *Therapeutic monitoring*

■ Monitor patients who take high doses for toxicity or skin disorders.

### *Special populations*

**Pregnant patients.** Safety of amounts exceeding 5,000 IU/day (oral) or 6,000 IU/day (parenteral) during pregnancy isn't known.
**Breast-feeding patients.** Vitamin A appears in breast milk. The RDA of vitamin A for breast-feeding women in the United States is 1,300 and 1,200 retinol equivalents for the first

---

6 months and second 6 months, respectively. Unless the maternal diet is grossly inadequate, infants can usually obtain sufficient vitamin A from breast-feeding. The effect of large maternal doses of vitamin A on breast-fed infants is unknown.

## Patient counseling

■ Instruct patient to avoid prolonged use of mineral oil while taking drug because mineral oil reduces vitamin A absorption in the intestine.

■ Tell patient not to exceed recommended dose.

■ Instruct patient to report promptly symptoms of overdose, such as nausea, vomiting, anorexia, malaise, drying or cracking of skin or lips, irritability, headache, or loss of hair.

■ Inform patient of the need to consume adequate protein, vitamin E, and zinc, which, along with bile, are needed for vitamin A absorption.

---

# vitamin E (alpha tocopherol)

Amino-Opti-E, Aquasol E, E-200 IU Softgels, E-400 IU in a water-soluble base, E-1000 IU Softgels, E-Complex-600, E-Vitamin Succinate, Vita-Plus E

*Pharmacologic classification:* fat-soluble vitamin
*Therapeutic classification:* vitamin
*Pregnancy risk category A (C if greater than RDA)*

## Available forms

Available without a prescription, as appropriate
*Capsules:* 100 IU, 200 IU, 400 IU, 600 IU, 1,000 IU
*Tablets:* 100 IU, 200 IU, 400 IU, 500 IU, 600 IU, 1,000 IU
*Oral solution:* 50 IU/ml

## Indications and dosages

*Vitamin E deficiency in premature infants and in patients with impaired fat absorption (including patients with cystic fibrosis); biliary atresia*
*Adults:* 60 to 75 IU P.O. daily, depending on severity. Maximum dose, 300 IU/day.
*Children:* 1 unit/kg P.O. daily.
*Premature neonates:* 5 units P.O. daily.
*Full-term neonates:* 5 units P.O. per L of formula.
*Prevention of vitamin E deficiency*
*Adults:* 30 units P.O. daily.
  The RDA for vitamin E is as follows.
*Infants through age 6 months:* 4 mg
*Children ages 7 months to 1 year:* 5 mg
*Children ages 1 to 3:* 6 mg
*Children ages 4 to 8:* 7 mg

*Children ages 9 to 13:* 11 mg
*Children ages 14 to 18:* 15 mg
*Adults ages 19 and older:* 15 mg
*Breast-feeding women:* 19 mg

## Mechanism of action

*Nutritional action:* As a dietary supplement, the exact biochemical mechanism is unclear, although it's believed to act as an antioxidant. Vitamin E protects cell membranes, vitamin A, vitamin C (ascorbic acid), and polyunsaturated fatty acids from oxidation. It also may act as a cofactor in enzyme systems, and some evidence exists that it decreases platelet aggregation.

## Pharmacokinetics

*Absorption:* GI absorption depends on the presence of bile. Only 20% to 60% of the vitamin obtained from dietary sources is absorbed. As dose increases, the fraction of vitamin E absorbed decreases.
*Distribution:* Distributed to all tissues and is stored in adipose tissue.
*Metabolism:* Metabolized in the liver by glucuronidation.
*Excretion:* Excreted primarily in bile. Some enterohepatic circulation may occur. Small amounts of the metabolites are excreted in urine.

| Route | Onset | Peak | Duration |
|-------|-------|------|----------|
| P.O. | Unknown | Unknown | Unknown |

## Contraindications and precautions

No known contraindications. Use cautiously in patients with liver or gallbladder disease.

## Interactions

**Drug-drug.** *Cholestyramine, colestipol, mineral oil, sucralfate:* Possible increased vitamin E requirements. Use together cautiously.
*Oral anticoagulants:* Possible risk of hemorrhage after large doses of vitamin E. Advise clinician to monitor patient closely for bleeding.
*Orlistat:* Possible decreased absorption of vitamin E. Drugs should be given at least 2 hours apart.
*Vitamin K:* Decreased therapeutic effect of vitamin K. Avoid use together.

## Adverse reactions

None reported with recommended doses. Hypervitaminosis E symptoms include fatigue, weakness, nausea, headache, blurred vision, flatulence, and diarrhea.

## Overdose and treatment

Signs of overdose include a possible increase in blood pressure. Treatment is generally supportive.

---

## Clinical considerations
- Drug should be given with bile salts if patient has malabsorption caused by lack of bile.

### Therapeutic monitoring
- Advise clinician to monitor patient for adverse drug events and for therapeutic effect.

### Patient counseling
- Tell patient to store vitamin E in a tight, light-resistant container.
- Instruct patient to swallow capsules whole and not to crush or chew them.

---

# vitamin K derivatives
## phytonadione
AquaMEPHYTON, Mephyton

*Pharmacologic classification:* vitamin K
*Therapeutic classification:* blood coagulation modifier
*Pregnancy risk category C*

---

### Available forms
Available by prescription only
*Tablets:* 5 mg
*Injection (aqueous colloidal solution):* 2 mg/ml, 10 mg/ml
*Injection (aqueous dispersion):* 2 mg/ml, 10 mg/ml

### Indications and dosages
*Hypoprothrombinemia secondary to vitamin K malabsorption or drug therapy, or when oral administration is desired and bile secretion is inadequate*
*Adults:* 5 to 10 mg P.O. daily, or titrated to patient's requirements.
*Hypoprothrombinemia secondary to vitamin K malabsorption, drug therapy, or excess vitamin A*
*Adults:* 2 to 25 mg P.O. or parenterally, repeated and increased up to 50 mg, if needed.
*Children:* 5 to 10 mg P.O. or parenterally.
*Infants:* 2 mg P.O. or parenterally.
*Hypoprothrombinemia secondary to effect of oral anticoagulants*
*Adults:* 2.5 to 10 mg P.O., S.C., or I.M., based on PT and INR, repeated, if needed, 12 to 48 hours after oral dose or 6 to 8 hours after parenteral dose. In emergency, give 10 to 50 mg slow I.V., rate not to exceed 1 mg/minute, repeated q 6 to 8 hours, p.r.n.
*Prevention of hemorrhagic disease in neonates*
*Neonates:* 0.5 to 1 mg S.C. or I.M. immediately after birth, repeated in 2 to 3 weeks, if needed, especially if mother received oral anticoagulants or long-term anticonvulsant therapy during pregnancy.

*Prevention of hypoprothrombinemia related to vitamin K deficiency in long-term parenteral nutrition*
*Adults:* 5 to 10 mg I.M. weekly
*Children:* 2 to 5 mg I.M. weekly
   The RDA for vitamin K is as follows.
*Infants up to age 6 months:* 5 mcg
*Children ages 6 months to 1 year:* 10 mcg
*Children ages 1 to 3:* 15 mcg
*Children ages 4 to 6:* 20 mcg
*Children ages 7 to 10:* 30 mcg
*Males ages 11 to 14:* 45 mcg
*Males ages 15 to 18:* 65 mcg
*Men ages 19 to 24:* 70 mcg
*Men over age 24:* 80 mcg
*Females ages 11 to 14:* 45 mcg
*Females ages 15 to 18:* 55 mcg
*Women ages 19 to 24:* 60 mcg
*Women over age 24:* 65 mcg
*Pregnant or breast-feeding women:* 65 mcg

### I.V. administration
- Drug may be diluted with preservative-free $D_5W$, normal saline, or dextrose 5% and normal saline.
- Advise clinician to give drug immediately after dilution.
- When I.V. administration is considered unavoidable, the drug should be injected very slowly, not exceeding 1 mg/minute.

### Incompatibilities
Incompatible with amino acid 2% with dextrose 12.5%, dextran 12%, ranitidine HCl, dobutamine HCl.

### Mechanism of action
*Coagulation modifying action:* Vitamin K is a lipid-soluble vitamin that promotes hepatic formation of active prothrombin and several other coagulation factors (specifically factors II, VII, IX, and X).
   Phytonadione (vitamin $K_1$) is a synthetic form of vitamin K and is also lipid-soluble. Vitamin K doesn't counteract the action of heparin.

### Pharmacokinetics
*Absorption:* Phytonadione requires the presence of bile salts for GI tract absorption. Once absorbed, vitamin K enters the blood directly. Onset of action after I.V. injection is more rapid, but of shorter duration, than that occurring after S.C. or I.M. injection.
*Distribution:* Concentrates in the liver for a short time. Hemorrhage is usually controlled within 3 to 6 hours, and normal prothrombin levels are achieved in 12 to 14 hours.
*Metabolism:* Metabolized rapidly by the liver; little tissue accumulation occurs.
*Excretion:* Data are limited. High levels occur in feces; however, intestinal bacteria can synthesize vitamin K.

---

| Route | Onset | Peak | Duration |
|---|---|---|---|
| P.O. | 6-12 hr | Unknown | Unknown |
| I.M., I.V., S.C. | 1-2 hr | Unknown | Unknown |

## Contraindications and precautions
Contraindicated in patients hypersensitive to drug.

## Interactions
**Drug-drug.** *Broad-spectrum antibiotics, especially cefamandole, cefoperazone, and cefotetan:* Possible interference with actions of vitamin K, producing hypoprothrombinemia. Use together cautiously.
*Mineral oil:* Inhibited absorption of oral vitamin K. Advise clinician to give drugs at well-spaced intervals and monitor result.
*Oral anticoagulants:* Antagonized anticoagulant therapeutic effect. Use vitamin K only for severe hypoprothrombinemia.
*Orlistat:* Possible decreased absorption of vitamin K. Advise clinician to give drugs at least 2 hours apart.

## Adverse reactions
**CNS:** headache, dizziness, convulsive movements.
**CV:** transient hypotension after I.V. administration, rapid and weak pulse, *arrhythmias.*
**GI:** nausea, vomiting.
**Hematologic:** *severe hemolytic anemia* in neonates.
**Hepatic:** hyperbilirubinemia, *fatal kernicterus.*
**Respiratory:** *bronchospasm,* dyspnea.
**Skin:** diaphoresis, flushing, erythema, urticaria, pruritus, allergic rash; pain, swelling, hematoma at injection site.
**Other:** cramplike pain, *anaphylaxis and anaphylactoid reactions* (usually after too-rapid I.V. administration).

## Overdose and treatment
Excessive doses of vitamin K may cause hepatic dysfunction in adults; in neonates and premature infants, large doses may cause hemolytic anemia, kernicterus, and death. Treatment is supportive.

## Clinical considerations
■ Excessive use of vitamin K may temporarily defeat oral anticoagulant therapy; higher doses of oral anticoagulant or interim use of heparin may be required.
■ Phytonadione for hemorrhagic disease in infants causes fewer adverse reactions than do other vitamin K analogues; phytonadione is the vitamin K analogue of choice to treat an oral anticoagulant overdose.
■ Patients receiving phytonadione who have bile deficiency require concurrent use of bile salts to ensure adequate absorption.

■ Drug should be discontinued if allergic or severe CNS reactions appear.
■ Phytonadione can falsely elevate urine steroid levels.

### Therapeutic monitoring
■ With I.V. administration, advise clinician to monitor patient for flushing, weakness, tachycardia, and hypotension. Shock may follow. Deaths have occurred.
■ Advise clinician to monitor PT and INR to determine effectiveness.
■ Advise clinician to monitor patient response and watch for adverse effects; failure to respond to vitamin K may indicate coagulation defects or irreversible liver damage.

### Special populations
**Pediatric patients.** Don't exceed recommended dose. Hemolysis, jaundice, and hyperbilirubinemia in neonates, particularly premature infants, may be related to vitamin K administration.
**Breast-feeding patients.** It isn't known if vitamin K appears in breast milk. Use with caution in breast-feeding women.

## Patient counseling
■ Explain rationale for drug therapy; stress importance of complying with medical regimen and keeping follow-up appointments.
■ Instruct patient to take a missed dose as soon as possible, but not if it's almost time for next dose, and to report missed doses.

# warfarin sodium
Coumadin

*Pharmacologic classification:* coumarin derivative
*Therapeutic classification:* anticoagulant
*Pregnancy risk category X*

## Available forms
Available by prescription only
*Tablets:* 1 mg, 2 mg, 2.5 mg, 3 mg, 4 mg, 5 mg, 6 mg, 7.5 mg, 10 mg
*Injection:* 5 mg/vial

## Indications and dosages
*Pulmonary emboli, deep vein thrombosis, MI, rheumatic heart disease with heart valve damage, atrial arrhythmias*
*Adults:* Initially, 2 to 5 mg P.O. or I.V.; then daily. PT and INR are used to establish optimal dose. Usual maintenance dose, 2 to 10 mg P.O. daily.

## I.V. administration
■ Reconstitute by adding 2.7 ml of sterile water for injection to 5 mg vial of drug. Resultant solution is 2 mg/ml.

■ After reconstitution, warfarin injection is stable for 4 hours at controlled room temperature.
■ Dose should be injected slowly (over 1 to 2 minutes) into peripheral vein.
■ I.V. warfarin provides an alternative for patients who can't tolerate or receive oral medication.

### Incompatibilities
None reported.

## Mechanism of action
*Anticoagulant action:* Warfarin inhibits vitamin K-dependent activation of clotting factors II, VII, IX, and X, which are formed in the liver; it has no direct effect on established thrombi and can't reverse ischemic tissue damage. However, warfarin may prevent additional clot formation, extension of formed clots, and secondary complications of thrombosis.

## Pharmacokinetics
*Absorption:* Rapidly and completely absorbed from GI tract.
*Distribution:* Highly bound to plasma protein, especially albumin; it crosses placental barrier but doesn't appear in breast milk.
*Metabolism:* Warfarin is hydroxylated by liver into inactive metabolites.
*Excretion:* Metabolites are reabsorbed from bile and excreted in urine. Half-life of parent drug is 1 to 3 days, but is highly variable. Because therapeutic effect is more dependent on clotting factor depletion (factor X has half-life of 40 hours), PT won't peak for 1½ to 3 days despite use of a loading dose. Duration of action—2 to 5 days—more closely reflects drug's half-life .

| Route | Onset | Peak | Duration |
|-------|-------|------|----------|
| P.O. | ½-3 days | Unknown | 2-5 days |
| I.V. | Unknown | Unknown | Unknown |

## Contraindications and precautions
Contraindicated in pregnant women; in patients with bleeding or hemorrhagic tendencies, GI ulcerations, severe hepatic or renal disease, severe uncontrolled hypertension, subacute bacterial endocarditis, aneurysm, ascorbic acid deficiency, history of warfarin-induced necrosis, threatened abortion, eclampsia, preeclampsia, regional or lumbar block anesthesia, polycythemia vera, and vitamin K deficiency; in those for whom diagnostic tests or therapeutic procedures have potential for uncontrolled bleeding; in unsupervised patients with senility, alcoholism, psychosis, or lack of cooperation; and after recent eye, brain, or spinal cord surgery.

Use cautiously in patients with diverticulitis, colitis, hypertension, hepatic or renal disease, drainage tubes in any orifice, infectious disease or disturbance of intestinal flora, trauma, surgery resulting in large exposed surface, indwelling catheters, known or suspected deficiency in protein C or S, HF, severe diabetes, vasculitis, polycythemia vera, concurrent use of NSAIDs, or risk of hemorrhage and during lactation.

## Interactions
**Drug-drug.** *Acetaminophen:* Possible increased bleeding with use of acetaminophen longer than 2 weeks and doses higher than 2 g/day. Advise clinician to monitor patient closely.

*Allopurinol, amiodarone, anabolic steroids, cephalosporins, chloramphenicol, cimetidine, ciprofloxacin, clofibrate, danazol, diazoxide, diflunisal, disulfiram, erythromycin, glucagon, heparin, ibuprofen, influenza virus vaccine, isoniazid, itraconazole, ketoprofen, lovastatin, metronidazole, methimazole, miconazole, neomycin (oral), norfloxacin, ofloxacin, omeprazole, pentoxifylline, propafenone, propoxyphene, propylthiouracil, quinidine, salicylates, simvastatin, streptokinase, sulfinpyrazone, sulfonamides, sulindac, tamoxifen, tetracyclines, thiazides, thyroid drugs, tricyclic antidepressants, urokinase, vitamin E:* Increased PT. Advise clinician to monitor patient closely for bleeding. Dose reduction of warfarin may be needed.

*Anticonvulsants:* Increased serum levels of phenytoin and phenobarbital. Advise clinician to monitor patient closely.

*Barbiturates:* Possible inhibited anticoagulant effect for several weeks after barbiturate withdrawal; possible fatal hemorrhage after cessation of barbiturate effect. Advise clinician to monitor patient closely. If barbiturates are withdrawn, reduce anticoagulant dose.

*Carbamazepine, corticosteroids, ethchlorvynol, glutethimide, griseofulvin, oral contraceptives, rifampin, vitamin K:* Decreased anticoagulant effect. Avoid use together.

*Chloral hydrate:* Possible increased or decreased anticoagulant effect of warfarin. Avoid use together.

*Cholestyramine:* Decreased anticoagulant effect of warfarin when used together. Advise clinician to give 6 hours after warfarin.

*Ethacrynic acid, indomethacin, mefenamic acid, phenylbutazone, sulfinpyrazone:* Increased anticoagulant effect of warfarin; severe GI irritation (possibly ulcerogenic). Avoid use together.

**Drug-herb.** *Angelica root, anise, arnica flower, asafoetida, bromelain, celery, chamomile, clove, Danshen, devil's claw, dong quai, fenugreek, feverfew, garlic, ginger, ginkgo biloba, horse chestnut, licorice, meadowsweet, onion, papain, parsley, passion flower, quassia, red clover, reishi mushroom, rue, sweet clover, tumeric:* Possible increased risk of bleeding. Discourage concurrent use.

---

*Ginseng, St. John's wort, ubiquinone:* Possible decreased anticoagulant effect. Discourage concurrent use.

*Green tea:* Decreased anticoagulant effect from vitamin K content of green tea. Patient should minimize variable consumption of green tea and other foods or nutritional supplements containing vitamin K.

*Motherwort, red clover:* Increased risk of bleeding. Discourage use together.

**Drug-food.** *Foods or enteral products containing vitamin K:* Possible impaired anticoagulation. Advise patient to maintain a consistent daily intake of leafy green vegetables.

**Drug-lifestyle.** *Alcohol use:* Possible enhanced anticoagulant effects. Advise patient to avoid alcohol.

## Adverse reactions

**GI:** anorexia, nausea, vomiting, cramps, *diarrhea,* mouth ulcerations, sore mouth.

**GU:** hematuria.

**Hematologic:** prolonged PT, INR, and PTT, *hemorrhage* (with excessive dosage).

**Hepatic:** hepatitis, elevated liver function test results, jaundice.

**Metabolic:** enhanced uric acid excretion.

**Skin:** dermatitis, urticaria, necrosis, gangrene, alopecia, *rash.*

**Other:** *fever.*

## Overdose and treatment

Signs and symptoms of overdose vary with severity and may include internal or external bleeding or skin necrosis of fat-rich areas, but most common sign is hematuria. Excessive prolongation of PT and INR or minor bleeding mandates withdrawal of therapy; withholding one or two doses may be adequate in some cases.

Treatment to control bleeding may include oral or I.V. phytonadione (vitamin $K_1$) and, in severe hemorrhage, fresh frozen plasma or whole blood. Use of phytonadione may interfere with subsequent oral anticoagulant therapy.

## Clinical considerations

■ Store drug in light-resistant containers at 59° to 86° F (15° to 30° C).

■ PT and INR are used to determine optimal dose.

■ Warfarin causes false-negative serum theophylline levels.

### Therapeutic monitoring

■ Advise clinician to monitor PT and INR closely.

■ Advise clinician to monitor patient for signs of bleeding.

### Special populations

**Pregnant patients.** Drug is contraindicated during pregnancy.

**Breast-feeding patients.** Although drug doesn't appear to accumulate in breast milk, use with caution in breast-feeding women.

**Pediatric patients.** Infants, especially neonates, may be more susceptible to anticoagulants because of vitamin K deficiency. Safety and efficacy haven't been established in children under age 18.

**Geriatric patients.** Geriatric patients are more susceptible to effects of anticoagulants and are at increased risk for hemorrhage; this may be caused by altered hemostatic mechanisms or age-related deterioration of hepatic and renal functions.

## Patient counseling

■ Tell patient to promptly report any unusual bruising or bleeding.

■ Warn patient to avoid taking OTC products containing aspirin, other salicylates, or drugs that may interact with the anticoagulant, causing an increase or decrease in action of drug, and to seek medical approval before stopping or starting drug.

■ Advise patient not to substantially alter daily intake of leafy green vegetables, such as asparagus, broccoli, cabbage, lettuce, turnip greens, spinach, or watercress, or of fish, pork or beef liver, green tea, or tomatoes. These foods contain vitamin K and widely varying daily intake may alter anticoagulant effect of warfarin.

■ Instruct patient to inform all prescribers (including dentists) about use of warfarin.

# xylometazoline hydrochloride
Otrivin, Otrivin Pediatric Nasal Drops

*Pharmacologic classification:* sympathomimetic
*Therapeutic classification:* decongestant, vasoconstrictor
*Pregnancy risk category C*

## Available forms
Available without a prescription
*Nasal drops:* 0.05% (pediatric use), 0.1%
*Nasal spray:* 0.1%

## Indications and dosages
*Nasal congestion*
*Adults and children ages 12 and older:* Apply 2 or 3 drops or sprays of 0.1% solution to nasal mucosa q 8 to 10 hours, not to exceed three times in 24 hours.
*Infants and children ages 6 months to 11 years:* Apply 2 or 3 drops of 0.05% solution to nasal mucosa q 8 to 10 hours, not to exceed three times in 24 hours.
*Infants under age 6 months:* 1 drop of 0.05% solution in each nostril q 6 hours, p.r.n.

## Mechanism of action
*Decongestant action:* Acts on alpha-adrenergic receptors in nasal mucosa to produce constriction, decreasing blood flow and nasal congestion.

## Pharmacokinetics
None reported.

| Route | Onset | Peak | Duration |
|-------|-------|------|----------|
| Nasal | 5-10 min | Unknown | 5-6 hr |

## Contraindications and precautions
Contraindicated in patients hypersensitive to drug or those with acute-closure glaucoma. Use cautiously in patients with hyperthyroidism, cardiac disease, hypertension, diabetes mellitus, and advanced arteriosclerosis.

## Interactions
**Drug-drug.** *Tricyclic antidepressants:* Possible potentiation of pressor effects of tricyclic antidepressants if significant systemic absorption occurs. Advise clinician to monitor patient closely.

## Adverse reactions
**EENT:** transient burning, stinging; dryness or ulceration of nasal mucosa; sneezing; rebound nasal congestion, irritation (with excessive or long-term use).

## Overdose and treatment
Signs and symptoms of overdose include somnolence, sedation, sweating, CNS depression with hypertension, bradycardia, decreased cardiac output, rebound hypotension, CV collapse, depressed respirations, coma.

Because of rapid onset of sedation, emesis isn't recommended in therapy unless given early. Activated charcoal or gastric lavage may be used initially. Advise clinician to monitor vital signs and ECG. Seizures should be treated with I.V. diazepam.

## Clinical considerations
■ Systemic absorption is less likely and drug is more effective if 3 to 5 minutes elapse between sprays and nose is cleared before next spray.

### Therapeutic monitoring
■ Advise clinician to observe carefully for adverse effects in patients with CV disease, diabetes mellitus, or hyperthyroidism.

### Special populations
**Pediatric patients.** Children may be prone to greater systemic absorption, with resultant increase in adverse effects.
**Geriatric patients.** Use with caution in geriatric patients with cardiac disease, diabetes mellitus, or poorly controlled hypertension.

## Patient counseling
■ Inform patient that drug should only be used for short-term relief of symptoms (3 to 5 days maximum).
■ Instruct patient on correct method of administration.
■ Caution patient not to exceed recommended dose to avoid rebound congestion.
■ Instruct patient to promptly report insomnia, dizziness, weakness, tremor, or irregular heartbeat.

---

Reactions may be *common*, uncommon, *life-threatening*, or COMMON AND LIFE-THREATENING.

# zafirlukast

Accolate

*Pharmacologic classification:*
leukotriene receptor antagonist
*Therapeutic classification:* antasthmatic
*Pregnancy risk category B*

## Available forms
Available by prescription only
*Tablets:* 10 mg, 20 mg

## Indications and dosages
*Prophylaxis and chronic treatment of asthma*
*Adults and children ages 12 and older:* 20 mg P.O. b.i.d. taken 1 hour before or 2 hours after meals.
*Children ages 5 to 11:* 10 mg P.O. b.i.d., 1 hour before or 2 hours after meals.
◊ *Prophylaxis for seasonal allergic rhinitis*
*Adults:* 20 to 40 mg P.O. single dose before environmental exposure.

## Mechanism of action
*Antasthmatic action:* Selectively competes for leukotriene receptor ($LTD_4$ and $LTE_4$) sites, blocking inflammatory action.

## Pharmacokinetics
*Absorption:* Rapidly absorbed.
*Distribution:* Over 99% is protein-bound to plasma proteins, predominantly albumin.
*Metabolism:* Extensively metabolized via cytochrome P-450 2C9 (CYP2C9) system. Also inhibits CYP 3A4 and CYP 2C9 isoenzymes.
*Excretion:* Primarily excreted in feces. Mean terminal half-life is about 10 hours.

| Route | Onset | Peak | Duration |
|-------|-------|------|----------|
| P.O. | Rapid | 3 hr | Unknown |

## Contraindications and precautions
Contraindicated in patients hypersensitive to drug or its components. Use cautiously in patients with hepatic impairment and in geriatric patients.

## Interactions
**Drug-drug.** *Aspirin:* Increased plasma levels of zafirlukast. Advise clinician to monitor patient closely.
*Erythromycin, theophylline:* Decreased plasma levels of zafirlukast. Advise clinician to monitor patient closely.
*Warfarin:* Increased PT and INR. Advise clinician to monitor PT and INR; dosage adjustment may be needed.

## Adverse reactions
**CNS:** asthenia, dizziness, *headache.*
**GI:** abdominal pain, diarrhea, dyspepsia, nausea, vomiting.

**Hepatic:** elevated liver enzyme levels.
**Musculoskeletal:** back pain, myalgia.
**Other:** accidental injury, fever, infection, pain.

## Overdose and treatment
There is no experience with zafirlukast overdose. If an overdose occurs, advise clinician to treat patient symptomatically and provide supportive measures, p.r.n. If indicated, unabsorbed drug should be removed from GI tract.

## Clinical considerations
■ Drug isn't indicated for the reversal of bronchospasm in acute asthma attacks.
■ Food reduces bioavailability; drug should be taken on an empty stomach.

### Therapeutic monitoring
■ Advise clinician to monitor patient for adverse reactions.

### Special populations
**Pregnant patients.** Use in pregnant women only if clearly indicated.
**Breast-feeding patients.** Drug appears in breast milk. Because of potential risk to infant, don't use in breast-feeding women.
**Pediatric patients.** Safety and efficacy in children under age 7 haven't been established.
**Geriatric patients.** Drug clearance is reduced in geriatric patients; use with caution.

## Patient counseling
■ Instruct patient to continue taking drug as prescribed even if symptoms resolve.
■ Advise patient to continue taking other antasthmatics as prescribed.
■ Instruct patient to take drug 1 hour before or 2 hours after meals.

# zalcitabine
(dideoxycytidine, ddC)
Hivid

*Pharmacologic classification:* nucleoside analogue
*Therapeutic classification:* antiviral
*Pregnancy risk category C*

## Available forms
Available by prescription only
*Tablets (film-coated):* 0.375 mg, 0.75 mg

## Indications and dosages
*Adjunctive therapy for advanced HIV infection in patients who have shown significant clinical or immunologic deterioration*
*Adults and children ages 13 and older:* 0.75 mg P.O. q 8 hours. Can be taken with zidovudine (200 mg P.O. q 8 hours).

≡*Dosage adjustment.* Patients with creatinine clearance of 41 to 55 ml/min may be at an increased risk of toxicity and should be closely monitored. For patients with creatinine clearance of 40 ml/min or less, refer to the table.

| Creatinine clearance (ml/min) | Adult dosage |
|---|---|
| 10-40 | 0.75 mg P.O. q 12 hours |
| < 10 | 0.75 mg P.O. q 24 hours |

## Mechanism of action
*Antiviral action:* Zalcitabine is active against HIV. Within cells, it's converted by cellular enzymes into its active metabolite, dideoxycytidine 5'-triphosphate. It inhibits the replication of HIV by blocking viral DNA synthesis. The drug inhibits reverse transcriptase by acting as an alternative for the enzyme's substrate, deoxycytidine triphosphate.

## Pharmacokinetics
*Absorption:* Well absorbed; however, absorption has considerable interindividual variation. Average oral bioavailability is 70% to 88%.
*Distribution:* Steady-state volume of distribution is $0.534 \pm 0.127$ L/kg. Drug enters the CNS.
*Metabolism:* Doesn't appear to undergo significant hepatic metabolism; phosphorylation to the active form occurs within cells.
*Excretion:* Primarily excreted by the kidneys; about 70% of a dose appears in urine within 24 hours. Mean elimination half-life is 2 hours.

| Route | Onset | Peak | Duration |
|---|---|---|---|
| P.O. | Unknown | ½-2 hr | Unknown |

## Contraindications and precautions
Contraindicated in patients hypersensitive to drug or its components. Use cautiously in patients with preexisting peripheral neuropathy, impaired renal function, liver failure, or history of pancreatitis, HF, or cardiomyopathy. Use with caution in patients at risk for developing peripheral neuropathy, including those with low CD4+ counts (less than 50 cells/mm³), diabetes, weight loss, or patients taking concurrent drugs that have the potential to cause peripheral neuropathy.

## Interactions
**Drug-drug.** *Aminoglycosides, amphotericin, foscarnet:* Increased risk of nephrotoxicity. Advise clinician to monitor renal function closely. Avoid use together when possible.
*Antacids containing aluminum or magnesium:* Decreased absorption of zalcitabine. Separate administration times.

*Chloramphenicol, cisplatin, dapsone, didanosine, disulfiram, ethionamide, glutethimide, gold salts, hydralazine, iodoquinol, isoniazid, metronidazole, nitrofurantoin, phenytoin, ribavirin, vincristine:* Increased risk of peripheral neuropathy. Advise clinician to monitor closely and avoid use together when possible.
*Cimetidine, probenecid:* Increased serum zalcitabine level. Advise clinician to monitor level closely.
*Didanosine, stavudine:* Overlapping toxicities. Don't use together.
*Pentamidine:* Increased risk of pancreatitis. Avoid use together.

## Adverse reactions
**CNS:** *peripheral neuropathy, headache, fatigue,* dizziness, confusion, **seizures,** impaired concentration, amnesia, insomnia, mental depression, tremor, hypertonia, anxiety.
**CV:** cardiomyopathy, **HF,** chest pain.
**EENT:** pharyngitis, ocular pain, abnormal vision, ototoxicity, nasal discharge.
**GI:** nausea, vomiting, diarrhea, abdominal pain, anorexia, constipation, stomatitis, esophageal ulcer, glossitis, **pancreatitis.**
**Hematologic:** anemia, **neutropenia, leukopenia, thrombocytopenia.**
**Hepatic:** AST, ALT, and alkaline phosphatase levels elevated; **hepatomegaly.**
**Metabolic:** *hypoglycemia,* LACTIC ACIDOSIS.
**Musculoskeletal:** myalgia, arthralgia.
**Respiratory:** cough.
**Skin:** pruritus, night sweats, *erythematous, maculopapular, or follicular rash,* urticaria.
**Other:** fever.

## Overdose and treatment
Inadvertent overdose in children has been treated with gastric lavage and activated charcoal without sequelae. Acute overdose from high doses hasn't been reported; sequelae are unknown. Advise clinician to treat by emptying stomach (gastric lavage or induced emesis) and providing supportive and symptomatic treatment. There's no known antidote; it isn't known if drug is removed by hemodialysis or peritoneal dialysis.

## Clinical considerations
■ The main dose-limiting toxicity is peripheral neuropathy, initially characterized by numbness and burning in the limbs. If drug isn't withdrawn, symptoms can progress to sharp, shooting pain or severe, continuous burning pain requiring narcotic analgesics and may or may not be reversible.
■ Drug should be stopped if symptoms indicating peripheral neuropathy are bilateral and persist beyond 72 hours. When symptoms subside, drug may be reintroduced at 0.375 mg P.O. every 8 hours. If symptoms worsen or persist beyond 1 week, drug should be permanently withdrawn.

■ If drug is discontinued because of toxicity, advise clinician to resume recommended dose for zidovudine alone, which is 100 mg every 4 hours.

**◢ALERT** Don't confuse this drug with other antivirals that may use initials for identification.

### Therapeutic monitoring

■ Advise clinician to monitor patient closely for signs of toxicity and CNS and CV symptoms.

■ CBC and chemistry should be performed before drug therapy and periodically thereafter.

### Special populations

**Pregnant patients.** Use drug in pregnancy only when potential benefits justify possible risks to fetus.

**Breast-feeding patients.** It isn't known if drug appears in breast milk. Because of risk of transmitting the virus, HIV-positive women shouldn't breast-feed.

**Pediatric patients.** Safety and efficacy in children under age 13 haven't been established. Drug has been used in children ages 6 months to 13 years (0.015 to 0.04 mg/kg every 6 hours) with adverse reactions similar to those reported for adults.

**Geriatric patients.** Dosage should be carefully selected and renal function monitored.

### Patient counseling

■ Inform patient that drug doesn't cure HIV infection and that HIV can still be transmitted.

■ Instruct patient to promptly report symptoms of peripheral neuropathy and pancreatitis.

■ Tell patient to take drug 1 hour before or 2 hours after meals.

# zaleplon

Sonata

*Pharmacologic classification:* pyrazolopyrimidine
*Therapeutic classification:* hypnotic
*Pregnancy risk category C*
*Controlled substance schedule IV*

### Available forms

Available by prescription only
*Capsules:* 5 mg, 10 mg

### Indications and dosages

#### Short-term treatment for insomnia

*Adults:* 10 mg P.O. daily immediately before bedtime; may increase dose to 20 mg if needed. Low-weight adults may respond to 5-mg dose.

*Elderly:* Initially, 5 mg P.O. daily immediately before bedtime; doses over 10 mg aren't recommended.

≡*Dosage adjustment.* For debilitated patients: Initially, 5 mg P.O. daily immediately before bedtime; doses over 10 mg aren't recommended.

≡*Dosage adjustment.* For patients with mild to moderate hepatic failure or those also receiving cimetidine: 5 mg P.O. daily immediately before bedtime.

### Mechanism of action

*Hypnotic action:* Although zaleplon is a hypnotic with a chemical structure unrelated to benzodiazepines, it interacts with the gammaaminobutyric acid-BZ receptor complex in the CNS. Modulation of this complex is hypothesized to be responsible for sedative, anxiolytic, muscle relaxant, and anticonvulsant effects of benzodiazepines.

### Pharmacokinetics

*Absorption:* Rapidly and almost completely absorbed.

*Distribution:* Distributed substantially into extravascular tissues. Plasma protein–binding is about 60%.

*Metabolism:* Extensively metabolized, primarily by aldehyde oxidase and, to a lesser extent, CYP3A4 to inactive metabolites. Less than 1% of dose is excreted unchanged in urine.

*Excretion:* Rapidly excreted, with a mean half-life of about 1 hour.

| Route | Onset | Peak | Duration |
|-------|-------|------|----------|
| P.O. | Rapid | 1-2 hr | Unknown |

### Contraindications and precautions

Don't use in patients with severe hepatic impairment. Use cautiously in geriatric and debilitated patients, in those with compromised respiratory function, and in those with signs and symptoms of depression.

### Interactions

**Drug-drug.** *Carbamazepine, phenobarbital, phenytoin, rifampin, other CYP3A4:* Possible reduced bioavailability and peak levels of zaleplon by about 80%. Consider an alternative hypnotic.

*Cimetidine:* Increased zaleplon bioavailability and peak levels by 85%. For patient taking cimetidine, use initial zaleplon dose of 5 mg.

*CNS depressants, such as imipramine and thioridazine:* Possible additive CNS effects. Use cautiously together.

**Drug-food.** *High-fat foods, heavy meals:* Prolonged absorption, delayed peak zaleplon levels by about 2 hours; possible delay in sleep onset. Drug shouldn't be given with meals.

**Drug-lifestyle.** *Alcohol use:* Possible increased CNS effects. Advise patient to avoid alcohol.

### Adverse reactions

**CNS:** *headache,* amnesia, dizziness, somnolence, depression, hypertonia, nervousness, de-

personalization, hallucinations, vertigo, difficulty concentrating, anxiety, paresthesia, hypoesthesia, tremor, asthenia, migraine, malaise.
**CV:** chest pain, peripheral edema.
**EENT:** abnormal vision, conjunctivitis, eye pain, ear pain, hyperacusis, epistaxis, parosmia.
**GI:** constipation, dry mouth, anorexia, dyspepsia, nausea, abdominal pain, colitis.
**GU:** dysmenorrhea.
**Musculoskeletal:** arthritis, myalgia, back pain.
**Respiratory:** bronchitis.
**Skin:** pruritus, rash, photosensitivity reaction.
**Other:** fever.

## Overdose and treatment
Signs and symptoms usually include exaggerated CNS-depressant effects of drug, ranging from drowsiness to coma. Advise clinician to use immediate gastric lavage when appropriate and general supportive measures for symptomatic management.

## Clinical considerations
■ Limit hypnotics use to 5 weeks.
■ Potential for drug abuse and dependence exists.
■ Because zaleplon works rapidly, it should only be ingested immediately before bedtime or after patient has gone to bed and has experienced difficulty falling asleep.
■ Adverse reactions are usually dose-related. The lowest effective dose should be used.

### Therapeutic monitoring
■ Advise clinician to closely monitor patient with compromised respiratory function caused by preexisting illness.
■ Advise clinician to closely monitor geriatric or debilitated patients.
■ Advise clinician to reevaluate patient if hypnotics are to be taken for longer than 5 weeks.

### Special populations
**Pregnant patients.** Drug isn't recommended for use during pregnancy.
**Breast-feeding patients.** A small amount of drug appears in breast milk. Breast-feeding women shouldn't take this drug because its effects on infants aren't known.
**Pediatric patients.** Safety and efficacy in children haven't been established.
**Geriatric patients.** Geriatric patients appear to be more sensitive to the effects of hypnotics. Advise clinician to monitor these patients closely.

## Patient counseling
■ Inform patient that dependence can occur, and that drug is recommended for short-term use only.
■ Advise patient that insomnia may recur for a few nights after stopping drug, but should resolve on its own.

■ Advise patient that zaleplon works rapidly and should only be taken when a 4-hour period of undisturbed sleep is possible.
■ Advise patient to avoid alcohol while taking drug and to notify prescriber before taking any prescription or OTC drugs.
■ Inform patient that a high-fat or heavy meal may delay onset of drug action.
■ Instruct patient to promptly report adverse events.

# zanamivir
Relenza

*Pharmacologic classification:* neuraminidase inhibitor
*Therapeutic classification:* antiviral
*Pregnancy risk category B*

## Available forms
Available by prescription only
*Powder for inhalation:* 5 mg per blister

## Indications and dosages
***Treatment of uncomplicated acute illness from influenza virus in patients who have been symptomatic for no longer than 2 days***
*Adults, adolescents, and children ages 7 and older:* Two oral inhalations (one 5-mg blister per inhalation for a total dose of 10 mg) b.i.d. using the Diskhaler inhalation device for 5 days. Two doses should be taken on the first day of treatment as long as there's at least 2 hours between doses. Subsequent doses should be about 12 hours apart (in the morning and evening) at about the same time each day.

## Mechanism of action
*Antiviral action:* Zanamivir most likely inhibits neuraminidase on the surface of the influenza virus, potentially altering virus particle aggregation and release. With the inhibition of neuraminidase, the virus can't escape from its host cell to attack others, inhibiting the process of viral proliferation.

## Pharmacokinetics
*Absorption:* About 4% to 17% of orally inhaled drug is systemically absorbed.
*Distribution:* Less than 10% plasma protein–bound.
*Metabolism:* Not metabolized and excreted by the kidneys as unchanged drug.
*Excretion:* Excreted unchanged in urine. Unabsorbed drug is excreted in feces. The serum half-life of zanamivir ranges from 2½ to 5 hours.

| Route | Onset | Peak | Duration |
|-------|-------|------|----------|
| Oral inhalation | Unknown | 1-2 hr | < 24 hr |

## Contraindications and precautions

Contraindicated in patients hypersensitive to drug or its components. Use cautiously in patients with severe or decompensated COPD, asthma, or other underlying respiratory disease.

## Interactions

None reported.

## Adverse reactions

**CNS:** headache, dizziness.
**EENT:** nasal signs and symptoms; sinusitis; ear, nose, and throat infections.
**GI:** diarrhea, nausea, vomiting.
**Respiratory:** bronchitis, *bronchospasm,* cough.

## Overdose and treatment

No reports of overdose exist. Signs and symptoms of overdose include exaggeration of adverse reactions of drug.

## Clinical considerations

■ Patients with underlying respiratory disease should have a fast-acting bronchodilator available in case of wheezing while taking zanamivir. Patients scheduled to use an inhaled bronchodilator for asthma should use their bronchodilator before taking zanamivir.
■ Safety and efficacy of zanamivir haven't been established for influenza prophylaxis.
■ Use of zanamivir shouldn't affect the evaluation of patients for their annual influenza vaccination.
■ Consider possibility of primary or concomitant bacterial infection before diagnosis of influenza is made.

### Therapeutic monitoring

■ Advise clinician to monitor patient for bronchospasm and decline in lung function. Drug should be stopped if these occur.

### Special populations

**Pregnant patients.** Use drug during pregnancy only when the potential benefits justify possible risk to fetus.
**Breast-feeding patients.** It isn't known if drug appears in breast milk. Use cautiously in breast-feeding women.
**Pediatric patients.** Safety and efficacy in children under age 7 haven't been established.
**Geriatric patients.** No overall differences in safety and efficacy were observed in clinical trials involving geriatric patients and younger patients.

## Patient counseling

■ Advise patient that zanamivir hasn't been shown to reduce the risk of transmitting influenza virus to others.
■ Advise patient with underlying respiratory disease who is scheduled to use an inhaled bronchodilator to do so before taking zanamivir.

Tell patient to have a fast-acting bronchodilator available if wheezing occurs while taking zanamivir.
■ Advise patient to always check inside the mouthpiece of the Diskhaler before each use to make sure it's free of foreign objects.
■ Instruct patient on proper administration technique and demonstrate when possible.
■ Advise patient to finish the entire 5-day course of treatment, even if symptoms improve before the fifth day.
■ Tell patient to promptly contact prescriber if increased respiratory symptoms (wheezing, dyspnea, signs or symptoms of bronchospasm) occur.

# zidovudine (AZT)
Retrovir, Retrovir IV

*Pharmacologic classification:* thymidine analogue
*Therapeutic classification:* antiviral
*Pregnancy risk category C*

## Available forms

Available by prescription only
*Capsules:* 100 mg
*Syrup:* 50 mg/5 ml
*Injection:* 10 mg/ml
*Tablets:* 300 mg

## Indications and dosages

### Treatment of HIV infection

*Adults and children over age 12:* 200 mg P.O. q 8 hours or 300 mg P.O. q 12 hours (600 mg daily dose). Or, 1 mg/kg I.V. five to six times daily.
*Children ages 3 months to 12 years:* 180 mg/m² q 6 hours (720 mg/m²/day). Don't exceed 200 mg q 6 hours. Some clinicians recommend 160 mg/m² P.O. q 8 hours, 120 mg/m² I.V. q 6 hours, or 20 mg/m²/hr by continuous I.V. infusion.

### Maternal-fetal transmission of HIV

*Adults:* Maternal dosing: Give 100 mg P.O. 5 times daily, or 200 mg t.i.d., or 300 mg b.i.d. until onset of labor. During labor and delivery, administer 2 mg/kg I.V. over 1 hour followed by a continuous infusion of 1 mg/kg/hour until clamping of the umbilical cord. Infant dosing: 2 mg/kg P.O. q 6 hours starting within 8 to 24 hours after birth and continuing until 6 weeks of age; alternatively, administer 1.5 mg/kg via I.V. infusion over 30 minutes q 6 hours.

◊ *Postexposure prophylaxis in health care workers or others following occupational exposure*

*Adults:* 600 mg P.O. daily in divided doses (300 mg b.i.d., 200 mg t.i.d., or 100 mg q 4 hours) with oral lamivudine.

≡*Dosage adjustment.* For patients with severe renal impairment, dosage may need to be reduced to 300 to 400 mg daily P.O. In patients with end-stage renal failure who are on dialysis, give 100 mg every 6 to 8 hours P.O., or 1 mg/kg I.V. every 6 to 8 hours. Dosage adjustment may also be needed in patients with decreased liver function.

## I.V. administration
■ Drug should be administered I.V. only until P.O. regimen can begin.
■ Dilute drug in $D_5W$ to concentration no greater than 4 mg/ml.
■ Infuse intermittent I.V. doses at a constant rate over 60 minutes.

### Incompatibilities
Incompatible with other biological or colloidal solutions; for example, blood products or solutions containing protein.

## Mechanism of action
*Antiviral action:* Zidovudine is converted intracellularly to an active triphosphate compound that inhibits reverse transcriptase (an enzyme essential for retroviral DNA synthesis), inhibiting viral replication. When used in vitro, drug inhibits certain other viruses and bacteria; however, this has undetermined clinical significance.

## Pharmacokinetics
*Absorption:* Absorbed rapidly from GI tract. Average systemic bioavailability is 65% of dose; drug undergoes first-pass metabolism.
*Distribution:* Preliminary data reveal good CSF penetration. About 36% of dose is plasma protein–bound.
*Metabolism:* Metabolized rapidly to an inactive compound.
*Excretion:* Parent drug and metabolite are excreted by glomerular filtration and tubular secretion in the kidneys. Urine recovery of parent drug and metabolite is 14% and 74%, respectively. Elimination half-life of these compounds is 1 hour.

| Route | Onset | Peak | Duration |
|-------|-------|------|----------|
| P.O., I.V. | Unknown | ½ -1½ hr | Unknown |

## Contraindications and precautions
Contraindicated in patients hypersensitive to drug. Use cautiously in patients in advanced stages of HIV and in those with severe bone marrow suppression, renal insufficiency, or hepatomegaly, hepatitis, or other risk factors for hepatic disease.

## Interactions
**Drug-drug.** *Acetaminophen, aspirin, indomethacin:* Possible impaired hepatic metabolism of zidovudine. Advise clinician to monitor patient closely.
*Acyclovir:* Possible seizures, lethargy, and fatigue. Use together cautiously.

*Amphotericin B, dapsone, flucytosine, ganciclovir, pentamidine:* Increased risk of nephrotoxicity and bone marrow suppression. Advise clinician to monitor patient closely.
*Fluconazole, methadone, valproic acid:* Increased zidovudine level. Advise clinician to monitor patient for toxicity.
*Ganciclovir, interferon-alpha:* Increased risk of hematologic toxicity. Advise clinician to monitor patient closely.
*Other cytotoxic drugs:* Additive adverse effects on bone marrow. Avoid use together.
*Probenecid:* Impaired elimination of zidovudine. Advise clinician to monitor patient for toxicity.
*Ribavirin:* Antagonized antiviral activity of zidovudine against HIV. Avoid use together.

## Adverse reactions
**CNS:** *headache, seizures,* paresthesia, *malaise, asthenia,* insomnia, *dizziness,* somnolence.
**GI:** *nausea, anorexia, abdominal pain, vomiting,* constipation, *diarrhea,* dyspepsia, taste perversion.
**Hematologic:** *severe bone marrow suppression (resulting in anemia), agranulocytosis, thrombocytopenia.*
**Musculoskeletal:** myalgia.
**Skin:** *rash,* diaphoresis.
**Other:** *fever.*

## Overdose and treatment
None reported.

## Clinical considerations
■ Optimum duration of treatment, as well as dose for optimum effectiveness and minimum toxicity, isn't known.
■ Drug doesn't cure HIV infection or AIDS but may reduce morbidity resulting from opportunistic infections.
■ Significant anemia (hemoglobin less than 7.5 g/dl or reduction of less than 25% of baseline) or significant neutropenia (granulocyte count less than 750 cells/mm$^3$ or reduction of less than 50% from baseline) may require suspension of zidovudine therapy until occurrence of bone marrow recovery. With less severe anemia or neutropenia, a reduction in zidovudine dose may be adequate.

### Therapeutic monitoring
■ Advise clinician to monitor CBC and platelet count at least every 2 weeks.
■ Advise clinician to monitor patient for adverse events.

### Special populations
**Pregnant patients.** Drug is given antepartum and intrapartum.
**Breast-feeding patients.** Drug appears in breast milk. CDC and most clinicians recommend that HIV-infected women not breast-feed infants regardless of antiretroviral therapy.

---

Reactions may be *common,* uncommon, *life-threatening,* or COMMON AND LIFE-THREATENING.

**Pediatric patients.** Drug is given to children of all ages. A study is in progress to evaluate dosing in premature neonates.

## Patient counseling

- Inform patient that drug frequently causes low RBC count, possibly requiring blood transfusions or epoetin alfa therapy during treatment.
- Stress importance of following prescribed dose schedule.
- Instruct patient to promptly report adverse effects.
- Inform patient that drug therapy doesn't reduce ability to transmit HIV infection.

# zileuton
Zyflo Filmtab

*Pharmacologic classification:*
5-lipoxygenase inhibitor
*Therapeutic classification:* antasthmatic
*Pregnancy risk category C*

## Available forms
Available by prescription only
*Tablets:* 600 mg

## Indications and dosages
*Prophylaxis and chronic treatment of asthma*
*Adults and children ages 12 and older:* 600 mg P.O. q.i.d.

## Mechanism of action
*Antasthmatic action:* Inhibits enzyme responsible for the formation of leukotrienes, reducing inflammatory response.

## Pharmacokinetics
*Absorption:* Rapidly absorbed with oral administration.
*Distribution:* Apparent volume of distribution is 1.2 L/kg. Drug is 93% bound to plasma proteins, primarily albumin.
*Metabolism:* Oxidatively metabolized by the cytochrome P-450 system. Several active and inactive metabolites of zileuton have been identified.
*Excretion:* Elimination is predominantly via metabolism with a mean terminal half-life of 2½ hours.

| Route | Onset | Peak | Duration |
|-------|-------|------|----------|
| P.O. | Rapid | 2 hr | Unknown |

## Contraindications and precautions
Contraindicated in patients hypersensitive to drug or its components and in those with active hepatic disease or transaminase elevations at least three times the upper limit of normal. Use with caution in patients with hepatic impairment or history of heavy alcohol use.

## Interactions
**Drug-drug.** *Propranolol, other beta blockers:* Increased beta-blocker effect. Advise clinician to monitor patient; beta-blocker dose may need to be reduced.
*Theophylline:* Decreased theophylline clearance; possible doubling of serum theophylline levels. Advise clinician to reduce theophylline dose and monitor serum levels.
*Warfarin:* Increased PT and INR. Advise clinician to monitor PT and INR; adjustment of anticoagulant dosage may be needed.

## Adverse reactions
**CNS:** malaise, asthenia, dizziness, *headache,* insomnia, nervousness, somnolence.
**CV:** chest pain.
**EENT:** conjunctivitis.
**GI:** abdominal pain, constipation, dyspepsia, flatulence, nausea.
**GU:** urinary tract infection, vaginitis.
**Hematologic:** *leukopenia.*
**Hepatic:** elevated liver enzyme levels.
**Musculoskeletal:** arthralgia, hypertonia, myalgia, neck pain and rigidity.
**Skin:** pruritus.
**Other:** accidental injury, fever, lymphadenopathy, pain.

## Overdose and treatment
Data on overdose are limited. Drug isn't removed by dialysis. If overdose occurs, advise clinician to treat patient symptomatically and provide supportive measures. If indicated, unabsorbed drug should be eliminated by emesis or gastric lavage.

## Clinical considerations
- Drug isn't indicated for use in the reversal of bronchospasm in acute asthma attacks.

### Therapeutic monitoring
- Advise clinician to obtain liver enzyme levels at baseline and then once a month for the first 3 months, then every 2 to 3 months for the remainder of the first year and periodically thereafter.

### Special populations
**Breast-feeding patients.** It isn't known if drug appears in breast milk. Use with caution in breast-feeding women.
**Pediatric patients.** Safety and efficacy in children under age 12 haven't been studied.

## Patient counseling
- Caution patient that drug isn't a bronchodilator and shouldn't be used to treat an acute asthma attack.
- Advise patient to continue taking all other antasthmatics.
- Tell patient to promptly report adverse drug events.

# zinc
Orazinc, Verazinc, Zinc 15, Zinc-220, Zincate

*Pharmacologic classification:* trace element, miscellaneous anti-infective
*Therapeutic classification:* nutritional supplement, topical anti-infective
*Pregnancy risk category C*

## Available forms
Available by prescription only
*Injection:* 10 ml (1 mg/ml), 30 ml (1 mg/ml with 0.9% benzyl alcohol), 5 ml (5 mg/ml), 10 ml (5 mg/ml), 50 ml (1 mg/ml)
*Capsules:* 220 mg (50 mg zinc)
Available without a prescription, as appropriate
*Tablets:* 10 mg (1.4 mg zinc), 15 mg (2 mg zinc), 50 mg (7 mg zinc), 66 mg (15 mg zinc), 78 mg (11 mg zinc), 110 mg (25 mg zinc), 200 mg (47 mg zinc)
*Capsules:* 110 mg (25 mg zinc), 220 mg (50 mg zinc)

## Indications and dosages
RDA of zinc is 15 mg/day P.O. for adults and 0.3 mg/kg/day P.O. for children.
*Metabolically stable zinc deficiency*
*Adults:* 2.5 to 4 mg/day I.V.; add 2 mg/day for acute catabolic states.
*Stable zinc deficiency with fluid loss from the small bowel*
*Adults:* Add 12.2 mg/L of total parenteral nutrition solution or 17.1 mg/kg of stool output.
*Zinc deficiency*
*Children under age 5:* 100 mcg/kg/day I.V.
*Premature infants:* 300 mcg/kg/day I.V.
*Dietary supplementation*
*Adults:* 25 to 50 mg P.O. daily.

## I.V. administration
▪ Because of potential for infusion phlebitis and tissue irritation, an undiluted direct injection must not be administered into a peripheral vein.

## *Incompatibilities*
None reported.

## Mechanism of action
*Metabolic action:* Zinc serves as a cofactor for more than 70 different enzymes. It facilitates wound healing, normal growth rates, and normal skin hydration and helps maintain the senses of taste and smell.

Adequate zinc provides normal growth and tissue repair. In patients receiving total parenteral nutrition with low plasma levels of zinc, dermatitis has been followed by alopecia. Zinc is an integral part of many enzymes important to carbohydrate and protein mobilization of retinal-binding protein.

Zinc sulfate ophthalmic solution exhibits astringent and weak antiseptic activity, which may result from precipitation of protein by the zinc ion and by clearing mucous from the outer surface of the eye. Drug has no decongestant action and produces mild vasodilation.

## Pharmacokinetics
*Absorption:* Absorbed poorly from GI tract; only 20% to 30% of dietary zinc is absorbed. After administration, zinc resides in muscle, bone, skin, kidney, liver, pancreas, retina, prostate, and, particularly, RBCs and WBCs. Zinc binds to plasma albumin, alpha-2 macroglobulin, and some plasma amino acids, including histidine, cysteine, threonine, glycine, and asparagine.
*Distribution:* Major zinc stores are in the skeletal muscle, skin, bone, and pancreas.
*Metabolism:* Zinc is a cofactor in many enzymatic reactions. It's required for the synthesis and mobilization of retinal binding protein.
*Excretion:* After parenteral administration, 90% is excreted in stool, urine, and sweat. After oral use, the major route of excretion is secretion into the duodenum and jejunum. Small amounts are also excreted in urine (0.3 to 0.5 mg/day) and sweat (1.5 mg/day).

| Route | Onset | Peak | Duration |
|-------|-------|------|----------|
| P.O., ophthalmic | Unknown | Unknown | Unknown |
| I.V. | Immediate | Immediate | Unknown |

## Contraindications and precautions
Parenteral use of zinc sulfate is contraindicated in patients with renal failure or biliary obstruction (and requires caution in all patients); advise clinician to monitor zinc plasma levels frequently. Don't exceed prescribed doses. In patients with renal dysfunction or GI malfunction, trace metal supplements may need to be reduced, adjusted, or omitted. Hypersensitivity may result. Routine use of zinc supplementation during pregnancy isn't recommended.

Administering copper in the absence of zinc or administering zinc in the absence of copper may result in decreased serum levels of either element. When only one trace element is needed, it should be added separately and serum levels monitored closely. To avoid overdose, multiple trace elements should be given only when clearly needed. In patients with extreme vomiting or diarrhea, extreme amounts of trace element replacement may be needed. Excessive intake in healthy persons may be deleterious.

## Interactions
**Drug-drug.** *Fluoroquinolones, tetracycline:* Impaired antibiotic absorption. Avoid use together.

---

Reactions may be *common*, uncommon, *life-threatening*, or COMMON AND LIFE-THREATENING.

*Methylcellulose suspensions (ophthalmic preparation):* Precipitation of methylcellulose. Avoid use together.

*Sodium borate (ophthalmic preparation):* Possible precipitation of zinc borate. Avoid use together; glycerin may prevent this interaction.

**Drug-food.** *Dairy products:* Possible reduced zinc absorption. Advise patient to avoid dairy products.

## Adverse reactions
**CNS:** restlessness.
**GI:** distress and irritation, nausea, vomiting with high doses, gastric ulceration, diarrhea.
**Skin:** rash.
**Other:** dehydration.

## Overdose and treatment
Signs and symptoms of severe toxicity include hypotension, pulmonary edema, diarrhea, vomiting, jaundice, and oliguria. Advise clinician to discontinue dose and begin support measures.

## Clinical considerations
■ Results may not appear for 6 to 8 weeks in zinc-depleted patients.
■ Calcium supplements may confer a protective effect against zinc toxicity.

### *Therapeutic monitoring*
■ Advise clinician to monitor patient for signs of toxicity.

## Patient counseling
■ Warn patient that GI upset may occur after oral administration but may be diminished if zinc is taken with food.

# ziprasidone
Geodon

*Pharmacologic classification:* atypical antipsychotic
*Therapeutic classification:* psychotropic drug
*Pregnancy risk category C*

## Available forms
*Capsules:* 20 mg, 40 mg, 60 mg, 80 mg

## Indications and dosages
**Symptomatic treatment of schizophrenia**
*Adults:* Initially, 20 mg b.i.d. with food. Dosages are highly individualized. Dosage adjustments, if needed, should occur no sooner than every 2 days; but to allow for lowest possible doses, the interval should be several weeks for symptom response. Effective dosage range is usually 20 to 80 mg b.i.d. Maximum recommended dosage is 100 mg b.i.d.

## Mechanism of action
*Psychotropic action:* Mechanism of action is unknown. The drug is thought to work through dopamine and serotonin antagonism. These two neurotransmitters are generally targeted for treatment of positive and negative symptoms of schizophrenia. Blocking these neurotransmitters allows symptomatic improvement with minimal adverse effects in the extrapyramidal system.

## Pharmacokinetics
*Absorption:* Serum levels peak in about 6 to 8 hours. Absorption is doubled when drug is taken with food; administration with food is recommended.
*Distribution:* Highly protein-bound.
*Metabolism:* Undergoes hepatic metabolism; no active metabolites. Less than one-third of drug is metabolized through the cytochrome P-450 system. CYP3A4 (major) and CYP1A2 (minor) are the pathways involving the cytochrome P-450 system.
*Excretion:* Half-life is about 7 hours.

| Route | Onset | Peak | Duration |
|-------|-------|------|----------|
| P.O. | 1-3 days | 6-8 hr | 12 hr |

## Contraindications and precautions
Contraindicated in patients hypersensitive to drug. Also contraindicated in patients taking other drugs known to prolong the QT interval and in those with a history of QT-interval prolongation, congenital QT syndrome, recent MI, or uncompensated HF. Advise clinician to discontinue drug in patients who have a QT interval greater than 500 msec.

Use cautiously in patients with a history of bradycardia, hypokalemia, or hypomagnesemia and in patients experiencing acute diarrhea.

Patients who experience dizziness, palpitations, or syncope should undergo further evaluation and monitoring. Patients taking antipsychotic drugs are at risk for developing neuroleptic malignant syndrome or tardive dyskinesia.

## Interactions
**Drug-drug.** *Carbamazepine:* Possible decreased levels of ziprasidone. Higher doses of ziprasidone may be needed to achieve desired effect.

*Drugs that increase dopamine, such as levodopa and dopamine agonists:* Possible antagonistic effect on ziprasidone. Use together cautiously.

*Drugs that lower serum potassium or magnesium, such as diuretics:* Possible increased risk of arrhythmias. Advise clinician to monitor serum potassium and magnesium levels if giving together.

*Drugs that prolong QT interval, including dofetilide, moxifloxacin, pimozide, quinidine, sotalol, sparfloxacin, thioridazine:* Possible increased risk of arrhythmias when used together. Don't give together.

*Ketoconazole:* Possible increased levels of ziprasidone. Lower doses of ziprasidone may be needed to achieve desired effect.

## Adverse reactions
**CNS:** *somnolence,* akathisia, dizziness, extrapyramidal symptoms, dystonia, hypertonia, asthenia.
**CV:** tachycardia, orthostatic hypotension.
**EENT:** rhinitis, abnormal vision.
**GI:** *nausea,* constipation, dyspepsia, diarrhea, dry mouth, anorexia.
**Musculoskeletal:** myalgia.
**Respiratory:** cough.
**Skin:** rash.

## Overdose and treatment
Symptoms of overdose included sedation, slurred speech, and hypotension. Also advise clinician to monitor patients for obtundation, seizure, extrapyramidal reactions, dystonia, and arrhythmias. There is no antidote, and dialysis isn't effective. Consider administration of activated charcoal or a laxative. If patient is unconscious, an I.V. line should be established. Otherwise, symptomatic monitoring and treatment is recommended, particularly ECG monitoring for arrhythmias.

## Clinical considerations
■ Don't adjust dosage any sooner than every 2 days. Longer intervals may be needed because symptom response may not be seen for 4 to 6 weeks.
■ Ziprasidone has caused prolongation of the QT interval. Consider other antipsychotic drugs instead of ziprasidone in patients with a history of QT prolongation, acute, congenital QT syndrome, and other conditions that place patient at risk for life-threatening arrhythmias.
■ Patients who develop symptoms of arrhythmias should undergo further CV monitoring.
■ Patients who develop symptoms of neuroleptic malignant syndrome should be treated immediately because this condition can be life-threatening.
■ Ziprasidone should be taken with food, which increases the effect.

### Therapeutic monitoring
■ Electrolyte disturbance, such as hypokalemia or hypomagnesemia, increases the risk of developing an arrhythmia. Advise clinician to monitor potassium and magnesium levels before starting therapy and correct imbalances.

■ Advise clinician to monitor QT interval for prolongation during therapy.
■ Advise clinician to monitor patient for development of tardive dyskinesia.

### Special populations
**Breast-feeding patients.** Patients who are breast-feeding shouldn't take ziprasidone.

## Patient counseling
■ Tell patient to take drug with food.
■ Tell patient to immediately report to prescriber symptoms of dizziness, fainting, irregular heart beat, or relevant cardiac problems.
■ Advise patient to report to prescriber any abnormal movements, recent episodes of diarrhea, sudden fever, muscle rigidity, or change in mental status.

---

# zolmitriptan
Zomig, Zomig-ZMT

*Pharmacologic classification:* selective 5-hydroxytryptamine receptor agonist
*Therapeutic classification:* antimigraine drug
*Pregnancy risk category C*

## Available forms
Available by prescription only
*Tablets:* 2.5 mg, 5 mg
*Orally disintegrating tablets:* 2.5 mg, 5 mg

## Indications and dosages
*Treatment of acute migraine headaches with or without aura*
*Adults:* Initially, 2.5 mg P.O. or lower. A dose lower than 2.5 mg can be achieved by manually breaking a 2.5-mg tablet in half; do not break the orally disintegrating tablets in half. If headache returns after initial dose, a second dose may be given after 2 hours. Maximum dose is 10 mg in 24-hour period.
≡*Dosage adjustment.* For patients with liver disease, use doses less than 2.5 mg. Don't use orally disintegrating tablets because they shouldn't be broken in half.

## Mechanism of action
*Antimigraine action:* Zolmitriptan binds with high affinity to human recombinant 5-HT$_{1D}$ and 5-HT$_{1B}$ receptors, aborting migraine headaches by causing constriction of cranial blood vessels and inhibition of pro-inflammatory neuropeptide release.

## Pharmacokinetics
*Absorption:* Well absorbed after oral administration. Mean absolute bioavailability is about 40%.
*Distribution:* Apparent volume of distribution is 7 L/kg. Drug is 25% plasma protein–bound.
*Metabolism:* Converted to an active *N*-desmethyl metabolite. Time to maximum concentration for the metabolite is 2 to 3 hours. Mean elimination half-life of zolmitriptan and the active *N*-desmethyl metabolite is 3 hours.
*Excretion:* Mean total clearance is 31.5 ml/minute/kg, of which one-sixth is renal clearance. The renal clearance is greater than the glomerular filtration rate, suggesting renal tubular secretion. About 65% of dose is excreted in urine and 30% in feces.

| Route | Onset | Peak | Duration |
|-------|-------|------|----------|
| P.O. | Unknown | 2 hr | 3 hr |
| S.L. | Unknown | 2 hr | Unknown |

## Contraindications and precautions
Contraindicated in patients hypersensitive to drug or its components and in those with uncontrolled hypertension, ischemic heart disease (angina pectoris, history of MI, or documented silent ischemia), or other significant heart disease (including Wolff-Parkinson-White syndrome).

Avoid use within 24 hours of other 5-HT$_1$ agonists or ergot-containing drugs or within 2 weeks of discontinuing MAO inhibitor therapy. Also avoid use in patients with hemiplegic or basilar migraine.

Use cautiously in patients with liver disease and in pregnant or breast-feeding women.

## Interactions
**Drug-drug.** *Cimetidine:* Doubled half-life of zolmitriptan. Advise clinician to monitor patient closely.
*Ergot-containing drugs:* Additive vasospastic reactions. Avoid use together.
*Fluoxetine, fluvoxamine, paroxetine, sertraline:* Weakness, hyperreflexia, and incoordination. Use together cautiously.
*MAO inhibitors, oral contraceptives:* Increased plasma levels of zolmitriptan. Avoid use together.

## Adverse reactions
**CNS:** somnolence, vertigo, *dizziness,* hyperesthesias, paresthesia, asthenia.
**CV:** *arrhythmias,* hypotension, palpitations, pain or heaviness in chest, *pain, tightness, or pressure in the neck, throat, or jaw.*
**GI:** dry mouth, dyspepsia, dysphagia, nausea.
**Musculoskeletal:** myalgia.
**Skin:** sweating.
**Other:** warm or cold sensations.

## Overdose and treatment
No specific antidote exists. If severe intoxication occurs, intensive care procedures are recommended, including establishing and maintaining a patent airway to ensure adequate oxygenation and ventilation, and monitoring and support of the CV system. Effect of hemodialysis or peritoneal dialysis on plasma levels of zolmitriptan is unknown.

## Clinical considerations
■ Drug isn't intended for prophylactic therapy of migraine headaches or for use in hemiplegic or basilar migraines.
■ Safety hasn't been established for cluster headaches.
■ Although not reported in clinical trials, serious cardiac events, including fatality, have occurred rarely following use of 5-HT$_1$ agonists. Events reported have included coronary artery vasospasm, transient myocardial ischemia, MI, ventricular tachycardia, and ventricular fibrillation.

### Therapeutic monitoring
■ Advise clinician to monitor blood pressure in patients with liver disease.

### Special populations
**Pregnant patients.** Use cautiously during pregnancy.
**Breast-feeding patients.** It isn't known if drug appears in breast milk. Use caution when giving to breast-feeding women.
**Pediatric patients.** Safety and efficacy in children haven't been established.
**Geriatric patients.** Although the pharmacokinetic disposition is similar to that seen in younger adults, there's no information in this population because patients over age 65 were excluded from clinical trials.

## Patient counseling
■ Advise patient to take drug only as prescribed.
■ Advise patient to immediately report pain or tightness in chest or throat, heart throbbing, rash, skin lumps, or swelling of the face, lips, or eyelids.
■ Caution patient not to take drug with other migraine drugs.
■ Instruct patient not to release the orally disintegrating tablets from their blister pack until just before administration. Tell him to open pack and dissolve tablets on tongue.
■ Advise patient not to break the orally disintegrating tablets in half.

# zolpidem tartrate
Ambien

*Pharmacologic classification:* imida-
zopyridine
*Therapeutic classification:* hypnotic
*Pregnancy risk category B*
*Controlled substance schedule IV*

## Available forms
Available by prescription only
*Tablets:* 5 mg, 10 mg

## Indications and dosages
***Short-term management of insomnia***
*Adults:* 10 mg P.O. immediately before bed-
time.
≡*Dosage adjustment.* For geriatric or debil-
itated patients or patients with hepatic insuffi-
ciency, 5 mg P.O. immediately before bedtime.
Maximum daily dose, 10 mg.

## Mechanism of action
*Hypnotic action:* While zolpidem is a hypnotic drug with a chemical structure unrelated to
benzodiazepines, barbiturates, or other drugs
with known hypnotic properties, it interacts
with a gamma-aminobutyric acid (GABA)-
benzodiazepine or omega-receptor complex
and shares some of the pharmacologic properties of the benzodiazepines. It exhibits minimal muscle relaxant or anticonvulsant properties.

## Pharmacokinetics
*Absorption:* Absorbed rapidly from GI tract.
Food delays drug absorption.
*Distribution:* Protein-binding is about 92.5%.
*Metabolism:* Converted to inactive metabo-
lites in the liver.
*Excretion:* Primarily eliminated in urine; elim-
ination half-life is about 2½ hours.

| Route | Onset | Peak | Duration |
|-------|-------|------|----------|
| P.O. | Rapid | ½-2 hr | Unknown |

## Contraindications and precautions
No known contraindications. Use cautiously
in patients with conditions that could affect
metabolism or hemodynamic response and in
those with decreased respiratory drive, depression, or history of alcohol or drug abuse.

## Interactions
**Drug-drug.** *Other CNS depressants:* Enhanced
CNS depression. Don't use together.
**Drug-lifestyle.** *Alcohol use:* Possible exces-
sive CNS depression. Advise patient to avoid
alcohol.

## Adverse reactions
**CNS:** daytime drowsiness, light-headedness,
abnormal dreams, amnesia, dizziness, head-
ache, hangover, sleep disorder, lethargy, de-
pression, asthenia, vertigo, falls.
**CV:** palpitations, chest pain.
**EENT:** sinusitis, pharyngitis, dry mouth.
**GI:** nausea, vomiting, diarrhea, dyspepsia, con-
stipation, abdominal pain.
**Musculoskeletal:** back pain, myalgia, arthral-
gia.
**Skin:** rash.
**Other:** flulike symptoms, hypersensitivity re-
actions.

## Overdose and treatment
Symptoms may range from somnolence to light
coma. CV and respiratory compromise also
may occur. Advise clinician to use general
symptomatic and supportive measures, with
immediate gastric lavage when appropriate.
Advise clinician to give I.V. fluids p.r.n;
flumazenil may be useful. Advise clinician to
monitor and treat hypotension and CNS depression. Sedatives should be withheld after
zolpidem overdose even if excitation occurs.

## Clinical considerations
■ Be aware of potential for hoarding or self-
overdosing by hospitalized patients who are
depressed, suicidal, or known to abuse drugs.
■ Drug therapy should be limited to 7 to 10
days; advise clinician to reevaluate patient if
drug is to be taken for longer than 2 weeks.
■ Zolpidem has CNS-depressant effects similar to other sedative-hypnotic drugs. Because
of its rapid onset of action, drug should be tak-
en immediately before going to bed.
■ Dosage adjustments may be needed when
drug is given with other CNS-depressants because of the potentially additive effects.

### Therapeutic monitoring
■ Advise clinician to observe patients with history of addiction to or abuse of drugs or alcohol because they're at risk for habituation and
dependence.

### Special populations
**Breast-feeding patients.** Use of drug in breast-
feeding women isn't recommended.
**Pediatric patients.** Safety and efficacy in children under age 18 haven't been established.
**Geriatric patients.** Impaired motor or cognitive performance after repeated exposure or
unusual sensitivity to sedative-hypnotics may
occur in geriatric patients. Recommended dose
is 5 mg rather than 10 mg.

## Patient counseling
■ Stress importance of taking drug only as prescribed; inform patient of potential drug dependency associated with hypnotics taken for
long periods.
■ Inform patient that tolerance may occur if
drug is taken for longer than a few weeks.

---

- Warn patient against use of alcohol or other sleep aids during therapy to avoid serious adverse effects.
- Caution patient to avoid activities that require alertness, such as driving a car, until adverse CNS effects of drug are known.

# zonisamide
Zonegran

*Pharmacologic classification:* sulfonamide
*Therapeutic classification:* anticonvulsant
*Pregnancy risk category C*

## Available forms
Available by prescription only
*Capsules:* 100 mg

## Indications and dosages
*Adjunct therapy for treatment of partial seizures in adults with epilepsy*
*Adults over age 16:* Initially, 100 mg P.O. as single daily dose for 2 weeks. After 2 weeks, dosage may be increased to 200 mg/day for at least 2 weeks. It can then be increased to 300 mg for at least 2 weeks; then 400 mg P.O. daily, with the dose stable for at least 2 weeks to achieve steady-state at each level. Doses can be given once or twice daily except for the daily dose of 100 mg at initiation of therapy. Drug can be taken with or without food.

≡*Dosage adjustment.* Use cautiously in patients with hepatic and renal disease because they may require slower adjustment and more frequent monitoring.

## Mechanism of action
*Anticonvulsant action:* Exact mechanism of action is unknown. Zonisamide is thought to produce its antiseizure effects through action at the sodium and calcium channels, thereby stabilizing neuronal membranes and suppressing neuronal hypersynchronization. Other models suggest that synaptically driven electrical activity is suppressed without potentiation of GABA synaptic activity. The drug may also facilitate dopaminergic and serotonergic neurotransmission.

## Pharmacokinetics
*Absorption:* Plasma levels peak in 2 to 6 hours. Food delays, but does not affect bioavailability.
*Distribution:* Extensively binds to erythrocytes. Drug is about 40% plasma protein–bound. Protein-binding is unaffected in the presence of therapeutic levels of phenytoin, phenobarbital, or carbamazepine.
*Metabolism:* Metabolized by cytochrome P-450 3A4. Clearance of drug increases in patients who are concurrently taking enzyme-inducing drugs.
*Excretion:* Excreted primarily in urine as parent drug and as glucuronide of a metabolite. Half-life in plasma is about 63 hours.

| Route | Onset | Peak | Duration |
|-------|-------|------|----------|
| P.O. | Unknown | Unknown | Unknown |

## Contraindications and precautions
Contraindicated in patients hypersensitive to sulfonamides or zonisamide. Use cautiously in patients with renal and hepatic dysfunction. Don't use in patients whose glomerular filtration rate is less than 50 ml/minute.

## Interactions
**Drug-drug.** *Drugs that induce or inhibit CYP3A4:* Possible alteration in serum zonisamide levels. Advise clinician to monitor patient.

## Adverse reactions
**CNS:** *headache, dizziness,* ataxia, asthenia, nystagmus, paresthesia, confusion, difficulties in concentration or memory, mental slowing, agitation or irritability, depression, insomnia, anxiety, nervousness, schizophrenic or schizophreniform behavior, *somnolence,* fatigue, tiredness, speech abnormalities, difficulties in verbal expression, tremor, *seizures,* abnormal gait, hyperesthesia, incoordination.
**EENT:** rhinitis, diplopia, pharyngitis, amblyopia, tinnitus.
**GI:** taste perversion, *anorexia,* nausea, diarrhea, dyspepsia, constipation, dry mouth, abdominal pain, vomiting.
**Hematologic:** ecchymosis.
**Metabolic:** weight loss.
**Respiratory:** increased cough.
**Skin:** rash, pruritus.
**Other:** flu syndrome, accidental injury.

## Overdose and treatment
No antidote available. Following a suspected overdose, advise clinician to induce emesis or perform gastric lavage with precautions to protect the airway. Recommend using supportive care with frequent monitoring of vital signs and close observation of the patient. Renal dialysis may not be effective. Contact a poison control center for information on management of zonisamide overdose.

## Clinical considerations
- Advise clinician to monitor patient for symptoms of hypersensitivity.
- Consider discontinuing zonisamide in patients who develop an unexplained rash.
- Advise clinician to monitor body temperature, especially in the summer, because decreased sweating has occurred (especially in patients ages 17 and younger), resulting in heatstroke and dehydration.

---

■ Abrupt withdrawal of zonisamide may precipitate increased frequency of seizures or status epilepticus; advise clinician to reduce dosage or discontinue drug gradually.
■ Fluid intake and urine output should be increased to help prevent kidney stones, especially in patients with predisposing factors.

### Therapeutic monitoring
■ Advise clinician to monitor renal function periodically. If acute renal failure or a clinically significant sustained increase in creatinine and BUN levels develops, drug should be stopped.

### Special populations
**Breast-feeding patients.** It isn't known if drug appears in breast milk. A decision should be made to discontinue either breast-feeding or drug, taking into account the importance of drug to the mother. Use drug only if the benefits outweigh the risk.
**Pediatric patients.** Safety and efficacy in children under age 16 haven't been established.
**Geriatric patients.** Use with caution; advise clinician to start at lower end of dosage range.

## Patient counseling
■ Advise patient to take drug with or without food and not to bite or break the capsule.
■ Tell patient to contact prescriber immediately if any of the following occurs: skin rash; fever, sore throat, mouth sores, or easy bruising; sudden back pain, abdominal pain, or pain when urinating; bloody or dark urine; decreased sweating or a rise in body temperature; depression; or speech or language problems.
■ Caution patient that drug can cause drowsiness. Tell him not to drive or operate dangerous machinery until effects of drug are known.
■ Warn patient not to stop drug without prescriber's approval.
■ Advise patient to drink six to eight glasses of water a day to help reduce risk of kidney stones.
■ Tell a woman to notify prescriber if she is pregnant or breast-feeding or plans to become pregnant or breast-feed.
■ Advise a woman of childbearing potential to use a contraceptive while taking this drug.

# Subcutaneous, intramuscular, and intravenous injection techniques

## Subcutaneous administration

S.C. injection allows slower, more sustained drug administration than I.M. injection.

### For single-dose ampules

Wrap the neck of the ampule in an alcohol sponge and snap off the top. If desired, attach a filter needle to the needle and withdraw the drug. Tap the syringe to clear air from it. Cover the needle with the needle sheath. Before discarding the ampule, check the label against the patient's medication record. Discard the filter needle and the ampule. Attach the appropriate needle to the syringe.

### For single-dose or multidose vials

Reconstitute powdered drugs according to the instructions on the label. Clean the vial's rubber stopper with an alcohol sponge. Pull the syringe plunger back until the volume of air in the syringe equals the volume of drug to be withdrawn from the vial. Insert the needle into the vial. Inject the air, invert the vial, and keep the bevel tip of the needle below the level of the solution as you withdraw the prescribed amount of drug. Cover the needle with the nee-

dle sheath. Tap the syringe to clear any air from it. Check the drug label against the patient's medication record before returning the multidose vial to the shelf or drawer or before discarding the single-dose vial.

### Implementation

- Select the injection site from those shown, and tell the patient where you'll be giving the injection.
- Put on gloves. Position and drape the patient, if necessary.
- Clean the injection site with an alcohol sponge. Loosen the protective needle sheath.
- With your nondominant hand, pinch the skin around the injection site firmly to elevate the S.C. tissue, forming a 1" (2.5 cm) fat fold, as shown on page 1274.
- Holding the syringe in your dominant hand (while pinching the skin around the injection site with the index finger and thumb of your nondominant hand), grip the needle sheath between the fourth and fifth fingers of your nondominant hand, and pull back to uncover the needle. Don't touch the needle.
- Position the needle with its bevel up.
- Tell the patient she'll feel a prick as the needle is inserted. Insert the needle quickly in one motion at a 45-degree or 90-degree angle, as

shown above, depending on needle length and the amount of S.C. tissue at the site. Some drugs, such as heparin, should always be injected at a 90-degree angle.

■ Release the skin to avoid injecting the drug into compressed tissue and irritating the nerves. Pull the plunger back slightly to check for blood return. If none appears, slowly inject the drug. If blood appears upon aspiration, withdraw the needle, prepare another syringe, and repeat the procedure.

■ After injection, remove the needle at the same angle used for insertion. Cover the site with an alcohol sponge, and massage the site gently.

■ Remove the alcohol sponge, and check the injection site for bleeding or bruising.

■ Don't recap the needle. Follow institutional policy to dispose of injection equipment.

■ Remove and discard gloves. Wash your hands.

### Clinical considerations

■ Don't aspirate for blood return when giving insulin or heparin. It's not necessary with insulin and may cause a hematoma with heparin.

■ Don't massage the site after administering heparin.

■ Repeated injections in the same site can cause lipodystrophy, a natural immune response. This complication can be minimized by rotating injection sites.

## Intramuscular administration

I.M. injections deposit the drug deep into well-vascularized muscle for rapid systemic action and absorption of up to 5 ml.

### Implementation

■ Wash your hands.

■ Select an appropriate injection site. Avoid a site that's inflamed, edematous, or irritated, or that contains moles, birthmarks, scar tissue, or other lesions. Dorsogluteal or ventrogluteal muscles are used most commonly.

**Dorsogluteal muscle**

- Posterior superior iliac spine
- Greater trochanter of femur
- Sciatic nerve

**Ventrogluteal muscle**

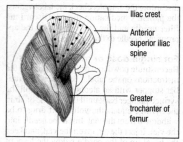

- Iliac crest
- Anterior superior iliac spine
- Greater trochanter of femur

**Deltoid muscle**

- Acromial process
- Deep brachial artery
- Radial nerve
- Humerus

**Vastus lateralis and rectus femoris muscles**

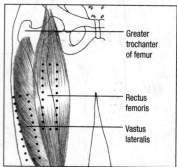

- Greater trochanter of femur
- Rectus femoris
- Vastus lateralis

- The deltoid muscle may be used for injections of 2 ml or less, as shown.
- The vastus lateralis is used most often in children; the rectus femoris may be used in infants, as shown.
- Rotate injection sites for patients who require repeated injections.
- Position and drape the patient appropriately.
- Loosen, but don't remove, the needle sheath.
- Gently tap the site to stimulate nerve endings and minimize pain.
- Clean the site by moving an alcohol sponge in circles increasing in diameter to about 2" (5 cm). Allow the skin to dry; alcohol stings in the puncture.
- Put on gloves.
- With the thumb and index finger of your nondominant hand, gently stretch the skin.
- With the syringe in your dominant hand, remove the needle sheath with the free fingers of your other hand.
- Position the syringe perpendicular to the skin surface and a couple of inches from the skin. Tell the patient that he'll feel a prick. Then quickly and firmly thrust the needle into the muscle.
- Pull back slightly on the plunger to aspirate for blood. If none appears, inject the drug slowly and steadily to let the muscle distend gradually. You should feel little or no resistance. Gently but quickly remove the needle at a 90-degree angle.
- If blood appears, the needle is in a blood vessel. Withdraw it, prepare a fresh syringe, and inject another site.
- Using a gloved hand, apply gentle pressure to the site with an alcohol sponge. Massage the relaxed muscle, unless contraindicated, to distribute the drug and promote absorption.
- Inspect the site for bleeding or bruising. Apply pressure, as necessary.
- Discard all equipment properly. Don't recap needles; put them in an appropriate biohazard container to avoid needle-stick injuries.
- Remove and discard gloves. Wash your hands.

## Clinical considerations

- To slow absorption, some drugs are dissolved in oil. Mix them well before use.
- Never inject into the gluteal muscles of a child who has been walking for less than 1 year.
- If the patient must have repeated injections, consider numbing the area with ice before cleaning it. If you must inject more than 5 ml, divide the solution and inject it at two sites.
- Urge the patient to relax the muscle to reduce pain and bleeding.
- I.M. injections can damage local muscle cells and elevate serum enzyme levels (creatine kinase), which can be confused with elevated levels caused by MI. Diagnostic tests can be used to differentiate between them.

# I.V. bolus administration

This method allows rapid I.V. drug administration to quickly achieve peak levels in the bloodstream. It may also be used for drugs that can't be given I.M. because they're toxic or the patient has reduced ability to absorb them, or to deliver drugs that can't be diluted.

Bolus doses may be injected directly into a vein or through an existing I.V. line.

## Implementation
*To give a direct injection:*
- Wash your hands and put on gloves.
- Select the largest vein suitable to dilute the drug and minimize irritation.
- Apply a tourniquet above the site to distend the vein, and clean the site with an alcohol or povidone-iodine sponge, working outward in a circle.
- If you're using the needle of the drug syringe, insert it at a 30-degree angle with the bevel up. The bevel should reach ¼" (0.6 cm) into the vein. Insert a steel needle-winged device bevel up, tape the wings in place when you see blood return, and attach the syringe containing the drug.
- Check for blood backflow.
- Remove the tourniquet, and inject the drug at the ordered rate.
- Check for blood backflow to ensure that the needle remained in place and all of the injected drug entered the vein.
- For a steel needle-winged device, flush the line with normal saline solution from the second syringe to ensure complete delivery.
- Withdraw the needle, and apply pressure to the site with a sterile gauze pad for at least 3 minutes to prevent hematoma.
- Apply an adhesive bandage when the bleeding stops.
- Remove and discard gloves. Wash your hands.
*To give an injection through an existing I.V. line:*
- Wash your hands and put on gloves.
- Check the compatibility of the drug.
- Close the flow clamp, wipe the injection port with an alcohol sponge, and inject the drug as you would a direct injection.
- Open the flow clamp and readjust the flow rate.
- Remove and discard gloves. Wash hands.
- If the drug isn't compatible with the I.V. solution, flush the line with normal saline solution before and after the injection.

## Clinical considerations

- If the existing I.V. line is capped, making it an intermittent infusion device, verify patency and placement of the device before injecting the drug. Then flush the device with normal saline solution, administer the drug, and follow with the appropriate flush.

■ Immediately report signs of acute allergic reaction or anaphylaxis. If extravasation occurs, stop the injection, estimate the amount of infiltration, and notify the clinician.
■ When giving diazepam or chlordiazepoxide hydrochloride through a steel needle-winged device or I.V. line, flush with bacteriostatic water to prevent precipitation.

# I.V. administration through a secondary I.V. line

A secondary I.V. line is a complete I.V. set connected to the lower Y-port (secondary port) of a primary line instead of to the I.V. catheter or needle. It features an I.V. container, long tubing, and either a microdrip or a macrodrip system, and can be used for continuous or intermittent drug infusion. When used continuously, it permits drug infusion and titration while the primary line maintains a constant total infusion rate.

A secondary I.V. line used only for intermittent drug administration is called a piggyback set. In this case, the primary line maintains venous access between drug doses. A piggyback set includes a small I.V. container, short tubing, and usually a macrodrip system, and it connects to the primary line's upper Y-port (piggyback port).

## Implementation

■ If the drug is incompatible with the primary I.V. solution, replace the primary solution with a fluid that's compatible with both solutions, and flush the line before starting the drug infusion.
■ Hang the container of the secondary set and wipe the injection port of the primary line with an alcohol sponge.
■ Insert the needle or needleless system from the secondary line into the injection port, and tape it securely to the primary line.
■ To run the container of the secondary set by itself, lower the primary set's container with an extension hook. To run both containers simultaneously, place them at the same height.
■ Open the clamp and adjust the drip rate.
■ For continuous infusion, set the secondary solution to the desired drip rate; then adjust the primary solution to the desired total infusion rate.
■ For intermittent infusion, wait until the secondary solution is completely infused; then adjust the primary drip rate, as required.
■ If the secondary solution tubing is being reused, close the clamp on the tubing and follow your institution's policy: Either remove the needle or needleless system and replace it with a new one, or leave it taped in the injection port and label it with the time it was first used.

■ Leave the empty container in place until you replace it with a new drug dose at the prescribed time. If the tubing won't be reused, discard it appropriately with the I.V. container.

## Clinical considerations

■ If institutional policy allows, use a pump for drug infusion. Put a time tape on the secondary container to help prevent an inaccurate administration rate.
■ When reusing secondary tubing, change it according to institutional policy, usually every 48 to 72 hours. Inspect the injection port for leakage with each use; change it more often, if needed.
■ Except for lipids, don't piggyback a secondary I.V. line to a total parenteral nutrition line because it risks contamination.

# Herbal medicines

Advise patient to consult with his health care provider before using an herbal preparation because a treatment with proven efficacy may be available. When a patient fills a new prescription, ask him if he is taking any herbal or dietary supplements. Caution patient that if he delays seeking medical diagnosis and treatment, his condition could worsen. Tell patient to store herbs in tightly sealed containers away from light and away from children and pets.

| Herb names | Reported uses | Clinical considerations | Patient counseling |
|---|---|---|---|
| **ALOE**<br>Aloe Gel, Aloe Latex, Aloe Vera, Cape | Aloe latex is used orally as a cathartic. It's used to treat constipation; to provide evacuation relief for patient with anal fissures, hemorrhoids, or recent anorectal surgery; and to prepare a patient for diagnostic testing of the GI tract.<br>Aloe gel is used to treat minor burns and skin irritation and to aid in wound healing. It may also be effective as an antibacterial. | • Aloe's laxative effects are apparent within 10 hours.<br>• Advise clinician to monitor patient for signs of dehydration. Geriatric patients are particularly at risk.<br>• Advise clinician to monitor electrolyte levels, especially potassium, after long-term use.<br>• If patient is using aloe topically, advise clinician to monitor wound for healing. | • If patient is taking digoxin or another drug to control his heart rate, a diuretic, or a corticosteroid, warn him not to take aloe without consulting his health care provider.<br>• Advise patient to reduce dosage if cramping occurs after a single dose and not to take aloe for longer than 1 to 2 weeks at a time without consulting his health care provider.<br>• Advise patient to notify his health care provider immediately if he experiences feelings of dehydration, weakness, or confusion, especially if he has been using aloe for a prolonged period. |
| **ANGELICA**<br>Nature's Answer Angelica Root Liquid | Angelica seed is used as a diuretic and diaphoretic. It's also used to treat conditions of the kidneys and the urinary, GI, and respiratory tracts as well as rheumatic and neuralgic symptoms. | • Advise clinician to monitor patient for persistent diarrhea, which may be a sign of something more serious.<br>• Advise clinician to monitor patient for dermatologic reactions.<br>• Photodermatosis is possible after contact with the plant juice or plant extract. | • Caution patient not to delay seeking medical treatment for symptoms that may be related to a serious medical condition.<br>• Advise patient not to take angelica if pregnant or if taking a gastric acid blocker or anticoagulant.<br>• Advise patient to notify his health care provider if he develops a rash. |
| **BETEL PALM**<br>Areca Catechu, Piper Betle | Used as a mild CNS stimulant, digestive aid, and to treat coughs, stomach complaints, diphtheria, middle ear inflammation, and worm infestation. | • Arecaine, a compound of the herb, is poisonous, and may affect respiration and heart rate, or cause seizures. Seed doses of 8 g can be fatal. | • Warn patient that chewing betel palm may cause cancerous lesions in the mouth, severe oral mucosal changes, or asthmalike symptoms and that he should consult his health care provider immediately if he develops any of these.<br>• Advise patient not to apply betel palm leaves as a facial dressing because of adverse dermatological reactions. |
| **BITTER MELON**<br>Bitter Melon, Bitter Melon Juice, Bitter Melon Power, Bitter Melon Tincture | Used to treat diabetes symptoms. May help treat GI disorders. | • The hypoglycemic effects of bitter melon are dose related, so dosage should be adjusted gradually.<br>• Bitter melon seeds contain vicine, which may cause an acute condition characterized by headache, fever, abdominal pain, and coma. | • Pregnant patients should avoid this herb because it can stimulate menstruation.<br>• Patients taking insulin or oral antidiabetics should consult their health care provider before using this herb. |

| Herb names | Reported uses | Clinical considerations | Patient counseling |
|---|---|---|---|
| **CAPSICUM** Capsin, Capzasin-P, Dolorac, No Pain-HP, Pain Doctor, Zostrix, ZostrixOHP, Cayenne Pepper Capsules and Alcoholic Extract | The FDA has approved topical capsaicin for temporary relief of pain from rheumatoid arthritis, osteoarthritis, post-herpetic neuralgia (shingles), and diabetic neuropathy. It's also used in personal defense sprays. Oral capsicum is used for various GI complaints, including dyspepsia, flatulence, ulcers, and stomach cramps. | • Alcoholic extract may be unsuitable for children, alcoholic patients, patients with liver disease, and those taking disulfiram or metronidazole. • Adverse skin reactions to topically applied capsaicin are treated by washing the area thoroughly with soap and water. Soaking the area in vegetable oil after washing provides a slower onset but longer duration of relief than cold water. Vinegar water irrigation is moderately successful. Rubbing alcohol may also help. • EMLA, an emulsion of lidocaine and prilocaine, provides pain relief in about 1 hour to skin that has been severely irritated by capsaicin. • Capsicum shouldn't be taken orally for longer than 2 days and then shouldn't be used again for 2 weeks. | • If patient is pregnant or is breast-feeding or is planning pregnancy, advise her not to use this herb. • If patient is applying capsicum topically, inform him that it may take 1 to 2 weeks for him to experience maximum pain control. • If patient is using capsicum topically, instruct him to wash his hands before and immediately after applying it and to avoid contact with eyes. Advise contact lens wearer to wash his hands and to use gloves or an applicator if handling his lenses after applying capsicum. Tell him not to use topical capsicum on broken or irritated skin and instruct him not to tightly bandage any area to which it is applied. |
| **CHAMOMILE** Azulon, Chamomile Flowers, Chamomile Tea, Kid Chamomile, Standardized Chamomile Extract, Wild Chamomile | Used orally to treat diarrhea, anxiety, restlessness, stomatitis, hemorrhagic cystitis, flatulence and motion sickness. Used topically to stimulate skin metabolism, reduce inflammation, encourage wound healing, and treat cutaneous burns. Also used for its antibacterial and antiviral effects. | • People sensitive to ragweed and chrysanthemums or other Compositae family members (arnica, yarrow, feverfew, tansy, artemisia) may be more susceptible to contact allergies and anaphylaxis. • Patients with hay fever or bronchial asthma caused by pollens are more susceptible to anaphylactic reactions. | • If patient is pregnant or is planning pregnancy, advise her not to use chamomile. • If patient is taking an anticoagulant, advise him not to use chamomile because of possible enhanced anticoagulant effects. • Advise patient that chamomile may enhance an allergic reaction or make existing symptoms worse in susceptible patients. • Instruct parent not to give chamomile to any child before checking with a knowledgeable practitioner. |
| **CHONDROITIN** CDS, Chondroitin Sulfate, Chondroitin Sulfate A, Chondroitin Sulfate C, Chondroitin Sulfuric Acid, Chonsurid | Used to decrease pain and inflammation after extravasation with ifosfamide, vindesine, doxorubicin, or vincristine. | • Chondroitin may alter the effects of conventional drugs. • Advise clinician to monitor patient for allergic reactions, such as shortness of breath or rash. | • Instruct patient not to discontinue other arthritis treatment without discussing it with his health care provider. • Little information exists about chondroitin's long-term effects. • Instruct patient to notify his health care provider if he experiences any allergic reactions, such as shortness of breath or rash. |
| **COENZYME Q10** Ubiquinone | Used to treat ischemic heart disease, hypertension, and heart failure, to guard against doxorubicin cardiotoxicity, and to protect the | • If patient has diabetes, advise clinician to monitor glucose levels regularly. • Adverse reactions are rare. • Coenzyme Q10 shouldn't be used during pregnancy. | • Warn patient not to treat signs and symptoms of heart failure—such as increasing shortness of breath, edema, or chest pain—with coenzyme Q10 before seeking appropriate medical evaluation. |

| Herb names | Reported uses | Clinical considerations | Patient counseling |
|---|---|---|---|
| **COENZYME Q10** (continued) | myocardium during invasive cardiac surgery. | | • Advise patient with heart failure that coenzyme Q10 shouldn't replace conventional drug therapy.<br>• Patient taking an antilipemic, anticoagulant, cardiac drugs, or insulin should discuss the use of coenzyme Q10 prior to use. |
| **COMFREY** Symphytum officinale, Ass Ear, Black Root, Blackwort, Boneset, Bruise wort, Consound, Gum Plant, Healing Herb, Knitback, Knitbone, Salsify, Slippery Root, Wallwort | Used to treat bruises, sprains, joint inflammation, swelling, ulcers, gastritis, cancer, angina, and diarrhea. Also used to help in wound healing. | • Comfrey preparations have been identified as potentially harmful because of reports of liver toxicity.<br>• Patients taking comfrey should be monitored for signs and symptoms of hepatotoxicity, including abdominal distention, nausea, and abdominal pain, and elevated liver function test results. | • If patient is pregnant or breast-feeding or is planning pregnancy, advise her not to use comfrey.<br>• Advise patient that the internal use of comfrey isn't recommended.<br>• Inform patient that external preparations shouldn't be applied to broken or abraded skin.<br>• Advise patient that many comfrey preparations don't indicate the amount of pyrrolizidine alkaloids they contain. These alkaloids are hepatotoxic.<br>• Advise patient to discontinue use if he experiences visual disturbances, changes in heart rhythm, or dry skin and mouth. |
| **CREATINE MONOHYDRATE** Creatine | Used as a dietary supplement to increase strength and endurance, produce energy, enhance muscle size, improve stamina, and promote faster muscle recovery. | • If muscle cramping occurs, patient should stop taking creatine and contact health care provider. A smaller dose may be needed.<br>• This product is useful only for intense exercise and short duration or when short bursts of strength are needed. | • If patient is a young athlete, discuss creatine's use and adverse effects with the parents and the patient. Advise parents to monitor young athlete's use of creatine and to promptly report adverse effects to the health care provider.<br>• If patient is taking cimetidine, probenecid, or an NSAID, advise him to consult his health care provider before taking creatine.<br>• Advise patient to drink plenty of fluids while taking creatine. |
| **DONG QUAI** Chinese Angelica, Dang-Gui, Tang-Kuei | Used to treat anemia, hepatitis, hypertension, migraines, neuralgias, rhinitis, and gynecologic disorders, including irregular menstruation, dysmenorrhea, PMS, and menopausal symptoms. | • Advise clinician to monitor patient for signs of easy bruising or bleeding.<br>• If dong quai must be used with another anticoagulant, advise clinician to closely monitor PT and INR.<br>• Advise clinician to monitor patient for photosensitivity reactions. | • If patient is pregnant or breast-feeding, advise her not to use dong quai.<br>• Instruct patient to avoid taking dong quai with an anticoagulant, unless otherwise instructed by his health care provider. |
| **ECHINACEA** Coneflower Extract, Echina-Care Liquid, Echinacea, Echinacea Angustifolia Herb, Echinacea Extract, Echinacea Fresh Freeze Dried, Echinacea Glycerite, Echinacea Herbal Comfort, | Used to stimulate the immune system and treat acute and chronic upper respiratory and urinary tract infections. Used also in wound healing, as an adjunct to a conventional antineoplastic therapy and to provide prophylaxis against the common cold. | • Daily dose depends on the preparation and potency but shouldn't exceed 8 weeks.<br>• Echinacea is considered supportive treatment for infection; it shouldn't be used in place of antibiotic therapy.<br>• Echinacea is usually taken at the first sign of illness and continued for up to 14 days. Regular prophylactic use isn't recommended.<br>• Herbalists recommend us- | • Advise patient not to delay seeking appropriate medical evaluation for a prolonged illness.<br>• Advise patient that prolonged use may result in overstimulation of the immune system and possible immune suppression. Echinacea shouldn't be used longer than 14 days for supportive treatment of infection.<br><br>*(continued)* |

| Herb names | Reported uses | Clinical considerations | Patient counseling |
|---|---|---|---|
| **ECHINACEA** *(continued)* Echinacea Red Root Supreme, Echinacea Root Complex | | ing liquid preparations because it's believed that echinacea functions in the mouth and should have direct contact with the lymph tissues at the back of the throat. | |
| **EPHEDRA** Available as combination products, including Chromemate, Escalation, Excel, Herbal Ecstasy, Herbal Fen-Phen, Herbalife, Metabolife, Power Trim, Up Your Gas | Used to treat respiratory tract diseases with mild bronchospasm. Allopathic practitioners have used it since the 1930s to treat asthma. Also used as a CV stimulant and to treat various other conditions, including chills, coughs, colds, flu, fever, headaches, edema, and nasal congestion; it's also used as an appetite suppressant. | • Compounds containing ephedra have been linked to several deaths and more than 800 adverse effects, many of which appear to be dose related. <br>• Patients with eating disorders may abuse this herb. <br>• Pills containing ephedra have been combined with other stimulants like caffeine and sold as "natural" stimulants in weight loss products. Deaths from overstimulation have been reported. <br>• Dosages high enough to produce psychoactive or hallucinogenic effects are toxic to the heart. | • Advise patient not to use this herb in place of getting the proper medical evaluation for a prolonged illness. <br>• Advise patient with thyroid disease, hypertension, CV disease, or diabetes to avoid using ephedra. <br>• Advise patient not to use ephedra-containing products for longer than 7 consecutive days because of the risk of anaphylaxis and dependence. <br>• Advise patient to watch for adverse reactions, particularly chest pain, shortness of breath, palpitations, dizziness, and fainting. |
| **FEVERFEW** Feverfew Extract, Feverfew Leaf, Feverfew Leaf and Flower, Feverfew LF and FL-GBE, Feverfew Power, Migracare Feverfew Extract, Migracin, MigraSpray, MygraFew | Used most commonly to prevent or treat migraine headaches and to treat rheumatoid arthritis. Used to treat asthma, psoriasis, menstrual cramps, digestion problems, and intestinal parasites; to debride wounds; and to promote menstrual flow. | • If patient is taking an anticoagulant, coagulation values, such as INR, PTT, and PT should be monitored. Also, advise clincian to observe patient for abnormal bleeding. <br>• Rash or contact dermatitis may indicate sensitivity to feverfew. Patient should discontinue use immediately. <br>• Abruptly stopping the herb may cause tension headaches, insomnia, joint stiffness and pain, and lethargy. | • If patient is pregnant, planning to become pregnant, or breast-feeding, advise her not to use feverfew. <br>• Educate patient about the potential risk of abnormal bleeding when combining herb with an anticoagulant. <br>• Caution patient that a rash or abnormal skin alteration may indicate an allergy to feverfew. Instruct patient to stop taking the herb if a rash appears. |
| **FLAX** Dakota Flax Gold, Flax Seed Oil, Flax Seed Whole | Used internally to treat diarrhea, constipation, diverticulitis, gastritis, enteritis, and bladder inflammation. Used externally to remove foreign objects from the eye. Also used as a poultice for skin inflammation. | • When flax is used internally, it should be taken with more than 5 oz of liquid per tablespoon of flaxseed. <br>• Even though flax may decrease a patient's cholesterol level or increase bleeding time, it isn't necessary to monitor cholesterol level or platelet aggregation. | • Warn patient not to treat chronic GI disturbances with flax before seeking appropriate medical evaluation. <br>• Instruct patient to drink plenty of water when taking flaxseed. <br>• Instruct patient not to take any drug for at least 2 hours after taking flax. |
| **GARLIC** Garlicin, Garlic Powermax, Garlinase 4,000, GarliPure, Garlique, Garlitrin 4,000, Kwai, Kyolic Liquid, Wellness Garlicell | Used most commonly to decrease total cholesterol and triglyceride levels and increase HDLs. Also used to help prevent atherosclerosis and platelet aggregation. Used to decrease the risk of | • Garlic isn't recommended for patients with diabetes, insomnia, pemphigus, organ transplants, and rheumatoid arthritis, and in postsurgical patients. <br>• Advise clinician to monitor patient for signs and symptoms of bleeding. | • Advise patient to consume garlic in moderation, to minimize the risk of adverse reactions. <br>• Discourage use of garlic before surgery. <br>• If patient is using garlic to lower his serum cholesterol levels, advise him to notify his health care provider and to have his serum cholesterol levels monitored. |

| Herb names | Reported uses | Clinical considerations | Patient counseling |
|---|---|---|---|
| **GARLIC** (continued) | cancer, stroke and heart attack and to treat coughs, colds, fevers, and sore throats. | • Garlic may lower blood glucose level. If patient is taking an antihyperglycemic, advise clinician to watch for signs and symptoms of hypoglycemia. | • Advise patient that using garlic with anticoagulants may increase the risk of bleeding. |
| **GINGER** Alcohol-Free Ginger Root, Caffeine Free Ginger Root, Ginger Aid Tea, Ginger Kid, GingerMax, Ginger Powder, Ginger Root, Quanterra Stomach Comfort, Travellers | Used as an antiemetic, to treat colic, flatulence, indigestion, hypercholesterolemia, burns, ulcers, depression, impotence, liver toxicity, as an anti-inflammatory, as an antispasmodic, and for its antitumorigenic activity in cancer patients. | • Advise clinician to monitor patient for signs and symptoms of bleeding. If patient is taking an anticoagulant, advise clinician to monitor PTT, PT, and INR carefully. • Use in pregnant patients is questionable. • Ginger may interfere with the intended therapeutic effect of conventional drugs. | • If patient is pregnant, advise her to consult with a knowledgeable practitioner before using ginger medicinally. • Educate patients to look for signs and symptoms of bleeding, such as nosebleeds or excessive bruising. |
| **GINKGO** Bioginkgo, Gincosan, Ginkgo Go!, Ginkgo Liquid Extract Herb, Ginkgo Nut, Ginkgo Power, Ginkgo Capsules, Ginkgo, Quanterra Mental Sharpness | Primarily used to manage cerebral insufficiency, dementia, and circulatory disorders. Also used to treat headaches, asthma, colitis, impotence, depression, altitude sickness, tinnitus, cochlear deafness, vertigo, PMS, macular degeneration, diabetic retinopathy, and allergies. | • Ginkgo extracts are considered standardized if they contain 24% ginkgo flavonoid glycosides and 6% terpene lactones. • Treatment may be for at least 6 to 8 weeks, but therapy beyond 3 months isn't recommended. • Seizures have been reported in children after ingestion of more than 50 seeds. • Patients must be monitored for possible adverse reaction such as GI problems, headaches, dizziness, allergic reactions, and serious bleeding. | • If patient is taking the herb for motion sickness, advise him to begin taking it 1 to 2 days before taking the trip and to continue taking it for the duration of his trip. • Inform patient that the therapeutic and toxic components of ginkgo can vary significantly from product to product. • Advise patient to discontinue use at least 2 weeks before surgery. |
| **GINSENG, ASIAN** American Ginseng, American Ginseng Root, Centrum Ginseng, Chikusetsu Ginseng, Chinese Red Panax Ginseng Concentrate, Ginseng Manchurian | Used to manage fatigue and lack of concentration and to treat atherosclerosis, bleeding disorders, colitis, diabetes, depression, and cancer. Also used to help recover health and strength after sickness or weakness. | • Use isn't recommended for longer than 3 months. • Ginseng is believed to strengthen the body and increase resistance to disease. • Reports have circulated of a severe reaction known as the ginseng abuse syndrome in patients taking large doses—more than 3 g per day for up to 2 years. | • Inform patient that the therapeutic and toxic components of ginseng can vary significantly from product to product. Advise him to obtain his ginseng from a reliable source. • Patients experiencing ginseng abuse syndrome report a feeling of increased motor and cognitive activity combined with significant diarrhea, nervousness, insomnia, hypertension, edema, and skin eruptions. |
| **GLUCOMANNAN** Koch, Konjac, Konjac Mannan | Used to manage constipation, diabetes, obesity, hypercholesterolemia, and hyperlipidemia. Used to induce weight loss. | • Glucomannan may result in a feeling of fullness that decreases appetite. • Advise clinician to monitor patient for adverse effects, such as esophageal obstruction, lower GI obstruction, flatulence, diarrhea, and hypoglycemia. • Advise clinician to monitor patient's weight and cholesterol and glucose levels. | • Advise patient to avoid using tablet form because it poses an increased risk of esophageal obstruction. • Inform patient that the therapeutic and toxic components of glucomannan may vary significantly from product to product. |

| Herb names | Reported uses | Clinical considerations | Patient counseling |
|---|---|---|---|
| **GREEN TEA** Chinese Green Tea Bags, Green Tea, Green Tea Extract, Green Tea Power, Green Tea Power, Caffeine Free, Standardized Green Tea Extract | Used to prevent cancer, hyperlipidemia, atherosclerosis, dental caries, and headaches, and to treat wounds, skin disorders, stomach disorders, and infectious diarrhea. Also used as a CNS stimulant, a mild diuretic, and antibacterial and, topically, as an astringent. | • Look for products standardized to 80% polyphenol and 55% epigallocatechin gallate. <br> • Prolonged high caffeine intake may cause restlessness, irritability, insomnia, palpitations, vertigo, headache, and adverse GI effects. <br> • The tannin content in tea increases the longer it's left to brew; this increases the antidiarrheal properties of the tea. | • Instruct patient not to consume more than 5 cups a day, or 300 mg of caffeine, to avoid or minimize adverse effects. <br> • Advise patient that heavy consumption may be associated with esophageal cancer secondary to the tannin content in the mixture. <br> • Tell patient that the adverse GI effects of chlorogenic acid and tannin can be avoided if milk is added to the tea mixture. <br> • Tell patient that the first signs of toxic reaction are vomiting and abdominal spasm. |
| **HAWTHORNE** Hawthorne Berry, Hawthorne Extract, Hawthorne Formula, Hawthorne Power | Used to regulate blood pressure and heart rate and to treat atherosclerosis. Used as a cardiotonic and as a sedative for sleep. Used in mild cardiac insufficiency, heart conditions not requiring digoxin, mild stable forms of angina pectoris, and mild forms of bradycardia and palpitations. | • High doses may cause hypotension and sedation. Advise clinician to monitor patient for CNS adverse effects, and monitor blood pressure. <br> • Hawthorne may interfere with digoxin's effects or serum monitoring. <br> • Advise clinician to observe patient closely for adverse reactions, especially adverse CNS reactions. | • Advise patient to avoid use because of toxic adverse effects and narrow therapeutic index. <br> • Warn patient to keep all herbal products away from children and pets. |
| **HORSE CHESTNUT** Arthro-Therapy, Cell-U-Var Cream, Varicare, Varicosin, VenoCare Ultra-Joint, Venastat | Used to treat chronic venous insufficiency, varicose veins, leg pain, tiredness, tension, and leg swelling. Extract is used as a conjunctive treatment for lymphedema, hemorrhoids, and enlarged prostate. <br> Horse chestnut has been used as an analgesic, anticoagulant, antipyretic, astringent, expectorant, and tonic. It has also been used to treat skin ulcers, phlebitis, leg cramps, cough, and diarrhea. | • The nuts, seeds, twigs, sprouts, and leaves of horse chestnut are poisonous. Standardized formulations remove most of the toxins and standardize the amount of aescin. <br> • Signs and symptoms of toxicity include loss of coordination, salivation, hemolysis, headache, dilated pupils, muscle twitching, seizures, vomiting, diarrhea, depression, paralysis, respiratory and cardiac failure, and death. <br> • Advise clinician to monitor patient for signs of toxicity and discontinue horse chestnut immediately if any occur. | • Inform patient that the FDA classifies horse chestnut as an unsafe herb and that deaths have occurred. <br> • Tell patient that this is only symptomatic treatment of chronic venous insufficiency and not a cure. <br> • Advise patient not to confuse horse chestnut with sweet chestnut, used as a food. <br> • Advise patient to keep the herb away from children. Consumption of amounts of leaves, twigs, and seeds equaling 1% of a child's weight may be lethal. |
| **KAVA** Alcohol-Free, Fava-Kava, Kavacin, Kava Kava Plus, Kava Kava Root, Fava Tone, St. John's Plus Kava Kava, and Standardized Kava Extract | Used to treat nervous anxiety, stress, and restlessness. It's used orally to produce sedation, to promote wound healing, and to treat headaches, seizure disorders, the common cold, respiratory tract infection, tu- | • Patient shouldn't use kava with conventional sedative-hypnotics, anxiolytics, MAO inhibitors, other psychopharmacologic drugs, levodopa, or antiplatelet drugs without first consulting a health care provider. <br> • Periodic monitoring of liver function test results and CBC may be needed. | • Encourage patients to seek medical diagnosis before taking kava. <br> • Advise patient that usual doses can affect motor function; caution him against performing hazardous activities. <br> • Tell patient oral use is probably safe for 3 months or less, but use for longer than 3 months may be habit forming. |

| Herb names | Reported uses | Clinical considerations | Patient counseling |
|---|---|---|---|
| **KAVA** (continued) | berculosis, and rheumatism. It's also used to treat urogenital infections, including chronic cystitis, veneral disease, uterine inflammation, menstrual problems, and vaginal prolapse. Some herbal practitioners consider kava an aphrodisiac. Kava juice is used to treat skin diseases, including leprosy. It's also used as a poultice for intestinal problems, otitis, and abscesses. | • Heavy kava users are more likely to complain of poor health, are underweight, and have puffy faces, scaly rashes, and some evidence of pulmonary hypertension. These symptoms resolve several weeks after the herb is stopped.<br>• Toxic doses can cause progressive ataxia, muscle weakness, and ascending paralysis, all of which resolve when herb is stopped.<br>• Extreme use (more than 300 g per week) may increase GGT levels. | • Warn patient to avoid taking herb with alcohol because of increased risk of CNS depression and liver damage. |
| **KHAT** Abyssinian Tea, Arabian Tea, Chaat, Gat, Kat, Kus es Salahin, Qut, Somali Tea, Tchaad, Tohai, Tohat, Tschut | Leaf is used for treating depression, fatigue, obesity, and gastric ulcers. The leaf and stem are chewed as a euphoriant or appetite suppressant. | • Advise cautious use in patients with diabetes, hypertension, tachyarrhythmias, glaucoma, migraines, GI disorders, or underlying psychotic disorders.<br>• Although khat doesn't cause physical dependence, it may cause psychological dependence and can cause serious adverse effects. | • Tell patient that the leaf isn't physically addicting but may cause psychological dependence.<br>• Caution women to notify health care provider about planned, suspected, or known pregnancy.<br>• Long-term use may lead to hypertension in young adults, increased susceptibility to infection, insomnia, and disturbed circadian rhythms. |
| **MELATONIN** Circadian (controlled-release, not available in U.S.), Mela-T, Melatonex | Used for treating insomnia, jet lag, shift-work disorder, blind entrainment, immune system enhancement, tinnitus, depression, and benzodiazepine withdrawal in geriatric patients with insomnia. Topically, it's used for skin protection against ultraviolet light. | • Monitor patient for excessive daytime drowsiness.<br>• May increase human growth hormone levels. | • Warn patient to avoid hazardous activities until full extent of CNS depressant effect is known.<br>• If patient wishes to conceive, tell her that melatonin may have a contraceptive effect. However, herb shouldn't be used as birth control.<br>• Warn patient about possible additive effects if taken with alcohol.<br>• Advise patient to use only the synthetic form (not the animal-derived product) because of concerns about contamination and viral transmission.<br>• Advise patient not to use melatonin for prolonged periods because safety data aren't available. |
| **MILK THISTLE** Liver Formula with Milk Thistle, Milk Thistle Extract, Milk Thistle Phytosome, Milk Thistle Plus, Milk Thistle Power, Milk Thistle Super Complex, Silybin Phytosome, Silymarin Milk Thistle, Simply | Used for dyspepsia, liver damage from chemicals, *Amanita* mushroom poisoning, supportive therapy for inflammatory liver disease and cirrhosis, loss of appetite, and gallbladder and spleen disorders. It's also used as a liver protectant. | • Mild allergic reactions may occur, especially in people allergic to members of the Asteraceae family, including ragweed, chrysanthemums, marigolds, and daisies.<br>• Don't confuse milk thistle seeds or fruit with other parts of the plant or with blessed thistle (*Cnictus benedictus*).<br>• Silymarin has poor water solubility; therefore, efficacy when prepared as a tea is questionable. | • Although no chemical interactions have been reported in clinical studies, advise patient that herb may interfere with therapeutic effect of conventional drugs.<br>• Warn patient not to take this herb while pregnant or breast-feeding.<br>• Tell patient to stay alert for possible allergic reactions, especially if allergic to ragweed, chrysanthemums, marigolds, or daisies.<br>• Warn patient not to take herb for liver inflammation or cirrhosis before seeking appropriate medical *(continued)* |

| Herb names | Reported uses | Clinical considerations | Patient counseling |
|---|---|---|---|
| **MILK THISTLE** *(continued)* Milk Thistle, Thisilyn | | | evaluation because doing so may delay diagnosis of a potentially serious medical condition. |
| **PASSION FLOWER** Passion Flower, Alcohol Free Passion Flower Liquid | Used as a sedative, a hypnotic, an analgesic, and an antispasmodic for treating muscle spasms caused by indigestion, menstrual cramping, pain, or migraines. Also used for neuralgia, generalized seizures, hysteria, nervous agitation, and insomnia. Crushed leaves and flowers are used topically for cuts and bruises. | • Monitor patient for possible adverse CNS effects.<br>• No adverse effects have been observed with recommended doses.<br>• A disulfiram-like reaction may produce nausea, vomiting, flushing, headache, hypotension, tachycardia, ventricular arrhythmias, and shock leading to death.<br>• Patients with liver disease or alcoholism shouldn't use herbal products that contain alcohol. | • Because sedation is possible, caution patient to avoid hazardous activities.<br>• Warn patient not to take herb for chronic pain or insomnia before seeking medical attention because doing so may delay diagnosis of a potentially serious medical condition.<br>• Caution pregnant patients to avoid this herb. |
| **ST. JOHN'S WORT** Alterra, Hypercalm, Kira, Quanterra Emotional Balance, St. John's Wort Extracts, Tension Tamer, various combination products | Used orally for mild to moderate depression, anxiety, psychovegetative disorders, sciatica, and viral infections, including herpes simplex virus types 1 and 2, hepatitis C, influenza virus, murine cytomegalovirus, and poliovirus. St. John's wort has also been used to treat bronchitis, asthma, gallbladder disease, nocturnal enuresis, gout, and rheumatism, although it hasn't proven effective in these cases. | • Recommended duration of therapy for depression is 4 to 6 weeks; if no improvement occurs, a different therapy should be considered.<br>• Clinical studies have used formulations of standardized 0.3% hypericin as well as hyperforin-stabilized version of the extract.<br>• Serotonin syndrome may cause dizziness, nausea, vomiting, headache, epigastric pain, anxiety, confusion, restlessness, and irritability.<br>• Because St. John's wort decreases the effect of certain prescription drugs, advise clinician to watch for signs of drug toxicity if patient stops using the herb. Drug dosage may need to be reduced.<br>• St. John's wort has mutagenic effects on sperm cells and oocytes and adverse effects on reproductive cells; therefore, it shouldn't be used by pregnant patients or those planning pregnancy.<br>• Topically, the volatile plant oil is an irritant. | • Instruct patient to consult a health care provider for a thorough medical evaluation before using St. John's wort.<br>• If patient takes St. John's wort for mild to moderate depression, explain that several weeks may pass before effects occur. Tell patient that a new therapy may be needed if no improvement occurs in 4 to 6 weeks.<br>• Inform patient that St. John's wort interacts with many other prescription and OTC products and may reduce their effectiveness.<br>• Patients taking an MAOI, an SSRI, digoxin, or a protease inhibitor should not use St. John's wort.<br>• Tell patient that St. John's wort may cause increased sensitivity to direct sunlight. Recommend protective clothing, sunscreen, and limited sun exposure.<br>• Inform patient that a sufficient wash-out period is needed after stopping an antidepressant before switching to St. John's wort.<br>• Tell patient to report adverse effects to a health care provider. |
| **SAW PALMETTO** Centrum Saw Palmetto, Herbal Sure Saw Palmetto, Permixon, PlusStrogen, Premium Blend Saw Palmetto, Proactive Saw Palmetto, | Used to treat symptoms of BPH and coughs and congestion from colds, bronchitis, or asthma. Also used as a mild diuretic, urinary antiseptic, and astringent. | • Herb should be used cautiously for conditions other than BPH because data about its effectiveness in other conditions is lacking.<br>• Advise clinician to obtain a baseline prostate-specific antigen (PSA) test before patient starts taking herb because it may cause a false-negative PSA result. | • Warn patient not to take herb for bladder or prostate problems before seeking medical attention because doing so could delay diagnosis of a potentially serious medical condition.<br>• Tell patient to take herb with food to minimize GI effects.<br>• Caution patient to promptly notify |

| Herb names | Reported uses | Clinical considerations | Patient counseling |
|---|---|---|---|
| **SAW PALMETTO** (continued) Propalmex, Quanterra Prostate | | | health care provider about new or worsened adverse effects.<br>• Warn women to avoid herb if planning pregnancy, if pregnant, or if breast-feeding. |
| **SHEPHERD'S PURSE** Blindweed, Capsella, Case-Weed, Lady's Purse, Mother's Heart Pepper-and-Salt, Pick-Pocket, Poor Man's Parma-cettie, Rattle Pouches, Shepherd's Heart, Shovelweed, St. James' Weed, Witches' Pouches | Used internally to treat dysmenorrhea, mild menorrhagia, and metrorrhagia. Also used for headache, mild cardiac insufficiency, arrhythmia, hypotension, nervous heart complaints, premenstrual complaints, hematemesis, hematuria, diarrhea, acute catarrhal cystitis, topically, as a styptic for nosebleeds and other superficial bleeding injuries. | • The use of shepherd's purse instead of ergot for uterine bleeding is inappropriate.<br>• Advise clinician to monitor blood pressure, which may increase or decrease, and thyroid function in patients taking thyroid hormones who were previously well controlled.<br>• Advise clinician to monitor patient for palpitations, especially if susceptible to arrhythmias, and for changes in menstruation. | • Warn patient not to use alcohol-containing forms if he takes disulfiram, metronidazole, or any other drug that interacts with alcohol.<br>• Inform women that shepherd's purse may cause abnormal menstruation.<br>• Tell patient that this herb may aggravate kidney stones, CV therapy, thyroid therapy, and antihypertensive or antihypotensive therapy.<br>• Caution patient to avoid hazardous tasks until full sedative effects of herb are known.<br>• Urge patient to promptly notify health care provider about new symptoms or adverse effects. |
| **TEA TREE OIL** Tea Tree Oil, Tea Tree Oil Lotion, Tea Tree Soap | Used topically for contusions, inflammation, myalgia, burns, hemorrhoids, and vitiligo. In traditional Chinese medicine, tea tree oil has been used as a gargle for tonsillitis and as a lotion for dermatoses. | • Because of systemic toxicity, tea tree oil shouldn't be used internally.<br>• Essential oil should be used externally only after being diluted, especially by people with sensitive skin.<br>• Tea tree oil shouldn't be used around nose, eyes, and mouth.<br>• Vaginal douches using concentrations as strong as 40% require extreme caution. | • Tell patient to use very dilute tea tree oil (0.25% to 0.5%) as topical anti-infective.<br>• Explain that a few drops are sufficient in mouthwash, shampoo, or sitz bath.<br>• Caution patient not to apply oil to wounds or to skin that's dry or cracked.<br>• Warn patient to keep all herbal products away from children and pets. |
| **VALERIAN** All-Heal, Amantilla, Baldrian, Belgium Valerian, Capon's Tail, Garden Heliotrope, Indian Valerian, Mexican Valerian, Pacific Valerian, Radix, Setewale, Setwall, Vandal Root | Used to treat menstrual cramps, restlessness and sleep disorders from nervous conditions, and other symptoms of psychological stress, such as anxiety, nervous headaches, and gastric spasms. Used topically as a bath additive for restlessness and sleep disorders. | • Valerian seems to have a more pronounced effect on those with disturbed sleep or sleep disorders.<br>• Evidence of valerian toxicity includes difficulty walking, hypothermia, and increased muscle relaxation.<br>• Withdrawal symptoms, such as increased agitation and decreased sleep, can occur if valerian is abruptly stopped after prolonged use.<br>• Advise clinician to monitor CNS status and patient response to herb. | • Explain that patient may not feel herb's effect for 2 to 4 weeks.<br>• Inform patient that most adverse effects occur only after long-term use.<br>• Patient shouldn't stop abruptly after long term use.<br>• Instruct patient to avoid hazardous activities until full CNS effects of herb are known. |

# Therapeutic drug monitoring guidelines

| Drug | Laboratory test monitored | Therapeutic ranges of test |
|------|---------------------------|----------------------------|
| aminoglycoside antibiotics (amikacin, gentamicin, tobramycin) | Serum amikacin peak<br>trough<br>Serum gentamicin/tobramycin peak<br>trough<br>Serum creatinine | 20 to 25 mcg/ml<br>5 to 10 mcg/ml<br><br>4 to 8 mcg/ml<br>1 to 2 mcg/ml<br>0.6 to 1.3 mg/dl |
| amphotericin B | Serum creatinine<br>BUN<br>Serum electrolytes (especially potassium and magnesium)<br><br><br><br>Liver function tests<br>CBC with differential and platelets | 0.6 to 1.3 mg/dl<br>5 to 20 mg/dl<br>Potassium: 3.5 to 5 mEq/L<br>Magnesium: 1.5 to 2.5 mEq/L<br>Sodium: 135 to 145 mEq/L<br>Chloride: 98 to 106 mEq/L<br>*<br>***** |
| antibiotics | WBC with differential<br>Cultures and sensitivities | ***** |
| biguanides (metformin) | Serum creatinine<br>Fasting serum glucose<br>Glycosylated hemoglobin<br>CBC | 0.6 to 1.3 mg/dl<br>70 to 110 mg/dl<br>5.5 to 8.5% of total hemoglobin<br>***** |
| clozapine | WBC with differential | ***** |
| digoxin | Serum digoxin<br>Serum electrolytes (especially potassium, magnesium, and calcium)<br><br><br><br>Serum creatinine | 0.8 to 2 ng/ml<br>Potassium: 3.5 to 5 mEq/L<br>Magnesium: 1.5 to 2.5 mEq/L<br>Sodium: 135 to 145 mEq/L<br>Chloride: 98 to 106 mEq/L<br>Calcium: 8.6 to 10 mg/dl<br>0.6 to 1.3 mg/dl |
| diuretics | Serum electrolytes<br><br><br><br><br>Serum creatinine<br>BUN<br>Uric acid<br>Fasting serum glucose | Potassium: 3.5 to 5 mEq/L<br>Magnesium: 1.5 to 2.5 mEq/L<br>Sodium: 135 to 145 mEq/L<br>Chloride: 98 to 106 mEq/L<br>Calcium: 8.6 to 10 mg/dl<br>0.6 to 1.3 mg/dl<br>5 to 20 mg/dl<br>2 to 7 mg/dl<br>70 to 110 mg/dl |
| erythropoietin | Hematocrit | Women: 36% to 48%<br>Men: 42% to 52% |
| ethosuximide | Serum ethosuximide | 40 to 100 mcg/ml |
| gemfibrozil | Serum lipids | Total cholesterol: < 200 mg/dl<br>LDL: < 130 mg/dl<br>HDL: Women: 40 to 75 mg/dl<br>Men: 37 to 70 mg/dl<br>Triglycerides: 10 to 160 mg/dl |

Note: ***** For those areas marked with asterisks, the following values can be used:

Hemoglobin: Women: 12 to 16 g/dl
Men: 14 to 18 g/dl
Hematocrit: Women: 37% to 48%
Men: 42% to 52%
RBCs: 4 to 5.5 x 10⁶/mm³
WBCs: 5 to 10 x 10³/mm³

Differential: Neutrophils: 45% to 74%
Bands: 0% to 8%
Lymphocytes: 16% to 45%
Monocytes: 4% to 10%
Eosinophils: 0% to 7%
Basophils: 0% to 2%

## Monitoring guidelines

Advise clinician to wait until the administration of the third dose to check drug levels. Advise clinician to obtain blood for peak level 30 minutes after I.V. infusion or 60 minutes after I.M. administration. For trough levels, advise clinician to draw blood just before next dose. Dosage may need to be adjusted accordingly and rechecked after three doses. Advise clinician to monitor serum creatinine and BUN levels and urine output for signs of decreasing renal function.

Advise clinician to monitor serum creatinine, BUN, and serum electrolyte levels at least weekly and also regularly monitor blood counts and liver function tests during therapy.

Specimen cultures and sensitivities will determine the cause of the infection and the best treatment. Advise clinician to monitor WBC with differential weekly during therapy.

Advise clinician to check renal function and hematologic parameters before initiating therapy and at least yearly thereafter. If the patient has impaired renal function, metformin shouldn't be used because it may cause lactic acidosis. Advise clinician to monitor response to therapy by periodically evaluating fasting glucose and glycosylated hemoglobin levels. A patient's home monitoring of blood glucose levels helps monitor compliance and response.

Obtain WBC with differential before therapy starts, weekly during therapy, and 4 weeks after discontinuing the drug.

Serum digoxin levels should be checked at least 12 hours, preferably 24, after the last dose is administered. For monitoring maintenance therapy, levels should be checked at least 1 to 2 weeks after therapy is initiated or changed. Adjustments in therapy should be made based on entire clinical picture, not solely on drug levels. Electrolytes and renal function should also be checked periodically during therapy.

Baseline and periodic determinations of serum electrolytes, serum calcium, BUN, uric acid, and serum glucose should be performed to monitor fluid and electrolyte balance.

With the initiation of therapy and after any dosage change, advise clinician to monitor the hematocrit twice weekly for 2 to 6 weeks until stabilized in the target range and a maintenance dose determined. The hematocrit should be monitored at regular intervals thereafter.

Advise clinician to check drug level 8 to 10 days after therapy is initiated or changed.

Therapy is usually withdrawn after 3 months if response is inadequate. Patient must be fasting to measure triglycerides.

---

\* For those areas marked with one asterisk, the following values can be used:

ALT: 7 to 56 U/L
AST: 5 to 40 U/L
Alkaline phosphatase: 17 to 142 U/L
LDH: 60 to 220 U/L
GGT: < 40 U/L
Total bilirubin: 0.2 to 1 mg/dl

| Drug | Laboratory test monitored | Therapeutic ranges of test |
|---|---|---|
| heparin | Activated partial thromboplastin time (aPTT) | 1.5 to 2 times control |
| HMG-CoA reductase inhibitors (fluvastatin, lovastatin, pravastatin, simvastatin) | Serum lipids | Total cholesterol: < 200 mg/dl<br>LDL: < 130 mg/dl<br>HDL: women: 40 to 75 mg/dl<br>men: 37 to 70 mg/dl<br>Triglycerides: 10 to 160 mg/dl |
| | Liver function tests | * |
| insulin | Fasting serum glucose<br>Glycosylated hemoglobin | 70 to 110 mg/dl<br>5.5% to 8.5% of total hemoglobin |
| lithium | Serum lithium<br>Serum creatinine<br>CBC<br>Serum electrolytes (especially potassium and sodium) | 0.5 to 1.4 mEq/L<br>0.6 to 1.3 mg/dl<br>*****<br>Potassium: 3.5 to 5 mEq/L<br>Magnesium: 1.5 to 2.5 mEq/L<br>Sodium: 135 to 145 mEq/L<br>Chloride: 98 to 106 mEq/L |
| | Fasting serum glucose<br>Thyroid function tests | 70 to 110 mg/dl<br>TSH: 0.2 to 5.4 microU/mL<br>$T_3$: 80 to 200 ng/dl<br>$T_4$: 5.4 to 11.5 mcg/dl |
| methotrexate | Serum methotrexate | Normal elimination:<br>< 10 micromol 24 hours post dose<br>< 1 micromol 48 hours post dose<br>< 0.2 micromol 72 hours post dose |
| | CBC with differential<br>Platelet count<br>Liver function tests<br>Serum creatinine | *****<br>150 to 450 x $10^3$/mm³<br>*<br>0.6 to 1.3 mg/dl |
| phenytoin | Serum phenytoin<br>CBC | 10 to 20 mcg/ml<br>***** |
| potassium chloride | Serum potassium | 3.5 to 5 mEq/L |
| procainamide | Serum procainamide<br>Serum N-acetylprocainamide<br><br>CBC | 4 to 8 mcg/ml (procainamide)<br>5 to 30 mcg/ml (combined procainamide and NAPA)<br>***** |
| quinidine | Serum quinidine<br>CBC<br>Liver function tests<br>Serum creatinine<br>Serum electrolytes (especially potassium) | 2 to 6 mcg/ml<br>*****<br>*<br>0.6 to 1.3 mg/dl<br>Potassium: 3.5 to 5 mEq/L<br>Magnesium: 1.5 to 2.5 mEq/L<br>Sodium: 135 to 145 mEq/L<br>Chloride: 98 to 106 mEq/L |
| sulfonylureas | Fasting serum glucose<br>Glycosylated hemoglobin | 70 to 110 mg/dl<br>5.5% to 8.5% of total hemoglobin |

Note: ***** For those areas marked with asterisks, the following values can be used:

Hemoglobin: Women: 12 to 16 g/dl
          Men: 14 to 18 g/dl
Hematocrit: Women: 37% to 48%
        Men: 42% to 52%
RBCs: 4 to 5.5 x $10^6$/mm³
WBCs: 5 to 10 x $10^3$/mm³

Differential: Neutrophils: 45% to 74%
       Bands: 0% to 8%
       Lymphocytes: 16% to 45%
       Monocytes: 4% to 10%
       Eosinophils: 0% to 7%
       Basophils: 0% to 2%

### Monitoring guidelines

When drug is given by continuous I.V. infusion, advise clinician to check aPTT every 4 hours in the early stages of therapy. When drug is given by deep S.C. injection, advise clinician to check aPTT 4 to 6 hours after injection.

Liver function tests should be performed at baseline, 6 to 12 weeks after therapy is initiated or changed, and periodically thereafter. If adequate response is not achieved within 6 weeks, a change in therapy should be considered.

Advise clinician to monitor response to therapy with evaluations of serum glucose and glycosylated hemoglobin levels. Glycosylated hemoglobin is a good measure of long-term control. A patient's home monitoring of blood glucose levels helps monitor compliance and response.

Checking blood lithium levels is crucial to the safe use of the drug. Advise clinician to obtain serum lithium levels immediately before next dose. Levels should be monitored twice weekly until stable. Once at steady state, levels should be checked weekly; when the patient is on the appropriate maintenance dose, levels should be checked every 2 to 3 months. Advise clinician to monitor serum creatinine, serum electrolyte, and fasting serum glucose levels; CBC; and thyroid function tests before therapy is initiated and periodically during therapy.

Advise clinician to monitor methotrexate levels according to dosing protocol. CBC with differential, platelet count, and liver and renal function tests should be monitored more frequently when therapy is initiated or changed and when methotrexate levels may be elevated, such as when the patient is dehydrated.

Advise clinician to monitor serum phenytoin levels immediately before next dose and 2 to 4 weeks after therapy is initiated or changed. Advise clinician to obtain a CBC at baseline and monthly early in therapy. Advise clinician to watch for toxic effects at therapeutic levels. The measured level should be adjusted for hypoalbuminemia or renal impairment, which can increase free drug levels.

Check level weekly after oral replacement therapy is initiated until stable and every 3 to 6 months thereafter.

Advise clinician to measure procainamide levels 6 to 12 hours after a continuous infusion is started, or immediately before the next oral dose. Combined (procainamide and NAPA) levels can be used as an index of toxicity when renal impairment exists. CBC should be obtained periodically during longer-term therapy.

Advise clinician to obtain levels immediately before next oral dose and 30 to 35 hours after therapy is initiated or changed. Advise clinician to obtain periodic blood counts, liver and kidney function test results, and serum electrolyte levels.

Advise clinician to monitor response to therapy by periodically evaluating fasting glucose and glycosylated hemoglobin levels. A patient's home monitoring of blood glucose levels helps monitor compliance and response.

---

\* For those areas marked with one asterisk, the following values can be used:

ALT: 7 to 56 U/L
AST: 5 to 40 U/L
Alkaline phosphatase: 17 to 142 U/L
LDH: 60 to 220 U/L
GGT: < 40 U/L
Total bilirubin: 0.2 to 1 mg/dl

| Drug | Laboratory test monitored | Therapeutic ranges of test |
|------|--------------------------|----------------------------|
| theophylline | Serum theophylline | 10 to 20 mcg/ml |
| thyroid hormone | Thyroid function tests | TSH: 0.2 to 5.4 microU/ml<br>$T_3$: 80 to 200 ng/dl<br>$T_4$: 5.4 to 11.5 mcg/dl |
| vancomycin | Serum vancomycin | 20 to 35 mcg/ml (peak)<br>5 to 10 mcg/ml (trough) |
| | Serum creatinine | 0.6 to 1.3 mg/dl |
| warfarin | INR | For an acute MI, atrial fibrillation, treatment of pulmonary embolism, prevention of systemic embolism, tissue heart valves, valvular heart disease, or prophylaxis or treatment of venous thrombosis: 2 to 3<br>For mechanical prosthetic valves or recurrent systemic embolism: 2.5 to 3.5 |

Note: ***** For those areas marked with asterisks, the following values can be used:

Hemoglobin: Women: 12 to 16 g/dl  
           Men: 14 to 18 g/dl  
Hematocrit: Women: 37% to 48%  
          Men: 42% to 52%  
RBCs: 4 to 5.5 x 10⁶/mm³  
WBCs: 5 to 10 x 10³/mm³

Differential: Neutrophils: 45% to 74%  
          Bands: 0% to 8%  
          Lymphocytes: 16% to 45%  
          Monocytes: 4% to 10%  
          Eosinophils: 0% to 7%  
          Basophils: 0% to 2%

**Monitoring guidelines**

Advise clinician to obtain serum theophylline levels immediately before next dose of sustained-release oral product and at least 2 days after therapy is initiated or changed.

Advise clinician to monitor thyroid function tests every 2 to 3 weeks until appropriate maintenance dose is determined.

Serum vancomycin levels may be checked with the third dose administered, at the earliest. Peak levels should be drawn ½ hour after the I.V. infusion is completed. Trough levels should be drawn immediately before the next dose is administered. Renal function can be used to adjust dosing and intervals.

Advise clinician to check INR daily, beginning 3 days after therapy is initiated. Advise clinician to continue checking it until therapeutic goal is achieved and monitor it periodically thereafter. Levels should also be checked 7 days after any change in warfarin dose or concomitant, potentially interacting therapy.

* For those areas marked with one asterisk, the following values can be used:
ALT: 7 to 56 U/L
AST: 5 to 40 U/L
Alkaline phosphatase: 17 to 142 U/L
LDH: 60 to 220 U/L
GGT: < 40 U/L
Total bilirubin: 0.2 to 1 mg/dl

# Cytochrome P-450 enzymes and common drug interactions

Cytochrome P-450 enzymes, identified by "CYP" followed by numbers and letters identifying the enzyme families and subfamilies, are found throughout the body (primarily in the liver), and are important in the metabolism of many drugs. The following table lists potential drug-drug interactions based on the substrates, inducers, and inhibitors that can influence drug metabolism. The table includes common drug interactions, and the absence of a drug from the table doesn't necessarily imply that it isn't metabolized by one of the CYP enzymes.

| CYP enzyme | Substrates |
|---|---|
| 1A2 | Amitriptyline, caffeine, chlordiazepoxide, clomipramine, clozapine, cyclobenzaprine, desipramine, diazepam, haloperidol, imipramine, olanzapine, ropinisole, tacrine, theophylline, warfarin, zileuto |
| 2C9 | Amitriptyline, carvedilol, clomipramine, dapsone, diazepam, diclofenac, flurbiprofen, fluvastatin, glimepiride, ibuprofen, imipramine, indomethacin, losartan, mirtazapine, naproxen, omeprazole, phenytoin, piroxicam, ritonavir, sildenafil, tolbutamide, torsemide, S-warfarin, zafirlukast, zileuton |
| 2C19 | Amitriptyline, carisoprodol, clomipramine, diazepam, imipramine, lansoprazole, mephenytoin, omeprazole, pentamidine, R-warfarin |
| 2D6 | Amitriptyline, carvedilol, chlorpheniramine, chlorpromazine, clomipramine, clozapine, codeine, cyclobenzaprine, desipramine, dextromethorphan, donepezil, doxepin, fentanyl, flecainide, fluoxetine, fluphenazine, fluvoxamine, haloperidol, hydrocodone, imipramine, loratadine, maprotiline, meperidine, methadone, metoprolol, mexiletine, morphine, methamphetamine, nortriptyline, oxycodone, paroxetine, perphenazine, propafenone, propoxyphene, propranolol, risperidone, thioridazine, timolol, tramadol, trazodone, venlafaxine |
| 3A4 | Alfentanil, alprazolam, amiodarone, amitriptyline, amlodipine, atorvastatin, bromocriptine, buspirone, carbamazepine, clarithromycin, clomipramine, clonazepam, cocaine, corticosteroids, cyclophosphamide, cyclosporine (neural), dapsone, delavirdine, doxorubicin, dexamethasone, diazepam, diltiazem, disopyramide, ergotamine, erythromycin, ethosuximide, etoposide, felodipine, fentanyl, fexofenadine, finasteride, flutamide, fluvastatin, ifosfamide, imipramine, indinavir, isradipine, itraconazole, ketoconazole, lidocaine, loratadine, losartan, lovastatin, midazolam, methadone, methylprednisolone, miconazole, nefazodone, nicardipine, nifedipine, nimodipine, nisoldipine, paclitaxel, pravastatin, prednisone, quinidine, quinine, rifabutin, ritonavir, saquinavir, sertraline, sildenafil, simvastatin, tacrolimus, tamoxifen, teniposide, testosterone, triazolam, troleandomycin, verapamil, vinca alkaloids, warfarin, zileuton, zolpidem |

| Inducers | Inhibitors |
|---|---|
| Cigarette smoking, phenobarbital, phenytoin, primidone, rifampin, ritonavir | Ciprofloxacin, cimetidine, clarithromycin, enoxacin, erythromycin, fluvoxamine, grapefruit juice, isoniazid, ketoconazole, levofloxacin, mexiletine, norethindrone, norfloxacin, omeprazole, paroxetine, tacrine, zileuton |
| Carbamazepine, phenobarbital, phenytoin, primidone, rifampin | Amiodarone, chloramphenicol, cimetidine, co-trimoxazole, disulfiram, fluconazole, fluoxetine, fluvastatin, fluvoxamine, isoniazid, itraconazole, ketoconazole, metronidazole, omeprazole, ritonavir, sulfinpyrazone, ticlopidine, zafirlukast |
| No information available. | Felbamate, fluconazole, fluoxetine, fluvoxamine, omeprazole, ticlopidine |
| Carbamazepine, phenobarbital, phenytoin, primidone | Amiodarone, chloroquine, cimetidine, fluoxetine, fluphenazine, fluvoxamine, haloperidol, paroxetine, perphenazine, propafenone, propoxyphene, quinidine, ritonavir, sertraline, thioridazine |
| Barbiturates, carbamazepine, glucocorticoids, griseofulvin, nafcillin, phenytoin, primidone, rifabutin, rifampin, troglitazone | Clarithromycin, cyclosporine (neural), danazol, delavirdine, diltiazem, erythromycin, fluconazole, fluoxetine, fluvoxamine, grapefruit juice, indinavir, isoniazid, itraconazole, ketoconazole, metronidazole, miconazole, nefazodone, nelfinavir, nicardipine, nifedipine, norfloxacin, omeprazole, prednisone, quinidine, quinine, rifabutin, ritonavir, saquinavir, sertraline, troleandomycin, verapamil, zafirlukast |

# Dosage equivalents for opioids

In this table, the second and third columns show starting dosages for opioids. Within these two columns, all dosages listed are equivalent. The fourth and fifth columns show the reference values needed to calculate equivalent dosages not listed in the second and third columns. All dosages and values are for opioid-naïve patients who weigh 50 kg (110 pounds) or more.

The values in the fourth and fifth columns allow for conversion from one administration route to another and for changes from one opioid to another. To use these values, first calculate the total daily dose of the current opioid by multiplying the dose with the frequency of administration in a 24-hour period. Look up the reference values on the table for both the current and the new therapy, noting their dosage form (P.O. or parenteral).

Follow this equation: (daily dose of current dosage form x reference value of new drug or new dosage form) ÷ reference value of current drug = daily dose of new dosage form.

Clinicians should start the new therapy at 75% of the calculated dose to minimize the potential for overdose or other untoward effects. Also, a rough calculation of a rescue dose, used for breakthrough pain that occurs between doses, is about 10% to 20% of the total daily dose.

## Example 1: Changing the administration route

A patient is being given 10 mg I.V. morphine every 4 hours around-the-clock. The patient is now able to take P.O. immediate-release morphine. What is the dose of P.O. immediate-release morphine?

The total daily dose of morphine is 60 mg I.V. The equianalgesic reference values of morphine are 10 mg for I.V. and 30 mg for P.O. administration. First, multiply the I.V. dose and oral reference values together, then divide by the I.V. reference value. Multiply the daily dose by 75%. (60 mg I.V. × 30 mg P.O. = 1800 mg, then divide by 10 mg I.V. = 180 mg daily of P.O. morphine) Divide 180 mg daily dose by number of doses given per day to calculate how much morphine is given per dose. If frequency is every 4 hours, the amount of morphine per dose is 30 mg P.O. Multiply 30 mg dose by 75% to get a 22.5 mg-starting dose.

## Example 2: Changing the opioid and administration route

A patient is receiving a total daily dose of 30 mg P.O. hydromorphone. A decision is made to change to morphine administered as an I.V. bolus. What is the dose of morphine?

The equianalgesic reference values are as follows: 7.5 mg for P.O. hydromorphone and 10 mg for I.V. morphine. (30 mg P.O. hydromorphone 210 mg I.V. morphine = 300 mg, then divide by 7.5 mg P.O. hydromorphone = 40 mg I.V. morphine daily.) Multiply 40 mg dose by 75% to get 30 mg total daily dose. Divide 30 mg I.V. daily dose into appropriate dosing frequency.

### Opioid agonist

morphine IR

morphine SR (MS Contin, Oramorph SR)

hydromorphone (Dilaudid)

levorphanol (Levo-Dromoran)

meperidine (Demerol)

methadone (Dolophine)

oxymorphone (Numorphan)

codeine

### Combination opioid preparations

codeine (with aspirin or acetaminophen)

hydrocodone (with acetaminophen)

oxycodone IR (with aspirin or acetaminophen)

### Opioid agonist-antagonist and partial agonist

buprenorphine (Buprenex)

butorphanol (Stadol)

nalbuphine (Nubain)

pentazocine (Talwin)

### Key

| | |
|---|---|
| NR | = Not Recommended |
| NA | = Not Available |
| IR | = Immediate Release |
| SR | = Sustained Release |
| ATC | = Around the Clock |
| I.M. | = Intramuscular injection |
| S.C. | = Subcutaneous injection |
| I.V. | = Intravenous injection |
| p.r.n. | = as needed |

| Usual starting doses for moderate to severe pain | | Equivalent reference values | |
| --- | --- | --- | --- |
| *Oral* | *Parenteral* | *Oral* | *Parenteral* |
| 10-30 mg q 3-4 h | 5-10 mg q 3-4 h (I.M.) 1-2.5 mg q 5 min p.r.n. (I.V.) | 30 mg q 3-4 h (around-the-clock dosing) 60 mg q 3-4 h (single or intermittent dosing) | 10 mg q 3-4 h (I.M., S.C., I.V.) |
| 90-120 mg q 12 h | NA | 90-120 mg q 12 h | NA |
| 2-4 mg q 4-6 h, or 6 mg q 3-4 h | 1-2 mg q 4-6 h (I.M.) 0.1-0.5 mg q 5 min p.r.n. (I.V.) | 7.5 mg q 3-4 h | 1.5 mg q 3-4 h (I.M., S.C., I.V.) |
| 2-4 mg q 6-8 h | 2 mg q 6-8 h (I.M., I.V.) | 4 mg q 6-8 h | 2 mg q 6-8 h (I.M., S.C.) |
| NR | 50-100 mg q 3-4 h (I.M.) 5-10 mg q 5 min p.r.n. (I.V.) | 300 mg q 2-3 h | 100 mg q 3 h (I.M., S.C., I.V.) |
| 5-20 mg q 6-8 h | 2.5-10 mg q 6-8 h (I.M.) | 20 mg q 6-8 h | 10 mg q 6-8 h (I.M.) |
| NA | 1 mg q 4-6 h (I.M.) | NA | 1 mg q 4-6 h (I.M., S.C.) |
| 15-60 mg q 3-4 h | 15-60 mg q 3-4 h (I.M., S.C., I.V.) | 200 mg q 3-4 h | 130 mg q 3-4 h (I.M., I.V., S.C.) |
| 60 mg q 3-4 h | NA | 180-200 mg q 3-4 h | NA |
| 5-10 mg q 3-4 h | NA | 30 mg q 3-4 h | NA |
| 5-10 mg q 3-4 h | NA | 30 mg q 3-4 h | NA |
| NA | 0.3 mg q 6 h (I.M., I.V.) | NA | 0.3 mg q 6 h (I.M., I.V.) |
| NA | 1-4 mg q 3-4 h (I.M.) | NA | 2 mg q 3-4 h (I.M.) |
| NA | 10 mg q 3-6 h (I.M.) | NA | 10 mg q 3-6 h (I.M.) |
| 50 mg q 4-6 h | NR | 150-180 mg q 3-4 h | 60 mg q 3-4 h (I.M., S.C.) |

# Guidelines for use of selected antimicrobials

The following table provides guidelines for the first-line (denoted by the numeral 1) and second-line (numeral 2) management of specific selected organisms and should be used as a general reference only. Use patient condition, sensitivities, institutional policies, and recent research when initiating new therapy.

| | Aminoglycosides | | | | Cephalosporins | | | | | | | | |
|---|---|---|---|---|---|---|---|---|---|---|---|---|---|
| | Amikacin | Gentamicin | Netilmicin | Tobramycin | Cefazolin | Cefepime | Cefixime | Cefotaxime | Cefoxitin | Ceftazidime | Ceftizoxime | Ceftriaxone | Cefuroxime |
| **Gram-negative aerobes** | | | | | | | | | | | | | |
| Acinetobacter | 1 | 2 | 2 | 2 | | | | | | | | | |
| Bacteroides fragilis | | | | | | | | | 2 | | | | |
| Chlamydia pneumoniae | | | | | | | | | | | | | |
| Chlamydia psittaci | | | | | | | | | | | | | |
| Chlamydia trachomatis | | | | | | | | | | | | | |
| Citrobacter fruendii | | 1 | | 1 | | | | | | | | | |
| Enterobacter sp. | 1 | 1 | 1 | 1 | | 2 | | | | | | | |
| Escherichia coli | 2 | 2 | 2 | 2 | 1 | | 1 | 1 | 1 | 1 | 1 | 1 | 1 |
| Haemophilus influenzae† | | | | | | | | 1 | | | 1 | 1 | |
| Haemophilus influenzae‡ | | | | | | | 2 | | | | | | 2 |
| Klebsiella pneumoniae (UTI) | | | | | 1 | | | 1 | 1 | 1 | 1 | 1 | 1 |
| Klebsiella pneumoniae (pneumonia) | 2 | 2 | 2 | 2 | | | 1 | 1 | 1 | 1 | 1 | 1 | 1 |
| Legionella pneumophila | | | | | | | | | | | | | |
| Moraxella catarrhalis | | | | | | 2 | 2 | 2 | 2 | 2 | 2 | 2 | 2 |
| Neisseria gonorrhoeae | | | | | | | 1 | | | | | 1 | |
| Proteus mirabilis | | | | | 2 | 2 | 2 | 2 | 2 | 2 | 2 | 2 | 2 |
| Proteus vulgaris | | | | | | | 1 | 1 | | | 1 | 1 | 1 |
| Pseudomonas aeruginosa | 2 | 2 | 2 | 1 | | 2 | | | | 1 | | | |
| Serratia marcescens | 2 | 2 | 2 | 2 | | | | 1 | | | 2 | 2 | 1 |
| Shigella sp. | | | | | | | | | | | | | |
| Vibrio cholerae | | | | | | | | | | | | | |
| **Gram-positive aerobes** | | | | | | | | | | | | | |
| Bacillus anthracis | | | | | | | | | | | | | |
| Campylobacter jejuni | | | | | | | | | | | | | |
| Clostridium difficile | | | | | | | | | | | | | |
| Clostridium perfringens | | | | | 2 | | | 2 | 2 | | 2 | 2 | |
| Enterococcus faecalis | | | | | | | | | | | | | |
| Enterococcus faecium | | | | | | | | | | | | | |
| Listeria monocytogenes | | 1 | | 1 | | | | | | | | | |
| Nocardia asteroides | | | | | | | | | | | | | |
| Staphylococcus aureus | | | | | 1 | | | | | | | | |
| Staphylococcus saprophyticus | | | | | | | | | | | | | |
| Streptococcus pneumoniae | | | | | | | | 2 | | | | 2 | |
| Streptococcus pyogenes (group A) | | | | | 1 | 1 | 1 | 1 | 1 | | 1 | 1 | 1 |
| Streptococcus (anaerobic sp.) | | | | | | | | | | | | | |
| Streptococcus (viridans group) | | 1 | | | | | | | | | | 2 | |
| **Other aerobes** | | | | | | | | | | | | | |
| Borrelia burgdorferi (skin) | | | | | | | | | | | | 2 | 2 |
| Mycoplasma pneumoniae | | | | | | | | | | | | | |
| Pneumocystis carinii | | | | | | | | | | | | | |

† life-threatening  ‡ non–life-threatening

| | Miscellaneous | | | | | | | | | | | | | Penicillins | | | | | | |
|---|---|---|---|---|---|---|---|---|---|---|---|---|---|---|---|---|---|---|---|---|
| | Azithromycin | Aztreonam | Chloramphenicol | Clarithromycin | Clindamycin | Eyrthromycin | Imipenem/Cilastatin | Meropenem | Metronidazole | Pentamidine | Rifampin | Trimethoprim/Sulfamethoxazole | Vancomycin | Amoxicillin | Ampicillin | Mezlocillin | Nafcillin | Penicillin G | Piperacillin | Ticarcillin |
| | | | | | | | 1 | 1 | | | | 2 | | | | | | | | |
| | | | | | 2 | | 2 | 2 | 1 | | | | | | | | | | | |
| | 2 | | | 2 | | 2 | | | | | | | | | | | | | | |
| | | | 2 | | | | | | | | | | | | | | | | | |
| | 1 | | | | | 2 | | | | | | | | | | | | | | |
| | | 2 | | | | | 1 | 1 | | | | | | | | | | | | |
| | | | | | | | 1 | 1 | | | | | | | | | | | | |
| | | 2 | | | | | 2 | 2 | | | | 2 | | | | | | | | |
| | | 2 | | | | | 2 | 2 | | | | | | | | | | | | |
| | 2 | | | 2 | | | | | | | | 1 | | | | | | | | |
| | | 2 | | | | | | | | | | 2 | | | | | | | | |
| | | 2 | | | | | 2 | 2 | | | | 2 | | | | | | | | |
| | 1 | | | 2 | | 2 | | | | | 2 | | | | | | | | | |
| | 2 | | | 2 | | | | | | | | 1 | | | | | | | | |
| | | | | | | | | | | | | | | | | | | | | |
| | | 2 | | | | | | | | | | 1 | | | | | | | | |
| | | | | | | | | | | | | 1 | | | | | | | | |
| | | 2 | | | | | 2 | 2 | | | | | | | | | 1 | | 1 | 1 |
| | | 2 | | | | | | | | | | 1 | | | | | | | | |
| | | | | | | | | | | | | 1 | | | | 2 | | | | |
| | | | | | | | | | | | | 2 | | | | | | | | |
| | | | | 2 | | 2 | | | | | | | | | | | | | 1 | |
| | 2 | | | 2 | 2 | 1 | | | | | | | | | | | | | | |
| | | | | | | | | | 1 | | | | 2 | | | | | | | |
| | | | | 2 | | | | | | | | | | | | | | | 1 | |
| | | | | | | | | | | | | | 2 | 1 | 1 | | | 1 | | |
| | | | 2 | | | | | | | | | | 1 | | | | | | | |
| | | | | | | | | | | | | 2 | | | | | 1 | 1 | | |
| | | | | | | | | | | | | 1 | | | | | | | | |
| | | | | | 2 | | | | | | 2 | 2 | 1 | | | | | 1 | | |
| | | | | | 2 | | | | | | | | | | | | | | | |
| | | | | | | | | | | | | | | 1 | 1 | 1 | | 1 | | |
| | 2 | | | 2 | 2 | 2 | | | | | | | | 1 | | | | 1 | | |
| | | | | | 2 | | | | | | | | | | | | | 1 | | |
| | 2 | | | 2 | 2 | 2 | | | | | | | | | | | | 1 | | |
| | 2 | | | 2 | 2 | 2 | | | | | | | | | 1 | | | | 2 | |
| | 2 | | | 2 | 2 | 1 | | | | | | | | | | | | | | |
| | | | | | | | | | | 2 | | 1 | | | | | | | | |

(continued)

| | | Combination with b-lactamase inhibitors | | | | Tetracy-clines | | Fluoroquinolones | | | |
|---|---|---|---|---|---|---|---|---|---|---|---|
| | | Amoxicillin/ Clavulanic acid | Ampicillin/ Sulbactam | Piperacillin/ Tazobactam | Ticarcillin/ Clavulanic acid | Doxycycline | Minocycline | Ciprofloxacin | Levofloxacin | Norfloxacin | Ofloxacin |
| **Gram-negative aerobes** | Acinetobacter | | 2 | | | | | 2 | | | 2 |
| | Bacteroides fragilis | 2 | 2 | 2 | 2 | | | | | | |
| | Chlamydia pneumoniae | | | | | 1 | | | 2 | | |
| | Chlamydia psittaci | | | | | 1 | | | | | |
| | Chlamydia trachomatis | | | | | 1 | | | | | 2 |
| | Citrobacter freundii | | | | | | | 1 | | | |
| | Enterobacter sp. | | | | | | | 1 | | | |
| | Escherichia coli | | | 2 | | | | 2 | 2 | 2 | 2 |
| | Haemophilus influenzae† | | 1 | 2 | 1 | | | 1 | 1 | | 1 |
| | Haemophilus influenzae‡ | 1 | 1 | | | | | 2 | | | 2 |
| | Klebsiella pneumoniae (UTI) | 2 | | | 2 | | | 1 | 2 | 2 | 2 |
| | Klebsiella pneumoniae (pneumonia) | 2 | 2 | 2 | 2 | | | 2 | 2 | | 2 |
| | Legionella pneumophila | | | | | 2 | | 1 | 1 | | 1 |
| | Moraxella catarrhalis | 1 | 1 | | | | | 2 | 2 | | 2 |
| | Neisseria gonorrhoeae | | | | | | | 2 | | | 2 |
| | Proteus mirabilis | | | | | | | | | | |
| | Proteus vulgaris | 2 | | | | | | 1 | 1 | 1 | 1 |
| | Pseudomonas aeruginosa | | | | | | | 2 | | | |
| | Serratia marcescens | | | | | | | 2 | 2 | | 2 |
| | Shigella sp. | | | | | 2 | | 1 | | 1 | 1 |
| | Vibrio cholerae | | | | | 1 | | 1 | | | 1 |
| **Gram-positive aerobes** | Bacillus anthracis | | | | | 1 | | | | | |
| | Campylobacter jejuni | | | | | | | 2 | | | 2 |
| | Clostridium difficile | | | | | | | | | | |
| | Clostridium perfringens | | | | | | | | | | |
| | Enterococcus faecalis | | | | | | | | | | |
| | Enterococcus faecium | | | | | 2 | | | | | |
| | Listeria monocytogenes | | | | | | | | | | |
| | Nocardia asteroides | | | | | | 2 | | | | |
| | Staphylococcus aureus | 2 | 2 | 2 | 2 | | | 2 | 2 | | 2 |
| | Staphylococcus saprophyticus | | | | | | | 2 | | 1 | 2 |
| | Streptococcus pneumoniae | | | | | 1 | | | 1 | | |
| | Streptococcus pyogenes (group A) | | | | | | | | | | |
| | Streptococcus (anaerobic sp.) | | | | | | | | | | |
| | Streptococcus (viridans group) | | | | | | | | | | |
| **Other aerobes** | Borrelia burgdorferi (skin) | | | | | 1 | | | | | |
| | Mycoplasma pneumoniae | | | | | 1 | | | 2 | | |
| | Pneumocystis carinii | | | | | | | | | | |

† life-threatening    ‡ non–life-threatening

# Selected narcotic analgesic combination products

Many common analgesics are combinations of two or more generic drugs. This table reviews common narcotic analgesics.

| Trade names and controlled substance schedule (CSS) | Generic drugs | Indications and adult dosages |
|---|---|---|
| Aceta with Codeine<br>*CSS III* | • acetaminophen 30 mg<br>• codeine phosphate 30 mg | For fever, mild to moderate pain. Give 1-2 tablets q 4 hours. Maximum, 12 tablets in 24 hours. |
| Alor 5/500 Tablets, Damason-P, Lortab ASA<br>*CSS III* | • aspirin 500 mg<br>• hydrodocone bitartrate 5 mg | For moderate to moderately severe pain. Give 1-2 tablets q 4 hours. Maximum, 8 tablets in 24 hours. |
| Anexsia 7.5/650, Lorcet Plus<br>*CSS III* | • acetaminophen 650 mg<br>• hydrocodone bitartrate 7.5 mg | For arthralgia, bone pain, dental pain, headache, migraine, moderate pain. Give 1-2 tablets q 4 hours. Maximum, 6 tablets in 24 hours. |
| Capital with Codeine, Tylenol with Codeine Elixir<br>*CSS V* | • acetaminophen 120 mg<br>• codeine phosphate 12 mg/5 ml | For mild to moderate pain. Give 15 ml q 4 hours. |
| Darvocet-N 50<br>*CSS IV* | • acetaminophen 325 mg<br>• propoxyphene napsylate 50 mg | For mild to moderate pain. Give 1-2 tablets q 4 hours. Maximum, 12 tablets in 24 hours. |
| Darvocet-N 100, Propacet 100<br>*CSS IV* | • acetaminophen 650 mg<br>• propoxyphene napsykate 100 mg | For mild to moderate pain. Give 1 tablet q 4 hours. Maximum, 6 tablets in 24 hours. |
| Lorcet 10/650<br>*CSS III* | • acetaminophen 650 mg<br>• hydrocodone bitartrate 10 mg | For moderate to moderately severe pain. Give 1 tablet q 4 hours. Maximum, 6 tablets in 24 hours. |
| Lortab 2.5/500<br>*CSS III* | • acetaminophen 500 mg<br>• hydrocodone bitartrate 2.5 mg | For moderate to moderately severe pain. Give 1-2 tablets q 4 hours. Maximum, 8 tablets in 24 hours. |
| Lortab 5/500<br>*CSS III* | • acetaminophen 500 mg<br>• hydrocodone bitartrate 5 mg | For moderate to moderately severe pain. Give 1-2 tablets q 4 hours. Maximum, 8 tablets in 24 hours. |
| Lortab 7.5/500<br>*CSS III* | • acetaminophen 500 mg<br>• hydrocodone bitartrate 7.5 mg | For moderate to moderately severe pain. Give 1 tablet q 4 hours. Maximum, 8 tablets in 24 hours. |
| Lortab 10/500<br>*CSS III* | • acetaminophen 500 mg<br>• hydrocodone bitartrate 10 mg | For moderate to moderately severe pain. Give 1 tablet q 4-6 hours. Maximum, 6 tablets in 24 hours. |
| Percocet 2.5/325<br>*CSS II* | • acetaminophen 325 mg<br>• oxycodone hydrochloride 2.5 mg | For moderate to moderately severe pain. Give 1-2 tablets q 4-6 hours. Maximum, 12 tablets in 24 hours. |
| Percocet<br>*CSS II* | • acetaminophen 325 mg<br>• oxycodone hydrochloride 5 mg | For moderate to moderately severe pain. Give 1-2 tablets q 4 hours. Maximum, 12 tablets in 24 hours. |
| Percocet 7.5/500<br>*CSS II* | • acetaminophen 500 mg<br>• oxycodone hydrochloride 7.5 mg | For moderate to moderately severe pain. Give 1-2 tablets q 4-6 hours. Maximum, 8 tablets in 24 hours. |

| Trade names and controlled substance schedule (CSS) | Generic drugs | Indications and adult dosages |
|---|---|---|
| Percocet 10/650 CSS II | • acetaminophen 650 mg • oxycodone hydrochloride 10 mg | For moderate to moderately severe pain. Give 1-2 tablets q 4-6 hours. Maximum, 6 tablets in 24 hours. |
| Percodan-Demi CSS II | • aspirin 325 mg • oxycodone hydrochloride 2.25 mg • oxycodone terephthalate 0.19 mg | For moderate to moderately severe pain. Give 1-2 tablets q 6 hours. Maximum, 8 tablets in 24 hours. |
| Percodan, Roxiprin CSS II | • aspirin 325 mg • oxycodone hydrochloride 4.5 mg • oxycodone terephthalate 0.38 mg | For moderate to moderately severe pain. Give 1 tablet q 6 hours. Maximum, 4 tablets in 24 hours. |
| Propoxyphene Napsylate/ Acetaminophen CSS IV | • acetaminophen 650 mg • propoxyphene napsylate 100 mg | For mild to moderate pain. Give 1 tablet q 4 hours. Maximum, 6 tablets in 24 hours. |
| Roxicet CSS II | • acetaminophen 325 mg • oxycodone hydrochloride 5 mg | For moderate to moderately severe pain. Give 1-2 tablets q 4 hours. Maximum, 12 tablets in 24 hours. |
| Roxicet 5/500, Roxilox CSS II | • acetaminophen 500 mg • oxycodone hydrochloride 5 mg | For moderate to moderately severe pain. Give 1-2 tablets q 4-6 hours. Maximum, 8 tablets in 24 hours. |
| Roxicet Oral Solution CSS II | • acetaminophen 325 mg • oxycodone hydrochloride 5 mg/5 ml | For moderate to moderately severe pain. Give 5-10 ml q 4-6 hours. Maximum, 60 ml in 24 hours. |
| Tylenol with Codeine No. 2 CSS III | • acetaminophen 300 mg • codeine phosphate 15 mg | For fever, mild to moderate pain. Give 1-2 tablets q 4 hours. Maximum, 12 tablets in 24 hours. |
| Tylenol with Codeine No. 3 CSS III | • acetaminophen 300 mg • codeine phosphate 30 mg | For fever, mild to moderate pain. Give 1-2 tablets q 4 hours. Maximum, 12 tablets in 24 hours. |
| Tylenol with Codeine No. 4 CSS III | • acetaminophen 300 mg • codeine phosphate 60 mg | For fever, mild to moderate pain. Give 1 tablet q 4 hours. Maximum, 6 tablets in 24 hours. |
| Tylox CSS II | • acetaminophen 500 mg • oxycodone hydrochloride 5 mg | For moderate to moderately severe pain. Give 1-2 tablets q 4 hours. Maximum, 12 tablets in 24 hours. |
| Vicodin CSS III | • acetaminophen 500 mg • hydrocodone bitartrate 5 mg | For moderate to moderately severe pain. Give 1-2 tablets q 4 hours. Maximum, 8 tablets in 24 hours. |
| Vicodin ES CSS III | • acetaminophen 750 mg • hydrocodone bitartrate 7.5 mg | For moderate to moderately severe pain. Give 1 tablet q 4-6 hours. Maximum, 5 tablets in 24 hours. |
| Wygesic CSS IV | • acetaminophen 650 mg • propoxyphene napsylate 65 mg | For mild to moderate pain. Give 1 tablet q 4 hours. Maximum, 6 tablets in 24 hours. |

# Index

---

*t refers to a table.*

---

---

---

t refers to a table.

---

t refers to a table.